Emergency Medicine

Volume I

Emergency Medicine

Second Edition

Editor in Chief

Harold L. May, M.D.
Assistant Professor of Surgery, Harvard Medical School; Associate in Surgery, Brigham and Women's Hospital, Boston

Associate Editors

Richard V. Aghababian, M.D.
Associate Professor of Medicine and Director, Division of Emergency Medicine, University of Massachusetts Medical School, Worcester

Gary R. Fleisher, M.D.
Associate Professor of Pediatrics, Harvard Medical School; Chief, Emergency Medicine, Children's Hospital, Boston

Little, Brown and Company
Boston/Toronto/London

Second Edition

Emergency medicine / editor in chief, Harold L. May; associate editors, Richard V. Aghababian, Gary R. Fleisher. — 2nd ed.
p. cm.
Includes bibliographical references and index.
ISBN 0-316-55185-6
1. Emergency medicine. I. May, Harold L. II. Aghababian, Richard. III. Fleisher, Gary R. (Gary Robert), 1951–
[DNLM: 1. Emergencies. 2. Emergency Medical Services. 3. Emergency Medicine—methods. WB 105 E536]
RC86.7.E57825 1992
616.02′5—dc20
DNLM/DLC 91-33723
for Library of Congress CIP

Printed in the United States of America

RRD-OH

Show me your ways, O Lord,
teach me your paths;
guide me in your truth . . .

Stretch out your hand to heal . . .

The Bible

Contents

Preface

In order to justify the time, effort, and expense involved in its production, a second edition of any textbook on emergency medicine should bring something special to the field. This edition does that. The first edition was well received and widely distributed, but the fact that it was not comprehensive limited its usefulness to the busy emergency physician. Although no textbook can encompass a medical specialty completely, this second edition of *Emergency Medicine* has been written with the hope that it will define the field of emergency medicine so comprehensively and usefully that it will become an indispensable resource for emergency medicine clinicians, teachers, and students.

The book presents authoritative discussions of the common conditions seen in the emergency department and also discusses many other conditions that are being seen with increasing frequency. For the student, it describes the details of assessment and management in clinically useful ways and gives practical help in decision making about admission or discharge of the patient, appropriate follow-up, and timing of referral. It provides detailed, carefully illustrated descriptions of the procedures that have to be performed. For the experienced practitioner, it presents up-to-date pathophysiologic discussions and epidemiologic information.

The scope of this edition has been expanded far beyond that of the first edition. The book has more than doubled in size. The organization of the book, which was one of the strengths of the first edition, is unchanged, but each chapter has been extensively revised or, in most cases, completely rewritten and expanded. Many of the chapters of the first edition have been replaced by multi-chapter sections, each of which has been edited by an authority in the field, making it possible to present much more complete discussions of each clinical condition. Here are a few of the new features of this edition:

- Acknowledging that many of the medical advances of recent years have resulted from an explosive increase in our understanding of molecular and cellular biology, we begin this edition with a review of some basic elements of molecular biology as they relate to life and death, starting with the cell itself.

- Because of the central role the body's immune defenses play in normal and pathologic processes, a section on body defense, immunity, and disorders of the immune system has been added.

- A section on pain control in the emergency department discusses physiologic mechanisms of pain, general approaches to pain control, and specific techniques, both for adults and children, including local and regional anesthesia.

- Because many patients with occupation-caused emergencies are presenting in emergency departments, a section on work-related emergencies has been added, including the recently described, but frequently seen, cumulative trauma syndrome.

- The 17-chapter section on infections discusses the emergency department presentation and management of a spectrum of infections, from the common cold to life-threatening infections of the central nervous system.
- Recognizing that there are identifiable groups of patients who require special considerations in the emergency department, regardless of their presenting emergency, we have added a new section to discuss general physiological, psychological, and management considerations that are special for each of these groups. The presenting groups range from such common ones as the pregnant patient, the elderly patient, and the hypochondriacal patient, to such an extraordinary one as the VIP patient.
- There are multi-chapter sections on acute disorders of each of the organ systems, injuries, pediatric emergencies, clinical pharmacology and toxicology, and organizational, medicolegal, and social considerations of emergency care.
- The procedure section has been expanded by the addition of new sections—most notably, techniques for providing field blocks and intravenous regional anesthesia and techniques for pediatric airway management and circulatory support.

One of the weaknesses of the first edition was that it did not include enough emergency physicians among its contributors to ensure its unfailing usefulness for them. It was written more for interns, residents, and moonlighters than for emergency medicine specialists. One of the great strengths of this edition is that its contributors include some recognized authorities in the field of emergency medicine and many highly experienced emergency physicians from all parts of the United States and Canada. The list of contributors also includes authorities in other medical specialties, some of whom have been responsible for the basic medical advances of recent years. An emergency medicine textbook that is written exclusively by emergency physicians has the advantage of relevance to medical practice in the emergency department but has the limitation of not being authoritative in many areas. One written only by specialists in fields other than emergency medicine may be authoritative but not always completely helpful in emergency department practice. We believe that the contributions of emergency physicians and authorities in other specialties are uniquely combined in this book so that it is comprehensive, useful, and authoritative to a degree that has never before been achieved.

A book of such scope and complexity can only be written and produced by the combined efforts of many individuals. I gratefully acknowledge the wise counsel and great help provided by the associate editors, Dr. Richard V. Aghababian and Dr. Gary R. Fleisher. I am also deeply grateful to the other section editors: Dr. Gregory L. Eastwood, Dr. Christopher H. Fanta, Dr. Richard H. Glew, Dr. David W. Lhowe, Dr. Michael A. McGuigan, Dr. Paul M. Paris, and Dr. Ronald D. Stewart. It is hard work to be a section editor for a book such as this, but I hope that each of the editors will find the book worthy of the significant investment of time and effort that they made in helping to produce it. They are responsible for its great range.

Others have contributed in other ways. I am grateful to Dr. Eugene Braunwald, Dr. Judah Folkman, and Dr. Charlotte Yeh for their helpful advice; to Dr. Harry Mellins, for instructive x-rays; and to Dr. Harry Kozakewich, for special pathology slides. We were saddened by the untimely deaths of Dr. Stephen E. Hedberg after the publication of the first edition and Dr. Charles Huggins after he had completed the chapter on the principles of emergency transfusion medicine for the second edition. I acknowledge with deep thanks the help that Dr. Huggins's colleague, Dr. James Harmon, gave in updating a portion of the final draft of his chapter. Laurel Cook illustrated the orthopedic injury section, Chapter 88, and portions of Chapter 89. Harriet Greenfield illustrated the procedure section and many of the other chapters. I am grateful to John Buckley for his patient and careful preparation of many of the photographs. Special thanks must go to Suzanne Gariepy for her unfailing helpfulness and her attention to details that make a book such as this possible. Carmen Christmas's assistance is also deeply appreciated. It has been a pleasure to work closely with the perfect production editor, Elizabeth Willingham, who has been relentless and, at the same time, very understanding. I am grateful, too, to Susan Pioli, for her encouragement and support throughout the long process of producing this book.

H.L.M.

Section Editors

Richard V. Aghababian, M.D.	Associate Professor of Medicine and Director, Division of Emergency Medicine, University of Massachusetts Medical School, Worcester
Gregory L. Eastwood, M.D.	Dean, School of Medicine, Medical College of Georgia, Augusta
Christopher H. Fanta, M.D.	Associate Professor of Medicine, Harvard Medical School; Clinical Director, Respiratory Division, Brigham and Women's Hospital, Boston
Gary R. Fleisher, M.D.	Associate Professor of Pediatrics, Harvard Medical School; Chief, Emergency Medicine, Children's Hospital, Boston
Richard H. Glew, M.D.	Professor of Medicine, Molecular Genetics, and Microbiology, University of Massachusetts Medical School; Chair, Department of Medicine, Medical Center of Central Massachusetts-Memorial, Worcester
David W. Lhowe, M.D.	Instructor, Department of Orthopedic Surgery, Harvard Medical School; Assistant in Orthopedic Surgery, Massachusetts General Hospital, Boston
Harold L. May, M.D.	Assistant Professor of Surgery, Harvard Medical School; Associate in Surgery, Brigham and Women's Hospital, Boston
Michael A. McGuigan, M.D., C.M.	Associate Professor of Pediatrics and Pharmacology, University of Toronto Faculty of Medicine; Medical Director, Poison Information Centre, Hospital for Sick Children, Toronto
Paul M. Paris, M.D.	Associate Professor of Medicine, University of Pittsburgh School of Medicine; Chief, Department of Emergency Medicine, Presbyterian-University Hospital, Pittsburgh
Ronald D. Stewart, M.D.	Professor of Anesthesiology, Dalhousie University Faculty of Medicine; Attending Physician, Department of Emergency Medicine, Victoria General Hospital, Halifax, Nova Scotia

Contributing Authors

Susan L. Abend, M.D.
Assistant Professor of Medicine and Psychiatry, University of Massachusetts Medical School, Worcester

Frederick W. Ackroyd, M.D.
Associate Professor of Surgery, Harvard Medical School; Visiting Surgeon, Massachusetts General Hospital, Boston

Richard V. Aghababian, M.D.
Associate Professor of Medicine and Director, Division of Emergency Medicine, University of Massachusetts Medical School, Worcester

David Allegra, M.D.
Instructor in Radiology, Harvard Medical School; Attending Radiologist, Brigham and Women's Hospital, Boston

Paul Allen, M.D., Ph.D.
Associate Professor of Anesthesia, Harvard Medical School; Senior Anesthesiologist and Associate Clinical Director, Department of Anesthesia, Brigham and Women's Hospital, Boston

E. Jackson Allison, Jr., M.D., M.P.H.
Professor and Chairman of Emergency Medicine, East Carolina University School of Medicine; Chief of Service, Emergency Department, Pitt County Memorial Hospital, Greenville, North Carolina

Joseph S. Alpert, M.D.
Edward Budnitz Professor of Cardiovascular Medicine, University of Massachusetts Medical School; Director, Division of Cardiovascular Medicine, University of Massachusetts Medical Center, Worcester

Alison B. Anderson, M.D.
Assistant Professor of Pediatrics, University of South Florida College of Medicine; Associate Director, Pediatric Emergency Care Center, Tampa General Hospital, Tampa

Ronald J. Anderson, M.D.
Associate Professor of Medicine, Harvard Medical School; Director of Clinical Training, Department of Rheumatology and Immunology, Brigham and Women's Hospital, Boston

Kenneth A. Arndt, M.D.
Professor of Dermatology, Harvard Medical School; Dermatologist-in-Chief, Beth Israel Hospital, Boston

Canan Avunduk, M.D., Ph.D.
Assistant Professor of Medicine, Division of Digestive Diseases and Nutrition, University of Massachusetts Medical School, Worcester

Brian J. Awbrey, M.D.
Instructor in Orthopedics, Harvard Medical School; Assistant in Orthopedics, Department of Orthopedic Surgery, Massachusetts General Hospital, Boston

David Bachman, M.D.
Assistant Professor of Pediatrics, University of Utah School of Medicine; Staff Physician, Emergency Department, Primary Children's Medical Center, Salt Lake City

M. Douglas Baker, M.D.
Associate Professor of Pediatrics, University of Pennsylvania School of Medicine; Associate Director, Emergency Medicine, Children's Hospital of Philadelphia, Philadelphia

Daniel T. Baran, M.D.
Associate Professor of Medicine and Orthopedics, University of Massachusetts Medical School, Worcester

Robert C. Basner, M.D.
Instructor of Medicine, Harvard Medical School; Associate in Medicine, Pulmonary Division, Beth Israel Hospital, Boston

Arthur E. Baue, M.D.
Professor of Surgery and Vice President for the Medical Center, St. Louis University Medical Center, St. Louis

Jerry Don Beavers, M.D., M.P.H.
Assistant Professor of Medicine, University of Massachusetts Medical School; Department of Community and Family Medicine, University of Massachusetts Medical Center, Worcester

Richard Clinton Becker, M.D.
Assistant Professor of Medicine, University of Massachusetts Medical School; Associate Director, Coronary Care Unit, and Director, Thrombosis Research Center, University of Massachusetts Medical Center, Worcester

Louis Bell, M.D.
Assistant Professor of Pediatrics, University of Pennsylvania School of Medicine; Division of Infectious Diseases, Children's Hospital of Philadelphia, Philadelphia

Joseph R. Benotti, M.D.
Associate Professor of Medicine, University of Massachusetts Medical Center; Director, Invasive and Interventional Cardiology, Saint Vincent Hospital, Worcester

Nicholas H. Benson, M.D.
Associate Professor of Emergency Medicine, East Carolina University School of Medicine; Medical and Program Director, EastCare Emergency Air Medical Service, Pitt County Memorial Hospital, Greenville, North Carolina

Charles B. Berde, M.D., Ph.D.
Assistant Professor of Anesthesia (Pediatrics), Harvard Medical School; Senior Associate in Anesthesia, Children's Hospital, Boston

Jeffrey Bernstein, M.D.
Instructor of Medicine, University of Massachusetts Medical School, Worcester

Daniel J. Berry, M.D.
Fellow, Department of Orthopedic Surgery, Mayo Clinic, Rochester, Minnesota

Don C. Bienfang, M.D.
Assistant Professor of Ophthalmology, Harvard Medical School, and Division of Ophthalmology, Department of Surgery, Brigham and Women's Hospital, Boston

William G. Bithoney, M.D.
Assistant Professor of Pediatrics, Harvard Medical School; Associate Chief, General Pediatrics, and Associate in Medicine, Children's Hospital, Boston

Joseph R. Bloomer, M.D.
Professor of Medicine and Director of Gastroenterology, Hepatology, and Nutrition, University of Minnesota Medical School; Attending Physician, University of Minnesota Hospital and Clinic, Minneapolis

Sergei Bogojavlensky, Ph.D., M.D.
Chairman, Department of Obstetrics and Gynecology, Burbank Hospital, Fitchburg, Massachusetts

Robert Bolte, M.D.
Associate Professor of Pediatrics, University of Utah School of Medicine; Co-Director, Emergency Services, Primary Children's Medical Center, Salt Lake City

Larry Borish, M.D.
Assistant Professor of Medicine, University of Colorado Health Sciences Center School of Medicine; Staff Physician, Department of Medicine, National Jewish Center for Immunology and Respiratory Medicine, Denver

G. Richard Braen, M.D.
Professor and Chairman, Department of Emergency Medicine, State University of New York at Buffalo School of Medicine and Biomedical Sciences, Buffalo

Lewis E. Braverman, M.D.
Professor of Medicine and Chief, Division of Endocrinology, University of Massachusetts Medical School, Worcester

Scott Breidbart, M.D.
Assistant Professor of Pediatrics, New York Medical College; Attending Pediatrician, Division of Pediatric Endocrinology, Westchester County Medical Center, Valhalla

David C. Brooks, M.D.
Assistant Professor of Surgery, Harvard Medical School; Associate Surgeon, Department of Surgery, Brigham and Women's Hospital, Boston

Linda Brown, M.D.
Assistant Professor of Medicine, Temple University School of Medicine; Attending Staff, Department of Nephrology, Germantown Hospital and Medical Center, Philadelphia

T. Edward Bynum, M.D.
Associate Professor of Medicine, Harvard Medical School; Director, Clinical Gastroenterology, Brigham and Women's Hospital, Boston

Edmund B. Cabot, M.D.
Instructor in Surgery, Harvard Medical School; Associate Surgeon, Division of General and Gastrointestinal Surgery, Brigham and Women's Hospital, Boston

William S. Carroll, J.D.
Boston, Massachusetts

Stuart R. Chipkin, M.D.
Assistant Professor of Medicine and Physiology, Boston University School of Medicine; Visiting Assistant Physician, Division of Endocrinology and Thorndike Memorial Laboratory, Boston City Hospital, Boston

Roger L. Christian, M.D.
Assistant Professor of Surgery, Harvard Medical School; Associate in Surgery, Brigham and Women's Hospital, Boston

Kathleen A. Cline, M.D.
Assistant Professor of Emergency Medicine, East Carolina University School of Medicine, Greenville, North Carolina

David M. Clive, M.D.
Associate Professor of Medicine, University of Massachusetts Medical School, Worcester

William E. Cobb, M.D.
Assistant Professor of Medicine, Brown University Program in Medicine; Associate Physician, Department of Medicine, Rhode Island Hospital, Providence

Alasdair K. T. Conn, M.D.
Assistant Professor of Surgery, Harvard Medical School; Chief, Emergency Services, Massachusetts General Hospital, Boston

Mary Ann Cooper, M.D.
Associate Professor and Education Director, Department of Emergency Medicine, University of Illinois College of Medicine, Chicago

William H. Cordell, M.D.
Clinical Assistant Professor of Emergency Medicine, Indiana University School of Medicine; Director of Emergency Medicine Research, Emergency Medicine and Trauma Center, Methodist Hospital of Indiana, Indianapolis

Howard M. Corneli, M.D.
Associate Professor of Pediatrics, University of Utah School of Medicine; Co-Director, Emergency Department, Primary Children's Medical Center, Salt Lake City

Ellen F. Crain, M.D., Ph.D.
Associate Professor of Pediatrics, Albert Einstein College of Medicine of Yeshiva University; Director, Pediatric Emergency Services, Bronx Municipal Hospital Center, Bronx, New York

Thomas Cropley, M.D.
Assistant Professor of Medicine (Dermatology), University of Massachusetts Medical School; Attending Dermatologist, University of Massachusetts Medical Center, Worcester

Malcolm DeCamp, Jr., M.D.
Clinical Fellow in Surgery, Harvard Medical School; Chief Resident Surgeon, Brigham and Women's Hospital, Boston

Jonathan T. Deland, M.D.
Associate Orthopedic Surgeon, Harvard Medical School and Brigham and Women's Hospital, Boston

Robert H. Demling, M.D.
Professor of Surgery, Harvard Medical School; Director, Longwood Area Trauma-Burn Center, Boston

Thomas G. DeWitt, M.D.
Associate Professor of Pediatrics, University of Massachusetts Medical School; Director, Division of General and Community Pediatrics, University of Massachusetts Medical Center, Worcester

Ronald A. Dieckmann, M.D., M.P.H.
Associate Clinical Professor of Pediatrics and Medicine, University of California, San Francisco, School of Medicine; Director, Pediatric Emergency Service, San Francisco General Hospital Medical Center, San Francisco

Gary V. Doern, Ph.D.
Professor of Medicine and Molecular Genetics and Microbiology, University of Massachusetts Medical School; Director, Department of Clinical Microbiology, University of Massachusetts Medical Center, Worcester

Magruder C. Donaldson, M.D.
Assistant Professor of Surgery, Harvard Medical School; Associate Surgeon, Brigham and Women's Hospital, Boston

Constance J. Doyle, M.D.
Clinical Instructor of Surgery, Section of Emergency Services, University of Michigan Medical School, Ann Arbor; Senior Attending Physician, Emergency Department, Foote Hospital, Jackson, Michigan

David E. Drum, M.D., Ph.D.
Associate Professor of Radiology, Harvard Medical School; Radiologist and Physician (Radiology), Brigham and Women's Hospital, Boston

Gary Dubin, M.D.
Assistant Professor of Medicine, Infectious Diseases Section, University of Pennsylvania School of Medicine and Hospital of the University of Pennsylvania, Philadelphia

David Dudgeon, M.D.
Professor of Surgery and Pediatrics, Johns Hopkins University School of Medicine; Attending Surgeon, Johns Hopkins Hospital, Baltimore

Lala Mathers Dunbar, M.D., Ph.D.
Assistant Professor of Medicine, Louisiana State University School of Medicine in New Orleans; Director, Major Emergency Room, Charity Hospital of Louisiana, New Orleans

Susan M. Dunmire, M.D.
Assistant Professor of Medicine, University of Pittsburgh School of Medicine; Academic Coordinator, Division of Emergency Medicine, Presbyterian-University Hospital, Pittsburgh

William Durbin, M.D.
Associate Professor of Pediatrics and Medicine, University of Massachusetts Medical School; Chief, Division of Pediatric Infectious Diseases, University of Massachusetts Medical Center, Worcester

Gregory L. Eastwood, M.D.
Dean, School of Medicine, Medical College of Georgia School of Medicine, Augusta

Harwood Egan, M.D.
Instructor of Pediatrics, Harvard Medical School; Assistant Pediatrician, Massachusetts General Hospital, Boston

Teddi F. Eisen, M.D.
Clinical Fellow, Harvard Medical School and Children's Hospital, Boston

Edward M. Eitzen, Jr., M.D., M.P.H.
Assistant Clinical Professor of Pediatrics, Uniformed Services University of the Health Sciences, Bethesda, Maryland; Assistant Clinical Professor of Pediatrics, University of Washington School of Medicine; Lieutenant Colonel, Medical Corps, and Chief, Operational Medical Branch, U.S. Army Medical Research Institute of Infectious Diseases, Fort Detrick, Frederick, Maryland

Roger H. Emerson, M.D.
Clinical Associate Professor of Orthopedic Surgery, University of Texas Health Science Center at Dallas Southwestern Medical School; Attending Surgeon, Department of Orthopedic Surgery, Presbyterian Hospital, Dallas

Daniel M. Epstein, M.D.
Instructor of Pediatrics and Psychiatry, Harvard Medical School; Assistant in Medicine, Children's Hospital, Boston

Lars C. Erickson, M.D.
Chief of Pediatric Cardiology, Naval Hospital, San Diego

John F. Erkkinen, M.D.
Maine Medical Center, Portland

Annmarie Errichetti, M.D.
Assistant Professor of Medicine, University of Massachusetts Medical School; Director, Noninvasive Cardiology, Medical Center of Central Massachusetts-Memorial, Worcester

Patrick G. Fairchild, M.D.
Assistant Professor of Medicine, University of Massachusetts Medical School; Director, HIV Clinical Center, University of Massachusetts Medical Center, Worcester

Christopher H. Fanta, M.D.
Associate Professor of Medicine, Harvard Medical School; Clinical Director, Respiratory Division, Brigham and Women's Hospital, Boston

Paul Feldon, M.D.
Clinical Associate Professor of Orthopedic Surgery, Tufts University School of Medicine; Chief, Hand Surgery Service, St. Elizabeth's Hospital, Boston

Lewis R. First, M.D.
Assistant Professor of Pediatrics, Harvard Medical School; Associate in Medicine and Director, Pediatric Group Associates Program, Children's Hospital, Boston

Edwin G. Fischer, M.D.
Assistant Professor of Surgery, Harvard Medical School; Director of Neurosurgery, New England Deaconess Hospital, Boston

Gary R. Fleisher, M.D.
Associate Professor of Pediatrics, Harvard Medical School; Chief, Emergency Medicine, Children's Hospital, Boston

Jacek B. Franaszek, M.D.
Medical Director, Department of Emergency Services, Hinsdale Hospital, Hinsdale, Illinois

Ian Frank, M.D.
Assistant Professor of Medicine, University of Pennsylvania School of Medicine, Philadelphia

Gerald H. Friedland, M.D.
Professor of Medicine, Yale University School of Medicine; Director, Yale AIDS Program, Yale-New Haven Hospital, New Haven, Connecticut

Ann Furtado, M.D.
Assistant Clinical Professor of Medicine, New York Medical College, Valhalla; Associate Director, Emergency Department, Metropolitan Hospital Center, New York

John Gaca, M.D.
Assistant Professor of Medicine, University of Massachusetts Medical School, Worcester; Emergency Room Physician, Norwood Hospital, Norwood, Massachusetts

Nelson M. Gantz, M.D.
Clinical Professor of Medicine, Pennsylvania State University College of Medicine, Hershey; Director, Department of Medicine, and Chief, Division of Infectious Disease, Polyclinic Medical Center, Harrisburg

Michael P. Gaudet, M.D.
Fellow, University of Massachusetts Medical School, Worcester

Pierre Gaudreault, M.D.
Clinical Associate Professor of Pediatrics, University of Montreal Faculty of Medicine; Director, Clinical Pharmacology and Toxicology Section, Sainte-Justine Hospital, Montreal

Joel Geiderman, M.D.
Assistant Clinical Professor of Medicine, University of California, Los Angeles, UCLA School of Medicine; Associate Director of Emergency Medicine, Cedars-Sinai Medical Center, Los Angeles

D. Gary Gilliland, Ph.D., M.D.
Instructor in Medicine, Harvard Medical School; Associate Physician, Brigham and Women's Hospital, Boston

David Gitlin, M.D.
Assistant Professor of Psychiatry, University of Massachusetts Medical School; Director of Consultation/Liaison Psychiatry, University of Massachusetts Medical Center, Worcester

Richard H. Glew, M.D.
Professor of Medicine, Molecular Genetics, and Microbiology, University of Massachusetts Medical School; Chair, Department of Medicine, Medical Center of Central Massachusetts-Memorial, Worcester

Stefan Goldberg, M.D.
Senior Fellow, Division of Pulmonary and Critical Care Medicine, University of Washington School of Medicine and Harborview Medical Center, Seattle

Don L. Goldenberg, M.D.
Professor of Medicine, Tufts University School of Medicine, Boston; Chief of Rheumatology, Newton-Wellesley Hospital, Newton, Massachusetts

Lee Goldman, M.D.
Professor of Medicine, Harvard Medical School; Vice-Chairman, Department of Medicine, Brigham and Women's Hospital, Boston

Rose H. Goldman, M.D.
Assistant Professor of Medicine, Harvard Medical School, Boston; Director, Occupational and Environmental Health, Cambridge Hospital, Cambridge

Robert C. Goldszer, M.D.
Assistant Professor of Medicine, Harvard Medical School; Associate Physician, Department of Internal Medicine, Brigham and Women's Hospital, Boston

Joel M. Gore, M.D.
Professor of Medicine, University of Massachusetts Medical School; Director, Coronary Care Unit, University of Massachusetts Medical Center, Worcester

Mark Greenwald, M.D.
Clinical Coordinator, Adverse Reaction Clinic, Division of Clinical Pharmacology, University of Toronto Faculty of Medicine and Hospital for Sick Children; Director, Toronto Asthma Program, Department of Pediatrics, Yorkfinch General Hospital, Toronto

Nicholas G. Guerina, M.D.
Instructor in Pediatrics, Harvard Medical School, Assistant in Newborn Medicine and Infectious Disease, Children's Hospital, Boston; Neonatologist, Brigham and Women's and Beth Israel Hospitals, Boston, and Newton-Wellesley Hospital, Newton, Massachusetts

Charles I. Haffajee, M.B., M.R.C.P.
Professor of Medicine, Tufts University School of Medicine; Director, Cardiac Electrophysiology and Pacing, Division of Cardiovascular Medicine, St. Elizabeth's Hospital, Boston

Stephen E. Hedberg, M.D.*
Clinical Assistant Professor of Surgery, Harvard Medical School; Associate Visiting Surgeon and Senior Endoscopist in Gastrointestinal Surgery, Massachusetts General Hospital, Boston

Gregory L. Henry, M.D.
Clinical Assistant Professor, Section of Emergency Medicine, Department of Surgery, University of Michigan Medical School, Ann Arbor; Chief, Department of Emergency Medicine, Beyer Hospital, Ypsilanti

Mark T. Herbert, M.D.
Clinical Assistant Professor of Medicine, Ohio State University College of Medicine; Attending Physician, Division of Infectious Diseases, Mount Carmel Medical Center, Columbus

Stephen T. Hickey, M.D.
Neurologist and Pain Fellow, Department of Anesthesiology, Pain Evaluation and Treatment Institute, University of Pittsburgh School of Medicine, Pittsburgh

Jay Himmelstein, M.D., M.P.H.
Associate Professor and Director, Occupational Health Program, University of Massachusetts Medical Center, Worcester

Dee Hodge III, M.D.
Assistant Professor of Pediatrics and Emergency Medicine, University of Southern California School of Medicine; Director, Pediatric Emergency Room, Los Angeles County-USC Medical Center, Los Angeles

John Holbrook, M.D.
Instructor in Emergency Medicine, University of Massachusetts Medical School, Worcester; Vice President, Medical Affairs, Mercy Hospital, Springfield, Massachusetts

Norman K. Hollenberg, M.D., Ph.D.
Professor of Medicine, Harvard Medical School; Brigham and Women's Hospital, Boston

Charles E. Horton, Jr., M.D.
Assistant Professor of Urology, Eastern Virginia Medical School, Norfolk

*Deceased

Charles Huggins, M.D.*
Associate Professor of Surgery, Harvard Medical School; Visiting Surgeon and Director, Blood Transfusion Service, Massachusetts General Hospital, Boston

Richard Hunt, M.D.
Assistant Professor of Emergency Medicine, East Carolina University School of Medicine; Attending Physician, Emergency Department, and Medical Director, EastCare Emergency Air Medical Service, Pitt County Memorial Hospital, Greenville, North Carolina

Martin E. Hurwitz, M.D.
Clinical Assistant Professor of Pediatrics and Clinical Instructor of Surgery, University of Michigan Medical School; Attending Pediatrician, St. Joseph Mercy Hospital, Ann Arbor

Robert W. Hussey, M.D.
Associate Professor of Orthopedic Surgery, Virginia Commonwealth University Medical College of Virginia School of Medicine; Chief, Spinal Cord Injuries, H.H. McGuire Veterans Administration Medical Center, Richmond

Ivor M.D. Jackson, M.R.C.P.
Professor of Medicine and Director, Division of Endocrinology, Brown University Program in Medicine; Physician-in-Charge, Division of Endocrinology, Rhode Island Hospital, Providence

Edward E. Jacobs, Jr., M.D.
Assistant Clinical Professor of Otolaryngology, Harvard Medical School; Surgeon, Massachusetts Eye and Ear Infirmary, Boston

Lenworth M. Jacobs, M.D.
Professor of Surgery, University of Connecticut School of Medicine, Farmington; Chief, Department of Emergency Medicine/Trauma, Hartford Hospital, Hartford

William J. Jaffurs, Jr., M.D.
Clinical Assistant Professor of Emergency Medicine, East Carolina University School of Medicine, Greenville, North Carolina; Director, Emergency Department, Cape Fear Memorial Hospital, Wilmington, North Carolina

Carol B. Jankowski, B.S.N., M.Ed.
Associate in Radiology, Harvard Medical School; Nurse Educator, Health Physics Department, Brigham and Women's Hospital, Boston

Peter J. Jederlinic, M.D.
Assistant Professor of Medicine, University of Massachusetts Medical School; Attending Physician and Director, Pulmonary Function Laboratory, University of Massachusetts Medical Center, Worcester

*Deceased

John C. Johnson, M.D.
Assistant Professor of Emergency Medicine, Indiana University School of Medicine, Indianapolis; Director, Center for Trauma and Emergency Care, Porter Memorial Hospital, Valparaiso, Indiana

Kirtly Parker Jones, M.D.
Associate Professor of Obstetrics and Gynecology, University of Utah School of Medicine; Chief, Division of Reproductive Endocrinology, University of Utah Medical Center, Salt Lake City

Leonard B. Kaban, D.M.D., M.D.
Professor and Chairman, Department of Oral and Maxillofacial Surgery, University of California, San Francisco, School of Dentistry; Attending Surgeon, Mofitt-Long Hospital, San Francisco

Edward L. Kazarian, M.D.
Assistant Professor of Surgery, University of Massachusetts Medical School; Director, Pediatric Ophthalmology, University of Massachusetts Medical Center, Worcester

Gary P. Kearney, M.D.
Assistant Clinical Professor of Surgery, Harvard Medical School; Associate in Surgery, Brigham and Women's Hospital, Boston

Mark A. Keroack, M.D.
Associate Professor of Medicine, University of Massachusetts Medical School; Chief, Division of Infectious Diseases, Medical Center of Central Massachusetts-Memorial, Worcester

Paul Klainer, M.D.
Assistant Professor of Medicine, University of Massachusetts Medical School, Worcester; Director, Emergency Services, Milford Whitinsville Regional Hospital, Milford, Massachusetts

Walter A. Koltun, M.D.
Assistant Professor of Surgery, Pennsylvania State University College of Medicine; Attending Surgeon, Milton S. Hershey Medical Center, Hershey, Pennsylvania

J. Kenneth Koster, Jr., M.D.
Associate Clinical Professor of Surgery, University of Florida College of Medicine, Gainesville; Chief, Thoracic and Cardiovascular Surgery, Baptist Medical Center, Jacksonville

Roy M. Kulick, M.D.
Assistant Professor of Pediatrics, University of Cincinnati College of Medicine; Associate Director, Division of Emergency Medicine, Children's Hospital Medical Center, Cincinnati

Peter G. Lacouture, Ph.D.
Instructor in Pediatrics, Harvard Medical School; Assistant in Medicine, Children's Hospital, Boston

Dennis M.D. Landis, M.D.
Professor of Neurology and Neuroscience, Case Western Reserve University School of Medicine; Neurologist, University Hospitals, Cleveland

Ira Landsman, M.D.
Assistant Director of Emergency Services, University of Missouri-Kansas City School of Medicine and Children's Mercy Hospital, Kansas City

Diane Panton Lapsley, M.S., R.N., C.S.
Cardiovascular Research Nurse and Clinical Specialist, Veterans Administration Medical Center, West Roxbury, Massachusetts

Thomas H. Lee, M.D.
Assistant Professor of Medicine, Harvard Medical School; Associate Physician, Department of Medicine, Brigham and Women's Hospital, Boston

David W. Lhowe, M.D.
Instructor of Orthopedic Surgery, Harvard Medical School; Assistant in Orthopedic Surgery, Massachusetts General Hospital, Boston

Craig Lillehei, M.D.
Instructor in Surgery, Harvard Medical School; Assistant in Surgery, Children's Hospital, Boston

James G. Linakis, Ph.D., M.D.
Assistant Professor of Pediatrics, Brown University Program in Medicine; Attending Physician, Emergency Department, Rhode Island Hospital, Providence

Neal Little, M.D.
Clinical Instructor of Surgery, University of Michigan Medical School; Attending Emergency Physician, St. Joseph Mercy Hospital, Ann Arbor

Robert E. Longden, Jr., J.D.
Suffolk University Law School, Boston

Harvey Louzon, M.D.
Attending Physician, Department of Emergency Medicine, Michael Reese Hospital and Medical Center, Chicago

Frederick H. Lovejoy, Jr., M.D.
William Berenberg Professor of Pediatrics, Harvard Medical School; Associate Physician-in-Chief, Children's Hospital, Boston

Janice A. Lowe, M.D.
Instructor in Pediatrics, Harvard Medical School; Assistant Pediatrician, Massachusetts General Hospital, Boston

Michael Lucca, M.D.
Assistant Professor of Surgery, Department of Emergency Medicine, Hahnemann University Hospital; Visiting Assistant Professor of Emergency Medicine, Medical College of Pennsylvania, Philadelphia

Stephen Ludwig, M.D.
Professor of Pediatrics, University of Pennsylvania School of Medicine; Division Chief, General Pediatrics, Children's Hospital of Philadelphia, Philadelphia

John D. MacArthur, M.D.
Associate Clinical Professor of Surgery, Yale University School of Medicine, New Haven, Connecticut; Senior Attending and Chairman, Department of Surgery, Bridgeport Hospital, Bridgeport, Connecticut

J. Dugan Mahoney, M.D.
Chief, Emergency Department, Quincy Hospital, Quincy, Massachusetts

Jacalyn S. Maller, M.D.
Clinical Assistant Professor of Pediatrics, University of Pennsylvania School of Medicine; Attending Physician, Emergency Department, Children's Hospital of Philadelphia, Philadelphia

Harold L. May, M.D.
Assistant Professor of Surgery, Harvard Medical School; Associate in Surgery, Brigham and Women's Hospital, Boston

Charles J. McCabe, M.D.
Assistant Professor of Surgery, Harvard Medical School; Associate Visiting Surgeon and Associate Chief, Emergency Services, Massachusetts General Hospital, Boston

Karin McCloskey, M.D.
Assistant Professor of Pediatrics, University of Alabama School of Medicine; Medical Director, Critical Care Transport, Children's Hospital of Alabama, Birmingham

Cynthia G. McGinn, M.D.
Instructor of Medicine, Harvard Medical School, Boston; Attending Physician, Emergency Medicine Department, Mount Auburn Hospital, Cambridge

Ann McGravey, M.D.
Instructor in Pediatrics, Harvard Medical School; Assistant in Medicine, Children's Hospital, Boston

Michael A. McGuigan, M.D., C.M.
Associate Professor of Pediatrics and Pharmacology, University of Toronto Faculty of Medicine; Medical Director, Poison Information Centre, Hospital for Sick Children, Toronto

Kevin M. McIntyre, M.D., J.D.
Associate Clinical Professor of Medicine, Harvard Medical School, Boston, and Veteran's Administration Medical Center, West Roxbury, Massachusetts

Michael L. McManus, M.D.
Instructor in Anesthesia (Pediatrics), Harvard Medical School; Assistant in Anesthesia, Children's Hospital, Boston

Marvin A. McMillen, M.D.
Associate Professor of Surgery, Yale University School of Medicine, New Haven, Connecticut; Director, Surgical Intensive Care Unit, West Haven Veterans Administration Medical Center, West Haven, Connecticut

Denise Sevigny McQuaide, R.N., M.S.N., G.N.P.
Senior Associate, A/D/S Consulting Group, Inc., Cambridge, Massachusetts; Former Manager, Gerontology Services, Burbank Hospital, Fitchburg, Massachusetts

Michael J. Miller, M.D., Ph.D.
Assistant Professor of Medicine, Harvard Medical School, Boston; Assistant Chief of Medicine, Brockton/West Roxbury Veterans Administration Medical Center, Brockton, Massachusetts

Cynthia Briede Molloy, M.D.
Assistant Professor of Clinical Pediatrics, University of Louisville School of Medicine; Attending Physician, Emergency Department, Kosair-Children's Hospital, Louisville, Kentucky

Thomas J. Moore, M.D.
Assistant Professor of Medicine, Harvard Medical School; Associate Physician, Brigham and Women's Hospital, Boston

Debra L. Motto, M.D.
Department of Infectious Disease, Kaiser Permanente, Stockton, California

John B. Mulliken, M.D.
Associate Professor of Surgery, Division of Plastic Surgery, Harvard Medical School; Attending Surgeon and Director, Craniofacial Center, Children's Hospital and Brigham and Women's Hospital, Boston

Edward A. Nalebuff, M.D.
Clinical Professor of Orthopedic Surgery, Tufts University School of Medicine; Director, Hand Surgery Service, New England Medical Center Hospital, Boston

Peter T. Nieh, M.D.
Senior Staff, Department of Urology, Lahey Clinic Medical Center, Burlington, Massachusetts

Nicholas O'Connor, M.D.
Assistant Professor of Surgery, Harvard Medical School; Plastic Surgeon, Brigham and Women's Hospital, Boston

Roger V. Ohanesian, M.D.
Attending Surgeon, University of California, Irvine, California College of Medicine and South Coast Medical Center, Laguna Beach, California

Patricia O'Malley, M.D.
Assistant Professor of Pediatrics, Harvard Medical School; Director, Pediatric Emergency Services, Massachusetts General Hospital, Boston

Dennis P. Orgill, M.D., Ph.D.
Chief Surgical Resident, Brigham and Women's Hospital, Boston

Robert T. Osteen, M.D.
Associate Professor of Surgery, Harvard Medical School; Vice Chairman, Department of Surgery, Brigham and Women's Hospital, Boston

H. Gregory Ota, M.D.
Clinical Instructor in Otology and Laryngology, Harvard Medical School; Assistant in Surgery, Massachusetts Eye and Ear Infirmary, Boston

Mary L. Palermo, M.D.
Associate Director, Pediatric Intensive Care Unit, Ochsner Medical Foundation Hospital, New Orleans

John A. Paraskos, M.D.
Professor of Medicine, University of Massachusetts Medical School; Associate Director, Cardiovascular Medicine, University of Massachusetts Medical Center, Worcester

Paul M. Paris, M.D.
Associate Professor of Medicine, University of Pittsburgh School of Medicine; Chief, Department of Emergency Medicine, Presbyterian-University Hospital, Pittsburgh

Robert C. Pascucci, M.D.
Instructor in Anesthesia (Pediatrics), Harvard Medical School; Associate Director, Multidisciplinary Intensive Care Unit, Children's Hospital, Boston

John D. Patrick, M.D.
Instructor in Medicine, Harvard Medical School, Boston; Associate Chairman, Department of Emergency Medicine, Mount Auburn Hospital, Cambridge

Thomas R. Pellegrino, M.D.
Professor and Chairman, Department of Neurology, Eastern Virginia Medical School; Attending Neurologist and Chief, Neurology Teaching Service, Sentara Norfolk General Hospital, Norfolk

David H. Perrott, D.D.S., M.D.
Assistant Professor, University of California, San Francisco, School of Dentistry; Attending Surgeon, Department of Oral and Maxillofacial Surgery, Mofitt-Long Hospital, San Francisco

Lynn M. Peterson, M.D.
Assistant Professor of Surgery, Harvard Medical School; Associate Surgeon, Brigham and Women's Hospital and Beth Israel Hospital, Boston

Bohdan Pichurko, M.D.
Associate Professor of Medicine, Wayne State University School of Medicine; Chief, Section of Pulmonary and Critical Care, Sinai Hospital, Detroit

Claus A. Pierach, M.D.
Associate Professor of Medicine, University of Minnesota Medical School; Department of Medical Education, Abbott-Northwestern Hospital, Minneapolis

David M. Poppel, M.D.
Senior Clinical Instructor, Tufts University School of Medicine (Western Campus) and Baystate Medical Center; Nephrologist, Western Massachusetts Kidney Center, Springfield

Glenn Pransky, M.D., M.Occ.H.
Associate Professor, Department of Family and Community Medicine, University of Massachusetts Medical School; Chief of Clinical Services, Occupational Health Program, University of Massachusetts Medical Center, Worcester

N. Heramba Prasad, M.D.
Assistant Professor of Emergency Medicine and Associate Medical Director, Division of Emergency Medical Services, East Carolina University School of Medicine; Physician, Emergency Department, Pitt County Memorial Hospital, Greenville, North Carolina

Jennifer Pratt, M.D.
Associate Director of Emergency Services, Miami Children's Hospital, Miami

Diana S. Preston, M.D.
Senior Medical Resident, Mount Auburn Hospital, Cambridge, Massachusetts

Frank F. Rand, M.D.
Department of Orthopedic Surgery, Harvard Medical School, Boston

Jeffrey M. Rank, M.D.
Assistant Professor of Medicine, Department of Gastroenterology, Hepatology, and Nutrition, University of Minnesota Medical School; Attending Physician, Department of Medicine, University of Minnesota Hospital and Clinic, Minneapolis

Peter Reich, M.D.
Professor of Psychiatry, Harvard Medical School, Boston; Chief of Psychiatry, Massachusetts Institute of Technology Medical Department, Cambridge

Donald T. Reilly, Ph.D., M.D.
Assistant Clinical Professor of Orthopedic Surgery, Harvard Medical School; Orthopedic Surgeon, Brigham and Women's Hospital, Boston

John Reilly, Jr., M.D.
Instructor in Medicine, Harvard Medical School; Associate Physician, Brigham and Women's Hospital, Boston

Francis P. Renzi, M.D.
Assistant Professor of Medicine, University of Massachusetts Medical School, Worcester

Marc Restuccia, M.D.
Instructor in Medicine, Department of Emergency Medicine, University of Massachusetts Medical School; Department of Emergency Medicine, University of Massachusetts Medical Center, Worcester

Mel Robinson, M.D.
Staff Physician, Emergency and Trauma Center, Memorial Hospital, Colorado Springs, Colorado

Malcolm P. Rogers, M.D.
Assistant Professor of Psychiatry, Harvard Medical School; Assistant Director, Psychiatry Division, Brigham and Women's Hospital

Alan Rosenbaum, Ph.D.
Associate Professor of Psychiatry, University of Massachusetts Medical School; Chief Psychologist, Outpatient Psychiatry Clinic, University of Massachusetts Medical Center, Worcester

David Rosenthal, M.D.
Henry K. Oliver Professor of Hygiene, Harvard University; Associate Physician, Brigham and Women's Hospital, Boston

Lanny J. Rosenwasser, M.D.
Professor of Medicine, University of Colorado Health Sciences Center School of Medicine; Head, Division of Allergy and Clinical Immunology, National Jewish Center for Immunology and Respiratory Medicine, Denver

Ronald N. Roth, M.D.
Assistant Professor of Medicine, University of Pittsburgh School of Medicine; Attending Physician, Emergency Department, Presbyterian-University Hospital, Pittsburgh

Donald H. Rubin, M.D.
Professor of Medicine, Vanderbilt University School of Medicine; Associate Chief of Staff for Research, Veterans Administration Medical Center, Nashville

Leslie Rubin, M.D.
Assistant Professor of Pediatrics, Harvard Medical School; Director of Pediatrics, Developmental Evaluation Center, Children's Hospital, Boston

John D. Rutherford, M.B.Ch.B.
Assistant Professor of Medicine, Harvard Medical School; Cardiologist and Co-Director, Clinical Cardiology Services, Brigham and Women's Hospital

Alfredo A. Sadun, M.D., Ph.D.
Professor of Ophthalmology and Neurological Surgery, University of Southern California School of Medicine and Estelle Doheny Eye Hospital, Los Angeles

Pradip Sahdev, M.D.
Trauma Fellow, University of Connecticut School of Medicine, Farmington, and Hartford Hospital

Andrew E. Sama, M.D.
Assistant Professor of Medicine, Cornell University Medical College, New York; Associate Director, Emergency Medical Services, North Shore University Hospital, Manhasset, New York

Jonathan E. Samuels, M.D.
Assistant Professor of Medicine, Albert Einstein College of Medicine of Yeshiva University; Division of Infectious Diseases, Montefiore Medical Center, Bronx, New York

John H. Sanders, Jr., M.D.
Associate Professor of Surgery, Northwestern University Medical School; Attending Surgeon, Division of Cardiothoracic Surgery, Northwestern Memorial Hospital, Chicago

Emmett Schmidt, M.D., Ph.D.
Assistant Professor of Pediatrics, Harvard Medical School; Assistant in Pediatrics, Massachusetts General Hospital, Boston

Eric W. Schmidt, M.D.
Clinical Instructor of Emergency Medicine, University of Massachusetts Medical School, Worcester

Robert Schoene, M.D.
Associate Professor, Division of Pulmonary and Critical Care Medicine, University of Washington School of Medicine; Director, Pulmonary Function Laboratory, Harborview Medical Center, Seattle

Earl Schwartz, M.D.
Associate Professor and Chairman, Department of Emergency Medicine, Bowman Gray School of Medicine of Wake Forest University and North Carolina Baptist Hospital, Winston-Salem, North Carolina

Richard M. Schwartzstein, M.D.
Instructor in Medicine, Harvard Medical School; Pulmonary Attending Physician and Medical Director, Emergency Unit, Beth Israel Hospital, Boston

Paula Schweich, M.D.
Clinical Assistant Professor of Pediatrics, University of Washington School of Medicine, Seattle; Pediatric Emergency Physician, Mary Bridge Children's Hospital, Tacoma

Ellen W. Seely, M.D.
Assistant Professor of Medicine, Harvard Medical School; Director, Clinical Research, Endocrinology-Hypertension Division, Brigham and Women's Hospital, Boston

Steven M. Selbst, M.D.
Associate Professor of Pediatrics, University of Pennsylvania School of Medicine; Director, Emergency Department, Children's Hospital of Philadelphia, Philadelphia

Andrew Selwyn, M.D.
Director of Cardiac Catheterization, Brigham and Women's Hospital, Boston

Gary S. Setnik, M.D.
Instructor in Medicine, Harvard Medical School, Boston; Chairman, Department of Emergency Medicine, Mount Auburn Hospital, Cambridge

Paul N. Seward, M.D.
Assistant Clinical Professor of Surgery, Medical College of Georgia School of Medicine; Medical Director, Emergency Department, University Hospital, Augusta

Michael Shannon, M.D., M.P.H.
Assistant Professor of Pediatrics, Harvard Medical School; Assistant in Medicine, Children's Hospital, Boston

Daniel J. Shea, M.D.
Assistant Professor of Medicine, Division of Emergency Medicine, University of Massachusetts Medical School, Worcester; Associate Director, Emergency Services, St. Luke's Hospital, New Bedford

Michael Shear, M.D.
Instructor in Medicine, Harvard Medical School, Boston; Attending Physician, Department of Emergency Medicine, Mount Auburn Hospital, Cambridge

Robert Shesser, M.D., M.P.H.
Professor of Emergency Medicine, George Washington University School of Medicine and Health Sciences; Vice Chairman, Department of Emergency Medicine, George Washington University Medical Center, Washington, D.C.

Sharon Silbiger, M.D.
Assistant Professor of Medicine, Albert Einstein College of Medicine of Yeshiva University; Attending Physician, Division of Nephrology, Montefiore Medical Center, Bronx, New York

John M. Siliski, M.D.
Instructor in Orthopedic Surgery, Harvard Medical School; Reconstructive Knee Unit, Department of Orthopedic Surgery, Massachusetts General Hospital, Boston

Robert W. Simms, M.D.
Assistant Professor of Medicine, Boston University School of Medicine; Assistant Visiting Physician, Boston City Hospital, Boston

John J. Skillman, M.D.
Professor of Surgery, Harvard Medical School; Chief, Division of Vascular Surgery, Beth Israel Hospital, Boston

Mark Smith, M.D.
Professor of Emergency Medicine, George Washington University School of Medicine and Health Sciences; Chairman, Department of Emergency Medicine, George Washington University Medical Center, Washington, D.C.

Robert J. Smith, M.D.
Associate Professor of Medicine, Harvard Medical School; Assistant Director of Research and Head of Section on Metabolism, Joslin Diabetes Center, Boston

Michael Sobel, M.D.
Associate Professor of Surgery, Virginia Commonwealth University Medical College of Virginia School of Medicine; Chief, Vascular Surgery Service, H.H. McGuire Veterans Administration Medical Center, Richmond

Harold S. Solomon, M.D.
Assistant Clinical Professor of Medicine, Harvard Medical School; Department of Medicine, Brigham and Women's Hospital, Boston

Edmund H. Sonnenblick, M.D.
Olson Professor of Medicine, Albert Einstein College of Medicine of Yeshiva University; Chief, Division of Cardiology, Jack D. Weiler Hospital of the Albert Einstein College of Medicine and Bronx Municipal Hospital Center, Bronx, New York

Peter L. Sosnow, M.D.
Assistant Professor of Emergency Medicine, University of Massachusetts Medical School, Worcester; Director, Emergency and Outpatient Services, Albany Memorial Hospital, Albany, New York

Robert S. Stern, M.D.
Associate Professor of Dermatology, Harvard Medical School; Dermatologist, Beth Israel Hospital, Boston

Lee Stevens, M.D.
Attending Physician, Emergency Department, Citizens Medical Center, Victoria, Texas

Ronald D. Stewart, M.D.
Professor of Anesthesiology, Dalhousie University Faculty of Medicine; Attending Physician, Department of Emergency Medicine, Victoria General Hospital, Halifax, Nova Scotia

Jeffrey Stoff, M.D.
Professor of Medicine and Physiology, University of Massachusetts Medical School; Director, Renal Medicine and Transplantation Medicine, University of Massachusetts Medical Center, Worcester

William Strauss, M.D.
Assistant Professor of Medicine, Harvard Medical School, Boston; Director, Preventive Cardiology, Veterans Administrations Medical Center, West Roxbury, Massachusetts

John E. Strobeck, M.D., Ph.D.
Clinical Assistant Professor of Medicine, Albert Einstein College of Medicine of Yeshiva University, Bronx, New York; Attending Cardiologist and Director, Cardiac Care, The Valley Hospital, Ridgewood, New Jersey

Richard M. Stromberg, M.D.
Chief, Emergency Medical Services, Baptist Medical Center, Jacksonville, Florida

Lewis Sudarsky, M.D.
Assistant Professor of Neurology, Harvard Medical School; Neurology Division, Brigham and Women's Hospital, Boston

David J. Sugarbaker, M.D.
Assistant Professor of Surgery, Harvard Medical School; Chief, Thoracic Surgery, Brigham and Women's Hospital, Boston

Fred W. Tecklenburg, M.D.
Assistant Professor of Pediatrics, Medical University of South Carolina College of Medicine, Charleston

Margaret Thompson, M.D.
Assistant Professor of Medicine, University of Toronto Faculty of Medicine; Emergency Physician, St. Michael's Hospital, Toronto

Susan B. Torrey, M.D.
Director, Emergency Department, Bath Memorial Hospital, Bath, Maine; Emergency Medicine Associates, Oxford, Maine

Stephen B. Trippel, M.D.
Assistant Professor of Orthopedic Surgery, Harvard Medical School; Department of Orthopedic Surgery, Massachusetts General Hospital, Boston

Robert D. Truog, M.D.
Instructor in Anesthesia (Pediatrics), Harvard Medical School; Associate Director, Multidisciplinary Intensive Care Unit, Children's Hospital, Boston

Pamela A. Turner, M.Ed.
Research Associate, Massachusetts Eye and Ear Infirmary, Boston

Henry D. Unger, M.D.
Assistant Professor of Surgery and Director, Department of Emergency Medicine, Hahnemann University Hospital; Visiting Assistant Clinical Professor, Department of Emergency Medicine, Medical College of Pennsylvania, Philadelphia

Joseph Upton, M.D.
Associate Professor of Surgery, Harvard Medical School; Department of Plastic Surgery, Beth Israel Hospital and Children's Hospital, Boston

Vincent P. Verdile, M.D.
Assistant Professor of Medicine, University of Pittsburgh School of Medicine; Director, Emergency Department, Presbyterian-University Hospital, Pittsburgh

David M. Vernick, M.D.
Assistant Professor of Otology and Laryngology, Harvard Medical School; Associate Surgeon in Otolaryngology, Brigham and Women's Hospital; Assistant Surgeon in Otolaryngology, Beth Israel Hospital; Assistant in Otolaryngology, Massachusetts Eye and Ear Infirmary, Boston

Ingrid M-O Vicas, M.D., C.M.
Clinical Associate Professor of Pharmacology and Clinical Assistant Professor of Internal Medicine, University of Calgary Faculty of Medicine; Director, Poison and Drug Information Service, Foothills Provincial General Hospital, Calgary

Maurice Victor, M.D.
Professor of Medicine (Neurology), Dartmouth Medical School, Hanover, New Hampshire; Distinguished Physician of the Veterans Administration Hospital, White River Junction, Vermont

Usha Vyas-Major, M.D.
Associate Director, Emergency Medical Services, Porter Memorial Hospital, Valparaiso, Indiana

Michael D. Wagoner, M.D.
Assistant Professor of Ophthalmology, Harvard Medical School; Co-Director, Cornea Service, Massachusetts Eye and Ear Infirmary, Boston

Thomas M. Walshe, M.D.
Assistant Professor of Neurology, Harvard Medical School, Boston; Neurologist, Brockton Veterans Administration Medical Center, Brockton, Massachusetts

Wayne S. Warren, M.D.
Clinical Instructor of Medicine, Yale University School of Medicine; Attending Physician, Department of Medicine, Yale-New Haven Hospital, New Haven, Connecticut

Peter Waters, M.D.
Instructor in Orthopedic Surgery, Harvard Medical School; Attending Orthopedic and Hand Surgeon, Children's Hospital and Brigham and Women's Hospital, Boston

Michael S. Weinstock, M.D.
Assistant Professor of Surgery, Cornell University College of Medicine, New York; Director, Emergency Medical Services, North Shore University Hospital, Manhasset, New York

Larry D. Weiss, M.D.
Clinical Assistant Professor of Medicine, Louisiana State University School of Medicine in New Orleans; Staff Physician, Department of Emergency Medicine, Charity Hospital of Louisiana, Jo Ellen Smith Medical Center, and Meadowcrest Hospital, New Orleans

Gil Wernovsky, M.D.
Instructor in Pediatrics, Harvard Medical School; Associate in Cardiology and Assistant Director, Cardiovascular Intensive Care Unit, Children's Hospital, Boston

Barry K. Wershil, M.D.
Assistant Professor of Pediatrics, Harvard Medical School; Assistant in Gastroenterology, Combined Program in Pediatric Gastroenterology/Nutrition, Children's Hospital, Boston

David L. Wessel, M.D.
Assistant Professor of Pediatrics, Harvard Medical School; Senior Associate in Cardiology, Associate in Cardiovascular Surgery, and Director, Cardiac Intensive Care Unit, Children's Hospital, Boston

Anthony D. Whittemore, M.D.
Associate Professor of Surgery, Harvard Medical School; Chief, Division of Vascular Surgery, Brigham and Women's Hospital, Boston

Kenneth A. Williams, M.D.
Assistant Professor of Emergency Medicine, University of Massachusetts Medical School; Medical Director, New England Life Flight, Emergency Department, University of Massachusetts Medical Center, Worcester

Paul H. Wise, M.D., M.P.H.
Assistant Professor of Pediatrics, Harvard Medical School; Assistant in Medicine, Children's Hospital, Boston

Lee A. Witters, M.D.
Eugene W. Leonard Professor of Medicine and Biochemistry, Dartmouth Medical School; Chief, Endocrine-Metabolism Division, Dartmouth-Hitchcock Medical Center, Hanover, New Hampshire

Alan C. Woodward, M.D.
Assistant Clinical Professor of Community Medicine, Tufts-New England Medical Center, Boston; Chief, Emergency Services, Emerson Hospital, Concord, Massachusetts

Alan D. Woolf, M.D., M.P.H.
Assistant Professor of Pediatrics, Harvard Medical School; Assistant in Medicine, Children's Hospital, Boston

Donald M. Yealy, M.D.
Assistant Professor of Emergency Medicine, Texas A&M University College of Medicine, College Station; Adjunct Clinical Assistant Professor of Emergency Medicine, University of Pittsburgh School of Medicine, Pittsburgh; Attending Physician, Department of Emergency Medicine, Darnall Army Community Hospital, Fort Hood, Texas

John K. Zawacki, M.D.
Associate Professor of Medicine, University of Massachusetts Medical School; Division of Digestive Diseases and Nutrition, University of Massachusetts Medical Center, Worcester

I. Life Support

A. Dying and Resuscitation

1. Life and Death

Harold L. May

Clinical death, the reversible transition between life and biologic death, is the ultimate emergency. It begins when the last agonal breath has been taken and the heart has stopped beating. The victim is unresponsive, with dilated pupils and without breath or heartbeat. If appropriate intervention is not immediate, resuscitation becomes impossible.

The idea that death can be reversed is not new. Since antiquity, people have struggled to find ways to resuscitate those who have died. Until relatively recently, many of the methods that were used were unchanged from those that had been practiced for more than 1,000 years, but during the past 5 decades, the pioneering work of Claude Beck, V.A. Negovsky, Peter Safar, and others has led to an increased understanding of the pathophysiology of cardiac arrest and to the development of clinically effective methods of its management. Direct compression and defibrillation of the heart through the open chest made resuscitation possible within the hospital during the 1940s under special conditions. But resuscitation for many potential victims of sudden death occurring outside the hospital was not possible until 1959, when Kouwenhoven, Jude, and Knickerbocker described successful external chest compression.

In 1985, there were 2,086,500 deaths in the United States. Of these, 771,000 (37.0%) were caused by heart disease, 461,500 (22.1%) by cancer, 153,000 (7.3%) by cerebrovascular disease, and 93,500 (4.5%) by accidents (Fig. 1-1). Many of these deaths were expected and unavoidable, either because of advanced age or irreparable pathology. But sudden cardiac arrest claims approximately 400,000 lives a year in the United States; about two-thirds of these deaths occur outside the hospital, usually within 2 hours after onset of symptoms. Most such deaths are caused by ventricular fibrillation. In these patients, clinical death is often the first symptom of disease.

Overall, only approximately 10 percent of the patients with prehospital cardiopulmonary resuscitation (CPR) attempts for cardiac arrest recover completely and are able to resume their former life-styles. The major reason for this poor outcome is permanent neurologic injury. In contrast, emergency resuscitation succeeds in 50 to 100 percent of patients who arrest during monitoring in the operating room or a hospital special care unit. Reports from communities with highly developed approaches to cardiac arrest victims—communities with large numbers of laypersons trained in CPR, a rapid emergency medical service response system, and well-trained paramedical personnel—have demonstrated that up to 40 percent of the patients documented to have ventricular fibrillation outside the hospital have been successfully resuscitated when bystanders started basic life support (BLS) within 4 minutes of collapse, and paramedics or physicians defibrillated the heart within 8 minutes. In selected subgroups of these reports, the success rate exceeds 60 percent. It is clear that BLS is a holding action, maintaining the victim for a limited period of time. It

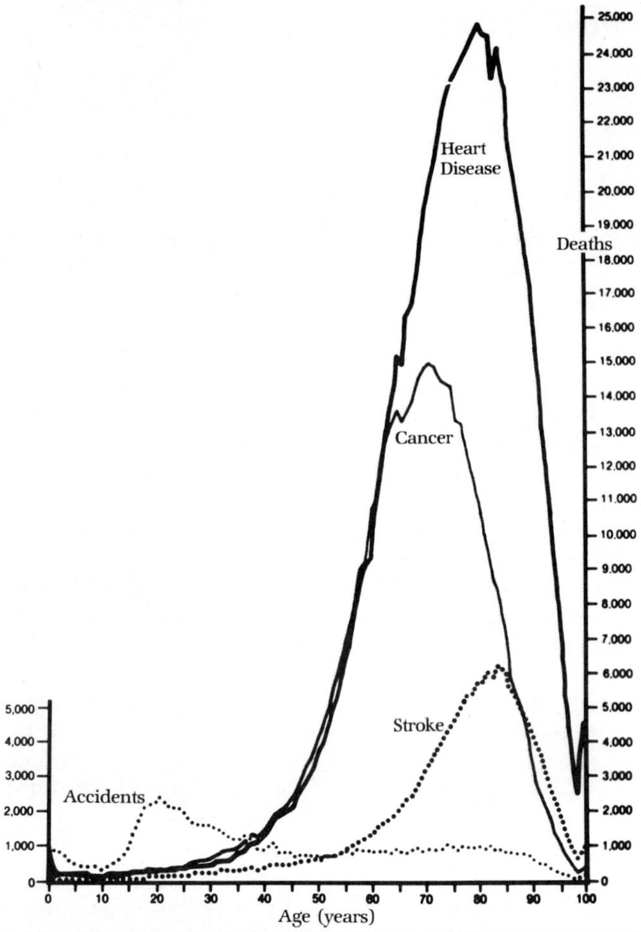

Fig. 1-1. Leading causes of death by age (1985). (From *Accident Facts.* Chicago: National Safety Council, 1988.)

must be followed by definitive therapy if the outcome is to be successful. Although initial efforts must focus on establishing adequate ventilation and circulation, the ultimate aim has to be to maintain the viability of the brain since life is defined by the viability of the brain.

BASIC MICROBIOLOGICAL CONCEPTS: NORMALLY FUNCTIONING CELLS

Cell Structure and Function

Many of the advances in medical practice that have occurred in the past 2 decades and the promise for further progress in the future have come and will come from our deepening understanding of the molecular biology of individual cells, the smallest units of life. Some of the central processes of cellular life, including homeostatic defense mechanisms, are reviewed here because many cells are driven by the same basic mechanisms, although their biological activity and functions vary widely. Despite the vastness of the assortment of noxious stimuli that confront the body, the repertoire of defenses with which it responds is usually limited. The same defense mechanisms are activated to a greater or lesser extent, for good and, sometimes, for ill, regardless of the stimulus.

In discussions here and in other chapters about acute illness, injury, and death caused by hypoxemia, trauma, chemical toxins, infections, and other noxious forces, many of the cellular forces and responses outlined below are at work.

Cytoplasm and Organelles

Each cell, bounded by a plasma membrane, contains intracellular membranes that concentrate and hold the set of enzymes that uniquely endow each compartment to carry out its special functions (Fig. 1-2). The membranes prevent the enzymatic reactions that are being carried out in adjacent compartments from interfering with each other, although they are often competing operations. Some proteins can be synthesized in the cytosol while others are being degraded in lysosomes; some fatty acids can be synthesized in the cytosol for use in the formation of the cell's membranes while other fatty acids are being broken down in the mitochondria to synthesize ATP.

The *nucleus,* with the body's genetic information stored in the DNA molecules of its chromosomes, determines the form, structure, and function of the cell as the DNA molecules direct the synthesis of the cell's specific proteins and pass on precise copies of the genetic code to daughter cells by cellular division. All the nuclei of the body contain identical genes; cell differentiation from one tissue to another occurs because the nuclei differentially control the use of the genetic information from cell to cell. The nuclear pores in the nuclear envelope allow passage of the genetic information from nucleus to cytoplasm. The outer surface of the nucleus is studded with ribosomes, large complexes composed of protein and molecules of ribonucleic acids, which together form a molecular framework on which protein molecules can be assembled.

The nucleus also contains at least one, sometimes two or three, nucleoli. In the *nucleolus,* the information that is encoded in the nucleus is translated into the synthesis of proteins by means of ribonucleic acids (RNAs), a group of nucleic acids that differ from DNA primarily in the composition of its bases. Three forms of RNA guide the synthesis of protein within the cell: ribosomal RNA (rRNA), messenger RNA (mRNA), and transfer RNA (tRNA).

Ribosomal RNA is continuously transcribed in the nucleolus to ensure a constantly adequate supply for the cell, and the newly synthesized rRNA is immediately packaged in the nucleus with ribosomal proteins, imported from the cell cytoplasm. The resulting ribosomes are thought to attain their final form only as they are individually transported through the nuclear pores into the cytoplasm.

The DNA information is transcribed to the second kind of RNA that is synthesized in the nucleolus, mRNA; one strand of the DNA double strand serves as the template for the synthesis of a complimentary single-stranded mRNA polymer. The filaments of mRNA leave the nucleolus by way of the nuclear pores and migrate into the cytoplasm, where both free and membrane-bounded ribosomes attach to them like beads on a necklace.

Amino acids cannot produce polypeptide chains without the help of tRNA. Once transfer RNA passes from the nucleolus and into the cytoplasm, the specific enzymatic terminals of its cloverleaf molecules serve as adapters as one end decodes the genetic message while the other end hooks up to specific amino acids only, thereby assembling the poly-

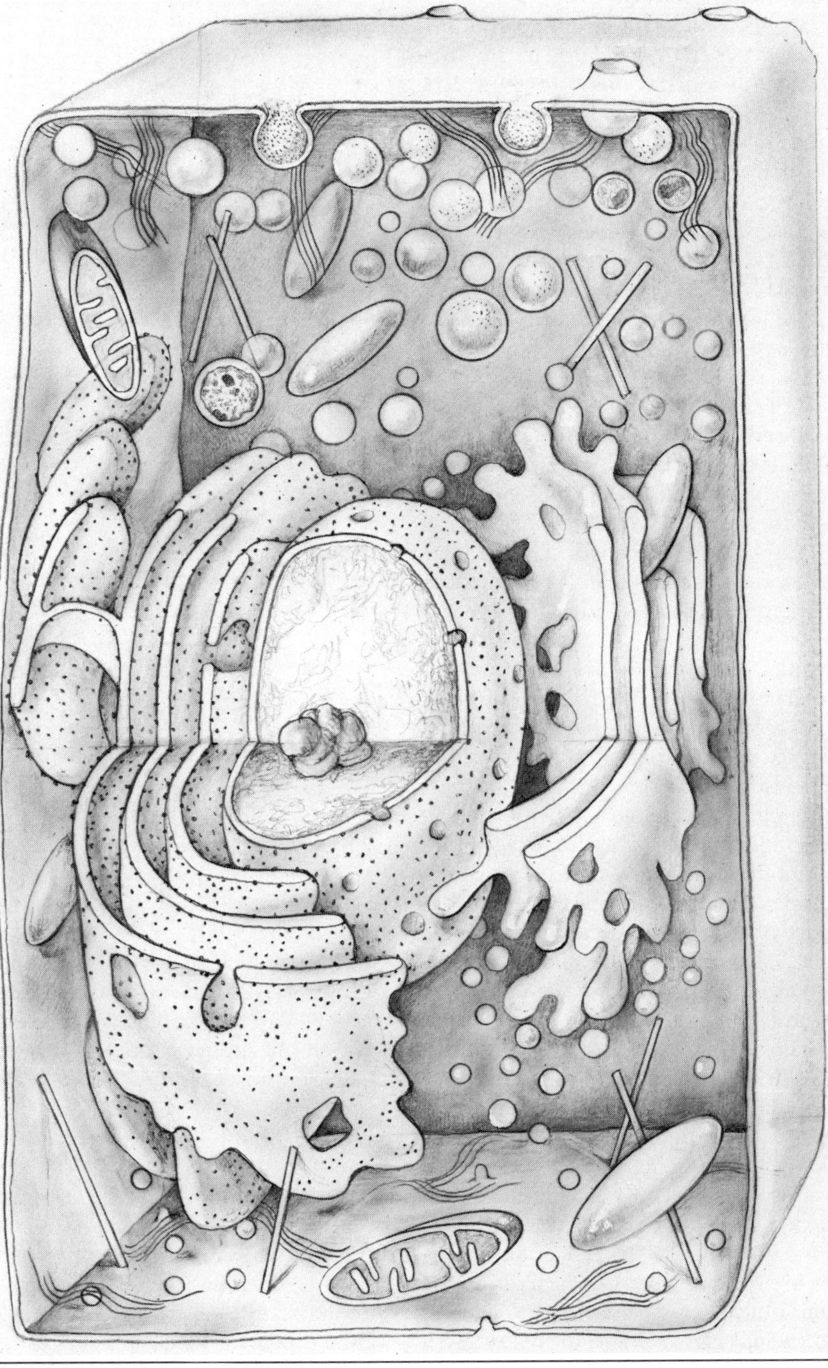

Fig. 1-2. The cell, showing the major organelles. Note intermediate filaments and sticklike microtubules. Actin filaments are not shown (see text). (Adapted from K.V. Krstic. *Ultrastructure of the Mammalian Cell.* Berlin: Springer-Verlag, 1979.)

peptide chains according to the genetically determined sequence. Amino acids are incorporated in polypeptides at a rate as fast as 20 per second, so that complete synthesis of an average-sized protein takes 20 to 60 seconds.

The *endoplasmic reticulum (ER),* a system of branching channels and passageways, typically constitutes more than half of the total membrane of the cell, sometimes amounting to as much as 25 times the surface of the plasma membrane. It is a membrane factory, producing nearly all the protein and lipid components for most of the cell's organelles as well as synthesizing proteins destined for export outside the cell. Lipids, proteins, and complex carbohydrates destined for transportation to the Golgi apparatus, plasma membrane, lysosome, or cell exterior are all synthesized in association with the ER. Rough ER, studded with ribosomes, is especially prominent in cells that specialize in protein secretion, such as antibody-secreting plasma cells. Smooth ER, which contains no ribosomes, is sometimes a predominant organelle in cells, such as hepatocytes, which specialize in lipid metabolism. Muscle cells have a specialized and elaborate ER, the sarcoplasmic reticulum, described in Chap. 16 (see Fig. 16-1).

The *Golgi apparatus,* usually located near the cell nucleus, consists of a stack of disk-shaped cisternae surrounded by swarms of small vesicles, which are required for the final steps in the synthesis and transport of many proteins. The Golgi apparatus is probably the principal director of macromolecular traffic in the cell, as vesicles shuttle rapidly and continually between the cell's organelles. The apparatus receives newly synthesized proteins and lipids from the ER and distributes them to the plasma membrane, secretory vesicles, and lysosomes, often modifying these molecules during their passage through the apparatus. Secretory cells concentrate and store products in Golgi-associated secretory vesicles for quick release to the cell's exterior when the cell is stimulated by a special signal.

The *mitochondria,* the respiratory organelles of the cell, produce the energy required for cellular metabolism. Each cell must satisfy its own energy needs at all times by continuously forming adenosine triphosphate (ATP) molecules, the body's principle immediate donor of free energy. This process occurs predominantly in the mitochondria. Cells with high energy requirements, such as the hepatocyte, may need as many as 1,000 to 1,500 mitochondria to meet their energy needs.

Since the ATP molecule is formed by the addition of a high-energy phosphate group to the adenosine diphosphate (ADP) molecule by the process of oxidative phosphorylation, oxygen and substrate must be transported continuously to the mitochondria to generate ATP. This requires the harmonious interplay of the cardiopulmonary system, the microcirculation, and cellular metabolism as the oxygen diffuses from one level to another, driven by the concentration gradient across membranes, finally reaching the mitochondria. The partial pressure of oxygen in pulmonary alveoli is normally approximately 104 mm Hg; in peripheral tissues, 95 mm Hg; in interstitial fluid, 40 mm Hg; normal intracellular PO_2 ranges from as low as 5 mm Hg to as high as 40 mm Hg. Since only 3 mm Hg of oxygen pressure is normally required in the mitochondrion for full support of the metabolic processes of the cell, it is clear that, under normal conditions, the circulatory system delivers an excess of substrate and oxygen to the cell and, under special physiologic conditions (such as exercise), it continuously couples blood flow and oxygen extraction to cellular oxygen need.

Although oxygen is the ultimate electron acceptor in aerobic cells, the electrons are not transferred directly from the fuel molecules to oxygen but are transferred along an electron transport chain to special carrier molecules (Fig. 1-3). The first step in oxidative phosphorylation in mitochondria is the ionization of the hydrogen atoms that have been removed from pyruvate, amino acids, and fatty acids, the breakdown products of carbohydrate, fat, and protein. The hydrogen atoms are peeled off in pairs, one becoming a hydrogen ion, and the other combining with a hydrogen receptor, nicotine adenine dinucleotide (NAD) to form NADH or with flavine adenine dinucleotide (FAD) to form $FADH_2$. The electrons that are removed from the hydrogen atoms enter molecules of the cytochrome system, an electron transport chain that is embedded in the inner membrane of the mitochondria. In the process of oxidative phosphorylation, the electrons that have been transported along the transport chain are transferred to molecular oxygen, thereby releasing a great deal of chemical energy to make the major

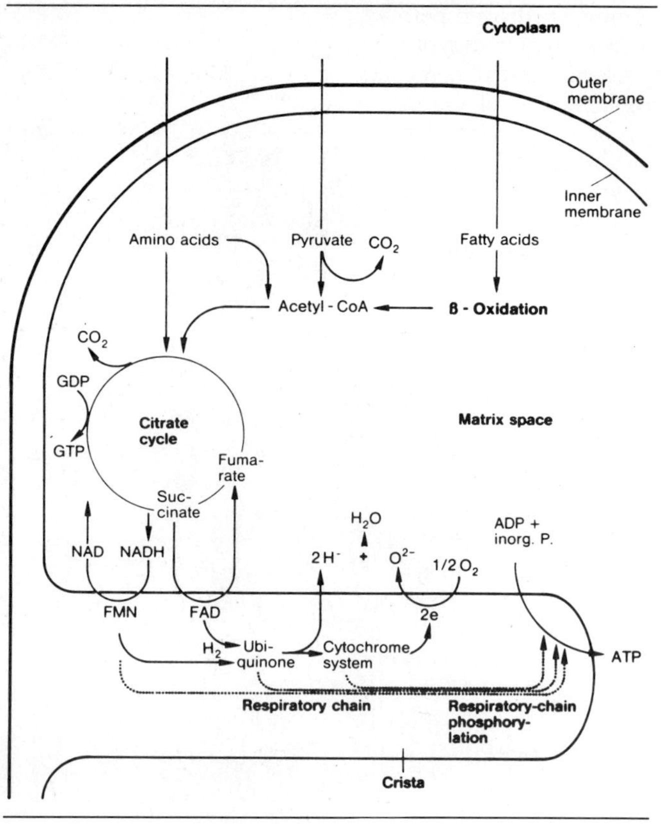

Fig. 1-3. Oxidative phosphorylation to form ATP in the mitochondrion. (From R.F. Schmidt and G. Thews. *Human Physiology* [2nd ed.]. Berlin: Springer-Verlag, 1989.)

portion of the cell's ATP by adding a high-energy phosphate group to ADP; the rest of the energy is liberated as heat.

ATP can also be formed by the creatine kinase reaction in which phosphocreatine (PCr) is used to phosphorylate ADP. This reaction is present in skeletal muscle, heart, and brain.

$$[PCr] + [ADP] + [H+] \leftrightarrow [ATP] + [AMP]$$

As is true of all metabolic reactions, there must be cutoff mechanisms for régulating the synthesis of ATP in order to prevent wasteful continued release of energy when the energy is not needed. The mechanisms for producing ATP anaerobically when the supply of oxygen is limited are discussed later in this chapter.

The *lysosomes,* the principal sites of intracellular digestion, contain powerful digestive enzymes—proteases, nucleases, lipases, phospholipases, phosphatases, sulfatases, and others. They provide a line of defense against invasion by bacteria and other foreign agents as they digest microorganisms and other contents that have been engulfed by the phagocytes. In most cells of the body, they participate in programmed cell death as organelles that have become worn out or exhausted and need to be replaced are incorporated into lysosomes and digested. Many of the cell components, such as receptors and membranes, are destroyed and recycled by this mechanism. Hepatocytes and macrophages contain as many as 200 lysosomes.

Peroxisomes, which are involved in peroxide metabolism, contain one or more enzymes that use molecular oxygen to produce hydrogen peroxide (H_2O_2). Like the mitochondria, they are major sites of oxygen utilization, normally accounting for at least 10 percent of total O_2 uptake in the liver. They contain most of the cell's catalase that converts hydrogen peroxide to water and oxygen when excess H_2O_2 accumulates in the cell. Although H_2O_2 is necessary in a number of cellular reactions and is capable of killing microorganisms, it is tolerated only in low concentrations in the cytosol.

Peroxisomes are relatively numerous in hepatocytes and in renal tubular cells, where they are thought to be important in detoxifying certain molecules. Almost half of the alcohol that is consumed is detoxified in the liver in this way. In the liver, peroxisomes also participate in gluconeogenesis, forming glucose from lipids and other noncarbohydrate precursors. They also catalyze one-fourth to one-half of fatty acid breakdown to feed the citric acid cycle in the mitochondria. Peroxisomes are also numerous in macrophages.

The *cytoplasm,* where all intermediary metabolism takes place, contains the thousands of enzymes that catalyze the reactions of protein synthesis, glycolysis, and gluconeogenesis, as well as the biosynthesis of sugars, fatty acids, nucleotides, and amino acids. Since approximately 20 percent of the weight of the cytosol is protein, it is more like a highly organized gel than a simple solution of enzyme molecules. Powered by ATP, the cell teems with activity as enzymes are switched on and off in response to intracellular messages, described below. The resulting conformational changes in the protein molecules contained in the cell regulate the biologic activity of the protein and, therefore, the functions of the cell, from muscle contraction for some cells to secretion of digestive enzymes for others.

The *cytoskeleton* is a group of cytoplasmic proteins that function as an integrated network to control and coordinate the movements and shapes of cells. It consists of three principal protein filaments: actin filaments, intermediate filaments, and microtubules. Actin, the most abundant protein in many cells, is distributed throughout the cytoplasm, but in most cells actin filaments are especially concentrated just beneath the plasma membrane, where they are often cross-linked with other proteins, giving mechanical strength to the cell's surface. Myosin, the most abundant protein in muscle, is found in most cells, although it is present in much lower concentrations than is actin. Actin filaments, interacting with myosin, are contractile, making possible movement of the cell and such changes in shape as invagination of the cell membrane. Intermediate filaments (intermediate between actin tubules and microtubules) are tough, ropelike, protein fibers in the cytoplasm of most cells. In most cells they extend outward in gentle curves from the nucleus to the periphery. They are particularly prominent in cells that are subjected to mechanical stress; they support or stiffen cells and play a role in organizing intracellular organelles for coordinated activity. Microtubules are hollow, nonbranching cylinders that give mechanical strength to the cell and permit asymmetry of shape of specialized cells and structures. As discussed in Chap. 16, the function of the cytoskeletal structures is controlled, at least in part, by cytosolic calcium ion concentration.

Cell Membranes

The cell membranes are intensely active metabolically. They consist of a lipid bilayer in which various proteins are incorporated as a mosaic of molecules (Fig. 1-4). About 50 percent of the mass of a typical plasma membrane is protein. Some membrane proteins function as receptors of extracellular signals; others serve to transport molecules or ions across the membrane. The kinds and amounts of proteins in a

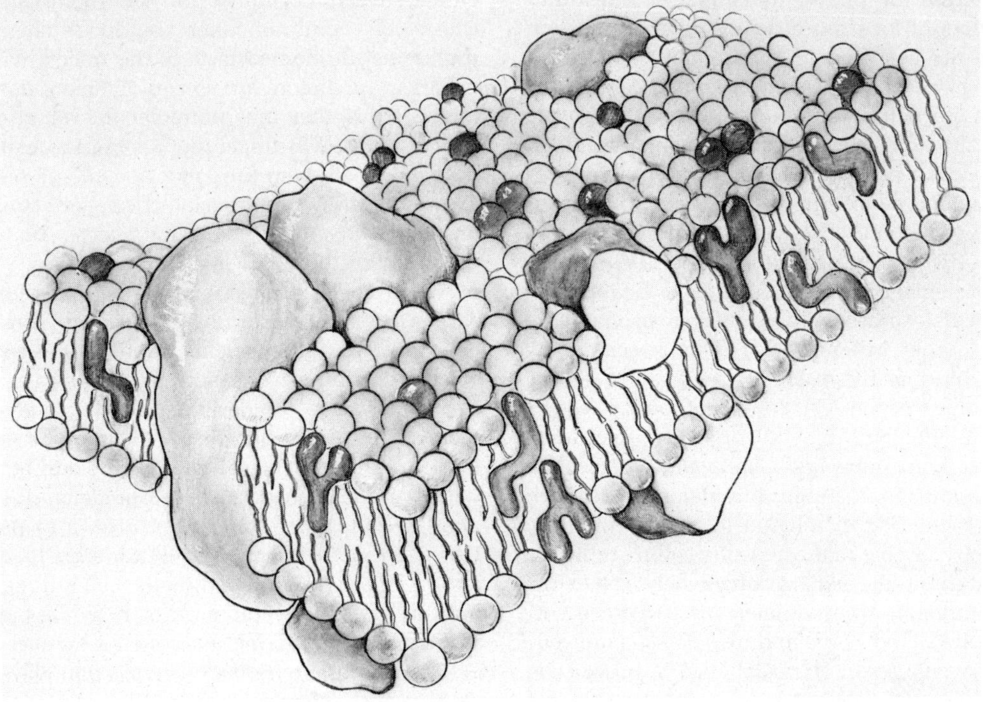

Fig. 1-4. The plasma membrane, showing the bilayer of phospholipids, the large protein molecules, and the smaller cholesterol and glycoprotein molecules.

membrane reflect its functions, since many of the specific functions of cellular membranes are carried out by their constituent proteins.

The most abundant lipids in cellular membranes are phospholipids, but glycolipids and cholesterol are also found, the relative proportion depending on the tissue. The lipid bilayer exists in a relatively fluid state, with the consistency of olive oil. Protein molecules are distributed on each surface of the lipid bilayer, whereas other proteins penetrate both layers, protruding from one or both of its surfaces. Because membrane lipids and many membrane proteins contain hydrophilic and hydrophobic regions in the same molecule, the membranes show selective permeability. Lipids determine the solubility of the plasma membrane; fat-soluble compounds readily enter cells, dissolving in the membrane, whereas fat-insoluble compounds enter by more complex mechanisms.

Transport Across Membranes

The plasma membrane and the membranes of the intracellular organelles function as dynamic, regulatory barriers to the entry and exit of molecules and particles. Small, uncharged molecules normally move selectively across membranes by passive transport along a concentration gradient, from higher to lower concentration, or by active transport, in which energy is expended to pump a molecule against its concentration gradient. In general, the smaller the molecule and the more soluble it is in oil, the more rapidly it will diffuse passively across a cellular membrane. Because the water molecule is small and uncharged, it diffuses rapidly, in spite of the fact that it is relatively insoluble in oil. In contrast, the cell membrane is highly impermeable to all charged molecules, no matter how small.

Some of the transporter proteins (*channel proteins*), act as though they were aqueous channels that traverse the membrane and permit molecules of appropriate size and charge to move across the bilayer by simple passive diffusion. Large numbers of ions move down the concentration gradient and into the cell through these channels. Certain channel proteins, *gated pores* or *gated channels*, open only in response to a particular stimulus and are otherwise closed. In electrically excitable cells, calcium channels open in response to an action potential triggered when a messenger molecule (usually a neurotransmitter) binds to a receptor on the surface of the cell. The channels are continually opening and closing in response to appropriate signals. Other transport proteins, *carrier proteins*, specifically bind and transfer molecules across the lipid bilayer, probably by a conformational change in the protein as the specific molecules attach to a binding site or sites.

More than one-third of the ATP consumed by the resting human is used in fueling the $Na^+ - K^+$ *pump*, a protein that pumps in two directions, pumping 3 Na^+ out of the cell for every 2 K^+ that it pumps in. It thereby maintains the negative charge of the cell's interior in relation to its environment, generating an electrical potential across the cell membrane. As the pump maintains the Na^+ gradient between extra- and intracellular fluids at approximately 10:1, the cell volume is also controlled, and nerve and muscle cells are rendered electrically excitable. In electrically active nerve cells that must continually reestablish their membrane potentials following depolarization, the $Na^+ - K^+$ pump consumes approximately 70 percent of the cell's total energy requirement.

The Ca^{2+} gradient in a typical cell is about 10,000:1. The almost infinitely low cytosolic Ca^{2+} concentration requires mechanisms for calcium removal. One of these, the *calcium pump*, an ATPase enzyme, responds to minute increases in intracellular calcium. More drastic swings in concentration activate the other calcium removal system, the so-called *sodium-calcium exchanger*, a protein that is particularly abundant in excitable cells (nerve and muscle cells), which repeatedly experience rapid influxes of calcium in response to electrical impulses. The exchanger serves mainly to remove large quantities of calcium from excitable cells following stimulation.

Whereas small molecules can be transported across cell membranes by transport proteins, large molecules, such as proteins, or polysaccharide can be transported only by *endocytosis*, the process by which substances can be brought into a cell by being enclosed in a small portion of plasma membrane. Under the control of cytoskeletal elements, a part of the membrane invaginates, then pinches off, forming an intracellular vesicle that contains the ingested material. By the reverse process, *exocytosis*, many kinds of cell secretions leave the cells in which they are synthesized.

Cell-to-Cell Signaling and Intracellular Communication

Cells must communicate with each other. Adjacent cells communicate directly through small gaps in the intercellular junctions; through these, small, water-soluble molecules can pass directly from one cell to another so that the adjacent cells are coupled electrically and metabolically. The size of these openings is so small that large molecules (proteins, polypeptides, and nucleic acids) cannot pass.

In addition to the long-distance communication that occurs between hormones or nerves and their target cells, cell-to-cell communication by local chemical mediators maintains the homeostasis of the microenvironment. These chemical mediators are so rapidly taken up or destroyed by the cells that they may not enter the bloodstream in significant amounts. Chemical mediators may act only on the cells that produced them (an autocrine effect), on cells in the immediate vicinity (a paracrine effect), or systemically, as with any other hormone (endocrine effect). These mediators are discussed in the following paragraphs.

As extracellular signals are sent and received, they alter cell function. The external signals, or first messengers, must be converted into internal signals, or second messengers, which will induce the biochemical changes within the cell that will lead to the desired physiologic effect(s). Few hormones are fat soluble; these, the steroids and thyroid hormones, penetrate the cell membrane and attach to receptors within the cell on or near the nucleus, directly interacting with DNA to alter messenger RNA and protein synthesis. However, most of the extracellular signals are water soluble and therefore never penetrate the cell membrane but instead bind to specific receptors on or near the membrane's outer surface, thus activating a second messenger inside the cell.

Two major second messenger pathways, calcium ions, and cyclic adenosine monophosphate (cyclic AMP or cAMP) interface with other compounds described below, which are also termed *second messengers.* These second messengers sometimes act directly, binding to the target protein as occurs in skeletal muscle when the calcium ion binds to a protein, triggering a change that leads to contraction of the muscle (see Chap. 16). More commonly, the second messengers act indirectly. Changes in the intracellular concentration of these second messengers activate enzymes, protein kinases, which modulate the activities of target proteins in cells by phosphorylating them. Since the addition of a high-energy phosphate group (obtained from the ubiquitous ATP molecule) to a selected protein activates it by inducing a change in its shape, phosphorylation is often the switch that turns the many enzymes of the cytosol on or off. The change in structure of the target intracellular proteins results in a change in their function and activity. The net result is an alteration of cell function.

The metabolism and functions of calcium and cAMP are intertwined, the calcium and the cAMP second messenger pathways nearly always functioning together to couple stimulus to response.

Cyclic AMP and G Protein

Cyclic AMP is formed from cytosolic ATP by the action of adenylate cyclase, an enzyme bound to the cytosolic surface of the membrane. Cyclic AMP can function as an intracellular mediator because its intracellular concentration is tightly controlled, and it can change fivefold within short seconds in response to extracellular signals.

The binding site for hormones and other first messengers (the receptor) extends from the outer layer of the cell membrane to the inner layer, but the effector (e.g., adenylate cyclase) is a separate protein. The vital bridge between the receptor and the effector is a third protein, termed *G protein* because it binds guanine nucleotide, such as guanosine triphosphate (GTP) (Fig. 1-5). G proteins are subdivided into three distinct subunits: α, β, and γ. The α subunits differ slightly from one G protein to another, thereby conferring receptor and effector specificity. G proteins have enormous physiologic and pathophysiologic significance because at least one of the G proteins is present in all cells and the G protein coupling systems are used by an astonishingly wide array of first messengers for conveying signals to cells.

When the receptor recognizes a specific first messenger, even when present in low concentrations in a mixture of many other molecules, it activates the G protein, which conducts the signal to the effector. Often, the effector is an enzyme of second messenger metabolism, such as adenylate cyclase or phospholipase C (discussed in the following paragraphs), but, in some cases, it is an ion channel involving calcium or potassium flux.

The major guanine nucleotide within cells is GTP, approximately 10 times the cytosolic concentration of the related guanosine diphosphate (GDP). When inactive, G proteins are tightly bound to GDP. When a receptor coupled to a G protein is activated by a first messenger, however, the G protein releases its GDP (Fig. 1-6). This permits the G protein to bind the more abundant GTP, thereby activating the G protein and causing it to dissociate from the receptor and then activate the effector. A shutoff mechanism is just as important for a regulator as its activating signal. The shutoff for G proteins is the enzyme, guanine triphosphatase

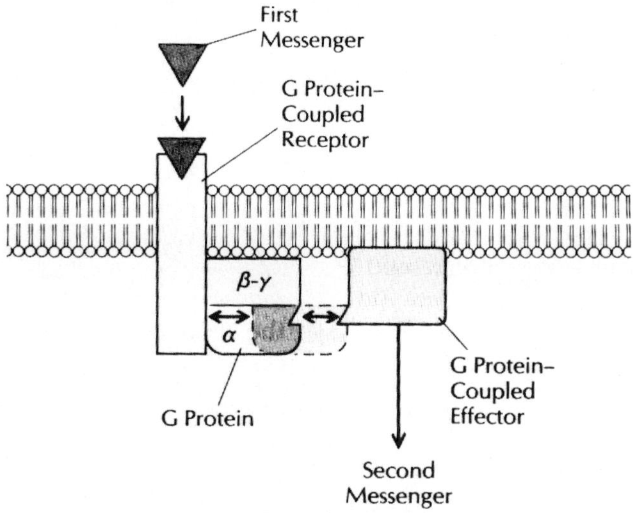

Fig. 1-5. The G protein-coupled receptor-effector system. (This figure and Figs. 1-6 through 1-8 are reproduced with permission from S.M. Spiegel. G proteins in clinical medicine. *Hospital Practice* Volume 23, issue 6, pages 95–100. Figs. 1d, 2, 4, 5. Illustration by Albert Miller 95, 97–100.)

(GTPase), which hydrolyses bound GTP to GDP, returning the G protein to its basal state and switching off the signaling system.

The G protein that regulates cAMP stimulation, designated G_S, is present in all cells. It can mediate many different kinds of physiologic effects by many different kinds of first messengers because the G_S protein is not coupled to one receptor alone but to multiple receptors, each apparently recognizing only a given first messenger. Some of these cell surface receptors (e.g., those for catecholamines) are found in many tissues, whereas others are more restrictively distributed. The beginning of the response, described previously, is similar in all cells. The production of cAMP sets off a biochemical chain reaction of protein kinase recruitment and cAMP-dependent phosphorylation. Since the protein substrates for phosphorylation vary among cell types, the physiologic effect(s) of phosphorylation also vary. In a thyroid cell, for example, G_S-coupled cAMP stimulation may lead to release of thyroid hormone (Fig. 1-7); the same second messenger may alter phosphate transport in a proximal renal tubular cell; vasopressin may use the G_S-regulated signaling system to induce water reabsorption in a renal medullary cell; and glucagon will use the same system to initiate glycogenolysis in a liver cell.

The adenylate cyclase–cAMP system is under dual regulation. G_S proteins lead to cAMP formation from stimulation of adenylate cyclase, but another important and ubiquitous G-protein system, termed G_i, inhibits cAMP formation when adenylate cyclase is stimulated. One of the G_i proteins stimulates membrane-bound phospholipase C, which appears to regulate another important signal system, termed the *phosphoinositide (PI) cycle,* based on molecules that are cannibalized from the cell membrane. Phospholipase C cleaves the membrane phospholipid, phosphatidylinositol biphosphate (PIP_2) into inositol triphosphate (IP_3) and diacylglycerol (DG or DAG) (Fig. 1-8). Each of these cleavage products modulates important signaling pathways. IP_3,

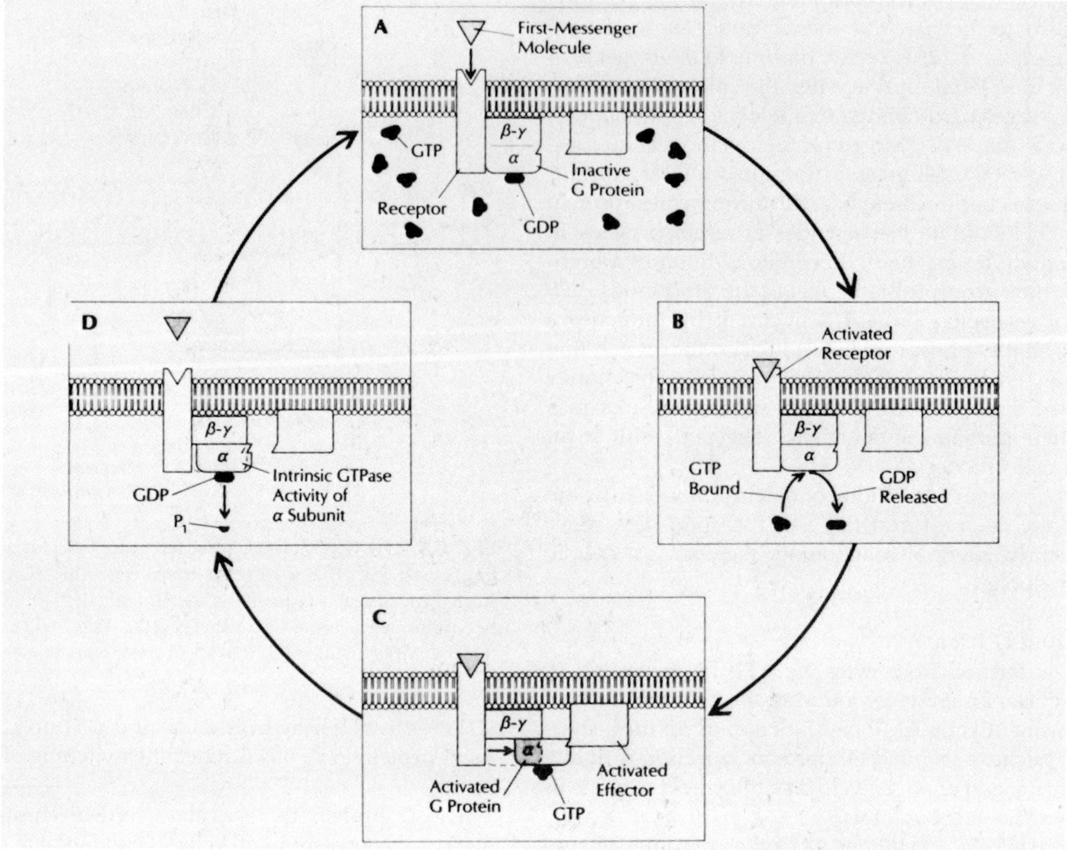

Fig. 1-6. Activation of the G protein system.

a water-soluble messenger, diffuses into the cytoplasm to initiate quick mobilization of calcium ions that are stored in the endoplasmic reticulum. This is a key event in signal transduction for a wide variety of cell types, including nerve and muscle cells. The other second messenger, DAG, is lipid soluble and remains within the lipid bilayer; there it facilitates the membrane attachment and activation of protein kinase C (PKC), a membrane-bound enzyme that phosphorylates various proteins.

Calcium Ions

If any ion had to be designated as the predominant intracellular messenger, it would have to be the calcium ion, which regulates neurotransmission and muscle contraction, influences membrane permeability, and modulates the activity of many other cellular processes. The changes in many intracellular enzyme activities, including phospholipases and protein kinases, and the polymerization of one form of actin to another and of the protein tubulin to form microtubules occur at different "set points" of cytosolic Ca^{2+} concentration. For all reactions, the normal regulation/modulation function of free intracellular Ca^{2+} requires that its concentration be maintained within a relatively narrow range. The steep calcium ion gradient is maintained by the cell membrane, which is ordinarily highly impermeable to the calcium ion, and by the cell's mechanisms for expelling excess calcium, either by an enzymatic pump to pump it out of the cell or into an intracellular organelle. As Rassmussen points out, all mammalian cells exist in a hostile, Ca^{2+}-rich environment, and we are faced with the continued threat of cellular Ca^{2+} intoxication. Preservation of the integrity of the cell membrane is vital.

The very low calcium level that is normal for cytosol means that relatively few ions need to be moved to regulate an enzyme. This requires a small expenditure of energy. In contrast, regulation by cAMP exacts a high energy cost since it must be synthesized and broken down each time it carries a message, and both steps require a significant investment of energy.

When the cell is stimulated by an electrical impulse or some other signal, calcium enters through calcium channels on the plasma membrane or from an intracellular organelle, and the influx of the ions is detected as a second messenger. Calmodulin, which is present in abundance in all mammalian cells, appears to be the most common conveyer of the intracellular calcium message. When cytosolic concentration of calcium ions rises above a certain threshold level, calcium ions bind to each molecule of calmodulin, inducing it to take on a new, more compact shape. This activates it and enables it, in turn, to activate protein kinases, which can phosphorylate other proteins. Calmodulin regulates many cellular functions by this mechanism.

Cell Injury—Inflammation

During the past 2 decades, it has become increasingly clear that among the body's many chemical messengers, many that act predominantly locally have a major influence on the

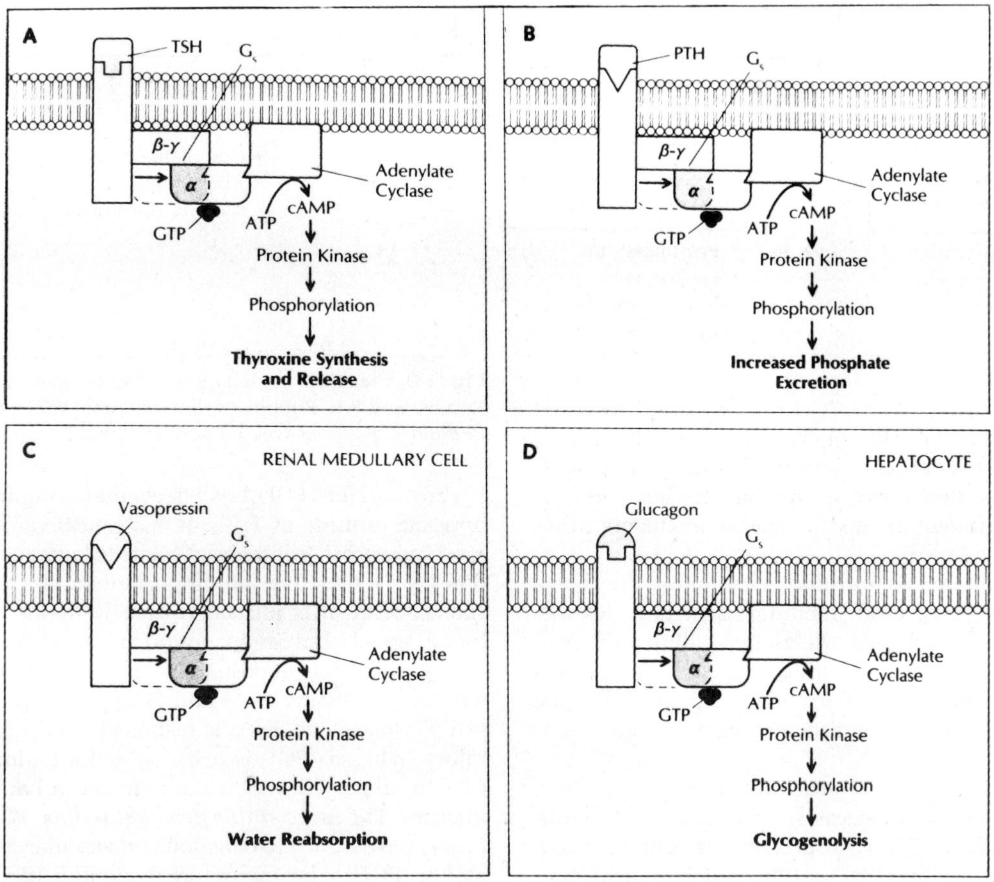

Fig. 1-7. The versatility and ubiquity of G_S-coupled cAMP stimulation.

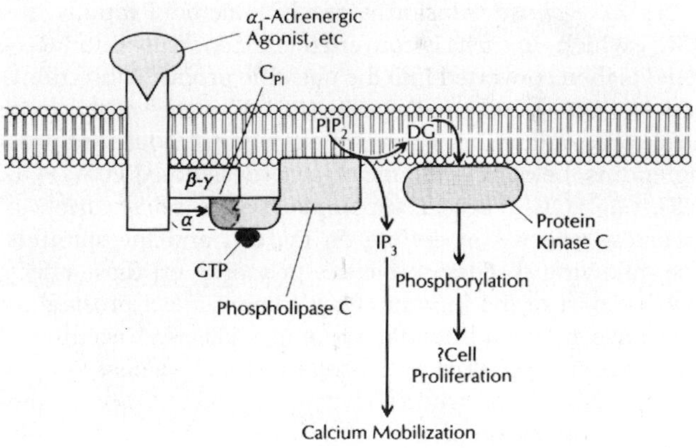

Fig. 1-8. The G protein coupled to phospholipase C, its effector.

body's metabolic responses. The mediators of inflammation have been called the hormones of the microenvironment because of their role in maintaining local homeostasis by their capacity to produce clinical inflammation in response to stimuli that cause cell injury—bacteria, burns, trauma, toxic chemical agents, necrotic tissue, ischemia, or immunologic reactions. As previously mentioned, the body responds to the vast assortment of noxious stimuli that confront it with a complex, but limited, repertoire of defenses, and many of the actions of the defense mediators are nonspecific. This lack of specificity is apparent in the inflammatory response, which acts to limit the spread of pathogens, mobilize the immune system, and regulate the metabolism of the host as the body fights invading organisms or responds to an injury or other noxious stimulus.

Some of the mediators of the inflammatory reaction are derived from cells; others are from plasma (Fig. 1-9). Some are secreted by cells that are specialized for that function; others can be produced by most of the cells of the body.

Inflammatory Mediators Synthesized by Cells

THE EICOSANOIDS. Arachidonic acid (eicosatetraenoic acid) does not occur free in the cell, but it can be synthesized by almost all the cells of the body when their membranes are perturbed by mechanical or chemical stimuli (even though the perturbance may be slight) or if their receptors are activated by appropriate mediators. This disturbance of normal homeostasis activates phospholipase A_2, often indirectly by first activating phospholipase C. As previously described, phospholipase C mediates the conversion of PIP_2 to IP_3 and DAG. Elevation of cytosolic calcium ion concentration activates phospholipase A_2; then, the activated phospholipase A_2 leads to cleavage of membrane phospholipids to form arachidonic acid. Within 5 to 50 seconds after the initial stimulus, arachidonic acid is metabolized by two distinct pathways. The cyclooxygenase pathway forms prostanoids

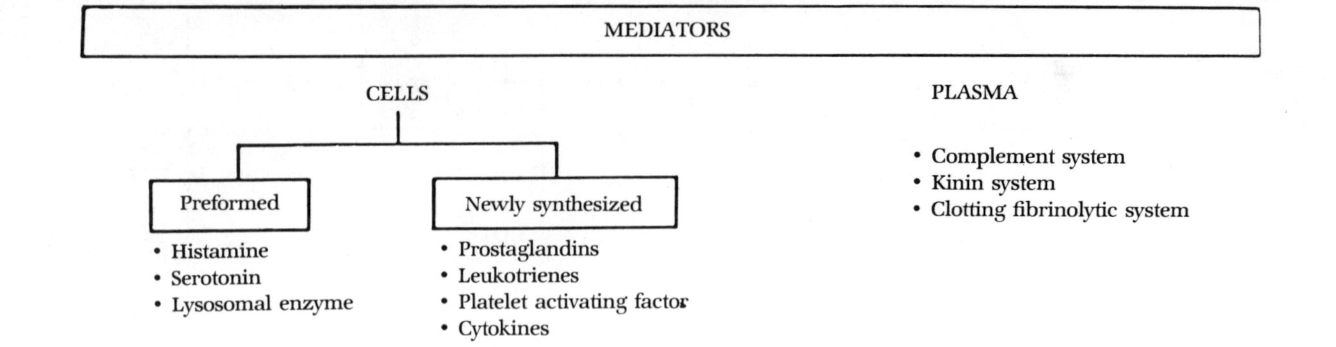

Fig. 1-9. Chemical mediators of infection. (From R.S. Cotran, V. Kumar, and S.L. Robbins. Inflammation and Repair. In *Robbins Pathologic Basis of Disease.* Philadelphia: Saunders, 1989.)

(prostaglandins, prostacyclin, or thromboxane); the lipoxygenase pathway produces leukotrienes and certain acids (Fig. 1-10). These derivatives of arachidonic acid, termed *eicosanoids,* are among the body's defense mediators in response to stress or injury.

Since their actions are so transitory, eicosanoids are generally considered as "fine-tune" modulators of host defense. They have a range of biological effects, depending on the cell type and on the physiologic setting; each cell type has a characteristic profile. For every action produced by one eicosanoid, there is an antagonistic action produced by another.

The fact that the release of arachidonic acid is potently blocked by glucocorticosteroids explains the anti-inflammatory actions of glucocorticosteroids. The action of cyclooxygenase is inhibited by aspirin, indomethacin, and other nonsteroidal anti-inflammatory drugs (NSAIDs). This ability of NSAIDs to inhibit prostaglandin biosynthesis explains all the biological actions of this group of drugs.

Cyclooxygenase transforms arachidonic acid rapidly into PGG_2, which, in turn, is converted enzymatically into PGH_2. PGH_2 is then converted into the unstable products thromboxane A_2 (TxA_2) and prostacyclin (PGI_2), or one of the more stable prostaglandins. There are more than 16 different prostaglandins, belonging to nine classes (designated PGA, PGB, PGC. . . .PGI). These compounds have a wide variety of biological effects, depending on the cell and the stimulus. The following discussion focuses primarily on those effects that are part of the inflammatory response, but prostaglandins have many additional metabolic effects. Virtually all cells, except for erythrocytes, contain cyclooxygenase and are thereby capable of synthesizing prostanoids. Once synthesized, the prostanoids are immediately extruded from the cytoplasm into the interstitium or the bloodstream. Since they are almost instantly inactivated in the tissue after local release, the paracrine action of these compounds is measured in seconds or less.

Thromboxane A_2 (TxA_2) is formed primarily by platelets, although it may also be synthesized in leukocytes and macrophages to a lesser degree. As a powerful platelet aggregator and vasoconstrictor of small and large blood vessels, it is a potent thrombogenic substance. Its effect is so strong that it contributes to ischemia in several shock states, thereby interfering with organ blood flow. Because its half-life is only 30 seconds, its actions are largely limited to the microenvironment into which it is released.

Prostacyclin (PGI) has effects that are almost completely opposite to those of TxA_2. It is a potent vasodilator and the most powerful inhibitor of platelet aggregation known to date; it is therefore an important antithrombogenic substance. Since it is formed primarily by the endothelium of blood vessels but is not found in platelets, it protects the vessel wall from deposition of platelet aggregates. The interactions between TxA_2 and PGI_2 play a major role in control of blood flow. TxA_2 is responsible for repair of vascular injury, whereas PGI_2 is responsible for maintenance of normal circulatory flow. Prostacyclin has a half-life of about 3 minutes. The more *stable prostaglandins, PGE_2, $PGF_{2\alpha}$,* and *PGD_2,* have a variety of actions on vascular tone and permeability. PGD_2, the major prostaglandin produced by mast cells, induces vasodilation in systemic resistance vessels and bronchoconstriction in the lungs. PgE compounds, produced in many organs, are vasodilators that are capable of inducing the classic local manifestations of inflammation—rubor, dolor, tumor, and calor. As described below, they also participate with cytokines in eliciting systemic manifestations of inflammation, such as fever and headache (see Fig. 1-11). Members of the PgF group are venoconstrictors that are thought to be involved in the termination of the inflammatory response.

The *lipoxygenase pathway* initially produces intermediate derivatives, hydroperoxyeicosatetraenoic acid (HPETE). 12-HPETE is formed in platelets; 5-HPETE and 15-HPETE are formed in leukocytes. HPETE may be metabolized to hydroxyeicosatetraenoic acid (HETE), a potent chemotactic stimulus for neutrophils. 5-HPETE also gives rise to the leukotrienes, designated thus because the capacity to synthesize them appears to be limited to certain leukocytes—notably, neutrophils, basophils, eosinophils, monocytes/macrophages, and some mast cells.

The *leukotrienes* are potent mediators of inflammation at the local level. *Leukotriene B_4 (LTB_4),* synthesized by neutrophils, monocytes, and macrophages, is the most potent natural chemotactic factor identified to date, with chemotaxis for neutrophils, eosinophils, and monocytes.

LTC_4, LTD_4, and LTE_4, formerly known as slow-reacting substances of anaphylaxis (SRS-A), are synthesized by basophils, eosinophils, and some mast cells. SRS-A is by far the most potent vasoactive and spasmogenic mediator known. It is discussed in Chap. 89.

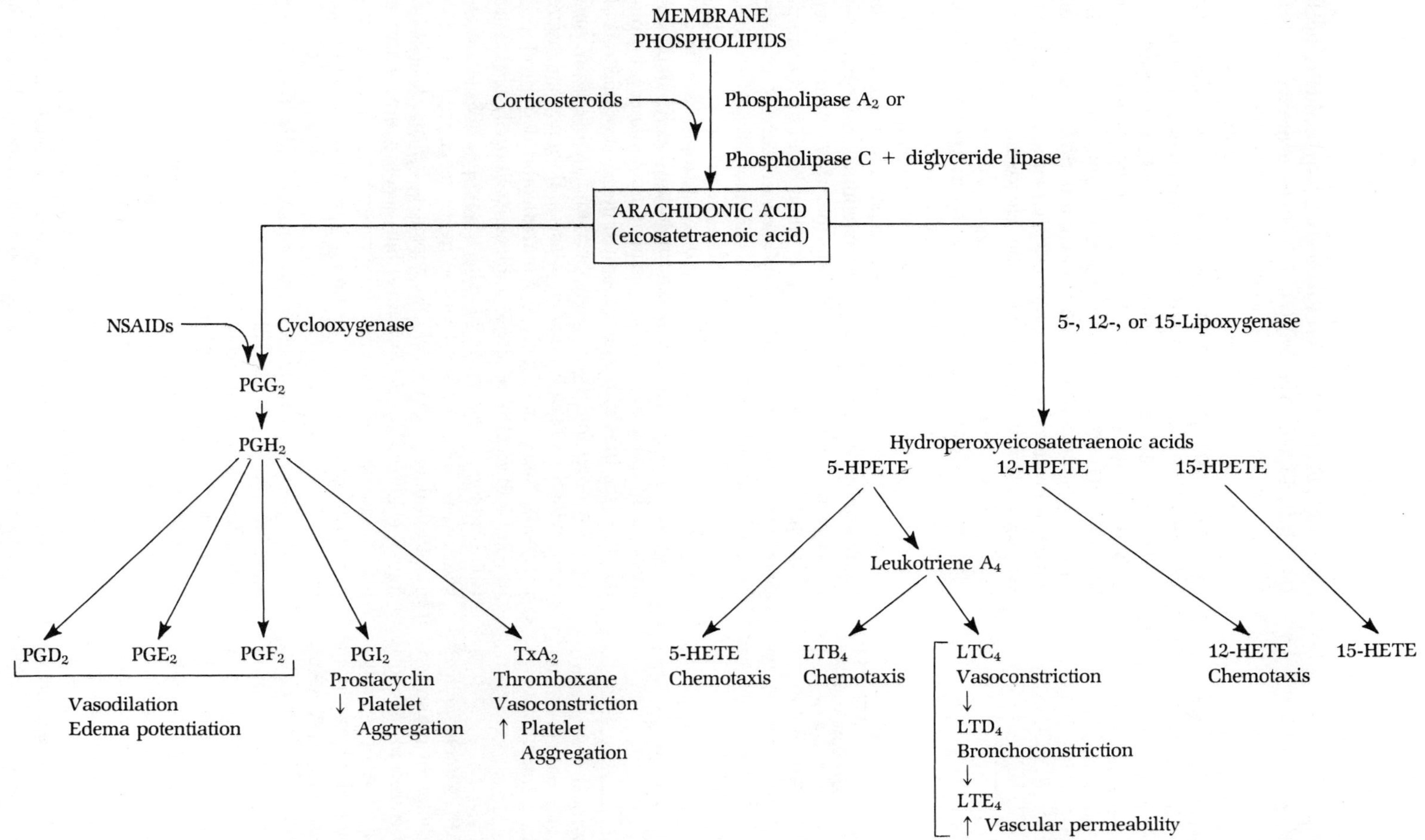

Fig. 1-10. The arachidonic acid cascade involved in inflammatory responses.

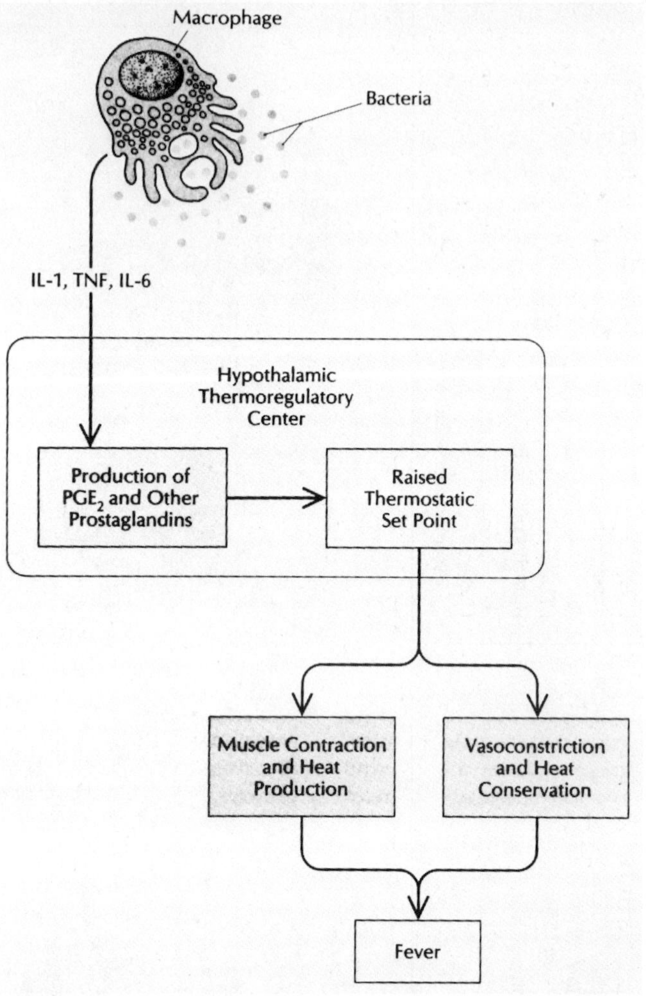

Fig. 1-11. The mechanism of action of endogenous pyrogens in inducing fever. (From C.A. Dinarello. The endogenous pyrogens in host-defense interactions. *Hosp. Pract.* 24:111, 1989.)

PLATELET-ACTIVATING FACTOR (PAF). Platelet-activating factor is a potent phospholipid mediator of inflammation, which, like the eicosanoids, is not stored in its active form within cells but is synthesized rapidly after phospholipase A_2 activation in response to immunologic, hypoxic, or other appropriate stimuli. It has been known for many years that PAF is released by IgE-sensitized mast cells/basophils, responding to antigen stimulation by causing aggregation of platelets and release of their active constituents, histamine and serotonin. It is now recognized that it is also released by neutrophils, endothelium, monocytes, platelets, and by other cells. It appears, too, that PAF modulates regional blood flow by complex mechanisms that are not completely understood. In addition to activating platelets, it causes vasoconstriction, bronchoconstriction, and increased leukocyte margination and adhesion to endothelium. It is also chemotactic for leukocytes. In low doses it produces vasodilation and increases venular permeability 100 to 10,000 times more strongly than does histamine and 2 to 3 times more powerfully than do the leukotrienes. PAF and tumor necrosis factor are able to elicit the release of each other, and PAF also stimulates the synthesis of prostaglandins and leukotrienes.

Although the information that is currently available about the PAF's vasoactive effects is incomplete, it already seems clear that it has the ability to amplify tissue injury during critical illness by perpetuation of perfusion deficits. It is considered a major mediator influencing the outcome of ischemia, as its actions are combined with those of TxA_2 and the leukotrienes.

OXYGEN-DERIVED FROM RADICALS. Superoxide radicals (O_2^-), hydrogen peroxide (H_2O_2), or the hydroxyl radicals ($OH\cdot$) are normally produced in limited amounts from molecular oxygen in the cytosol, mitochondria, lysosome, peroxisome, or plasma membrane of some cells. These cells also produce protective enzymes. Superoxide dismutase (SOD) in the cytosol and mitochondria scavenges the superoxide radical by catalyzing its conversion to hydrogen peroxide and oxygen, and if H_2O_2 migrates into the cytoplasm or is formed there by the action of SOD, it is broken down into water and molecular oxygen by the enzyme catalase (most of which is located in the peroxisome), or various peroxidases.

As noted later in this chapter, oxygen-derived free radicals are important weapons used by activated neutrophils and macrophages in fulfilling their roles. If these metabolites are released extracellularly, they cause endothelial damage with resultant increased vascular permeability, and they can damage any other cell membrane that they contact. They also inactivate antiproteases, potentially leading to unopposed protease activity with increased destruction of cytoskeletal components of tissue.

CYTOKINES. Gram-negative organisms can produce broad-scale physiologic derangements, including such manifestations as diffuse intravascular coagulation, acute renal tubular necrosis, interstitial pneumonitis, necrosis of portions of the gastrointestinal tract, high fever and hypotension, and other evidence of gram-negative sepsis and inadequate tissue perfusion. Since most of these features could be reproduced by the infusion of a single molecule, lipopolysaccharide (LPS), found in the bacterial cell membrane, LPS, an endotoxin, was once regarded as the agent responsible for the manifestations of gram-negative sepsis. It was also suspected that the anorexia and wasting that accompanied chronic infections and malignancies were caused by soluble factors produced by organisms, by tumors, or by the cells of the host.

Ultimately, it became clear that endotoxin, by itself, is not harmful to most cells and tissues of the host, but many of the deleterious distant effects were caused by factors elaborated by the host's immune system in response to the endotoxin. During the past few years, some of these substances have been identified and termed *cytokines*. These are soluble proteins that may induce systemic as well as local effects on the microenvironment in response to injury and critical illness.

Tumor necrosis factor (TNF), also termed *cachectin,* was identified as the lethal mediator that was capable of inducing a shock state very similar to that induced by endotoxin; it was also able to provoke a state of wasting very similar to that observed in cancer patients. There is no current evidence that cachectin/TNF exists in the tissue in stored form, but it is released from tissue macrophages and circulating monocytes within 15 minutes of activation, reaching a peak at 90 minutes, and disappearing within 3 to 4 hours as it binds to its widespread plasma membrane receptor.

The term *interleukin* defines a white cell product that acts on other white cells. In fact, *TNF, interleukin-1* (IL-1), and weaker acting *IL-6*, are cytokines that are synthesized by a variety of cell types in addition to macrophages, including endothelial cells, lymphocytes, epithelial cells, fibroblasts, keratinocytes, and astrocytes. Also, they act not only on leukocytes, but also on many other cell types. They are key mediators of the body's response to microbial invasion, inflammation, immunological reactions, and tissue injury.

Because of their role in eliciting fever, these cytokines have been termed *endogenous pyrogens*. There is no current evidence that they are produced in health, but their production can be stimulated by nearly all infections, immune complexes, toxins, physical injury, and a variety of inflammatory processes. They act synergistically and they induce the same spectrum of biologic effects. Once released into the circulation, they have local effects at sites of inflammation or tissue injury as well as systemic effects on target tissues and distant organs. They thus may act as a link between inflammatory and metabolic processes.

As they reach the hypothalamic thermoregulatory center, they induce fever by stimulating the abrupt release of arachidonic acid, which is metabolized to prostaglandins, particularly PGE_2, in the anterior hypothalamus (Fig. 1-11). The prostaglandins raise the thermostatic set point and drive the mechanisms of heat conservation (vasoconstriction) and heat production (shivering) until the blood and core temperature are elevated to match the hypothalamic set point.

Fever is associated with other metabolic changes, the acute-phase responses, which represent primary actions of cytokines on tissues in which they originate. In the liver, they induce increases in synthesis of a number of proteins, including ceruloplasmin, a protein that is important in clearing oxygen radicals from injured and infected tissues, complement components, fibrinogen, and alpha$_2$-macroglobin, a protease inhibitor that may play an important role at the site of infection or injury by inhibiting the proteases that are released by leukocytes and macrophages. Other acute-phase proteins bind to lipids or directly to bacterial surfaces, perhaps acting as nonspecific opsonins. It is thought that the burst of energy and the amino acids that are required for the hepatic protein synthesis of the acute phase may be provided by an IL-1–mediated increase in protein degradation and amino acid release from skeletal muscle. As the host defenses are marshalled against infection or injury, the acute-phase response also includes the release of ACTH and corticosteroids and the stimulation of neutrophilia.

Some of the local actions of IL-1 and TNF contribute to homeostasis, but others have a great pathogenic potential. One of their nonleukocytic targets is the endothelial cell, in which they orchestrate a cascade of biochemical events that can lead to vascular changes associated with inflammation and tissue injury. They stimulate the synthesis and release of the vasodilatory prostaglandins PGI_2 and PGE_2, but they also enhance production of PAF, the leukotrienes, and other factors that alter the endothelial surface in such a way that leukocytes and platelets adhere avidly (Table 1-1). This readily leads to vascular congestion and clot formation.

Current evidence suggests that TNF elaboration is an essential initial step for subsequent cellular damage seen during sepsis and that it has direct effects on cellular function, but much of its effects are indirect, mediated by other inflammatory molecules. By inducing the production of numerous additional mediators, such as eicosanoids, PAF, activated neutrophils, tissue macrophages, and lymphocytes, cytokines amplify and extend the inflammatory response (Fig. 1-12). By redundant pathways, they also activate the complement, kinin, and coagulation and fibrinolytic systems. These are discussed in following sections.

Table 1-1. Mediators stimulated by tumor necrosis factor

Peptide regulatory factors
Interleukin-1 (IL-1)
Interleukin-6 (IL-6)
Granulocyte-macrophage colony-stimulating factor (GM-CSF)
Tumor necrosis factor (TNF)
Platelet-derived growth factor (PDGF)
Transforming growth factor-β (TGF-β)
Eicosanoids
Prostaglandins
Leukotrienes
Platelet-activating factor
Hormones
Corticotropin/cortisol
Epinephrine
Norepinephrine
Glucagon

Source: K.J. Tracey, H. Vlassara, and A. Cerami. Peptide regulatory factors: Cachectin/tumour necrosis factor. *Lancet* 1:1122, 1989. © by The Lancet Ltd.

Preformed Inflammatory Mediators Derived from Cells

THE VASOACTIVE AMINES. *Histamine* is stored primarily in mast cells in tissue and basophils in blood, but it is also stored in gastric mucosa, neurons, platelets, and epidermis. It produces vasodilatation (confined to the venules) and increased vascular permeability. It is present in early inflammation, but its content diminishes within the first hour.

Serotonin (5-hydroxytryptamine [5-HT]), which is released from platelets and cells of the gastrointestinal tract, is a neurotransmitter that acts primarily on nerve endings and smooth muscle. It increases platelet aggregation and is a potent vasoconstrictor (acting primarily as a venoconstrictor rather than an arterial constrictor). It is also a powerful bronchoconstrictor.

These vasoactive amines are released from mast cells by many agents, including trauma, cold, immunologic reactions, fragments of complement, IL-1, and factors from neutrophils, monocytes, and platelets. They are released from platelets when platelets are stimulated by PAF, as previously described, and also when platelet aggregation occurs, as discussed later in this chapter.

LYSOSOMAL ENZYMES. Neutrophils, monocytes, and tissue macrophages may release lysosomes as part of the inflammatory response. Acid proteases act primarily within the lysosome of the phagocyte, where the pH is acidic. Neutral proteases can degrade extracellular components, such as collagen, fibrin, elastin, and cartilage. If unchecked, these and other lysosomal constituents can cause considerable tissue damage while increasing vascular permeability. They

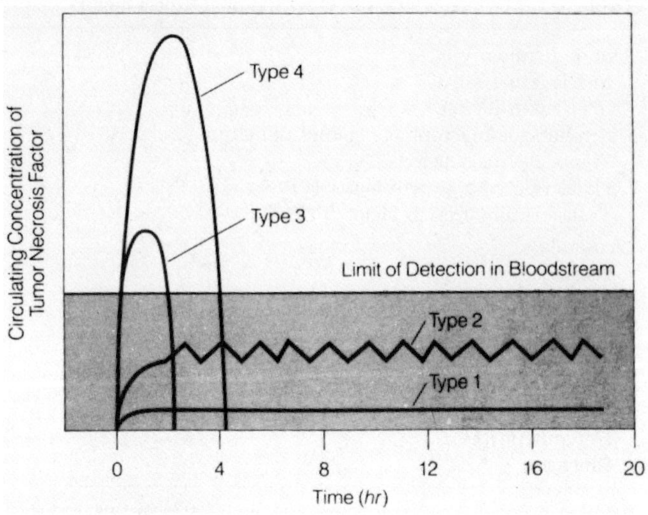

Fig. 1-12. Differing patterns of cytokine release in different infections. Type 1 represents localized cellulitis. TNF and other cytokines are produced locally, inducing local responses that aid host defense and tissue repair. Overspill into the circulation is minimal. Type 2 is the type of response that might result from an appendiceal abscess. There is local generation of cytokines, and as bacteria or their endotoxins leak into the circulation, circulating mononuclear cells also synthesize cytokines and give rise to moderate systemic response. Because only a small number of cytokine-producing cells are stimulated at any one time, the response of these cells, although of long duration, is not strong enough to be detectable in the bloodstream. However, the signal is sufficient to generate systemic manifestations of the localized infection. Type 3 infection response might follow manipulation of a catheter in the urinary bladder to relieve an obstruction. A few cytokine-producing cells simultaneously elaborate TNF to produce a high-amplitude signal. Because the endotoxemia is transient, both the signal and the host response are short-lived. The cytokine response is too short and of insufficient amplitude to give rise to life-threatening, irreversible host alterations. Type 4 infection might result from meningococcal septicemia. An acute, massive entry of endotoxins into the circulation activates virtually all of the cytokine-producing cells of the body. Because the half-life of cytokines is short, they disappear from the circulation quickly, but the high amplitude of the initial signal is so explosive that it is misinterpreted by the host, causing the entire body to behave as if it were a massive wound. The entire vascular tree shows increased permeability and vasodilatation. (From P.Q. Bessey. Metabolic Response to Critical Illness. In D.W. Wilmore, et al. [eds.], *Care of the Surgical Patient,* Section II, Chapter 11. © 1989 Scientific American, Inc. All rights reserved.)

are normally held in check by a system of antiproteases in the serum and tissue fluids.

Inflammatory Mediators Derived from Plasma

Three interrelated and interacting systems of plasma proteases are active in the inflammatory process—the complement, clotting, and kinin systems.

THE COMPLEMENT SYSTEM. The complement system consists of 18 serum proteins that are crucial in generating the inflammation response, supplementing the humoral immune system of immunoglobulins. As described in Chap. 89, the complement system is activated through a cascade that may take either of two pathways. The classical pathway, activated by antigen–antibody complexes, leads to formation of the third component of complement, C3, which fragments into C3a, a potent mast cell degranulator that increases vascular permeability, and C3b, which binds to and opsonifies the target cell surface. Since the alternate pathway does not require antibody for its activation, it is a major contributor to the inflammatory reaction, forming the powerful inflammatory agent C5a, which activates leukocytes, and, like C3a, induces mast cell degranulation. C5b sequentially binds other fragments—C6, C7, C8, and C9—finally forming C5b-9, the membrane attack complex (MAC), which inserts into the lipid bilayers, increasing cell permeability and causing cell lysis. It also stimulates arachidonic acid metabolism and production of reactive oxygen metabolites by macrophages and other cells.

THE CLOTTING/FIBRINOLYTIC SYSTEM. The blood clotting factors, a series of plasma proteins, circulate in inactive form until they are activated in stepwise fashion to form a clot in response to injury to a blood vessel wall. Blood clotting involves two pathways: the extrinsic pathway (activated within seconds) begins with trauma to the endothelium; the intrinsic pathway (activated within minutes) begins within the bloodstream (Fig. 1-13).

As described later in this chapter, platelets are quickly activated by, and attracted to, exposed collagen at the site of vessel injury, aggregating and adhering to the surface and releasing thromboxane A_2 and other mediators that promote strong vasoconstriction and formation of a platelet plug. At the same time, the negatively charged structures of exposed subendothelium activate the intrinsic pathway by partially activating factor XII (Hageman factor) as it is adsorbed onto the damage site. Activated factor XII (factor XIIa), a trypsin-like protease, has two important substrates. One is factor XI, which when cleaved by factor XIIa acts as a trigger of the intrinsic coagulation pathway. The other substrate is prekallikrein, the activation of which leads to the release of bradykinin, one of the most potent vasodepressors and endothelial cell activators (discussed below). Both the intrinsic and extrinsic coagulation pathways lead to a final common pathway, with increase in effect from step to step so that there is overall biologic amplification as one factor after another is activated. This coagulation cascade produces prothrombin activator that splits prothrombin to form thrombin. Thrombin cleaves plasma fibrinogen into fibrin monomers, soluble molecules that polymerize with other fibrin monomers to form insoluble fibrin macromolecules; these are long threads that build a reticulum for a clot as they run in all directions, entrapping blood cells, platelets, and plasma and holding the clumps in place. With activation of factor XIII by thrombin, firmer chemical bonds are formed and the clot is toughened, as cross links are introduced between polymerized fibrin molecules.

The fibrinolytic system, which serves to prevent the formation of intravascular fibrin or to remove it, is just as important as the coagulation system. It can be rapidly activated, preventing fibrin from forming in disastrous excess or forming where it is not needed. Plasmin (also called fibrinolysin) is a strong proteolytic enzyme that breaks fibrin down into smaller, soluble fragments. Its inactive precursor, plasminogen, adsorbs onto fibrin polymers as they form. When plas-

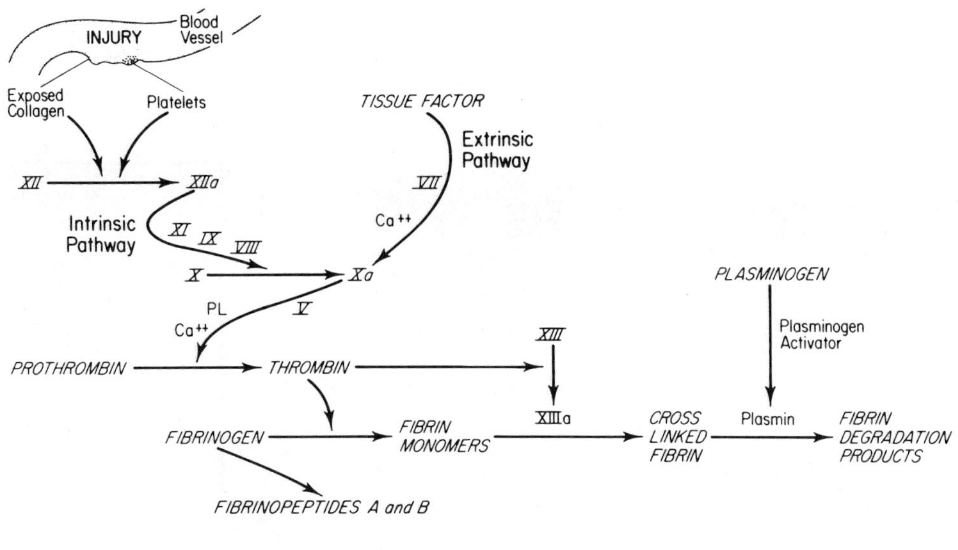

Fig. 1-13. Coagulation and fibrinolytic system (see text). (Ca^{++} = calcium ions; PL = phospholipid; a = activated factor.) (From D.S. Rosenthal. Hematologic Oncologic Disorders and Heart Disease. In E.B. Braunwald [ed.], *Heart Disease.* Philadelphia: Saunders, 1980. P. 1973.)

minogen activator is released from lysosomes of injured endothelial and tissue cells, it enters the bloodstream and binds selectively to fibrin polymers, where it hydrolyzes plasminogen to plasmin on the fibrin strands. Here the plasmin can break down the fibrin into much smaller soluble fragments, the fibrin-split products.

Since plasmin is a powerful protease and is relatively nonspecific, any plasmin that is generated in the circulating blood instead of on fibrin will not only digest and inactivate fibrin but will also degrade fibrinogen, other coagulation factors, some hormones, and complement. To prevent this, plasmin inhibitors are present in normal circulation.

Coagulation is partly an inflammatory event. The coagulation system interacts at several levels with two other systems of circulating protein inflammatory mediators, the kinin system and the complement system.

THE KININ SYSTEM. The kinin system is one of the three mediator systems triggered by activation of factor XII of the intrinsic clotting system (Hageman factor) (Fig. 1-14). Hageman factor, activated by contact with surface-active agents, such as collagen, basement membrane, and endotoxin, produces prekallikrein, which converts plasma prekallikrein activator into an active proteolytic form, the enzyme kallikrein. This cleaves high-molecular–weight kininogen (HMWK) to produce short-acting bradykinin. HMWK is also a catalyst in the activation of Hageman factor. Bradykinin is a potent vasodilator that increases vascular permeability, evokes pain, and increases bronchial resistance. Kallikrein has chemotactic activity and also causes aggregation of neutrophils. Since it is also an activator of Hageman factor by feedback, it makes profound amplification of the initial stimulus possible.

Inflammatory Cells

MAST CELLS. Mast cells have been termed "sentinels" by Austin because of their distribution in the body on cutaneous and mucosal surfaces and around venules, points of constant exposure to potentially noxious agents. Moreover, of all the immunologically active cells, they are the only ones that possess a recognition system that is already in the tissues. The system can recognize "nonself" the moment it enters the body. All exogenous antigens and most noxious stimuli that penetrate the body must enter through the skin or through the gastrointestinal or other mucosa. If penetration to the circulation does occur, the mast cell guards the interface between the venous vasculature and arterial circulation.

The stimulus releases some mast cell mediators that are preformed and initiates the synthesis of others. Preformed histamine and serotonin, which are stored in large secretory vesicles, are released rapidly when the mast cell is stimulated by injury, local infection, or certain immunologic reactions. In addition, the mast cell's prepackaged granules contain heparin and powerful neutral trypsin-like proteases that are capable of digesting proteins in the surrounding tissues. Histamine causes venules to dilate and become leaky, thereby facilitating the access of the mediators of the inflammatory reaction—serum proteins such as antibodies and components of the complement system and phagocytic white blood cells—to the injury sites. These leukocytes are attracted to the scene by potent chemotactic factors that are released during mast cell degranulation. Recruiting of these protective proteins and cells to the inflammatory site is critical to a fully developed local host response.

LEUKOCYTES. Accumulation of leukocytes—principally neutrophils and monocytes—is the central feature in the inflammatory reaction. In normally flowing blood, the layer of plasma in contact with endothelial lining of the microvessels is relatively cell-free since the red and white blood cells flow in the central column. As the blood flow slows and stagnates, the white cells move from the central column to posi-

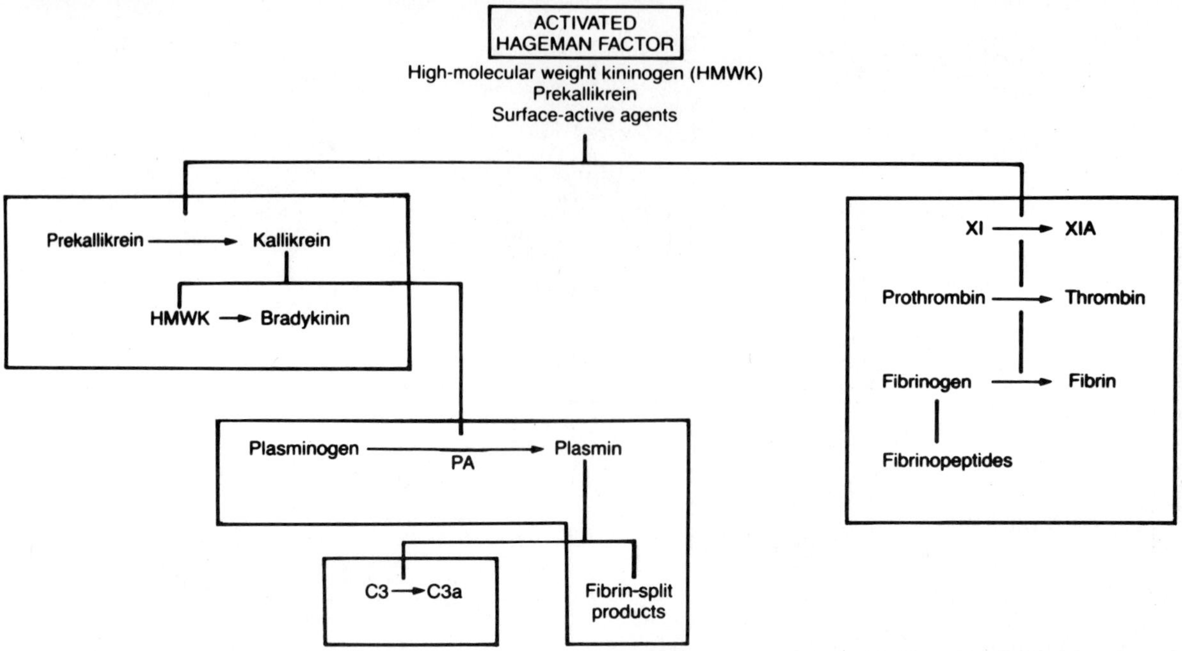

Fig. 1-14. Plasma mediator systems triggered by activation of Hageman factor. (PA = plasminogen activator.) (From R.S. Cotran, V. Kumar, and S.L. Robbins. Inflammation and Repair. In *Robbins Pathologic Basis of Disease.* Philadelphia: Saunders, 1989.)

tions in contact with the endothelium, slowing and finally coming to rest, lining the endothelial surface and sticking to it, partially, at least, because of such agents as PAF, which enhance this adhesion. Attracted by chemotactic factors—bacterial products, components of the complement system (particularly C5a), products of lipoxygenase pathway, immune complexes, or necrotic tissue—the leukocytes crawl through widened interendothelial junctions to the site of injury or infection.

Although the leukocyte's functions are highly specialized, it is basically a secretory cell and shares many of the same basic mechanisms as other secretory cells. Its plasma membrane contains specific receptors for chemotactic agents. If these receptors are occupied, phospholipase C is activated, resulting in hydrolysis of PIP_2 to IP_3 and DAG (previously described). IP_3 causes release of calcium from intracellular stores, and the increased cytosolic Ca^{2+} concentration triggers the assembly of contractile elements that are responsible for cell movement and also activates phospholipase A_2, which converts membrane phospholipids to arachidonic acid.

In less than 1 minute after the triggering stimulus has been received, NADPH oxidase, an enzyme on the surface of the white cell's plasma membrane, induces molecular oxygen (dissolved in the serum) to pick up an electron from the electron-carrier NADPH (reduced nicotinamide adenine dinucleotide), thereby converting the O_2 to the superoxide anion (O_2^-). Most of the superoxide is further converted by the enzyme SOD (discussed previously) into H_2O_2, which is intensely active. By the process of endocytosis, the O_2^- and H_2O_2 are carried into the cell as more is produced by the inside surface of the vacuole membrane. (Any hydrogen peroxide that migrates into the cytoplasm of the leukocyte is rapidly broken down into water and molecular oxygen by the intracellular enzyme catalase.) Within the vacuole, some of the H_2O_2 reacts with the chloride ion to form hypochlorite ($Cl_2O_2^{--}$), a potent bacteriocidal agent.

Some of the superoxide radical that was released into the immediate neighborhood of the leukocyte reacts with the membrane lipids of nearby cells, damaging or even destroying some of them while they stimulate other cells to produce arachidonic acid. The lipoxygenase pathway products of this reaction include strong chemotactic substances that attract additional neutrophils to the invasion site; the cyclooxygenase pathway produces TxA_2, which leads to platelet aggregation and vasoconstriction as the body attempts to wall off and localize the invasion.

Neutrophil aggregation is a sign of these intracellular events and the prelude to degranulation and release of the tissue destructive enzymes. The neutrophils are able to attach to and engulf some bacteria or necrotic debris and ultimately attempt to kill or degrade the organism or necrotic tissue by the release of the superoxide radicals and by release of their granules containing powerful cytolytic enzymes.

ENDOTHELIAL CELLS. Both endothelial cells and circulating blood cells are negatively charged and therefore repel each other; intact vessel walls do not interact with platelets. Because of this, intact endothelium is nonthrombogenic. On the other hand, the endothelial cells that cover the basement membrane and collagen lining the normal blood vessel walls synthesize and secrete factor VIII–related von Willebrand factor (factor VIII:vWF), a plasma glycoprotein that facilitates platelet adhesion under conditions of high shear stress by forming a bridge between platelet membrane receptors and the vascular subendothelium. (It also serves as the plasma carrier for factor VIII, the antihemophilic factor, a critical blood coagulation protein.) When a blood vessel is injured, the exposed subendothelial structures therefore become highly attractive for platelets and for other blood cells and are therefore thrombogenic. When cell injury or another appropriate stimulus perturbs the endothelial cell's plasma membrane, arachidonic acid is synthesized and rapidly metabolized to produce PGI_2, the vasodilator that powerfully inhibits platelet aggregation, counteracting the effect of TxA_2.

As noted below, during the process of clot formation, when thrombin interacts with endothelial cells, plasminogen activator is released from endothelial cells, promoting plasmin formation and clot lysis.

PLATELETS. Normal intact endothelium prevents blood cells and coagulation factors from attaching to the vessel wall. However, within a few seconds after a vessel is injured, platelets are activated as they cover and adhere to exposed subendothelial collagen, thereby triggering the coagulation cascade (see Fig. 1-13). The activated platelets release ADP and serotonin from their dense granules and release other mediators, including fibrinogen, fibronectin, and factor VIII:vWF, from other granules. The outer layer of the platelet plasma membrane contains receptors for extracellular fibrinogen and other adhesive proteins that mediate the adhesion of platelets to the wall of the injured vessel and the subsequent formation of platelet aggregates. These aggregates are formed chiefly through platelet–platelet bridging by fibrinogen. ADP induces other platelets to absorb fibrinogen from plasma and aggregate onto the platelets that are already adherent to the injured vessel wall.

Although platelets have no nuclei, they have many of the functional characteristics of whole cells, and platelet activation follows the same basic pattern that is used by so many other cells: The elevation of cytosolic Ca^{2+} concentration is one of the mechanisms for the synthesis of arachidonic acid from membrane phospholipids. In the platelet, arachidonic acid is rapidly metabolized to TxA_2, the strong stimulus for platelet aggregation and for vasoconstriction. ADP and TxA_2 act synergistically to recruit circulating platelets and promote aggregation.

Collagen activates the intrinsic coagulation cascade, leading to the formation of thrombin, which joins ADP and TxA_2 is causing platelet aggregation and clot formation, as previously described.

The cytoplasm of platelets contains more actin and myosin than most nonmuscle cells. The contractile proteins in the activated platelets induce calcium-dependent changes in platelet shape as the platelet extends long pseudopods along fibrin strands. Within a few minutes after a clot has formed, it begins to contract, usually expressing most of the fluid from the clot within 30 to 60 minutes. This retraction requires the presence of platelets.

MACROPHAGES/MONONUCLEAR PHAGOCYTES. These are the scavenger cells of the body. In the presence of inflammation, they engulf and digest debris from injured or dead cells, including neutrophils, bacteria, and foreign particles. They are mobile in the bloodstream as the monocyte but are also resident in the tissues and organs as the resident macrophages. Because of their large repertoire of hydrolytic enzymes, they are able to degrade a variety of materials quickly. This versatile cell can produce arachidonic acid metabolites, oxygen-free radicals, chemotactic factors for leukocytes, neutral proteases that degrade connective tissue components, complement components, coagulation factors, plasminogen activator, cytokines, and PAF. The secretion of these products is regulated by cell-to-cell communication.

Host Defense Regulation

The mediators of acute inflammation are summarized in Tables 1-2 and 1-3. Host defense homeostasis with regard to the acute inflammatory response requires not only that the humoral and cellular defense mechanisms be activated effectively, but, just as important, cutoff mechanisms must inactivate them at an appropriate time to minimize the damage that they themselves can cause.

The price that the body pays for the local protection provided by the inflammatory reaction is a certain amount of tissue destruction. However, if the homeostatic mechanisms escape regulatory control, generalized tissue injury results. This generalized injury is minimized under normal conditions by the host's ability to limit the acute inflammatory response by such mechanisms as the mobilization of antiproteases, SOD, catalase, and other scavengers of oxygen-free radicals, and by many other mechanisms, some of which were described previously.

It is beyond the scope of this chapter to discuss the roles of the neuroendocrine system in host defense. These are discussed in other chapters. Attention here is focused on the liver, which plays a central role in coordinating host regulation of the inflammatory response since it contains so many of the fixed macrophages of the body, as Kupffer cells lining its sinusoidal network. These cells, along with splenic macrophages, clear the blood of bacteria, vasoactive substances, and particulate matter that would otherwise stimulate the inflammatory response. The accompanying hepatocytes synthesize acute-phase reactants and also antiproteases that are necessary to down-regulate the inflammatory response.

DEATH

Pathophysiology

If they are severe enough, hypoxia, trauma, chemical toxin infection, or other noxious agents directly cause injury or death. But the body's defense mediators that are summoned to maintain the body's homeostasis sometimes cause additional injury and hasten death if wave on wave of inflammatory mediators overwhelm regulatory mechanisms and the response becomes uncontrolled.

The body's response depends on the type and severity of the stimulus and the type and condition of the tissue The discussion that follows focuses on the disintegration of the normal cellular mechanisms that result from hypoxia and, ultimately, circulatory arrest.

Hypoxia and Circulatory Arrest

HYPOXIA. Under normal conditions, the circulatory system delivers a surplus of oxygen and substrate to the tissues. But when oxygen delivery decreases below a critically low level, O_2 extraction is insufficient to meet the energy demands of the cell aerobically. As the production of ATP lags behind cellular energy needs, cytosolic AMP accumulates. This

Table 1-2. Summary of mediators of acute inflammation

Mediator	Source	Action		
		Vascular leakage	Chemotaxis	Other
Histamine and serotonin	Mast cells, basophils, and platelets	+	—	
α				
Bradykinin	Plasma substrate	+	—	Pain
α				
C3a	Plasma protein via liver; macrophages	+	—	Opsonic fragment (C3b)
C5a		+	+	Leukocyte adhesion
Prostaglandins	Most cells, from membrane phospholipids	Potentiate other mediators	—	Vasodilation, pain, fever
α				
Leukotriene B_4	Leukocytes	—	+	Leukocyte adhesion
Leukotriene C_4, D_4, E_4	Leukocytes, mast cells	+	—	Bronchoconstriction, vasoconstriction
Lysosomal components				
Cationic proteins	Leukocytes	+	+	Immobilization of neutrophils
Neutral proteases	Leukocytes	+	—	Tissue damage
Oxygen metabolites	Leukocytes	+		Endothelial damage, tissue damage
PAF	Leukocytes; other	+	+	Bronchoconstriction
IL-1 and TNF	Macrophages; other	—	+	Acute phase reactions Leukocyte adhesion

Source: R.S. Cotran, V. Kumar, and S.L. Robbins. Inflammation and Repair. In *Robbins Pathologic Basis of Disease.* Philadelphia: Saunders, 1989.

Table 1-3. Most likely mediators in inflammation

Vasodilation
- Prostaglandins

Increased vascular permeability
- Vasoactive amines
- C3a and C5a (through liberating amines)
- Bradykinin
- Leukotriene C_4, D_4, E_4, PAF

Chemotaxis
- C5a
- Leukotriene B_4
- Other chemotactic lipids
- Bacterial products

Fever
- IL-1; TNF
- Prostaglandins

Pain
- Prostaglandins
- Bradykinin

Tissue damage
- Neutrophil and macrophage lysosomal enzymes
- Oxygen metabolites

Source: R.S. Cotran, V. Kumar, and S.L. Robbins. Inflammation and Repair. In *Robbins Pathologic Basis of Disease.* Philadelphia: Saunders, 1989.

stimulates the process of anaerobic glycolysis, with the production of lactate and the generation of ATP

Glucose + 2Pi + 2ADP → 2 lactate + 2ATP + 2H20*

This increase in glycolytic rate with hypoxia has been termed the *Pasteur effect.* In the presence of hypoxemia, glucose is metabolized preferentially because the ratio of moles of ATP produced per mole of O_2 consumed is higher with glucose than with other metabolic fuels. Although glucose consumption maximizes the utilization of available O_2 during conditions of anaerobic glycolysis, the yield of ATP during that time, 2 moles of ATP per mole glucose, is dramatically lower than its normal yield during oxidative phosphorylation, 36 moles of ATP per mole glucose. The increased cytosolic lactate concentration is an additional disadvantage of glycolysis. This glycolytic production of lactic acid is one of the first metabolic reactions to hypoxia; in itself, it is not a threat to cell viability unless it is exaggerated.

Unlike the heart and other vital organs that can get energy from metabolizing fat and proteins, the brain's energy requirements must be met by the metabolism of glucose. In the hypoxic brain, glucose has to be broken down anaerobically. If the systemic arterial pressure is not drastically decreased, severe degrees of hypoxemia may be present without causing a significant decrease in brain ATP because of the compensatory cerebral vasodilatation and active anaerobic glycolysis triggered by anoxia. If perfusion is maintained at near-normal levels, even in the presence of moderately severe

*Pi = high-energy phosphate group.

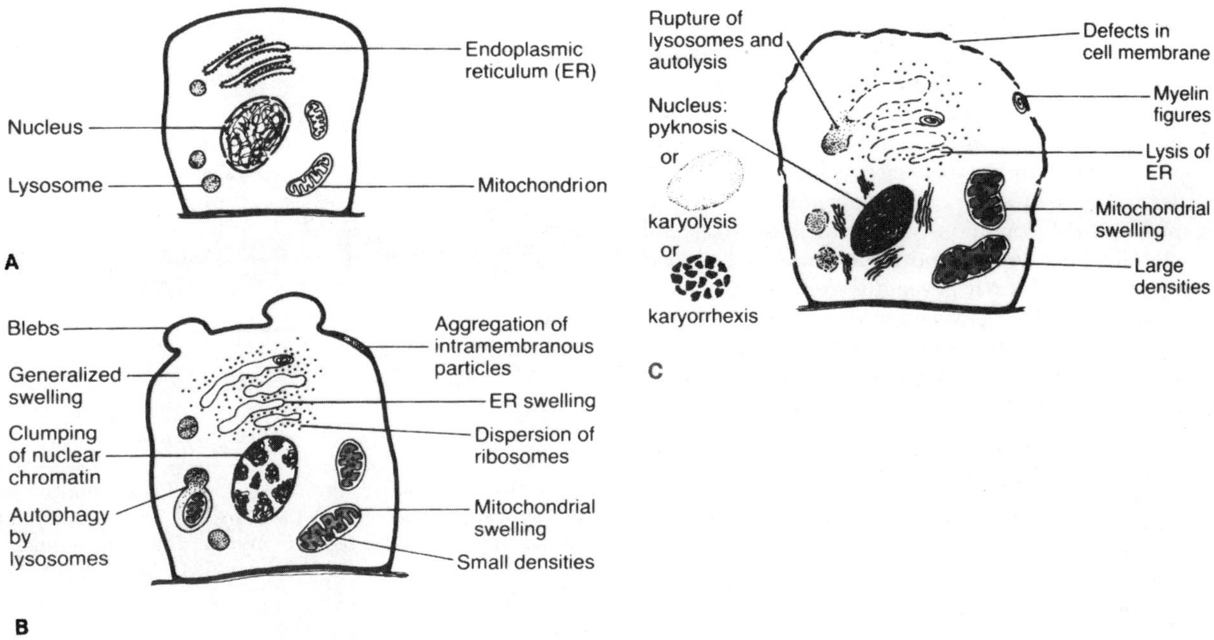

Fig. 1-15. A. Schematic representation of the normal cell. B. Ultrastructural changes in reversible injury. C. Changes in irreversible injury. (From R.S. Cotran, V. Kumar, and S.L. Robbins. Cellular Injury and Adaptation. In *Robbins Pathologic Basis of Disease.* Philadelphia: Saunders, 1989.)

hypoxemia, total energy production is not severely reduced and neuronal survival is not threatened. But anaerobic glycolysis alone cannot produce enough ATP to maintain the viability of the neurones of the brain for a prolonged period of time.

If there is a combination of severe hypoxemia and severe hypoperfusion, with the blood flow reduced below a critical threshold level, cerebral arterial oxygen transport is reduced to the point of threatening the viability of cerebral neurons. In the presence of hypoperfusion, the body attempts to compensate, partly by the mechanism of autoregulation, shunting blood away from the splanchnic region and other parts of the body while protecting the flow to the heart, brain, and kidney (see Chap. 40). Under such conditions as these, the body is not homogeneous. Some vital structures may receive enough oxygen to maintain aerobic metabolism while others are receiving insufficient oxygen. Depending on the cause of pathology and the severity of the oxygen deficit, when enough cells in a tissue sustain such ischemic injury, tissue function becomes impaired and an inflammatory process is triggered. Under such circumstances, release of inflammatory mediators accentuates the ischemia and further limits the delivery of oxygen and substrate to the tissues, causing further organ damage.

CIRCULATORY ARREST. Brain oxygen stores are depleted within less than 10 seconds of circulatory arrest (the time that it takes for unconsciousness to develop), and the brain glucose stores and ATP will last only about 5 minutes for subsequent anaerobic energy metabolism. Because of this, until recently, it has been believed that cessation of circulation for longer than about 5 minutes almost always resulted in irreversible brain damage. It is now known that individual neurons in vivo can survive up to 60 minutes of normothermic anoxia and that full recovery has occasionally occurred after up to 20 minutes of normothermic anoxia. However, although such exceptions have been observed, it is unlikely that complete functional restoration of all neurons can occur after circulatory arrest of more than 5 minutes (under normal conditions) unless effective resuscitative measures are utilized.

When the glucose supply in the brain or glycogen supply in other cells is depleted, the levels of ATP and creatine phosphate fall, triggering a cascade of reactions. As the energy-dependent sodium/potassium pump fails, K^+ leaks out of the cells, slowly at first, then rapidly floods the interstitium, while Na^+ moves into the cells; cell membranes are depolarized as the ion gradient that had been preserved by the membrane-bound ATPases is dissipated. Acute cellular swelling occurs as sodium enters the cells, and the intracellular osmotic load is further raised by the accumulation of catabolic metabolites, such as inorganic phosphates and lactates (Fig. 1-15).

These ion exchanges are accompanied by the sudden influx of Ca^{2+} into the cell, possibly because of opening of voltage-dependent Ca^{2+} gates, combined with the disabling of the mechanism for pumping Ca^{2+} out of the cell. The rise in cytosolic Ca^{2+} triggers the unraveling of many Ca^{2+}-supported mechanisms, leading to lipolysis, proteolysis, and disassembly of microtubules. Blebs may form at the cell surface as cytosolic skeletal components break down. Cells, such as intestinal epithelium, that possess microvilli begin to lose the microvillous structure. Protein synthesis stops as the ribosomes become detached from the endoplasmic reticulum. The endoplasmic reticulum and the mitochondria swell as the cell swelling increases.

Stasis of blood flow and low arterial PO_2 and pH cause derangement of blood elements, with sludging of red blood cells, aggregating of platelets and leukocytes, and adhering of these cells to capillary endothelium. Phospholipase A_2 is activated, triggering the arachidonic acid cascade, which, among other things, leads to the synthesis and release of oxygen-free radicals from the leukocytes. Although the recruitment of inflammatory mediators has not been studied extensively, it must be hypothesized that many, if not all, of the inflammatory mediators that have been described previously are activated under such circumstances and play critical roles in the body's responses, depending on the underlying pathological conditions. Some of these roles are understood, but others require study. For example, the blood may be hypercoagulable or hypocoagulable in a given area, depending on the balance between the forces of the coagulation cascade and those of the fibrinolysin system. The blood vessels in a given area may be dilated or constricted, depending on the balance between the effects of the vasoactive mediators. Up to a certain point, all the above disturbances are reversible if oxygenation and adequate perfusion are restored soon enough.

As the cell's supply of ATP is rapidly depleted, it is replaced by ADP. The ADP in turn is replaced by adenosine monophosphate (AMP). The AMP is further catabolized to adenosine, inosine, and hypoxanthine, which will subsequently serve as a substrate for the reoxygenation reperfusion injury (Fig. 1-16).

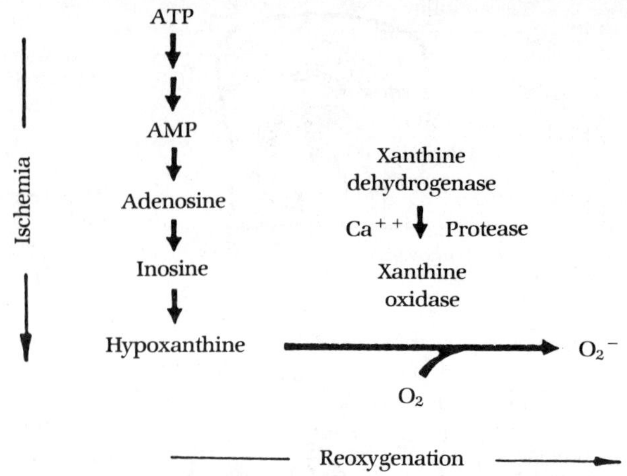

Fig. 1-16. Hypothesized mechanism for ischemia-induced production of superoxide. (From J.M. McCord. Oxygen-derived free radicals in postischemic tissue injury. Reprinted by permission of *The New England Journal of Medicine,* [312:159, 1985].)

Reperfusion—Reoxygenation Injury

Ischemia, by itself, will ultimately produce tissue death if it lasts long enough and is severe enough. However, it is now clear that a substantial part of the tissue injury that in the past was termed *ischemic injury* does not actually occur during the period of ischemia but during the period of reperfusion and reoxygenation, when molecular oxygen is reintroduced to the tissue.

Hypoxanthine, which accumulates during ischemia, is the substrate for the enzyme xanthine oxidase, which is widely distributed among tissues in the form xanthine dehydrogenase. Xanthine dehydrogenase appears to be the major source of superoxide in postischemic tissue. The intestines, lung, and liver are particularly rich sources, the mucosal villi of the intestine containing the highest concentration of any tissue. In light of this finding, it seems to be highly significant that the intestinal mucosa is probably the tissue most exquisitely sensitive to ischemic injury. There is considerable evidence that the elevated cytosolic calcium concentration activates a protease capable of converting xanthine dehydrogenase to xanthine oxidase. Hence, during ischemia, a new enzyme, xanthine oxidase, appears, along with one of its two required substrates, hypoxanthine (or xanthine). It is hypothesized that when molecular oxygen is supplied during the reperfusion of the tissue, it produces a burst of superoxide radical and hydrogen peroxide production (McCord). (This sequence is diagrammed in Fig. 1-16). As previously discussed, substantial quantities of oxygen radicals are also generated by activated leukocytes.

In the same way that oxygen radicals kill microorganisms and degrade necrotic tissue, they can also destroy normal cells. They cause peroxidation of membrane phospholipids, with consequent cell injury from disruption and lysis of intracellular organelles and of the cell as a whole. The hydroxyl radical (OH^-) oxidizes parts of proteins and nucleic acids, thereby causing enzyme inactivation and DNA strand-breaks. Oxygen radicals cause secondary damage from the effects of increased concentration of cytosolic Ca^{2+}. If membranes are severely damaged, the scene is set for a flooding of calcium ions into the cells when the ischemic tissue is reperfused.

Irreversible Injury

Complete circulatory arrest without reperfusion leads to necrosis of different organs at different times. Heart muscle stops contracting within 60 seconds of coronary occlusion, but this noncontractility does not mean that the muscle cell has died. In the myocardium, indications of irreversible injury—large flocculent amorphous densities—can be seen in the mitochondria as early as 30 to 40 minutes after ischemia (Table 1-4). In the liver, between 1 and 2 hours of ischemia are required to produce irreversible damage to the liver cells. In the brain, neurons suffer irreversible damage after 3 to 5 minutes. In the kidney, 20 minutes of ischemia fails to produce cell death, whereas 30 minutes of ischemia induces widespread death among epithelial cells in the proximal tubules. Many cells that show resistance to hypoxic injury are those that are able to generate ATP anaerobically or conserve ATP by reducing its consumption. Fibroblasts, epidermis, and skeletal muscle that is put at complete rest can survive many hours of ischemia.

The boundary line dividing reversible injury from cell death is seldom sharp. Figure 1-15C illustrates some of the most basic findings in irreversibly injured cells. By the time that cell injury is irreversible, cellular swelling, one of the earliest signs of cell damage, has increased markedly. One of the most basic of all the changes is the membrane damage, which leads to a fatal loss of permeability of the membrane and loss of volume regulation for the cell. Phospholipid degradation leads to accumulation of free fatty acids (FFA), much of it arachidonic acid. The FFAs have a detergent effect on membranes, potentially causing changes in permeability and electrophysiologic alterations. There is a constant turnover of phospholipids in normally functioning cells; degradation of phospholipids that is required for maintenance of body homeostasis is normally balanced by resynthesis of

Table 1-4. Susceptibility of cells to ischemic necrosis

High	Neurons (3–5 min)
Intermediate	Myocardium, hepatocytes, renal epithelium (30 min–2 hr)
Low	Fibroblasts, epidermis, skeletal muscle (many hours)

Source: R.S. Cotran, V. Kumar, and S.L. Robbins. Cellular Injury and Adaptation. In *Robbins Pathologic Basis of Disease*. Philadelphia: Saunders, 1989.

these molecules so that the integrity of the membranes is always maintained. This system finally breaks down in the severely hypoxic cell as phospholipids are lost and phospholipases continue to be activated by a number of possible mechanisms: increase in cytosolic Ca^{2+}, detergent action of free fatty acids, decreased synthesis of membrane phospholipids, and release of toxic free radicals by ischemic cells. Some of the cell membrane damage is due to Ca^{2+}-mediated activation of intracellular proteases, which leads to disassembly of intermediate filaments of the cytoskeleton. This, in the presence of cell swelling, results in detachment of the cell membrane from the cytoskeleton and makes the membrane vulnerable to stretching and rupture.

The mitochondria are swollen and contain large amorphous densities, evidence of massive calcium influx. The injury to lysosomal membranes (caused, at least in part, by the falling pH caused by glycolysis, lactate accumulation, and breakdown of phosphate esters) allows leakage of their enzymes—RNAases, DNAases, proteases, phosphatases, and others—into the cell, and the lysosomes ultimately rupture and are autolyzed with enzymatic digestion of cell components. The nuclei swell, rupture, or shrink, with irreparable damage to the cell's genetic apparatus.

The molecular events associated with irreversible cell damage are complex, and current understanding is incomplete, but it is clear that if hypoxia is severe enough and prolonged enough, there are at least three interrelated systems whose malfunction plays central roles in tissue and organ death: (1) Oxidative phosphorylation to synthesize ATP ceases; (2) membranes are irreparably damaged; and (3) calcium ions flood the cytosol. It is also clear that oxygen, which is central to life, can contribute to death if it is supplied too late, and that inflammatory mediators, which are essential in maintaining the body's homeostasis, can also lead to death if they are recruited in such force that they overpower the mechanisms that normally modulate their effects.

Regardless of the initiating cause, cell injury quickly involves more than the cell to include its environment and the adjoining cells. As cascade upon cascade of inflammatory mediators are recruited, damage that may have been local initially spreads. Damage that was initially reversible sooner or later becomes irreversible.

The Terminal Patient

There is wide variation in the sequence of events that accompanies death and in the duration of its stages, depending on the underlying pathology and the physiologic state of the person before the terminal event (Fig. 1-17). Sudden cardiac arrest caused by ventricular fibrillation leads within seconds to clinical death, in which neither pulse nor respiration can be detected in the unresponsive patient. In the patient dying in shock from loss of blood or progressive respiratory insufficiency, however, clinical death is preceded by a preterminal state that may last for many hours. In spite of the differences of mechanisms, there are many similarities and characteristic stages, which have been well described by Negovsky and by Safar.

Preagonal Period

In victims of sudden cardiac arrest from ventricular fibrillation (e.g., as a result of electrical shock), there is virtu-

Fig. 1-17. Stages and reversibility of dying. (From P. Safar. The Mechanisms of Dying and Their Reversal. In G. Schwartz, et al. [eds.], *Principles and Practice of Emergency Medicine*. Philadelphia: Saunders, 1986.)

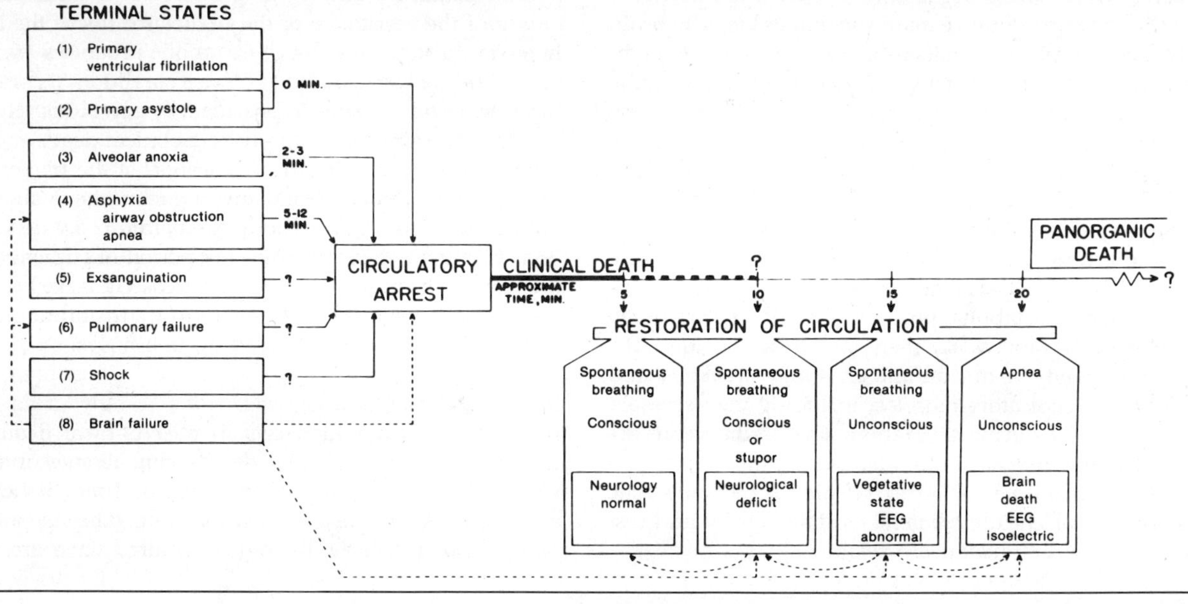

ally no preagonal period, but in other conditions in which death is not instantaneous, the hemodynamic and respiratory disorders that are predominating influences during the preagonal period lead to hypoxia and tissue acidosis. The energy supply during this time is basically aerobic, but functional impairment of the body organs aggravates the disturbance of circulation as ventilation/perfusion relationships in the lungs deteriorate, the ability of the liver to excrete toxic wastes is disrupted, and the kidneys eventually stop functioning. Hypoxia causes reflex stimulation of life-ensuring systems—chemoreceptors, angioreceptors, the respiratory and vasomotor centers, and the reticular formation of the brain stem—in an effort to compensate for failing functions and to preserve the higher centers in the central nervous system (CNS). The rate and depth of breathing, heart rate, and cardiac output increase while the arterial blood pressure rises in response to constriction of the peripheral and splanchnic blood vessels. At the same time, the capillary network of the brain dilates in an effort to increase the blood supply to the vital structures of the brain. However, in the dying patient, the activation of the compensatory mechanisms is followed by the equally important inhibition of the brain cortex, which defends the higher structures of the central nervous system from maximum exhaustion. The cortical neurons, the most sensitive of all the cells of the body to hypoxia, are the first to go out of action. The energy expenditure of the CNS is lessened; cortical functions are suspended while energy resources are concentrated on the vital regulation of function of the internal organs. The patient first loses rational mentation and then loses consciousness.

Terminal Pause

The sudden cessation of respiration after a period of tachypnea—the terminal pause—is a response to an increase in the tone of the vagus nerves as they are stimulated by hypoxia. Oxidative processes are repressed and glycolytic processes increase. The duration of the terminal pause varies from 5 or 10 seconds to 3 or 4 minutes.

Agonal State

The agonal state, which begins after the terminal pause, is the last chaotic and primitive manifestation of life. The brain has switched completely to anaerobic glycolysis and its highest function has failed, relieving the bulbar centers from the regulatory influence of the cerebral cortex. Thus free, these lower centers organize one last effort in the dying patient's struggle for life. The almost extinct processes of respiration and circulation are temporarily reactivated. Sometimes there is a short-term regaining of consciousness. Decerebrate rigidity and general tonic spasms may be observed. Because of the anaerobic glycolysis that energizes this period, incompletely oxidized metabolic products rapidly accumulate. Respiration is at first weak, then increases considerably, and, after reaching a maximum, gradually weakens and ceases. All the respiratory muscles, including the accessory ones, are involved during inhalation. The cardiac contractions temporarily increase in frequency, and the blood pressure may reach a level of 30 to 40 mm Hg. If energetic therapy is not started immediately, cardiac activity and respiration cease and clinical death sets in.

Clinical Death

Clinical death has been defined by Negovsky as "the period of respiratory, circulatory, and brain arrest during which initiation of resuscitation can lead to recovery with prearrest central nervous system (CNS) function." It begins either with the last agonal inhalation or the last cardiac contraction. The patient is without pulse or blood pressure and is completely unresponsive to the most painful stimulus; the pupils are widely dilated. Some reflex reactions to external stimulation are preserved. During intubation, for example, respiration may be restored in response to stimulation of the receptors of the superior laryngeal nerve, the nucleus of which is located in the medulla oblongata near the respiratory center.

The duration of clinical death depends on the length of time the cerebral cortex survives in the absence of circulation and respiration. Under normal temperature conditions, this period does not, as a rule, exceed 3 to 6 minutes. Signs of the alteration of cells begin the moment clinical death sets in, and, with time, disorders increase. The character and length of the preceding period of dying have considerable effect on the duration of clinical death. In sudden death from ventricular fibrillation in a previously healthy person, the period of clinical death is usually 4 to 6 minutes; however, when the pathologic process has been tempestuous, the period of clinical death is shortened, even though the preceding events may have progressed rapidly. When the terminal stage has been lengthy, the period of clinical death shortens even more; if the patient spends a long time (several hours) in severe hypotension, resuscitation becomes impossible even a few seconds after the cessation of cardiac activity because of exhaustion of all energy resources, severe morphologic damage, and the flood of toxic metabolites that are circulated during attempts to reperfuse and reoxygenate the tissues.

For the same reason, age also affects the length of the period of clinical death. Resuscitation is much more likely to be successful after the cardiac arrest of a young, healthy person than after that of an elderly person. Isolated cases have been described in which it has been possible to resuscitate children after 10 or even 12 minutes of clinical death, resulting in complete restoration of vital functions.

Terminal states that develop in cases of hypothermia have specific features. The main property of hypothermia—increase of the resistance of the higher sectors of the brain to hypoxia through slowing of metabolic processes and reduction of the energy demand—creates conditions for prolonged brain survival on energy provided by glycolysis. Hypothermia is successfully used to prolong clinical death and is also a factor favorably affecting restoration of the higher sectors of the brain. Experimental investigations have shown that moderate hypothermia (body temperature 24–26°C, 75.2–78.8°F) during dying enables the period of clinical death to be prolonged up to 1 hour (Negovsky). On a background of deep hypothermia (8–10°C, 46.4–50°F), the duration of clinical death has been prolonged up to 2 hours.

Biological Death and Brain Death

Biological death, which sets in after clinical death, is an irreversible state of cellular destruction. Tissues of the body vary in their ability to survive anoxic and metabolic insults, and hence some organs irretrievably "die" sooner than others. During early biological death, when irreversible changes have already occurred in the brain cortex and full restoration of the function of the CNS is impossible, it is occasionally possible to restore the activity of the heart and of the respiratory and certain subcortical centers. Successful cardiopulmonary resuscitation may thus occur despite less successful brain resuscitation, leading to the survival of a person with significant brain damage or, in the worst cases, to the condition of *brain death.*

The determination of when biological death has occurred may frequently fall to the emergency physician and in some circumstances is difficult. Legal criteria for certification of death vary from state to state and nation to nation, and many jurisdictions lack a definition compatible with modern techniques of life support. The President's Commission for the Study of Ethical Problems in Medicine and Biomedical and Behavioral Research, recognizing the need for a uniform statute to provide a clear and socially accepted basis for making determinations of death, in July 1981 proposed this model:

Uniform Determination of Death Act

An individual who has sustained either (1) irreversible cessation of circulatory and respiratory functions, or (2) irreversible cessation of all functions of the entire brain, including the brain stem, is dead. A determination of death must be made in accordance with accepted medical standards.

The fulfillment of the first criterion is generally the easier to determine. If, despite optimal cardiopulmonary resuscitation and support for a reasonable period of time, the patient is unable to develop and sustain spontaneous circulation, the patient is dead. Most determinations of death in the emergency setting will be made on this basis.

Fulfillment of the second criterion is more problematic. Guidelines to assist in the medical determination of cessation of brain function have been published, including those of the Ad Hoc Committee of the Harvard Medical School (1968) (Table 1-5), the United States Collaborative Study of Cerebral Death (1976) (Table 1-6), and the Conference of Royal Colleges and Faculties of the United Kingdom (1976) (Table 1-7). A more recent 1981 statement of currently accepted medical standards has been published as a supplement to the recommendations of the President's Commission. An outline of these guidelines is presented in Table 1-8. All have their limitations, and all should be recognized as guidelines for the exercise of good medical judgment rather than as absolute criteria to be used in a blind "checklist" fashion. The essence of the determination is satisfactory assurance that

Table 1-5. Harvard criteria for brain death

1. *Unreceptive and unresponsive.* "Even the most intensely painful stimuli evoke no vocal or other response. . . ."
2. *No movements or breathing.* "Observation covering a period of at least one hour by physicians is adequate to satisfy the criteria of no spontaneous muscular movements or spontaneous respiration or response to stimuli. . . . The total absence of spontaneous breathing may be established by turning off the respirator for three minutes and observing whether there is any effort on the part of the subject to breathe. . . ." (This requires that carbon dioxide tension be normal and the patient be breathing room air for 10 minutes before the test.)
3. *No reflexes.* "The pupil will be fixed and dilated and will not respond to a direct source of bright light. . . . Ocular movement (to head turning and to irrigation of ears with ice water) and blinking are absent. . . . There is no evidence of postural activity (decerebrate or other). . . . Swallowing, yawning, vocalizing are in abeyance. . . . Corneal and pharyngeal reflexes are absent. . . . As a rule the stretch or tendon reflexes cannot be elicited."
4. *Flat electroencephalogram.* "Of great confirmatory value is the flat or isoelectric electroencephalogram. . . ." (Technical guidelines including 5 μV/mm or higher gains, absence of response to pinch or noise, and 10-minute minimum recording time are added.) "All of the above tests shall be repeated at least 24 hours later with no change." Hypothermia (temperature below 32.2°C, 90°F) and central nervous system depressants such as barbiturates must be excluded. "In situations where . . . electroencephalographic monitoring is not available, the absence of cerebral function has to be determined by purely clinical signs . . . or by the absence of circulation as judged by standstill of blood in the retinal vessels, or by absence of cardiac action. . . ."

Source: A definition of irreversible coma: Report of the Ad Hoc Committee of the Harvard Medical School to examine the definition of brain death. *J.A.M.A.* 205:337, 1968.

Table 1-6. Criteria for cerebral death (brain death) proposed by the Collaborative Study of Cerebral Death

PREREQUISITE

All appropriate diagnostic and therapeutic procedures have been performed.

CRITERIA

Each criterion must be present for 30 minutes at least 6 hours after the onset of coma and apnea.

1. Coma with cerebral unresponsivity (see definition 1)
2. Apnea (see definition 2)
3. Dilated pupils
4. Absent cephalic reflexes (see definition 3)
5. Electrocerebral silence (see definition 4)

CONFIRMATORY TEST

Absence of cerebral blood flow

DEFINITIONS

1. *Cerebral unresponsivity.* A state in which the patient does not respond purposively to externally applied stimuli, obeys no commands, and does not phonate spontaneously or in response to a painful stimulus
2. *Apnea.* The absence of spontaneous respiration, manifested by the need for controlled ventilation (i.e., the patient makes no effort to override the respirator) for at least 15 minutes
3. *Cephalic reflexes.* Pupillary, corneal, oculoauditory, oculovestibular, oculocephalic, ciliospinal, snout, cough, pharyngeal swallowing
4. *Electrocerebral silence.* An electroencephalogram with an absence of electrical potentials of cerebral origin over 2 μV from symmetrically placed electrode pairs over 10 cm apart and with interelectrode resistance between 100–10,000 Ω

Source: An appraisal of the criteria of cerebral death: A summary statement: A collaborative study. *J.A.M.A.* 237:982, 1976.

Table 1-7. Criteria for the diagnosis of brain death

A. Conditions under which the diagnosis of brain death should be considered
   1. The patient is deeply comatose.
      a. There should be no suspicion that this state is due to depressant drugs.
      b. Primary hypothermia as a cause of coma should have been excluded.
      c. Metabolic and endocrine disturbances that can be responsible for or can contribute to coma should have been excluded.
   2. The patient is being maintained on a ventilator because spontaneous respiration had previously become inadequate or had ceased altogether. Relaxants . . . and other drugs should have been excluded as a cause of respiratory failure.
   3. There should be no doubt that the patient's condition is due to irremediable structural brain damage. The diagnosis of a disorder that can lead to brain death should have been fully established.

B. Diagnostic tests for confirmation of brain death
   All brainstem reflexes are absent.
   1. The pupils are fixed in diameter and do not respond to sharp changes in the intensity of incident light.
   2. There is no corneal reflex.
   3. The vestibulo-ocular reflexes are absent.
   4. No motor responses within the cranial nerve distribution can be elicited by adequate stimulation of a somatic area.
   5. There is no gag reflex or reflex response to bronchial stimulation by a suction catheter passed down the trachea.
   6. No respiratory movements occur when the patient is disconnected from the mechanical ventilator for long enough to ensure that the arterial carbon dioxide tension rose above the threshold for stimulation of respiration.

C. Other considerations
   1. *Repetition of testing.* The interval between tests must depend upon the primary pathology and the clinical course of the disease. . . . In some conditions the outcome is not so clearcut, and in these cases it is recommended that the tests should be repeated. The interval between tests depends upon the progress of the patient and might be as long as 24 hours. . . .
   2. *Integrity of spinal reflexes.* It is well established that spinal cord function can persist after insults that irretrievably destroy brainstem functions. . . .
   3. *Confirmatory investigation.* It is now widely accepted that electroencephalography is not necessary for the diagnosis of brain death. . . . Other investigations such as cerebral angiography or cerebral blood-flow measurements are not required for the diagnosis of brain death.
   4. *Body temperature.* . . . It is recommended that it should not be less than 35°C before the diagnostic tests are carried out.
   5. *Specialist opinion and the status of the doctors concerned.* Only when the primary diagnosis is in doubt is it necessary to consult with a neurologist or neurosurgeon. Decision to withdraw artificial support should be made after all the criteria presented above have been fulfilled and can be made by any of the following combination of doctors:
      a. A consultant who is in charge of the case and one other doctor.
      b. In the absence of a consultant, his [or her] deputy, who should have been registered for 5 years or more and who should have had adequate experience in the care of such cases, and one other doctor.

Source: Conference of Royal Colleges and Faculties of the United Kingdom: Diagnosis of brain death. *Lancet* 2:1069, 1976.

there is no cerebral or brain stem function remaining, that complicating conditions have been ruled out, and that the patient can no longer survive as an individual, independent being. Satisfactory resolution of these issues frequently requires an extended period of observation, and determination of death on a neurologic basis can rarely be attained in the emergency department setting.

MECHANISMS OF RAPID DEATH

There are two broad categories into which cardiac arrest can be divided—*primary cardiac arrest,* in which sudden cessation of cardiac function is the first manifestation of acute decompensation, and *secondary cardiac arrest,* in which factors external to the heart cause cardiac arrest as a complication of some other process.

Primary Cardiac Arrest

A number of disease states predispose to sudden cardiac dysrhythmias or loss of cardiac function. Poor coronary perfusion accompanied by imbalance of myocardial oxygen supply and demand is the most common cause of such an arrest. This mechanism, unfortunately, is seen in patients who have reasonably healthy hearts. Electrical shock, for example, can cause death from a sudden cardiac dysrhythmia even if the damage it causes to other body systems is minimal. Chronic congestive heart failure from valvular disease, myocarditis, or other disease of heart muscle, and ventricular scarring and fibrosis from previous infarction can all lead to primary cardiac arrest. In many such cases, the pumping function of the heart is so weakened that resuscitation from arrest is impossible.

Sudden loss of cardiac pumping function occurs in association with several patterns of cardiac electrical activity. Ventricular fibrillation, ventricular standstill or asystole, and electromechanical dissociation are three patterns associated with clinical death.

Ventricular Fibrillation

Ventricular fibrillation causes the majority of sudden deaths in patients with preexisting myocardial ischemia. Electrical activity is random and uncoordinated; there is no sequencing of atrial, nodal, and ventricular depolarization. Although the fibrillating myocardium is quite active and its

Table 1-8. Criteria for determination of death

An individual presenting the findings in *either* section A (cardiopulmonary) *or* section B (neurologic) is dead. In either section, a diagnosis of death requires that *both* cessation of functions, as set forth in subsection 1, *and* irreversibility, as set forth in subsection 2, be demonstrated.

A. An individual with irreversible cessation of circulatory and respiratory functions is dead.
   1. Cessation is recognized by an appropriate clinical examination.
   2. Irreversibility is recognized by persistent cessation of function during an appropriate period of observation and/or trial of therapy.

B. An individual with irreversible cessation of all functions of the entire brain, including the brain stem, is dead.
   1. Cessation is recognized when evaluation discloses findings of a *and* b:
      a. Cerebral functions are absent.
      b. Brain stem functions are absent.
   2. Irreversibility is recognized when evaluation discloses findings of a *and* b *and* c:
      a. The cause of coma is established and is sufficient to account for the loss of brain functions.
      b. The possibility of recovery of any brain functions is excluded.
      c. The cessation of all brain functions persists for an appropriate period of observation and/or trial of therapy.

Source: Guidelines for the determination of death: Report of the medical consultants on the diagnosis of death to the President's Commission for the Study of Ethical Problems in Medicine and Biomedical and Behavioral Research. *J.A.M.A.* 246:2184, 1981.

metabolic demands remain high, there is no effective cardiac output and no coronary perfusion; ischemia intensifies as the condition persists. Although myocardial ischemia and spontaneous ectopy are the most common causative factors, external influences on the heart, including electrical shock, electrolyte abnormalities, hypothermia, drugs, and excess circulating catecholamines, can precipitate ventricular fibrillation.

Ventricular Asystole

Ventricular asystole, a less commonly seen condition, is a pulseless state with cardiac standstill and an isoelectric electrocardiogram (ECG). Its presence usually indicates a severe condition with widespread myocardial damage, and resuscitation is often difficult or impossible. Asystole may develop as the end point of a prolonged period of ventricular fibrillation. Less commonly, it may result from increased parasympathetic tone from extraordinary vagal stimulation, with consequent depression of rhythm and conduction. Predisposing conditions, aside from generalized ischemic disease, include Stokes-Adams syndrome (focal ischemia in the conduction system) and dependence on an electrical pacemaker. Electrocution, massive drug overdose, and electrolyte abnormalities may also result in asystole.

Electromechanical Dissociation

Electromechanical dissociation, in which relatively normal cardiac electrical activity is present but is not accompanied by appropriate mechanical contraction, is unusual as a presenting rhythm but frequently appears during resuscitative efforts. Inadequate perfusion pressure is present, and volume and pharmacologic support may be required to restore normal circulation. Cardiomyopathy, severe hypocalcemia, and intravascular volume depletion may lead to electromechanical dissociation. Pericardial tamponade may mimic electromechanical dissociation, but it is easily diagnosed and treated by surgical drainage of pericardial fluid.

Secondary Cardiac Arrest

Although the heart may be quite healthy, failure or dysfunction in another organ system may, after a variable period of time, lead to secondary cardiac arrest. Correction of the primary problem must occur simultaneously with the resuscitation of the heart; the severity of the primary disease and the length of time it has been present will determine the ultimate prognosis of the patient.

Respiratory failure, whatever its cause, may lead to arterial hypoxemia and hypercarbia. Cardiac activity may initially be stimulated by such abnormalities, but, if they remain uncorrected, the patient becomes acidotic, the myocardium is unable to sustain tone or contraction, and asystole ensues. Acute hypoxia or anoxia causes a very rapid deterioration to cardiac arrest, usually within 2 to 3 minutes. If hypoxia is prevented by administration of oxygen but ventilation is interrupted and the victim is allowed to become hypercarbic and acidotic, the process is somewhat prolonged; cardiac arrest will not usually occur until the arterial pH falls below 6.8.

Sudden loss of blood volume, such as in massive traumatic hemorrhage, will result in cardiac arrest. The initial circulatory compensation for such loss is by vasoconstriction and tachycardia; peripheral vascular beds are shut down, and the reduced blood volume is circulated more and more rapidly to the essential organs. Although an adequate perfusion pressure can be maintained by such adjustments for a short period of time, this pressure gradually diminishes as losses continue and intravascular volume is depleted. Cardiac output is no longer able to meet metabolic demands of the vital organs, including the heart itself, and cardiac arrest ensues.

CNS failure may occur acutely from trauma, intracranial hemorrhage, or rapid increases in intracranial pressure. Brain stem output to the heart and respiratory muscles is altered, and their function becomes erratic, depressed, and ultimately terminated.

Metabolic derangements, embolic phenomena, extremes of temperature, toxins, and *acute anaphylactic reactions* can all lead to sudden cessation of cardiorespiratory function. It is the goal of the rescuer to begin resuscitation as early as possible in this period of clinical death in order to avoid the onset of irreversible organic changes and to prevent progression to biologic death.

SELECTED READING

History and Epidemiology

American Heart Association. Standards and guidelines for cardiopulmonary resuscitation and emergency cardiac care. *JAMA* 255:2841, 1986.

Beck, CS, Pritchard, H, and Feil, HS. Ventricular fibrillation of long duration abolished by electric shock. *JAMA* 135:985, 1947.

Black, PM. Brain death. *N Engl J Med* 299:338–344, 393–401, 1978.

Black, PM. Guidelines for the diagnosis of brain death. In AK Ropper, SK Kennedy, and NT Zervas (eds.), *Neurologica-Neurosurgical Intensive Care*. Baltimore: University Park Press, 1983.

Breivik, H, and Abramson, N, et al. Reversibility of clinical death patients: the myth of the 5 minute limit. *Abst Emerg Med* 16:496, 1987.

Cobb, LA, Werner, JA, and Trobaugh, GB. Sudden cardiac death: I. A decade's experience with out-of-hospital resuscitation. II. Outcome of resuscitation: Management and future directions. *Mod Concepts Cardiovasc Dis* 49:37, 1980.

Earnest, MP, et al. Long term survival and neurological status after resuscitation from out-of-hospital cardiac arrest. *Neurology* 30: 1298, 1980.

Guidelines for the determination of death. *JAMA* 246:2184, 1981.

Jude, JR, Kouwenhoven, WB, and Knickerbocker, GG. Cardiac arrest: Report of application of external cardiac massage on 118 patients. *JAMA* 178:1063, 1961.

Kouwenhoven, WB, Jude, JR, and Knickerbocker, GG. Closed-chest cardiac massage. *JAMA* 173:1064, 1960.

Kouwenhoven, WB, and Langworthy, OR. Cardiopulmonary resuscitation. An account of forty-five years of research. *JAMA* 226:877, 1973.

Kuller, LH. Sudden death—definition and epidemiologic considerations. *Prog Cardiovasc Dis* 23:1, 1980.

Myerburg, RJ, et al. Clinical, electrophysiologic and hemodynamic profile of patients resuscitated from prehospital cardiac arrest. *Am J Cardiol* 68:568, 1980.

President's Commission for the Study of Ethical Problems in Medicine and Biomedical and Behavioral Research. *Defining Death: Medical, Legal, and Ethical Issues in the Determination of Death.* Washington, DC: Government Printing Office, 1981.

The Cell

Alberts, B, et al. *Molecular Biology of the Cell* (2nd ed.). New York: Garland, 1989.

Carafoli, E, and Penniston, JT. The calcium signal. *Sci Am* 253(5): 70, 1985.

Cotran, RS, Kumar, V, and Robbins SL. Cellular Injury and Adaptation. In *Robbins Pathologic Basis of Disease.* Philadelphia: Saunders, 1989.

Eisenberg, MS, et al. Sudden cardiac death. *Sci Am* 254:37, 1986.

Hossmann, KA, and Kleihues, P. Reversibility of ischemic brain damage. *Arch Neurol* 29:375, 1973.

Krstic, KV. *Ultrastructure of the Mammalian Cell.* New York: Springer-Verlag, 1979.

Moosy, J (moderator). Pathophysiologic limits to the reversibility of clinical death. *Crit Care Med* 16:1022, 1988.

Negovsky, VA. *Current Problems of Reanimatology.* Moscow: Mir Publishers, 1975.

Rassmussen, H, and Barrett, PQ. Calcium messenger system: An integrated view. *Physiol Rev* 64:238, 1984.

Safar, P. *Cardiopulmonary Cerebral Resuscitation.* Philadelphia: Saunders, 1981.

Safar, P. The mechanisms of dying and their reversal. In G Schwartz, et al. (eds.), *Principles and Practice of Emergency Medicine.* Philadelphia: Saunders, 1986.

Safar, P. Resuscitation from clinical death: Pathophysiologic limits and therapeutic potentials. *Crit Care Med* 16:923, 1988.

Shier, WT. The final steps to toxic cell death. *J Toxicol Toxin Rev* 4(2):191, 1985.

Spiegel, SM. G proteins in clinical medicine. *Hosp Pract* 23:93, 1988.

Weinman, EJ, Dubinsky, WP, Jr., and Shenolikar, S. Regulation of the renal $Na^+ - H^+$ exchanger. *Hosp Pract* 24:157, 1989.

Weiss, L (ed.). The Cell. In *Histology Cell and Tissue Biology* (5th ed.). New York: Elsevier, 1983.

Pathophysiology of Clinical Death

Shier, WT. Why study mechanisms of cell death? *Methods Achiev Exp Pathol* 13:1, 1988.

Siesjo, BK. *Brain Energy Metabolism.* New York: Wiley, 1978.

Siesjo, BK, and Wieloch, T. Cerebral metabolism in ischemia: neurochemical basis for therapy. *Br J Anaesth* 57:47, 1985.

Trump, BF, Berezesky, IK, and Osornio-Vargas, AR. Cell death and the disease process. The role of calcium. In ID Bowen and RA Lockshin (eds.), *Cell Death in Biology and Pathology.* London: Chapman & Hall, 1981.

Inflammation

Bessey, PQ. Metabolic Response to Critical Illness. In DW Wilmore, et al (eds), *Care of the Surgical Patient.* New York: Scientific American, Inc., 1989.

Beutler, B. Cachectin in tissue injury, shock, and related states. *Crit Care Clin.* 5:353, 1989.

Cotran, RS, Kumar, V, and Robbins, SL. Inflammation and Repair. In *Robbins Pathologic Basis of Disease.* Philadelphia: Saunders, 1989.

Dinarello, CA. The endogenous pyrogens in host-defense interactions. *Hosp Pract* 24:111, 1989.

Lefer, AM. Induction of tissue injury and altered cardiovascular performance by platelet-activating factor: Relevance to multiple systems organ failure. *Crit Care Clin* 5:331, 1989.

Pinsky, MR, and Matuscak, GM. Multiple systems organ failure: Failure of host defense homeostasis. *Crit Care Clin* 5:353, 1989.

Weissman, G, Smolen, JE, and Korchak, MM. Release of inflammatory mediators from stimulated neutrophils. *N Engl J Med* 303:27, 1980.

Reoxygenation Injury

Ernster, L. Biochemistry of reoxygenation injury. *Crit Care Med* 16:947, 1988.

McCord, JM. Oxygen-derived free radicals in postischemic tissue injury. *N Engl J Med* 312:159, 1985.

2. Resuscitation: Current Concepts

John A. Paraskos

Since the development of cardiopulmonary resuscitation (CPR), death can no longer be equated with the loss of the vital signs of spontaneous respiration and pulse. For some individuals with adequately preserved cardiopulmonary and neurologic systems, the cessation of breathing and cardiac contraction can be reversed if CPR and definitive care are available. If other systems are also spared, prolonged and vigorous life may ensue. The short period during which loss of vital signs can be reversed is often referred to as *clinical death*. For clinical death to be reversed, however, restoration of ventilation and circulation must intervene before irreversible damage to vital structures occurs. The state of irreversible death is referred to as *biological death*. In difficult circumstances, the best single criterion (medical and legal) for the ultimate death of the functioning integrated human individual (i.e., the person) is brain death.

In the past 30 years, considerable advances have been made in the emergency care of victims of profound circulatory collapse and cardiac arrest; nevertheless, the current techniques of CPR seem to be far from optimal. Sporadic accounts of attempted resuscitations are recorded from antiquity, but until 1960 successful resuscitation was largely limited to occasional victims of respiratory arrest. Emergency thoracotomy with "open heart massage" was described in the 1950s and was often successful if definitive therapy was readily available [1]. Electrical reversal of ventricular fibrillation by externally applied electrodes was described by Zoll and colleagues [2] in 1956. The ability to reverse a fatal arrhythmia without opening the chest challenged the medical community to develop a method of sustaining ventilation and circulation long enough to bring the electrical defibrillator to the patient's aid. In 1958, adequate rescue ventilation with the mouth-to-mouth technique was described by Safar and coworkers [3] and Elam and associates [4]. In 1960, Kouwenhoven [5] described "closed chest massage," thereby introducing the modern era of CPR. The simplicity of this technique (". . . all that is needed are two hands") has led to its widespread dissemination.

The interaction of closed-chest compression with mouth-to-mouth ventilation was developed as basic CPR. The first national conference on CPR was sponsored by the National Academy of Sciences in 1966. Members of this conference recommended that all training programs adhere to American Heart Association standards [6]. The second national conference on CPR was cosponsored in 1973 by the American Heart Association and the National Research Council of the National Academy of Sciences. Members of this conference recommended that instruction in CPR should be extended to the general public [7]. Instruction in CPR of both professionals and the public soon followed through community programs in basic life support (BLS). The American Red Cross has also played an important role in instructing the public through its wide-reaching programs in CPR. In addition, the American Heart Association supports professional teaching programs in advanced cardiac life support (ACLS) that emphasize the interaction of basic CPR with emergency stabilization and transport, ventilatory support, intravenous access, pharmacotherapy, and electrical therapy. Standards for both BLS and ACLS were set in the 1973 National Conference on Cardiopulmonary Resuscitation and Emergency Cardiac Care [7]. These standards were updated in 1979 and again in 1985 [8, 9]. The last National Conference was cosponsored by the American College of Cardiology, the American Red Cross, and the National Heart, Lung, and Blood Institute.

The efficacy of standardized CPR has been given considerable scrutiny in recent years. Unfortunately, its success does not go beyond Kouwenhoven's [5] modest goal of short-term sustaining of viability until definitive therapy can be administered. The benefit of rapid initiation of CPR has been demonstrated in numerous studies [10, 11]. Data from prehospital care systems in Seattle showed that 43% of patients found in ventricular fibrillation (VF) were discharged from the hospital if CPR (i.e., BLS) was applied within 4 minutes and defibrillation (i.e., ACLS) within 8 minutes. If either was delayed, survival rates were much lower. For patients in asystole or electrical mechanical dissociation, survival rates were much smaller [12, 13]. In a study in Miami [14], none of the patients found in bradyarrhythmia or asystole survived, whereas 23% of those in VF were eventually discharged. It has been suggested [13] that one of the benefits of the early initiation of CPR is the prolongation of VF, thereby increasing the possibility that defibrillation will be successful. When onset of CPR has been delayed or the time to defibrillation is greater than 10 minutes, the likelihood is increased that the patient will be in asystole or in "fine" VF and that the condition will convert to asystole. Patients who suffer cardiac arrest in the hospital can be expected to receive CPR and definitive therapy well within the 4- and 8-minute time frame noted in Seattle. Nevertheless, their chances of being discharged alive are generally worse than for out-of-hospital victims because of serious underlying medical problems [15–17].

Soon after the dawning of the modern era of CPR over two decades ago, Pantridge introduced the mobile intensive care unit in Belfast, Ireland [18]. Since then emergency medical transport programs have spread throughout the world. In recent years there has been a move to further approximate Pantridge's mobile intensive care unit by adding the capability of defibrillation to the emergency medical services (EMS) system. This capability is already available in some metropolitan areas where full paramedics are employed. Emergency medical technicians (EMTs) who can perform defibrillation (EMT-Ds) and EMTs equipped with automatic or semiautomatic defibrillators will allow more EMS systems to provide this necessary service.

Thus, the present approach to CPR is modestly successful for ventricular fibrillation. However, CPR has most likely not yet been optimized and further improvement is greatly needed [19]. Research continues to evaluate new approaches and techniques. While further refinements in the delivery of CPR can be expected and enthusiastically encouraged, assiduous attention to research methods and applicability to humans is required to prevent an overly hasty and potentially injurious change in the present standards. The evaluation of apparently contradictory research results is made difficult by the wide variety of experimental methods and models. Animal preparations for research in resuscitative techniques have limited application to the human, largely because of the differences in size and configuration of the thoracic cage. Before changes in CPR can reasonably be entertained, the new techniques must have been demonstrated to improve either survival or neurologic outcome; they must be simple to apply in an arrest and, optimally, they should be simple to teach and applicable by one rescuer without undue effort.

MECHANISMS OF BLOOD FLOW DURING CPR

An understanding of the mechanism by which blood flows during the performance of CPR would seem to be a prerequisite to any significant improvement in the delivery of CPR. However, there is no unanimity among the researchers in this area. Indeed, significant advances seem to have been made by research groups holding very different ideas concerning the basic mechanism of blood flow during CPR. It is even possible that several mechanisms are operative; one or the other may be more important in individuals of different size and chest configuration.

Cardiac Compression Theory

Initially, when closed-chest cardiac massage was described, it was generally believed that blood flow during sternal compression was caused by cardiac compression [5]. That is, the blood was thought to be propelled by the compression of the heart as it is trapped between the sternum and the vertebral column. If this mechanism were operative, the pressures in the ventricles of the heart would be expected to rise higher during sternal compression than the transmural thoracic pressure. With each sternal compression, the semilunar valves would be expected to open as the atrioventricular valves closed; indeed, an echocardiographic study using minipigs has shown such valve motion [20]. During sternal release, the pressure in the ventricles would be expected to fall and the atrioventricular valves to open, allowing the heart to fill from the lungs and systemic veins. While some studies in animals have demonstrated such pressure changes during CPR [21], most have not [22]. If the cardiac compression mechanism were operative, ventilation would best be interposed between sternal compressions so as not to interfere with cardiac compression; also, the faster the sternal compression, the higher the volume of blood flow, assuming that the ventricles had enough time to fill.

The mechanism of cardiac compression was first brought into question in 1962 when Weale and Rothwell-Jackson [23] demonstrated that during chest compression the rise in venous pressure was almost equal to that of arterial pressure. The following year, Wilder and associates [24] showed that ventilation performed synchronously with chest compression produced higher arterial pressures than did alternating ventilation and compression. It was over a decade later, however, before more data confirmed these initial findings.

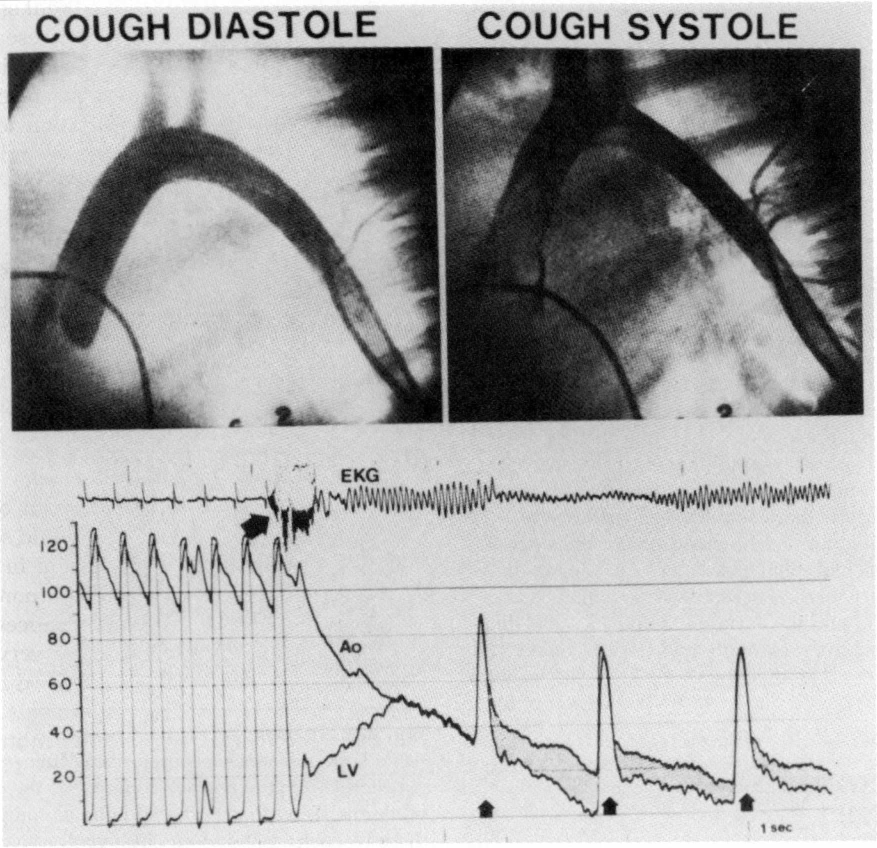

Fig. 2-1. Experimental cough CPR during ventricular fibrillation in a dog. Top: A left lateral aortagram before and during the first induced cough. Bottom: Aortic and left ventricular pressures before and after the induction of ventricular fibrillation (*slanted arrow*). With each cough (*vertical arrows*) a pulse wave is recorded. The aortic valve opens and with each cough contrast medium is washed out of the aortic root. Between coughs there is a coronary pressure gradient (*shaded*) between the aorta and the intracardiac pressures. (From J.M. Criley, et al. Modifications of CPR based on the cough. *Circulation* 74 (Suppl IV):45, 1986. By permission of the American Heart Association, Inc.)

Thoracic Pump Theory

Criley [25] reported in 1976 that during cardiac arrest, repeated forceful coughing was capable of generating systolic pressures comparable to those of normal cardiac activity (Fig. 2-1). This finding suggested that high intrathoracic pressures could sustain blood flow, independent of sternal compression. Subsequently, Neimann and associates [26] proposed that the flow of blood occasioned by sternal compression was also caused by increased intrathoracic pressure. Studies using pressure measurements [27, 28], angiography [29], and echocardiography [30, 31] support this hypothesis and suggest that during CPR the heart serves only as a conduit. According to the thoracic pump theory, flow is generated by a pressure gradient between intrathoracic and extrathoracic vascular structures (Figs. 2-2 and 2-3). Forward flow to the arterial side is favored by functional venous valves, and greater compressibility of veins as compared to arteries at their exit points from the thorax [22, 29, 32, 33]. The thoracic pump theory provides the rationale for experimental attempts at augmenting forward flow by increasing intrathoracic pressure.

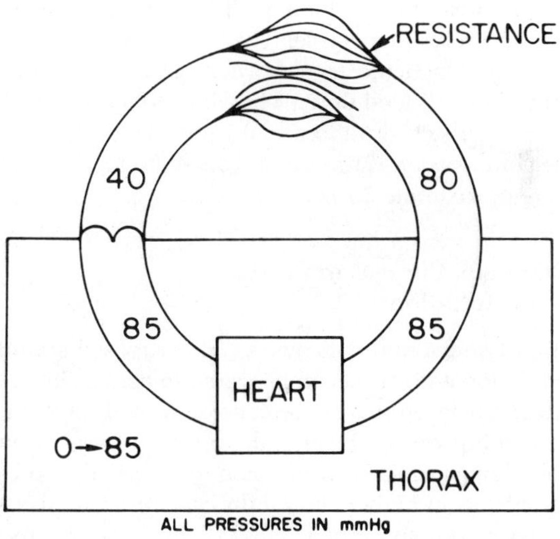

Fig. 2-2. Transmission of pressures by the thoracic pump. The increased intrathoracic pressure during sternal compression is transmitted to the aorta rather than to the venae cavae. (From M.L. Weisfeldt and N. Chandra. Physiology of CPR. Reproduced with permission, from the *Annual Review of Medicine*, Vol. 32. © 1981 by Annual Reviews, Inc.)

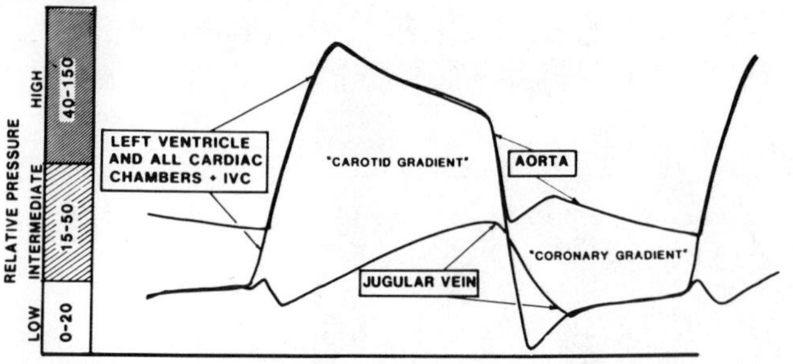

Fig. 2-3. Pressure events during CPR. Intracardiac pressures during external thoracic compression based on actual pressures measured during clinical and experimental CPR. The systolic pressure in all cardiac chambers and the inferior vena cava (IVC) rises to a level equal to the thoracic pressure during application of force to the chest. The "systolic" pressure in the jugular vein (as well as other brachiocephalic veins) is of lesser magnitude because of closure of venous valves at the thoracic inlet. The gradient between the aorta and the jugular and brachiocephalic veins drives the blood through the brachiocephalic vascular bed. During diastole, there is a gradient between the systemic veins and cardiac chambers on the one hand and the aorta on the other. This "diastolic gradient" is responsible for coronary and visceral blood flow. (From J.M. Criley, et al. Modifications of CPR based on the cough. *Circulation* 74 (Suppl IV): 43, 1986. By permission of the American Heart Association, Inc.)

EXPERIMENTAL AND ALTERNATE TECHNIQUES OF CPR

Longer Compression Duration

In 1977, Taylor and associates [34] proposed the use of longer compression duration to 40 or 50 percent of the compression-relaxation cycle. This technique prolongs the time during which the transthoracic gradient is operative and should favor blood flow. While it is difficult to maintain longer compression durations at a rate of 60 cycles per minute, the compression duration at rates of 90 to 100 naturally tends to approximate 50 percent.

Simultaneous Chest Compression and Lung Inflation

In 1980, Chandra and colleagues [35] proposed simultaneous ventilation with chest compression. In conventional CPR, the intrathoracic pressures are considerably dissipated during chest compression through the open airways. Sustained inflation during chest compression prevents this pressure loss and results in higher carotid flow and arterial pressures. High airway pressures of 60 to 110 mm Hg are used to augment carotid flow, requiring intubation and a mechanical ventilator. This technique therefore is an advanced life-support method that requires sophisticated skills and equipment. Furthermore, its use has not met with universal success even in canine preparations [36].

Abdominal Binding

Harris and associates [37] anticipated the thoracic pump theory as early as 1967, by demonstrating that blood flow was augmented during CPR when continuous pressure was applied to the abdomen. In 1971, Redding [38] also reported on continuous or static abdominal binding, as did Chandra and colleagues [39] in 1981. Abdominal binding clearly increases intrathoracic pressure and redistributes blood flow during CPR. The technique also increases aortic diastolic pressure; unfortunately, it also raises right atrial pressure, so that coronary perfusion may be adversely affected [40]. The central venous and intracranial pressures are also raised and, although cerebral blood flow increases, studies have also demonstrated diminished cerebral oxygenation [41]. In another study, simultaneous ventilation and compression with abdominal binding decreased the percentage of dogs that were successfully resuscitated [42].

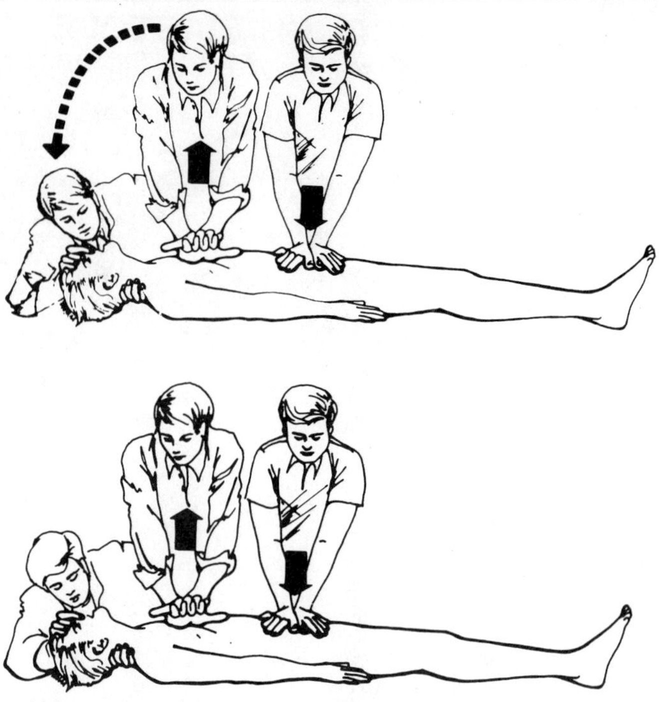

Fig. 2-4. Rescuers performing interposed abdominal compression CPR. Top: Two rescuers performing interposed abdominal compression CPR. One rescuer compresses the chest and ventilates while the second performs abdominal compression. Bottom: With three rescuers, ventilation, chest compression, and abdominal compression are each performed by a single individual. For clarity, rescuers are shown on the same side of the victim. (From C.F. Babbs. CPR with interposed abdominal compression. *Circulation* 74 (Suppl IV):38, 1986. By permission of the American Heart Association, Inc.)

Interposed Abdominal Compression

In 1982, Ralston and associates [43] reported a variation on the abdominal binding technique, whereby the adominal compression is released when the sternum is being compressed. This technique promises to improve coronary flow by augmenting aortic pressure during the "diastole" of sternal rebound. Higher oxygen delivery and higher cerebral and myocardial blood flows have been reported [44]. Unfortunately, this method requires a second or third rescuer to apply the abdominal compression (Fig. 2-4). The instructions are somewhat complex and do not adapt themselves to teaching the lay public. The potential for liver and gastric injury is apparently less than with continuous abdominal

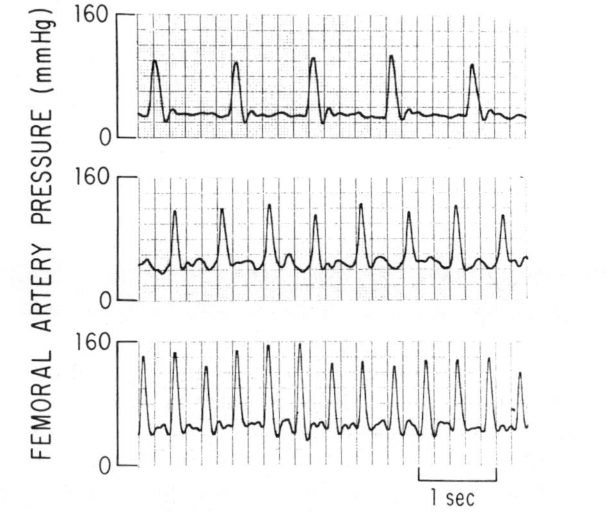

Fig. 2-5. Effect of compression rate on femoral artery pressure from a patient undergoing manual sternal compression early after cardiac arrest. The upper panel represents a rate of 60 per minute, the center panel a rate of 100 per minute, and the lower panel a rate of 150 per minute. (From G.W. Maier, et al. The physiology of external cardiac massage: High-impulse cardiopulmonary resuscitation. *Circulation* 70:86, 1984. By permission of the American Heart Association, Inc.)

binding [45]. One study has failed to demonstrate an improvement in outcome for patients given standard CPR or CPR with interposed abdominal compression [46].

High-Impulse CPR

Data of Maier and colleagues [21] suggest that in their chronically instrumented dog model, the mechanism of direct cardiac compression is operative. In this model, peak cardiac and vascular pressures were consistently two to four times greater than the corresponding intrathoracic pressures. In addition, stroke volume and coronary blood flow were maximized with chest compressions of moderate force and brief duration. By increasing the rate of compression to a high of 150 per minute, the cardiac output continued to increase as the coronary flow remained as high as 75 percent of pre-arrest values (Fig. 2-5). Unfortunately, rapid fatigue of a single rescuer maintaining high impulse and high compression rates is expected. The potential for increased injury also exists.

Compression-Ventilation Sequence

Placing compression before ventilation in the CPR sequence has been advocated by Crul and associates [47] and has been recommended and taught by the Dutch Heart Association. Crul argues that most cardiac arrests are caused by ventricular fibrillation or tachycardia and that arterial blood oxygen is usually adequate at the onset of such arrests. In a canine preparation, it was shown that thoracic compression could be performed for up to 30 seconds before arterial blood oxygen saturation fell to unacceptable levels. The standard sequence of airway, breathing, and compression would, they argued, cause an unnecessary delay in brain perfusion. They also suggested that early sternal compression might trigger heart contraction in a manner similar to that of a sternal thump. Lesser and colleagues [48] have argued that no data exist to support the clinical value of the compression-ventilation sequence, and, moreover, current standards allow no more than a 30-second delay in compression. In cases of asphyxial arrest, initial ventilation may reverse profound hypoxia and hypotension, whereas initial compression might even trigger ventricular fibrillation. In addition, airway obstruction would not be recognized at the outset. It could also be argued that initial attention to breathing makes a false diagnosis of cardiac arrest less likely in instances of vasovagal syncope with a small pulse that may be difficult to find. In summary, there is little to warrant a change in the conventional sequence without a clear demonstration of its clinical superiority.

Open-Chest CPR

Open-chest CPR was one of the first forms of successful CPR [49–51] and was shown to be effective when definitive care was available. Survival rates, largely in operating room arrests, ranged from 16 to 37 percent [52, 53]. Mechanistically, open-chest CPR clearly involves cardiac compression without use of a thoracic gradient; Weale [23] demonstrated lower venous pressures and higher arterial pressures than with closed-chest compression. There is considerable evidence that open-chest CPR may be more efficacious than closed-chest CPR in terms of cardiac output as well as cerebral and myocardial preservation [54, 55]. Clearly, some patients with penetrating chest trauma are not likely to respond to chest compression and are candidates for open-chest CPR [56–58]. Several studies suggest a benefit from thoracotomy in these patients [59–61].

INFECTIOUS DISEASES AND CARDIOPULMONARY RESUSCITATION

The fear provoked by the spread of human immunodeficiency virus (HIV) is understandable and warranted, given the seriousness of the infection. This anxiety has in some instances led to excessive caution when dealing with strangers who might be carriers of the virus. Its effect on the willingness of both the lay public and health professionals to learn or perform CPR is serious and must be addressed at some length.

We will discuss the scientific evidence concerning the risk of infection associated with both CPR training and actual rescue procedures. However, before doing so, it is worth stepping back and trying to place the whole issue in perspective. It is easy to blame the lay public's concern about the infectiousness of HIV on ignorance or mass hysteria. However, is it so unreasonable for the lay public to maintain a respectful distrust of scientific authorities when dealing with a public-health issue whose existence was not even suspected a decade ago? In the public's view, these were the same scientific authorities who were giving the blood transfusions and factor VIII infusions during the late 1970s and early 1980s that caused a significant number of HIV infections. The public's fear is reasonable and can only be counteracted by continued education and stressing of the facts. While health-care professionals may have less of an excuse to be unnecessarily frightened, their opportunity for exposure to patients with HIV is greater and must be adequately addressed [62].

Cardiopulmonary resuscitation with mouth-to-mouth ventilation was first introduced over a quarter of a century ago. Widespread instruction of lay people in CPR occurred after the 1973 standards conference on CPR. Historically, these years coincided with a truly unique "golden period" of relative freedom from fear of severe respiratory contagion. The CPR effort would have been unthinkable during earlier decades of constant public fear of bacterial pneumonia, influenza, diphtheria, syphilis, tuberculosis, and poliomyelitis, to name a few of the deadly diseases that could have been spread by mouth-to-mouth ventilation. The age of powerful antibiotics and immunizations allowed us to exchange saliva with strangers and even victims of sudden death with an almost carefree abandon. The greatest concern seemed to be that of catching a cold or at worst the flu. It is ironic that this freedom from fear has been dispelled by a disease that has not been shown to be transmitted by either respiratory aerosol or by saliva.

It is clear that mouth-to-mouth ventilation results in the exchange of saliva between the victim and the rescuer. However, saliva has not been implicated in the transmission of HIV even after bites, percutaneous inoculation, or contamination of open wounds with saliva from HIV-infected patients [63–68]. Hepatitis B–positive saliva has also not been demonstrated to be infectious when applied to oral mucous membranes or through contamination of shared musical instruments or CPR training mannequins used by hepatitis B carriers. It is possible, however, that the mouth-to-mouth technique could result in the exchange of blood between victim and rescuer if there are open lesions or trauma to the buccal mucosa or lips. It should be mentioned that diseases such as tuberculosis, herpes, or respiratory viral infections are potentially spread during mouth-to-mouth ventilation. The impact of these facts is different for lay people and health-care professionals, and different for those carrying infection and for those at risk of infection.

Implications for Rescuers with Known or Suspected Infections

Potential rescuers who know or highly suspect that they are infected with a serious pathogenic organism should not perform mouth-to-mouth ventilation if another rescuer is available who is less likely to be infectious or if the circumstances allow for any other immediate and effective method of ventilation, such as mechanical ventilation devices.

Implications for Health-Care Professionals

Even though the probability of a rescuer becoming infected with HIV during CPR seems to be minimal, all those called on to provide CPR in the course of their employment should have ready access to mechanical ventilation devices. Bag-valve mask devices should be available as initial ventilation equipment, and early endotracheal intubation should be encouraged when equipment and trained professionals are available. Masks with one-way valves and plastic mouth and nose covers with filtered openings are available and provide some protection from transfer of oral fluids and aerosols. S-shaped mouthpieces, masks without one-way valves, and handkerchiefs provide little, if any, barrier protection and should not be considered for routine use. With these guidelines in mind, health-care professionals are reminded that they have a moral and ethical obligation, and in some instances a legal obligation, to provide CPR, especially in the setting of their occupational duties.

Implications for Lay Rescuers

A trained lay person is not legally obligated to provide CPR. The obligation is an individual moral and ethical one. The informed lay person should be motivated to perform CPR by the knowledge that a delay in initiating ventilation could result in death or disablement for an otherwise salvageable person. The potential rescuer should also recognize that the risk, even with a known HIV-positive victim, is considered to be very low. Lay persons should also be motivated to become trained in CPR by the knowledge that they will most often be called on to provide CPR to members of their own family or to close friends. A seemingly useful strategy would be to target family members of patients at increased risk of sudden cardiac death for CPR training [69, 70].

Implications for Mannequin Training in CPR

The American Hospital Association guidelines specify that students or instructors should not actively participate in CPR training sessions with mannequins if they have dermatologic lesions on their hands or in oral or circumoral areas, if they are known to be infected with hepatitis or HIV, or if they have reason to believe that they are in the active stage of any infectious process. In routine training of ventilation, instructors should not allow participants to exchange saliva by performing mouth-to-mouth ventilation in sequence without barrier mouthpieces. Special plastic mouthpieces and specialized mannequins are now available that allow protection from such interchange of mucus.

Training in CPR for Persons with Chronic Infections

If a potentially infectious person is to be trained in CPR, common-sense precautions should be taken to protect other participants from any risk of infection. The chronically infected individual should be given a separate mannequin for practice that is not to be used by anyone else until it has been adequately disinfected. The chronically infected trainee should be made aware of the preceding guidelines for potential rescuers with infections. Additionally, counseling should not ignore the potential risk of infection for the immunocompromised rescuer.

If an employing agency requires successful completion of a CPR course as a prerequisite for employment, it is up to that agency to decide whether to waive its requirement for an employee who is unable to complete a CPR course for whatever reason. That agency also must determine whether a chronically infected individual should continue to work in a situation in which the administration of CPR is a duty of employment.

REFERENCES

1. Stephenson, HE, Jr, Reid, C, and Hinton, JW. Some common denominators in 1200 cases of cardiac arrest. *Ann Surg* 137: 731, 1953.
2. Zoll, PM, et al. Termination of ventricular fibrillation in man by externally applied electrical countershock. *N Engl J Med* 254: 727, 1956.
3. Safar, P, Escarraga, L, and Elam, JO. A comparison of the mouth to mouth and mouth to airway methods of artificial respiration with the chest pressure arm-lift method. *N Engl J Med* 258:671, 1958.
4. Elam, JO, et al. Oxygen and carbon dioxide exchange and energy cost of expired air resuscitation. *JAMA* 167:328, 1958.
5. Kouwenhoven, WB, Jude, JR, and Knickerbocker, GG. Closed chest cardiac massage. *JAMA* 173:1064, 1960.
6. Cardiopulmonary resuscitation: Statement by the Ad Hoc Committee on Cardiopulmonary Resuscitation of the Division of Medical Sciences, National Academy of Sciences–National Research Council, *JAMA* 198:372, 1966.
7. Standards for cardiopulmonary resuscitation (CPR) and emergency cardiac care (ECC). *JAMA* 227 (Suppl):833, 1974.
8. Standards and guidelines for cardiopulmonary resuscitation (CPR) and emergency cardiac care (ECC). *JAMA* 244:453, 1980.
9. Standards and guidelines for cardiopulmonary resuscitation (CPR) and emergency cardiac care (ECC). *JAMA* 255:2843, 1986.
10. Cummins, RO, et al. Survival of out-of-hospital cardiac arrest with early initiation of cardiopulmonary resuscitation. *Am J Emerg Med* 3:114, 1985.
11. Weaver, WD, et al. Considerations for improving survival from out-of-hospital cardiac arrest. *Ann Emerg Med* 15:1181, 1986.
12. Eisenberg, MS, Bergner, L, and Hallstrom, A. Cardiac resuscitation in the community: Importance of rapid provision and implications for program planning. *JAMA* 241:1905, 1979.
13. Weaver, WD, et al. Improved neurologic recovery and survival after early defibrillation. *Circulation* 69:943, 1984.
14. Myerburg, RJ, et al. Clinical electrophysiologic and hemodynamic profile of patients resuscitated from prehospital cardiac arrest. *Am J Med* 68:568, 1980.
15. Bedell, SE, et al. Survival after cardiopulmonary resuscitation in the hospital. *N Engl J Med* 309:569, 1983.
16. DeBard, ML. Cardiopulmonary resuscitation: Analysis of six years' experience and review of the literature. *Ann Emerg Med* 10:408, 1981.
17. Lemire, JG, and Johnson, AL. Is cardiac resuscitation worthwhile? A decade of experience. *N Engl J Med* 286:970, 1972.
18. Pantridge, JF, and Geddes, JS. A mobile intensive care unit in the management of myocardial infarction. *Lancet* 2:271, 1967.
19. Paraskos, JA. External compression without adjuncts. *Circulation* 74 (Suppl IV):33, 1986.
20. Deshmukh, HG, et al. Echocardiographic observations during cardiopulmonary resuscitation: A preliminary report. *Crit Care Med* 13:904, 1985.
21. Maier, GW, et al. The physiology of external cardiac massage: High-impulse cardiopulmonary resuscitation. *Circulation* 70: 86, 1984.
22. Weisfeldt, ML, and Chandra, N. Physiology of CPR. *Ann Rev Med* 32:435, 1981.
23. Weale, FE, and Rothwell-Jackson, RL. The efficiency of cardiac massage. *Lancet* 1:990, 1962.
24. Wilder, RJ, et al. Methods of coordinating ventilation and closed chest cardiac massage in the dog. *Surgery* 53:186, 1963.
25. Criley, JM, Blaufuss, AJ, and Kissel, GL. Cough induced cardiac compression. *JAMA* 236:1246, 1976.
26. Niemann, JT, et al. Cough-CPR: Documentation of systemic perfusion in man and in an experimental model—a "window" to the mechanism of blood flow in external CPR. *Crit Care Med* 8:141, 1980.
27. Rudikoff, MT, et al. Mechanisms of blood flow during cardiopulmonary resuscitation. *Circulation* 61:345, 1980.
28. Weisfeldt, ML, Chandra, N, and Tsitlik, J. Increased intrathoracic pressure—not direct heart compression—causes the rise in intrathoracic vascular pressures during CPR in dogs and pigs. *Crit Care Med* 9:377, 1981.
29. Niemann, JT, et al. Pressure-synchronized cineangiography during experimental cardiopulmonary resuscitation. *Circulation* 64:985, 1981.
30. Rich, S, Wix, HL, and Shapiro, EP. Clinical assessment of heart chamber size and valve motion during cardiopulmonary resuscitation by two dimensional echocardiography. *Am Heart J* 102:368, 1981.
31. Werner, JA, et al. Visualization of cardiac valve motion in man during external chest compression using two-dimensional echocardiography: Implications regarding the mechanism of blood flow. *Circulation* 63:1417, 1981.
32. Babbs, CF. New versus old theories of blood flow during CPR. *Crit Care Med* 8:191, 1980.
33. Fisher, J, et al. Determinants and clinical significance of jugular venous valve competence. *Circulation* 65:188, 1982.
34. Taylor, GJ, et al. Importance of prolonged compression during cardiopulmonary resuscitation in man. *N Engl J Med* 296:1515, 1977.
35. Chandra, N, Rudikoff, M, and Weisfeldt, ML. Simultaneous chest compression and ventilation at high airway pressure during cardiopulmonary resuscitation. *Lancet* 1:175, 1980.
36. Bircher, N, and Safar, P. Comparison of standard and "new" closed-chest CPR and open-chest CPR in dogs. *Crit Care Med* 9:384, 1981.
37. Harris, LC, Jr, Kirimli, B, and Safar, P. Augmentation of artificial circulation during cardiopulmonary resuscitation. *Anesthesiology* 28:730, 1967.
38. Redding, JS. Abdominal compression in cardiopulmonary resuscitation. *Anesth Analg* 50:668, 1971.
39. Chandra, N, Snyder, LD, and Weisfeldt, ML. Abdominal binding during cardiopulmonary resuscitation in man. *JAMA* 246: 351, 1981.
40. Neimann, JT, et al. Hemodynamic effects of continuous abdominal binding during cardiac arrest and resuscitation. *Am J Cardiol* 53:269, 1984.
41. Bircher, N, and Safar, P. Cerebral preservation during cardiopulmonary resuscitation. *Crit Care Med* 13:185, 1985.
42. Sanders, AB, et al. Failure of one method of simultaneous chest compression, ventilation, and abdominal binding during CPR. *Crit Care Med* 10:509, 1982.
43. Ralston, SH, Babbs, CF, and Niebauer, MJ. Cardiopulmonary resuscitation with interposed abdominal compression in dogs. *Anesth Analg* 61:645, 1982.
44. Voorhees, WD, Babbs, CF, and Niebauer, MJ. Improved oxygen delivery during cardiopulmonary resuscitation with interposed abdominal compressions. *Ann Emerg Med* 12:128, 1933.
45. Babbs, CF, Schoenlein, WE, and Lowe, MW. Gastric insufflation during IAC-CPR and standard CPR in a canine model. *Am J Emerg Med* 3:99, 1985.
46. Mateer, JR, et al. Prehospital IAC-CPR versus standard CPR: Paramedic resuscitation of cardiac arrests. *Am J Emerg Med* 3:143, 1985.
47. Crul, JF, Neursing, BTJ, and Zimmerman, AHE. The ABC sequence of cardiopulmonary resuscitation (CPR). *J World Assoc Emerg Disaster Med* 1–4 (Suppl):236, 1985.
48. Lesser, R, et al. Sternal compression before ventilation in cardiopulmonary resuscitation (CPR). *J World Assoc Emerg Disaster Med* 1–4 (Suppl):239, 1985.

49. Hake, TG. Studies on ether and chloroform from Professor Schiff's physiological laboratory. *Practitioner* 12:241, 1874.
50. Boehm, R. Ueder Wiederbelebung nach Vergiftungen und Asphyxie. *Arch Exp Pathol u Pharmacol* 8:68, 1878.
51. Pike, FH, Guthrie, CC, and Stewart, GN. Studies in resuscitation. I. The general conditions affecting resuscitation, and the resuscitation of blood and the heart. *J Exp Med* 10:371, 1908.
52. Stephenson, HE, Jr. *Cardiac Arrest and Resuscitation.* St. Louis: Mosby, 1958.
53. Turk, LN, and Glenn, WW. Cardiac arrest—results of attempted resuscitation in 42 cases. *N Engl J Med* 251:795, 1954.
54. Bartlett, RL, et al. Comparative study of three methods of resuscitation: Closed-chest, open-chest manual, and direct mechanical ventricular assistance. *Ann Emerg Med* 13:773, 1984.
55. Bircher, N, and Safar, P. Manual open-chest cardiopulmonary resuscitation. *Ann Emerg Med* 13:770, 1984.
56. Del Guercio, LRM, et al. Comparison of blood flow during external and internal cardiac massage in man. *Circulation* 31 (Suppl 1):171, 1965.
57. Shocket, E, and Rosenblum, R. Successful open cardiac massage after 75 minutes of closed chest massage. *JAMA* 200:157, 1967.
58. Sykes, MK, and Ahmed, N. Emergency treatment of cardiac arrest. *Lancet* 2:347, 1963.
59. Bodai, BI, et al. Emergency thoracotomy in the management of trauma—a review. *JAMA* 249:1891, 1983.
60. Cogbill, TH, et al. Rationale for selective application of emergency department thoracotomy in trauma. *J Trauma* 23:453, 1983.
61. Danne, PD, Finelli, F, and Champion, HR. Emergency bay thoracotomy. *J Trauma* 24:796, 1984.
62. Block AJ. The physician's responsibility for the care of AIDS patients: An opinion. *Chest* 94:1283, 1988.
63. Fox, PC, et al. Saliva inhibits HIV-1 infectivity. *J Amer Dental Assn* 116:635, 1988.
64. Freidland, GH, et al. Lack of transmission of HTLV III/LAV infection to household contacts of patients with AIDS or AIDS related complex with oral candidiasis. *N Engl J Med* 314:344, 1986.
65. Marcus, R, et al. Surveillance of health care workers exposed to blood from patients infected with the human immunodeficiency virus. *N Engl J Med* 319:1118, 1988.
66. Sande, MH. Transmission of AIDS: The case against casual contagion. *N Engl J Med* 314:380, 1986.
67. Recommendations for prevention of HIV transmission in health care settings. *MMWR* 36(2S):3S, 1987.
68. Update: Universal precautions for prevention of transmission of human immunodeficiency virus, hepatitis B virus, and other bloodborne pathogens in health care settings. *MMWR* 37(24): 377, 1988.
69. Dracup, K, et al. Can family members of high-risk cardiac patients learn cardiopulmonary resuscitation? *Arch Intern Med* 149:61, 1989.
70. Goldberg, RJ. Training of family members of high-risk cardiac patients in cardiopulmonary resuscitation: Skills performance and need for physician recommendations. *Arch Intern Med* 149:25, 1989.

SELECTED READING

An appraisal of the criteria of cerebral death: A summary statement: A collaborative study. *JAMA* 237:982, 1976.

Copley, DP, et al. Improved outcome for prehospital cardiopulmonary collapse with resuscitation by bystanders. *Circulation* 56: 902, 1977.

A definition of irreversible coma. Report of the Ad Hoc Committee of the Harvard Medical School to examine the definition of brain death. *JAMA* 205:337, 1968.

Guidelines for the determination of death: Report of the medical consultants on the diagnosis of death to the President's Commission for the Study of Ethical Problems in Medicine and Biomedical and Behavioral Research. *JAMA* 246:2184, 1981.

Harris, LC, Jr, Kirimli, B, and Safar, P. Ventilation–cardiac compression ratios in CPR. *Anesthesiology* 28:806, 1967.

Koehler, RC, et al. Augmentation of cerebral perfusion by simultaneous chest compression and lung inflation with abdominal binding after cardiac arrest in dogs. *Circulation* 67:266, 1983.

Luce, JM, et al. Regional blood flow during cardiopulmonary resuscitation in dogs using simultaneous and nonsimultaneous compression and ventilation. *Circulation* 67:258, 1983.

Lund, I, Skulberg, A. Resuscitation of cardiac arrest outside hospitals: Experience with a mobile intensive care unit in Oslo. *Acta Anaesthesiol Scand* 53 (Suppl):13, 1973.

Tweed, WA, Bristow, G, and Donen, N. Resuscitation from cardiac arrest: Assessment of a system providing only basic life support outside of hospital. *Can Med Assoc J* 122:297, 1980.

Vertesi, L, Wilson, L, and Glick, N. Cardiac arrest: Comparison of paramedic and conventional ambulance services. *Can Med Assoc J* 128:809, 1983.

Voorhees, WD, Ralston, SH, and Babbs, CF. Regional blood flow during cardiopulmonary resuscitation with abdominal counterpulsation in dogs. *Am J Emerg Med* 2:123, 1984.

3. Resuscitation Management

CARDIAC ARREST: UNOBSTRUCTED AIRWAY

John A. Paraskos

The skills necessary to perform adequately during a cardiac (or respiratory) arrest and to interface smoothly with advanced cardiac life support (ACLS) techniques cannot be learned from reading texts and manuals. The basic life support (BLS) program and other cardiopulmonary resuscitation (CPR) courses taught according to American Heart Association (AHA) standards allow hands-on experience that at least approximates the real situation and tests the psychomotor skills needed in an emergency situation. All those who engage in patient care should be trained in BLS. If their duties require a higher level of performance, they should be trained in ACLS as well. It is wise to keep in mind that these skills deteriorate with disuse and need to be updated. It is also worth repeating that "certification" in BLS or in ACLS is neither a license to perform these techniques nor a guarantee of skill. Certification is simply an acknowledgment that an individual attended a specific course and passed the required tests. If employers or government agencies require such certification of certain health workers, it is by their own mandate.

The following discussion of BLS and ACLS techniques reviews standards and guidelines that have been established by the AHA and were presented in the 1986 *Journal of the American Medical Association* supplement, which acknowledged the twenty-fifth anniversary of contemporary CPR [1]. Guidelines for advanced cardiac care are presented in greater detail in the AHA's 1987 *Textbook of Advanced Cardiac Life Support* [2].

BASIC LIFE SUPPORT FOR ADULTS: UNOBSTRUCTED AIRWAY

Basic life support is meant to externally support the circulation and respiration of a victim of cardiac or respiratory arrest. After recognizing and ascertaining the need, CPR is initiated and definitive help is summoned in the form of emergency providers of ACLS.

Respiratory arrest may be caused by such accidents as airway obstruction, drowning, stroke, smoke inhalation, drug overdose, electrocution, or physical trauma. The heart may continue to circulate blood for several minutes and the residual oxygen in lungs and blood may keep the brain viable. Early intervention by opening the airway and providing ventilation may prevent cardiac arrrest and be all that is required to restore respiration.

Cardiac arrest results in rapid depletion of oxygen in vital organs. After 4 to 6 minutes without circulation, brain damage can occur. After 6 minutes brain damage is expected to occur except in hypothermia (e.g., drowning in cold water). Therefore, early bystander CPR (within 4 minutes) and rapid ACLS with attempted defibrillation (within 8 minutes) are essential in improving survival and neurological recovery rates [3, 4].

The sequence of steps in CPR is often summarized by the mnemonic "ABCs of CPR." This refers to the three broad areas of Airway, Breathing, and Circulation. While this device is useful in teaching the public, it should be remembered that each step is preceded by assessment of the need for intervention. Opening the airway is preceded by *determining unresponsiveness;* breathing is preceded by *determining breathlessness;* circulation is preceded by *determining pulselessness.*

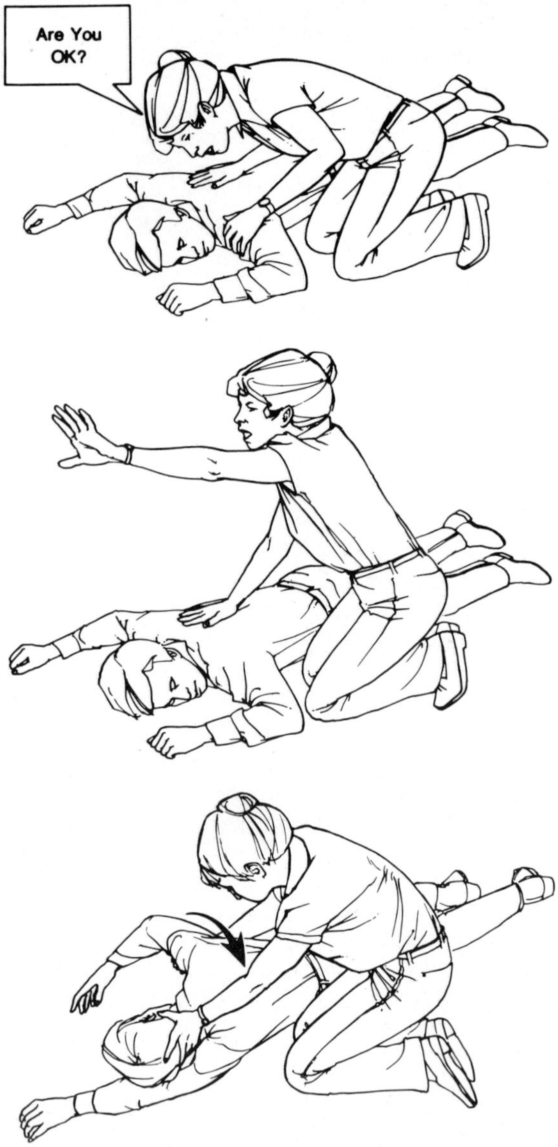

Fig. 3-1. Initial steps in cardiopulmonary resuscitation. Top: Determine unresponsiveness. Center: Call for help. Bottom: Position the victim. (This figure and Figs. 3-2, 3-3, 3-6, 3-11 through 3-16, 3-18 through 3-22, and 3-40 and 3-42 are from W. H. Montgomery, J. Donegan, and K. M. McIntyre. Standards and guidelines for cardiopulmonary resuscitation and emergency cardiac care. *J.A.M.A.* 225:2916, 1986. Reproduced with permission. Standards and Guidelines for Cardiopulmonary Resuscitation and Emergency Cardiac Care. American Heart Association.)

Assessment and Determination of Unresponsiveness

A victim of a cardiac arrest may be found in an apparently unconscious state—an "unwitnessed arrest"—or a victim may be observed to suddenly lapse into unconsciousness—a "witnessed arrest." In either case, the rescuer must react promptly to assess responsiveness by attempting to wake and communicate with the victim—"tap or gently shake and shout." The rescuer should call for help to summon nearby persons (Fig. 3-1). When another individual arrives, he or she should be asked to call immediately for emergency medical services (EMS) (dial 911 in many localities) and identify the location and nature of the emergency. If no other person has arrived within the first minute, the rescuer should interrupt CPR to call or phone for assistance, assuming this can be done without delay.

For witnessed arrests, health-care professionals may assess the pulse as the next step. If the carotid pulse cannot be palpated in a 5- to 10-second period, a precordial thump may be attempted at this time by striking the lower third of the victim's sternum with the fist, from a height of approximately 8 inches (or the span of the stretched fingers). If the pulse does not return, the rescuer proceeds with establishing the airway, as discussed in the following paragraph. To facilitate learning and skills retention, the lay public is not taught to differentiate between witnessed and unwitnessed arrests.

Opening the Airway and Determination of Breathlessness

After establishing unresponsiveness and positioning the victim, the next step in an unwitnessed arrest is to open the airway and check for spontaneous breathing. As was noted previously, in a witnessed arrest this step is often taken after the initial attempts to defibrillate. The *head tilt–chin lift maneuver* (Figs. 3-2 and 3-3) is most frequently successful in opening the airway. In this technique, the head is tilted backward by a hand placed on the forehead. The fingers of the other hand are positioned under the mandible and the chin is lifted upward. While the teeth are almost approximated, the mouth should not be allowed to close. Considerable cervical hyperextension occurs with this method; therefore, it should be avoided, if possible, in patients with cervical injuries. The *jaw-thrust maneuver* (Fig. 3-4) provides the safest initial approach to opening the airway of a patient with a cervical spine injury; it allows excellent airway opening with a minimum of cervical extension. This maneuver is accomplished by grasping the angles of the mandible with both hands and lifting upward, thus tilting the head gently backward. If mouth-to-mouth ventilation is required while the jaw thrust is being performed, the vic-

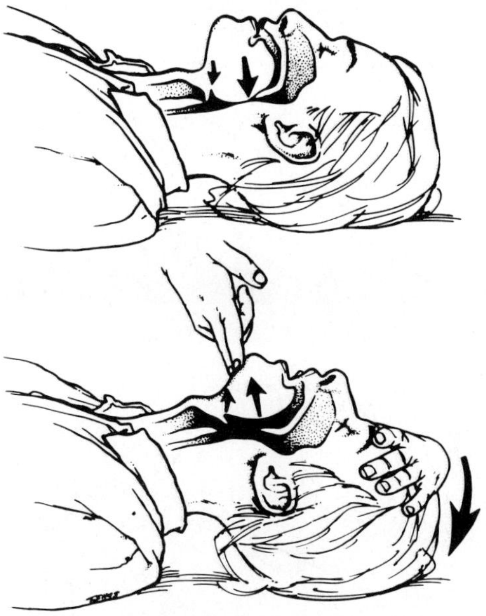

Fig. 3-2. Opening the airway. Top: Airway obstruction caused by tongue and epiglottis. Bottom: Opening the airway with the head tilt–chin lift maneuver.

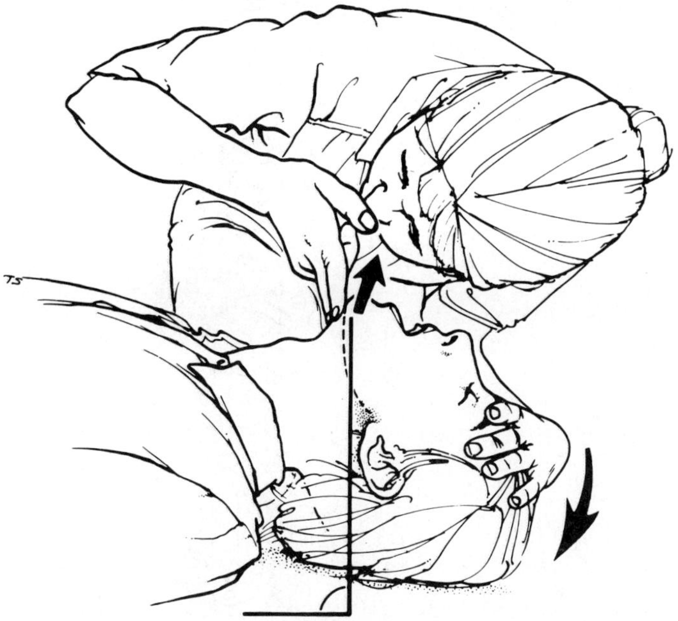

Fig. 3-3. Determining breathlessness. Open the airway and "look, listen, and feel."

tim's nostrils must be occluded by the fleshy aspect of the rescuer's cheek.

After opening the airway, the rescuer takes three to five seconds to determine whether there is spontaneous air exchange. This is accomplished by placing an ear over the patient's mouth and nose while watching to see if the patient's chest and abdomen rise and fall ("look, listen, and feel"; see Fig. 3-3). If the rescuer fails to see movement and fails to hear the respiration and feel the rush of air against the ear and cheek, rescue breathing should be initiated.

Rescue Breathing

If spontaneous breathing is absent, rescue breathing must be initiated (Fig. 3-5). If equipment is immediately available and the rescuer is trained, intubation and ventilatory adjuncts may be used initially; otherwise, the victim's nostrils are pinched with thumb and forefinger and *mouth-to-mouth ventilation* is begun. The rescuer takes a deep breath and makes a tight seal over the victim's mouth. The rescuer breathes into the victim's mouth twice, completely refilling his or her lungs after each breath. Each breath should be delivered over 1.0 to 1.5 seconds, allowing the victim's lungs to deflate between breaths. Thereafter, the rate of 12 breaths per minute is maintained for as long as is necessary, with tidal volumes of 800 to 1,200 cc. The reason for delivering the breath over a full second or more is to prevent gastric insufflation. Melker [5] has demonstrated airway pressures well in excess of those required to open the lower esophageal sphincter when quick breaths are used to ventilate patients. As soon as possible, airway adjuncts with 100 percent delivered oxygen are substituted for mouth-to-mouth ventilation. If the victim wears dentures, they are usually best left in place to assist in forming an adequate seal.

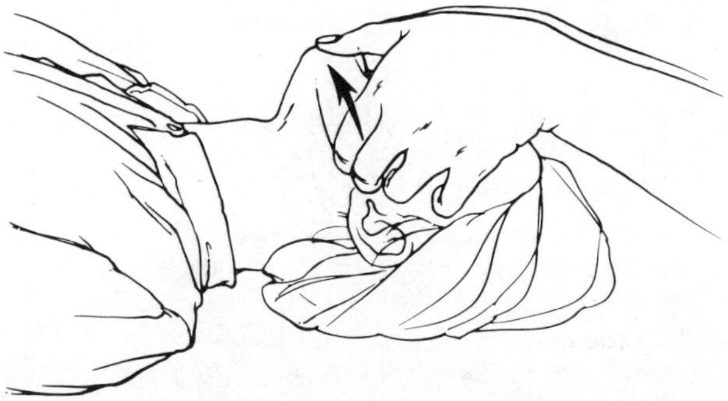

Fig. 3-4. Jaw-thrust maneuver. Opening the airway with minimum extension of the neck. (Reproduced with permission. © *Healthcare Provider's Manual for Basic Life Support.* Dallas: American Heart Association, 1988. P. 37.)

If air cannot be passed into the victim's lungs, another attempt at opening the airway should be made. Use of the jaw-thrust maneuver may be necessary. If subsequent attempts at ventilation are still unsuccessful, the victim should be considered to have an obstructed airway, and attempts should be made to dislodge a potential foreign-body obstruction (see the Obstructed Airway section of this chapter).

Mouth-to-nose ventilation may be necessary in cases of severe facial trauma or trismus (see Fig. 3-5, center). In this technique, the head tilt–chin lift maneuver is used to open the airway while the rescuer's mouth forms a seal over the victim's nose; during delivery of the air, the victim's mouth is occluded, by using the palm of the hand if necessary. During exhalation, the mouth is allowed to reopen so that the soft palate does not obstruct the air flow through the nasopharynx.

If a tracheostomy tube is in place, direct application of

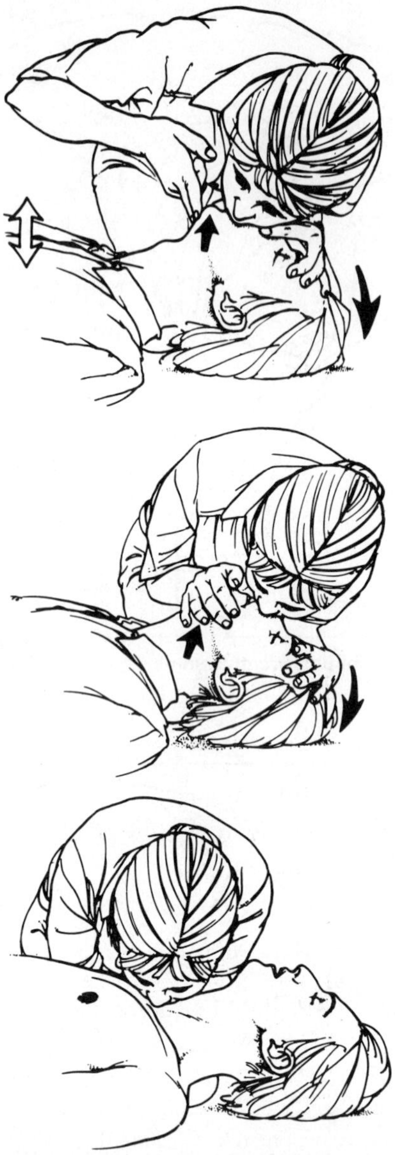

Fig. 3-5. Rescue breathing. Top: Mouth-to-mouth. Center: Mouth-to-nose. Bottom: Mouth-to-stoma. (From *Cardiopulmonary Resuscitation,* 1981. Courtesy of the American Red Cross.)

mouth-to-stoma ventilation is necessary until ventilatory adjuncts are available (see Fig. 3-5, bottom). Unless there is a cuff on the tracheostomy tube that can be inflated, the victim's mouth will have to be occluded with one hand throughout the ventilatory cycle. Mouth-to-stoma ventilation is also preferable if the victim has an established tracheostomy stoma.

Establishing Pulselessness

In the adult, the absence of a central pulse is best established by palpating the carotid artery (Fig. 3-6), although, rarely, the carotid pulse is absent because of localized obstruction. If a pulse is not felt after 10 seconds of careful searching, chest compression is initiated, unless electrical countershock for ventricular arrhythmia or artificial pacing for asystole is immediately available.

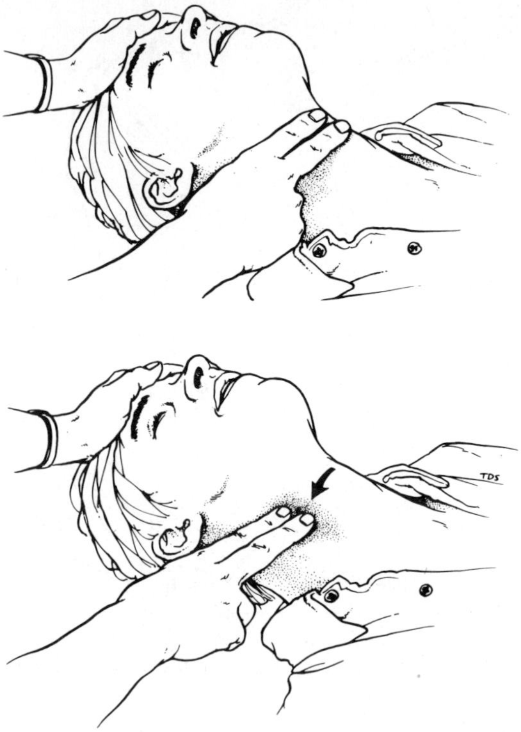

Fig. 3-6. Determining pulselessness. Top: Feeling the laryngeal cartilage. Bottom: Fingers slid into groove between trachea and sternomastoid muscle, searching for carotid pulse.

Chest Compression

Artificial circulation depends on adequate chest compression through sternal depression. The safest manner to depress the sternum is with the heel of the rescuer's hand on the lower half of the sternum, with the fingers kept off the rib cage (Fig. 3-7). It is usually most effective to cover the heel of one hand with the heel of the other, the heel being parallel to the long axis of the sternum. If the rescuer's hands are placed either too high or too low, or if the fingers are allowed to lie flat, broken ribs and organ laceration can result.

The rescuer's elbows should be kept locked, the arms straight within the shoulders directly over the patient's sternum (Fig. 3-7). This position allows the rescuer's upper body to provide a perpendicular force for sternal depression. The sternum is depressed 1.5 to 2.0 inches at a rate of 80 to 100 per minute.

Ventilation and sternal compression should not be interrupted for longer than seven seconds to check on the return of a pulse, except under special circumstances. Within the first minute of basic life support, if ACLS assistance has not already been summoned, CPR may have to be interrupted long enough to dial the hospital or clinic "arrest code" or outside EMS number (e.g., 911). Other warranted interruptions include taking time to execute ACLS procedures (e.g., endotracheal intubation, placement of central venous lines) or because of an absolute need to move the patient. Even in

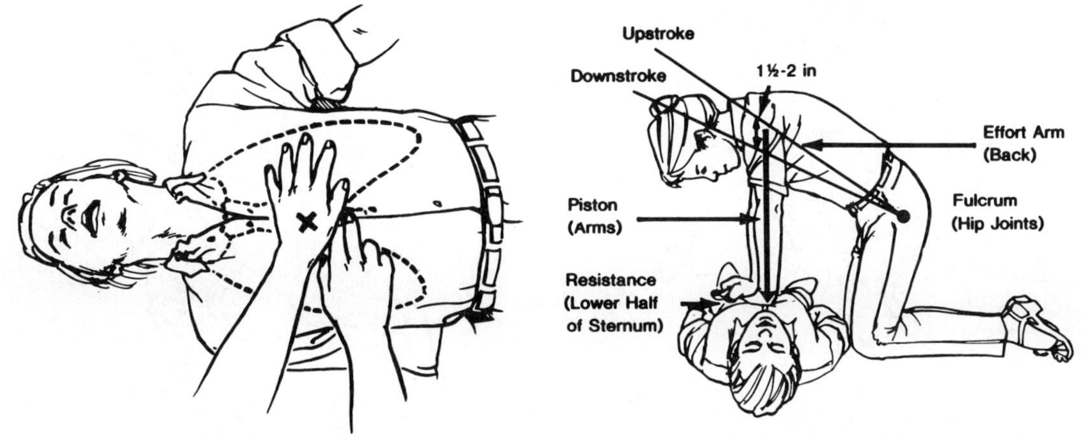

Fig. 3-7. External chest compression. Left: Locating the proper hand position on the lower half of the sternum. Right: Proper position of the rescuer, with shoulders directly over the victim's sternum and elbows locked. (From *Cardiopulmonary Resuscitation*, 1981. Courtesy of the American Red Cross.)

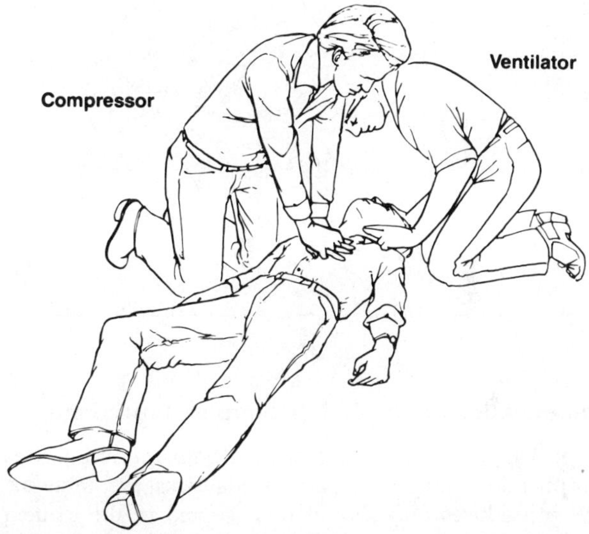

Fig. 3-8. Two-rescuer CPR. The ventilator assesses the condition of the victim while the compressor assumes the proper position for external chest compressions. (Reproduced with permission. © *Healthcare Provider's Manual for Basic Life Support*. Dallas: American Heart Association, 1988. P. 51.)

these limited circumstances, CPR should not be interrupted for longer than 30 seconds.

Two-Rescuer Cardiopulmonary Resuscitation

The combination of artificial ventilation and circulation can be delivered more efficiently and with less fatigue by two rescuers. One rescuer, positioned at the victim's side, performs sternal compressions while the other rescuer, positioned at the victim's head, maintains an open airway and performs ventilation (Fig. 3-8). This technique should be mastered by all health-care workers who are called on to perform CPR. Lay persons have not been routinely taught the method in the interest of improving retention of basic skills. The compression rate for two-rescuer CPR, as for one-rescuer CPR, is 80 to 100 per minute. To ensure adequate time (1.0–1.5 seconds) for filling the lungs, a pause for a breath should be allowed after each fifth compression.

As soon as the second rescuer arrives, he or she should immediately determine if the EMS system has been accessed. If not, the second rescuer calls the EMS system and then enters the sequence as soon as the original rescuer completes a cycle of 15 compressions and two breaths. One rescuer moves to the victim's head, opens the airway, and checks for a pulse. The other rescuer has taken a position at the victim's side and has found the proper hand position for sternal compressions. The rescuer at the victim's head informs the other as to the presence or absence of a pulse. If no pulse is present, the ventilator gives a single breath and the compressor begins external chest compressions at a rate of 80 to 100 per minute, counting aloud, "one and, two and, three and, four and, five." The compressor pauses after the fifth compression just long enough to allow the other rescuer to ventilate (taking 1.0–1.5 seconds to fill the lungs). The compression-to-ventilation ratio then continues at 5:1.

If CPR is not in progress when the two rescuers arrive, one should ensure that the EMS system is activated immediately. The other goes to the head of the victim and proceeds to (1) determine unresponsiveness; (2) position the victim; (3) open the airway and check for breathing; (4) if breathing is absent, say "no breathing" and give two ventilations; (6) check for a pulse; and (7) if no pulse is present, inform the other rescuer. The other rescuer has assumed the proper hand position and begins sternal compression after the first rescuer states "no pulse."

When the rescuer performing compressions has fatigued and desires to switch responsibilities, the signal for change can be incorporated in the mnemonic (Fig. 3-9). After the ventilator has delivered the breath at the end of the fifth compression, he or she moves to the victim's chest and finds the correct hand position for compression. The other rescuer moves to the victim's head and checks the pulse and breathing. In the absence of spontaneous pulse or breathing, the new ventilator delivers a breath, signaling a new cycle of five compressions to one ventilation.

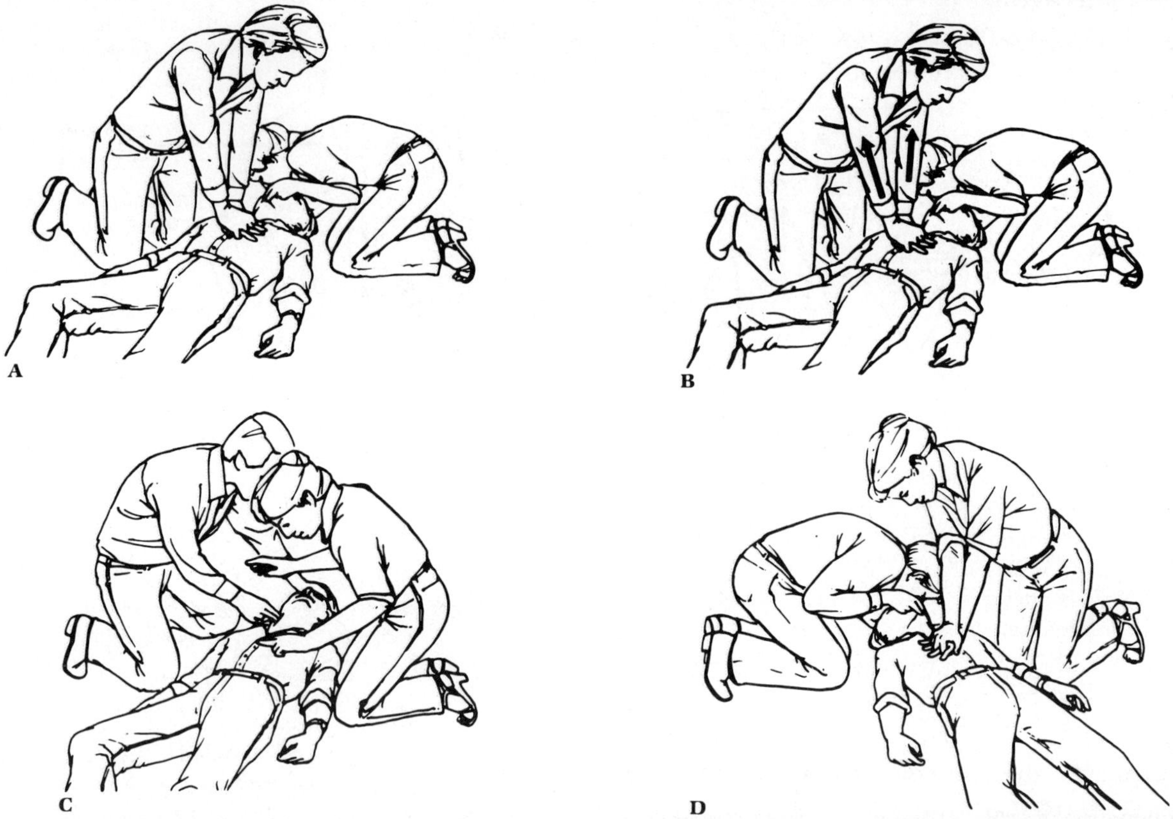

Fig. 3-9. Switching responsibilities in two-rescuer CPR. A. Compressor indicates desire to switch: "Change and, two and, three and, four and, five." B. Ventilator delivers a rescue breath after the fifth compression. C. Ventilator moves to the victim's chest and finds proper position, while the compressor moves to the victim's head and checks for spontaneous breathing and pulse. D. The new ventilator delivers a breath, signaling need for a new cycle of compressions and ventilations in a 5:1 ratio. (Reproduced with permission. © *Healthcare Provider's Manual for Basic Life Support.* Dallas: American Heart Association, 1988. P. 42.)

Complications of Basic Life Support Procedures

Proper application of CPR should help minimize serious complications. Nevertheless, serious risks are inherent in BLS procedures and should be accepted in the context of cardiac arrest. Awareness of these potential complications is of great importance in the post-resuscitative care of the arrest victim.

Gastric distention and regurgitation are common complications of artificial ventilation without endotracheal intubation. They are more likely to occur when ventilation pressures exceed the opening pressure of the lower esophageal sphincter [6, 7]. Mouth-to-mouth ventilation should allow 1.0 to 1.5 seconds for air delivery to the lungs to prevent airway pressures from exceeding 20 to 25 cm of H_2O. *Staircase ventilation,* or breathing rapidly without allowing full exhalation, should also be avoided for the same reason. No attempts should be made to relieve gastric distention to avoid causing regurgitation and aspiration, unless the distention is so severe that it is interfering with adequate ventilation. If ventilation appears to be severely compromised, BLS should be interrupted briefly while the victim is rolled on the side and moderate pressure is applied over the epigastrium to expel some of the accumulated air. If regurgitation occurs, the vomitus should be allowed to drain from the mouth while the victim is lying on the side. After residual vomitus is removed and the mouth is cleared, the victim is repositioned and CPR should be reinstituted immediately. While an esophageal obturator airway (EOA) may decrease the threat of distention and regurgitation during its use, there exists an increased risk at the time of its removal. To obviate this risk, the trachea should be intubated and protected with an inflated cuff before the esophageal cuff is deflated and the EOA is removed.

Complications of sternal compression and manual thrusts include rib and sternal fractures, costochondral separation, flail chest, pneumothorax, hemothorax, hemopericardium, subcutaneous emphysema, mediastinal emphysema, pulmonary contusions, bone marrow and fat embolism, as well as lacerations of the esophagus, stomach, inferior vena cava, liver, or spleen [8–10]. While rib fractures are common during CPR, especially in the elderly, no serious sequelae are likely to develop unless tension pneumothorax occurs and is ignored. The more serious complications are unlikely to occur in CPR if proper hand position is maintained and exaggerated depth of sternal compression is avoided. Unfortunately, overzealous or repeated abdominal or chest thrusts for relief of airway obstruction are more likely to cause fractures or lacerations. For this reason, the abdominal thrust is not recommended for the infant less than one year of age.

Monitoring Effectiveness of Basic Life Support

The victim should be monitored for resumption of spontaneous breathing and circulation after the first minute of CPR and every few minutes thereafter. To determine if the victim has resumed spontaneous breathing and circulation, chest compression must be stopped for 5 seconds and breathlessness and pulselessness rechecked as noted previously.

The effectiveness of the rescue effort is assessed regularly by the ventilator, who notes the chest motion and escape of expired air. The adequacy of circulation is assessed by noting an adequate carotid pulse with sternal compressions.

Pupillary response, if present, is a good indicator of cerebral circulation. However, fixed and dilated pupils should not be accepted as evidence for irreversible or biological death. Ocular disorders, such as cataracts, and a variety of drugs (e.g., atropine and ganglion-blocking agents) will interfere with the pupillary light reflex. The decision to cease CPR should be made only by the physician in charge of the resuscitation effort, when it is obvious that the victim's spontaneous circulation will not respond to adequate administration of ACLS with attempts at drug and electrical therapy. Remediable problems such as airway obstruction, severe hypovolemia, and pericardial tamponade should also have been reasonably excluded by careful attention to ACLS protocols.

ADVANCED CARDIAC LIFE SUPPORT IN ADULTS

The use of adjunctive equipment, more specialized techniques, and pharmacologic and electrical therapy in the treatment of the victim of cardiac or respiratory arrest is generally referred to as *advanced cardiac life support,* or *ACLS.* ACLS techniques and their interface with BLS and the EMS system are the subject of the American Heart Association's ACLS teaching program [11]. An improvement in survival after in-hospital cardiac arrest has been demonstrated after medical house officers were trained in ACLS [12]. An in-depth discussion is available in the ACLS text published by the AHA [2].

The following sections focus on the techniques and medications used in the initial resuscitative efforts. The demarcation from therapies more commonly reserved for the critical care unit is often indistinct; indeed, it is expected to vary with the experience of the prehospital team and the degree of physician supervision. In general, most ACLS measures should be applied by trained individuals operating within an EMS system in the community, in transport as well as in the hospital setting.

Airway and Ventilatory Support

Oxygenation and optimal ventilation are prerequisites of successful resuscitation. Ventilation with the rescuer's exhaled breath, which provides 16 to 17 percent oxygen, may produce an alveolar partial pressure of oxygen (P_{AO_2}) of 80 mm Hg. Arterial hypoxemia is inevitable because of diminished cardiac output, intrapulmonary shunting, and ventilation-perfusion ($\dot{V}/\dot{Q}$) mismatch. Therefore, supplemental oxygen should be administered as soon as it is available, beginning with 100 percent. In the postresuscitation period, the amount of administered oxygen may be decreased as guided by the arterial blood partial pressure of oxygen (PaO_2).

Emergency ventilation in the hospital or by EMS personnel commonly begins with the combined use of a mask and oral airway. *Mouth-to-mask ventilation* is a very effective form of ventilation, as long as an adequate seal is maintained between the mask and face. Most masks are best applied by flaring the top and molding it over the bridge of the nose. The inflated rim is then carefully molded to the cheeks as the mask is allowed to recoil. Relatively firm pressure is required to maintain the seal. Masks with one-way valves also provide a measure of isolation from the victim's saliva and breath aerosol. *Bag-valve-mask ventilation* requires strong hands for adequately compressing the self-inflating bag. The bag should be connected to a gas reservoir and to oxygen so that 100 percent oxygen delivery can be approximated. It cannot be overemphasized that the success of this method depends on airway patency and an adequate seal between the mask and face. Equally important to the successful use of the bag and mask is adequate compression of the bag to deliver the required tidal volume. It is advisable that all individuals who use this technique practice on a recording ventilating mannequin to assess the adequacy of the method in their hands. Many people will discover that their hands are not large enough or strong enough to deliver 800 to 1,200 cc of air. Some may have to squeeze the bag between their elbow and chest wall to supply adequate ventilation. If two people are available to ventilate, one should secure the mask while the other uses both hands to attend to the bag (Procedure 1).

Desirable features in mask design include the following:

1. *Transparent material,* allowing the rescuer to assess lip color and to observe vomitus, mucus, or other obstructing material in the patient's airway
2. *Cushioned rim* around the mask's perimeter to conform to the patient's face and to facilitate a tight seal
3. *Standard 15-mm/22-mm connector,* allowing the use of additional airway equipment
4. *Comfortable fit* to the rescuer's hand
5. *Oxygen insufflation inlet,* allowing oxygen supplementation during mouth-to-mask ventilation
6. *One-way valve,* allowing some protection from patient's breath and aerosol during mouth-to-mask ventilation
7. *Availability in appropriate sizes and shapes,* for various-sized faces; most adults will be accommodated by a standard, medium-sized (no. 4) oval-shaped mask

Necessary features in ventilating bags include the following:

1. *Self-refilling feature,* allowing operation independent of a fresh gas source. These are often referred to as *Ambu bags.* Non–self-refilling units should not be used.
2. *Fresh-gas inlet,* allowing either ambient air or supplemental oxygen to flow into the reservoir bag through a valve inlet.
3. *Nipple for oxygen connection,* located close to the gas inlet valve.

4. *Reservoir bag* that is easy to clean and sterilize without damage to its material.
5. *Availability in pediatric and adult sizes.*
6. *Non-rebreathing valve,* directing flow to the patient during inhalation and to the atmosphere during exhalation. The valve casing should be transparent to allow visual inspection of its function. It should be easy to clean and assemble. A pop-off feature is often present to prevent inadvertently high airway pressures. Such a valve, however, should have provision to override the pop-off feature since higher airway pressures are sometimes required to ventilate lungs with unusually high resistances.
7. *Reservoir tubing* that can be attached to the fresh-gas inlet valve, allowing an accumulation of oxygen to refill the reservoir bag during the refill cycle. Such a reservoir allows delivered oxygen to approach 100%; without it the self-refilling bag can deliver only 40 to 50 percent oxygen.

Oxygen-powered resuscitators allow the pressure of compressed oxygen tanks at 50 psi to drive lung inflation. They are usually triggered by a manual control button and can be delivered through a mask or tube for ease of ventilation. These devices have, in the past, delivered oxygen at a flow rate of 100 liters per minute and allowed airway pressures of 60 cm H_2O. Unfortunately, such devices, when used with masks and unprotected airways (not separated from the esophagus by an inflated cuff), are likely to cause gastric distention and poor ventilation. Furthermore, they are not as reliable as mouth-to-mask or valve-bag-mask ventilation; if they are to be used in adults, they should be recalibrated to deliver flows of no more than 40 liters per minute so as to avoid opening the lower esophageal sphincter and causing gastric insufflation. A relief valve should be present that opens at approximately 60 cm H_2O and vents any excess volume into the atmosphere. In addition, an audible alarm should sound whenever the relief valve pressure is exceeded. This alarm is needed to warn the rescuer that the victim is requiring higher inspiratory pressures and may not be adequately ventilated. Barotrauma is likely to occur in infants and children. Children often have high airway resistances and are difficult to ventilate with these resuscitators. In general these devices should not be used with infants or children.

Endotracheal intubation is required if the patient cannot be rapidly resuscitated or when adequate spontaneous ventilation does not resume quickly. Attempts at intubation should be made by experienced personnel. The patient should be hyperventilated before each attempt, and resuscitative efforts should not be interrupted by more than 30 seconds with each attempt. Cricoid pressure should be applied, when possible, by a second person during endotracheal intubation to protect against regurgitation of gastric contents. The prominence inferior to that of the thyroid cartilage is the cricoid cartilage. Downward pressure should be applied here with the thumb and index finger (Fig. 3-10) until the cuff of the endotracheal tube is inflated [6, 13]. Once an endotracheal tube is in place, ventilation need no longer be synchronized with chest compressions but may be performed asynchronously at 12 or more ventilations per minute. (See Procedure 4.)

Once the victim is intubated and the trachea is protected from regurgitation, faster inspiratory flow rates are possible,

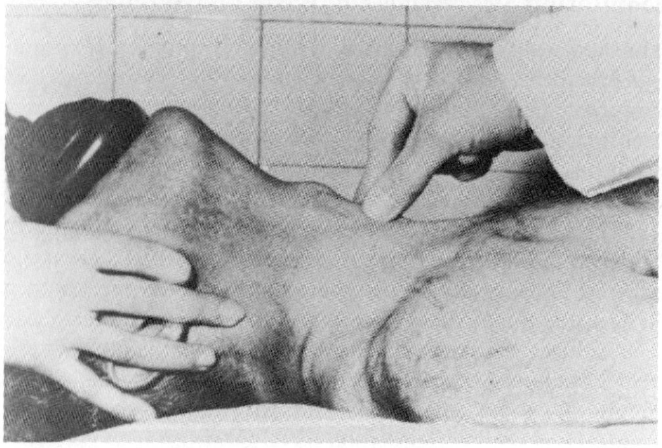

Fig. 3-10. Cricoid pressure. Application of downward pressure over the cricoid with neck extended. (From B.A. Sellick. Cricoid pressure to control regurgitation of stomach contents during induction of anesthesia. *Lancet* 2:405, 1961.)

the ventilations may be more frequent, and ventilations may be asynchronous with the compressions. Under these circumstances, more rapid ventilations than 12 to 15 per minute are advisable in an attempt to hyperventilate and improve carbon dioxide removal.

Esophageal obturator airways are used by some prehospital emergency medical services. They are designed to be inserted blindly through the victim's mouth into the esophagus. Once the device has been positioned into the esophagus, the distal balloon is inflated, occluding the esophagus. The lungs are ventilated through proximal holes in the pharynx. Several modifications are available. The *esophageal gastric tube airway* allows decompression of the stomach through a gastric lumen. Should a patient arrive in the emergency department with either of these devices in place, endotracheal intubation should be accomplished and the cuff inflated before the esophageal obturator is removed. Vomiting is common after removal of such a device.

Circulatory Support

Chest compression should not be unduly interrupted while adjunctive procedures are instituted. The rescuer coordinating the resuscitation effort must ensure that adequate pulses are generated by the compressor. The carotid or femoral pulse should be evaluated every few minutes during the resuscitative effort.

Mechanical chest compressors are available and seem useful in the hands of experienced resuscitators. It is important that such devices be correctly calibrated to provide a stroke of 1.5 to 2.0 in. The position of the press on the sternum must be checked frequently to assure adequate compression with a minimum of damage. The press may be a manually operated hinged device or may be powered by compressed gas (usually 100 percent oxygen). The plunger is mounted on a backboard and is associated with a time-pressure cycled ventilator. This device is programmed to deliver CPR in a 5:1 compression to ventilation ratio using a compression duration that is 50 percent of the cycle length. Such units allow the patient to be harnessed to the backboard, fixing the location of the plunger. When it is used properly, with careful monitoring of patient position, such a device facilitates CPR during transport. An acceptable electrocardiogram (ECG) can often be recorded with the compressor in operation, and defibrillation can be delivered during the downstroke of chest compression, without delays in CPR.

Electrocardiographic monitoring is necessary during resuscitation to guide appropriate electrical and pharmacologic therapy. Until such monitoring allows diagnosis of the rhythm, the patient should be assumed to be in ventricular fibrillation.

Most defibrillators currently marketed have built-in monitoring circuitry in the paddles ("quick-look" paddles). On application of the defibrillator paddles, the patient's ECG is displayed on the monitor screen. Such a system allows initial therapy to be administered appropriately. For continuous monitoring beyond the first few minutes, a standard ECG monitoring unit should be employed.

Electrocardiographic monitoring must never be relied on without frequent reference to the patient's pulse and clinical condition. What appears to be ventricular fibrillation or asystole on the monitor screen must not be treated as such unless the patient is found to be pulseless. An apparently satisfactory rhythm seen on the monitor must not be a source of self-congratulation unless it is accompanied by an adequate pulse and blood pressure.

Defibrillation is the definitive treatment for the vast majority of cardiac arrests. It should be delivered as early as possible and repeated frequently until a pulse returns.

If an electrical defibrillator is not immediately available, a *precordial thump* may be employed. Conversion of ventricular tachycardia and ventricular fibrillation by a precordial thump has been well documented [14–16]. A solitary precordial thump, therefore, is warranted in monitored ventricular fibrillation or pulseless ventricular tachycardia in the absence of a defibrillator. If the thump successfully leads to a rhythm with a pulse, a bolus of lidocaine should be given. In patients with ventricular tachycardia who have a pulse, a precordial thump should not be used unless an electric defibrillator is available since a thump can induce ventricular fibrillation [17].

Electrical defibrillation involves passing an electric current through the heart and causing synchronous depolarization of the myocytes. As the myocytes repolarize, the opportunity arises for the emergence of organized pacemaker activity.

Proper use of the defibrillator requires special attention to several items (Procedure 13):

1. *Selection of proper energy levels* lessens myocardial damage and arrhythmias occasioned by unnecessarily high energies. Inadequate energies will not terminate the arrhythmia. An initial energy of 200 joules appears to be safer than higher energies [18] and equally effective [18, 19]. If the patient remains pulseless after the initial shock, the next defibrillation attempt should be at 200 to 300 joules, and the third and subsequent attempts should be at no higher than 360 joules. If ventricular fibrillation recurs after successful defibrillation, the prior successful energy level should be tried again.

2. *Proper asynchronous mode.* If the rhythm is ventricular fibrillation, the synchronizing switch must be deactivated or the defibrillator will dutifully await the nonforthcoming R wave. For rapid, pulseless ventricular tachycardia (approximately 150–200 beats per minute), it is best not to attempt synchronization with the R wave, since this increases the likelihood of delivering the shock on the T wave. If the countershock falls on the T wave and induces ventricular fibrillation, another unsynchronized countershock is delivered promptly after confirming pulselessness.

3. *Proper position of the paddles,* allowing the major energy of the electric arc to traverse the myocardium. The anterolateral position requires that one paddle be placed to the right of the upper sternum, just below the clavicle. The other paddle is positioned to the left of the nipple in the left midaxillary line. In the anteroposterior position, one paddle is positioned under the left scapula with the patient lying on it. The anterior paddle is positioned just to the left of the lower sternal border.

4. *Adequate contact between paddles and skin* should be assured, using just enough electrode paste to cover the paddle face, without spilling over the surrounding skin. The rescuer should hold the paddles with firm (approximately 25 lbs) pressure. The pressure should be delivered using the forearms; leaning into the paddles should be avoided lest the rescuer slip.

5. *No contact must be present with anyone other than the victim.* The rescuer must be sturdily balanced on both feet, not standing on a wet floor. CPR must be discontinued, with no one remaining in contact with the patient. It is the responsibility of the person holding the paddles to check the patient's surroundings, assure the safety of all participants, loudly announce the intention to countershock, and depress both buttons.

6. *If no skeletal muscle twitch or spasm has occurred,* recheck the equipment, contacts, and synchronizer switch used for elective cardioversions.

7. *Assess the pulse and rhythm after each countershock,* before proceeding with therapeutic interventions. If the patient remains pulseless, resume CPR, place an intravenous line, administer epinephrine, and reshock at 360 joules.

Pacemaker therapy requiring positioning of transvenous or transthoracic electrodes is time consuming, technically demanding, and usually interferes with adequate performance of CPR. Recent improvements in external pacing equipment often allow myocardial capture with greatly reduced pain and skeletal muscle contraction [20]. Unfortunately, pacing is not effective in producing a perfusing rhythm in most cases of cardiac arrest [21, 22]. Patients who are helped with emergency pacing are those with severe bradycardias or conduction block who have reasonably well-preserved myocardial function [23] (Procedure 15).

Venous access with a reliable intravenous route must be established early in the course of the resuscitative effort to allow for the administration of necessary drugs and fluids. However, initial defibrillation attempts and CPR should not be delayed while waiting for the placement of an intravenous line. *Peripheral venous access* through antecubital veins is often more convenient because it is less likely to interfere with other rescue procedures. Cannulation of such veins may be difficult, however, because of venous collapse or constriction. A large-bore catheter system should be used since needles in the vein are apt to become dislodged during CPR. A long catheter may be threaded into the central circulation. Alternatively, the extremity may be elevated and a large volume of flush solution used to help entry of the drug into the central circulation. Lower-extremity peripheral veins should be avoided since entry of drugs into the central circulation from such veins during CPR is questionable [24].

Central venous access offers a more secure route for drug administration and should be attempted if initial resuscitative efforts are not successful. Femoral vein cannulation is apparently difficult to achieve during CPR [25] and flow into the thorax is slower than in upper-torso access. If the femoral vein is successfully cannulated, a long line should be placed into the vena cava above the level of the diaphragm. Internal jugular or subclavian routes are preferable, but their placement should not be allowed to delay defibrillation attempts or to interfere with CPR. They should be placed by experienced operators (Procedure 9).

Drugs such as epinephrine, atropine, and lidocaine can be administered via the endotracheal tube if there is delay in achieving venous access. Intracardiac injection of epinephrine is indicated only if intravenous and endotracheal routes are not available.

Drug Therapy

Correction of hypoxemia should be attempted early during CPR with administration of the highest possible oxygen concentration. Inadequate perfusion, decreased pulmonary blood flow, pulmonary edema, atalectasis, and ventilation-perfusion mismatch all contribute to the difficulty in maintaining adequate tissue oxygenation. Inadequate tissue oxygenation results in anaerobic metabolism, the generation of lactic acid, and the development of metabolic acidosis. (See the previous section on airway and ventilatory support.)

Correction of acidosis is difficult during cardiac arrest, and acidosis is inevitable if the arrest has lasted for more than several minutes. Metabolic acidosis develops, as was noted previously, because of tissue hypoxia and conversion to anaerobic metabolism. Respiratory acidosis occurs because of the apnea or hypoventilation accompanying intrapulmonary ventilation-perfusion abnormalities; it is also contributed to by the marked decrease in pulmonary blood flow that exists even with well-performed CPR. The exhaled carbon dioxide during CPR is markedly diminished [26–29] and cannot be adequately increased even with endotracheal intubation and increased volume of moved air; as a result the $PaCO_2$ rises. Hyperventilation should be attempted to achieve as much removal of carbon dioxide as possible under the unfavorable circumstances of CPR. Early intubation should be an important goal so that large volumes of gas can be moved in and out of the lung without causing gastric insufflation. Once the airway is protected, ventilation can proceed asynchronously with sternal compression and at a faster rate than the 5:1 ratio would allow.

Sodium bicarbonate reacts with hydrogen ions to buffer metabolic acidosis by forming carbonic acid, which dissociates into carbon dioxide and water. Each 50 mEq sodium bicarbonate will generate 260 to 280 mm Hg carbon dioxide, which can be eliminated only through the expired air. As the carbon dioxide concentration in exhaled gas during CPR is markedly decreased, the carbonic acid generated by sodium bicarbonate cannot be effectively eliminated. Paradoxical intracellular acidosis is likely to result and arterial blood gases may not correctly reflect the state of tissue acidosis [30]. The sodium and osmolar load of bicarbonate is high, and excessive administration will result in hyperosmolarity, hypernatremia, and worsened cellular acidosis. With these concerns in mind, the AHA guidelines suggest that sodium bicarbonate be avoided until successful resuscitation has reestablished a perfusing rhythm [31]. In the postresuscitative state, the degree of acidosis can be better estimated from blood gases and the acidemia corrected with hyperventilation and possibly bicarbonate administration. Sodium bicarbonate is of questionable value in treating metabolic acidosis during cardiac arrest; it has not been shown to facilitate ventricular defibrillation or survival in cardiac arrest [32]. In any case the option of using bicarbonate during cardiac arrest should not be exercised until at least 10 minutes have passed and the patient has not responded to initial defibrillatory and drug intervention.

Volume replacement is often required during CPR, especially if the initial attempts at defibrillation have failed. Electromechanical dissociation is particularly likely to be caused either by acute severe hypovolemia (e.g., exsanguination) or by a cardiovascular process for which volume expansion may be a life-saving temporizing measure (e.g., pericardial tamponade, pulmonary embolism, septic shock). The usual clues for hypovolemia, such as collapsed jugular and peripheral veins and evidence of peripheral vasoconstriction, are unavailable during cardiac arrest; furthermore, dry mucous membranes and absence of normal secretions (tears, saliva) are unreliable indicators in acute hypovolemia. Most physical findings of tamponade, pulmonary embolism, or septic shock are absent during arrest. Therefore, one must be guided by an appropriate clinical history and have a low threshold to administer volume during CPR.

Simple crystalloids such as 5% dextrose in water are inappropriate for rapid expansion of the circulatory blood volume. Isotonic crystalloids (0.9% saline, Ringer's lactate), colloids, or blood are necessary for satisfactory volume expansion. Crystalloids are more readily available, easier to administer, and cost less than colloids. Furthermore, crystalloids do not cause allergic reactions or infections. Colloids, on the other hand, are more likely to sustain intravascular volume and oncotic pressure. Some studies [33] have suggested shorter resuscitation times and better survival with colloids as opposed to crystalloids.

If the patient has a weak pulse, simple elevation of the legs may help by encouraging venous return to the central circulation. In profound hypovolemia with subsequent arrest, military antishock garments (MAST suits) may ameliorate the hypovolemia until fluid administration or surgical intervention has supervened. Volume challenges should be given as needed until pulse and blood pressure have been restored or until there is evidence of volume overload. In the post-resuscitative phase, pulmonary artery and central venous catheterization are usually needed to adequately monitor volume replacement. Fluid replacement is guided by the patient's clinical course, urine output, and catheterization data. The goal is to achieve optimal cardiac output and perfusion pressure without excessive fluid expansion or pulmonary congestion. A further discussion of the use of volume in treating shock and other cardiovascular problems can be found in the chapters on The Critically Injured Patient (Chaps. 40–43).

Sympathomimetic Drugs and Vasopressors
Sympathomimetic drugs and vasopressors either act directly on adrenergic receptors or act indirectly by releasing catecholamines from nerve endings. The agents most useful during cardiac emergencies are the adrenergic agents, which include the endogenous biogenic amines epinephrine, norepinephrine, and dopamine, and the synthetic agents isoproterenol and its derivative dobutamine [34]. The effects of these adrenergic agents can be divided into several broad categories: stimulation of certain peripheral smooth muscles, inhibition of other peripheral smooth muscles, cardiac stimulation, metabolic effects, and central nervous system effects. The variable effects of different agents appear to be caused by the presence of several species of adrenergic receptors. The classification of adrenergic receptors into *alpha* and *beta* was first proposed by Alquist [35] in 1948. The concept was based on the variable activity of a series of sympathomimetic agents at effector sites. The functions associated with alpha receptors are vasoconstriction, mydriasis, and intestinal relaxation. The functions associated with beta receptors are vasodilatation, cardioacceleration, positive inotropism, bronchial relaxation, and intestinal relaxation. Metabolic effects of adrenergic agents are largely beta and include glycogenolysis and fatty acid release. Insulin release is increased by beta agents and inhibited by alpha agents.

Beta receptors are of two types: beta-1 and beta-2. The beta-1 receptors are responsible for cardiac stimulation and lipolysis. The beta-2 receptors are responsible for vasodilatation and bronchodilatation. Alpha-1 and alpha-2 receptors are also present, but refer to postsynaptic (alpha-1) and presynaptic (alpha-2) location.

Norepinephrine acts on both alpha and beta-1 receptors, but its alpha effects often predominate. Epinephrine also acts on both receptors, with its beta effects more prominent. The synthetic agent isoproterenol is a pure beta agonist and its actions are blocked by beta blockers such as propranolol. The synthetic agents methoxamine and phenylephrine are pure alpha agonists and their effects are blocked by phenoxybenzamine or phentolamine.

Dopamine has beta activity and (at higher dosages) alpha activity. At all dosages, it has a vasodilator activity on renal, mesenteric, coronary, and intracerebral arteries that cannot be blocked by beta blockers. This effect can be attenuated by haloperidol and phenothiazines, suggesting the presence of specific dopaminergic receptors in these vascular beds.

EPINEPHRINE. Epinephrine is the most frequently used pressor agent during CPR. As was mentioned previously, epinephrine is a naturally occurring catecholamine that has both alpha and beta activity. *Indications* for the use of epinephrine include all forms of cardiac arrest, since its alpha vasoconstrictive activity is important in raising the perfusion pressure of myocardium and brain. The importance of the alpha-adrenergic activity during resuscitation has been pointed out in several studies, whereas administration of pure beta agonists (such as isoproterenol or dobutamine) has been shown to be ineffective. The beta action of epinephrine has theoretical usefulness in asystole and bradycardiac arrests through increasing the heart rate. The beta effect is also touted to convert asystole to ventricular fibrillation (VF) or "fine" VF to "coarse." Coarse or wide-amplitude VF is easier to convert to a perfusing rhythm than is fine or small-amplitude VF.

Administration of epinephrine is best performed intravenously. An adult in cardiac arrest should promptly be given a 0.5-mg dose at a 1:10,000 dilution (5 ml). It should be given in the upper extremity or centrally (see section on circulatory support) and may be repeated every five minutes. It should not be administered in the same intravenous line as an alkaline solution. If an intravenous line has not been established, 1 mg epinephrine (10 ml of 1:10,000 dilution) can be administered into the endotracheal tube and distributed through the tracheobronchial mucosa. This route gives rapid onset and sustained duration of action. Atropine and lidocaine can also be administered by the endotracheal route. The intracardiac route of injection should be avoided, since it can lead to serious complications such as intramyocardial injection, coronary laceration, and pneumothorax. This technique should be considered a last resort. An intravenous titration of 1 to 4 μg per minute can also be given for inotropic and pressor support. Some researchers suspect that doses much higher than those just mentioned may be more advantageous during arrest. Until the results of ongoing research become available, currently advised doses should be used. *Precautions* in the use of epinephrine and other alpha agonists include tissue necrosis from extravasation and inactivation from admixture with bicarbonate.

NOREPINEPHRINE. Norepinephrine is a potent alpha agonist with beta activity. Its salutary alpha effects during CPR are similar to those of epinephrine. It is not known whether it is more effective than epinephrine during arrest, but ongoing research should answer this question before long.

The major effect of norepinephrine is on the blood vessels. Initial coronary vasoconstriction usually gives way to coronary vasodilatation, probably as a result of increased myocardial metabolic activity. In a heart with compromised coronary reserve, this may cause further ischemia. During cardiac arrest, its usefulness, like that of epinephrine, is most likely due to peripheral vasoconstriction with increase in perfusion pressure. During cardiogenic shock (when peripheral vasoconstriction is often already extreme) its effect is more difficult to predict. Norepinephrine produces a slightly more rapid vasoconstrictive response than do other catecholamines. It also causes considerable renal and mesenteric vasoconstriction, whereas dopamine, at low infusion rates, causes vasodilatation in these vascular beds. *Indications* for the use of norepinephrine during cardiac arrest are similar to those for epinephrine, although there is no apparent reason to prefer it to epinephrine. Norepinephrine appears to be most useful in the treatment of shock caused by inappropriate decline in peripheral vascular resistance, such as septic and neurogenic shock.

Administration is by intravenous infusion, titrated to an adequate perfusion pressure. Four to 8 mg of the bitartrate (2–4 mg of the base) should be diluted in 500 ml D_5W or 5% dextrose in normal saline. If 8 mg of the bitartrate is diluted to 500 ml, 1 ml will contain 16 μg/ml; a microdrip administration set may be used to deliver 1 ml in 60 drops. After observing the response to an initial dose of 2 μg/kg per minute, adjust the dose to maintain a low normal blood pressure (85–90 mm Hg systolic, or somewhat higher in a previously hypertensive individual). An average effective adult dose is 2 to 12 μg per minute. Higher doses are needed in some patients. It should not be administered in the same intravenous line as an alkaline solution. After the patient has been transferred to a critical care unit, the drug may be continued for several days but should be gradually tapered when possible. Abrupt termination of the infusion (as may occur in transport) can lead to sudden severe hypotension.

Precautions to the use of norepinephrine include its inappropriate use in hypovolemic shock and in cases with already severe vasoconstriction. Intraarterial pressure monitoring is strongly recommended when norepinephrine is used, since indirect blood measurement is often incorrect in patients with severe vasoconstriction. In patients with myocardial ischemia or infarction, the myocardial oxygen requirements are increased by all catecholamines, but especially by norepinephrine through its marked afterload increasing properties. Unless the need for perfusion pressure outweighs the afterload increase, norepinephrine is likely to be deleterious. Heart rate, rhythm, direct systemic and pulmonary pressures, and cardiac output should be closely monitored when using this drug in the patient with myocardial ischemia or infarction. If extravasation of norepinephrine occurs in superficial tissues, ischemic necrosis and sloughing are apt to develop. Norepinephrine, therefore, should be administered through a catheter well advanced into the vein. If extravasation does occur, 5 to 10 mg phentolamine in 10 to 15 ml saline should be infiltrated as soon as possible into the area of extravasation.

ISOPROTERENOL. Isoproterenol is a synthetic catecholamine with almost pure beta-adrenergic activity. Its cardiac activity includes potent inotropic and chronotropic effects, both of which will increase the myocardium's oxygen demand. Bronchodilatation occurs and the arterial beds of skeletal muscle, kidneys, and gut dilate, resulting in a marked drop in systemic vascular resistance. The cardiac output can be expected to increase markedly, unless enough myocardial ischemia is caused by the increased myocardial oxygen demand. Systolic blood pressure is usually maintained because of the rise in cardiac output; however, the diastolic and mean pressures usually decrease. As a result, coronary perfusion pressure drops at a time when myocardial oxygen requirement is increased. This combination can be expected to have deleterious effects in patients with ischemic heart disease, especially in the situation of a cardiac arrest. The main clinical usefulness of isoproterenol is in its ability to stimulate pacemakers within the heart. *Indications* for isoproterenol are primarily in the setting of atropine-resistant, hemodynamically significant bradyarrhythmias. These include profound sinus and junctional bradycardia as well as various forms of high-degree atrioventricular block. It should be used as an interim solution until a temporary pacemaker can be inserted. Isoproterenol is not indicated in cardiac arrest.

Administration of isoproterenol is by titration of an intravenous solution. Isoproterenol (Isuprel), 1 mg, is diluted with either 250 ml D_5W (4 μg/ml) or 500 ml D_5W (2 μg/ml). The infusion rate should be only rapid enough to effect an adequate perfusing heart rate. The infusing rate may be from 2 to 20 μg per minute (0.05–0.5 μg/kg per minute). Depending on the adequacy of cardiac reserve, a target heart rate as low as 50 to 55 beats per minute may be satisfactory. Occasionally, more rapid rates are necessary. *Precautions* in the use of isoproterenol are largely due to the increase in myocardial oxygen requirement, with its potential of provoking ischemia. The marked chronotropic effects cause tachycardia and may provoke serious ventricular arrhythmias, including ventricular fibrillation. The drug must be used with extreme caution in patients with coronary artery disease, especially those who have had a recent myocardial infarction. Its use is generally contraindicated if tachyarrhythmia is already present, especially if the arrhythmia is secondary to digitalis toxicity. If significant hypotension develops with its use, it may be combined with or switched to dopamine or epinephrine.

DOPAMINE. Dopamine hydrochloride is a naturally occurring precursor of norepinephrine that has alpha, beta, and dopamine receptor stimulating activity. The dopamine receptor activity dilates renal and mesenteric arterial beds at low doses (1–2 μg/kg per minute), which may not produce an increase in heart rate or blood pressure. These effects cannot be blocked with either beta or alpha blocking agents. At doses from 2 to 10 μg/kg per minute, dopamine exerts primarily beta-adrenergic activity, with an increase in contractile force and heart rate. At doses of 10 μg/kg per minute and above, the alpha-adrenergic activity becomes more and more prominent, causing peripheral vasoconstriction and constriction of renal and splanchnic arterial beds. Above 20 μg/kg per minute, alpha activity is likely to overcome dopaminergic effects and lower renal and mesenteric blood flow. *Indications* for the use of dopamine are primarily significant hypotension and cardiogenic shock. Its dopaminergic effects may be useful in early shock with decreasing urine output; it may be started at low doses along with volume expansion.

Administration is by intravenous titration. A 200-mg ampul is diluted to 250 or 500 ml in D_5W or D_5NS for a concentration of 800 μg/ml or 400 μg/ml. It should not be administered in the same intravenous line as an alkaline solution. For hypotension, the initial infusion rate is usually 2 to 5 μg/kg per minute, which is increased until a satisfactory response is achieved in blood pressure and urine output. As with all infusions of catecholamines, the lowest infusion rate that results in a satisfactory perfusion should be the goal of therapy. Rarely, a patient may need greater than 20 μg/kg per minute. Monitoring of urine output, cardiac output, systemic vascular resistance, and left ventricular filling pressure is necessary for optimal control of the hemodynamic response. *Precautions* are similar to those for other catecholamines. Tachycardia or ventricular arrhythmias may require reduction in dosage or discontinuation of the drug. If significant hypotension occurs from the dilating activity of dopaminergic or beta-active doses, small amounts of an alpha-active drug may be used as well as dopamine. Dopamine may increase myocardial ischemia. Sloughing can occur if dopamine extravasates into subcutaneous tissues.

DOBUTAMINE. Dobutamine is a potent, synthetic beta-adrenergic agent that differs from isoproterenol in that tachycardia is less of a problem. Unless ischemia supervenes, cardiac output will increase, as will renal and mesenteric blood flow. *Indications* for dobutamine are primarily in the short-term enhancement of ventricular contractility in the patient with heart failure. It may be used in the postresuscitative stabilization of the arrest victim or in the patient with heart failure that is refractory to other drugs. It also may be used in combination with intravenous nitroprusside, which lowers peripheral vascular resistance and thereby the left ventricular afterload. While nitroprusside lowers peripheral resistance, dobutamine maintains the perfusion pressure by augmenting the cardiac output.

Administration is by slow, titrated intravenous infusion. As low a dose as 0.5 μg/kg per minute may prove to be effective. However, the usual dose range is 2.5 to 10.0 μg/kg per minute. The contents of a 250-mg vial are dissolved in 10 ml sterile water and then to 250 or 500 ml D_5W for a concentration of 1 mg/ml or 0.5 mg/ml. It should not be administered in the same intravenous line as alkaline solutions. *Precautions* are similar to those for other beta agonists. Dobutamine may cause tachycardia, ventricular arrhythmias, myocardial ischemia, and extension of infarction. Caution must be exercised in its use in patients with coronary artery disease.

Antiarrhythmic Agents

Antiarrhythmic agents play an important role in stabilizing the rhythm in many resuscitation situations. Lidocaine has proved the most useful in counteracting the tendency to ventricular arrhythmias. Bretylium has a similar use. Procainamide is occasionally used in the postresuscitative care of the patient.

LIDOCAINE. Lidocaine is an antiarrhythmic agent that often proves effective against ventricular arrhythmias, such as premature ventricular complexes (PVCs) and ventricular tachycardia (VT). PVCs are not unusual in apparently healthy people and most often are benign. Even in the patient with chronic heart disease, PVCs and nonsustained runs of VT are usually asymptomatic, and controversy exists concerning the need to treat under these circumstances. The situation is very different for patients with myocardial ischemia or recent myocardial infarction, since their condition is much more likely to progress from PVCs to sustained VT or VF. Such patients should be treated promptly with antiarrhythmic agents such as lidocaine. The efficacy of prophylactic lidocaine in reducing primary ventricular fibrillation in patients with acute myocardial infarction has been established. *Indications* are primarily to suppress ventricular arrhythmias in patients with myocardial ischemia and recent myocardial infarction. The prophylactic use of lidocaine is recommended for patients who are highly suspected of having a myocardial infarction. The drug is also of use in ventricular tachycardia and in VF that has recurred after successful defibrillation or that has been refractory to defibrillation. It is used after successful conversion of VT or VF to protect against recurrence. Correction of the underlying cause of the ventricular irritability (myocardial ischemia, hypoxemia, hypercarbia, electrolyte imbalance, and so forth) must also be addressed if the arrhythmia is to be managed successfully.

Administration of lidocaine begins with an intravenous bolus. The onset of action is rapid and the duration of action is brief, although it may be prolonged by use of a continuous infusion of the drug. A solution of lidocaine, typically 20 mg/ml (2 percent), should be prepared for intravenous administration. Prefilled syringes of lidocaine are available for bolus injection. Several dosage schedules are in use, but the most common is a bolus of 1 mg/kg, followed by a continuous infusion of 2 to 4 mg per minute (15–50 μg/kg per minute). If the patient has suffered an acute myocardial infarction, the infusion is continued for a period of hours to days and tapered slowly. If the cause of the arrhythmia has been corrected, the infusion may be tapered more rapidly.

Precautions should be taken against excessive accumulation of the drug. Dosage should be reduced in patients with low cardiac output, congestive failure, hepatic failure, or age greater than 70 years because of decreased liver metabolism of the drug. Toxic manifestations are usually neurologic and can vary from slurred speech, tinnitus, sleepiness, and dysphoria to localizing neurologic symptoms. Frank seizures can occur with or without preceding neurologic symptoms and can be controlled with short-acting barbiturates or diazepam. Conscious patients should be warned about the possible symptoms of neurologic toxicity and asked to report them immediately if they occur. Enlisting the patient's aid also allays the fear that would otherwise develop from unexpected neurologic symptoms. The fear surrounding intensive cardiac care is great enough without allowing the patient to assume the worst should such symptoms develop. Excessive blood levels can significantly depress myocardial contractility.

BRETYLIUM. Bretylium tosylate is an adrenergic blocking agent that initially causes a release of norepinephrine from peripheral adrenergic nerve terminals. It subsequently prevents further release of norepinephrine from these same terminals or their uptake of norepinephrine. The latter effect potentiates the actions of circulating catecholamines. Bretylium has been demonstrated to be effective in suppressing ventricular arrhythmias in a variety of conditions, including acute myocardial infarction and ischemia. It has been demonstrated in animal studies to have a primary antifibrillatory effect [36, 37]. Clinically, bretylium has been found effective in the treatment of ventricular tachycardia and ventricular fibrillation. It has not been found to be more effective than lidocaine in direct comparisons. Based on animal work [38] higher dosages than are currently recommended may be needed for improved efficacy, but investigation in the field is still preliminary.

Bretylium's initial release of norepinephrine from nerve endings causes an increase in cardiac output and mean systemic pressure, which lasts 10 to 20 minutes after parenteral administration. This initial action is followed by a delayed hypotensive effect secondary to peripheral adrenergic blockade. Hypotension is the most common side effect but is generally mild and does not require discontinuation of the drug. Hypotension is most marked in patients with volume depletion or limited myocardial reserve. Paradoxically, hypotension is more often produced by low doses (less than 5 mg/kg), which are apt to cause peripheral dilatation without augmentation of cardiac output. *Indications* for bretylium are ventricular tachycardia and fibrillation, especially if they prove refractory to lidocaine and electrical countershocks. Bretylium may also be used to suppress recurrent VT or VF and has been used for arrhythmia prophylaxis in acute myocardial infarction.

Administration is by intravenous bolus. Bretylium is available in 10-ml ampuls that contain 500 mg. For unresponsive VF, 5 mg/kg undiluted is given in a rapid bolus, followed by additional attempts at electrical defibrillation. If this dose fails, a 10-mg/kg bolus is administered and is repeated if necessary every 15 to 30 minutes up to a maximum total initial dose of 30 mg/kg. Each bolus should be followed by an attempt at electrical defibrillation at maximum delivered energy (or at previously successful energy level). For slow drips, 500 mg should be diluted to 50 ml with saline. An intravenous drip of 5 to 10 mg/kg over 10 to 20 minutes may be given for recurrent or refractory VT and repeated, as needed, every 6 to 8 hours. Alternatively, a 1- to 2-mg per minute drip may be administered. *Precautions* include the production of nausea and vomiting, especially by rapid infusions. There is a high incidence of mild orthostatic hypotension. However, more severe hypotension may occur, requiring the placing of the patient in Trendelenburg's position and the administration of fluids. Rarely, low dosages of pressor agents may be required. Digitalis toxic ventricular arrhythmias are likely to be worsened during the early transient norepinephrine release. Bretylium is relatively contraindicated in patients who have a marked restriction in their ability to increase their stroke volume; these patients include those with severe aortic or pulmonic stenosis and those with severe pulmonary hypertension.

PROCAINAMIDE. Procainamide hydrochloride is an antiarrhythmic agent with quinidine-like activity. Like quinidine it is useful in suppressing a wide variety of both ventricular and supraventricular arrhythmias. It is effective against reentrant as well as ectopic arrhythmogenic mechanisms. It has somewhat less vagolytic effect than quinidine and does not cause the rise in digoxin level seen with quinidine. Procainamide is sometimes useful in the critical care setting for the suppression of ventricular arrhythmias that cannot be effectively treated by lidocaine or bretylium, or in patients who cannot be treated with either of these two agents. *Indications* include the suppression of ventricular arrhythmias that are refractory to lidocaine or to both lidocaine and bretylium (Figs. 3-11, 3-12). It may also be used in patients with supraventricular arrhythmias that cause hemodynamic compromise.

Administration is either oral or by intravenous injection. For serious arrhythmias in the critical care setting, intravenous injection is preferable. An infusion of 20 mg per minute (0.3 mg/kg per minute) is given up to a loading dose of 1 gm (15 mg/kg) or until the arrhythmia is suppressed, hypotension develops, or the QRS interval widens by 50 percent of its original width. A maintenance infusion may then be started at 1 to 4 mg per minute. The dosage should be lowered in the presence of renal failure. Blood levels of procainamide and its metabolite N-acetylprocainamide should be monitored in patients with renal failure or in patients who are receiving more than 3 mg per minute for over 24 hours. Infusions as low as 1.4 mg/kg per hour may be needed in patients with renal insufficiency.

Precautions to the use of procainamide include its production of systemic hypotension, disturbance in atrioventricular conduction, and decreased ventricular contractility. Its infusion intravenously must be monitored carefully with frequent blood pressure determinations and measurement of

Assess for need for acute suppressive therapy

↓

→ Rule out treatable cause
→ Consider serum potassium
→ Consider digitalis level
→ Consider bradycardia
→ Consider drugs

Lidocaine, 1 mg/kg

↓

If not suppressed,
repeat lidocaine, 0.5 mg/kg, every 2–5 min,
until no ectopy, or up to 3 mg/kg given

↓

If not suppressed,
procainamide, 20 mg/min,
until no ectopy, or up to 1,000 mg given

↓

If not suppressed
and not contraindicated,
bretylium, 5–10 mg/kg, over 8–10 min

↓

If not suppressed,
consider overdrive pacing

Once ectopy resolved, maintain as follows:
- After lidocaine, 1 mg/kg → Lidocaine drip, 2 mg/min
- After lidocaine, 1–2 mg/kg → Lidocaine drip, 3 mg/min
- After lidocaine, 2–3 mg/kg → Lidocaine drip, 4 mg/min
- After procainamide → Procainamide drip, 1–4 mg/min (check blood level)
- After bretylium → Bretylium drip, 2 mg/min

Fig. 3-11. Ventricular ectopy. Acute suppressive therapy according to a sequence developed to assist in teaching how to treat a broad range of patients with ventricular ectopy. Some patients may require therapy not specified herein. This algorithm should not be construed as prohibiting such flexibility.

ECG intervals PR, QRS, and QT. Hypotension usually responds to slowing of the infusion rate. If the QRS interval increases by more than 50 percent of its initial width, procainamide infusion should be discontinued. Widened QRS signifies toxic blood levels and may herald serious atrioventricular conduction abnormalities and asystole. This is particularly true of patients with digitalis intoxication and those with antecedent atrioventricular conduction abnormalities. Marked increase in QT interval may predispose a patient to ventricular arrhythmias of the "torsade de points" variety. Patients who have ventricular arrhythmias of the torsade variety or who have ventricular arrhythmias associated with bradycardias should not be treated with procainamide.

Other Agents

Other agents occasionally found useful or necessary during resuscitation or in the immediate postresuscitation period include atropine, calcium, nitroprusside, and nitroglycerin. Many other emergency drugs may be required in particular circumstances and are discussed in other parts of this text; an incomplete list of these drugs includes antibiotics, thiamine, thyroxin, morphine, naloxone, adrenocorticoids, calcium channel blockers, fibrinolytic agents, anticoagulants, and dextrose.

ATROPINE. Atropine sulfate is a vagolytic drug that is useful in increasing heart rate by stimulating pacers and facilitating atrioventricular (AV) conduction suppressed by excessive vagal tone. *Indications* for its use are primarily in bradycardias that are causing hemodynamic difficulty or are associated with ventricular arrhythmias (Fig. 3-13). At-

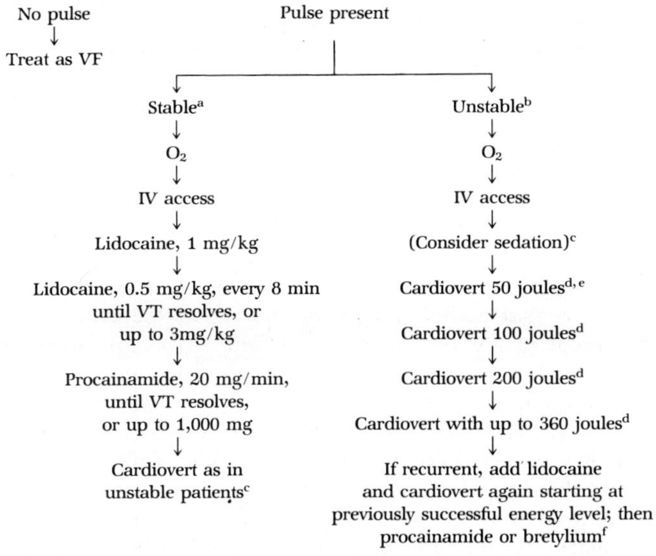

Fig. 3-12. Sustained ventricular tachycardia. This sequence was developed to assist in teaching how to respond to a broad range of patients with sustained VT. Some patients may require therapy that is not specified herein. This algorithm should not be construed as prohibiting such flexibility. [a] If a patient becomes unstable (see [b]) at any time, move to "unstable" arm of the algorithm. [b] "Unstable" indicates symptoms (e.g., chest pain, dyspnea), hypotension, congestive heart failure, ischemia, or infarction. [c] Sedation should be considered for all patients except those who are unconscious or who cannot wait because of severe hemodynamic instability. [d] For patients in shock or marked pulmonary edema, unsynchronized cardioversion should be performed if sychronization would cause a delay; for patients with rapid VT greater than 150 beats per minute, unsynchronized cardioversion is preferable to avoid synchronizing on the T wave. If VF appears to result on the monitor and the patient is pulseless, countershock immediately without synchronization. [e] A precordial thump may be employed before cardioversion. [f] If VT resolves, begin intravenous infusion of the antiarrhythmic drug that aided resolution of VT; if cardioversion is unsuccessful, use intravenous lidocaine, followed by bretylium. Procainamide may also be considered.

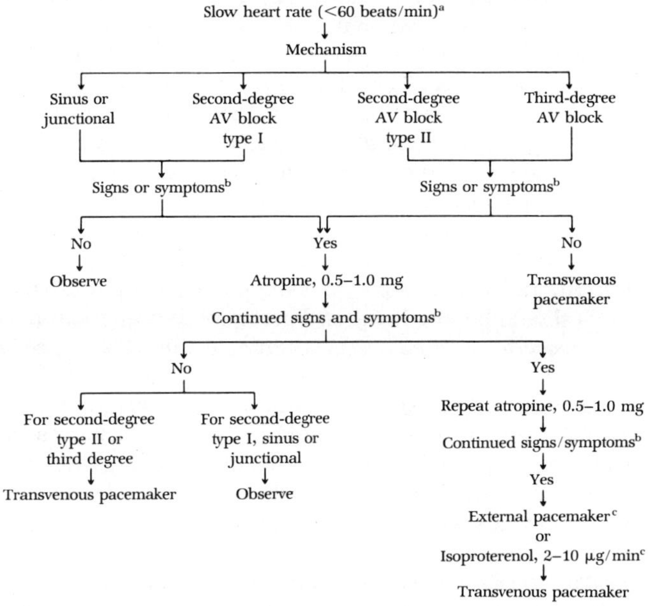

Fig. 3-13. Bradycardia with a pulse. This sequence was developed to assist in teaching how to treat a broad range of patients with bradycardia. Some patients may require therapy not specified herein. This algorithm should not be construed as prohibiting such flexibility. [a] A solitary chest thump or cough, which may stimulate cardiac electrical activity and result in improved cardiac output, may be used at this point. [b] Hypotension, ventricular ectopy, altered mental status, ischemia, infarction, or symptoms (e.g., chest pain or dyspnea). [c] Temporizing therapy. (AV = atrioventricular.)

ropine may be useful in AV block at the nodal level. It is also used in asystole and bradycardic arrests in the hope that decreased vagal tone will allow the emergence of an effective pacemaker [39].

Administration is by intravenous bolus. If a full vagolytic response is desired rapidly, as in asystole or bradycardic arrest, 1 mg should be administered intravenously at once. If a satisfactory response has not occurred within two to five minutes, an additional 1 mg should be given in a bolus. For bradycardias with a pulse, initial dose should be 0.5 mg, repeated every five minutes until the desired effect is obtained, to a maximum dose of 2 mg. Atropine is well absorbed by the endotracheal route. *Precautions* include concern that an inordinately rapid rate not be provoked. Patients with ischemic heart disease are likely to have worsened ischemia or ventricular arrhythmias if the rate is too rapid. Uncommonly, a patient will have a paradoxical slowing of rate with atropine; this is more likely to occur with smaller first doses and is caused by a central vagal effect. This effect is rapidly counteracted by additional atropine. If this situation is encountered, the next dose of atropine should be given immediately. If additional atropine does not correct the problem, the patient may require judicious use of isoproterenol or pacemaker therapy, or both.

CALCIUM. Calcium has a positive inotropic effect, which has led to its use in patients with cardiac arrest. The contractile state of the myocardium in part depends on the intracellular concentration of the calcium ion. Transmembrane calcium flux serves an important regulatory function in both active contraction and active relaxation. The use of calcium in cardiac arrest is based on an early report by Kay and Blalock [40] in which several pediatric cardiac surgical patients were successfully resuscitated, apparently with the aid of calcium. Several recent field studies [41, 42] have failed to demonstrate an improvement in survival or neurologic outcome with the use of calcium versus a control. In addition, many patients during arrest are found to have severely hypercalcemic blood levels with the conventional doses of calcium [43, 44]. This apparently is due to the markedly contracted volume of distribution of the ion in the arrested organism. In addition, calcium has the theoretical disadvantage of facilitating postanoxic tissue damage, especially in brain and heart. Digitalis toxicity may be exacerbated by the administration of calcium. *Indications* for the use of calcium should be restricted to those circumstances in which it has been shown to be of benefit [39, 45]: in calcium channel blocker toxicity, severe hyperkalemia, severe hypocalcemia, arrest after multiple transfusions with citrated blood, fluoride toxicity, and coming off heart-lung bypass after cardioplegic arrest.

Administration of calcium may be by any of its three available salts: calcium chloride, calcium gluceptate, and calcium gluconate. The gluconate salt is unstable and less frequently available. The chloride salt provides the most direct source of calcium ion and produces the most rapid effect. The gluceptate and gluconate salts require hepatic degradation to release the free calcium ion. Calcium chloride is, therefore, the best choice. It is highly irritating to tissues and must be injected into a large vein, with precautions to avoid extravasation. Calcium chloride is available in a 10% solution. An initial dose of 250 to 500 mg may be administered, and it should be slowly injected over several minutes. It may be repeated as necessary at 10-minute intervals if strong indications exist. *Precautions* include slow injection without extravasation. If bicarbonate has been administered through the same line, it must be cleared before the calcium is introduced. If the patient has a rhythm, rapid injection can result in bradycardia. Calcium salts must be used with caution in patients who are receiving digitalis.

SODIUM NITROPRUSSIDE Sodium nitroprusside is a rapid-acting dilator of both arteries and veins. Systemic arterial dilatation decreases impedance to left ventricular outflow (afterload reduction), thereby diminishing resistance to left ventricular ejection and improving cardiac output. Venous dilatation simultaneously provides preload reduction by withholding blood from the central circulation and reducing left ventricular filling pressure and volume. Myocardial oxygen consumption drops and subendocardial blood flow may rise as the ventricular wall stress is lowered. In addition, the lowered left ventricular filling pressures bring about a decrease in pulmonary capillary pressure and pulmonary congestion. Although vasodilators are most commonly used in the critical care unit setting, they are occasionally needed in the emergency department to aid in the stabilization of the resuscitated patient with severe left ventricular dysfunction. *Indications* for nitroprusside include any situation in which cardiac output is severely reduced, causing either cardiogenic shock with elevated systemic vascular resistance or pulmonary congestion from elevated left ventricular filling pressure. Patients with aortic or mitral regurgitation or a left-to-right shunt from a ventricular septal rupture are apt to respond especially well to nitroprusside infusion. Nitroprusside has also become a preferred treatment for patients in hypertensive crisis.

Administration is by intravenous infusion. The onset of action is rapid so that the effects of dose change become apparent within several minutes. For patients with severe left ventricular failure, infusion should begin at 10 μg per minute with increments of 5 to 10 μg per minute at 5-minute intervals. Most patients will respond to a 50 to 100 μg per minute total dose, although an occasional patient will require a significantly higher dose. Patients in hypertensive crisis may be started at 50 μg per minute and may require as much as 400 to 1,000 μg per minute. Nitroprusside is available in 50-mg vials of dihydrate. The drug should be dissolved in 5 ml D_5W and diluted to a volume of 250 to 1,000 ml D_5W. Because of the instability of the reconstituted solution, it is recommended that it be used within a period of 4 hours. The solution should be wrapped in opaque material since nitroprusside will deteriorate more rapidly with light exposure. *Precautions* include hypotension, generally secondary to excessive dosage. Some patients with hypotension at the start cannot tolerate nitroprusside. Many can be given nitroprusside with volume repletion. Nitroprusside is converted to thiocyanate by a hepatic enzyme and the thiocyanate is cleared by the kidneys. Signs and symptoms of thiocyanate toxicity include nausea, tinnitus, blurred vision, and delirium. Blood levels of thiocyanate can be measured and should be obtained in patients with renal dysfunction and in patients who receive high doses for a prolonged period.

NITROGLYCERIN. Nitroglycerin, like nitroprusside, is a vasodilator that sometimes proves useful in the emergency treatment of the postresuscitation patient. It can be given sublingually, transdermally, or intravenously, depending on the situation and the dose desired. Unlike nitroprusside, nitroglycerin is a more potent dilator of venous capacitance vessels than arterioles; therefore, it is more of a preload reducer than an afterload reducer. Coronary dilatation does occur and may be particulary beneficial in patients with coronary spasm and acute ischemia. Myocardial ischemia is reversed both through the lowering of preload and myocardial oxygen consumption and by coronary dilatation. *Indications* include sublingual or transdermal nitroglycerin for angina. The sublingual route is preferable for an episode of angina. For persistent or frequently recurring ischemia unrelieved by other routes of administration, an infusion of nitroglycerin is often effective. It is a useful drug if coronary spasm is suspected. An infusion of nitroglycerin may also be used for preload reduction in patients with left ventricular failure. It may be given together with an infusion of nitroprusside, especially if ischemia has not been reversed by the hemodynamic effects of nitroprusside alone.

Administration is by a sublingual tablet or spray (0.3–0.4 mg) or a transdermal patch or ointment. For rapid effect the sublingual route should be used. It may be repeated every 3 to 5 minutes if pain relief or correction of ST segment deviation has not occurred. If ischemia persists, an infusion should be begun and titrated to achieve the desired result. A 50-μg bolus of nitroglycerin may be given before the initiation of an intravenous drip. Two 20-mg vials may be diluted in 250 ml D_5W for a concentration of 160 μg/ml. The infusion is started at 10 to 20 μg per minute and increased by 5 to 10 μg every 5 to 10 minutes until the desired effect is achieved (e.g., fall in left ventricular pressure to 15–18 mm Hg or relief of chest pain and ST segment deviation). While most patients respond to 50 to 200 μg per minute, an occasional patient will require 500 μg per minute or more; however, the maintenance of high plasma levels of nitroglycerin may induce tolerance. Intermittent dosing, with nitrate-free periods, and the use of the lowest possible effective dose are recommended. *Precautions* include hypotension and syncope, especially if the patient has had an acute myocardial infarction, is volume depleted, or has restriction to left ventricular outflow, as in aortic stenosis, pulmonic stenosis, pulmonary hypertension, or hypertrophic obstructive cardiomyopathy. The rapid titration of intravenous nitroglycerin in patients with left ventricular failure necessitates careful hemodynamic monitoring to assure efficacy and safety. The hypotensive patient may be placed in Trendelenburg's position and given volume replacement. Rarely, a patient with severe obstructive coronary disease develops worsened ischemia with nitroglycerin through a coronary steal mechanism.

If ischemia is persistent in spite of maximal tolerated nitroglycerin dose, the dose should be decreased and thought given to other modalities of therapy, including heparin or cardiac catheterization, with a view to early revascularization. There is evidence that heparin anticoagulation may be of use in persistent unstable angina. Early reports of the efficacy of fibrinolytic therapy in unstable angina are intriguing and warrant further investigation.

Clinical Settings

The procedures involved in the resuscitation of a victim of cardiovascular or respiratory collapse are all part of a continuum that progresses from the initial recognition of the problem and the institution of CPR to intervention with drugs, defibrillators, pacemakers, transport, and postresuscitative evaluation and care. The following sections focus on the pharmacologic and electrical intervention appropriate to various clinical settings common in cardiac arrest.

Ventricular Fibrillation

Ventricular fibrillation is the initial rhythm encountered in 50 to 70 percent of prehospital cardiac arrests and in 30 to 40 percent of hospital cardiac arrests. In a significant percentage of hospital cardiac arrests and a smaller number of prehospital arrests, *pulseless ventricular tachycardia* is the first rhythm encountered by rescue personnel. Attempts at electrical defibrillation are the most important interventions in treating these arrhythmias (Fig. 3-14). The sooner they are administered, the more likely they are to succeed. If a defibrillator is not immediately available and an adult cardiac arrest is witnessed, a precordial thump should be delivered after pulselessness is determined [14, 15]. Many witnessed arrests in the emergency department will be in monitored patients; the rescuer, however, must never rely solely on the monitored signal but must always confirm the need for CPR by determining the absence of a pulse. If, after the precordial thump, a pulse has not returned, CPR is continued. In unmonitored cases, where a defibrillator is readily available, "quick-look" paddles should confirm the diagnosis of VF or VT, and countershock should be attempted at an energy level of 200 joules without delay. If the patient remains pulseless and VF or VT persists, a second shock at 200 to 300 joules should be delivered immediately. A third countershock at 360 joules is to be given if pulseless ventricular arrhythmia persists. Pulse and rhythm must be checked after each shock. If VF or VT recurs after transiently converting (rather than persisting without converting), the energy level that had previously been successful should be used in the next attempt to defibrillate.

In cases that persist in pulseless VT or fibrillation despite three attempts at countershock, CPR is initiated, supplemental oxygen is added when available, intravenous access is established, and epinephrine, 5 ml of a 1:10,000 dilution, should be administered as a bolus. It is best if the drug is administered into the central circulation; if the antecubital vein is used, the arm should be elevated and the drug flushed with 50 ml fluid to facilitate access to the central circulation. During CPR drugs should not be given into more peripheral venous access or below the level of the diaphragm, as access into the thoracic circulation may be sluggish [46, 47]. Early intubation is preferable if it can be performed without delay-

Witnessed arrest
↓
Check pulse—If no pulse
↓
Precordial thump
↓
Check pulse—If no pulse

Unwitnessed arrest
↓
Check pulse—If no pulse

↓
CPR until a defibrillator is available
↓
Check monitor for rhythm—If VF or VT[a]
↓
Defibrillate, 200 joules[b]
↓
Defibrillate, 200–300 joules[b]
↓
Defibrillate with up to 360 joules[b]
↓
CPR if no pulse
↓
Establish IV access
↓
Epinephrine, 1:10,000, 0.5–1.0 mg IV push[c]
↓
Intubate if possible[d]
↓
Defibrillate with up to 360 joules[b]
↓
Lidocaine, 1 mg/kg IV push
↓
Defibrillate with up to 360 joules[b]
↓
Bretylium, 5 mg/kg IV push[e]
↓
(Consider bicarbonate)[f]
↓
Defibrillate with up to 360 joules[b]
↓
Bretylium, 10 mg/kg IV push[e]
↓
Defibrillate with up to 360 joules[b]
↓
Repeat lidocaine or bretylium
↓
Defibrillate with up to 360 joules[b]

Fig. 3-14. Ventricular fibrillation and pulseless ventricular tachycardia. This sequence was developed to assist in teaching a broad range of patients with VF or pulseless VT. Some patients may require therapy not specified herein. This algorithm should not be construed as prohibiting such flexibility. The flow of the algorithm assumes that VF or pulseless VT is continuing. [a]Treat VF or pulseless VT identically. [b]Check for pulse after each shock; if VF or VT converts transiently, use that prior successful energy level. [c]Epinephrine should be repeated every five minutes. [d]Defibrillation and epinephrine should not be delayed to intubate, unless the patient cannot be ventilated otherwise. Early intubation is preferable if it can be accomplished simultaneously with other necessary interventions. (Endotracheal epinephrine may be used if an intravenous line cannot be established.) [e]Some may prefer repeated doses of lidocaine, which may be given in 0.5-mg/kg boluses every eight minutes to a total of 3 mg/kg. [f]Value is questionable; however, its use after the victim has failed to respond to this point is not inappropriate. Dose is 1 mEq/kg. Half the dose may be repeated every 10 minutes.

ing defibrillation attempts and administration of epinephrine. Within two to three minutes of epinephrine administration, defibrillation is again attempted at 360 joules. If VF or VT has not responded, or has responded only transiently, lidocaine hydrochloride, 1 mg/kg, should be administered as an intravenous push. Since large clinical studies [48, 49] of refractory VF have failed to demonstrate any differential advantage between bretylium and lidocaine, one may choose to use either repeated doses of lidocaine (at 0.5 mg/kg boluses every 8 minutes for a total of 3 mg/kg) or bretylium (initially at 5 mg/kg, then at 10 mg/kg). Repeated doses of epinephrine (5–10 ml of a 1:10,000 dilution) should also be administered at five-minute intervals in an attempt to maintain an adequate coronary perfusion pressure during CPR.

Adequacy of ventilation should be assessed with an arterial blood gas determination, if possible. Sodium bicarbonate is of questionable value during cardiac arrest but may be administered at 1 mEq/kg if at least 10 minutes have passed.

Repeated countershocks at 360 joules should be administered after each major drug intervention. If a perfusing supraventricular rhythm develops, a lidocaine infusion should be started at 2 mg to 4 mg per minute. A lidocaine bolus should be administered if one had not yet been given during the sequence of interventions. In addition, blood gas determination and sodium bicarbonate administration are more likely to be of value once a perfusing rhythm has been restored and the carbon dioxide pressure (PCO_2) of expired air has risen.

Asystole or Pulseless Bradyarrhythmia

Asystole or pulseless bradyarrhythmia (Fig. 3-15) is the first rhythm encountered in 30 to 40 percent of prehospital as well as hospital cardiac arrests. Asystole is obviously the end result of any pulseless rhythm and is probably most often the termination of VF. In the prehospital setting, many cases of asystole are related to delayed response time in initiating BLS or ACLS, or both. Primary asystole or bradycardic arrest associated with increased parasympathetic tone is less common but does occur. Whether this rhythm occurs as the initial rhythm or whether it follows defibrillation of VT/VF, it carries a very poor prognosis, with fewer than 1 to 2 percent of patients expected to successfully revert to a perfusing rhythm. Even more rarely will such a patient leave the hospital with reasonable neurologic integrity or significant long-term survival. Such a patient's best hope lies in the early discovery and treatment of a reversible cause for cardiovascular collapse, such as hypovolemia. Occasionally, asystole develops as a result of excessive vagal tone, such as is seen with induction of anesthesia, during surgical procedures, or with stimulation of the carotid body, bladder, or gastrointestinal tract. Unfortunately, most patients with asystole or bradycardic arrest suffer from severe coronary artery disease and are unlikely to be salvageable.

In patients with apparent asystole or bradycardic arrest, CPR is initiated; as soon as possible an intravenous line should be established and epinephrine administered, as in VT/VF. If a perfusing rhythm is not promptly restored, a full vagolytic dose of atropine should be given, with 1 mg initially and another within several minutes. Additional doses of epinephrine should be given at no longer than five-minute intervals if a favorable response has not yet occurred.

If rhythm is unclear and possibly ventricular fibrillation, defibrillate as for VF—If asystole is present[a]

↓

Continue CPR

↓

Establish IV access

↓

Epinephrine, 1:10,000, 0.5–1.0 mg IV push[b]

↓

Intubate when possible[c]

↓

Atropine, 1.0 mg IV push (repeated in 5 min)

↓

(Consider bicarbonate)[d]

↓

Consider pacing

Fig. 3-15. Asystole. This sequence was developed to assist in teaching a broad range of patients with asystole. Some patients may require therapy not specified herein. This algorithm should not be construed as prohibiting such flexibility. The flow of this algorithm assumes that asystole is continuing. [a]Asystole should be confirmed in two leads. [b]Epinephrine should be repeated every five minutes. [c]CPR and the administration of epinephrine and atropine should not be delayed by attempts at intubation, unless the victim cannot be ventilated otherwise. Early intubation is preferable if it can be accomplished along with other necessary interventions. (Endotracheal epinephrine and atropine may be used if an intravenous line cannot be established.) [d] Value is questionable; however, its use after the victim has failed to respond to this point is not inappropriate. Dose is 1 mEq/kg. Half the dose may be repeated every 10 minutes.

It has been demonstrated that VF can masquerade as asystole in several leads for minutes at a time [50]. Given this possibility, it is important to check at least two different lead configurations at 90-degree orientation to confirm the diagnosis of asystole. If the diagnosis is still in question, early attempts at defibrillation are warranted [51].

As in other forms of arrest, sodium bicarbonate has not been shown to be of benefit until a perfusing rhythm has been reestablished. Calcium has also not been shown to be of value and may be detrimental (see previous section).

Temporary artificial pacing is of no likely benefit in primary or postcountershock asystole or bradycardic arrests. The use of pacing with endocardial, percutaneous transthoracic, or external cutaneous electrodes has led to pitifully few long-term survivals in these cases [22, 23].

The use of isoproterenol in an attempt to stimulate pacemakers through its beta-adrenergic agonist effects has not proved beneficial. Indeed, its peripheral beta stimulation produces a decrease in arterial resistance and perfusion pressure that is likely to be detrimental, whereas alpha agonists appear to increase myocardial and cerebral perfusion [52–54].

Electromechanical Dissociation

Electromechanical dissociation (EMD) is present when an arrest victim is found to have organized, electrocardiographic ventricular complexes (QRS) unassociated with effective ventricular contraction (Fig. 3-16). Pulseless VT and wide-complex bradyarrhythmias are not considered here as they are likely to be of a different pathophysiology than

Continue CPR
↓
Establish IV access
↓
Epinephrine, 1:10,000, 0.5–1.0 mg IV push[a]
↓
Intubate when possible[b]
↓
(Consider bicarbonate)[c]
↓
Consider: Hypovolemia
Cardiac tamponade
Tension pneumothorax
Hypoxemia
Acidosis
Pulmonary embolism

Fig. 3-16. Electromechanical dissociation. This sequence was developed to assist in teaching a broad range of patients with electromechanical dissociation. Some patients may require therapy not specified herein. This algorithm should not be construed as prohibiting such flexibility. The flow of this algorithm assumes that electromechanical dissociation is continuing. [a]Epinephrine should be repeated every five minutes. [b]CPR and the administration of epinephrine should not be delayed by attempts at intubation, unless the victim cannot be ventilated otherwise. Early intubation is preferable if it can be accomplished along with other necessary interventions. (Endotracheal epinephrine may be used if an intravenous line cannot be established.) [c]Value is questionable; however, its use after the victim has failed to respond to this point is not inappropriate. Dose is 1 mEq/kg. Half the dose may be repeated every 10 minutes.

pulseless narrow-complex EMD. When narrow-complex EMD is encountered, the following causes should be considered: severe hypovolemia, cardiac tamponade, massive pulmonary embolism, tension pneumothorax, and severe myocardial contractile dysfunction.

With the diagnosis of EMD, CPR is initiated and as soon as possible, volume is administered in the form of intravenous crystalloid or colloid. If EMD is indeed caused by intravascular volume depletion, a fluid challenge may return a pulse. Epinephrine or dopamine should be administered as in other forms of arrest, and doses should be repeated if a pulse has not returned. In patients at high risk of pericardial effusions—that is, in patients hospitalized with recent myocardial infarction, in those with known malignancy, in patients with severe renal failure, or in those recently subjected to cardiac catheterization—pericardiocentesis should be attempted early in the course of CPR. In prehospital arrests pericardial tamponade is rare, but an attempt at pericardiocentesis is warranted if there is no favorable response to volume or alpha agonists.

SPECIAL SITUATIONS

Near-drowning victims may recover after prolonged periods of submersion, especially in cold water. Apparently, the hypothermia and the bradycardia of the diving reflex protect against organ damage [55, 56]. Successful resuscitation has been described after 40 minutes or more of submersion in cold water [56, 57]. Since it is often difficult for bystanders and rescuers to estimate the duration of submersion, CPR should usually be initiated at the scene, unless there exists physical evidence of irreversible death, such as putrefaction. (See the section of this chapter on near-drowning.)

Hypothermia can occur with environmental exposures other than cold-water drowning. The body's ability to maintain temperature is diminished by alcohol, sedation, antidepressants, neurologic problems, and advanced age. Because of the associated bradycardia and oxygen sparing effects, prolonged hypothermia and arrest may be tolerated with complete recovery. A longer period may be needed to establish breathlessness and pulselessness because of the profound bradycardia and slowed respiratory rate. Thoracotomy with open-chest CPR has also been advocated in resistant cases of hypothermic arrest, as will be discussed further. Resuscitative efforts should not be abandoned until near normal temperature has been reestablished [58] (see Chap. 34).

Electric shock can lead to tetanic spasm of respiratory muscles or convulsion causing respiratory arrest. Ventricular fibrillation or asystole can occur from the electric shock or after prolonged respiratory arrest. Before initiating assessment and CPR, the potential rescuers must ascertain that the victim is no longer in contact with the electrical energy and that "live wires" are not in dangerous proximity. If the victim is located at the top of a utility pole, CPR is best instituted after the victim is lowered to the ground [59] (see Chap. 77).

Open-chest CPR with thoracotomy should be applied early in cases of penetrating chest trauma associated with cardiac arrest, as was mentioned previously. In such patients, thoracotomy by trained personnel will allow for the relief of pericardial tamponade and possible control of exsanguinating hemorrhage. Well-equipped trauma centers should have multidisciplinary teams that can provide early definitive surgical treatment. The unanswered question is whether another subgroup of patients who have not responded to conventional ACLS techniques (including defibrillation attempts and drugs) would be benefited by thoracotomy and open-chest CPR. Results of animal studies suggest that survival may be improved over closed-chest compression if open-chest CPR is used within the first 15 minutes of arrest [60–62]. If open-chest CPR is delayed until 20 minutes or more after closed-chest CPR has been in progress, there is no improvement in outcome despite improved hemodynamics [62]. In patients with out-of-hospital arrest in whom open-chest CPR was attempted after 30 minutes of conventional CPR, survival did not improve [63].

Other instances in which open-chest CPR may be considered include: (1) cardiac arrest in patients with chest deformity in whom closed-chest CPR is not providing a pulse; (2) penetrating abdominal trauma with deterioration and cardiac arrest in which aortic cross-clamping may provide temporary control of abdominal hemorrhage; (3) blunt trauma with cardiac arrest; and (4) cardiac arrest due to hypothermia, pulmonary embolism, pericardial tamponade, or abdominal hemorrhage in which initiation of conventional therapy and closed-chest CPR is not proving effective. In these cases, the decision for open-chest CPR should be made quickly, within the first quarter-hour of arrest if possible. This decision presupposes quick availability of definitive surgical intervention.

REFERENCES

1. Montgomery, WH, Donegan, J, and McIntyre, KM (eds.). Standards for cardiopulmonary resuscitation (CPR) and emergency cardiac care (ECC). *JAMA* 255:2905, 1986.
2. *Textbook of Advanced Cardiac Life Support*. Dallas: American Heart Association, 1987.
3. Abramson, N, et al. An international collaborative clinical study mechanism for resuscitation research. *Resuscitation* 10: 141, 1982.
4. Longstreth, WT, Diehr, P, and Inui, TS. Prediction of awakening after out-of-hospital cardiac arrest. *N Engl J Med* 308:1378, 1983.
5. Melker, RJ, and Banner, MJ. Ventilation during CPR: Two-rescuer standards reappraised. *Ann Emerg Med* 14:397, 1985.
6. Salem, MR, et al. Efficacy of cricoid pressure in preventing gastric inflation during bag-mask ventilation in pediatric patients. *Anesthesiology* 40:96, 1974.
7. Melker, RJ. Alternative methods of ventilation during respiratory and cardiac arrest. *Circulation* 74 (Suppl IV):63, 1986.
8. Krischer, JP, et al. Complications of cardiac resuscitation. *Chest* 92:287, 1987.
9. Nagel, EL, et al. Complications of CPR. *Crit Care Med* 9:424, 1981.
10. Powner, DJ, Holcombe, PA, and Mello, LA. Cardiopulmonary resuscitation–related injuries. *Crit Care Med* 12:54, 1984.
11. Carveth, SW, et al. Training in advanced cardiac life support. *JAMA* 235:2311, 1976.
12. Lowenstein, SR, et al. Benefits of training physicians in advanced cardiac life support. *Chest* 89:512, 1986.
13. Sellick, BA. Cricoid pressure to control regurgitation of stomach contents during induction of anaesthesia. *Lancet* 2:404, 1961.
14. Caldwell, G, et al. Simple mechanical methods of cardioversion: A defense of the precordial thump and cough version. *Br Med J* 291:627, 1985.
15. Pennington, JE, Taylor, J, and Lown, B. Chest thump for reverting ventricular tachycardia. *N Engl J Med* 283:1192, 1970.
16. Wei, JY, Green, HL, and Weisgeldt, ML. Cough facilitated cardioversion of ventricular tachycardia. *Am J Cardiol* 45:174, 1980.
17. Yakaitis, RW, and Redding, JS. Precordial thumping during cardiac resuscitation. *Crit Care Med* 1:22, 1973.
18. Weaver, WD, et al. Ventricular defibrillation: A comparative trial using 175-J and 320-J shocks. *N Engl J Med* 207:1101, 1982.
19. Kerber, RE, et al. Determinants of defibrillation: Prospective analysis of 183 patients. *Am J Cardiol* 52:739, 1983.
20. Zoll, PM, et al. External noninvasive temporary cardiac pacing: Clinical trials. *Circulation* 71:937, 1985.
21. Falk, RH, et al. External non-invasive cardiac pacing in out-of-hospital cardiac arrest. *Crit Care Med* 11:779, 1983.
22. Hedges, JR, Syverud, SA, and Dalsey, WC. Developments in transcutaneous and transthoracic pacing during bradyasystolic arrest. *Ann Emerg Med* 13:822, 1984.
23. Clinton, JE, et al. Emergency noninvasive external pacing. *J Emerg Med* 2:155, 1985.
24. Niemann, JT, et al. Pressure-synchronized cineangiography during experimental cardiopulmonary resuscitation. *Circulation* 64:985, 1981.
25. Jastremski, MS, Matthias, HD, and Randell, PA. Femoral venous catheterization during cardiopulmonary resuscitation: A critical appraisal. *J Emerg Med* 1:387, 1984.
26. Falk, JL, Rackow, EC, and Weil, MH. End-tidal carbon dioxide concentration during cardiopulmonary resuscitation. *N Engl J Med* 318:607, 1988.
27. Garnett, AR, et al. End-tidal carbon dioxide monitoring during cardiopulmonary resuscitation. *JAMA* 257:512, 1987.
28. Trevino, RP, et al. End-tidal CO_2 as a guide to successful cardiopulmonary resuscitation: A preliminary report. *Crit Care Med* 13:910, 1985.
29. Weil, MH, et al. Cardiac output and end-tidal carbon dioxide. *Crit Care Med* 13:907, 1985.
30. Weil, MH, et al. Arterial blood gases fail to reflect acid-base status during cardiopulmonary resuscitation: A preliminary report. *Crit Care Med* 13:884, 1985.
31. Jaffe, A. Cardiovascular pharmacology I. *Circulation* 74 (Suppl IV):70, 1986.
32. Guerci, AD, et al. Failure of sodium bicarbonate to improve resuscitation from ventricular fibrillation in dogs. *Circulation* 74 (Suppl 4):75, 1986.
33. Shoemaker, WC, et al. Fluid therapy in emergency resuscitation: Clinical evaluation of colloid and crystalloid regimens. *Crit Care Med* 9:367, 1981.
34. Otto, CW. Cardiovascular pharmacology II: The use of catecholamines, pressor agents, digitalis, and corticosteroids in CPR and emergency cardiac care. *Circulation* 74 (Suppl 4):80, 1986.
35. Alquist, RP. A study of adrenotropic receptors. *Am J Physiol* 153:586, 1948.
36. Anderson, JL, et al. Kinetics of antifibrillatory effects of bretylium: Correlation with myocardial drug concentration. *Am J Cardiol* 46:583, 1980.
37. Babbs, CF, et al. Elevation of ventricular defibrillation threshold in dogs by antiarrhythmic drugs. *Am Heart J* 98:345, 1979.
38. Bacaner, MB. Treatment of ventricular fibrillation and other acute arrhythmias with bretylium tosylate. *Am J Cardiol* 21: 530, 1968.
39. Paraskos, JA. Cardiovascular pharmacology III: Atropine, calcium, calcium blockers, and beta blockers. *Circulation* 74 (Suppl IV):86, 1986.
40. Kay, JH, and Blalock, A. The use of calcium chloride in the treatment of cardiac arrest in patients. *Surg Gynecol Obstet* 93:97, 1951.
41. Stueven, HA, et al. Use of calcium in prehospital cardiac arrest. *Ann Emerg Med* 12:136, 1983.
42. Harrison, EE, and Amey, BD. Use of calcium in electromechanical dissociation. *Ann Emerg Med* 13:844, 1984.
43. Carlon, GC, et al. Calcium chloride administration in normocalcemic critically ill patients. *Crit Care Med* 8:209, 1980.
44. Dembo, DH. Calcium in advanced life support. *Crit Care Med* 9:358, 1981.
45. Thompson, BM, Stueven, HA, and Tonsfeldt, DJ. Calcium: Limited indications, some danger. *Circulation* 74 (Suppl IV):90, 1986.
46. Barsan, WG, Levy, RC, and Weir, H. Lidocaine levels during CPR: Differences after peripheral venous, central venous, and intracardiac injections. *Ann Emerg Med* 10:73, 1981.
47. Hedges, JR, et al. Central versus peripheral intravenous routes in cardiopulmonary resuscitation. *Am J Emerg Med* 2:385, 1984.
48. Haynes, RE, et al. Comparison of bretylium tosylate and lidocaine in management of out of hospital ventricular fibrillation: A randomized clinical trial. *Am J Cardiol* 48:353, 1981.
49. Olson, DW, et al. A randomized comparison study of bretylium tosylate and lidocaine in resuscitation of patients from out-of-hospital ventricular fibrillation in a paramedic system. *Ann Emerg Med* 13:807, 1984.
50. Ewy, GA, et al. Ventricular fibrillation masquerading as ventricular standstill. *Crit Care Med* 9:841, 1981.
51. Ornato, JP, et al. Treatment of presumed asystole during prehospital cardiac arrest: Superiority of electrical countershock. *Am J Emerg Med* 3:395, 1985.
52. Michael, JR, et al. Mechanisms by which epinephrine augments cerebral and myocardial perfusion during cardiopulmonary resuscitation in dogs. *Circulation* 69:822, 1984.

53. Redding, JS, and Pearson, JW. Evaluation of drugs for cardiac resuscitation. *Anesthesiology* 24:203, 1963.
54. Sanders, AB. The roles of methoxamine and norepinephrine in electromechanical dissociation. *Ann Emerg Med* 13:835, 1984.
55. Scholander, PF. The master switch of life. *Sci Am* 209:92, 1963.
56. Siebke, H, et al. Survival after 40 minutes submersion without cerebral sequelae. *Lancet* 1:1275, 1975.
57. Southwick, FS, and Dalgish, PH. Recovery after prolonged asystolic cardiac arrest in profound hypothermia. A case report and literature review. *JAMA* 243:1250, 1980.
58. Steinman, AM. The hypothermic code: CPR controversy revisited. *J Emerg Med Serv* 10:32, 1983.
59. Gordon, AS, Ridolpho, PF, and Cole, JE. *Definitive Studies on Pole-Top Resuscitation.* Camarillo, Calif.: Research Resuscitation Laboratories, Electric Power Research Institute, 1983.
60. Bircher, NG, and Safar, P. Cerebral preservation during cardiopulmonary resuscitation. *Crit Care Med* 13:185, 1985.
61. Sanders, AB, et al. Improved resuscitation from cardiac arrest with open-chest CPR in dogs. *Crit Care Med* 9:384, 1981.
62. Sanders, AB, et al. Importance of the duration of inadequate coronary perfusion pressure in resuscitation from cardiac arrest. *J Am Coll Cardiol* 6:113, 1985.
63. Geehr, EC, Lewis, FR, and Auerbach, PS. Failure of open-heart massage to improve survival after prehospital non-traumatic cardiac arrest (letter). *N Engl J Med* 314:1189, 1986.

SELECTED READING

Adjuncts for artificial circulation. In *Textbook of Advanced Cardiac Life Support.* Dallas: American Heart Association, 1987. P. 43.

Eisenberg, MS, et al. Treatment of out-of-hospital cardiac arrest with rapid defibrillation by emergency medical technicians. *N Engl J Med* 302:1379, 1980.

Healthcare Provider's Manual for Basic Life Support. Dallas: American Heart Association, 1988.

Hedges, JR, et al. Prehospital trial of emergency transcutaneous cardiac pacing. *Circulation* 76:1337, 1987.

Melker, R, Cavallaro, D, and Krischer, J. One-rescuer CPR—A reappraisal of present recommendations for ventilation. *Crit Care Med* 9:423, 1981.

Melker, RJ. Asynchronous and other alternative methods of ventilation during CPR. *Ann Emerg Med* 13:758, 1984.

Myerburg, RJ, et al. Survivors of prehospital cardiac arrest. *JAMA* 247:1485, 1982.

Stueven, HA, et al. Calcium chloride: Reassessment of use in asystole. *Ann Emerg Med* 13:820, 1984.

Weil, MH, et al. Acid-base determinants of survival after cardiopulmonary resuscitation. *Crit Care Med* 13:888, 1985.

CARDIAC ARREST: OBSTRUCTED AIRWAY

N. Heramba Prasad
E. Jackson Allison, Jr.
Nicholas H. Benson

ADULT BASIC LIFE SUPPORT

Complete upper-airway obstruction can cause unconsciousness and cardiopulmonary arrest and thus needs immediate attention and expert management.

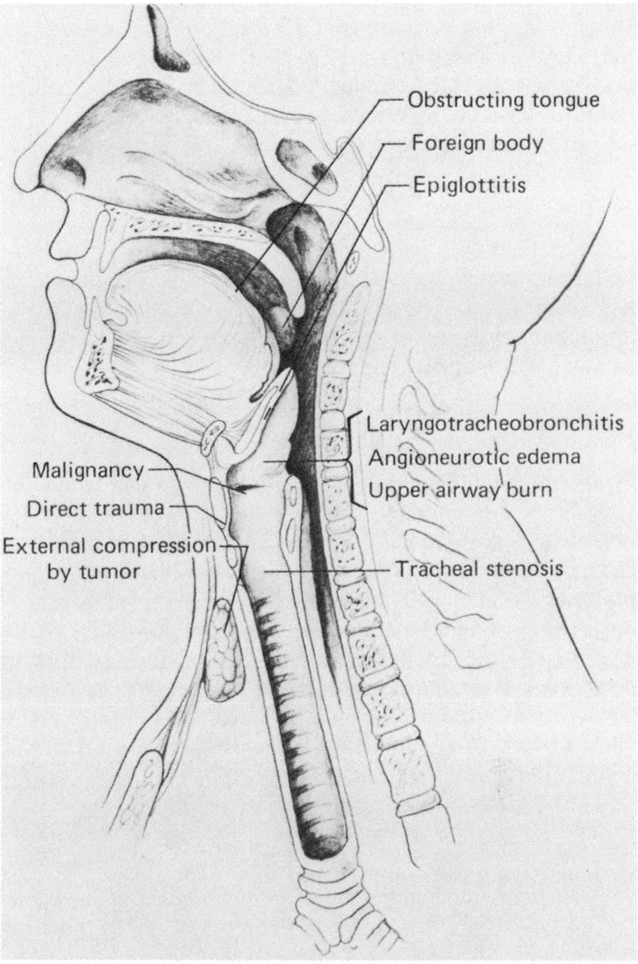

Fig. 3-17. Causes of upper airway obstruction.

Causes of Airway Obstruction

Obstruction due to the tongue falling backward in an unconscious person and the aspiration of a foreign body (e.g., food bolus or other nonorganic materials) are the most common causes of complete airway obstruction. Some other common causes of airway obstruction are shown in Fig. 3-17. Although these conditions do not usually cause complete airway obstruction, the emergency physician must be alert to a possible rapid deterioration requiring immediate airway intervention. Such conditions include infections such as epiglottitis, croup, and abscesses; trauma; burns; allergic reactions resulting in angioneurotic edema; malignancies; and tracheal stenosis.

Obstruction by the Tongue

The most common cause of airway obstruction that an emergency physician encounters is the tongue falling backward against the hypopharynx and obstructing the upper airway in an unconscious victim. Cardiac arrest, drug overdose, and trauma are also common causes. In the unconscious patient, muscle flaccidity causes the mandible and the tongue to sag backward against the hypopharynx. This condition can be corrected by either the head tilt–chin lift (Fig. 3-18) or jaw-thrust maneuvers.

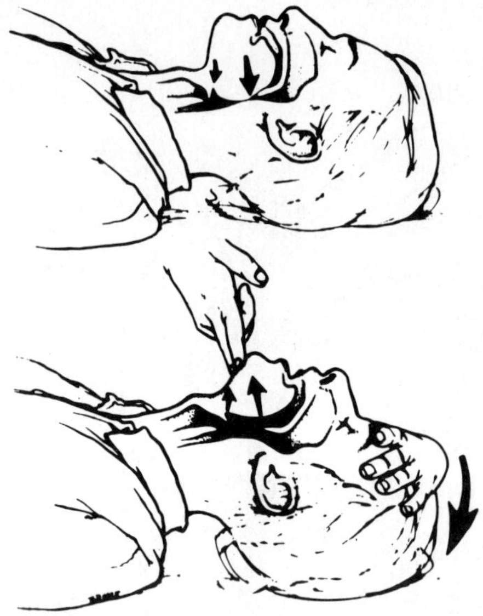

Fig. 3-18. Head tilt–chin lift maneuver.

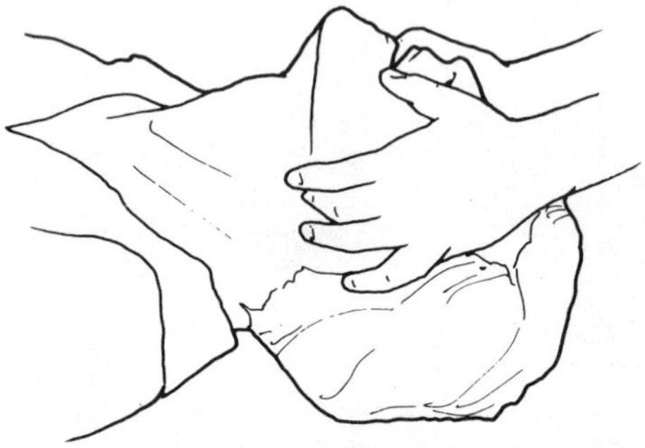

Fig. 3-19. Mandible or jaw thrust method for opening the airway.

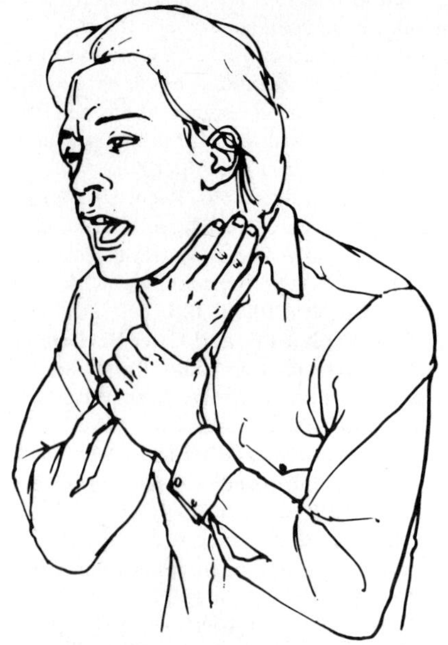

Fig. 3-20. Universal distress signal.

The modified jaw thrust is especially useful in trauma victims when the status of the cervical spine is uncertain. In this maneuver, the jaw is displaced forward without extending the neck. The rescuer positions himself or herself at the head of the victim and places the fingers of both hands behind the angles of the mandibles, as shown in Fig. 3-19. The rescuer displaces the jaw anteriorly without tilting the head. Thus, the neck is held in a neutral position. If jaw thrust is unsuccessful in opening the airway, the head can be tilted backward very slightly. Quite frequently these maneuvers alone are sufficient to open an obstructed airway. The airway can be supported further by the use of an oropharyngeal or nasopharyngeal tube to prevent the tongue from falling backward again (see Procedures 2 and 3). If these measures fail, further advanced measures such as endotracheal intubation may be necessary.

Foreign Bodies

Choking on meat is a common cause of airway obstruction in adults. Factors associated with adults' choking on food include ingestion of alcohol or other drugs, especially anticholinergics; dentures and poor chewing habits; rapid eating; and laughing and talking while eating. This emergency, when it occurs in restaurants, has been mistaken for a heart attack, and hence it is sometimes called a "café coronary." Approximately 3,000 deaths caused by foreign-body obstruction are reported annually.

Recognition of Foreign-Body Airway Obstruction

The sequence of events during airway obstruction progresses rapidly. Three stages have been described. In the first stage the patient senses the obstruction and is in obvious distress. He or she is unable to speak, breathe, or cough if there is complete obstruction and may grasp the neck with the thumb and fingers (universal distress signal) (Fig. 3-20). There may be attempts at respiration, but no air exchange occurs. Marked supraclavicular and intercostal retractions are present and the patient becomes cyanotic. In the second phase the victim becomes unconscious, respiratory movements cease, and blood pressure and pulse start to fall. In the last stage the pulse and blood pressure disappear and the patient goes into cardiac arrest.

The clinical manifestation of an aspirated foreign body depends on the degree of airway obstruction, and is classified as partial or complete obstruction. During partial obstruction, the patient is able to breathe and cough forcibly. He or she may experience wheezing and stridor during the bouts of coughing.

Management

The degree of intervention necessary depends on the adequacy of air exchange. In the presence of good air exchange to the lungs, it is preferable to encourage the person to continue coughing efforts in order to dislodge the foreign body. The rescuer may do more harm by trying to intervene. The emergency medical services (EMS) system should be activated. The air exchange may be poor initially or good air exchange may progress to poor exchange. The cough may

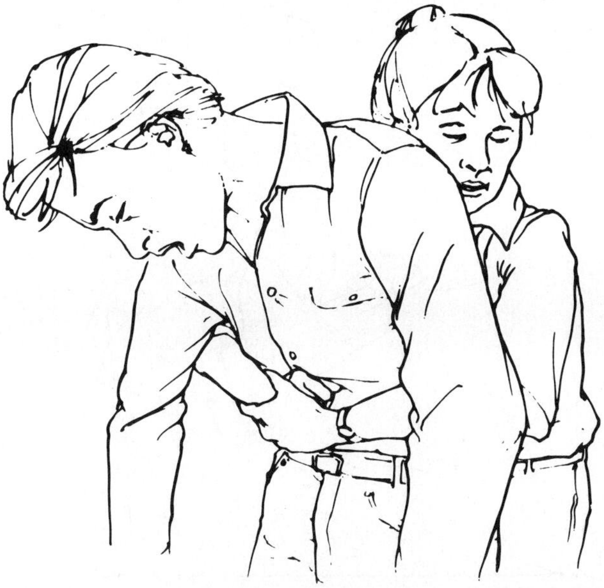

Fig. 3-21. Subdiaphragmatic abdominal thrust (Heimlich maneuver) for relieving foreign body airway obstruction.

become ineffective; increasing inspiratory difficulty and cyanosis may prevail. With complete airway obstruction the victim is unable to speak, breathe, or cough and may clutch the neck with thumb and fingers, the universal distress signal. The public should be encouraged to use this sign so that bystanders will be able to distinguish choking from heart attack, stroke, seizures, fainting, or drug overdose.

Heimlich Maneuver

The subdiaphragmatic abdominal thrust (Heimlich maneuver) is recommended for relieving foreign body airway obstruction. If the person is conscious and standing, the rescuer stands behind the victim, wrapping his or her arms around the waist, and places the clenched fist of one hand between the umbilicus and the xiphoid process in the upper abdomen. The fist is placed with the thumb pointing toward the abdomen. The rescuer then cups the fist with the other hand and presses the victim's abdomen with a quick upward thrust (Fig. 3-21). The clenched fist should be well below the xiphoid process in order to avoid injury to internal organs. If the attempt is unsuccessful, it may be repeated as needed. Each individual thrust should be a separate and distinct movement. The abdominal thrust can also be self-administered. The victim makes a fist with one hand and places the thumb side on the abdomen above the navel and below the xiphoid process. The victim then cups the fist with the other hand and quickly presses inward and upward. Several thrusts may be necessary to clear the airway.

Currently, the American Heart Association (AHA) does not recommend back blows. It has been suggested that, as a single method, back blows may not be as effective as the Heimlich maneuver in adults. Because of this and in an effort to simplify training, the AHA recommends the Heimlich maneuver as the only method to be used.

If the person becomes unconscious, he or she is placed in the supine position. The rescuer then straddles the thighs and places the heel of one hand against the victim's abdomen and, with the help of the other hand, delivers quick upward thrusts (Fig. 3-22).

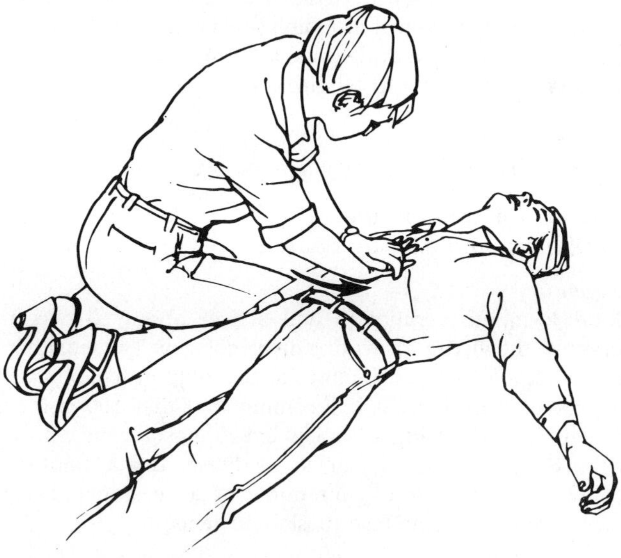

Fig. 3-22. Heimlich maneuver for the unconscious victim.

Chest thrusts can be used in the advanced stages of pregnancy or in the markedly obese victim. In these circumstances the subdiaphragmatic abdominal thrust is replaced with the backward chest thrust. If the victim is conscious, the rescuer stands behind him and places the arms around the victim's chest. The rescuer then places the thumb side of the fist in the middle of the breastbone, taking care not to injure the xiphoid process and the margins of the rib cage. The rescuer cups the fist with the other hand and performs backward thrusts until the foreign body is expelled. The chest-thrust technique can also be used in an unconscious victim. He or she is placed in the supine position and the rescuer straddles the abdominal area and administers backward thrusts at midsternal level.

Finger Sweep

The finger sweep technique can be used in an unconscious victim to clean the pharynx and mouth. With the patient lying supine, the mouth is opened by grasping both the tongue and the lower jaw and lifting the mandible (tongue-jaw lift). This alone may partially relieve the obstruction. Placing the index finger of the other hand down along the side of the cheek and deep into the throat, the posterior pharyngeal area is swept. A hooking action is used to dislodge the foreign body and maneuver it into the mouth so that it can be removed. Caution must be taken not to force the object deeper into the airway.

If the initial attempt to ventilate the victim is unsuccessful, the rescuer repositions the victim's head and again attempts to ventilate. Improper positioning of the chin and head is the most common cause of difficulty with ventilation. If the victim still cannot be ventilated, the rescuer should proceed with the foreign-body airway obstruction maneuvers described earlier.

In certain situations, the mouth-to-nose technique may be more effective. This technique is recommended when it is impossible to ventilate through the victim's mouth, the mouth cannot be opened (trismus), the mouth is seriously injured, or a tight mouth-to-mouth seal is difficult to achieve. In patients who have undergone a laryngectomy, mouth-to-stoma ventilation should be attempted.

ADULT ADVANCED LIFE SUPPORT

Adjuncts for Oxygenation, Ventilation, and Airway Control

Oxygen

Mouth-to-mouth ventilation will deliver about 16 percent oxygen to the victim, providing an alveolar oxygen tension of 80 mm Hg. Because of the low cardiac output, hypoxia will be present; therefore, it is recommended that 100 percent oxygen be used during advanced life support for the cardiac victim. Supplemental oxygen can be delivered to a spontaneously breathing person by a number of devices, including a nasal cannula, plastic face mask, and tents.

Masks

Before attempts are made to intubate, it is important to oxygenate by mouth-to-mouth, mouth-to-mask, or bag-valve-mask ventilation. (Mouth-to-mouth ventilation should be avoided, if possible, because of the risk of contagious disease.) A well-fitting mask is an effective, simple adjunct for providing artificial ventilation by appropriately trained personnel. The mask should have the following characteristics: It should be transparent, it should fit snugly on the face, it should have an oxygen inlet, and it should be available in many sizes. Some masks are equipped with a one-way valve that provides diversion of the victim's exhaled air away from the rescuer. The rescuer positions himself or herself at the top of the patient's head and opens the airway using a jaw-thrust maneuver. The mask is fitted onto the victim's mouth and nose and an adequate seal is assured. The rescuer uses both hands to hold the mask over the face of the victim, at the same time using the jaw-thrust maneuver. The rescuer, after taking a deep breath, blows air through the coupling unit of the mask. Bag-valve-mask ventilation (BVMV) can also be used in this instance by experienced personnel in providing oxygenation before intubation (Fig. 3-23) (see Procedure 1). Some studies have shown that in a prehospital setting, mouth-to-mask ventilation when used with an oxygen inlet provides better oxygenation and mask seal than BVMV. However, BVMV is always the preferred method of ventilation in the hospital.

The delivered fractional oxygen percentage (FDO_2) of the resuscitation bag depends on the rate of ventilation, the volume delivered from the bag, the flow of oxygen into the bag, the refilling time of the bag after compression, and the type of reservoir used. Corrugated tubes are not as effective as reservoir bags. It is possible to deliver oxygen concentration of 90 percent or greater with BVMV devices. This requires a tight face seal, a reservoir bag, and an oxygen inlet with a flow rate sufficient to keep the reservoir bag filled (usually 15 liters/min). A demand valve might be useful if a reservoir bag is not available. Bag-valve-mask ventilation, instituted early after chin lift–head tilt maneuvers to open the airway, along with the introduction of an oropharyngeal or a nasopharyngeal tube, can sustain patients for an extended period of time. On some occasions no other airway intervention may be necessary.

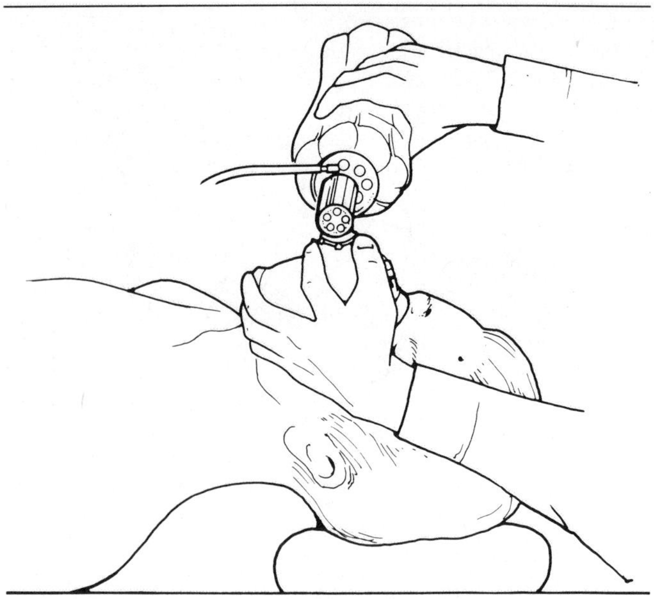

Fig. 3-23. Bag and mask unit. Note position of hands.

The major advantage of BVMV is that it can provide a sense of compliance to the rescuer, indicating the need for change in pressure and alerting the rescuer to the presence of airway obstruction, pneumothorax, and so forth. The device is readily available and can be used with an enriched oxygen mixture.

Bag-valve-mask ventilation has several disadvantages. First, the effectiveness of ventilation depends on the rescuer's level of experience. Frequently, two rescuers are needed, one to hold the mask firmly on the victim's face and the other to compress the bag. Even experienced anesthesiologists have found it difficult to hold the mask with one hand and compress the bag with the other. Second, gastric distention can occur. This can be controlled by adjusting the force of the compressions on the bag. Third, in a person with a full stomach, BVMV can cause regurgitation of gastric contents. It is preferable not to use BVMV in these instances. Cricoid pressure during BVMV may help prevent this problem in an unconscious victim.

Intubation Using the Esophageal Obturator Technique

In the search for easier and simpler intubation that can be used in the prehospital setting, numerous devices have been developed in the past two decades. In 1968 the esophageal obturator airway (EOA) was introduced (see Procedure 4B). A few years later modifications were made to the original tube, resulting in the esophageal gastric tube airway. The principle of the esophageal obturator is as follows: The tube has a blind end; it is inserted into the esophagus; there is no need to extend the neck; once the tube is in the esophagus, the balloon is inflated and the esophagus is occluded; with a tightly sealed mask on the face, ventilation is accomplished through side ports in the tube; the holes open into the retropharynx and, because of the occlusion of the esophagus, air enters the trachea.

This technique is relatively simple and has been used extensively in various EMS systems. The EOA has enjoyed generalized acceptance as well as harsh criticism. One original problem was an ill-fitting mask, but this was subsequently corrected by design changes. Other criticisms toward the EOA have been: concern over injury to the esophagus, since excessive cuff inflation can cause pressure and damage to the esophagus distal to the cuff; rupture of the esophagus as a result of forceful retching against an occluded esophagus; the fact that the EOA does not address the issue of secretions, foreign bodies, and excessive bleeding in the upper airway that can potentially be aspirated into the trachea; and fear of improper placement of the airway into the trachea.

Despite all of these problems, the EOA has enjoyed enormous popularity all across the nation with numerous EMS systems. It has been thought that the skill needed to introduce the EOA is minimal compared to that required for orotracheal intubation and that the training time is also less. However, recently both of these beliefs have been challenged.

The incidence of endotracheal intubation with the EOA is reported to be between 2 and 20 percent; unrecognized, prehospital endotracheal intubation is perhaps more frequent. Rupture of the esophagus is estimated to occur in as many as two percent of patients.

Because of the disadvantages mentioned, the EOA was later modified. The blind esophageal obturator was replaced by a tube with openings at both ends so that gastric contents could be aspirated with a nasogastric tube. A separate opening was made in the face mask, through which ventilation could be accomplished. The esophagus was occluded with a balloon on the open-ended tube. The modified version of the tube came to be known as an esophageal gastric tube airway (EGTA). This particular modification still does not eliminate the danger of aspiration from upper-airway secretions and foreign bodies, or from accidental endotracheal intubation. Because of these concerns various other tubes are being field tested. One such modification is the tracheal esophageal airway (TEA), modified in such a way that if it enters the trachea, it can be used as an endotracheal tube and ventilated accordingly. If the tube goes into the esophagus, it essentially acts as an EOA.

The pharyngeal tracheal lumen (PTL) airway is gaining acceptance. This device addresses the issue of upper-airway secretions. The airway consists of a long tube and a short tube (Fig. 3-24). The long endotracheal-type tube is located within the shorter tube. The tip of the long tube enters either the trachea or the esophagus while the short tube enters the retropharynx above the epiglottis. Both tubes are fitted with balloons. The balloon on the short tube, when inflated, will fill the oropharynx and control upper-airway hemorrhage and aspiration. The airway is inserted until the block contacts the patient's teeth. The long tube presumably will have entered the esophagus. Both balloons are then inflated and ventilation is attempted by blowing into the short tube. If the chest rises, the long tube has entered the esophagus and ventilation is carried out through the short tube. If the chest does not rise, the long tube has presumably entered the trachea and ventilation is carried out through it in the same manner as with the endotracheal tube. Both the long and short tubes are fitted with standard adapters for connection with ventilation devices. Initial studies indicate that the PTL can successfully contain hemorrhage and secretions from the upper airway. The reliability and the acceptability of the PTL in the field remain to be seen.

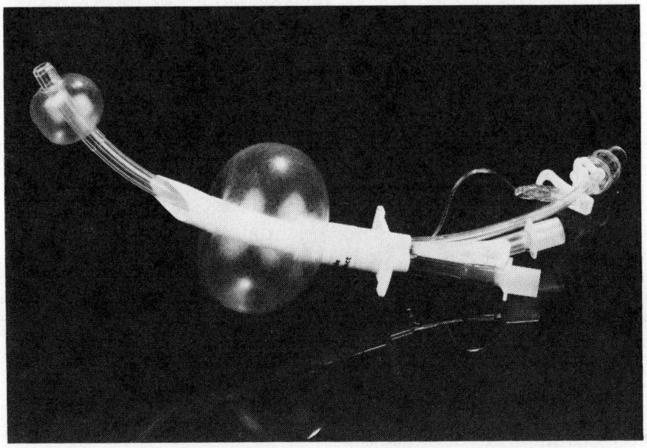

Fig. 3-24. Pharyngeal tracheal lumen airway.

Another modification is the esophageal tracheal combitube (ETC tube), which is similar to the PTL in design and principle. The proximal balloon is smaller than that of the PTL, however, and is placed between the tongue and soft palate. A plastic twin-lumen tube, with one lumen resembling an EOA and the other an endotracheal tube (ETT), is used. Ventilation is possible after either esophageal or tracheal placement. The proximal balloon eliminates the need for a face mask. A study of the ETC in 24 patients undergoing elective surgery, and 21 patients receiving cardiopulmonary resuscitation, indicates that the ETC is as effective as the ETT.

Orotracheal Intubation

Orotracheal intubation (see Procedure 4A) is the most common and definitive method of establishing and managing the airway. It is safe, requires no surgery, and is performed under direct vision. In experienced hands the procedure is rapid and accurate. There are, however, some disadvantages to the use of orotracheal intubation. The most important is the danger to the cervical spine in a victim of blunt trauma. The level of consciousness of the patient may be a limiting factor. In patients with head injuries, excessive trismus makes it impossible to open the mouth unless muscle relaxants are used. Careful judgment and proper technique are needed under these circumstances.

Certain measures can be employed to ensure success of intubation. The use of a stylet in the endotracheal tube is not always necessary but may help direct the tip of the tube into the trachea. The Sellick maneuver (applying direct pressure over the cricoid cartilage) can also help visualize the glottic opening when the larynx is located far anteriorly.

Complications of endotracheal intubation are numerous. In a prospective study of 150 critically ill patients, 62 percent of the patients who underwent endotracheal intubation had complications related to the airway. Some of the common complications reported are:

1. Cervical fracture and subluxation
2. Damage to the teeth by applying force through the laryngoscope blade
3. Injuries to the retropharyngeal structures such as hematomas and lacerations, later causing infection
4. Perforation of the pyriform sinus
5. Emphysema of the mediastinum and subcutaneous tissues
6. Pneumothorax
7. Aspiration of blood, teeth, and laryngoscope bulb
8. Improper intubation (bronchial, esophageal)
9. Tracheal perforation
10. Damage to vocal cords
11. Overinflation of the cuff, resulting in tracheitis and ulcers leading to necrosis
12. Tracheoesophageal or tracheopleural fistula

In an attempt to overcome the difficulties in a patient with potential cervical spine injury, other techniques have been described. Tactile orotracheal intubation may be helpful in these situations. The physician stands to the left side of the patient facing his or her right shoulder and places the index and middle finger of the gloved left hand into the patient's mouth. By sliding the finger down, the epiglottis is palpated. Using the fingers as a guide, the physician inserts an endotracheal tube with the stylet inside and the tip curved to form a hook just posterior to the epiglottis and guides it through the epiglottic opening. During this procedure, the danger of being bitten on the fingers is of obvious concern to the physician. Tactile orotracheal intubation can be accomplished in an unconscious person irrespective of the length of the physician's index and middle fingers.

Use of a lighted stylet to facilitate endotracheal intubation has also been described. The rationale is that this allows the procedure to be accomplished without undue extension of the neck. A flexible surgical light acts as a stylet and is inserted into a standard endotracheal tube. The tip of the endotracheal tube is carefully bent at a slightly acute angle to form a hook. The patient's jaw and tongue are pulled forward and the tube is introduced in the midline along the tongue to hook up the epiglottis. When the tube is placed correctly, transillumination of the soft tissue of the neck is clearly discernible in the midline. Right or left pyriform sinus placement is seen as a transilluminated area lateral to the midline. When the tube is in the esophagus, the light is subdued and diffused. Once correct placement is established, the tube is advanced over the lighted stylet. Care is taken not to pull back on the stylet before advancing the tube into the trachea. Three hundred intubations have been reported using this procedure, during elective surgery as well as in emergency situations, with very few failures or complications.

Other measures that have been used to facilitate orotracheal intubation in a difficult situation, when the neck cannot be moved, include attaching a prism to the handle of the laryngoscope blade to enable visualization of the areas beyond the curve of the blade. A word of caution regarding orotracheal intubation: A common error during intubation is failure to visualize the tip of the tube passing between the vocal cords. This can be prevented by guiding the tube sideways from the right side of the mouth so that the performer's hand does not obstruct the view of the larynx. Another common error is pushing the tube too far down toward the carina or into the right main-stem bronchus. The average distance from the lips to the carina is 28.5 cm in men and 25.2 cm in women. The 20- to 23-cm mark on the endotracheal tube usually is a good length when placed at the corner of the mouth. The margin of safety in children is less. The child's age divided by 2 plus 12 cm will ensure a good position.

Nasotracheal Intubation

Nasotracheal intubation is a blind procedure. The endotracheal tube is introduced through either nostril, passed through the nasal cavity into the nasopharynx, and pushed down further into the oropharynx and larynx. Because of the natural curvature of the pharynx, the tube is likely to enter the trachea. By subtly altering the direction of the tube and listening for breath sounds through it, the tube is maneuvered into the trachea.

It is possible to place the endotracheal tube with a success rate of approximately 90 percent. Care should be taken not to use undue force in pushing the tube through the posterior pharyngeal area. A common complication of nasotracheal intubation is epistaxis. Injury has been reported to retropharyngeal structures by the tip of the tube, resulting in hematoma and subsequent infection. One of the prerequisites for blind nasotracheal intubation is that the patient be breathing; without respirations, the proper placement of the tube cannot be assessed. In certain circumstances the tube can be guided through the epiglottic opening by digital manipulation inside the mouth (the patient should be unconscious and, hence, unable to bite). A laryngoscope blade can be used through the mouth to visualize the tube in the pharynx and the tube can be guided into the trachea with the help of Magill forceps.

A flexible fiberoptic laryngoscope can be used to aid in direct visualization and intubation through the nasotracheal route. The endotracheal tube is placed on the scope before endoscopy. The scope with the endotracheal tube is inserted through the nostril and, under direct visualization, the tube can be slipped into the trachea. An obvious limitation is that bleeding and aspirated material can make visualization difficult.

Nasotracheal intubation offers some advantages over orotracheal intubation. It can be used in individuals with an injured cervical spine since the movements of the neck can be kept to an absolute minimum. The patient may also tolerate the procedure better. In situations in which laryngoscopy is difficult or contraindicated because of congenital abnormalities around the oropharyngeal area, or when the patient is uncooperative, nasotracheal intubation is a good alternative. In conditions that can result in trismus, such as closed head injury, decerebrate rigidity, seizures, and facial injuries, nasotracheal intubation may be helpful. Caution should be taken in patients with maxillofacial injury. In the presence of basilar skull fracture, any object introduced through the nostrils theoretically can go through the cribriform plate of the ethmoid and enter the frontal lobe of the brain. This has been reported in the literature with nasogastric tubes. Nasotracheal tubes, being bigger in size and more rigid, are unlikely to enter through the cribriform plate if care is taken in directly guiding the tube posteriorly and then downward. If there is doubt, the procedure should be discontinued. A blind nasal approach is clearly contraindicated in any person with suspected foreign-body obstruction because of the fear of pushing the foreign body further down. Blind nasotracheal intubation is also contraindicated in acute epiglottitis. Another problem with nasotracheal intubation is an increase in the associated risk of meningitis or encephalitis. The bacteria resulting from this procedure may be unacceptable in certain patients, especially those with cardiovascular valve abnormalities or prostheses.

Before intubation, the standard endotracheal tube can be formed into a circle by inserting the distal end into the proximal adapter for about 10 to 20 seconds. This ensures proper anterior curving of the distal end. Insertion through the nose is accomplished without disturbing the curve by aiming the tip toward the ipsilateral ear initially and later rotating the tube toward the midline. One author (NHP) has used this technique successfully for a number of years.

A recently introduced modification is the Endotrol tube. A finger-operated ring controls the tip of the tube. By pulling on this ring, the tip can be moved forward, aiding in successful tracheal entry.

Another tool that has been used to facilitate nasotracheal intubation is a lighted stylet.

Retrograde Intubation of the Trachea

Retrograde intubation of the trachea has been described as another useful adjunct in establishing airway control. When orotracheal or nasotracheal intubation is not feasible, or is contraindicated as in circumstances described previously, retrograde tracheal intubation may be performed. Retrograde intubation requires little operator experience and can be performed without moving the patient's neck or head; therefore, it presents an attractive alternative to cricothyrotomy. However, it should be emphasized that airway control must be obtained quickly in most of these circumstances, and that when there is a compromise of speed, a different procedure would be more useful.

In 1960 Butler and Cirillo reported retrograde intubation after removal of a tracheostomy tube from the operative field in neck surgery. In 1963 Waters described guided, blind endotracheal intubation when severe oral deformity due to nutritional disorders precluded orotracheal intubation.

The equipment for retrograde intubation includes a flexible-tip guide wire, standard endotracheal tube, syringe, and hemostats. The cricothyroid membrane is punctured in the usual manner, care being taken to aim the needle slightly caudad in order to avoid injury to cricothyroid arteries. After correct placement into the airway is determined, the needle is angled cephalad and the guide wire is inserted through the needle. The guide wire is passed through the needle until it comes out through the mouth or the nose. If this does not occur, the wire should be retrieved from the oropharynx with forceps. The guide wire is then fed through the side port at the distal end of the endotracheal tube. This allows an extra centimeter of the tube to be placed below the vocal cords before removal of the guide wire. With the guide wire held tightly at the neck, the endotracheal tube is threaded over the guide into the trachea. Slight pressure and twisting of the tube may be necessary to overcome resistance. Once the tube is felt to "pop" into the trachea and cannot be moved any further, the guide is removed. It is preferable to cut the wire at skin level and pull it proximally through the endotracheal tube to avoid contamination of the subcutaneous tissues in the neck. The endotracheal tube is advanced slightly further down and placement is confirmed.

Percutaneous Transtracheal Ventilation

Percutaneous transtracheal ventilation (PTV) (see Procedure 5), involves insertion of a catheter through the cricothyroid membrane into the trachea. The catheter is then attached to a high-pressure oxygen source and oxygen is delivered intermittently into the trachea. Although endotracheal intubation and ventilation are unquestionably the treatment of choice, PTV offers a viable alternative when intubation cannot be accomplished rapidly. Hence, the indications for PTV are essentially similar to those of cricothyrotomy. Even though reports indicate that adequate oxygenation and elimination of carbon dioxide can be maintained with PTV for extended periods of time (i.e., 30 minutes), it should be remembered that this is a temporizing measure and that a definite airway should be secured as soon as possible. PTV can be established while awaiting radiographic results of the status of the cervical spine. After the cervical spine has been "cleared," orotracheal intubation can be accomplished. On the other hand, if a surgical airway is mandated, a cricothyrotomy or a semielective tracheostomy can be performed under more controlled situations. Because cricothyrotomy is a surgical procedure, some emergency physicians view it with trepidation. Under these circumstances, PTV is a possible alternative.

Percutaneous transtracheal ventilation was first described in 1954. Since then modifications have been made. The efficacy of ventilation using intermittent jets of oxygen delivered through a bronchoscope has been demonstrated. By making the oxygen delivery intermittent, it is possible to allow time for the carbon dioxide to escape and viable respiratory status to be maintained.

Various catheter sizes and oxygen delivery systems have been studied to determine which methods provide better oxygenation. Using a catheter and ventilating with a self-inflating bag is not satisfactory. A high-pressure oxygen source is necessary for successful PTV. Some studies suggest that by means of PTV proximal airway secretions and partial obstruction can be cleared by propelling the objects cephalad. However, a definite danger of PTV in complete airway obstruction exists: High-pressure oxygen ventilation without means for air to escape from the lungs has resulted in tension pneumothoraxes and massive subcutaneous emphysema.

There is no specific apparatus for PTV. Earlier methods of PTV involved complicated machinery that precluded safe and rapid application in emergencies. Recently, various models have been described that are simple to use and for which materials are readily available in the emergency department. Oxygen can be provided by a 50-psi wall oxygen source coupled to a standard flowmeter. Setting the flowmeter at the wide-open position (15 liters per minute) provides the high flow rate necessary. Standard oxygen tubing is used to connect the oxygen source to the catheter. The cricothyroid membrane is punctured using an over-the-needle catheter (14-gauge). The needle is withdrawn and a three-way plastic stopcock is attached to the catheter. The plastic oxygen tubing is connected to the three-way stopcock. A small hole is then cut near the distal end of the oxygen tubing. By occluding this hole with the thumb, high-pressure oxygen can be delivered through the cannula into the trachea. Removing the thumb diverts the oxygen stream through the side hole and allows the patient to exhale passively. Using this device, Levinson, et al., determined that the endothoracic pressure was kept well below the danger level that would cause lungs to rupture (80–150 cm water). With this device they provided a tidal volume of 400 cc at a rate of six respirations per minute. The inspiratory flow rate was 110 cc per second. The inspiratory time averaged two to three seconds. Others have described inspiration for one second followed by a four-second expiration, thereby closely resembling the respiratory cycle of a deeply breathing adult. Alternatively, a second 14-gauge catheter can be placed in the cricothyroid membrane to allow better elimination of carbon dioxide; the lumen of this catheter is covered while oxygen is being jet-insufflated in the primary catheter.

PTV is a useful device as a temporizing measure during preparation for definitive airway procedures. This author (NHP) has had occasion to use PTV before cricothyrotomy. The PTV can be instituted rapidly during the time it takes to set up the cricothyrotomy tray. Care should be taken while making the incision for cricothyrotomy; the PTV catheter through the cricothyroid membrane should not be cut. While a semiemergent tracheostomy is being performed, the catheter in the cricothyroid membrane acts as a landmark to assure the midline. It is well known that in emergency situations an assistant holding the retractors can pull on one side or the other, distorting the midline considerably.

The reported complications of PTV are essentially due to barotrauma. Tension pneumothorax and pneumomediastinum have also been reported, and subcutaneous emphysema is a problem. Catheter dislodgment has been known to occur. Care should be taken to avoid these complications. Coughing, which may be induced during the procedure in patients with intact reflexes, can be prevented by the instillation of lidocaine (2 ml of a 4% solution) through the catheter before ventilation.

Cricothyrotomy

Cricothyrotomy (see Procedure 7) is a valuable tool for airway control in difficult situations. The procedure had fallen into disfavor after having been the subject of controversy for over 60 years. Because of the risk of subglottic stenosis, excessive bleeding, high infection rates, and damage to the vocal cords, the procedure was condemned by surgeons in the past. It should be remembered that tracheostomy is certainly a more useful procedure than cricothyrotomy under elective conditions. However, in emergencies, cricothyrotomy has a definite role. The procedure is easier to perform. It does have a higher complication rate, but this may be acceptable when one considers the catastrophic nature of the alternative. Emergency cricothyrotomy as a lifesaving procedure is becoming more and more accepted. It should be converted to a tracheostomy by an experienced surgeon later. There is some evidence in the current literature that adequately performed cricothyrotomy can be used for long-term management of the airway without fear of subglottic stenosis.

Indications for cricothyrotomy include inability to establish an airway by other methods, such as endotracheal intubation; relief of complete airway obstruction when it is not possible to use an endotracheal airway or retrieve the foreign body through a scope; and severe facial trauma that renders techniques of intubation impossible.

The difficulty for the emergency physician arises in deciding when to perform a cricothyrotomy. Indications are clear in circumstances in which the patient is in obvious respiratory distress and obtaining airway access through intubation becomes impossible. In situations in which cervical spine fracture is suspected, the question exists as to whether inline immobilization and intubation are preferable to cricothyrotomy. Recent data seem to indicate that even with the best possible cervical immobilization, cervical spine movement can occur. However, when nasotracheal intubation fails, and if the patient does not have a cervical spine fracture, current consensus favors orotracheal intubation with inline immobilization. If available, a flexible fiberoptic laryngoscope can be used. Conversely, the patient with a known cervical spine injury should have a cricothyrotomy done if nasotracheal intubation fails.

Cricothyrotomy should not be undertaken in children. Fortunately, the number of cases of children in need of surgical airway intervention is very small. Whenever possible, these children should be intubated orally with inline immobilization. Needle cricothyrotomy is an alternate choice. In blunt and penetrating trauma to the neck, the anatomic landmarks may be obscured by swelling and distortion. In these circumstances, a cricothyrotomy is almost impossible to perform. A tracheostomy is preferred if the possibility of injury exists below the cricothyroid level.

In the presence of laryngeal pathology or after a prolonged intubation, cricothyrotomy is not advisable because the complication rate increases. The incidence of subglottic stenosis is higher in these situations. However, studies now indicate that the risk of subglottic stenosis is not as great as was previously thought in properly performed emergency cricothyrotomy.

Percutaneous cricothyrotomy kits are available. These work on the principle that with a percutaneous trocar puncture and serial dilators an adequate cricothyrotomy can be performed. A blind puncture by inexperienced hands may cause an alarmingly high rate of complications. Familiarity with the device becomes essential. Simple needle cricothyrotomy with percutaneous transtracheal ventilation may be safer under certain circumstances. Cricothyrotomies are relatively new and, therefore, have not yet been studied enough for definitive opinions to be formed.

Tracheostomy

Tracheostomy continues to be the definitive surgical management for the airway. Once a very popular procedure, it is being performed less and less as the success rate in endotracheal intubation has increased. Tracheostomy was performed in ancient times. During the last century, tracheostomy gained favor as a dramatic operation to relieve upper-airway obstruction caused by diphtheria. Commonly, tracheostomy is an elective surgical procedure performed in the operating room; thus, the emergency physician seldom has any reason to become familiar with this procedure. The technique of tracheostomy is more complicated than cricothyrotomy. Every emergency physician should be familiar with cricothyrotomy. However, some basic information about tracheostomy is necessary as occasionally an emergency physician may see a patient with complications from tracheostomy and be called on to replace a dislodged tracheostomy tube.

The major advantage of tracheostomy is that it provides the best route for long-term airway management. The patient is able to swallow secretions and nourishment, thereby avoiding the problems of malnutrition associated with translaryngeal intubation. However, tracheostomy is accompanied by a high rate of complications, especially when it is performed on an emergency basis under suboptimal conditions.

Controversy exists as to how long an endotracheal tube can be left in place before tracheostomy is performed. In 1951, this period was said to be 8 to 12 hours. By 1969, it had reached 3 days and by 1976, it was 11 days. Clearly, no specific time limit can be set forth to decide when to perform a tracheostomy. This decision must be individualized depending on the following conditions:

1. Estimated temporal need for the airway
2. Tolerance of the endotracheal tube
3. The likelihood of improvement of care after tracheostomy
4. The likelihood of lessening morbidity and mortality with tracheostomy

Complications of tracheostomy can occur during the procedure itself, when the tube is in place, during removal of the tube, or after removal of the tube. These complications include subcutaneous or mediastinal emphysema in 13 percent of tracheostomies. Hemorrhage has been known to occur in about 10 percent and pneumothorax in 5 percent. Injury to the thyroid gland, recurrent laryngeal nerve, or carotid sheath has been reported. Cardiac arrest during the procedure can also occur. Mortality during tracheostomy is reported as 3 percent (range, 0–5.3 percent).

The most common complication while the tracheostomy tube is in place relates to cuff problems. Tracheitis and ischemia leading to ulceration and necrosis of the cartilage have been reported. There is a 15 percent incidence of pneumonia and 3 percent incidence of atelectasis after tracheostomy. Impairment of the cough reflex is perhaps the causative factor. Complications during and after decannulation usually occur in the intensive care unit.

Medications During Intubation

Although it is usually not necessary to use medications to intubate a patient, at times their use is warranted and essential. Some of these situations include: when intubating an alert patient, when intubating a trauma victim suffering from severe head injury, when the patient has a full stomach, or when the patient is combative or uncooperative. The medications used in these circumstances are described in Chapter 9.

SELECTED READING

Abman, SH, Fan, LL, and Cotton, EK. Emergency treatment of foreign-body obstruction of the upper airway. *J Emerg Med* 2:7, 1984.

American Heart Association. *Advanced Cardiac Life Support Course.* Dallas: American Heart Association, 1987.

Ampel, L, et al. An approach to airway management in the acutely head-injured patient. *J Emerg Med* 6:1, 1988.

Asensio, JA, et al. Trauma: A systematic approach to management. *Am Fam Physician* 38:97, 1988.

Auerbach, PS, and Geehr, EC. Inadequate oxygenation and ventilation using the EGTA in the prehospital setting. *JAMA* 250:3067, 1983.

Barriot, P, and Riou, B. Retrograde technique for tracheal intubation in trauma patients. *Crit Care Med* 16:712, 1988.

Bartlett, RL, et al. The pharyngeo-tracheal lumen airway: An assessment of airway control in the setting of upper airway hemorrhage. *Ann Emerg Med* 16:343, 1987.

Bjoraker, DG, Kumar, NB, and Brown, ACD. Evaluation of an emergency cricothyrotomy instrument. *Crit Care Med* 15:157, 1987.

Brantigan, CO, and Grow, JB Sr. Cricothyroidotomy revisited again. *Ear Nose Throat J* 59:26, 1980.

Brantigan, CO, and Grow, JB Sr. Subglottic stenosis after cricothyroidotomy. *Surgery* 91:217, 1982.

Bryson, TK, Benumof, JL, and Ward, CF. The esophageal obturator airway. *Chest* 74:537, 1978.

Butler, FS, and Cirillo, AA. Retrograde tracheal intubation. *Anesth Analg Curr Res* 39:333, 1960.

Cardiopulmonary Resuscitation Committee. Standards for cardiopulmonary resuscitation (CPR) and emergency cardiac care (ECC). *JAMA* 255:2915–2936, 2961–2964, 1986.

Clinton, JE, and Ruiz, E. Emergency Airway Management Procedures. In JR Robert and JR Hedges (eds), *Clinical Procedures in Emergency Medicine.* Saunders: Philadelphia, 1985. P. 126.

Dailey, RH. Acute upper airway obstruction. *Emerg Med Clin North Am* 1:261, 1983.

Davis, HW, et al. Acute upper airway obstruction: Croup and epiglottitis. *Pediatr Clin North Am* 28:859, 1981.

Delaney, KA, and Hessler, R. Emergency flexible fiberoptic nasotracheal intubation: A report of 60 cases. *Ann Emerg Med* 17:919, 1988.

Deweese, DD, and Saunders, WH. *Textbook of Otolaryngology.* St. Louis: Mosby, 1982.

Dickison, AE. The normal and abnormal pediatric upper airway—recognition and management of obstruction. *Clin Chest Med* 8:583, 1987.

Don Michael, TA, and Gordon, AS. The oesophageal obturator airway: A new device in emergency cardiopulmonary resuscitation. *Br Med J* 281:1531, 1980.

Don Michael, TA, Lambert, EH, and Mehran, A. Mouth-to-lung airway for cardiac resuscitation. *Lancet* 2:1329, 1968.

Frass, M, et al. The esophageal tracheal combitube: Preliminary results with a new airway for CPR. *Ann Emerg Med* 16:768, 1987.

Gold, MI, and Buechel, DR. Translaryngeal anesthesia: A review. *Anesthesiology* 20:181, 1959.

Goldthorn, J, and Badgwell, JM. Upper airway obstruction in infants and children. *Int Anesthesiol Clin* 24:133, 1986.

Haponik, EF, et al. Acute upper airway injury in burn patients—serial changes of flow-volume curves and nasopharyngoscopy. *Am Rev Respir Dis* 135:360, 1987.

Hardwick, WC, and Bluhm, D. Digital intubation. *J Emerg Med* 1:317, 1984.

Harrison, RR, et al. Mouth to mask ventilation: A superior method of rescue breathing. *Ann Emerg Med* 11:74, 1982.

Heimlich, HG. A life saving maneuver to prevent food-choking. *JAMA* 234:398, 1975.

Iserson, KV. Blind nasotracheal intubation. *Ann Emerg Med* 10: 468, 1981.

Jackson, C. High tracheotomy and other errors the chief causes of chronic laryngeal stenosis. *Sing Gynecol Obstet* 32:392, 1921.

Jorden, RC. Airway management. *Emerg Med Clin North Am* 6:671, 1988.

Leo, JD, and Simon, RR. Upper Airway Obstruction and Procedures and Techniques in Airway Management. In BE Brenner (ed), *Comprehensive Management of Respiratory Emergencies.* Rockville, MD: Aspen, 1985.

Levinson, MM, et al. Emergency percutaneous transtracheal ventilation (PTV). *JACEP* 8:396, 1979.

Kilany, SM. Complications of tracheostomy. *Ear, Nose & Throat J* 59:123, 1980.

McEwen, W. Clinical observations on the introduction of tracheal tubes by the mouth, instead of performing tracheotomy or laryngotomy. *Br Med J* 2:122–124, 163–165, 1880.

Meislin, HW. The esophageal obturator airway: A study of respiratory effectiveness. *Ann Emerg Med* 9:54, 1980.

Mlinek, EJ Jr, Clinton, JE, and Ruiz, E. Limitations of emergency fiberoptic scope intubation. *Ann Emerg Med* 17:439, 1988.

Montoya, D. Management of the choking victim. *Can Med Assoc J* 135:305, 1986.

Niemann, JT, et al. The pharyngeo-tracheal lumen airway: Preliminary investigation of a new adjunct. *Ann Emerg Med* 13:591, 1984.

Rice, DH. General principles of airway management. *Otolaryngol Clin North Am* 14:735, 1981.

Ruddy, J. Bacterial tracheitis in a young adult. *J Laryngol Otol* 102:656, 1988.

Ryckman, F, and Rodgers, BM. Obstructive airway disease in infants and children. *Surg Clin North Am* 65:1663, 1985.

Safar, P, and Penninck, J. Cricothyroid membrane puncture with special cannula. *Anesthesiology* 28:943, 1967.

Shea, SR, MacDonald, JR, and Gruzinski, G. Prehospital endotracheal airway or esophageal gastric tube airway: A critical comparison. *Ann Emerg Med* 14:102, 1985.

Smith, JP, et al. A field evaluation of the esophageal obturator airway. *J Trauma* 23:317, 1983.

Stewart, RD. Tactile orotracheal intubation. *Ann Emerg Med* 13: 175, 1984.

Stoelting, RK. Endotracheal Intubation. In RD Miller (ed), *Anesthesia.* New York: Churchill Livingstone, 1981.

Tintinalli, JE, and Claffey, J. Complications of nasotracheal intubation. *Ann Emerg Med* 10:142, 1981.

Tove, FJ, and Weinstein, JD. Clinical experience with percutaneous tracheostomy and cricothyroidotomy in 100 patients. *J Trauma* 26:1034, 1986.

Waters, DJ. Guided blind nasotracheal intubation. *Anesthesiology* 18:158, 1963.

Weiss, S. A new emergency cricothyroidotomy instrument. *J Trauma* 23:155, 1983.

Weymuller, EA Jr, and Cummings, CW. Cricothyroidotomy: The impact of antecedent endotracheal intubation. *Ann Otol Rhinol Laryngol* 91:437, 1982.

NEAR-DROWNING

Mary L. Palermo
Robert D. Truog

Drowning and *near-drowning* are the terms commonly used to describe submersion-immersion injuries. *Drowning* is defined as death resulting from asphyxia that occurs within 24 hours of the event. It is responsible for approximately 150,000 deaths worldwide and 8,000 deaths in the United States annually. *Near-drowning* is defined as survival of victims for at least 24 hours after a submersion-immersion event and is estimated to affect nearly 50,000 individuals per year. The presence of complications, especially those of pulmonary, cardiovascular, neurologic, and infectious causes, contributes significantly to the prognosis of near-drowning victims, with ultimate outcome dependent on the extent of hypoxic injury and recovery.

The majority of near-drowning victims are less than 25 years of age, and approximately 40 percent are under the age of 4 years. Drowning is currently the third most common cause of death in infants and children. Swimming pools are the most common site of drowning for children under 5 years, with bathtubs, in which infants and children are frequently left unattended, the next most common. Fluid-filled containers such as buckets also pose a significant risk, especially to toddlers. Older victims are often engaged in various sporting activities such as swimming and diving in pools, rivers, and creeks, or water-skiing and surfing. Of recent note is the association of alcohol consumption and drug usage with water-related injuries, which in some studies has been found to be as high as 50 percent in both drowning and near-drowning victims.

Reduction of submersion-immersion injuries may best be accomplished by prevention. Toddlers and young children must be supervised constantly in and near all potential accident sites. Pool owners should provide sufficient barriers to access and, without question, be certified in cardiopulmonary resuscitation. Older individuals need to exercise greater caution and act responsibly while involved in water activities in an effort to minimize the possibility of a tragic occurrence.

Early, quality on-site cardiopulmonary resuscitation is crucial in the treatment of near-drowning victims. Resuscitation must be carried out aggressively in the field, and continued as well in the emergency department, where further evaluation and stabilization may be accomplished. This early effective intervention appears to be the best predictor of survival in near-drowning victims.

PATHOPHYSIOLOGY

Drowning and near-drowning injuries involve two major pathophysiologic pathways: hypoxia and hypothermia. Drowning events can be categorized as wet versus dry, fresh versus salt water, and cold versus warm water.

In the usual sequence of events, the drowning victim is quickly overcome by fright and panic, which is followed by a period of struggling, fatigue, and breath-holding. Large amounts of water may be swallowed and later vomiting may occur with subsequent aspiration. This is known as *wet drowning* and occurs in 80 to 90 percent of all drowning victims. The remaining 10 to 20 percent of patients do not aspirate and are referred to as *dry drowning* victims. These patients experience the initial reflex laryngospasm that prevents water from entering the trachea, but as they become progressively hypoxic and lose consciousness, the laryngospasm abates and water passively enters the trachea and subsequently the lungs. The presence of any fluid or particulate matter in the lungs, regardless of the mechanism of

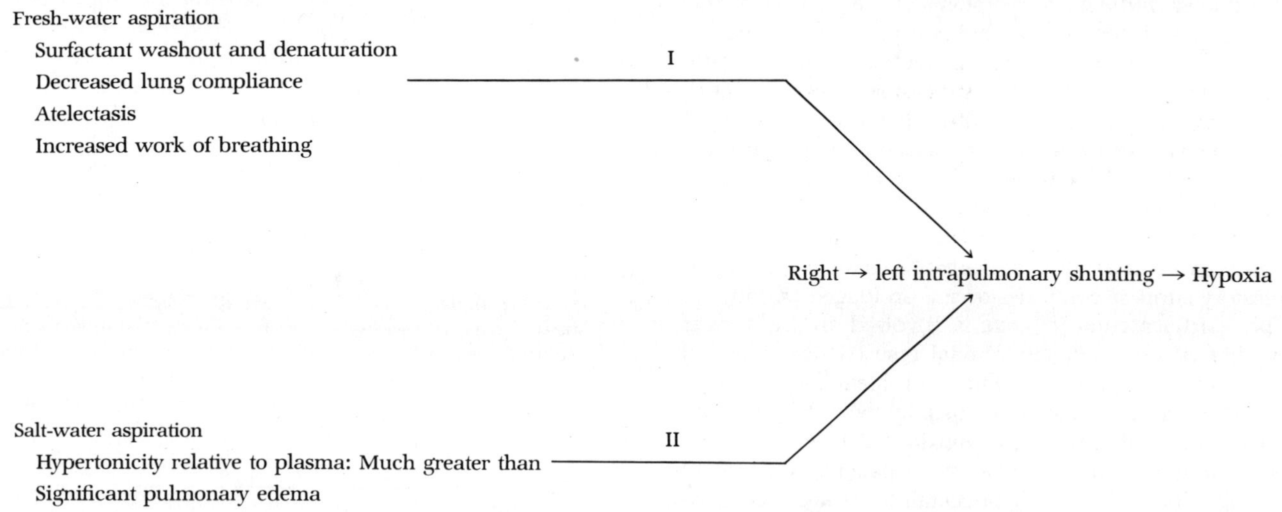

Fig. 3-25. Mechanisms of hypoxia in fresh- and salt-water aspiration.

entry, poses a significant risk to the patient for pulmonary complications, such as airway obstruction, inflammatory reactions, adult respiratory distress syndrome, and infection.

The composition and quantity of the fluid involved in drowning and near-drowning events have historically received a great deal of attention, especially in regard to pathophysiologic and clinical differences. Recently, however, emphasis has been directed toward the final common insult: hypoxia. The hypoxia produced is a result of right-to-left intrapulmonary shunting via two very different mechanisms, depending on whether fresh or salt water is aspirated (Fig. 3-25).

Fresh-water aspiration results in movement of fluid from the involved pulmonary space into the intravascular space, as fresh water is hypotonic to plasma. Since relatively small amounts of fluid are actually aspirated, usually less than 22 ml/kg, no significant changes in intravascular volume, electrolyte composition, or hemolysis occur. However, both surfactant washout and denaturation take place. This leads to decreased lung compliance, atelectasis, increased work of breathing, and eventually intrapulmonary right-to-left shunting and severe hypoxia.

Salt-water aspiration, like that of fresh water, results in surfactant washout. Although, as previously mentioned, only small amounts of fluid are actually aspirated by near-drowning victims, large amounts of fluid shift from the intravascular space into the pulmonary space because of the hypertonicity of salt water compared to plasma. This leads to the development of significant pulmonary edema over a relatively short period of time (minutes to hours). As a result, a right-to-left intrapulmonary shunt is established and severe hypoxia rapidly follows.

Recent emphasis on the effects of water temperature in drowning and near-drowning victims has centered on cold-water environments and the development of hypothermia. The effects of hypothermia are rapid heat loss, death, dysrhythmias, and neuroprotection. *Hypothermia* is defined as a core temperature less than 35°C and may in itself be the cause of death. It is associated with dysfunction of various organ systems, the most important of which are the cardiovascular and central nervous systems. In submersion events, hypothermia quickly develops as heat is rapidly lost to a cold, wet environment. Children are at greater risk for the development of hypothermia as they possess greater surface area to mass ratio than adults.

The effect of hypothermia on the cardiovascular system is mainly one of dysrhythmias. Occasionally, direct vagal stimulation by cold water onto the larynx may produce immediate ventricular fibrillation and rapid death. However, in general, as core temperature is gradually reduced, various atrial and ventricular arrhythmias develop. It is also important to keep in mind that hypothermia may mask the presence of underlying cardiovascular involvement and that such involvement is apparent only as rewarming is accomplished. Treatment of the near-drowning victim should therefore include the anticipation and aggressive management of dysrhythmias.

Whether or not hypothermia in the drowning or near-drowning victim is neuroprotective, such as is the case for hypothermic arrest during cardiovascular surgery, depends on when hypothermia develops. It appears that the mechanism for neuroprotection maximally occurs only when hypothermia precedes hypoxia and hypoperfusion. Evidence for this can be found in reports of near-drowning victims who survive with normal neurologic outcomes after up to 40 minutes of submersion in ice water. In the presence of a hypothermic near-drowning victim who arrives in the emergency department, one must always think positively in terms of neurologic outcome and thus continue to proceed aggressively with all resuscitative efforts.

CLINICAL PRESENTATIONS

A wide variety of clinical presentations are encountered in near-drowning victims, ranging from no symptoms or only mild respiratory distress to pulselessness and apnea. These differing clinical features depend on a variety of factors, including water temperature, duration of submersion, occurrence of aspiration, and, most important, promptness and effectiveness of treatment.

Pulmonary, cardiovascular, and neurologic involvement

predominates. Pulmonary symptoms range from tachypnea and cough in mild cases to fulminant pulmonary edema in severely affected patients. Many individuals require ventilatory assistance in their initial on-site resuscitation, with eventual endotracheal intubation and mechanical ventilation. Of these patients, some will progress to adult respiratory distress syndrome and its associated respiratory failure. Additional pulmonary complications, including inflammatory reactions, infections, and pneumothoraxes and pneumomediastinum secondary to barotrauma, frequently develop as respiratory support continues over a prolonged period.

The cardiovascular system is involved in most near-drowning victims and, thus, initial resuscitative efforts include cardiac evaluation. The main problem encountered is that of dysrhythmias, which are usually the result of a combination of hypothermia and hypoxia. Often these arrhythmias become evident as hypothermic patients undergo rewarming but acidosis and hypoxia fail to resolve. Therefore, continuing evaluation and appropriate cardiac management are mandated in all near-drowning victims at the scene and on arrival to the emergency department.

Central nervous system presentations in the near-drowning victim range from the asymptomatic, alert, and oriented patient to one who is comatose and in need of cardiopulmonary resuscitation. Special consideration must be given to the possibility of head and neck trauma and necessary precautions taken to prevent further injury. Many near-drowning victims exhibit seizure activity, an early sign of hypoxic cerebral injury, and this often complicates the resuscitative effort. Others will experience differing neurologic deficits, especially in speech and motor function, with varying degrees of recovery encountered over time. It appears that prompt and effective resuscitation, beginning at the scene, is critical in effecting survival with the best neurologic outcome in the near-drowning victim.

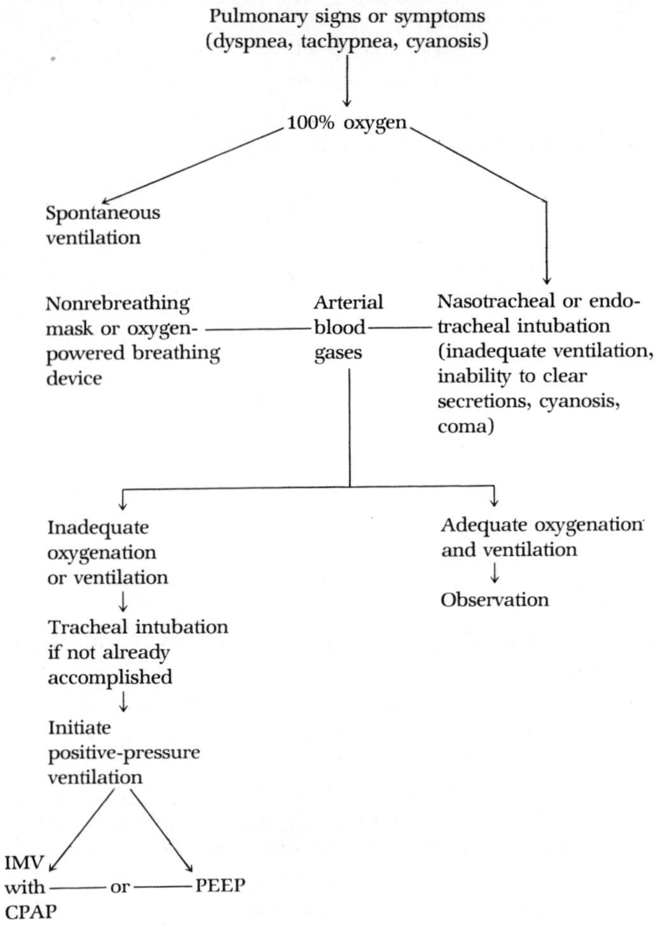

Fig. 3-26. Pulmonary management. (IMV = intermittent mandatory ventilation; CPAP = continuous positive airway pressure; PEEP = positive end-expiratory pressure.) (From R. Knopp. Near drowning. *J.A.C.E.P.* 7:249, 1978.)

MANAGEMENT

Treatment of drowning and near-drowning victims must begin immediately at the scene, with the initiation of cardiopulmonary resuscitation (CPR) in the water if necessary. The restoration of adequate ventilation and circulation through early and effective CPR with appropriate consideration of possible cervical spine involvement reduces potential hypoxic injury and correlates with improved survival and neurologic outcome. All efforts initiated on-site should continue throughout transport of the victim to the emergency department, where further evaluation and treatment can take place. On-site and initial hospital management includes the following:

Airway, breathing, and circulation (ABC) assessment
CPR, if indicated, with cervical spine protection
Supplemental oxygen
Intravascular access
Continuous evaluation of respiratory, cardiovascular, and central nervous systems with specific interventions
Basic diagnostic studies
- Arterial blood gas
- Serum electrolytes
- Hematocrit
- Chest x-ray
- Cervical spine films

Respiratory System Support

A priority in initial hospital management of near-drowning victims involves pulmonary resuscitation, including the use of 100 percent oxygen and positive-pressure ventilation with positive end-expiratory pressure (PEEP) (Fig. 3-26). Even patients who are asymptomatic should receive supplemental oxygen until an arterial blood gas determination demonstrates no evidence of hypoxia. Although these patients may initially appear clinically and radiographically normal, pulmonary decompensation may develop up to 72 hours after the precipitating event. Therefore, inhospital observation for at least 24 hours after a significant submersion is recommended.

In patients who are mildly symptomatic (i.e., tachypneic, coughing) and who are able to maintain adequate airway patency with spontaneous ventilation, the application of continuous positive airway pressure (CPAP) via a tight-fitting face mask may be attempted in an effort to prevent the collapse of additional alveoli. However, in the majority of near-drowning victims, a significant right-to-left intrapulmonary shunt is established, leading to the development of hypoxia. In general, an arterial oxygen tension (PaO_2) less than 100 mm Hg in 40 percent or more oxygen necessitates endotracheal intubation and the use of positive-pressure ventilation with PEEP. This serves to improve ventilation-perfusion ratios by reinflating atelectatic areas of lung and better aerating lungs affected by pulmonary edema. It is necessary to titrate PEEP to a level where intrapulmonary shunt is decreased without inordinate reductions in cardiac output. Once this level is achieved, it is important that PEEP not be rapidly decreased or suddenly discontinued, as this would result in a significant decrease in PaO_2 secondary to the accumulation of additional pulmonary edema fluid and in an increase in the intrapulmonary shunt.

Cardiovascular System Support

The attainment of hemodynamic stability is essential early in the management of near-drowning victims. Dysrhythmias, hypothermia, large and rapid volume shifts, and significant metabolic acidosis are all factors that contribute to the difficult and often prolonged cardiac resuscitation. Adequate intravascular access must be rapidly established to provide routes of administration for volume and resuscitative medications. Intravenous sodium bicarbonate should be given to correct existing and persistent acidosis. A variety of pharmacologic agents to support the cardiovascular system and the establishment of central venous access for monitoring purposes are frequently necessary during resuscitation, especially in severely affected near-drowning victims.

Central Nervous System Support

An additional priority in initial management is that of neurologic resuscitation. The neurologic injury that occurs in near-drowning victims is a diffuse encephalopathy resulting from hypoxia and hypoperfusion. Continuation or establishment of effective CPR provides the oxygenation and perfusion necessary to minimize this potential hypoxic injury and effect the best neurologic outcome.

A number of methods have been attempted to reliably identify near-drowning victims in terms of intact neurologic survival. In general, patients who are awake and alert at the scene or who are arousable on arrival in the emergency department despite requiring resuscitation have the best neurologic prognosis. Patients with the worst prognosis are those who arrive comatose in the emergency department with evidence of significant hypoxic injury (i.e., seizures, posturing, flaccidity). However, intact survivors have occasionally been reported even from the group of presenting near-drowning victims with the most unstable conditions. As a result, all severely affected near-drowning patients should receive full, aggressive cerebral resuscitation, including controlled hyperventilation, attempts at alleviating existing hypothermia through rewarming methods, fluid management through both restriction and the use of osmotic and loop diuretics, and the administration of sedatives, muscle relaxants, and barbiturates. The cerebral resuscitation protocol is as follows:

- Controlled hyperventilation
- Controlled hypothermia
- Fluid management
  - Restriction
  - Osmotic and loop diuretics
- Sedatives
- Muscle relaxants
- Barbiturates
- Monitoring
  - Central venous pressure
  - Arterial blood pressure
  - Urine output

Other Issues

Basic diagnostic studies should be obtained on all near-drowning victims and include an arterial blood gas, serum electrolytes, hematocrit, and chest x-ray. Cervical spine films are necessary if head or neck trauma, or both, are evident or suspected. Fluid and electrolyte imbalance requires correction and careful monitoring. Placement of an arterial line allows evaluation of pulmonary therapy by frequent blood gas determinations and provides an accurate measurement of blood pressure.

The use of antibiotics in near-drowning victims should be determined on an individual basis, with prophylaxis advocated by many clinicians for presumed aspiration. It is important to culture any fluid or material obtained from the oropharynx and lungs in an effort to identify potential pathogens, with appropriate antibiotic therapy reserved for evidence of infection. The use of steroids in an attempt to minimize the pulmonary injury of near-drowning has not been proved effective, and some studies suggest that they may even interfere with normal pulmonary healing. Therefore, the administration of steroids for this purpose in near-drowning victims is not recommended. Finally, the use of intracranial pressure monitoring and aggressive therapy to reduce elevated intracranial pressure, if present, is controversial. The current approach to cerebral resuscitation remains hyperventilation, dehydration, sedation, and muscle relaxation. Hypothermia and barbiturates have been used in the treatment of refractory intracranial hypertension.

DISPOSITION

All victims of significant submersion events, including those who are asymptomatic, should be admitted to the hospital for at least 24 hours. This inhospital observation is recommended because a risk for the development of pulmonary insufficiency and neurologic depression exists for a period of time after an event. The degree of neurologic involvement in near-drowning victims varies and neurologic function and recovery range from normal and complete to a vegetative state in approximately 3 percent of victims. In general, near-drowning victims who arrive in the emergency department either awake or with a blunted level of consciousness (i.e., lethargic, agitated, confused) have an excellent neurologic prognosis. Comatose victims with signs of significant hypoxic injury (i.e., posturing, seizures, flaccidity) have the worst prognosis, although even among these patients survivors with normal neurologic functions have been reported.

The practice of early resuscitation, including aggressive cerebral resuscitation, as well as intensive care management has undoubtedly improved overall near-drowning survival, but it also may well increase the number of neurologically devastated victims. Therefore, despite the crucial role of early effective resuscitation in determining both survival and neurologic outcome in near-drowning victims, the key issue that must continue to be addressed is that of prevention of drowning and near-drowning injuries.

SELECTED READING

Conn, AW, and Barker, FA. Fresh water drowning and near-drowning—an update. *Can Anaesth Soc J* 31:538, 1984.
Hoff, BH. Multisystem failure: A review with special reference to drowning. *Crit Care Med* 7:310, 1979.
Modell, JH. The pathophysiology and treatment of drowning. *Acta Anaesthesiol Scand* 29(Suppl):263, 1968.
O'Rourke, PP. Outcome of children who are apneic and pulseless in the emergency room. *Crit Care Med* 14:466, 1986.
Pearn, J. The management of near drowning. *Br Med J* 291:1447, 1985.
Pearn, JH, Bart, RD, and Yamaoka, R. Neurologic sequelae after childhood near-drowning. *Pediatrics* 64:187, 1979.
Young, RS, Zaneiaitis, EL, and Dooling, EC. Neurologic outcome in cold water drowning. *JAMA* 244:1233, 1980.

RESUSCITATION OF THE PREGNANT PATIENT

Sergei Bogojavlensky

Resuscitation in late pregnancy is complicated by profound changes in physiology and the demands of two patients at once. Sudden catastrophes, including highway accidents, violence, overdosage, and burns; general medical mishaps, such as respiratory collapse, aspiration, stroke, and septic shock; and purely obstetric events, including amniotic fluid embolism, torrential placental bleeding, or rarities such as spontaneous splenic vein rupture, account for half of maternal deaths in industrialized countries.

PHYSIOLOGIC CHANGES DURING PREGNANCY

The key to effective intervention is a familiarity with the major physiologic phenomena to which the growing fetal-placental unit gives rise. The uterus grows, becomes an abdominal organ (vulnerable to traumatic injury), compresses the inferior vena cava and abdominal aorta, and receives 20 percent of total maternal cardiac output. Maternal oxygen consumption increases by 20 percent, hormonal changes occur, and nutritional demands rise. In addition, the uterine-placental-umbilical exchange system is supported by the mother and has unique features important for resuscitation.

Physiologic changes begin almost immediately after conception. However, it is mainly in the third trimester—24 weeks plus—that certain maneuvers are unique to the pregnant patient, as will be detailed in this chapter.

Respiratory

Oxygen consumption increases up to 20 percent, achieved by a rise in minute ventilation to 40 percent at term (partly due to progesterone), and is accomplished by an increase in tidal volume of 40 percent and in respiratory rate of 15 percent. Alveolar and arterial oxygen saturation rise, while CO_2 falls. This increases the CO_2 gradient between the fetal and maternal circulations, facilitating diffusion across the epithelioid syncytiotrophoblast from the umbilical capillaries to the intervillous space. Maternal arterial pH is maintained by renal excretion of buffer base. Normal bicarbonate levels are 18 to 31 mEq/liter, markedly lower than nonpregnant values. The enlarging uterus elevates the diaphragm and widens the thorax. Vital capacity remains unchanged, but residual volume and expiratory reserve volume are diminished by 20 percent. The volume of air in the lungs at resting expiration, functional residual capacity, decreases by 15 percent, so that the shunt fraction increases and leads to less oxygen reserve. In an acute clinical setting that produces decreased or increased closing volumes, rapid hypoxemia may ensue.

Cardiovascular

Plasma volume increases by 45 to 50 percent, and red blood cell volume by 20 percent, bringing about the so-called dilution "anemia" of pregnancy, with a normal hematocrit that is 15 percent below nonpregnant values. Increased mineralocorticoid activity causes sodium retention, increased body water, and increased plasma volume.

Pregnancy increases metabolic demands. Oxygen consumption rises by 20 percent and cardiac output increases 35 to 50 percent in response. Changes in pregnancy can be summarized as follows:

Cardiac output	Increases by 40 percent
Stroke volume	Increases by 30 percent
Heart rate	Increases by 15 percent
Systolic blood pressure	Midtrimester decrease, 0 to 5 mm Hg; normal at term
Diastolic blood pressure	Decreases 10 to 20 mm Hg
Total peripheral resistance	Decreases 15 percent

Decreased total peripheral resistance is partly a result of increased prostacyclin and the smooth-muscle relaxing effect of progesterone.

The uterus grows 20-fold—70 gm to 1,100 gm. Uterine blood flow increases about 40 times as a result of increased cardiac output and decreased vascular resistance. In this way, the maternal circulatory system is coupled in parallel to an added low-resistance circulation, sharply lowering total peripheral resistance. A vital repercussion is that any decrease in cardiac output will quickly bring down systemic arterial pressure, and fetal hypoxia may ensue rapidly.

The enlarged uterus makes maternal cardiac output sensitive to position. When the gravida is supine, the uterus may compress and even completely occlude the inferior vena cava and compress the abdominal aorta as well. Venous return to the heart is diminished and cardiac output falls. The effect of the supine position is most dramatic toward term, dropping cardiac output by up to 30 percent. Even at 24 weeks' gestation, the effect may be significant.

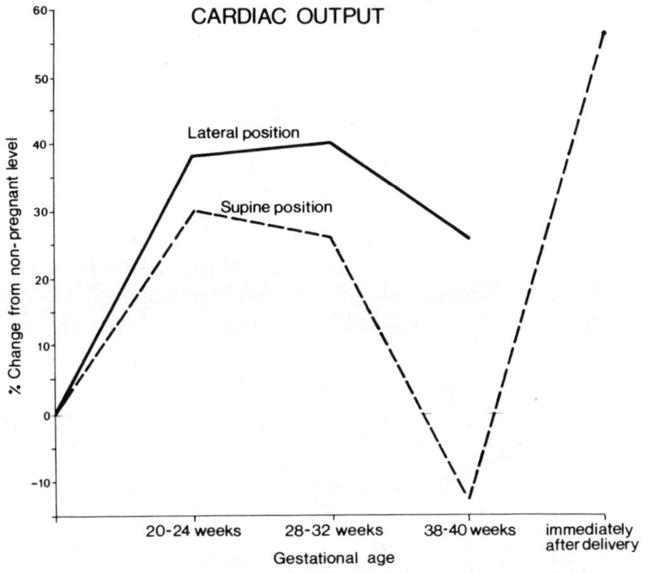

Fig. 3-27. The negative effect of the supine position on cardiac output during pregnancy. (Adapted from G.W. Ostheimer. *Manual of Obstetric Anesthesia.* New York: Churchill Livingstone, 1984.)

Figure 3-27 charts the negative effect of the supine position on cardiac output during pregnancy and highlights the dramatic increase in cardiac output immediately after birth. The uterus is empty and the myometrium has contracted and obliterated the pregnant uterine vasculature, so that the parallel, low-resistance circulation is eliminated. The total increase in cardiac output is much greater than what is gained from eliminating caval and aortic compression alone. For resuscitation, timely and efficient emptying of the uterus therefore becomes an essential life-saving move, quickly resurrecting cardiac output.

Uteroplacental Circulation

In late pregnancy, 10 percent, or 500 to 700 ml per minute, of the maternal cardiac output flows to the uteroplacental unit through the uterine and ovarian arteries from the abdominal aorta. In the muscle wall of the uterus, these form a densely collateralized network, eventually branching down to the spiral arteries, which penetrate the placenta to perfuse a septated segment of the intervillous space where exchange with the capillaries of the fetal chorionic villi occurs. Flow through the myometrial vessels is regulated by smooth muscle. The spiral arteries are not muscled and are more susceptible to occlusion. Venous drainage begins in the decidual layer and ultimately collects in the inferior vena cava.

On the other side of the placental circulation, 50 percent of fetal cardiac output enters the umbilical capillaries and exchanges with maternal blood, to return cleansed and oxygenated. As can be seen in the following formula, uteroplacental blood flow is directly determined by maternal blood pressure since the uterine vascular bed is normally fully dilated:

$$\text{Uterine blood flow} = \frac{\text{maternal blood pressure} - \text{uterine venous pressure}}{\text{vascular resistance of the uterus}}$$

Resistance in the uterine vasculature is a function of the muscle tone of the myometrium and vasoconstriction from alpha effects of catecholamines.

Compression of the aorta will drop perfusion pressure. Inferior vena cava compression increases uterine venous pressure. Intervillous perfusion pressure falls. Any hypotension immediately reduces intervillous perfusion with rapid fetal hypoxia.

Intermittent increases in the tone of the myometrium, particularly with normal contractions in labor, are well tolerated by the fetus. Prolonged uterine hypertonicity from any cause markedly decreases intervillous blood flow. In the clinical setting, two common causes of uterine tetany are placental abruption and uterine trauma. Severe maternal hypoxia, alkalosis, or acidosis will also increase resistance in the uterine vessels. (Of all the therapeutic catecholamines, only ephedrine, because of its central mechanism of cardiac stimulation, does not diminish the intervillous circulation and may be used at times to treat maternal hypotension.)

On the fetal side of this system, fetal cardiac output determines adequate perfusion. It must be clearly held in mind that the fetus in late pregnancy responds to asphyxia with bradycardia.

In summary, the following maternal parameters will lead to fetal asphyxia via inadequate placental perfusion:

Hypotension	Hemorrhage, sepsis, impaired venous return, supine aortocaval compression, cord trauma, cardiopulmonary catastrophes (including amniotic fluid embolism)
Uterine hypertonus	Catecholamines, abruption of the placenta, direct uterine trauma
Respiratory impairment	Maternal hypoxia, respiratory and metabolic alkalosis, hyperventilation, increased thoracic pressure

MONITORING OF THE FETUS

During a cardiopulmonary crisis in late pregnancy, continuous surveillance of fetal heart activity is the only way to evaluate the state of the umbilical-placental-uterine circulation. This can be done by auscultation, vascular Doppler devices, or, most handily, by electronic fetal monitoring equipment. The conventional criteria, currently still in vogue, of continuous electronic fetal monitoring can be relied on only to confirm fetal viability if enlisted in the resuscitation setting. Persistent fetal bradycardia, 60 to 100 beats per minute or less, that is unresponsive to measures of maternal resuscitation is a trustworthy sign of possible developing fetal asphyxia. Knowledgable obstetric expertise should be enlisted immediately. If continued resuscitation of the mother in the left lateral position maintains stable maternal vital signs but does not improve such profound fetal bradycardia, then rapid operative delivery is the next responsibility of the resuscitation team. In cases of persistent fetal heart rate of 60 beats per minute or less, immediate delivery is the only fetal resuscitation move left. This approach should help eliminate many fetal deaths in situations where the degree of trauma to the mother has not been judged to be critical. (In this context, the nonobstetrician especially is concerned about how one determines whether a fetus is not hopelessly premature. Survival rates depend on both birth weight and gestational age. Modern neonatal care yields survival rates at 24 weeks' gestation of between 20 and 40 percent. A rule of thumb is that when the uterine fundus is even just barely above the umbilicus, survival is a definite possibility.)

A cautionary note about electronic fetal monitoring is imperative. Currently, widely used electronic signs of fetal "distress" have come under increasing skepticism as to their validity for intervention. Even though such signs might be expected to have a high sensitivity (true positive rate) in the kind of maternal cardiovascular collapse situation discussed here, there is no solid scientific evidence that any pattern except continuing bradycardia of 60 beats per minute or less is correlated with ongoing fetal asphyxia. Extrapolation and analogy from routine electronic fetal monitoring practices to the catastrophic setting of maternal cardiopulmonary arrest and resuscitation are not advised. Operative intervention for dubious "fetal distress" (e.g., for such electronic chimeras as "decreased variability") in a clinical situation where the resuscitation team has just managed to maintain and stabilize the mother's crashing cardiac output is to be avoided.

MANEUVERS FOR RESUSCITATION OF THE MOTHER

The preceding summary of the changes in maternal physiology produced by the growing fetus has been intended as background for the current position that immediate delivery by cesarean section may be the only possible successful maneuver for cardiopulmonary collapse in late pregnancy. Standard external cardiac compression is performed with the patient supine on a hard surface. In advanced pregnancy, the supine position causes aortocaval compression, so that successful resuscitation may be impossible (Figs. 3-28 and 3-29).

Initially, resuscitation should proceed with the pregnant patient tilted to her left, via a wedge under the right hip or by

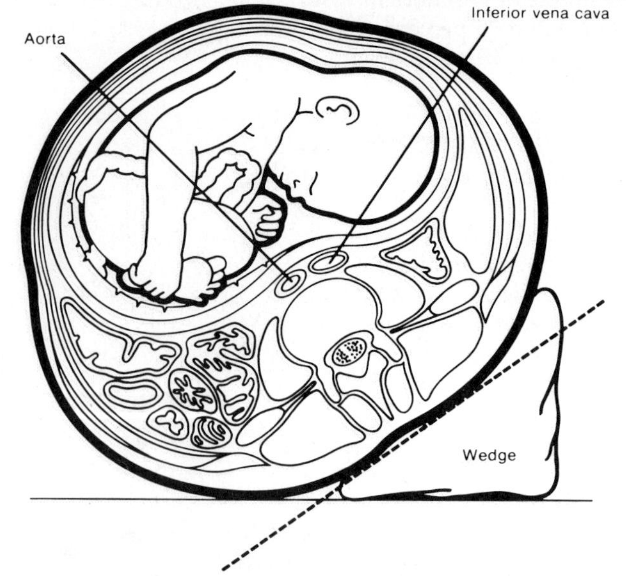

Fig. 3-29. With the mother in the left lateral decubitus position, the uterus is off the aorta and inferior vena cava. Thus, cardiac output is restored. (From G. W. Ostheimer. *Regional Anesthesia Techniques in Obstetrics*. New York: © Breon Laboratories, 1980.)

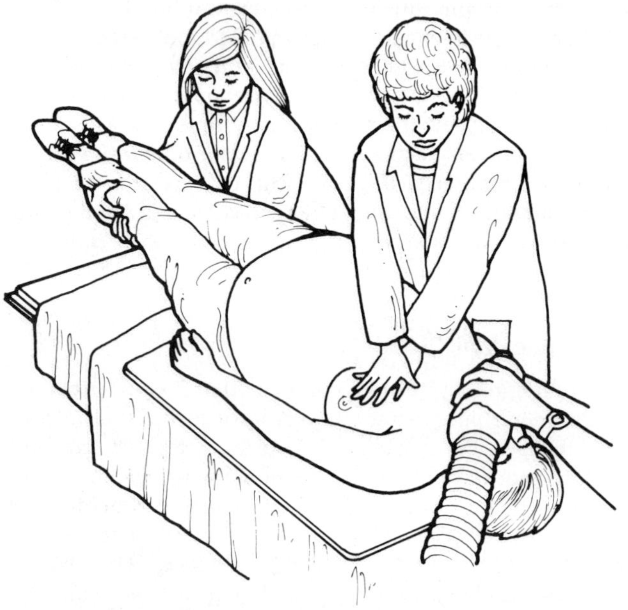

Fig. 3-30. Cardiopulmonary resuscitation in late pregnancy. Note left lateral tilt and raised legs.

Fig. 3-28. The effect of maternal position on cardiac output. With the mother supine, the uterus compresses the aorta and inferior vena cava, causing a drop in cardiac output. (From G.W. Ostheimer. *Regional Anesthesia Techniques in Obstetrics*. New York. © Breon Laboratories, 1980.)

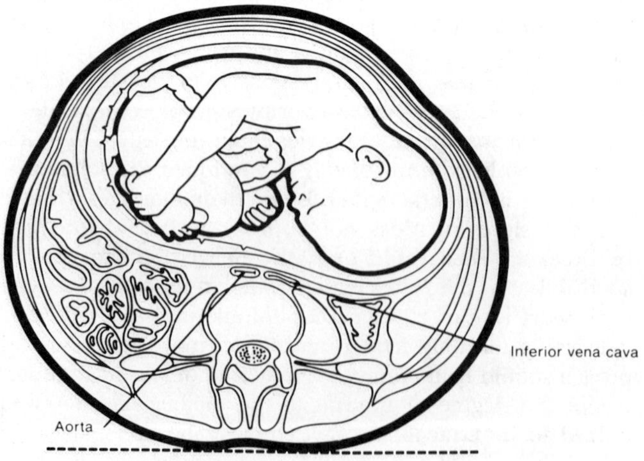

tilting the table to thirty degrees. Endotracheal intubation is difficult due to breast enlargement, but very important because of slow gastric emptying time. If tilting is not possible, one member of the team should pull the uterus to the patient's left and lift it upward toward the patient's head. It is also helpful to elevate the patient's legs (Fig. 3-30). If these efforts do not restore maternal perfusion after five minutes, the uterus must be emptied in order to restore cardiac output. Such cesarean delivery is done for the survival of the mother, but the infant will also benefit. In a recent review of reports of perimortem cesarean section, Katz, et al., concluded that 70 percent of living babies delivered within five minutes of maternal death developed normally.

EMERGENCY CESAREAN SECTION FOR MATERNAL CARDIOVASCULAR COLLAPSE

If the cardiac output of the third-trimester pregnant patient does not respond after five minutes of external cardiac compression, adequate ventilation, volume replacement, and correction of cardiac arrhythmias, metabolic abnormalities, central hypothermia, and so forth, immediate emptying of the uterus is urgent. External cardiac compression should continue as well as all other measures. This procedure should be done in the emergency room by the person with the most surgical experience. Speed is essential; aseptic technique is important but not a priority. Hemostasis is left for after the fetus and placenta are extracted.

The directions outlined here are not only for nonobstetricians but for all nonsurgeons: Open the abdominal wall in midline between the navel and the pubic symphysis (Fig. 3-31). Cut through to the peritoneal cavity at the umbilicus with a scalpel (Fig. 3-32). The enlarged uterus will keep the bowel away. Then extend the incision downward, cutting in a firm continuous motion. After this, make the classic incision in the uterus (Fig. 3-33); this method is quick and safe for the nonobstetrician. Start in the midline at the fundus and cut downward as far as the yellow fat where the bladder is attached over the lower segment of the uterus (Fig. 3-34). As soon as the amniotic cavity is entered, use the fingers of the other hand to guide the scissors or scalpel from the inside of the uterine muscle out to make an incision long enough to extract the fetus (Fig. 3-35).

The chance of injuring small bowel is minimal, and the likelihood of cutting or tearing into the bladder is minor. Both are easily repaired and fear of such complications should not cause hesitation.

Clamp the umbilical cord (use two snaps, Kelly's or even one ligature on the fetal side of the cord as it is cut) even

Fig. 3-31. Emergency cesarean section: abdominal skin incision.

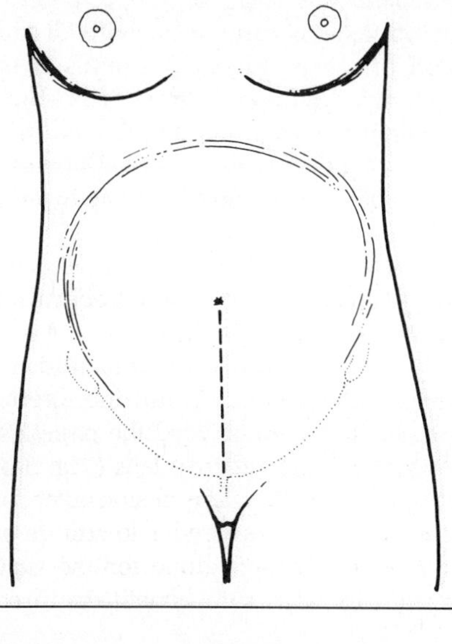

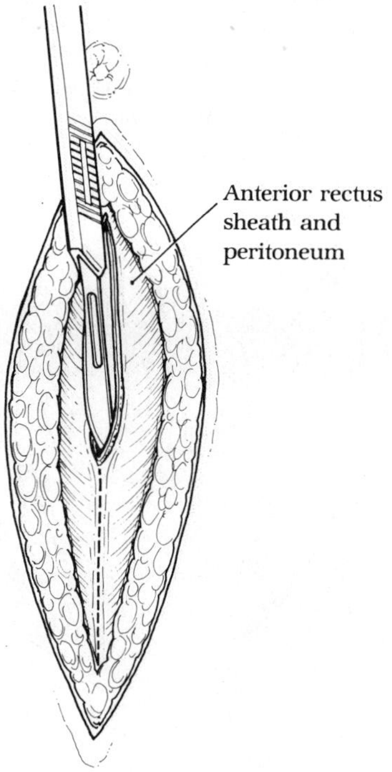

Fig. 3-32. Abdominal wall incision. The blade may be used up through all layers. This incision is quick and avoids bowel and uterus.

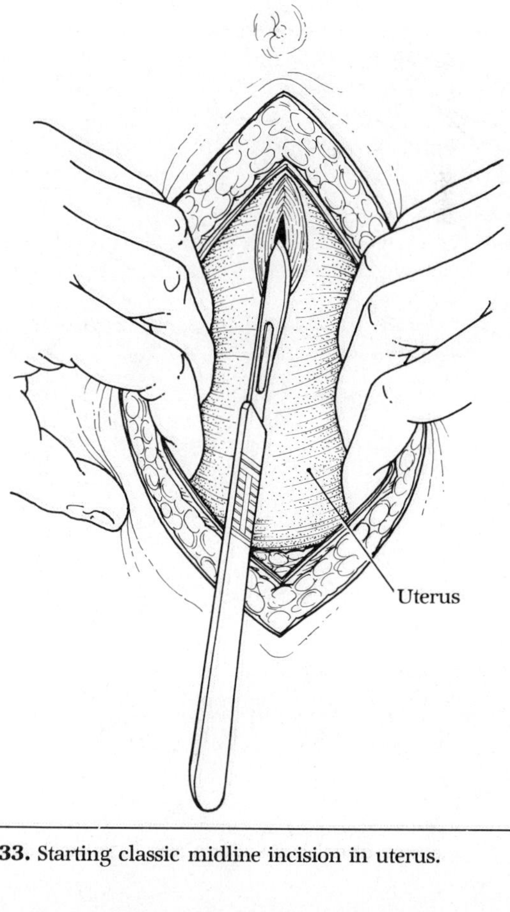

Fig. 3-33. Starting classic midline incision in uterus.

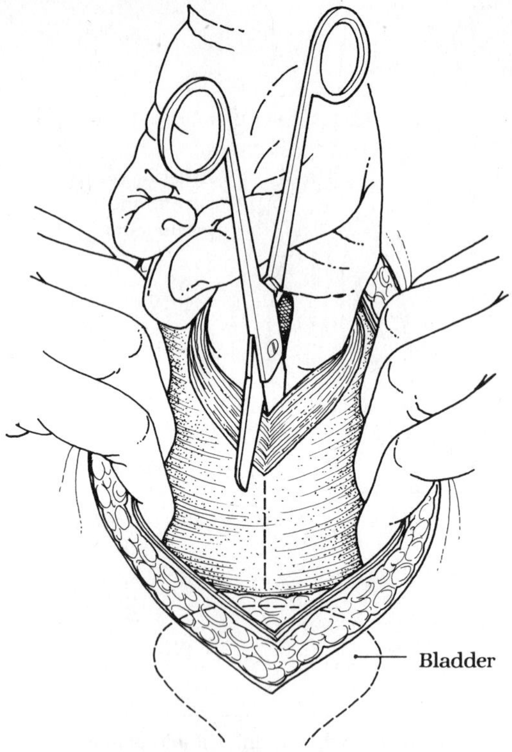

Fig. 3-34. Uterine myometrial incision. Stop at fat over bladder.

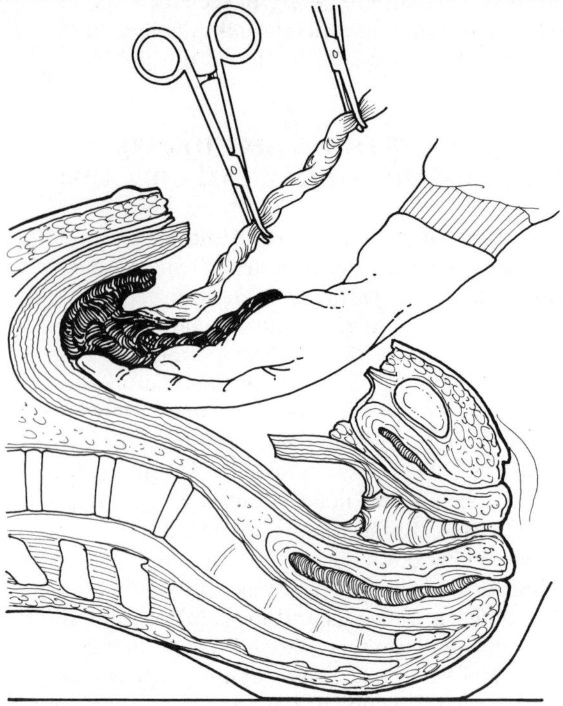

Fig. 3-36. Remove placenta.

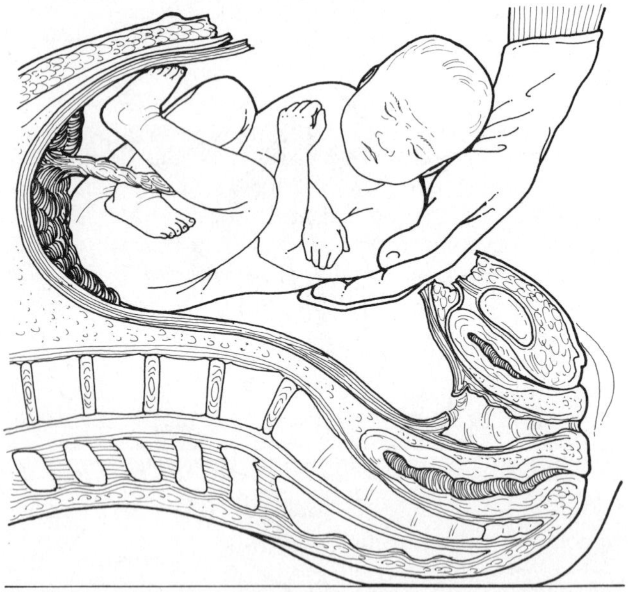

Fig. 3-35. Shoehorn delivery of infant.

before delivering the baby. The placenta will usually extrude spontaneously; removal will be quicker with bimanual massage of the uterus (Fig. 3-36). The placenta is easily removed by twisting. Even if it does not come out, immediate control of bleeding is accomplished by taking a large (Penrose) rubber drain and tightening it around the isthmus of the uterus. The ovarian blood supply will also be included and occluded. Twist the rubber as a tight tourniquet and secure it with a hemostat (Fig. 3-37).

During this procedure (two minutes perhaps), the team should continue cardiopulmonary resuscitation. Postdelivery uterine bleeding responds to intravenous oxytocin and to methylergonovine. Oxytocin should not be given as an undiluted intravenous bolus as it will cause hypotension, tachycardia, and even serious arrhythmias. It is best given with intravenous solutions; it is compatible with all such solutions and with blood products. Mix two ampuls of oxytocin (10 units each) with any amount of intravenous solution already infusing. Intravenous oxytocin is deactivated in minutes, so that a continuous infusion must be maintained. (Two ampuls in a liter of solution is standard.) Methylergonovine, in the face of hypotension and hemorrhage, may be given as an intravenous bolus (0.2 mg), or in any intravenous solution as a drip at any convenient rate. It is more effective than oxytocin for bleeding from uterine atony.

Closing of the uterus and abdomen should preferably be done by a surgeon, who should first make certain that the bladder and intestines need no repair. (Insert a Foley catheter if this was not done already.) The uterus should be inspected to make certain that it is empty of placenta, membranes, and clots. The myometrium is most easily closed with through-and-through, simple, or figure-of-eight (or running) sutures with sufficient strength to withstand

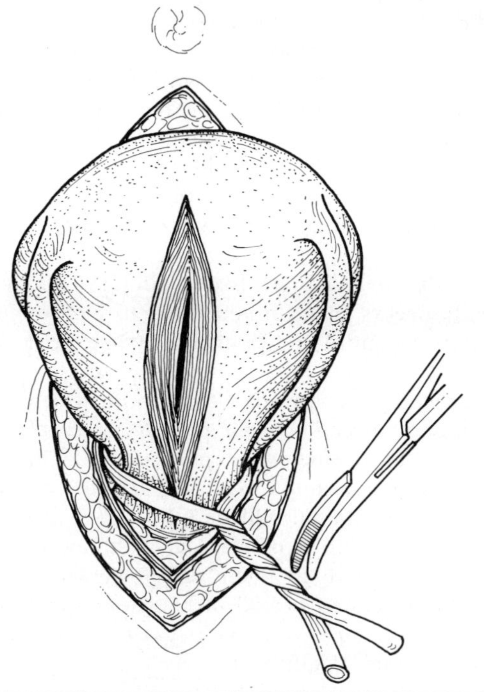

Fig. 3-37. Rubber tourniquet to occlude ovarian and uterine arteries.

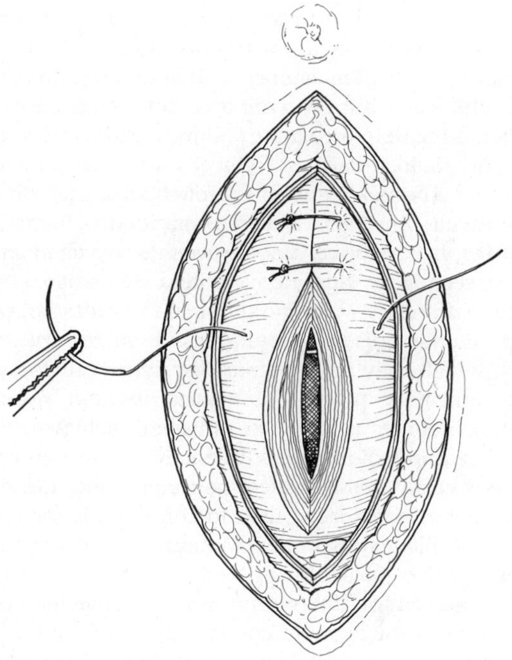

Fig. 3-38. Closure of myometrium. Oversew individual bleeding vessels.

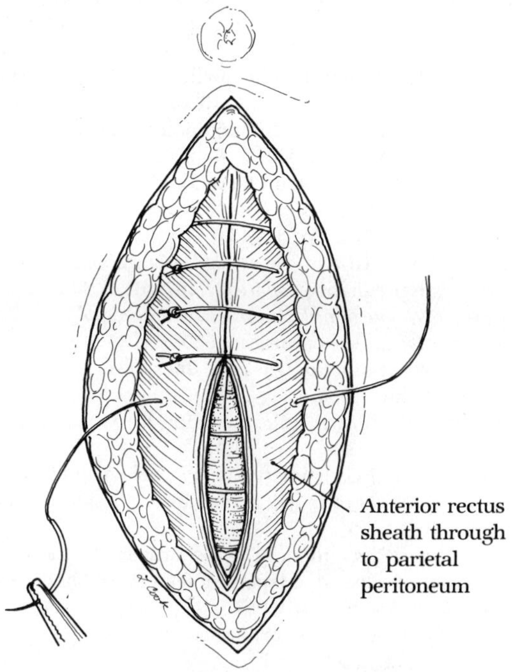

Fig. 3-39. Mass closure of abdominal wall (excluding skin).

enough tension to compress bleeding myometrium. (Number 0 or 1 absorbable sutures such as Chromic, Vicryl, Dexon, or PDS will work well.) Each pole of the uterine incision should be first sutured just beyond the incision to occlude any retracted vessels. Any spot that continues to bleed should be oversewn once again (Fig. 3-38). Keep tension on the myometrial sutures. Clear the abdomen of blood and clot, and vernix and meconium, with large surgical sponges.

Close the abdominal wall with Vicryl, PDS or Dexon (Number 0 or 1) sutures, using a mass closure technique (Fig. 3-39). Take wide bites, either interrupted or running, through the rectus fascia, and muscle into the parietal peritoneum. Close the skin with whatever is convenient. Give an intravenous bolus of antibiotic—for example, ampicillin, cefazolin, cefoxitin, or any other antibiotic with broad (both gram-positive and gram-negative) coverage—as soon as the decision to operate is made, but do not delay because of this. If not confident of hemostasis, leave a large drain (Penrose, Jackson-Pratt, large-bore Foley catheter) in the pelvis and bring it out through the abdominal incision. It may be attached to gentle suction. Designate one attendant to keep track of sponges. Average blood loss at elective cesarean section is 600 ml minimally. This should be taken into account in immediate postoperative care.

SELECTED READING

DePace, NL, Betesh, SS, and Kolter, MM. Postmortem cesarean section with recovery of both mother and offspring. *JAMA* 248:971, 1982.

Gabbe, SG, Niebyl, JR, and Simpson, JL (eds). *Obstetrics: Normal and Problem Pregnancies.* New York: Churchill Livingstone, 1986.

Kasten, GW, and Martin, ST. Resuscitation from bupivacaine induced cardiovascular toxicity during partial vena cava occlusion. *Anesth Analg* 65:341, 1986.

Katz, VL, Dotters, D, and Droegemueller, W. Perimortem cesarean delivery. *Obstet Gynecol* 68:571, 1986.

Marx, GF. Cardiopulmonary resuscitation of late pregnant women. *Anesthesiology* 56:156, 1982.

McFadzean, I. Maternal Blood Flow to the Uterus. In GVP Chamberlain and AW Wilkinson (eds.), *Placental Transfer*. Kent, England: Pitman, 1979. Pp. 31–43.

Oates, S, Williams, GL, and Rees, GAD. Cardiopulmonary resuscitation in late pregnancy. *Br Med J* 297:404, 1988.

Ostheimer, GW. *Regional Anesthesia Techniques in Obstetrics*. New York: Breon Laboratories, 1980.

Ostheimer, GW. *Manual of Obstetric Anesthesia*. New York: Churchill Livingstone, 1984.

Rees, GAD, and Willis, BA. Resuscitation in late pregnancy. *Anesthesia* 43:347, 1988.

Skaredoff, MN, and Ostheimer, GW. Physiological changes during pregnancy: Effects of major regional anesthesia. *Reg Anaesth* 6: 28, 1981.

Thacker, SB, and Berkelman, RL. Assessing the diagnostic accuracy and efficacy of selected antepartum fetal surveillance techniques. *Obstet Gynecol Surv* 41:1, 1986.

Ueland, K, et al. Maternal cardiovascular dynamics. *Am J Obstet Gynecol* 104:856, 1969.

Weber, CE. Postmortem cesarean section: Review of the literature case reports. *Am J Obstet Gynecol* 110:158, 1971.

Wheeler, AS, and Harris, BA. The uterus, placenta, and fetus. *Semin Anesth* 1:101, 1982.

RESUSCITATION OF THE NEWBORN, INFANT, AND CHILD

Robert C. Pascucci

The cause of cardiopulmonary arrest in infants and children is different from that in adults, and the differences affect not only the conduct of resuscitation but also the long-term outlook for the patient. The typical adult arrest victim is first seen after a sudden collapse, the cause of which is likely to have been an acute ventricular dysrhythmia related to coronary or other preexisting cardiac disease. This is termed a "primary" or "cardiogenic" cardiac arrest. If resuscitation is provided promptly and recovery of spontaneous circulation is rapid, the adult patient has an excellent chance of good survival.

Children do not usually have preexisting cardiac disease and are rarely seen with primary cardiac arrest. In the previously healthy child, cardiac arrest is likely to be secondary to some other primary disturbance. These other causes are multiple. The clinical history is of great importance in sorting out the cause; an accurate and complete review of the antecedent events will often suggest a specific diagnosis that is not apparent from the examination alone.

Most often, a noncardiac primary event leads to loss of the airway or respiratory insufficiency; progressive hypoxemia and acidosis ensue and, over an extended period of time, lead to a secondary cardiac arrest. Examples of major events that may necessitate resuscitation include:

1. *Aspiration of foreign bodies.* Aspiration of toys, peanuts, balloons, hot dogs, plastic sheeting, or similar materials all may cause suffocation.
2. *Infection.* Airway infection (croup, epiglottitis, or severe lower airway disease) can directly cause respiratory insufficiency; other infections (meningitis, sepsis) can lead to central respiratory depression.
3. *Trauma.* Direct trauma to the airway, multiple trauma, near-drowning, and the like can cause a respiratory arrest.
4. *Sudden infant death syndrome (SIDS).* This syndrome typically occurs in an infant three to four months old, although the entire first year of life carries risk.

As resuscitation progresses, attention must be directed to evaluation and correction of the primary cause of the arrest as well as to its result. Often, particularly if the primary cause is respiratory, simple restoration of the airway, oxygenation, and ventilation will be all that are needed to restore cardiac function. Unfortunately, although cardiopulmonary resuscitation is often easily achieved in these children, the extended period of hypoxemia and ischemia before presentation may ultimately result in a poor outcome, especially in neurologic function.

Because of the poor outcome for children after resuscitation from a full cardiac arrest, pediatric advanced life support training places major emphasis on the early recognition of impending cardiorespiratory failure. There is good reason for this. Children often are first seen in the emergency department with a disease process that is known to progress to hypoxemia or cardiac decompensation if it is unrecognized or untreated. There is often time to forestall this decompensation, however. Early assessment, anticipatory support, and timely intervention may allow treatment of the primary disease before progression can occur. It is unquestionably true, in these children, that prevention is better than cure.

It is not difficult to recognize children in severe respiratory distress or obvious cardiac failure, and these patients are usually treated quickly and effectively by most practitioners. More difficult, however, is the recognition of more subtle signs of respiratory or cardiac distress during an emergency visit for a seemingly unrelated problem. The astute clinician must be vigilant to avoid missing such warning signs. Primary pulmonary disease results in altered respiratory mechanics, which may only be manifest by grunting or a prolonged expiratory phase. Tachypnea without respiratory distress, sometimes referred to as "silent tachypnea," is an excellent example of a more subtle finding. A rapid respiratory rate is easily missed unless one specifically looks for it, yet it is a common mechanism to compensate for a developing metabolic acidosis in early shock, severe dehydration, or some forms of poisoning.

Early intervention for circulatory insufficiency requires appreciation of the signs of poor perfusion: Coolness of the skin, slow capillary refill, and decreased urine output are straightforward indicators of inadequate cardiac output. Subtle changes in the level of consciousness, with alternating confusion, lethargy, and agitation; failure to recognize parents; or simply a child who "just doesn't act right" are warning signs of brain, and therefore systemic, hypoperfusion. Tachycardia, with a normal or even elevated blood pressure, is often the early warning of insufficient cardiac output; hypotension is a late and sudden complication, often an immediate precedent of frank cardiac arrest.

The progression from these early signs of distress to complete cardiopulmonary arrest can occur with frightening speed, particularly in infants and small children. Rapid attention to and alleviation of airway disease, restoration of lost intravascular volume, and general supportive care provided in a timely fashion will usually prevent or minimize hypoxic or ischemic damage, avoiding a secondary cardiac arrest. Unless the primary disease is itself devastating, the prognosis for children so managed is reasonably good. If the child is allowed to progress to a true cardiac arrest, the prognosis for good outcome is markedly decreased.

RESUSCITATION: BASIC LIFE SUPPORT

As an arbitrary convention, the resuscitation literature has defined a newborn baby as a newborn, anyone younger than one year as an infant, anyone one to eight years old as a child, and anyone over eight years old as an adult. We shall use those conventions here, with the caveat that, although adult techniques of resuscitation may be applied to a nine-year-old child, medication dosages should continue to be based on a "per kilogram" basis until true adult size and weight are achieved (Table 3-1). Standards and guidelines for cardiopulmonary resuscitation (CPR) are updated and published approximately every six years by national research and consensus conferences; the following recommendations are based on the 1985 conferences and the 1986 revision of the guidelines.

The Physiology of Cardiopulmonary Resuscitation

The mechanism of blood flow and its distribution during CPR have been extensively investigated over the past decade. The assumption, prevalent since Kouwenhoven's initial description of closed-chest CPR in 1960, has been that forward blood flow during CPR is generated by compression of the heart between the sternum and spine. Recent investigation has proposed that, in larger animals and probably in humans, thoracic rather than direct cardiac compression is the driving force for blood flow: A general increase in intrathoracic pressure, generated by chest compression, forces blood outward through the aorta. Flow is predominantly in a forward direction because of valves in the jugular venous system, which prevent retrograde flow through that system. The forward flow also results from collapse of the veins at the thoracic inlet, and perhaps from the reduced compliance (and, thus, greater pressure development) in the arterial tree as compared to the venous system.

Table 3-1. Pediatric resuscitation: Average weights for age

Age	Weight (kg)	Weight (lb)
Term newborn	3–4	6–9
6 mo	7–8	15–18
1 yr	9–11	20–24
18 mo	10–12	22–26
2 yr	11–14	24–30
3 yr	15	33
5 yr	20	44
8 yr	25	55
10 yr	30	66
15 yr	50	110

Investigation continues into the distribution of this blood flow, with special attention to the generation of adequate coronary and cerebral perfusion. It has become apparent that coronary perfusion depends on the generation of an adequate aortic diastolic (i.e., the relaxation phase of chest compression) pressure; a sufficient aortic-to-right-atrial pressure difference is necessary to allow flow. Cerebral blood flow has been more problematic: It is more difficult to quantify, and some techniques that have been suggested to increase intrathoracic pressure, thereby improving forward blood flow, may actually impede cerebral perfusion.

It is possible that circulation of blood during CPR occurs by both thoracic-pump and cardiac-pump mechanisms, with the dominant one being determined by the individual patient's size and anatomy. Chest compression in newborns and infants, because of their smaller and more compliant thoracic cavity, may well generate flow by direct cardiac compression. Older children may be more like adults, with a predominance of the thoracic-pump mechanism. The best method for CPR may also vary, then, from individual to individual; in some instances, open-chest resuscitation with direct cardiac compression may return to clinical practice as the preferable technique.

Basic Life Support Techniques

Assessment of the patient's responsiveness is accomplished easily: Vigorous stimulation (shake and shout) should produce awakening and a cry. If not, further therapy is needed and help should be summoned. In the field, the circumstances in which a child is found will often suggest whether trauma has occurred. If there is any question of trauma, caution must be taken in positioning the child to avoid further damage. If head or neck injury is suspected, axial cervical traction must be maintained until cervical spine injury is excluded or the neck is immobilized. If the child is face down, he or she must be rolled over as a unit, carefully avoiding twisting or tilting of the spinal column. To ensure effective CPR, the child should be supine on a firm, flat surface.

Airway

Loss of the airway is frequently the primary cause of a pediatric arrest; thus, the first step in resuscitation is the establishment of an open airway. Soft-tissue obstruction, as from loss of pharyngeal muscle tone, can be relieved by the head tilt–chin lift maneuver (Fig. 3-40) or by a jaw-thrust maneuver (Fig. 3-41). In our experience, this straight anterior thrust of the jaw by forceful dislocation of the mandible at the angles of the jaw seems to work best and, if neck injury is suspected, has the additional advantage of minimizing spinal motion. One should avoid hyperextension of the neck, which may stretch and occlude the trachea. These maneu-

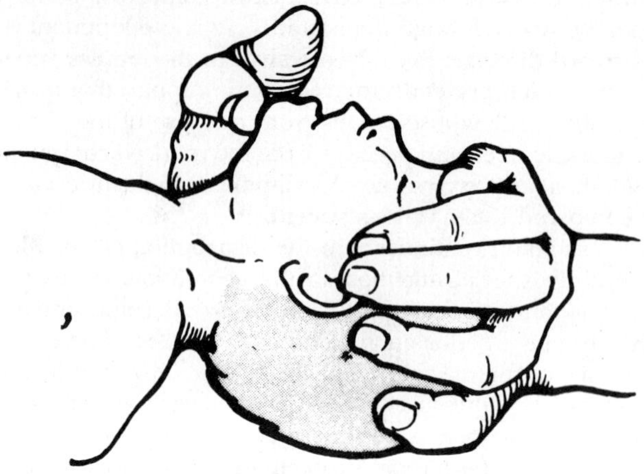

Fig. 3-40. The head tilt–chin lift method for opening the airway. Care must be taken to avoid extreme hyperextension of the neck.

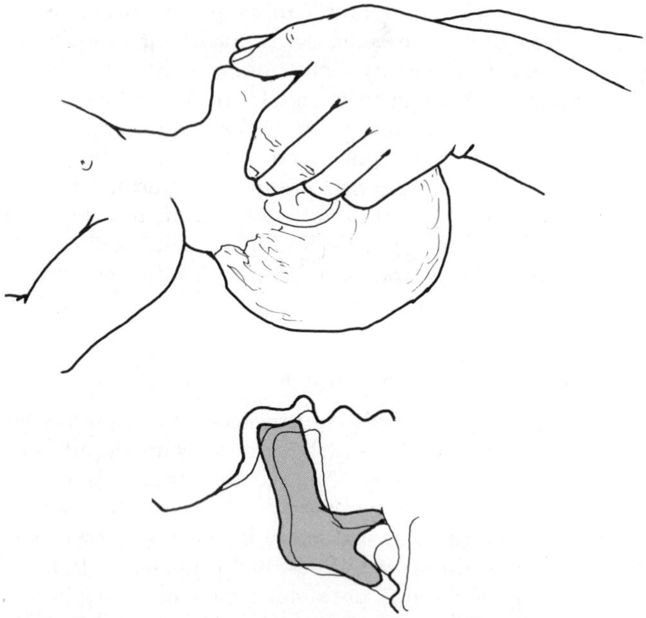

Fig. 3-41. Jaw-thrust maneuver. Anterior motion of the jaw by forceful dislocation of the mandible at the temporomandibular joint; a click is felt as the jaw moves forward. This is a particularly effective way to open the airway.

vers will relieve soft-tissue airway obstruction in most children. If necessary, oral or nasal airway adjuncts may be inserted; their use is discussed further in this chapter and in the Procedures section of this text (see Procedures 2, 3, and 41).

Foreign material (toys, food, loose teeth) should be removed from the oropharynx under direct vision. Airway obstruction secondary to an aspirated foreign body may be partial or complete. *Complete* foreign-body airway obstruction in the child may be relieved with subdiaphragmatic abdominal thrusts (the Heimlich maneuver) in a manner analogous to that used in adults. Because of concern for potential intraabdominal injury resulting from this maneuver in infants, a combination of back blow and chest thrusts

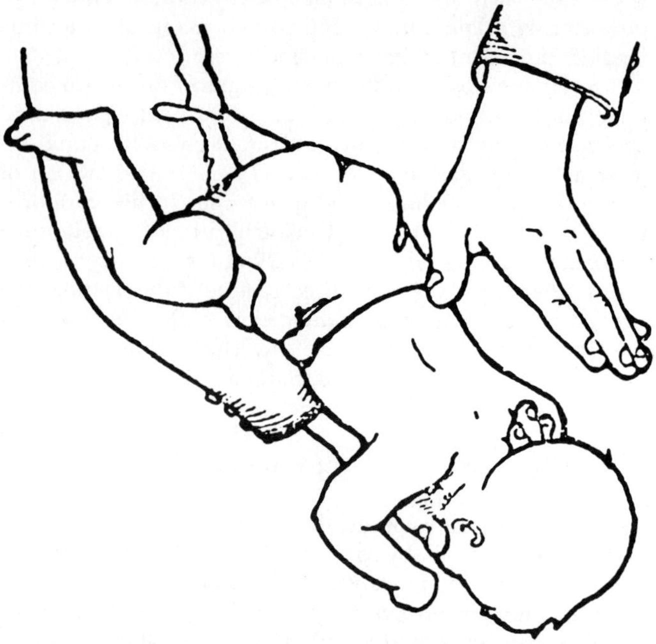

Fig. 3-42. Back blows in the infant. The lowered head allows gravity to assist in expulsion of foreign material.

is recommended for relief of airway obstruction in this age group. The infant should be placed face down on the rescuer's forearm, head lower than trunk, to allow gravity to assist in expulsion of the object (Fig. 3-42). Four back blows are forcefully given with the heel of the hand between the infant's shoulder blades; the infant is then turned as a unit to a face-up position, and four chest thrusts are delivered in the same location to that detailed later for chest compressions. If the object is dislodged into the upper airway, it can be removed carefully.

If the foreign body is causing *partial* airway obstruction but the child has adequate spontaneous air movement and cough, it is best not to attempt dislodgment of the foreign body (which may then totally occlude the airway) but rather to arrange for more sophisticated management such as bronchoscopy. Oxygen should be administered as soon as it is available since, despite severe airway obstruction, hypoxemia may be averted by increasing the fractional concentration of inhaled oxygen (FiO_2).

Breathing

Successful relief of airway obstruction will be signified by the return of air flow through the nose and mouth of the victim who is still attempting to breathe; this is assessed by "look, listen, and feel" as in adult resuscitation. If the infant or child does not ventilate adequately, rescue breathing must begin.

An airtight seal must be secured between the rescuer's mouth and the victim's mouth or, in an infant, over the mouth and nose (Fig. 3-43). Two breaths, of sufficient volume to make the chest rise, are given slowly (1.0–1.5 seconds per inflation) with a pause between breaths. Care should be taken to avoid excess pressure and volume; gastric distention may occur, hindering lung expansion and making regurgitation more likely. If adequate chest expansion is not

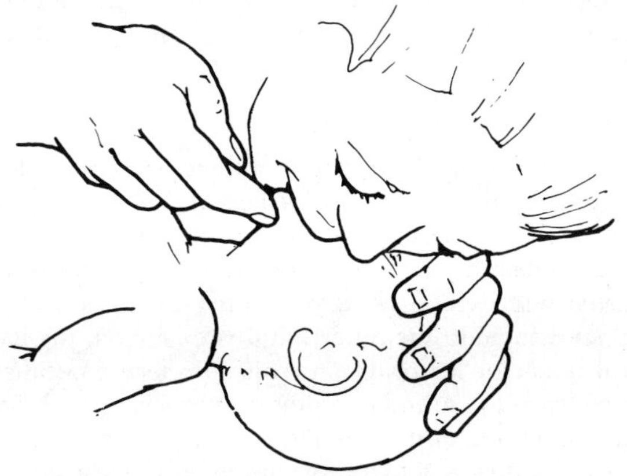

Fig. 3-43. Mouth-to-mouth ventilation. The rescuer may cover either just the mouth or the mouth and nose, depending on the child's size. Care must be taken to maintain anterior jaw displacement throughout the breathing cycle.

obtained, airway obstruction persists, and the rescuer should repeat the procedure of opening the airway and attempting to ventilate. If the airway remains obstructed, the presence of a foreign body should be suspected, and management should be begun as previously discussed.

Once chest expansion is attained, the pulse is checked (see the following section). If adequate circulation is present, rescue breathing alone is continued. The younger infant requires a faster ventilatory rate than the older child; typical rates are 30 to 40 breaths per minute for the newborn and infant, 20 to 30 breaths per minute for the young child, and 12 to 20 breaths per minute for the older child.

Circulation

As soon as the patient is ventilated effectively, the pulse should be palpated to determine if cardiac compression will also be required. In the infant the pulse can best be felt by palpating the brachial or femoral artery; in the child, the carotid artery is used. If the pulse is absent, weak, or very slow, closed-chest cardiac compression should begin immediately.

The child is placed on a firm surface, and the chest is compressed by applying pressure over the lower third of the sternum, just below the level of the nipples, depressing it approximately one-third of the anterior-posterior diameter of the chest (1.5–2.5 cm in the infant, 2.5–3.0 cm in the small child, and 4–5 cm in the adolescent). In the older child, two-hand compression is used as in the adult. In the younger child, one hand will provide adequate compression; in the infant, two or three fingers may be sufficient (Fig. 3-44A). For the newborn or small infant, better compression may be accomplished by placing both thumbs over the midsternum and encircling the chest with both hands so that the fingers provide a firm base beneath the back (Fig. 3-44B). This technique is only used when two rescuers are available. The rate of cardiac compression should be a minimum of 80 beats per minute (bpm) for older children, 80 to 100 bpm for younger children, and 100 to 120 bpm for infants, with a compression-relaxation ratio of 1:1. The compression-ventilation ratio is 5:1 (even if there is only one rescuer), with a pause after every fifth compression to allow the breath to be delivered over approximately 1.0 to 1.5 seconds. If two rescuers are working together, the compression cadence should be counted aloud by the rescuer who is performing chest compression. With effective cardiac compression, pulses should be palpable in major arteries.

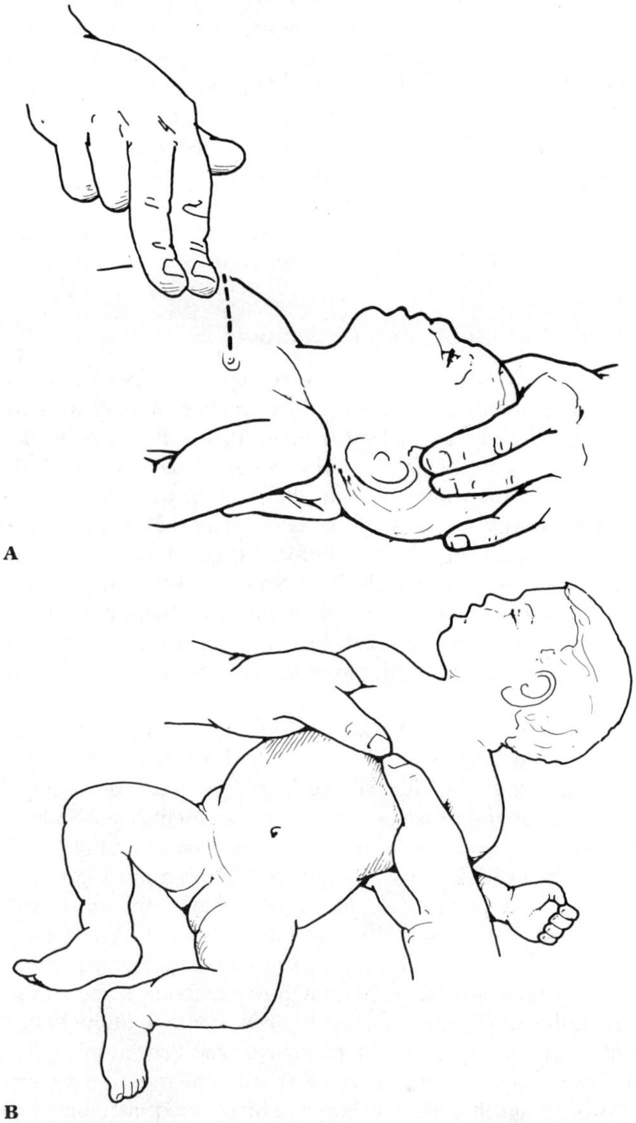

Fig. 3-44. Chest compression in the infant and child. A. Working from the side, the rescuer uses two fingers, compressing the chest in the midline at approximately one finger's width below an imaginary line drawn between the nipples. B. An alternate technique for the newborn or small infant, useful when two rescuers are present. The fingers support the child from the vertebral column behind; the thumbs provide compression over the lower third of the sternum.

RESUSCITATION: ADVANCED LIFE SUPPORT

Advanced life support must be provided on the background of continued effective basic CPR. This point cannot be overemphasized since, often, the basics are forgotten in the excitement of the moment. As anyone who has been involved in a resuscitation in a hospital setting can attest, a frequent problem in delivering life support is the presence of too many people, with resulting confusion and inefficiency. Control and coordination of efforts are important. One physician should take on the role of director of the resuscitation. This individual should oversee the performance of all team members, not personally performing tasks but assigning duties as needed, thus allowing him- or herself to stand back and evaluate the progress of the resuscitation as a whole.

Airway, Breathing, and Circulation

Details of advanced airway management in infants and children are presented in the Procedures section of this text, and will be touched on only briefly here. Most soft-tissue airway obstruction can be successfully relieved by careful positioning and firm anterior jaw dislocation, as noted previously. If necessary, oral or nasal airway adjuncts can be inserted. The oral airway should be sized carefully and placed so as to just encircle the tongue; if it is too long or too short, it will worsen rather than improve the obstruction. Nasal airways can be used, but must be placed gently to avoid trauma and bleeding from the child's vascular adenoid bed.

If the patient is not breathing, bag-mask ventilation with 100 percent oxygen should be begun as soon as possible. The mask is chosen by the rescuer's preference. For infants, triangular-shaped masks such as the Rendell-Baker-Soucek will allow a good mask fit and seal with minimal dead space; older children can be ventilated with a more conventional-shaped ovoid mask (Fig. 3-45). Ideally, the mask will be transparent. A self-inflating bag-valve system is useful because of its ability to function without a fresh-gas source, but most experienced rescuers will prefer to use some variation on the Mapleson or Ayre's T-piece system to allow better control of FIO_2 and airway pressures (see Procedure 41A). The rate, volume, and force of ventilation must be varied according to the patient's size to achieve adequate chest expansion without causing gastric distention. An orogastric or nasogastric tube will relieve this distention should it occur; placement of such a tube should be a routine part of resuscitation in infants and children.

Ventilation should be continued with bag and mask until everything is prepared for intubation. A common mistake, particularly in the less controlled surroundings of the emergency department, is to rush to intubate the patient without adequate equipment, preparation, or assistance. Ventilation and oxygenation come first, with intubation following as a relatively elective procedure. Time is required to assemble the correct endotracheal tube, laryngoscope and blade, suction apparatus, and related materials; skilled assistance from a respiratory therapist or other trained individual is invaluable. An oral endotracheal tube is best in most emergency situations (see Procedure 41B); it can be exchanged for a nasal tube when the child's condition is more stable. Once intubation is achieved, the adequacy of bilateral ventilation must be confirmed and frequently reassessed. If adequate bilateral air entry is not present, one must quickly run through a differential diagnosis: Malposition or obstruction of the endotracheal tube, excess leak through the glottis, other leaks in the system, gastric distention, pneumothorax, and hemothorax must all be considered and excluded.

Venous Access

Venous access is needed to allow volume and drug administration. Many details of venous access techniques are reviewed in the Procedures section of this text. The clinician who is establishing this access should use the approach and technique with which he or she is most experienced. Suggested sites include the antecubital, saphenous, jugular, or femoral veins; the femoral vein is often preferred because it is relatively easy to cannulate without interfering with the resuscitation effort. Although the security of a well-placed deep venous line is reassuring, fluids and medications can be administered through peripheral catheters, and undue delay should not be generated by repeated attempts at central access.

If venous access is delayed, the standard doses of epinephrine, atropine, lidocaine, and naloxone can be diluted in sterile water and administered through the endotracheal tube. Recently, there has been interest in an older technique—intraosseous administration of fluids using a bone-marrow needle placed through the anterior surface on the tibia. This technique has been demonstrated to be excellent for emergency infusion of fluids, blood products, and medications.

Volume

The child who is first seen in arrest may be hypovolemic. It is important to remember that the child subjected to ongoing loss of circulatory volume responds somewhat differently than the adult. As losses continue, the adult will become tachycardic and hypotensive over some time; the hypotension can be used as an indicator of the need for volume replacement. The infant or child will also become tachycardic; blood pressure, however, is much better preserved than in the adult, because of the child's highly responsive vascular circuit and ability to vasoconstrict. A child can be drastically hypovolemic and still have a relatively normal blood pressure. When the volume loss finally exceeds the ability to compensate, however, the subsequent loss of blood pressure is catastrophic, and loss of cardiac output with subsequent cardiac arrest occurs within minutes.

It is inappropriate, then, to be reassured that a child is doing well and is not hypovolemic simply because the blood pressure is adequate. Volume replacement must be begun early, guided by clinical history, physical examination, degree of tachycardia, and response to volume challenge. The usual maintenance solution for children is 5% dextrose in quarter-normal saline. This may be used as a "keep-open" solution during resuscitation but is not appropriate for use in volume restoration because of its potential for inducing hyponatremia if given rapidly or in large quantity. Volume infusion is given in aliquots of 10 ml/kg of an isotonic solution: normal saline, Ringer's lactate, or colloid, with the latter reserved for specific indications or for use once greater than 30 to 40 ml/kg crystalloid has been given. If a coagulopathy exists, fresh-frozen plasma, platelets, or cryoprecipitate may be administered. The normal hematocrit in new-

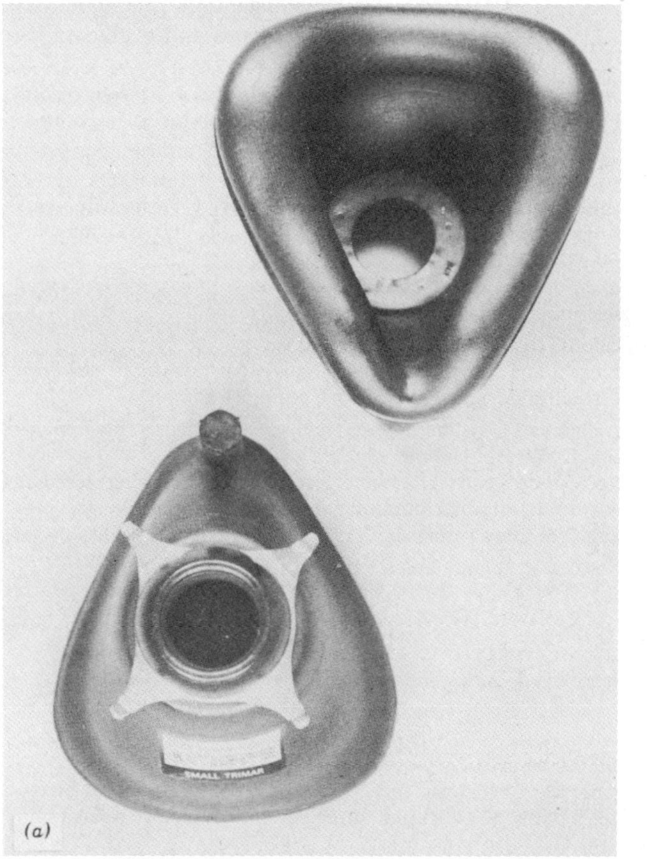

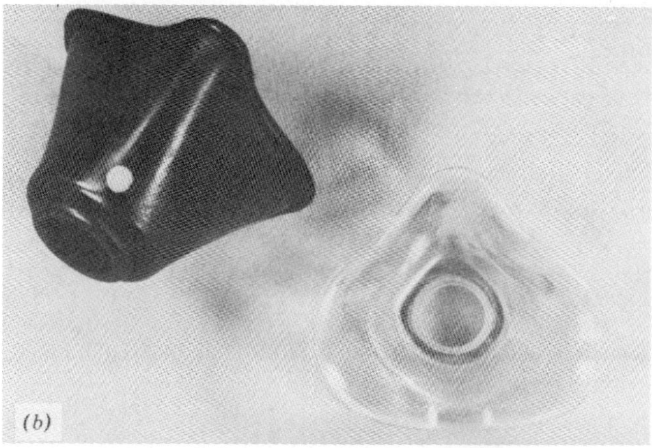

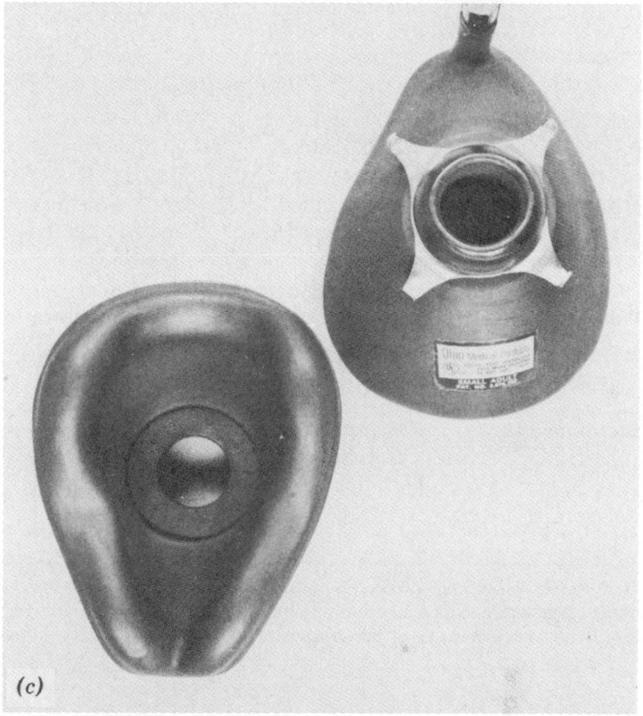

Fig. 3-45. *Masks.* The Trimar (a) and the Rendell-Baker-Soucek (b) masks are triangular in shape and will fit an infant or small child well. The conventional mask (c) has a more oval shape that is suitable for older children and adults. The rescuer should choose one that will allow a good fit and be comfortable to use.

borns is in the range of 45 to 50 percent; by three months of age, it may have dropped to 30 percent, but rises again to 35 percent by one year of age and remains there until puberty, when it rises to adult levels. If the patient's hematocrit is low, red blood cells can be given as a portion of the volume replacement.

Temperature

Temperature should be measured during resuscitation with a thermometer capable of registering temperatures as low as 20°C. The hypothermic child will be difficult to resuscitate until he or she is warmed past 30°C; in such a case, it is best to continue good basic CPR, refrain from repeated drug administration, and direct attention to rewarming, using warming lights, warmed respiratory gases and intravenous fluids, gastric or colonic irrigation with warmed solutions, warmed peritoneal dialysis, or heat exchange by an extracorporeal circuit.

Most significant from the viewpoint of resuscitation are the effects of cold on the cardiovascular system. As cooling proceeds through the 28° to 30°C range, progressive bradycardia ensues. Ventricular fibrillation can occur in response to stimulation (as from the placement of a central venous catheter into the heart) in the 28° to 32°C range; lower temperatures give rise to spontaneous ventricular fibrillation and, ultimately, asystole. These dysrhythmias are often resistant to standard therapy, but may spontaneously convert as temperature is returned to normal.

Abnormalities of Rate and Rhythm

The child should receive electrocardiographic (ECG) monitoring as soon as possible; the ECG will guide further therapy. The most common patterns seen in pediatric cardiac arrests are asystole or a very slow, idioventricular rhythm. These patterns probably reflect the long prodrome of hypoxia and ischemia that precede the actual arrest. Ventricular tachycardia or fibrillation at presentation is decidedly uncommon; blind defibrillation is therefore not indicated in children.

A rhythm disturbance is treated as an emergency if it compromises the cardiac output or if it has the potential to

Table 3-2. Pediatric resuscitation drugs

Drug	Dose and route*	How supplied	Comments
Epinephrine	10 μg/kg IV, IT (0.1 ml/kg 1:10,000 solution)	1:1,000 (1 mg/ml) 1:10,000 (0.1 mg/ml)	Indications: asystole; fine ventricular fibrillation, to coarsen before electroshock; to increase vascular tone and perfusion pressure
Atropine	0.02 mg/kg IV, IT	0.4 mg/ml 1 mg/ml 1 mg/10 ml	Indications: bradycardia with hypotension, bradycardia with ventricular ectopy; severe bradycardia (HR < 90–100 in infants, < 60–70 in children) *Cautions:* tachycardia not well tolerated in coronary disease; small doses may paradoxically worsen bradycardia
Sodium bicarbonate ($NaHCO_3$)	1–2 mEq/kg IV	8.4% (1 mEq/ml)	Indications: significant metabolic acidosis *Cautions:* dilute 1:1 with D_5W or sterile water for use in newborns and small infants; avoid excessive administration
Calcium chloride ($CaCl_2$)	10–30 mg/kg (0.1–0.3 ml/kg) IV	10% solution (100 mg $CaCl_2$/ml)	Indications: hypotension; hypocalcemia, hyperkalemia, hypermagnesemia; calcium channel blocker overdose *Cautions:* not effective in asystole; extravasation may yield tissue necrosis; rapid administration may produce bradycardia; may precipitate coronary vasospasm in susceptible patients
Calcium gluconate	30–90 mg/kg (0.3–0.9 ml/kg) IV	10% solution (100 mg/ml)	Same as $CaCl_2$; slightly less sclerotic
Dextrose	0.5–1.0 gm/kg (2–4 ml/kg of 25% solution) IV	50% (500 mg/ml) and 25% (250 mg/ml) solution	Indications: hypoglycemia (documented or suspected) *Cautions:* hypertonic solution; administer slowly
Lidocaine	1 mg/kg IV, IT	1% (10 mg/ml) or 2% (20 mg/ml) without epinephrine	Indications: ventricular tachycardia *Cautions:* metabolism slowed in congestive failure; avoid in high degrees of AV block; rapid administration can cause seizures
Bretylium	5 mg/kg; 10 mg/kg (repeat dose) IV	50 mg/ml	Useful in refractory ventricular fibrillation
Naloxone (Narcan)	10 μg/kg IV, IT	0.4 mg/ml 0.02 mg/ml	Indications: suspected narcotic overdose

*Intravenous drugs may also be given intraosseously. Intratracheal drugs should be diluted to 5–10 ml with sterile water. Drugs may be administered via intracardiac injection as a last resort, but this route carries significant risk of myocardial damage.
Key: IV = intravenous; IT = intratracheal; HR = heart rate; AV = atrioventricular.

degenerate into a lethal rhythm. In general, the clinician is faced with three types of dysrhythmias: too fast, too slow, or disorganized. Although specific therapy must be available for specific dysrhythmias in more stable circumstances, all tachydysrhythmias associated with cardiovascular decompensation are treated with synchronized cardioversion. The initial electrical charge for cardioversion is 0.5 to 1.0 joules/kg; if unsuccessful, the dose may be increased to 2.0 joules/kg. Bradydysrhythmias are treated by ensuring good oxygenation and ventilation, performing basic CPR, and administering medications as detailed in the following section. Ventricular fibrillation is treated by nonsynchronized defibrillation, using an initial dose of 2 joules/kg, with increases to 4 to 6 joules/kg if subsequent attempts are necessary.

Should cardioversion or defibrillation be required, pediatric paddles should be used; the largest electrode size allowing good contact with the skin over the entire electrode area is best. An appropriate electrically conductive gel and firm pressure should be used to ensure good transmission of the current between paddle and skin. Paddle placement is ideally in an anterior-posterior pattern, with one paddle on the anterior chest over the heart and the second (often larger) under the back. An alternative placement is with one paddle lateral to the apex of the heart in the midaxillary line and the other on the upper anterior surface of the contralateral chest.

Medications

Restoration of oxygenation and ventilation, with a short period of good basic CPR, may be all that is required to restore spontaneous cardiac function. Pharmacologic therapy may be needed, however, and is generally similar to that used in the adult; doses are shown in Table 3-2. Although the intravenous route of administration is preferred, certain drugs (atropine, epinephrine, lidocaine, and naloxone) can be given via the endotracheal tube. Medications are well absorbed from the bone marrow and, thus, the intraosseous route may also be useful.

Epinephrine

Aside from oxygen, epinephrine is clearly the most important of all resuscitation drugs for children as well as adults.

Although the drug has both alpha- and beta-adrenergic stimulating effects, there is much evidence to suggest that the alpha (vasoconstrictive) effect is the one of greatest importance in restoring cerebral and coronary perfusion. Enhanced myocardial blood flow allows removal of waste products and reoxygenation of the heart muscle. Epinephrine should be one of the first drugs given for cardiac arrest; specific indications include asystole, bradyarrhythmias, fine ventricular fibrillation, and (as an infusion) for pressor support after resuscitation.

Atropine
Infants and small children have little ability to increase stroke volume because of their small, relatively noncompliant ventricles and depend on heart rate for cardiac output. Atropine is useful to increase heart rate in bradycardic children, and also to provide protection from the vagal stimulation of laryngoscopy and intubation. One must be careful to give an adequate dose (0.02 mg/kg or more); smaller doses may actually worsen bradycardia by a central mechanism.

Bicarbonate
The acid-base status of patients undergoing resuscitation is unclear and the subject of ongoing investigation. The administration of sodium bicarbonate in an effort to correct acidosis has been a long-standing practice, with little documentation of benefit and increasing evidence of possible risk. It is no longer recommended in adult CPR, where, if resuscitation is reasonably prompt, little lactic acidosis occurs, and where respiratory acidosis is rapidly corrected by successful resuscitation. The pediatric arrest, as noted previously, has a different cause; the child often is first seen after a prolonged prodrome and a significant component of metabolic acidosis has developed. A small initial dose of bicarbonate (1 mEq/kg or less) may be indicated in these children after adequate ventilation is assured; subsequent doses should be administered based on results of blood gas determinations. The drug still carries risks of generating hyperosmolarity, hypernatremia, and metabolic alkalosis if given in large quantity.

Calcium
The role of calcium in resuscitation is also in question. There is little documentation of its efficacy and some concern about its potential for aggravation of postresuscitation disease. Calcium is indicated for hypocalcemia, hyperkalemia, hypermagnesemia, and calcium channel blocker overdose; it is occasionally useful for transient circulatory support in hypotension. Evidence has been found that there may be developmental changes in calcium flux and its relation to myocardial function, perhaps making the infant more dependent on extracellular calcium concentration. The infant who is less than one year of age seems particularly sensitive to the effect of calcium channel blocking agents. Whether these differences will indicate a more important role for calcium in sustaining myocardial performance in infants than in adults remains to be seen.

Dextrose
Hypoglycemia is not uncommon during acute illness in smaller children because of their limited glycogen stores. The presence of hypoglycemia during resuscitation is easily detected with a blood glucose test strip; if blood glucose is low, glucose administration may dramatically improve the child's condition. Empiric glucose administration once during resuscitation is acceptable, but one should be cautious not to induce hyperglycemia, which carries risks of hyperosmolarity and which may worsen the cerebral outcome in the postresuscitation period. Glucose is most often administered as 25% dextrose in water; this solution is hyperosmolar and must be administered slowly, especially in small infants.

Antiarrhythmics
Lidocaine is useful for management of ventricular ectopy and as an adjunct to defibrillation in the child with an unstable rhythm. Persistent dysrhythmias are uncommon in the postresuscitation period, presumably because of the lack of coronary disease in children. If present, they suggest the presence of a metabolic or toxic cause. Thus, a lidocaine infusion is required only infrequently in children.

Bretylium may be effective in terminating serious arrhythmias, including ventricular fibrillation, where other agents have failed. It should be administered to patients with refractory ventricular tachycardia or fibrillation; rapid infusion in the conscious patient may induce nausea and vomiting.

Continued Cardiovascular Support
Infusions of catecholamines and other agents are often required to maintain perfusion in the postresuscitation period. A full discussion of the various agents used is beyond the scope of this chapter, but typical doses and dilutions are given in Table 3-3. The drugs differ in inotropic and vascular effect. *Dopamine* is very commonly used, both for its special effect on renal blood flow and urine output in lower doses (2–5 μg/kg per minute) and for its support of myocardial contractility at moderate doses (5–20 μg/kg per minute). At high doses, however, dopamine causes prominent peripheral vasoconstriction, which may be undesirable. *Dobutamine* offers a similar increase in contractility, but without a significant increase in peripheral vascular tone; it has no selective renal effect. *Epinephrine* is the most potent direct-acting catecholamine and is most beneficial when used as a low-dose infusion (<0.3 μg/kg per minute) to provide inotropic support; significant peripheral vasoconstriction is seen at higher doses. *Isoproterenol* is a very potent, positive inotropic and chronotropic agent; it is most useful in settings where a large increase in heart rate and contractility is de-

Table 3-3. Pediatric drug infusions*

Drug	Dilution	Factor	Dose range (μg/kg/min)
Dopamine	40 mg/50 ml	0.075	2–20
Dobutamine	25 mg/50 ml	0.12	2.5–15
Isoproterenol	2 mg/50 ml	1.5	0.1–1.0
Epinephrine	2 mg/50 ml	1.5	0.1–1.0
Norepinephrine	2 mg/50 ml	1.5	0.1–1.0
Lidocaine	100 mg/50 ml	0.03	15–50
Nitroprusside	25 mg/50 ml	0.12	1–10

*Infusion rate (ml/hr) = weight (kg) × desired dose (μg/kg/min) × factor.
Source: Modified from chart prepared by Judy Shaw, R.N., Coordinator, Nursing Education, Multidisciplinary Intensive Care Unit, The Children's Hospital, Boston.

sired and where peripheral vasodilation will be acceptable or beneficial.

Stabilization and Transfer

Once stabilization of the child has been attained, arrangements should be made for transfer to an intensive care unit. Many tertiary-level pediatric hospitals can provide an experienced transport team to accompany the child, providing ongoing care en route. Experience has shown that such provision of intensive care in transport has resulted in a better long-range outcome for the children involved.

As was discussed earlier, primary cardiac arrest is uncommon in the child. An underlying disease process, frequently of the respiratory system, is usually present. Attention to its accurate diagnosis and swift correction are essential in the postresuscitative period to avoid recurrence of cardiopulmonary collapse. Proper application of measures such as mechanical ventilation should be begun during acute resuscitation and continued in later support. Organ-system support and prevention of further damage are begun as early as possible. Renal failure may be averted or ameliorated by judicious volume administration and the use of dopamine or diuretics. Prevention of cerebral swelling and intracranial hypertension may avert secondary central nervous system damage and allow a good outcome.

The decision to terminate unsuccessful resuscitative efforts is particularly difficult in the child, from both medical and emotional viewpoints. The most certain basis for this decision is sustained cardiovascular unresponsiveness despite prolonged resuscitation, which usually implies massive prior insult. Assessment of cerebral damage and function is more difficult. Clear-cut absence of cerebral circulation for prolonged periods of time at normal temperatures, a physical examination that demonstrates deep unconsciousness, lack of spontaneous respiration, lack of all brainstem reflexes, and fixed and dilated pupils for more than 30 minutes despite adequate cardiorespiratory support are ominous signs that may support a decision to cease resuscitation. Unfortunately, even these conditions are not foolproof indicators of cerebral death. If there is any doubt, it is best to complete cardiorespiratory resuscitation and, if stability is attained, to assess neurologic function more carefully over the succeeding 24 hours.

Whether or not the resuscitation is successful, support of the family must be provided throughout the resuscitation period and into the subsequent hours, days, and months. Parents will often feel great guilt over the illness or loss of their child. "If only we had brought him to the doctor sooner . . ." is a universal thought and fear of every parent whose child is seriously ill. Young siblings, too, will feel guilt over the child's illness: Somehow, it must have been their fault. The family unit and its individual members must be sustained; if this is not accomplished successfully, resuscitation of the child has been, in a real way, incomplete.

SPECIAL CONSIDERATIONS: THE NEWBORN

Newborn delivery and resuscitation may occur in settings outside the obstetric suite, where conditions may be less than optimal. Although every effort should be made to delay the birth and to speed the mother to a delivery room, the emergency department must be prepared to deal with an occasional neonate in distress.

Preparation

Anticipation and preparation for newborn resuscitation are critical. If possible, a special area of the emergency ward should be set aside for this purpose. An appropriate table on which the infant can be placed, facilities for warming and drying the baby, and a resuscitation tray with all necessary equipment should be readily available.

All newborns, but particularly premature and asphyxiated babies, have difficulty in tolerating a cold environment. If a delivery is immediately anticipated, the room should be warmed and a radiant warmer focused on the newborn resuscitation area. Heat loss may be prevented by this environmental warming and by rapid drying of the infant, especially the head.

Initiation

When the neonate has been delivered, he or she is placed on the resuscitation table in a slight Trendelenburg's position. Vigorous towel drying and gentle bulb suctioning of the nose and oropharynx provide stimulation. If thick or particulate meconium is present in the amniotic fluid, the baby's hypopharynx must be thoroughly suctioned. Ideally, this will occur immediately after delivery of the head, before the onset of respiration. If adequate clearing has not been possible before delivery is complete, the baby's pharynx and trachea must be suctioned under direct vision. This is best accomplished by tracheal intubation and, as meconium is viscous, by applying suction directly to the endotracheal tube as it is withdrawn. Several attempts may be necessary to remove as much of this material as possible.

Assessment of the baby's status is begun immediately. Respiratory effort, heart rate, color, and activity are scored by the standard Apgar system (Table 3-4) at one and five minutes after birth. Respiratory effort can be determined by simple observation and auscultation. Heart rate is obtained by auscultation, by feeling femoral or brachial pulses, or—most

Table 3-4. The Apgar score*

Sign	0	1	2
Heart rate	Absent	Below 100	Over 100
Respiratory effort	Absent	Slow, irregular	Good, crying
Muscle tone	Limp	Some flexion of extremities	Active motion
Response to catheter in nostril (tested after oropharynx is clear)	No response	Grimace	Cough or sneeze
Color	Blue, pale	Body pink, extremities blue	Completely pink

*Infant is scored at one and five minutes of age.
Source: Modified from V. Apgar. A proposal for a new method of evaluation of the newborn infant. *Current Res. Anesth. Analg.* 32:260, 1953.

rapid and unique to the newborn—by palpation of the pulse in the umbilical cord remnant. If the 5-minute Apgar score is less than 7, additional scores are recorded every 5 minutes for a total of 20 minutes. Resuscitation, of course, is not delayed to complete these assessments, but is begun as indicated in the following section.

Airway, Breathing, and Circulation

Spontaneous breathing, with increasing depth and rate, should begin immediately. If the respiratory effort is inadequate, the administration of oxygen and positive-pressure ventilation is begun. Indications for positive-pressure ventilation include apnea, a heart rate less than 100 bpm, or persistent generalized cyanosis despite a maximal FIO_2. Care must be taken to clear the airway, to maintain a good mask seal, and to assess the adequacy of ventilation by observing bilateral chest wall movement and by auscultation. If gastric distention ensues, an orogastric tube should be placed.

Once adequate ventilation has been established for 15 to 30 seconds, heart rate is assessed. If the heart rate is greater than 100 bpm and spontaneous respiratory efforts begin, one may stop positive-pressure ventilation and observe. If spontaneous breathing has not begun, positive-pressure ventilation must be continued. Endotracheal intubation is indicated if bag-mask ventilation is ineffective, if prolonged mechanical ventilation is necessary, or if there is suspicion of a congenital diaphragmatic hernia (scaphoid abdomen and unilateral decrease of breath sounds, both secondary to the presence of intestine in the chest). If the heart rate is less than 60 bpm or 60 to 80 bpm and not rapidly increasing, chest compressions should be begun.

Chest compressions are performed as previously discussed; either the standard two-finger technique or the modified technique with both thumbs on the sternum and the rescuer's hands surrounding the chest (see Fig. 3-44B) may be used. A rate of 120 compressions per minute is recommended; a palpable femoral pulse should be generated. Compressions are continued until a spontaneous heart rate of 80 or greater, with adequate perfusion, is attained.

Volume and Drug Administration

Rapid access to the circulation may be obtained by cannulation of the umbilical vessels. The umbilical vein is a large, thin-walled, single vessel easily located in the cord; details of the cannulation technique may be found in the Procedures section of this text. In general, these catheters are not left in place for extended periods of time. The umbilical arteries may also be used and offer the advantage of monitoring arterial blood pressure and gases. Arterial cannulation is usually more time consuming, however, and is generally deferred until the infant's condition is more stable. If vascular access is not readily available, certain medications may be given through the endotracheal tube as discussed previously.

Volume expansion with isotonic crystalloid, albumin, or (if red cells are thought necessary) O-negative blood cross-matched against the mother's blood may be given in aliquots of 10 ml/kg. Hypovolemia should be suspected if there has been evidence of acute bleeding from the fetus or placenta and especially if pallor, tachycardia, or faint pulses are present.

Medications are administered as discussed previously. Epinephrine, again, is the most important drug in resuscitation. Bicarbonate may be useful if there is a prolonged resuscitation or severe metabolic acidosis. A rapid strip test for blood glucose will indicate a need for dextrose administration. Naloxone may be particularly useful to counteract the effect of maternal narcotic administration; it is possible to induce a withdrawal reaction in the infant born to a chronically drug-addicted mother, however, and one should proceed with caution in this circumstance.

SELECTED READING

Chameides, L (ed). *Textbook of Pediatric Advanced Life Support.* Dallas: American Heart Association, 1988.

Dean, JM, et al. Age-related changes in chest geometry during cardiopulmonary resuscitation. *J Appl Physiol* 62:2212, 1987.

Eisenberg, M, Bergner, L, and Hallstrom, A. Epidemiology of cardiac arrest and resuscitation in children. *Ann Emerg Med* 12:672, 1983.

Finholt, DA, et al. The heart is under the lower third of the sternum. *Am J Dis Child* 140:646, 1986.

Koehler, RC, et al. Beneficial effect of epinephrine infusion on cerebral and myocardial blood flows during CPR. *Ann Emerg Med* 14:744, 1985.

Montgomery, WH, Donegean, J, and McIntyre, KM (eds). Standards and guidelines for cardiopulmonary resuscitation (CPR) and emergency cardiac care (ECC). *JAMA* 255:2905, 1986.

Nakanishi, T, and Jarmakani, JM. Developmental changes in myocardial mechanical function and subcellular organelles. *Am J Physiol* 246:H615, 1984.

O'Rourke, PP. Outcome of children who are apneic and pulseless in the emergency room. *Crit Care Med* 14:466, 1986.

Otto, CW, Eisenberg, MS, and Bircher, NG (eds). Wolf Creek III Conference on Cardiopulmonary Resuscitation. *Crit Care Med* 13:881, 1985.

Rogers, MC. New developments in cardiopulmonary resuscitation. *Pediatrics* 71:655, 1983.

Sanders, AB, Ewy, GA, and Taft, TV. Prognostic and therapeutic importance of the aortic diastolic pressure in resuscitation from cardiac arrest. *Crit Care Med* 12:871, 1984.

Sanders, AB, Meislin, HW, and Ewy, GA. The physiology of cardiopulmonary resuscitation. *JAMA* 252:3283, 1984.

Schleien, CL, et al. Effect of epinephrine on cerebral and myocardial perfusion in an infant animal preparation of cardiopulmonary resuscitation. *Circulation* 73:809, 1986.

Von Seggern, K, Egar, M, and Ruhrman, BP. Cardiopulmonary resuscitation in a pediatric ICU. *Crit Care Med* 14:275, 1986.

Zaritsky, A. Cardiopulmonary resuscitation in children. *Clin Chest Med* 8:561, 1987.

4. Postresuscitation Care

Marc Restuccia
Richard V. Aghababian

Patients who survive a catastrophic event because of medical intervention require intensive monitoring and evaluation in the emergency department. Resuscitation must be viewed as a continuum. The process begins when the patient suffers a catastrophic event and the emergency medical system is activated. The immediate resuscitation phase either in the field or in the emergency department is followed by stabilization of the patient. If the individual can be temporarily stabilized, postresuscitative care begins. This stage, which involves assessing the cause of the patient's deterioration, continued observation, and initiation of corrective treatment, ends when the patient is admitted to the hospital from the emergency department or is transferred to another facility. Although the focus in this chapter is on the care rendered in the emergency department, it is necessary to remember that this is only a portion of the care that the patient requires.

The initial steps in stabilizing the patient are done rapidly, with minimal time taken out for contemplation. Such courses as advanced cardiac life support (ACLS) and advanced trauma life support (ATLS) have taught emergency medical technicians (EMTs), nurses, and physicians to rapidly resuscitate the victim using rigid protocols. Growth in our understanding of hypoxic injury and the enlarging body of knowledge concerning the pathophysiology of reoxygenation injury have led to the realization that this is a time of critical importance in determining clinical outcome. In addition one must keep in mind that factors such as acute ischemia, injury, or hypoxia, which initially led to the patient's deterioration, may still be present and are likely to recur.

PATHOPHYSIOLOGY

Much research is being conducted on hypoxic cellular injury and death. The most critical organs during resuscitation are the brain and the heart. The central nervous system (CNS) has limited stores of adenosine triphosphate (ATP) and oxygen; thus, hypoxia from whatever cause will quickly lead to cell dysfunction and death. Likewise, the myocardium cannot easily increase its extraction of oxygen from the coronary arteries. It, too, has only limited stores of energy and interruption of its blood supply will quickly lead to first ischemic injury and then to frank necrosis. With ischemia the cell quickly loses its ability to regulate its internal and external milieu. Ion homeostasis is soon lost, with extracellular potassium rising first, followed by an increase in intracellular sodium, chloride, and, most important, calcium. In addition, the brain experiences profound acid-base changes as it is forced to rely increasingly on anaerobic glycolysis. Before the cell itself dies, the intracellular organelles show signs of ischemic change. Mitochondria are the major producers of intracellular ATP. In the face of anaerobic conditions, they rapidly lose their ability to generate the ATP that is necessary for membrane pumps and protein synthesis. Multiple events take place in the cell when this energy depletion occurs. Communication within the cell rapidly ceases, macromolecules and intracellular assemblies break down, and ionic gradients are disrupted.

Although loss of ATP will inevitably lead to cell death, the final, terminal event for the cell is loss of the integrity of the cellular membrane with cellular disruption. At what point intracellular changes go from partially to totally irreversible is not clear. It is reasonable to assume, however, that the longer the period of impaired or absent oxygen delivery, the greater the likelihood of cellular death or impairment and the greater the number of cells lost. Based on this assumption, it is believed that the more rapid the restoration of normal respiratory and circulatory function and, hence, oxygenation, the better the odds for functional recovery. Lowering the metabolic rate of the brain's cells has been shown to afford some protection from ischemic induced injury. It has been known for some time that a hypothermic patient who undergoes a hypoxic event quite often has a better outcome than a normothermic patient. This has led to attempts to control cerebral metabolism with medications such as barbiturates. To date these studies have been disappointing. Other studies using such medications as calcium channel blockers are ongoing and may affect clinical care in the future. At this point, the best treatment for hypoxic injury is zealous attention to optimizing tissue oxygenation.

Another interesting entity of recent interest is the phenomenon of postresuscitation injury. Some patients seem to deteriorate even after adequate restoration of respiratory and circulatory function. Studies have shown that destructive cerebral changes occur during the first 5 to 15 minutes after arrest, occasionally even with restoration of cerebral blood flow. At this time the most likely explanation for this appears to lie in the generation of free radicals; recently, it has been explained via the production of oxygen radicals. Superoxide radical can be formed enzymically or nonemzymically. This radical probably interacts with iron to lead to lipid peroxidation and then to cell-membrane reduction. Also, oxygen radicals may mediate cellular destruction through disruption of calcium homeostasis. Ischemia followed by recirculation seems to be a potent stimulus for the formation of these free radicals. Current research includes the use of calcium blocking agents, superoxide dismutase, or an iron chelator. These interventions may be used clinically in the future to minimize reoxygenation injury. At this time we are limited to maximizing cardiac, pulmonary, and circulatory function to minimize the damage to the CNS.

PHASE 1: STABILIZATION

With these considerations in mind, the practical aspects of current postresuscitative stabilization will now be addressed. The physician should continue to be guided by the well-known "ABCs" of advanced life support.

The continued adequacy of oxygenation is the key consideration in *airway management*. In the intubated patient, the airway, be it oral, nasal, or a cricothyroidotomy, must be confirmed in place. A chest x-ray, preferably upright although a supine one will suffice, is needed to assess the position of the airway. Ideally, the airway should be at least 2 cm above the carina. Once the airway is in position, its location should be noted via the centimeter gradations located along the tube and it should be well secured. Most commonly this means taping it securely around the head of the victim.

Difficulty in *ventilating* a patient with a well-situated tube or continued gurgling with respiration could indicate the need for suctioning secondary to mucus or blood in the airway. A good wall- or stand-mounted suctioning device must be immediately available should the need arise. If not already in place, a nasogastric tube should be passed to decompress the stomach and help avoid aspirations. This is also the time to assess the integrity of the thoracic wall and cavity. Listen for evidence of a pneumothorax, fractured ribs, or subcutaneous emphysema secondary to either the initial event or the resuscitation itself. In addition, positive-pressure ventilation itself can lead to subcutaneous emphysema and pneumothorax. Thus, the clinician must be constantly assessing the patient for the development of such complications. Except in cases of known chronic lung disease in patients who have histories of carbon dioxide retention, it is most appropriate to initially oxygenate these patients with 100 percent inspired oxygen. A quick and easy way to assess adequacy of oxygenation is via pulse oximetry. This should not take the place of the more traditional arterial blood gas (ABG) determination. An ABG will yield information on acid-base status as well as $PaCO_2$ and PaO_2. However, the ease of use and immediate information on oxygenation saturation available with the pulse oximeter make its early use in resuscitation advisable.

Interstitial fluid (such as occurs with pulmonary edema) of any cause must be cleared so that oxygen can easily diffuse from the functioning alveoli to hemoglobin in the pulmonary capillaries. Blood flow through the pulmonary circulation must be adequate to allow the exchange of oxygen for carbon dioxide.

After ensuring the adequate function of respiratory systems, attention should turn to the *circulatory system*. This phase of stabilization requires attention to cardiac rate, rhythm, and overall function as well as total-body circulatory status. A cardiac monitor should be placed on the patient as soon as practicable to observe heart rate and rhythm in a continuous manner and treat potentially lethal arrhythmias rapidly. Reliable external pacing devices are now available to assist in the management of bradyarrhythmias. In addition a 12-lead electrocardiogram (ECG) should be obtained and, if possible, compared to previous tracings. Studies clearly show that in the ischemic myocardium, time is of the essence and consideration for thrombolytic therapy should be accomplished early.

Ongoing loss of blood needs to be identified and treated. Hemorrhage will usually manifest itself as an increase in heart rate and a decrease in blood pressure and urinary output. Control of external hemorrhage is accomplished with direct pressure to the bleeding site. In some instances of internal hemorrhage, surgical intervention will be needed. Continued crystalloid and blood product replacement is necessary to assure adequate cardiac output and tissue perfusion. A Foley catheter is indispensible for monitoring urinary flow and, hence, renal perfusion. External monitoring of pulse and blood pressure is usually adequate in the emergency department. In a few instances, such as if thrombolytic therapy is being considered, it may be advisable to place an intraarterial monitoring line before a thrombolytic state is induced. More frequently, a central line may be placed either to assess central venous pressure or preparatory to placement of a Swan-Ganz catheter. Although all of these monitoring systems are useful, in general they can be deferred during the stabilization phase to the observation and diagnosis stage.

After assuring the stability of the respiratory and circulatory systems, attention should turn to the rest of the body. For victims of trauma, skeletal injuries should be evaluated both with inspection and palpation and with appropriate radiologic studies. In patients who have immobilized cervical spines, a minimum study at this time should include a lateral x-ray of the cervical vertebrae. All seven cervical vertebrae should be well visualized. Suspected fractures and dislocations should be splinted and stabilized, if at all possible in an anatomically correct position. This will lessen the likelihood of neurovascular compromise, perhaps reduce some of the patient's discomfort, and it is hoped, avoid further injury. All other portions of the body including the abdomen, back, rectum, genitalia, skin, and nervous system should also be evaluated for additional clues of underlying medical conditions or unforeseen injuries.

Constant monitoring of vital signs is imperative since changes in the clinical condition of the patient will be reflected in a change in pulse or blood pressure. Temperature also must be monitored. Hypothermia, although somewhat protective to the cells of the brain during hypoxic insults, is very arrhythmogenic and must be treated. Likewise, hyperthermia has undesirable side effects, such as increasing metabolic demands on an organism not able to meet them. Causes of the change from normal body temperature must be sought and treated.

Ongoing fluid needs can be assessed via such parameters as mental status, vital signs, and urine output. A Foley catheter, if not already present, should be inserted and the urine flow measured. An acceptable minimum urinary output is 30 to 50 ml per hour in an adult and 1 to 2 ml/kg per hour in a child.

Also, at this time attention should be paid to the acid-base status of the patient. An arterial blood gas, as mentioned previously, is invaluable, since it will yield information both on the respiratory status and the arterial pH of the patient. The need for this information is clear. Patients with prolonged "down-time" or coexisting medical illnesses such as diabetes may be profoundly acidotic, and this condition will seriously impair the cardiac status of the patient and may lead to long-term sequelae. In addition persons with suspected increased intracranial pressure require hyperventilation to decrease the PCO_2 and produce a mildly alkalotic pH. Because of these considerations the pulse oximeter, although useful for rapid and continued assessment of oxygenation, should not be used in place of an arterial blood gas determination, especially in patients suspected of having increased intracranial pressure. The two tests are complementary.

As the secondary survey and stabilization phase draws to a close, one should begin to think of diagnostic testing. If it was not already done when intravenous lines were placed initially, laboratory work should be obtained. At a minimum one should obtain a complete blood count, electrolytes, blood urea nitrogen (BUN), creatinine, chemistry screen, blood for the blood bank, and perhaps extra tubes for unforeseen needs, such as a toxicology screen or prearrest medication levels. A platelet count as well as a prothrombin time and partial thromboplastin time are helpful, especially if oozing is noted from puncture sites or there is some difficulty in controlling hemorrhage. In addition a urinalysis should be obtained. Consideration should be given to obtaining a toxicology screen in any patient suspected of substance abuse or unexplained coma. If any other specialized radiologic studies are contemplated, such as a KUB (kidneys, ureters, bladder), intravenous pyelogram, computed tomographic scan, or coronary angiogram, arrangements for their performance should be made.

PHASE 2: OBSERVATION AND DIAGNOSIS

At this time members of the medical team taking care of the patient can step back and reassess what has been done to the patient, their response, and the potential for other interventions. Continuous monitoring is a must. Continuous rhythm monitoring and repeat ECGs may help determine the cause of the acute event. Modern automated pulse and blood pressure monitors are available and free doctors and nurses for more pressing matters. Consideration should once again be given to the need for more specialized or invasive monitoring techniques, such as central venous hemodynamic measurements, an intraarterial line, or, rarely, a Swan-Ganz catheter. Likewise, in a patient suspected of having an increase in intracranial pressure (ICP), ICP pressure monitoring bolts may be placed after appropriate neurosurgical consultation.

This raises the issue of emergency department consultations. Every emergency department should have a list of available subspecialists. Conferring with a surgeon, neurologist, or cardiologist for appropriate cases will not only engender better patient care but may prove invaluable when it comes time for a decision on disposition.

Physicians and nurses must also consider the patient's family. When the patient is stabilized and it is safe to do so, the physician or nurse should confer with the patient's family, especially if they are present in the emergency department. The family should be apprised of the situation in honest, nonfrightening, and understandable terms. In return the physician or nurse can obtain valuable information about the patient's past medical history, medication history, and any allergies. The family should also be questioned concerning the patient's and their wishes about further treatment. In particular, attention should be paid to their wishes about continued mechanical support. The patient's private physician should be consulted and involved if at all possible. His or her knowledge of the patient and the family, as well as the appearance of a familiar physician may do much to help the situation. The family may wish to have a clergy member involved for support and guidance. During this extremely stressful time, all efforts should be made to aid the family both in coping with the situation and potentially arriving at some extremely difficult decisions.

The ongoing monitoring, management, and care of the patient in the emergency department may prove to be problematic. Discussion with nurses and other physicians can do much to maximize efficiency and avoid either inadequate coverage or overly stressed personnel. The most appropriate place in the emergency department for the patient should be considered. For example, the patient may not require the trauma-resuscitation area and can be just as well monitored in another portion of the department. This policy makes for the best use of the department's personnel and facilities.

Finally, any loose ends must be addressed. If fractures can but have not yet been reduced, set, or stabilized, this should be accomplished. Any repairable laceration or other wound that requires care should be treated. Tetanus toxoid and antibiotics should be administered if indicated. The need to continue long-term medications during the postresuscitative phase should be considered as well. At the end of this phase, the patient should be ready for admission or transport. As far as is possible, the physician taking care of the patient should have a reasonably clear understanding of what happened to the victim and what facilities and interventions will be necessary.

PHASE 3: DISPOSITION

After the patient has been stabilized and evaluated, arrangements must be made for inpatient care. A determination of the needed level of care and its availability should be made. Is an intensive care unit necessary or will simple telemetry on a ward suffice? Is telemetry necessary or will an "unmonitored" bed be sufficient? The answer to these questions will vary not only with the disease process that is causing the present situation but also with other comorbid illnesses. It may be entirely appropriate to admit a terminally ill cancer patient to a regular ward if heroic measures are no longer indicated or desired. Conversely, a young asthmatic patient may require the services of an intensive care unit, at least during the initial phase of care. If the required level of care is not available, transfer to another acceptable facility is required. Can trauma victims receive adequate care at a community hospital or would it be more appropriate to transfer them to either a level I or II trauma center? In an overcrowded hospital, transfer to another comparable facility with available beds is perhaps in the patient's best interests. Such referral patterns and the means to implement them are best worked out in advance by a regionally approved protocol.

When transporting a patient either to a more comprehensive hospital level via ground ambulance or by air ambulance over many miles, certain steps must be considered.

1. *Mode of transport.* Transport of the patient can be as simple as a gurney going up the elevator to as complex as a helicopter transfer to a referral center. What is needed, what is available, and how to go about implementing it are the questions that need to be addressed in advance.

2. *Access.* Can you get the patient there from here? Again, a vast range of answers can be given to this question. Can the patient fit on the elevator with a monitor, ventilator, and IVs? How do you air-transport someone when you have no helipad? Can you air-evacuate a patient who is on an intraaortic balloon device? Again, individual situations will require individual answers.

3. *Personnel.* Who must accompany the patient? Can an orderly take the patient to the floor or is a nurse or a physician needed? Considerations that will go into this decision are the seriousness of the patient's condition, length of the trip, availability of personnel, and level of professional expertise needed to ensure the patient's safety.

4. *Equipment.* What will be needed to safely transport/transfer the patient? Any items that may possibly be needed should be available. Seizures in a helicopter or elevator, cardiac arrest en route, or sudden hemorrhage can have tragic consequences if no provision is made for them. At the very least a transportation kit containing such code medications as epinephrine, lidocaine, diazepam, and other drugs should be made up in advance. Other items such as oxygen, suction, monitors, defibrillators, and laryngoscope may be required and should be available.

5. *Tests.* Will the patient be going to the radiology department or the catheterization laboratory for further testing before going to his or her room? If so, what personnel will be required to be with the patient and what equipment will be needed?.

6. *Problems.* What difficulties might be encountered en route and how can they be avoided or managed? Will the patient become agitated and require sedation; is the airway tenuous; should the patient be intubated now for safety's sake? Anticipating problems and avoiding them is much easier than trying to deal with them when they arise.

7. *Packaging.* The patient must be packaged to allow easy access to such crucial items as IVs, the airway, and monitors for vital signs. Loose tubing or lines must be secured to avoid inadvertent accidents. The patient must be securely wrapped before transport for security. Attention should be given to the environment. During the winter months attention must be paid to keeping the patient warm; this can be accomplished with thermal or regular blankets. The burn patient may require sterile sheets for transfer. A small amount of planning can make any transport safer and easier.

8. *Transfer.* At this point the patient is handed over to the responsibility of an equally or higher-qualified caregiver. The sending physician must ensure that the receiving physician or facility is aware of the patient and have a good grasp of the patient's condition. In addition, all documentation that can go with the patient should be sent. The chart, clearly and completely filled out so that it is easy to follow what the patient's condition was at presentation and what was done for him or her, should remain with the patient. If the patient is being transferred to another facility, copies of the chart should be sent as well. If the person is being admitted to the same hospital, such items as laboratory and x-ray results will be available to the admitting physician. If, however, the patient is being sent elsewhere, it is necessary for copies of the laboratory results and, if at all possible, the x-rays to go with the patient. Any changes from previous ECGs, laboratory tests, or x-rays should be noted. This not only makes good medical sense but, in today's climate makes good economic sense also. The responsibility for the patient shifts when he or she is actually transferred to the care of the receiving physicians and nurses.

The problems of postresuscitative care have become increasingly complex as our ability to preserve and sustain life improves. Technology and training have become more sophisticated. Victims of catastrophic illness and accidents are more often being successfully resuscitated and are in need of advanced postevent treatment. All too often, even with the best of care, the outcome is suboptimal. The patient may survive only temporarily or may be left with significant impairment. Future issues that need to be addressed are improvement in our interventions and diagnoses. New technologies and interventions are likely to greatly enhance the abilities of clinicians to successfully resuscitate victims of catastrophic illness.

The ethics of resuscitation and postresuscitation care will also need to be addressed. Not infrequently the resuscitated patient is left with some degree of impairment. In an era of shrinking health-care funds, can all patients continue to receive our all-out interventions? Will society be willing to pay the cost or will some individuals be deemed beyond our ability to provide medical care? What criteria should be used to decide whom we should treat? What criteria should be met by those gaining access to advanced health care? These questions and society's answers to them will, in large part, determine the future of emergency medical care.

SELECTED READING

Ernster, L. Biochemistry of reoxygenation injury. *Crit Care Med* 16:949, 1988.

Negovsky, VA. Post resuscitation disease. *Crit Care Med* 16:943, 1988.

Siesjo, BK. The mechanism of ischemic brain injury. *Crit Care Med* 16:955, 1988.

5. Medicolegal Aspects of Cardiopulmonary Resuscitation and Emergency Cardiac Care

Kevin M. McIntyre

Medicolegal aspects of resuscitation may be divided into decision-making aspects and performance aspects. Decision making is far more likely to result in legal problems, primarily because of the wide variety of patient circumstances and the time pressure for immediate decisions that characterizes the emergency-care setting. The emergency-care provider is confronted with questions of whether to initiate resuscitative efforts and, having started, when to terminate. Judgment is a critical ingredient and one that is not easily taught. The primary concern must be protection of the patient's rights and well-being as opposed to avoidance of legal actions. Fortunately, the latter intention is best served by optimal protection of the patient's interests in the vast majority of cases. Execution of appropriate life-prolonging and life-saving actions is much easier to standardize than decision-making aspects, as is evident in publications that have defined and updated "standards" for cardiopulmonary resuscitation and emergency cardiac care since 1974.

We will take for granted the published reality of standards for the execution of resuscitative efforts and concentrate on the more difficult issue—that of decision making. At the outset, we must affirm the verity that underlies all considerations of medical care and its legal implications—that is, that the patient's right to an opportunity to recover, to live, is paramount. The process by which that right is defended begins within the mind-set of the emergency-care provider and proceeds inextricably from that mind-set through the medical realities of uncertainty of prognosis, implications of biological survival without neurologic recovery, potential long-term emotional costs to the patient's family, and impact on the medical and professional staff who may be obliged to provide continuing care. The implications of the often immense costs of long-term care must be considered as well. These issues and their implied burdens are as trying as any in medicine; however, unlike the standards for resuscitation just alluded to, there are few neurologic, ethical, sociologic, religious, or legal guidelines that assure us of an outcome that would predictably comport with the patient's wishes or even reflect a unanimity of attitude among emergency-care providers. Accordingly, this chapter initially considers general concepts of legal liability and then goes on to discuss specific aspects of resuscitation that need to be addressed in the emergency-care setting.

Just as the preferred approach to the problem of sudden death is prevention, the preferred approach to potential liability in cardiopulmonary resuscitation (CPR) and emergency cardiac care (ECC) is prevention. This implies a definition of foreseeable problem areas and appropriate strategies to deal with identified points of legal vulnerability. As alluded to earlier, the touchstone for prevention of legal liability in CPR and ECC, as in other forms of medical-care delivery, is good-quality medical care.

In considering the quality of ECC, it is important to emphasize that the provider is not obliged to render the best possible care to the patient. Rather, the provider must provide care appropriate to the patient's condition and desires. Increasingly, attention is focused on the patients' rights, and an awareness and respect for them is part of the obligation of care providers. The physician's decision to withhold or withdraw life-sustaining care should not be arbitrary but should reflect the best possible assessment of the condition of the patient (diagnostic certainty), the patient's prognosis to the extent that this can be determined (including appropriate protection of the patient's life and well-being while diagnosis and prognosis remain in doubt), the desires of the patient, and the availability of certain medical-care capabilities.

THE EMERGENCY PHYSICIAN'S DUTY OF CARE

General Concepts of Legal Liability

As with physicians in other specialties, the emergency physician's duty to the patient is generally considered by the courts as contractual in nature. It is established when the physician-patient relationship is established. The contract is implied since no actual terms of agreement are usually expressed. The physician's duty begins when the patient presents him- or herself for medical care and the physician undertakes to provide that care. In certain circumstances, such as in an emergency facility that represents itself as such, the physician responsible may not have the option of refusing to undertake the care of the patient.

While the basis of the physician-patient relationship may be considered contractual, the legal action is usually based on the claim that the physician failed to exercise "reasonable care" in treatment of the patient and that the physician's failure was the direct cause of the patient's injury. The duty to exercise reasonable care is imposed by the law on every individual with regard to his or her dealings with every other person. When failure to exercise reasonable care results in injury, the injured party has a legal right to an action for recovery or compensation. In legal parlance, this is known as a *tort*, a civil wrong based on the violation of the duty to exercise reasonable care, a violation that results in the injury of another.

Elements of a Malpractice Action

Four elements must be established if a malpractice claim is to be successful. The plaintiff (i.e., the patient) or his or her representative making the claim against the physician must establish (1) that a duty to provide care existed on the part of the physician—that is, that a physician-patient relationship existed; (2) that a breach of the duty to provide reasonable care was committed—that is, that the physician was negligent; (3) that the patient suffered an injury; and (4) that there was a cause-and-effect relationship between the breach of medical practice or duty and the injury that the patient sustained—that is, that the physician's negligence was the proximate cause of the patient's injury.

The Physician-Patient Relationship and the Duty of Care

The physician-patient relationship establishes the duty to provide care that conforms to accepted standards of medical practice and can be established in a number of ways. It is most frequently instituted when a physician accepts an individual as a patient. When a patient seeks medical care at a hospital emergency facility, the duty to perform in the best interests of the patient may be established by the patient arriving at the emergency facility and indicating in one way or another that he or she is seeking care. The duty to perform in the patient's best interests may be established even when the patient is unconscious. For example, the arrival of a cardiac-arrest victim at an emergency department will establish a duty to perform in the best interests of the patient because the law considers that, were the patient able to communicate, he or she would request appropriate medical care.

Negligence and the Standard of Care

How are the patient, the physician, and the court to establish the kind of care that the patient should have received in order to decide whether the care provided by the physician (or the nurse, the paraprofessional, or the hospital) was adequate or negligent? The courts have defined the physician's duty to the patient in specific terms: "The physician is required to possess that degree of knowledge and skill, and to exercise that degree of care, judgment, and skill which other physicians of good standing of the same school or system of practice usually exercise in the same or similar localities under like or similar circumstances" (Lane vs. Calvert, Md. 138A.2d 902 [1958]).

The physician's performance is measured against the medical knowledge and professional performance of the average reputable physician in his or her community, not against that of the most skillful physician. This standard of conduct can usually be defined only through the use of expert testimony and the opinions of the defendant's colleagues unless the physician's performance was so obviously negligent as to be recognized as such by the common knowledge of the layperson. Usually, the physician's peers, by their testimony ("the expert witness"), inform the judge or jury what constitutes the usual performance of a physician under the same or similar circumstances. In the last analysis, therefore, the physician is judged to a large extent by colleagues through their testimony, although the judge or the jury has the final say in deciding whether the physician's performance measured up to the standard offered by the medical experts.

Increasingly, the standard of care for the physician is based on a nationwide rather than on a local standard. This is particularly the rule for medical specialists and would generally be so for emergency physicians, particularly in view of the nationally accepted standards that have been defined in such areas as trauma treatment and resuscitation. The reference in the previously stated definition to "the same or similar localities" is generally left out when the legal duty of the medical specialist is stated.

The heart of the legal duty imposed on the physician is expressed by the following portions of the quotation: "The physician is required . . . to exercise that degree of care, judgment, and skill which other physicians . . . usually exercise . . . under like or similar circumstances." The physician is not required to effect a cure and he or she is not obligated to obtain a good result in every instance. The failure to effect a cure or obtain a good result does not, of itself, imply negligence. The physician promises, by implication, only that he or she will use that degree of skill, knowledge, and care that would be used by the average reputable physician and will exert his or her best judgment in an effort to bring about a good result. Thus, the legal duty is measured by the degree of skill and care that would have been exercised by the average physician under the same or similar circumstances. The fact that the physician's peers will ultimately pass judgment on the appropriateness of his or her treatment should a lawsuit ensue dramatizes the importance of judicious use of consultants by the physician who is managing difficult, complex, and potentially controversial cases.

Standard of Care for the Emergency Physician

It is important to emphasize that the physician staffing an emergency department is expected to have certain capabilities, one of which is the ability to mobilize a resuscitation effort. The emergency physician will be judged according to the way a physician staffing an emergency department would be expected to perform. There are objective expressions of training and performance, listed by specialty groups such as the American College of Emergency Physicians, which can be used to help establish a standard of care within such an emergency facility. It is particularly important that the physician be aware that he or she is likely to be judged according to the average performance of the expert in the field of therapy that the doctor undertook to apply, rather than the performance of a physician in his or her own specialty. Thus, if the general practitioner is staffing an emergency department and undertakes to treat a fracture, he or she may be expected to treat that fracture to the standard of the average orthopedic surgeon. When a general practitioner is performing as the emergency-facility physician, he or she will generally be expected to provide care to the standard of the average emergency physician.

Injury and Causation

The patient who claims that malpractice was committed must show that injury occurred, whether it was physical or emotional, or both. However negligent the physician, litigation cannot be sustained without evidence of injury. Further, the injury must be shown to be the direct result of the substandard care of the physician. This means that it must be demonstrated that the injury would not have occurred unless the doctor either failed to act or acted improperly.

Great Danger and Due Diligence

When the danger of serious injury or death is great, the physician's obligation to exercise diligence in his or her effort to protect the patient must be proportionately high. When cardiac arrest or any other serious cardiac or pulmonary problem is present or suspected, the risk to the patient of death or brain damage is high, and reasonable steps to protect the patient from such foreseeable consequences must be taken.

Brain Death

Criteria for the definition of brain death were first developed by an ad hoc committee of the Harvard Medical School. Since then, brain-death statutes have been passed in Kansas, then in other states. The brain-death criteria developed by the Harvard Medical School were recognized by the Massachusetts court in the Golston case and by other courts as a medically and legally acceptable definition of death. In fact, in every case in which the definition of death was made according to such criteria, the courts, in Curran's words, "have uniformly upheld the physician's actions as medically proper, ethically justified and legally sound." Approaches to severe brain damage that fell short of those strict criteria continued to be dealt with by the physician, family, prognosis committee, or all three, but rarely by the court, up to the time of the Quinlan decision.

PERFORMANCE VERSUS DECISION MAKING IN CARDIOPULMONARY RESUSCITATION AND EMERGENCY CARDIAC CARE

Successful resuscitation is generally thought to require the reestablishment of effective cardiovascular functions and complete neurologic recovery. The fact that serious brain damage is the consequence of resuscitation efforts in some cases has led to efforts to predict the likelihood of full neurologic recovery. This practice has in the past influenced, and continues to influence, decision making in CPR, including the decision of whether to initiate and whether to discontinue CPR. Accordingly, the legal implications of making such decisions on this basis need to be considered.

The Question of Brain Recoverability

As was alluded to previously, the decision to initiate resuscitation for the cardiac arrest victim is based on the fundamental presumption that the brain may still be viable even though the heart has stopped. The accepted medical standard assumes that when the possibility exists that the brain is viable, and there are no compelling medical or legal reasons to act otherwise, resuscitation should be initiated. As a result of this presumption and the implementation of resuscitation, many patients who would have been declared dead in the traditional sense have survived. The fact that there are a number of people alive with residual brain damage, some mild and some severe, is equally true, but the number of individuals with severe neurologic sequelae represents a small percentage of total resuscitative attempts. Under most circumstances it is not possible to determine the likelihood of brain recovery at the time the decision to initiate or withhold resuscitation needs to be made. Furthermore, there are undoubtedly patients who might have recovered completely but who are now dead because CPR was not provided in a timely manner, or was improperly or ineffectively performed, implying the necessity for clear guidelines in both decision making and in the quality of performance in the area of resuscitation.

The extent to which improper decision making, including improper omission or termination of CPR and inappropriate maintenance or suspension of life support, affects outcome is a question that continues to be among the most significant in this area. All too often, the conscientious physician finds that guidelines may be very difficult to apply to the circumstances of a particular patient. Thus, a reappraisal of medical and legal concepts that bear on decisions to provide or withhold resuscitation, the cessation of resuscitative efforts, the standard of care in resuscitation, and associated practices is timely. There are several sets of circumstances that are both frequent and recurrent and, accordingly, will continue to present the CPR-ECC care provider with difficult medical, ethical, and legal decisions.

Initiating CPR: To Start or Not to Start

The current standard of care as is applied to resuscitative efforts requires that resuscitation be implemented by a responsible person or agency when two conditions are fulfilled: (1) the possibility exists that the brain is viable, and (2) there is no legally or medically legitimate reason to withhold it. It is clear that persistent, severe brain damage is a more dreaded outcome than death for both care provider and, in most cases, family and loved ones. The possibility of brain recovery implies as well the possibility of permanent brain damage. Since accurate prognostication of postresuscitation brain status is not possible at present, resuscitation efforts should be implemented promptly when these two conditions are present. One important situation discussed in the following section, in which the decision to initiate or withhold CPR must be made over and over again is the case of a cardiac-arrest victim who arrives at the emergency facility in a condition that was once referred to as "dead on arrival."

"Dead on Arrival"

Resuscitation of the out-of-hospital cardiac-arrest victim has met with increasing success, undoubtedly because of broad-based improvement in emergency medical services along with the education and training of laypersons and first responders. Still too frequently, however, a cardiac-arrest victim is rushed to the emergency facility without benefit of resuscitation efforts. Before the time resuscitation became a standard procedure, this patient would qualify as "dead on arrival," or "DOA."

Although it is usually impossible to determine accurately the duration of complete cessation of cardiovascular function because of the lack of competent and reliable observers at the scene, efforts to do so are often made. For the responsible physician to make a decision not to initiate CPR in this setting, however, he or she must be confident, at the least, of the ability of the observer to recognize cardiac arrest, of the reliability of that observer in documenting the time elapsed, that the observer is acting in good faith, and that no independent influences such as drugs or cold are operative.

The argument that the patient could have collapsed as a result of a cardiac or noncardiac cause, and continued to have cardiac activity at a level sufficient to sustain the brain until he or she was rushed through the door of the emergency facility, may be an insurmountable one. Armed with the knowledge that weak or slow pulses may be missed by inexperienced observers, a plaintiff's attorney may inquire as to the person on whom the physician should reasonably rely as a witness to the onset and progression of the process of brain death. And do the care and interest of the family, however positive and legitimate, render them sufficiently expert at recognizing cardiac arrest so that the physician can rely on them? The same questions can be asked about a friend, neighbor, or police officer, unless that person had received special training in recognition of cardiac arrest as part of a resuscitation course. And even then, should the physician rely on the expertise of a person claiming to be practiced in the recognition of cardiac arrest who is either unable or unwilling to provide CPR? In short, the physician or other responsible care provider is usually obliged to initiate resuscitative measures and may be held liable if he or she elects not to do so on an arbitrary basis. One justifiable basis for withholding resuscitation would be, for example, the certain knowledge that the patient would have qualified for a "do not resuscitate" designation, which will be discussed in a later section of this chapter.

Emergency medical technicians (EMTs) and the paramedics who staff mobile emergency units, have comparable areas of potential vulnerability. When these medical-care personnel respond to the cardiac-arrest victim in the field, they often find themselves in the same predicament as the emergency-department physician, attempting to determine how long circulatory arrest has been present. The history provided by witnesses is generally not a reliable basis for withholding resuscitation in such settings. Furthermore, the number of case reports of complete recovery after extended periods of unsupported cardiac arrest, particularly as a result of cold-water immersion, is growing. When brain viability is in doubt, the EMT or paramedic should initiate CPR.

Manifestations of Brain Damage as a Basis for Withholding Cardiopulmonary Resuscitation

Is the suspicion of irreversible brain damage or brain death a valid basis for withholding CPR? The absence of a pupillary response to light is not a reliable sign of brain death since certain disease states and certain drugs can render the pupil nonreactive, as do some cataract operations. Perhaps more important, initially unreactive pupils may become reactive in the course of resuscitation, demonstrating the unreliability of this sign as a prognosticator of brain nonrecoverability.

The use of a single observation of a "flat" electroencephalogram (EEG) to document irreversible brain damage is unacceptable for a number of reasons: (1) The duration over which electrocerebral silence by EEG should exist before it can be assumed that all possibility of resuscitation is past remains to be defined; (2) to take the 10 to 20 minutes to perform the EEG is to assure brain death since resuscitative efforts must be withheld during this procedure; (3) drugs may affect the EEG independently, resulting in a flat response; and (4) a single flat EEG does not meet the current legal or medical brain-death standards.

"Boxcars" in the fundi have been recognized as indicators of cessation of cerebral perfusion and, therefore, indicators of brain death. However, the acceptability of this sign, assuming its validity, depends on the reliability of the observer. Since there is no permanent record, how many observers should verify it? For how long should fundi be explored while the brain remains hypoxic for lack of resuscitative efforts? One is left with the reality that there are no practically useful, reliable signs of brain death that can be applied in a timely manner to the cardiac-arrest victim, with the exception of decapitation, rigor mortis (in the absence of extreme cold), and perhaps established dependent lividity.

Case law supports the medical priority for supporting cardiovascular and ventilatory function before attempting to assess brain status. In the case of *Dubry vs. Gardena Medical Center*, neurologic experts found that generalized, irreversible brain damage had occurred and, based on this finding, recommended that life support be withheld. However, the court, based on expert testimony, found this unacceptable because support of cardiovascular and respiratory function, both of which were severely impaired, was not performed before neurologic evaluation. Furthermore, misdiagnosis of irreversible cessation of all brain function has been reported in the case of brain contusion in association with reduced cerebral function due to hypovolemia. Vigorous treatment of hypovolemic shock resulted in recovery despite that misdiagnosis. In short, therefore, since it is usually not possible to predict nonrecoverability of a brain acutely insulted by cardiac arrest, and since attempts to do so increase anoxia time and the likelihood of further permanent brain damage, the responsible physician, nurse, or paramedic is usually obligated to commence CPR. Evaluation of brain status and the difficult decisions that may be forthcoming in this regard should be deferred until the issue of cardiovascular responsiveness has been determined (as discussed in an earlier section). The designation "DOA" is in large measure an anachronism and an invitation to legal as well as medical sanctions.

Termination of Cardiopulmonary Resuscitation: When to Stop

A number of criteria for deciding to discontinue CPR have been offered. Clearly, the physician has the primary responsibility for this decision. It has been recommended that the nonphysician continue basic life support as long as it is needed or until the rescuer is exhausted or relieved by a physician, another rescuer, or a rescue team. The often-discussed liability risk of the layperson, functioning in good faith in this capacity, has been shown not to be supported by facts. With increasing frequency the lay rescuer or other first responder who provides manual support is relieved by a rescue team capable of providing advanced cardiac life support (ACLS) with definitive drug and electrical therapy. The decision to terminate ACLS at this level also must be made with increasing frequency. Practical, workable guidelines for terminating ongoing resuscitative efforts have not been available.

The duration of resuscitation has been considered as a possible criteria for the decision to terminate. It is well known that the longer resuscitative efforts continue to be unsuccessful, the less likely it is that the victim will recover fully. On the other hand, it is also well known that complete recovery has followed resuscitative efforts that lasted two or three hours or more. Thus, duration of resuscitative effort as the sole criteria for a decision to terminate CPR is arbitrary and legally unacceptable. Suspicion of permanent brain damage has been based on estimates of duration of unattended cardiac arrest, lack of pupillary response to light, and lack of any neurologic signs of life. These criteria, too, are unreliable for reasons previously discussed. The need for guidelines for the cessation of CPR has been strengthened by the reality that litigation is more likely to follow when the patient survives with permanent brain damage than when the patient dies. The troubling awareness on the part of the physician that the risk of permanent brain damage increases with the duration of the resuscitative effort may also favor the decision to terminate.

An additional difficulty arises when a physician makes the decision to terminate resuscitation contrary to the feelings of trained paramedical personnel who initiated resuscitative efforts, a circumstance that at times belies the shared medical and legal responsibilities of the emergency-facility physician and the out-of-hospital emergency team. But what medically and legally sound guidelines can be used to decide on termination of CPR?

Cardiovascular Unresponsiveness as a Basis for the Termination of Cardiopulmonary Resuscitation

It is well known that the heart tolerates hypoxemia far better than the brain, so that in many circumstances cardiovascular function may be reestablished while the brain may not recover. Since CPR is initiated because both brain and heart may recover, and since there is presently no reliable means of defining "brain death" during resuscitation, the decision to discontinue resuscitative efforts should be based on cardiovascular unresponsiveness. The major thrusts of resuscitation include the reestablishment of circulation and oxygenation of brain, heart, and other organs; correction of metabolic disturbances such as hypoxemia and acidosis; stimulation of electrical activity in a depressed heart or suppression of excessive electrical activity in a heart that is electrically hyperexcitable; and application of appropriate electrical therapy such as defibrillation. In the critically important though infrequent circumstances in which cardiovascular collapse occurs as the result of a readily reversible process such as cardiac tamponade, therapy must be directed toward that cause. The use of therapeutic modalities in appropriate combination and sequence, from administration of basic life support through the application of ACLS, will often result in the establishment of effective cardiovascular activity. When these techniques have been properly applied, and yet the cardiovascular system fails to respond, the cardiovascular system can be said to be unresponsive to standard resuscitative therapy. Accordingly, the decision to terminate a resuscitative effort that was initiated because of the possibility of brain and heart viability may be reasonably based on the determination that death in traditional terms has supervened—that is, cardiac death as defined by cardiovascular unresponsiveness to acceptable resuscitative techniques. At this point, the issue of brain viability becomes, at least for the present, an academic concern.

Proof of the medical and legal validity of the definition of death by "cardiovascular unresponsiveness" in a particular case many depend on the care providers' ability to demonstrate that therapeutic techniques appropriate to test the "unresponsiveness" of the cardiovascular system were employed, should the question arise subsequently. The possibility that the question may arise in litigation underscores the importance of adequate documentation.

Withholding Resuscitation and "Do Not Resuscitate" Orders

It is held by most within the medical, religious, philosophical, and legal communities that resuscitation is a form of medical therapy that, as with most other forms of therapy, is indicated in some situations but not in others. This conviction was clearly enunciated at the National Conferences on CPR and ECC in 1973, 1979, and 1985. As was discussed previously, when there is doubt, resuscitation should be instituted; in the emergency department setting, this decision must be made without delay. One of the situations in which it is usually not indicated is in the case of the terminally ill patient for whom no further therapy for the underlying disease process remains available and death appears imminent. Of particular importance to the emergency-care provider is the question of the validity of information provided that the patient in the emergency department, now unconscious or incompetent, has elected, with the agreement of physician and family, not to be resuscitated. It is of particular concern to the emergency-care provider that a method for supplying such information be developed so that it is immediately available. In the absence of a credible expression of the patient's "do not resuscitate" status, the care provider is usually obliged to initiate resuscitative efforts.

CONCLUSIONS

With regard to the "standard of care" performance in CPR and ECC, a National Conference on Cardiopulmonary Resuscitation and Emergency Cardiac Care was held in Washington in 1973. Standards for CPR and ECC were developed and subsequently published. These standards were updated by national conferences in 1979 and 1985 and reflected a consensus among experts who represented the American Heart Association, American College of Emergency Physicians, American College of Cardiology, American Society of Anesthesiologists, and the National Heart, Lung, and Blood Institute, among many others. These materials provide a definition of the current standard of care at virtually every level of performance in CPR and ECC.

A responsible physician or other medical or paramedical person has a duty to provide CPR to the cardiac-arrest victim as a form of routine and ordinary care unless there is a medically or legally justifiable reason to withhold that care. "Do not resuscitate" orders or their equivalent should be written in such cases and a legally valid method for getting this information into the hands of emergency-care personnel needs to be implemented broadly.

Termination of CPR should be based on cardiovascular unresponsiveness to competently delivered basic life support and ACLS unless there is another medically or legally justifiable reason to terminate. Life-support mechanisms and efforts can and should be suspended when the patient's status meets brain-death criteria.

SELECTED READING

Commonwealth of Massachusetts vs Golston, 336 NE 2d 744, 1977.

Curran, WJ. Setting the medicolegal issues concerning brain-death statutes: Matters of legal ethics and judicial precedent. *N Engl J Med* 299:31, 1978.

Derr vs Bonney, 231 P 2d 637, 1951.

De Villota, ED, et al. Recovery from profound hypothermia with cardiac arrest after immersion. *Br Med J* 4:394, 1973.

Dubry vs Gardena Medical Center, California Superior Ct, Los Angeles Co, Docket No. SWC 1098, 1972.

Eliastam, M, et al. Cardiac arrest in the emergency medical service system: Guidelines for resuscitation. *JACEP* 6:525, 1977.

Grenvik, A, et al. Cessation of therapy in terminal illness and brain death. *Crit Care Med* 6:284, 1978.

Kansas Session Laws of 1970, Chap 378.

Lambrew, C. Medical control (editorial). *JACEP* 6:66, 1977.

Lane vs Calvert, 138 A 2d 902, 1958.

Lund, I, and Skulberg, A. Cardiopulmonary resuscitation by lay people. *Lancet* 2:702, 1976.

In the matter of Karen Quinlan, 70 NJ 10, 335 A 2d 647, 1976.

McIntyre, KM. Medicolegal aspects of cardiopulmonary resuscitation (CPR) and emergency cardiac care (ECC). *JAMA* 244:511, 1980.

McIntyre, KM. Medicolegal Aspects of Cardiopulmonary Resuscitation (CPR) and Emergency Cardiac Care (ECC). In *Textbook of Advanced Cardiac Life Support.* Dallas: American Heart Association, 1987. Pp. 271–284.

McIntyre, KM, and Hampton, AG. Status of liability risk for out-of-hospital (OH) cardiopulmonary resuscitation (CPR). *Circulation* 54 (Suppl 2):II–224, 1976.

Rabkin, MT, Gilerman, G, and Rice NR. Orders not to resuscitate. *N Engl J Med* 295:364, 1976.

Report of the Ad Hoc Committee of the Harvard Medical School to Examine the Definition of Brain Death. A definition of irreversible coma. *JAMA* 205:337, 1968.

Sandoe, E, Flensted-Jensen, E, and Dupont, B. Long-term prognosis in patients resuscitated from cardiac arrest. *Isr J Med Sci* 5:769, 1969.

Seibke, H, et al. Survival after 40 minutes; submersion without cerebral sequelae. *Lancet* 1:1275, 1975.

Silverman, D, et al. Cerebral death and the electroencephalogram. Report of the Ad Hoc Committee of the American Electroencephalographic Society on EEG criteria for determination of cerebral death. *JAMA* 209:1505, 1969.

Sims, JK, and Penick, M. How much CPR is enough CPR? *JACEP* 7:218, 1978.

Standards for cardiopulmonary resuscitation (CPR) and emergency cardiac care (ECC). *JAMA* 227 (Suppl):833, 1974.

Standards and Guidelines for Cardiopulmonary Resuscitation (CPR) and Emergency Cardiac Care (ECC). *JAMA* 244 (Suppl):453, 1980.

Standards and Guidelines for Cardiopulmonary Resuscitation (CPR) and Emergency Cardiac Care (ECC). *JAMA* 255:2843, 1986.

Thompson, RG, Hallstrom, AP, and Cobb, LA. Beneficial effort of bystander-initiated CPR in out-of-hospital ventricular fibrillation (abstract). *Circulation* 56 (Suppl 3):111, 1977.

B. Acute Disorders of the Respiratory System

6. Normal and Pathologic Physiology of the Respiratory System

Christopher H. Fanta

The primary gas-exchanging functions of the lungs are oxygenation of the blood and excretion of carbon dioxide. Under resting conditions, approximately 360 liters per day of oxygen are needed to support oxidative metabolism in an adult, with approximately 288 liters per day of carbon dioxide released as an end product of these enzymatic pathways. To achieve these needs of the body, one must breathe approximately 8,000 liters per day of air. Under conditions of physical stress, the respiratory system may for short periods of time be called on to increase the volume of gas that is breathed by as many as 10 times.

It is clear that for normal functioning, the respiratory system must first of all act as an effective bellows, continually pumping gas into and out of the lungs. The bellows, or pump, function of the respiratory system requires muscles to expand the chest and a skeletal framework (the thoracic cage) on which these muscles can act. In addition, a control mechanism (respiratory center in the brainstem) must be in place to regulate the rate and magnitude of the pumping action, and neural pathways must interconnect this "controller" with the lungs, thoracic cage, and respiratory muscles so that afferent and efferent neural traffic can pass between them. Together, these components of the respiratory system subserve the function of ventilation; by convention, the units of ventilation are liters per minute, and the total amount of gas moved in and out of the lungs (total ventilation) is designated $\dot{V}_E$.*

An inability to sustain adequate ventilation can result from disorders in any of these components of the respiratory system. Examples include depression of the controller (e.g., narcotic drug overdose), neuromuscular weakness (e.g., amyotrophic lateral sclerosis), distortion of the thoracic cage (e.g., kyphoscoliosis), and various diseases of the lungs (e.g., chronic obstructive pulmonary disease). The primary consequence of inadequate ventilation is the accumulation of carbon dioxide in the blood (hypercapnia).

It is not sufficient, however, for the purpose of exchanging gases between blood and the outside environment, simply to have air (or other inhaled gas mixtures) be moved in and out of the thorax. The gas-exchanging function of the lungs requires that the ventilated air† be delivered to alveoli (of

*V is used to indicate volume; $\dot{V}$ is used to designate volume per unit time. Total ventilation is generally measured as the exhaled volume per unit time, hence $\dot{V}_E$.

†Under special circumstances individuals may breathe gas mixtures other than air. However, for the sake of simplicity, the term *air* is used alone here and subsequently to indicate the gas or gases that are being inspired.

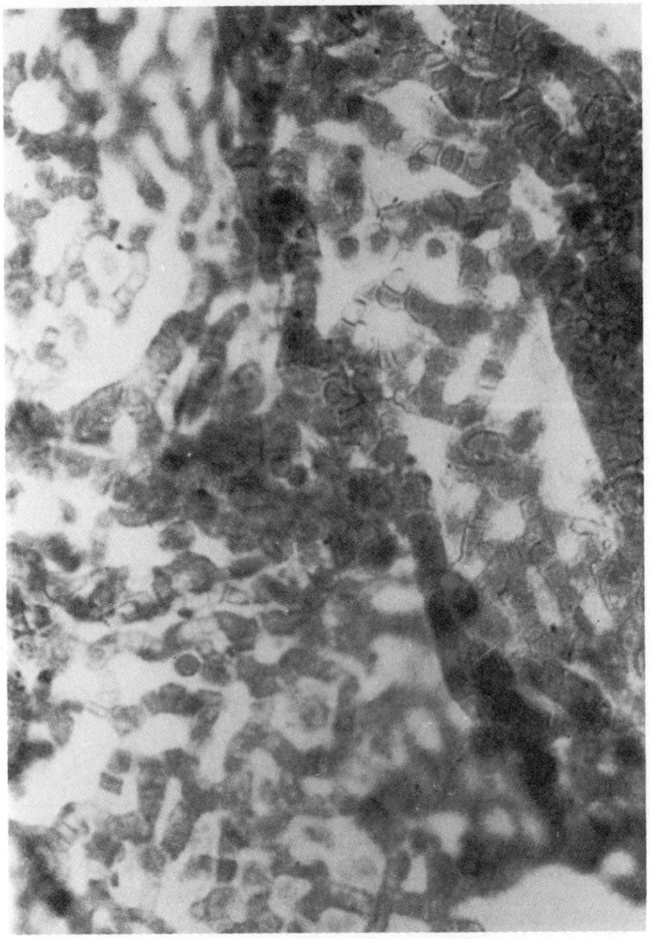

Fig. 6-1. A dense network of pulmonary capillaries within the interalveolar septum envelop pulmonary alveoli with blood. This hematoxylin and eosin-stained section from human lung is magnified 650 times. (From V.E. Krahl. Anatomy of the Mammalian Lung. In W.O. Fenn and H. Rahn [eds.], *Handbook of Physiology*. Washington, D.C.: American Physiological Society, 1964. P. 259.)

which the mature lung has approximately 300 million) while venous blood is being perfused through the pulmonary capillary network surrounding them (Fig. 6-1). Gas exchange takes place at the delicate interface between alveolus and capillary—across alveolar epithelium and its basement membrane, a thin interstitial space, and vascular endothelium and its basement membrane, which are together referred to as the "alveolar-capillary membrane" (Fig. 6-2). Air that enters the lungs but does not reach functioning alveolar-capillary units is "wasted" from the point of view of exchanging gases with the blood; it enters portions of the lung considered "dead space" with respect to gas exchange. That portion of the total ventilation ($\dot{V}_E$) that does not participate in gas exchange is referred to as "wasted ventilation" or "dead-space ventilation," abbreviated $\dot{V}_D$.

Conversely, that portion of the total ventilation that reaches perfused alveoli and is available for oxygen and carbon dioxide transfer is called the "alveolar ventilation," or $\dot{V}_A$. Total ventilation is simply the sum of dead-space ventilation and alveolar ventilation ($\dot{V}_E = \dot{V}_D + \dot{V}_A$). Insufficient elimination of carbon dioxide from pulmonary capillary blood and consequent hypercapnia result whenever alveolar ventilation is inadequate for the metabolic rate of the body (i.e., the rate at which carbon dioxide is being produced). Alveolar ventilation can be reduced because of a decrease in total ventilation or because of an increase in dead-space ventilation for which a compensatory increase in total ventilation does not occur. Under normal resting conditions, during which total ventilation equals approximately 6 liters per minute, approximately 4.0 to 4.5 liters per minute of alveolar ventilation eliminates approximately 200 ml per minute of carbon dioxide and maintains the arterial carbon dioxide tension equal to 40 ± 4 mm Hg.

Like carbon dioxide elimination, effective transfer of oxygen into pulmonary capillary blood requires adequate ventilation and, in particular, adequate alveolar ventilation. However, oxygenation differs from the process of carbon dioxide removal in that oxygen transfer is also critically dependent on the relatively uniform *distribution* of alveolar ventilation throughout the lungs. Besides the overall amount of alveolar ventilation, one must consider the distribution of the alveolar ventilation on a local or regional basis throughout the lungs, and also the regional distribution of pulmonary arterial blood flow. Adequate oxygenation of the mixed venous blood that enters the pulmonary vascular bed requires that alveolar units receive ventilation appropriate to their rate of perfusion with blood; underventilated units can cause hypoxemia even in the presence of normal or increased overall alveolar ventilation. Thus, another important task of the respiratory system is the matched distribution of ventilation and blood flow throughout the lungs, delivering more air to alveoli that receive relatively larger amounts of blood flow and less air to alveoli that are relatively less perfused. Normal lungs do an excellent job of matching ventilation and perfusion by delivering most of the ventilation to the lung bases, which also receive the greatest amount of blood flow. In addition, in the presence of disease, compensatory mechanisms exist to redistribute ventilation or blood flow away from regions of low perfusion or ventilation, respectively. Local hypocapnia causes constriction of airways and local alveolar hypoxia induces pulmonary arteriolar constriction. Nonetheless, focal or diffuse diseases of the airways or lung parenchyma can interfere with the balanced distribution of ventilation and perfusion, causing hypoxemia; examples include foreign-body aspiration, asthma, focal pneumonia, and pulmonary edema. In each example, overall alveolar ventilation is usually normal to increased, so that carbon dioxide tensions are typically normal or low.

To understand how regional mismatching of alveolar ventilation and pulmonary blood flow can cause hypoxemia, as well as why oxygen and carbon dioxide behave differently in this respect, one must consider the way in which each gas is transported in the blood. For oxygen, approximately 98 to 99 percent of the gas is carried in the blood bound to hemoglobin (Hb); the remainder is dissolved in plasma. When fully saturated (i.e., when all sites on the hemoglobin molecule that are available for binding oxygen are occupied by oxygen molecules), a gram of hemoglobin carries 1.34 ml oxygen. This value is referred to as the *oxygen-carrying capacity* of blood. The amount of oxygen transported in a liter of blood

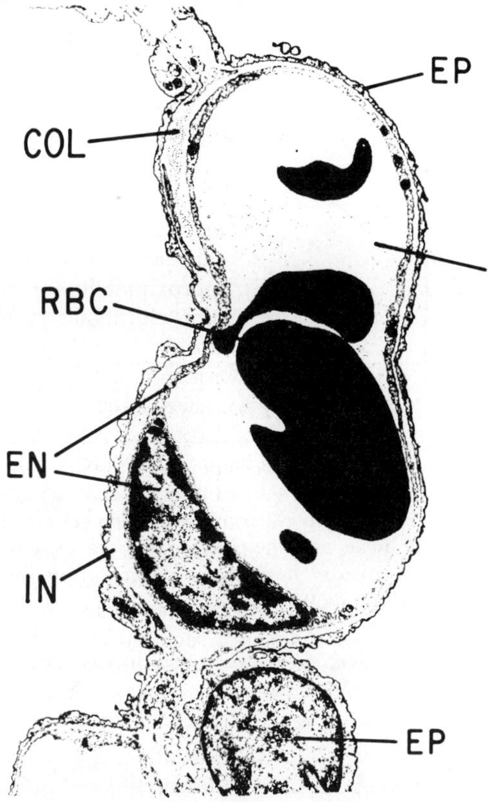

Fig. 6-2. This transmission electron micrograph of an alveolar septum demonstrates the structures through which gases must diffuse from alveolus to red blood cell, the so-called alveolar-capillary membrane. (EP = epithelial cell; COL = collagen fibers; RBC = red blood cell; EN = endothelial cell; IN = interstitial space; PL = plasma.) (From E.R. Weibel. Morphological basis of alveolar-capillary gas exchange. *Physiol. Rev.* 53:419, 1973.)

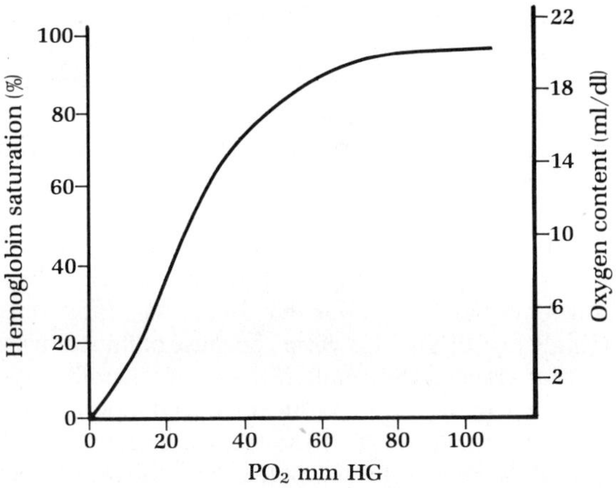

Fig 6-3. The oxygen-hemoglobin dissociation curve, relating the partial pressure of oxygen in the blood (in mm Hg) to the percent saturation of hemoglobin with oxygen (expressed as a percent of 100), is sigmoidal in shape. The percent saturation of hemoglobin with oxygen is directly correlated with the oxygen content of blood (expressed in ml O_2/dl blood or "volumes percent"). (Adapted from J.B. West. *Respiratory Physiology—The Essentials* [2nd ed.]. Baltimore: Williams & Wilkins, 1979. P. 71.)

is principally determined by the concentration of hemoglobin and the degree to which the hemoglobin molecules are saturated with oxygen. In vitro and in vivo methods are now available to measure directly the percent saturation of hemoglobin with oxygen (O_2 saturation). Oxygen saturation normally declines slightly with age; it is approximately 97 percent in a healthy young adult. Thus, in a healthy young male adult, one can calculate the amount of oxygen in 100 ml blood (the oxygen content of blood) as follows:

O_2 content = O_2-carrying capacity × O_2 saturation × Hb concentration

= 1.34 ml O_2/gm Hb × 97% × 15 gm Hb/dl blood

= 19.5 ml O_2/dl blood*

This calculation omits the small amount of oxygen dissolved in plasma, equal to 0.003 ml O_2 × arterial partial pressure of oxygen (PO_2), or approximately 0.3 ml/dl blood. The actual amount of oxygen in blood is not directly measured but must be calculated.

The extent to which hemoglobin is saturated with oxygen varies with the partial pressure of oxygen in the blood.† The relationship between the O_2 saturation of hemoglobin and the PO_2 of blood is sigmoidal rather than direct, as given by the oxygen-hemoglobin dissociation curve (Fig. 6-3). The shape and position of the normal oxygen-hemoglobin dissociation curve have several important implications, including the following: At normal values for arterial PO_2 (approximately 95 mm Hg in young adults), hemoglobin is nearly fully saturated with oxygen; further increments in arterial PO_2 cause only small increases in the O_2 saturation of hemoglobin and, therefore, in the amount of oxygen transported in arterial blood.‡ Conversely, the arterial PO_2 can fall quite significantly, to as low as 60 mm Hg, with only small resultant decrements in the amount of oxygen carried in the blood. Under normal circumstances, a PO_2 of approximately 60 mm Hg and an O_2 saturation of approximately 90 percent identify the top of the "shoulder" or "steep portion" of the oxygen-hemoglobin dissociation curve. Below approximately 60 mm Hg, even relatively small decreases in arterial

*The unit of measure used here, ml O_2/dl blood, is also referred to as "volumes percent."

†The partial pressure of a gas dissolved in a liquid (such as blood) is equal to the partial pressure of that gas in the gas phase with which it is in equilibrium, such that the liquid neither gives up nor takes up additional gas.

‡For instance, if a normal person breathes a gas mixture with 40 percent oxygen, the arterial PO_2 will rise from approximately 95 mm Hg to greater than 200 mm Hg. Arterial O_2 saturation will increase from 97 to 100 percent and the amount of hemoglobin-bound oxygen will rise by only 3 percent, from 19.5 to 20.1 ml O_2/dl blood. (Dissolved oxygen will increase from 0.3 to 0.6 ml O_2/dl blood; the overall O_2 content of blood therefore rises from 19.8 to 20.7 ml/dl blood, only a 5% increase.)

PO_2 cause comparatively large changes in O_2 saturation of hemoglobin and the O_2 content of blood.

In the presence of respiratory disease, when an imbalance in the relative distribution of alveolar ventilation and pulmonary blood flow creates areas of the lung with low ventilation relative to perfusion (referred to as areas of low $\dot{V}/\dot{Q}$), blood leaving those areas will have a relatively low PO_2 (and a relatively high partial pressure of carbon dioxide, or PCO_2). Other lung regions may receive excess ventilation relative to their perfusion (areas of high $\dot{V}/\dot{Q}$); blood leaving these latter zones will have a relatively high PO_2 (and a correspondingly low PCO_2). However, because of the nature of the hemoglobin-oxygen dissociation curve, areas with high $\dot{V}/\dot{Q}$ cannot compensate for the reduced oxygenation that has occurred in areas of low $\dot{V}/\dot{Q}$. Despite the higher arterial PO_2 of blood leaving high $\dot{V}/\dot{Q}$ areas of the lung, the oxygen content of the blood from these regions is minimally increased, and in balance the admixture of blood exiting high and low $\dot{V}/\dot{Q}$ zones results in arterial blood with reduced O_2 content, O_2 saturation, and PO_2. This point is worth emphasizing since regional ventilation-perfusion mismatching with areas of low $\dot{V}/\dot{Q}$ is the most common cause of hypoxemia.

By contrast, the relationship between the PCO_2 in blood and the carbon dioxide content of that blood is far simpler; the curve relating the two is nearly linear within the physiologic range (Fig. 6-4). As a result, blood leaving areas of the lung with high $\dot{V}/\dot{Q}$ will have a reduced carbon dioxide content in direct proportion to the reduced PCO_2 in those alveoli and can compensate for hypercarbic blood exiting areas of low $\dot{V}/\dot{Q}$. Thus, an equal mixture of blood from comparable high and low $\dot{V}/\dot{Q}$ areas will result in normal carbon dioxide content and partial pressure, despite a reduced PO_2.

The disparate transport mechanisms for oxygen and carbon dioxide and their physiologic consequences are of paramount importance in understanding the gas-exchanging function of the lungs. To reiterate, overall alveolar ventilation is the principal determinant of arterial PCO_2; arterial PO_2 depends not only on overall alveolar ventilation, but also on the regional distribution of alveolar ventilation with respect to pulmonary capillary perfusion. An extreme *hypothetical* example is offered to help clarify the distinction. Consider a person with total right-lung atelectasis due to mucous plugging who maintains normal perfusion (approximately 50% of pulmonary blood flow) to that nonventilated lung and a constant total ventilation. In this example, the entire right lung represents a zone of low $\dot{V}/\dot{Q}$ (or, more precisely, $\dot{V}/\dot{Q} = 0$). Blood with a low PO_2 (45 mm Hg) and O_2 content (15 ml O_2/dl blood) would exit the right lung; blood leaving the left lung, which would now receive twice its usual amount of ventilation, would have a high PO_2 (125 mm Hg) and O_2 content (20 ml O_2/dl blood). The admixed arterial blood would contain approximately 17.5 ml O_2/dl blood [(15 + 20)/2] and have a PO_2 of approximately 53 mm Hg. On the other hand, because in this example total ventilation and alveolar ventilation are maintained normally, arterial PCO_2 would remain normal. Blood draining from the right lung would contain excess carbon dioxide; blood draining from the left lung would have a reduced carbon dioxide content. The mixture of the two would result in an average carbon dioxide content that is normal, yielding eucapnia. (In actual practice, compensatory pulmonary arteriolar vasoconstriction in response to alveolar hypoxia would decrease perfusion to the atelectatic right lung, whereas total alveolar ventilation would increase in response to hypoxemia and other stimuli.)

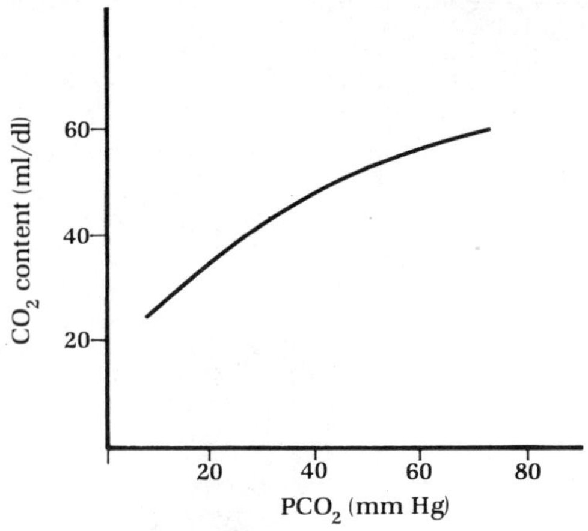

Fig. 6-4. The carbon dioxide dissociation curve, relating the partial pressure of carbon dioxide in the blood (in mm Hg) to the carbon dioxide content of blood (in ml CO_2/dl blood or "volumes percent"), is nearly linear over the physiologic range. (Adapted from J.B. West. *Respiratory Physiology—The Essentials* [2nd ed.]. Baltimore: William & Wilkins, 1979. P. 77.)

HYPERCAPNIA

Arterial PCO_2 is directly proportional to the rate at which carbon dioxide is produced by metabolizing tissues and released into systemic capillaries ($\dot{V}CO_2$); it is inversely proportional to alveolar ventilation ($\dot{V}A$). The following equation describes these relationships and includes a corrective factor used so that all values are expressed in units of body temperature and ambient pressure saturated with water (BTPS):

$$PCO_2 = 0.863 \times \dot{V}CO_2/\dot{V}A$$

One useful aspect of this equation is that it identifies the hyperbolic relationship between arterial PCO_2 and alveolar ventilation (Fig. 6-5): For any given metabolic rate of the patient, arterial PCO_2 will double if alveolar ventilation is halved, and, conversely, arterial PCO_2 can be reduced by 50% if alveolar ventilation is doubled. Also, one can see in graphic form that the slope of the curve is steep at elevated values of PCO_2. As a result, small changes in alveolar ventilation cause relatively large changes in arterial PCO_2 when hypercapnia is present.

Alveolar ventilation cannot be measured directly. In clinical practice we routinely estimate alveolar ventilation from total ventilation. The latter is the product of respiratory rate and tidal volume and can be measured or, more often, estimated by inspection. Thus, the apneic or hypopneic patient brought to the emergency department with a phenobarbital overdose is observed to have a reduced total ventilation and is consequently assumed to have a decreased alveolar ventilation and hypercapnia. Reduced alveolar ventilation and hypercapnia can also occur in clinical situations where total ventilation is normal or increased. For instance, during a

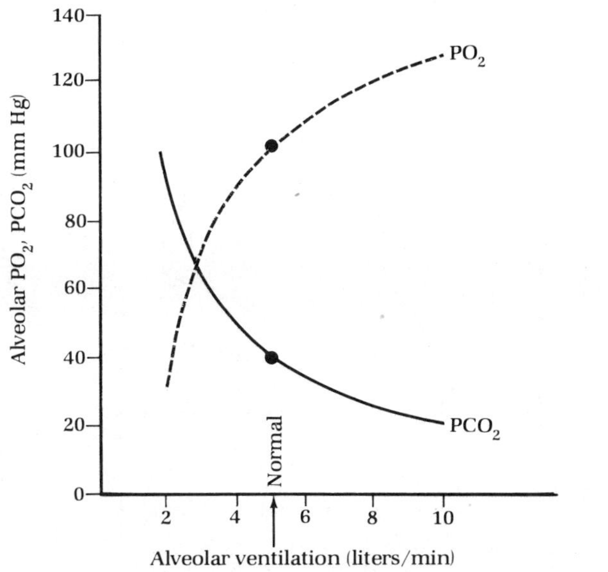

Fig. 6-5. The relationships between alveolar ventilation and the alveolar gas tensions for oxygen and carbon dioxide. Alveolar (and arterial) PCO_2 varies inversely with alveolar ventilation in a hyperbolic relationship. (Adapted from J.B. West. *Pulmonary Pathophysiology—The Essentials* [3rd ed.]. Baltimore: Williams & Wilkins, 1987. P. 24.)

very severe asthmatic attack, despite rapid and labored breathing, carbon dioxide retention can develop, in large measure because dead-space ventilation has increased at the expense of alveolar ventilation (recall that $\dot{V}_E = \dot{V}_A + \dot{V}_D$).

The clinical manifestations of hypercapnia depend on its severity and rapidity of development. Acute rises in arterial PCO_2 to above approximately 50 mm Hg cause symptoms of sympathetic stimulation (e.g., restlessness and palpitations) and of arteriolar vasodilation (e.g., headache and flushing). The effect of hypercapnia on the motor system may include a fine tremor, arterixis, clonic jerking of the limbs, and occasional generalized convulsions. However, chronic elevations of arterial PCO_2 to as high as 80 mm Hg or greater may remain asymptomatic if accompanying hypoxemia is averted by administration of supplemental oxygen and if severe acidemia is prevented because of renal compensation. The major adverse consequences of hypercapnia are central nervous system depression and acidosis. In the absence of other sedating influences, the narcotizing effect of carbon dioxide is generally not observed until arterial PCO_2 exceeds 90 mm Hg. Acidemia can contribute to cardiovascular instability and metabolic disturbances at pH values less than 7.30, and especially when less than 7.20. It is worth noting that the effects of hypercapnia on the central nervous system are fully reversible, whereas hypoxia can cause permanent damage to brain tissue.

HYPOXEMIA

At sea level the two most important causes of hypoxemia are alveolar hypoventilation and mismatching of the distribution of alveolar ventilation with pulmonary capillary blood flow ($\dot{V}/\dot{Q}$ mismatch). The fall in arterial PO_2 that occurs with alveolar hypoventilation is directly proportional to the rise in PCO_2. This relationship reflects the effect of increased PCO_2 on the mixture of gases within alveoli. As alveolar PCO_2 rises, the alveolar PO_2 falls proportionately, maintaining the sum total of partial pressures of all alveolar gases at atmospheric pressure. The change in alveolar PO_2 for a given change in PCO_2 is not a 1:1 ratio, but is given by the equation $\Delta PO_2 = \Delta PCO_2/R$, where R, the respiratory exchange ratio, is equal to approximately 0.8 under normal metabolic conditions. Thus, in the absence of intrinsic lung disease, if alveolar hypoventilation (such as can be caused by a tranquilizer overdose) causes alveolar and arterial PCO_2 to rise from 40 mm Hg to 60 mm Hg, one would predict that alveolar and arterial PO_2 will fall by 20 mm Hg/0.8, or 25 mm Hg (e.g., arterial PO_2 from 95 mm Hg to 70 mm Hg). The effect of varying PCO_2 on the alveolar PO_2 is shown graphically in Fig. 6-5.

As was discussed previously, regional imbalances between the rates of alveolar ventilation and pulmonary capillary perfusion produce hypoxemia because blood leaving zones with low (or zero) $\dot{V}/\dot{Q}$ has a reduced oxygen saturation. The impact of lung regions with absent ventilation ($\dot{V}/\dot{Q} = 0$) is distinct from regions with low $\dot{V}/\dot{Q}$. Not only does the arterial blood leaving alveolar zones where $\dot{V}/\dot{Q} = 0$ have a lower PO_2 (equal to that of mixed venous PO_2), but also the PO_2 of that blood is minimally improved by the administration of supplemental oxygen. This pathologic circumstance in which some lung regions receive pulmonary blood flow but are not ventilated at all is referred to as a "physiologic shunt" (as opposed to an anatomic right-to-left shunt). The greater the fraction of cardiac output that passes through unventilated regions of the lung (i.e., the greater the "shunt fraction" or "venous admixture"), the more severe is the resultant hypoxemia and the less will the patient's arterial PO_2 improve when supplemental oxygen is provided. Clinical disorders in which significant physiologic shunting develops usually involve diffuse parenchymal lung diseases such as pulmonary edema or *Pneumocystis* pneumonia. Because of the diffuse nature of these diseases, compensatory hypoxia-induced vasoconstriction cannot redirect pulmonary blood flow away from unventilated lung zones. The differing responses of arterial PO_2 to the administration of 100 percent oxygen for patients with hypoxemia caused primarily by low $\dot{V}/\dot{Q}$ regions in the lungs ("$\dot{V}/\dot{Q}$ mismatching") versus patients with hypoxemia predominantly due to physiologic shunting are shown in Fig. 6-6.

Hypoxemia also develops when the PO_2 in the air (or other inhaled gas mixture) is reduced. The most common example of this cause of hypoxemia is breathing at high altitudes. For example, at 7,000 ft (the altitude to which airplane cabins are pressurized during most commercial air flights), the barometric pressure is approximately 590 mm Hg and the PO_2 in the inspired air is only approximately 114 mm Hg. The arterial PO_2 in a normally functioning lung would be approximately 65 mm Hg (assuming unchanged alveolar ventilation). Two equations are used to make these calculations. In the first equation the PO_2 in the inspired air (P_IO_2) is equal to atmospheric pressure (P_{atm}) minus the partial pressure of water vapor (P_{H_2O}) times the fraction of oxygen in the inspired air (F_IO_2), or

$$P_IO_2 = (P_{atm} - P_{H_2O}) \times F_IO_2$$

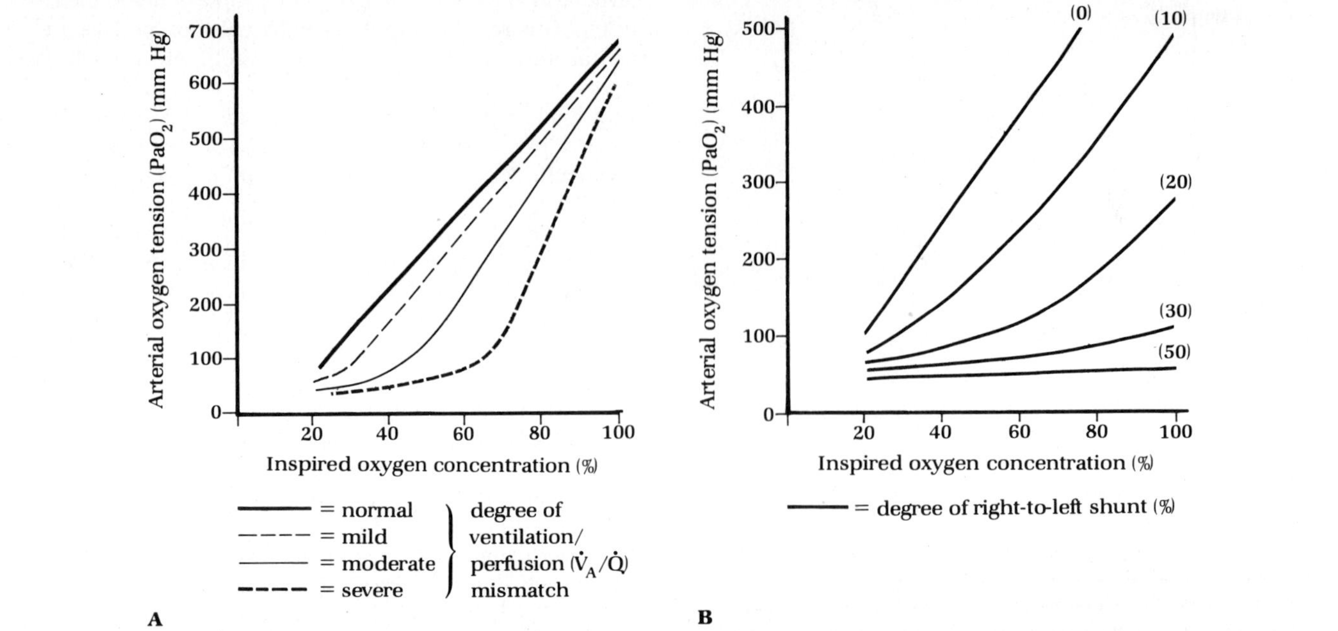

Fig. 6-6. The increase in arterial oxygen tension (PaO_2) in response to varying concentrations of inspired oxygen is shown for different degrees of ventilation-perfusion mismatch (A) and shunt (B). Unlike ventilation-perfusion mismatch, in right-to-left shunting the inhalation of 100 percent oxygen does not correct the PaO_2 to normal. The greater the shunt fraction, the smaller the impact of supplemental oxygen on the resultant PaO_2. (From R.H. Ingram, Jr., and C.H. Fanta. Respiratory Failure. In E. Rubenstein and D.D. Federman [eds.], Subsection 14, *Scientific American Medicine*, a loose-leaf medical information service in internal medicine. New York: Scientific American, 1988. Pp. 1, 2.)

Note that this equation can also be used to determine the PO_2 of inspired gas when supplemental oxygen is administered (i.e., when F_IO_2 is greater than 0.21). In the second equation ideal alveolar PO_2 is equal to the inspired PO_2 minus alveolar PCO_2 divided by R, or

$$P_AO_2 = P_IO_2 - (PCO_2/R)$$

This latter equation is a slightly simplified form of what is called the "ideal alveolar gas equation." It permits estimation of a single theoretical value for alveolar PO_2 in a lung with ideal distribution of pulmonary blood flow. Determination of the difference between this calculated value for alveolar PO_2 (P_AO_2) and the measured arterial PO_2 (PaO_2) proves to be clinically useful in some situations. The difference between P_AO_2 and PaO_2 is referred to as the *alveolar-to-arterial (A-a) gradient* for oxygen. In healthy persons breathing room air, the A-a gradient is 5 to 10 mm Hg in young adults and increases with age. The presence of a small A-a gradient in normal persons reflects slight imperfections in the matched distribution of ventilation and perfusion as well as small anatomic right-to-left shunts (e.g., the thebesian veins drain directly into the left atrium). Patients with hypoxemia due to low inspired oxygen tension or alveolar hypoventilation have a normal A-a gradient for oxygen; patients with hypoxemia due to $\dot{V}/\dot{Q}$ mismatching or physiologic shunt have an increased A-a gradient, which constitutes evidence for intrinsic lung disease (in the absence of intracardiac right-to-left shunt).

In the following clinical example, a 52-year-old patient, a heavy cigarette-smoker, is seen in the emergency ward with a depressed level of consciousness. Arterial blood gases, with the patient breathing room air at sea level (P_{atm} = 760 mm Hg), reveal the following: PO_2 = 50 mm Hg, PCO_2 = 72 mm Hg, pH = 7.18. Do these blood gas results reflect the presence of significant chronic obstructive pulmonary disease? Using the ideal alveolar gas equation given previously (and assuming a value of 0.8 for the respiratory exchange ratio, R), one can calculate the ideal alveolar PO_2 to be 60 mm Hg, as follows:

$$\begin{aligned} P_AO_2 &= (P_{atm} - P_{H_2O}) \times F_IO_2 - PCO_2/R \\ &= (760 - 47) \times 0.21 - 72/0.8 \\ &= 150 - 90 \\ &= 60 \text{ mm Hg} \end{aligned}$$

The A-a gradient for oxygen ($P_AO_2 - PaO_2$) is 60 mm Hg − 50 mm Hg, or 10 mm Hg, a normal value for a 52-year-old person. Thus, there is no evidence for any intrinsic lung disease in this patient; the observed hypoxemia can be accounted for entirely on the basis of alveolar hypoventilation.

It was formerly thought that diseases characterized by thickening of the pulmonary interstitium (e.g., sarcoidosis) might cause hypoxemia by impairing diffusion of oxygen from alveolus to pulmonary capillary—the so-called alveolar-capillary block. It now appears that although diffusion of oxygen may be slowed in such circumstances, in persons at rest with a normal circulation time the delay is not sufficient to prevent complete equilibration of oxygen tensions across the alveolar-capillary membrane. Thus, impaired diffusion is generally not a significant mechanism for hypoxemia in patients assessed at rest.

Anemia does not cause hypoxemia; it does, however, reduce the oxygen content of blood. In the absence of lung disease, a young person with a hemoglobin concentration of 10 gm/dl would have a normal arterial PO_2 of approximately 95 mm Hg and a reduced oxygen content of approximately 13 ml O_2/dl blood. In an anemic patient who is hypoxemic despite maximal oxygen supplementation, one can improve oxygen delivery to metabolizing tissues by increasing the hemoglobin concentration with red blood cell transfusions.

Finally, cardiac output can have an indirect impact on oxygenation of arterial blood. When cardiac output is low, mixed venous oxygen tension falls because of increased extraction of oxygen in peripheral tissues. In the presence of physiologic shunt, a low cardiac output induces a further depression of arterial PO_2, because of the effect of venous admixture in which mixed venous blood has a reduced PO_2. In general, the effect of a reduced cardiac output on arterial oxygenation is small.

Like excess carbon dioxide, low oxygen tensions in arterial blood have both hemodynamic and central nervous system consequences. Manifestations of hypoxemia include vasoconstriction, hypertension, and increased cardiac output. Severe hypoxemia, especially in conjunction with hypercapnia and acidosis, produces vasodilation, with consequent hypotension and cardiovascular collapse. Cardiac arrhythmias, particularly ventricular premature beats, are common in the profoundly hypoxemic patient ($PO_2 < 40$ mm Hg). Central nervous system effects of hypoxemia include headache, irritability, confusion, drowsiness, and profound fatigue. Generalized seizures can develop at very low oxygen tensions. Compensatory mechanisms to protect against tissue hypoxia include increased cardiac output, increased red blood cell mass in response to erythropoietin secretion by the kidneys, rightward shift of the oxygen-hemoglobin dissociation curve due to increased concentrations of 2,3-diphosphoglycerate, and biochemical adaptations at the level of the mitochondrion.

CONTROL OF VENTILATION

The unconscious generation of a regular, rhythmic pattern of breathing is basic to species along the entire evolutionary tree from primitive sea animals (Aplysius) to mammals. Neurons grouped in the dorsal and ventral medulla appear to serve this "pacemaker" function in humans, and even in some deeply comatose patients, normal breathing may continue uninterrupted.

On the other hand, abnormalities in the normal breathing pattern can give clues to the site of brainstem dysfunction in comatose patients. For instance, apneustic breathing, characterized by deep inspirations followed by pauses at full inspiration ("inspiratory gasps"), is indicative of lesions in the pons. Biot's respirations, in which totally chaotic, patternless breathing is found, usually indicates injury in the region of the reticular formation in the medulla. The most commonly encountered disturbance of respiratory rhythm is Cheyne-Stokes respiration, in which apneas of 20 to 30 seconds are followed by breaths of crescendo-decrescendo rate and depth. Although found with certain brainstem lesions, Cheyne-Stokes respiration is far more often a manifestation of congestive heart failure. The delayed circulation time present in congestive heart failure prolongs the time necessary to complete the feedback loop connecting peripheral chemoreceptors (discussed later) and the central respiratory controller, making possible an oscillatory pattern of output and overcorrection from the respiratory center.

The respiratory system is capable of effecting rapid adjustments in ventilation to meet the needs of a changed metabolic rate (e.g., during exercise), to correct acute deviations in acid-base status, and to protect the body (especially the brain) from hypoxia. In addition, normal respiratory rhythm can be modified to coordinate breathing with other involuntary acts (e.g., sneezing) as well as voluntary acts (e.g., singing) that involve the respiratory muscles. To accommodate these various functions, the respiratory control center in the medulla receives input from various sites and of various types. This information includes signals from sensory nerve endings in the airways, lung parenchyma, respiratory muscles, and chest wall as well as chemoreceptors in the carotid and aortic bodies (sensitive to changes in oxygen tension) and in the brainstem (sensitive to changes in pH, reflecting fluctuations in PCO_2).

Motor neurons from the medullary centers descend via cranial nerves to activate upper-airway muscles (e.g., abductor muscles of the larynx and genioglossus muscle of the tongue) at the initiation of inspiration; neural pathways also descend into the ventrolateral spinal cord to connect with phrenic motor neurons (C3–C5) to innervate the diaphragm and with motor neurons of the thoracic cord to innervate the intercostal muscles. Separate pathways in the dorsolateral portion of the spinal cord connect centers in the cerebral cortex responsible for the voluntary control of respiration with motor neurons in the spinal cord.

Both the hypoxic and hypercapnic drives to ventilation can be tested and quantified. Although there is considerable interindividual variability, the general shapes of these curves, relating level of ventilation to gas tension in the arterial blood, are shown in Fig. 6-7. Several clinically relevant points regarding these ventilatory response curves bear emphasis. First, small increases in arterial PCO_2 (e.g., above 45 mm Hg) are a stimulus to increased ventilation, whereas hypoxemia provokes little increase in ventilation until the arterial PO_2 falls to approximately 55 to 60 mm Hg (O_2 saturation to approximately 90%). Second, adaptation to chronically abnormal blood gas tensions alters the ventilatory response to acute changes. Thus, in the presence of chronic hypercapnia (with accompanying rises in the bicarbonate concentrations in cerebrospinal fluid and medullary extracellular fluid), the ventilatory response to acute rises in arterial PCO_2 is blunted. Likewise, with chronic exposure to hypoxia, such as occurs during acclimatization to high altitude, the increase in ventilation is less than during acute hypoxia. Third, the PCO_2–$\dot{V}_E$ curve is shifted by associated changes in arterial PO_2, and the PO_2–$\dot{V}_E$ curve is similarly shifted by alterations in PCO_2 and pH. Thus, hypoxemia and hypercapnia are additive stimuli to ventilation; normoxia lessens the increase in ventilation observed in response to hypercapnia, and alkalosis decreases the ventilatory response to hypoxemia.

Clinical application of these observations is illustrated in the following example. A patient with severe chronic obstructive pulmonary disease and chronic carbon dioxide retention is brought to the emergency department wearing face mask oxygen (inspired oxygen concentration of approximately 50%). He is somnolent and difficult to arouse; his respirations are only 12 per minute and relatively shallow.

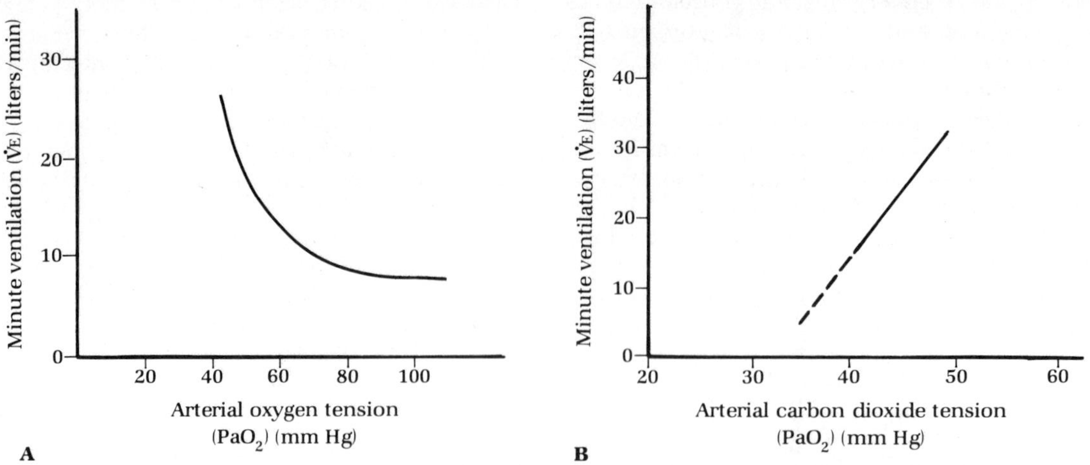

Fig. 6-7. The effect of lowering the inspired oxygen tension (A) and raising the inspired carbon dioxide tension (B) on the level of ventilation. These demonstrate the hypoxic and hypercapnic ventilatory drives, respectively. The curves are representative of a typical response, but great interindividual variability exists within the normal population. (From R.H. Ingram, Jr., and C.H. Fanta. Ventilatory Control and Disturbances During Wakefulness and Sleep. In E. Rubenstein and D.D. Federman [eds.], Subsection 14, *Scientific American Medicine*, a loose-leaf medical information service in internal medicine. New York: Scientific American, 1987. Pp. 2, 3.)

Arterial blood gases reveal the following: $PO_2 = 95$ mm Hg, $PCO_2 = 78$ mm Hg, and pH = 7.40. What can be done to increase his ventilation, besides correcting the underlying lung disease and possibly administering respiratory stimulants? It can be assumed that this ventilatory response to hypercapnia has been blunted by chronic hypercapnia. However, it may be possible to stimulate his drive to ventilation by lowering his inspired oxygen concentration such that the arterial PO_2 is reduced to approximately 55 mm Hg. In addition, correction of his metabolic alkalosis (pH 7.40 with $PCO_2 = 78$ mm Hg indicates a mixed acid-base disorder with respiratory acidosis and metabolic alkalosis) will increase his responsiveness to hypoxemia and hypercapnia. Finally, it must be remembered that there are independent motor pathways from the cerebral cortex to the respiratory muscles. If he can be aroused to follow simple commands, it may be possible to exhort him to take more rapid and deeper breaths, taking advantage of the voluntary control of ventilation.

Rarely, patients can have defective ventilatory drives to both hypoxia and hypercapnia. Such individuals typically come to medical attention because of ventilatory failure, manifested as hypoxemia, hypercapnia, cor pulmonale, or secondary erythrocytosis. Characteristic of this condition, called *primary alveolar hypoventilation syndrome,* is the ability of the patient transiently to lower the arterial PCO_2 to normal by voluntary hyperventilation, such as on coaching from a physician. Treatment with respiratory stimulants such as medroxyprogesterone may be successful in correcting this disorder of ventilatory drive.

Far more common are the ventilatory disturbances that occur primarily during sleep. Foremost among these is the sleep apnea syndrome. Patients with this disorder have repetitive periods of apnea during sleep, sometimes exhibiting as many as several hundred apneas during an eight-hour period, with apneic episodes that last up to 60 seconds or longer. The most common mechanism causing these apneas is upper-airway obstruction occluding airflow despite the generation of respiratory efforts by the inspiratory muscles. An anatomically narrowed upper airway plus an abnormal, sleep-induced decrease in the tonic and phasic activation of the upper-airway muscles (normally responsible for maintaining airway patency during inhalation) contribute to these *obstructive* apneas. Obesity is a common finding in sleep apnea syndrome, perhaps at least in part because excess fat deposition in the posterior pharynx causes upper-airway narrowing. Relatively small amounts of weight loss (e.g., lowering weight from 350 to 300 lbs) can significantly ameliorate the condition in some obese patients.

Far less often, apneas during sleep occur because of the periodic absence of any inspiratory effort; these apneas presumably result from failure of the central (medullary) centers for respiration and are called *central* apneas. *Mixed* apneas combine features of both central and obstructive apneas; they begin as absent inspiratory effort and conclude with inspiratory efforts against an occluded upper airway.

Repetitive and prolonged apneas induce recurrent hypoxemia and hypercapnia. The apneas are terminated by arousals (to a lighter stage of sleep) or frank awakenings, fracturing the night's sleep. Some of the common clinical manifestations of sleep apnea syndrome can be directly related to the disordered sleep pattern and the cyclic derangements in blood gases. These signs and symptoms include restless, thrashing sleep; snoring; somnambulism; daytime hypersomnolence; changes in personality and intellectual functioning; cor pulmonale; secondary erythrocytosis; and sleep-related cardiac arrhythmias. Other manifestations include systemic hypertension; extreme sensitivity to the respiratory depressant effects of sedatives, hypnotics, and narcotic analgesics; enuresis; and daytime dreamlike hallucinations.

Other than weight loss, traditional treatment for severe obstructive sleep apnea syndrome has been tracheostomy. A tracheostomy tube kept patent during sleep bypasses an obstructed upper airway and permits normal ventilation. In this way one can potentially achieve complete reversal of the signs and symptoms of the sleep apnea syndrome. Alternative forms of therapy have been attempted with varying degrees of success. These include medications to stimulate ventilatory drive and upper-airway muscle tone during sleep (e.g., medroxyprogesterone and protryptyline), surgical correction of upper-airway structural abnormalities (e.g., tonsillectomy and adenoidectomy in children and uvulopalatopharyngoplasty), and pneumatic splinting of the upper airway during sleep using nasally applied, continuous, positive airway pressure (nasal CPAP). This latter device has proved highly successful and is currently the treatment of first choice in the majority of cases. It can be applied immediately in the hospitalized patient, offering a potential alternative to intubation in the individual with severe ventilatory failure due to obstructive sleep apnea.

ASSESSMENT OF LUNG FUNCTION

With the exception of measurements of expiratory flow such as spirometry and peak expiratory flow determination, pulmonary function testing is infrequently performed in the emergency department. Nonetheless, knowledge of the common tests of pulmonary function, the relevant nomenclature, and the information that can be derived from these tests is often necessary so that the emergency department physician can meaningfully interpret available data and determine which tests might be useful in the subsequent evaluation of patients with respiratory complaints. For this reason, we will briefly review here some of the fundamental tests used to assess lung function.

Spirometry is the most commonly performed pulmonary function test. It involves a timed maximal forced exhalation. Patient cooperation and maximal effort are required for meaningful results. Thus, delirious or stuporous patients or patients with significant chest pain are unable to perform reliable spirometric testing. The test provides a record of the entire volume of gas that the patient is able to exhale (the forced vital capacity, or FVC) and the rate at which this gas is exhaled, on a scale of seconds (Fig. 6-8). In this way, measurements of expiratory flow (volume/time = flow) can be made. The rate of exhalation varies over the vital capacity range; it is greatest soon after the initiation of exhalation and slows progressively thereafter until the exhalation is completed. The most widely used measure of expiratory flow is the rate of exhalation during the first second of exhalation (the one-second forced expiratory volume, or FEV_1). Although expressed in units of liters, the FEV_1 is a measure of flow, since a unit of time is implied in its definition (volume in the first *second* of exhalation). Another commonly used measure of expiratory flow derived from spirometry is the rate of exhalation during the midportion of the vital capacity, between 25 and 75 percent of the vital capacity volume. This parameter has two names: It is alternately called the *forced expiratory flow between 25 and 75 percent of the vital capacity* (FEF_{25-75}) and the *maximal midexpiratory flow* (MMF).

Spirometry, sometimes in combination with complete measurement of lung volumes (discussed later in this section), is used to categorize ventilatory disorders into obstructive, restrictive, or mixed patterns and to determine the severity of the deviation from normal. Assessment of severity is based on a comparison with results obtained from healthy persons of the same age, height, sex, and preferably, race.

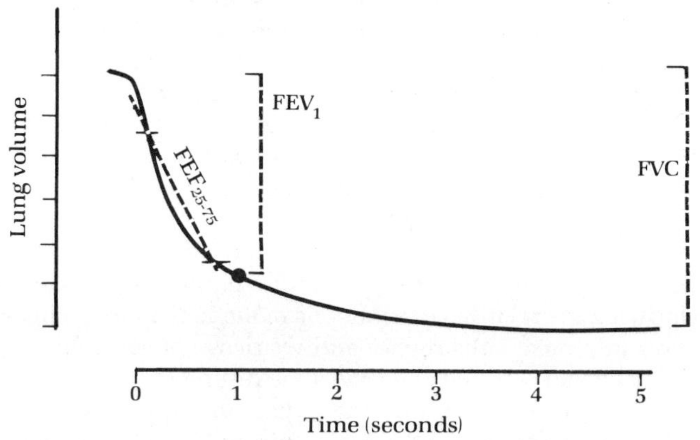

Fig. 6-8. A spirogram depicts the volume of exhaled gas over time during a maximal forced exhalation. The total volume of exhaled gas is the forced vital capacity (FVC); the volume exhaled in the first second is the one-second forced expiratory volume (FEV_1); and the flow in the midportion of the vital capacity, between 25 percent and 75 percent of the vital capacity, is the FEF_{25-75}, which is expressed in liters per second.

The results of testing in a particular patient can be expressed as a percentage of the predicted normal value.

Obstructive patterns on pulmonary function testing (i.e., obstruction to the flow of gas during exhalation) are characterized by decreased values for FEV_1 and FEF_{25-75} with relatively preserved values of FVC. As severe airflow obstruction develops, it becomes impossible to exhale the normal volume of gas and so FVC also declines. However, whenever airflow obstruction is present, the ratio of FEV_1 to FVC will always be reduced. Diseases in which obstruction of expiratory flow is the primary pathophysiologic derangement include asthma, chronic bronchitis and emphysema, and bronchiolitis. Obstructive deficits are often part of the ventilatory abnormalities found in congestive heart failure, sarcoidosis, bronchiectasis, and lymphangioleiomatosis.

By contrast, restrictive ventilatory abnormalities (i.e., restriction to the volume of gas that the lungs can contain) are characterized by reduction of the FVC with preservation of a normal ratio of FEV_1 to FVC. Thus, although the FEV_1 is reduced in restrictive deficits, the decrease is in proportion to the reduction in FVC. The simplest example of a restrictive abnormality is the pulmonary function of a patient who has undergone pneumonectomy and has normal function of the remaining lung. The FVC and FEV_1 would both be approximately 50 percent of normal, with FEV_1/FVC maintained at a normal level. In restrictive abnormalities due to diffuse parenchymal lung disease, such as asbestosis, a small *increase* in the FEV_1/FVC may be observed. This observation is explained at least in part by the following: The increased force required on inspiration to expand these stiff lungs is returned as an increased driving pressure during exhalation, forcing gas out of the lungs more rapidly than normal.

Although one can measure the maximal volume of gas that can be exhaled from the lungs (FVC) with spirometry, one cannot determine the volume of gas that remains within the lungs at the end of a complete exhalation, called the "residual volume" (RV). This volume, and other so-called "static lung volumes" to be discussed shortly, require for their measurement more extensive pulmonary testing by a gas dilution technique or plethysmography, routine tests performed in most pulmonary function testing laboratories. Using these techniques, one can measure not only RV but also the total volume of gas that can be contained within the lungs (total lung capacity, or TLC, equal to RV plus FVC) and the volume of gas within the lungs at the end of exhalation during tidal breathing (functional residual capacity, or FRC). Measurement of these static lung volumes is helpful in defining the nature of restrictive ventilatory abnormalities and determining their severity; it is also particularly useful in clarifying the relative contributions of the individual components in a mixed obstructive and restrictive abnormality.

Functional residual capacity is the resting lung volume; it is the volume of gas in the lungs when no respiratory efforts are being made (e.g., after the administration of a paralyzing agent such as pancuronium). At FRC the tendency of the lungs to recoil to a smaller volume (inward recoil pressure of the lungs) is exactly balanced by the opposing tendency of the chest wall to recoil to a larger volume (outward recoil pressure of the thoracic cage). Thus, FRC can be altered not only by disorders that reduce the volume of gas within alveolar spaces (e.g., pulmonary edema) but also by changes in the elastic properties of the lungs or chest wall (e.g., massive obesity).

By contrast, maximal muscular effort is required to achieve TLC and RV. Inspiratory muscle strength (predominantly of the diaphragm) is needed to overcome the elastic properties of the lungs and thoracic cage as the respiratory system is expanded to TLC; expiratory muscle strength (predominantly of the abdominal wall musculature and intercostals) is required to compress the thoracic cage when approaching RV. TLC and RV may be abnormal if the elastic properties (compliance) of the lungs or chest wall, or both, are altered or if neuromuscular diseases affect respiratory muscle strength. Examples include emphysema, in which a decrease in the elastic recoil pressure of the lungs can lead to an increase in TLC; diffuse fibrous thickening of the pleurae (fibrothorax), in which increased stiffness (decreased compliance) of the respiratory system causes a reduction in TLC; and Guillain-Barré syndrome, in which respiratory muscle weakness can cause both a decreased TLC and increased RV.

Other divisions of TLC besides FRC, RV, and FVC can be measured or calculated. Their names and the corresponding subdivisions are shown in Fig. 6-9. These measurements are less often needed in defining patterns of pulmonary function abnormalities, and thus they are not discussed further here.

A variety of disorders of the lungs, pleura, chest wall, and "ventilatory pump" can cause restrictive abnormalities of pulmonary function. Restriction results from collapse, filling, or destruction of alveolar spaces or from an inability to expand the thoracic cage fully. In the former instances (e.g., diffuse pulmonary fibrosis or massive pleural effusion), all lung volumes (i.e., TLC, FRC, RV, and FVC) tend to be symmetrically reduced. In neuromuscular diseases, restriction may be manifested as a reduction in TLC (because of inspiratory muscle weakness) but an elevation in RV (because of expiratory muscle weakness). By contrast, restriction in certain conditions that affect the thoracic cage (in particular, massive obesity and late pregnancy) is characterized by decreases in RV and FRC with relative preservation

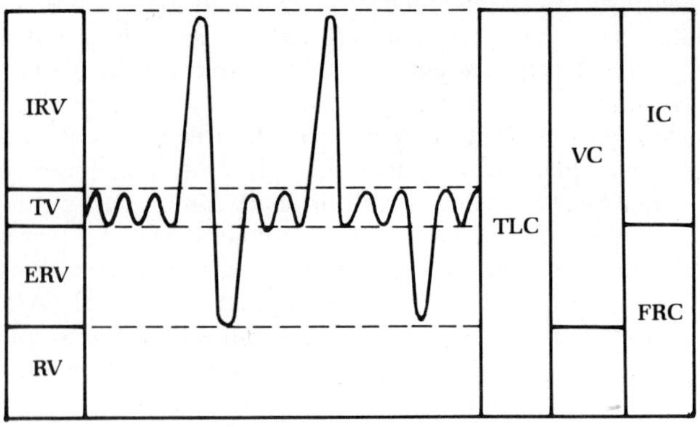

Fig. 6-9. The various subdivisions of total lung capacity, which is the amount of gas contained within the lungs at the end of a maximal inhalation. By convention, "capacities" are portions of the total lung capacity that can be formed by combination of two or more "volumes."

of TLC and FVC. These differing patterns of restriction are illustrated in Fig. 6-10.

In suspected or known disorders of respiratory neuromuscular function, it is sometimes useful to measure respiratory muscle strength directly. For instance, in patients with Guillain-Barré syndrome, assessment of respiratory muscle strength may prove more sensitive than measurement of lung volumes in determining the extent of respiratory system involvement or the response to treatment. The pressure that can be generated at the mouth when one attempts to inhale or exhale maximally against a closed shutter is referred to as the *maximal static inspiratory or expiratory pressure* (MIP or MEP), respectively. The former is usually measured after a maximal exhalation (i.e., MIP is recorded at RV); the latter is usually measured after a maximal inhalation (i.e., MEP is recorded at TLC). Normal values vary with age and sex; typical values for a young male adult are 100 to 140 cm H_2O for MIP and 160 to 190 cm H_2O for MEP. Respiratory muscle reserve is such that when the lungs and thoracic cage are normal, decreases in vital capacity do not reliably occur until respiratory muscle strength has declined to approximately 40 percent of normal.

One other test of pulmonary function is the diffusing capacity for carbon monoxide (D_{LCO}). In this much misunderstood test, the amount of carbon monoxide taken up by the blood is measured after inhalation with a breath-hold of a gas mixture that contains a known concentration of carbon monoxide. The purpose of the test is to assess the amount and function of alveolar-capillary membrane available for gas exchange between ventilated alveoli and perfused pulmonary capillaries. However, other variables will affect the results and so must be taken into consideration. These variables include the alveolar volume, the pulmonary capillary blood volume, the hemoglobin concentration, and the presence of carboxyhemoglobin (e.g., in cigarette smokers). Uptake of carbon monoxide from alveoli depends not only on the integrity of the alveolar-capillary membrane but also on the volume of blood into which the carbon monoxide can diffuse, the amount of hemoglobin to which it can bind, and the pressure difference for carbon monoxide between alveoli

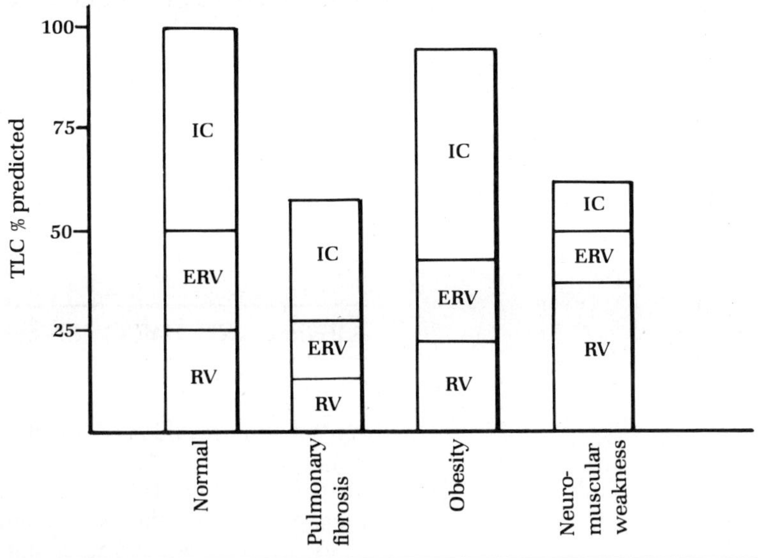

Fig. 6-10. Three different patterns of restrictive lung volume abnormalities. In pulmonary fibrosis (and other causes of diffuse parenchymal lung disease) lung volumes are symmetrically reduced. In obesity, the expiratory reserve volume and residual volume (and consequently, functional residual capacity) are reduced while total lung capacity is relatively preserved. In neuromuscular weakness involving both inspiratory and expiratory muscles, total lung capacity is reduced, residual volume is increased, and functional residual capacity remains normal. (Adapted from E.H. Bergofsky. Respiratory failure in disorders of the thoracic cage. *Am. Rev. Respir. Dis.* 119:643, 1979.)

and blood. Normally, the concentration of carbon monoxide in blood is zero, but in the presence of carboxyhemoglobinemia, the pressure gradient between alveoli and blood is reduced due to significant "back pressure" from carbon monoxide in the blood.

Since any disease in which the total lung capacity is reduced will also have a decreased amount of alveolar-capillary membrane participating in gas exchange, the diffusing capacity is generally corrected for reductions in alveolar volume. Thus, in a patient who has undergone pneumonectomy and has a normal remaining lung, the uncorrected DLCO will be approximately 50 percent of normal but the DLCO corrected for alveolar volume will be normal. Similarly, the DLCO should be corrected for hemoglobin concentration. After these corrections have been made, residual reductions in the DLCO must be attributable to decreased alveolar-capillary surface area, diminished pulmonary blood volume (e.g., in large pulmonary emboli), or carboxyhemoglobinemia. The DLCO is elevated in the presence of increased pulmonary blood volume (e.g., left-to-right shunt) and diffuse alveolar hemorrhage. In the latter condition, blood in the alveolar spaces binds the inhaled carbon monoxide, reducing its concentration in the exhaled gas and mimicking an increased uptake by the pulmonary circulation.

The DLCO is most commonly used to assess the presence and severity of diffuse parenchymal lung diseases such as sarcoidosis or cytotoxic drug-induced diffuse lung injury. In some instances the DLCO is an early indicator of lung involvement, becoming reduced at a time when lung volumes are still within the normal range. It can sometimes be useful in distinguishing restrictive ventilatory abnormalities due to diffuse parenchymal lung disease from restrictive deficits of other causes (e.g., respiratory muscle weakness or thoracic cage abnormalities), since in the latter conditions the corrected DLCO remains normal. In the obstructive diseases, a reduced DLCO suggests the presence of emphysema; chronic bronchitis and asthma are associated with normal values for DLCO. In patients with emphysema, a DLCO less than or equal to 55 percent of predicted is said to be predictive of oxygen desaturation with exercise. Finally, a decreased DLCO with a normal chest radiograph may be a useful clue to the presence of occult thromboembolic disease or early *Pneumocystis* pneumonia.

SELECTED READING

Cherniack, RM. *Pulmonary Function Testing.* Philadelphia: Saunders, 1977.

Fishman, AP, Goldring, RM, and Turino, GM. General alveolar hypoventilation: A syndrome of respiratory and cardiac failure in patients with normal lungs. *Q J Med* 35:261, 1966.

Guilleminault, C, and Dement, WC (eds). *Sleep Apnea Syndromes* (Kroc Foundation Series, vol 11). New York: Liss, 1978.

Sicker, HO, and Hickam, JB. Carbon dioxide intoxication: The clinical syndrome, its etiology and management with particular reference to the use of mechanical respirators. *Medicine* (Baltimore) 35:389, 1956.

Sullivan, CE, et al. Reversal of obstructive sleep apnea by continuous positive airway pressure applied through the nares. *Lancet* 1:862, 1981.

Weinberger, SE, Johnson, TS, and Weiss, ST. Clinical significance of pulmonary function tests: Use and interpretation of the single-breath diffusing capacity. *Chest* 78:483, 1980.

West, JB. Pulmonary Pathophysiology—The Essentials (3rd ed). Baltimore: Williams & Wilkins, 1987.

Williams, MH. Disturbance of respiratory control. *Clin Chest Med* 1:1, 1980.

7. Symptoms and Signs of Respiratory Disorders

Christopher H. Fanta

APNEA AND HYPOVENTILATION

Apnea is the cessation of breathing. During apnea the arterial oxygen tension (PO_2) falls and the arterial carbon dioxide tension (PCO_2) rises at approximately 3 to 5 mm Hg per minute during conditions of normal resting metabolic rate. Thus, within a few minutes vital organs (most notably the brain and heart) are exposed to significant hypoxemia and acidemia; within 20 to 30 minutes, death ensues. Brief periods of apnea (usually <10 seconds in duration) occur during normal sleep. Longer periods of apnea can result from the voluntary control of ventilation (e.g., breath-holding during underwater swimming) or as a compensatory mechanism after hyperventilation. In the emergency department, however, prolonged apnea is usually evidence for respiratory system failure ("respiratory arrest") and requires urgent intervention.

Hypoventilation is breathing of a rate and depth that are inadequate to achieve normal elimination of carbon dioxide; an elevated arterial PCO_2 indicates the presence of hypoventilation. As was noted in Chap. 6, the determinants of arterial PCO_2 are the rate at which carbon dioxide is released from metabolically active tissues and the level of alveolar ventilation. Thus, if the wasted (dead-space) ventilation is large, it is possible to have rapid and labored breathing that fails to eliminate adequate amounts of carbon dioxide because of alveolar hypoventilation. In this section, however, we will address the problem of global hypoventilation—that is, reduced respiratory rate, tidal volume, or both, resulting in hypercapnia despite normal rates of dead-space ventilation and carbon dioxide production. Patients with hypoventilation are at risk of progressing to apnea; their emergency management is directed at preventing or reversing that process.

PATHOPHYSIOLOGY

Apnea can result from complete obstruction of the upper airways or, more often, from cessation of activity in the respiratory centers in the medulla. Respiratory center output can be interrupted by profound hypotension ("cardiopulmonary arrest"), depressant medications and toxins, and diseases that directly injure the brainstem. On the other hand, comatose patients with bilateral cerebral cortical disease may continue with normal respirations, indicating intact medullary function.

Defined as cessation of breathing for 10 seconds or more, apneas can occur in the context of certain distinctive breathing patterns in which, following apneas, respiration resumes spontaneously without physician intervention. In adults, the most common of these circumstances are Cheyne-Stokes respirations and sleep-disordered breathing (sleep apnea syndrome). The former, crescendo-decrescendo breathing cycles interrupted by 20- to 30-second apneas, occurs in patients with congestive heart failure or primary brainstem disease. The latter, which includes apneas due to upper-airway occlusion (obstructive apnea), absent respiratory drive (central apnea), or a combination of both (mixed apnea), occurs exclusively during sleep. Both Cheyne-Stokes respirations and sleep-disordered breathing are discussed in Chap. 6. Their importance in this context is that resuscitative measures (i.e., intubation and mechanical ventilation) are generally not indicated.

Hypoventilation may represent a normal respiratory compensatory mechanism for metabolic alkalosis. In this setting, the arterial pH is always greater than 7.40 and the arterial PCO_2 generally does not exceed 55 mm Hg. In the absence of metabolic alkalosis, hypoventilation produces a respiratory acidemia, normally a potent stimulus to increased ventilation. Failure to increase minute ventilation despite hypercapnia and acidemia implies either a mechanical failure of the respiratory system or impaired central drive to ventilation. Phrased in another way, some patients hypoventilate because they "can't breathe" more, others because they "won't breathe" more. In the former category are patients with failure of the respiratory pump (e.g., severe kyphoscoliosis, neuromuscular diseases with respiratory muscle weakness, or generalized tonic-clonic seizure) and some patients with severe obstructive lung disease. In the latter category are patients with depressed brainstem function due to drugs, toxins, hypotension, or structural injury; some patients with severe obstructive lung disease and abnormal ventilatory drive; and patients with rare, idiopathic conditions that affect ventilatory drive, such as primary alveolar hypoventilation. Conscious patients with impaired output of the medullary respiratory center (*involuntary* drive to respiration) often have preserved a normal *voluntary* ventilatory drive. Thus, for instance, patients with primary alveolar hypoventilation characteristically have the ability to lower their elevated arterial PCO_2 to normal by voluntary hyperventilation. By contrast, patients who cannot breathe more because of mechanical impairment are unable to reduce significantly their PCO_2 regardless of effort.

DIFFERENTIAL DIAGNOSIS

Like asystole, prolonged apnea is a final common pathway for death of the organism; its differential diagnosis includes all fatal diseases. From a practical standpoint, apnea that occurs in the absence of prior respiratory disease is usually due to drug overdose, particularly of narcotics, sedatives, or hypnotics; brainstem injury (infarct, hemorrhage, or compression); or severe cerebral hypoxia, most often in the setting of cardiac arrest. As was noted previously, the differential diagnosis of apnea includes temporary cessation of breathing in Cheyne-Stokes and sleep-disordered breathing.

The differential diagnosis of hypoventilation is discussed in detail in Chap. 15. A brief checklist of potential causes of hypoventilation is given in Table 7-1, divided into central (respiratory drive) and peripheral (lungs and ventilatory pump) disorders. It should be noted that although hypoxemia and hypercapnia usually stimulate increased ventilation, in the extreme ($PO_2 < 30–40$ mm Hg, $PCO_2 > 80–90$ mm Hg) they cause central nervous system depression and hypoventilation. Also, in patients with chronically elevated arterial PCO_2 with compensatory metabolic alkalosis, hypercapnia has a blunted effect on respiratory drive. In this setting, relief of hypoxemia with high inspired oxygen concentrations can precipitate more severe hypoventilation by removing the hypoxic stimulus to breathing. Finally, patients with chronic hypoventilation are often exquisitely sensitive to the respiratory depressant effects of sedatives, hypnotics, and narcotic analgesics. Thus, in patients with acute-on-chronic hypercapnia, a detailed history of medication use should always be obtained.

Table 7-1. Causes of hypoventilation

Central (decreased ventilatory drive)
Drugs, toxins
Brainstem disease
Severe hypoxemia, severe hypercapnia
Metabolic alkalosis
Sleep apnea syndrome
Primary alveolar hypoventilation
Peripheral (normal or increased ventilatory drive)
Lungs and pleura
COPD of the "blue bloater" type
Severe bronchiectasis (e.g., cystic fibrosis)
Upper-airway obstruction
Fibrothorax
Chest wall and respiratory muscles
Kyphoscoliosis
Primary myopathies (e.g., muscular dystrophy)
Disorders involving innervation of respiratory muscles (e.g., myasthenia gravis, poliomyelitis, cervical spinal cord injury)

APPROACH TO THE PATIENT WITH APNEA OR HYPOVENTILATION

History

In a patient with apnea or profound hypoventilation, one must undertake immediate intervention to restore ventilation, deferring history-taking until later. When time is available to obtain a history, useful information may be provided by the person(s) who accompany the patient to the emergency department. One should inquire about antecedent illnesses, complaints expressed by the patient before apnea, and the patient's appearance when first discovered, as well as all medications taken by the patient. Also, one should attempt to determine the duration of apnea before resuscitation efforts, a factor that will influence prognosis for full neurologic recovery.

Another important piece of information in evaluating hypoventilation is the duration of the abnormality. Chronicity may be suggested by symptoms, such as long-standing exercise intolerance. It can also be extracted from the medical records: for example, prior hypercapnia; erythrocytosis, which can indicate chronicity since chronic hypercapnia is frequently accompanied by chronic hypoxemia sufficient to stimulate erythropoietin secretion; and elevated serum bicarbonate concentration, which reflects renal compensation for chronic hypercapnia. In a patient with unexplained chronic hypercapnia who has no evidence for primary pleuropulmonary disease, sleep apnea syndrome is frequently an important diagnostic consideration. Symptoms that indicate this diagnosis include snoring, restless sleep, and daytime hypersomnolence. Other symptoms and signs of sleep apnea syndrome are discussed in Chap. 6. The differential diagnosis of *acute* hypoventilation is relatively circumscribed, including mainly causes of acute respiratory center depression and acute neuromuscular disorders.

Physical Examination

Brief observation of the apneic patient allows identification of apnea due to upper-airway obstruction, Cheyne-Stokes respirations, and sleep apnea syndrome. Patients with upper-airway obstruction (as in the so-called "café coronary," when solid food becomes lodged in the hypopharynx, glottis, or trachea) desperately struggle for breath and usually gesture to their throats to indicate the perceived site of obstruction. In Cheyne-Stokes respirations, apneas last only 20 to 30 seconds and are interspersed with cycles of crescendo-decrescendo breathing. In sleep apnea syndrome, sleeping patients can have cessation of breathing for as long as 60 to 90 seconds. Obstructive and mixed apneas (the most common forms) usually terminate with a sudden snorting inspiration as the tongue is protruded forward, out of the air passageway. In severe sleep apnea syndrome (such as might cause a patient to fall asleep while being evaluated in the emergency department), apneas occur repetitively as often as 50 times an hour.

A detailed neurologic examination is an important part of the evaluation of the apneic patient. Special attention should be paid to evidence for brainstem dysfunction and cranial nerve deficits. Pupillary size may be a clue to narcotic drug overdose.

In evaluating hypoventilation, inspection of the rate and depth of breathing is particularly important in the unconscious patient. It may be necessary to act on a clinical impression of hypoventilation without awaiting the results of arterial blood gas determination. An obvious example is the patient with agonal respirations—the shallow, ineffective, and erratic breathing that is often a harbinger of apnea.

Partial upper-airway obstruction can contribute to hypoventilation; this mechanism is particularly common in a comatose patient unable to protect the upper airway by cough or control of the tongue. In a patient with depressed respiratory drive, one may have to listen carefully at the mouth to appreciate the stridorous breathing of partial upper-airway obstruction.

Finally, it is important to observe the pattern of abdominal and chest wall excursions during breathing in a patient who is hypoventilating. Inspiratory expansion of the thorax accompanied by paradoxical inward movement of the abdomen suggests diaphragmatic weakness, paralysis, or fatigue. On the other hand, inward displacement of the anterior chest wall during inspiration, with synchronous outward movement of the abdomen, is found in lower-cervical and upper-thoracic spinal cord injuries that cause paralysis of intercostal muscles.

Laboratory Studies

In virtually all patients with apnea or hypoventilation, arterial blood gases and a chest x-ray are indicated to assess the severity of the blood gas derangement and to evaluate for cardiopulmonary disease, respectively. Hypercapnia is the sine qua non of these disorders and oximetry is therefore inadequate for measurement of the gas exchange abnormality.

The most common cause of hypercapnia in most emergency department settings is severe chronic obstructive pulmonary disease (COPD). One should be cautious about ascribing hypercapnia to COPD simply on the basis of a patient's long-standing history of cigarette smoking. Chronic airflow obstruction develops in only a minority of cigarette smokers and hypercapnia develops in only a small fraction of patients with chronic airflow obstruction. Hypercapnia is rarely due to COPD unless the one-second forced expiratory volume (FEV_1) is less than 1.5 liters (and usually less than 1.0 liter). Thus, pulmonary function testing can be valuable in assessing the cause of hypoventilation in the emergency department.

Additional studies are warranted in patients without severe airflow obstruction or primary pleuropulmonary disease. Most important, a toxic screen for respiratory depressant drugs should be sent on urine or blood samples, or both. Repeat arterial blood gas measurement at the end of 30 to 60 seconds of voluntary hyperventilation helps to identify patients with intact voluntary drive to ventilation (e.g., central alveolar hypoventilation). In certain cases, elective work-up should include measurement of respiratory muscle strength, usually assessed in the pulmonary function laboratory in terms of the maximal inspiratory pressure (MIP) and maximal expiratory pressure (MEP) that can be generated at the mouth, and polysomnography ("sleep study") to evaluate for sleep apnea syndrome.

Management

The patient with prolonged apnea ("respiratory arrest") requires immediate respiratory resuscitation. This procedure, discussed in Chaps. 2 and 3, includes ensuring a patent upper airway and providing assisted ventilation. In patients with aspirated solid food, providing a patent upper airway may simply involve performing the Heimlich maneuver. In other patients, unconscious and with vomitus in the pharynx, suctioning material from the mouth and pharynx, turning the patient to the decubitus position (to avoid having the tongue occlude the oropharynx), and placing an oral airway into the mouth will be indicated. In still other patients with mechanical obstruction of the upper airway, emergency cricothyroidotomy may be necessary.

Assisted ventilation can be provided in a number of ways. Because of the risk of transmission of disease from oropharyngeal secretions and blood, mouth-to-mouth resuscitation should not be performed in the emergency department; alternative methods should be readily available. Disposable one-way valve mouth-to-mask resuscitation devices (Fig. 7-1) obviate the need for direct physical contact, but even these instruments should be unnecessary because of the availability of mechanical devices for ventilation. In a patient with a patent upper airway, ventilation can usually be supported for many minutes with a tight-fitting face mask

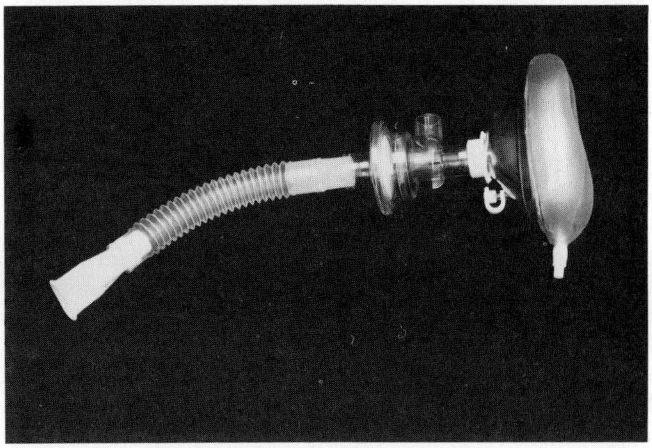

Fig. 7-1. A one-way valve mouth-to-mask resuscitation device. It should be used in situations in which mouth-to-mouth resuscitation would have been performed previously.

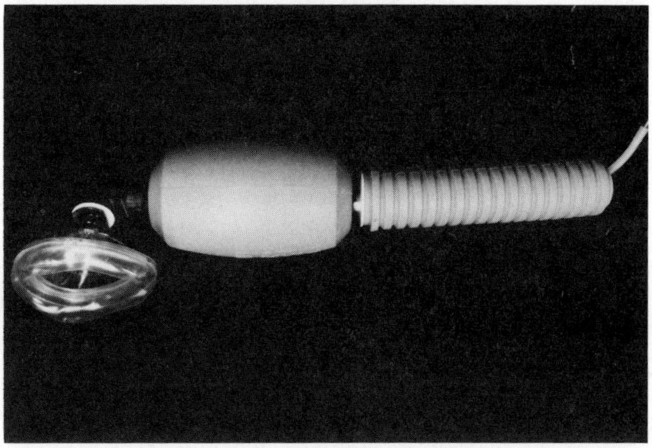

Fig. 7-2. Manually assisted ventilation can be provided with this self-filling reservoir bag (Ambu bag) and tight-fitting face mask. Usually, 100 percent inspired oxygen is administered through the attached tubing.

attached to a self-filling reservoir bag (Ambu bag), through which high-flow oxygen can be supplied (Fig. 7-2). A potential complication of prolonged mechanical ventilation by Ambu bag is overdistention of the stomach with gas. Therefore, intubation with mechanical ventilation is preferred if ventilation needs to be supported for more than 10 to 15 minutes. General guidelines for initiating assisted ventilation with a mechanical ventilator are given in Chap. 15.

In managing the patient with hypoventilation, an initial clinical judgment must be made as to whether the observed level of ventilation is sufficient to support life. If respirations are clearly agonal and a forerunner of respiratory arrest, assisted ventilation should be begun promptly, as described previously. On the other hand, if it appears that apnea is not imminent, the physician can send a sample of blood for arterial blood gas analysis and, while awaiting the results, make interventions that will lead to increased spontaneous ventilation and improved oxygenation. In general, if blood gas analysis indicates hypercapnia with an arterial pH less than approximately 7.20, assisted ventilation should be provided.

Conservative measures that may increase the level of spontaneous ventilation depend on the underlying cause of hypoventilation. In narcotic drug overdose, naloxone (Narcan) will reverse the respiratory depressant effect of the drug and thereby stimulate ventilation. In myasthenia gravis, intravenous edrophonium (Tensilon) will usually improve respiratory muscle strength acutely. For patients with obstructive lung diseases, bronchodilators and possibly corticosteroids are indicated. In some patients with preserved voluntary drive to ventilation, including some patients with severe COPD, exhortation to breathe deeper and faster will lead to increased ventilation for as long as the patient's attention can be focused on breathing. Central respiratory stimulants such as doxapram (Dopram) have had limited success and are not widely available.

The cause of hypercapnia is hypoventilation and, as emphasized here, its treatment focuses on methods to increase ventilation. However, hypercapnia is always accompanied by a reduced arterial PO_2 (in the absence of oxygen supplementation), sometimes to an extent that is life-threatening. Thus, supplemental oxygen is indicated in some patients with hypoventilation-induced hypoxemia. Oxygen supplementation must be given cautiously, however, because of concern over inducing worsening hypercapnia; the concentration of administered oxygen should be limited to 1 to 2 liters per minute by nasal cannulas or 24 to 28 percent by Venturi face mask. If even this low oxygen concentration leads to more severe hypercapnia and respiratory acidosis, assisted ventilation will need to be instituted. Nonetheless, withholding supplemental oxygen from the severely hypoxemic patient with hypercapnia has the potential for a worse outcome (myocardial injury or hypoxic encephalopathy) and should be eschewed. In a patient receiving assisted ventilation, oxygen can be administered without fear of precipitating worse ventilatory failure.

For the long-term management of hypoventilation due to neuromuscular weakness or kyphoscoliosis, a number of alternatives to conventional positive-pressure ventilation via tracheostomy are available. These include negative-pressure ventilators such as the "iron lung," cuirass, and "raincoat," rocking beds, and positive-pressure ventilation via a tight-fitting nasal mask. In general, however, the complexity involved with setting up these devices precludes their usefulness in an emergency situation. Further discussion of the management of respiratory failure is provided in Chap. 15.

DYSPNEA

Dyspnea is an unpleasant awareness of breathing, an uncomfortable feeling that breathing is labored. It is a frequent manifestation of most serious cardiopulmonary diseases and as such is a common presenting complaint of patients seen by an emergency service. Synonyms often employed by patients and physicians include "shortness of breath," "breathlessness," and "air hunger." Probably the most common stimulus that evokes the symptom of dyspnea is exercise, because of the increased demand for ventilatory output that it necessitates. However, one cannot simply equate the mechanical act of rapid breathing with dyspnea. In a well-trained athlete, the increased level of ventilation that accompanies even strenuous exercise is not perceived as unpleasant and so the athlete does not complain of dyspnea. However, if an athlete is asked to perform the same exercise task with an added respiratory load (e.g., the resistive load of breathing through a partially obstructed nose), he or she may well experience dyspnea. Prolonged breath-holding, although not a stimulus directly applicable to clinical medicine, is another way in which normal persons can experience dyspnea.

Patients with a variety of cardiopulmonary diseases experience dyspnea on exertion; this symptom is a major cause of disability due to respiratory and cardiac diseases. In general, the more severe the derangement in cardiopulmonary function, the greater the exercise limitation. One commonly cited system for classifying patients according to the severity of their exercise limitation resulting from dyspnea was proposed by the New York Heart Association in reference to patients with congestive heart failure:

Class I	No limitation: no dyspnea with ordinary physical activity.
Class II	Slight limitation: dyspnea with ordinary physical activity; comfortable at rest.
Class III	Marked limitation of physical activity: dyspnea on minimal activity; comfortable at rest.
Class IV	Discomfort on any physical activity: dyspnea present at rest and intensifies with any physical exertion.

Dyspnea at rest is particularly distressful: It is often acute and severe (e.g., in pulmonary embolism or pneumothorax) and it cannot be escaped by reducing one's activity level. Management of patients with this problem is discussed separately in Chap. 8. Patients with dyspnea at rest due to cardiopulmonary disease inevitably experience more severe breathlessness with increased activity. The occasional patient who reports shortness of breath while sitting quietly but no exercise limitation due to breathlessness has either primary hyperventilation or is describing another uncomfortable breathing sensation with the same terms used to describe dyspnea.

Sometimes dyspnea is positional. Orthopnea, or dyspnea brought on by lying supine, is typical of congestive heart failure, severe obstructive lung disease, and diaphragmatic weakness. Platypnea is shortness of breath that occurs in the upright posture and is ameliorated by lying supine; it is an uncommon symptom reported by some patients with pulmonary arteriovenous malformations, severe liver disease, or weakness of the abdominal muscles. Platypnea is usually associated with hypoxemia that develops on assuming the upright position (orthodeoxia). Extensive unilateral lung disease can present with trepopnea—that is, dyspnea that develops in the lateral decubitus position. Finally, many patients with advanced COPD report that bending over, such as in order to tie one's shoes, is a particularly troublesome cause of their dyspnea. The act of bending presumably causes dyspnea by putting the respiratory muscles at an increased mechanical disadvantage.

PATHOPHYSIOLOGY

None of the current theories regarding the mechanism(s) of dyspnea fully explains all of the pertinent observations. One can, however, identify stimuli that commonly trigger dyspnea as well as receptors and neural pathways involved in the generation and transmission of signals important in the perception of breathing and probably of dyspnea. Based on this information and extensive experimentation, some involving psychophysical grading of the intensity of dyspnea, theories have been developed that examine dyspnea in terms of the length-tension relationship of respiratory muscles and the central respiratory output (respiratory effort).

Hypoxemia, hypercapnia, and acidosis are commonly recognized chemical stimuli for increased ventilation and, thus, potentially for dyspnea. Receptors are situated both peripherally (carotid bodies) and centrally (medulla). Any disease that results in the acute development of severe hypoxemia or respiratory acidosis can be expected to produce dyspnea. In most healthy persons hypoxemia does not stimulate a significant increase in ventilation until the arterial PO_2 falls below 55 to 60 mm Hg; thus, mild hypoxemia (PO_2 maintained at greater than 60 mm Hg) would not be expected to cause dyspnea. Likewise, although ventilation increases linearly with rising arterial PCO_2 above approximately 45 mm Hg, persons with normal respiratory systems generally do not perceive an increase in their level of ventilation in response to hypercapnia until minute ventilation has approximately doubled.

Perhaps for the same reason, persons with normal cardiopulmonary function can develop hyperpnea in response to metabolic acidosis without experiencing dyspnea. Patients with diabetic ketoacidosis and Kussmaul's respiration may not report a sensation of breathlessness. On the other hand, in an exercising individual, the development of lactic acidosis results in a disproportionate increase in ventilation (beyond the metabolic requirements for oxygen delivery and carbon dioxide excretion), usually accompanied by dyspnea.

With *chronic* hypoxemia and hypercapnia, compensatory mechanisms come into play that improve tissue oxygen delivery and uptake and that buffer the excess blood carbon dioxide content. In addition, adaptive mechanisms may operate for dyspnea as for other sensations, such that prolonged application of the stimulus results in a decrease in the sensory intensity with which it is perceived. As a consequence, patients with chronic derangements in PO_2 and PCO_2 (measured at rest) may experience no or minimal resting dyspnea. A curious example of this phenomenon is found when comparing the two clinical types of patients with advanced COPD, the "pink puffer" and the "blue bloater" (see Chap. 10 for a more detailed discussion of these clinical types). By maintaining an increased level of ventilation, the pink puffer achieves relatively normal gas exchange but tends to experience more marked dyspnea with exertion; on the other hand, the blue bloater has chronic hypoxemia and hypercapnia and yet is generally less troubled by dyspnea.

A common misconception is that correction of hypoxemia

can be equated with relief of dyspnea. Routinely encountered clinical examples to the contrary are patients with pulmonary edema or pulmonary embolism who may be seen in the emergency department with profound hypoxemia and dyspnea, receive supplemental oxygen such that their arterial PO_2 corrects to normal, and yet remain severely breathless. As will be discussed next, mechanical stimuli from the airways, lung parenchyma, and chest wall also contribute to the sensation of dyspnea and would not be expected to respond to oxygen administration.

Sensory information regarding respiration is derived from receptors in the airways (irritant and stretch receptors) and lungs (called J-receptors because of their juxtaposition to pulmonary capillaries within the interstitium of the lung) and is carried centrally via the vagus nerve. In addition, muscle spindles within intercostal muscles and tendon organs within the diaphragm send afferent input regarding length and tension changes from these respiratory muscles. The importance of these mechanoreceptors in modifying the sensation of dyspnea is illustrated by a breath-holding experiment. If after prolonged breath-holding and the development of dyspnea a subject breathes from a gas mixture with low oxygen and high carbon dioxide, chosen so as to match the alveolar gas mixture and not alleviate hypoxemia or hypercapnia, the sensation of dyspnea is ameliorated and breath-holding can be prolonged. The same outcome can be achieved by isovolumic expansion of the chest—that is, contraction of the diaphragm with downward displacement of the abdominal contents, but no air entry into the lungs. In clinical medicine, it has long been observed that patients with pleural effusions who undergo thoracentesis may experience relief of dyspnea out of proportion to increases in lung volume or improvement of gas exchange achieved by removal of pleural fluid. This effect is presumed to be achieved by restoring respiratory muscle length and length-tension relationships toward normal.

One theory of the mechanism of dyspnea, the *length-tension inappropriateness theory* of respiratory sensation, focuses on the dyspnea-producing signals that originate in muscle receptors. According to this theory, dyspnea develops when expansion of the chest is less than would be expected (based on a subject's previous experience) for a given amount of inspiratory muscle tension. Because muscle afferents project to the cerebral cortex, dyspnea may be experienced as a result of a direct action of this input on higher brain centers.

Other investigators postulate that respiratory center motor output plays an important role in creating the sensation of dyspnea. In this construct, dyspnea is an expression of the sense of effort to breathe. It is a function of the following ratio: inspiratory muscle pressure during breathing divided by maximal inspiratory muscle pressure achievable (under the particular conditions of muscle length, tension, and velocity of shortening). Thus, for instance, in COPD with severe airflow obstruction and pulmonary hyperinflation, dyspnea increases with increasing levels of exercise (as inspiratory muscle force increases) and develops sooner than in healthy persons, in part because of the added resistive load to breathing (necessitating greater than normal inspiratory pressures) and in part because of impaired contractile ability of the foreshortened inspiratory muscles (reducing the maximal capacity for force generation).

It is possible that diverse signals regarding gas exchange, lung inflation and muscle tension, and respiratory force and effort may all contribute to our awareness of breathing and to the perception that it is unpleasant. In addition, psychological factors can modify one's response to dyspnea, just as they do with other sensations, such as pain. Thus, anxiety, depression, dependency, and hysteria may be characteristics that heighten the sense of dyspnea for any given degree of sensory input.

DIFFERENTIAL DIAGNOSIS

The differential diagnosis of dyspnea is too broad to consider in terms of individual diseases; instead, general consideration will be given here to disease categories that need to be considered when evaluating the patient with dyspnea (Table 7-2). A more detailed discussion of respiratory disorders that may manifest with respiratory distress (i.e., acute dyspnea at rest) can be found in Chap. 8.

Dyspnea is a common complaint among patients with *obstructive lung diseases.* Patients with chronic airflow obstruction (e.g., emphysema and chronic bronchitis, cystic fibrosis, and bronchiolitis) exhibit dyspnea on exertion that is roughly proportional to the severity of the obstructive deficit, although there is enormous interindividual variability. Acute exacerbations (e.g., due to superimposed acute bronchitis) are typically characterized by worsening exercise limitation due to dyspnea. Patients with asthma also experience dyspnea during episodes of acute airflow obstruction, but they are usually asymptomatic between episodes. Dyspnea due to upper-airway obstruction is usually, although not always, accompanied by stridorous or wheezy breathing. Clues to the diagnosis of obstructive lung diseases are a prolonged expiratory phase of the respiratory cycle and expiratory wheezing on chest auscultation. It should be noted

Table 7-2. Causes of dyspnea

Respiratory disorders
Obstructive lung disease (e.g., COPD, asthma, bronchiolitis, bronchiectasis)
Parenchymal lung disease (e.g., pulmonary edema, atelectasis, pneumonia)
Pulmonary vascular disease (e.g., pulmonary embolism, primary pulmonary hypertension)
Pleural disease (e.g., pleural effusion, pneumothorax, fibrothorax)
Chest wall abnormalities (e.g., kyphoscoliosis, massive obesity)
Neuromuscular disease (e.g., Guillain-Barré syndrome, diaphragmatic paralysis, muscular dystrophy)
Cardiac and pericardial disorders
Cardiac disease (e.g., ischemic heart disease, valvular heart disease, cardiomyopathy)
Pericardial disease (e.g., pericardial tamponade, constrictive pericarditis)
Noncardiopulmonary disorders
Septic shock
Anemia
Obesity
Aging
Physical deconditioning

that in many of the obstructive lung diseases, results of chest radiography are frequently entirely normal.

Parenchymal lung diseases that cause dyspnea include a great variety of acute and chronic conditions. Focal pneumonias can cause dyspnea in patients with preexisting respiratory disease; multifocal and diffuse pneumonias, most notoriously *Pneumocystis* pneumonia, produce dyspnea even among persons without previous respiratory compromise. Atelectasis and aspiration (see Chap. 14) and pulmonary edema (see Chap. 11) are other parenchymal lung diseases that can lead to the development of dyspnea suddenly or over the course of a few hours to days. Chronic diffuse parenchymal lung diseases include some disease processes that are primarily alveolar (e.g., alveolar proteinosis) and others that are primarily interstitial (e.g., idiopathic pulmonary fibrosis). The pathologic process can involve infection (e.g., miliary tuberculosis), inflammation (e.g., sarcoidosis), neoplasm (e.g., lymphangitic carcinomatosis), vasculitis (e.g., Wegener's granulomatosis), or hemorrhage (e.g., Goodpasture's syndrome with diffuse alveolar hemorrhage). The diagnosis of parenchymal lung disease is often suggested on chest auscultation by detection of inspiratory rales; the chest radiograph is usually abnormal and serves as a guide to the subsequent evaluation. Normal results on chest radiography do not exclude this diagnosis, however: It has been recognized that in the early but symptomatic stages of *Pneumocystis* pneumonia, the chest radiograph may be normal, and in a large series of patients with chronic diffuse lung diseases proven by lung biopsy, 10 percent were diagnosed at a time when their chest x-rays were still normal.

The most common *pulmonary vascular disease* causing dyspnea is pulmonary thromboembolism (see Chap. 13). Other, rarer causes of embolic vascular obstruction, also likely to include dyspnea as a presenting symptom, are tumor embolism, fat embolism, amniotic fluid embolism, septic embolism, and air embolism. In each case the physical findings tend to be nonspecific. (An exception is the petechial rash over the upper thorax sometimes seen in fat embolism.) The diagnosis is usually suggested by the historical context: metastatic carcinoma in tumor embolism, long-bone fracture in fat embolism, complicated delivery in amniotic fluid embolism, intravenous drug abuse or septic thrombophlebitis in septic embolism, and trauma or invasive medical intervention in air embolism. Primary pulmonary hypertension, multiple arteriovenous malformations, and pulmonary venoocclusive disease are additional, rare vascular causes of dyspnea.

Pleural diseases can induce acute (e.g., pneumothorax) or chronic (e.g., pleural effusion, mesothelioma) dyspnea. Physical findings generally are distinctive (unless pneumothorax complicates emphysema, in which case chest hyperexpansion, hyperresonance to percussion, and distant breath sounds are also found over the contralateral lung); chest radiography confirms the presence of pleural disease. *Chest wall abnormalities* such as kyphoscoliosis are obvious on inspection and do not require extensive diagnostic evaluation. Similarly, examination should reveal the presence of abdominal distention, which can cause dyspnea by compromising diaphragmatic excursion and chest wall expansion. Finally, *neuromuscular diseases* that impair respiratory muscle function (e.g., myasthenia gravis) are usually made obvious by the simultaneous involvement of peripheral muscle groups. However, unilateral diaphragmatic paralysis can occur as an isolated disorder (idiopathic or secondary to injury of the ipsilateral phrenic nerve) and can be manifested as exertional dyspnea. On chest radiography the involved hemidiaphragm is elevated but maintains its domed contour; fluoroscopic examination during a sudden inspiration ("sniff test") reveals paradoxical cephalad movement of the involved side.

Dyspnea rather than chest pain may be the dominant manifestation of any *cardiac or pericardial disease* that impairs left ventricular function. Dyspnea and often orthopnea are prominent symptoms when left atrial pressure (and consequently pulmonary venous pressure) is elevated, and left atrial pressure increases further during exercise in the failing heart. In patients with impaired forward cardiac output as the primary abnormality (e.g., constrictive pericarditis, restrictive cardiomyopathy, or right ventricular infarction), both fatigue and dyspnea develop with exertion. Despite what may be a normal arterial oxygen content, limited oxygen delivery to exercising peripheral tissues because of decreased blood flow results in the premature onset of anaerobic metabolism with generation of lactic acid, stimulating increased ventilation and dyspnea. By a similar mechanism, *septic shock* may cause acute and profound dyspnea. If the *anemia* is severe enough (the absolute value of hemoglobin depending on the rapidity of development of the anemia), oxygen delivery is reduced despite normal or increased cardiac output. Patients may complain that tiredness, dyspnea, or a combination of these two symptoms restricts their activities.

Finally, aging, obesity, and poor physical conditioning are common conditions that predispose to the development of breathlessness with exertion. Under these circumstances patients generally come to anticipate and accept their exercise limitation because of its very gradual evolution. Often, patients will use one of these conditions as an incorrect explanation for dyspnea that is actually caused by a more serious underlying medical problem.

APPROACH TO THE PATIENT WITH DYSPNEA

History

A useful distinction that can often be made on the basis of historical information alone is the separation of patients into those with acute or new-onset dyspnea from those with acute-on-chronic dyspnea. Patients who were previously well and in whom dyspnea develops suddenly or within a period of a few hours to days have a relatively limited differential diagnosis that includes (but is not restricted to) pulmonary embolism, pneumothorax, new onset of asthma, aspiration or diffuse pneumonia, septic shock, and congestive heart failure. On the other hand, patients with long-standing dyspnea who are acutely short of breath when seen in the emergency department may have any of a broad spectrum of chronic cardiac or pulmonary diseases, with deterioration due to an exacerbation of the underlying illness (e.g., infectious flare of bronchiectasis) or a superimposed cardiac or pulmonary illness (e.g., congestive heart failure complicating COPD). In determining the chronicity of dyspnea, it is useful to inquire about the patient's ability at some earlier date to perform specific tasks (e.g., climbing one flight of stairs without stopping). Objective data such as prior chest radiographs or pulmonary function tests, if available, also can delineate the chronicity of the underlying problem.

Physical Examination

Tachypnea is the hallmark of the dyspneic patient regardless of cause. However, if the patient has dyspnea only on exertion, breathing observed at rest may be normal. Other physical findings can help to narrow the differential diagnosis, particularly in the patient with a normal chest radiograph. For example, stridor points to a diagnosis of upper-airway obstruction; diffuse wheezing suggests asthma or asthmatic bronchitis; bilateral inspiratory rales raise consideration of radiographically occult diffuse interstitial lung disease or pneumonia; a pleural friction rub indicates pleural inflammation and possible pulmonary embolism; generalized muscle weakness alerts one to possible respiratory muscle weakness; and pallor indicates probable anemia.

Laboratory Evaluation

In a patient for whom dyspnea is a major complaint, initial evaluation in the emergency department should involve arterial blood gases and chest radiography. Arterial blood gas analysis (or pulse oximetry) permits identification of the hypoxemic patient, helps to define the severity of the problem (influencing patient triage), and determines the need for immediate supplemental oxygen administration. The chest radiograph is a useful screening test for a broad array of cardiopulmonary disorders. In some cases the radiographic findings will be diagnostic; in others they will be nonspecific but will serve to focus the subsequent evaluation (e.g., diffuse pulmonary infiltrates with bilateral hilar adenopathy may direct one toward subsequent fiberoptic bronchoscopy and transbronchial lung biopsy for tissue diagnosis of suspected sarcoidosis). In still other cases, results of the chest x-ray will be abnormal but the findings will be unrelated to the problem that is causing the dyspnea (e.g., apical pleural cap or solitary pulmonary nodule).

Additional tests may be necessary to elucidate the cause of dyspnea, but in many instances these tests are best pursued electively in the outpatient setting. Pulmonary function testing is probably the most helpful initial test, since it can be used to screen for a multitude of cardiopulmonary diseases and to categorize an abnormality into obstructive, restrictive, or both, categories. Multiple pulmonary emboli may be a cause of chronic dyspnea, usually with hypoxemia and "subacute cor pulmonale"; suspicion of this diagnosis should lead to perfusion lung scanning. Echocardiography is an excellent tool for evaluating suspected cardiac causes of dyspnea. Myocardial contractile function, valvular competence, pericardial disease, and pulmonary artery hypertension can all be assessed by this technique. To evaluate the complaint of dyspnea on exertion only, it may be necessary to assess oxygenation during exercise; this is most easily achieved by oximetry either during simple walking or more formally with treadmill or stationary-bicycle ergometry. Patients with early diffuse interstitial lung disease of any cause may have normal resting gas exchange but characteristically exhibit a fall in arterial oxygen saturation with exercise. Finally, in some patients with unexplained dyspnea, formal cardiopulmonary exercise testing may prove helpful. This procedure usually involves an incremental exercise challenge during which heart rate, minute ventilation, oxygen saturation, and in some cases oxygen consumption and carbon dioxide production are measured. Cardiopulmonary exercise testing can be used to help distinguish cardiac from pulmonary limitations to exercise and to suggest a pattern of response characteristic of physical deconditioning.

Management

In managing acute, severe dyspnea, the first goal must be the correction of severe hypoxemia or hypercapnia, if present. To a variable extent, treatment of the underlying disease may promptly achieve this goal (e.g., diuresis in pulmonary edema or bronchodilation in asthma). However, because a favorable response to treatment may be delayed or unachievable, supplemental oxygen will usually be necessary to alleviate hypoxemia initially. Various methods available to deliver oxygen supplementation are discussed in Chap. 8.

Often more difficult is the decision to perform intubation and mechanically assisted ventilation in the hypercapnic patient. Factors guiding that decision include the severity of the hypercapnia, its chronicity and the degree of renal compensation (as reflected in the arterial pH), the reversibility of the underlying disease, and the trend of the arterial pH in response to initial therapy. A gestalt that the patient "looks tired" or is "about to fatigue" is not adequate justification for invasive ventilatory support. Methods for initiating mechanically assisted ventilation are discussed in Chap. 15.

Relief of chronic dyspnea almost always must be achieved by treating the underlying cause. Symptomatic treatments of dyspnea are poorly developed. Narcotic analgesics alleviate dyspnea and are often used for palliation of the terminally ill patient with severe dyspnea. However, serious adverse side effects such as sedation and respiratory depression are common and usually unacceptable for patients who are not premorbid. Other techniques that have been used to improve exercise tolerance in dyspneic patients include oxygen supplementation in patients in whom oxygen desaturation develops with exercise, breathing retraining exercises, and pulmonary rehabilitation programs (exercise training), particularly in advanced COPD. Unlike pain management, our resources to palliate severe dyspnea are at present quite limited when the underlying cause cannot be corrected.

WHEEZING AND STRIDOR

Wheezing and stridor are physical signs of airway narrowing. Wheezing is a continuous musical sound that originates from intrathoracic airways; stridor is a continuous but far harsher sound that emanates from the upper airways, usually the glottis or trachea. Snoring is similar to stridor in that it is a continuous inspiratory sound generated in the upper airways, specifically the oropharynx. The sound of snoring is distinctive and resolves with arousal of the patient from sleep, and so it is not readily confused with stridor.

Because diffuse wheezes are the hallmark of asthma, and

because asthma is a disease frequently encountered in the emergency department, one is apt to assume that a patient seen in the emergency department with wheezing has asthma. However, it is worth remembering the adage "all that wheezes is not asthma," and to remain alert to the possibility of alternative diagnoses in the wheezing patient. This critical thinking is particularly important in patients who lack a prior history of asthma or whose wheezing is in some way atypical for asthma, as will be discussed in this section.

PATHOPHYSIOLOGY

The flow of gas through the larynx and tracheobronchial tree is normally quiet. The rapid flow of gas through a narrowed portion of this system, however, sets up vibrations in the adjacent tissues that generate sounds much like the reed of a wind instrument. These conditions can be created in some normal persons at the end of a complete, forceful exhalation to residual volume. At these low lung volumes, airways are narrowed in the lung periphery and end-expiratory wheezes can be produced. In asthma, diffuse narrowing of intrathoracic airways is caused by a combination of tracheobronchial smooth-muscle constriction, bronchial wall thickening, and intraluminal secretions and debris. The resultant wheezing may be heard during some or all of expiration or throughout the entire respiratory cycle. Wheezes are characteristically heard in all lung fields, have a high-pitched and musical quality, and are variable from breath to breath. When recorded and subjected to frequency analysis, these wheezes are found to be made up of multiple tones that start and stop at variable points throughout the wheezing sound. Identical wheezing can be heard in COPD, particularly asthmatic bronchitis, and its presence in COPD has been shown to correlate with the likelihood of a bronchodilator response on pulmonary function testing.

Two other types of wheezing can be distinguished on analysis of recorded lung sounds as well as on careful auscultation. One pattern, expiratory polyphonic wheezing, is heard in some patients with emphysema; it is a diffuse, multitoned wheeze heard late in the expiratory phase and reproducible with each breath. The other pattern is fixed monophonic wheezing, heard in focal airway narrowing. Although the sound can be heard from all points of auscultation around the chest, its loudness is asymmetric, and one can usually perceive a localized zone from which it appears to emanate. Fixed monophonic wheezing is one reproducible tone; it starts and stops at the same point with each respiratory cycle. The more central the focal obstruction (especially tracheal lesions), the more likely is the sound to be mistaken for the wheezing of asthma, because of relatively uniform transmission of the sound to all lung fields. The differential diagnosis of fixed monophonic wheezing includes lesions within the tracheobronchial lumen, such as mucous plugs, neoplasms, and aspirated foreign bodies, and extrinsic compression of an airway by lymph nodes, neoplasms, or anomalous or aneurysmal blood vessels. It is clear that the finding of fixed monophonic wheezing has clinical implications that are very different from those derived from auscultation of the diffuse, multitoned wheezing of asthma.

Intrathoracic airways are subjected to pleural pressure swings as they occur throughout the respiratory cycle. For this reason wheezes are most easily elicited during exhalation, during which an increased pleural pressure is transmitted to the interstitial space surrounding the airways, contributing to their compression. By contrast, the glottis is an extrathoracic structure not under the influence of pleural pressure, and stridor is most commonly heard on inspiration, when intraluminal pressure at the glottis falls below the surrounding atmospheric pressure, leading to its narrowing. Stridor is audible to the unaided ear, and usually both patient and physician can readily identify its site of origin as the throat. Loudness of stridorous breathing is proportional to the rate of flow of gas across the narrowed upper-airway segment. Thus, stridor can be accentuated by having the patient hyperventilate slightly.

DIFFERENTIAL DIAGNOSIS

The differential diagnosis of wheezing is shown in Table 7-3, divided according to the focal or diffuse nature of the wheezes. A few specific points will be emphasized. First, the severity of airflow obstruction in an asthmatic attack cannot be reliably judged on the basis of the loudness or timing of wheezing. Some measure of airflow obstruction such as spirometry or peak expiratory flow determination is required for accurate assessment of severity. Second, in some patients with congestive heart failure, wheezing is the manifestation of their pulmonary edema ("cardiac asthma"). The mechanism of wheezing appears to be in part the accumulation of edema fluid in the perivascular interstitial space, with resulting bronchial compression. A component of bronchospasm may also play a role. It is unknown why only some patients with pulmonary edema exhibit this finding, although a predisposition to airway hyperreactivity may contribute. Wheezing has also been reported as a manifestation of pulmonary embolism, but it should be considered an uncommon physical finding in this disorder. Herpetic tracheobronchitis is a newly described entity among immunocompetent hosts. The few cases described to date involved middle-aged and elderly persons without prior history of obstructive lung disease who developed wheezing and severe airflow obstruction that was unresponsive to conventional bronchodilator therapy. Bronchoscopic examination of the airways in

Table 7-3. Differential diagnosis of wheezing

Focal wheezing
Mucous plugging
Aspirated foreign body
Endobronchial neoplasm
Extrinsic bronchial compression (e.g., by lymph nodes, vascular anomalies, or neoplasm)
Tracheobronchial amyloidosis
Diffuse wheezing
Asthma
COPD
Bronchiolitis
Congestive heart failure ("cardiac asthma")
Sarcoidosis
Pulmonary embolism
Herpetic tracheobronchitis

herpetic tracheobronchitis revealed severe inflammatory and necrotic changes, and viral cultures were positive for herpes simplex virus. Acyclovir provides effective therapy.

The differential diagnosis of stridor can be considered in terms of acute and chronic causes. The acute onset of stridor is usually due to foreign-body aspiration or infection. In adults, among whom croup is rare, the most common infectious cause of acute stridor is epiglottitis, with *Hemophilus influenzae* as the most common pathogen (see Chap. 9). Typical manifestations of epiglottitis include fever, sore throat, shortness of breath, painful swallowing, and drooling.

Rarely, vocal cord discoordination with adduction on inspiration or expiration, or both, causes stridorous breathing. If limited to expiration, the sound made by vocal cord dysfunction can be confused with asthma. This disorder is usually found in association with serious psychiatric disease and requires direct visualization of the vocal cords during respiration for diagnosis.

Stridor of subacute or chronic duration has a broader differential diagnosis that includes laryngeal cancer, vocal cord polyps, bilateral vocal cord paralysis, cricoarytenoiditis associated with rheumatoid arthritis, and rare laryngeal infections such as tuberculosis and leprosy. In the patient who has had prior intubation, especially if prolonged, vocal cord paralysis and laryngeal stricture are important diagnoses to be considered.

APPROACH TO THE PATIENT WITH WHEEZING OR STRIDOR

The approach to the patient with diffuse wheezing due to obstructive lung disease, such as asthma, COPD, bronchiectasis, or bronchiolitis, is outlined in detail in Chap 10. In the occasional patient in whom pulmonary edema mimics asthma because of the presence of diffuse wheezing, the correct diagnosis will usually be suspected on the basis of history (antecedent history of cardiac disease and congestive heart failure) and physical examination (possible inspiratory rales, jugular venous distention, and S_3 cardiac gallop). The correct diagnosis will be confirmed by chest x-ray findings consistent with congestive heart failure. Bronchodilators may be somewhat effective in alleviating wheezing in cardiac asthma, but optimal therapy consists of diuretics, inotropic agents, and possible afterload reduction (see Chaps. 11 and 21).

A chest radiograph should be obtained in any patient with focal wheezing. An example of an abnormal finding in such a setting is shown in Fig. 7-3. In this patient focal left anterior and retrosternal wheezing was due to tracheal compression by a thoracic aortic aneurysm. In some patients with focal wheezing, results of chest radiography will be inconclusive, and elective fiberoptic bronchoscopy should be scheduled for further evaluation. Treatment will vary depending on the cause of the tracheobronchial narrowing. Examples of potential therapeutic interventions include rigid bronchoscopy to extract a foreign body, radiation therapy and chemotherapy to shrink lymphomatous adenopathy, and surgery, radiation therapy, or laser bronchoscopy to treat a bronchogenic carcinoma.

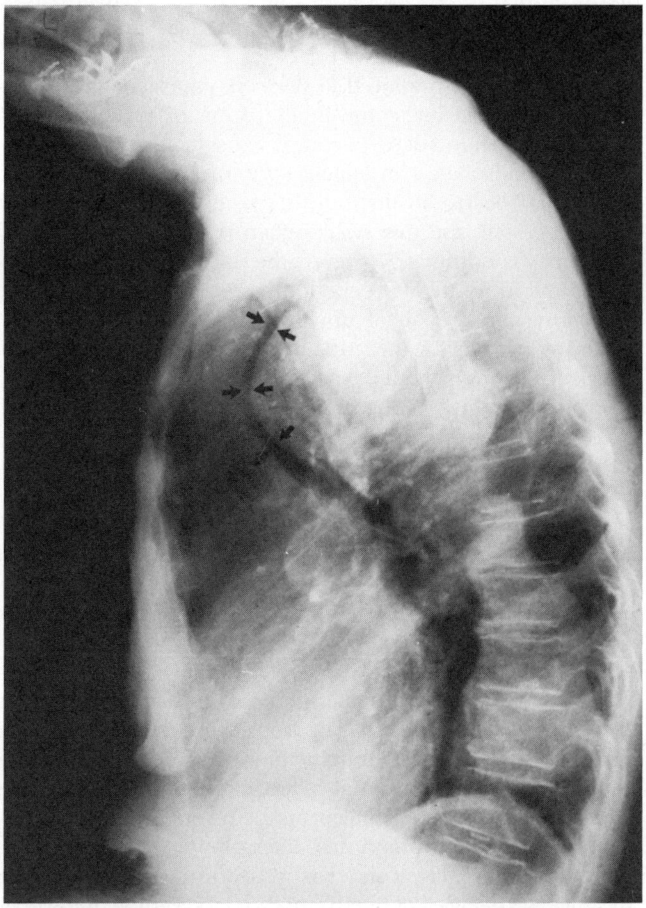

Fig. 7-3. Lateral chest radiograph of an elderly woman who came to an emergency department with wheezing. A large thoracic aortic aneurysm can be seen compressing the trachea, displacing it forward and narrowing its lumen.

Patients with the acute onset of stridor require close monitoring because they are at risk for the development of complete upper-airway obstruction. Initial assessment in most patients will include arterial blood gas determination, chest x-ray, and lateral soft-tissue x-ray views of the neck.

In pure upper-airway obstruction, ventilation-perfusion matching throughout the lungs is well maintained so that hypoxemia only develops when alveolar hypoventilation is present. Thus, the adequacy of gas exchange in a patient with upper-airway obstruction is determined primarily by the level of arterial PCO_2 An elevated PCO_2 generally calls for immediate intervention. A normal or low PCO_2 is not cause for reassurance, however, since complete or near-complete upper-airway occlusion can develop quite suddenly.

Lateral neck films are frequently helpful in defining the site of airway obstruction, in identifying the presence of a radiopaque foreign body, and, in patients with epiglottitis, revealing epiglottic swelling. Visual inspection of the upper airway by indirect or direct laryngoscopy often provides the greatest amount of information but poses some hazard because of the risk of inducing further edema in response to the trauma of the procedure. Thus, direct inspection of the airway should be undertaken only by an individual who is highly skilled in the procedure, and should be avoided altogether in patients with disorders such as angioneurotic edema or severe epiglottitis.

One should be prepared to perform emergency cricothyroidotomy or tracheostomy in the event of progression of upper-airway narrowing to complete occlusion. Some physicians have advocated an anticipatory tracheostomy in severe epiglottitis because of the morbidity and potential mortality associated with the procedure when it is performed under emergency conditions. However, the role of prophylactic tracheostomy in adults with epiglottitis remains controversial.

Airflow across a focal upper-airway narrowing can be increased by having the patient breathe a low-density gas mixture, such as oxygen, 20 percent, and helium, 80 percent. Occasionally, this approach proves useful as a temporizing measure while the underlying abnormality is being corrected.

CYANOSIS

Cyanosis is a bluish discoloration of the skin or mucous membranes, usually resulting from increased amounts of deoxygenated hemoglobin in the blood and occasionally due to the presence of abnormal blood pigments caused by the accumulation of abnormal forms of hemoglobin. Until recently, when rapid blood gas determinations became routinely available, cyanosis was relied on to indicate the presence and degree of hypoxemia and to regulate the use of supplemental oxygen. This physical finding remains an important potential sign of hypoxemia and a strong indication that the patient's arterial oxygen saturation should be determined.

PATHOPHYSIOLOGY

Under optimal conditions for observation, cyanosis can be detected by most observers when the concentration of deoxygenated hemoglobin in the capillary blood of superficial tissues such as the skin, mucous membranes, and nail beds equals or exceeds 5 gm/dl blood. Less often, cyanosis is caused by methemoglobinemia ($\geq$1.5 gm/dl blood) or sulfhemoglobinemia ($\geq$0.5 gm/dl blood); these conditions will be discussed separately. It should be noted that hemoglobin in *capillary* (C) blood, as it courses, for instance, through the subpapillary venous plexus of the dermis, will be less saturated with oxygen than *arterial* (A) blood, although more fully saturated than *venous* (V) blood. As a rough estimate of the oxygen saturation of capillary blood, one can calculate the average oxygen contents of the arterial and venous blood, as given by the equation $C = (A + V)/2$. In a person with a normal hemoglobin concentration and rate of tissue extraction of oxygen, capillary blood would be expected to contain 5 gm/dl deoxygenated hemoglobin when the arterial oxygen saturation is approximately 80 percent, corresponding to an arterial PO_2 of 45 mm Hg under normal conditions of oxygen-hemoglobin dissociation. Thus, under the conditions specified, cyanosis that is due to deoxygenated hemoglobin is a sign of quite marked hypoxemia. Conversely, clinically significant hypoxemia can exist in the absence of detectable cyanosis.

Besides the degree of oxygen saturation of blood as it leaves the lungs, the other important determinants of cyanosis due to deoxygenated hemoglobin are the hemoglobin concentration, the amount of oxygen consumption by the tissues, and the presence of right-to-left shunting of blood. For any given capillary blood oxygen saturation, more desaturated hemoglobin will be present at a higher hemoglobin concentration, less at a lower concentration. Thus, polycythemia, which commonly develops in the setting of chronic hypoxemia, causes cyanosis to be visible at a higher oxygen saturation, whereas anemia has the opposite effect. For instance, one would predict that cyanosis would become detectable in a patient with a hemoglobin concentration of 10 gm/dl and normal tissue oxygen extraction only when the arterial oxygen saturation fell to approximately 70 percent (arterial $PO_2 = 37$ mm Hg).

Even in the presence of a normal arterial oxygen saturation, the amount of deoxygenated hemoglobin in capillary blood will rise if oxygen consumption by tissue is increased. In the skin and mucous membranes, oxygen consumption increases under conditions of decreased perfusion or stasis of blood. A major impairment of cardiac output can cause diffuse cyanosis by this mechanism. Altered vasomotor function can impair venous drainage of the skin diffusely (e.g., in septic shock), in the hands and feet only (e.g., in Raynaud's phenomenon), or locally (e.g., in superior vena cava syndrome). A common example is the cyanosis that develops in an arm distal to a tourniquet or blood pressure cuff left in place too long.

The impact of increased tissue extraction of oxygen in causing cyanosis will be magnified in the presence of right-to-left shunting of blood. For instance, when cardiac output decreases, mixed venous oxygen falls. A right-to-left shunt will allow admixture of this desaturated venous blood into the arterial circulation, exacerbating arterial hypoxemia.

Other factors influence how readily one can detect in the dermal capillaries the presence of blood that contains deoxygenated hemoglobin. Skin pigmentation is important: In dark-skinned persons cyanosis is usually more readily detected in the oral mucous membranes, tongue, conjunctivae, and nail beds than in the skin. Other modifying factors are the thickness of the epidermis and the density of blood-filled capillaries in the skin. It is perhaps these latter influences, as well as regional differences in oxygen extraction, that account for the fact that even in cases of cyanosis due to arterial hypoxemia, bluish discoloration of the skin is not uniform and is often best revealed in the fingers and toes, tip of the nose, and lobes of the ears.

Cyanosis due to deoxygenated hemoglobin in the blood can be categorized into *central* and *peripheral* types. Central cyanosis refers to cyanosis due to hemoglobin desaturation of the arterial blood of any cause; peripheral cyanosis is used to describe cyanosis that results from increased tissue oxygen consumption (and therefore develops "in the periphery"). These two terms are not meant to distinguish the site at which the cyanosis is detected, and often these types of cyanosis are indistinguishable except by determination of arterial oxygen content. Rarely, cyanosis that results from certain forms of congenital heart disease may involve the upper or lower half of the body to a greater extent ("differential cyanosis"), as may occur in patent ductus arteriosus with transposition of the great vessels or patent ductus and preductal coarctation of the aorta, respectively.

Methemoglobinemia and Sulfhemoglobinemia

Hemoglobin that contains iron in an oxidized (ferric) state is called *methemoglobin.* Normally, in the adult only approximately 1 percent of hemoglobin exists as methemoglobin, in which form it is incapable of transporting oxygen. The remaining 99 percent of hemoglobin is maintained in the ferrous state by reducing agents within the erythrocyte. When present in excess of approximately 1.5 gm/dl blood (equivalent to approximately 10% methemoglobinemia in a person without anemia), methemoglobin confers a chocolate-brown discoloration to the blood that is detectable in the skin.

Methemoglobinemia is occasionally congenital in origin. A number of different single amino acid substitutions in the alpha or beta hemoglobin chains can create an abnormal hemoglobin, hemoglobin M, in which iron is fixed in the ferric state. Persons heterozygous for hemoglobin M have concentrations of methemoglobin no greater than approximately 25 percent; homozygosity for hemoglobin M is fatal. Another cause of congenital methemoglobinemia is an inherited deficiency of an enzyme, nicotinamide adenine dinucleotide (NADH)-dependent methemoglobin reductase, which is important in reducing iron within the heme moiety to its normal ferrous state. Persons homozygous for this reductase deficiency have methemoglobin concentrations of 10 to 50 percent.

More often, methemoglobinemia is acquired on exposure to certain chemical compounds that oxidize hemoglobin either directly or indirectly through metabolites. Medications most often implicated in causing acquired methemoglobinemia are nitrates (converted to nitrites in the intestines), sulfonamides, and lidocaine or benzocaine. In industrial exposures, cyanosis due to methemoglobinemia can be caused by ingestion, inhalation, or even absorption through the skin of aniline and related compounds, used in the manufacture of dyestuffs, plastics, pesticides, and pharmaceuticals. In the home aniline and its derivatives can be found in paints, varnishes, inks, and shoe polishes.

Many of these same amino and nitro compounds can also cause sulfhemoglobinemia, in which as little as 0.5 gm/dl blood of the abnormal hemoglobin can cause cyanosis. In one series of cases, phenacetin and acetanilid were the drugs that were implicated most often. Once formed, sulfhemoglobin, which cannot transport oxygen, persists in that form for the life of the red blood cell; it cannot be converted back to normal hemoglobin.

DIFFERENTIAL DIAGNOSIS

The broad differential diagnosis of cyanosis can be simplified into three major categories based on the mechanisms discussed previously, as outlined in Fig. 7-4. Cyanosis due to hypoxemia can be the result of any respiratory, cardiac, or central nervous system disorder that produces low arterial oxygen tensions. Respiratory conditions span the gamut, including parenchymal abnormalities (e.g., pneumonia), airway disorders (e.g., upper-airway obstruction, asthma), pulmonary vascular diseases (e.g., pulmonary embolism), chest wall abnormalities (e.g., flail chest or kyphoscoliosis), and neuromuscular disorders (e.g., amyotrophic lateral sclerosis). Except in cases of diffuse parenchymal lung disease, in which right-to-left shunting of blood through unaerated portions of the lungs occurs, cyanosis due to these respiratory conditions would be expected to resolve rapidly with the supplemental administration of oxygen. In contrast, cyanosis due to congenital heart disease with intracardiac right-to-left shunting is usually refractory to supplemental oxygen, since the portion of blood that is shunted through the heart does not come in contact with alveolar gas, while the portion of blood that passes through the lungs is nearly fully saturated with oxygen even in the absence of oxygen enrichment (if the lungs are normal). Acquired right-to-left intracardiac shunts are uncommon, but can occur in the setting of pulmonary arterial hypertension and, rarely, right ventricular infarction. Far more commonly, heart disease causes cyanosis on the basis of pulmonary edema. Central nervous system disorders can be a cause of cyanosis due to profound hypoventilation; a common example is stupor or coma after a narcotic or sedative drug overdose.

Cyanosis in the absence of hypoxemia belongs to one of two categories. It can result from the presence of abnormal hemoglobins in the blood or from decreased flow or stasis of blood in the peripheral circulation. Congenital abnormalities of hemoglobin include hemoglobin M (causing methemoglobinemia) and hemoglobins with low oxygen affinity, such as Hb_{Kansas}, which are associated with oxygen desaturation of hemoglobin even at normal arterial oxygen tensions. The acquired hemoglobinopathies that cause cyanosis are methemoglobinemia and sulfhemoglobinemia, as was discussed previously.

Stasis of blood with increased extraction of oxygen in the capillaries can occur on a "global" basis as a result of impaired cardiac output (e.g., myocardial infarction), profound hypotension (e.g., sepsis), or increased blood viscosity (e.g., polycythemia). Stasis with cyanosis can occur exclusively in exposed surfaces such as the extremities and parts of the face (acrocyanosis). The differential diagnosis includes vasospastic disorders such as Raynaud's phenomenon, circulating cold-agglutinating antibodies (as can form in infectious mononucleosis), and use of vasoactive drugs (e.g., dopamine). Localized cyanosis due to stasis usually results from fixed venous obstruction, such as in superior vena cava syndrome or subclavian steal syndrome. Rarely, cyanotic spells can occur from the episodic release of vasoactive substances into the circulation, as has been described in carcinoid tumors.

APPROACH TO THE PATIENT WITH CYANOSIS

As suggested by the flow diagram in Fig. 7-4, the crucial first step in the management of a cyanotic patient is arterial blood gas determination. When cyanosis is due to hypoxemia, treatment is focused on correction of this abnormality with supplemental oxygen and, in some cases of hypoventilation, with mechanically assisted ventilation. Patients with large

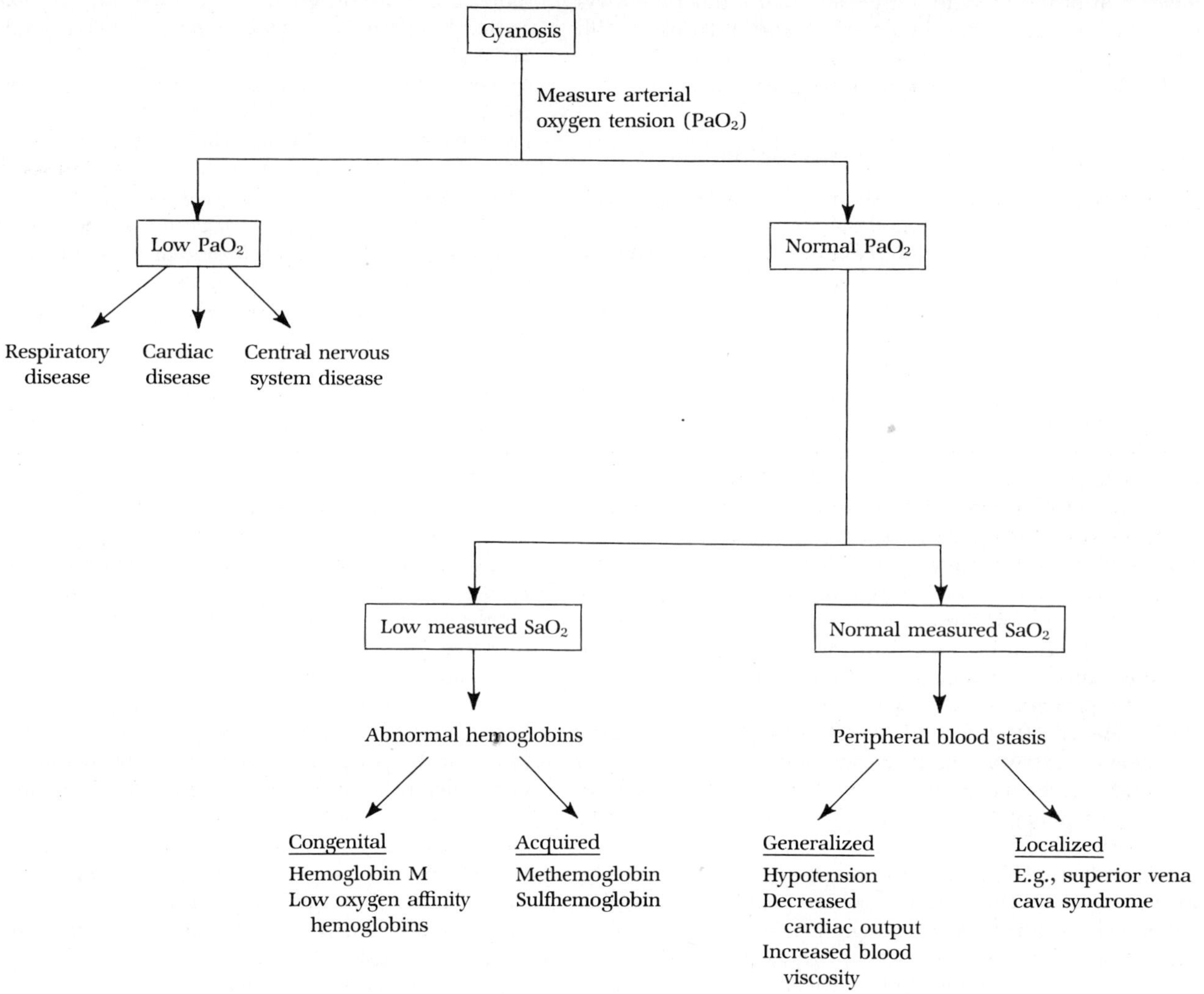

Fig. 7-4. Flow-diagram for the evaluation of the cyanotic patient.

intrapulmonary shunts resulting from diffuse parenchymal lung disease (e.g., pulmonary edema) may not correct their hypoxemia with supplemental oxygen alone; positive airway pressure during expiration may be required to decrease the amount of venous admixture.

In the patient who is cyanotic but not hypoxemic, it is important to measure the arterial oxygen saturation (SaO_2). As part of arterial blood gas analysis, some laboratories report a calculated SaO_2 based on the arterial oxygen tension (PO_2) and assume normal oxygen-hemoglobin association properties. The calculated SaO_2 is overestimated in the presence of some abnormal forms of hemoglobin, such as methemoglobin and sulfhemoglobin. On the other hand, a measured SaO_2 will be found to be inappropriately low for the arterial oxygen tension, alerting one to the possibility of methemoglobinemia, sulfhemoglobinemia, and, rarely, abnormal low-affinity hemoglobins. The presence of methemoglobinemia and sulfhemoglobinemia can then be confirmed and quantitated by spectroscopic techniques in most blood gas laboratories. An alternative clue to the presence of these abnormal forms of hemoglobin is the failure of venous blood to turn pink rapidly when oxygen is bubbled through it. Two other bedside tests can be applied in the diagnosis of methemoglobinemia and sulfhemoglobinemia. In one, a drop of blood allowed to dry on filter paper will leave a brown spot and can be contrasted with the red color of normal blood. In the other, the addition of potassium cyanide solution to blood containing methemoglobin causes the blood to turn pink immediately as a result of the formation of cyanomethemoglobin.

Most patients with less than 20 percent methemoglobinemia will have few if any symptoms, and treatment is indicated only for cosmetic reasons. In concentrations greater than 20 to 30 percent, symptoms due to decreased tissue oxygenation, including headache, weakness, lightheadedness, and chest discomfort, begin to develop. At very high concentrations, cardiovascular collapse occurs, with death at concentrations in the range of 70 to 80 percent. Severe cases of methemoglobinemia can be treated with methylene blue, which serves as a cofactor to accelerate the activity of a methemoglobin reductase. The usual dose is 1 to 2 mg/kg of a 1% solution administered intravenously over 5 minutes; this dose may be repeated after one hour if cyanosis and signs of tissue hypoxia have not resolved. Excess amounts of methylene blue can have a number of adverse effects, including, paradoxically, direct oxidation of hemoglobin to methemoglobin and bluish discoloration of the skin. Rarely, in severe or refractory cases, blood transfusions or exchange transfusions are needed. In milder cases of methemoglobinemia, as in sulfhemoglobinemia, it is probably sufficient simply to withdraw the offending toxin, if one can be identified.

Finally, patients with cyanosis and normal arterial oxygen saturation have cyanosis caused by increased oxygen extraction (so-called peripheral cyanosis). When due to hypoperfusion, cold-precipitating or agglutinating antibodies, or vasospastic phenomena, cyanosis is usually accompanied by cold, clammy, often mottled skin. Therapy is directed at raising the blood pressure or warming the affected body parts. Localized cyanosis should prompt a search for focal venous obstruction.

SHARP CHEST PAIN

Because chest pain of acute onset can be a symptom of several very serious diseases—including such varied conditions as myocardial infarction, pulmonary embolism, pneumothorax, and aortic dissection—the prompt and systematic evaluation of this symptom in the emergency department is mandatory. Most often, in patients with acute chest pain one is called on to establish or exclude the diagnosis of myocardial infarction or unstable angina. In this section we focus specifically on *sharp* chest pain. Most patients with myocardial infarction describe the quality of their chest pain as "pressure," "aching," or "burning/indigestion." (For a detailed discussion of myocardial ischemia and myocardial infarction, see Chaps. 18 and 19.) It should be noted, however, that the descriptions "sharp" or "stabbing" do not exclude a diagnosis of myocardial infarction. In one series, 8 of 104 patients with acute myocardial infarction described their chest pain in these terms. In this same study, the combination of three clinical features—a sharp or stabbing chest pain, the absence of prior angina or myocardial infarction, and pain that could be reproduced with chest wall palpation or had a pleuritic or positional component to it—reliably excluded myocardial ischemia. In all other circumstances, however, an electrocardiogram was indicated to evaluate further the potential myocardial cause of the chest pain.

PATHOPHYSIOLOGY

Defining the quality of chest pain, its location, its onset and duration, and the stimuli that exacerbate or alleviate it is fundamental to formulating a differential diagnosis. In most instances, however, this information is useful not because of a detailed understanding of pathophysiologic mechanisms for pain sensation, but because of accumulated experience based on clinical observation. Unfortunately, patients' reporting of their perception of chest (and other) pain is highly variable; differences in use of language and in pain threshold, as well as differences in the actual disease process, account for much of this variability. In addition, whereas pain originating in skin is usually discrete and well localized, pain sensation that derives from internal organs is often more difficult to localize and characterize. Thus, any generalizations about different types of chest pain and the diseases that cause them are certain to have major variations and exceptions associated with them.

Sharp chest pain can originate from chest wall structures, parietal pleural and pericardial membranes, mediastinal structures, and upper-abdominal organs. The lungs and visceral pleura are anesthetic; thus, pneumonias and lung cancers cause no chest pain until they extend to the parietal pleura. As a general rule, pain that emanates from viscera deep to the skin is perceived as coming from those dermatomes that send afferent nerves to spinal roots that also innervate the involved viscera. This concept of referred pain is well illustrated by pain of pleural origin. Costal portions of the parietal pleura are innervated by intercostal nerves that enter the spinal cord in thoracic dorsal nerve roots, the same nerve roots that supply the overlying skin. Thus, a patient who perceives a pain of pleural origin in an area of the lateral chest wall usually correctly identifies the underlying zone of pleural inflammation or stretching. On the other hand, sensory nerve fibers from the central portion of the diaphragmatic pleura are carried via the phrenic nerve and enter the spinal cord at the C3–C5 dorsal roots, nerve roots that also receive sensory input from skin overlying the neck and upper part of the shoulder. Thus, disease involving the central diaphragmatic pleura causes neck and shoulder pain. By the same mechanism, pain sensation that originates from the peripheral aspects of the diaphragmatic pleura (T7–T12 nerve roots) may be perceived in the lower thorax, upper-abdominal, or lumbar areas.

Pain of pleural origin characteristically worsens on deep inspiration. When severe, this aspect of the pain can restrict comfortable breathing and result in a sensation of dyspnea; when mild, it can only be elicited at maximal inhalation. Although chest pain that worsens with deep inspiration is referred to as pleuritic, it should be remembered that chest wall and pericardial pain can also be exacerbated on inspiration, and that pleural pain can sometimes be a steady, aching pain unrelated to the respiratory cycle. In one series of young (<40 years old) patients seen in an emergency department for pleuritic chest pain, 89 of 97 patients (92%) were diagnosed as having one of three causes of pleural irritation: viral or idiopathic pleurisy, pulmonary embolism, or infectious pneumonia. However, the diversity of other causes of pleuritic pain was striking even in this limited series of young patients. These diagnoses were sickle cell crisis, tuberculous pleurisy, pancreatitis, ruptured aortic aneurysm, fractured rib, and bronchial asthma.

Pain that is easily elicited by movement or palpation of the thoracic cage usually originates in the skin or musculoskeletal structures of the chest wall. An example that is usually obvious diagnostically is chest wall trauma, with patients sustaining direct injury to one or more of the following: skin, muscles, ribs, sternum, or vertebrae. Light palpation over the area of injury typically reproduces or intensifies the pain. Pain of pleural origin can also be made worse if forceful compression of the chest with deformation of its contours is employed by the examiner; a diagnosis of pulmonary embolism, for instance, should not be excluded if forceful palpation causes the chest pain to worsen somewhat. Chest pain that radiates circumferentially from the back around anteriorly and is aggravated by percussion of the vertebrae is likely to be nerve root or "radicular" pain, such as is caused by a vertebral compression fracture or displacement of an intervertebral disk.

The perception of noxious stimuli that originate in mediastinal structures is described in terms of a variety of pain sensations. Besides the squeezing, heavy discomfort of myocardial ischemia, patients may speak of a burning retrosternal discomfort, often described with an accompanying vertical movement of the hand in esophageal reflux, a raw anterior chest discomfort in acute tracheobronchitis with repetitive coughing, a sharp, searing pain radiating to the back or abdomen in aortic dissection, and a sometimes sharp, sometimes squeezing retrosternal chest discomfort that improves on bending forward in pericarditis. These are, however, classic descriptions and consideration of these diagnoses should not depend on the patient's ability to call forth these particular adjectives. Disorders of the heart, esophagus, trachea, great vessels, and pericardium should be considered simply because of the retrosternal location of the pain.

Finally, patients may experience chest pains that are neither angina-like nor pleuritic; these pains often localize to one side of the chest or the other and may vary in location over time. If occasional and fleeting, such pains are often part of the normal life experience; if repetitive and prolonged, they are referred to as "atypical" chest pains and can be a symptom of serious disease. Mitral valve prolapse and sarcoidosis are two examples of diseases that, when associated with chest pains, characteristically cause atypical chest pains. The pathophysiologic mechanisms involved in the pain are completely unknown.

Table 7-4. Differential diagnosis of sharp chest pain

Musculoskeletal chest pain
Chest wall trauma/strain
Vertebral compression fracture
Costochondritis (Tietze's syndrome)
Herpes zoster infection (shingles)
Chest wall infection (e.g., actinomycosis)
Chest wall neoplasm
Pleuritic chest pain
Pneumonia
Viral or idiopathic pleurisy
Pulmonary embolism
Pneumothorax
Pleural neoplasm
Sickle cell crisis
Pericarditis
Rib fracture
Retrosternal chest pain
Myocardial infarction
Pericarditis
Esophagitis
Esophageal rupture
Dissecting thoracic aortic aneurysm
Tracheitis
Subdiaphragmatic causes of chest pain
Gastritis
Cholecystitis
Pancreatitis
Hepatic or splenic abscess
Atypical chest pains
Mitral valve prolapse
Sarcoidosis
"Fibromyalgia"

DIFFERENTIAL DIAGNOSIS

The differential diagnosis of sharp chest pain is given in Table 7-4, presented under the categories of musculoskeletal pain, pleuritic chest pain, retrosternal chest pain, subdiaphragmatic causes of chest pain, and atypical chest pains. It is recognized that these categories are not mutually exclusive. Thus, pericarditis can cause a chest pain that is pleuritic in quality and retrosternal in location, and the pain of a rib fracture typically intensifies with deep inspiration. Most often, however, history and physical examination allow one to assign a patient with chest pain to at least one of these categories, which then can be useful in formulating a differential diagnosis. The first three of these categories are discussed here in greater detail.

Musculoskeletal Chest Pain

Localized traumatic injury to the chest wall is a common example of musculoskeletal chest pain. Blunt or penetrating trauma is usually an obvious cause for chest wall lacerations, contusions, or rib fractures. However, other, more subtle activities, such as violent coughing or vomiting, heavy lifting, or sudden twisting movements can also cause fractures or costochondral subluxation, even in patients without underlying osteoporosis. The chest pain can usually be localized by the patient to a discrete area that is exquisitely tender to palpation. Often the pain is made worse by movement of the thorax, including the displacement of the rib cage that results from a deep inhalation. Chest radiography is usually not helpful in establishing this diagnosis unless an actual fracture has occurred.

An acute perichondritis involving the sternal costochondral juncture (Tietze's syndrome) causes a sharp, often pleuritic chest pain in the parasternal area, sometimes associated with localized costosternal swelling. Light pressure applied to the area reproduces the pain. Plain films of the area are typically normal; the diagnosis can usually be made on clinical grounds alone.

Primary chest wall infections (e.g., actinomycosis) and neoplasia (e.g., chondrosarcoma) are fortunately rare. They may be suggested by pain associated with localized swelling and sometimes erythema and warmth of the chest wall.

Dermatomal distribution of chest pain suggests origin of the pain in a nerve root, typically in association with vertebral or intervertebral disk disease, or both. In this case, tenderness to palpation or light percussion may be appreciated not over the lateral or anterior chest wall but over the spine. Occasionally, the chest pain of recurrent herpes zoster infection (shingles) antedates the appearance of the typical vesicular skin rash by a day or two, posing a diagnostic dilemma until the rash appears.

Pleuritic Chest Pain

Any pneumonia that extends to the pleural surface is likely to cause pleuritic chest pain. In air space pneumonias, which begin in the lung periphery and spread centrifugally, pleuritic chest pain characteristically develops early in the course. For instance, pleuritic chest pain is not infrequently a presenting symptom of pneumococcal pneumonia. In this circumstance, pleural effusion may or may not be present, and if present, it may be infected (empyema) or sterile (parapneumonic effusion).

Acute inflammation of the pleural space in the absence of an underlying pneumonia is usually referred to as pleurisy. Often the cause remains unproved and a viral infection is presumed. Patients with acute viral (or idiopathic) pleurisy tend to experience the abrupt onset of pleuritic chest pain, sometimes associated with low-grade fever, headache, and myalgia. The white blood cell count is usually normal; in a minority of patients, mild leukocytosis is present. In one series, a small pleural effusion was found in 12 percent of patients with viral pleurisy. The illness is self-limited and can be treated symptomatically with nonsteroidal antiinflammatory drugs. However, the diagnosis is one of exclusion and, most important, pulmonary embolism must not be overlooked. Other causes of pleural (and pericardial) inflammation include collagen-vascular diseases, particularly systemic lupus erythematosus and rheumatoid arthritis; uremia; and postpericardiotomy syndrome (Dressler's syndrome).

The possibility of pulmonary embolism must at least be considered in any patient with the sudden onset of pleuritic chest pain in the absence of pneumonia. The nonspecific symptoms of dyspnea, cough, chest pain, and apprehension are the most common complaints in pulmonary embolism; hemoptysis occurs in only approximately one-third of patients. A low-grade fever and mild leukocytosis may be found, mimicking an acute infection. Results of chest radiography are most often normal or nonspecific; abnormal findings most frequently encountered include pleural effusion, atelectasis, and pleural-based infiltrate. The wedge-shaped, pleural-based opacity referred to as Hampton's hump, though characteristic, is a rare finding. The results of arterial blood gas analysis can neither establish nor exclude a diagnosis of pulmonary embolism; hypoxemia is common but nonspecific and an arterial $PO_2 > 80$ mm Hg can be found in as many as 10 percent of patients. An electrocardiogram that shows evidence of P pulmonale or right heart strain in the absence of prior cardiopulmonary disease suggests pulmonary embolism but is an infrequent finding, usually restricted to patients with massive embolism.

Because of the nonspecific nature of these routine tests, when the diagnosis of pulmonary embolism is seriously considered, radionuclide lung scanning is usually needed for further diagnostic evaluation. This test is particularly appropriate when the history reveals a predisposing factor for venous thrombosis (e.g., oral contraceptive use, postpartum period, obesity, recent surgery or leg immobility, or strong family history), when there is a prior history of deep venous thrombosis or pulmonary embolism, when the physical examination reveals signs of phlebitis in a lower extremity, or when acute chest pain is accompanied by otherwise unexplained hypoxemia, electrocardiographic evidence of right heart strain, or pleural effusion or atelectasis on chest radiography. A normal perfusion lung scan excludes the diagnosis of recent pulmonary embolism. The presence of segmental or lobar perfusion defects with corresponding normal ventilation on ventilation scanning virtually establishes the diagnosis in a clinically high-risk patient. A detailed discussion of pulmonary embolic disease appears in Chap. 13.

Acute pleuritic chest pain poses a common and often difficult diagnostic problem in patients with sickle cell anemia. Adult patients tend to be functionally asplenic and at increased risk for pneumonia, which may have a pleuritic involvement; at the same time, sickle crises are commonly manifested with pleuritic chest pain, thought due to in situ microvascular thromboses in the pulmonary arterial circulation. The distinction is often difficult to make clinically and patients frequently are treated for both possibilities.

Another important cause of pleuritic chest pain is pneumothorax. Some patients with pneumothorax experience a sudden onset of excruciating chest pain and associated shortness of breath; others have a less dramatic inception of pain that may then wax and wane over hours or even days before intensifying sufficiently to prompt an emergency department visit. It is common for this chest pain to be felt in the upper chest, anteriorly or posteriorly, and sometimes in the shoulder. The diagnosis is supported by the finding on physical examination of unilateral chest hyperexpansion with ipsilateral hyperresonance but distant or absent breath sounds; tracheal deviation to the contralateral side is found in tension pneumothorax. Chest radiography usually suffices to establish or exclude the diagnosis. Further discussion of pneumothorax can be found in Chap. 12.

Finally, neoplasia of the pleura, whether primary (i.e., mesothelioma) or metastatic, generally causes a steady, aching chest pain that intensifies on deep inspiration. Work-up is usually directed at further evaluating the pleural effusion or lobulated pleural thickening found on chest radiography.

Retrosternal Chest Pain

Sharp retrosternal chest pain can be caused by diseases of the esophagus, pericardium, aorta, or trachea. Reflux esophagitis is particularly common. One can often elicit a history of pain ascending from epigastrium to xiphoid, brought on by eating large meals or by assuming a recumbent position. A barium swallow may confirm the diagnosis, but this is not a sensitive test for acid reflux. Sometimes more extensive diagnostic procedures may be necessary, such as esophagoscopy, the Bernstein test (application of dilute hydrochloric acid to the distal esophagus), or continuous monitoring of pH with a probe positioned in the distal esophagus. Often, however, in the emergency department setting a therapeutic trial of antacids is used; prompt relief of the chest pain supports a diagnosis of acid-peptic disease. Esophageal rupture, such as can occur after severe vomiting (Boerhaave syndrome), gastrointestinal endoscopic procedures, or trauma, provokes a severe retrosternal pain. Mediastinal widening and pleural effusion are frequent radiographic findings. Leakage of swallowed radiocontrast material outside of the esophagus establishes the diagnosis of esophageal rupture; a small amount of barium sulfate is the radiographic agent of choice. Also, characteristic findings on pleural fluid analysis are an acidic pH and an elevated concentration of amylase of the salivary isoenzyme.

The chest pain of acute pericarditis can be very severe,

have a pleuritic component, and radiate to the neck and arms. Other patients experience a more steady chest heaviness that can be mistaken for myocardial infarction. Detection of a pericardial friction rub on auscultation virtually clinches the diagnosis. The electrocardiogram may show diagnostic diffuse ST-segment elevations or may have only nonspecific ST-segment and T-wave abnormalities. Normal results on echocardiography do not exclude the diagnosis of pericarditis.

Thoracic aortic dissection commonly results in a severe anterior chest pain that rapidly reaches peak intensity. Pain can extend to the back, lumbar area, or abdomen. A disparity in the blood pressure between the arms or other signs of arterial occlusion should bring this diagnosis to mind. The chest radiograph is a good initial screening test; it often reveals widening of the mediastinum due to increased aortic diameter. However, a normal chest radiograph does not exclude the diagnosis of acute aortic dissection. Confirmatory tests include computed tomography with intravenous contrast, magnetic resonance imaging, or angiography.

Patients with acute tracheobronchitis may describe a chest discomfort that is aggravated by repetitive coughing. The discomfort is often described as a raw or harsh sensation, but it is generally not severe. The diagnosis must be made on the basis of clinical findings and the response to treatment since no specific laboratory test can be applied.

APPROACH TO THE PATIENT WITH SHARP CHEST PAIN

Because sharp chest pain, particularly if sustained and severe, can be a symptom of life-threatening disease, a thorough and expeditious evaluation is necessary. If profound hypotension or hypertension accompanies the chest pain, initial management needs to be directed at hemodynamic stabilization. At the same time, the major, potentially fatal, nontraumatic illnesses that must be considered immediately are myocardial infarction (with an atypical presentation of *sharp* chest pain), tension pneumothorax, pulmonary embolism, and aortic dissection (Fig. 7-5).

History and physical examination alone may strongly suggest one of these diagnoses. In most cases, an electrocardiogram and chest radiograph are also indicated. Normal results on electrocardiography in a patient with sharp chest pain virtually exclude myocardial infarction; likewise, a normal chest x-ray rules out pneumothorax. A normal electrocardiogram and chest x-ray cannot, however, exclude the possibility of pulmonary embolism, so that if clinical suspicion of this diagnosis is high, additional studies are needed. Perfusion and ventilation lung scans are usually the procedures of choice to evaluate further for pulmonary embolism; in some circumstances venous ultrasonography or other noninvasive tests for deep venous thrombosis in the lower extremities may prove useful adjuncts to testing (see Chap. 13). Emergency department management of the patient found to have a myocardial infarction, tension pneumothorax, pulmonary embolism, or aortic dissection is dealt with in other sections of this text (see Chaps. 19, 12, 13, and 51, respectively). The treatments for these diseases differ radically, and the use of analgesics alone would be inappropriate management.

In patients with a normal chest radiograph and electrocardiogram, a number of diagnostic possibilities besides pulmonary embolism persist. If the physical examination reveals upper-abdominal tenderness to palpation, gastrointestinal diseases such as pancreatitis or cholecystitis need to be considered. Blood analysis (e.g., serum amylase and lipase) or imaging studies (e.g., abdominal ultrasound) can help to establish these diagnoses. On the other hand, if heartburn, belching, or symptoms of regurgitation suggest esophageal reflux, a therapeutic trial of antacids may provide the most useful and immediate information. One generally must rely on history and physical examination alone to diagnose musculoskeletal causes of chest pain (other than rib fracture) or viral/idiopathic pleurisy. Other differential diagnostic possibilities are identified in Fig. 7-5.

Symptomatic treatment of sharp chest pain that is not considered to be gastrointestinal in origin primarily relies on nonsteroidal antiinflammatory drugs and analgesics. Thus, for idiopathic or viral pleurisy, nonsteroidal antiinflammatory drugs such as ibuprofen or indomethacin are commonly prescribed; aspirin is often used to treat idiopathic or viral pericarditis. Similar treatment is appropriate for acute costochondritis (Tietze's syndrome). Because these are self-limited illnesses, patients should be informed that persistence of pain beyond approximately two weeks should lead to further evaluation of its cause.

Chest wall injury such as a rib fracture often requires more potent analgesia with narcotic drugs such as codeine or related compounds (e.g., oxycodone or hydrocodone). Because these drugs also act to suppress cough, they help to minimize this aggravating stimulus for chest wall pain, but they must be used with caution in patients with mucous hypersecretion (e.g., chronic bronchitis) or chronic hypercapnia. Immobilization of the chest wall such as with circumferential bandages is not recommended because of the potential predisposition to atelectasis with hypoxemia and the risk of superinfection.

In patients with chronic underlying respiratory conditions and borderline ventilatory reserve, acute chest pain can trigger respiratory failure if it restricts comfortable inhalation or effective cough. In such patients, arterial blood gases need to be measured and hospitalization is often warranted so that analgesia can be titrated to pain relief without depression of respiratory drive. In this circumstance localized chest wall pain can often best be managed by local injections of anesthetic agents or by appropriate intercostal nerve blocks (see Chap. 44).

COUGH

Cough is a powerful protective mechanism for removal of material from the tracheobronchial tree. Under normal con-

Fig. 7-5. Flow-diagram for the evaluation of the patient with acute sharp chest pain. The top row suggests an initial evaluation for four common and potentially life-threatening causes of acute sharp chest pain; the bottom row lists potential causes of sharp chest pain according to the type of pain.

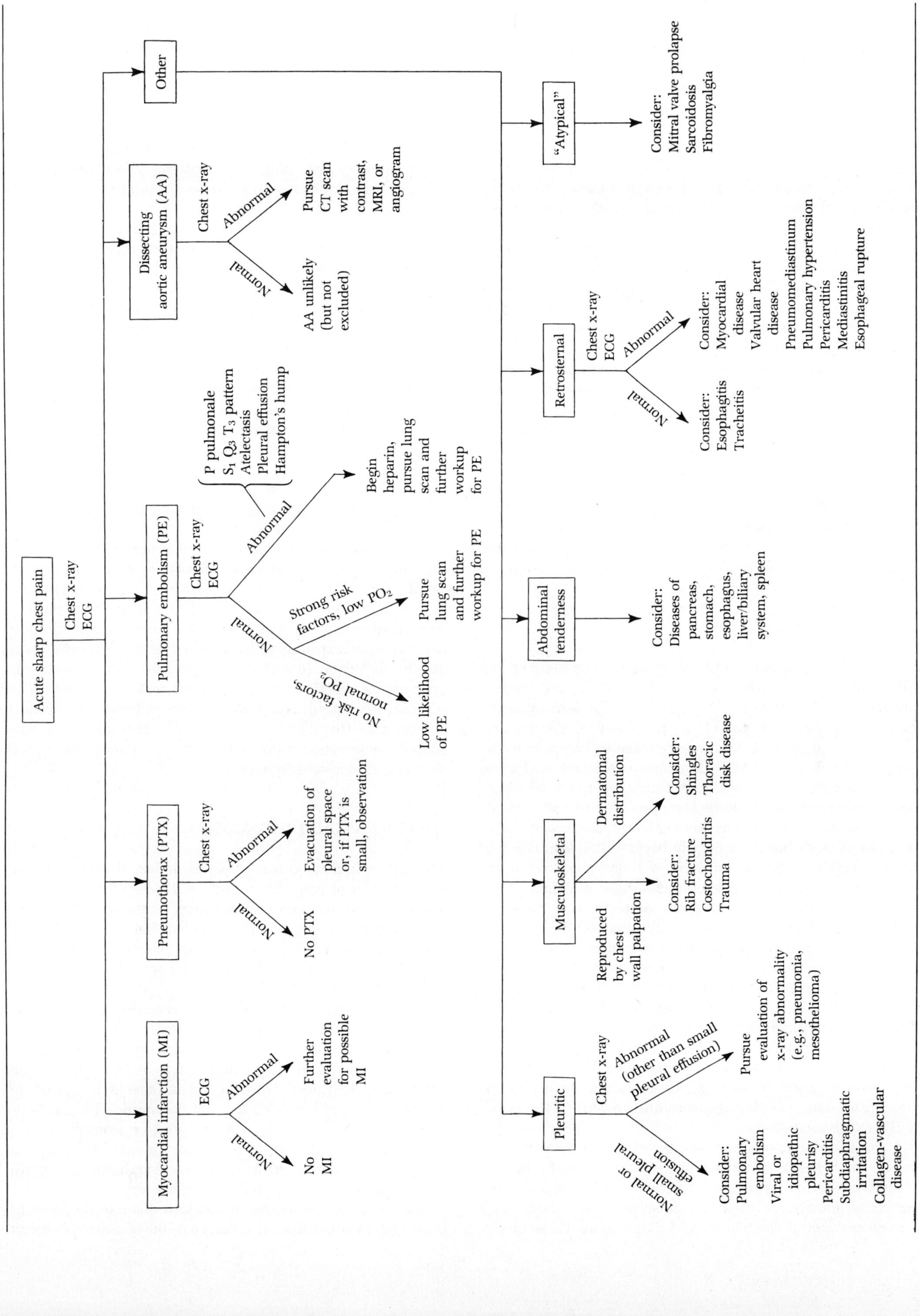

Acute sharp chest pain
Chest x-ray
ECG
Myocardial infarction (MI)
ECG
Normal
Abnormal
No MI
Further evaluation for possible MI
Pneumothorax (PTX)
Chest x-ray
Normal
Abnormal
No PTX
Evacuation of pleural space or, if PTX is small, observation
Pulmonary embolism (PE)
Chest x-ray
ECG
Normal
Abnormal
No risk factors, normal PO2
Strong risk factors, low PO2
Low likelihood of PE
Pursue lung scan and further workup for PE
P pulmonale
S1 Q3 T3 pattern
Atelectasis
Pleural effusion
Hampton's hump
Begin heparin, pursue lung scan and further workup for PE
Dissecting aortic aneurysm (AA)
Chest x-ray
Normal
Abnormal
AA unlikely (but not excluded)
Pursue CT scan with contrast, MRI, or angiogram
Other
Pleuritic
Chest x-ray
Normal or small pleural effusion
Abnormal (other than small pleural effusion)
Consider: Pulmonary embolism Viral or idiopathic pleurisy Pericarditis Subdiaphragmatic irritation Collagen-vascular disease
Pursue evaluation of x-ray abnormality (e.g., pneumonia, mesothelioma)
Musculoskeletal
Reproduced by chest wall palpation
Dermatomal distribution
Consider: Rib fracture Costochondritis Trauma
Consider: Shingles Thoracic disk disease
Abdominal tenderness
Consider: Diseases of pancreas, stomach, esophagus, liver/biliary system, spleen
Retrosternal
Chest x-ray
ECG
Normal
Abnormal
Consider: Esophagitis Tracheitis
Consider: Myocardial disease Valvular heart disease Pneumomediastinum Pulmonary hypertension Pericarditis Mediastinitis Esophageal rupture
"Atypical"
Consider: Mitral valve prolapse Sarcoidosis Fibromyalgia

ditions, mucus secreted by tracheobronchial mucous glands onto the luminal surfaces of airways is swept mouthward by synchronized beating of the cilia that protrude from the surface of the epithelial lining cells; the airways are protected from foreign material by the protective actions of the epiglottis and larynx. However, airway secretions in excessive amounts or of abnormal viscoelastic properties cannot be effectively cleared by this "mucociliary escalator" alone. Were it not for a forceful cough mechanism, airway lumina would become narrowed or occluded by these accumulating secretions, resulting in airflow obstruction, atelectasis, increased work of breathing, and abnormal gas exchange. These are the potential consequences, for example, of a simple tracheobronchitis in a patient with impaired cough due to respiratory muscle weakness, such as in muscular dystrophy. Likewise, cough is essential in defending the respiratory system from aspirated particulate matter after failure of the upper-airway defenses.

At other times, cough serves no functional purpose; however, because of its repetitive nature, it is a cause of morbidity as well as a symptom of disease. When little or no sputum is raised, the cough is described as "dry," "nonproductive," or "irritative." In some cases such a cough is simply a mild nuisance to the patient and is not, of itself, likely to prompt an emergency department visit. However, in other cases forceful coughing can cause soreness and pain in the chest and abdominal musculature, disturb sleep, and culminate in emesis, rib fracture, or syncope, consequences of sufficient concern to the patient to warrant emergency evaluation.

PATHOPHYSIOLOGY

Cough can be initiated voluntarily by neural signals originating in the cerebral cortex. More often, however, it is the end product of a reflex arc that originates with sensory nerve endings ("cough receptors"), is composed of afferent and efferent neural pathways, and is coordinated centrally in the brainstem ("cough center"). The larynx, trachea, and main bronchi are richly endowed with cough receptors; teleologically, these proximally situated receptors guard the entrance to the respiratory tract. Receptors extend to more peripheral bronchi as well, but their density becomes far less. Some of these receptors ("irritant receptors") are situated superficially, just deep to the interepithelial tight junctions. They can be triggered by irritant gases, aerosols, and fumes as well as chemical mediators of inflammation (e.g., histamine). In the presence of airway inflammation, these sensory nerve endings can become more openly exposed to inhaled substances, and their firing threshold may be reduced. It is likely that excessive airway secretions also somehow stimulate these receptors. Other receptors are thought to be situated more deeply within the tracheobronchial walls and to be sensitive to mechanical deformation of the airways, such as occurs, for instance, during bronchoconstriction. Afferent impulses are carried via the vagus nerve to the medulla.

Clinical observations have suggested that in disease states cough can result from stimulation of a number of other intrathoracic and extrathoracic structures, including the nose, ear canal, pharynx, and paranasal sinuses; pleura; stomach and esophagus; pericardium; and diaphragm. These observations have led to speculation that cough receptors may also be present in these locations and that afferent impulses may reach the medulla via other neural pathways, such as the trigeminal or phrenic nerves.

From the cough center in the medulla, a highly coordinated message is sent to the larynx and respiratory muscles via the vagus, phrenic, intercostal, and lumbar nerves. The motor output of a cough involves the following sequence: inspiration to a variable lung volume above resting lung volume (functional residual capacity), brief (approximately 0.2 seconds) closure of the glottis with contraction of the expiratory muscles against the closed glottis, and reflex opening of the glottis with continued forceful exhalation. Cough may be forceful even in the laryngectomized patient, but glottic closure augments the positive intrathoracic pressures achieved during cough, commonly raising pressures to greater than 200 cm H_2O. With the sudden release of these pressures, high expiratory flows are achieved. Airway walls and gas within airways are made to oscillate, giving rise to the noise we commonly associate with cough. In addition, the large intrapleural pressures cause dynamic compression of airways, and as these airways narrow, the linear velocity of gas moving through them increases. Velocities as high as 60 miles per hour can be achieved during coughing. The force generated by these high linear velocities helps to strip adherent mucus from airway walls and to propel it mouthward.

Cough is impaired by any of the following abnormalities: weakness of the inspiratory muscles (preventing an adequate inhalation before the expiratory phase of cough), inability to achieve glottic closure (e.g., vocal cord paralysis), expiratory muscle weakness, severe obstructive lung disease (limiting the maximal expiratory flows that can be achieved), and airway distortion (e.g., in bronchiectasis). In addition, abdominal or chest wall pain, such as after operation or trauma, can inhibit cough to the point of serious respiratory compromise (for instance, in the cigarette smoker with mucous hypersecretion who sustains blunt trauma to the chest during a motor-vehicle accident).

DIFFERENTIAL DIAGNOSIS

The differential diagnosis of cough is broad and spans the entire gamut of respiratory and cardiovascular diseases. In addition, rhinitis with postnasal drip, esophageal reflux, and occasionally diaphragmatic or pericardial irritation can be associated with cough. Cough is usually one of a complex of symptoms that, taken as a whole, supports consideration of a specific diagnosis.

In general, the quality of the sound associated with coughing is not helpful in narrowing the differential diagnosis. A bark-like cough preceded by an inspiratory whoop may suggest pertussis ("whooping cough"), but more often the tone, resonance, amplitude, and perceived site of origin of the cough are nonspecific, or at least indecipherable, with respect to diagnosis. In a cigarette smoker over the age of approximately 40 years, a persistent change in the type of cough or the development of a new cough should always raise consideration of possible lung cancer.

If a cough is productive of sputum, one can derive diagnostic information from the nature of the sputum produced.

Purulent sputum generally indicates a respiratory tract infection, although one not necessarily bacterial in cause. Asthmatic sputum may appear purulent on gross inspection in the absence of respiratory infection; microscopic examination, however, will reveal predominantly eosinophils rather than neutrophils. Cough productive of pink, frothy sputum suggests pulmonary edema. The presence of mucoid sputum production is of limited use diagnostically, since cough associated with a variety of infections (e.g., viral, mycoplasmal, and *Pneumocystis* pneumonias), inflammatory disorders (of the airways or lung parenchyma), and neoplasms can give rise to it. Cough productive of blood is discussed in the next subsection, Hemoptysis.

A common diagnostic problem is posed by the patient with a persistent, nonproductive cough—in the absence of fever, chest pain, wheezing, or shortness of breath—and a normal chest radiograph. In this circumstance one should inquire about exposure to inhaled irritants (e.g., cigarette smoke, paint fumes, chemicals in the workplace, contaminated humidifiers, and so forth) and about symptoms of possible aspiration or regurgitation of gastric contents. If responses to these inquiries are negative, the most common conditions that give rise to this scenario are persistent airway irritation after a tracheobronchitis (so-called "postviral tussive syndrome"), rhinitis with postnasal drip, and asthma. The latter, sometimes referred to as "cough-variant asthma," is an example of cough as a manifestation of bronchoconstriction; it typically responds to treatment with bronchodilators. The diagnosis of asthma is supported by the finding of airflow obstruction on pulmonary function testing or the demonstration of airway hyperreactivity on bronchoprovocation challenge (see Chap. 10). A radiographically occult, endobronchial neoplasm is a rare cause of cough when the chest x-ray is normal.

APPROACH TO THE PATIENT WITH COUGH

History and physical examination are useful in evaluating a patient with cough mainly to elicit other, related symptoms or physical findings. Detailed questioning about the cough sometimes provides helpful information; for example, its onset suddenly after choking on food would alert one to a likely aspiration, and its occurrence during the work week and remission on the weekend would suggest a work-related environmental stimulus. More often, however, the specific characteristics of the cough do not elucidate its cause.

In general, if a cough is sufficiently severe to bring a patient to the emergency department with that symptom as chief complaint, chest radiography should be performed to evaluate it. Infiltrates, mass lesions, and pulmonary vascular disease undetectable by physical examination may become manifest on radiography. If the chest x-ray is abnormal, further work-up is directed at the finding on chest film. If the chest x-ray is normal, chronic bronchitis should be considered in a long-term cigarette smoker and foreign-body aspiration should be suspected in a patient with gastroesophageal disease (e.g., achalasia), loss of consciousness, or pharyngeal dysmotility. Postnasal drip can contribute to cough in patients with rhinosinusitis, and asthma should be suspected if associated wheezing is present, if the symptom is intermittent, and if there is a personal or family history of atopic diseases.

Cough is best treated by addressing the underlying condition that is causing it. Thus, in some patients antibiotics will be the treatment of choice for an underlying bronchitis or pneumonia; in other patients diuretics and cardiac inotropes will be indicated for left ventricular failure. Symptomatic treatment of cough with suppressant drugs is generally reserved for patients in whom the cough is nonfunctional (i.e., raising no more than scant amounts of sputum) and in whom its cause cannot be identified or, if identified, cannot be promptly corrected. Cough suppression is particularly appropriate in patients with severe complications of coughing, such as cough-induced emesis, syncope, or rib fractures. Codeine or the related compounds oxycodone and hydrocodone are generally effective in ameliorating cough if given in adequate doses (up to 30–60 mg every four to six hours). Adverse effects of these agents include constipation and psychological disturbances such as nightmares and confusion, especially in the elderly; furthermore, their addictive potential is high. Cough suppression is contraindicated in patients with increased airway secretions at risk for mucous plugging, and in patients with marginal respiratory reserve, at risk for hypercapnic respiratory failure secondary to the respiratory depressant effects of these narcotic drugs.

Expectorants are medications intended to stimulate cough, usually for the purpose of promoting clearance of excess airway secretions. Since cough normally occurs in this situation, it is difficult to identify a therapeutic indication for an expectorant. On the other hand, it would be highly desirable to have available drugs that improve the viscoelastic properties of mucus, facilitating its clearance by ciliary action and cough. A number of medications are marketed as mucolytic agents with this purpose, including guaifenesin, glycerol guaiacolate, acetylcysteine, and supersaturated potassium iodide. The benefit accrued from these medications is rarely dramatic, however, and most often it is difficult to demonstrate any therapeutic effect.

Finally, in patients with mucous hypersecretion and an ineffective cough (e.g., due to expiratory muscle weakness), a number of techniques can be used to assist in removal of airway secretions. These include postural drainage and chest physiotherapy, nasotracheal suctioning, and manually assisted cough. The latter technique involves a sudden, forceful upward compression of the upper abdomen akin to a Heimlich maneuver in a supine patient. In some severely compromised patients, intubation with suctioning through an endotracheal tube proves necessary to maintain adequate gas exchange.

HEMOPTYSIS

Expectoration of blood from the chest must always be considered a potential sign of serious lung disease. Massive hemoptysis is usually terrifying to both patient and physician and is not likely to be ignored, but even mild blood-streaking of the sputum can be a clue to important underlying pathology (e.g., lung cancer) and in most cases requires an attempt at etiologic diagnosis. A chest radiograph is the pivotal diagnostic test in the assessment of hemoptysis.

PATHOPHYSIOLOGY

If one considers that virtually the entire cardiac output passes through the pulmonary capillary bed within a few microns of alveolar epithelium, it is perhaps surprising that bleeding into the respiratory tract does not occur more often. Probably because the pulmonary circulation is a low-pressure system and pulmonary arterial vasoconstriction occurs in areas of lung injury associated with alveolar hypoxia, hemorrhage from the pulmonary vasculature is relatively rare. Most episodes of hemoptysis, and particularly most cases of massive hemoptysis, involve bleeding from the bronchial circulation. Bronchial arteries have a variable anatomy but usually arise from the descending aorta at approximately the level of T5 to T6 and from the first right intercostal artery. They supply the tracheal wall and the bronchial tree to the level of the terminal bronchioles. Disruption of inflamed superficial vessels along the tracheobronchial mucosa, as occurs, for instance, in chronic bronchitis, is one of the most common causes of hemoptysis. Massive hemoptysis can ensue when there is erosion into larger bronchial arteries or arterioles (e.g., in neoplastic disease), when the bronchial vessels become dilated in response to surrounding chronic inflammation (e.g., in bronchiectasis), or when bronchial arteries empty into anastomotic pulmonary arteries (e.g., in bronchiectasis). Occasionally, arteriovenous malformations or ectopic deposition of highly vascular tissue (e.g., pulmonary endometriosis) is the source of bleeding.

DIFFERENTIAL DIAGNOSIS

A differential diagnosis of hemoptysis based on pathophysiologic mechanisms is not practical, since one cannot determine the source of the bleeding (bronchial vs. pulmonary circulation) based on clinical grounds, including analysis of the expectorated blood. Rather, it is more useful to consider a dichotomy based on the chest radiograph: hemoptysis with a pertinent radiographic abnormality versus hemoptysis with a normal chest x-ray or one in which no relevant abnormality is found.

Hemoptysis with a Pertinent Radiographic Abnormality

Pulmonary infections are a common cause of hemoptysis, especially when necrosis or bronchiectasis is involved. Usually purulent sputum is mixed with blood, giving a clue to the presence of infection. Classic examples include the rusty-colored sputum of pneumococcal pneumonia and the "currant jelly" appearance of sputum in some cases of *Klebsiella* pneumonia. Hemoptysis can occur in lung abscess of any cause. Bleeding can result from a number of manifestations of tuberculous disease: (1) Hemoptysis can be part of active pulmonary tuberculosis (primary or reactivation disease); (2) it can originate at a site of inactive tuberculosis, particularly with cavitary or bronchiectatic disease; (3) a calcified tuberculous lymph node can erode into a bronchus (broncholith) with associated bleeding; and (4) fungal colonization of a tuberculous cavity (mycetoma) frequently leads to hemoptysis. Atypical mycobacterial infections are also often associated with hemoptysis. Invasive fungal infections can erode directly into pulmonary or bronchial vessels; invasive aspergillosis would be a typical example in immunocompromised hosts. Bronchiectasis of any cause can cause recurrent hemoptysis, often but not exclusively in association with acute infectious flares. In most instances, radiographic evidence for bronchiectasis is present even on plain chest films. Worldwide, one of the most common infectious causes is paragonimiasis, in which larval forms of *Paragonimus westermani* migrate out of the small bowel and enter the lungs, maturing into adult flukes within the pulmonary parenchyma, where they cause a granulomatous response, suppuration, and necrosis. Characteristic bubble-like cystic shadows, 0.5 to 2.0 cm in diameter, superimposed on ill-defined parenchymal infiltrates, may suggest the diagnosis radiographically.

Common neoplastic causes of hemoptysis include bronchogenic carcinoma, bronchial adenoma, and pulmonary metastases. Single or multiple pulmonary mass lesions are the most common presentation, but endobronchial lesions can be manifested instead as atelectasis (segmental, lobar, or entire lung) or postobstructive pneumonia. In bronchioloalveolar carcinoma, an air space infiltrate may be the radiographic finding. Nodular densities associated with hemoptysis may also lead to consideration of Wegener's granulomatosis, lung abscesses, and pulmonary infarcts.

Diffuse radiographic abnormalities can be found in hemoptysis due to pulmonary vasculitides, the most commonly encountered of which are Goodpasture's syndrome, Wegener's granulomatosis, and systemic lupus erythematosus. When direct injury to the alveolar-capillary membrane causes diffuse alveolar hemorrhage, the chest radiograph has a characteristic appearance and evolution. Initially, one finds signs of air space filling, with acinar shadows and air bronchograms. As blood is taken up into the lymphatic channels over the ensuing 2 to 3 days, the pattern changes to one of reticulonodular infiltrates, sometimes with Kerley B lines. In the absence of further bleeding, the chest x-ray usually clears entirely over 10 to 12 days. In pulmonary edema, extravasation of blood can cause the frothy sputum to be pink-tinged, but the diagnosis is rarely confused with other causes of hemoptysis.

Tracheobronchial bleeding of any cause, if sufficiently brisk, can lead to aspiration of blood into dependent portions of the lung and an accompanying radiographic abnormality. This "blood pneumonitis" is nonspecific and should not be mistaken for evidence regarding the primary site of the hemoptysis. Other, rarer considerations include arteriovenous malformations, endometriosis (catamenial hemoptysis), and tracheobronchial amyloid.

Hemoptysis with a Normal or Noncontributory Chest Radiograph

If no pertinent abnormality is seen on chest radiography, the diagnosis is most often chronic bronchitis, usually in association with an acute infectious exacerbation. However, other causes must be considered, most important a radiographically occult lung cancer. Even in selected patients evaluated bronchoscopically, the frequency of this latter abnormality varies widely among reported series, from 0 to 22 percent. The significance of these studies is simply to indicate that in a patient with hemoptysis who is at risk for lung cancer, a normal chest radiograph does not fully exclude that diagnosis. Other potential causes of hemoptysis in this setting include pulmonary embolism, mitral stenosis, and bronchiectasis.

Massive Hemoptysis

Although important in determining patient management, the amount of blood expectorated in general aids little in the differential diagnosis. However, when bleeding becomes massive (defined here as >200 ml blood over ≤24 hours), certain causes can be suspected more highly. The four most common causes of massive hemoptysis are cancer of the lung, tuberculosis, lung abscess, and bronchiectasis. Less often, mycetoma, arteriovenous malformation, pulmonary vasculitis, or mitral stenosis will be found.

APPROACH TO THE PATIENT WITH HEMOPTYSIS

History

Although it is usually apparent from the patient's initial description whether or not the source of the bleeding that is being reported is the chest, occasionally one must clarify an imprecise complaint of "spitting up blood." Sometimes oral, nasal, or gastrointestinal bleeding is mistaken for hemoptysis. Most often one can discriminate among these possibilities by inquiring about gingival bleeding, nosebleeds, or vomiting; sometimes it is helpful to have the patient mimic or duplicate the process by which the blood was produced. A frothy sample of expectorated blood indicates hemoptysis rather than hematemesis; microscopic demonstration of alveolar macrophages in the sample would clinch the distinction.

The amount of blood expectorated should be documented as carefully as possible. One should also inquire about additional sites of bleeding, entertaining the possibility of a systemic bleeding dyscrasia or of one of the pulmonary-renal hemorrhage syndromes (e.g., Goodpasture's syndrome). Questions about the use of aspirin, other nonsteroidal antiinflammatory drugs, or anticoagulants would be appropriate; these drugs can exacerbate hemoptysis as a result of some other cause although they do not induce hemoptysis per se. On the other hand, profound thrombocytopenia can be associated on occasion with diffuse pulmonary hemorrhage in the absence of any other identifiable predisposition.

Additional history-taking should be directed toward elucidating a specific cause from among the various diagnostic possibilities. A few examples include the following: Fever and purulent sputum production suggest an infectious cause, chronic bronchitis would not be likely in the absence of active or former cigarette smoking, associated dyspnea and pleuritic chest pain of sudden onset can indicate pulmonary embolism, and cyclic hemoptysis on a monthly basis in a woman of childbearing age raises consideration of catamenial hemoptysis due to endometriosis.

Physical Examination

Physical examination can help to localize the site of bleeding to one or the other lung and to narrow the differential diagnosis. For instance, persistent focal wheezing would suggest partial endobronchial obstruction, such as by a lung cancer or bronchial adenoma. Likewise, unilateral dullness to percussion, tactile fremitus, or inspiratory rales can help to lateralize the likely bleeding source. Physical findings outside the thorax can give clues as to cause. For example, clubbing of digits should alert the physician to the possibility of lung cancer or chronic suppurative lung disease (e.g., bronchiectasis). Multiple telangiectases over the lips and oral mucosa suggest the diagnosis of hereditary telangiectases (Osler-Rendu-Weber syndrome), which is associated with pulmonary arteriovenous malformations. An opening snap and diastolic rumble heard over the cardiac apex call attention to the presence of mitral stenosis. It should be noted that the physical examination is often normal or noncontributory in patients with hemoptysis, even during a period of active bleeding.

Laboratory Studies

Immediate studies appropriate to all patients with hemoptysis include an assessment of hemostatic mechanisms and a chest radiograph. Hemostasis can be investigated with blood studies for prothrombin time, partial thromboplastin time, and platelet count; if a qualitative defect in platelet function is a consideration (e.g., in uremia or recent aspirin use), a bleeding time should be ordered as well. As was noted previously, the chest radiograph is the crucial test in evaluating a patient with hemoptysis. An abnormality found on chest film may be sufficiently characteristic as to indicate both the site and the cause of the hemoptysis. Three examples are shown in Fig. 7-6: Based on the respective chest x-rays, one could suspect the diagnoses of lung cancer, mycetoma, and bronchiectasis and, in the first two examples, localize the probable site of bleeding.

Even when the chest radiograph is not specific, an abnormality can direct the nature of the subsequent evaluation. If one finds diffuse alveolar and interstitial infiltrates (diffuse alveolar hemorrhage), additional work-up will differ entirely from evaluation of the patient whose chest x-ray reveals a rounded opacity with central cavitation suggestive of a lung abscess or possibly a cavitary neoplasm. Thus, once a relevant radiographic abnormality is identified, additional diagnostic studies are directed at elucidating the nature of that abnormality and are tailored to the appropriate radiographic differential diagnosis. Most often this further evaluation will take place outside of the emergency department setting; an urgent bronchoscopy performed in the emergency department is almost never indicated.

If the chest x-ray is normal or noncontributory, depending on the clinical circumstances (amount of bleeding, presence of risk factors for lung cancer, presence of tracheobronchitis, and so forth), one may choose to monitor the patient with serial chest x-rays, to perform fiberoptic bronchoscopy, or

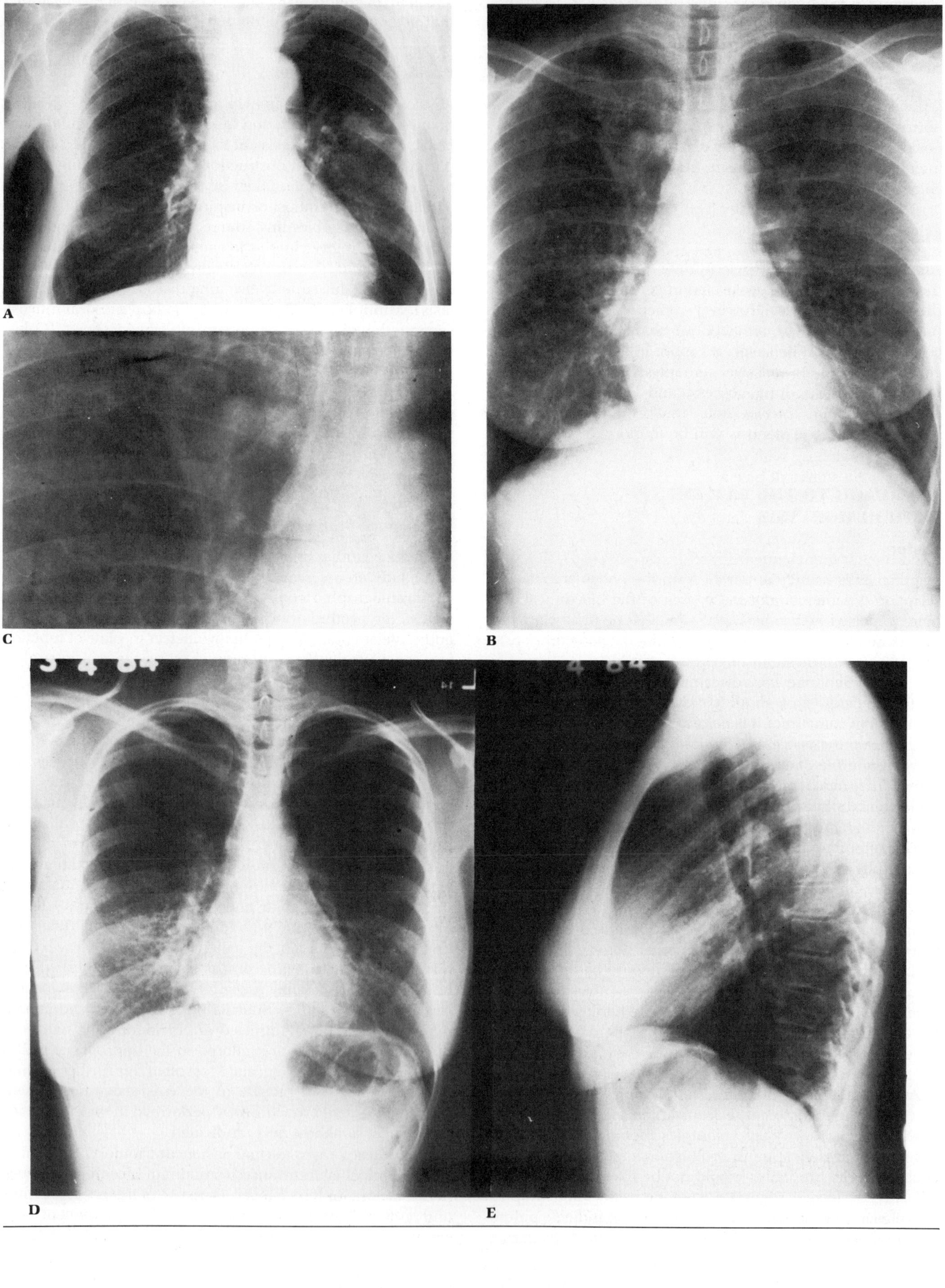

A B C D E

occasionally to obtain a computed tomographic scan of the chest. Again, this work-up will take place after the patient leaves the emergency department.

Patient Management

The patient with massive hemoptysis (≥200 ml blood/24 hours) will require hospital admission for close observation and often for surgical intervention. The major risk to the patient is not exsanguination but asphyxiation if the blood cannot be cleared sufficiently rapidly from the airways. One must ensure adequate oxygenation, if possible with supplemental oxygen delivered by nasal cannulas rather than by face mask so as not to interfere with expectoration of blood. If the patient has a depressed level of consciousness or cannot clear blood from his or her airways rapidly enough to prevent asphyxiation, endotracheal intubation is required so that endotracheal suctioning can be provided. The endotracheal tube should be as large as possible to avoid plugging of the tube with clotted blood. In addition, adequate intravenous access should be established immediately, the hematocrit measured, and blood sent to the blood bank for typing and cross matching with units of red blood cells. If one can lateralize the source of bleeding to one lung by examination or chest radiograph, the patient should be positioned with that lung dependent in order to reduce the risk of spillage or apiration of blood into the uninvolved lung.

Additional management strategies depend on the cause of the hemoptysis and the respiratory reserve of the patient. Therapeutic options include bronchoscopic tamponade of a bleeding airway, thoracotomy with resection of focally involved lung, and angiographic bronchial artery embolization. Fiberoptic bronchoscopy is almost never indicated in massive hemoptysis: Because of the narrow diameter of the suction channel, one cannot clear the blood from the airways effectively through the fiberscope and visualization is rapidly lost. If it is necessary to localize the source of bleeding endoscopically before operation (e.g., bilateral abnormalities on chest radiograph), rigid bronchoscopy is usually necessary. In most patients with sufficient respiratory reserve to survive thoracotomy and lung resection, surgery offers improved survival compared to conservative measures when hemoptysis is massive. Thus, thoracic surgical consultation is generally warranted. In recent years, angiographic techniques have made possible the selective catheterization and embolization of bronchial arteries for the treatment of massive hemoptysis. This approach is particularly effective in patients with dilated bronchial arteries, such as occurs in bronchiectasis. This therapeutic option can be considered for patients in whom thoracic surgery is contraindicated (e.g., in those with extensive bilateral disease or limited ventilatory reserve) and may require transfer of the patient to a specialized center with expertise in this procedure.

In patients with smaller amounts of hemoptysis, such as a few teaspoonfuls, one is often faced with a difficult decision regarding the disposition of the patient from the emergency department. Some patients are at risk for more massive bleeding and should be observed in the hospital; other patients can safely receive appropriate therapy at home (e.g., antibiotics for acute respiratory tract infection). The decision may be complicated by the patient's considerable fear. No single recommendation can be made that is appropriate to all patients. In general, one should be guided by whether treatment of the underlying lung condition necessitates hospitalization, by a history of prior episodes of hemoptysis, by the patient's ventilatory reserve, and by a knowledge of those conditions most often associated with massive hemoptysis. Thus, a patient with advanced COPD who has a small amount of hemoptysis in association with a lung abscess should be admitted for intravenous antibiotics and observation of the rate of hemoptysis; another patient with a similar amount of hemoptysis who has known bronchiectasis and who has expectorated blood many times in the past may not require hospitalization.

Fig. 7-6. Chest radiographs from three patients with hemoptysis. In each example, the radiographic findings suggest a potential cause for the hemoptysis. A. Left mid-lung zone mass is suspicious for lung cancer. B. Right upper lobe cavity with intracavitary mass is characteristic of a mycetoma. C. Enlarged view of mycetoma. D, E. Right middle lobe and lingular infiltrates are consistent with a diagnosis of bronchiectasis.

SELECTED READING

Apnea and Hypoventilation

Cherniack, NS, and Longobardo, GS. Cheyne-Stokes breathing. *N Engl J Med* 288:952, 1973.

Strohl, KP, Cherniack, NS, and Gothe, B. Physiologic basis of therapy for sleep apnea. *Am Rev Respir Dis* 134:791, 1986.

Dyspnea

Cherniack, NS, and Altose, MD. Mechanisms of dyspnea. *Clin Chest Med* 8:207, 1987.

Epler, GR, et al. Normal chest roentgenograms in chronic diffuse infiltrative lung disease. *N Engl J Med* 298:934, 1978.

Estenne, M, Yernault, JC, and DeTroyer, A. Mechanism of relief of dyspnea after thoracocentesis in patients with large pleural effusions. *Am J Med* 74:813, 1983.

Mahler, DA. Dyspnea: Diagnosis and management. *Clin Chest Med* 8:215, 1987.

Wasserman, K, and Casaburi, R. Dyspnea: Physiological and pathophysiological mechanisms. *Ann Rev Med* 39:503, 1988.

Woolcock, AA, et al. Effects of dihydrocodeine, alcohol, and caffeine on breathlessness and exercise tolerance in patients with chronic obstructive lung disease and normal blood gases. *N Engl J Med* 305:1611, 1981.

Wheezing and Stridor

Cabanes, LR, et al. Bronchial responsiveness to methacholine in patients with impaired left ventricular function. *N Engl J Med* 320:1317, 1989.

Christopher, KL, et al. Vocal-cord dysfunction presenting as asthma. *N Engl J Med* 308:1566, 1983.

Forgacs, P. *Lung Sounds*. London: Bailliere Tindall, 1978.

Sherry, MK, et al. Herpetic tracheobronchitis. *Ann Intern Med* 109:229, 1988.

Cyanosis

Blount, SG Jr. Cyanosis: Pathophysiology and differential diagnosis. *Prog Cardiovasc Dis* 13:595, 1971.

Brandenburg, RO, and Smith, HL. Sulfhemoglobinemia: A study of 62 clinical cases. *Am Heart J* 42:582, 1951.
Comroe, JH Jr, and Bothelho, S. The unreliability of cyanosis in the recognition of arterial anoxemia. *Am J Med Sci* 214:1, 1947.
Curry, S. Methemoglobinemia. *Ann Emerg Med* 11:214, 1982.
Lundsgaard, C, and van Slyke, DD. Cyanosis. *Medicine* 2:1, 1923.

Sharp Chest Pain

Branch, WT Jr, and McNeil, BJ. Analysis of the differential diagnosis and assessment of pleuritic chest pain in young adults. *Am J Med* 75:671, 1983.
Donat, WE. Chest pain: Cardiac and noncardiac causes. *Clin Chest Med* 8:241, 1987.
Lee, TH, et al. Acute chest pain in the emergency room: Identification and examination of low-risk patients. *Arch Intern Med* 145:65, 1985.

Cough

Irwin, RS, Corrao, WM, and Pratter, MR. Chronic persistent cough in the adult: The spectrum and frequency of causes and successful outcome of specific therapy. *Am Rev Respir Dis* 123 (Pt 1): 413, 1981.
McCool, FD, and Leith, DE. Pathophysiology of cough. *Clin Chest Med* 8:189, 1987.
McFadden, ER Jr. Exertional dyspnea and cough as preludes to acute attacks of bronchial asthma. *N Engl J Med* 292:555, 1975.

Hemoptysis

Crocco, JA, et al. Massive hemoptysis. *Arch Intern Med* 121:495, 1968.
Remy, J, et al. Treatment of hemoptysis by embolization of bronchial arteries. *Radiology* 122:33, 1977.
Weaver, LJ, Solliday, N, and Cagell, DW. Selection of patients with hemoptysis for fiberoptic bronchoscopy. *Chest* 76:7, 1979.

8. Respiratory Distress: Initial Assessment and Patient Management

Christopher H. Fanta

Respiratory distress is both a symptom and the manner in which a patient manifests that symptom. The symptom is breathlessness at rest—the sensation of not being able to obtain a satisfying breath despite labored breathing. At its worst, it is the feeling of suffocation. Respiratory distress is present when the patient reports that he or she "can't breathe" and conveys discomfort or distress in his or her breathing. It is understandably associated with a sense of panic, so that the urgency of the situation is usually readily communicated to the physician in attendance. Respiratory distress is usually but not always associated with arterial blood gas abnormalities, yet severe derangements in PO_2 and PCO_2 may not be accompanied by respiratory distress if they are chronic and accompanied by compensatory adaptations. Similarly, the chest radiograph or pulmonary function test is often helpful in determining the cause of respiratory distress, but it cannot be used to establish the presence of respiratory distress or to assess its severity.

In some instances, respiratory distress is one of a constellation of signs and symptoms, the diagnosis is obvious, and treatment of the underlying disease alleviates the distress. An example is the patient who presents to the emergency department with an acute exacerbation of asthma. Respiratory distress is only one of the symptoms, although if severe enough, it is usually the dominant complaint; treatment with bronchodilators alleviates the respiratory distress along with other features of the disease. At other times, however, respiratory distress is a chief complaint in the absence of an immediately obvious explanation, and one must then work through its differential diagnosis to come to a specific etiology.

The differential diagnosis of respiratory distress will be considered here according to anatomic categorization. When a patient presents with respiratory distress of unknown cause, one should rapidly consider as diagnostic possibilities diseases of the following components of the respiratory system: airways, lung parenchyma, pulmonary vasculature, pleura, and thoracic cage. In the absence of any detectable abnormalities, the possibility of primary hyperventilation should be considered. Another heuristic model, based on the results of arterial blood gases and chest radiograph, will be discussed in the section concerning patient management.

Upper airway obstruction is a common cause of respiratory distress, a particularly well-known example being foreign body aspiration such as occurs in the so-called café coronary, when a piece of food becomes lodged in the posterior pharynx or glottis. Other disorders that can cause acute obstruction of the upper airway include anaphylaxis, epiglottitis, and laryngospasm. Subacute or chronic narrowing may culminate in respiratory distress—for instance, in pa-

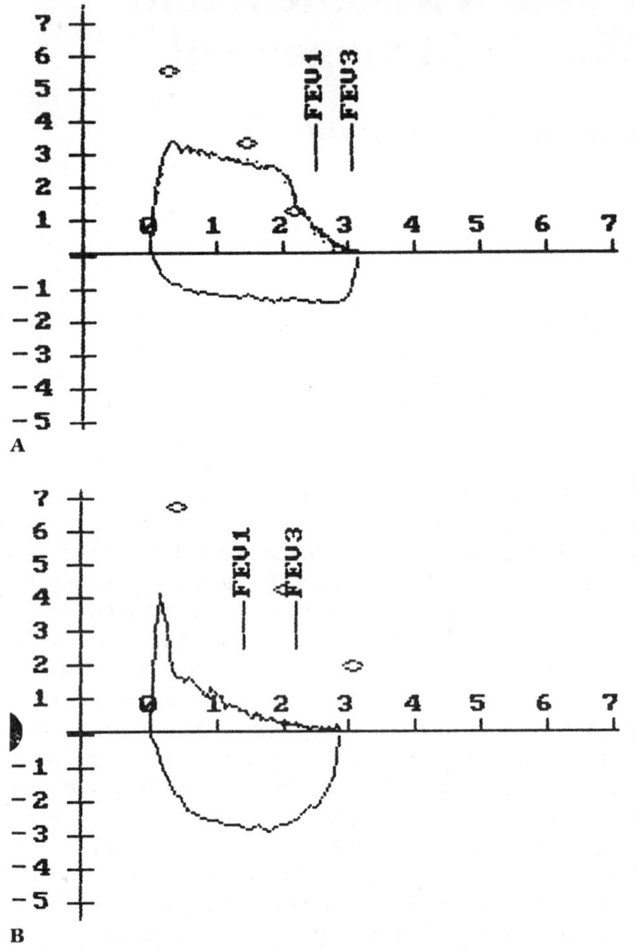

Fig. 8-1. The flow–volume loop displays flow (on the ordinate) over the vital capacity range (on the abscissa) during a maximal forced exhalation followed by a maximal forced inhalation. Expiratory flow appears above the horizontal line and inspiratory flow below it. A. The flow–volume loop in a patient with a fixed upper airway obstruction has plateau-like flattening of both the expiratory and inspiratory portions of the loop. B. The flow–volume loop in a patient with diffuse intrathoracic airways obstruction (e.g., COPD) has a characteristic scooped contour on its expiratory portion; the inspiratory portion has a normal shape.

tients with cricoarytenoiditis owing to rheumatoid arthritis or in those with an enlarging tracheal tumor, but the long antecedent history of related symptoms helps to distinguish entities such as these from the acute illnesses just noted. Patients will frequently localize the site of their distress to their upper airway by pointing to or clutching their throats. Stridor is often a powerful clue to the upper airway location of the problem, and hoarseness indicates involvement of the glottis. A plateau pattern on a flow–volume loop obtained in the pulmonary function laboratory implies a localized area of flow limitation, indicative of focal upper airway obstruction (Fig. 8-1A). Specific methods used to image or visualize the upper airways include lateral neck films, computed tomography (CT) scan, indirect or direct (fiberoptic) laryngoscopy, and fiberoptic bronchoscopy. Conditions causing obstruction of the upper airway are discussed in more detail in Chap. 9.

Diffuse airways obstruction characterizes asthma, chronic bronchitis and emphysema, bronchiolitis, and, when involvement of airways is sufficiently widespread, bronchiectasis (e.g., cystic fibrosis). Respiratory distress is a common manifestation of acute exacerbations of these obstructive lung diseases—the exacerbations being characterized physiologically by acute worsening of airflow obstruction. The severity of the expiratory airflow obstruction can be gauged by the extent of reduction in 1-second forced expiratory volume (FEV_1), but the presence or absence of respiratory distress cannot be reliably predicted from the FEV_1 or any other measure of lung function. If severe airflow obstruction develops over a short period of time, it is more likely to be accompanied by respiratory distress than if the same degree of airflow obstruction has been present chronically. For instance, an asthmatic patient who when well has normal lung function is likely to experience respiratory distress if his or her FEV_1 falls abruptly to 25 to 30 percent of normal, whereas a patient with chronic obstructive pulmonary disease (COPD) who persistently maintains an FEV_1 of the same magnitude (25–30% of normal) probably experiences dyspnea on exertion but not respiratory distress.

The shape of the expiratory flow–volume curve exhibits a characteristic scooped or concave appearance that is distinct from the pattern of upper airway obstruction (Fig. 8-1B). This contour of the flow–volume curve is found in all diseases with diffuse airways obstruction and is not specific for any one entity; furthermore, it does not localize the predominant site of airflow obstruction to either the central or peripheral airways. The diffuse obstructive lung diseases are discussed further in Chap. 10.

Note that in patients with respiratory distress owing to upper airway obstruction and, in some cases, diffuse airways obstruction, the chest radiograph can be entirely normal.

Widespread involvement of the *pulmonary parenchyma* can cause respiratory distress and, as in the obstructive diseases, the tempo of the underlying illnesses can vary from sudden in onset (e.g., congestive heart failure) to indolent and chronic (e.g., asbestosis). The parenchyma (interstitium or alveoli) can become filled with edema, inflammatory cells, blood, neoplastic tissue, or fibrosis. Examples include pulmonary edema, *Pneumocystis* pneumonia, diffuse alveolar hemorrhage (e.g., Goodpasture's syndrome), lymphangitic carcinomatosis, and idiopathic pulmonary fibrosis. In each instance, the lungs become stiff (poorly compliant), and, to minimize the work of breathing, respirations tend to be rapid and shallow. When airway obstruction (and increased resistive work of breathing) is combined with diffuse parenchymal involvement (and increased elastic work of breathing), such as occurs in aspiration of gastric contents, acute pulmonary edema, bronchopneumonias, and diffuse pulmonary hemorrhage, the likelihood of producing respiratory distress is increased. With rare exceptions (e.g., early *Pneumocystis pneumonia*), the chest radiograph is abnormal and reflects the widespread involvement with diffuse opacities involving both lungs.

In general, focal abnormalities of the pulmonary parenchyma, such as a segmental or even lobar pneumonia or atelectasis, do not cause respiratory distress. In part, the respiratory system has sufficient ventilatory reserve to accommodate minor losses of functioning lung tissue, and, in part, compensatory pulmonary arteriolar vasoconstriction preserves matching of perfusion to ventilation, minimizing hypoxemia. However, in the presence of severe underlying respiratory disease, such as advanced COPD or neuromuscular weakness, even a limited area of disease in the pulmonary parenchyma may provoke respiratory distress. Thus, in this regard, coexistent respiratory abnormalities are likely to have additive effects in triggering respiratory compromise.

Diffuse disorders of the lung parenchyma and atelectasis are discussed in greater detail in Chap. 14.

Acute obstruction of the *pulmonary vasculature*, such as occurs in pulmonary embolism, is frequently accompanied by respiratory distress. Dyspnea and apprehension are found in more than half of patients with acute pulmonary thromboemboli. Curiously, their presence cannot be correlated with the size (massive vs. submassive) of the vascular occlusion. It is possible that coexistent chest pain contributes to respiratory distress in some patients; pain with each deep breath is likely to synergize with the sensation of being unable to get a fully satisfying breath in causing distress. Embolization of the pulmonary vessels with amniotic fluid, tumor cells, foci of infection (septic emboli), and air, although causing distinct clinical syndromes, can equally provoke respiratory distress. Although a variety of x-ray abnormalities can be found in acute pulmonary thromboembolism, including atelectasis, pleural effusion, and pleural-based infiltrates (representing areas of pulmonary infarction), it should be noted that a normal chest radiograph is also consistent with this diagnosis. More extensive discussion of pulmonary embolism appears in Chap. 13.

Pneumothorax is the most common of the *pleural diseases* causing respiratory distress. Again, the combination of dyspnea and chest pain can synergize to produce this manifestation. A patient who presents to the emergency department with respiratory distress and chest pain and who, on physical examination, has hypotension, a unilaterally hyperexpanded and hyperresonant chest with ipsilateral absence of breath sounds, and tracheal deviation to the contralateral side, should rapidly be suspected of having a tension pneumothorax. Less dramatic instances of pneumothorax can also be accompanied by respiratory distress and may require a chest radiograph for diagnosis.

Pleural effusions are generally well tolerated but can cause respiratory distress if they become massive or bilateral and large, especially if accompanied by pleuritic chest pain. If the effusions are mobile, respiratory distress can be positional, occurring when the pátient is supine and alleviated when the patient sits up. Encasement of the lungs by pleural fibrosis or neoplasm develops slowly and so is likely to cause respiratory distress only in the terminal phases of disease. Diseases of the pleura are discussed in Chap. 12.

Thoracic cage abnormalities cause respiratory distress primarily because of failure of the ventilatory pump. However, additional contributing factors may include focal areas of atelectasis because of the mechanical inability to expand those areas of the lung and retained airway secretions owing to ineffective cough. Certain positions, especially the supine position, can put an already compromised respiratory system at further mechanical disadvantage, precipitating respiratory distress.

The thoracic cage is considered here to comprise all those elements that surround the lungs and pleura and contribute to their movement, including skeletal components (ribs, vertebrae, and sternum), respiratory muscles (and their innervation), and the abdomen. Acute disorders in each of these categories that commonly lead to respiratory distress include thoracic trauma with a flail chest, high spinal cord transection, and severe abdominal pain and distention (e.g., in severe pancreatitis), respectively. Patients with more chronic disorders, such as kyphoscoliosis or amyotrophic lateral sclerosis (ALS), generally develop respiratory distress only when an acute insult supervenes. In patients with a weak cough and marginally compensated respiratory function at baseline, that added respiratory stress can be as minimal as an acute tracheobronchitis.

Disorders of the thoracic cage that can culminate in ventilatory failure are considered in more detail in Chap. 15.

Finally, the patient with *primary* or *psychogenic hyperventilation* also experiences respiratory distress. In the absence of significant respiratory disease, he or she perceives air hunger and an accompanying sense of panic. The drive to hyperventilation appears to originate in the central nervous system. Stimuli provoking anxiety or fear may trigger the hyperventilation; at other times, the precipitating event may be obscure. By contrast, hyperventilation in response to exercise or metabolic acidosis is functional or compensatory and is generally not associated with respiratory distress.

Although the diagnosis is one of exclusion, primary hyperventilation may be suggested by the following features: a history of panic disorder or prior bouts of psychogenic hyperventilation, respiratory alkalosis with a normal alveolar-to-arterial gradient for oxygen (arterial PO_2 often greater than 100 mm Hg), and symptoms of acute alkalemia such as numbness around the lips and fingertips.

ASSESSMENT AND MANAGEMENT

History

The diversity of etiologies for respiratory distress makes a detailed review of all potentially pertinent historic data impossible. Often, however, one can use clinical clues to narrow the relevant differential diagnosis and to focus one's questioning. For instance, the sudden onset of respiratory distress in the postoperative patient raises consideration of pulmonary thromboembolism, pneumonia, or atelectasis, whereas respiratory distress with a similarly acute onset occurring while the patient was eating at a restaurant is more likely to suggest aspiration, anaphylaxis, or, in the asthmatic patient, possibly acute bronchospasm owing to ingested allergens or sulfites. Associated symptoms often help to guide the evaluation. For example, cough and wheezing in a patient with respiratory distress are usually indicative of airway diseases, whereas pleuritic chest pain points to diseases such as pulmonary embolism, pneumonia, pneumothorax, and pleural effusion. In the absence of any detectable cardiopulmonary disease, the symptoms of light-headedness and circumoral numbness suggest primary or psychogenic hyperventilation.

Respiratory distress that occurs in the supine position usually raises suspicion of congestive heart failure, but it should be remembered that obstructive lung diseases such as asthma or COPD can have similar presentations and that respiratory distress associated with diaphragmatic weakness can likewise be alleviated by sitting upright. The patient's past medical, especially cardiopulmonary, history is particularly relevant in evaluating respiratory distress. One searches for sudden and catastrophic illness in the previously healthy patient, whereas relatively minor events may trigger respiratory distress in a chronically compromised patient. A past history of similar events is always revealing.

Physical Examination

The physical examination in a patient with respiratory distress may be as varied as the causes. In some patients, the physical findings will rapidly establish a specific diagnosis or at least define a category of diseases. For instance, stridor is evidence for upper airway obstruction; widespread musical wheezing suggests diffuse airways diseases such as asthma or asthmatic bronchitis; paradoxical inward movement of the anterior abdominal wall on inspiration indicates diaphragmatic weakness; and bilateral basilar inspiratory rales together with jugular venous distention, peripheral edema, cardiomegaly, and a left ventricular early diastolic (S3) gallop are diagnostic of congestive heart failure. The physical examination can at least be expected to help focus the evaluation to one of the anatomic categorizations offered previously, that is, to distinguish airways diseases from parenchymal lung diseases, from pleural diseases, from disorders of the thoracic cage. The physical examination in patients with acute pulmonary vascular obstruction is admittedly generally nonspecific, and there are usually no abnormal physical findings in patients whose sole abnormality is primary hyperventilation.

Laboratory Evaluation

In patients with respiratory distress of uncertain etiology, a chest radiograph and arterial blood gas determination are indicated. The chest x-ray is often helpful in determining the cause of the respiratory distress, and the arterial blood gases define the severity of the associated disturbances in oxygenation and ventilation. Taken together, the results of these two tests have been used to categorize patients with acute respiratory failure in a dichotomous schema, as shown in Fig. 8-2, and this model can be used in formulating the differential diagnosis of respiratory distress. According to this conceptualization, patients are considered to have "white lungs" on chest radiograph if large or diffuse opacifications are present, and "black lungs" if they are absent. Blood gas abnormalities are divided into hypoxemia with hypercapnia and hypoxemia with eucapnia or hypocapnia. It should be emphasized that not all patients with respiratory distress have respiratory failure (e.g., primary hyperventilation, some patients with upper airway obstruction, asthma, or acute pulmonary embolism) and that patients with *chronic* respiratory failure often do not exhibit respiratory distress.

Nonetheless, with this schema one can use the initial chest x-ray and arterial blood gas results to help narrow one's differential diagnosis in a patient with respiratory distress. Thus, if the chest radiograph reveals clear lung fields ("black [image of the] lungs") and the arterial blood gases demonstrate hypoxemia with a normal or reduced arterial PCO_2, pulmonary embolism, pneumothorax, and intracardiac shunt are leading diagnostic considerations. On the other hand, clear lung fields on chest x-ray associated with *hypercapnic* respiratory failure suggest upper airway obstruction, neuromuscular disorders involving the respiratory system, and severe obstructive lung diseases.

Similarly, the pattern of blood gas abnormalities helps to differentiate among patients with respiratory distress and extensive opacification on chest x-ray ("white [image of the] lungs"). Hypoxemia with eucapnia or hypocapnia is the more common blood gas finding, typical of the diffuse parenchymal lung diseases (such as pulmonary edema), atelectasis, and massive pleural effusions. In this setting, carbon dioxide retention is usually found only in severe or terminal phases of disease or in patients with underlying respiratory muscle weakness. As noted earlier, respiratory distress with a normal arterial-to-alveolar gradient for oxygen and a normal chest x-ray is probably due to primary or psychogenic hyperventilation. However, a normal arterial PO_2 does not rule out pulmonary embolism.

With the information derived from history taking, physical examination, arterial blood gases, and chest radiograph, one often has sufficient information to make a specific diagnosis and to initiate appropriate therapy in a patient who presents with respiratory distress of uncertain cause. In other cases, additional diagnostic tests will be needed—the choice of the further examination being determined by these initial results. For instance, in a 40-year-old, cigarette-smoking woman on birth control pills who develops the sudden onset of chest pain and respiratory distress and has hypoxemia, hypocapnia, and a normal chest radiograph, perfusion lung scanning should be obtained to evaluate for suspected pulmonary embolism. In other patients, pulmonary function testing will be indicated if airflow obstruction is the suspected but not proven cause of respiratory distress. Given the urgency of the situation, the patient will often receive an initial "therapeutic trial" to relieve the respiratory distress pending more definitive diagnostic studies, for example, nitrates and diuretics in a patient suspected of having congestive heart failure, bronchodilators if the suspected diagnosis is diffuse airways obstruction.

Certain principles of management apply to all patients with respiratory distress. The first is that the patient should receive continuous medical attention until the distress at least begins to abate, if not completely resolve. The sense of asphyxiation is so noxious and terrifying that no patient should be left to struggle with it alone while less urgent matters are addressed.

The second principle, as during a resuscitative effort, is that the upper airway must be maintained patent. In some patients with respiratory distress owing to upper airway obstruction, this dictum may involve emergent intubation or even tracheostomy. If observation is elected in the patient with partial upper airway obstruction and adequate gas exchange, very close monitoring is mandated, since hypercapnic respiratory failure and total airway occlusion can develop very rapidly in almost all diseases involving the upper airway.

The third principle is that adequate oxygenation must be ensured. Unrelieved hypoxemia threatens the brain and myocardium with permanent damage and may induce complications, such as seizures, myocardial infarction, and cardiac arrhythmias, that can cause death. Thus, *at the same time* that initial patient assessment is taking place, arterial

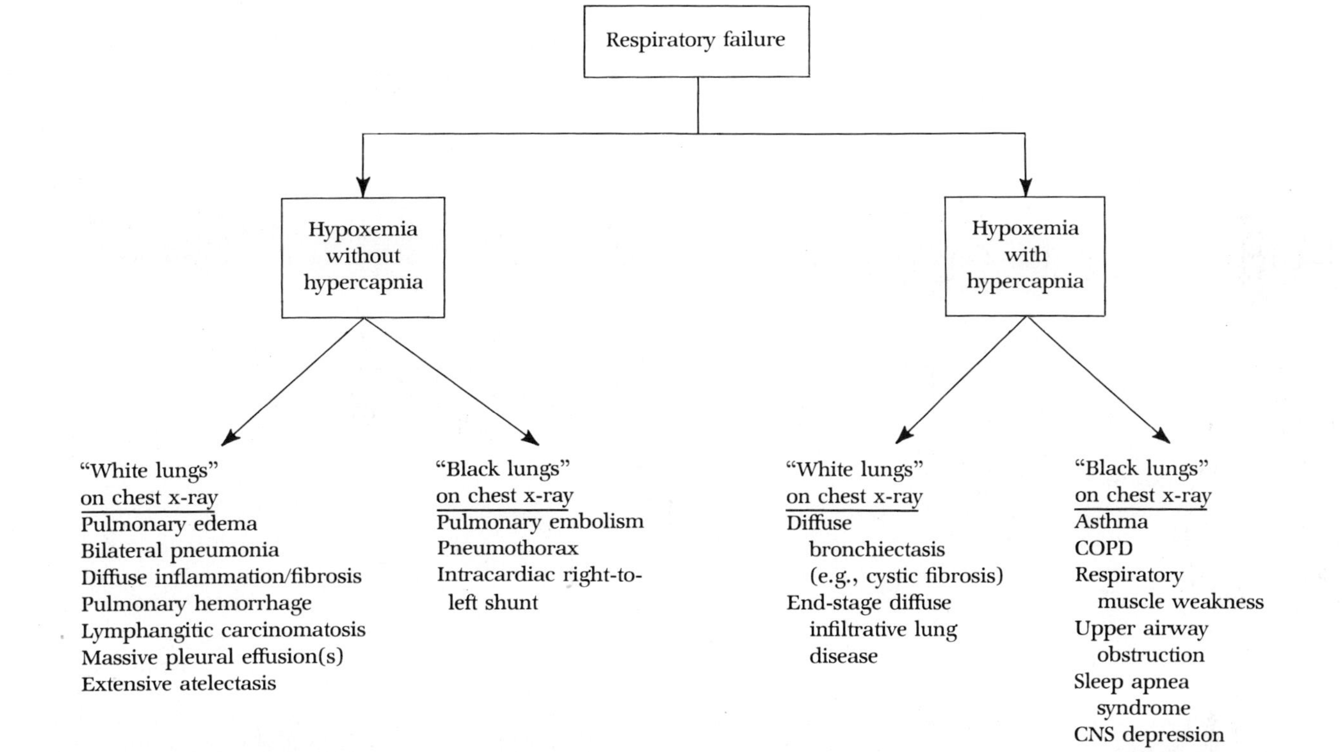

Fig. 8-2. The "black lungs-white lungs" dichotomous model of respiratory failure. "Black lungs" is used to refer to lucent or hyperlucent lung fields on chest x-ray; "white lungs" have diffuse or multifocal opacities on chest x-ray.

oxygen saturation must promptly be determined and supplemental oxygen administered, if needed. Cyanosis is not a sensitive clinical clue to the presence of hypoxemia (see Chap. 7), and so the absence of detectable cyanosis cannot be relied on to exclude hypoxemia. In any patient with respiratory distress not immediately reversible with specific treatment (e.g., bronchodilators for acute exacerbation of asthma), oxygenation must be directly measured by arterial blood gas determination or by oximetry. The availability of highly accurate finger or ear pulse oximeters has greatly facilitated both the rapid determination and the continuous monitoring of arterial oxygen saturation in acutely ill patients.

The immediacy of the threat posed by hypoxemia depends on the presence or absence of compensatory mechanisms that may have developed in response to chronic hypoxemia. For instance, correction of an arterial PO_2 of 50 mm Hg is less urgent in the chronically hypoxemic patient with accompanying secondary erythrocytosis than in a previously healthy individual lacking this compensatory adaptation. As a general rule, the goal of therapy is to maintain the arterial oxygen saturation at greater than or equal to 90 percent, which corresponds to an arterial PO_2 of $\geq$58 mm Hg under conditions of normal body temperature and pH. In patients with acute myocardial infarction or pregnancy, a target of 90 to 100 mm Hg may be more appropriate. In some patients who, while breathing room air, are able to maintain their oxygen saturation at approximately 90 percent only by profound hyperventilation with associated increased work of breathing, supplemental oxygen administration may help to reduce respiratory work and the oxygen cost of breathing.

If instantaneous results via oximetry are not available, supplemental oxygen should be given pending results of arterial blood gas analysis and response to therapy directed at the underlying disease. The short-term risk of excessive oxygen administration is limited to patients with chronic carbon dioxide retention, in whom worsened hypercapnia may be precipitated. If chronic hypercapnia is suspected (e.g., severe COPD, neuromuscular weakness, or sleep apnea syndrome), low-flow oxygen supplementation should be given initially. Controlled oxygen supplementation can be achieved using nasal cannulae at 1 to 2 liters/minute flow of oxygen or an air entrainment (Venturi) face mask with a jet orifice adaptor that delivers 24 percent oxygen (Fig. 8-3A, C). The advantage of the former is good patient comfort and acceptance; the latter offers more precise control over the concentration of oxygen actually delivered.

In patients without chronic hypercapnia, high inspired oxygen concentrations can be given initially, with subsequent adjustments in the delivered oxygen concentration based on follow-up measurements of arterial oxygen saturation or PO_2. A simple face mask with oxygen flow set between 5 and 8 liters/minute will deliver an inspired oxygen concentration of 40 to 60 percent (Fig. 8-3B). This represents appropriate initial therapy for patients with acute respiratory distress not suspected of chronic CO_2 retention, pending results of arterial blood gases. If additional oxygen supplementation is needed, options include partial rebreathing masks, nonrebreathing masks, and high-flow "cascade" systems (Fig. 8-3D–F). The first two masks include a 750- to 1000-ml bag, connected to the base of the mask, that is meant to serve as a reservoir for oxygen, minimizing rebreathing of exhaled

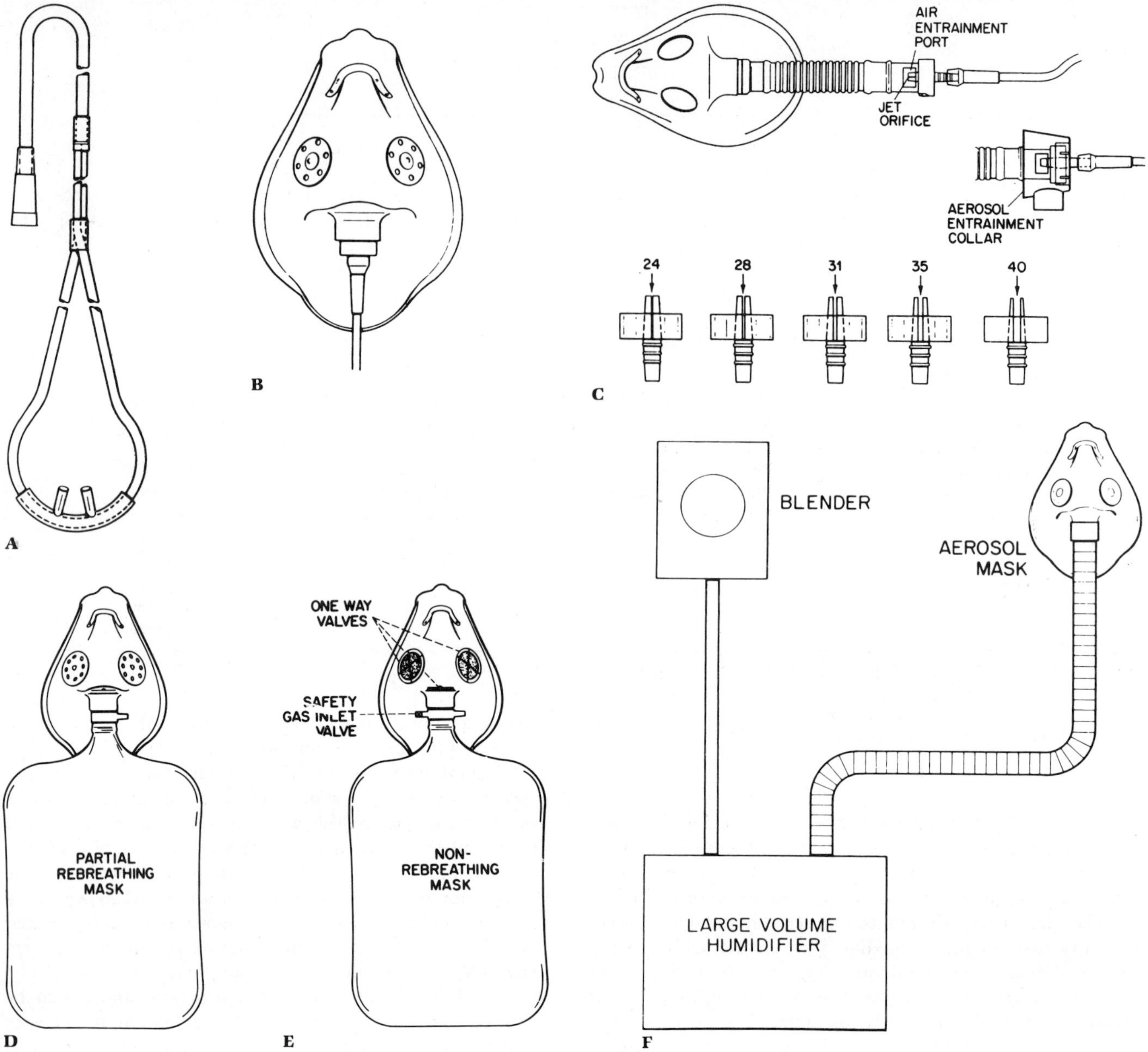

Fig. 8-3. Methods of delivery of supplemental oxygen. A. Nasal cannulae. B. Simple face mask. C. Air entrainment (Venturi) mask. The numbers shown above the jet orifice adaptors refer to the percentage of oxygen delivered. D. Partial rebreathing mask. E. Nonrebreathing mask. F. High-flow cascade system. (From R.M. Kacmarek and J.K. Stoller [eds.]. *Current Respiratory Care.* Philadelphia: B.C. Decker, 1988. Pp. 2, 3, 5, 6.)

carbon dioxide. The nonrebreathing mask also includes one-way flap valves to reduce entrainment of room air into the system during inspiration. Partial rebreathing masks, run at 8 to 10 liters/minute oxygen flow, deliver approximately 60 percent inspired oxygen; nonrebreathing masks can achieve approximately 80 percent inspired oxygen at flows of 10 to 15 liters/minute oxygen. The high-flow cascade system with tight-fitting face mask can deliver more than 100 liters/minute of pure oxygen, satisfying the gas delivery requirements of even the most breathless and tachypneic patient. With this system, nearly 100 percent oxygen can be administered as a humidified gas.

Some patients remain hypoxemic despite maximal oxygen supplementation by nonrebreathing mask or high-flow cascade because of the presence of large shunt fractions (i.e., large fraction of the cardiac output passing through the lungs without coming in contact with ventilated alveoli). Most often, intubation with mechanical ventilation and possibly positive end-expiratory pressure (PEEP) is necessary in such patients. PEEP reduces the shunt fraction primarily by raising the lung volume at which tidal breathing occurs (i.e., raising functional residual capacity [FRC]), thereby reexpanding areas of microatelectasis. Rarely, in the emergency department, one might attempt to achieve the same beneficial effect of PEEP without requiring an artificial airway. This objective can be attempted with continuous positive airway pressure (CPAP) applied through a tight-fitting face mask. Face mask CPAP should be considered a temporizing measure while definitive treatment takes effect (e.g., diuresis for pulmonary edema). Its disadvantages include the cumbersome head gear used to secure the mask to the face, making application and removal difficult. In addition to inconvenience, this drawback increases the risk of aspiration of gastric contents if the patient were to vomit.

In summary, oxygen therapy should be tailored to the particular needs of the patient with respiratory distress, as determined by oximetry or arterial blood gas analysis. Adequacy of oxygenation should be reassessed after administration of supplemental oxygen (allowing approximately 15–20 min for equilibration at the new inspired oxygen tension), and, where necessary, the concentration of inspired oxygen should then be adjusted up or down to achieve the target arterial PO_2 of 60 to 80 mm Hg. Intubation and mechanical ventilation, 100 percent inspired oxygen, and possibly PEEP are indicated if adequate oxygen delivery cannot be achieved via face mask or if the work of breathing required to maintain a satisfactory PO_2 is excessive and nonsustainable (e.g., respiratory rate $\geq$ 40 breaths/min). It is important to remember that the causes of dyspnea and respiratory distress are often complex and multiple, such that relief of hypoxemia may not always alleviate the patient's distress. For instance, in patients with acute pulmonary embolism or pulmonary edema, respiratory discomfort often persists after arterial oxygen saturation has been corrected to normal.

Finally, in the management of patients with respiratory distress, adequate ventilation must also be ensured. Toward this end, arterial PCO_2 must be measured; also, renal compensation for hypercapnia can be assessed by measurement of arterial pH. In some patients, therapy directed at the underlying pathophysiologic process (e.g., bronchodilator administration in COPD or suction of upper airway secretions in diseases of respiratory muscle weakness) may alleviate respiratory distress and correct the hypercapnia. In other patients, mechanical ventilatory support is needed, usually necessitating intubation and positive-pressure ventilation. The indications for and practical application of mechanical ventilation for ventilatory failure are considered in detail in Chap. 15.

SELECTED READING

Cowley, DS, and Roy-Byrne, PP. Hyperventilation and panic disorder. *Am J Med* 83:929, 1987.

Kacmarek, RM. In-Hospital Administration of Oxygen. In RM Kacmarek and JK Stoller (eds.), *Current Respiratory Care.* Philadelphia: Decker, 1988.

Kryger, M, et al. Diagnosis of obstruction of the upper and central airways. *Am J Med* 61:85, 1976.

Sasahara, AA, et al. Clinical and physiologic studies in pulmonary thromboembolism. *Am J Cardiol* 20:10, 1967.

Smith, RA, et al. Continuous positive airway pressure (CPAP) by face mask. *Crit Care Med* 8:483, 1980.

9. Partial Obstruction of the Upper Airway

N. Heramba Prasad
E. Jackson Allison, Jr.
Nicholas H. Benson

Management of complete airway obstruction is detailed in Chap. 3. This chapter focuses on the etiology and management of partial upper airway obstruction.

There are numerous causes for upper airway obstruction. Trauma, infectious diseases, foreign bodies, and inflammatory conditions are common etiologic agents. It has been estimated that 25 to 40 percent of patients with penetrating neck injury have associated airway obstruction. The majority of blunt upper airway trauma is caused by acceleration/deceleration forces from motor vehicle accidents. Other causes include contact sports, assault with blunt objects such as fists, blunt trauma by a wire or tree branch when riding a motorcycle, strangulation, and child abuse. Steering wheel injuries can also cause blunt upper airway trauma. Most upper airway injuries seen in clinical practice are due to blunt trauma.

Infections constitute about 80 percent of the causes of airway obstruction in children. In adults, the most likely cause is due to aspirated foreign bodies or vomitus. The incidence of acute epiglottitis is estimated to be 1 to 3 per 1000 pediatric admissions. More than 70 percent of all pediatric stridor is caused by croup.

The causes of airway obstruction can broadly be classified into acute and chronic, traumatic and nontraumatic. Some of the common causes of airway obstruction follow:

1. Unconsciousness, which may cause the tongue to fall backward against the hypopharynx, thus obstructing the airway. This is the most common cause of airway obstruction encountered by the emergency physician.
2. Foreign bodies in the airway.
3. Infection—acute epiglottitis, peritonsillar and retropharyngeal abscesses, croup, diphtheria, Ludwig's angina.
4. Trauma—direct and indirect trauma to the larynx and surrounding structures.
5. Allergic and anaphylactic reactions.
6. Corrosives, toxins, and burns.
7. Space-occupying lesions such as tumors and hematomas.
8. Paralysis of the vocal cord(s).

ANATOMY AND PATHOPHYSIOLOGY

Functional Anatomy of the Airway

The airway extends from the nostrils and the nasal passages downward to the bronchi and their terminal branches. It can be divided further into the portion above and below the vocal cords: supraglottic and subglottic areas, respectively.

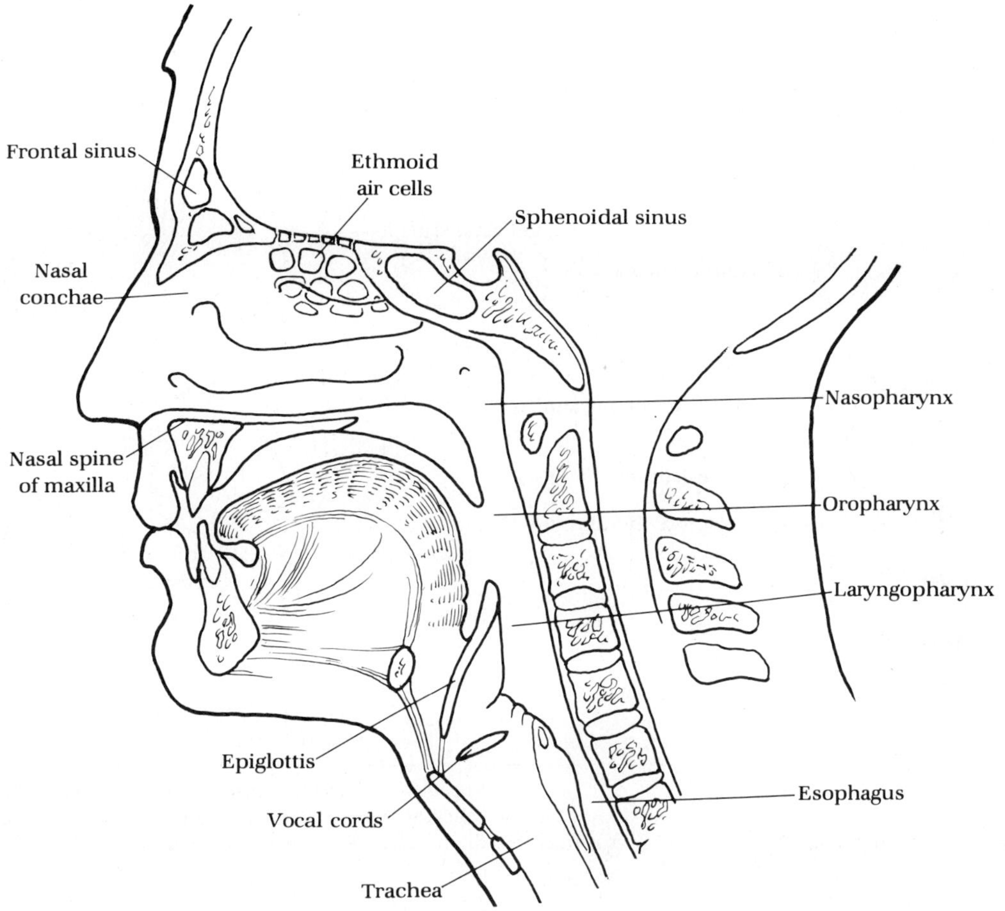

Fig. 9-1. Sagittal view of the upper airway.

The supraglottic area consists of the nasal passages, the nasopharynx, oropharynx, and laryngopharynx. The subglottic area is comprised of the trachea, the mainstem bronchi, and their branches.

The nasal cavity starts at the opening of the nostrils and curves posteriorly toward the nasopharynx. The nostrils are divided by a septum in the midline. Deviations of the septum are common. Each nostril is surrounded by a roof, a floor, and medial and lateral walls. Anteriorly, the roof is formed by the nasal bones and the spine of the frontal bone. The cribriform plate of the ethmoid forms the roof posteriorly (Fig. 9-1). It is important to note that in traumatic situations, where a fracture of the cribriform plate of the ethmoid might exist, an object introduced into the nose may traverse through the base of the skull and into the frontal lobe.

The pharynx is a fibromuscular tube that extends from the base of the skull to the lower border of the cricoid cartilage where it becomes continuous with the esophagus. The nasopharynx starts from behind the nasal cavity and ends at the tip of the uvula. The oropharynx extends from the soft palate to the tip of the epiglottis below. The laryngopharynx extends from the epiglottis to the lower border of the cricoid cartilage. The larynx bulges posteriorly into the laryngopharynx (sometimes referred to as the retropharynx).

The larynx is composed of cartilages and ligaments. The thyroid, cricoid, and arytenoid cartilages form the bulk of the larynx in addition to corniculate, cuneiform, and epiglottis (Fig. 9-2). The larynx extends from its oblique entrance or aditus (formed by the aryepiglottic folds, the tip of the epiglottis, and the posterior commissure), to the lower border of the cricoid cartilage. It is suspended from the hyoid bone by the thyrohyoid membrane.

The trachea starts at the lower border of the cricoid cartilage and ends at the carina. The length of the trachea varies from 10 to 14 cm (vocal cords to the carina). The distance from the lips to the carina averages 28.5 cm in men and 25.2 cm in women.

The larynx functions essentially as a valve, open during respiration, partially closed during phonation, and closed during deglutition. The function of the epiglottis is not quite clear. It seems that in the neonate, there is some physiologic role in separating the respiratory and alimentary tracts, but adults without an epiglottis have been known to swallow without aspiration.

The narrowest part of the upper airway is at the vocal cords in adults and at the cricoid cartilage in children. These are the most common sites in which foreign bodies may become lodged.

The airway conducting system, which is comprised of the upper and lower airways, forms the anatomic dead space. The average volume of this space in adults is 150 ml. At rest, the anatomic dead space equals the physiologic dead space, measuring approximately 30 percent of the tidal volume.

The important factor in airflow through the upper airway is the airway's diameter. As the airway diameter decreases,

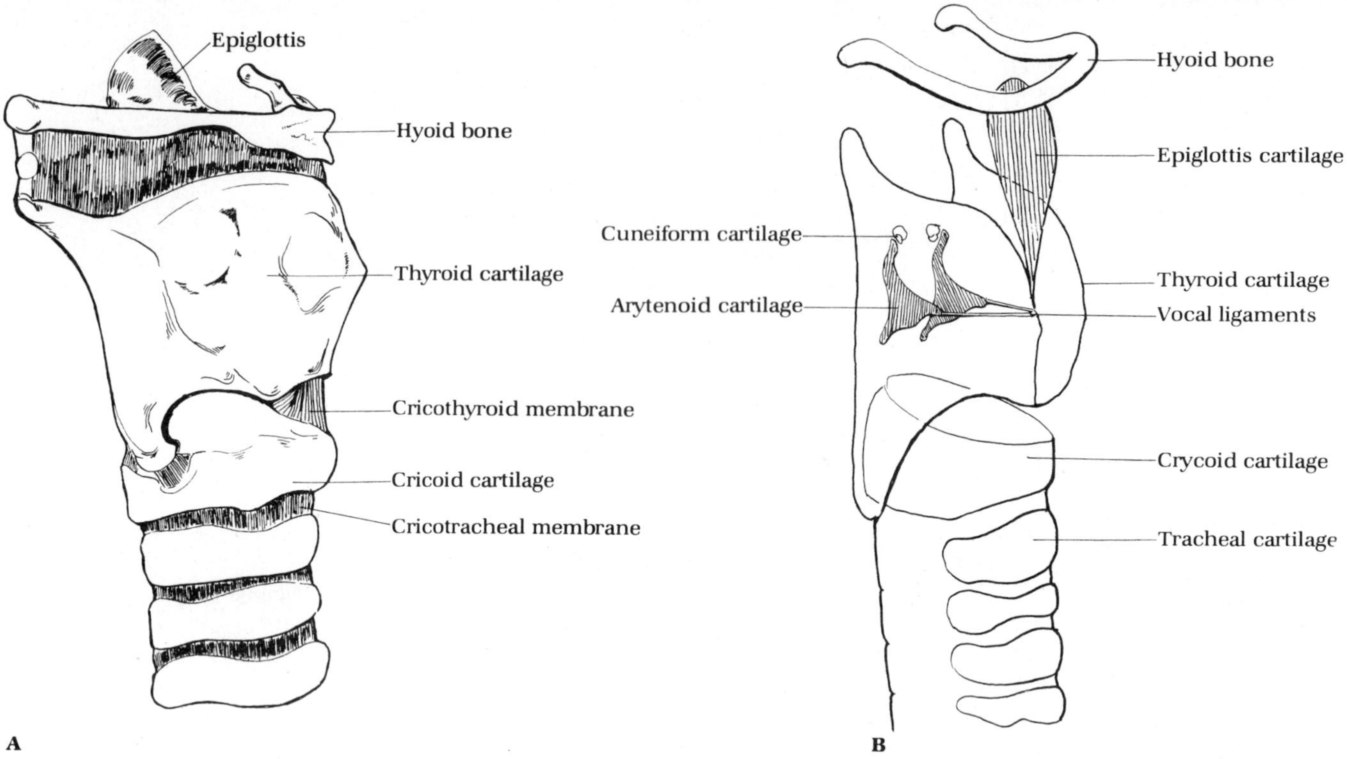

Fig. 9-2. A. Larynx—lateral view. B. Laryngeal cartilages—schematic view. Note that the vocal ligaments move according to the position of the arytenoid cartilages.

the resistance to airflow increases by a factor of approximately four.

Pathophysiology

Acute and complete obstruction will rapidly lead to death. In the presence of obstruction, initially there will be an increase in sympathetic outflow (increase in blood pressure, pulse, and respiratory rate). Later, as the PaO_2 falls and the $PaCO_2$ rises, the blood pressure and pulse will start to fall. Vital signs disappear and death ensues in a few minutes. If the obstruction is relieved during the critical first 4 or 5 minutes, there is usually prompt and spontaneous resolution of the abnormalities.

The movement of the intrathoracic and extrathoracic trachea during inspiration and expiration has been studied. During inspiration, the intrathoracic trachea widens under the influence of the negative intrathoracic pressure, while the extrathoracic trachea narrows. The reverse is true during expiration where pleural pressure becomes positive relative to atmospheric pressure. A foreign body causing partial obstruction of the extrathoracic trachea, for example, may cause difficulty during inspiration but not during expiration. The opposite occurs when the intrathoracic trachea is partially obstructed. This knowledge has been used clinically to detect subacute and chronic obstructions in various portions of the trachea, but, in acute situations, where time is of the essence, it is not helpful.

In the presence of partial airway obstruction owing to an aspirated foreign body, the victim may be capable of some air exchange ranging from good to poor. With good air exchange, the patient can cough forcefully, although he or she wheezes or has stridor between coughs. The American Heart Association recommends that if there is good air exchange, the victim should be encouraged to persist with spontaneous coughing, and the helper should stand by but not interfere until necessary.

EVALUATION

History

Evaluation of the patient who is in respiratory distress is discussed in Chap. 8. The history may provide a diagnostic clue when evaluating a patient with upper airway obstruction. Age of the patient, time of onset of illness, prodromal symptoms, and fever may suggest an infectious cause. History of allergies and past medical illnesses such as tumors or bleeding disorders may be helpful in steering the clinician toward a proper diagnosis.

Physical Examination

Depending on the severity and acuteness of the obstruction, the patient may show signs of respiratory distress, panic, and hypoxia. Inspiratory or expiratory stridor may be present. Drooling may be evident. Air entry into the lungs may be diminished; cyanosis may prevail.

A lateral neck roentgenogram may be helpful in evaluation if time permits. Soft tissue densities such as the epiglottis or posterior pharyngeal swellings can be seen. An occluding foreign body with air trapped around it may be visualized.

PRINCIPLES OF MANAGEMENT

There are numerous options available to the emergency physician in order to obtain airway control. Some of these techniques involve complicated procedures. The search for a simple and effective airway for prehospital care has been long-standing, and numerous ingenious devices are being tested and introduced. The principles described in Chap. 3 for complete airway obstruction can also be applied to partial obstruction.

In the prehospital setting, opening the airway by head-tilt–chin-lift or modified jaw-thrust methods can be carried out in an unconscious victim. If the victim has good air exchange, the emergency medical technician (EMT) should stand by and not interfere. Supplemental oxygen can be provided by means of nasal cannulae or a plastic face mask with a reservoir. If the patient's sensorium deteriorates, ventilatory assistance may become necessary. This can be accomplished effectively by mouth-to-mask or by bag-valve-mask ventilation. An oropharyngeal or a nasopharyngeal airway may be used to ensure patency of the upper airway.

A cardiac arrest victim can be intubated in the prehospital setting. Attempts at any form of intubation are contraindicated in (1) infections of the upper respiratory tract causing stridor, (2) trauma victims with significant maxillofacial or cervical injuries, and (3) victims who have ingested corrosives. Depending on the level of training and local guidelines, the EMT may be able to use an EOA, EGTA, PTL, or ETC airway (Fig. 9-3). The reader is referred to Chap. 3 and the procedure section for details of these airways.

The "gold standard" for managing the airway is endotracheal intubation either orally or nasally; however, this requires a considerable amount of training and expertise. In the emergency department, when the integrity of the airway is compromised, immediate measures should be undertaken to relieve the obstruction. Bag-valve-mask ventilation should be used to assist ventilation as needed. A quick assessment should be made looking for the cause of the airway compromise. Orotracheal intubation should be attempted if no contraindication exists. In trauma victims, the cervical spine should be immobilized prior to attempting intubation. In these situations, nasotracheal intubation may be attempted if the patient is breathing spontaneously. The emergency physician should be familiar with various adjuncts used in facilitating intubation of the trachea. These include the use of a lighted stylet, fiberoptic flexible laryngoscope, and tactile and retrograde intubation. These are described in Chap. 3. If these procedures cannot be performed or if they take an undue amount of time, the next rational step is to initiate transtracheal percutaneous ventilation using high-flow oxygen. This "buys time" during which further assessment of the airway can be made. Depending on the circumstances, either nasotracheal intubation or a semielective cricothyrotomy can be performed.

Medications During Intubation

It is rarely necessary to use medication(s) to accomplish endotracheal intubation in the emergency department (see Procedure 4). Occasionally, however, sedation may be required. In some instances, muscle relaxants used in conjunction with sedatives are needed. A situation may arise when an alert individual has to be intubated. In addition, trauma victims with severe head injuries have been known to develop an increase in intracranial pressure following any therapeutic manipulation. Hypoxia, injuries, or drug abuse may cause combativeness or uncooperative behavior. It is also important to realize that the majority of victims presenting to the emergency department with airway obstruction probably have full stomachs. Therefore, the emergency physician must be familiar with certain medications used to facilitate intubation. Some of the commonly used medications are as follows:

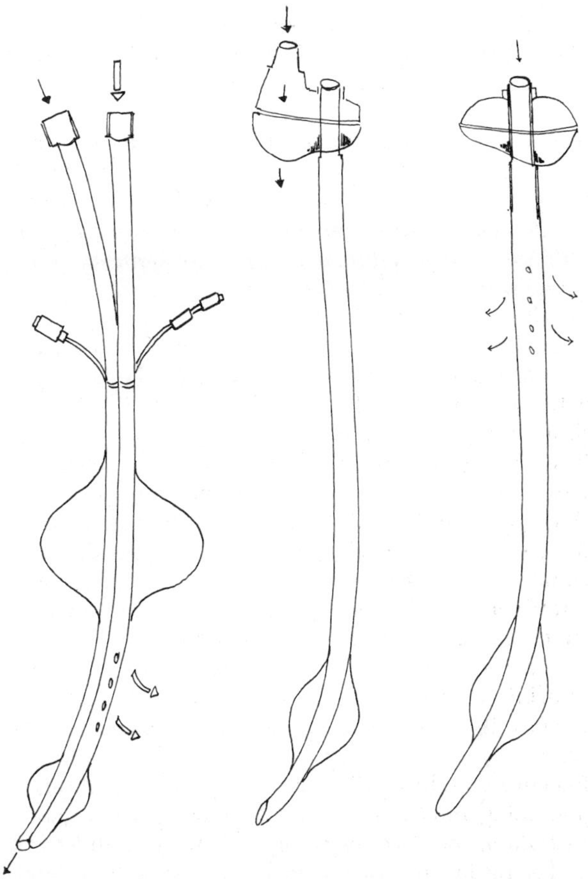

Fig. 9-3. Schematic diagram comparing the esophageal-tracheal combitube (ETC), esophago-gastric tube airway (EGTA), and the esophageal obturator airway (EOA). Note that in the esophageal mode, ventilation is accomplished through the esophageal port of the ETC (broad arrows). The open lumen of the EGTA is used for gastric decompression. The distal end of EOA is blind.

Sedatives

1. Minor tranquilizers—diazepam (0.2 mg/kg given in increments of 2.5 mg IV), midazolam (0.05–0.1 mg/kg titrated slowly in increments of 1–2 mg every 2 min).
2. Major tranquilizers—droperidol (2.5–5 mg IV titrated to achieve the desired effect).
3. Fentanyl (1–2 µg/kg; average adult dose 0.025–0.05 mg IV). After intravenous injection, effects are usually seen in 3 to 4 minutes, with a peak effect at 10 to 15 minutes.
4. Morphine sulphate (titrated in increments of 2–3 mg IV to a maximum of 10–15 mg IV).

Muscle Relaxants

1. Depolarizing agent—succinylcholine
2. Nondepolarizing agents—pancuronium bromide, vecuronium bromide, atracurium besylate

The use of muscle relaxants during emergency intubation is hazardous. They should be administered only by physicians who are thoroughly familiar with their use. *The physician must be absolutely certain that he or she can establish a definitive airway within a few precious moments of inducing respiratory paralysis and apnea.*

Succinylcholine (SCh), causes depolarization at the neuromuscular junction. This results in brief uncoordinated muscle fasciculations followed by paralysis. Following intravenous injection of SCh (1–2 mg/kg), onset of action is seen within 60 seconds; it lasts for 5 to 10 minutes.

The rapid onset and the short duration of action of SCh makes it preferable to nondepolarizing muscle relaxants such as pancuronium. However, muscle fasciculations are a definite disadvantage. These may lead to hyperkalemia (especially in a muscle damaged trauma victim), myoglobinemia, and myoglobinuria. Abdominal wall muscle fasciculations can lead to regurgitation and possible aspiration of stomach contents. Its acetylcholine (ACh)-like activity at muscarinic receptors can cause bradydysrhythmias, excessive salivation, and increased secretions in the respiratory tract.

Pancuronium bromide and vecuronium bromide are nondepolarizing muscle relaxants. Following intravenous administration, the onset of paralysis is seen in about 3 minutes, lasting for an hour or more. The slow onset and the long duration of action make it less desirable for use in emergency situations. Because of their longer duration of action, these agents are helpful in maintaining paralysis *after* intubation. Nondepolarizing agents have minimal cardiovascular side effects. A primary dose followed by a paralyzing dose in 4 or 5 minutes has been used by anesthesiologists to reduce the onset time of paralysis in situations in which the use of SCh is contraindicated.

The effects of muscle relaxants can be partially "neutralized" by the use of an anticholinesterase (e.g., neostigmine). It acts by increasing the amounts of ACh available to compete at the receptor site.

Local Anesthesia

The commonly used topical anesthetic agents are lidocaine, cocaine, and tetracaine. Cocaine has been used extensively to produce topical analgesia to the nares. The onset of anesthesia is almost immediate, with the duration lasting for 30 minutes to an hour. Clinically, concentrations of 4 to 10 percent are used. Cocaine, being an astringent, induces local vasoconstriction, thereby minimizing bleeding. The safe clinical dose is about 3 to 4 mg/kg.

Lidocaine, when applied to the mucous membranes in the form of a liquid solution, viscous solution, or aerosol, produces anesthesia in approximately 1 minute. The effect peaks in 2 to 5 minutes. Lidocaine aerosol spray contains 10 mg of lidocaine per spray. By simply spraying over the relevant structures, anesthesia can be accomplished. Viscous lidocaine or liquid lidocaine in concentrations of 2 to 4 percent can be used topically. Lidocaine aerosol can be used sequentially, using direct laryngoscopy as one proceeds into the airway.

Rapid Sequence Induction

The term *rapid sequence induction* refers to a specific method of general anesthesia that can be used in emergency situations. It is especially helpful in conditions of increased intracranial pressure or when a patient has a full stomach. A brief summary follows:

1. The essential aspect of intubation is preoxygenation. Preoxygenation with 100 percent oxygen administered to a patient results in "nitrogen washout" of the lungs, creating an oxygen reservoir of approximately 34 ml/kg (functional residual capacity [FRC]). This offers protection against hypoxia for approximately 6 or 7 minutes.
2. As preoxygenation is being carried out, the following supplies should be obtained and readily available: necessary drugs, endotracheal tubes, laryngoscope blades, suction equipment, fiberoptic laryngoscope, and cricothyrotomy tray. Be sure that assistants are available.
3. Talk to the patient in a calm voice, even if the patient is obtunded. It is helpful to explain the procedure in a conversational tone.
4. Use of sedation may be helpful; however, remember that excessive sedation may depress respiratory efforts. Furthermore, the sedated patient may become more distressed and develop hypoxia and combativeness. Midazolam (0.1 mg/kg IV), is useful as a sedative. The brief half-life of midazolam makes it preferable over diazepam. Fentanyl, at the dosage range of 1 to 2 μg/kg can be used intravenously. Fentanyl is a short-acting synthetic opiate that is approximately 100 times more potent than morphine and has the advantage of being reversed easily with naloxone.
5. An assistant should be ready to perform the Sellick maneuver, which is accomplished by direct compression of the trachea at the cricoid cartilage. The purpose is twofold: It prevents regurgitation of stomach contents, and it helps in visualization of the laryngeal structures during intubation. The Sellick maneuver should *not* be used when the patient is still awake. It may in itself induce regurgitation and aspiration.
6. A priming dose of pancuronium or vecuronium can be used at this time. These are nondepolarizing muscle relaxants, and they help in reducing muscle fasciculations that occur following SCh injection. The priming dose of the agent is approximately 10 percent of the paralyzing dose. This should be given approximately 3 minutes before the actual intubation. A dose of 0.01 mg/kg of either agent has been shown to be effective. The mode of action of priming with pancuronium is not clearly understood.
7. Lidocaine (1.0–1.5 mg/kg) may now be administered intravenously. Lidocaine, given 2 minutes before intubation, has been shown to blunt the rise in intracranial pressure. Some anesthesiologists use atropine or glycopyrrolate at this stage to reduce secretions; however, in emergency situations, this is not necessary.
8. General anesthesia is induced using a calculated dose of thiopental sodium (3–4 mg/kg) given by rapid IV injection. This is followed by SCh (1–2 mg/kg IV). As the patient loses consciousness, cricoid pressure should be

applied (Sellick maneuver). From this point on, cricoid pressure should be maintained until intubation is completed. Bag-valve-mask ventilation should not be performed during rapid sequence induction because of the fear of gastric distention and regurgitation. If the intubation attempt fails, mask ventilation (with cricoid pressure maintained) may be performed. A second attempt at intubation or the use of adjuncts such as a fiberoptic laryngoscope may be undertaken. Measures should be available for immediate cricothyrotomy in case this becomes necessary.

SPECIFIC CAUSES OF UPPER AIRWAY OBSTRUCTION

Epiglottitis

Acute epiglottitis or supraglottitis is a life-threatening condition because it may rapidly progress to complete airway obstruction. This condition is most common in children, but cases have been reported in adults. The clinical manifestations vary according to age (see Chap. 160). In the adult, the symptoms are somewhat less acute than in children. Usually, the patient presents to the emergency department complaining of sore throat and dysphagia. The diagnosis of epiglottitis in adults is commonly overlooked in the emergency department. Drooling is not seen as commonly in adults as in children. Respiratory distress and stridor are present. Whereas in children, any attempted maneuver to visualize the epiglottis may precipitate total airway obstruction, in adults, this is usually not the case. Adults tolerate examination better. However, because of the seriousness of the infection, immediate measures must be available to protect the airway. An ear-nose-throat (ENT) consultation should be obtained. Although it is recommended that the child not be sent to the x-ray department for soft tissue and lateral neck films without medical supervision and life-saving equipment, in the adult, this can be done safely to facilitate diagnosis.

Once the diagnosis of epiglottitis is suspected, the child should never be left alone; a physician should always remain. Equipment should be available to perform emergency intubation or tracheostomy. An ENT consultant should be called immediately. There is some controversy regarding the proper management of the airway. At this time, the consensus seems to favor nasotracheal intubation rather than tracheostomy. This should be done by an ENT specialist, preferably in the operating room.

There are case reports of epiglottitis in children being treated conservatively with steroids and antibiotics under close observation, but this has not been accepted universally. However, ill adults can be admitted to the intensive care unit and managed under close medical supervision; those less ill may be managed as outpatients with scrupulously close follow-up.

Other infections that may cause upper respiratory tract obstruction include croup (laryngotracheobronchitis) and peritonsillar and retropharyngeal abscesses. The treatment for abscess is incision and drainage by an ENT specialist. Croup should be differentiated from epiglottitis. The treatment for croup is medical management with nebulization, oxygenation, and humidification. Occasionally, a patient may need endotracheal intubation.

Trauma

Direct or indirect trauma to the larynx or surrounding structures may precipitate partial or complete airway obstruction (see Chap. 59). The trauma can lead to bleeding or avulsion of teeth or tissues that may lead to aspiration. Localized swelling and hematomas can also cause obstruction. Attempts to intubate have been known to precipitate laryngospasm. Laryngotracheal injuries resulting from blunt trauma are becoming more and more common. Usually, the injury is a result of direct impact against an automobile dashboard or steering wheel, or from "clothesline injuries" incurred while riding motorcycles. Tracheostomy is the recommended treatment for complete laryngeal obstruction. Cricothyrotomy is usually not feasible because there is damage to the airway at a lower level. Blind nasotracheal intubation should *not* be attempted. With complete transection of the trachea or cricotracheal disruption, retraction of the distal trachea into the mediastinum may occur. Repeated blind nasotracheal intubation attempts can further traumatize an already damaged trachea. Recently, percutaneous transtracheal insufflation has been advocated for emergency airway management in these patients. In situations in which a person trained in tracheostomy is not available, a judicious attempt at controlled orotracheal intubation may be the procedure of choice.

Other causes for concern in trauma include the integrity of the cervical spine and the patient's level of consciousness and combativeness, either secondary to the injury or to hypoxia. Patients with severe head injuries should be hyperventilated in order to reduce the risk of increased intracranial pressure, and an adequate airway must be established without causing further injury to the cervical spine. Usually, orotracheal or nasotracheal intubation can be accomplished successfully in the presence of partial airway obstruction. Use of medications such as sedatives and muscle relaxants are helpful to prevent increase in intracranial pressure and to improve patient comfort.

Foreign Bodies

Foreign body aspiration causing complete airway obstruction is discussed in Chap. 3. If there is partial airway obstruction, the patient is able to breathe and cough forcibly. There may be wheezing and stridor. In the presence of good air exchange to the lungs, it is preferable not to intervene in the prehospital setting. The EMS system should be activated. The rescuer should stand by and be alert for increasing respiratory distress and deteriorating air exchange. Emergency medical service (EMS) personnel may be able to apply supplemental oxygen via nasal cannulae or face mask, depending on how well the patient tolerates the procedure. According to local guidelines and approval, the paramedic may be able to use direct laryngoscopy and retrieve the foreign body with the use of Magill forceps. Once the patient reaches the hospital, direct rigid or flexible fiberoptic laryngoscopy can be used to determine the degree of obstruction, and retrieval of the foreign body can be attempted.

Space-Occupying Lesions

Space-occupying lesions, such as benign or malignant tumors, hematomas, and inflammatory swellings, may cause upper airway obstruction. Hematomas have been known to develop secondary to bleeding disorders (hemophilia) or anticoagulant therapy. The treatment depends on the degree and rapidity of progression of the obstruction. Endotracheal intubation should be performed if necessary. Transfusion of appropriate clotting factors, reversal of anticoagulation therapy, or emergency irradiation of malignant tumors may be required.

Allergic Reactions

Angioneurotic edema can cause swelling and obstruction of the airway. Nontraumatic causes of accumulation of edema fluid and swelling of the upper airway include anaphylaxis, preeclampsia or eclampsia, and hereditary angioneurotic edema.

Anaphylaxis is an IgE mast cell response to specific allergens (haptens). Virtually any material can be an allergen. Hymenoptera venom, certain enzymes, shellfish, nuts, chocolate, beer, radiographic contrast material, and antisera are commonly recognized allergens. The allergen-hapten combines with a protein complex. This complex bonds to the IgE receptors on the surface of the mast cell and results in the release of a slow-reacting substance of anaphylaxis (SRS-A), eosinophil and neutrophil chemotactic factors (ECF, NCF), histamine, kallikreins, and platelet activating factor (PAF). The resultant increase in capillary permeability causes localized edema. Smooth muscle tone changes (e.g., vasodilatation, bronchoconstriction).

The patient may present with symptoms such as wheezing, hoarseness, hypotension, stridor, abdominal cramping and diarrhea, urticaria, and pruritus. The treatment consists of supplemental oxygen, correction of intravascular volume depletion as needed, and parenteral administration of epinephrine, diphenhydramine hydrochloride, and steroids. Anaphylactic airway obstruction usually responds to subcutaneous administration of epinephrine, 0.3 ml of a 1:1000 solution (0.01 ml/kg for children). If the patient is in shock and has decreased peripheral perfusion, the epinephrine can be administered intravenously as a 1 : 10,000 solution. Diphenhydramine hydrochloride (0.5–1.0 mg/kg IV, up to 50 mg) may also be given. If the patient's condition deteriorates rapidly, endotracheal intubation or surgical intervention may be necessary. If the blood pressure cannot be maintained with volume expansion, vasopressors such as dopamine, dobutamine, or epinephrine may be needed. Intravenous corticosteroids (e.g., hydrocortisone, methyl prednisolone) can be helpful and should be given early. There is a delay of several hours before their effects are noted. Anaphylaxis is discussed further in Chap. 90.

Corrosives, Toxins, and Burns

Corrosives, because of the direct damaging effect to the mucosa, can cause considerable tissue destruction to the pharynx and larynx (see Chap. 156). The danger to the structures is directly proportional to the concentration and toxicity of the agent. Strong acids and alkalis can cause severe burns to the mucosa. The immediate tissue destruction and inflammatory edema can cause varying degrees of acute airway obstruction. Scarring and deformity secondary to the destruction of the tissues will cause delayed stenosis of the airway. Acids usually cause coagulation necrosis and superficial burns; alkalis cause liquifaction necrosis, producing deep burns. Attempts at blind intubation are contraindicated. Endoscopy by a specialist, or surgical airway intervention such as cricothyrotomy may be required.

Smoke inhalation is a common cause of laryngeal edema (see Chap. 75). Severe pain and hoarseness should prompt immediate indirect laryngoscopic evaluation and airway intervention. Endotracheal intubation or cricothyrotomy or tracheostomy may be needed.

Paralysis of the Recurrent Laryngeal Nerve

The recurrent laryngeal nerve may be paralyzed because of tumor involvement, viral infections, multiple sclerosis, surgical procedures, or trauma. In approximately 10 to 20 percent of cases, the paralysis is bilateral. When the nerve is paralyzed, the vocal cord assumes a midline position; seldom is there complete obstruction because of bilateral vocal cord paralysis.

If the patient's airway is completely obstructed, an attempt should be made to insert an orotracheal tube. If this fails, cricothyrotomy is indicated.

SELECTED READING

Leo, JD, and Simon, RR. Upper Airway Obstruction and Procedures and Techniques in Airway Management. In BE Brenner (ed), *Comprehensive Management of Respiratory Emergencies.* Rockville, MD: Aspen, 1985.

Morris, IR. Functional anatomy of the upper airway. *Emerg Med Clin North Am* 6(4):639, 1988.

Jorden, RC. Airway management. *Emerg Med Clin North Am* 6:671, 1988.

Morris, IR. Pharmacologic aids to intubation and to rapid sequence induction. *Emerg Med Clin North Am* 6:753, 1988.

Basmajian, JV. *Grant's Method of Anatomy* (8th ed.). Baltimore: Williams & Wilkins, 1971.

Graney, DO. Basic Science: Anatomy. In CW Cummings, et al (eds), *Orolaryngology—Head and Neck Surgery.* St. Louis: Mosby, 1986.

Stoelting, RK. Endotracheal Intubation. In RD Miller (ed), *Anesthesia.* New York: Churchill Livingstone, 1981.

American Heart Association. *Advanced Cardiac Life Support Course,* 1987.

Lennon, RL, Olson, RA, and Gronert, GA. Atracurium or vecuronium for rapid sequence endotracheal intubation. *Ann Emerg Med* 15:1243, 1986.

Tintinalli, JE, and Claffey, J. Complications of nasotracheal intubation. *Ann Emerg Med* 10:142, 1981.

Tove, FJ, and Weinstein, JD. Clinical experience with percutaneous tracheostomy and cricothyroidotomy in 100 patients. *J Trauma* 26:1034, 1986.

Delaney, KA, and Hessler, R. Emergency flexible fiberoptic nasotracheal intubation: A report of 60 cases. *Ann Emerg Med* 17: 919, 1988.

Asensio, JA, et al. Trauma: A systematic approach to management. *Am Fam Phys* 38:97, 1988.

Ruddy, J. Bacterial tracheitis in a young adult. *J Laryngol Otol* 102:656, 1988.

Ampel, L, et al. An approach to airway management in the acutely head-injured patient. *J Emerg Med* 6:1, 1988.

Dickison, AE. The normal and abnormal pediatric upper airway—recognition and management of obstruction. *Clin Chest Med* 8:583, 1987.

Haponik, EF, et al. Acute upper airway injury in burn patients—serial changes of flow-volume curves and nasopharyngoscopy. *Am Rev Respir Dis* 135:360, 1987.

Montoya, D. Management of the choking victim. *Can Med Assoc J* 135:305, 1986.

Goldthorn, J, and Badgwell, JM. Upper airway obstruction in infants and children. *Int Anesthesiol Clin* 24:133, 1986.

Ryckman, F, and Rodgers, BM. Obstructive airway disease in infants and children. *Surg Clin North Am* 65:1663, 1985.

Abman, SH, Fan, LL, and Cotton, EK. Emergency treatment of foreign-body obstruction of the upper airway. *J Emerg Med* 2:7, 1984.

Dailey, RH. Acute upper airway obstruction. *Emerg Med Clin North Am* 1:261, 1983.

Davis, HW, et al. Acute upper airway obstruction: Croup and epiglottitis. *Pediatr Clin North Am* 28:859, 1981.

Rice, DH. General principles of airway management. *Otolaryngol Clin North Am.* 14:735, 1981.

Don Michael, TA, Lambert, EH, and Mehran, A. Mouth-to-lung airway for cardiac resuscitation. *Lancet* 2:1329, 1968.

Cardiopulmonary Resuscitation Committee. Standards for cardiopulmonary resuscitation (CPR) and emergency cardiac care (ECC). *JAMA* 255:2915, 2961, 1986.

Shea, SR, MacDonald, JR, and Gruzinski, G. Prehospital endotracheal airway or esophageal gastric tube airway: A critical comparision. *Ann Emerg Med* 14:102, 1985.

Auerbach, PS, and Geehr, EC. Inadequate oxygenation and ventilation using the EGTA in the prehospital setting. *JAMA* 250:3067, 1983.

McEwen, W. Clinical observations on the introduction of tracheal tubes by the mouth, instead of performing tracheotomy or laryngotomy. *Br Med J* 2:122, 163, 1880.

Brantigan, CO, and Grow, JB. Cricothyroidotomy revisited again. *Ear Nose Throat J* 59:26, 1980.

Brantigan, CO, and Grow, JB. Subglottic stenosis after cricothyroidotomy. *Surgery* 91:217, 1982.

Jackson, C. High tracheotomy and other errors—the chief causes of chronic laryngeal stenosis. *Surg Gynecol Obstet* 32:392, 1921.

Heimlich, HG. A lifesaving maneuver to prevent food choking. *JAMA* 234:398, 1975.

Deweese, DD, and Saunders, WH. *Textbook of Otolaryngology.* St. Louis: Mosby, 1982.

Clinton, JE, and Ruiz, E. Emergency airway management procedures. In JR Robert and JR Hedges (eds), *Clinical Procedures in Emergency Medicine.* Philadelphia: Saunders, 1985.

Gold, MI, and Buechel, DR. Translaryngeal anesthesia: A review. *Anesthesiology* 20:181, 1959.

10. Obstructive Lung Diseases

Christopher H. Fanta

This chapter discusses diseases that may present with acute airflow obstruction owing to diffuse narrowing of airways. With the exception of emphysema, which secondarily involves airways because of loss of elasticity of the lung parenchyma, the disorders reviewed here are primarily airway diseases. Airways may be compromised because of bronchial smooth muscle constriction, airway wall inflammation, accumulation of secretions within the bronchial lumens, or combinations of these elements. The airflow obstruction may be fully reversible, as in asthma, or may have a fixed component that cannot be corrected, as in emphysema and chronic bronchitis. If airflow is sufficiently impaired, gas exchange is disturbed owing to mismatching of ventilation and perfusion and ultimately to global hypoventilation. The goal of therapy, therefore, is to improve airflow so as to alleviate dyspnea and restore adequate ventilation. Although treatment is often stereotypic, with bronchodilators being the mainstay, the precise choice of therapy and the anticipated outcome will depend to a large extent on the underlying disease and the specific cause of the acute exacerbation.

ASTHMA

Asthma is a very common disease, with an estimated prevalence in the United States of 3 to 5 percent. Because severe exacerbations frequently require emergent care, asthma results in hundreds of thousands of emergency department visits each year. Most cases are diagnosed in early childhood, but the estimated annual incidence of new cases of asthma remains relatively stable after age 20 at approximately 3 cases per 1000 persons in the general population. Thus, the onset of asthma in adulthood, while raising a number of differential diagnostic possibilities, should not be looked on as uncommon. Of persons older than 40 years who develop asthma, many are current or former cigarette smokers without any associated atopic diseases. Those cigarette-smoking patients with evidence of chronic bronchitis and emphysema who develop episodic wheezing and shortness of breath are probably best characterized as having "asthmatic bronchitis," although the distinction from asthma may be largely semantic, since treatment is essentially identical in both cases.

PATHOPHYSIOLOGY

A definition of asthma proposed by the American Thoracic Society describes the condition as "a disease characterized by an increased responsiveness of the trachea and bronchi to various stimuli manifested by a widespread narrowing of the airways that changes in severity either spontaneously or as a result of therapy." Two essential features of this definition are the concepts of reversible airflow obstruction and airway hyperreactivity. Asthma manifests as expiratory obstruction to airflow that varies widely over time or improves greatly (that is, more than 15–20%) following administration of inhaled bronchodilator. Typically (although not uniformly) lung function returns to normal or near normal when the disease is inactive. The wide swings in airway caliber that characterize asthma result from an underlying abnormal reactivity of the tracheobronchial tree: Stimuli that have negligible influence on normal airways trigger diffuse narrowing of asthmatic airways. This bronchial hyperreactivity is fundamental to asthma; it persists even when patients are asymptomatic and lung function is normal. Airway hyperreactivity can be demonstrated in the pulmonary function laboratory by administering nonspecific stimuli such as methacholine or histamine by inhalation or by the eucapnic hyperventilation of cold air. These stimuli cause little or no change in pulmonary function among normal persons but induce significant airflow obstruction (a greater than 20% fall in one-second forced expiratory volume [FEV_1]) in persons with airway hyperreactivity. Such bronchoprovocation testing is usually reserved for patients with a history suggestive of asthma who are seen at a time when they are free of wheezing on examination and have no airflow obstruction on baseline pulmonary function testing.

The etiology and precise mechanism of airway hyperreactivity in asthma are unknown, although many potential pathogenetic factors have been identified. In some patients, asthma develops as part of a constellation of allergic diseases, including allergic rhinitis and conjunctivitis ("hay fever") and atopic dermatitis (eczema). The abnormality that unifies these conditions is atopy—the tendency to respond to environmental allergens with the formation of specific antibodies of the immunoglobulin E class, which bind to receptors on the surface of mast cells. Reexposure to allergen with resultant allergen-IgE interaction leads to activation of the mast cell. The activated mast cell undergoes the explosive release of preformed chemical mediators present within cytoplasmic granules as well as the new synthesis of mediators derived from membrane phospholipids. Among the preformed mediators are histamine, eosinophil chemotactic factor, neutrophil chemotactic factor, and platelet activating factor; among the newly generated mediators are thromboxanes, prostaglandins, and leukotrienes. These chemicals have a variety of effects on the bronchi, all of which favor the development of inflammation and bronchoconstriction. They directly stimulate bronchial smooth muscle cells to contract, and they indirectly cause bronchoconstriction via an autonomic nervous system reflex pathway (chemical mediators stimulate sensory nerve endings, resulting in afferent impulses and then reflex efferent traffic via cholinergic [excitatory] pathways). They induce leakiness in the bronchial microcirculation, allowing plasma proteins to exude into the airway wall and facilitating cellular migration out of the circulation. Chemotactic factors attract and activate eosinophils and neutrophils, thereby amplifying the inflammatory process. Eosinophils are found in abundance in asthmatic airways and can often be identified in expectorated sputum. They can be stimulated to release important proinflammatory substances, including major basic protein, a potent mediator that disrupts ciliary function and promotes sloughing of epithelial cells along the respiratory tract mucosal surface. Further amplification of the inflammatory response may occur when stimulation of the sensory nerve endings of C fibers induces local release of peptide neurotransmitters (tachykinins). These peptides, such as substance P and neurokinin, are potent stimulants of bronchoconstriction, vasodilation, and mucus secretion.

Sensitized asthmatic subjects exposed to certain allergens may develop not only immediate airflow obstruction, developing within 5 to 10 minutes and resolving over approximately 1 hour, but also a late asthmatic response, typically occurring 4 to 8 hours after the exposure and slowly abating over the ensuing 12 to 24 hours. This delayed and often more severe airflow obstruction is associated with an influx of inflammatory cells into the airways, with a second wave of mediator release, and with a measurable increase in airway reactivity as demonstrated by bronchoprovocation testing.

Thus, the necessary elements have been identified whereby an immunologic response to inhaled allergen might elicit not only bronchoconstriction but also an inflammatory state of the airways associated with nonspecific hyperreactivity (i.e., hyperreactivity that may be provoked by a variety of stimuli, many of which are not antigens). Certain forms of occupational asthma would seem to support this model for the etiology and pathogenesis of asthma. Repetitive exposure to inhaled allergens (such as animal danders among animal handlers or wheat antigens among bakers) may over time cause sensitization even among workers without prior atopy. Continued exposure then triggers asthmatic symptoms. Symptoms often begin with the workweek ("Monday morning" asthma) and may be particularly troublesome at night after a day of work, suggestive of the late asthmatic response. Persons with asthma acquired in the workplace have nonspecific hyperreactivity; stimuli other than the initial sensitizing allergen may exacerbate their condition, just as in other forms of asthma. Occupational asthma often but not always remits upon withdrawal from the offending antigen.

It must be noted, however, that many persons with asthma have no evidence for atopic disease. They have normal total circulating levels of IgE antibody, absence of detectable circulating IgE antibodies to a broad panel of specific antigens, negative skin test reactions to intradermal injection of antigen, and no blood eosinophilia. Nonetheless, their disease behaves in every way identically to that of asthma in atopic individuals except that inhaled allergens do not trigger bronchoconstriction in them. This suggests that (1) there may be a heterogeneity of mechanisms by which persons acquire airway hyperreactivity and the syndrome that we recognize as asthma, or (2) airway hyperreactivity may be an abnormality intrinsic to bronchial musculature or to the autonomic innervation of airways, with the allergen-induced immediate hypersensitivity reaction being only one of many pathways that can elicit the abnormal response.

For many years it has been convenient to categorize asthmatic patients according to the dichotomy of "extrinsic" and "intrinsic" asthma. The distinction is based on the presence of atopy and sensitivity to inhaled or intradermal allergens among persons with "extrinsic" asthma and the absence of these features among those with "intrinsic" asthma. The utility of this distinction is probably overrated, however, since nonspecific airway hyperreactivity is present in all asthmatic patients, the clinical manifestations of asthma are indistinguishable between the two types, and treatment is, for the most part, identical.

Airflow obstruction in asthma is caused by circumferential constriction of bronchial smooth muscle, inflammatory thickening of the airway wall, and encroachment of the bronchial lumen by airway secretions (mucus, plasma exudate, and cellular debris). The presence and severity of the airflow obstruction are reflected in decreases in expiratory flow during the forced expiratory maneuver: peak expiratory flow rate (PEFR), FEV_1 and forced expiratory flow between 25 and 75 percent of the vital capacity (FEF_{25-75}, also referred to as the maximal midexpiratory flow [MMF]). In the asymptomatic asthmatic patient, expiratory flow may be entirely normal; in some asymptomatic patients, ongoing inflammation in the lung periphery may manifest as an isolated reduction in FEF_{25-75}. During an asthmatic attack, however, expiratory flow may become severely impaired, with FEV_1 falling to as low as 20 percent of normal or even less. In the presence of an asthmatic attack, lung volumes will also change acutely: There is an increase in the lung volume at which tidal breathing occurs (i.e., functional residual capacity [FRC]) as well as increases in residual volume (RV) and often total lung capacity (TLC). The hyperinflation at FRC, while helping to decrease expiratory flow limitation, puts the inspiratory muscles at a mechanical disadvantage and may contribute to the sensation of dyspnea experienced by patients during an asthmatic attack.

Dyspnea and tachypnea typify exacerbations of asthma even in the absence of hypoxemia. The resulting alveolar hyperventilation accounts for the arterial hypocapnia (e.g., $PCO_2 =$ 30–35 mm Hg) that is observed in moderately severe attacks of asthma. As airflow obstruction worsens, however, the arterial PCO_2 may begin to rise. Despite continued hyperventilation, wasted ventilation rises disproportionately and so alveolar ventilation (the determinant of PCO_2) decreases. Thus, in the setting of an attack of asthma, a normal PCO_2 (i.e., approximately 40 mm Hg) indicates severely disordered gas exchange and impending respiratory failure. Still worse airflow obstruction, possibly combined with fatigue of the respiratory muscles, ultimately leads to a decrease in total ventilation, hypercapnia, and respiratory failure. In the absence of sedation, hypercapnia rarely develops unless the FEV_1 falls to less than 25 percent of normal.

Hypoxemia is common in asthmatic attacks, but in the absence of respiratory failure, it is rarely severe. In one large series of patients (studied at sea level) in whom arterial blood gases were drawn on their presentation to an emergency department, the average PO_2 was 69 mm Hg. The correlation between the degree of airflow obstruction (e.g., FEV_1) and the PO_2 is poor, making it difficult to predict which patients might be significantly hypoxemic. Chronic hypoxemia is not a feature of asthma and so cor pulmonale is not one of its sequelae.

CLINICAL EVALUATION

History

In general, patients with asthma who present to an emergency department for treatment of an exacerbation of their disease pose no diagnostic dilemma. Most often they volunteer the information that they have asthma and are suffering increased symptoms of their disease. History taking is usually directed at determining the cause, duration, and severity of the present attack, as well as screening for any complicating conditions. Common triggering events include the following: respiratory tract infections (usually viral); vigorous exertion, especially when performed in cold air; exposure to aeroallergens, such as animal danders; and exposure to inhaled irritants such as dust, fumes, cigarette smoke, or high concentrations of air pollutants. All patients with asthma will develop airflow obstruction if given nonselective beta-adrenergic blocking drugs, such as propranolol or timolol; the latter may be encountered in the form of eyedrops used to treat glaucoma. Some asthmatic patients exhibit "aspirin sensitivity": Within minutes to a few hours of ingestion of aspirin or other nonsteroidal anti-inflammatory drugs, they may develop a severe exacerbation. Other patients may exhibit food allergies. The most widely recognized sensitivity, occurring in perhaps 5 percent of asthmatic patients, is to sulfiting agents, such as sodium bisulfite. These chemicals are encountered in fruits and vegetables that have been sprayed to prevent oxidation, in certain wines and beers, in avocadoes (e.g., guacamole), and peeled potatoes. A very small percentage of asthmatic patients react to Food, Drugs, and Cosmetics (FD&C) yellow dye #5, tartrazine, an artificial coloring ubiquitously distributed among foods, drinks, medicines, and products for oral hygiene. As for any chronic disease, a common precipitating event is the omission of medicines that had previously been taken regularly to prevent symptoms. In particular, patients who have recently been withdrawn from corticosteroids are especially at risk for a recurrent flare of their disease. Finally, in many instances, no specific cause can be elicited to explain the acute deterioration.

Determining the duration of the present attack of asthma may provide prognostic information about the anticipated rate of improvement. A prolonged exacerbation, especially if it occurs despite use of medications at home to treat asthma, is less likely to remit rapidly. A useful question asks when the patient was last able to get a full night's sleep. The answer will indicate how long symptoms have been sufficiently severe to wake the patient from sleep.

Symptoms that are not typical of asthma and thus, if present, would suggest a complicating or comorbid illness include fever, hemoptysis, and sharp chest pain. Respiratory tract infection, allergic bronchopulmonary aspergillosis, or pneumothorax/pneumomediastinum might account for these symptoms. On the other hand, chest tightness is a common sensation during an asthmatic attack not to be confused with angina, and discolored sputum may be caused by sputum eosinophilia and should not be equated with purulence owing to infection. Wheezing, cough, and shortness of breath are, of course, the cardinal symptoms of an asthmatic attack.

Physical Examination

Physical findings include tachycardia and tachypnea. The expiratory phase of respiration is prolonged, as in all of the obstructive lung diseases. Chest examination usually reveals diffuse high-pitched musical wheezes, either during expiration or throughout the respiratory cycle. Often wheezing can be appreciated even without the benefit of the stethoscope. Occasionally, extremely severe airflow obstruction may result in a "silent chest," in which breath sounds are distant and air movement is insufficient to generate wheezes. Other physical findings that correlate with the presence of severe airflow obstruction (FEV_1 usually < 1.5 liters) are (1) pulsus paradoxus (fall in systolic blood pressure of more than 12 mm Hg during inspiration); (2) use of accessory muscles of respiration, in particular the sternocleidomastoid muscles, to assist in inspiration; and (3) diaphoresis and the refusal to lie supine on the examining table because of breathlessness. However, the absence of any of these signs does not rule out the possibility of severe airflow obstruction.

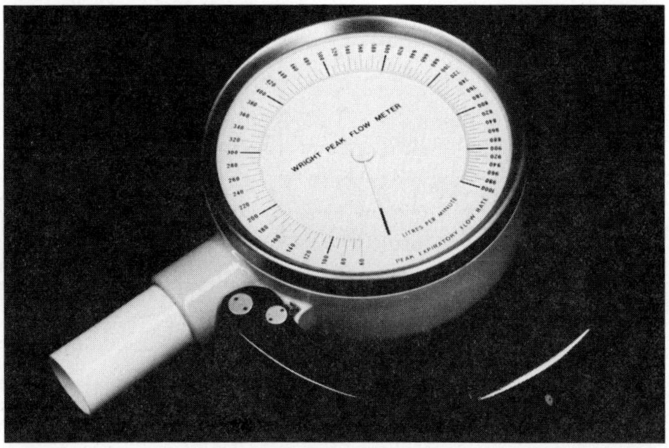

Fig. 10-1. Expiratory airflow obstruction can be assessed quickly and objectively using a peak flow meter such as the Wright peak flow meter shown here (Armstrong Medical Industries Inc., Lincolnshire, IL). Usually, three maximal forced exhalations are performed, and the best result is recorded. Expiratory flow is displayed in liters per minute.

Laboratory Data

The diagnosis of asthma is made on the basis of history and physical examination; no laboratory test will establish the diagnosis in the emergency department setting, although a large (≥20%) increase in expiratory flow following bronchodilator administration is supportive evidence. The role of laboratory testing in an acute attack of asthma is primarily to assess disease severity and to evaluate for potential complications. The most important measurement with respect to severity is some determination of expiratory flow, usually either spirometry (from which FEV_1 is derived) or peak flow measurement (giving PEFR). The two values correlate well. Both depend on good patient cooperation and a maximal expiratory effort, so that careful patient coaching during performance of either test is of paramount importance. Spirometry or peak flow determination can be performed either immediately on presentation or, in the patient who is very breathless, after initial bronchodilator therapy; it can then be repeated periodically to assess the response to treatment. A peak flow meter (Wright) is shown in Fig. 10-1. Normal predicted values for PEFR, based on patient age, height, and sex, are shown in nomogram form in Fig. 10-2.

Arterial blood gases are used primarily to identify patients who are developing hypercapnic respiratory failure, since such patients require particularly close monitoring and intensive therapy, often best delivered in an intensive care unit. Except for the patient who is cyanotic or has obviously shallow and ineffective respirations on presentation, arterial blood gases can be reserved until after intial bronchodilator treatment. Furthermore, pulmonary function testing can be used to screen patients who need arterial blood sampling, since hypercapnia is unlikely to develop (in the absence of sedating drugs) unless the FEV_1 is less than approximately 25 percent of predicted. The patient who is not making satisfactory improvement and who has an FEV_1 or PEFR less than or equal to 25 percent of normal after initial bronchodilator therapy should have arterial blood gases measured. Indiscriminant measurement of blood gases in all asthmatic patients should be discouraged, since fear of the discomfort involved in this procedure is one reason that some patients inappropriately delay seeking needed treatment for their asthma in the emergency department.

Assessing for hypoxemia is more problematic, since arterial PO_2 may vary during the course of treatment and correlates poorly with the degree of airflow obstruction. Continuous monitoring of arterial oxygen saturation by oximetry would be ideal but is not often readily available. Alternative approaches include measuring arterial blood gases in patients older than 50 to 55 years or persons of any age with known cardiac disease if they fail to improve rapidly with treatment, or administering low flow oxygen (e.g., 2 liters/minute oxygen by nasal cannulae) to such patients until obvious improvement is observed.

Chest radiographs are routinely obtained in the evaluation of acute exacerbations of asthma, although their utility in routine cases is questionable. A number of studies have demonstrated that the frequency with which clinically significant radiographic abnormalities are found is very low (approximately 2%); pneumonia, pneumothorax/pneumomediastinum, and segmental or lobar collapse are the most common findings. It can be argued that chest films should be reserved for unusual cases, such as patients with chest pain, fever, new onset of asthma, multiple recent exacerbations, atypical physical findings, or failure to respond to treatment.

Blood studies that may be of use include a complete blood count and in patients taking a theophylline preparation prior to presentation, a serum theophylline level. The clinical utility of the eosinophil count has probably been overemphasized. An elevated eosinophil count simply is consistent with the presence of an allergic disease; a normal count neither argues against the diagnosis of asthma nor diminishes the likelihood of a response to corticosteroid therapy.

Finally, examination of expectorated sputum may be helpful in an asthmatic patient with fever and discolored sputum. Inspection of sputum under the microscope permits distinction between purulent sputum indicative of an acute tracheobronchitis (characterized by abundant neutrophils) and sputum typical of an asthmatic exacerbation (characterized by abundant eosinophils). Other microscopic findings in asthmatic sputum include clumps of shed epithelial lining cells (Creola bodies), crystalline material (lysophospholipase) from degenerated eosinophils (Charcot-Leyden crystals), and spirals of fibrin and mucus in the shape of bronchial casts (Curschmann's spirals) (Fig. 10-3).

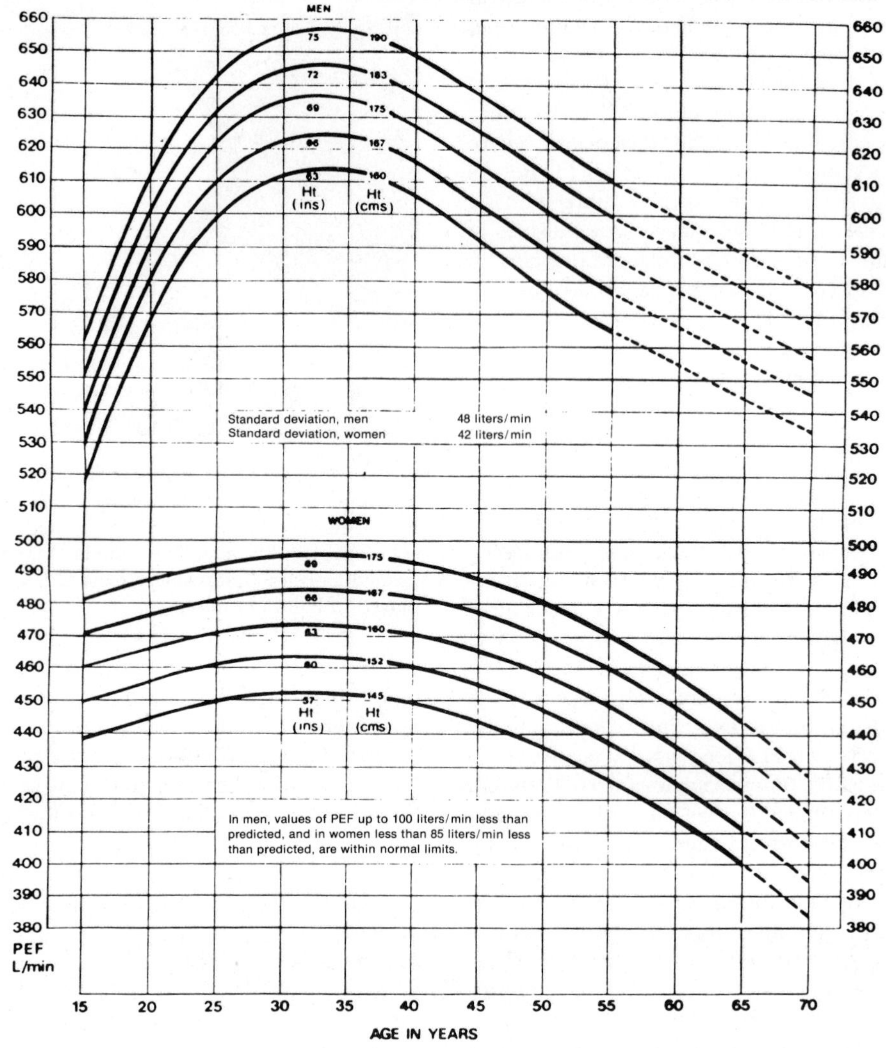

Fig. 10-2. Nomogram for normal values of peak expiratory flow based on sex, age, and height. The normal range encompasses two standard deviations above and below the normal value. (From Armstrong Medical Industries Inc., Lincolnshire, IL.)

DIFFERENTIAL DIAGNOSIS

Most patients with asthma relate *episodic* shortness of breath and wheezing, with intervening asymptomatic or minimally symptomatic periods. Patients who report persistent, invariant symptoms should be suspected of having an alternative diagnosis, such as bronchiolitis obliterans or sarcoidosis with endobronchial involvement. Persistent wheezing may also be unilateral, emanating from a focal source. In focal tracheobronchial obstruction, wheezing is characteristically monophonic—that is, the wheeze consists of one sound that starts and stops at essentially the same point in each respiratory cycle. Typical causes might include an endobronchial obstructing lesion, such as a neoplasm or aspirated foreign body, or extrinsic compression of an airway, such as by an aortic aneurysm or enlarged hilar lymph node.

Asthmatic symptoms often become manifest or worsen at night during sleep ("nocturnal asthma"). The differential diagnosis of nocturnal asthma includes congestive heart failure and esophageal reflux with aspiration. Occasionally, myocardial ischemia may be associated with transient left ventricular dysfunction and pulmonary venous hypertension, resulting in wheezing and shortness of breath as a variant manifestation of angina. Wheezing has also been described as a presenting symptom in patients with pulmonary embolism, although the frequency with which this manifestation occurs appears to be very small.

Rarely, upper airway obstruction may mimic asthma. A few patients have been reported with dysfunctional vocal cord movements resulting in inappropriate adduction during inspiration or expiration; usually, psychiatric disturbances are also present. In such cases, wheezing would be heard best over the trachea; laryngoscopy performed during an attack establishes this uncommon diagnosis.

TREATMENT

The primary goal of treatment in most instances of an asthmatic exacerbation is the prompt reversal of airflow obstruction, with accompanying relief of dyspnea. Only in the most

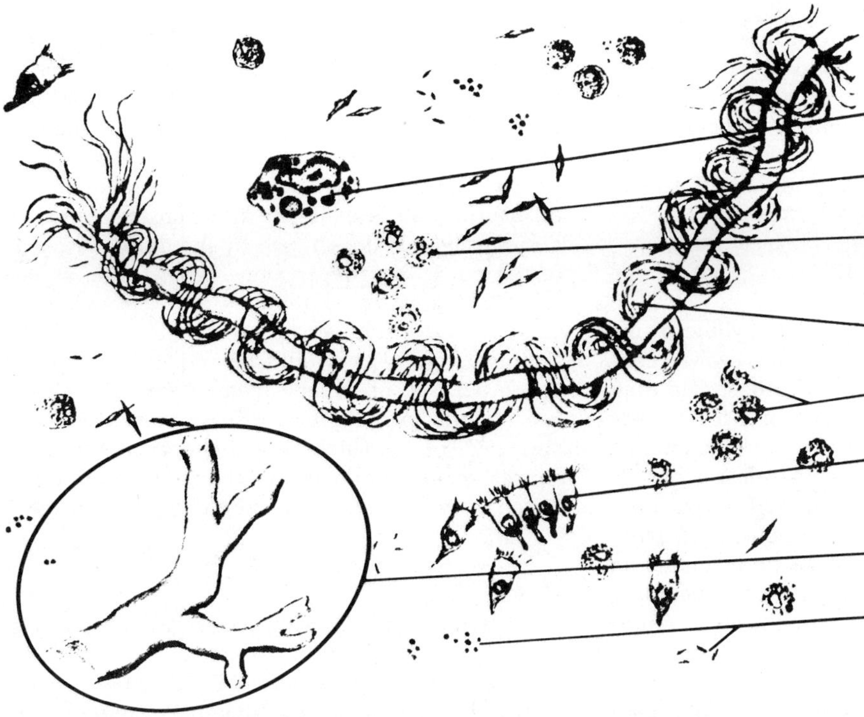

Fig. 10-3. Schematic drawing of elements that may be seen on microscopic examination of asthmatic sputum. (Copyright 1979, Ciba-Geigy Corporation. Reproduced with permission from the Ciba Collection of Medical Illustrations by Frank H. Netter, M.D. All rights reserved.)

severe cases in which acute respiratory failure has supervened does the focus of management shift to ventilatory support and correction of hypoxemia, and this circumstance will be considered separately.

Beta-Adrenergic Agonists

Airflow obstruction can be corrected most rapidly by the administration of bronchodilators—that is, drugs that have as their principal mode of action the relaxation of tracheobronchial smooth muscle. Beta-adrenergic agonists are the bronchodilators of choice. Their rapid onset of action and potency exceed those of the methylxanthines and anticholinergics. The beta-agonists are best given by inhalation in all adult patients except those who are apneic. Compared to oral or subcutaneous administration, the inhalational route achieves a more rapid onset of action and greater bronchodilation while causing fewer side effects. The bronchodilator effect of the inhaled beta-agonists is dose-dependent, and sequential administration of standard recommended doses leads to incremental bronchodilation. Finally, the optimal means of delivering inhaled bronchodilators continues to be debated. Over the last 10 years, the intermittent positive pressure breathing (IPPB) machines that had been widely used for nebulization of bronchodilator solutions have given way to simpler handheld nebulizers driven by compressed air or oxygen. More recently, it has been suggested that a beta-agonist bronchodilator delivered by metered-dose inhaler from a pressurized cannister, especially when used in combination with a spacer device, may be as effective as the nebulized bronchodilator solution. However, until additional investigations are performed using metered-dose inhalers in the emergency department setting, the efficacy of this method of administration for severe asthmatic exacerbations should be considered unproved.

In sum, for the young asthmatic patient without concomitant cardiac disease, we routinely administer isoetharine 5.0 mg (0.5 ml of a 1.0% solution diluted in approximately 2.5 ml of normal saline) by handheld nebulizer every 20 to 30 minutes, for three doses as the initial bronchodilator therapy. Isoetharine is a relatively selective, beta$_2$-specific agonist with a short (approximately 60–90 min) duration of action, suitable for repetitive administration. Other beta-agonists available for wet aerosol administration include isoproterenol, metaproterenol, and albuterol. Side effects related to systemic sympathetic stimulation are common, including tremulousness, heart pounding, anxiety, and headache. Although some patients develop a significant tachycardia, *on average* heart rate does not significantly change after the initial three doses; blood pressure tends to fall slightly.

In older patients with known or potential cardiac disease, particularly coronary-artery disease or cardiac arrhythmias, the potential chronotropic and inotropic stimulation from even the beta$_2$-selective bronchodilators poses some risk for cardiac morbidity. Optimal treatment in this setting has yet to be defined. One reasonable approach is to continue to use the inhaled beta-agonists as first-line bronchodilator therapy but to reduce by 50 percent the dose given with each treatment and to administer the drug with close cardiac monitoring.

Beta-agonist bronchodilators have proved to be effective in treating asthmatic exacerbations even among patients chronically receiving sympathomimetic bronchodilators for treatment of their asthma. Clinically significant tolerance to their activity does not appear to develop (unlike the response of myocardial tissue to chronic administration of sympathomimetic drugs). In addition, severe airflow obstruction does not preclude use of the inhaled bronchodilators. Despite concern that in severely obstructed patients one might be unable to deliver medication to the lung periphery by this route of administration, maximal achievable bronchodilation is obtained with the inhaled beta-agonists even among patients with an initial FEV_1 less than 1 liter.

Theophylline

Over the last several years, the role of theophylline in the emergency department treatment of asthma has evolved considerably. Controlled clinical trials have demonstrated that, when used alone, intravenous aminophylline is a relatively weak bronchodilator, 3 to 4 times less effective than inhaled beta-agonists administered in the repetitive dose schedule described previously. Furthermore, when used in combination with the inhaled beta-agonists, intravenous aminophylline provides an insignificant increment in bronchodilation while causing additional adverse side effects, including tremor, nausea, anxiety, and palpitations. Effects of aminophylline other than bronchodilation, such as delaying diaphragmatic muscle fatigue, stimulating ventilatory drive, and improving ventricular contractile function, might constitute theoretic indications for the use of aminophylline in the emergency treatment of asthma, but there is no evidence to indicate actual clinical benefit from any of these nonbronchodilator activities.

By contrast, among stable asthmatic patients in the *outpatient* setting, the combination of theophylline and beta-agonists (the latter given in conventional doses by oral administration or by metered-dose inhaler) has repeatedly been demonstrated to effect additive bronchodilation. The differing responses observed in the outpatient setting and in the emergency department may reflect differences in the type or degree of bronchoconstrictor stimulation in the two circumstances or (more likely) may be a consequence of the much larger doses of inhaled beta-agonist medications that are delivered in the emergency department.

These observations suggest that the methylxanthines, if they have any role in the emergency care of asthmatic attacks, should be considered to play a relatively minor role. Some patients, in anticipation of their discharge home, will be given maintenance or loading doses of a methylxanthine; other patients will also receive a methylxanthine prior to their hospitalization for further treatment of their asthma. It should be emphasized, however, that the acute relief of airflow obstruction in the emergency department is not dependent on the use of a methylxanthine and bears no significant relation to the serum theophylline level.

In the patient who is not vomiting, maintenance and loading doses of methylxanthines can be achieved as well by oral as by intravenous administration. The rapidly absorbed elixirs of theophylline (e.g., Elixophyllin, 7 mg/kg as a full loading dose) give serum theophylline concentrations 1 hour after administration that are comparable to those achieved following intravenous aminophylline (5.6 mg/kg by bolus infusion over 20 minutes as a full loading dose). The loading doses of theophylline and aminophylline should be reduced by 50 percent or more in patients who were taking theophylline preparations within the 12 to 24 hours prior to presentation to the emergency department; loading doses should be omitted entirely in patients at risk for theophylline toxicity (e.g., patients who have taken large doses of theophylline, who have ingested theophylline-containing medications immediately prior to presentation, or who have symptoms suggestive of theophylline toxicity). The usual maintenance dose of theophylline is 8–10 mg/kg given in divided doses (the dosing schedule determined by the timed-release properties of the particular preparation chosen). For aminophylline, 0.6 mg/kg/hour by continuous intravenous infusion is the recommended maintenance dose in nonsmoking adults. Maintenance doses should be reduced in patients with a decreased rate of hepatic metabolism owing to congestive heart failure, primary liver disease, or coincident use of certain medications (including cimetidine, erythromycin, and ciprofloxacin); it may need to be increased in the (rare, it is hoped) patient who is an active cigarette smoker.

Anticholinergics

Plant derivatives with anticholinergic properties, including atropine and stramonium, are ancient remedies for asthma. Although atropine is an effective bronchodilator and can be given by inhalation, near complete systemic absorption across the respiratory tract mucosa causes problems with systemic anticholinergic side effects; atropine may also impede mucociliary clearance, predisposing to the development of mucus plugging. In 1987 a quaternary ammonium derivative of atropine, ipratropium bromide, was released in metered-dose inhaler form. This atropine congener has minimal systemic absorption and does not impede mucociliary function. However, the bronchodilator activity of ipratropium bromide, even when delivered in an experimental wet aerosol form, is less than that of the beta-adrenergic agonists for patients with asthma, and the onset of action is considerably slower (peak activity at approximately 60 min). Ipratropium bromide has not been approved for use in the treatment of asthma. It remains to be determined whether a particular subset of asthmatic patients can be identified who might benefit from anticholinergic therapy in the emergency treatment of their disease.

Oxygen

Supplemental oxygen by nasal cannulae should be administered to patients with arterial oxygen saturation less than 90 percent by oximetry or arterial blood gas determination. In some circumstances, it may be most practical to give empiric oxygen supplementation at 2 liters/minute to all patients older than 50 years with severe asthmatic exacerbations until initial improvement from bronchodilator therapy is observed.

Reassessment and Continued Treatment

After the initial bronchodilator treatments have been administered, repeat assessment of lung function should be performed, including measurement of arterial blood gases in patients with persistent respiratory distress and an FEV_1 or

PEFR less than or equal to 25 percent of normal. Despite continued administration of bronchodilators, in most asthmatic patients the rate of improvement in airflow obstruction slows after the initial 60 to 90 minutes of intensive therapy. If, after this initial therapy, asthmatic symptoms and severe airflow obstruction persist (e.g., $FEV_1 \leq 40\%$ of predicted), one can anticipate that a prolonged course of treatment will probably be needed, often necessitating hospitalization. At the other end of the spectrum, some patients will be free of symptoms and audible wheezing and on repeat assessment will manifest expiratory flows in excess of 60 to 65 percent of predicted; such patients can probably be discharged home with little likelihood of a recurrent flare of asthma soon after discharge (i.e., a "relapse"). Most patients will fall in between these two ends of the spectrum, having some persistent asthmatic symptoms and values of FEV_1 or PEFR between 40 and 60 percent of predicted. These patients should receive additional bronchodilator therapy in the emergency department, anticipating some further although slowed improvement. We recommend continuing with the inhaled beta-agonist bronchodilators; the frequency of administration is generally reduced to *hourly* treatments in order to minimize toxic side effects.

Corticosteroids

In patients whose asthma proves refractory to bronchodilator therapy, corticosteroids are the most potent treatment modality available. An important mechanism of their action is the suppression of the inflammatory component of asthma—the bronchial edema, cellular infiltration, and mucous hypersecretion that contribute prominently to airway narrowing. Thus, it is not surprising that this benefit derived from corticosteroids may not be observed for several hours to days following administration. In severe asthmatic attacks, corticosteroids supplement but do not replace intensive bronchodilator therapy.

Given the delay in onset of action of corticosteroids, it is questionable whether their administration has any impact on the outcome of treatment in the emergency department. On the other hand, for the same reason, their early administration is desirable in patients who manifest no or inadequate improvement with bronchodilators alone. A set of indications for the use of corticosteroids in the emergency treatment of asthma based on this reasoning is as follows: (1) patients who, after initial intensive bronchodilator therapy, remain symptomatic with an FEV_1 or PEFR less than or equal to 40 percent of predicted, (2) patients who present with an exacerbation of their asthma despite an optimal outpatient bronchodilator regimen and do not achieve values for FEV_1 or PEFR greater than or equal to 60 to 65 percent of predicted after inital emergency department treatment, (3) patients who present with an exacerbation of their asthma despite outpatient oral corticosteroid therapy, and (4) patients at particularly high risk for a poor outcome because of prior respiratory failure or recent frequent emergency department visits or hospitalizations for their asthma.

The optimal dose of corticosteroids is unknown. A common regimen is methylprednisolone, 60 to 125 mg as an intravenous bolus, repeated every 6–8 hours. Comparable oral doses appear to be equally effective. Potential adverse consequences from even the acute, short-term use of corticosteroids include gastrointestinal distress, blurring of vision, sleeplessness, potentiation of tremor induced by sympathomimetic drugs, hyperglycemia, fluid retention, psychosis, and aseptic necrosis of bone.

Ancillary Measures

The importance of adequate hydration to permit mobilization of tenacious secretions has been emphasized in the pediatric population, because small children are at risk of dehydration during severe exacerbations of their asthma. In adults with adequate access to water, increased fluid intake is not a necessary component of their treatment regimen.

Other measures designed to facilitate clearance of tenacious airway secretions, including chest physiotherapy, expectorants, and mucolytic agents, are generally not beneficial in the treatment of severe asthma and in some cases are potentially detrimental.

Antibiotics are probably prescribed too frequently in the treatment of asthmatic exacerbations. Most infectious exacerbations are viral in etiology and many exacerbations are not caused by infectious agents. Controlled studies have shown no improvement in outcome when patients with asthmatic exacerbations are treated with antibiotics irrespective of presenting symptoms. We would reserve empiric, broad-spectrum antibiotic treatment (e.g., ampicillin, erythromycin, tetracycline, or trimethoprim-sulfamethoxazole) for febrile patients with sputum purulence (in whom neutrophils rather than eosinophils account for the discolored sputum).

MANAGEMENT OF RESPIRATORY FAILURE IN ASTHMA

As noted previously, most patients with an exacerbation of their asthma present with hypocapnia. The finding of eucapnia (PCO_2 = 40 mm Hg) during an acute attack is an ominous sign indicating impending ventilatory failure. Hypercapnia that persists despite initial aggressive bronchodilator therapy should be considered a life-threatening emergency, usually requiring hospital admission into an intensive care unit setting. Besides very close monitoring of hemodynamics and gas exchange, such patients require maximal bronchodilator therapy plus immediate institution of corticosteroids. Inhaled beta-agonist bronchodilators can be administered as often as once every hour in patients who remain severely obstructed; some physicians have used continuous bronchodilator nebulization and delivery by face mask to ensure continued maximal bronchodilation. In children, intravenous isoproterenol has been used to achieve a maximal bronchodilator effect; in adults, this approach is to be discouraged because of the unacceptably high risk of myocardial injury even in the absence of preexisting coronary artery disease. Parenteral beta-agonists (epinephrine, 0.3 mg or terbutaline, 0.25 mg) are best given by subcutaneous injection; in the desperate circumstance of a hypotensive and apneic patient, epinephrine can also be squirted into the airways via the endotracheal tube. Once effective ventilation has been achieved with mechanical ventilation, beta-agonist bronchodilators should again be nebulized in-line with the ventilator tubing.

It is difficult to specify precise values for arterial PCO_2 at which intubation and mechanical ventilation become indicated in the asthmatic patient. Any patient with a PCO_2 greater than or equal to 50 mm Hg should be managed in a location where emergent intubation can be performed promptly. Important considerations in the decision to support ventilation mechanically are (1) the trend in serial PCO_2 values, (2) the patient's ability to cooperate with administration of inhaled bronchodilator therapy, (3) the bronchodilator response to initial therapy, and (4) the work of breathing. One would proceed more quickly toward mechanically assisted ventilation in patients who have rising PCO_2 values on serial determinations, are unable to cooperate with administration of medications (e.g., because of agitation or sedation), have had little response to initial intensive bronchodilator treatment, and have very labored breathing (e.g., diaphoretic, breathing $\geq$30 breaths/minute despite treatment).

In some extremely obstructed asthmatic patients, achieving adequate ventilation (i.e., correction of PCO_2 toward normal) proves difficult even by mechanical means owing to severely impaired expiratory flow and gas trapping. During mechanical ventilation, high inflation pressures may preclude increases in delivered tidal volume, and the long time required for exhalation may prevent increases in respiratory rate. In this extreme circumstance, the best initial strategy is "controlled mechanical hypoventilation": correct hypoxemia with supplemental oxygen, tolerate an elevated PCO_2 value despite mechanical ventilation, and avoid excessive inflation pressures during positive pressure breathing. As the airflow obstruction gradually improves with treatment, it will become possible to correct the hypercarbia safely.

DISPOSITION FROM THE EMERGENCY DEPARTMENT

The decision whether to admit a patient with asthma to the hospital or discharge him or her home is usually made on the basis of symptoms (wheezing and breathlessness) and physical examination (auscultation of wheezes). These criteria are imperfect, however, since as many as 15 to 20 percent of patients who are discharged home when free of symptoms and audible wheezes are likely to return to the emergency department with a relapse of their disease within 7 to 10 days. It should be remembered that the potent beta-agonist bronchodilators administered in the emergency department have a duration of action of only a few hours. To prevent a recurrence of asthmatic symptoms, it is usually necessary to intensify the treatment regimen that the patient was taking at the time of the exacerbation. For some, this may simply mean instituting a program of oral theophylline and inhaled beta-adrenergic agonists (e.g., slow-release theophylline, 300 mg by mouth twice daily, and albuterol by metered-dose inhaler, 2 puffs inhaled by mouth 4 times daily); in others already on these medications, a short course of oral corticosteroids is usually indicated (e.g., prednisone, 60 mg/day, tapered by 10-mg decrements every 3–4 days). In one controlled clinical trial, administration of methylprednisolone, 64 mg/day, tapered to zero over 8 days, reduced the rate of relapse from 21 percent to 6 percent. Follow-up medical contact should be scheduled for a short interval (e.g., within 5–7 days) following discharge home, especially in the steroid-treated patient, since the risk of recurrent symptoms is highest during this period.

CHRONIC OBSTRUCTIVE PULMONARY DISEASE

A variety of diseases may cause chronic airflow obstruction as their predominant pathophysiologic manifestation, but in this century, the term *chronic obstructive pulmonary disease* (COPD) has been used to refer to two particular pathologic processes, chronic bronchitis and emphysema. The use of one encompassing term is appropriate, since in any given patient, chronic bronchitis and emphysema almost always occur together in varying degrees, and our ability to distinguish the contribution of one or the other component to the overall clinical picture is quite limited. In addition, chronic bronchitis and emphysema account for the vast majority of cases of chronic obstructive diseases of the lung. An estimated 10 million Americans suffer chronic bronchitis and emphysema, with a high rate of associated disability. More than 60,000 deaths each year are attributable to these diseases.

PATHOPHYSIOLOGY

Chronic bronchitis is an inflammatory disease of the airways characterized by mucous hypersecretion and in some patients, chronic airflow obstruction. For the purpose of epidemiologic surveys, it is defined as the presence of cough and sputum production for at least 3 months of the year in at least 2 consecutive years. Although chronic exposure to certain dusts and irritant gases may cause occupational forms of chronic bronchitis (e.g., in miners or textile workers), cigarette smoking accounts for the vast majority of cases. The prevalence of chronic bronchitis among persons older than 45 years who smoke more than 20 cigarettes per day exceeds 50 percent. The prevalence of chronic bronchitis among cigar and pipe smokers is intermediate between that of cigarette smokers and nonsmokers.

The chronic productive cough of chronic bronchitis is caused by increased secretion of mucus into the airways. This mucous hypersecretion results predominantly from hyperplasia and hypertrophy of mucous glands in the central airways and may occur in the absence of significant limitation to expiratory airflow. However, in the bronchioles and smallest bronchi, inflammatory changes, including squamous metaplasia, edema, increased muscle mass, and submucosal fibrosis, do compromise the airway lumen. These pathologic findings in the peripheral airways are among the earliest changes detectable in young cigarette smokers; they are in large measure reversible with smoking cessation. On the other hand, with continued cigarette smoking, progression of these abnormalities can lead to clinically significant airflow obstruction.

Some patients with chronic bronchitis develop airway hyperreactivity, which manifests as episodic bronchoconstriction with wheezing. For instance, an acute tracheobronchitis may trigger a period of shortness of breath, wheezing, and reversibly increased airflow obstruction. This subset of patients can best be described as having "asthmatic bronchitis," since their disease behaves like asthma superimposed on the fixed airflow obstruction of chronic bronchitis and emphysema.

Unlike chronic bronchitis, emphysema is a disease not of the airways but of the lung parenchyma. It is defined in pathologic terms: permanent dilatation of airspaces with accompanying destruction of their walls. An important consequence of this degradative process is a diminution in the elasticity of the lungs. Lung elasticity determines the force with which the lungs tend to recoil to a smaller volume. The loss in elastic recoil that characterizes emphysema limits expiratory airflow by decreasing the driving pressure for exhalation (i.e., the pressure difference between alveolar pressure and atmospheric pressure) and by reducing the forces acting to hold airways open during exhalation.The expiratory airflow obstruction caused by emphysema, in which the primary site of the pathologic processes is the acinus, is indistinguishable from that caused by diseases principally involving the airways, such as chronic bronchitis and asthma.

Although some emphysematous changes are commonly found at postmortem examination in older persons, the severe, widespread emphysema that causes clinical illness is almost exclusively found in cigarette smokers. The only other known cause of clinically significant emphysema is the rare genetic disorder alpha$_1$-antitrypsin deficiency (also called alpha$_1$-protease inhibitor deficiency). This latter diagnosis may be suspected if emphysema develops in a nonsmoker, has its onset at an unusually young age (average age at onset of dyspnea in patients with alpha$_1$-antitrypsin deficiency who smoke cigarettes is 35–40 years), or is associated with a strong family history of emphysema. It can be diagnosed by blood test: The alpha$_1$-antitrypsin level is markedly reduced (usually less than 50% of normal). Confirmation can be obtained by electrophoretic identification of the abnormal alpha$_1$-antitrypsin protein in the peripheral blood; the most common variant form is referred to as protease inhibitor Z (PiZZ phenotype).

Recognition of the association between a deficiency of protease inhibitor function in the blood and the development of severe emphysema has served to shape current concepts of the pathogenesis of emphysema in cigarette smokers (with normal alpha$_1$-antitrypsin phenotype). Toxic components of cigarette smoke and its metabolic derivatives have been shown to inactivate the alpha$_1$-antitrypsin enzyme while at the same time recruiting elastase-secreting neutrophils. The resultant protease-antiprotease imbalance permits enzymatic degradation of lung tissue at the acinar level. The unique susceptiblity that explains why only 10 to 15 percent of cigarette smokers develop clinically significant emphysema remains to be elucidated.

Because emphysema is defined in terms of its pathology, this diagnosis can rarely be made with complete certainty antemortem. Clinical clues to the presence of emphysema in a patient with a long history of cigarette smoking (usually at least 30–40 years) and persistent airflow obstruction include (1) a reduced diffusing capacity for carbon monoxide (not found in chronic bronchitis or asthma), (2) persistently increased total lung capacity, and (3) radiographic demonstration of an increased total lung capacity (pulmonary hyperinflation). The latter finding is best recognized as flattening of the normal curvature of the domes of the diaphragm. Other radiographic signs of emphysema are hyperlucent lung zones and, in a small percentage of cases, bullae. Because of the uncertainties inherent in making these clinical correlations and also the tremendous fear that the diagnostic label "emphysema" evokes in the minds of some patients, one should be appropriately cautious in its application.

Patients with advanced chronic bronchitis and emphysema (FEV_1 <1.5 liters) may follow distinct paths in their gas exchange and hemodynamic responses to severe airflow obstruction. One group of patients (type A) will increase their resting level of ventilation despite the increased work of breathing that this act requires. As a result, they maintain PCO_2 values at or below normal, typically in association with only modest hypoxemia (PO_2 >60 mm Hg). Pulmonary hypertension, if present, is generally mild; cor pulmonale develops only very late in the natural history of this syndrome. Such patients are called "pink puffers," "pink" because of their adequate oxygenation, "puffers" because of the dyspnea and tachypnea that accompany their increased levels of ventilation.

Another group of patients (type B), in the face of identical degrees of airflow limitation, respond with more modest increases in ventilation—to levels that are insufficient to meet resting metabolic needs for excretion of carbon dioxide. The consequence is chronic hypercapnia (PCO_2 ≥45 mm Hg), respiratory acidosis, and, because of associated ventilation/perfusion mismatching, often profound hypoxemia. Acidosis and especially alveolar hypoxia are potent stimuli for pulmonary arteriolar vasoconstriction, which may lead in turn to the development of pulmonary hypertension and right heart failure (cor pulmonale). Patients who follow this path are called "blue bloaters," "blue" because of cyanosis, "bloaters" because of the fluid retention that characterizes right heart failure.

The precise cause(s) that accounts for these divergent patterns of chronic respiratory failure in COPD is (are) uncertain. In general, "pink puffers" have predominantly emphysematous COPD, whereas "blue bloaters" have predominantly chronic bronchitis or a mixture of chronic bronchitis and emphysema. It is possible that the work of breathing imposed by the two pathologic processes differs sufficiently so as to evoke two divergent ventilatory responses. Alternatively, the hypercapnia observed in type B patients may reflect a familial depression of the central (medullary) drive to respiration that becomes manifest only in the presence of a marked increase in the work of breathing. Regardless of the underlying mechanism(s), it is important to note that patients with severe COPD and chronic carbon dioxide retention are prone to worsening hypercapnia and respiratory acidosis with sleep, medications that depress respiratory drive, and any stress that further increases the work of breathing (e.g., respiratory tract infection, congestive heart failure, pneumothorax).

CLINICAL EVALUATION

History

Patients with symptomatic COPD typically have cough (often with mucoid sputum production), exertional dyspnea, or both, on a daily basis. Emergency department visits are frequently prompted by exacerbations of these symptoms: increased cough, increased sputum production or a change in the character of the sputum that is expectorated, or increased dyspnea. At other times, the presenting symptom may be the consequence of disordered gas exchange (hypoxemia with or without hypercapnia): confusion, anxiety, restlessness, headache, or, in the extreme, seizures or coma. In patients with cor pulmonale, an exacerbation of COPD may present with symptoms of worsening right heart failure, including lower extremity swelling, abdominal distention, or right upper quadrant abdominal discomfort owing to hepatic congestion. As in asthma, chest tightness and orthopnea are common symptoms during exacerbations in COPD and should not be misinterpreted as evidence for myocardial ischemia or pulmonary edema.

As with any chronic disease, evaluation of an exacerbation of COPD should focus on a search for potentially correctable precipitating events. Particularly common are respiratory tract infections, either viral or bacterial; fever, if present, strongly points to this diagnosis. However, an increase in sputum volume or the development of sputum purulence may also occur in the absence of demonstrable infection, perhaps in response to nonspecific airway irritants (e.g., air pollution). Thus, many exacerbations, although reversible, are triggered by events that cannot be specifically identified. Patients with COPD are at increased risk of spontaneous pneumothorax, which usually presents with increased dyspnea and chest pain. Sometimes, comorbid diseases may exacerbate COPD, causing patients to present with worsening dyspnea as their predominant symptom. Common among these illnesses are congestive (left ventricular) heart failure, pulmonary embolism, and any condition causing upper abdominal pain or distention, with consequent compromise of diaphragmatic function. Adverse effects of medications are another important cause of deterioration in COPD. Analgesics, cough suppressants, tranquilizers, and sleeping pills are common offenders, causing diminished central drive to respiration and, either directly or indirectly as a result of sedation, impaired cough reflex. Drugs with atropinic effects or side effects, including many over-the-counter cold remedies, may adversely affect mucociliary clearance; retained secretions and worsened airflow obstruction may ensue. Finally, some patients with COPD, especially those with asthmatic bronchitis, develop bronchoconstriction in response to beta-blocking drugs in the same manner as asthmatic patients, as described earlier.

Physical Examination

Physical findings common to all patients with obstructive lung diseases are prolongation of the expiratory phase of respiration and, with severe airflow obstruction, pulsus paradoxus. Other signs vary depending on the predominant underlying pathology (emphysema versus chronic bronchitis) and on the precipitating event. Patients with principally emphysematous COPD exhibit hyperinflation and hyperresonance on chest examination; breath sounds are generally distant and may be totally absent over bullous regions. On the other hand, in chronic bronchitic patients, hyperinflation is absent and signs of airway disease are common—that is, low- and high-pitched wheezes (commonly referred to as rhonchi and wheezes, respectively). These findings are particularly prevalent when respiratory tract infection and mucus hypersecretion have caused the deterioration. Inspiratory rales are occasionally heard at the lung bases in COPD, probably reflecting a component of atelectasis; care should be taken not to misinterpret this finding as indicative of congestive heart failure without additional supportive evidence.

The emergency department physician is often faced with the dramatic presentation of respiratory failure in patients with COPD. In some cases, the picture is that of severe respiratory distress: profound air hunger associated with cyanosis, tachypnea, tachycardia, and sometimes hypertension. Supplemental oxygen corrects the cyanosis but may not alleviate the dyspnea, which results mostly from the severe airflow obstruction and associated increased work of breathing. In other cases of respiratory failure, acute-on-chronic carbon dioxide retention is associated with a blunted respiratory drive: Respirations are inappropriately slow or shallow, or both, for the severity of blood gas derangement; at times only agonal respirations will be found. Cyanosis is likely and hypotension may be present. This latter presentation with respiratory depression is often associated with right heart failure in the "blue bloater" type of patient, giving rise to findings of jugular venous distention, hepatomegaly, hepatojugular reflux, peripheral edema, and ascites.

Laboratory Data

The diagnosis of COPD can be suspected on the basis of history—cough and dyspnea in a long-term cigarette smoker—and whenever possible should be confirmed with demonstration of airflow obstruction on pulmonary function testing. Since the majority of cigarette smokers never develop significant airflow obstruction, it is erroneous to assume a priori that dyspnea in a smoker is universally the result of COPD.

Spirometry in COPD typically reveals an obstructive pattern that is minimally improved following acute administration of a bronchodilator. In a large series of patients with COPD, the average immediate response to inhaled bronchodilator was a 15 percent increase in FEV_1. Note that any increase in expiratory flow that is expressed as a percentage increase will be magnified by a low initial value for expiratory flow.

Although there is a rough correlation between the severity of airflow obstruction and the degree of respiratory disability in COPD, individual adaptation to chronic airflow obstruction varies so widely that in any given patient one cannot accurately predict the degree of obstruction based on how dyspneic the patient is at presentation. It is useful to remember, however, that hypercapnia owing to COPD alone develops only when the FEV_1 falls below 1.5 liters, and usually to less than 1 liter. If hypercapnia is present in a patient with COPD and an FEV_1 greater than 1.5 liters, alternative causes for the carbon dioxide retention should be sought.

Arterial blood gases are a mandatory part of the evaluation of all significant exacerbations of COPD. Because cyanosis is an unreliable sign for the early detection of hypoxemia and because hypercapnia can be suspected based on physical examination only when it is extreme (causing asterixis and respiratory depression), arterial blood gases are needed to assess the extent of derangement in gas exchange. Determination of the presence of carbon dioxide retention is particularly important. If hypercapnia is present on the initial determination, arterial PCO_2 must be closely monitored throughout the course of treatment, since such patients are at risk for worsening hypercapnia, consequent respiratory depression, and apneic respiratory arrest. On the other hand, if hypercapnia is absent on the initial blood gas determination, the subsequent development of carbon dioxide retention during the course of treatment is generally uncommon unless respiratory depressant drugs are administered or an adverse event (e.g., pneumothorax or mucous plugging) supervenes.

Chest radiography is appropriate in the evaluation of patients with marked dyspnea or cough, or both, even in the presence of known COPD; the principal value is detection of any complicating cardiopulmonary diseases. For instance, pneumonia, pneumothorax, atelectasis, and congestive heart failure may be difficult to diagnose with certainty by physical examination in patients with severe COPD but could be identified on chest x-ray. In uncomplicated chronic bronchitis, the chest x-ray is unremarkable. There may be thickening of bronchial walls (seen as a parahilar ring shadow on the posteroanterior film) and a nonspecific increase in bronchovascular markings at the lung bases, but most often the chest x-ray is entirely normal. As noted previously, radiographic features suggestive of emphysema include hyperlucent lung fields, bullae, and signs of hyperinflation (flattened diaphragms, a narrow, vertically oriented cardiac silhouette, and increased retrosternal airspace on the lateral film). With the development of pulmonary arterial hypertension, one finds dilatation of central pulmonary arteries with rapid pruning of peripheral arterial branches ("winter tree" effect). If right heart failure ensues, the cardiac silhouette increases in diameter and the azygos vein may be enlarged. Pleural effusions are *not* caused by right heart failure alone.

An electrocardiogram is generally indicated, especially in patients who complain of chest tightness or heaviness as part of their presentation. In severe COPD, electrocardiographic abnormalities may be present even in the absence of myocardial ischemia. In right heart strain, one may find prominent R waves in the right precordial leads ($R > S$ in lead V_1), persistent S waves in leads I and V_5 or V_6, and peaked P waves in the inferior leads ("P pulmonale"). In some emphysematous patients, altered positioning of the heart in the thorax may cause poor R wave progression in the right precordial leads—changes that may be mistaken for anterior myocardial infarction.

DIFFERENTIAL DIAGNOSIS

There are numerous differential diagnoses to be considered in a patient with severe dyspnea and cough; these have been addressed in Chap. 7. Two particular circumstances deserve further mention here. First, patients with exacerbations of their COPD (e.g., secondary to an acute tracheobronchitis) are sometimes misdiagnosed as having acute pulmonary edema and are treated emergently with morphine sulfate (and diuretics) with adverse consequences. The confusion is not surprising when one considers some of the features that may characterize the acute presentation in COPD—namely, orthopnea, jugular venous distention, peripheral edema, and, occasionally, bibasilar inspiratory rales. A left ventricular early diastolic (S_3) gallop would indicate congestive heart failure but may be difficult to detect reliably in the tachypneic and tachycardic patient. Often the history of similar previous events allows rapid determination of the likely cause of this episode. In other ambiguous cases, one may be able to temporize until a chest radiograph can permit distinction between COPD and pulmonary edema.

Second, differentiation between pneumothorax and bullous lung disease may be difficult in patients with emphysematous COPD. More than one patient has had a chest tube mistakenly placed into an apical bulla in an urgent effort to relieve dyspnea thought secondary to a pneumothorax. Before making the diagnosis of pneumothorax, one must be confident that the visceral pleural line, with its typical convex curvature, can be identified. An incomplete line or one oriented horizontally or concave to the lung apex may represent the inferior margin of a bulla. If the distinction cannot be made with certainty on plain chest x-ray, computer-assisted tomography is often useful.

The differential diagnosis of hypercapnic respiratory failure is considered in detail in Chap. 15.

TREATMENT

The initial management decision in treating a patient with a severe exacerbation of COPD is whether mechanically assisted ventilation must be provided immediately. If the patient is comatose with agonal or absent respirations, the decision is straightforward: immediate ventilatory support must be instituted with either manual ventilation and a tightly held face mask (Ambu bag and mask) or with endotracheal intubation and manual or mechanical ventilation. In other patients, clinical judgment is necessary. An experienced physician will on clinical inspection alone be able to identify patients who have hypopneic respirations that are clearly too shallow and slow to maintain adequate ventilation. In addition, such patients generally have a depressed level of consciousness that makes cooperation with bronchodilator administration and other therapeutic maneuvers difficult. These patients have impending respiratory arrest; they, too, should receive immediate ventilatory support. In the majority of cases, however, especially when the patient is alert and cooperative, a decision regarding mechanical ventilation can await the results of arterial blood gas determination and response to initial therapeutic measures.

A specific numerical value for arterial PCO_2 that denotes inadequate spontaneous ventilation and a need for mechanical ventilation is difficult to define for patients who may have chronic hypercapnia and renal compensation for respiratory acidosis. Thus, a patient with chronic elevation of PCO_2 to 65 mm Hg who presents with an acute decompensation and blood gas results of $PCO_2 = 75$ mm Hg and pH $= 7.26$ can probably be managed initially with bronchodilator therapy and close blood gas monitoring rather than immediate intubation and mechanical ventilation despite the extreme hypercapnia. In the presence of hypercapnia, factors that would favor prompt institution of ventilatory support include a depressed mental status (impairing cough and impeding cooperation with administered therapies), severe acidemia (pH < 7.20–7.25), a very rapid (and therefore unsustainable) respiratory rate (≥ 30 breaths/min), and lack of improvement with initial bronchodilator treatment.

Severe hypoxemia can cause irreversible cerebral and myocardial injury. Thus, another immediate goal of emergency department treatment in severe COPD is correction of potentially life-threatening hypoxemia. Following sampling of arterial blood, low-flow supplemental oxygen should be administered. If, on blood gas analysis, the PO_2 is found to be 60 mm Hg or greater, supplemental oxygen can then be discontinued.

A key principle of oxygen administration in COPD is use of low inspired concentrations. Delivery of high inspired oxygen concentrations, such as uncontrolled face mask oxygen, is both unnecessary and potentially dangerous. It is unnecessary for two reasons: First, because ventilation/perfusion mismatching rather than shunt is the predominant mechanism of hypoxemia, relatively small increases in the inspired oxygen tension generally suffice to raise arterial PO_2 into a safe range; and second, because chronically hypoxemic patients have compensatory mechanisms that help them to adapt to their chronic hypoxemia, correction of the arterial PO_2 to normal is unnecessary. Uncontrolled oxygen administration is potentially dangerous in those patients with severe COPD and chronic hypercapnia because of the risk of inducing worsening carbon dioxide retention. The arterial PCO_2 may be caused to rise to levels that produce dangerous acidemia and central nervous system depression ("CO_2 narcosis") with resultant respiratory arrest. The risk of this outcome is minimized by use of supplemental oxygen in low concentrations.

A typical, empirically chosen initial method of administration is by nasal cannulae at 2 liters/minute or by Venturi mask at 24 percent oxygen concentration. The latter has the advantage of more precise control of the inspired oxygen concentration, whereas the former is often better tolerated by patients, who may experience a sense of suffocation with a mask that covers nose and mouth. It is important to repeat the measurement of arterial blood gases following oxygen administration (allowing approximately 20 minutes for establishment of equilibrium at the new oxygen concentration) to ensure that the PO_2 has increased to approximately 55 to 70 mm Hg (the high end of this range being the target in patients with concomitant coronary artery disease) and that the PCO_2 has not risen excessively.

Patients who remain profoundly hypoxemic despite low-flow oxygen supplementation should receive small increments in the delivered oxygen concentration, monitoring the arterial blood gas response. It is not acceptable to withhold further oxygen supplementation in the hypoxemic patient ($PO_2 < 50$ mm Hg) because of concern that arterial PCO_2 will rise too high. If adequate oxygenation cannot be achieved without inducing severe hypercapnia, mechanically assisted ventilation must be instituted. The prevention of severe hypoxemia takes therapeutic precedence.

This same principle applies to the patient brought to the emergency department having been misguidedly given uncontrolled supplemental oxygen (e.g., by ambulance personnel). The delivery system providing oxygen at a high concentration should be replaced by low-flow oxygen; it should not be simply removed entirely. Allowing the severely hypercapnic patient to breathe room air would potentially result in dangerous degrees of hypoxemia more rapidly than in correction of the elevated PCO_2.

At the same time that the patient's ventilatory status is being assessed and adequate oxygenation ensured, treatment of airflow obstruction should be instituted. Bronchodilators are the mainstay of therapy, and inhaled beta-adrenergic agonists provide the most potent bronchodilation with the most rapid onset of action. Side effects are minimized when beta-agonists are given by inhalation as opposed to parenteral administration, but even by the inhaled route, cardiac stimulation is common. Because COPD is generally a disease of middle-aged and older patients, who may have known cardiac disease or who, by virtue of their age, are at risk for occult coronary artery disease, beta-agonist bronchodilators cannot be given with the same impunity as in the young patient with asthma. Which drugs in which doses provide effective bronchodilation with the least risk of cardiovascular toxicity remains to be defined. Based on knowledge currently available, it seems reasonable to administer aerosolized beta-agonists as first-line therapy in COPD, but to reduce the standard nebulized dose of medication by 25 to 50 percent in patients with known or suspected coronary artery disease. Where available, continuous electrocardiographic monitoring should be performed in such patients.

Anticholinergic therapy offers a potential alternative to sympathomimetics for acute bronchodilation. In studies of patients with COPD, anticholinergic drugs have proved equipotent to beta-agonists in terms of bronchodilation, and in some circumstances, the two types of drugs appear to have an additive bronchodilator effect. Because it is poorly absorbed across the respiratory tract mucosa, the atropine congener ipratropium bromide causes minimal cardiac stimulation when given by inhalation. The major disadvantage of ipratropium bromide is its delayed onset of action (15 minutes) and time to peak effect (approximately 60 minutes). A solution of ipratropium bromide suitable for nebulization is not currently available in the United States. When it does become approved for use in this country, nebulized ipratropium bromide may come to play an important role in emergency department treatment of COPD.

When used in combination with beta-adrenergic agonists, theophylline adds little if any bronchodilation. Some controlled clinical trials have shown no advantage to the use of theophylline together with beta-agonists in hospitalized patients with COPD, and an acute bronchodilator benefit in the emergency department seems unlikely. If toxic side effects prevent administration of full doses of inhaled beta-agonists, it is possible that theophylline in combination with reduced sympathomimetic doses might provide additive bronchodilation with reduced toxicity.

A theoretic indication for the use of theophylline in COPD is its stimulatory effect on diaphragmatic contractility. Experimental evidence indicates that theophylline delays the onset of diaphragmatic muscle fatigue; in theory, by this mechanism it might forestall the development of hypercapnic respiratory failure in some patients with exacerbations of COPD. It remains conjectural, however, whether this observed effect of theophylline is clinically beneficial.

Based on the nature of the underlying disease processes, one might predict that corticosteroids would be of little benefit in purely emphysematous COPD, whereas they might exert a beneficial anti-inflammatory effect in chronic bronchitis, and especially in asthmatic bronchitis. Sometimes it is possible to identify patients who are likely to be steroid responsive. Clinical studies suggest that patients with a large reversible component to their airflow obstruction on pulmonary function testing before and after bronchodilator and patients with a history of episodic wheezing and bronchospasm (asthmatic-like attacks) are most likely to derive improvement in airflow obstruction from a brief course of corticosteroids. At other times, among severely ill patients with COPD who require hospitalization for respiratory failure, all patients without a firm contraindication should receive corticosteroids. An accelerated rate of improvement has been demonstrated in this situation, and it is impossible to determine which patients will not derive benefit from use of corticosteroids. One regimen for steroid administration in this setting is 0.5 mg/kg of methylprednisolone by intravenous bolus every 6 hours.

Patients with exacerbations of their COPD characterized by increased cough and sputum production, especially when accompanied by fever and a change in the character of the sputum from mucoid to purulent, should receive antibiotic therapy. Admittedly, many such exacerbations are not caused by a bacterial or mycoplasma infection, but our ability to determine which patients do have treatable infections is poor, and withholding antibiotics in those with bacterial or mycoplasma infection leads to increased morbidity and possibly mortality. *Streptococcus pneumoniae* (pneumococcus) and *Hemophilus influenzae* are common isolates from the sputa of patients with COPD, and antibiotics such as ampicillin, tetracycline, trimethoprim-sulfamethoxazole, and some cephalosporins (e.g., cefaclor) provide good coverage. In the absence of pneumonia, any one of these antibiotics can be given empirically—that is, without the benefit of sputum gram stain and culture results.

Finally, diuretic therapy may be of help in patients who present with right heart failure and peripheral edema. By reducing pulmonary capillary blood volume, diuretics may improve gas exchange acutely. Oxygen administration facilitates this process by reducing pulmonary arterial hypertension, with consequent improvements in right heart output and left ventricular filling. On the other hand, digitalis is not indicated for treatment of right heart failure, since it is minimally effective as a right ventricular inotrope and carries an increased risk of toxicity in the presence of hypoxemia and electrolyte and acid–base shifts, to which patients with COPD are susceptible.

DISPOSITION FROM THE EMERGENCY DEPARTMENT

When available, information about the extent of airflow obstruction and gas exchange derangement at a time when the patient is at a baseline level of function proves extremely valuable in deciding which patients with COPD exacerbations can be safely managed at home following emergency department treatment. Thus, for one patient, an $FEV_1 = 0.7$ liters and $PCO_2 = 52$ mm Hg may represent an acute decompensation with severe breathlessness and respiratory failure necessitating hospitalization, whereas, for another patient, these same values may indicate a chronic level of function being maintained satisfactorily at home. In the absence of baseline data, judgments must be made based on the severity of the patient's symptoms, descriptions of the patient's functional status at baseline, and the patient's capacity for independent or assisted self-care.

A common misconception is that supplemental oxygen can be prescribed for use at home on an as-needed basis in the outpatient management of episodic bouts of dyspnea. In most cases, dyspnea indicates worsened airflow obstruction, not primarily hypoxemia; and bronchodilators are the treatment of choice for the acute relief of airflow obstruction, not oxygen. Supplemental oxygen at home is indicated for relief of *chronic* hypoxemia (defined as a $PO_2 \leq 55$ mm Hg, or ≤ 59 mm Hg in the presence of cor pulmonale or secondary erythrocytosis) and should be prescribed on a continuous or at least nocturnal (8–12 hours/day) basis. Determination of the need for long-term oxygen supplementation should be made after optimization of the patient's medical regimen and clinical status, not during an acute flare of illness.

BRONCHIECTASIS

Bronchiectasis is a localized irreversible dilatation of the bronchi owing to inflammation and necrosis in the bronchial walls. If the bronchiectatic changes are widespread, the disease may be characterized by chronic airflow obstruction, usually with an associated restrictive component resulting from atelectasis and peribronchial inflammation. Bronchiectasis is also a chronic suppurative lung disease: Bronchiectatic airways are usually permanently infected with bacteria (or occasionally mycobacteria). Owing to loss of the integrity of the bronchial mucosa and the normal bronchial clearance mechanisms, antibiotics can suppress but not eradicate the persistent infection. As a result, many patients with bronchiectasis have chronic purulent sputum production. Two complications commonly precipitate emergency department visits: acute febrile exacerbations characterized by increased cough and sputum production, and hemoptysis.

Bronchiectasis is generally caused by a necrotizing bronchopneumonia that receives no or inadequate treatment; permanent destruction and dilatation of the bronchial wall is the sequela. Staphylococcus and gram-negative bacilli can produce bronchiectasis; pneumococcus does not. Extensive reactivation tuberculosis is commonly associated with bronchiectasis, but because of effective gravitational drainage of secretions from the upper lobes, chronic suppuration does not develop ("dry bronchiectasis"). Bronchiectasis may also occur when infection develops distal to an obstructing endobronchial mass or foreign body. This possibility should be ruled out by bronchoscopy when focal bronchiectasis develops de novo in an adult. Important causes of diffuse bronchiectasis include cystic fibrosis, the immotile cilia syndrome (including Kartagener's syndrome), and hypogammaglobulinemia.

Bronchiectasis is suggested by the presence of daily cough with purulent sputum, often in prodigious amounts. If left undisturbed in a container for several hours, the sputum will often settle into three separate layers: frothy on top, purulent in the middle, and mucoid at the bottom. A history of repetitive intermittent hemoptysis is common. Sinusitis is a frequent associated finding. Physical findings often include the presence of focal inspiratory rales in the area of bronchiectasis. These rales may suggest the presence of an acute pneumonia, but they can be heard chronically, even when the patient is free of acute symptoms. Clubbing may be present.

The diagnosis of bronchiectasis may be suggested by abnormalities on the plain chest radiograph. Most often one finds increased markings in the orientation of bronchovascular bundles; partial segmental or lobar atelectasis may be associated. The clue to the correct diagnosis is the chronicity of these findings: Bronchiectatic changes will be present on old films obtained prior to the acute illness that prompted the emergency department visit. Certain radiographic findings, if present, point specifically to a diagnosis of bronchiectasis. These include parallel linear opacities ("tram-lines") representing thickened bronchial walls seen in longitudinal section and grouped cystic structures, representing cystic bronchiectasis.

Prior sputum culture results may also give a clue to the presence of bronchiectasis, since the pathogens that infect bronchiectatic airways tend to be relatively limited. Staphylococcus, *Hemophilus influenzae*, and pseudomonas are the most common bacteria. Isolation of pseudomonas species in this setting is particularly telling, since in the absence of neutropenia or a tracheostomy, this organism is otherwise rarely found in the sputa of ambulatory patients.

In the past, definitive diagnosis of bronchiectasis required bronchography, during which an oil-based iodinated contrast agent was used to coat the airways prior to fluoroscopic examination. The morbidity of this procedure contributed to its decline from contemporary use. Computed tomography (CT) using current generation scanners has proved sufficiently sensitive to detect most cases of bronchiectasis. As a result, CT scanning has almost entirely replaced bronchography when radiographic confirmation of the clinical diagnosis is sought.

Patients with bronchiectasis typically present to the emergency department not with a bronchospastic exacerbation, as in asthma and COPD, but with worsening pulmonary infection. The chest radiograph may show denser or more extensive infiltrate in areas of previous (chronic) abnormality. Such a patient is often diagnosed as having recurrent pneumonia, and, as such, the cause may seem mysterious. In fact, the infection represents an exacerbation of chronic pulmonary suppuration. As noted, hemoptysis is common in bronchiectasis; empyema and bronchopleural fistula are rare complications.

The mainstays of treatment in bronchiectasis are antibiotics and postural drainage; bronchodilators are added when significant airflow obstruction is present. The choice of antibiotics should be guided by the pathogen isolated from the sputum. It is only recently that an oral antibiotic, ciprofloxacin, has become available for ambulatory treatment of pseudomonas infections. Severe exacerbations in which pseudomonas plays a role should be treated with two synergistic antipseudomonas antibiotics, which usually requires at least initial hospitalization for intravenous antibiotic administration.

Hemoptysis associated with bronchiectasis usually subsides within a few days of initiation of effective antibiotic treatment. Occasionally, bronchiectasis may cause massive and life-threatening hemoptysis. Until recently, bronchoscopic identification of the bleeding site and prompt surgical resection was the preferred management of massive hemoptysis. More recently, an alternative, nonsurgical approach has become available in the form of bronchial artery embolization. In the hands of skilled and experienced interventional radiologists, this angiographic technique has proved highly successful in terminating hemoptysis without sacrificing functional lung tissue. It is particularly suited for the patient who is a poor surgical candidate because of extensive bilateral bronchiectasis and limited ventilatory reserve.

SELECTED READING

Asthma

Boushey, HA, et al. Bronchial hyperreactivity. *Am Rev Respir Dis* 121:389, 1980.

Brenner, BE, Abraham E, and Simon, RR. Position and diaphoresis in acute asthma. *Am J Med* 74:1005, 1983.

Fanta, CH, Rossing, TH, and McFadden, ER, Jr. Glucocorticoids in acute asthma: A critical controlled trial. *Am J Med* 74:845, 1983.

Fiel, SB, et al. Efficacy of short-term corticosteroid therapy in outpatient treatment of acute bronchial asthma. *Am J Med* 75:259, 1983.

Martin, TG, Elenbaas, RM, and Pingleton, SH. Use of peak expiratory flow rates to eliminate unnecessary arterial blood gases in acute asthma. *Ann Emerg Med* 11:70, 1982.

McFadden, ER, Jr. Pathogenesis of asthma. *J Allergy Clin Immunol* 73:413, 1984.

McFadden, ER, Jr, and Lyons, HA. Arterial-blood gas tension in asthma. *N Engl J Med* 278:1027, 1968.

Rossing, TH, et al. Emergency therapy of asthma: Comparison of the acute effects of parenteral and inhaled sympathomimetics and infused aminophylline. *Am Rev Respir Dis* 122:365, 1980.

Siegel, D, et al. Aminophylline increases the toxicity but not the efficacy of an inhaled beta-adrenergic agonist in the treatment of acute exacerbations of asthma. *Am Rev Respir Dis* 132:283, 1985.

Zieverink, SE, et al. Emergency room radiography of asthma: An efficacy study. *Radiology* 145:27, 1982.

Chronic Obstructive Pulmonary Disease

Albert, RK, Martin, TR, and Lewis, SW. Controlled clinical trial of methylprednisolone in patients with chronic bronchitis and acute respiratory insufficiency. *Ann Intern Med* 92:753, 1980.

Anthonisen, NR, et al. Antibiotic therapy in exacerbations of chronic obstructive pulmonary disease. *Ann Intern Med* 106:196, 1987.

Anthonisen, NR, Wright, EC, and the IPPB Trial Group. Bronchodilator response in chronic obstructive pulmonary disease. *Am Rev Respir Dis* 113:814, 1986.

Bone, RC, Pierce, AK, and Johnson, RL, Jr. Controlled oxygen administration in acute respiratory failure in chronic obstructive pulmonary disease: A reappraisal. *Am J Med* 65:896, 1978.

Ishikawa, K, Eddleman, EE, Jr, and Pipberger, HV. Electrocardiograms in pulmonary emphysema mimicking myocardial infarction: A frequent dilemma. *Med Ann DC* 39:20, 1970.

Nocturnal Oxygen Therapy Trial Group. Continuous or nocturnal oxygen therapy in hypoxemic chronic obstructive lung disease: A clinical trial. *Ann Intern Med* 93:391, 1980.

Rebuck, AS, et al. Nebulized anticholinergic and sympathomimetic treatment of asthma and chronic obstructive airways disease in the emergency room. *Am J Med* 82:59, 1987.

Rice, KL, et al. Aminophylline for acute exacerbations of chronic obstructive pulmonary disease: A controlled trial. *Ann Intern Med* 107:305, 1987.

U.S. Public Health Service. The Health Consequences of Smoking: Chronic Obstructive Lung Disease. A Report of the Surgeon General, 1984. US DHHS Publication No. (PHS) 84-50205.

Bronchiectasis

Barker, AF, and Bardana, EJ, Jr. Bronchiectasis: Update of an orphan disease. *Am Rev Respir Dis* 137:969, 1988.

Grenier, P, et al. Bronchiectasis: Assessment by thin-section CT. *Radiology* 161:95, 1986.

Remy, J, et al. Treatment of hemoptysis by embolization of bronchial arteries. *Radiology* 122:33, 1977.

Rivera, M, and Nicotra, MB. *Pseudomonas aeruginosa* mucoid strain: Its significance in adult chest diseases. *Am Rev Respir Dis* 126:833, 1982.

11. Pulmonary Edema

CARDIOGENIC PULMONARY EDEMA

John Gaca

Pulmonary edema, the result of extravascular fluid accumulation in the pulmonary interstitial and alveolar air spaces, causes abnormal lung mechanical function and altered respiratory gas exchange. Hypoxia and tissue hypoxemia are the consequence.

Acute or chronic left ventricular failure is probably the most common cause of pulmonary edema. Other etiologies, however, can produce pulmonary edema. They do so by distinctly different pathophysiologic processes than those operational in left ventricular decompensation.

A review of the pathogenesis of cardiogenic pulmonary edema (CPE) will clarify the relationship among several abnormalities of left heart function and the common pathway to the development of pulmonary edema–elevated pulmonary capillary pressure. This will be contrasted to the processes in noncardiogenic pulmonary edema (NCPE).

A clear understanding of the pathogenesis of pulmonary edema will allow for a rational approach to all types of pulmonary edema. In this chapter, guidelines for the diagnosis and optimal management of the cardiovascular abnormalities resulting in CPE are presented.

PATHOGENESIS

Efficient oxygen and carbon dioxide exchange requires anatomic proximity of the pulmonary capillaries and the alveoli. Fluid flux occurs between these two structures. This exchange is governed by factors described in the Starling equation (see below). Normally, a small amount of fluid is filtered from the pulmonary capillaries into the interstitium. Net fluid exchange is controlled by the balance between the hydrostatic and protein oncotic pressures within the pulmonary vasculature relative to the same pressures in the surrounding interstitial tissue. The alveolar membrane is relatively impermeable to this fluid under normal circumstances. Therefore, the rate at which fluid exits the pulmonary capillaries and the rate of its lymphatic drainage determines whether pulmonary edema develops (Fig. 11-1).

The alveolar membrane's "impermeability" has a pressure limit, and edema fluid in severe CPE gains access to this space. Moreover, injuries that increase the endothelial and epithelial permeability as seen in some forms of NCPE may produce much more severe abnormalities in pulmonary function than would result if only the endothelial lining were affected.

The Starling equation enables an understanding of the factors that regulate the exchange of fluid across the capil-

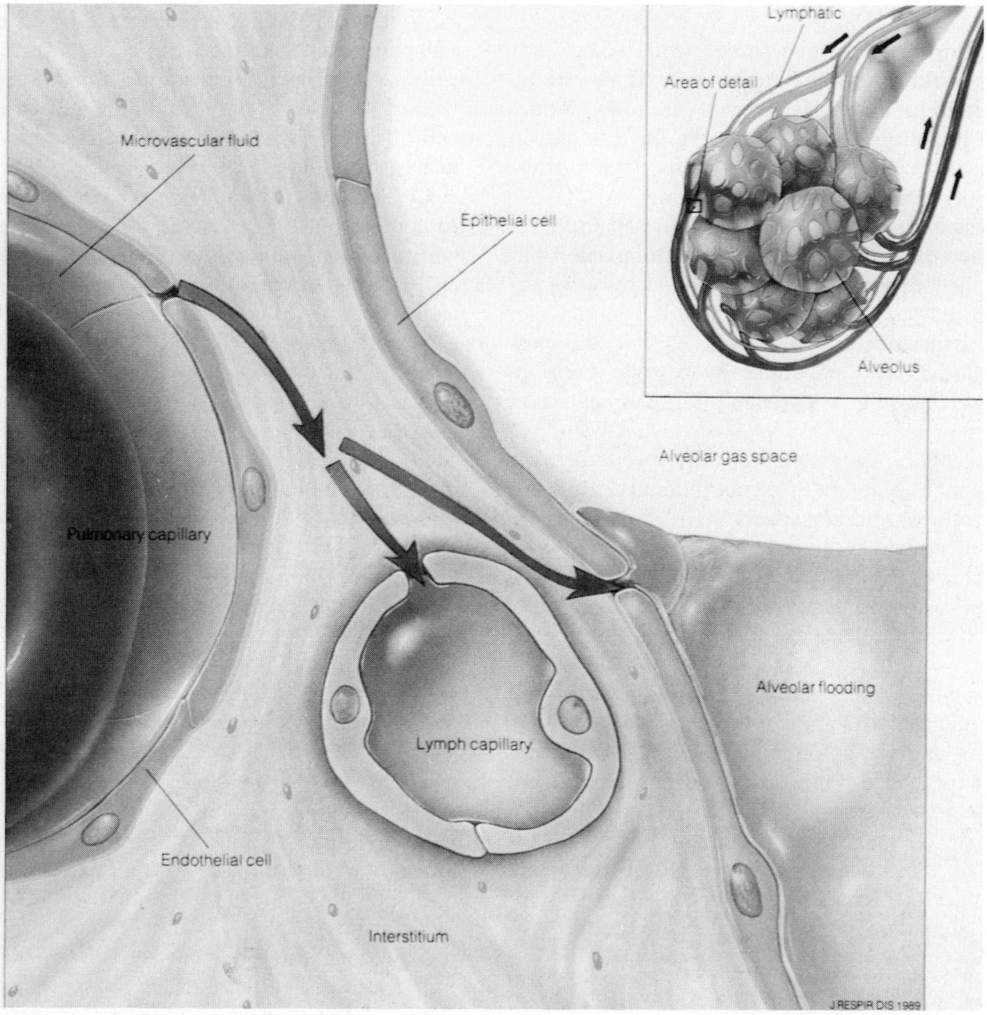

Fig. 11-1. Elevated pulmonary capillary pressure secondary to heart failure causes an increased flow of microvascular fluid through the endothelial cell barrier. Pulmonary lymphatics are unable to drain the excess fluid, causing alveolar flooding and pulmonary edema. Normally, the fluid drains through the interstitium along a hydraulic gradient to the lymph capillaries; little or no fluid enters the alveoli because of the relative impermeability of the alveolar wall. Elevated pulmonary capillary pressure may also interact with increased membrane permeability or reduced plasma osmotic pressure to increase microvascular fluid flow sufficiently to produce pulmonary edema. (From A.H. Gradman and E. Mostoufi-Moab. Cardiogenic pulmonary edema: Multiple causes and therapies. *J. Resp. Dis.* 10:68, 1989.)

lary membrane:

$$Q = K(S) \cdot [(P_c - P_i) - \sigma(\pi_c - \pi_i)]$$

where:

Q: the net flow out of the pulmonary capillaries into the interstitium.

K: a constant; the hydraulic conductance. It is a function of capillary permeability.

P_c: the hydrostatic pressure inside the capillary.

P_i: the hydrostatic pressure inside the interstitium.

σ: the reflection coefficient characterizing the ease with which proteins cross the capillary membrane.

π_c: the intracapillary plasma oncotic pressure.

π_i: the interstitial oncotic pressure.

Usually, P_c is directly related to pulmonary capillary pressure and *is the primary factor involved in the genesis of CPE.*

σ, the reflection coefficient, represents the effective gradient across the pulmonary capillary *for a given protein.* It is another indication of membrane permeability. If the membrane is abnormally permeable, the difference between capillary and interstitial oncotic pressure ($\pi_c - \pi_i$) is reduced and fluid flows more freely into the interstitial space at any level of hydrostatic driving pressure.

Analysis of the Starling equation shows that the formation of pulmonary edema is controlled by three important factors: pulmonary capillary pressure, membrane permeability, and plasma oncotic pressure.

Any increase of hydrostatic pulmonary capillary pressure, typically occurring with left ventricular failure, increases fluid flow out of the pulmonary capillaries. Equally important vis à vis the pathogenesis of NCPE, any increase in membrane permeability or reduction in plasma oncotic pressure has a similar effect. The development of pulmonary edema is not solely the responsibility of disordered left heart function.

It is particularly important that some of the factors may interact to increase fluid flow sufficiently to produce pulmonary edema; mild to moderate elevation of pulmonary capillary pressure in the clinical situation where there is associated low plasma oncotic pressure or increased membrane permeability could result in pulmonary edema.

The pulmonary lymphatics drain the increased fluid deposited in the interstitium. Any increase in pulmonary capillary pressure is accompanied by a parallel increase in the production of pulmonary lymph. As interstitial lung water increases, active lymphatic flow increases. As fluid is deposited into the interstitium, interstitial hydrostatic pressure rises. This tends to offset the heightened pulmonary capillary pressure.

When the capacity of these compensatory mechanisms is exceeded, peribronchial and perivascular edema occurs. Alveolar flooding follows at a later time.

As a corollary, any impediment of lymphatic drainage, such as carcinomatous lymphatic obstruction or elevated pressure in the systemic venous system where it is joined by the thoracic duct, will facilitate the formation of pulmonary edema.

At the onset of CPE, the increase in interstitial fluid will not seriously impair gas exchange. Once alveolar "flooding" occurs, there are more pronounced ventilation/perfusion mismatches and increased pulmonary shunting. Significant hypoxemia is the consequence.

The pulmonary stretch receptors are stimulated with interstitial edema. This causes respiratory distress and tachypnea. Pulmonary compliance is decreased. At the alveolar flooding stage, these abnormalities are more pronounced.

CLINICAL PRESENTATION AND ASSESSMENT

Several pathophysiologic events result in the physical signs of acute cardiogenic pulmonary edema:

1. Increased pulmonary capillary hydrostatic pressure
2. Desaturation of arterial blood
3. Diminished cutaneous blood flow
4. Intense sympathetic nervous system activity
5. Bronchiolar edema

Increased pulmonary capillary hydrostatic pressure causes the net deposition of fluid in the compliant pulmonary capillary–alveolar interstitium. The progression to frank alveolar edema causes breathlessness, tachypnea, orthopnea, and wet rales.

Desaturation of arterial blood develops as alveolar edema forms. The decreased cutaneous blood flow is a compensatory mechanism to preserve blood flow to more vital organs. Cyanosis results.

Intense sympathetic nervous system activity causes diaphoresis, peripheral vasoconstriction, cool moist skin, and tachycardia.

Bronchiolar edema can result in bronchospasm, causing wheezes and rhonchi.

The initial clinical presentation of CPE is somewhat similar to that of NCPE. Extreme breathlessness is apparent, and the patient is cyanotic, diaphoretic, and tachypnic. Moist rales, as well as wheezes and rhonchi, are auscultated. Accessory muscles of respiration are maximally utilized to accomplish the increased work of breathing required by the decreased lung compliance.

CPE is a low flow state with a cool and mottled periphery. In contrast, NCPE is usually a hyperdynamic illness with a warm and vasodilated periphery. This is due to the fact that NCPE is usually associated with an underlying disease (e.g., trauma, sepsis, pancreatitis). CPE is usually associated with a distinct acute cardiac event such as an acute myocardial infarction or endocarditis.

Auscultation may aid in the diagnosis. CPE is usually associated with traditional evidence of left ventricular failure such as the S_3 gallop. The presence of characteristic murmurs may indicate an etiology. Patients with NCPE do not manifest an S_3 unless volume is overloaded.

It should be emphasized that the history and physical examination cannot be relied on to distinguish CPE from NCPE. S_3 can be heard in the overhydrated patient with adult respiratory distress syndrome (ARDS); in those patients with NCPE who have inadequate filling pressures or associated cardiac disease, vasoconstriction with cool mottled extremities may prevail.

CHEST ROENTGENOGRAPHY

In pulmonary edema, fluid does not collect uniformly throughout the lungs. The radiographic distribution is determined by the cause of pulmonary edema. A principally basal and perihilar pattern is most typical of CPE. A peripheral patchy distribution is characteristic of ARDS. There are reasons for these pathoanatomic differences.

The lungs include a range of anatomic compartments. Blood flow in the lungs includes both pulmonary and bronchial circulations. The pulmonary circulation is a relatively compliant high-capacity system.

When the fluid filtration exceeds removal across the pulmonary lymphatic circulation in CPE, edema fluid collects in the perivascular and peribronchiolar interstitial spaces. Before this happens, however, the compliant pulmonary arterial system attempts adjustment. There is redistribution of intrapulmonary blood flow to the upper lobes of the lungs, causing apical plumping of pulmonary vessels. With increasing venous pressure, there is decreased flow to the lower lobes, caused by increasing basilar interstitial edema. Apparent blood flow to the upper zones increases. At this point, the compensatory mechanisms have been overwhelmed. The increasing interstitial edema gains access to the alveolar spaces.

The sequence of roentgenographic changes that occur with CPE are as follows:

1. *Perivascular cuffing:* The well-defined pulmonary arteries lose their definition and become blurred.
2. *Perihilar hazing:* With increasing interstitial edema, the hilar borders become ill-defined (Fig. 11-2A).
3. *Septal lines:* The edema collected in the lymphatics causes the normally nonvisible channels to become distended and form sharp linear densities that extend from

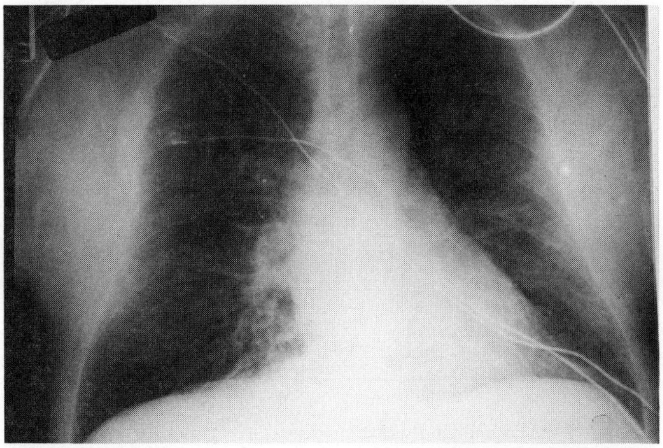

A

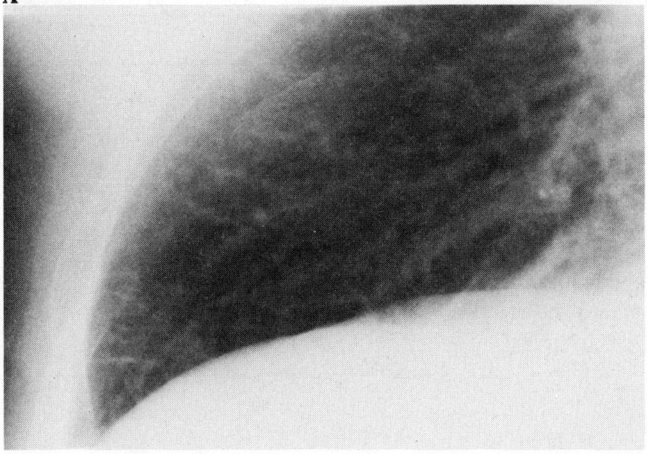

B

Fig. 11-2. Portable anteroposterior chest radiograph in a patient with congestive heart failure. The cardiac silhouette is enlarged, the bilateral infiltrates are predominantly perihilar, and Kerley B lines (horizontal lines extending to the pleural margin) are present at the lung periphery (B).

the pleural surface toward the center of the chest (Kerley B lines) (Fig. 11-2B).

4. *Subpleural fluid:* Fluid may accumulate in the subpleural spaces.
5. *Alveolar pulmonary edema:* As the volume and pressure of interstitial fluid becomes greater than the ability of the pulmonary lymphatics to cope with it, fluid moves into the alveolus. The density of the fluid appears the same as that of pneumonia but is highly gravity-dependent and will vary with the patient's position (Fig. 11-3A).

NCPE that results from primary alveolar–capillary membrane damage causes pulmonary edema that is pathophysiologically and roentgenographically different from CPE. Here it is not a primary alteration in the hydrostatic Starling forces but a diffuse injury to the alveolar–capillary membrane. This results in abnormally increased alveolar–capillary membrane permeability in the presence of a low or normal pulmonary capillary hydrostatic pressure. The diffuse nature of the injury causes the peripheral, patchy distribution of edema in the chest x-ray of NCPE (Figs. 11-3B and 11-4).

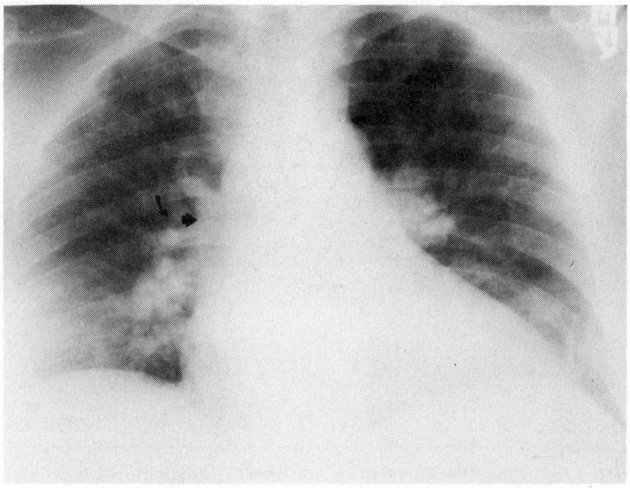

A

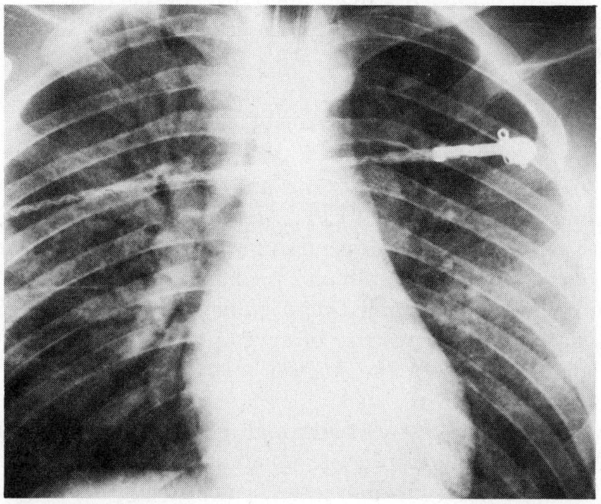

B

Fig. 11-3. A. Heart failure. The heart is large, and the pulmonary circulation appears engorged. The vascular pedicle width, delineated by the horizontal arrows, is increased. On the right, the margin occurs where the superior vena cava crosses the upper margin of the right main-stem bronchus. On the left, the pedicle is delineated by the margin of the left subclavian artery at the aorta. The angle formed by the right superior pulmonary vein crossing the descending artery (curved arrow) is obliterated. A relatively uniform haze is apparent in the lower lung field. B. Adult respiratory distress syndrome, with diffuse pulmonary edema and air bronchograms. The vascular pedicle is small. There are no signs of interstitial fluid, but uniform, diffuse, widespread haziness in the lung field reflects extensive cortical involvement. (From F. Mishkin. Radiological findings in acute pulmonary edema. *IM: Internal Medicine for the Specialist* 1986.)

However, in the majority of cases, chest roentgenography proves to be of little help in differentiating between the types of pulmonary edema. Patients are frequently too ill to be subjected to anything other than a portable technique. Maximal inspiration and elimination of motion artifact are difficult to achieve. The chest x-ray can usually confirm the presence of clinically suspected pulmonary edema but cannot be relied on to distinguish the type.

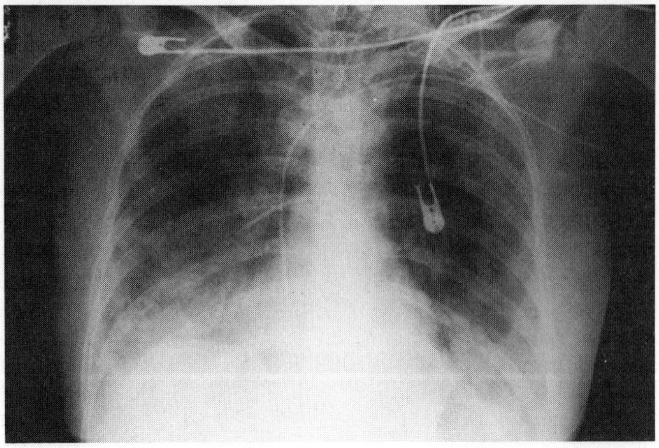

Fig. 11-4. Portable anteroposterior chest radiograph in a patient with adult respiratory distress syndrome. Extensive bilateral alveolar filling is present with air bronchograms; the cardiac silhouette is normal in size. An endotracheal tube and Swan-Ganz catheter are in place.

OTHER DIAGNOSTIC PROCEDURES

The electrocardiogram (ECG) is an important component in the clinical evaluation of CPE. Any arrhythmia that results in a marked increase in ventricular rate (>200 beats/minute) may precipitate pulmonary edema, even in otherwise healthy persons. Sustained ventricular tachycardia may present as CPE. The presence of new Q waves or ST-segment elevation or depression suggest myocardial infarction or ischemia or both.

M-mode and two-dimensional echocardiography and Doppler ultrasonography are invaluable aids in identifying and quantitating valvular lesions, measuring systolic performance, and estimating left ventricular size and degree of hypertrophy.

The sine qua non of CPE is a persistent elevation of pulmonary capillary hydrostatic pressure greater than 18 to 20 mm Hg. A close approximation of this can be obtained with the Swan-Ganz balloon flotation catheter. Pulmonary arterial "wedge" pressure is a reflection of pulmonary capillary pressure. For details of its insertion see Procedure 16.

DIFFERENTIAL DIAGNOSIS

Acute cardiogenic pulmonary edema is most likely to be confused with a number of other possible diagnoses listed in Table 11-1. Acute exacerbations of chronic obstructive lung disease usually occur in patients with long-established severe lung disease. Auscultation of the lungs often reveals reduced breath sounds, whereas patients with CPE usually have wet rales. Blood gas analysis is essential in differentiating patients with CPE from those with chronic obstructive pulmonary disease (COPD). Patients with CPE usually have a respiratory alkalosis unless they are so critically ill that they have a metabolic acidosis. Patients with acute exacerbation of COPD retain carbon dioxide, resulting in a respiratory acidosis.

Episodes of bronchial asthma are usually characterized by a history of similar episodes, and the patient is aware of the diagnosis. There is usually no profound diaphoresis, profound hypoxemia, or cyanosis. Rhonchi and rales are not prominent. The chest x-ray does not show pulmonary edema.

Acute pulmonary embolism may mimic pulmonary edema. Auscultation and chest x-ray show clear lung fields. The pulmonary arterial wedge pressure is frequently normal or even low in massive pulmonary embolism.

As described, NCPE may be difficult to distinguish clinically from acute CPE. Table 11-2 provides a list of historic, clinical, and laboratory discriminants. Measurement of the pulmonary artery "wedge" pressure provides the only definitive distinction.

Table 11-1. Differential diagnosis of cardiogenic pulmonary edema

Diagnosis	Supportive evidence
Acute exacerbation of COPD	CO_2 retention, history of COPD
Acute asthma	History of asthma, less diaphoresis and decreased PaO_2; chest x-ray clear
Pulmonary embolism	Wedge pressure low or normal, no rales, and a normal chest x-ray
Noncardiogenic pulmonary edema	See Table 11-2

Table 11-2. Discriminants of cardiogenic pulmonary edema from noncardiogenic pulmonary edema

CPE	NCPE
HISTORY	
Acute cardiac event	Acute cardiac event not typical
	Another disease
PHYSICAL EXAMINATION	
Low flow state (cool extremities)	Typically high flow state (warm extremities)
S_3/large heart	No S_3
Neck vein distention	No jugular venous distention
	Presence of another severe disease
LABORATORY	
ECG with ischemia/infarct	No acute changes on ECG
Chest x-ray with basilar and perihilar distribution	Chest x-ray with peripheral distribution
Cardiac enzymes may be increased	Cardiac enzymes normal
Wedge pressure >18 mm Hg	Wedge pressure <18 mm Hg

CARDIOGENIC ABNORMALITIES CAUSING PULMONARY EDEMA

Elevation of the pulmonary capillary pressure secondary to left heart failure is the most common cause of pulmonary edema. A comprehensive discussion of congestive heart failure can be found in Chap. 21. This elevated pulmonary capillary pressure, the common denominator for cardiac conditions that result in pulmonary edema, is closely approximated clinically by the pulmonary artery wedge pressure.

Experimental work has shown that pulmonary edema occurs when this wedge pressure exceeds 25 mm Hg, assuming normal membrane permeability, plasma oncotic pressure, and lymphatic drainage. It is important, however, to recall that the net transcapillary flow represents the interaction of multiple factors.

A pulmonary wedge pressure as low as 14 mm Hg may produce pulmonary edema in the presence of a significant abnormality in alveolar–capillary membrane permeability or decrease in plasma oncotic pressure, or both. Generally, though, CPE is due solely to increased pulmonary capillary pressure.

The categories of left heart abnormalities that cause pulmonary edema are:

1. Left ventricular systolic dysfunction
2. Left ventricular diastolic dysfunction
3. Left ventricular volume overload
4. Increased left ventricular afterload
5. Left heart valvular disorders

Left Ventricular Systolic Dysfunction

Systolic function directly relates to myocardial contractility. Many cardiac conditions impair left ventricular contractility. The most common cause is coronary artery disease. Ventricular function is reduced by either segmental infarction or gradual ischemic necrosis. Other causes of systolic dysfunction include dilated cardiomyopathy and hypertension.

Acute ischemic syndrome regularly results in regional left ventricular wall motion abnormalities and reduced ventricular contractility. At times, left ventricular dysfunction may be severe or prolonged enough to result in acute CPE.

To compensate for the deficient cardiac output, the heart adjusts in several ways. By the Frank–Starling mechanism, an increase in stroke volume results from an increase in left ventricular diastolic volume and muscle fiber length. The immediate benefit of ventricular dilatation is augmented cardiac output. The cost, however, is an increase in pulmonary capillary pressure. Any increase in left ventricular volume causes an automatic increase in left ventricular end-diastolic pressure, which is transmitted to the pulmonary venous system and elevates pulmonary capillary pressure.

The heart has the capacity of adapting after a myocardial infarction. Remodeling occurs. This involves ventricular dilatation, increased ventricular compliance, hypertrophy, and hypercontractility of the remaining normal myocardium. The end result is an enlarged ventricle with a somewhat reduced ejection fraction but near-normal cardiac output. This compensation of altered left ventricular function is possible provided that the initial ischemic insult was not so large as to overwhelm the remaining normal myocardium in its attempt to compensate.

Left Ventricular Diastolic Dysfunction

Contractile dysfunction is matched by relaxation dysfunction in the left heart's ability to cause pulmonary edema. The rate at which left ventricular muscle relaxes during diastole and the degree of diastolic left ventricular compliance are the elements of diastolic dysfunction.

In diastole, the normal left ventricular volume and pressure increase concurrently. The left ventricular end-diastolic pressure rarely exceeds 12 mm Hg. In diastolic dysfunction, the ventricle is stiff and poorly compliant. When the ventricle fills, pressure rises disproportionately compared to volume. This abnormal pressure–volume relationship may be such that a left ventricular end-diastolic pressure of greater than 25 mm Hg is achieved, despite a normal left ventricular end-diastolic volume. Although the cardiac silhouette on chest x-ray and the ejection fraction may be normal, pulmonary edema can develop.

The most common cause of diastolic dysfunction is left ventricular hypertrophy resulting from any type of stress that stimulates myocardial thickening, including afterload stresses of aortic stenosis, coarctation, and severe hypertension. Primary or secondary myocardial disorders resulting in a restrictive cardiomyopathy cause diastolic dysfunction.

Volume Overload

Acute pulmonary edema can be a consequence of volume overload. Although not truly cardiogenic in the sense that some form of left ventricular dysfunction is responsible, edema can occur because the normal myocardium's emergent compensatory mechanisms are overwhelmed.

When clinical conditions effect an acute or chronic increase in venous return (preload) that exceeds the left ventricle's ability to accept and pump it, pulmonary edema can occur. The contractile and relaxation mechanisms are "normal"; they are simply overwhelmed.

Volume overload frequently occurs in patients with renal failure and recipients of inordinate volumes of intravenous fluid or blood products during surgery. An "intrinsic" form of volume overload occurs in such situations as anemia and hyperthyroidism, where there are greater requirements placed on the heart to produce greater outputs to meet metabolic demands. The need is, in some way, recognized. However, the heart's ability to meet the demand is exceeded. In this phenomenon of "high output" failure, chronic volume overload may ultimately lead to systolic dysfunction.

Increased Afterload

Increased afterload is the outflow resistance that the left ventricle must pump against to eject blood. Arterial pressure and systemic vascular resistance are utilized as clinical estimates of afterload. Severe hypertension may cause pulmonary edema despite normal left ventricular contractility. In an attempt to contract against high outflow resistance, the left ventricle may be unable to empty completely at end systole. The result is left ventricular dilatation and increased end-diastolic pressure.

Hypertension is the most common clinical cause of abnormally elevated afterload. Prolonged elevation of blood pressure results in increased left ventricular wall stress. This results in the compensatory process of hypertrophy, which tends to normalize wall stress. Hypertrophy, however, leads to diastolic dysfunction and, ultimately, a reduction in contractility—systolic dysfunction.

Valvular Disorders

Valvular abnormalities can belong in the aforementioned subsets of cardiac abnormalities. In aortic stenosis, the hemodynamic abnormality is the ultimate "increased afterload." Left ventricular hypertrophy occurs, and, eventually, ventricular contractility diminishes and left ventricular end-diastolic volume increases. With hypertrophy, diastolic dysfunctional abnormalities also exist. These serve to independently elevate left ventricular end-diastolic pressure and pulmonary venous pressure.

Aortic regurgitation imposes a volume overload on the left ventricle. Reflux of blood into the left ventricle in diastole increases both left ventricular end-diastolic pressure and volume. Ventricular compensation may occur for a long period of time before increased left ventricular end-diastolic pressure develops with consequent heart failure.

Acute aortic regurgitation is poorly tolerated. Chest trauma or endocarditis resulting in massive aortic insufficiency causes an abrupt volume overload on a left ventricle unable to undergo adequate compensatory changes. Pulmonary edema rapidly develops.

The narrow valvular orifice in mitral stenosis is a mechanical impediment to left ventricular filling. Left atrial pressure has to increase in order to fill the left ventricle. Besides this mechanical obstruction, any increase in heart rate will reduce the duration of diastole and interfere with atrial emptying, thus elevating the left atrial pressure. This can cause pulmonary edema.

Blood under high pressure refluxes into the left atrium in systole in mitral regurgitation. This high pressure is transmitted directly to the pulmonary circulation. Moreover, mitral regurgitation imposes a volume overload on the left ventricle.

EMERGENT THERAPY

The management strategy depends on the underlying pathology and is shown in Table 11-3. All forms of CPE gain expression in the elevation of pulmonary capillary pressure; diuretics and other measures to reduce intravascular volume are utilized.

Patients with severe renal impairment may require dialysis or plasma ultrafiltration. Rotating tourniquets or phlebotomy, although cumbersome, time consuming, and of questionable efficacy, may be required in extreme situations.

Another avenue is the dilatation of the systemic venous circulation and the pharmacologic reduction of venous return. Intravenous morphine sulfate at a dose of 2 to 5 mg infused over 2 minutes and repeated over 15-minute intervals up to a total dose of 15 to 20 mg and furosemide 20 to 80 mg intravenously are useful. Morphine, in addition to reducing venous and arteriolar tone, relieves patient distress, eases the work of breathing, and decreases central and peripheral stimulation. Left ventricular filling pressure falls, and heart rate and blood pressure decrease.

Nitroglycerin, 0.3 to 0.6 mg sublingually, may provide prompt reduction in preload. Because it can be given quickly and has almost immediate onset and short duration of action, sublingual nitroglycerin may be given while a venous line is being readied and blood is drawn.

Table 11-3. Therapeutic strategy for cardiogenic pulmonary edema

Abnormality	Cause	Therapy
Left ventricular systolic dysfunction	CAD, MI, ischemic necrosis, dilated cardiomyopathy, hypertension	Digitalis, catecholamines amrinone; if ischemia, nitrates, calcium channel blockers; revascularize if recurrent ischemic edema
Left ventricular diastolic dysfunction	Hypertension, restrictive cardiomyopathy, anything causing systolic dysfunction	Diuretics, nitrates, morphine; if renal impairment, dialysis
Volume overload	Renal failure, large fluid intake, anemia	As for diastolic dysfunction
Increased afterload	Hypertension	Nitroprusside, nitroglycerin, counterpulsation for depressed LV
Valvular disorders	Aortic stenosis	Inotropics, diuretics, valve repair or replacement
	Aortic regurgitation	Diuretics, inotropics, nitroprusside; valve replacement
	Mitral stenosis	Diuretics, digoxin, valve repair or replacement
	Mitral regurgitation	Diuretics, inotropics, nitroprusside, and counterpulsation

Key: CAD = coronary artery disease; MI = myocardial infarction; LV = left ventricle.

Intravenous nitroglycerin may be administered at a dose of 5 to 10 μg/minute and increased by 10 μg every 2 to 5 minutes until dyspnea improves or the pulmonary artery wedge pressure is reduced to less than 17 mm Hg.

It is important to monitor the effect of diuresis on pulmonary gas exchange with periodic arterial blood gas analysis. Reducing left ventricular filling pressure also reduces cardiac output. Therefore, both blood pressure and urine output should be monitored. Reduction in systolic blood pressure to less than 100 mm Hg should be avoided. A urinary output less than 30 ml/hour implies either a low cardiac output or intravascular volume depletion. Other general measures include maximizing oxygenation, reversing acidosis, and treating serious arrhythmias (see Chap. 21).

ADJUNCTIVE THERAPY

Based on the specific cardiogenic abnormality, other specific therapy is used. In patients with systolic dysfunction, therapy is further aimed at improving ventricular contractility. Any intervention that increases contractility will improve ejection fraction and reduce left ventricular end-diastolic pressure and volume. Inotropic agents (see Chap. 21), including digitalis glycoside, catecholamines and amrinone, may be used.

Intravenous digoxin, 0.25 mg every 4 to 6 hours to a total dose of 1 mg, is the digitalis glycoside of choice.

Intravenous dopamine and dobutamine are the least arrhythmogenic of the sympathomimetic amines. The usual dose of dopamine is 1 to 5 μg/kg/minute. Doses higher than this may produce undesirable vasoconstriction. The dosage of dobutamine is 2.5 to 10.0 μg/kg/minute.

Amrinone is both an inotropic agent and a vasodilator. An initial bolus of 0.75 mg/kg is followed by an infusion of 5 to 10 μg/kg/minute.

Another approach in managing systolic dysfunction is the reduction of afterload with intravenous vasodilator drugs. Nitroprusside (initial dosage of 40–80 μg/min, with dosage increased by 5 μg/min every 5 minutes until dyspnea is relieved or blood pressure decreases to below 150/90 mm Hg) and intravenous nitroglycerin have been used to acutely lower left ventricular preload and afterload.

Intra-aortic balloon counterpulsation pumping is a mechanical approach to afterload reduction that is used in patients with severely depressed ventricular function. This approach is indicated in acute myocardial infarction where ventricular function is severely depressed or in severe mitral regurgitation with reasonably preserved left ventricular function.

With systolic dysfunction, there is heightened sensitivity to increases or decreases in afterload. A reduction in afterload may have a beneficial effect on the failing left ventricle and result in a significant increase in stroke volume. Afterload reduction also increases the left ventricular ejection fraction and reduces left ventricular end-diastolic pressure and volume.

Patients with pure diastolic dysfunction do not benefit from either inotropic agents or afterload reducing agents. Treatment is directed at reducing intravascular volume with diuresis or reducing systemic venous pressure.

Anti-ischemic therapy is indicated for patients with coronary artery disease and acute ischemic episodes. Transient reduction in contractility during anginal episodes or more prolonged contractile abnormalities, referred to as "stunned myocardium," may be manifest. Drugs such as intravenous nitroglycerin and calcium channel blockers are extremely useful in treating acute ischemic events. Of the calcium channel blockers, either nifedipine (10–30 mg PO tid) or diltiazem (30–90 mg PO qid) may be used. Utilization of verapamil is discouraged in patients with left ventricular failure because of its negative inotropic effect. Recurrent bouts of ischemia and pulmonary edema require aggressive treatment. Urgent cardiac catheterization and revascularization, either bypass grafting or angioplasty, should be performed.

Patients with critical aortic stenosis in whom pulmonary edema develop should be stabilized with intravenous diuretics and inotropic agents. Swan-Ganz catheter monitoring is required to avoid overdiuresis. Once the patient is stabilized, cardiac catheterization is done. Depending on the hemodynamics and the overall condition of the patient, a palliative percutaneous aortic valvuloplasty or the more definitive aortic valve replacement is performed. More recently, percutaneous partial cardiopulmonary bypass has been utilized in the patient with severe aortic stenosis presenting in extremis. This provides the necessary and safe hemodynamic support so that emergent valvuloplasty can be performed safely.

In the patient with mitral stenosis, therapy is aimed at reducing heart rate and decreasing intravascular volume by diuresis. The reduction in heart rate is particularly important in atrial fibrillation with a rapid ventricular response. The shortened diastolic filling time and the loss of atrial contraction quickly result in pulmonary edema. Intravenous digoxin should be administered in 0.25-mg boluses until the ventricular rate is below 100 beats/minute. Intravenous verapamil (5–10 mg over 2 minutes, repeated at 20- to 30-minute intervals up to a maximum dose of 20 mg) may be used to control the rate. Left ventricular function in mitral stenosis is generally preserved so that the negative inotropic risk of using verapamil is minimal. When the patient is stable, catheterization should be done.

Mitral valve replacement or repair or closed mitral valvuloplasty can then be done in the appropriate patient.

Patients with mitral or aortic regurgitation are treated with inotropic agents and diuretics. Afterload reduction may be particularly beneficial. Intravenous nitroprusside is the therapy of choice; if there is associated symptomatic coronary artery disease, intravenous nitroglycerin may be preferable.

In those patients who develop pulmonary edema secondary to acute/subacute endocarditis-induced valvular abnormalities, urgent catheterization and valve replacement are required.

SELECTED READING

Dalen, JE, and Alpert, JS. Natural history of pulmonary embolism. *Prog Cardiovasc Dis* 17:259, 1975.

Diener, CF, and Burrows, B. Further observation on the course and prognosis of chronic obstructive lung disease. *Am Rev Respir Dis* 11:719, 1975.

Gradman, AH, and Mostoufi-Moab, E. Cardiogenic pulmonary edema: Multiple causes and therapy. *J Respir Dis* 10:68, 1989.

Ingram, RH. Pulmonary Edema: Cardiogenic and Noncardiogenic. In E. Braunwald (ed.), *Heart Disease*. Philadelphia: Saunders, 1988.

Rinaldo, JE, and Rogers, RM. Adult respiratory distress syndrome. *N Engl J Med* 306:900, 1982.

Sibbald, WJ, and Cunningham, DR. Noncardiac or cardiac pulmonary edema. *Chest* 84:452, 1982.

Snapper, JR, and Brigham, KL. Pulmonary edema. *Hosp Prac* 21: 87, 1986.

NONCARDIOGENIC PULMONARY EDEMA (ADULT RESPIRATORY DISTRESS SYNDROME)

Richard M. Schwartzstein

Critically ill patients with a wide variety of medical and surgical problems may present with a syndrome of hypoxemia, diffuse pulmonary infiltrates, and normal cardiac function. This clinical picture constitutes what is commonly referred to as the adult respiratory distress syndrome (ARDS). It is characterized pathophysiologically by diffuse injury to the pulmonary alveolar–capillary membrane, which leads to exudation of protein-rich fluid from the vascular space to the interstitial and alveolar spaces of the lung. The patient appears to have "pulmonary edema" radiographically, but cardiac function is normal—that is, the pulmonary edema is "noncardiogenic," or not the result of left ventricular dysfunction.

ARDS was first described as a clinical entity in 1967, although it was recognized in retrospect to have accompanied severe trauma in many individuals wounded during World War II and the Korean War. There are now an estimated 150,000 cases of ARDS per year in the United States. Despite improvements in the technology of ventilators and in our ability to support critically ill patients in medical and surgical intensive care units, the mortality rate associated with ARDS remains between 40 and 60 percent.

Physicians practicing emergency medicine must be familiar with ARDS in order to recognize patients at risk for this form of respiratory failure and to optimize initial therapy in those patients already exhibiting increased pulmonary capillary permeability.

Table 11-4. Medical conditions associated with the adult respiratory distress syndrome

Inhalational route of injury to lung
Near-drowning
Smoke inhalation/toxic chemicals
Oxygen toxicity
Aspiration
Vascular route of injury to lung
Sepsis
Drug overdose
Fat embolism
Pancreatitis
Multiple trauma
Uremia
Multiple transfusions
Direct injury to lung
Thoracic trauma
Reexpansion pulmonary edema

PATHOPHYSIOLOGY

There appear to be three different clinical mechanisms by which the alveolar-capillary membrane may suffer damage leading to increased permeability and the syndrome of noncardiogenic pulmonary edema. First, the lung may be damaged by the inhalation of toxic substances. Smoke inhalation or aspiration of gastric contents, for example, brings noxious substances to the alveolus via the airways. Second, the alveolar-capillary membrane may be injured as the result of toxins delivered to the capillaries through the circulation. This is the mechanism by which ARDS is thought to develop in patients with sepsis or pancreatitis. Third, the lung may suffer direct physical injury (e.g., thoracic trauma). Table 11-4 lists the common medical conditions associated with ARDS and groups them according to the most likely route by which the lung is injured.

When one examines a list of conditions associated with ARDS, one is struck by the great variety of medical and surgical problems that appear. What does smoke inhalation have in common with fat embolism or thoracic trauma such that all of these conditions produce similar pathologic and physiologic changes in the lung? Although numerous investigations have been designed in an effort to answer this question, the puzzle is not yet complete.

Attempts have been made to define clinically patients at risk for developing noncardiogenic pulmonary edema. Eight conditions have been identified: sepsis; trauma resulting in multiple fractures; aspiration of gastric contents; drug overdose involving aspirin, narcotics, or sedatives resulting in admission to an intensive care unit; near-drowning; head injury with prolonged loss of consciousness or intracranial hemorrhage; multiple emergency transfusions; and pulmonary contusion. The presence of any one of these disorders is said to result in a 25 percent chance of the patient developing ARDS. If two or more of these conditions are present, the risk of ARDS is thought to be doubled.

Researchers have also sought to define the biochemical mediators of lung injury. There are increasing data to support the role of inflammatory cells, the complement pathway, and intravascular coagulation in producing damage at the level of the alveolar-capillary membrane. The pulmonary circulation contains a large population of marginated polymorphonuclear leukocytes, which, when activated, release toxic metabolites and proteolytic enzymes leading to endothelial injury. Stasis in pulmonary capillaries may result in activation of the clotting cascade, the products of which may also produce endothelial damage and further augment the inflammatory process. Specific mediators of lung injury in experimental preparations have included substances such as prostaglandins, platelet-activating factor, interleukin 1, cachectin, and leukotrienes. Despite these data, attempts to prevent ARDS by blocking the release or action of one or more of these mediators have largely been unsuccessful, and clinical cases have been identified that seem to confound the hypothetical mechanisms of lung injury (e.g., the presence of ARDS in patients who are neutropenic).

The lung of a patient with noncardiogenic pulmonary edema may be characterized by one of three pathologic stages: exudative, proliferative, or fibrotic. In the exudative stage, one sees interstitial and alveolar edema with proteinaceous material in the alveoli. This material may organize into hyaline membranes. In the proliferative stage, much of the alveolar fluid appears to be reabsorbed and fibrin deposition becomes prominent. There is also extensive infiltration with inflammatory cells and fibroblasts. The third pathologic stage is notable for fibrosis with destruction of alveoli and loss of lung units.

These pathologic changes in the lung are translated into a number of abnormalities in pulmonary physiology. The presence of fluid, inflammatory cells, and fibrin in the interstitium of the lung leads to a decrease in compliance—that is, the lung becomes more stiff. This reduction in lung compliance may first be apparent as "small lungs" on a chest radiograph and, later, if respiratory failure develops, is evidenced by the high airway pressures required to deliver an adequate tidal volume to the patient with a mechanical ventilator. The combination of reduced pulmonary compliance and fluid-filled alveoli leads to the second major physiologic abnormality, increased shunt. As patients with ARDS exhale and lung volume becomes smaller, individual lung units tend to collapse. If these units fail to reexpand on the next inspiration, no gas exchange can take place and the red blood cells flowing through the capillaries to these units are not oxygenated. The result is hypoxemia that is relatively refractory to increases in the concentration of inspired oxygen. The collapse of alveoli in ARDS is further exacerbated by loss of surfactant or changes in surfactant function resulting from chemical interactions with proteins in the alveolar exudate.

A third physiologic abnormality seen in patients with ARDS involves the pulmonary vasculature. In normal individuals, the pulmonary arterioles respond to local areas of hypoxia in the lung by constricting, thereby redirecting blood flow to areas of the lung that are better ventilated. This reflex vasoconstriction is not fully operative in patients with ARDS. Consequently, there is greater mismatching of ventilation and perfusion in the lung, which leads to further hypoxemia.

CLINICAL ASSESSMENT

Physicians practicing emergency medicine must be able to identify patients at risk of developing noncardiogenic pulmonary edema and must be able to recognize the early signs of the syndrome. In the first instance, identification of a patient in a high-risk group may alter the decision to discharge the patient from the emergency department or lead to arrangements for early follow-up. On the other hand, ability to diagnose ARDS may alter initial therapy in a critically ill patient.

History

The respiratory symptoms of a patient presenting with an illness complicated by noncardiogenic pulmonary edema are quite nonspecific. Patients usually complain of increasing dyspnea on exertion, which, over time, progresses to dyspnea at rest. Cough and wheezing may also be present. Once the lung has been injured and the pulmonary capillaries begin leaking fluid and protein into the interstitial and alveolar spaces, symptoms develop quickly and the patient may progress to hypoxic respiratory failure within 24 hours. Early in the course of the illness, however, the clinical picture is dominated by the primary disease process. Recognition of the *potential* for pulmonary damage is critical. In some cases—for example, patients with smoke inhalation—manifestations of the capillary injury may be delayed for 24 to 48 hours, and, although the patient is otherwise feeling well, the potential for complications may dictate that the patient be observed closely. In most other patients in whom ARDS develops, one is dealing with a seriously ill individual with derangements in multiple organ systems.

Physical Examination

Inspiratory rales is the most common finding and is generally most prominent in the dependent portions of the lung. Rales are probably a manifestation of the reexpansion of previously collapsed alveoli. Rhonchi and wheezes may also be heard. Physical findings of pulmonary consolidation (e.g., bronchial breath sounds and egophony) may be present in more advanced cases in which there is extensive alveolar collapse with patent central airways. Tachypnea is invariably present if the patient's respiratory centers have not been adversely affected by the underlying illness (e.g., drug overdose). What is often most impressive about the physical examination of a patient with ARDS is the relative paucity of chest findings present when contrasted with the severe abnormalities of the chest radiograph and arterial blood gases.

One of the primary objectives of the physical examination in a patient with pulmonary edema is to determine whether the patient has cardiac dysfunction—that is, whether there is evidence of left ventricular failure. Although patients with noncardiogenic pulmonary edema may have an elevated pulmonary capillary wedge pressure in addition to leaky capillaries, this combination is generally not found at the time that the patient presents to the emergency ward. Therefore, the presence of an S_3 gallop, jugular venous distention, and peripheral edema (along with a history of orthopnea and paroxysmal nocturnal dyspnea) should suggest to the physician the diagnosis of congestive heart failure rather than ARDS.

Laboratory Data

As discussed previously, the clinical picture of a patient with ARDS is often dominated by the features of the primary illness responsible for the damage to the lung. The laboratory data generally reflect this point as well. For example, patients with the sepsis syndrome may have a leukocytosis with a large number of "bands" as well as evidence of disseminated intravascular coagulation. A patient with severe pancreatitis, on the other hand, may present with an elevated serum amylase and hypocalcemia. The focus of this discussion will be on those aspects of the laboratory investigation that provide information about the respiratory system in a patient with ARDS. These findings are common to most patients with noncardiogenic pulmonary edema regardless of the primary illness.

The chest radiograph in patients with mild ARDS shows diffuse interstitial infiltrates. In more severe cases, there is patchy alveolar consolidation distributed fairly uniformly throughout both lung fields. Air bronchograms may be seen. As the disease progresses over days to weeks, one may see clearing of the alveoli with residual fibrosis. In the most severe cases, there may be frank "honeycombing" of the lung. In contrast to the chest radiograph in congestive heart failure, the heart size is usually normal, pleural effusions are absent, and there is no evidence of vascular redistribution from the bases to the apices. Furthermore, the pattern of the alveolar infiltrates is central or perihilar in congestive heart failure, whereas it tends to be more diffuse and patchy in ARDS (see Figs. 11-2, 11-3, and 11-4).

Arterial blood gases typically reveal a large alveolar-arterial oxygen gradient—that is, significant hypoxemia when the patient is breathing "room air"—and a primary respiratory alkalosis—that is, a low PCO_2. The provision of high concentrations of inspired oxygen will often have little impact on the arterial PO_2. This finding is an indication of the high shunt fraction found in most patients with ARDS.

(For a review of the concept of intrapulmonary shunting as a cause of hypoxemia, see Chap. 6.) In those patients with more severe ARDS who develop significant fibrosis of the lung, hypercapnia may arise as the amount of physiological dead space increases. The development of hypercapnia refractory to high minute ventilations is often a harbinger of irreversible respiratory failure in these patients. In addition to the primary respiratory acid–base disturbances that result from the exudation of protein and fluid into the interstitial and alveolar spaces of the lung, the underlying illness responsible for the lung injury may also lead to a primary metabolic or respiratory acidosis or alkalosis. For example, patients with sepsis or hypotension owing to hemorrhage or pancreatitis may have a lactic acidosis. Patients with toxic levels of salicylates may demonstrate both a primary metabolic acidosis and a primary respiratory alkalosis independent of the acid–base abnormalities arising from pathology in the lung itself.

Most individuals with noncardiogenic pulmonary edema are too ill to undergo formal pulmonary function testing. However, the increased lung water present in these patients is likely to result in reduced lung volumes (a "restrictive" pattern) and reduced diffusing capacity. Forced expiratory flows are usually normal to mildly reduced.

DIFFERENTIAL DIAGNOSIS

As noted previously, the differential diagnosis of a patient with diffuse pulmonary infiltrates and hypoxemia primarily includes ARDS and congestive heart failure. The findings on chest radiograph and physical examination help distinguish these entities. Less commonly, infectious processes will produce diffuse infiltrates and hypoxemia. Viral pneumonias and *Pneumocystis carinii* pneumonia are most frequently seen with this combination of findings. The latter is restricted primarily to patients with the acquired immunodeficiency syndrome (AIDS) and to patients with other causes of altered T-cell function (e.g., lymphoma). Bacterial pneumonias are classically more focal on chest radiograph than would be expected with noncardiogenic pulmonary edema. The distinction between severe diffuse pulmonary infection and ARDS, which may develop secondary to the infection, is often blurred. If the patient has refractory hypoxemia, the general principles of therapy for ARDS are usually followed in conjunction with the administration of antimicrobial therapy, when available. Rarer causes of diffuse pulmonary infiltrates and hypoxemia include diffuse alveolar hemorrhage (e.g., Goodpasture's syndrome), alveolar proteinosis, and hypersensitivity reactions in the lung.

THERAPY: GENERAL PRINCIPLES

When treating patients with noncardiogenic pulmonary edema, it is important to remember that the majority of patients who die with this disorder succumb to the underlying disease; they do not die respiratory deaths. Therefore, it is critical that one aggressively treat the primary process while supporting the patient's respiratory system.

Most patients with ARDS have significant hypoxemia. The use of supplemental oxygen to ensure an oxygen-hemoglobin saturation of 90 percent is crucial to maintaining optimal organ system function throughout the body. A fear associated with use of high concentrations of inspired oxygen is the potential for oxygen toxicity. Inhalation of high concentrations of oxygen is thought to result in production of oxygen radicals, which may lead to significant damage to the lung. When inspiring 100 percent oxygen, a patient may develop evidence for plumonary oxygen toxicity within 24 hours. At lower concentrations of oxygen, the time to the development of oxygen toxicity is prolonged. With an inspired concentration of oxygen at or below 60 percent, it appears that there is no significant risk of oxygen toxicity—that is, the patient may stay on this level of supplemental oxygen indefinitely without fear of causing further damage to the lung. The "bottom line" for physicians practicing in an emergency ward is that patients with ARDS must be given sufficient oxygen to raise the oxygen-hemoglobin saturation to 90 percent (a PaO_2 of approximately 60 mm Hg). Venturi masks, which allow for careful regulation of the inspired concentration of oxygen, may be used in patients with COPD and a history of chronic hypercapnia. Although one always tries to use the lowest concentration of oxygen necessary to achieve an oxygen-hemoglobin saturation of 90 percent, one should not be concerned with the danger of oxygen toxicity in the first several hours of the patient's therapy. Methods to minimize the inspired concentration of oxygen such as positive end-expiratory pressure (PEEP) and inverse ratio ventilation are best left to the critical care specialist in the intensive care unit.

Patients with noncardiogenic pulmonary edema or those at risk for this syndrome frequently develop hypotension. Management of hemodynamic instability in these patients can be extremely difficult. The first response of most physicians when faced with a patient who is hypotensive is to administer volume expanders (e.g., saline or Ringer's lactate solution). However, in the setting of a damaged alveolar-capillary membrane, increases in left ventricular filling pressures will ultimately be translated into an increased hydrostatic pressure in the pulmonary capillaries and will exacerbate the flooding of the interstitial and alveolar spaces with fluid. Thus, one will increase the pulmonary edema and worsen the hypoxemia of the patient. Depending on the specifics of the clinical situation, one may use pharmacologic agents to support the patient's hemodynamics, either vasopressors such as dopamine, phenylephrine, or norepinephrine, or inotropic agents such as dobutamine or amrinone, rather than volume expanders. One must remember, however, that the ultimate goal of therapy in a critically ill patient is to deliver oxygen to the tissues. Oxygen delivery depends on the patient's hemoglobin, cardiac output, and PaO_2. Thus, pharmacologic interventions that increase blood pressure at the expense of cardiac output by severely constricting the peripheral vasculature may actually be detrimental to tissue perfusion.

In managing the hemodynamics of a patient with ARDS, one must continually balance tissue perfusion and oxygen delivery to the tissues with the need to minimize hydrostatic pressure in the pulmonary capillaries. In many of these patients, to optimize therapy one requires the information obtained from a pulmonary artery catheter (Swan-Ganz catheter), in particular, the pulmonary capillary wedge pressure, cardiac output, and mixed venous oxygen saturation. When faced with a critically ill patient in the emergency ward who is hypotensive and possibly at risk for ARDS or already noted to be hypoxemic, volume expanders are still the appropriate initial first line of therapy. Generally, if volume expanders are needed and the patient is anemic, it is best to give blood products. Ultimately, however, one may be compelled to switch to pharmacologic means to support the patient's circulation rather than be faced with an inability to oxygenate the blood.

Inflammation appears to play a major role in the pathophysiology of noncardiogenic pulmonary edema. Consequently, much attention has been given to the possible efficacy of anti-inflammatory agents as a treatment for this syndrome. A multi-center, randomized, placebo-controlled trial of methylprednisolone (30 mg/kg every 6 hours for 24 hours) in patients with ARDS showed that there were no significant differences in mortality or reversal of ARDS between the steroid and placebo groups. Therefore, steroids *cannot* be recommended as treatment for noncardiogenic pulmonary edema.

Finally, it is important to note that most patients who survive ARDS will regain relatively normal pulmonary function within 12 months of the original injury. Despite severe gas exchange abnormalities and the need for mechanical ventilation at the time of the acute illness, survivors generally do not have chronic respiratory symptoms.

SPECIFIC SYNDROMES

The number of clinical conditions associated with ARDS is too large to deal with each in detail. However, there are four conditions of particular importance to physicians practicing emergency medicine: smoke inhalation, near-drowning, drug overdose, and neurogenic pulmonary edema.

Smoke Inhalation

An individual trapped in a burning building is subject to at least four types of respiratory injury. The heat from the fire may cause a thermal injury to the respiratory mucosa, although the damage is usually confined to the upper airway. If steam, which has 4000 times the heat capacity of dry air, is inhaled, thermal injury can extend to the lower respiratory tract. Second, particulate matter in smoke may transport heat and toxic chemicals to the lower airways as well as induce local inflammation. Third, toxic gases released largely from burning plastics may dissolve in the liquid layer lining the upper and lower respiratory tracts and may result in a chemical injury to the alveoli. Fourth, a patient may suffer the effects of carbon monoxide poisoning. Patients with smoke inhalation and thermal injuries frequently present with signs of upper-airway obstruction as well as bronchospasm. They are also at risk for noncardiogenic pulmonary edema. The onset of ARDS, however, may be delayed 24 to 48 hours after the exposure. One can often predict the risk to the patient of developing ARDS based on historical information. Exposure to smoke in an enclosed space, unconsciousness or inebriation associated with smoke inhalation, fires involving plastics, and steam explosions all increase one's risk for serious respiratory complications. Furthermore, 85 percent of patients with serious smoke inhalation will have carboxyhemoglobin levels greater than 15 to 20 percent. Treatment of these patients includes close attention to the patency of the upper airway (if stridor is present, the patient usually requires prophylactic intubation to prevent sudden upper airway occlusion), bronchodilators for wheezing, and high concentrations of inspired oxygen to reduce the half-life of carboxyhemoglobin. There is no role for steroids or prophylactic antibiotics. Because of the delayed onset of ARDS in these patients, individuals with a history of carboxyhemoglobin level consistent with a significant smoke exposure should be admitted for observation. (For additional discussion of smoke inhalation injuries, see Chap. 75.)

Near-Drowning

There are approximately 8,000 deaths each year in the United States due to drowning. Aspiration of either fresh or salt water can lead to noncardiogenic pulmonary edema. Inhalation of even small quantities of fresh water appears to result in a loss of surfactant with resulting atelectasis and hypoxemia. Similarly, sea water will fill alveoli, may lead to disruption of the alveolar-capillary membrane, and produce intrapulmonary shunting. Respiratory arrest generally precedes cessation of cardiac activity in these patients, and, if the drowning has occurred in cold water, the attendant hypothermia will slow metabolism and preserve tissue viability for up to 40 minutes. Thus, resuscitative efforts should be continued until the patient has been warmed to usual body temperature, and the patient should not be declared dead until resuscitation maneuvers are unsuccessful at the higher body temperature. One should not attempt to physically empty fluid from the lungs. In the case of freshwater drowning, the fluid is rapidly absorbed into the blood stream. With salt water aspiration, absorption is slower, but the alveolar fluid is not readily removed by mechanical means. A nasogastric tube should be placed to remove water that has been swallowed to prevent regurgitation and further aspiration. As in cases of smoke inhalation, there is no role for steroids or prophylactic antibiotics, and since the onset of ARDS may be delayed several hours after an episode of near-drowning, it is prudent to observe such patients for 24 hours in the hospital. (See Chap. 3 for further discussion.)

Drug Overdose

Drug-induced noncardiogenic pulmonary edema has most commonly been associated with heroin use and aspirin overdose. The mechanisms by which these drugs damage the alveolar-capillary membrane remain obscure. The drugs may have a direct toxic effect on the alveolar-capillary membrane, or they may trigger an unexplained immunologic reaction leading to aggregation of polymorphonuclear leukocytes in the lung and release of toxic metabolites. In some cases of heroin-induced ARDS, there may be stimulation of the central nervous system leading to a "neurogenic" type of pulmonary edema (see below). In the case of salicylate toxicity, there is some evidence to suggest that inhibition of prostaglandin synthesis leads to loss of the normal integrity of the pulmonary microcirculation. Risk factors for the development of ARDS in association with salicylate toxicity include age (older patients are more likely to develop ARDS), chronic use of salicylates, a history of smoking, and a salicylate level greater than 40 mg/dl. These risk factors should be kept in mind when using sodium bicarbonate therapy to enhance elimination of salicylates from the blood. The volume load associated with bicarbonate therapy could exacerbate the amount of fluid leaking into the lung if noncardiogenic pulmonary edema develops. Treatment of these patients is in keeping with the general principles of therapy previously outlined. The radiographic findings of pulmonary edema usually clear within 3 days from diagnosis.

Neurogenic Pulmonary Edema

Noncardiogenic pulmonary edema has been associated with a wide variety of injuries to the brain, including head trauma, intracerebral hemorrhage, seizures, strokes, and tumors. The respiratory findings are believed to emerge within minutes of the damage to the central nervous system. The mechanism by which brain injury leads to disruption of the alveolar-capillary membrane is poorly understood. There is some evidence to suggest that the injury is mediated through the sympathetic nervous system. For example, in animal models of neurogenic pulmonary edema, rats pretreated with adrenergic blocking agents either did not develop pulmonary edema or developed milder forms of pulmonary edema than did the untreated animals. A sudden and massive discharge from the sympathetic nervous system is believed to result in acute pulmonary hypertension, which leads to injury of the pulmonary capillaries and exudation of fluid and protein into the interstitial and alveolar spaces. There is no specific treatment for neurogenic pulmonary edema. Therapy is directed at the primary neurologic process and on support for the patient's respiratory status as previously outlined.

SELECTED READING

Alberts, WM, Priest, GR, and Moser, KM. The outlook for survivors of ARDS. *Chest* 306:900, 1982.

Bernard, GR, et al. High dose corticosteroids in patients with the adult respiratory distress syndrome. *N Engl J Med* 317:1565, 1987.

Heffner, JE, and Sahn, SA. Salicylate-induced pulmonary edema. *Ann Intern Med* 95:405, 1981.

Montgomery, AB, et al. Causes of mortality in patients with the adult respiratory distress syndrome. *Am Rev Respir Dis* 132:485, 1985.

Pepe, PE, et al. Clinical predictors of the adult respiratory distress syndrome. *Am J Surg* 144:124, 1982.

Rinaldo, JE, and Rogers, RM. Adult respiratory distress syndrome. *N Engl J Med* 306:900, 1982.

Tate, RM, and Repine, JE. Neutrophils and the adult respiratory distress syndrome. *Am Rev Respir Dis* 125:552, 1983.

12. Disorders of the Pleural Space

Bohdan Pichurko

The pleural space in the healthy individual contains no air and only a thin film of fluid. When the normal condition is disturbed, fluid or gas or both may accumulate at varying rates, compressing and displacing respiratory and cardiovascular structures within the thorax. Small and slowly developing collections of intrapleural fluid (pleural effusion) or air (pneumothorax) typically cause limited disability and are often evaluated in an office setting. In contrast, rapidly advancing effusions and pneumothoraces may cause rapid deterioration, particularly in patients with antecedent cardiopulmonary disease. These unstable patients will seek urgent medical care and require prompt recognition and initial treatment by the emergency department physician.

ANATOMY

The pleura is a continuous membrane that covers the structures of the thoracic cavity. Its parietal component lines the interior rib cage, diaphragm, and mediastinum. The visceral pleura extends over the surface of the entire lung parenchyma, including the interlobar fissures and joins the parietal pleura at the lung root or hilum. The visceral and parietal pleurae are in direct apposition along their costal (rib cage), diaphragmatic, and mediastinal surfaces, separated by a fluid layer measuring only 10 microns in thickness. This fluid-lined area surrounded by pleurae constitutes the normal pleural space. The right and left pleural spaces are distinct and separated by the mediastinum with no direct communication between them.

Pleural tissue consists of a one-cell thick surface layer of mesothelial cells resting on several layers of elastin and collagen-rich connective tissue. The metabolically active and pleomorphic mesothelial cells are studded with microvilli that extend into the pleural fluid layer, assisting in fluid absorption and in concentrating a lubricating glycoprotein mixture to reduce surface friction. Mesothelial cells are regularly shed into the pleural space where they either remain intact or can transform into phagocytic macrophages.

The connective tissue components offer structural support and are particularly thick and dense in the visceral pleura where they help to regulate lung expansion. In addition, the visceral and parietal pleurae contain a loose layer of connective tissue located adjacent to the underlying lung or chest wall. Rich networks of lymphatics and arterial, venous, and capillary channels traverse this area.

The pleural blood and lymphatic circulations are important determinants of the movement and composition of pleural fluid. The parietal pleura receives its blood supply from the systemic circulation and specifically from branches of arteries supplying adjacent chest wall structures. For example, the large costal surface shares the intercostal and internal mammary arteries; the mediastinal parietal pleura is perfused by mediastinal, internal mammary, and bronchial artery branches; and the diaphragmatic pleura receives branches of the thoracic and abdominal aorta and internal mammary and celiac arteries. Venous drainage is via the bronchial circuit for all segments of the parietal pleural circulation except the diaphragmatic, which empties into the inferior vena cava and the brachiocephalic venous trunk. Due to limitations associated with human investigation and to differences between mammalian animal models, there is still some controversy about the pulmonary versus bronchial contributions to the arterial perfusion of the visceral pleura. Today, many investigators accept the bronchial circulation as the origin of its arterial blood supply. The terminal arteries supply an extensive network of oversized subpleural capillaries that are 5 to 10 times the usual capillary diameter. Notably, these capillaries then feed into veins of the pulmonary circulation.

The lymphatic circulation is important in the clearance of both pleural fluid and formed elements such as blood cells and foreign particulates. The visceral pleura is richly endowed with lymphatic channels arranged in two networks that both ultimately direct lymph toward the pulmonary hilum. Lymph vessels that course over the surface of the lung within the subpleural layers are most densely distributed over the lower lobes. Other lymphatics pierce the visceral pleural surface and enter the parenchyma, coursing alongside interlobular and peribronchial blood vessels on their way toward the lung root. Unlike visceral pleural lymphatics, the lymphatic circulation of the parietal pleura communicates directly with the pleural space via distinct 2 to 5 μ round or semilunar openings in the mesothelial layer called *stomas*. Each stoma is joined to a dilated lymphatic vessel (lacuna) and serves to remove large particles from the pleural cavity. Stomas are situated along the mediastinal and costal surface with a density of roughly 1 per square millimeter but are relatively sparse in other areas. Lymph from the parietal circulation is drained regionally, with the sternal nodes receiving anterior thoracic and anterior diaphragmatic flow, intercostal nodes draining the costal surface, and anterior mediastinal nodes collecting lymphatic flow from the mediastinal parietal pleura.

The parietal pleura receives sensory innervation to its costal and peripheral diaphragmatic surfaces from adjacent intercostal nerves. The central portion of the diaphragmatic pleura is innervated by the phrenic nerves. Thus, irritation of this surface produces referred pain in the ipsilateral shoulder area. In contrast, the visceral pleura receives no sensory nerve supply whatsoever and so is completely anesthetic.

PNEUMOTHORAX

INTRODUCTION AND EPIDEMIOLOGY

Pneumothorax may be categorized according to its etiology and the type of patient in whom it occurs. If a pneumothorax occurs in the absence of overt injury to the chest, it is referred to as a *spontaneous pneumothorax*. Patients enjoying otherwise good health are said to suffer a *primary spontaneous pneumothorax*. Chronic obstructive pulmonary disease (COPD), varieties of interstitial disease, and other acute and chronic lung disorders predispose to a *secondary* variety of spontaneous pneumothorax. Distinct from these is the presence of pleural air in a trauma victim. *Traumatic pneumothorax* may take several forms: (1) penetrating chest wounds allowing direct entry of atmospheric air into the pleural space, (2) blunt chest wall trauma resulting in alveolar rupture and release of its gaseous content into the pleural cavity, and (3) medical diagnostic and therapeutic procedures such as central venous catheter placement, mechanical ventilation, or thoracentesis creating an air leak into the pleural space. This last category may involve either ambient air or alveolar gas and is termed an *iatrogenic pneumothorax*.

Patterns in the incidence of primary spontaneous pneumothorax are influenced by a strong representation of reports from the military and by the likely omissions of mild cases that did not come to medical attention. Available data indicate an incidence of approximately 10 per 100,000 population with a male-female ratio of 3:1. The peak incidence is between 20 and 30 years of age or soon after full growth is achieved, and cigarette smokers have a higher incidence than nonsmokers. The incidence of spontaneous pneumothorax secondary to preexisting lung disease is more evenly distributed among age groups. Pneumothorax in the newborn is largely related to meconium aspiration or to hyaline membrane disease. Cystic fibrosis, often causing recurrent pneumothoraces, affects adolescents and young adults. COPD leads the list of etiologies in the middle and senior age groups and accounts for more than half of all secondary spontaneous pneumothoraces. Although the relative incidence of primary pneumothorax outnumbers secondary pneumothorax by a 3:1 ratio among all patients, the ratio is nearly reversed (1:2) in patients older than 40 years of age. Together, spontaneous pneumothorax accounts for approximately 0.3 percent of hospital admissions.

Traumatic pneumothorax varies widely in incidence, depending on the frequency of exposure to potential injury and, in the iatrogenic cases, on the experience and skill of the responsible physician. Representative figures for various medical interventions include a 5 to 10 percent risk associated with transbronchial lung biopsy, 20 to 30 percent risk following a transthoracic needle aspiration of the lung, and less than 5 percent associated with mechanical ventilation. The complication rate of positive pressure ventilation increases with peak airway pressures exceeding 60 cm H_2O, particularly when coupled with preexisting subpleural cysts or with alveolar distention owing to gas trapping.

PATHOPHYSIOLOGY

The exact etiology of primary spontaneous pneumothorax remains controversial. Speculation has focused on congenital or acquired structural deficiences of lung and pleural tissue. This hypothesis is supported by the radiographic and intraoperative findings of multiple subpleural cysts or blebs concentrated around the lung apex of affected patients and not seen in healthy individuals. Whether the blebs are the end result of inflammatory or ischemic processes or of alveolar rupture owing to increased distending pressures that affect the lung apex is uncertain. Each competing hypothesis draws considerable support from clinical and pathologic investigation. In the end, it is likely that we will recognize a pathogenesis that is multifactorial and variable among patients.

Clinically apparent pulmonary disorders predispose to spontaneous pneumothorax in a variety of ways. For example, bullous emphysema involves the dual risk factors of producing thin-walled blebs while also destroying the interstitial support structures of the lung. Granulomatous diseases such as tuberculosis as well as benign or carcinomatous infiltrative processes may stud the subpleural lung, producing local tissue necrosis and rupture through the adjacent visceral pleura. Alternatively, freed alveolar gas may migrate medially along bronchovascular structures toward the hilum, where entry is gained into the mediastinum and also by dissection into the pleural space.

Regardless of etiolgy, the accumulation of intrapleural air disrupts intrathoracic mechanics in a similar fashion and so produces generally predictable changes in cardiopulmonary function. Normally, the pressure within the pleural space is slightly negative, or below that of ambient air. This pressure is created by the hydraulic coupling of the inwardly recoiling lung with the outwardly recoiling chest wall. If the lung and thoracic cage could be separated, the lung would contract to a nearly gasless tissue mass the size of an adult fist or about 5 percent of total lung capacity (TLC), whereas the volume of the isolated thoracic cage would be 70 percent of TLC. Thus, throughout the entire range of restful breathing, the thin film of pleural fluid supplies outward traction on the lung and inward traction on the chest wall. The introduction of air into the pleural space uncouples the lung from the chest wall, producing a variable degree of lung collapse and rib cage expansion as the intrapleural pressure rises to less negative or positive levels.

The most common effects of a pneumothorax are (1) a reduction in vital capacity, (2) increased pulmonary vascular resistance, and (3) hypoxia owing to a disruption of ventilation/perfusion (V/Q) balance. Hypercapnia is avoided in the majority of cases as the decrease in ventilation of the affected lung is offset by a hyperventilation of the contralateral lung. A particularly severe and refractory hypoxia and circulatory collapse follow the development of a tension pneumothorax. In this situation, air enters the pleural space from the lung or through the chest wall but is prevented from escaping, occupying an increasing volume at progressively higher pressures. Consequently, the ipsilateral lung, heart, and intrathoracic vessels are compressed while the diaphragm and chest wall are displaced outwardly with their movement restricted. The severe hypotension and hypoxia that attend a tension pneumothorax are inevitably fatal unless the built-up positive intrathoracic pressure is promptly relieved.

INITIAL ASSESSMENT

History

The appreciation of patients' signs and symptoms can be traced to Laennec's first published description of pneumothorax in the early nineteenth century. Nearly all patients who have sustained a spontaneous pneumothorax will describe ipsilateral chest or shoulder pain. It is typically of sudden onset and is continuous in character but occasionally will vary with respiration. A majority of patients will complain of dyspnea, particularly if the pneumothorax is large or if there is an underlying respiratory impairment. Occasionally, a patient will desrcibe a dry cough. A presentation that involves hemoptysis and syncope indicates intrapleural bleeding (hemopneumothorax) from a torn vascularized pleural adhesion. One in four patients will relate the onset of symptoms to strenuous activity, but, in most cases, the pneumothorax occurs during ordinary daily activities or sleep.

A history of fever and weight loss and of chronic respiratory symptoms such as exertional dyspnea, cough, or wheezing should be sought to determine whether a chronic pulmonary disorder underlies the acute event. A pattern of chronic arthritis, occupational exposure to inorganic dusts, or a temporal association with menses support preexisting lung or pleural pathology associated with connective-tissue disease, pneumoconioses, or a catamenial pneumothorax, respectively. Often the patient will have suffered previous episodes and so will offer the diagnosis as the admitting complaint.

Physical Examination

An initial glance will reveal the patient exhibiting a shallow, rapid pattern of respiration. In some cases, severe air hunger, diaphoresis, cyanosis, and hypotension will be evident and should alert the physician to a tension pneumothorax or an associated pneumomediastinum. In a trauma victim, a penetrating chest wound with an audible inspiratory "hiss" should be quickly identified as the portal of air entry.

Inspection of the chest wall may reveal an asymmetric thorax with an increased volume and a dampened respiratory excursion on the affected side. Palpation will reveal decreased fremitus over the pneumothorax—less commonly, a contralaterally shifted trachea and, rarely, subcutaneous emphysema. Percussion produces a hyperresonant tone relative to the unaffected lung. In cases of pneumothorax under high pressure (tension), the tympanitic quality can be detected across the midline. Cardiac impulses and sounds will be displaced toward the contralateral hemithorax. Breath sounds are typically diminished or absent and, when elicited, have a bronchial or tubular quality. A rhythmic crepitation in synchrony with cardiac systole may occasionally be heard along the left sternal border and may indicate an associated pneumomediastinum.

Laboratory Data

Arterial blood gas determinations should be done promptly to evaluate the patient's oxygenation and ventilation and to assess the urgency and choice of therapeutic interventions. Serum chemistries and a complete blood count (CBC) are of modest diagnostic value on a routine basis, but a leukocytosis or anemia in a febrile or obviously toxic and debilitated patient may support an infectious etiology.

Electrocardiographic changes associated with a pneumothorax include a reduction in amplitude of the QRS complexes and T wave inversion in the precordial leads, mimicking a nontransmural myocardial infarction. Partial or complete reversal in the upright posture will help to distinguish these etiologies.

Electromechanical dissociation in a pulseless patient alerts the physician to consider the diagnosis of tension pneumothorax.

Radiology

The demonstration on chest x-ray of an outwardly convex visceral pleural line separated from the adjacent thoracic wall by a hyperlucent gas shadow without vascular markings is diagnostic of a pneumothorax (Fig. 12-1). An associated pleural effusion may occur in 10 to 25 percent of cases and will produce a distinct linear air-fluid level. Tension pneumothorax produces a marked contralateral shift of the mediastinum, expansion of the ipsilateral rib cage detected as a widening of the intercostal spaces, and a depression of the diaphragm (Fig. 12-2). Occasionally, anatomic landmarks such as skin folds, rib margins, or lung bullae may be mistaken for a pleural line producing false-positive diagnoses and inappropriate treatment. This error can be avoided by following each linear density over its entire length and noting that a skin fold line will extend outside the thorax. To distinguish a pleural line from rib periosteum, one can follow normal pulmonary vascular markings peripherally to determine whether they extend beyond the line in question. Comparison of a posteroanterior (PA) x-ray with a contralateral decubitus chest film will reveal a shift of a pleural air collection from an apical to a lateral position and thus a change in the contour of a pleural line, whereas no change will be found in the configuration of a rib shadow.

Perhaps the most important and difficult distinction to make involves the fibrous wall of a large lung cyst or bulla. A patient with bullous emphysema experiencing an exacerbation will exhibit many of the signs and symptoms of a pneumothorax, including dyspnea, tachypnea, decreased fremitus, hyperresonance, and absent breath sounds. In such a setting, the finding of a hyperlucent and nonperfused lobe or lung can be misinterpreted by even expert physicians and lead to potentially harmful needle aspiration or thoracotomy tube insertion. The wall of a bullous lesion is typically outwardly concave rather than convex, is less regular, and is not easily identifiable as a continuous line if followed from the apex to the base (Fig. 12-3). In addition, older chest films that disclose the same findings would be invaluable in resolving this often worrisome dilemma.

False-negative results occasionally attend a small pneumothorax if an inspiratory PA film is ordered. In contrast, the positive pleural pressure of an expiratory chest x-ray selectively reduces the lung size and so increases the relative dimension of a small pneumothorax. Additionally, compressing the lung increases lung density facilitating detection of the more lucent pleural air. These features favor the use of an expiratory PA chest x-ray to detect small pneumothoraces.

The size of a pneumothorax can be roughly quantitated in order to monitor a patient's progress and often to guide the choice of therapy. Given that the volume of the thoracic cavity (TH) and of the lung (L) are proportional to the cube of their respective diameters, the percent (%) pneumothorax equals: 100 minus $\text{diameter}_L{}^3/\text{diameter}_{TH}{}^3$. The diameters are measured as the horizontal distances from the mediastinum medially to the pleural line (lung [L]) or to the chest wall (thorax [TH]), laterally.

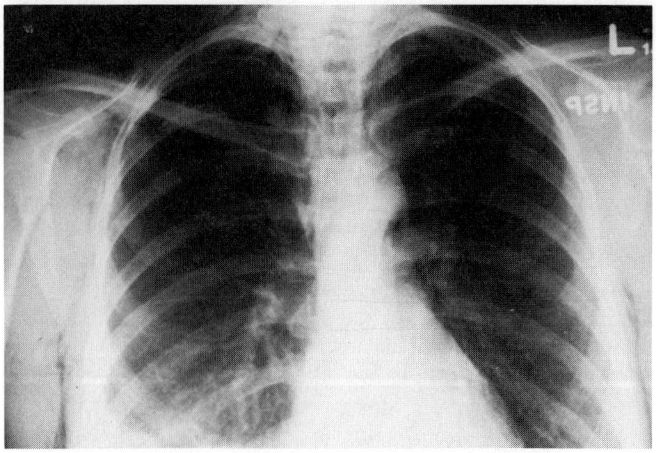

Fig. 12-1. Posteroanterior chest radiograph demonstrates various forms of spontaneous pulmonary barotrauma, including pneumothorax, pneumomediastinum, and subcutaneous emphysema.

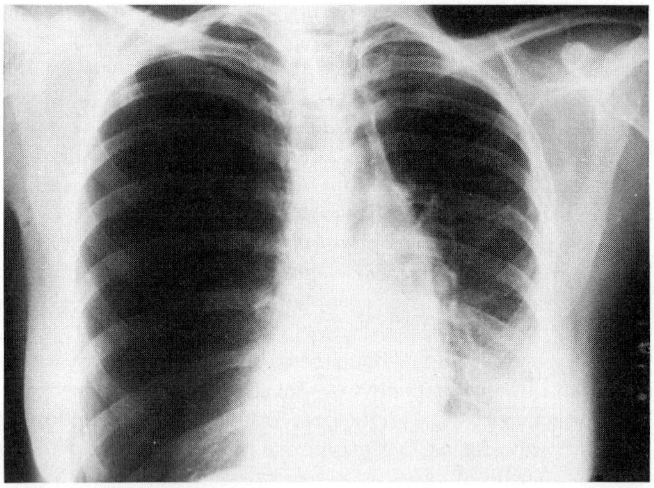

Fig. 12-2. Left-sided tension pneumothorax with its characteristic radiographic features: contralateral displacement of the mediastinum, flattening of the diaphragm, and widening of the intercostal spaces on the affected side.

DIFFERENTIAL DIAGNOSIS

The symptoms and signs of a pneumothorax are nonspecific and, as a result, life-threatening processes such as aortic dissection, pulmonary embolism, and myocardial infarction must also be initially considered—particularly in aortic dissection, which, like primary spontaneous pneumothorax, may affect the young man with a tall, thin (Marfanoid) habitus. Other diagnoses with similar presentations include pericarditis and pleuritis of any etiology, thoracic neuralgias (herpes zoster), acute cholecystitis, and esophageal rupture. If the history and examination are supportive, an expiratory chest radiograph should be considered early to avoid extensive additional testing and delay in therapy.

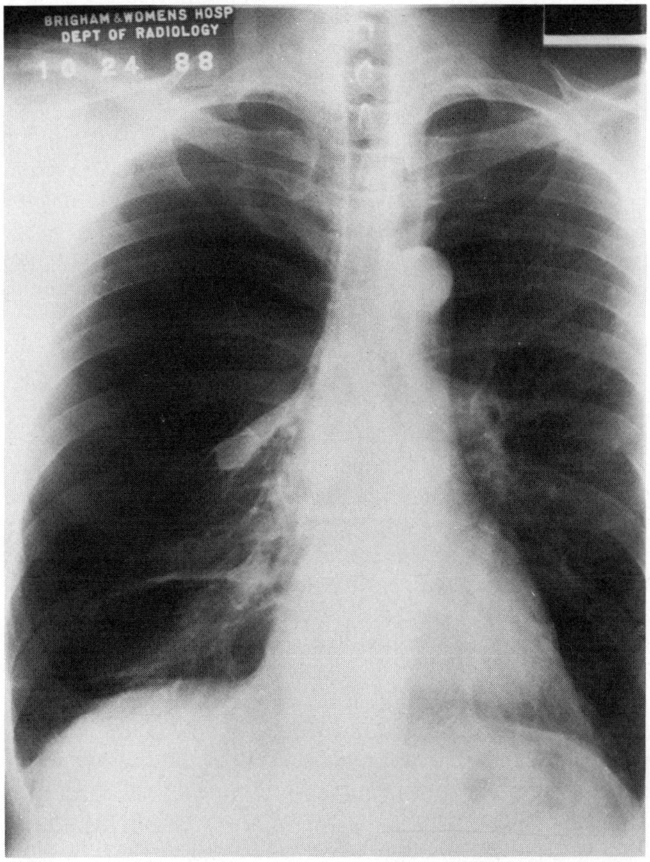

Fig.12-3. Giant right-sided bulla masquerading as a pneumothorax. The thin irregular medial border of the lung cyst can easily be mistaken for the visceral pleural border of a collapsed lung.

MANAGEMENT

The goals of treatment are essentially the same for all episodes of pneumothorax regardless of etiolgy. Therapy is designed to reexpand the lung by evacuating the pleural air at a rate commensurate with the level of disability and to prevent recurrence. The method selected to achieve these goals is individualized based on the following considerations: (1) severity of symptoms and disability, (2) size of the pneumothorax, (3) presence of a persistent air leak, (4) associated intrapleural bleeding, (5) underlying cardiopulmonary health, (6) history of previous pneumothoraces, and (7) mechanism of lung collapse.

Primary Spontaneous Pneumothorax

In a young, healthy individual a small (less than 20%) pneumothorax that produces no respiratory disability may be observed on an outpatient basis under certain conditions. The physician must determine by repeat x-ray that the air leak has sealed and that there will be no progressive lung collapse. Further, the physician should explain that the rate of spontaneous resolution is slow (1.25% of the hemithoracic volume is resorbed daily; thus, a 20% pneumothorax would be expected to resolve in approximately two weeks) and that following the first episode, there is a 50 percent chance of a future recurrence. Finally, the patient should understand the nature of the problem and the need for limiting activity during recovery and committing to close follow-up.

Any uncertainty about either the stability of the pneumothorax or the patient's understanding and ability to comply with instructions mandates admission and inpatient observation. In the asymptomatic patient, a high inspired oxygen fraction (F_IO_2 of 0.9 to 1.0) applied by face mask will increase the pleural space-to-capillary gradient for nitrogen and so will expedite the resorption of the pleural air collection.

Large or symptomatic pneumothoraces require evacuation. Aspiration of a pneumothorax by a 16-gauge needle placed in the anterior second intercostal space is controversial. While it spares the more invasive procedure of chest tube insertion and may convert the pneumothorax to a size that can then be managed conservatively, it has significant limitations. Specifically, it is not suitable for use in the setting of a persistent air leak and carries the risk of lung puncture, bleeding, and pleural infection. Even in the limited setting in which aspiration is suitable treatment (as discussed below under iatrogenic pneumothorax), insertion of a needle has been replaced by use of less hazardous thin flexible tubes (e.g., McSwain Dart).

The primary modality in treating a spontaneous pneumothorax is tube thoracostomy. The tube (usually 28 French) is generally placed arteriorly in the second intercostal space or in the midaxillary line as discussed in detail elsewhere in this text (see Procedure 20). This positioning is suitable for evacuation of air as it moves cephalad within a free pleural space. The presence of adhesions may trap the pleural air into one or more focal loculations requiring chest tube(s) to be directed at the specific collections. The chest tube is connected to a water seal unit, commonly a one-piece plastic disposable version of a three-bottle collection system. Frequently, this alone is sufficient to facilitate expansion of the collapsed lung. If, on inspection, air bubbles continue to pass through the water seal chamber either continuously or with a patient's cough, a persistent bronchopleural air leak is likely present. The chest tube and its insertion site must be examined, however, to ensure that atmospheric air is not being drawn in at the site of the incision or through a chest tube portal left outside the thorax during insertion. If the lung fails to expand or a bronchopleural leak is present, the thoracostomy tube–water seal unit is attached to continuous suction. This method provides complete lung reexpansion in more than 90 percent of cases, with an average hospital stay of 5 days. Serial x-rays and regular bedside observations of the water seal unit for air leaks aid in assessing the patient's response to therapy.

The desire to avoid the cost and inconvenience of hospitalization in otherwise healthy individuals with primary spontaneous pneumothorax has spurred the development of ambulatory models of tube thoracostomy. This approach involves the placement of a chest tube fitted with a one-way flutter (Heimlich) valve that allows the steady evacuation of pleural gases but prohibits entry of outside air. The exact approach varies from immediate application of the Heimlich valve to initial water seal treatment with flutter valve insertion after lung reexpansion has been documented. With careful outpatient follow-up and proper selection of patients (e.g., excluding those with concomitant pleural fluid or blood that will occlude the system), up to three fourths of the patients will respond over a period of 1 to 3 weeks with no further therapy required.

Secondary Spontaneous Pneumothorax

Unlike the typically stable status of the healthy patient who suffers a pneumothorax, the condition of the patient with underlying pulmonary disease is usually critical, with a mortality rate of nearly 20 percent. Thus, the diagnosis must be considered and confirmed without delay and tube thoracostomy drainage implemented promptly. There is no role for outpatient observation in this setting. Even in the patient who initially appears stable, evacuation of intrapleural air will improve oxygenation and eliminate the risk of a subsequent decline resulting from an occult persistent air leak. The success rate of tube thoracostomy in achieving full lung expansion is less than that for the primary variety. Approximately one-fourth of patients will require placement of additional chest tubes to re-expand the lung fully or thoracotomy to close the air leak and resect the bullae.

Traumatic Pneumothorax

The pneumothorax associated with trauma represents a higher level of complexity and risk to the patient. In all cases, chest tube evacuation should be initiated when the diagnosis has been confirmed. In addition, several complications must be ruled out, including an open chest wound, flail chest, tracheobronchial fracture, and esophageal rupture.

The detection of an open chest wound requires immediate closure, establishment of a secure airway, and arrangements for thoracotomy. Emergency treatment of associated tension physiology is discussed in the following paragraphs.

A flail chest owing to multiple rib fractures renders the patient's spontaneous respiratory efforts ineffectual. Prompt intubation and controlled ventilation with sedation and paralysis as necessary will restore ventilatory efficiency and facilitate healing of the unstable chest wall.

Tracheobronchial fracture is suggested by a pneumothorax associated with fracture of the uppermost ribs, hemoptysis, or hemopneumothorax. In addition to chest tube drainage of pleural air and blood, a diagnostic bronchoscopy should be performed with a thoracic surgeon in attendance.

Esophageal rupture typically presents a left-sided pleural effusion but is associated with pneumothorax in more than 50 percent of cases. The diagnosis is supported by noting a high amylase level and a pH less than 7.0 on chemical analysis of the fluid. Pneumomediastinum and subcutaneous emphysema are common associated findings. Oral contrast studies are confirmatory as a preliminary to surgical repair.

Iatrogenic Pneumothorax

Pneumothorax associated with diagnostic or therapeutic procedures range in severity from the introduction of small amounts of ambient air during a thoracentesis to a massive bronchopleural leak in a ventilator-dependent patient. Asymptomatic, small pleural air collections may be treated conservatively with bed rest, observation, and supplemental oxygen. In those situations in which ambient air was introduced along a needle tract and in which no visceral pleural tear exists, tube or catheter aspiration of the pleural air as discussed earlier—in an effort to avoid disability and more invasive therapy—is appropriate.

Pneumothorax resulting from barotrauma in the patient ventilated with positive airway pressure represents an emergency indication for tube thoracostomy with 15 to 25 cm H_2O suction applied to enhance pleural evacuation. Most bronchopleural fistulae will seal with this management. In some patients, despite appropriate therapy, the positive pressure generated by the ventilator prevents healing or even enlarges the pleural defect, warranting modified ventilator modalities such as independent lung ventilation or high-frequency ventilation, occasionally coupled with lifesaving attempts at surgical closure.

Tension Pneumothorax

Pleural air accumulating under positive pressure poses a grave risk to the patient, irrespective of its pathogenesis. In the extreme case of shock and cyanosis, the urgency of the situation precludes a confirmatory chest x-ray. In the presence of the characteristic physical findings (see above), a large-bore needle attached to a saline-filled cylinder from a large syringe is introduced in the anterior second intercostal space on the affected side. If the diagnosis is correct, air will bubble through the column of sterile saline until the intrathoracic pressure approaches that of the outside atmosphere. As this is only a temporizing measure, arrangements for thoracostomy tube placement should urgently be made. This could then be followed by chest x-ray and other diagnostic studies.

PLEURAL EFFUSION

INTRODUCTION AND EPIDEMIOLOGY

More than 1.5 million new patients present annually for evaluation of a pleural effusion. They represent a broad range of etiologies, including cardiopulmonary as well as extrathoracic and systemic disorders. Nearly one-third of the total number is associated with congestive heart failure, while an equal number is evenly divided between neoplastic and infectious causes. Direct sampling and chemical analysis of the pleural fluid can distinguish effusions that arise owing to a disruption of the normal mechanical forces that govern fluid movement (transudates) from those caused by a direct alteration of the pleural tissue or its vasculature (exudates). This distinction is of central importance in beginning the search for a specific diagnosis.

PATHOPHYSIOLOGY

The nearly fluid-free state of the normal pleural space is maintained by the dynamic equilibrium between fluid formation at the surface of the parietal pleura and fluid resorption principally by pleural lymphatic channels. Earlier concepts of fluid movement as governed by a net hydrostatic and colloid osmotic pressure gradient from the parietal pleura to pleural space to visceral pleura were reassessed in light of evidence that the visceral pleura, like the parietal pleura, receives its blood supply from systemic arteries rather than from the lower pressure pulmonary circulation. Current data still support fluid formation by the parietal (and, rarely, visceral) pleura in accordance with Starling's law of transcapillary exchange but have reassigned the primary role in fluid removal from the visceral pleural capillaries to the lymphatic vessels located in the submesothelial layer of the parietal pleura. The lymphatic circulation is also responsible for removing high–molecular weight proteins and particulate material such as blood cells and cellular debris shed by the pleural surfaces.

Abnormal collections of pleural fluid are due to one or more of the following causes: (1) lymphatic blockage, (2) increased capillary permeability, (3) increased capillary hydrostatic pressure involving the systemic or pulmonary circulations or both, (4) reduction in colloidal osmotic (plasma oncotic) pressures, and (5) reduction (greater negativity) in pleural pressure as occurs in extensive atelectasis.

Two prominent clinical features are impaired gas exchange and a subjective sense of dyspnea. Hypoxia results from the compression of lung tissue that accompanies moderate to large pleural fluid accumulations. The resulting reduction in ventilation coupled with the relatively preserved perfusion produce a low $\dot{V}/\dot{Q}$ relationship in the involved region. Particularly noteworthy is the observation that immediate removal of the pleural effusion does not restore normal gas exchange and, paradoxically, may produce worsening hypoxia within the first 24 to 36 hours. A prompt increase in regional blood flow but a more delayed reexpansion of lung tissue transiently worsens the $\dot{V}/\dot{Q}$ impairment.

Pleural fluid evacuation will often improve dyspnea despite an absence of commensurate improvement in gas exchange or in pulmonary function, particularly in patients with large effusions and those who have limited reserve owing to an underlying cardiopulmonary limitation. It is likely that the cause of the dyspnea is related to the distorting effect of the effusion on the diaphragm and respiratory muscles in the chest wall. With reduction in the size and weight of the pleural fluid, the previously flattened diaphragm will resume its preferred domed configuration, and pleural pressure will tend toward its physiologic range. These changes will improve respiratory mechanics and decrease the work of breathing.

INITIAL ASSESSMENT

History

Of the known causes of pleural effusion, relatively few produce acute symptomatology or deterioration of such severity as to bring about an emergency department visit. Among these few are infection, pulmonary embolism, trauma, and cardiac disease (including pericardial); initial questioning should be directed at these etiologies in an acutely ill patient.

Most patients will describe a pattern of dyspnea, cough, and, less often, local or referred pleuritic pain. The last-mentioned symptom has relatively greater diagnostic significance because, unlike the others, it requires direct pleural irritation by infection, neoplasm, or infarction, and so militates against congestive heart failure, nephrosis, and other causes of a bland (and painless) transudative effusion. The patient should be questioned about signs and symptoms of infection, including fever, night sweats, cough productive of discolored sputum, or hemoptysis. Previous exposure to tuberculosis, results of any past PPD (purified protein derivative) skin test, and a history of travel should be elicited when the patient describes features of infection. To evaluate the possibility of pulmonary thromboembolism, the patient should be questioned about lower extremity pain or swelling, recent surgery, oral contraceptive use when applicable, hemoptysis, near syncope, and an episodic or recurring character of the dyspnea.

The presence of a malignancy should be considered in a chronically ill–appearing patient and, accordingly, a history of a past neoplasm or of recent weight loss, hemoptysis, adbominal pain, change in bowel habits, hematochezia, hematuria, or breast lumps must be sought in the appropriate patients. A pattern of arthralgias, dermal eruptions and changes in skin coloration or thickness support an immunologic systemic disorder as a possible etiology.

Physical Examination

The characteristic thoracic examination consists of reduced tactile fremitus and dullness to percussion compared to the unaffected lung. Auscultation over the effusion reveals reduced voice transmission and distant or nearly absent breath sounds. Near the top of the fluid, bronchial breath sounds and enhanced conduction of sound (egophony) suggesting consolidation may be generated by the lung tissue compressed by the fluid collection. Leather-like or crepitant pleural rubs can be auscultated in a minority of instances. In the setting of a massive effusion, signs of a high pleural pressure, including asymmetric expansion of the thorax and contralateral displacement of the trachea and apical cardiac pulsation will be noted. Focal areas of ecchymoses over the thorax and a dyskinetic rib cage suggest one or more rib fractures and, possibly, a related hemothorax. Cardiac examination is of central importance in evaluating the presence of congestive heart failure, pericarditis, or pulmonary embolization. In the last case, the constellation of distended neck veins, left parasternal lift, and an accentuated pulmonic second heart sound (P_2) in the absence of left ventricular dysfunction indicates repeated or massive embolization producing acute right heart failure.

In addition to the cardiopulmonary examination, physical findings of arthritis, lymphadenopathy, deep vein thrombosis, breast nodule, or adnexal mass on pelvic examination will offer important clues as to the probable etiology of the pleural effusion.

Laboratory Data

An initial assessment of the patient's gas exchange should be made by arterial blood gas measurement or by oximetry. A CBC is pertinent in a patient who exhibits fever or hypotension. An urgent prothrombin time, partial thromboplastin time, and a platelet count, will screen for a hemorrhagic diathesis prior to thoracentesis.

A diagnostic thoracentesis is important in determining the etiology of a pleural effusion. Consequently, in the absence of contraindications (e.g., anticoagulation), it should be performed prior to therapy in any cooperative patient who presents with an effusion of unknown origin. One exception to this would be a patient with a long history of congestive heart failure who presents with a constellation of supportive clinical and radiographic findings. Before a thoracentesis is undertaken at the bedside, fluid should be free flowing as assessed by upright and decubitus x-ray and accessible—that is, not loculated nor subpulmonic.

Clear yellow pleural fluid should be submitted routinely for cell count and differential; for chemistry values, including total protein, lactate dehydrogenase (LDH), and glucose; and in many cases for cytology. Fluid that is turbid, thick, or malodorous should be sent for pH, Gram's stain, and aerobic and anaerobic cultures. Hemorrhagic pleural fluid should also be sent for cytology and acid-fast bacillus (AFB) stain and culture as should fluid of any character when the clinical setting suggests tuberculosis or neoplasia. Pleural fluid amylase levels are indicated in a patient with possible pancreatitis or in a chest trauma victim with a suspected esophageal tear. Additional fluid should be stored for follow-up studies as indicated. Concomitant serum protein and LDH will facilitate characterization of the fluid as a transudate or exduate.

Transudates are those fluids that meet the following criteria:

1. Pleural fluid protein to serum protein ratio of less than 0.5
2. Pleural fluid LDH to serum LDH ratio of less than 0.6
3. Pleural fluid LDH value of less than 200

Pleural fluid that exceeds one or more of the aforementioned limits is designated an *exudate*.

Radiology

Pleural fluid of any etiology that moves freely within the pleural space characteristically presents as a homogeneously dense opacity within the affected hemithorax. When viewed on an upright film, its superior border is curvilinear, with the apex at its lateral margin where it adjoins the chest wall (Fig. 12-4). On a decubitus film, the fluid shifts and settles along the new inferior margin of the hemithorax. Large effusions produce a shift of the mediastinum to the opposite side. Small amounts of fluid (less than 300 ml) may settle into the "posterior gutter" formed by the posterior costophrenic angle and may be evident on a lateral upright film but undetected on a PA upright. Occasionally, fluid will be trapped between the diaphragm and the diaphragmatic surface of the lung. The subpulmonic effusion is suggested on PA film by the lateral displacement of the point at which the inferior margin of the lung curves caudad into the costophrenic recess and is confirmed by a layering of fluid on a lateral decubitus film.

Pleural fluid that does not exhibit the aforementioned characteristics of free fluid should be evaluated in light of earlier films if possible. The discovery of chronicity suggests a chronic pleural thickening rather than fluid. However, the same pleural pattern in a febrile patient with an ipsilateral pulmonary infiltrate (Fig. 12-5) strongly supports a complicated parapneumonic or infected pleural effusion that de-

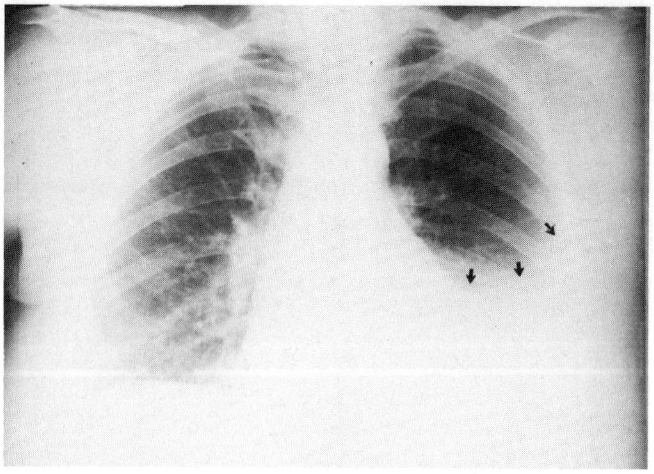

Fig. 12-4 Posteroanterior chest radiograph illustrates the features of a freely flowing left pleural effusion. Note the fluid's uniform density and the curvilinear superior margin with its concave upward configuration.

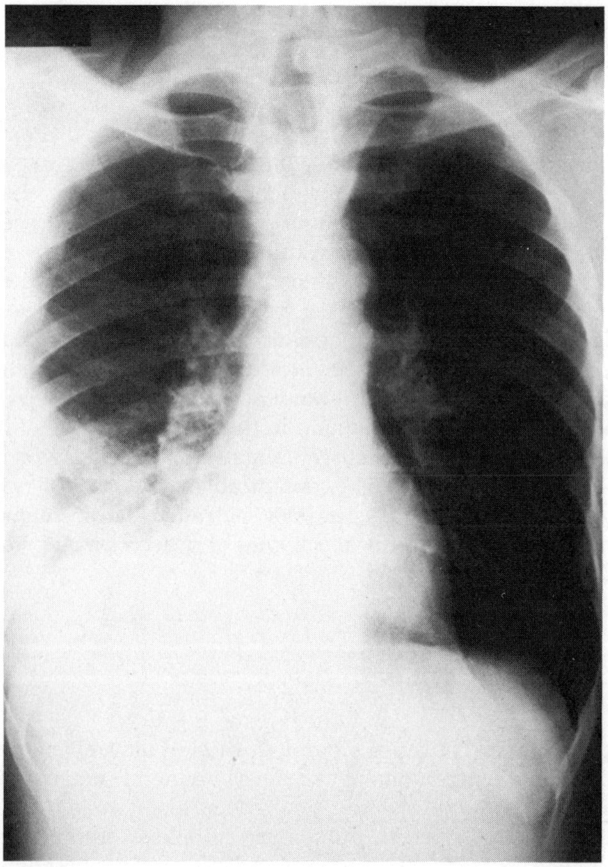

Fig. 12-5. Posteroanterior upright chest x-ray reveals a right lower lobe infiltrate, hilar adenopathy, and a pleural effusion that does not collect along the dependent surface as expected of an uncomplicated, aseptic effusion. Diagnostic thoracentesis yielded grossly purulent fluid confirming an empyema.

mands prompt sampling and drainage usually under ultrasound guidance.

DIFFERENTIAL DIAGNOSIS

The clinical presentation of pleural effusions mimics other pulmonary and cardiac causes of dyspnea, tachypnea and cough, such as COPD, pneumothorax, pneumonia, and congestive heart failure. When chest pain is a prominent feature, costochondritis, neuralgias, and myocardial infarction are to be considered. Once the presence of pleural fluid is confirmed by chest radiography, further inquiry is guided by the laboratory characterization of the pleural fluid. The chief causes of transudative effusions are congestive heart failure and hypoalbuminemia owing to either nephrosis or advanced liver disease. A specific etiology for transudative effusion can usually be determined in an urgent care setting by a review of history, physical findings, serum chemistry, and urinalysis.

The etiologic spectrum of exudative effusions is considerably wider and more difficult to establish during an initial evaluation. General categories include infection (bacterial, tuberculous, virus), malignancy (lung, breast, ovarian), collagen-vascular disorders (systemic lupus erythematosus, rheumatoid arthritis), traumatic (hemothorax, chylothorax), occupational (benign asbestos effusion), and miscellaneous sources of inflammation (pulmonary embolism, radiation, uremia).

MANAGEMENT

While much of the workup and treatment of pleural effusions occurs outside the urgent care setting, acute insults such as trauma, pulmonary embolism, and aggressive infection can precipitate a rapid deterioration in status. Emergency management typically begins before a specific etiology has been determined and focuses on initial stabilization of the patient. When present, hypoxia is corrected with supplenental oxygen, and hypotension owing to sepsis or blood loss is supported with intravenous fluids, blood products, and pressors as required. Subsequent treatment is individualized based on an assessment of the underlying cause.

Trauma

A common posttraumatic pleural complication is a *hemothorax*. In a stable, cooperative patient with an uncertain medical history, a thoracentesis may be initially performed. The finding of hemorrhagic fluid with a hematocrit greater than one-half that of the peripheral blood is confirmatory and mandates tube-thoracostomy drainage to prevent fibrothorax and a trapped lung. More commonly, the patient's tenuous status and the high index of suspicion support placement of a thoracostomy tube as the initial diagnostic and therapeutic procedure. Continued bleeding complicated by hypotension despite red cell transfusion is best managed by emergent thoracotomy. In contrast to the placement of chest tubes for evacuation of air, the optimal location for fluid drainage is posteriorly and inferiorly in the thoracic cage.

The discovery of pleural fluid that is milky white in color is indicative of a *chylothorax* owing to traumatic rupture of the thoracic duct. Here too, prompt placement of a chest tube is appropriate for both diagnosis and therapy, as the thoracic duct defect may heal with up to 2 weeks of conservative management via tube drainage. Persistent leakage warrants surgical repair. During the course of therapy, intensive nutritional support is required to offset the loss of lipid-rich fluid and to prevent malnutrition.

Esophageal or tracheal rupture may complicate blunt chest trauma and are discussed in the section concerning pneumothorax.

Parapneumonic Effusions and Empyema

The distinction between a bland, sterile parapneumonic effusion and a complicated or frankly infected pleural fluid is crucial when deciding on a course of treatment. In the former case, the treatment consists of antibiotic therapy of the underlying pneumonia (usually *Streptococcus pneumoniae* or *Staphylococcus aureus*) with no specific treatment of the effusion. In contrast, the treatment of a complicated effusion or empyema requires prompt drainage via chest tube in addition to antibiotic therapy. Numerous reports have confirmed that patient survival is jeopardized by a delay in drainage of a pleural infection. The decision regarding chest tube placement begins with a visual evaluation of the aspirated pleural fluid and also includes the results of Gram's stain, pH, and glucose measurements. Any fluid that appears purulent and thick to visual inspection or that demonstrates organisms on Gram's stain should be drained by tube thoracostomy, regardless of etiology. In addition, parapneumonic effusions with a pH of less than 7.0 or a glucose level of less than 50 mg/dl or both are associated with a high incidence of infection or loculation and warrant chest tube drainage. If fluid with these chemical characteristics appears nonviscous, initial complete drainage of the involved pleural space may be attempted by thoracentesis.

The choice of empiric antibiotics rests on Gram's stain results of sputum and pleural fluid and a familiarity with the pattern of commonly involved bacteria. Empyemas are most commonly infected by a mix of aerobic and anaerobic bacterial strains, but up to one-third involve anaerobes alone. Consequently, anaerobic cultures must be included when processing the diagnostic sample of fluid on a patient with suspected infection. If Gram's stains are not revealing, a combination of agents designed to cover anaerobes and gram-positive and -negative aerobes should be selected until culture and sensitivity results are available.

Pulmonary Embolism

Pleural effusions accompany pulmonary emboli in approximately 40% of cases. The effusions are typically serous or bloody exudates owing to either ischemia and infarction of the pleura or, less commonly, are secondary to associated atelectasis and so are transudative in character. Workup should proceed with a ventilation/perfusion lung scan. If the study is not diagnostic and if sufficient suspicion still exists, pulmonary angiography is indicated. Treatment of the effusion consists of therapy directed at the underlying embolism. Continuous heparin infusion is the cornerstone of therapy in this setting and may be initiated as the diagnostic workup proceeds when clinical suspicion is high and the risk of bleeding complications is not prohibitive.

SELECTED READING

Chretien, J, and Hirsch, A (ed). *Diseases of the Pleura*. New York: Masson, 1983.

Light, RW. *Pleural Diseases*. Philadelphia: Lea & Febiger, 1983.

Chretien, J, Bignon, J, and Hirsch, A (eds). *The Pleura in Health and Disease*. New York: Dekker, 1985.

Rothberg, AD, Marks, KH, and Maisels, MJ. Understanding the pleurevac. *Pediatrics* 67:482, 1981.

Sahn, SA. Spontaneous pneumothorax: A common emergency. *J Respir Dis* 4:12, 1983.

Steier, M, et al. Pneumothorax complicating continuous ventilatory support. *J Thorac Cardiovasc Surg* 67:17, 1974.

Sahn, SA. The differential diagnosis of pleural effusions. *West J Med* 137:99, 1982.

Light, RW, et al. Parapneumonic effusions. *Am J Med* 69:507, 1980.

Bartlett, JG, et al. Bacteriology of empyema. *Lancet* 1:338, 1974

Himmelman, RB, and Callen, PW. The prognostic value of loculations in parapneumonic pleural effusions. *Chest* 90:852, 1986.

13. Disorders of the Pulmonary Vasculature

Robert C. Basner

PULMONARY THROMBOEMBOLISM

Pulmonary thromboembolism (PTE) is estimated to be responsible for 300,000 annual hospitalizations per year in the United States, with a case fatality rate approaching 25 percent over the past decade. Immediate mortality from PTE is most often the result of acute pulmonary artery hypertension and resultant cardiogenic shock. Late morbidity and mortality secondary to unresolved or recurrent emboli is characterized by impairment of gas exchange function of the lung, chronic pulmonary hypertension, and chronic cor pulmonale.

There are no symptoms or signs specific for pulmonary thromboembolism. Moreover, the initial presentation of acute PTE is quite variable. At one extreme is the virtually asymptomatic individual with, perhaps, significant risk factors for thromboembolism and subtle physical findings such as tachypnea and tachycardia. At the other extreme is the patient with massive PTE and cardiovascular collapse in whom the diagnosis may be confused with other cardiovascular catastrophes. It is evident, then, that the clinician in the emergency unit not only must be able to recognize and treat immediately life-threatening episodes of PTE but also must be vigilant to the possibility of underlying PTE in the patient who is less acutely ill in order to avoid the consequences of a missed or delayed diagnosis.

PATHOPHYSIOLOGY AND RISK FACTORS

Pulmonary emboli most commonly result from the migration of thrombi formed in the deep venous system of the lower extremities. Thrombogenic stimuli such as venous stasis, hypercoagulability, and damage to vascular endothelium may all play a role in the initiation of the fibrin and platelet aggregates that these thrombi represent. Resultant venous outflow obstruction or inflammation or both may produce lower extremity pain, swelling, or even a palpable cord, but the majority of deep venous thrombi cannot be detected by clinical examination. Most deep venous thrombi undergo spontaneous lysis or organization, but up to 20 percent of untreated calf vein thrombi may propagate to more proximal veins of the lower extremity and from there embolize to the pulmonary circulation.

The major risk factors associated with PTE are essentially those for deep venous thrombosis (DVT). Immobility of the lower extremities is probably the most important of these factors. Prolonged bed rest (especially for a week or more) is associated with a high frequency of DVT, but pulmonary thromboembolism may be seen in otherwise healthy individuals who have been immobile during automobile or plane trips of only several hours' duration. Orthopedic surgery of the lower limb, particularly the hip, knee, or tibia, is associated with a greater than 50 percent incidence of subsequent DVT if no prophylaxis againt DVT is given; nonorthopedic surgery also creates significant risk, particularly operations lasting longer than 30 minutes and those necessitating prolonged postoperative immobility. Nonsurgical trauma to the lower extremity is associated with the same thrombogenic risks as surgical trauma, with hip fracture being the most commonly found traumatic condition associated with DVT. Other documented risk factors for DVT/PTE include underlying malignancy, advancing age, previous venous thromboembolism, congestive heart failure, obesity, and estrogen therapy. Although there is some controversy as to whether pregnant patients are at greater risk for DVT and PTE than nonpregnant control populations, postpartum patients definitely have a substantially increased incidence of DVT and PTE compared with age-matched controls. Pulmonary thromboembolism may also result from thrombi formed in the pelvic veins (typically following gynecologic or prostate procedures) or at the site of catheters placed in the central venous circulation for hemodynamic monitoring, cardiac pacing, or hyperalimentation.

Acute embolization involving more than 50 percent of the cross-sectional area of the pulmonary arterial circuit typically results in a sudden increase in pulmonary vascular resistance, which may be severe enough to induce right ventricular overload and failure. Less massive emboli are more likely to present with acute effects on lung function and gas exchange. Maldistribution of ventilation and perfusion with resultant ventilation/perfusion inequality, increased alveolar dead space with an increased physiologic dead space to tidal volume ratio (V_D/V_T), and atelectasis have all been associated with acute PTE and may contribute to the dyspnea and hypoxemia so commonly found in this disorder.

CLINICAL PRESENTATION AND INITIAL ASSESSMENT

The clinician in the emergency unit is often faced with assessing an ambulatory patient with pleuritic chest pain and other nonspecific respiratory signs and symptoms; many such patients undergo some workup for PTE, as well as expectant anticoagulation. Large series have identified PTE in approximately 20% of all such patients. The age of the patient is an important factor in assessing the likelihood of PTE. Ambulatory patients with pleuritic chest pain who are *younger than 40 years of age* and have neither predisposing factors for DVT/PTE (as previously outlined) nor clinical evidence of DVT, carry an extremely low likelihood of having had a documentable pulmonary thromboembolus. The risks, discomforts, and costs of proceeding with anticoagulation and workup for acute PTE in such patients are difficult to justify based on available data. On the other hand, in patients with pleuritic chest pain who are *older than 40 years of age* the absence of the aforementioned clinical variables does not rule out a diagnosis of PTE; 18 percent of such patients were subsequently found to have PTE in a recent series of ambulatory patients.

The major clinical entities that most commonly must be differentiated from PTE in the emergency unit include ischemic heart disease, pleural inflammation from causes other than PTE (such as viral pleurisy), costochondritis, and viral or bacterial pneumonia. Most patients with symptomatic PTE will note either new or worsened dyspnea. Pleuritic chest pain and hemoptysis actually occur much less frequently; these reflect underlying pulmonary infarction or congestive atelectasis. Syncope may occur in the setting of massive PTE secondary to a suddenly decreased cardiac output. Tachycardia and tachypnea are the most frequent initial physical findings of acute PTE; a low-grade fever may also be present. Common (albeit nonspecific) chest findings include splinting, chest wall tenderness, a pleural friction rub, and signs of pulmonary consolidation, atelectasis, pleural effusion, or bronchospasm. When pulmonary vascular resistance is significantly elevated following acute PTE, any or all of the following may be found: pulsus paradoxus, elevated jugular venous pulse, right ventricular gallop, prominent pulmonary component of the second heart sound, and a murmur of tricuspid insufficiency. Systemic hypotension and impaired consciousness are generally the result of massive embolism.

There are no laboratory abnormalities consistently found following acute PTE. Arterial blood gases may fail to demonstrate significant hypoxemia, particularly in young ambulatory patients. Furthermore, the finding of arterial hypoxemia does not differentiate acute PTE from other entities causing similar presenting signs and symptoms.

The chest radiograph may be entirely normal or may demonstrate a parenchymal infiltrate, atelectasis, or an elevated hemidiaphragm. Regional oligemia with proximal vessel cutoff (Westermark sign) or a pleural-based density convex toward the hilum (Hampton hump) may also be seen, but none of these findings is sensitive or specific for acute PTE. The presence of a small unilateral pleural effusion in young ambulatory patients with pleuritic chest pain has been shown to be a fairly sensitive, although nonspecific indicator of acute PTE. The main importance of the chest radiograph in PTE is to enable one to rule out other diagnoses, as well as to aid in the interpretation of subsequent lung scintigraphy.

The electrocardiogram most commonly will be normal or will exhibit a sinus tachycardia; acute pulmonary thromboembolism is a relatively uncommon cause of atrial arrhythmia. In massive PTE, a pattern of acute cor pulmonale may develop; this pattern includes the commonly referred to "$S_1Q_3T_3$" changes of a new Q wave with inverted T wave in limb lead III, along with a "reciprocal" S wave in limb lead I. Inverted T waves may also be present across the anterior precordium. Such an electrocardiogram (ECG) must be differentiated from that of acute myocardial infarction, particularly since these two entities may cause closely similar clinical presentations (Fig. 13-1).

DIAGNOSTIC EVALUATION

If the clinician is considering the diagnosis of acute pulmonary thromboembolism based on the aforementioned criteria and principles, the next procedure of choice, typically, is lung scintigraphy (ventilation/perfusion scanning). Antico-

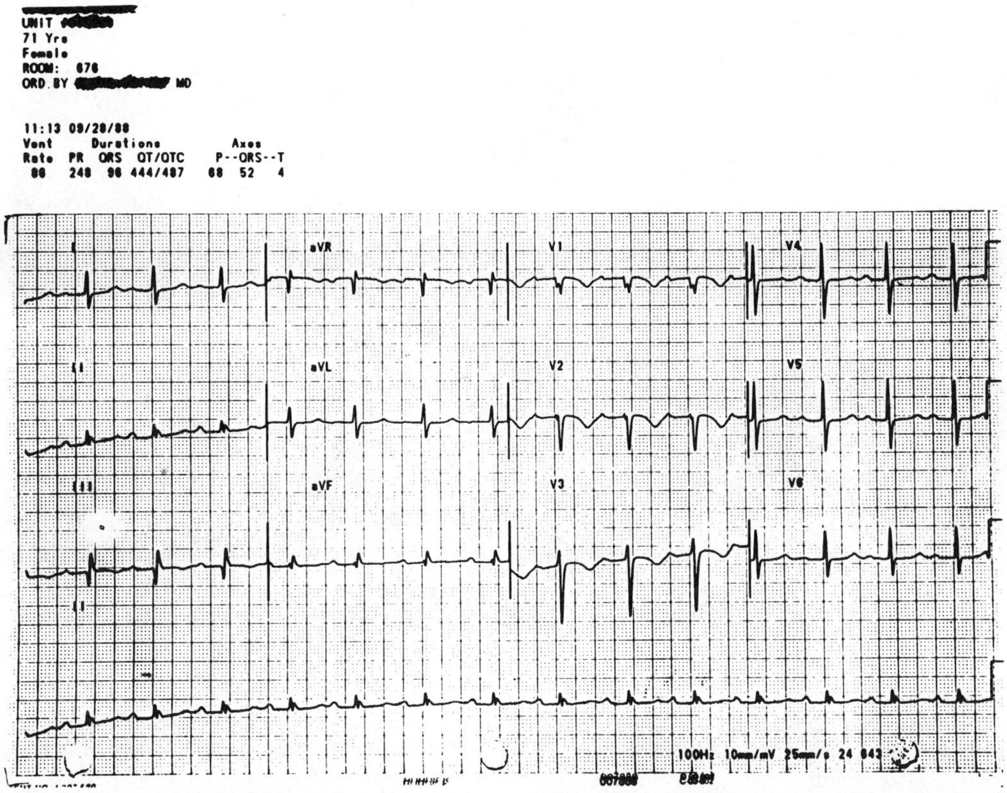

Fig. 13-1. Electrocardiogram from a 71-year-old woman with sudden onset of dyspnea, chest pain, and systemic hypotension, who was being ruled out for acute myocardial infarction. She was subsequently proved to have massive pulmonary thromboembolism. The electrocardiogram is consistent with acute cor pulmonale (see text).

agulation therapy with intravenous heparin should be initiated while awaiting lung scanning in this situation, provided that there are no contraindications to such therapy (see below). Perfusion lung imaging involves intravenous injection of ^{99m}Tc-labeled macroaggregated albumin; multiple view scanning of activity in the lungs is ideally carried out with the patient in the upright position. Under such circumstances, the absence of perfusion defects can be assumed to effectively rule out acute PTE, and another diagnosis must be entertained. The presence of a perfusion defect will usually mandate ventilation scintigraphy. If xenon-133 gas is to be used for ventilation scanning, it is best administered prior to perfusion scanning because of the possibility of image degradation by the technetium. Posterior views, along with left and right posterior oblique views on wash out, should be obtained. Aside from the normal perfusion scan, three categories of PTE "probability" are currently recognized; patterns of perfusion and ventilation defects are grouped within these categories based on their association with angiographically documented PTE:

1. *The "low probability" scan.* This includes small (occupying less than 25% of a bronchopulmonary segment) or nonsegmental perfusion defects regardless of their number, ventilation status (i.e., "matched" or "mismatched"), or correlation with the chest radiograph. Such a scan is associated with a 10 percent or less incidence rate of angiographically proven PTE. Further, a patient with such a scan, if discharged, is unlikely to return with a documented PTE.

2. *The "high probability" scan* (Fig. 13-2). This carries a greater than 90 percent incidence of angiographically proven PTE. Such a scan would include the following patterns:

- **a.** Two or more segmental (occupying at least 75% of a bronchopulmonary segment) perfusion defects in the presence of normal ventilation and a normal chest radiograph.
- **b.** One segmental or greater perfusion defect with two or more moderate size defects in the presence of normal ventilation and chest radiograph.
- **c.** Four or more moderate size perfusion defects with normal ventilation and chest radiograph.

3. *The "intermediate probability" scan.* Quite simply, such a scan includes any pattern of abnormalities that cannot be defined as either "high" or "low" probability. The "indeterminate" scan—one in which a perfusion defect exactly matches an area of radiographic opacity—falls into this category and has been estimated to neither lower or raise the posttest probability of PTE being present. The clinician must be wary of assessing all perfusion defects that occur in the same general distribution as radiographic abnormality as "indeterminate," however. A perfusion defect that is substantially smaller than a corresponding x-ray abnormality carries the same significance as a low-probability scan, whereas the presence of two or more segmental perfusion defects that are substantially larger than corresponding radiographic or ventilation abnormalities should be considered a pattern of high probability.

It must be recognized that the results of lung scanning need to be interpreted in light of the clinician's pretest suspicion of

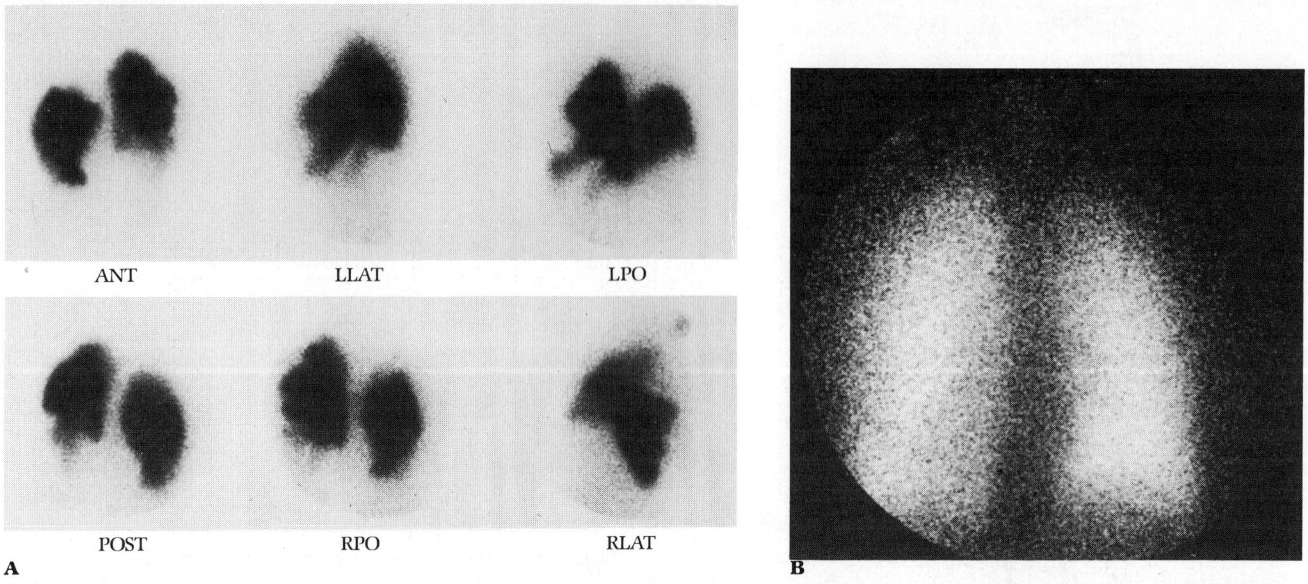

Fig. 13-2. Ventilation/perfusion lung scans in a pattern interpreted as having a high probability for pulmonary embolism. A. Six views of the lungs are shown on perfusion scan: there are multiple segmental perfusion defects in both lungs. (ANT = anterior view; LLAT = left lateral view; LPO = left posterior oblique view; POST = posterior view; RPO = right posterior oblique view; RLAT = right lateral view.) B. A single frame from the ventilation scan demonstrates uniform distribution of ventilation throughout both lungs. Thus, multiple segmental ventilation/perfusion mismatches exist.

acute PTE. In general, a normal or "low probability" scan in the setting of a low clinical likelihood of PTE requires no further workup or therapy. Similarly, a high index of suspicion for PTE prior to scanning plus a "high probability" scan pattern may be taken as acceptable evidence of acute PTE; no further documentation is necessary to justify initiation and maintenance of anticoagulation therapy in this circumstance. Data from the ongoing Prospective Investigation of Pulmonary Embolism Diagnosis (PIOPED) trial should help clarify the validity of these conclusions.

Whereas most other combinations of clinical and lung scan findings will require the definitive evaluation provided by pulmonary angiography, additional noninvasive tests are usually available that may help confirm the diagnosis, thus potentially eliminating the need for angiography. Noninvasive imaging of the lower extremities may be used to document the presence of deep venous thrombosis. Impedance plethysmography (IPG) has correlated well with venography-proven DVT in the ambulatory setting. Indeed, the combination of IPG and ventilation/perfusion lung scanning achieved nearly 100 percent diagnostic sensitivity and specificity for PTE in a series of ambulatory patients with pleuritic chest pain. Conditions that cause elevation of central venous pressure, such as congestive heart failure or decompensated chronic obstructive pulmonary disease (COPD), may lead to a false-positive result. Ultrasound imaging as been reported to be highly sensitive for thombi located in the common femoral and popliteal veins. The accuracy of both these techniques is considered to be somewhat operator-dependent.

Echocardiography with pulsed Doppler recordings can suggest the presence of acute PTE by providing evidence of tricuspid regurgitation or right ventricular hypokinesis or dilation. Further, these parameters may be followed to assess hemodynamic responses during the course of therapy.

Utilizing multiple oblique projections (similar to lung scintigraphy) and subselective injections (guided by the previously obtained scintigram), pulmonary angiography can definitively visualize thrombi as filling defects within the vessels and remains the "gold standard" for the diagnosis of acute PTE. Pulmonary artery pressures should always be measured prior to dye injection in order to avoid right ventricular overload and failure in the presence of significant pulmonary hypertension. A history of allergy to or bronchospasm following injection of contrast material must also be ruled out. The decision to proceed with angiography in these settings must be made in light of the urgency for definitive documentation of acute PTE (see below). The mortality rate for selective pulmonary angiography is estimated to be much less than 1 percent overall. Most morbidity from the procedure is associated with venous catheterization, usually accomplished via femoral vein approach; the incidence of such complications, particularly bleeding and hematoma, is increased if thrombolytic agents are subsequently used.

MANAGEMENT

Differentiating massive from submassive PTE on clinical grounds allows for a rational approach to management options. Massive PTE is diagnosed in the setting of acute cor pulmonale and clinically significant hemodynamic compromise; syncope, shock, or outright cardiorespiratory arrest are the usual manifestations. Such a definition identifies a group of patients with PTE for whom anticoagulation therapy alone is associated with a particularly poor outcome. Submassive PTE, by definition, occasions no such clinically apparent hemodynamic compromise.

When submassive PTE has been diagnosed, anticoagulation with heparin is generally the next therapeutic maneuver if no contraindications to its use exist. As noted earlier, anticoagulation should be undertaken as soon as the diagnosis is strongly suspected. The rationale for such therapy is to prevent recurrence of embolism while allowing the endogenous fibrinolytic system to dissolve the remaining clot. A continuous infusion of heparin to maintain the partial thromboplastin time (PTT) between 1.5 and 2.5 times control values is begun following an initial intravenous bolus. Doses are initially determined based on the patient's weight: A 70-kg patient will receive a bolus in the range of 5,000 units and a subsequent infusion in the range of 1,000 units per hour. The maintenance infusion is adjusted according to repeat determinations of the PTT. The prompt use of heparin in this manner has been shown to lower mortality from PTE in both controlled and uncontrolled studies.

Prior to initiating anticoagulation, careful attention must be paid to the presence of factors associated with increased risk of bleeding with heparin. Examination of the stool for occult blood should be considered mandatory in this regard. Signs, symptoms, or laboratory evidence of active internal bleeding should alert the clinician to the likelihood of serious hemorrhagic complications from heparinization; the presence of a coagulopathy or a history of recent internal surgery or trauma should likewise be considered relative contraindications to heparinization. In such circumstances, anticoagulation is generally deferred until definitive diagnosis by pulmonary angiography (or venography for DVT) has been made.

Treatment for such patients, as well as for patients with a history of heparin-induced thrombocytopenia, will usually involve some form of interruption of the inferior vena cava (IVC) without anticoagulation. Placement of a transvenous Kimray-Greenfield filter via venotomy is currently the preferred method of IVC interruption in this setting.

Heparinized patients in whom significant risk for recurrent thromboembolism remains are maintained on warfarin (Coumadin) for a minimum of 3 months; subsequent evaluation of risk for recurrence is generally made at that time. Warfarin should be initiated early in the clinical course. While the standard for warfarin therapy in this setting calls for maintenance of the prothrombin time (PT) at approximately 1.5 to 2.0 times the control value, recent work suggests that "low-dose" warfarin therapy, in which the PT is maintained between 1.2 and 1.4 times the control value, is as effective as "full-dose" warfarin in the prevention of recurrent proximal DVT and produces significantly fewer hemorrhagic complications. Whichever warfarin dosage regimen is chosen, the PT should be documented to be in the desired therapeutic range for at least 3 to 5 days (thus ensuring therapeutic anticoagulation for a full week) prior to discontinuing heparin. Warfarin crosses the placental barrier and is contraindicated in the pregnant patient; adjusted-dose subcutaneous heparin is useful to prevent a recurrence of DVT and PTE in this situation.

The indications for the use of thrombolytic agents in acute PTE remain controversial. In contrast to heparin, these agents promote active dissolution of recently formed clot; they are also associated with a higher frequency of hemorrhagic complications. Streptokinase and urokinase are currently approved by the Food and Drug Administration (FDA) for the treatment of acute PTE. Both of these agents have been shown to lyse clot in the pulmonary arteries more quickly and completely than does heparin alone, but no reduction in mortality has been proved with the use of these drugs, even in the setting of massive PTE. Further, follow-up ranging from 1 week to 6 months after thrombolytic therapy has generally failed to show continued improvement in clot lysis over that observed with heparin alone.

Tissue plasminogen activator (tPA) is a newer thrombolytic agent, which, by virtue of its specificity for fibrin, is expected to achieve comparable clot lysis without the fibrinogen depletion and hemorrhagic risk associated with the other agents. Recent trials have shown tPA to be actually more efficacious in lysing pulmonary artery clot than urokinase, while indeed causing fewer hemorrhagic complications. Open-label studies have demonstrated the ability of tPA to achieve significantly lowered pulmonary artery pressures and increased right ventricular function in patients hemodynamically compromised following acute PTE. Further controlled studies are planned to better define the role of tPA versus heparin alone for the treatment of both massive and submassive PTE; at the present time, this medication remains experimental for this indication.

Thrombolytic therapy is currently recommended for patients with either anatomically or hemodynamically manifested massive PTE; clinicians familiar with the administration and monitoring of thrombolytic agents should participate in the care of such patients. Heparin should not be infused concomitantly with lytic medications and, in general, is discontinued just prior to initiation of lytic therapy and restarted when either the PTT or thrombin time is less than twice the control value.

When thrombolytic therapy is contraindicated in massive PTE (e.g., recent internal surgery, biopsy, or trauma; parturition; any history of cerebrovascular accident, central nervous system [CNS] tumor, or recent CNS trauma; uncontrolled hypertension; coagulopathy), emergent pulmonary embolectomy may be lifesaving. Interruption of the IVC is generally carried out along with embolectomy in these patients. Indications for IVC interruption also include any situation in which serious bleeding has occurred or may occur with anticoagulation, recurrent PTE despite documented therapeutic anticoagulation, and septic embolization.

Respiratory management of the patient with massive PTE always includes supplemental oxygen; mechanical ventilation with or without positive end-expiratory pressure (PEEP) may be necessary to support such a patient. Aggressive pain and fever control should be initiated in order to decrease metabolic and circulatory demand. Volume expansion and vasopressor therapy may be necessary to support the systemic circulation while efforts to actively lyse pulmonary artery clot, or to prevent further emboli, are undertaken.

OTHER FORMS OF PULMONARY EMBOLISM

While bland deep venous thrombosis is by far the most common source of pulmonary emboli, other types of emboli must be considered in the appropriate clinical setting, since the management of each of these is usually quite different from that of PTE. The most important of these other forms of pulmonary emboli are discussed briefly in the following sections.

SEPTIC EMBOLISM

Septic thrombi may result from either bacterial invasion of a formed sterile thrombus or after blood-borne bacteria have caused venous wall injury and thrombosis. Typically, such infected thrombi are formed in the setting of intravenous drug abuse, indwelling venous catheter infection, or pelvic thrombophlebitis following obstetric and gynecologic procedures. A septic thrombus may embolize to the pulmonary circulation just as a bland thrombus may; symptoms of pulmonary septic embolism are generally similar to those of bland embolism, although fever tends to be more prominent in septic embolism.

A distinguishing feature of pulmonary septic embolism may be found on the chest radiograph, which often demonstrates multiple small nodules within hours of the initial event. These nodules tend to cavitate while new nodules continue to develop.

Empiric therapy with intravenous antibiotics should be begun as soon as the diagnosis is suspected; this should include coverage for penicillinase-producing staphylococci, as well as for gram-negative organisms. All potential sources of septic emboli must be removed or isolated; this may necessitate surgical ligation proximal to the site of a septic phlebitis. Concomitant tricuspid valve endocarditis should also be sought by echocardiography. Anticoagulation is generally not indicated early in the course of treatment but has been reported to be efficacious as an alternative to surgical ligation.

FAT EMBOLISM

Fat embolism to the pulmonary circulation should be suspected in the patient who becomes suddenly dyspneic following long bone fracture or orthopedic surgery. Nontraumatic fat embolism has been reported in patients with fatty liver or systemic lupus erythematosus and in immunocompromised patients in the setting of corticosteroid therapy. Fat droplets embolized to the circulation can cause mechanical obstruction of pulmonary blood flow, thus resulting in a syndrome similar to that of PTE. Additionally, the fatty acids released from degradation of these fat droplets are believed to be directly toxic to the lungs, resulting in a spectrum of disease ranging from mild chemical pneumonitis to adult respiratory distress syndrome (ARDS). In addition to dyspnea, the characteristic clinical features of fat embolism syndrome include mental status changes; evanescent petechiae of the neck, axillae, and upper torso; thrombocytopenia; and progressive hypoxemia. Most patients who manifest signs and symptoms of fat embolization do so within 48 hours of bone trauma or surgery. Mild dyspnea may progress quite quickly to respiratory failure, just as initial confusion or irritability or both may quickly progress to coma.

The diagnosis of this syndrome is based on clinical findings in a compatible setting. The chest radiograph is often normal at the time of initial symptoms. Aggressive supportive therapy ideally includes monitoring in an intensive care unit. Supplemental oxygen, with mechanical ventilation and PEEP as necessary to correct hypoxemia, should be initiated early. Infectious or hemorrhagic complications are managed as they occur. There is some experimental evidence suggesting that corticosteroids given prophylactically to patients at high risk for fat embolism may decrease the incidence of developing the syndrome.

AIR EMBOLISM

Symptomatic pulmonary air embolism most often occurs in the setting of central venous catheter placement; such catheters, subjected to negative intrathoracic pressure, may allow a large volume of air under atmospheric pressure to enter the venous circulation. Thoracic surgery and transthoracic needle biopsy or aspiration similarly predispose to air embolism. Air may also reach the venous system under positive pressure, as during head and neck surgery and obstetric/gynecologic procedures (particularly those that induce pneumoperitoneum).

To produce symptoms, air emboli must be of large enough volume to cause pulmonary blood flow obstruction; an air bolus on the order of 200 ml has been estimated to be a lethal dose in humans. Signs and symptoms of pulmonary air embolism are thus similar to those described previously for massive PTE and may include systemic hypotension, unresponsiveness, and arterial hypoxemia. Noncardiogenic pulmonary edema has been described following pulmonary air embolization.

The chest radiograph may demonstrate air-fluid levels within the central pulmonary arteries; regional oligemia may be apparent distal to the site of the air embolus. If the diagnosis is suspected, immediate supportive measures should include placing the patient in the left lateral decubitus position (to allow the air embolus to move above the right ventricular outflow tract), supplemental oxygen, removal of all possible sites of air entry, and consideration of positive pressure mechanical ventilation.

TUMOR EMBOLISM

Pulmonary tumor emboli typically result from intravascular metastases of solid tumors; lung and breast cancers are the most common underlying malignancies, but tumor emboli from renal, cervical, prostate, gastric, and parotid gland cancers, as well as those from choriocarcinoma and hepatoma, have been reported. The differentiation of pulmonary tumor emboli from thromboemboli can be exceedingly difficult, particularly since the presence of such underlying malignancies predisposes to both types of pulmonary emboli, and signs and symptoms are closely similar. The importance of such differentiation lies in the potential to treat the patient with tumor emboli with cytotoxic chemotherapy acutely while avoiding the significant risks that anticoagulation would involve in such a patient. Lung scintigraphy in the setting of pulmonary tumor emboli characteristically demonstrates multiple small, subsegmental perfusion defects rather than the larger defects (segmental or greater) typical of pulmonary thromboembolism. The diameter of these tumor emboli is often below the resolution of pulmonary angiography, and lung biopsy rather than pulmonary angiogram should be considered when the clinical setting combined with the findings of lung scintigraphy strongly suggest the diagnosis of pulmonary tumor embolism.

AMNIOTIC FLUID EMBOLISM

Amniotic fluid embolism is a rare and catastrophic complication of labor and delivery in which obstruction of the pulmonary circulation by amniotic fluid occurs. Prolonged labor, unusually strong uterine contractions, and premature separation of the placenta are all conditions that predispose to this syndrome. The sudden onset of severe shortness of breath, hypoxemia, or cardiovascular collapse in such situations should cause the clinician to consider amniotic fluid embolism. As previously noted, PTE may also occur in this setting; thus, the differentiation may be difficult. Examination of a central venous aspirate has been reported to be diagnostically useful. Amniotic fluid debris may be identified in the top layer of a centrifuged sample.

Both disseminated intravascular coagulation (DIC) and ARDS are likely to develop in patients who survive the initial event. Treatment is supportive, and anticoagulation is generally not indicated unless deemed necessary for treating related DIC. The short-term mortality rate for pulmonary amniotic fluid embolism approaches 90 percent.

SELECTED READING

Alderson, PO, and Martin, EC. Pulmonary embolism: Diagnosis with multiple imaging modalities. *Radiology* 164:297, 1987.

Branch, WT, and McNeil, BJ. Analysis of the differential diagnosis and assessment of pleuritic chest pain in young adults. *Am J Med* 75:671, 1983.

Faer, MJ, and Messerschmidt, GL. Nonfatal pulmonary air embolism: Radiographic demonstration. *Am J Roentgenol* 131:705, 1978.

Goldhaber, SZ. *Pulmonary Embolism and Deep Venous Thrombosis.* Philadelphia: Saunders, 1985.

Goldhaber, SZ, et al. Clinical suspicion of autopsy-proven thrombotic and tumor pulmonary embolism in cancer patients. *Am Heart J* 114:1432, 1987.

Hirsh, J, Genton, E, and Hull, R. *Venous Thromboembolism.* New York: Grune & Stratton, 1981.

Hull, RD, et al. Pulmonary embolism in outpatients with pleuritic chest pain. *Arch Intern Med* 148:838, 1988.

Marriott, HJL. *Practical Electrocardiography* (7th ed.). Baltimore: Williams & Wilkins, 1983.

McNeil, BJ. Ventilation-perfusion studies and the diagnosis of pulmonary embolism. *J Nucl Med* 21:319, 1980.

Peltier, LF. Fat embolism. A perspective. *Clin Orthop* 232:263, 1988.

Sperry, K. Amniotic fluid embolism. To understand an enigma. *JAMA* 255:2183, 1986.

Thrombolytic therapy in thrombosis. A National Institute of Health Consensus Development Conference. *Ann Intern Med* 93:141, 1980.

The Urokinase Pulmonary Embolism Trial: A national cooperative study. *Circulation* (suppl 2): 47 and 48, 1973.

Yu, PN. *Pulmonary Blood Volume in Health and Disease.* Philadelphia: Lea & Febiger, 1969.

14. Disorders of the Pulmonary Parenchyma

John Reilly, Jr.

ASPIRATION

The term *pulmonary aspiration* refers to a spectrum of abnormalities unified by the feature that material from or intended for the digestive tract is inhaled into the tracheobronchial tree. Aspiration may occur when the normal physiologic defenses designed to keep foreign material out of the respiratory system, including pharyngeal, glottic, and cough mechanisms, are depressed, deficient, or overwhelmed. During deep sleep, most normal individuals can be demonstrated to aspirate small amounts of oropharyngeal material if sensitive tests using dyes or radiolabeled particulates are used. On the other hand, the clinical syndrome of disease related to aspiration occurs only in subjects who for some reason aspirate an amount large enough to cause clinically evident disease. Thus, patients at risk for aspiration include (1) patients with depression of consciousness, such as caused by seizures, general anesthesia, or sedative (often alcohol) intoxication; (2) patients with neurologic disease causing an impaired gag reflex or swallowing mechanism, such as amyotrophic lateral sclerosis or myasthenia gravis; (3) patients with general debilitation, possibly with a nasogastric tube in place; and (4) patients with gastrointestinal disorders predisposing to gastric reflux, disordered swallowing, or repeated or prolonged vomiting.

There are three different clinical syndromes grouped under the heading of pulmonary aspiration, with some patients exhibiting features of more than one syndrome. The three syndromes can conveniently be termed (1) chemical injury, (2) bacterial infection, and (3) foreign body aspiration. In this section, the three clinical aspiration syndromes will briefly be described and the approach to the patient presenting to the emergency department will be outlined, highlighting important historical and physical features, followed by laboratory tests and suggestions for management.

CHEMICAL INJURY

Regurgitation of acidic gastric contents followed by their inhalation into the tracheobronchial tree results in a syndrome of chemical injury to the lungs. The classic description of the clinical entity is generally attributed to Mendelson, who in 1946 described its occurrence in obstetric patients observed to aspirate gastric contents while under the influence of anesthetic agents. It is best described as a chemical burn to the lungs. The principal determinant in the development of this injury pattern is the acidity of the aspirated material. Significant injury occurs when the pH of the aspirated material is 2.4 or below, whereas little damage occurs at pH 2.5 or greater.

In the published series describing this entity, the majority of cases occur in patients who have suffered from a depression in consciousness, usually as a result of general anesthesia or sedative (including alcohol) intoxication. The clinical presentation develops 1 to 12 hours after the aspiration event. It consists of the development of tachypnea, dyspnea, and fever; some patients also have significant wheezing. The chest x-ray frequently shows a diffuse bilateral abnormality consistent with noncardiogenic pulmonary edema (adult respiratory distress syndrome); alternatively, patchy alveolar infiltrates may develop. The abnormality is usually bilateral but can be unilateral.

Management of the patient consists of supportive therapy. Supplemental oxygen, aggressive pulmonary drainage, and bronchodilators are the mainstays of management. Older references recommended the use of corticosteroids to minimize lung injury. Animal studies demonstrated that steroids are effective in preventing such injury, but only when administered *prior to* the aspiration. Trials in humans suffering aspiration with chemical injury have demonstrated no benefit of steroid treatment and in fact have indicated that such treatment increases the risk of developing a superimposed bacterial pneumonia.

Most patients with this syndrome recover, but overall the mortality rate has been reported to be as high as 25 percent. Patients who present in shock or with hypoxemia severe enough to warrant mechanical ventilatory support have a considerably higher mortality. Approximately 25 percent of the patients who present with this syndrome will later develop a superimposed infectious pneumonia—on average 3 to 5 days after presentation. Of those destined to survive, most have recovered by 10 to 12 days.

INFECTIOUS PNEUMONIA

Infectious pneumonia owing to aspiration is clinically quite distinct from the chemical injury syndrome just discussed. In this instance, patients present several days to weeks after the aspiration of oropharyngeal contents. Rather than a chemical burn with capillary leak, the pathophysiology is that of bacterial pneumonia, and the bacteriology reflects the oropharyngeal flora. Patients often present with a subacute course characterized by malaise, fatigue, fever, and cough productive of purulent and foul-smelling sputum. Some may have pleuritic chest pain, but this is not typical. In many instances, given the time elapsed between the presumed event and the presentation to medical attention, it may not be possible to establish precisely when the aspiration occurred. As mentioned previously, a history of impairment of consciousness or other predisposing factor such as recent dental work strongly suggests this diagnosis in a patient who presents with what appears to be a bacterial pneumonia.

On evaluation, the patient often appears chronically ill; fever is commonly but not uniformly present. Examination of the oropharynx may reveal poor dentition and periodontal disease, factors predisposing to the overgrowth of anaerobic bacteria in the oral cavity. Focal rales or signs of consolidation may be heard on auscultation of the chest. Findings suggestive of pleural effusion are occasionally present. Neurologic examination may reveal an underlying neurologic disorder predisposing to aspiration.

Laboratory data may include a leukocytosis, but a normal white blood cell count by no means rules out this diagnosis. Chest x-ray shows either an infiltrate or lung abscess, often with cavitation. The location of the abnormality on chest radiograph can be predicted from the anatomy of the lung. Disease is more often present in the right lung than the left because of the fact that the right mainstem bronchus continues in a relatively straight line from the trachea. In both lungs, the pneumonia is more likely to be in the dependent segments of the lung. In patients who aspirate while in the supine position, the superior segment of the lower lobe is often the site of disease. Occasionally, a pleural effusion may be present.

The bacteriology of infectious aspiration pneumonia closely reflects that of the oropharynx. In those patients with community-acquired infection (i.e., not resident in a medical or nursing home facility), anaerobic bacteria are the predominant pathogens (except in edentulous persons); polymicrobial isolates are common. Anaerobic infection progresses to putrefaction over 7 to 10 days, causing the sputum to have the characteristic foul smell associated with anaerobes. *Klebsiella pneumoniae* infection is reported to occur with greater frequency in alcoholics. In hospitalized or institutionalized patients, aerobic organisms such as *Staphylococcus aureus* and gram-negative bacilli assume a larger role in the pathogenesis of the infection.

Once a presumptive diagnosis of infectious aspiration pneumonia has been made, the choice of antibiotics depends largely on whether the pneumonia can be considered community-acquired. For patients who have been "in the community," penicillin has for many years been the mainstay of therapy because of its excellent activity against normal oropharyngeal flora, particularly anaerobes. One report has suggested that clindamycin may be more efficacious than penicillin in treating anaerobic lung infections because of fewer treatment failures. Either choice is acceptable.

For patients brought to the emergency department from a nursing home or other institutional setting in whom gram-negative bacillary or *S. aureus* involvement becomes more likely, therapy should consist of an aminoglycoside and either a semisynthetic penicillin or a cephalosporin with acceptable *S. aureus* coverage.

In all instances, if a significant pleural effusion is present (i.e., a layer of pleural liquid more than 10 mm thick on lateral decubitus chest x-ray), it must be further evaluated with a thoracentesis to determine whether the patient has an empyema or merely a parapneumonic effusion. Patients with anaerobic empyema are notorious for presenting with an indolent course, so that the lack of fever or an acutely ill appearance should not dissuade the physician from performing the thoracentesis. In most instances, chest tube drainage is required for management of anaerobic empyema.

FOREIGN BODY

The third syndrome subsumed under the general heading of aspiration is aspiration of a foreign body into the tracheobronchial tree. The spectrum of symptoms related to the presence of a foreign body ranges from stridor and potential suffocation (the "cafe coronary") when the object occludes the larynx or trachea to recurrent focal pneumonias when a segmental airway becomes partially occluded.

As with the other syndromes previously discussed in this section, aspiration of a foreign body tends to occur in patients with neurologic disorders or some impairment of consciousness. In addition, it frequently occurs in young children. Except for the unusual instances in which the aspirated object is radiopaque, the diagnosis of a foreign body in the airways rests on the clinical history and indirect signs on physical examination and radiography. Although sometimes one can obtain a history of an object that has been aspirated (such as a peanut in children), often the mental status of the patient precludes a reliable clinical history. Other clues in the presentation to suggest foreign body aspiration may include a history of recurrent pneumonias in the same anatomic location; the occurrence of hemoptysis; the presence of a localized monophonic wheeze suggesting obstruction of an airway; segmental or lobar atelectasis on the chest x-ray; and failure of a pneumonia to clear on antibiotic therapy.

Symptoms of loud inspiratory wheezing or respiratory distress should suggest the possibility of partial occlusion of the larynx or trachea. Further supportive evidence is provided by the presence on physical examination of stridor heard over larynx or trachea. In this setting, urgent evaluation of the upper airway is required. If available, this is best done with direct laryngoscopy or rigid bronchoscopy, or both. The rigid bronchoscope is preferred to the flexible in this setting because of the superior ability of the rigid scope to provide protection of the airway and to pass larger instruments for the removal of the object.

When the presence of a foreign body is suspected in a more distal airway, the situation does not carry the same urgency. It should, however, be evaluated promptly, because the longer an object remains in place, the more likely it is to elicit an inflammatory response that will complicate removal of the object. Supportive evidence for the presence of such an object can sometimes be obtained with inspiratory and expiratory chest films, which may demonstrate that the area of lung distal to the occluded airway fails to decrease in size with expiration. When suspected, direct inspection of the tracheobronchial tree should be performed to establish whether a foreign body is present. This does not have to be done emergently but should be done in a timely fashion because of the considerations outlined previously. The manner in which the object is removed will depend on its size and location. Options include fiberoptic bronchoscopy, rigid bronchoscopy, and surgical excision via thoracotomy.

INTERSTITIAL LUNG DISEASE

Interstitial lung disease refers to a group of entities that share the common feature of involving the pulmonary interstitium. The interstitium consists of the structures between the alveolar walls in the pulmonary parenchyma. It contains the collagen, elastin, glycoproteins, lymphatics, and vasculature. In clinical terms, the interstitial lung diseases are usually so termed because of their appearance on chest x-ray. The x-ray is characterized by the presence of a "reticular" or "reticulonodular" pattern of increased fine linear or nodular markings believed to represent increased tissue density in the interstitium of the lung. The number of diseases causing this appearance is vast, and a comprehensive discussion is beyond the scope of this text. In this section, I attempt to provide a strategy for assessing whether a particular patient has a problem that requires urgent treatment and suggest guidelines for initial evaluation and decision regarding hospitalization.

Once it appears that the patient has a chest x-ray suggestive of interstitial lung disease, it is incumbent upon the emergency physician to attempt to make a determination as to whether the patient is presenting with a slowly progressive *chronic* problem or whether the visit is indeed precipitated by an emergency—that is, a rapidly progressive *acute* process.

The history should attempt to elucidate the rate of progression of the disease, with an emphasis on establishing an objective measure of progress (e.g., a rough quantitation of the exercise tolerance using commonly performed tasks as a measure such as flights of stairs or city blocks of walking or physical activity associated with the patient's occupation). In addition, a careful occupational history is particularly important in this setting.

ACUTE INTERSTITIAL LUNG DISEASE

A list of the entities causing acute interstitial lung disease is given in Table 14-1. History taking pertinent to these conditions should include detailed questions about current symptoms (including fever), recent trauma, occupational or industrial exposure to fumes or chemicals, and drug use (both prescription and illicit). In addition, it is critical to elicit information about any past cardiac disease or risk factors, the presence of illness in other household members or close contacts, recent travel, and illnesses or medications that may cause impaired immune defenses. Common examples include underlying malignancy, recent chemotherapy, and the acquired immunodeficiency syndrome (AIDS). Attempts should be made to establish whether the patient is a member of a demographic group at risk for the development of infection caused by the human immunodeficiency virus (HIV)—namely, homosexual, user of intravenous drugs, prostitute, or a hemophiliac or other recipient of blood products.

The physical examination should include assessment for signs of respiratory compromise: tachypnea, cyanosis, use of accessory muscles of respiration, and retraction of the intercostal muscles. Examination of the thorax in interstitial lung diseases usually reveals bilateral inspiratory crackles; other findings may indicate the comorbid presence of thoracic trauma, consolidation, or pleural effusions. Cardiovascular examination should include evaluation for jugular venous distention, hepatic engorgement, and peripheral edema, suggesting congestive heart failure. In addition, heart murmurs or gallops may provide clues pointing to a possible cardiac etiology for the patient's symptoms. The skin should be examined for the presence of signs of intravenous drug use, lesions of Kaposi's sarcoma, lesions of viral infections such as varicella or measles, petechiae consistent with fat

Table 14-1. Causes of acute interstitial lung disease

- Common
  - Hemodynamic
    - Left ventricular failure
    - Fluid overload
  - Capillary leak (adult respiratory distress syndrome)
    - Trauma
    - Sepsis
    - Aspiration
  - Infection
    - *Pneumocystis carinii* pneumonia
- Uncommon
  - Capillary leak
    - Fat emboli
  - Infection
    - Viral (e.g., measles, adenovirus, herpes viruses)
    - Mycobacterial (miliary tuberculosis)
    - Fungal (e.g., histoplasmosis, invasive aspergillosis)
  - Chemical injury
    - Inhalation (e.g., chlorine, NO_2, smoke)
    - Cytotoxic drugs (bleomycin, cyclophosphamide)
  - Allergic reaction
    - Drugs (penicillin, gold salts, nitrofurantoin)
    - Fungi (allergic bronchopulmonary aspergillosis)
    - Parasitic infections
  - Hemorrhage
    - Idiopathic pulmonary hemosiderosis
    - Goodpasture's syndrome
    - Behçet's syndrome
    - Systemic lupus erythematosus
  - Idiopathic
    - Eosinophilic pneumonia
    - Churg-Strauss vasculitis
    - Acute rheumatoid lung disease
    - Acute systemic lupus erythematosus

Source: Adapted from M. Turner-Warwick. Infiltrative and Interstitial Lung Diseases: General Principles and Diagnostic Approach. In J.F. Murray and J.A. Nadel (eds.), *Textbook of Respiratory Medicine*. Philadelphia: Saunders, 1988.

emboli or disseminated intravascular coagulation, and papular, pustular, or ulcerative lesions suggestive of disseminated bacterial or fungal infection. Fundoscopic examination may also be useful, revealing petechial hemorrhages or disseminated fungal infection. The remainder of the examination should include evaluation of any alteration in mental status, evidence for trauma (e.g., long bone fractures), and signs of deep-seated infection.

The chest x-ray may hold clues as to the specific etiology of the diffuse interstitial process based on its distribution (central versus peripheral; upper lobe predominant versus lower lobe predominant) and on the presence of coexistent adenopathy or pleural disease. If available, old x-rays are invaluable in attempting to establish the rate of progression of the abnormality. A complete blood count should be checked, including a differential. If possible, sputum should be collected for cultures and staining. An arterial blood gas should be checked to assess adequacy of oxygenation, acid–base status, and adequacy of ventilation.

Once the history, physical examination, and aforementioned laboratory studies have been performed, the clinician should be able either to make a clinical diagnosis or at least to narrow the number of possibilities responsible for the patient's problem. Once this is done, a plan for timely diagnostic evaluation and therapy can be formulated. In the following paragraphs, the most common entities presenting in this fashion are discussed, highlighting the pertinent historic, physical, and laboratory findings and suggesting initial evaluation and therapy.

Congestive heart failure with interstitial edema is certainly not a difficult diagnosis to make in the patient with a long cardiac history who presents with orthopnea, increasing edema, an elevated jugular venous pressure, and third heart sound. Given its prevalence, particularly in older patients, it should be carefully considered in the differential diagnosis of every patient presenting with acute interstitial abnormality to the emergency department. The patient should be questioned carefully for symptoms of ischemic heart disease, orthopnea, paroxysmal nocturnal dyspnea, increasing peripheral edema, exertional dyspnea or wheezing, increased salt intake, and any prior cardiac disease. Similarly, the physical examination should include a systematic assessment for the presence of signs of left ventricular failure. The presence of early alveolar filling in dependent portions of the lung or pleural effusions, seen early on as blunting of the costophrenic angles or widening of the interlobar fissures, is suggestive of the diagnosis. Fever and leukocytosis are unusual and should prompt consideration of alternative diagnoses. The electrocardiogram may reveal signs of ischemia, previous myocardial infarction, left ventricular hypertrophy, or arrhythmias that may precipitate congestive symptoms. Therapy is discussed in more detail in Chap. 11; it includes the administration of diuretics, supplemental oxygen, morphine (as needed), and agents to treat any ongoing ischemia or arrhythmia. Response to therapy is often quite prompt, and a beneficial response can often be taken as supporting evidence for the accuracy of the initial diagnosis.

In the current era, particularly in larger urban areas, pneumonia caused by *Pneumocystis carinii* is an increasingly common cause of symptomatic interstitial lung disease, particularly in younger patients. This protozoal infection was previously reported only as a rare cause of lung disease in immunosuppressed or extremely malnourished patients, such as survivors of World War II internment camps. In recent years, however, it has become the most common infectious diagnosis associated with the rapidly spreading AIDS epidemic (see Chap. 91). The initial symptoms of pneumocystis pneumonia can be subtle, with low-grade fever and a dry cough often being the only manifestations of the disease. All patients with acute interstitial lung disease, and particularly younger patients, should be questioned to determine whether they are a member of any of the demographic groups at increased risk for HIV infection. In addition, they should be asked about constitutional symptoms such as weight loss, lymphadenopathy, new skin lesions, unexplained diarrhea, or any prior unusual infections. On physical examination, the stigmata of intravenous drug use, the presence of widespread lymphadenopathy, cutaneous lesions of Kaposi's sarcoma, and oral candidiasis all suggest the possibility of an AIDS-related infection.

The chest x-ray may have minimal interstitial disease or may have some areas of alveolar or nodular opacities. Pleural effusions are extremely uncommon in this entity and should prompt a search for an alternative diagnosis. Serum chemistry determination may reveal an elevated lactate dehydrogenase (LDH). The hematology profile may show a lymphopenia and an anemia. Arterial blood gases usually reveal hypoxemia and signs of hyperventilation. None of the aforementioned signs is specific for pneumocystis pneumonia, however, and demonstration of the organism in pulmonary secretions or lung tissue is required to establish the diagnosis. Obtaining an appropriate sample usually requires either induction of sputum with nebulized hypertonic saline or a bronchoscopy with bronchoalveolar lavage. Toluidine blue or methenamine silver stain permits identification of the characteristic boat-shaped cysts.

The decision whether to hospitalize the patient suspected of having pneumocystis pneumonia while a diagnostic workup is being performed depends on the available resources and the clinical condition of the patient. In patients with minimal symptoms or x-ray abnormalities who have adequate oxygenation, outpatient evaluation beginning with attempts at sputum induction is often appropriate. Among patients who seem unreliable and unlikely to participate in an outpatient evaluation or in whom the disease is more advanced as manifested by more severe symptoms, x-ray changes, or hypoxemia, hospitalization with plans for prompt diagnostic evaluation is the more prudent course.

Because patients with AIDS experience a high incidence of adverse reactions to the antibiotics used to treat this infection, it is generally not recommended that antibiotics be administered based only on a clinical suspicion of pneumocystis pneumonia. If the patient is very ill and the infection is apparently progressing at a rapid rate, it is appropriate to institute therapy immediately and plan for a diagnostic procedure within 48 hours. Initial therapy is usually with trimethoprim/sulfamethoxazole (TMP/SMX), which can be administered orally or intravenously, or with intravenous pentamidine. Because of the high incidence of adverse reactions to these agents in this population, often taking the form of a rash (with TMP/SMX) or leukopenia (with either drug), patients should be monitored carefully while on therapy.

In addition to pneumocystis pneumonia, there are other less common infectious causes of acute interstitial disease. These include disseminated viral infections such as varicella, measles, respiratory syncitial virus, and adenovirus, miliary tuberculosis, and disseminated fungal infections such as histoplasmosis and aspergillosis. In many but by no means all instances, the presence of fever and leukocytosis offers an important clue to the infectious etiology of the underlying illness.

A diagnosis of acute viral pneumonia is most often suggested either by recent exposure to a person with a viral illness or by a characteristic eruption. Although uncommon, miliary tuberculosis is a cause of acute or subacute interstitial lung disease that is critically important to recognize and treat appropriately, given the potentially life-threatening consequences of untreated disease. Miliary tuberculosis occurs with increased frequency in the elderly, particularly in those with chronic disease or malnutrition resulting in a compromise in immune function, and in persons with AIDS. The subtlety of the presenting symptoms may disguise the severity of the disease. Although some patients will experience fever, weight loss, anemia, and cough, the majority will have little or no acute history other than malaise and "failure to thrive." The chest x-ray will reveal a diffuse pattern of very small nodular densities, which approximate the size of millet seeds (1–3 mm in diameter), hence "miliary" tuberculosis. There may be radiographic signs of preexisting tuberculosis exposure as well, usually in the form of apical scarring. Nervous system involvement is not infrequent in patients with disseminated tuberculosis, so that patients should be questioned carefully for the presence of even subtle neurologic symptoms. Among patients in whom an altered mental status makes it difficult to assess symptoms, careful consideration should be given to a lumbar puncture if miliary tuberculosis is in the differential diagnosis. There may be hepatic and bone marrow involvement as well, and if initial examination of sputum and cerebrospinal fluid does not establish the diagnosis, liver and bone marrow biopsy may be needed to obtain additional tissue for culture and histopathology. All patients with a compatible x-ray should have sputum examined for acid-fast bacilli and be hospitalized for further evaluation if tuberculosis remains a reasonable possibility to explain the patient's presentation. Because sputum smears are positive for acid-fast bacilli in only approximately one-third of patients with miliary tuberculosis, a negative sputum smear by no means rules out the diagnosis.

Other, less common causes of acute diffuse lung disease may be suggested by the specific clinical setting and the patient's clinical presentation. For instance, a history of recent antecedent long bone fracture, fever, mental status changes, tachypnea, and petechiae suggest the diagnosis of fat embolism, which may be supported by the finding of fat droplets in the sputum. Diffuse interstitial infiltrates on chest x-ray in a patient with hypotension and multiple sites of trauma evoke the possibility of the adult respiratory distress syndrome (ARDS). Similarly, the constellation of fever, tachypnea, and hemodynamic instability should suggest the presence of sepsis and ARDS and prompt a search for the underlying infection so that appropriate antibiotic therapy may be rapidly instituted.

The presence of a peripheral blood eosinophilia or eosinophils in the sputum may be a clue to the presence of one of the eosinophilic lung disorders. These include a reaction to drugs such as nitrofurantoin, gold, and penicillin. In addition, pulmonary infiltrates with eosinophilia (PIE syndrome) can also be seen with helminthic infections or allergic reaction to aspergillus (allergic bronchopulmonary aspergillosis). The latter diagnosis is usually made in patients with a history of asthma.

An antecedent history of exposure to chemical fumes in either an industrial setting or, not uncommonly, at home when working with cleaning solutions suggests the possibility of toxic injury to the lungs. The same is true if there is recent exposure to chemotherapeutic agents such as bleomycin or cyclophosphamide.

If the patient with diffuse lung infiltrates presents with a history of hemoptysis, several entities need to be considered in the differential diagnosis. One is pulmonary hemorrhage associated with renal disease, such as Goodpasture's syndrome. Consequently, renal function should be checked and a urinalysis performed in all such patients. Other diagnoses that can present in this manner include Wegener's granulomatosis, idiopathic pulmonary hemosiderosis, systemic lupus erythematosus, and Behçet's syndrome.

CHRONIC INTERSTITIAL PNEUMONIA

The differential diagnosis for chronic interstitial lung disease is vast, and a detailed discussion is beyond the scope of this chapter (Table 14-2). As outlined in the introductory remarks to this section, the critical distinction to make on patient presentation is whether the patient has symptoms of progression of a chronic syndrome or a new, acute process. Acute disease usually requires a rapid evaluation and therapy, often necessitating urgent hospital admission. In chronic disease, however, it is often possible to initiate the diagnostic evaluation as an outpatient. The evaluation of chronic interstitial lung disease frequently involves specialized diagnostic testing and procedures, including pulmonary function testing and some type of lung biopsy. In this instance, the role of the emergency physician should be (1) to rule out acute, reversible causes of symptoms (e.g., superimposed congestive heart failure or infection); and (2) to determine whether the patient's condition is sufficiently stable to permit outpatient evaluation or sufficiently unstable to require hospitalization for diagnosis and initiation of therapy. Once again, the importance of obtaining old chest x-rays cannot be overemphasized in helping to establish whether the process under consideration is an acute or chronic one.

As with acute interstitial lung disease, the patient should be carefully questioned about occupational and environmental exposure to dusts and fumes. This inquiry should encompass the entire employment history of the patient, since certain diseases such as those caused by asbestos or silica exposure develop only after many years of exposure and may become manifest after the patient has withdrawn from the exposure. Similarly, patients should be questioned carefully for constitutional symptoms such as fever, arthralgia, and weight loss.

While it is true that many of the chronic interstitial lung diseases require some form of invasive procedure for a definitive diagnosis, in some cases the etiology may sometimes be suggested by the specific features of the patient's presentation. For instance, symptoms of fever, arthralgias, erythema nodosum, or uveitis, coupled with the presence of hilar or mediastinal adenopathy on chest x-ray, makes sarcoidosis the likely diagnosis. Long-standing left ventricular failure or rheumatic heart disease such as mitral stenosis, coupled with the lack of fever or extrapulmonic manifestations, suggests the diagnosis of interstitial fibrosis owing to chronic pulmonary venous hypertension.

Similarly, hypersensitivity pneumonias resulting from organic dust exposure (e.g., farmer's lung and pigeon breeder's lung disease) may have constitutional symptoms such as fever. Eliciting a history of suitable exposure is critical to making the diagnosis. The presence of clubbing and a positive rheumatoid factor, in the absence of a history of rheumatoid arthritis or systemic lupus erythematosus, suggests the presence of idiopathic pulmonary fibrosis.

A past history of the use of certain drugs such as bleomycin, amiodarone, methotrexate, nitrofurantoin, or practolol raises the probability of drug-induced lung disease, whereas prior radiation therapy suggests radiation-induced pneumonitis, which often produces sharp demarcations on the chest radiography corresponding to the borders of the radiation therapy ports. A prior history of carcinoma or lymphoma makes consideration of lymphangitic spread of malignancy necessary, although this entity may develop in the absence of a previously known malignancy.

Table 14-2. Causes of chronic interstitial lung disease

Infection:	Viral pneumonias
Hemodynamic:	Mitral stenosis Uremia Chronic left ventricular failure
Radiation	
Neoplasms:	Lymphangitic carcinomatosis (often metastatic carcinoma) Lymphoma Alveolar cell carcinoma
Inhalation:	
Inorganic dusts: Silica, talc, beryllium, asbestos, coal, etc.	
Organic material: Foreign proteins/fungal organisms: farmer's lung, bird breeders, miller's lung, etc.	
Other:	Lipoid pneumonia Aspiration pneumonia
Drug reaction:	Amiodarone, bleomycin, nitrofurantoin, methotrexate, practolol
Idiopathic:	
Granulomatous: Sarcoidosis	
Necrotizing granulomas: Wegener's granulomatosis, eosinophilic granuloma, lymphomatoid granulomatosis	
Associated with connective tissue disease: Rheumatoid arthritis, systemic lupus erythematosus, dermatomyositis, scleroderma, ulcerative colitis, chronic active hepatitis	
Dysplastic cell accumulation:	
Muscle: Lymphangioleiomyomatosis, fibromuscular dysplasia	
Xanthomatous: Hand-Schüller-Christian disease, Letterer-Siwe disease, cholesterol pneumonia	
Neurofibrous: Neurofibromatosis	
Musculofibrous: Tuberous sclerosis	
Lymphatic: Lymphangectasia	
Protein accumulation: Alveolar proteinosis	
Other:	Idiopathic pulmonary fibrosis Lymphocytic interstitial pneumonia Bronchiolitis obliterans

Source: Adapted from M. Turner-Warwick. Infiltrative and Interstitial Lung Diseases: General Principles and Diagnostic Approaches. In J.F. Murray and J.A. Nadel (eds.), *Textbook of Respiratory Medicine.* Philadelphia: Saunders, 1988.

Most of the collagen vascular diseases can have pulmonary involvement in the form of interstitial lung disease. Although patients occasionally present initially with lung disease, more often there is an antecedent history of the connective tissue disorder. In this setting, the challenge for the clinician lies in differentiating pulmonary involvement owing to underlying disease from a drug reaction (e.g., methotrexate-associated pneumonitis) or pulmonary infection owing to the patient's possibly immunocompromised status (either as a result of the disease process itself or immunosuppressive therapy).

The chronic use of preparations containing mineral oil (e.g., certain laxatives) can often be overlooked unless the patient is specifically questioned about such use. Aspiration of these preparations, symptomatically or asymptomatically, can cause chronic interstitial disease in the form of lipoid pneumonia. In this setting, computed tomography (CT) scanning of the chest can be virtually diagnostic if areas of the infiltrates are found to be of fat density.

Skin lesions, renal involvement, gastrointestinal symptoms, or neurologic signs or symptoms should raise the possibility of a vasculitis involving the lung. In this instance, the patient should undergo prompt evaluation, given the virulence of some of these entities and the fact that they potentially have a favorable response to therapy.

For most patients with chronic interstitial lung disease, however, the diagnosis remains unclear after the initial history, physical examination, and review of chest x-ray. It is then up to the emergency physician to assess whether the rate of progression is sufficiently slow and the patient well enough to pursue the evaluation as an outpatient. If so, referral to a pulmonologist and scheduling of pulmonary function tests will serve to initiate the workup. If the patient has rapidly progressive symptoms or hypoxemia or is unable to meet the physical demands of an outpatient workup, he or she should be hospitalized.

Table 14-3. Causes of atelectasis

Impaired diaphragmatic mobility
Splinting
Pain owing to chest trauma
Pain owing to intra-abdominal process
Diaphragmatic paralysis
Neuromuscular disease
Phrenic nerve paralysis
Thermal injury from cardioplegia
Entrapment by lung/mediastinal malignancy
Entrapment by benign mediastinal adenopathy
Trauma
Bronchial obstruction
Extrinsic compression
Lymphadenopathy
Parenchymal mass
Endobronchial lesion
Bronchial secretions
Endobronchial tumor (primary or metastatic)
Foreign body
Associated with vascular obstruction
Embolic disease
Thromboemboli
Tumor emboli

ATELECTASIS

Atelectasis refers to the condition in which a portion of the lung has suffered a loss in volume. Cough and shortness of breath may be symptoms of atelectasis, or it may present as an asymptomatic finding on examination and chest radiograph. Even if asymptomatic, atelectasis should prompt careful consideration about the etiology. The common causes of atelectasis are listed in Table 14-3.

Atelectasis has a variety of presentations on chest x-ray. The most dramatic cases are total collapse of one or more lobes of the lung (lobar atelectasis). Associated radiographic manifestations, indicative of volume loss, include displacement of the major fissure, elevation of a hemidiaphragm, or shift of the mediastinal structures toward the side with volume loss. If the atelectasis is more limited in extent, the only manifestation on x-ray may be the linear stranding of "plate-like" atelectasis, representing the loss of alveolar volume and hence increased tissue density of a small (subsegmental) portion of the lung.

The chest x-ray may also give potential clues for the etiology of the atelectasis. A common cause of lobar atelectasis is the presence of obstruction in the airway supplying the affected part of the lung. This obstruction may result from extrinsic compression or an endobronchial process. Perhaps the most common example of extrinsic compression leading to atelectasis is right middle lobe syndrome, often the result of hilar adenopathy compressing the right middle lobe bronchus. Endobronchial obstruction can be the result of an aspirated foreign body, tenacious secretions (mucus plugging), or an endobronchial mass such as primary lung cancer or metastatic disease. The chest radiograph may give evidence of an endobronchial lesion, suggested by a visible cutoff of an airway, proximal mass lesion, or radiopaque foreign body. Hemoptysis may also be a clue to an endobronchial lesion. If the history suggests that impacted secretions may be responsible for the observed atelectasis, a trial of vigorous physical therapy and bronchodilator treatment is warranted to attempt lung reexpansion. Otherwise, when atelectasis is suspected to be the result of an endobronchial process, the patient should have a bronchoscopic examination of the airways to assess the etiology. Therapeutic interventions via the bronchoscope include aspiration of viscid secretions, removal of foreign bodies (usually performed via rigid bronchoscopy), and laser vaporization of endobronchial cancer.

One special instance of atelectasis resulting from impacted secretions deserves further mention. Patients with a history of asthma who present with episodes of segmental or lobar atelectasis may have allergic bronchopulmonary aspergillosis, a process characterized by recurrent occlusion of airways by mucus plugs containing inflammatory cells and *Aspergillus fumigatus*. In the advanced form of the syndrome, the patient may have signs of central bronchiectasis on chest x-ray. Peripheral eosinophilia is commonly associated with this syndrome. If suspected, total serum IgE level and radioallergosorbent (RAST) testing for IgE specific for aspergillus should be checked. In addition, mucus plugs produced by the patient should be processed as a tissue specimen and stained for fungus. Treatment is with oral corticosteroids.

Subsegmental or plate-like atelectasis may result from loss of diaphragmatic excursion on the affected side. Two of the potential causes are splinting owing to pain from the chest wall or an abdominal process and ipsilateral phrenic nerve paralysis. Phrenic nerve injury is most often due to disruption of the phrenic nerve by malignant tumor. An increasingly common cause of both temporary or permanent phrenic paralysis is thermal injury from the cold cardioplegia used during cardiac bypass surgery. Uncommonly, the paralysis may result from compression from mediastinal adenopathy arising from a benign cause, such as granulomatous disease (fibrosing mediastinitis). CT scan of the chest may be helpful in assessing the presence of mediastinal pathology to explain diaphragmatic paralysis and associated atelectasis.

The third possible etiology of atelectasis arises in the setting of the interruption of blood flow to the affected area. This is usually the result of occlusion of a portion of the pulmonary vasculature by embolic disease, usually thromboembolism. In patients presenting with symptoms consistent with pulmonary embolism, often the only abnormality on the chest x-ray is a small area of atelectasis. The presentation and diagnostic evaluation of patients with pulmonary embolic disease is discussed in Chap. 13.

SELECTED READING

Aspiration

Bartlett, JG, and Gorbach, SL. The triple threat of aspiration pneumonia. *Chest* 68:560, 1975.

Huxley, EJ, et al. Pharyngeal aspiration in normal adults and patients with depressed consciousness. *Am J Med* 64:564, 1978.

Mendelson, CL. The aspiration of stomach contents into the lungs during obstetric anesthesia. *Am J Obstet Gynecol* 52:191, 1946.

Murray, HW. Antimicrobial therapy in pulmonary aspiration. *Am J Med* 66:188, 1979.

Wolfe, JE, Bone, RC, and Ruth, WE. Effects of corticosteroids in the treatment of patients with gastric aspiration. *Am J Med* 63:719, 1977.

Wynne, JW, and Modell, JH. Respiratory aspiration of stomach contents. *Ann Intern Med* 87:466, 1977.

Interstitial Disease

Crystal, RG, et al. Interstitial lung diseases of unknown cause. Disorders characterized by chronic inflammation of the lower respiratory tract. *N Engl J Med* 310:154–166, 235–244, 1984.

Clement, MJ, Luce, JM, and Hopewell, PC. Diagnosis of pulmonary diseases. *Clin Chest Med* 9:497, 1988.

Levine, SJ, and White, DA. *Pneumocystis carinii. Clin Chest Med* 9:395, 1988.

Turner-Warwick, M. Infiltrative and Interstitial Lung Diseases. In JF Murray and JA Nadel (eds.), *Textbook of Respiratory Medicine*. Philadelphia: Saunders, 1988.

Atelectasis

Fraser, RC, et al. *Diagnosis of Diseases of the Chest* (3rd ed.). Philadelphia: Saunders, 1989.

Naidich, DP, et al. Computed tomography of lobar collapse: 1. Endobronchial obstruction. *J Comput Assist Tomogr* 7:745, 1983.

Naidich, DP, et al. Computed tomography of lobar collapse: 2. Collapse in the absence of endobronchial obstruction. *J Comput Assist Tomogr* 7:758, 1983.

Woodring, JH. Determining the cause of pulmonary atelectasis: A comparison of plain radiography and CT. *Am J Radiol* 150:757, 1988.

15. Ventilatory Failure

Michael J. Miller

Ventilatory failure is a medical emergency that exists when ventilation becomes inadequate for the gas exchange needs of the tissues. The hallmark of the condition is alveolar hypoventilation, resulting in arterial hypercapnia, severe acidemia, and varying degrees of hypoxemia. Ventilator failure may be precipitated by a disturbance in one or more of the following: the respiratory control system, the neural apparatus linking the control system to the respiratory muscles, the respiratory muscles, or the gas exchanger itself. Prompt recognition of the condition is essential if the patient is to be saved from irreversible tissue damage due to progressive hypoxia and acidemia.

In the cyanotic patient who is gasping for breath, the need for an accurate assessment of the adequacy of ventilation is obvious. In the patient with central nervous system (CNS) or neuromuscular disease, however, signs of respiratory distress may be minimal or lacking, and a high degree of clinical suspicion is necessary to direct the diagnostic strategy. It is important to note that the estimation of alveolar ventilation from clinical observation alone has been studied and found to be highly inaccurate; thus, analysis of arterial blood gases is essential to both the diagnosis and management of ventilatory failure.

PATHOPHYSIOLOGIC MECHANISMS

Failure of the Control of Ventilation

Although a variety of causes for central ventilatory failure exists (e.g., primary alveolar hypoventilation, hypothyroidism, severe obstructive sleep apnea syndrome, head trauma), perhaps the most common cause of this disorder in the emergency department setting is drug overdose, with resultant central depression of ventilation. The possibility of ventilatory failure should be suspected in any patient who is first seen with coma or obtundation. Since the cerebral cortex is, in general, more sensitive to the effects of depressant drugs than are brainstem respiratory centers, alteration of the sensorium will almost certainly be present by the time ventilatory failure has developed. Miosis may provide a clue to narcotic abuse. Breath sounds may be diminished and adventitious sounds absent. Respiratory efforts and chest wall displacement may appear reduced, but the magnitude of ventilatory depression is difficult to quantify from physical examination. Unless the patient has coexisting lung disease, results of the chest x-ray will be normal.

The diagnosis is established by the finding of arterial hypercapnia and a primary respiratory acidosis (with or without metabolic compensation, depending on the duration of hypoventilation), and hypoxemia with a normal A-aDO_2 (Table 15-1). (For additional discussion of the alveolar-to-arterial difference for oxygen [A-aDO_2] see Chap. 6.) This latter finding indicates that the patient's hypoxemia can be

Table 15-1. Use of the A-aDO_2 in the evaluation of ventilatory failure

Blood gas measurement	Narcotic-induced hypoventilation[a]	COPD[b]
pHa	7.19	7.22
$PaCO_2$	72	65
PaO_2	53	39
HCO_3^-	26	27
FIO_2	0.21	0.21
A-aDO_2[c]	6	29

[a]With normal lungs (i.e., A-aDO_2 < 20 mm Hg).
[b]From a patient with an acute exacerbation of chronic obstructive pulmonary disease (COPD).
[c]Calculation of the A-aDO_2: A = alveolar PO_2, a = measured arterial PO_2. $A = (PB - PH_2O) \times FIO_2 - PaCO_2/R$ where PB is the barometric pressure = 760 mm Hg, PH_2O = 47 mm Hg at 37°C, and R is the normal respiratory quotient = 0.8.
Key: $PaCO_2$ = partial pressure of carbon dioxide in arterial blood; PaO_2 = partial pressure of oxygen in arterial blood.

accounted for entirely by alveolar hypoventilation, and that hypoxemia is not due to lung disease. Except for the finding of a normal A-aDO_2, the arterial blood gas example shown in Table 15-1 resembles closely the pattern that might be seen in a patient with advanced chronic obstructive pulmonary disease (COPD) and acute respiratory failure. Therefore, failure of the physician to calculate the A-aDO_2 may lead to the faulty inference that the cause of the blood gas abnormality is lung disease rather than central depression of ventilation. Treatment of such a patient with bronchodilators and intravenous methylxanthines would be singularly unrewarding. The patient requires attempts to reverse CNS depression (e.g., naloxone for narcotic overdose) and mechanical ventilation if a dangerous level of respiratory acidemia develops (generally, pHa < 7.25–7.28). In patients with underlying lung disease and baseline arterial blood gas abnormalities, recognition of central ventilatory depression may be difficult, since the A-aDO_2 will be abnormal. In these instances, the history of drug ingestion is crucial, since the only clue to the presence of central ventilatory depression may be the finding of more severe hypercapnia without antecedent worsening of the patient's pulmonary symptoms.

Failure of the Innervation of Respiratory Muscle

From a pulmonary perspective, disorders in which there is failure of the innervation of respiratory muscle can be classified into two groups: primary neuromuscular diseases and diseases or processes in which the innervation of respiratory muscle fails as a result of metabolic disturbances or toxic effects of substances on them. Failure of the respiratory muscles due to disease or excessive workloads will be discussed in the following section.

Examples of primary neuromuscular disorders that may be seen with ventilatory failure in the emergency department are Guillain-Barré syndrome, myasthenia gravis, amyotrophic lateral sclerosis (ALS), poliomyelitis, transverse myelitis, and traumatic paralysis of the respiratory muscles due to spinal cord injury. The hallmark of these disorders is weakness; in Guillain-Barré syndrome, the weakness is usually symmetric, ascending, accompanied by minimal sensory complaints, and rapidly progressive (hours to days). Myasthenia gravis usually affects oculomotor, facial, and pharyngeal musculature before severe weakness is seen in respiratory muscle and other muscle groups. Loss of coordination of pharyngeal muscles, however, places these patients at an additional risk for aspiration. Amyotrophic lateral sclerosis is usually slowly progressive, with respiratory failure occurring only after a prolonged course of muscle weakness. Transverse myelitis can progress rapidly, producing paralysis of muscles below the site of the lesion, and should be suspected in patients who have had recent radiation therapy involving the spinal cord. In processes such as traumatic quadriplegia that denervate the intercostal muscles, ventilation is further compromised by chest wall instability and partial thoracic collapse during inspiration.

As a rule, any patient with diffuse and profound muscle weakness should have an arterial blood gas drawn to assess the adequacy of ventilation. In the nontraumatic examples, the onset of ventilatory failure can be insidious or subacute, and arterial blood gas analysis may show a partially compensated or compensated respiratory acidosis. In patients with previously normal lungs, the A-aDO_2 may be normal; with severe weakness, however, aspiration or atelectasis can contribute to hypoxemia with an elevated A-aDO_2. Although the expiratory muscles have been shown to be more severely impaired than inspiratory muscles in patients with ALS, the implications of differential weakness for the development of atelectasis, impaired cough, or ventilatory failure are speculative.

Examples of the production of ventilatory failure by toxic agents through interference with neuromuscular transmission are botulism, insecticide poisoning, and therapy with aminoglycosides. Botulinum toxin blocks the release of acetylcholine, producing rapidly progressive weakness, mydriasis, and respiratory failure; treatment is with antitoxin. Insecticides, such as those possessing anticholinesterase properties (organophosphates), can produce either central ventilatory depression or cause depolarization blockade at the neuromuscular junction. Aminoglycoside antibiotics can cause weakness through curarelike actions and can potentiate the effects of neuromuscular blocking agents or aggravate muscle weakness in patients with myasthenia gravis. These actions have been implicated in the development and persistence of ventilatory failure in patients with underlying lung disease. With the increasingly frequent use of parenteral antibiotics in the outpatient setting, the emergency physician should be aware that aminoglycoside therapy could contribute to the development of respiratory muscle weakness and ventilatory failure.

Failure of the Respiratory Muscles

Increased activity of the respiratory muscles is a nearly universal response of the respiratory system to lung injury, whether injury be in the form of pneumonia, pulmonary embolism, asthma, pulmonary edema, or any of a myriad of other forms of pulmonary pathology. The stimulus for this increased activity is derived from pulmonary receptors and chest wall mechanoreceptors, as well as from the central and

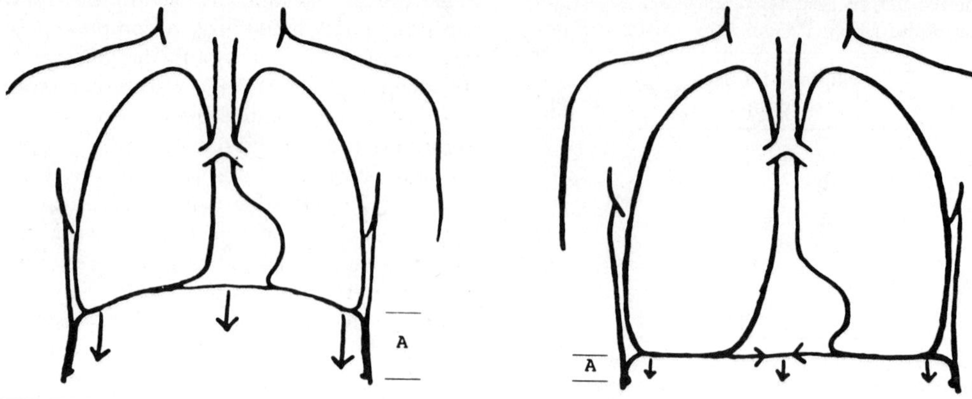

Fig. 15-1. The normal configuration of the lungs, chest wall, and diaphragm is shown schematically in the left panel. With normal lungs, the diaphragm has a considerable area of aposition (A) with the chest wall. The diaphragm can shorten along this area of aposition, allowing the dome of the diaphragm to move downward like a piston. The right panel illustrates the situation in conditions of pulmonary hyperinflation, such as asthma or chronic obstructive pulmonary disease. With hyperinflation, the diaphragm becomes shorter and much of the area of aposition is lost.

peripheral chemoreceptors that respond to blood gas abnormalities. The purpose of this increased respiratory muscle activation is to maintain adequate ventilation in the face of increasing respiratory workloads, or to increase minute ventilation above normal values, as seen during an acute asthmatic attack or with pulmonary emboli. This latter response may be an attempt to compensate for pulmonary gas exchange dysfunction and defend against arterial hypoxemia.

Inevitably, the burden imposed by lung disease falls heavily on the inspiratory muscles. In disease processes that cause a decrease in pulmonary compliance (i.e., "stiff lungs," as in pulmonary fibrosis, adult respiratory distress syndrome, or pulmonary edema), it is obvious that the inspiratory muscles must work substantially harder to stretch and thus ventilate the lungs. Less intuitive, however, is the fact that even with obstructive airways disease (e.g., asthma, COPD), in which the static compliance of the lung is normal or increased, and where the major consequence of the derangement is obstruction to expiratory airflow, inspiratory muscle function, again, may be severely compromised. This situation arises primarily because severe airway obstruction (as well as loss of elastic recoil in COPD) results in pulmonary hyperinflation.

Two major consequences of hyperinflation are illustrated in Fig. 15-1. First, the diaphragm, the major muscle of inspiration, is forced to operate at a shorter length. Because of the length-tension relationship of skeletal muscle, the ability of the shortened diaphragm to develop force is reduced. Second, hyperinflation changes the geometry of the diaphragm, making it much less effective at inflating the lungs. With severe hyperinflation, the geometric derangement can become such that part of the diaphragm's action becomes expiratory, as evidenced by the finding on chest examination of Hoover's sign, an inward displacement of the lower rib cage with inspiration.

This discussion would be of little interest in a textbook of emergency medicine were it not for the fact that inspiratory muscle fatigue and failure have but one outcome—ventilatory failure. It is essential, therefore, that in caring for patients in the emergency department, the physician assesses the impact of lung disease on inspiratory muscle function and reserve. Pertinent physical findings indicative of increased inspiratory muscle workload include an increased breathing frequency, intercostal retractions due to large negative inspiratory pleural pressures, and active recruitment of accessory muscles of inspiration (sternocleidomastoids and scalenes). In patients with COPD, accessory muscle hypertrophy may be apparent, and patients may insist on bracing the arms and maintaining an upright ("tripod") posture to facilitate accessory muscle function.

Hyperinflation (as suggested by decreased diaphragmatic excursion, increased anteroposterior chest diameter, or, on chest x-ray, flattened diaphragm contours and the finding of Hoover's sign, indicate a mechanically disadvantaged diaphragm. An ominous finding on physical examination is paradoxical thoracoabdominal motion (i.e., inward excursion of the abdomen during inspiration). This finding indicates that the diaphragm is profoundly fatigued and moving passively in response to the negative inspiratory pleural pressure generated by the intercostals and accessory muscles alone. While this pattern of respiratory muscle use may allow the diaphragm a period of rest, recovery can be prolonged and one must presume that ventilatory failure is imminent.

Patients with dyspnea who exhibit signs of severe inspiratory muscle-loading or dysfunction should be followed closely with arterial blood gas measurements, since failure to rapidly ameliorate the underlying airway obstruction or decreased static compliance often leads to respiratory muscle fatigue and ventilatory failure.

Although pharmacologic agents such as theophylline, caffeine, and certain beta-adrenergic agonists have been reported to improve diaphragmatic "contractility" and "reverse fatigue," no convincing evidence has been reported that they can be relied on to avert ventilatory failure in an emergency department setting. If ventilatory failure develops as a consequence of respiratory muscle fatigue, mechanical ventilation should be promptly instituted to support ventilation and allow respiratory muscles to recover.

Respiratory muscle weakness has also been reported in

a variety of systemic disorders, including polymyositis, alcoholic myopathy, steroid-induced myopathy, lipid storage myopathy, acid maltase deficiency, and Duchenne's muscular dystrophy. Profound respiratory muscle weakness has been precipitated by hypophosphatemia, as a result of depletion of substrate for high-energy phosphate production. Respiratory muscle weakness has been documented in association with viral upper-respiratory infections, possibly because of a direct viral myositis or interleukin-1–induced muscle proteolysis. Any of these disorders could increase the likelihood of ventilatory failure developing during acute respiratory infection.

Failure of Gas Exchange

Finally, ventilatory failure can occur in the absence of respiratory muscle fatigue, as a result of an overwhelming disturbance of the gas exchange function of the lung, which cannot be overcome by increased respiratory muscle activation. An example of this occurrence is hypercapnic respiratory failure due to a very severe acute asthma attack. Again, treatment must consist of mechanical ventilation if severe respiratory acidemia intervenes, since both acidemia and hypoxemia are detrimental to diaphragmatic contractile function, and subsequent diaphragmatic failure in the patient already severely compromised by lung disease would be disastrous.

Emergency Department Management of Ventilatory Failure

Ventilatory failure that results in a dangerous degree of respiratory acidemia (generally, pH < 7.25) and that is not rapidly reversible is an indication for intubation and mechanical ventilation. While awaiting endotracheal tube placement, the patient should be ventilated manually with a resuscitation bag and mask connected to high-flow oxygen. Orotracheal tube placement, guided by direct laryngoscopy, allows the use of large-bore endotracheal tubes and is routinely employed for emergency intubation. If this method fails, nasotracheal intubation using a smaller tube (<No. 8) can be used. In difficult cases, intubation can be accomplished by passing the endotracheal tube over a flexible fiberoptic bronchoscope that has been advanced into the trachea. After intubation, the endotracheal tube cuff is inflated and tracheal intubation is verified by auscultation over the chest and stomach during manual ventilation with a resuscitation bag. A chest x-ray should be obtained to define tube position and detect possible complications of intubation, such as aspiration. Usual initial ventilator orders include:

Inspired oxygen concentration (FIO_2)	All patients should receive 100 percent oxygen initially since complications of intubation are relatively common (aspiration, malpositioning of the endotracheal tube, leakage of the endotracheal cuff)
Ventilator mode	IMV or assist/control
Ventilator rate	8–14 breaths per minute
Tidal volume	10–15 ml/kg

In general, patients with obstructive airways disease (COPD, asthma) are best managed with respiratory rates at the low end of the previously stated range to provide adequate time for expiration. In patients with decreased static compliance (stiff lungs), ventilation using a high-frequency, low tidal volume pattern may be necessary to avoid excessive (>50 cm H_2O) peak airway pressures.

An arterial blood gas measurement should be obtained within 10 to 15 minutes after initiation of ventilation, and the concentration of inspired oxygen and the minute ventilation should be adjusted based on blood gas results. The inspired oxygen concentration can be modified to achieve the desired arterial PO_2, and respiratory rate and tidal volume, the determinants of minute ventilation, can be adjusted to achieve the target arterial PCO_2. In patients with chronically elevated arterial carbon dioxide tension ($PaCO_2$) and metabolic compensation, rapid correction of $PaCO_2$ to normal values should be avoided to prevent severe alkalemia. When stable, all patients who require mechanical ventilation should be expeditiously transferred from the emergency department to an intensive care area.

SELECTED READING

Belman, MJ (ed). Respiratory muscles: Function in health and disease. *Clin Chest Med* 9:175, 1988.

Belman, MJ, Sieck, GC, and Mazar, A. Aminophylline and its influence on ventilatory endurance in humans. *Am Rev Respir Dis* 131:226, 1985.

Bennett, DA, and Bleck, TP. Diagnosis and treatment of neuromuscular causes of acute respiratory failure. *Clin Neuropharm* 11:303, 1988.

Derenne, J-P, Fleury, B, and Pariente, R. Acute respiratory failure in chronic obstructive pulmonary disease. *Am Rev Respir Dis* 138:1006, 1988.

Grum, CM, and Chauncey, JB. Conventional mechanical ventilation. *Clin Chest Med* 9:37, 1988.

Murciano, D, et al. A randomized, controlled trial of theophylline in patients with severe chronic obstructive pulmonary disease. *N Engl J Med* 320:1521, 1989.

Weinberger, SE, Schwartzstein, RM, and Weiss, JW. Hypercapnia. *N Engl J Med* 321:1223, 1989.

C. Acute Cardiac Disorders

16. Normal and Pathologic Physiology of Heart Muscle Contraction

John E. Strobeck
Edmund H. Sonnenblick

ULTRASTRUCTURAL BASIS OF MYOCARDIAL CONTRACTION

Cardiac Muscle Cells

In general, the architecture of all the components of the ventricle, including the endocardium, conduction cells, capillaries, arteries, nerves, and veins, is similar in both left and right ventricles. The mass and thickness of the two ventricles differ owing to the different pressures under which they function. Atrial architecture is also similar between the two atria except that both the sinoatrial (SA) and atrioventricular (AV) nodes are located in the right atrium near the superior vena cava and the portion of the atrial septum closest to the AV junction, respectively.

Muscle cells spread from the apex of the heart in a fan-like fashion and occupy several layers oriented at varying angles to each other. This geometry provides transmural strength to the wall of the ventricle and promotes an apex to base force vector for efficiently reducing ventricular volume during contraction. Cardiac muscle cells are excited by an impulse originating in the SA node and invading all cells through low-resistance connections (nexuses) that exist between them. Therefore, electrical current distribution in the heart is defined by the equivalent network geometry of all myocytes combined (Fig. 16-1). Although bundles of myocytes may be seen to branch, myocytes themselves rarely branch (Figs. 16-1A and 16-2). Branching, however, does occur at intercalated disks where cells take off from their neighbors. Light microscopic analysis of serial sections through myocyte bundles at approximately 1-μm intervals has revealed that individual cardiac myocytes in a bundle are connected to at least two neighbors longitudinally and at least one laterally. The average distance between lateral connections among cells was of the order of one cell length. Most bundles are connected laterally to other bundles at least every 200 μm down the bundle. Bundle geometry is maintained by junctional complexes that are specializations of the plasma membrane and function as adhesion points between cells.

Intercalated disks form the points of apposition of cardiac myocytes. These structures are mosaics of three kinds of junctional complexes (desmosomes, nexuses, and intermediate junctions; Fig. 16-3). The intercalated disks are mainly located at the cell ends, where a Z-line would be expected. Actin filaments actually insert on the intercalated disk. Every cardiac myocyte has several ends producing an overall geometry that is cylindrical with exterior sculpturing suggestive of the skyline of a major city. The step-like plateaus of the facade are each occupied by an intercalated

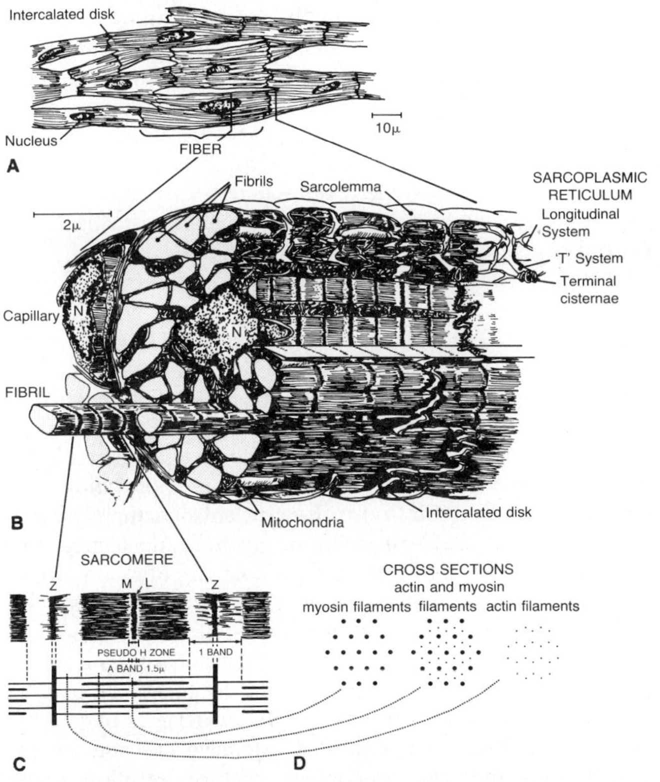

Fig. 16-1. Overview of the microscopic structure of heart muscle. A. Myocardium as seen under the light microscope. Branching of fibers is evident. Each fiber or cell contains a centrally located nucleus. B. Myocardial cell reconstructed from electron micrographs. Each cell is composed of multiple parallel fibrils. Each fibril is composed of serially connected sarcomeres (N = nucleus). C. Sarcomere from a myofibril, with diagramatic representation of myofilaments. Thick filaments (1.5 μm long, composed of myosin) form the A band and thin filaments (1.0 μm long, composed primarily of actin) extend from the Z-line through the I band into the A band. The overlapping of thick and thin filaments is seen only in the A band. D. Cross sections of the sarcomere indicate the specific lattice arrangements of the myofilaments. In the center of the sarcomere, only the thick, or myosin, filaments arranged in a hexagonal array are seen. In the distal portions of the A band, both thick and thin filaments are found, with each thick filament surrounded by six thin filaments. In the I band, only thin, or actin, filaments are found. (From E. Braunwald, J. Ross, Jr., and E.H. Sonnenblick. *Mechanisms of Contraction of the Normal and Failing Heart* [2nd ed.]. Boston: Little, Brown, 1976.)

disk. As a result of this peculiar shape of cardiac myocytes, cell lengths and diameters vary within a single cell and can range from 10 to 20 μm in diameter and 50 to 150 μm in length. In addition, attempts to isolate a population of single cells have not been successful at severing the connections between cells cleanly. In most instances, both halves of the nexus will remain with one of the cells, leaving a hole in the other.

Plasma Membrane

The plasma membrane displays a unit membrane construction and a number of specialized regions, including the in-

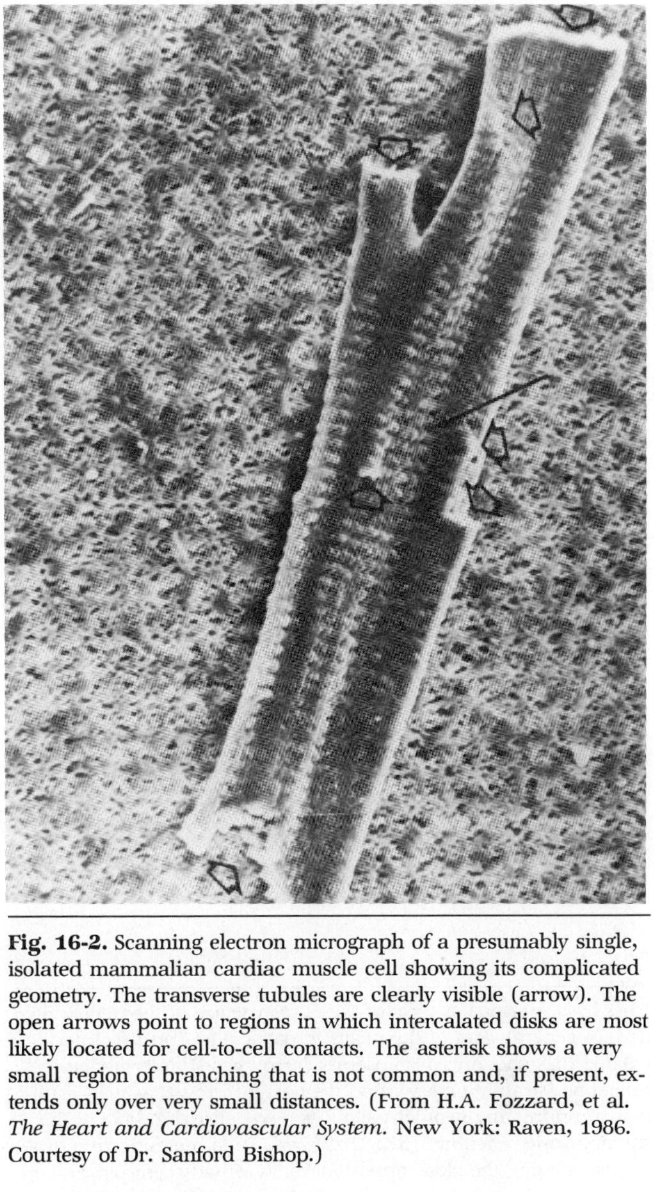

Fig. 16-2. Scanning electron micrograph of a presumably single, isolated mammalian cardiac muscle cell showing its complicated geometry. The transverse tubules are clearly visible (arrow). The open arrows point to regions in which intercalated disks are most likely located for cell-to-cell contacts. The asterisk shows a very small region of branching that is not common and, if present, extends only over very small distances. (From H.A. Fozzard, et al. *The Heart and Cardiovascular System.* New York: Raven, 1986. Courtesy of Dr. Sanford Bishop.)

tercalated disks and transverse tubular system. It is covered by a laminar coat separable into two layers, the lamina densa and lamina lucida. A synonym for the laminar coat is the glycocalyx. Extracellular collagen fibers are separated from the plasma membrane by the laminar coat, whereas microfibrils, which insert on the plasma membrane, actually traverse the laminar coat before mingling with collagen fibrils and fibers. Plasmalemma plus laminar coat plus collagen is termed *sarcolemma.*

The plasmalemma is anchored to an intracellular cytoskeleton by fibers approximately 10 nm in diameter. These fibers are located mainly at the Z-lines and, in contracted muscle, pull in the plasmalemma to create a scalloped surface and grooves, called *Z-grooves.* It is from these grooves that the transverse tubules emanate.

The transverse tubules are tubular extensions of the plasmalemma into the interior of the cardiac muscle cell. The majority of transverse tubules are oriented transversely to the longitudinal axis of the myocyte and extend to the center of

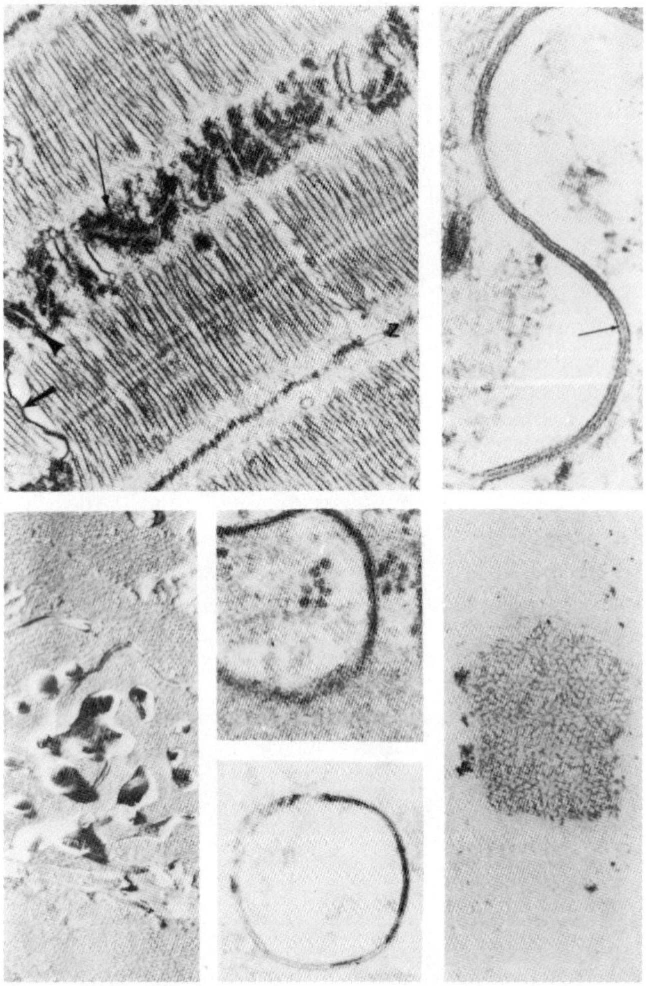

Fig. 16-3. Various aspects of the ultrastructure of the intercalated disk in general, and of the nexus in particular. *Top left.* Intercalated disk showing desmosomes (arrowhead), intermediate junctions (straight arrow), and the nexus (arrow), as well as the typical undulating geometry. At Z is a so-called Z-tubule of the sarcoplasmic reticulum (SR). *Top right.* High magnification of the nexus showing the close apposition between adjacent plasmalemmas, which leaves a narrow gap in the center (arrow) indicating the gap junction. *Bottom left.* Freeze-fracture of intercalated disk showing its geometry in three dimensions. *Bottom right.* Lanthanum space around the connections of the nexus. This space is continuous with the extracellular space but not with the center of the connections. *Center top.* Nexus with the gap contrasted with a special stain. *Center bottom.* Nexus contrasted with lanthanum showing the lanthanum space in both transverse and tangential section. The circular geometry is common. (From J.R. Sommer. The ultrastructure of the mammalian cardiac muscle cell, with special emphasis on the tubular membrane systems. A review. *Am. J. Pathol.* 82:192, 1976.)

the cell (see Fig. 16-1B). However, there are many longitudinal extensions producing a tubular network that is continuous with the extracellular space. The ratio of total plasmalemmal surface area (free surface plus T-tubules) to the total cell volume is a constant in cardiac muscle of many species and correlates directly with heart rate.

One of the functions of the transverse tubules is presumably the propagation of the action potential to the interior of the cardiac muscle cell. However, since the average diameter of the cardiac myocyte is small (10–20 μm), many investigators believe that a major role of the T-tubules is not apparent until the cardiac muscle cell undergoes the adaptive process of hypertrophy. This process of cell enlargement is very effective compensation, in the early stages, for many forms of myocardial and valvular heart disease and requires additional T-tubules for efficient cellular depolarization as well as necessary reductions of diffusion distances to maintain central oxygenation and metabolic stability.

The plasmalemma contains three kinds of *junctional complexes* that are often combined in intercalated disks: (1) the desmosome, (2) the intermediate junction, and (3) the nexus (gap junction) (see Fig. 16-3). The desmosomes and intermediate junctions probably serve an adhesive function. For example, desmosomes are particularly numerous between Purkinje's cells, so as to maintain the crucial intercellular clefts that separate them. Desmosomes are morphologically distinguished by their more discrete substructures, which are both intra- and extracellular. By immunoelectron microscopy, intermediate junctions contain vinculin and alpha-actinin, whereas desmosomes do not. Desmin is mostly localized to interfibrillary spaces near but not in desmosomes.

The nexuses are the anatomic substrate of the electrical coupling of all cardiac muscle cells. Nexuses are usually located parallel to the long axis of the myocyte as part of the intercalated disk. As a result of extensive electron microscopic study incorporating freeze-fracture techniques, the nexus consists of connections that are composed of six subunits, which form a hydrophilic channel in their center extending from one cell to the next across a narrow extracellular gap of about 3 nm. The protein composition of the nexus and therefore its coupling resistance may be modified by different functional states or changes in concentrations of intracellular Ca^{2+} or H^+. Thus, the known morphology of the nexus is consistent with its function of spreading excitation to all cells. The overall size of the nexus in cardiac muscle shows a distinct inverse relationship to the size of the coupled cells. This is consistent with the effective coupling resistance, which is anticipated as a function of the input resistance and suggests that the conductance of the nexus increases with its size.

Sarcoplasmic Reticulum

The sarcoplasmic reticulum (SR) in cardiac muscle is a tubular network surrounding the myofibrils and has the function of sequestering Ca^{2+} for muscle relaxation. The SR network has two main components: (1) the junctional SR (JSR) existing in three forms—the junctional SR proper, the extended junctional SR (EJSR), and the corbular SR; and (2) the free SR, which forms the Z retes, the M retes, the Z-tubules, and longitudinal SR segments (Figs. 16-1B and 16-4).

The junctional SR in cardiac muscle is a flat tubule containing electron-dense material. On the outside, the JSR carries small periodic processes or feet that emanate from the JSR's junctional membrane proper and often appear to make direct contact with the plasmalemma of either the transverse tubule or the cell surface. The junctional processes are also present on the portion of the junctional membrane toward the free cytoplasm.

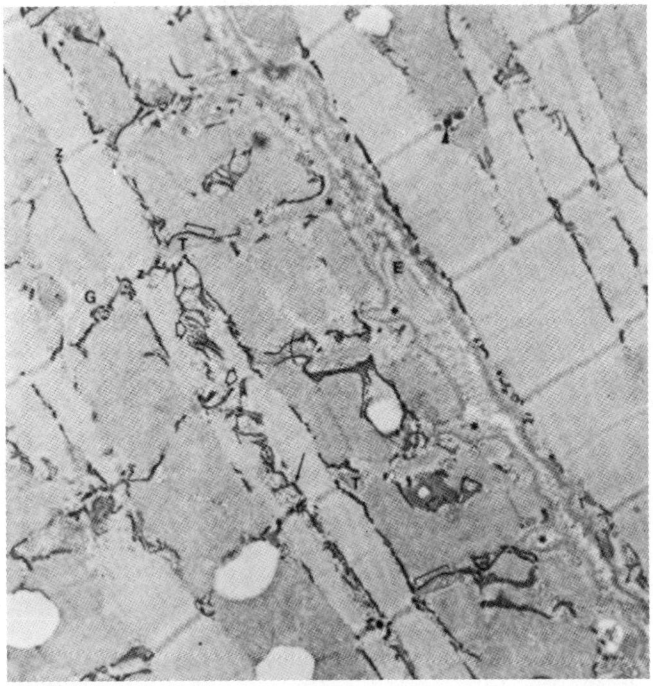

Fig. 16-4. Longitudinal section through mammalian cardiac muscle in which the SR has been differentially stained in black contrast medium. The extracellular space contains collagen. One of the cells has prominent Z-grooves (asterisks) from which transverse tubules emanate into the interior of the cells (T). The laminar coat of the plasmalemma extends into the transverse tubules. The SR forms a tubular network around the contractile material and is composed of free SR with M and Z retes (open arrows), with the Z rete often represented only by a single Z tubule (z). There are interior couplings of the SR (brackets) composed of junctional SR and plasmalemma forming diads (brackets) or triads (curved bracket) with transverse tubules, and peripheral couplings (brace) subjacent to the surface plasmalemma. Mitochondria are plentiful and tend to be confined to each sarcomere, defined by the space between two Z-lines. Corbular SR (arrowhead) is prominent in regions where transverse tubules are sparse. Golgi zones are multiple and may be found adjacent to or away from the perinuclear region (G). (From J.R. Sommer. *Handbook of Physiology. Section 2, The Cardiovascular System, Vol. I, The Heart.* Washington, D.C.: American Physiological Society. Pp. 113–186; 1979.)

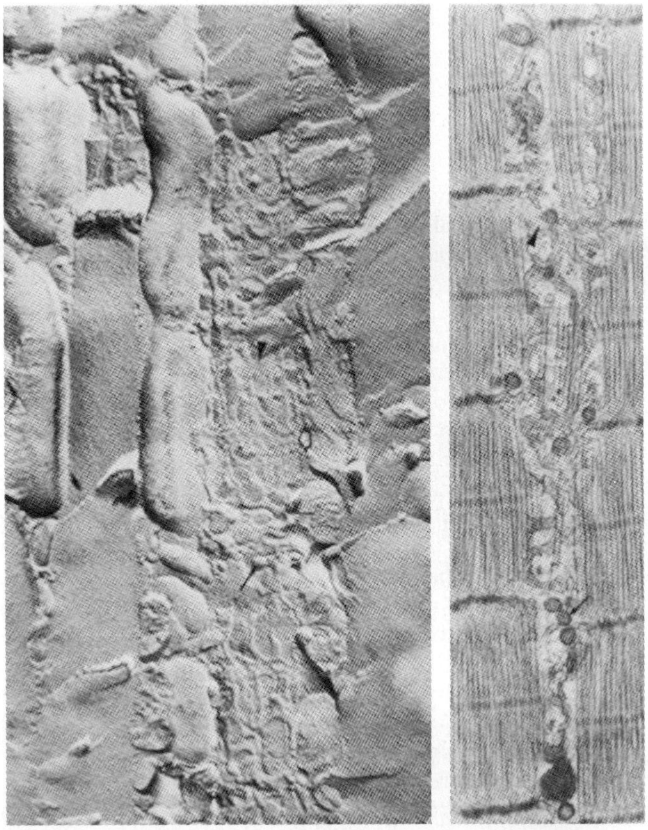

A B

Fig. 16-5. A. Mammalian cardiac muscle showing the overall geometry of the SR and, especially, of the corbular SR. Freeze-fracture preparation shows mitochondria, free SR with M retes (open arrow), corbular SR (arrow), and cisternal SR (arrowhead). (From P.C. Dolber and J.R. Sommer. Corbular sarcoplasmic reticulum of rabbit cardiac muscle. *J. Ultrastruct. Res.* 87:190, 1984.) B. Section showing free SR, corbular SR (arrow), and anchor fibers (arrowhead). (From J.R. Sommer. *Handbook of Physiology. Section 2, The Cardiovascular System, Vol. I, The Heart.* Washington, D.C.: American Physiological Society. Pp. 113–186; 1979.)

The extended junctional SR, in its continuous form, arises from the JSR by losing contact with the plasmalemma, extending from a peripheral coupling into the interior of the cardiac myocyte but without ever losing either the granular material in its lumen or the junctional processes. In its discontinuous form, EJSR is intercalated at Z-lines into the smooth tubular network of the free SR such that the continuity between EJSR and JSR proper (at the plasmalemma) is maintained by segments of free SR.

Corbular SR is a form of EJSR because it also has no contact with the plasmalemma (Fig. 16-5). Its structure is identical to JSR except that it is round in shape and has only one connection with the free SR. Corbular SR is located at Z-lines where it buds from the Z-tubule, which is a rudiment of the Z rete. Corbular SR is usually found in regions of myocytes where T-tubules failed to develop.

Freeze-fracture of the JSR shows the P-faces to be filled with particles that are representative of the Ca^{2+} pump protein. This is in agreement with the fact that isolated JSR has considerable ATPase activity. The detailed functions of the JSR remain to be sorted out, but there is strong evidence that the JSR stores and releases Ca^{2+}. The JSR's topographic relations to the plasmalemma and to the actin filaments have crucial functional implications and ensure rapid diffusion of Ca^{2+} to the regulatory proteins. The results of studies with Ca^{2+} and calsequestrin provide strong evidence that the JSR is capable of storing Ca^{2+}, but do not answer the question of whether the JSR is a Ca^{2+} release site for contraction. More recent data suggest that Ca^{2+} release is possible through the entire SR and that the junctional processes may act as receptors for "trigger Ca^{2+}" entering the cell as a result of surface membrane depolarization. The chemical transduction of the inward Ca^{2+} current by the junctional processes may in turn lead to the release of activator Ca^{2+} by the SR. No open connection between the SR and the extracellular space has ever been demonstrated.

Myofibrils

The contractile material in cardiac muscle on cross section appears to be widely branching, often creating dead-end crevices containing cytoplasm, mitochondria, and other intracellular organelles, including the cytoskeleton. In cardiac muscle, all contractile material is within 0.5 μm of SR tubules and mitochondria.

The myofibrils are assembled into small repeating units called sarcomeres, each stretching between two Z-lines. The sarcomere represents the structural basis of contraction (see Fig. 16-1C). The diastolic length of the cardiac sarcomere under normal physiologic conditions is between 2.0 and 2.2 μm. Sarcomere lengths less than 1.6 μm at peak contraction are unusual in cardiac muscle. The striations are produced by the thin actin filaments forming the light I bands and by the thick myosin filaments forming the dark A bands. In agreement with the sliding filament theory of muscle contraction, the actin and myosin filaments overlap in tandem with the state of contraction. High-resolution electron microscopy has revealed periodic extensions, the cross-bridges, from the myosin to the actin filaments. They represent the head pieces of the myosin molecule and display ATPase activity. Current data suggest that activation of muscle fibers causes conformational changes in these cross-bridges, which, through a rapid sequence of alternating attachments to and detachments from the actin filaments, pull them into the hexagonal A band lattice and thus cause shortening of the sarcomere. When actin filaments are completely pulled into the A band, the I band disappears. Active sequestration of intracellular Ca^{2+} by the SR reduces the number and intensity of activity of the cross-bridges allowing reextension of the actin filaments and the overall sarcomere length.

Cytoskeleton

The cytoskeleton is an intracellular scaffold serving to stabilize the topography of intracellular components and to control cell size and shape. Whereas the former is important for biochemical processes and to maintain diffusion distances, the latter is crucial for defining surface to volume ratios, which influence the electrical properties in a fundamental way.

Cardiac muscle contains three main classes of cytoskeletal fibers: (1) microtubules (25 nm); (2) actin or microfilaments (6 nm), which form cytoplasmic stress fibers; and (3) intermediate filaments (10 nm). Microtubules are composed mainly of tubulin and are found in the interfibrillary and perinuclear spaces, especially in the vicinity of the centrioles. Both microtubules and microfilaments serve some motile function and exist independently from the contractile apparatus.

Intermediate filaments can be separated into several subclasses, such as tonofilaments, vimentin, desmin, or skeletin. In adult cardiac muscle, the main intermediate filament protein is desmin. The intermediate filaments form a network that is oriented in longitudinal and transverse directions. They attach to Z-disk protein, to organelles such as the SR, nuclei, mitochondria, as well as the plasmalemma, and loosely divide the cytoplasm into transverse and longitudinal quasicompartments (Fig. 16-6).

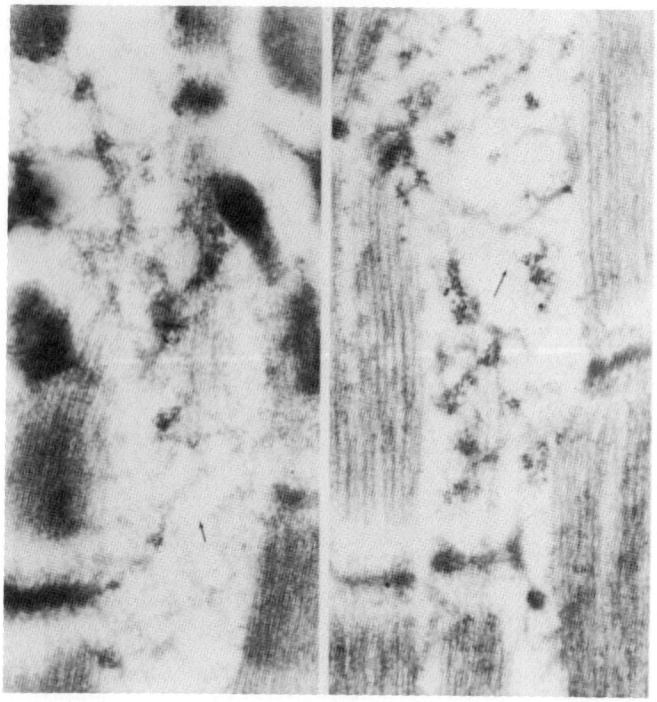

A B

Fig. 16-6. A. Cytoskeleton consisting of desmin filaments is identified by specific ferritin-labeled antibodies (arrow). B. Control section in which myosin is labeled with appropriate antibodies but not the desmin filaments (arrow). (From K.T. Tokuyasu. Visualization of longitudinally oriented intermediate filaments in frozen sections of chick cardiac muscle by a new staining method. Reproduced from the *Journal of Cell Biology* 1983, 97:562, by copyright permission of the Rockefeller University Press.)

EXCITATION-CONTRACTION-RELAXATION COUPLING

In cardiac muscle, the monophasic action potential describes the activity of several specific ion channels (Fig. 16-7). When activated, the sodium channel carries the positive charges of sodium ions into the cell causing depolarization of the membrane potential from approximately −90 mV at rest to an overshoot potential of +20 mV. This is followed by a phase of slow repolarization owing largely to the effect of an inwardly directed calcium channel and then a fast repolarization with return of the membrane potential to a normal level by the activity of an outwardly directive potassium channel. The adenosine triphosphate (ATP)–dependent sodium-potassium pump maintains the proper gradient of sodium and potassium between inside the cell and out. These channels for sodium, calcium, and potassium are all voltage-dependent and can be activated and inactivated. The transient states of channel activity are currently thought to be the result of voltage-regulated gating of each of the channels.

When the calcium channel is activated, positive charges are carried by calcium ions into the cell and in some way alter the properties of a distinct calcium release channel located in the internal couplings of the SR (Fig. 16-8). A

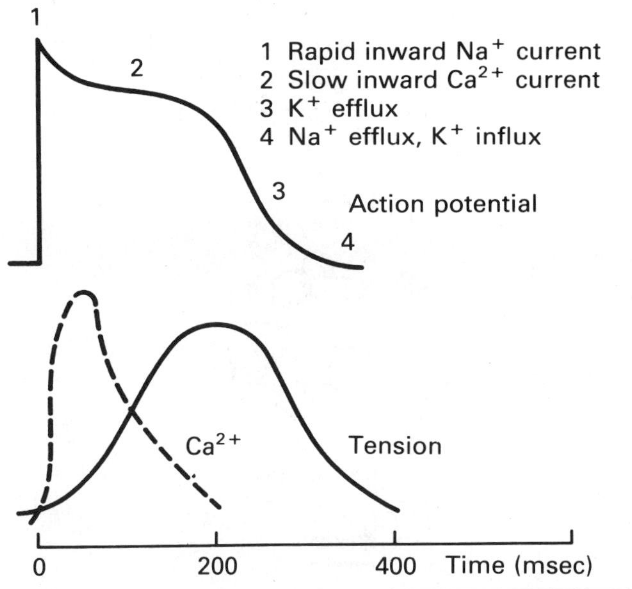

Fig. 16-7. The time course of changes of membrane potential, intracellular free Ca^{2+}, and isometric tension during a twitch contraction of cardiac ventricular muscle. (From J.S. Williams. *Treatment of Cardiovascular Diseases by Nifedipine.* Stuttgart: Schattauer, 1986. Pp. 4–30.)

Fig. 16-8. A representation of ion transport and excitation-contraction-relaxation coupling in heart muscle. (AMP = adenosine monophosphate; CAM = calmodulin; Mito = mitochondria; PDE = phosphodiesterase; SR = sarcoplasmic reticulum.) (From A. Schwartz. Calcium antagonists: Review and perspective on mechanism of action. *Am. J. Cardiol.* 64:31–91, 1989.)

relatively large amount of calcium is then released from the storage couplings and reacts with specific sites on troponin C. Troponin C represents one of three regulatory proteins located on the thin filament (actin). Binding of calcium to troponin C alters the conformation of troponin C, which in turn causes troponin I, troponin T, and tropomyosin to change positions so that the cross-bridges, containing the Sl myosin ATPase, can readily attach to specific sites on actin. Repetitive movement of the cross-bridges propels the thin filaments past the thick filament creating motion in each sarcomere (Fig. 16-9). Although the above description represents an oversimplification, there is considerable evidence to support this concept of muscle behavior. The activity of the SR calcium-ATPase, located specifically in the SR, pumps calcium from troponin C into the lumen of the SR. Muscle relaxation ensues when levels of calcium ions return to about 100 nM, the so-called diastolic calcium level. The calcium that was pumped into the SR moves into the internal coupling storage sites and is presumably re-released through the calcium release channels once again during the next electrically coupled contractile event. The calcium release channel is currently thought to be part of a very large protein commonly called the *junctional feet* protein because it appears to connect the internal coupling of the SR to the transverse tubule.

During the coupled process of excitation-contraction-relaxation, the calcium concentration intracellularly rises from a diastolic concentration of about 100 nM to about 1 μm and then returns to the diastolic level before the completion of the contractile cycle. The regulation of this calcium "transient" is interesting and complex. There is now little doubt that a series of protein kinases plays a major role in the regulation of the calcium transient. For example, a cyclic adenosine monophosphate (AMP)–dependent protein kinase is activated secondary to an increase in cyclic AMP. An increase in cyclic AMP could occur either by stimulation of

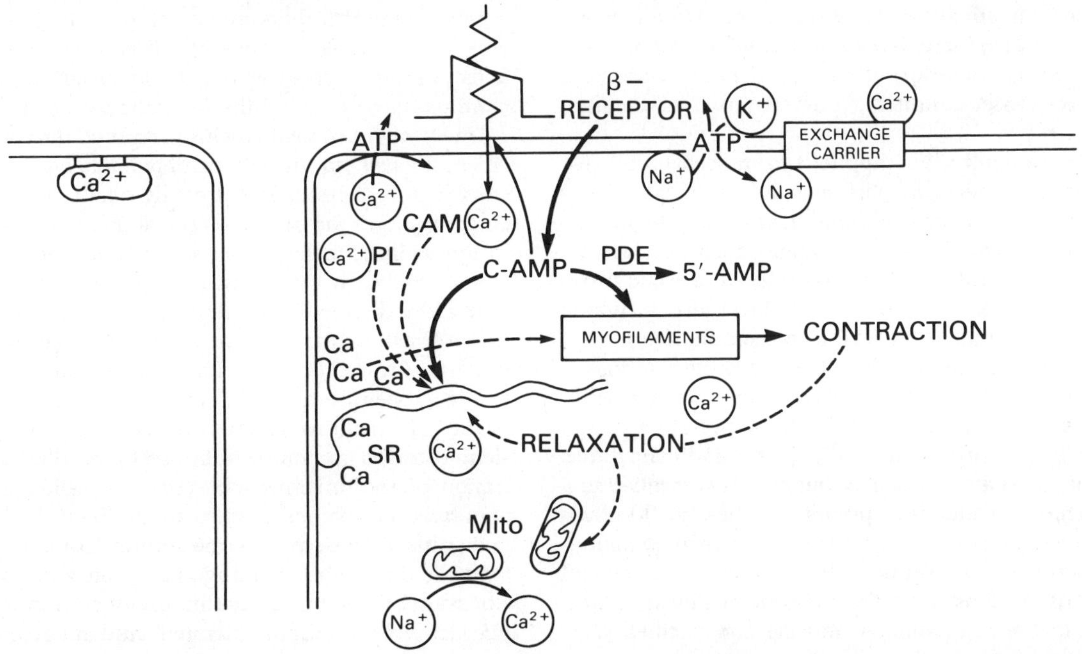

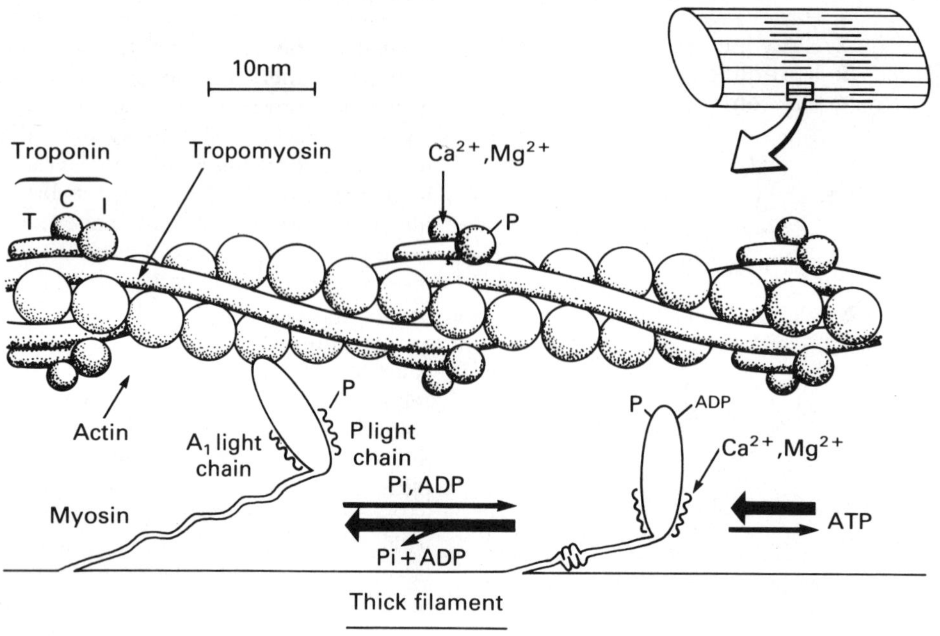

Fig. 16-9. Molecular structure of the thick and thin filaments of cardiac myofibrils and the mechanism of action of the calcium ion. (ADP = adenosine diphosphate; ATP = adenosine triphosphate.) (Modified from M.A. Matlib. *Calcium Antagonists*. Boston: Martinus Nijhoff, 1984. Pp. 79–93.)

the beta-adrenergic system or by inhibition of phosphodiesterases, which hydrolyze the cyclic nucleotide. Protein kinase B, which depends on calmodulin and calcium, is activated by calcium that enters via the calcium channel; protein kinase C is also activated by calcium. These enzymes catalyze the transfer of phosphate from ATP to various substrates. In the heart, the most important of these substrates is phospholamban, a small molecular-weight protein located in the SR close to the SR calcium-ATPase. The protein, in its nonphosphorylated form, inhibits the activity of the SR calcium-ATPase pump. When phospholamban is phosphorylated by any of the kinases, a deinhibition of the pump occurs, leading to an enhancement of relaxation. Enhancement of relaxation leads to increased levels of calcium stored in the SR that can be released during the next depolarization and contractile response, producing augmentation of contraction.

When catecholamine is applied to a heart cell (or when endogenous norepinephrine is released), the beta-adrenergic receptor is activated, initiating a cascade of reactions involving G proteins, guanylyl nucleotides, and adenylate cyclases. The result is an increase in levels of cyclic AMP. Cyclic AMP releases a subunit of protein kinase A, which transfers the phosphate from ATP to phospholamban.

Calcium entering the cell also activates protein kinase B and C, which also phosphorylate phospholamban. Troponin I is also phosphorylated by kinase A. This results in a lowering of the affinity of troponin C for calcium and contributes to relaxation. Cardiac contraction therefore is controlled in a complex fashion through the operation of these well-known regulatory mechanisms. The newly investigated phosphoinositide pathway that leads to the formation of inositol phosphates as well as activation of protein kinase C also contributes to the regulation of muscle contractility. Currently, there is much research activity in this field, and the results may prove as important as any of the aforedescribed mechanisms.

Thus, the process of excitation-contraction-relaxation in cardiac muscle involves biochemical and physiologic events that are coupled by calcium. Contraction and relaxation should be viewed as separate biochemical and physiologic events regulated differently, yet operating together. It is therefore possible to envision disease states in which the defect in these processes may be localized exclusively to the contraction or possibly the relaxation process.

The amount of total calcium required for contraction that enters the cell via the voltage-dependent calcium channel in cardiac sarcolemma is extremely small. This "trigger calcium" initiates the processes previously described. Increases in intracellular calcium caused by entry of trigger calcium are managed in one of two ways. The first method is an outwardly directed calmodulin-calcium–sensitive sarcolemmal ATPase that has recently been sequenced and plays an important role. The second method is a sodium-calcium exchange system, which is electrogenic in nature and located in the cell membrane. This system is very sensitive to transient changes in intracellular sodium. When the concentration of sodium ions increases intracellularly, as during depolarization or secondary to inhibition of the sodium-potassium ATPase pump, the sodium gradient from outside to inside diminishes, leading to a significant inhibition of the extrusion of calcium, providing more calcium availability to interact with contractile filaments and augment contraction.

The exchange system, which is reversible, plays a great role in regulating intracellular calcium concentrations.

DETERMINANTS OF VENTRICULAR CONTRACTILE PERFORMANCE

Preload

When isolated cardiac muscle is stimulated and held at a fixed length, the resultant contraction is termed *isometric*. In contrast to the situation with skeletal muscle, in which the force of contraction is nearly independent of muscle length over a wide range, and in which contraction is generally of a tetanic nature, the strength of individual isometric twitches in cardiac muscle is markedly length-dependent. An increase in the initial muscle length, induced by a change in passive stretch of the muscle, produces a resting load that has been termed *preload*.

The effects of length on resting and developed force are well established and are expressed by the resting and active length–tension curves. For reasons that are not completely understood, heart muscle is less compliant than skeletal muscle at rest, so that resting tension rises more rapidly as heart muscle is stretched. It is also not known to what extent resting force is borne by passive elastic elements of the muscle and to what extent it is maintained by active processes within the muscle. Whatever the relationship, the relatively high resting stiffness of cardiac muscle must be correlated with the inability to stretch the cardiac sarcomere beyond a length of about 2.2 μm. It is at that sarcomere length (Lmax) that the degree of overlap between actin and myosin filaments is optimal for contraction and muscle isometric force is maximal.

An increase in preload (resting muscle length and sarcomere length) produces an increase in muscle force over the physiologic range and is responsible for the increase in stroke volume of the ventricle when end-diastolic volume is increased. The mechanism of length-dependent muscle contractile behavior is still not completely understood. Between the optimum cardiac sarcomere length of 2.2 μm and 1.6 μm, muscle force declines to zero. Sarcomere length cannot be passively shortened below 2.0 μm.

If a cardiac muscle cell is skinned of its sarcolemma, thus ensuring maximal myofilament activation and possibly removing internal loads, and the contractile apparatus is activated by applying external Ca^{2+}, the decline in force with shortening sarcomere length is less pronounced than in skeletal muscle (Fig. 16-10). In a skinned cardiac fiber, the relation between muscle force and sarcomere length is shifted upward and to the left by increasing the extracellular Ca^{2+} concentration. When muscle force is corrected for passive resting force, borne presumably by noncontractile elements of the muscle, the muscle force–sarcomere length relation has a significantly steeper slope as calcium concentration is increased. These data support the concept of a length-dependent activation process as the basis of the length–tension relation in cardiac muscle.

The exact nature of the length-dependent activation process remains unsettled. It is not likely that the length–tension relation in cardiac muscle depends on length-dependent release of calcium to the myofilaments, because it has been shown that released calcium does not vary over a wide range of muscle and sarcomere lengths. However, there is convincing evidence that myofilament sensitivity to calcium decreases with decreasing sarcomere length in cardiac muscle. The data are not conclusive enough to rule out some effect of an internal load, because the nature of passive load-bearing structures in cardiac muscle is not completely understood. Structures such as axially oriented collagen fibers or intracellular microtubules or microfilaments might restrict shortening or elongation of sarcomeres and contribute to internal loads. However, the bulk of evidence suggests that, if present, the force of an internal load is small and will produce very slight effects at physiologic lengths.

Developed force, as noted earlier, is highly dependent on initial muscle length and, hence, sarcomere length; however, because of serial elasticities, peak muscle isometric force is obtained only with some obligatory sarcomere shortening during contraction. This shortening takes place at the expense of a series compliance, largely at the muscle ends. The question as to whether observed sarcomere shortening alters the amount of isometric force that would have been generated at any myofilament overlap if no sarcomere shortening had occurred has been answered. Sarcomere length can be

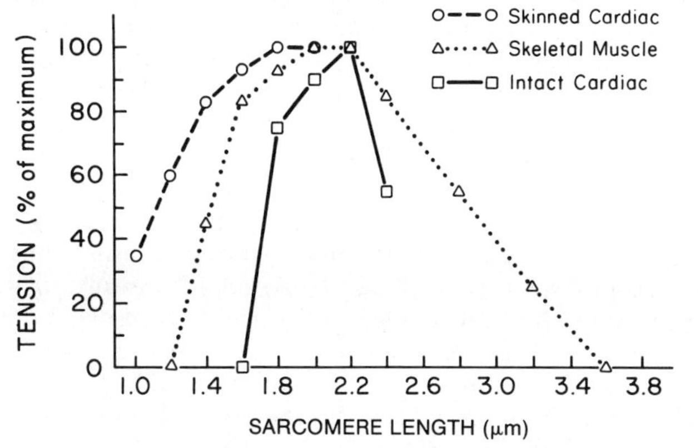

Fig. 16-10. Sarcomere length–tension relations are depicted for skinned cardiac muscle, skeletal muscle, and intact cardiac muscle. The data from intact cardiac muscle were obtained by fixing cat papillary muscles with glutaraldehyde at various diastolic lengths and recording the tension immediately prior to fixation. The average sarcomere length within the tissue was determined by electron microscopic methods. The relation between tension development and sarcomere length obtained with skeletal fibers (see A.M. Gordon, et al., *J. Physiol. (Lond.)* 184:170, 1966) has been superimposed for comparison. The data from skinned cardiac muscle are adapted from A. Fabiato, *Nature* 256:54, 1975, and have also been superimposed. In intact cardiac muscle, peak tension occurs with a diastolic sarcomere length of 2.2 μm. Whereas in skeletal muscle there is a plateau of developed tension between sarcomere lengths 2.2 and 2.0 μm, in intact cardiac muscle this is not the case, and developed tension falls as sarcomere length is decreased below 2.2 μm. Tension from skinned cardiac muscle that is maximally activated falls slower than tension in skeletal muscle. As intact cardiac muscle is stretched beyond 2.2 μm, resting tension rises substantially, while actively developed tension falls abruptly. In skeletal muscle, actively developed tension falls in a linear fashion between a sarcomere length of 2.2 and 3.6 μm.

held reasonably constant by appropriate stretch of the muscle during the course of contraction. This method, which eliminates uncertainties owing to series elasticity external to the sarcomere, proves that muscle force critically depends on a unique sarcomere length at the peak of contractile activity.

When considering the effect of muscle length on the mechanics of cardiac muscle in the ventricular wall, the concepts of isolated cardiac muscle mechanics take on new dimensions. Increasing the length of ventricular muscle fibers is accomplished by a filling or distending pressure in the ventricular chamber that is created by inflow of blood during diastole. This pressure at end-diastole, termed *ventricular preload,* is a function of chamber shape and size and the stiffness of the ventricular wall. The distending pressure in the ventricular chamber must be countered by an equal wall force that is generated by passive stretch of the muscle itself. The net wall force, which is the summated force from all the muscle fibers in the thickness of the wall, can be calculated for a spherical chamber as the product of intraventricular pressure and the cross-sectional area of the chamber at a given point along the long axis (net wall force = $P \times Ri^2$, where Ri is the internal radius of the spherical chamber). Wall stress (gm/cm^2), the force borne by a unit thickness area (cm^2) of myocardium, is calculated by dividing wall force by $(Ro - Ri)^2$ where Ro is the outside radius of a spherical chamber, and Ri is the internal radius noted earlier. A midwall length of the "average" circumferential fiber is calculated as 2π Rm, where Rm is the midwall radius of the spherical chamber.

If ejection of blood from the ventricle during systole is prevented, an isovolumic contraction is generated. A series of isovolumic contractions from a variety of midwall circumferential lengths generates a pressure–length diagram that is analogous to the length–tension relation in isolated cardiac muscle.

Starling's observation that "the mechanical energy set free on passage from the resting to the contracted state is a function of the muscle fibers' length, i.e., the area of chemically active surfaces" underlies our current concepts of the relation between the length–active-tension curve in isolated muscle and the effect of end-diastolic pressure on stroke volume or stroke work in the intact ventricle (the Frank Starling relationship). Shifts in the ventricular function curve, as shown in Fig. 16-11, can also be used to demonstrate changes in contractility of the ventricle. Thus, the concept of ventricular function curves is useful in evaluating changes owing to either load or contractility in clinical settings. In the heart, ventricular end-diastolic wall stress is analogous to the preload of an isolated muscle that, for physiologic loads, ultimately determines the resting length of sarcomeres in the ventricular wall. However, unlike the relation between muscle length and developed force in isolated muscle, where developed force reaches a maximum at a particular length (Lmax) and then declines to form a "descending limb," in the normal ventricle an ascending limb of ventricular function (i.e., the curve relating the increase in stroke volume with each increment in end-diastolic volume) continues above the range of normal end-diastolic pressures (i.e., 12–14 mm Hg). Furthermore, at end-diastolic pressures greater than 20 mm Hg, or in certain disease states, the predicted relation between midwall sarcomere lengths and diastolic wall stress is not always found.

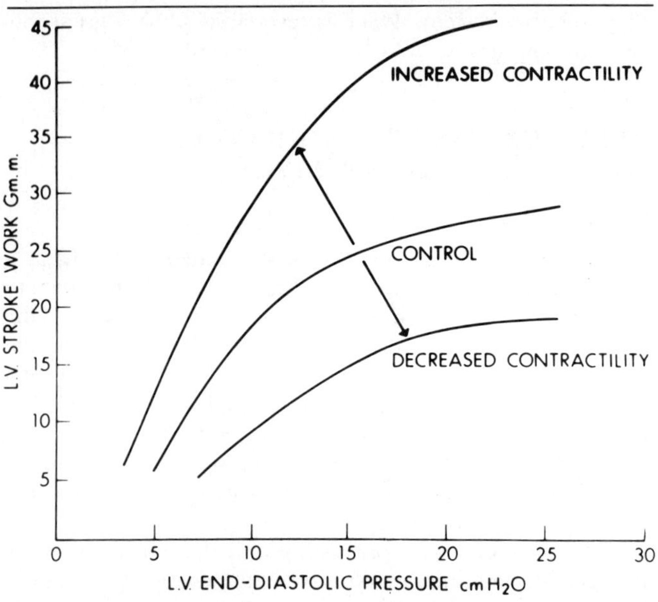

Fig. 16-11. Diagrammatic representation of ventricular function curves expressed as the relation between left ventricular end-diastolic pressure and stroke work. Note that increasing underlying myocardial contractility shifts the entire curve and changes its shape. It should be noted that the afterload, which can also change the shape and position of these curves, was kept constant during the experimental determination of these curves.

Sarcomere lengths vary considerably across the thickness of the ventricular wall. In the subendocardium, when studied at zero distending pressure, sarcomere lengths were longer than midwall or epicardial sarcomere lengths. As distending pressure was increased over the range of pressure defining the ascending limb of the length–tension curve in the intact left ventricle in open-chest dogs (2–20 Hg), sarcomere lengths approached their maximum (2.25 μm) at filling pressures of 10 to 12 mm Hg, but shorter sarcomeres from both the inner and outer layers lengthened near 2.25 μm as filling pressure approached 20 mm Hg. These findings may explain the apparent discrepancy between the observation that midwall sarcomere lengths in in situ hearts are near maximum when filling pressure is at the upper limit of normal (10–12 mm Hg), whereas an ascending limb of the ventricular isovolumic pressure–volume relation is observed until even higher filling pressures are reached. Thus, recruitment of short sarcomeres from across the ventricular wall constitutes the functional reserve (preload reserve) of the Frank Starling mechanism in the left ventricle at filling pressures above normal.

It has been shown that the relative degree of sarcomere shortening during ejection in the left ventricle is also not the same in all layers of the ventricular wall (Fig. 16-12). Thus, with 12 percent shortening in the midwall, epicardial fibers will shorten about 5 percent and endocardial layers will need to shorten approximately 20 percent of their initial lengths. Moreover, only the midwall fibers have been shown to shorten in a circumferential manner, whereas fibers in both the superficial and endocardial layers shorten in an apex-to-base direction. Angiographic studies have shown that circumferential shortening exceeds that of the apex-to-base direction and that large infoldings occur in the en-

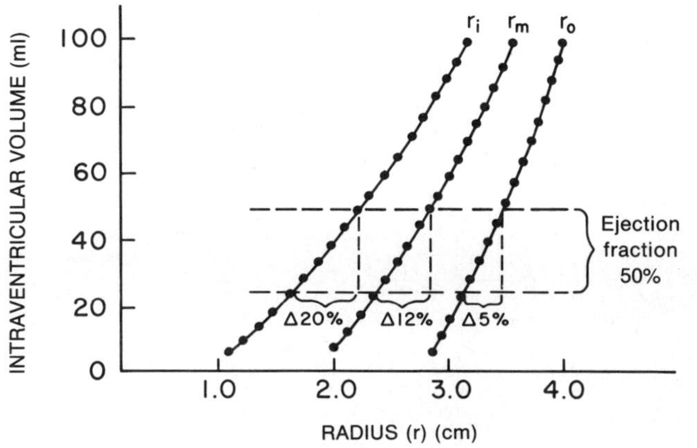

Fig. 16-12. Relation between intraventricular volume and changes in circumference in the inner (i), middle (m), and outer (o) layers of the left ventricular wall. The dashed horizontal lines demark a change in volume from 50 to 25 ml, which represents a left ventricular ejection fraction of 50 percent. Such an ejection fraction would require a 5 percent change in the outer circumference of the heart, a 12 percent change in the midwall layers, and a 20 percent change in the inner circumference.

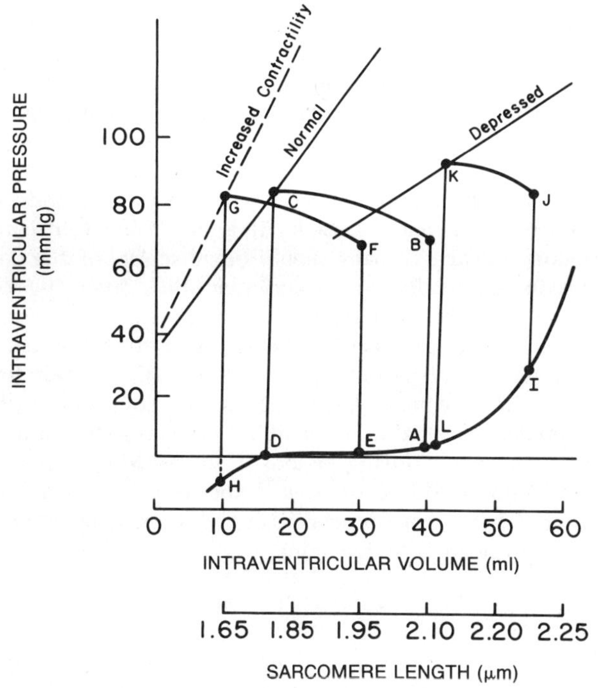

Fig. 16-13. Relationship of ventricular performance, in terms of ventricular pressure–volume relationships, to average midwall sarcomere length. These relationships are depicted under conditions of depressed, normal, or increased contractility.

docardial surfaces at end-systole; thus, models directly relating fiber shortening in multiple layers of the heart to stroke volume must be considered to be oversimplified.

Data obtained from fixed segments of cardiac muscle and from perfused intact heart, in addition to the findings from recent studies of sarcomere motion, permit construction of a diagram relating ventricular performance to sarcomere dimensions (Fig. 16-13). On the ordinate, intraventricular pressure is shown. This could be translated into wall stress using the formula given earlier. On the abscissa, intraventricular volume is shown. Volume, in turn, can be translated into circumferential fiber length in the midwall using the formula presented earlier. Accordingly, this diagram represents the pressure–volume relationship of the intact heart, as well as the approximate length–tension relation for the muscle composing the ventricular wall. Moreover, because diastolic sarcomere length is determined by diastolic ventricular volume and, hence, diastolic muscle length, midwall diastolic sarcomere lengths measured at these volumes are shown below the pressure–volume curve. These sarcomere lengths were obtained using rapid fixation methods that could produce as much as 5 percent shrinkage relative to the length occurring in vivo. Thus, a fixed sarcomere length of 2.0 μm might be translated into a sarcomere length of 2.1 μm in living muscle.

In Fig. 16-13, hypothetical pressure–volume loops have been portrayed on pressure–volume and pressure–sarcomere length axes. Loop ABCD represents contraction of the normal heart, loop EFGH shows a contraction potentiated by an inotropic stimulus, and loop IJKL illustrates a hypothetical loop for a failing ventricle.

Relative to the diastolic pressure–volume curve shown by connecting points, I,L,A,E,D, and H, volume is not zero when filling pressure is zero. Moreover, to empty the ventricle completely, a substantial negative pressure (H) is required. In an intact heart at zero filling pressure, sarcomere lengths range from 1.90 to 2.00 μm, and sarcomere lengths shorter than 1.9 μm are not observed in the relaxed ventricular wall. As noted earlier, diastolic sarcomere lengths in isolated cardiac muscle at slack muscle length also approximate 1.9 to 2.0 μm. Shorter sarcomere lengths are attained during contraction, but sarcomeres reextend their lengths on relaxation. When contracting freely, with minimal or zero load, muscle cells in the ventricular wall will be expected to shorten to sarcomere lengths as short as 1.5 to 1.6 μm and then reextend to an equilibrium length of 2.0 μm on the basis of restoring forces alone.

Returning to the pressure–volume (sarcomere) curve, we note that a normal ventricle starts to contract from a sarcomere length of about 2.1 μm. During isovolumic systole, sufficient force is generated to open the aortic valve (point B), following which ventricular ejection occurs (B to C). During ejection, the stress in the wall of the heart actually falls because of the progressive decline in ventricular volume, as predicted by the Laplace relation (tension = pressure × (Ri/2h), where Ri is the internal radius and h is the wall thickness). Shortening continues until the end-systolic pressure (force)–volume (length) curve is reached. The position and slope of this curve are determined by the underlying contractility, and to a lesser degree by the afterload of the ventricle. During systole, a normal heart ejects approximately two-thirds of its initial volume; this corresponds to an end-systolic sarcomere length of approximately 1.8 to 1.9 μm. Thus, a normal heart begins its ejection from a sarcomere length that has a small but significant distending force and completes ejection at a sarcomere length at which elastic restoring forces will be relatively small. Accordingly, in a normal ejecting heart, working at low heart rates, elastic recoil and early diastolic suction may make only a relatively small contribution to ventricular filling.

In a heart in which contractility is increased, ventricular ejection begins at point E in Fig. 16-13. The heart develops pressure and ejects volume to a midwall end-systolic sarcomere length of 1.65 μm. At this sarcomere length, a substantial amount of elastic energy will be stored during the process of systolic shortening and will provide a significant elastic recoil in early diastole. It is clear that ventricular "suction" in early diastole should be most apparent and effective in augmenting early ventricular filling during periods when contractility is augmented and heart rate is increased, such as physical exercise. In a failing heart, the advantage of elastic recoil will be diminished because of relatively long end-systolic sarcomere lengths. This may contribute to the inordinately elevated diastolic filling pressures seen in heart failure, especially during periods of increased demands for cardiac output. The loss of this elastic recoil will also make the failing heart more dependent on the contribution of atrial contraction to ventricular filling.

Afterload

Afterload, simply defined, is the load that the ventricular muscle senses and works against after it has begun to contract. In experimental systems in which the load placed on an isolated muscle, or against which an isolated ventricle contracts, can be controlled, the effects of varying the afterload on systolic performance can be clearly seen. However, when the intact circulation is considered as a ventricular pump that is coupled to a peripheral circulation with a characteristic input impedance, delineation of the factors contributing to the afterload on the ventricular muscle becomes more complex. It has been argued that the arterial input impedance best represents ventricular afterload, but others consider systolic ventricular pressure or wall tension as more appropriate indices of afterload. It is now clear that in a coupled cardiocirculatory system, there is a combination of factors, cardiac and vascular, some of which are independent, that contribute to the generation of ventricular afterload. A schematic diagram illustrating some of the more important factors affecting ventricular afterload is shown in Fig. 16-14. This diagram shows that cardiac-dependent ventriculoarterial coupling factors are independent of the vascular-dependent arterial afterload system. However, despite this theoretical independence, changes in arterial resistance and characteristic impedance have been shown to alter factors in the ventriculoarterial coupling system, such as wall stress and ventricular volume during systole. The degree of independence also lessens significantly in disease states with myocardial failure.

If one considers the afterload determinants of ventricular muscle, wall stress (force per unit area) is clearly the most important factor. The ventricular wall stress during ejection (ventricular muscle afterload) importantly influences the quantity of blood ejected by the ventricles. For example, abrupt increases or decreases in ejection pressure inversely alter the stroke volume and do so even when end-diastolic volume is independently controlled. Afterload is never constant during ventricular ejection but continually declines as ventricular volume and midwall radius decrease, as predicted by the Laplace relation (see above). This type of con-

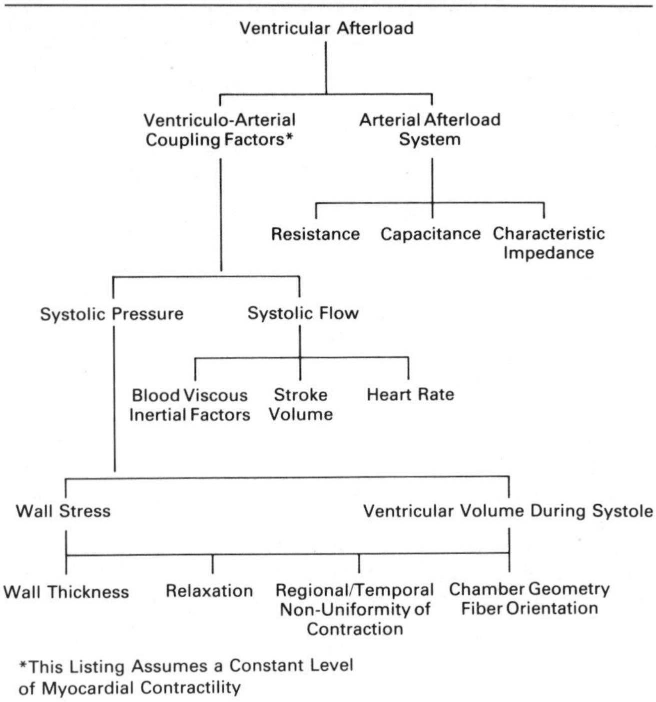

Fig. 16-14. Factors affecting ventricular afterload.

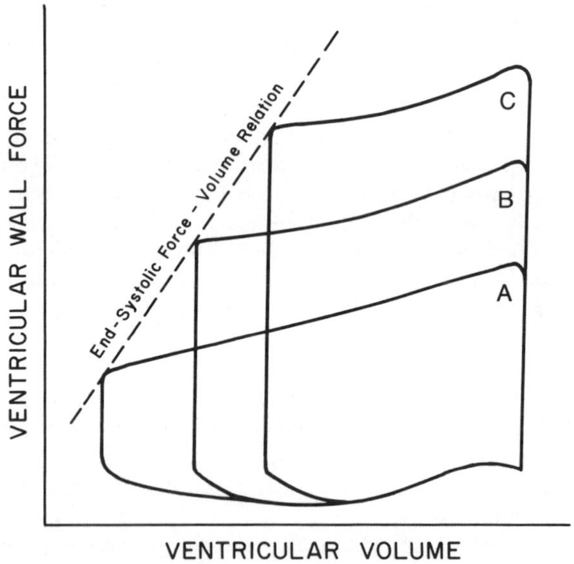

Fig. 16-15. Effects of changes in afterload created by increasing the impedance to ejection on the midwall–radius–wall force relations during normal contraction with preload held constant. Contractions A, B, and C show decreasing midwall radius and wall force during the ejection of three levels of afterload. There is an inverse relation between wall force during ejection and the extent of midwall shortening. Not shown, but occurring simultaneously, were reciprocal changes in the rate of midwall shortening with load (force–velocity relation). Note that at end-ejection, wall force and radius coincide with the isovolumic–radius–wall force line describing underlying myocardial contractility.

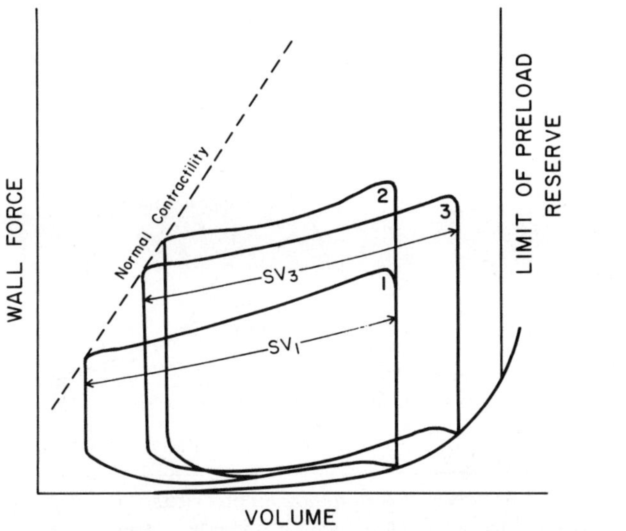

Fig. 16-16. Response of the normal heart to increases in ventricular afterload that occur during functioning in the physiologic portion of the wall–force–volume relationship. Note that loop 1, originating from a normal end-diastolic volume, ejects a normal quantity of blood for the basal level of contractility. With an afterload increase, the initial result is loop 2, and a diminished stroke volume. However, through the redistribution of total load and a slight increase in end-systolic volume, the heart uses its preload reserve and moves its functioning to loop 3. This beat originates from a slightly larger end-diastolic volume and contracts with slightly less afterload than loop 2 but ejects the same or nearly the same quantity of blood as loop 1. This sequence of events describes the process of afterload matching that is within the capability of the normal heart. Note that the relation between end-systolic wall force and volume is a unique relation describing underlying myocardial contractility.

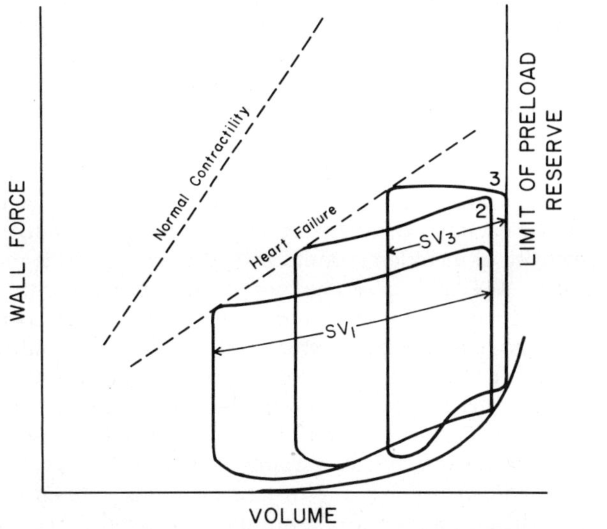

Fig. 16-17. Result of increased afterload occurring in a dilated, failing ventricle operating at a point in the wall–force–volume plane that is very near the limit of preload reserve (loop 1). With an increase in afterload, a significant reduction in stroke volume occurs. The heart attempts to compensate by using preload reserve but quickly reaches the limit without the addition of a significant increment of diastolic volume. Only a small increment of diastolic volume contributes further to the added afterload (loop 3) and produces a further decline in stroke volume. Thus, the failing heart, operating at the limit of preload reserve, is severely afterload-dependent for its stroke volume. At this level of functioning, very small reductions in ventricular afterload will produce a significant increase in stroke volume because of the relatively flat relationship between wall force and volume in the failing ventricle.

traction with continuously varying load is termed an *auxotonic contraction.* Increasing the afterload results in a reduction in stroke volume, as well as reductions in the extent and velocity of wall shortening, as shown in the end-systolic pressure–volume diagram in Fig. 16-15. If the afterload is rapidly varied during the course of a single ejection, an instantaneous force–velocity–length relation can be determined. Decreasing or increasing afterload causes immediate inverse changes in the velocity and extent of midwall shortening as well as the ejected volume. Also, in a manner analogous to what occurs in isolated muscle, the intact left ventricle reaches a point at end-systole that is near the isovolumetric length–active–tension curve, regardless of the imposed afterload or the time course of its application (Fig. 16-15). This relationship has been refined and presented as a specific index of ventricular contractility.

A low impedance to ventricular ejection, as is produced by mitral regurgitation, patent ductus arteriosus, ventricular septal defect, or arteriovenous shunt, can increase ejection fraction through a reduction in ventricular afterload in patients with normal ventricular contractility. Increases in afterload, such as that produced when an infusion of angiotensin elevates the systemic blood pressure, lead to compensatory alterations in preload, early diastolic ventricular function, and the contribution of ventricular volume to afterload, which allow maintenance of stroke volume in the normal heart (Fig. 16-16). In diseased hearts, however, when these compensatory mechanisms are impaired, stroke volume and stroke work fall, with similar elevations in afterload. This response of the diseased heart depends on the degree of reduction of ventricular contractility, as well as the capability for making adjustments in preload (Fig. 16-17). Thus, in the intact circulation, when there is relative hypovolemia or depressed ventricular contractility, or both, a given increase in afterload will cause a reduction in stroke volume, which does not occur when contractility is higher or when preload can increase adequately.

An understanding of the effects of afterload on ventricular muscle and ventriculoarterial coupling is crucial to an appreciation of the effects of chronic systemic or pulmonary arterial hypertension, the consequences of obstruction to ventricular ejection by valvular disease such as aortic or pulmonic stenosis, and the effects on hemodynamics of mitral or aortic regurgitation. Pharmacologic or surgical manipulation of afterload in these conditions constitutes the primary mode of therapy.

Contractility

Contractility is a concept derived from isolated cardiac muscle studies that defines the intensity of activation of the myofibrils during contraction (i.e., the processes leading to formation of force-generating sites and attachment of cross-bridges). Contractility can be influenced by membrane excitation, myoplasmic Ca^{2+}, interaction of Ca^{2+} with contractile proteins, and other properties of the contractile apparatus. Furthermore, contractility represents the integrated effects of various cellular mechanisms that are involved in the initiation and regulation of contractile activity, such as processes that change intracellular Ca^{2+} concentration (see excitation–contraction coupling above), change the sensitivity of myofilaments of Ca^{2+}, or produce shifts in the myosin ATPase isoenzyme population. Contractility has been defined in a variety of ways, most of which are specific to a given experimental preparation and experimental purpose. In mechanical terms, contractility can be described in isolated heart muscle as a unique surface that is generated during the first two-thirds of the contraction phase and defined by the interrelated variables of muscle force, velocity, and length. Thus, for any instantaneous fiber length and total load on the muscle during the first two-thirds of contraction, there is a unique velocity of shortening; the greater the contractility, the greater this velocity will be. From another point of view, at a given level of contractility and total load, the muscle will shorten to a particular end-systolic length predicted by the interrelationship. When load is changed, velocity and extent of shortening change, but the maximum rate of shortening at the lowest load is set by the level of contractility. Thus, the term *ventricular contractility* has a different connotation from the term *ventricular performance.* The former defines the properties of the muscle, the latter their expression as cardiac work. Practically, it is useful to identify a change in contractility as an alteration in cardiac function that is independent of changes in ventricular performance, which in general are changes produced by alterations in either preload or afterload or both.

Calcium ions play a central role in the excitation–contraction coupling sequence of cardiac muscle cells, and calcium homeostasis in muscle cells involves a large number of separate processes. The individual parts involved in cellular Ca^{2+} homeostasis include the contractile proteins, intracellular Ca^{2+} levels, sarcolemmal processes, and intracellular organelles involved in calcium turnover. The binding of Ca^{2+} to troponin C on the thin filaments causes the activation of contraction. Troponin C interacts with troponin I and T and tropomyosin to uncover actin sites on the thin filament to which the myosin heads of the thick filaments can bind and perform work. The amount of Ca^{2+} required to activate contraction depends on that bound to calcium-specific sites on troponin C, but because other structures in muscle cells also bind Ca^{2+}, it is generally assumed that for troponin C to be saturated fully, a total rise in intracellular calcium of 100 μm/liter is required. The maximal activation of intact mammalian heart cells measured as force generation is less than 50 percent of that which can be achieved by direct activation of mechanically skinned preparations, suggesting that only 25 to 50 μm/liter of calcium may be made available during each heartbeat. Measurements of intracellular calcium activity at rest and during contraction have been accomplished using ion-sensitive intracellular microelectrodes, as well as by using the light-emitting Ca^{2+}-sensitive protein aequorin, injected into cells of mammalian cardiac muscle. Experiments using aequorin as a Ca^{2+} indicator in mammalian ventricular muscle have confirmed that most inotropic interventions lead to increases in either the amplitude or duration of the accompanying Ca^{2+} transients (Fig. 16-18). These interventions include elevations of the external Ca^{2+} concentration and increasing heart rate and exposure of the muscle to cardiac glycosides. A second class of interventions has been shown to lead to changes in developed tension that are not accompanied by proportional changes in the aequorin light transient. Thus, in addition to any changes in the Ca^{2+} transient that may occur, these interventions lead to changes in the sensitivity of the contractile proteins to Ca^{2+} and therefore exert their effects on contractility through a different mechanism. Examples of this type of intervention are the actions of catecholamines, caffeine, and hypoxia with acidosis.

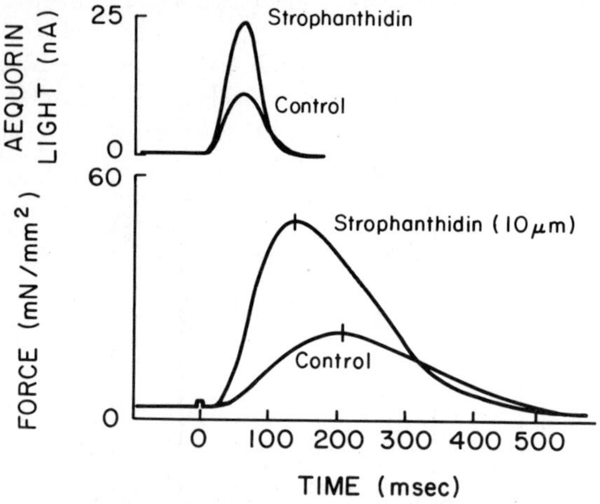

Fig. 16-18. Effects of strophanthidin on calcium transients and developed tension from an aequorin-injected ferret papillary muscle. Aequorin light current measured by a photomultipliertube is shown in the figure. The current output is a nonlinear function of the intracellular calcium concentration. The two superimposed contractions represent the average aequorin light (upper tract) and tension (lower tract) before and in the presence of 10 μm of strophanthidin.

It is well known that changes in the contractile state of cardiac muscle are of physiologic and pathologic significance. Although the concept of contractile state is not difficult, important difficulties have developed in its definition and measurement because contractile state is not a single measured variable but, instead, is a description of the muscle's overall mechanical capabilities at that level. These capabilities encompass the capacity of the muscle to both develop force and shorten. The extent to which the muscle will shorten is inversely related to the force it must develop in order to shorten. Similarly, the speed with which the muscle shortens will also be inversely related to the load against which it shortens. This inverse relationship between velocity of shortening and load is defined by the classic force–velocity curve, which can be seen as a way of relating the force-generating and shortening capabilities of the muscle at any given level of contractile state.

The mechanical behavior of heart muscle can be understood more simply with isolated muscle preparations in which force generation and shortening are unidirectional and can readily be normalized for differences in muscle thickness and length. The force–velocity curve of an isolated muscle preparation is generally constructed using peak velocity values measured in a series of contractions in which shortening occurred at different loads. When considered in terms of a simple analogue model of muscle in which the contractile element is in series with an elastic element, the course of isotonic shortening reflects solely the characteristics of the contractile element, because the length of the series elastic element is constant at any level of afterload. As the afterload is increased, the peak velocity of isotonic shortening is reduced, and when the load is so great that no contractile-element shortening occurs, peak isometric force is produced. When the curve relating load and velocity is extrapolated to zero load, the maximum velocity of shortening (Vmax) is obtained.

The force–velocity relationship obtained from afterloaded isotonic contractions has been of interest because it helps distinguish two major ways in which cardiac performance can be altered—that is, changing the initial muscle length (the basis of the Frank Starling phenomenon) and changing the contractile state through inotropic intervention. When the initial muscle length is increased, increases in the rate of force development (dF/dt) and peak isometric force (Po) are noted, with slight but significant increases in the time to peak tension (Fig. 16-19). The force–peak–velocity curves are shifted to the right, so that both Po and the velocity of shortening with a given load are augmented. However, when the force–velocity curves have been extrapolated to zero load, Vmax has been shown to vary little with changes in initial muscle length over a physiologic range, although at shorter initial lengths, Vmax will fall.

In Fig. 16-20, the force–velocity–length relationship has been plotted using data derived from recordings of shortening relative to muscle length in a series of afterloaded contractions. The base of this diagram shows a length–tension relationship; the projection to the rear illustrates the length–velocity relationship for the unloaded muscle; the projection to the left shows the force–velocity relationship. Point A on the base corresponds to the preload starting point. With activation, the contractile elements develop force along a hypothetical force–velocity curve, with force increasing until afterload is reached at point B, after which shortening proceeds across the surface until point C is reached. In any given contraction, the muscle moves in a predictable manner across the surface describing this relationship among force, length, and velocity.

Although the midportion of the force–velocity–length relationship characterizes the range of normal physiologic performance, analysis of this portion of the surface is complex. Thus, the mechanical limits to both shortening and force development, representing either extreme of the surface, are of both theoretical and practical interest. Because measurements of velocity during a series of afterloaded isotonic contractions are, of necessity, made later during contraction and at progressively shorter contractile-element lengths as afterload is increased, an extrapolated Vmax might be misleading. Unloading the muscle to near zero external load soon after contraction has begun has largely overcome this difficulty in determining Vmax (Fig. 16-21). In this manner, it has been suggested that Vmax can be measured directly in isolated muscle.

Utilizing these concepts, left ventricular chamber mechanics have been further investigated using isolated animal hearts studied in a servocontrolled apparatus in which ventricular volume and pressure could be completely controlled. Using assumptions from either a spherical or ellipsoidal model of the ventricle, ventricular force–midwall length–circumferential velocity relations were determined that agreed qualitatively with previously determined results in isolated ventricular muscle. Analyzing the three-dimensional surface created by the interrelation of these variables in the ventricle produced a clear mechanical description of ventricular contractility that was very sensitive to changes in the underlying contractile state. However, most of the key measurements required mathematical derivation from pressure and volume data only after a multitude of assumptions were made, careful measurements were taken of wall thickness, and independent control of preload and afterload was accomplished. An easier, phenomenologic method was sought to measure alterations in ventricular contractility that would be reflective of underlying myocardial strength yet would take into account the measured ventricular volume and the ventriculoarterial coupling factors outlined earlier.

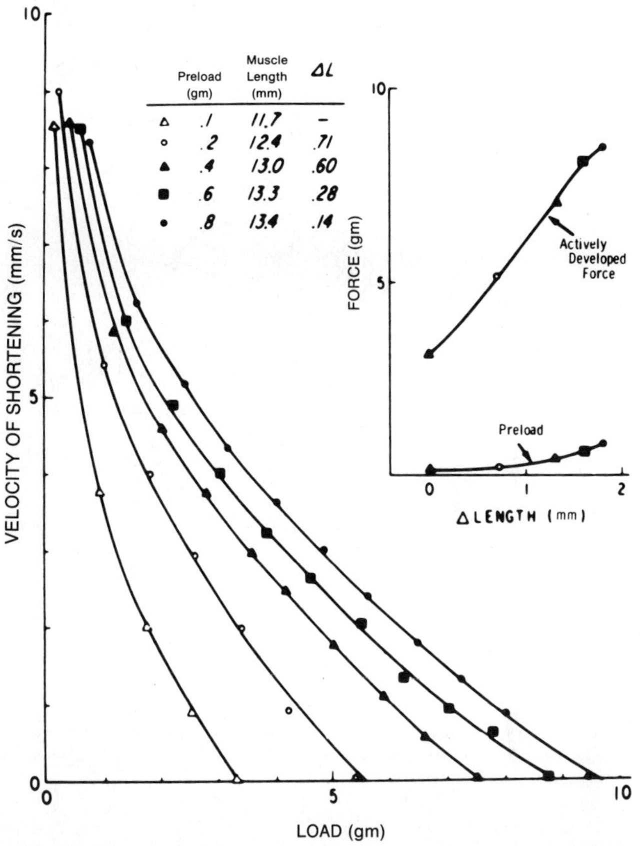

Fig. 16-19. Effects of increased initial muscle length on the force–velocity relationship and the length–tension relationship (inset). The relationship between peak velocity of afterloaded isotonic shortening and total load is shown for several initial muscle lengths of a cat papillary muscle. The inset shows the resting and developed active forces at these various lengths. When initial muscle length is increased, the actively developed force is augmented, as is the velocity of shortening with any individual load. Nevertheless, the maximum velocity of shortening is little altered with changes in preload alone. Moreover, if these curves were extrapolated back to zero load (Vmax), this value would show little, if any, change.

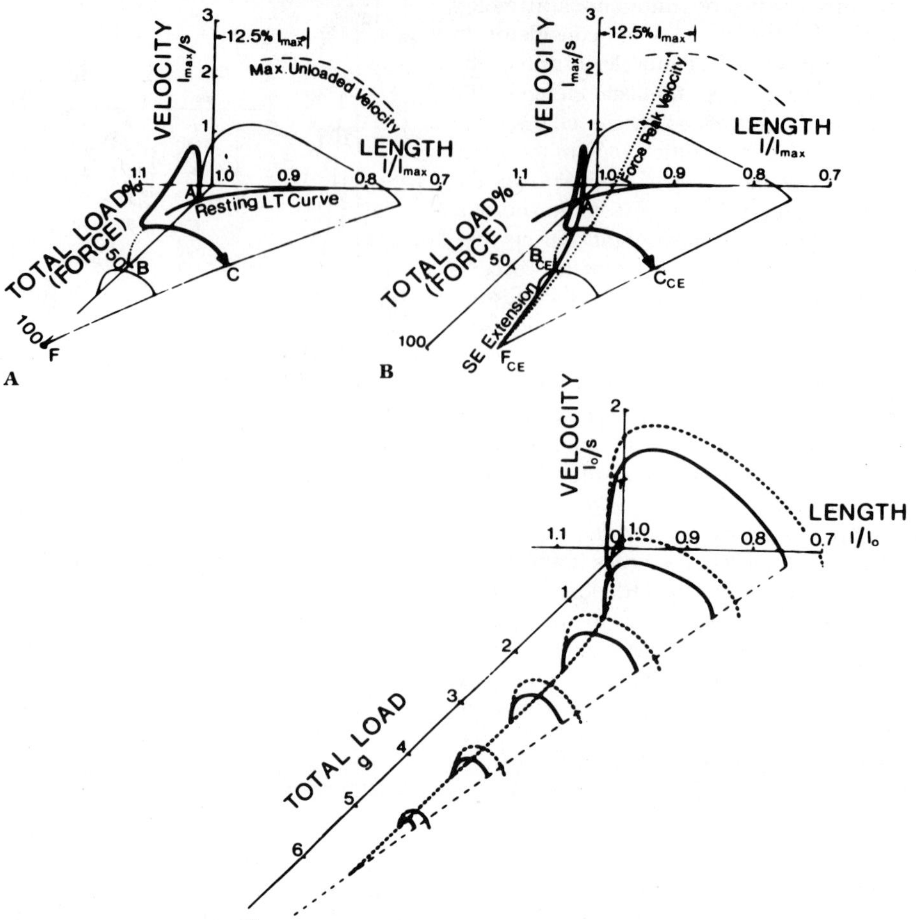

Fig. 16-20. Three-dimensional representation of simultaneous force, velocity, and length during contraction of papillary muscle. A. Velocity–length relations of isotonic contractions obtained at Lmax have been replotted as a function of total load (thin-line curves). Such a reconstruction can be obtained by plotting the velocity–length relations at various loads. As the load is increased, velocity and change in length decrease. The course of velocity of a hypothetical afterloaded isotonic contraction is superimposed (thick line). The velocity of shortening during the isometric phase of the contraction has been theoretically derived from a two-component muscle model. Velocity rises rapidly from point A to the appropriate level for the plane of this three-dimensional diagram. This plane also described the entire surface relating the three mechanical variables (length, load, and velocity) that define the contractility of the muscle. During isometric contraction, the contractile-element velocity falls as force rises. This velocity is not observed but is expressed in terms of the rate of force development, that is, dP/dt. At level B, the force development equals the load; the external shortening can then proceed between points B and CC. Velocity of shortening between B and C depends on the level of the force–velocity–length plane. The two-dimensional velocity–length relation is projected to the right (A-1), and the maximum unloaded velocity of shortening (Vmax) is also shown (dashed line). The force–velocity–length relation of the same muscle is shown in panel A after correction for extension of the series elastic component. The entire curve is moved to the right. The dotted line shown on the plane created by the force–velocity–length relation represents the force–velocity curve as obtained from afterloaded contraction. C. The effect of a positive inotropic intervention (dotted lines) on the force–velocity–length relation. The velocity of shortening at any given muscle length is augmented so that the entire surface relating force, velocity, and length is increased, and the extent of shortening is augmented. The projection of this surface to the right would be characterized by an increased Vmax.

This process has led to examination of chamber elastance, the ratio of ventricular pressure to volume during contraction. In analyzing the systolic pressure–volume relationship, end-systole can easily be determined as the point of maximum elastance (Emax equals the maximum P/V), and if two contractions at different preloads or different afterloads are studied, the volume intercept (Vo) at zero pressure can be determined (Fig. 16-22A). If elastance (P/V) is analyzed with respect to time, the curves in Fig. 16-22B are obtained. Notice that changes in afterload do not affect the time course or the peak elastance measured. Changes in contractility, however, produce a shorter time course and higher peak elastance, making Emax a useful indicator of contractility alterations.

Although a linear relation has been shown to exist between points of peak elastance in a series of contractions at a given contractility originating from different preloads, there is still debate as to whether the slope of this line or the volume intercept (Vo) is altered independently by changes in afterload. Evidence in isolated hearts and conscious animals

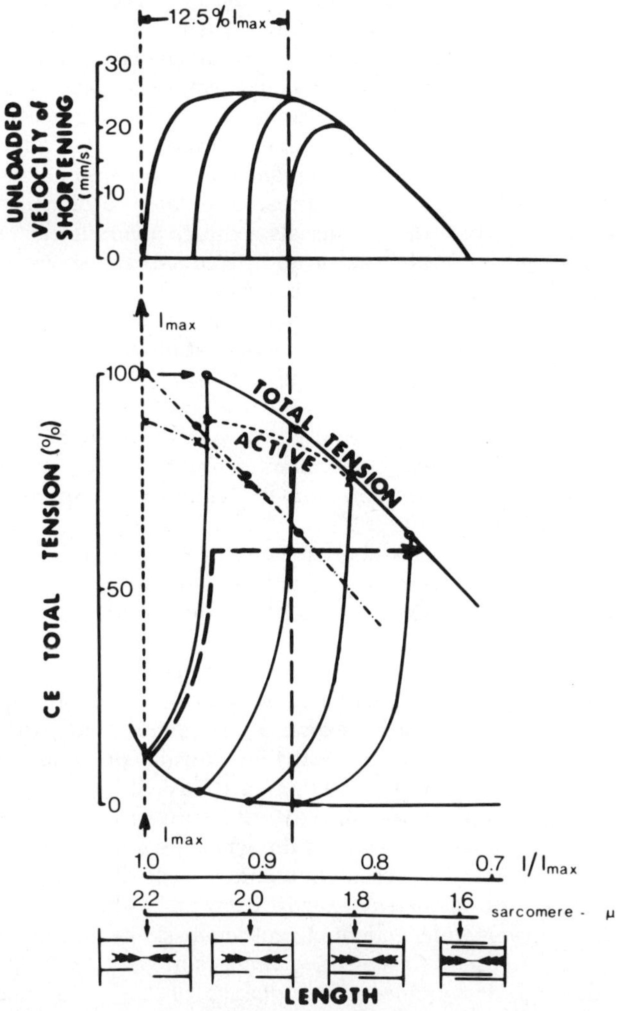

Fig. 16-21. The upper panel shows the velocity–length relations of unloaded muscle; the lower panel shows the length–active-tension relations of the contractile element in the papillary muscle of the cat. These relations are shown for contractions beginning from four different initial muscle lengths from Lmax to 12.5 percent of Lmax. At the bottom are shown the approximate sarcomere lengths related to the diastolic muscle lengths shown on the resting tension curve. When a contraction is initiated and then the preload removed (quick release), velocity rises to its peak level very rapidly and then shows a constant velocity (upper panel). As shortening progresses, velocity of shortening decreases. When initial muscle length is decreased, velocity rises onto the same plateau and follows the same pathway, with velocity ultimately declining. Only with the shortest initial muscle length does the velocity fail to rise onto the same plateau of velocity of shortening. When the load is zero, the plateau approximates Vmax. In the lower panel, the contractile-element length–active-tension curve shows a shift to the right with diminishing initial length. The heavy dashed line shows a hypothetical afterloaded isotonic contraction. Clearly, unloaded velocity of shortening, shown in the upper panel, occurs at longer contractile-element length than does the ultimate isometric force development, shown in the lower panel. This is due to the shortening of the contractile element when isometric force is generated. (From E. Braunwald, J. Ross, Jr., and E.H. Sonnenblick. *Mechanisms of Contraction of the Normal and Failing Heart.* Boston: Little, Brown, 1976.)

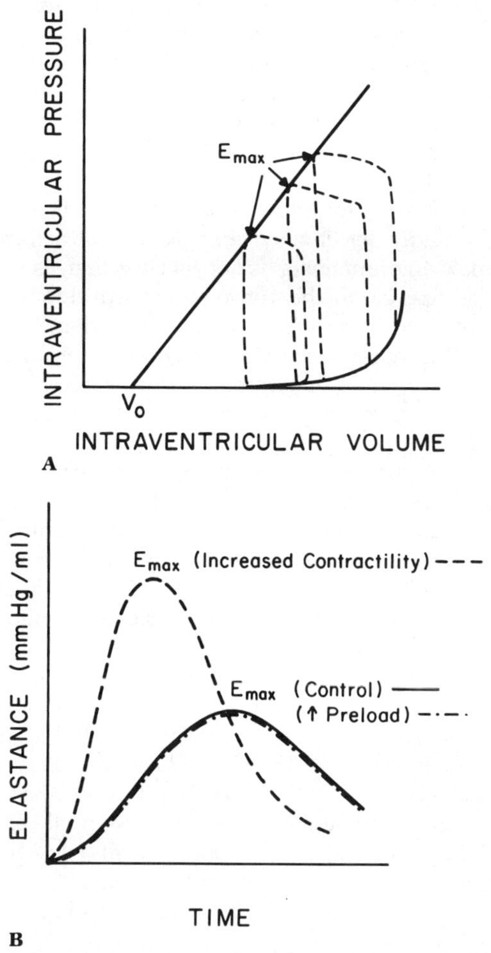

Fig. 16-22. A. Relationship between intraventricular pressure and volume during left ventricular contraction. Contractions in this figure originated at three different preloads with a constant afterload. End-systole is defined as the point at which the ratio of pressure to volume is maximal in each of the contractions. These points are illustrated at points of Emax. The end-systolic pressure–volume points are linearly related by a line that describes underlying myocardial contractility. The slope of this line and the volume intercept (Vo) are used to detect changes in intrinsic contractility. B. Plot of the ratio pressure/volume (elastance) in a series of contractions that demonstrate the sensitivity of this index to increases in contractility (dashed line) and insensitivity of the index to increases of preload (dot-dash line). Notice that the amplitude of peak elastance in a given contraction increases with increases in contractility and that the time to peak elastance is also shortened.

indicates that although the slope of the end-systolic pressure–volume relation is unchanged by varying preload, higher levels of afterload produce a leftward, parallel shift in the relation and lower the Vo without an increase in contractility. Also, different slopes and intercepts may result when end-systolic pressure–volume relations are constructed by varying venous return as opposed to changing arterial resistance or afterload. The reason that elevations in afterload exert an effect that effectively increases the end-systolic pressure at a given end-systolic volume may relate to ventricular resistance during ejection. In this model, end-systolic pressure is a function of end-systolic flow and end-systolic volume. At lower afterloads and higher flows, end-systolic pressure is lower than that predicted by a pure elastance model. At higher afterloads, end-systolic flow is lower, resulting in a higher peak end-systolic pressure–volume ratio. Thus, end-systolic pressure is not only a function of end-systolic volume and inotropic state but is also influenced by the resistance, capacitance, and characteristic impedance of the arterial circulation. Although the end-systolic pressure–volume relation will reliably detect acute changes in contractility in intact animals and humans, it is not yet clear that, as a clinical tool, it is superior to the conventional isovolumic indices such as peak dP/dt or dP/dt/P at 40 mm Hg developed pressure (DP). Ejection-phase indices such as the mean or maximum circumferential shortening velocity or ejection fraction are relatively insensitive to preload but are affected by changes in afterload.

Premature depolarization of the intact ventricle, whether by atrial or ventricular extrasystole, results in a contraction whose strength decreases with increasing prematurity of the extrasystole. The contraction following the extrasystole is more forceful than normal because of an increase in the level of contractility. This phenomenon, postextrasystolic potentiation, has been shown to be independent of variations in diastolic filling of the ventricle. Use has been made of this phenomenon in the cardiac catheterization laboratory, where application of timed premature beats has demonstrated motion in previously motionless areas of the ventricular wall, where contractility is reduced but not absent. This technique gives a reliable estimate of myocardial contractility reserve, and in conditions associated with regional abnormalities of myocardial contractility, such as ischemic heart disease, it provides useful prognostic information.

Heart Rate

Heart rate can be considered the fourth major determinant of cardiac performance. Increasing the frequency of contraction exerts a positive inotropic effect through operation of the interval–strength relation, although this effect is less prominent in intact conscious animals than in anesthetized animals or depressed hearts. In a normal subject, increasing the heart rate between 60 and 160 beats per minute has little effect on cardiac output, despite increases in contractility. Tachycardia reduces the duration of diastolic filling, but increases in contractility, induced by the frequency change, tend to restore normal filling dynamics through contractility-mediated reductions in the duration of systole.

DIASTOLIC PROPERTIES OF THE LEFT VENTRICLE

Before considering the diastolic properties of the intact ventricle, it is important to differentiate the factors responsible for alterations in chamber stiffness, as derived from left ventricular diastolic pressure–volume data, and the factors affecting myocardial stiffness, as derived from the stress–strain characteristics of the left ventricular wall.

The intrinsic physical properties of cardiac muscle are described by calculating myocardial stiffness constants from muscle stress–strain data. Stress is the force per unit cross-sectional area. Strain results from the application of the stress and is the fractional or percent change in dimension or size from the unstressed dimension; elasticity is a property of recovery of a deformed material after removal of a stress. Use of the terms *stress* and *strain* allows normalization of values so that the property of tissues obtained from organs of different sizes and shapes can be compared. Isolated cardiac muscle, like most biological materials, exhibits a curvilinear relation between diastolic stress and strain and is responsible for the nonlinear pressure–volume curve of the intact ventricle. Stiffness is defined by the instantaneous ratio of stress to strain at any given point on the curve relating stress to strain. The stiffness constant is the slope of the straight line relating these stress-strain ratios to the corresponding stress. The term *stiffness* has also been used when referring to the stiffness of the whole ventricular chamber and may be expressed in its simplified form as the ratio of change in pressure (dP) to a change in volume (dV).

Chamber stiffness is characterized by analyzing the curvilinear diastolic pressure–volume relation. The normal ventricle typically has a small slope at low ventricular end-diastolic pressures, and this slope becomes steeper at the upper limit of normal end-diastolic pressure and above (10–20 mm Hg). The relation between diastolic pressure and volume approximates an exponential relation, and as the chamber becomes progressively filled during each diastole, instantaneous ventricular compliance (dV/dP) decreases. The slope of the line relating dV/dP to pressure represents the elastic stiffness constant of the whole chamber, and although it does not represent the stiffness constant of the muscle of the ventricular wall exactly, its slope has been shown to be relatively independent of ventricular shape and therefore may be useful for detecting changes in wall stiffness.

Although instantaneous compliance of the ventricular chamber varies as the heart fills, an alteration in the compliance of the whole chamber can be identified by a change in the shape and position of the entire curve relating ventricular diastolic volume to pressure. It has been demonstrated that when incomplete relaxation owing to tachycardia is ruled out, acute interventions that alter myocardial contractility (other than myocardial ischemia) do not significantly shift the pressure–volume relation of the left ventricle. Volume loading and elevation of arterial pressure cause no apparent shift in the ventricular diastolic pressure–diameter relationship during the slow phase of ventricular filling. However, during the rapid phases of ventricular filling, under some circumstances, inertial and viscous properties appear to influence the resulting shape of the curve, and therefore compliance, significantly.

In the intact heart, alterations in the filling of one ventricle can substantially alter the diastolic pressure–volume relation of the opposite ventricle. Therefore, when right ventricular volume is changing significantly, changes in left ventricular end-diastolic pressure may not be a reliable guide, even to directional changes of the diastolic pressure–volume curve of the ventricle. Studies in which the pericardium is left intact have shown that not only the end-diastolic pressure but also the shape of the left ventricle is altered by increased right ventricular filling with encroachment of the interventricular septum on the left ventricular cavity.

Table 16-1. Primary etiologies of myocardial failure

Hemodynamic overloads	
Pressure overload	
High "central" resistance (e.g., valvular stenosis)	
High "peripheral" resistance (e.g., hypertension)	
Volume overload	
Valvular regurgitation (e.g., mitral regurgitation)	
High cardiac output state (e.g., A-V shunt, thyrotoxic)	
Oxygen deprivation	
Hypoxia and ischemia	Akinesis Asynergy Dyssynergy
↓ Infarction and/or fibrosis	(remodeling)
Cardiac muscle disease	
Idiopathic, hereditary, or acquired	
Viral	
Metabolic (e.g., ethanol, cobalt)	

THE FAILING HEART

Congestive heart failure has been considered a clinical syndrome characterized by pulmonary or systemic venous congestion accompanied by a low cardiac output. It has become clear, however, that such a broad definition has made full understanding of this syndrome difficult. The term *congestive* itself ensures that venous congestion is present, but we now know that severe heart failure may exist with normal or even low ventricular filling pressures. Also, pulmonary or systemic venous congestion may be severe in some patients with perfectly normal hearts. Thus, making a distinction between myocardial failure on the one hand and congestive heart failure on the other has provided a clearer understanding of this syndrome and has aided in the development of rational therapeutic modalities.

For this discussion, heart failure will be considered the pathophysiologic state in which an abnormality of systolic myocardial function is responsible for the failure of the heart to pump blood at a rate commensurate with the body's metabolic requirements during exercise. Reductions in myocardial systolic function leading to depression of the cardiac output may result from a primary abnormality in the heart muscle (i.e., cardiomyopathy) or may be secondary to ischemia produced by obstructive coronary artery disease. Myocardial failure may result secondarily from anatomic lesions of the cardiac valves or pericardium that interfere with cardiac filling or emptying, diastolic ventricular dysfunction, pulmonary embolism, or severe or prolonged disorders of cardiac rate or rhythm.

In the presence of a defect in myocardial contraction induced by one or more of the factors outlined in Table 16-1, the heart depends on three principle compensatory mechanisms to maintain its normal function as a pump (Table 16-2). First, the Frank Starling phenomenon is activated and an increased preload (i.e., elevated end-diastolic volume) acts to sustain cardiac stroke volume. Second, myocardial hypertrophy occurs, which increases the mass of contractile tissue. Third, neurohormonal activation occurs, resulting in increased catecholamine release by adrenergic cardiac nerves and the adrenal medulla, and increased production of renin-angiotensin and vasopressin occurs, which serves to augment myocardial contractility and increase blood pressure and cardiac filling pressures. Initially, these compensatory mechanisms can improve circulatory dynamics, but their potential is limited, and for a variety of reasons, they ultimately fail. The development of the syndrome of heart failure is thus a direct consequence of the limited ability and ultimate failure of these compensatory mechanisms.

Contractility of Hypertrophied and Failing Myocardium

When an excessive load, either a volume or a pressure load, is imposed on the ventricle, the development of myocardial hypertrophy provides for the reduction of stress per unit area of muscle toward normal values through an increase in myocardial mass and permits the ventricle to sustain the burden. However, with prolonged overloads and greater degrees of hypertrophy, the ventricle ultimately fails. Results of early studies of myocardial contractility in patients and experimental animals with various forms of ventricular overload were variable and inconclusive because of limitations inherent in assessing intrinsic contractility of the intact heart. For this reason, there has been substantial interest in the analysis

Table 16-2. Secondary compensations of myocardial failure

Compensation	Mechanism	Limiting factors
↑ Volume	Length–tension	Structure of sarcomere
	Sarcomere extension	"Fibril slippage," remodeling? LaPlace relation (T = P × r)*
↑ Hypertrophy	↑ Muscle mass	↑ Total force, but ↓ force/unit mass, ↓ actomyosin ATPase
↑ Neurohormonal activation	↑ Norepinephrine	↑ Norepinephrine depletion ↑ B-receptor down-regulation
	↑ Renin-angiotensin	↑ Sodium retention ↑ Vasoconstriction
	↑ Vasopressin	↑ Fluid retention

*T = wall tension; P = pressure; r = radius of the ventricle.

of isolated muscle behavior in experimental models of pressure or volume overload.

Pulmonary artery banding in a variety of mammalian species, producing right ventricular pressure overload and hypertrophy with progression to overt ventricular failure, has been studied extensively. Right ventricular hypertrophy and failure both reduced the Vmax, an index of contractility, below values obtained in muscles from normal animals. The changes were more marked in muscles from animals with heart failure than in those that had hypertrophy alone (Fig. 16-23). Heart failure clearly depressed maximum isometric tension, but hypertrophy without failure produced only mild depressions of peak force. Thus, ventricular hypertrophy in the absence of failure in this experimental model was associated with a depression of contractility per unit area of myocardium. Ventricular compensation preventing development of signs of heart failure was maintained by an increase in muscle mass. The precise alterations in subcellular function regulating myocardial contraction during the development of hypertrophy and failure have been studied in detail. Multiple defects appear to occur, including defects in energy production, calcium metabolism, and membrane function.

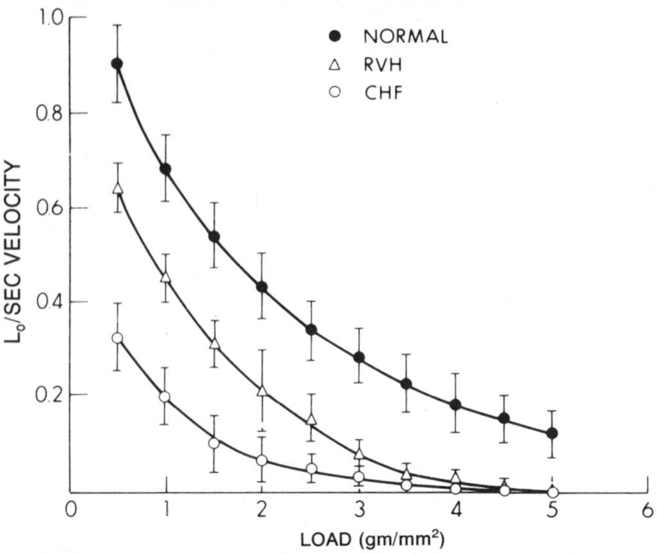

Fig. 16-23. Force–velocity relations in three groups of cat papillary muscles: (1) normal, (2) right ventricular hypertrophy without failure (RVH), and (3) right ventricular hypertrophy with congestive heart failure (CHF). Velocity is expressed in muscle lengths per second (Lo/s). Note the parallel depression of the lower load velocity with the development of hypertrophy and failure. (Adapted from J. Spann, et al. Contractile state of cardiac muscle obtained from cats with experimentally produced ventricular hypertrophy and heart failure. *Circ. Res.* 21:341, 1967.)

The contractile performance of the intact right ventricle of the same animals revealed depressions of function that paralleled the muscle function studies. Wall force developed by the right ventricle at equivalent end-diastolic fiber lengths was significantly lower than normal in animals with heart failure. Reducing or augmenting the end-diastolic volume in the heart failure group demonstrated that the relation between end-diastolic volume and stroke volume or stroke work was shifted downward and to the right of the normal curves, indicating a depression of performance. Thus, during the development of heart failure, ventricular volume increases and the performance of the ventricle returns to near-normal values through movement to the right and upward along a depressed ventricular function curve. Ventricular performance is thus preserved in the face of a reduction in overall contractility at the expense of an increased end-diastolic pressure, volume, and fiber length.

More recently, experimental models of pressure overload hypertrophy and failure have been reexamined and the results of muscle studies have been related to the type, duration, and severity of the overload, as well as to the degree of abruptness with which it was applied to the ventricle. Other models, such as renal vascular hypertension in rats, provide more clinically relevant temporal relationships between the application of the overload and the development of myocardial hypertrophy, consequent alterations in ventricular function, and their reversibility on relief of the overload.

In studies of muscle removed from animals with chronic volume overload (atrial septal defect), contractility was normal and exhibited none of the changes in the force–velocity or length–tension curves noted in muscles obtained from animals with pressure overload hypertrophy. Thus, the nature of the stress responsible for inciting the hypertrophy appears to play a critical role in determining whether hypertrophy is detrimental to myocardial contractility. Following the development of an arteriovenous fistula, the left ventricular end-diastolic pressure rises and stabilizes while the left ventricular end-diastolic diameter increases progressively and the wall thickens. With chronic adjustment to the shunt and to the elevated diastolic filling, myocardial function, as reflected in measurements of mean velocity of circumferential fiber shortening, remains normal. However, worsening of the shunt and, hence, the development of signs of congestive failure are uniformly associated with depressions of myocardial contractility. Thus, the development of hypertrophy with primary chamber enlargement in volume overload alters ventricular geometric relations in a way that allows maintenance of normal wall stress as well as optimal sarcomere length, permitting an enhancement of overall myocardial performance while contractility remains normal. With further overload, however, these mechanisms of compensation are inadequate.

As a result of the compensatory mechanisms serving the heart, ventricular performance usually is not markedly affected until the development of signs and symptoms of congestive heart failure. Therefore, indices of ventricular contractility, reflecting the intrinsic state of the myocardium itself, have been sought to define more precisely the course of myocardial deterioration in various myocardial diseases, as well as to provide an early indication of the need for either pharmacologic or surgical therapy. The search for the ideal index of ventricular contractility, defined in mechanical terms, has been hampered by both incomplete understanding of ventricular contraction and significant assumptions required before analysis of ventricular function in terms of isolated muscle mechanics can be undertaken. When studied, nearly all indices of ventricular contractility are performance-dependent, which means that their sensitivity in detecting a change in contractility is diminished to the extent that they are influenced by preload, afterload, and heart rate—important determinants of ventricular performance. However, despite these obstacles, ejection-phase indices such as the ejection fraction (ratio of stroke volume to end-diastolic volume) and the velocity of circumferential fiber shortening have clinical usefulness. By definition, these indices remain incomplete, and their limitations require continual consideration when they are applied to a clinical problem. With more precise information on ventricular contraction dynamics, it is hoped that more sensitive indices will emerge, permitting the early detection of myocardial failure and allowing therapy to begin before compensatory mechanisms are exhausted.

Adrenergic Nervous System in Heart Failure

The third form of compensation for failure of myocardial contraction involves augmented sympathetic nervous system activity with increased release of norepinephrine into the myocardium. It is well known that an increase in norepinephrine release augments myocardial contractility and participates in the regulation of cardiac performance during acute stress or exercise in the normal state. During early stages of heart failure, urinary excretion of catecholamines is elevated. However, during sustained loads on the myocardium with developing myocardial failure, the myocardium becomes depleted of its catecholamine stores. This depletion is related to failure of the adrenergic nerves of the heart.

Thus, with chronic failure, the myocardium becomes effectively denervated owing to progressive failure of the sympathetic nerve endings of the heart to synthesize, store, and release catecholamines. The myocardial catecholamines are most depleted in situations where the myocardium is most depressed. This does not mean, however, that a loss of myocardial catecholamine stores per se leads directly to heart failure, since pharmacologic depletion of myocardial catecholamine stores in the normal state does not alter basal contractility.

However, in heart failure with depression of myocardial contractility, the ability to augment contractility by localized catecholamine release is lost even though the responsiveness of the myocardium is normally sustained. Although there is an augmentation of the circulating catecholamines from peripheral nerves and the adrenal glands in the presence of heart failure, the degree to which this circulating store of catecholamines serves to support contractility of the heart is unknown. Evidence exists that persistent elevations of circulating catecholamines lead to a down-regulation of beta-receptors producing reductions in catecholamine effect on myocardial contractility and vascular tone. In fact, it is now recognized that the use of beta-adrenergic blocking agents in severe myocardial failure may actually result in improved circulatory dynamics, which could be related in part to an up-regulation of beta-receptors produced by the use of these agents.

Chronic elevations of circulating catecholamines also affect the peripheral vascular resistance in patients with congestive heart failure, often producing a significant increase in order to maintain blood pressure. This results in an increased impedance to ventricular ejection, which, in combination with a dilated heart, results in significant elevations of afterload and worsening ventricular performance.

Table 16-3. The myocardial and systemic components of heart failure

Myocardial failure
Decrease in force development and shortening secondary to myocyte loss and compensatory hypertrophy leading to pump failure (decreased cardiac output on demand)
Congestive heart failure
Peripheral effects of failure of pump to meet peripheral needs
↑ Sympathetic tone and renin-angiotensin activity
↑ Peripheral congestion, edema, and/or fatigue

Pathophysiology of Heart Failure

Myocardial failure resulting in ventricular dysfunction and ultimate depression of cardiac pump performance remains a fundamental, unsolved clinical problem. It invariably leads to a limitation of normal activities and early death of the patient. Indeed, the presence of myocardial failure appears to be the primary determinant of short- or long-term patient survival, independent of the etiology or whether treatment is medical or surgical.

The syndrome of heart failure may be considered in relation to two conditions (Table 16-3). The first condition is myocardial failure, either diffuse or segmental, characterized by a decrease in speed and force of muscle contraction. When the amount of myocardial depression is great enough, it is translated into a decrease in the reserves of pump function and ultimately into pump failure. Pump failure is then defined as the inability to provide a cardiac output on demand that is adequate to meet the peripheral needs during exercise. The second condition is congestive heart failure, which reflects systemic responses to an inadequate pump, characterized by augmented sympathetic nervous system activity, renal vasoconstriction, and activation of the renin-angiotensin system with peripheral congestion and edema.

Experimental heart failure has been studied in several animal models, all of which are characterized by hemodynamic pressure or volume overload. In these models, the time between the creation of the hemodynamic overload and the appearance of myocardial failure depends on the type of overload created (pressure or volume), the abruptness with which it is applied, and the severity of the overload created. Whereas initial hypertrophy in response to the hemodynamic overload tends to normalize the load per unit of myocardium and maintain pump performance early in the course, myocardial failure ultimately develops in most, but not all, instances. Whether depression of myocardial function ensues has correlated significantly with the severity of the overload and the extent of resultant myocardial hypertrophy. The contribution of other factors, such as age of the host when the overload occurs and concurrent vascular disease, is not clear.

From early studies of the mechanical correlates of acute pulmonary artery banding in the cat, it is clear that moderate degrees of obstruction of the pulmonary artery lead to right ventricular hypertrophy but not to ventricular failure. With more severe obstruction, a greater systolic pressure overload is produced and more severe hypertrophy occurs, as well as right ventricular failure. Studies of papillary muscles removed from hypertrophied hearts without congestive failure showed decrements in the maximum velocity of shortening of unloaded myocardium (Vmax), but not in peak force development (Po). Ultrastructural and biochemical studies done in the same preparation showed little histologic change aside from cell enlargement, little or no change in mitochondrial function, an increase in connective tissue, and a significant decrease in the rate-limiting enzymatic step for muscle shortening, namely actomyosin ATPase. A slowing of calcium binding by the sarcoplasmic reticulum from such preparations has also been found. As the systolic overload was increased further, additional myocardial failure as well as ventricular failure occurred, characterized by a fall in force production as well as a further decrease in velocity of the isolated papillary muscle. In addition to a further decline in actomyosin ATPase, catecholamine depletion occurred in the heart with failure of cardiac nerves to synthesize, store, or release norepinephrine.

Not all experimental systolic overloads have resulted in a clear-cut depression of myocardial function. This may be explained, at least in part, by variations in the severity and duration of the overload. Moreover, most studies of hypertrophy have involved the acute imposition of the load. This may produce initial pump failure with focal myocardial damage and subsequent recovery with residual scarring and hypertrophy. In studies of a more physiologic model of systolic pressure overload, renal vascular hypertension, it has been found that Vmax falls as a function of hypertrophy, yet force development is well maintained. Thus, systolic (renal) hypertension in the rat, which mimics hypertensive hypertrophy of humans, is associated with changes in contractile properties of the myocardium characterized by a decrease in Vmax, a prolongation of the duration of contraction, and a decrease in relaxation rate. Actomyosin ATPase rates fall along with these mechanical events. Of greater importance is the fact that all of these contractile changes are reversible when the hypertension is corrected.

It has also been shown that experimental diabetes mellitus in the rat leads to contractile changes characterized by a decrease in Vmax and slowed relaxation. Once again, this has been associated with a decrease in actomyosin ATPase and reduced rates of calcium binding by isolated sarcoplasmic reticulum. These alterations are reversed by treatment of a diabetic rat with insulin.

Diastolic overloads (volume overload) impose a change in diastolic volume without an increase in the systolic load on the myocardium. An increase in ventricular mass occurs but does not produce the same fall in contractility as is observed following systolic overloads. The reason for this discrepancy is not known, but one explanation is that diastolic overload may not lead to the same degree of cell enlargement during hypertrophy. However, with substantial volume overloads, sarcomeres in the wall of the heart are stretched to the limit of their length–tension curve, and "plastic" or "remodeling" alterations occur, leading to further dilatation. Furthermore, when volume is increased, without unloading of tension in the wall by increased ventricular emptying, the tension in the wall rises as a result of the LaPlace relation and hypertrophy ensues. This may then lead to late declines in contractility from this secondary tension overload. All the changes in mechanics described are subject to reversal on removal of the overload.

Of essential pathophysiologic importance to the problem of myocardial failure is the understanding of what factors lead to irreversible depression of myocardial function and ultimate pump failure in the face of a compensatory hypertrophic response to various pump overloads. Studies in different forms of cardiomyopathy have produced some insight into this question. These forms of cardiomyopathy include the hereditary cardiomyopathy that occurs in the Syrian hamster; the cardiomyopathy that develops in the hypertensive-diabetic heart; human diabetic hearts; and renal vascular hypertension. Histologic studies in each type of myopathy have all shown regions of fibrosis, myocytolysis, and even calcification adjacent to regions of severely hypertrophied but normal-appearing muscle. This has been interpreted to represent a process of microvascular hyperreactivity leading to microvascular spasm and focal myocytolysis, fibrosis, and hypertrophy of adjacent normal muscle cells.

Most human forms of cardiomyopathy also have focal myocardial fibrosis as their most significant pathologic feature. Because adult myocardial cells do not proliferate, microvascular spasm with focal myocytolytic necrosis will result in decreased numbers of ventricular myocytes. This will increase the load borne by the remaining myocytes, leading to their compensatory hypertrophy. Subsequently, in later stages of the cardiomyopathy, one would expect to find areas of focal necrosis and fibrosis intermingled with hypertrophied myocardium. Severe hypertrophy that results from this underlying microvascular process and the persistent hemodynamic overload results in extremely large cells in which activation is impaired and actomyosin ATPase activity is reduced. Widespread fibrosis also has substantial effects on overall ventricular compliance and produces diastolic ventricular dysfunction. Dilatation of the heart may then be superimposed in an attempt to compensate for decreased myocardial function. Thus, what began as widespread focal and even unrecognized myocyte necrosis, secondary to microvascular hyperreactivity and spasm, may terminate as hypertrophic myopathy characterized by large ventricular myocytes with impaired contractility, ultimately producing myocardial failure.

CONCLUSION

The current concept of the systemic response to myocardial failure is summarized in Fig. 16-24. Myocardial failure eventually ensues after cardiac compensatory mechanisms have been exhausted. An essential consideration relative to therapy and outcome of the process leading to myocardial failure depends on what is reversible and what is irreversible (Table 16-4). Reversible factors include hypertrophy when the load is removed prior to substantial cell loss. Ischemia is reversible until necrosis and cell loss occur, whether the result of large vessel obstruction or spasm. Once myocyte loss has occurred, an irreversible process develops that depends on the extent of further cell loss and ventricular "remodeling" for its progression.

Current therapy for the treatment of myocardial failure, as well as the systemic response to myocardial failure (congestive heart failure), has traditionally involved medication aimed at improving the contractile function of myocardial cells, as well as relieving the hemodynamic effects of the

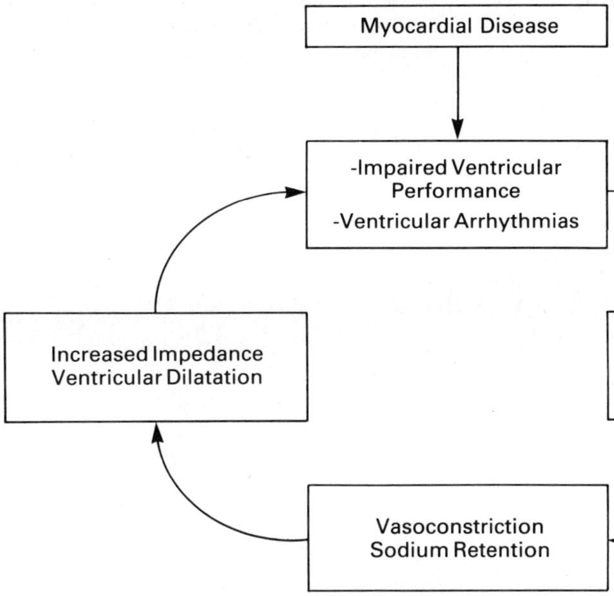

Fig. 16-24. The vicious circle of the pathophysiology of heart failure. As cardiac output falls, compensatory responses produce vasoconstriction and elevate systemic vascular resistance, which perpetuates myocardial failure.

Table 16-4. Reversible and irreversible factors in heart failure

Reversible
Hypertrophy
Volume increase—elastic
Ischemia*
Large vessel (coronary artery disease)
Small vessel (microvascular spasm)
Irreversible
Myocardial cell loss and fibrosis
Segmental
Diffuse focal
Volume increase—dilation with "plastic" or "remodeling" changes
Catecholamine depletion (?)
Defective transmembrane signal transduction (?)

*Ischemia includes both large-vessel obstructive disease with microvascular spasm prior to myocardial necrosis.

systemic response to myocardial failure. However, these medications provide palliative relief and in no way reverse the abnormality of the activating system or contractile proteins of the myocardium that are observed in the presence of severe hypertrophy. Moreover, the process of microvascular spasm and loss of cardiac cells with further fibrosis may be proceeding and may possibly be worsened by inotropic therapy. Although the need for palliative therapy in heart failure is not questioned, we must remain critically aware that the initial lesion, namely myocyte loss, causing an ultimate downhill course for the myocardium, is not being approached directly by these medications. Alternatively, it is possible that agents that affect microvascular spasm and perhaps other yet unknown factors may ultimately improve myocardial performance by preventing progression of the primary disease. These considerations strongly suggest that interest should shift from continued therapeutic attempts to bolster the already irreversibly damaged heart to attempts to identify patients with certain forms of cardiomyopathy at an earlier stage of the disease, where an opportunity to truly affect the long-term outcome exists.

SELECTED READING

Cardiac Ultrastructure

Dolber, PC, and Sommer, JR. Corbular sarcoplasmic reticulum of rabbit cardiac muscle. *J Ultrastruct Res* 87:190, 1984.

Sommer, JR, and Johnson, EA. The Ultrastructure of Cardiac Muscle. In RM Berne (ed), *Handbook of Physiology, Section 2, The Cardiovascular System, Vol. I, The Heart.* Pp 113–186. Washington, DC: American Physiological Society, 1979.

Sommer, JR, and Waugh, RA. The ultrastructure of the mammalian cardiac muscle cell, with special emphasis on the tubular membrane systems. A review. *Am J Pathol* 82:192, 1976.

Tokuyasu, KT. Visualization of longitudinally oriented intermediate filaments in frozen sections of chick cardiac muscle by a new staining method. *J Cell Biol* 97:562, 1983.

Excitation–Contraction–Relaxation Coupling

Blinks, JR. Sarcoplasmic Reticulum Function in Intact Cells: Information from Intracellular Ca^{++} Indicators. In ML Entman and WB Van Winkle (eds), *The Sarcoplasmic Reticulum in Normal and Diseased Muscles.* London: CRC Press, 1985.

Matlib, MA, and Schwartz, A. Action of Calcium Slow Channel Inhibitors on Cardiac and Vascular Smooth Muscle Membranes. In N Sperelakis and JB Caulfield (eds), *Calcium Antagonists.* Boston: Martinus Nijhoff, 1984. Pp. 79–93.

Williams, JS, Solaro, RJ, and Schwartz, A. The Role of Calcium in Cardiovascular Disease. In R Krebs (ed), *Treatment of Cardiovascular Diseases by Adalat (Nifedipine).* Stuttgart, New York: Schattauer, 1986. Pp. 4–30.

Myocardial Contraction in Normal and Failing Hearts

Braunwald, E, Ross, J, Jr, and Sonnenblick, EH. *Mechanisms of Contraction in the Normal and Failing Heart* (2nd ed). Boston: Little, Brown, 1976.

Ross, J, Jr. Afterload mismatch and preload reserve: A conceptual framework for analysis of ventricular function. *Prog Cardiovasc Dis* 18:255, 1967.

Sasayama, S, et al. Adaptations of the left ventricle to chronic pressure overload. *Circ Res* 38:172, 1977.

Sonnenblick, EH. Implications of muscle mechanics in the heart. *Fed Proc* 21:975, 1962.

Sonnenblick, EH, et al. The Pathophysiology of Heart Failure: The Primary Role of Microvascular Hyperreactivity and Spasm in the Development of Congestive Cardiomyopathies. In E Braunwald (ed), *Congestive Heart Failure: Current Research and Clinical Applications.* New York: Grune & Stratton, 1982. Pp. 87–97.

17. Symptoms and Signs of Cardiac Dysfunction

CHEST PAIN

Thomas H. Lee
Lee Goldman

The patient with acute chest pain poses one of the most common and most difficult problems for clinicians in the emergency department. The differential diagnosis is long and the presentations of many of the potential causes are notoriously varied. Thus, physicians often cannot reach a definitive diagnosis during the emergency department evaluation, and triage and management decisions must be based on probable diagnoses and their natural histories.

Because the potential clinical consequences of an inappropriate discharge of a patient with ischemic heart disease, pulmonary embolism, or aortic dissection are severe, physicians tend to admit patients, usually to intensive or coronary care units, if these diagnoses are suspected at all. We have found that about 96 percent of patients with acute myocardial infarction are admitted to the hospital. However, this excellent sensitivity for admitting such patients has been achieved at the expense of also admitting many patients without these life-threatening syndromes.

In this age of cost containment, the pressures for increasing the efficiency of the health-care system have led to considerable interest in reducing these "rule-out" admissions. However, this goal will be difficult to accomplish without also sending home patients who might benefit from hospitalization unless physicians can improve diagnostic accuracy in the emergency department. Thus, this chapter will review the pathophysiology and presentation of the most common and most important causes of acute chest pain, and then outline strategies for the evaluation and management of emergency department patients.

PATHOPHYSIOLOGY

Because so many organs or organ systems are in or near the chest, the potential causes of chest pain are remarkably varied (Table 17-1). However, when evaluating the emergency department patient who has just had an episode of pain and whose condition must therefore be considered potentially unstable, the physician's first priority is to exclude life-threatening syndromes, particularly ischemic heart disease, pulmonary embolism, and aortic dissection.

About 500,000 patients with *acute myocardial infarction* are seen in the emergency department every year in the United States. Recognizing these cases is especially important, since such patients have about a 25 percent mortality

Table 17-1. Differential diagnosis of chest pain

Cardiac
Ischemic heart disease
Aortic stenosis
Hypertrophic cardiomyopathy
Pericarditis
? Mitral valve prolapse
Vascular
Aortic dissection
Pulmonary embolism
Pulmonary hypertension
Pulmonary
Infection
Pneumothorax
Tumor
Mediastinal emphysema
Gastrointestinal
Esophageal reflux
Esophageal spasm
Peptic ulcer
Biliary disease
Pancreatitis
Neuromusculoskeletal
Cervical disk disease
Tietze's syndrome (costochondritis)
Bursitis
Intercostal muscle cramp
Herpes zoster
Tumor

over the next 72 hours if they are sent home, but only about a 10 percent mortality if they are admitted to the hospital. The standard of care for patients with recognized acute myocardial infarction is admission to the coronary care unit because of the high risk of ventricular tachycardia and fibrillation, particularly in the early hours of infarction. If patients without severe heart failure can be promptly resuscitated from these arrhythmias, their prognoses are similar to those of other patients with acute infarction who have not required resuscitation.

The importance of recognizing acute infarction has increased with the development of thrombolytic therapy. Agents such as streptokinase and recombinant tissue plasminogen activator can be administered intravenously in the emergency department and have been shown to improve postinfarction ventricular function and to reduce mortality. Because these agents must be given relatively soon after the onset of infarction to achieve meaningful myocardial salvage, the physician must make a prompt decision in the emergency department regarding the patient's probability of having an acute infarction. Since, in some series, more than 20 percent of the patients who received thrombolytic agents were found to have had major or minor bleeding complications, the consequences of administering these drugs to patients who are not having infarctions must be considered in this decision.

Even if a patient is not in the midst of an acute myocardial infarction, he or she may have *unstable angina* due to progression of fixed stenoses or nonocclusive thrombi, or from coronary artery spasm from a transient increase in vasoreactivity. Classically, exertional angina has been considered to be the result of fixed stenoses of the coronary arteries, while variant angina has been attributed to coronary artery spasm. However, it is now appreciated that many and perhaps even most patients with coronary artery disease have a mixture of these pathophysiologic processes. Thus, some patients whose chest pain is usually precipitated by walking up a hill will also have episodes while sitting at rest.

Pulmonary embolism is another important cause of sudden death and thus must always be considered when evaluating a patient with chest pain. Rough estimates suggest that about 650,000 cases occur in the United States each year, of which about 10 percent are fatal within one hour. The diagnosis is not made in approximately 75 percent of the remaining cases. Overall, about 200,000 people die from pulmonary emboli each year in this country.

Pulmonary emboli usually originate from thrombi in the venous circulation of the lower extremities, but thrombosis can begin in any part of the venous tree. Factors associated with the development of venous thrombosis include stasis or slowing of blood flow in the lower extremities due to inactivity or impedance to venous return, damage to the vessel wall, and alterations of the coagulation system such as deficiencies of antithrombin III, protein C, or protein S.

When these thrombi embolize to the pulmonary artery bed, they produce hemodynamic consequences beyond those attributable to mechanical obstruction of a single vessel. The role of humoral factors has been demonstrated by experiments showing that the left or right main pulmonary artery can be totally occluded by a balloon without adverse hemodynamic consequences, while obstruction of 30 percent of the pulmonary tree with emboli produces significant symptoms and elevations of pulmonary artery pressure.

These observations have led to the conclusion that humoral agents such as histamine, serotonin, and prostaglandins cause vasoconstriction and elevated pulmonary vascular resistance after pulmonary embolization. This vasoconstriction leads to hypoxemia and, occasionally, right heart failure. If the right heart cannot overcome the elevated pulmonary vascular resistance, cardiac output falls and sudden death can result.

Acute aortic dissection is an uncommon but challenging problem in the emergency department because specific tests, oftentimes invasive, may be required to establish or exclude the diagnosis. In this syndrome, which is also known as *dissecting aortic aneurysm,* no true aneurysm is present. Rather, a tear has developed in the intima of the aorta, allowing blood to push into the media of the vessel. Driven by arterial pulsations, the column of blood strips the intima of the aorta away from the adventitia. Antegrade advancement of this hematoma can lead to occlusion of major branches off the aorta, while retrograde spread can occlude the coronary arteries or unseat the aortic valve annulus, causing acute aortic valve insufficiency, or lead to rupture into the pericardial space with accompanying pericardial tamponade.

Other components of the differential diagnosis (see Table 17-1) may present with symptoms similar to those of acute ischemia, pulmonary embolism, or aortic dissection, because of related pathophysiologies. Patients with left ventricular hypertrophy due to *aortic stenosis* or *hypertrophic cardiomyopathies* may have true ischemia in the absence of atherosclerotic coronary stenoses as a result of inadequate perfusion of subendocardial tissue. Similarly, ischemic pain may develop in patients with right ventricular hypertrophy

Table 17-2. Characteristics of ischemic chest pain

Quality	Pressure or tightness
Onset	Angina is often associated with exertion, while acute myocardial infarction commonly occurs at rest; both may have a gradual increase in intensity and a gradual resolution
Location	Anywhere between epigastrium and neck, occasionally limited to left arm or shoulder, jaw, or upper back
Radiation	To left shoulder, left arm, neck, or jaw
Duration	Angina usually lasts at least 1 minute and less than 30 minutes; the pain of acute myocardial infarction may last considerably longer
Precipitating factors	Exertion, especially with upper extremities; cold; emotion; or eating
Relief	Angina is usually relieved within five minutes by rest or nitroglycerin, whereas symptoms of acute myocardial infarction may not respond to these measures

secondary to *pulmonary hypertension.* The pathophysiologic basis of chest pain associated with mitral valve prolapse is unclear, and some studies dispute any association between the two.

Irritation of pleural and pericardial surfaces is found not just in pulmonary embolism and pulmonary infarction, but also in *pericarditis, pulmonary infections* (e.g., pleurisy, pneumonia, and so forth), *pneumothorax,* and *pulmonary tumors.* Not surprisingly, these entities may be difficult to distinguish on the basis of the history alone.

The pathophysiologies of gastrointestinal and neuromusculoskeletal causes of chest pain are diverse, but the pain associated with them may mimic the symptoms of cardiovascular disorders. Because these diseases are less likely to cause life-threatening complications, their chronicity and precipitating factors may provide clues to their origin.

PRESENTATION

The classic symptoms of acute ischemic heart disease (Table 17-2) are well known to most clinicians; however, the manifestations of coronary disease may vary markedly for individual patients, and no single factor should be used to exclude this diagnosis. As is shown in Table 17-3, acute myocardial infarction or unstable angina, or both, occur occasionally even among patients with atypical symptoms such as pain that is sharp in quality, that seems to be reproduced by chest-wall palpation, or that is described as pleuritic or positional. Furthermore, the absence of diagnostic electrocardiographic findings is no guarantee against acute ischemic disease.

Nevertheless, data from the history, including the quality of pain, its location and patterns of radiation, and the associated symptoms, can be combined with findings from the electrocardiogram to estimate the probability of acute myocardial infarction or unstable angina. We have found that one of the most important issues to be addressed is whether the patient has a prior history of coronary artery disease. If so, the physician should focus on how the pain compares to earlier episodes of angina or infarction to determine whether the current episode represents an acute exacerbation. If the patient does not have a prior history of angina or myocardial infarction, the clinician faces the more difficult challenge of trying to decide whether the current symptoms represent the new onset of symptomatic cornary artery disease.

Although results of the physical examination may be completely normal in patients with evolving infarction, the physician should search for evidence of risk factors, such as hypertension and diabetes, and of complications of ischemic heart disease, such as congestive heart failure. In addition, the examination may reveal a nonischemic cause of chest pain, such as costochondritis or pericarditis.

The electrocardiogram is perhaps the single most important piece of clinical information. ST-segment elevation may reflect a new transmural infarction, repolarization abnormalities, or pericarditis, but myocardial infarction should be the primary working diagnosis until proved otherwise if the ST segments are concave downward, if there are accompanying Q waves or T-wave abnormalities, or if "reciprocal" changes are noted in other leads (Fig. 17-1). ST-segment depression also can be a nonspecific finding, but in the patient with acute chest pain, it should be considered indicative of ischemia until proved otherwise, especially if the ST segment is still depressed by 1 mm or more at 0.08 seconds after the beginning of the ST segment and if the ST segment is horizontal or downsloping.

Just as important as knowing which variables may be helpful in the emergency department is knowing the limitations of other pieces of clinical data. "Diagnostic trials" of nitroglycerin and antacids, for example, are unreliable indicators of whether a patient has ischemic heart disease or pain of gastrointestinal origin. Ischemic pain may not respond to sublingually administered nitroglycerin, particularly if the patient is in the midst of a myocardial infarction, while esophageal pain may respond rapidly. An apparent response to antacids also is not a reliable justification for a decision to discharge a patient, because ischemic pain waxes and wanes, and may thus abate coincident with a therapeutic maneuver, and because patients in pain are susceptible to a placebo effect from any intervention.

Pulmonary embolism also poses diagnostic difficulties in the emergency department, because its classic clinical features are so nonspecific. Patients with acute pulmonary embolism almost always have dyspnea, and, especially if the embolism has resulted in pulmonary infarction, the patient usually also complains of chest pain, which is generally described as pleuritic (that is, sharp in quality and worsened by inspiration or coughing). However, similar complaints may be described by many patients with other pulmonary diseases, musculoskeletal pain, or anxiety. Other symptoms that are less commonly encountered but suggestive of pulmo-

Table 17-3. Final diagnosis in patient subsets defined by emergency department clinical characteristics

Characteristic	Number of patients	Acute myocardial infarction (%)	Unstable angina (%)	Other (%)
Sex				
Male	286	22	25	53
Female	310	14	23	63
Age (yr)				
25–29	30	3	3	94
30–39	66	5	3	92
40–49	119	13	13	74
50–59	126	15	29	56
60–69	135	27	29	44
70–79	71	25	35	40
80+	49	22	49	29
Pain quality				
Pressure	253	24	30	46
Aching	79	13	19	68
Burning	43	23	21	56
Sharp or stabbing	157	5	17	78
Other	64	23	25	52
History of angina or prior infarction				
No	297	14	7	79
Yes	299	20	41	39
Pain reproduced by chest-wall palpation				
No	438	22	31	47
Partially	34	6	18	76
Fully	124	5	2	93
Pain pleuritic				
No	464	21	29	50
Partially	96	6	7	87
Fully	36	0	0	100
Pain positional				
No	460	20	29	51
Partially	112	9	9	82
Fully	24	4	4	92
Electrocardiogram				
Normal	114	1	4	95
Nonspecific changes	150	3	23	74
Abnormal but not suggestive of ischemia	72	4	21	75
Ischemic changes known to be old	60	7	48	45
Ischemic changes not known to be old	114	25	43	32
ST elevation not known to be old	86	73	13	14

Source: Derived from data published in T.H. Lee, et al. Acute chest pain in the emergency room. Identification and examination of low-risk patients. *Arch. Intern. Med.* 145:65, 1985.

nary embolism include apprehension, cough, hemoptysis, diaphoresis, and syncope.

Careful examination of the patient with pulmonary embolism will show respiratory rates greater than 16 per minute in more than 90 percent of cases. Other important clues from the physical examination include tachycardia, low-grade fever, rales, and an increased pulmonic second heart sound. Evidence of deep-vein thrombosis of the lower extremities is detectable in only about one-third of patients, so its absence should not be used to exclude pulmonary embolism.

Pulmonary embolism can cause a variety of electrocardiographic findings, the most common of which is sinus tachycardia. However, it can also cause atrial premature beats and new onset of atrial fibrillation, complete or incomplete right bundle branch block, and evidence of right heart strain. The heart will often be rotated as a result of acute right ventricular dilatation (Fig. 17-2), producing poor R-wave progression in leads $V_{1\text{-}3}$ and persistent S waves in the lateral chest leads. This rotation may also lead to the $S_1Q_3T_3$ complex that is also frequently encountered in normal patients or those with chronic lung disease. Thus, an $S_1Q_3T_3$ is highly suggestive of acute pulmonary embolism only if it is known to be new.

A chest x-ray should be obtained in all cases of suspected pulmonary embolism, even though pulmonary embolism commonly occurs without causing roentgenologic abnormalities. However, embolization may produce oligemia, alterations in vessel size, and loss of lung volume on the affected side, while cases in which pulmonary infarction has occurred may show parenchymal consolidation, often as a wedge-shaped pleural-based density, instead of oligemia.

Because the clinical presentations and routine laboratory findings associated with pulmonary embolism are so nonspecific, arterial blood gas sampling should be performed when this diagnosis is at all suspected. A normal PaO_2 does not exclude pulmonary embolism, as in some trials, about 10

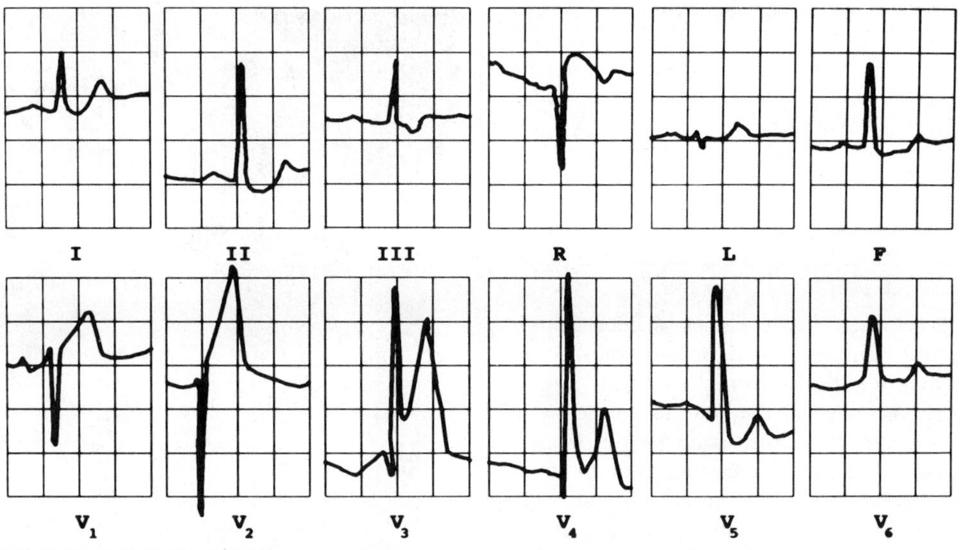

Fig. 17-1. Electrocardiogram of a patient with acute myocardial infarction. Note the ST-segment elevation and hyperacute (>15 mm) T waves in the anterior leads, as well as the reciprocal depression of ST segments in inferior and lateral leads.

percent of patients have had PaO_2 levels greater than or equal to 80 mm Hg. However, in cases in which there is an abnormally low PaO_2, further testing with ventilation-perfusion scintigraphy is usually warranted.

Aortic dissection should be suspected in patients with severe chest pain and any of the known risk factors for this entity (Table 17-4). The pain usually begins abruptly and reaches its peak intensity immediately. The patient's description of the pain is frequently an accurate reflection of the underlying pathophysiologic process, as adjectives such as "tearing" or "ripping" are commonly invoked. Furthermore, the pain location tends to indicate the site of the dissection—that is, patients who experience anterior chest pain usually have proximal aortic dissections, whereas patients in whom posterior thoracic pain develops usually have dissections of the descending aorta.

Other clinical findings may result from the complications of the dissection. Patients may have symptoms and signs of congestive heart failure due to acute aortic valve insufficiency, or syncope may develop because of acute pericardial tamponade. Occlusion of the great vessels off the aortic arch can lead to cerebrovascular accidents or pulse loss. An important physical finding is the difference in arterial blood pressures between the two arms or between the upper and lower extremities.

The most helpful radiologic finding is an abnormally widened aortic contour (Fig. 17-3), but even this sign can also occur in many older patients with nondissecting atherosclerotic disease of the aorta. Thus, further testing is usually required when this diagnosis is suspected (see the later section on laboratory tests).

Fig. 17-2. Electrocardiogram of a patient with a massive pulmonary embolism. Note the evidence of acute cor pulmonale (poor R-wave progression, ST-segment strain pattern in $V_{1\text{-}3}$, lateral S waves, and $S_1Q_3T_3$).

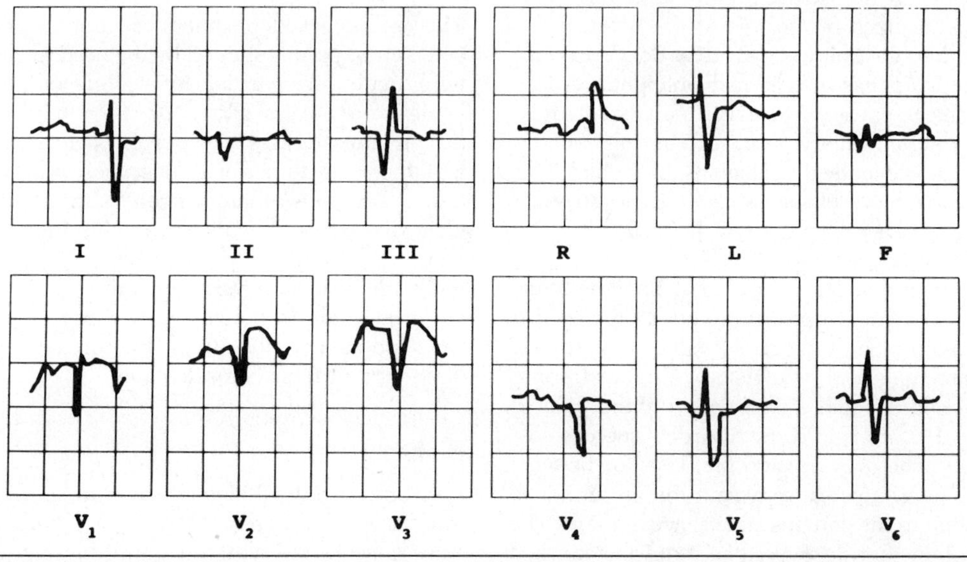

Table 17-4. Risk factors for acute aortic dissection

Marfan's syndrome
Advanced atherosclerosis
Ehlers-Danlos syndrome
Coarctation of the aorta
Bicuspid aortic valve
Pregnancy
Blunt chest trauma
History of hypertension

As was noted previously, aortic stenosis, hypertrophic cardiomyopathies, and pulmonary hypertension may be associated with pain that is indistinguishable from the angina of coronary artery disease because they are also ischemic in origin. In such cases, heart murmurs and other abnormalities seen on physical examination may suggest the structural abnormalities responsible for the chest pain, although echocardiography is often required to make the diagnosis.

Pericarditis is associated with two types of pain. Most common is pleuritic pain that is caused by irritation of the adjacent diaphragm and thus is often worsened when the patient lies down and is improved by sitting or standing. Pericarditis can also cause a steady substernal pressure that may be due to irritation of the relatively insensitive afferent nerve endings in the parietal pericardium or myocardium, or both.

Pulmonary parenchymal diseases, such as pneumonia and pneumothorax, usually produce a pleuritic pain attributable to irritation of the pleural surfaces. This pain may be located in the lateral or posterior chest, depending on the associated pathology. These processes are also likely to cause dyspnea. The pain of pneumothorax is distinctive in the abruptness of its onset.

Burning discomfort is the hallmark of acid-induced gastrointestinal disease. When this pain is substernal, it suggests hiatal hernia, whereas an epigastric location is typical of gastric or duodenal ulcer disease. This burning discomfort is often exacerbated by aspirin, alcohol, and certain foods, and may be relieved by antacids. Symptoms of a hiatal hernia tend to be worse when the patient lies down to sleep, whereas all forms of acid-induced disease may be worse in the early morning when the gastric secretions of an empty stomach are not neutralized by food.

However, not all gastrointestinal disorders produce "burning" pain. Reflux of gastric acid may precipitate esophageal spasm, which can cause a squeezing pain that is indistinguishable from angina. Biliary pain, such as that encountered in cholecystitis, is usually described as an "ache." This pain may be epigastric or substernal, and its occurrence about an hour after meals rather than after exertion may be the only clue that it is not ischemic.

Musculoskeletal disorders may not be associated with any visual signs, but their pain symptoms are often precipitated by movements or palpation of the chest wall or extremities. These diagnoses are suggested by a history of minor trauma or a new physical activity, and a description of the pain as sharp and fleeting. However, in some disorders such as costochondritis, a dull ache may develop that lasts for hours.

Intercostal muscle cramps cause a pain that is similar to cramps in calves that many patients experience at night. The patient may complain that deep breaths requiring marked

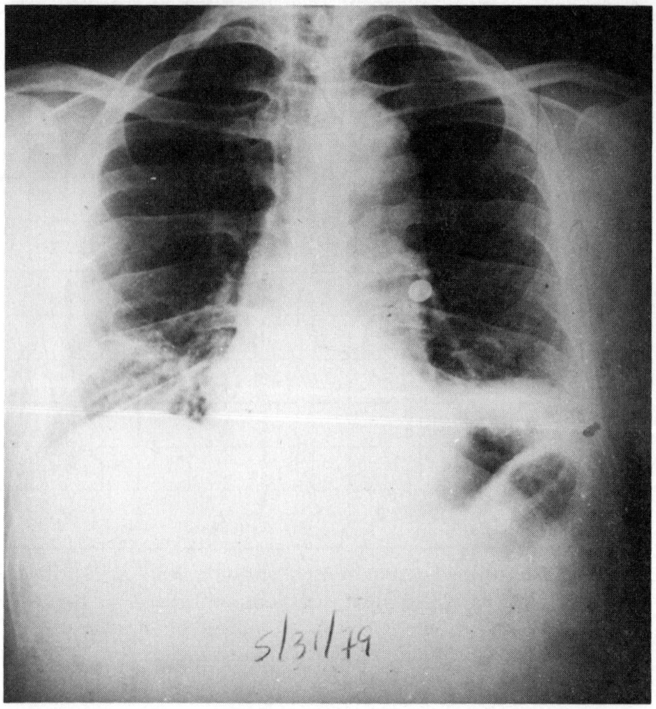

Fig. 17-3. Chest x-ray showing the widened superior mediastinum that may be the only evidence of an acute aortic dissection.

expansion of the chest wall are difficult during episodes. These cramps commonly occur when the patient is at rest.

While these clues may be helpful in diagnosing chest pain in the outpatient setting where the clinician has the opportunity to observe the patient on multiple occasions over a long period, in the emergency department, the clinician must be aware that these conditions can coexist with ischemic heart disease. Thus, demonstration that a hiatal hernia is present does not exclude acute myocardial infarction as the cause of the current episode of chest pain.

EVALUATION AND INITIAL MANAGEMENT

The emergency department evaluation of the patient with acute chest pain is shaped by the need to ensure that patients with acute myocardial infarction, pulmonary embolism, acute aortic dissection, or any other potentially life-threatening illnesses are appropriately triaged. Thus, it is not a high priority to perform tests, such as an upper gastrointestinal x-ray, to evaluate a strong clinical suspicion of peptic ulcer disease until acute myocardial infarction and unstable angina are eliminated as reasonable possibilities. Accordingly, the history, physical examination, and routine laboratory evaluation in the emergency-department setting should focus on acute, potentially life-threatening cardiovascular diseases and their complications.

History

In taking a medical history, the clinician should try to determine several features of the chest pain, including the time since onset of the symptoms and the rate of onset. Pain that has persisted continuously for several days without producing electrocardiographic changes is unlikely to represent ischemic heart disease, which is more likely to cause episodes of pain that build up to peak intensity over a few minutes. In contrast, the pain of pulmonary embolism or aortic dissection is usually abrupt in onset and immediately reaches peak intensity.

Other characteristics, such as the quality and location of pain and pattern of radiation (see Table 17-2), can be used to classify patients into groups at high and low risk for these conditions. While angina and acute myocardial infarction are pathophysiologically related and thus have qualitatively similar symptoms, some distinctions can be drawn. Transient ischemia that produces angina is classically induced by exertion and lasts less than 30 minutes; in contrast, myocardial infarction and its symptoms often begin while the patient is at rest and the pain may persist for much longer periods.

While data from the history are of critical importance in the assessment of the patient, relying too heavily on any single clinical feature is inadvisable. As is demonstrated in Table 17-3, acute myocardial infarction sometimes has initial symptoms of sharp, pleuritic chest pain, and atypical presentations of pulmonary embolism and aortic dissection are also not uncommon. Any of these three entities can produce diaphoresis, dyspnea, or syncope, but while these symptoms may not help differentiate among these diagnoses, they are often important clues that a serious illness is present.

Cardiac risk factors (i.e., hypertension, hypercholesterolemia, cigarette smoking, diabetes, or a family history of heart disease) are more common in patients with coronary artery disease. However, after consideration of the clinical variables listed above, they are not particularly helpful for evaluating the patient with acute chest pain in the emergency department and thus should not be allowed to dominate decision making.

Physical Examination

The physical examination should include vital signs taken by the physician. Blood pressure should be checked in both arms, particularly if aortic dissection is considered a possibility. If dissection is suspected, a large cuff should be used to measure blood pressure in the lower extremities, where systolic pressure is usually about 10 to 20 mm Hg higher than in the arms. Tachycardia (heart rate $>$ 100 beats per minute) and tachypnea (respiratory rate $>$ 16 per minute) are important warning signs of hemodynamic or respiratory dysfunction.

Since the causes of chest pain may begin or have manifestations outside of the chest, the examination of the patient with acute chest pain is not restricted to the thorax. The skin should be examined for evidence of cyanosis or for xanthelasma, which would suggest a hyperlipidemia that might cause severe coronary disease. Since tumors can present with chest discomfort, adenopathy should be sought in the usual locations. Potential gastrointestinal causes of chest pain, such as peptic ulcer disease or cholecystitis, should also be evaluated with a careful abdominal examination. If acute myocardial infarction is a reasonable possibility, however, a rectal examination to test for blood in the stool should be deferred unless there are specific reasons to suspect a serious gastrointestinal problem for which immediate detection is important.

The cardiovascular examination also begins outside of the thorax and should include a careful evaluation of the peripheral arterial and venous systems. Asymmetry of arterial pulses may reflect an aortic dissection or obstruction of a vessel due to atherosclerosis. The contour of the carotid pulse may reveal pulsus parvus et tardus, the weak, delayed upstroke typical of critical aortic stenosis, which can cause anginal pains in the absence of coronary artery disease. Congestive heart failure, including right heart failure from a pulmonary embolism or pericardial tamponade, should be suspected if the jugular veins are distended, and the presence of lower-extremity edema would further support these suspicions. The lower extremities should also be examined for signs of phlebitis, although the absence of detectable deep-vein thrombosis does not exclude pulmonary embolism.

Examination of the chest begins with inspection and palpation, measures that are especially important in the detection of costochondritis. When the patient's chest pain is reproduced by pressure on the chest wall, acute myocardial infarction is unlikely (see Table 17-3). The classic costochondral disorder, Tietze's syndrome, is characterized by swelling and inflammation of one or more of these joints, and an occasionally helpful diagnostic maneuver is injection of the area of inflammation with lidocaine to see if the pain resolves. However, because patients may be susceptible to a placebo effect, this test should not be used in the emergency department to exclude myocardial infarction.

Auscultation of the lungs should not only be directed at detecting rales as evidence of congestive heart failure but also should seek to identify signs of pneumonia or pleurisy; thus, auscultation of the bases alone is insufficient. Similarly, auscultation of the heart should not only include careful searches for murmurs but also attempt to identify the pericardial rub of pericarditis, a third heart sound from left ventricular dysfunction, or increased pulmonic second sounds that might indicate elevated pulmonary artery pressures.

It should be stressed that the physical examination can be entirely unremarkable in patients with acute myocardial infarction, pulmonary embolism, or aortic dissection. Usually, the examination does not substantially alter the probability of the presence of these entities as determined by data from the history. Thus, normal results of physical examination should not be used alone to justify a decision to send a patient home.

Laboratory Tests

The use of laboratory tests in the emergency department evaluation of patients with acute chest pain is shaped by several factors, including accessibility, cost, and test performance characteristics. Some tests, such as nuclear medicine studies, may not be available on a 24-hour basis. Others, such as aortography, are invasive and expensive and require specialized personnel. In addition, many readily available tests, such as cardiac enzymes, have limited predictive value.

At least two tests, however, should be ordered almost routinely. We recommend an electrocardiogram and chest x-ray for all patients in whom acute cardiovascular conditions are suspected. The only subgroup in whom we have

Table 17-5. Prevalence of acute myocardial infarction according to emergency department electrocardiographic findings*

Electrocardiographic finding	Approximate prevalence of acute myocardial infarction (%)
≥1 mm ST elevation or Q waves in two or more leads	75
Other new ST- or T-wave changes of ischemia or strain	25
Changes of infarction, ischemia, or strain known to be old	10
Other new or old abnormality (e.g., nonspecific ST-T wave abnormalities)	5
Normal tracing	2

*Estimates are based on experience with emergency department patients with acute chest pain who were evaluated at three university and four community hospitals from 1984 to 1986 in the Multicenter Chest Pain Study.

identified such a low risk of acute myocardial infarction that electrocardiograms might be unnecessary are patients with all three of the following: no prior history of coronary artery disease; pain that was sharp in quality; and pain that was pleuritic, positional, or reproduced by chest-wall palpation. However, this combination of low risk factors is encountered in only 10 percent of patients seen in the emergency department with acute chest pain.

While a markedly abnormal electrocardiogram is of obvious value in identifying patients at high risk of having acute myocardial infarction, a normal or near-normal tracing does not exclude myocardial infarction (Table 17-5). However, recent data indicate that the short-term complication rate of acute myocardial infarction may be lower in patients who are first seen with normal or nonspecific electrocardiograms than among those with more diagnostic initial tracings. These findings have led to preliminary recommendations that patients with suspected myocardial infarction and normal or nonspecific tracings often can be safely triaged to a monitored bed in a non–intensive care facility, such as an intermediate care unit.

Although we recommend electrocardiograms for essentially all adults with acute chest pain, the role of assays for cardiac enzymes such as creatine kinase (CK) and creatine kinase-MB (CK-MB) is less certain. These assays have become automated in recent years, and their results can now be obtained during the emergency department evaluation. Experience with serial enzyme sampling has shown these assays to be so sensitive for detecting acute myocardial infarction that they are used as the "gold standard" for making this diagnosis. However, when only a single sampling is available, as is the case in the emergency department, they are less reliable.

We have found that only about one-third of patients with acute myocardial infarction have abnormal CK and CK-MB levels at the time of their emergency department evaluations. Most of the other infarction patients are seen before the rise in CK and CK-MB levels, which usually occurs six to eight hours after the onset of myocardial necrosis, while a smaller subset is seen more than 18 hours after the onset of infarction, when enzyme levels may have declined to normal. In addition, we have found that commonly used CK-MB assays have about a 10 percent false-positive rate in patients who are not actually having acute myocardial infarction.

Thus, the sensitivity of a single sampling of CK and CK-MB is too low for these assays to be used to exclude myocardial infarction in the emergency department, and an abnormal CK-MB result does not necessarily mean that a patient is having an infarction. Therefore, we do not recommend routine sampling of cardiac enzymes. Instead, the decision to admit or discharge the patient should be made on the basis of other clinical data. If enzyme results are obtained, a patient should never be sent home because CK and CK-MB assays are normal, although unexpectedly high values might encourage a reevaluation of the patient and consideration of hospitalization for observation.

When pulmonary embolism is suspected on the basis of data from the history, physical examination, and routine laboratory tests including arterial blood gas sampling, the patient should undergo radionuclide ventilation-perfusion scanning, also known as lung scanning. This technology is considered highly sensitive for detecting disruptions of normal pulmonary blood flow, and a normal scan provides strong evidence against pulmonary embolization. However, an abnormal scan can result from almost any condition that alters local blood flow.

Various indexes are used to help assess these abnormalities, including the size and distribution of the abnormalities, correlation with the chest x-ray, relationship between ventilation and perfusion patterns, and changes in perfusion patterns over time. Lung or lobar perfusion defects constitute "high-probability" scans; in one series, 80 percent of patients with such scans had pulmonary emboli. Multiple segmental perfusion defects without matching ventilation defects also are high-risk findings, whereas subsegmental mismatches are less predictive of pulmonary embolism.

A matched loss of ventilation and perfusion suggests other processes, such as other lung diseases or congestive heart failure. Furthermore, patients with chronic obstructive lung disease are less likely to have conclusive results on lung scans since their chances of having a perfusion defect without a matching ventilation defect are reduced. However, a test result has limited value unless its clinical context is considered; thus, integration of lung-scan findings with other clinical data is discussed in the following section.

While aortography is the test of choice for diagnosing or excluding aortic dissection, this test is invasive and is therefore usually used only when the suspicion of dissection is moderate or high. Noninvasive technologies such as echocardiography and computed axial tomography (CT) scanning can frequently be used to make the diagnosis, but a negative test result should not be used to exclude aortic dissection. Thus, a decision to discharge a patient must be based on other clinical data. In the future, it is possible that

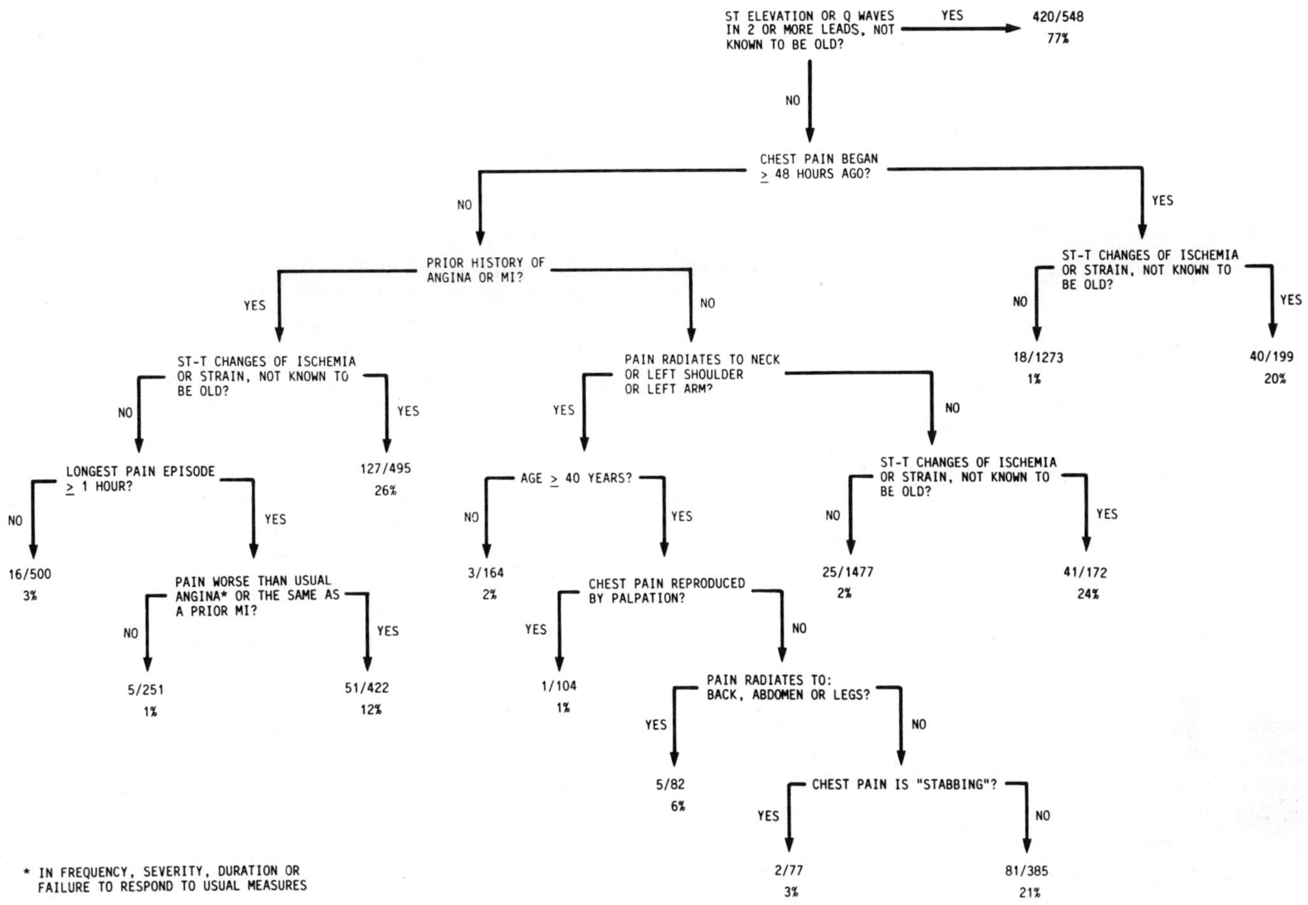

Fig. 17-4. A computer-derived algorithm for estimating the probability of acute myocardial infarction in emergency department patients with acute chest pain. (From T.H. Lee and R.T. Lee. *Cardiology: Problems in Primary Care.* Oradell, NJ: Medical Economics, 1989.)

magnetic resonance imaging technology will allow reliable noninvasive diagnosis of aortic dissection.

Integration of Clinical Data

Because no single clinical feature can be used to diagnose or exclude the most important causes of chest pain, the assessment of the probability of these diseases must be made by integrating multiple pieces of data. Clinicians perform such an integration subconsciously each time they see a patient, but in recent years, considerable investigative effort has focused on the development of prediction rules via multivariate statistical analysis of clinical data from large numbers of patients.

The algorithm that Goldman and associates have developed for predicting acute myocardial infarction (Fig. 17-4) has been prospectively validated in an independent set of patients and was found to have the same sensitivity for diagnosing acute myocardial infarction and significantly higher specificity than the triage decisions of the emergency department physicians who actually evaluated the patients. This algorithm allows clinicians to estimate the probability of acute myocardial infarction within individual patient subsets. Decisions based solely on the protocol would have reduced the admission of noninfarction patients to the coronary care unit by 11.5 percent without decreasing the admission of patients who developed emergent complications that required intensive care. Another algorithm, developed by Pozen and colleagues to predict acute ischemic heart disease (i.e., acute myocardial infarction or unstable angina) has been shown to reduce admission rates of patients without acute ischemic heart disease when the results are given by a research assistant to the physician during the emergency department evaluation.

An algorithm predicting the probability of pulmonary embolism on the basis of routine clinical and lung-scan data has recently been developed (Table 17-6) and prospectively tested on relatively small numbers of patients. However, because this algorithm has been applied only to this small group of patients, it requires further testing before it can be recommended for routine clinical use.

A more general approach has been described by Branch and McNeil. As shown in Table 17-7, if the patient's risk of pulmonary embolism can be determined from routine clinical data to be low (5 percent), moderate (15 percent), or

Table 17-6. Decision rule for diagnosis of pulmonary embolism

Clinical characteristic	Points
Age <65 yr	+3
Diagnosis of cancer	+4
Leg pain	+3
Substernal chest pain	−3
Heart rate >90 beats/min	+4
Heart rate increased by >20 beats/min	+4
New S3 or S4 gallop	−4
Positive lung scan	+5
Correction factor*	+8
Total score	1–31

*Added to make all scores positive. To use this algorithm, the point score for each patient is calculated. In an independent testing set of 68 patients, pulmonary embolism was found in 0 (0%) of 15 patients with 1–10 points, 15 (38%) of 40 patients with 11–18 points, 8 (89%) of 9 patients with 19–23 points, and 4 (100%) of 4 patients with 24–31 points.
Source: Adapted from V.L. Hoellerich and R.S. Wigton. Diagnosing pulmonary embolism using clinical findings. *Arch. Intern. Med.* 146:1699, 1986.

high (50 percent), the probability of pulmonary embolism for patients with individual lung-scan findings can be estimated. The authors caution, however, that the risk of pulmonary embolism is never actually zero, as demonstrated by reports of cases in which pulmonary emboli were angiographically demonstrated in the presence of ventilation-perfusion matching defects. Thus, even if results of a lung scan are "negative," angiography should be considered if the prior clinical suspicion is very high.

Initial Management

The development and proven benefit of thrombolytic agents now forces clinicians in the emergency department to make rapid decisions about which patients should receive this powerful but potentially toxic therapy. Patients who are more than six hours after the onset of their symptoms will receive less benefit from treatment; precise guidelines for such patients are still evolving. Because bleeding complications from these agents are common, they should be used only in patients with a high probability of acute transmural myocardial infarction, such as those with 1 mm or greater ST-segment elevation in two or more leads. Due to the risk of bleeding complications, these agents currently should be used selectively in patients more than 75 years of age. Other contraindications include cerebrovascular accident, cancer, recent surgery, recent gastrointestinal bleeding, and uncontrolled hypertension.

When a patient has a definite or probable acute myocardial infarction, management in the emergency department traditionally focuses on stabilizing the patient's condition until he or she can be transferred to the coronary care unit. This effort should include measures to reduce ongoing ischemia and prevent life-threatening arrhythmias. Lidocaine is indicated for patients who have hemodynamically significant ventricular arrhythmias but generally is no longer recommended routinely for patients with suspected or definite myocardial infarction. In deciding for individual patients, the physician should be guided by data indicating that the risk of primary ventricular fibrillation is higher in younger patients and in the first several hours after the onset of pain. Aggressive measures to treat congestive heart failure in the emergency department should be reserved for patients with marked hemodynamic impairment, such as pulmonary edema or incipient cardiogenic shock, who would otherwise be too unstable to be transferred.

Thus, the usual measures for a patient with probable acute myocardial infarction include:

1. Nasal oxygen
2. Establishment of intravenous access with a D_5W drip
3. Electrocardiographic monitoring
4. Treatment of ongoing ischemia with antianginal drugs or intravenously administered morphine sulfate
5. Rapid transfer to a monitored setting with full resuscitative capabilities

If the suspicion of acute myocardial infarction is low and the most likely diagnosis is unstable angina, the patient can often be treated in an intermediate care or step-down unit.

Table 17-7. Probability of pulmonary embolism in patient subsets

	Prior probability		
Scan pattern	Low (5%)	Moderate (15%)	High (50%)
No ventilation study performed			
Subsegmental perfusion defects	0.01	0.02	0.09
Segmental perfusion defects	0.10	0.27	0.68
Lobar perfusion defects	0.26	0.54	0.87
Ventilation-perfusion study performed			
Subsegmental mismatches	0.01	0.03	0.17
Segmental or lobar mismatches	0.54	0.80	0.96
Matching defects	0.00	0.00*	0.00*
Indeterminate	0.04	0.13	0.47

*Although the authors reported a 0.00 risk of pulmonary embolism, it is likely that the probability is finite but small.
Source: Adapted from W.T. Branch and B.J. McNeil. Analysis of the differential diagnosis and assessment of pleuritic chest pain in young adults. *Am. J. Med.* 75:671, 1983.

While the need for electrocardiographic monitoring is a major reason for admitting such patients, the risk of ventricular fibrillation in patients without acute myocardial infarction is low and the prophylactic administration of intravenous lidocaine is not indicated. The management of acute myocardial ischemia and myocardial infarction is discussed in greater detail in Chaps. 18 and 19.

In a small number of morbidly ill patients with clinical findings highly suggestive of pulmonary embolism, therapy with intravenous heparin may be initiated without lung scanning. Similarly, in instances in which the lung scan cannot be obtained until the next day, anticoagulation can be initiated while awaiting the test if the patient is considered to be at low risk for bleeding complications. However, in most cases of suspected pulmonary embolism, major management decisions come after the lung scan. The major choices are to observe the patient without performing further therapy, to perform pulmonary angiography, to begin anticoagulation at once, and to consider use of an inferior vena caval filter to prevent further emboli (see Chap. 13, section on Pulmonary Embolism). The first strategy is reserved for patients who have normal or near normal scans. The second strategy should be applied to patients with moderate to high probabilities of pulmonary embolism based on clinical characteristics and lung-scan data or patients whose lung-scan results are in conflict with other clinical data. The last two strategies, in which treatment is initiated, are directed at patients with high-probability lung scans and other clinical data that are strongly suggestive of pulmonary embolism. The inferior vena caval filter should be used in patients who have a high risk of bleeding with anticoagulation therapy, but the decision to place a filter is usually made after the patient has been admitted and has had serious thromboembolic disease documented definitively, and his or her risks of anticoagulation have been evaluated.

The use of noninvasive tests for deep-vein thrombosis of the lower extremities, such as Doppler ultrasound technology and impedance phlethysmography, is still in evolution. These techniques do not exclude thrombosis of pelvic veins and thus cannot be used to exclude the diagnosis of pulmonary embolism at this time. Thus, their role in the emergency-department evaluation of acute chest pain is limited.

The current gold-standard test for diagnosing or excluding aortic dissection is invasive aortography. If clinical suspicion of aortic dissection is high, aortography should be performed even if noninvasive studies such as echocardiography are not diagnostic. To stabilize the patient's condition before angiography, the clinician in the emergency department should provide adequate analgesia and attempt to prevent advancement of the aortic dissection by reducing blood pressure if the patient is not hypotensive. Blood pressure readings taken from the arms may be unobtainable or misleadingly low if the dissection has compromised the origins of their arterial supply. In such cases, pressure should be monitored with a femoral artery catheter. Treatment should be initiated without delay, since untreated acute dissections are frequently fatal, and more than one-fourth of patients die within 24 hours.

In lowering blood pressure, the clinician also has the goal of reducing the rate of rise of the arterial pulse (dP/dT), which is considered an important stress on the aortic wall. Thus, beginning therapy with a vasodilator drug, which might raise dP/dT, is inadvisable. Instead, a reasonable regimen might include intravenous beta-adrenergic blockade followed by intravenous sodium nitroprusside. Systolic blood pressure should be reduced to 100 to 120 mm Hg or to the lowest level that allows adequate renal and cerebral perfusion.

DISPOSITION

The standard of care for patients with definite acute myocardial infarction is admission to the coronary care unit. Although two randomized trials in England did not show a significant mortality difference between home care and coronary care units for patients with acute myocardial infarction, these studies excluded the high-risk patients who were most likely to benefit from coronary care and had too few patients to demonstrate the anticipated benefit. Other data suggest that the coronary care unit reduces mortality of acute infarction by about four percent.

In the last two decades, the coronary care unit has often been used as the initial level of care for patients with any suspicion at all of having acute myocardial infarction; thus, only about 30 percent of patients admitted to some coronary care units with this suspected diagnosis subsequently meet criteria for infarction. A clinically reasonable and cost-effective alternative to the coronary care unit for patients who are at sufficient risk for complications of acute ischemic heart disease to warrant admission but at relatively low (about 5–15 percent) risk for acute myocardial infarction is an intermediate care unit, where such patients can be electrocardiographically monitored while infarction is diagnosed or excluded with serial enzyme studies.

Patients with pulmonary embolism can usually be managed in intermediate care units or general medical beds if their hemodynamic and respiratory statuses are stable. However, if it appears that intubation or intravenous vasopressor support may be necessary, they should be triaged to the intensive or coronary care unit.

Patients with suspected aortic dissection should not be triaged until this diagnosis is made or excluded. If aortic dissection is present, they should be admitted to intensive or coronary care units, where they can undergo invasive hemodynamic monitoring and receive intravenous therapies as appropriate while decisions are made regarding the timing of surgery.

SELECTED READING

Branch, WT, and McNeil, BJ. Analysis of the differential diagnosis and assessment of pleuritic chest pain in young adults. *Am J Med* 75:671, 1983.

DeSanctis, RW, et al. Aortic dissection. *N Engl J Med* 317:1060, 1987.

Fineberg, HV, Scadden, D, and Goldman, L. Care of patients with a low probability of acute myocardial infarction. Cost effectiveness of alternatives to coronary-care unit admission. *N Engl J Med* 310:1301, 1984.

Goldman, L, et al. A computer protocol to predict myocardial infarction in emergency department patients with chest pain. *N Engl J Med* 318:797, 1988.

Hoellerich, VL, and Wigton, RS. Diagnosing pulmonary embolism using clinical findings. *Arch Intern Med* 146:1699, 1986.

Jaffe, AS. Acute myocardial infarction. State of the art. *Circulation* 74 (Suppl IV):IV-120, 1986.

Lee, TH, and Goldman, L. The coronary care unit turns 25: Historical trends and future directions. *Ann Intern Med* 8:887, 1988.

Lee, TH, et al. Acute chest pain in the emergency room: Identification and examination of low-risk patients. *Arch Intern Med* 145:65, 1985.

Lee, TH, et al. Clinical characteristics and natural history of patients with acute myocardial infarction sent home from the emergency room. *Am J Cardiol* 60:219, 1987.

Lie, KI, et al. Lidocaine in the prevention of primary ventricular fibrillation. *N Engl J Med* 291:1324, 1974.

Pasternak, RC, Braunwald, E, and Sobel, BE. Acute Myocardial Infarction. In E. Braunwald (ed), *Heart Disease: A Textbook of Cardiovascular Medicine* (3rd ed). Philadelphia: Saunders, 1988. Pp. 1222–1313.

Pozen, MW, et al. A predictive instrument to improve coronary-care-unit admission practices in acute ischemic heart disease. A prospective multicenter clinical trial. *N Engl J Med* 310:1273, 1984.

Tierney, WM, et al. Predictors of myocardial infarction in emergency room patients. *Crit Care Med* 13:526, 1985.

PALPITATIONS

John D. Rutherford

The term *palpitations* means either an awareness of heartbeat or an unpleasant sensation associated with the heartbeat. This sensation may be described as a forceful heartbeat; abrupt onset of a rapid heartbeat; a throbbing, pounding, or racing in the chest; or merely as skipped heartbeats.

More than 150 years ago, John Calthrop Williams, M.D., noted that palpitations are

> . . . frequently, by a careless observer, regarded as symptomatic of some serious organic and structural change being established, either in the coverings of the heart, its muscular tissue, or in some of its valvular appurtenances. A careful and deliberate inquiry, however, will, in the generality of cases, enable us to strip them of their apparent obscurity and reduce them to their true place in nosological arrangement.

HISTORY AND EXAMINATION

In the patient who is first seen with symptoms of "palpitations," it is important for the physician or nurse attending the patient to make certain inquiries (Table 17-8). These include: When did the palpitations first begin? Were they continuous or merely an occasional forceful beat or perhaps a skipped beat? Were they irregular or regular? What were the shortest and longest durations of the episodes? What were the shortest and longest time intervals between the episodes of palpitations? Were they associated with a feeling of faintness or in fact have they been associated with syncope? It is also important to ask if anyone counted the patient's pulse during an episode of tachycardia.

An irregularity of the pulse at a relatively normal rate may suggest either isolated atrial or premature ventricular contractions. Sinus tachycardia between a rate of 100 and 150 usually has a gradual onset and a gradual offset. A regular heart rate between 100 and 140 beats per minute may either be due to normal sinus tachycardia or possibly supraventricular tachycardia. A regular heart rate between 150 and 250 beats per minute that has an abrupt onset suggests either atrial flutter or supraventricular tachycardia. An irregular heart rate between 100 and 200 beats per minute indicates atrial fibrillation, although often patients are not aware of this abnormal rhythm.

It is also important to inquire whether the patient has any previous history of heart or thyroid disease; antiarrhythmic therapy or therapy with diuretics, adrenal steroids, digitalis, or psychotropic drugs; or an abnormal electrocardiogram (e.g., Wolff-Parkinson-White syndrome). Many cardiovascular drugs, particularly antiarrhythmic drugs, are proarrhythmic. The relationship between arrhythmic events and symptoms can be imprecise, as is demonstrated by comparison of diaries of patient's symptoms with 24-hour continuous monitoring of cardiac rhythm. Patients may complain of

Table 17-8. Characteristics of history of palpitations

Does the palpitation occur:	If so, suspect:
As isolated "jumps" or "skips"?	Extrasystoles
In attacks known to be of abrupt beginning, with a heart rate of 120 beats per minute or over, with regular or irregular rhythm?	Paroxysmal rapid heart action
Independent of exercise or excitement adequate to account for the symptom?	Atrial fibrillation, atrial flutter, thyrotoxicosis, anemia, febrile states, hypoglycemia, anxiety state
In attacks that develop rapidly though not absolutely abruptly, unrelated to exertion or excitement?	Hemorrhage, hypoglycemia, tumor of the adrenal medulla
In conjunction with the taking of drugs?	Tobacco, coffee, tea, alcohol, epinephrine, aminophylline, atropine, thyroid extract, monoamine oxidase inhibitors
On standing?	Postural hypotension
In middle-aged women, in conjunction with flushes and sweats?	Menopausal syndrome
When the rate is known to be normal and the rhythm regular?	Anxiety state

Source: From E. Braunwald. Chest Discomfort and Palpitations. In E. Braunwald, et al. (eds), *Harrison's Principles of Internal Medicine* (11th ed). New York: McGraw-Hill, 1987. P. 22. Reproduced with permission.

symptoms of palpitations when their cardiac rhythm is entirely normal or when they have sinus tachycardia related to some external event. It is also true that serious arrhythmias, such as ventricular tachycardia, can occur entirely in the absence of symptoms.

The importance of arrhythmias is always increased if the patient in question has documented cardiac disease, especially if there is evidence of ventricular dysfunction or abnormalities of the valves of the heart. Isolated ventricular premature beats, ventricular couplets, or even bigeminal or trigeminal rhythms may be relatively benign if the patient has no history of heart disease, the physical examination is otherwise normal, and there is no evidence of abnormalities of the myocardium, valves, or coronary arteries. On the other hand, in the presence of abnormal ventricular function (e.g., after myocardial infarction or untreated valvular abnormalities), such arrhythmias should be carefully assessed, provocative factors eliminated, and possibly antiarrhythmic therapy instituted. As Dr. Willis Hurst has noted, "The degree of abnormal sensation that the patient feels is not in any way directly related to the severity of underlying cardiac disease." In situations in which palpitations are associated with an abnormal, full-volume pulse, the patient is likely to feel increased sensation (e.g., anemia, aortic regurgitation, mitral regurgitation, patent ductus arteriosus, ventricular septal defect, or atrial septal defect).

Palpitations may be a prominent manifestation of acute or chronic anxiety states. In some patients a chronic anxiety disorder is manifested as persistent ill health and intractable symptoms with sighing respiration, palpitations, exhaustion, aches and pains in the thorax, nervousness, dizziness, faintness, and, at times, tremor and sweating, all occurring without overt endocrine or autonomic dysfunction. Such patients are usually readily identified and prove resistant to therapy and counseling.

DIFFERENT COMMON RHYTHMS ASSOCIATED WITH PALPITATIONS

Sinus Tachycardia

In general, sinus tachycardia, a normal rapid rhythm, has a gradual onset and offset and the heart rate is felt between 100 and 150 beats per minute. It is associated with anxiety, fever, anemia, thyroid heart disease, cardiac failure, pulmonary embolus, and high-output states (e.g., left-to-right shunt at the great-vessel, atrial, or ventricular level). In general, such symptoms are accompanied by other obvious findings, suggesting primary pathology associated with the cardiovascular, respiratory, gastrointestinal, genitourinary, or central nervous systems. The presence of sinus tachycardia will initiate a search for an underlying causal condition.

Isolated Ventricular Premature Beats or Atrial Premature Beats

These are probably the most common abnormalities of rhythm associated with the symptoms of palpitations. The sensation is usually due to the forceful beat noted after a premature beat. This post-extrasystolic potentiation is contributed to by the increased filling of the heart during the compensatory pause following an atrial or ventricular beat and is associated with an abnormal motion of the heart in the chest during the next ventricular systole. Causes of atrial extrasystoles include alcohol, tobacco, coffee, and pathologic conditions that affect the atrial pressures or size, including cardiac failure or ischemia. Ventricular premature beats are the most common form of rhythm disturbance found in health and disease. Precipitants include caffeine, tobacco, alcohol, sympathomimetic drugs, and hypoxia. Ventricular premature beats have been demonstrated in the majority of healthy subjects over 60 years of age.

In the absence of other symptoms of heart disease and in the presence of a normal cardiac examination and a structurally normal heart, a conservative approach to isolated ventricular or atrial premature beats is usually adopted. In patients with coronary artery disease who have symptomatic ventricular premature beats, it is common practice to arrange an exercise test to see whether the ventricular premature beats become more frequent or disappear during exercise. If they disappear, the condition of "overdrive suppression of the arrhythmia" is said to exist and often no further therapy is initiated. On the other hand, if the arrhythmia is exacerbated by exercise, it is not uncommon for beta-blocker therapy to be prescribed.

Atrial Fibrillation

Many patients with atrial fibrillation are asymptomatic. A rapid irregular pulse at a rate of 100 to 200 beats per minute suggests the presence of this heart rhythm. The common associated conditions contributing to the onset of atrial fibrillation include infection (e.g., pneumonia), thyroid heart disease (e.g., thyrotoxicosis), valvular heart disease (e.g., mitral valve stenosis), cardiomyopathy (e.g., alcoholic heart disease), and pericardial disease (e.g., chronic constrictive pericarditis). Atrial fibrillation is relatively common and is the most common of the atrial tachyarrhythmias. The arrhythmia may occasionally be precipitated by an alcoholic spree. Ventricular or valvular dysfunction and secondary abnormalities in left atrial pressure or size may contribute to the onset of atrial fibrillation but the onset of atrial fibrillation may precipitate heart failure.

Supraventricular Tachycardia

The term *supraventricular tachycardia* refers to tachyarrhythmias in which the impulse formation or reentry circuit is above the His bundle bifurcation. In recent years, it has been appreciated that the majority of such tachyarrhythmias are caused by a circulating or reentrant wave front. The minority of supraventricular tachyarrhythmias are due to enhanced automaticity. Two-thirds of the reentrant supraventricular tachycardias are caused by reentry within the atrioventricular (AV) node and almost one-third involve a bypass tract. The healthy heart may tolerate such arrhythmias for hours, days, or even weeks, and if they are paroxysmal and not clinically troublesome or persistent, they are usually well tolerated.

Usually, a 12-lead electrocardiogram will allow reentrant and ectopic supraventricular tachycardias to be distinguished. An ectopic mechanism is suggested by progressive acceleration for the first few beats (i.e., warm-up), all P waves looking the same, or the tachycardia being reset by a premature stimulus. On the other hand, in a reentrant tachycardia there is no warm-up, the initial ectopic P wave differs from the subsequent retrograde P waves, and a premature stimulus does not reset but actually may terminate the tachycardia, and prolongation of the first PR interval is the rule.

Ventricular Tachycardia

By definition, a run of ventricular tachycardia is said to occur when three or more ectopic ventricular beats occur at a rate equivalent to or more than 100 per minute. In general, with ventricular tachycardia, the complex is wide, rapid, and bizarre, and the finding that independent atrial activity is present suggests that the tachycardia is of ventricular origin.

Sudden Bradycardia or Heart Block

Sinoatrial block due to failure, or late emergence, of impulses from the sinus node is recognized by the absence of an expected P wave. Since the sinus impulse is not present, no ventricular response is provoked and the entire P-QRS-T sequence is missing. When a sinus beat is dropped, the resultant pause is equal to two cycles. Most causes of sinoatrial block are either structural disease of the heart or drug toxicity (e.g., digitalis, quinidine). Different degrees of AV block can occur. In first-degree AV block, the PR interval is prolonged but all impulses are conducted to the ventricles. With second-degree AV block, the conduction of some impulses to the ventricle is blocked, and with third-degree block or complete block, no impulses can reach the ventricles.

In any AV conduction disorders, it is important to ascertain the atrial and ventricular rates from the 12-lead electrocardiogram. A prolonged PR interval may be a normal finding or may occur with vagal stimulation or a variety of drugs, including digitalis, quinidine, procainamide, propranolol, or verapamil. Myocardial infarction, especially inferior infarction, is a common cause of AV block. Complete AV block may be congenital but the most common cause is either ischemic heart disease or primary disease of the specialized conducting tissues.

Sick sinus syndrome includes any form of sinus node depression, including marked sinus bradycardia, prolonged sinus pauses, sinus arrest, or sinoatrial block in association at times with bursts of ectopic atrial tachyarrhythmias. Atrial fibrillation may alternate with prolonged periods of sinus node dysfunction or abnormalities of AV conduction. The diagnosis of sick sinus syndrome usually requires continuous rhythm recording with 24-hour Holter monitoring.

SUMMARY

In patients who are first seen with "palpitations," a careful history will often provide clues to the significance and cause of the symptoms. Tachyarrhythmias should be documented, if possible, with a 12-lead electrocardiogram. If a patient has a structurally abnormal heart, a more aggressive approach to investigation and treatment should be adopted.

SELECTED READING

Braunwald, E. Chest Discomfort and Palpitations. In *Harrison's Principles of Internal Medicine* (11th ed). New York: McGraw-Hill, 1987. Pp 21–23.

Braunwald, E. The History. In E Braunwald (ed), *Heart Disease: A Textbook of Cardiovascular Medicine* (3rd ed). Philadelphia: Saunders, 1988. Pp 8–9.

Chatterjee, K. The History. In WW Parmley and K Chatterjee (eds), *Cardiology* (vol 1). Philadelphia: Lippincott, 1988. Pp 1–12.

Constant, J (ed). The Evolving Check List in History Taking. In *Bedside Cardiology* (3rd ed). Boston: Little, Brown, 1985. Pp 1–22.

EDEMA

David M. Poppel

Edema represents interstitial fluid in excess of normal levels. It occurs either locally, as in allergic reactions with focal alterations in capillary permeability, obstruction of specific veins or lymphatics, accumulation of excess peritoneal fluid (ascites), or more generally throughout the body (anasarca). Particularly in the latter case, the patient will gain weight and may be found to have swelling of the legs, which may "pit" when pressure is applied, or demonstrate periorbital puffiness or difficulty wearing rings or shoes that have previously fit normally. Generalized edema may tend to localize, based primarily on hydrostatic forces, thereby increasing in dependent areas.

PATHOPHYSIOLOGY

Body Compartments and Capillary Hemodynamics

Edema represents an excess of body fluids. Total body water (and contained solutes) is apportioned between two major compartments—about two-thirds within cells, and one-third in the extracellular "space," which is divided between plasma volume (about 25% of extracellular fluid) and interstitial fluid. The exchange of fluid between the vascular space and the interstitium is regulated by Starling forces, the hydrostatic and oncotic pressures of each compartment (Fig. 17-5). Increased intravascular hydrostatic pressure or decreased intravascular oncotic pressure (generated primarily by plasma proteins) or both favor movement of fluid out of the vascular space. This tendency is opposed by similar changes in interstitital hydrostatic and oncotic pressures. Movement of fluid into the interstitium tends to raise interstitial hydrostatic pressure while lowering oncotic pressure and thus mitigates further movement of plasma volume from the vessels. These changes may be offset by removal of interstitial fluid via the lymphatics. Even under normal circumstances, there is a small net tendency for fluid to leave the vascular space at the arteriolar capillaries, but edema will not form, provided that lymphatic channels remain patent. When excessive movement of fluids into the interstitium overwhelms the normal capacity of the lymphatics to clear

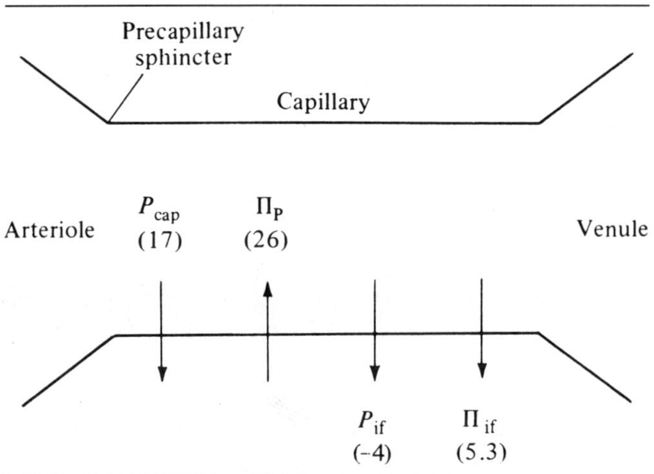

Fig. 17-5. Schematic respresentation of the hemodynamic factors controlling fluid movement across the capillary wall in skeletal muscle. The numbers in parentheses represent the approximate normal values, in mm Hg, for each of the factors. The negative value for P_{if} is probably generated by the removal of interstitial fluid by lymphatic vessels. The net effect is a small gradient favoring filtration of 0.3 mm Hg. These values for skeletal muscle do not apply to all visceral capillaries. (Key: P = hydrostatic pressure; π = oncotic pressure; cap = capillary; if = interstitial fluid; p = plasma.) (Modified from B.D. Rose. *Clinical Physiology of Acid–Base and Electrolyte Disorders* [2nd ed.]. New York: McGraw-Hill, 1984.)

extracellular fluid and return it to the vascular compartment, edema results.

Hydrostatic pressure in the arterial circulation is generated by the force of ventricular systole as it fills the great vessels and by the intrinsic wall tension of these vessels. Hydrostatic pressure in the more compressible venous side is influenced by the "back pressure" generated as blood attempts to return to the heart through the splanchnic, hepatic, and thoracic venous beds, as well as the competence of venous valves. Hydrostatic pressure in the interstitium depends on the local character of the tissues, which may be quite "loose," as in periorbital areas, or more "firm," as in muscular areas. As noted previously, lymphatics also play a role in regulating interstitial hydrostatic pressure.

Oncotic pressure is primarily the result of the proteins located respectively in the vascular and interstitial spaces. The quantity of these proteins is influenced by their synthesis (which depends primarily on adequate nutrient supply and liver function) and by their degradation and elimination (which can be amplified in catabolic states or conditions of protein loss, such as nephrotic syndrome or protein-losing enteropathies).

ETIOLOGY

Although edema can result from any one of several abnormalities that influence the balance of Starling forces, it most often results from increased capillary hydrostatic pressure or from decreased plasma oncotic pressure. In addition, the normal barrier to fluid movement from the vascular space to the interstitium, the capillary wall, may be damaged in a number of clinical settings and thus becomes more permeable, favoring movement of fluid from the vascular space, which may exceed the capacity of lymphatics to drain interstitial fluid. The major causes of edema are listed in Table 17-9.

Increased Capillary Hydrostatic Pressure

Major causes of increased hydrostatic pressure are ventricular failure, portal hypertension, and renal sodium retention.

Increased Blood Volume Due to Renal Na^+ Retention

HEART FAILURE. Ventricular function can be impaired by ischemia, inflammatory or infiltrative changes in the myocardium, valvular abnormalities, or restrictive pericardial processes. As a result, the ejection fraction of either ventricle may be compromised, leading to a fall in cardiac output and pulmonary or systemic venous congestion as "backward failure" develops. The latter process will affect venous hydrostatic pressures and thus lead to edema; it will manifest by increases in interstitial fluid in the lung or peripheral sites—for example, the splanchnic regions and lower extremities. In addition, the deterioration of cardiac output may be sufficient to initiate a series of responses that ultimately lead to renal salt retention (see next section). For a further discussion of heart failure, refer to Chaps. 11 and 21.

PRIMARY RENAL NA^+ RETENTION. Generalized edema results from sodium retention by the kidneys, a process often associated with, and in many cases, preceded by alterations in the hemodynamics of capillaries, favoring fluid movement into the interstitium from the vascular space. Regardless of the primary etiology of edema—for example, ventricular failure, liver disease, or nephrotic syndrome—renal salt retention plays a critical role in the development and maintenance of edema.

The sensors and effectors controlling sodium balance favor sodium retention in edematous states. These include activation of signals from several areas within the vascular bed (heart, aorta, and carotids) that are sensitive to vascular filling with the capacity to activate the renin-angiotensin-aldosterone axis and sympathetic nervous system, release antidiuretic hormone, decrease natriuretic hormones, and alter glomerular filtration rate (see Chap. 35). Activation of these mechanisms results in renal sodium avidity and volume overload.

The primary precipitant of what would appear to be inappropriate sodium retention is the subject of controversy. According to one theory, the "underfill hypothesis," the escape of a portion of total body fluid volume from the vascular space into the interstitial space or peritoneal cavity is perceived as inadequate filling of the vascular space and promotes renal sodium retention in an attempt to restore intravascular volume. A vicious cycle results in which retained sodium and water continue to escape the vascular space secondary to persistence of the primary process—for example, elevated hydrostatic pressure behind a failing ventricle, accumulation of ascites in portal hypertension, or ineffective plasma oncotic pressure in nephrotic syndrome. The volume sensors are thus continuously activated, signaling for renal sodium retention to restore the perceived volume defi-

Table 17-9. Etiology of edematous states

I. Increased capillary hydrostatic pressure
  A. Increased blood volume due to renal Na^+ retention
    1. Heart failure
    2. Primary renal Na^+ retention
      a. Renal failure
      b. Drugs: minoxidil, diazoxide, calcium-channel blockers (especially nifedipine), nonsteroidal anti-inflammatory drugs, fludrocortisone, estrogens
      c. Refeeding edema
      d. ?Hepatic cirrhosis
      e. ?Idiopathic edema
    3. Pregnancy and premenstrual edema
  B. Venous obstruction
    1. Hepatic cirrhosis or hepatic venous obstruction
    2. Acute pulmonary edema
    3. Local venous obstruction
II. Decreased plasma oncotic pressure
  A. Protein loss
    1. Nephrotic syndrome
    2. Protein-losing enteropathy
  B. Reduced albumin synthesis
    1. Liver disease
    2. Malnutrition
III. Increased capillary permeability
  A. Burns
  B. Trauma
  C. Inflammation
  D. Allergic reactions
  E. Adult respiratory distress syndrome
  F. ?Idiopathic edema
  G. ?Malignant ascites
IV. Increased interstitial oncotic pressure
  A. Lymphatic obstruction
  B. Increased capillary permeability
  C. Hypothyroidism

Source: B.D. Rose. *Clinical Physiology of Acid–Base and Electrolyte Disorders* (2nd ed.). New York: McGraw-Hill, 1984. Reproduced with permission.

cit, despite the presence of total body volume (salt and water) overload.

An alternative view, referred to as the "overflow hypothesis," proposes that renal salt retention is the primary event in edema formation and is precipitated not by ineffective filling of the vascular space but by more direct pathologic activation of afferent mechanisms to the kidney via, for example, hepatic pressure sensors in cirrhosis secondary to early portal hypertension, prior to the formation of ascites and intravascular volume depletion. Later, when volume depletion occurs, even more profound sodium avidity, as well as renal failure, may ensue. The "overflow hypothesis" could apply as well to congestive heart failure, and in fact, these theories are not mutually exclusive. The failure of the diseased left ventricle to perfuse the kidneys and other vascular beds may, without prior loss of fluid to the interstitium, promote a fall in glomerular filtration and an increase in sodium retention. Subsequent to the primary rise in intravascular volume and pressure, the forces favoring movement of fluid out of vessels are enhanced, and edema and vascular "underfilling" result (Fig. 17-6).

Venous Obstruction

The hydrostatic pressure in veins can be increased by functional or mechanical obstruction resulting in an increased tendency for fluid to leave the vascular space and enter the interstitium of areas drained by these vessels. For example, obstruction of the inferior vena cava by extension of a renal carcinoma will result in lower extremity edema. This, by the way, may ultimately lead to more generalized edema secondary to renal salt retention as poor venous return from the legs causes decrease in cardiac output with subsequent systemic hypoperfusion and activation of renal mechanisms that increase sodium avidity. Obstruction of the lymphatic channels by tumor invasion, scarring, or extrinsic compression will exacerbate localized edema by impairing the escape of interstitial fluid from the tissues. Another example of venous obstruction is hepatic vein occlusion, which can result in portal hypertension and ascites. Pulmonary venous hypertension in heart failure is a form of functional venous obstruction causing increased intracapillary hydrostatic pressure resulting in increased interstitial fluid.

Abnormal Oncotic Pressure

Decreased Plasma Oncotic Pressure

The major causes of decreased plasma oncotic pressure are urinary protein loss in nephrotic syndrome, gastrointestinal losses in some enteropathies, or decreased albumin synthesis, as in liver disease or severe malnutrition. Albumin pro-

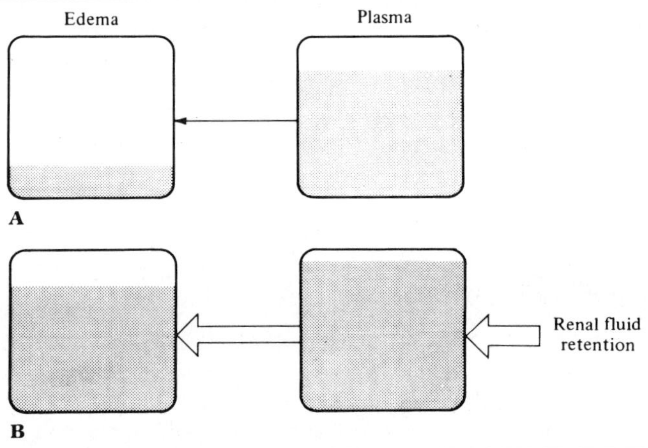

Fig. 17-6. Pathophysiology of edema formation when there is an alteration in capillary hemodynamics favoring the movement of fluid out of the plasma into the interstitium—for example, because of hypoalbuminemia in the nephrotic syndrome. The normal plasma volume is depicted as the full size of the plasma square. The shaded area in the edema square represents the increase in the interstitial fluid volume as edema. The initial reduction in the plasma volume produced by the loss of fluid into the interstitium (A) stimulates renal Na^+ and water retention (B). This appropriately restores the plasma volume toward normal, but because of the altered capillary hemodynamics, much of the retained fluid enters the interstitium and becomes apparent as edema. (From B.D. Rose. *Clinical Physiology of Acid–Base and Electrolyte Disorders* [2nd ed.]. New York: McGraw-Hill, 1984. Reproduced with permission.)

vides the major component of plasma oncotic pressure, and any chronic liver disease in which albumin synthesis is impaired can result in hypoalbuminemia sufficient to effectively lower oncotic pressure within the vascular space and thus decrease one of the forces tending to retain fluid within the vessels. A similar situation applies in the nephrotic syndrome, in which significant urinary loss of albumin and other proteins may lead to severe hypoalbuminemia (albumin less than 2.5 gm/dl). The escape of fluid from the vascular space continues as long as plasma oncotic pressure is insufficient and the compromise of vascular filling is sensed by the volume receptors in the large vessels that signal the kidney to retain salt and water. However, the vascular space can never be effectively repleted until opposing forces (increasing interstitial hydrostatic pressure and decreasing interstitial oncotic pressure) are sufficient to oppose further escape from the vessels resulting from persistent hypoproteinemia. The resultant edema will occur particularly in dependent areas where hydrostatic pressure is greatest.

Increased Interstitial Oncotic Pressure

If plasma proteins that normally escape into the interstitium in small amounts are not cleared, as with lymphatic obstruction owing to chronic lymphangitis or lymph node resection or radiation-induced damage, tissue oncotic pressure may rise, inducing a localized tendency favoring edema.

Increased Capillary Permeability

A variety of usually localized conditions can alter the integrity of capillaries and thereby change their permeability to intracellular fluids and proteins. Loss of the latter from intravascular fluid may lead to further efflux of fluids owing to decreased intravascular oncotic pressure. Such changes in capillaries may be due to direct trauma, which may be blunt (see Chap. 40), thermal (see Chap. 75), inflammatory (see Chap. 1), or allergic (see Chap. 90). These changes may be partly structural, as in trauma or burns, or functional, as in allergic reactions, in which humoral mediators—for example, histamine—alter local blood flow and the characteristics of capillary walls. More generalized alteration of capillary permeability may occur in systemic syndromes often related to trauma or infection in which a systemic capillary "leak" may be most pronounced clinically in the lungs, resulting in the adult respiratory distress syndrome (ARDS), a form of noncardiogenic pulmonary edema unrelated to ventricular failure (see Chap. 11).

Idiopathic Edema

Edema may also present without underlying cardiac, renal, or hepatic disease. Idiopathic edema, a diagnosis of exclusion, is a condition almost exclusively of women of childbearing age who demonstrate significant edema with weight gain, facial puffiness, extremity edema, and even abdominal wall edema, often associated with headaches, irritability, and depression. The pathogenesis of this condition remains unclear. Edema is often episodic, varying with respect to menses, stress, environmental heat, self-induced weight changes, and use of medications such as nonsteroidal anti-inflammatory drugs and diuretics. This condition is rarely incapacitating and as it apparently has no basis in significant organ system failure, has no effect on mortality. Some authorities have noted a relatively heightened sensitivity to postural changes with greater than normal falls in blood pressure and rise in leg volume in patients with idiopathic edema and have attributed this to a subtle capillary leak syndrome or possibly a heightened sensitivity to the renin-angiotensin-aldosterone axis or inhibition of natriuretic factors, or both. Others propose that in at least some patients, diuretic abuse causes persistent or intermittent stimulus for aldosterone secretion and development of adrenal hyperplasia. Cyclic carbohydrate and sodium binging have been proposed as stimuli of glucoregulatory hormones, which may have antinatriuretic action. Since many patients with idiopathic edema manifest excessive weight consciousness, such a theory is attractive, particularly as numerous cases have resolved with discontinuation of diuretics and control of cyclic eating patterns.

Iatrogenic Causes of Edema

Estrogen therapy, vasodilators, and nonsteroidal anti-inflammatory drugs can produce edema, especially in dependent areas, and must be considered in any patient without apparent organic cause for volume overload. In addition, these agents may exacerbate edema in patients with other problems—for example, congestive heart failure and renal failure. These drugs may directly affect renal sodium handling.

DIAGNOSIS

Presentation

Very soft pitting edema may be seen secondary to hypoalbuminemic states—for example, nephrotic syndrome or protein malnutrition. Pulmonary edema secondary to left ventricular failure may be florid, without coincident findings of right heart failure—for example, jugular venous distention or hepatomegaly and dependent edema, although the patient with severe left ventricular failure may have significant generalized edema secondary to avid salt retention (see previous discussion). Patients with congestive heart failure may complain of orthopnea, paroxysmal nocturnal dyspnea, and dyspnea on exertion, or may manifest arrhythmias secondary to valvular disease, coronary artery disease, or cardiomyopathies. They may be tachypneic and demonstrate gallop rhythms and rales on examination.

Patients with cirrhosis and portal hypertension may develop generalized edema owing to renal salt retention prior to development of significant ascites and further aggravation of lower extremity edema secondary to venous and lymphatic compression. They may manifest numerous stigmata of portal hypertension—for example, telangiectasia, jaundice, palmar erythema, gynecomastia, hepatomegaly, or a firm, shrunken liver. Signs and symptoms of hypothyroidism may be seen and should be sought in appropriate situations.

Mild edema, especially of the lower extremities, may be seen in pregnancy or in the premenstrual setting. Other conditions that may be associated with edema may be the presenting complaint—for example, hematuria (nephritis), diabetes and hypertension (common causes of renal failure), or drug use for hypertension (vasodilators) or pain (nonsteroidal anti-inflammatory drugs).

Evaluation

History
Careful history taking and physical examination will often indicate one of the major causes of edema—that is, congestive heart failure secondary to valvular or coronary artery disease, liver disease, renal failure, or nephrotic syndrome. A thorough medication history may reveal use of nonsteroidal anti-inflammatory drugs, converting enzyme inhibitors, and antibiotics that may impair renal function by vasomotor alterations or interstitial nephritis.

Physical Examination
Significant generalized edema, gross pulmonary edema, or ascites will be obvious on casual examination, whereas volume overload of lesser degrees may be more subtle and apparent only on close observation—for example, dependent areas, including the presacral area in recumbent patients.

Laboratory Examination
Further evaluation in the emergency department may be necessary to determine the specific etiology and extent of complications. Determination of serum creatinine and a carefully performed urinalysis may indicate renal disease and begin to clarify the specific pathogenesis. Presentation with hypertension, edema, and red and white cells and cellular casts in the urine indicate possible glomerulonephritis or interstitial nephritis, often resulting from medications. An active urinary sediment, with white cells and white cell casts, would favor the latter. High-grade proteinuria (3–4+ on dipstick) may indicate nephrotic syndrome, often accompanied by hypoalbuminemia and hypercholesterolemia. Semiquantitation of proteinuria with a spot urine protein to creatinine ratio (mg/dl:mg/dl, expressed as grams of proteinuria) provides useful confirmation. The presence of lipid (oval fat bodies or "Maltese crosses" on polarized light microscopy) in the urine is also helpful in indicating nephrotic syndrome.

Liver "function" tests and prothrombin time may indicate hepatic disease. Thyroid function tests, especially TSH (thyroid-stimulating hormone), may be helpful, if available in the emergency department.

RADIOLOGIC EVALUATION AND SPECIAL TESTING. Chest radiographs and electrocardiograms are helpful in evaluating cardiac problems. The chest radiograph will be abnormal with possible cardiomegaly, pulmonary congestion, and Kerley B lines. Modest amounts of ascites might require radiographic or ultrasonic imaging for detection. Localized edema should direct attention to causes of venous or lymphatic occlusion and may require specialized noninvasive or radiographic testing, such as impedance plethysmography, venography, or computed scanning or magnetic resonance imaging.

DISPOSITION

Often, full evaluation of edema will require hospitalization or extended outpatient work-up with appropriate referrals—for example, a nephrologist for nephrotic syndrome. The role of the emergency physician is to triage patients whose underlying condition is severe enough to require in-hospital care and evaluation and to decide who to treat acutely, and in which manner. Clues to the severity of the patient's condition can be obtained from the physical examination and evaluation of electrolyte, acid–base, and oxygenation status. Attention should also be paid to initial care for areas of skin breakdown, because edema is a risk factor for this. The emergency physician would be wise to record, if possible, the patient's weight as reference for assessment of therapy over time. Such a simple maneuver is often forgotten.

The emergency physician must intervene immediately in cases of edema associated with significant acute morbidity and mortality—for example, pulmonary edema, possibly cirrhosis with massive ascites or hepatorenal syndrome, and renal failure with significant volume overload. Such patients will generally require admission. The emergency physician must stabilize the patient and attempt volume removal, usually via diuretics and other measures to reduce pulmonary congestion in cases of deteriorating blood gases and respiratory distress (see section on congestive heart failure for details of acute therapy). Immediate follow-up care in the hospital must be ensured.

Other patients with edema who are in stable condition but need admission do not require emergent therapy for volume overload, and the emergency physician can focus on the appropriate initial evaluations of cardiac, hepatic, and renal functions. Many patients with volume overload but without significant acute illness (mild congestive heart failure, compensated cirrhosis, nephrotic syndrome, stable chronic renal failure, or idiopathic edema) may not require hospitalization; in such cases, the emergency physician need only ensure appropriate initial therapy and outpatient follow-up.

Adjustments of medications, including diuretics, as well as antinatriuretic agents, such as nonsteroidals and vasodilators, may be required. Dietary and activity instructions should be clarified.

SELECTED READING

DeWardener, HE. Idiopathic edema: Role of diuretic abuse. *Kidney Int* 19:881, 1981.

Epstein, M, and Perez, GO. Pathophysiology of Edema-Forming States. In MH Maxwell, et al. (eds), *Clinical Disorders of Fluid and Electrolyte Metabolism* (4th ed). New York: McGraw-Hill, 1987.

Reineck, HJ, and Stein, JH. Sodium Metabolism. In MH Maxwell, et al. (eds), *Clinical Disorders of Fluid and Electrolyte Metabolism* (4th ed). New York: McGraw-Hill, 1987.

Rose, BD. *Clinical Physiology of Acid–Base and Electrolyte Disorders* (2nd ed). New York: McGraw-Hill, 1984.

Schrier, RW. Pathogenesis of sodium and water retention in high output and low output cardiac failure, nephrotic syndrome; cirrhosis and pregnancy. *N Engl J Med* 319:1065, 1127–1136, 1988.

Skorecki, KL, and Brenner, BM. Body fluid homeostasis in man: A contemporary overview. *Am J Med* 70:77, 1981.

18. Myocardial Ischemia in Coronary Artery Disease

Andrew Selwyn

There is a growing appreciation that transient myocardial ischemia is usually a functional expression of coronary artery disease and is an invaluable indication that increased risk is eminently reversible by many currently available therapies. Myocardial ischemia is most commonly caused by atherosclerotic coronary stenosis. The syndrome can occur in patients who have no obvious history of coronary artery disease, in those with a history of chronic stable angina or unstable angina, or in those who have had myocardial infarction. Ischemia is frequently asymptomatic or it can be seen with atypical symptoms such as the abrupt onset of pulmonary edema or arrhythmias. Myocardial ischemia can complicate aortic stenosis and left ventricular hypertrophy, and occur after cocaine abuse, tachyarrhythmias, a gastrointestinal bleed, trauma, pheochromocytoma, or other stressful medical conditions, which will be discussed in more detail.

This chapter reviews the effects of ischemia on ventricular myocardium as a basis for describing the clinical presentations. A description of the most important ischemic syndromes is given as they are encountered in the emergency department. Finally, recommendations are presented regarding diagnosis, management, and the organized facilities that are needed to provide timely and effective treatment.

THE ISCHEMIC MYOCARDIUM

Transient ischemia results from a fall in the myocardial tissue oxygen content due to deficient blood supply or excessive myocardial demands with restricted blood supply. When tissue oxygen content falls, diastolic relaxation will fail and failure of systolic performance will follow within seconds. The intracellular compartmental movement of calcium is disturbed and anaerobic metabolism results, with the accumulation of protons, acidosis, and lactate. Failure of energy-dependent aerobic metabolism results in the leak of potassium from cells and an increase in the intercellular potassium concentration. Within minutes all energy metabolism fails and adenosine triphosphate and glycogen stores begin to fall. Electrical potentials are generated between ischemic and normal myocardium and the left-ventricular–end-diastolic pressure increases, while mitral regurgitation results if a papillary muscle is involved. The ventricle becomes more susceptible to arrhythmias, ventricular tachycardia, and even ventricular fibrillation. Pulmonary edema and hypotension ensue if the ischemic segment is big enough. If the imbalance between supply and demand is corrected, the affected segment of myocardium will recover but will exhibit prolonged disturbances of contractile function, energetic metabolism, and probably glycogen storage (stunning), which leave the heart poorly equipped for the next episode.

If ischemia extends beyond 20 minutes, membrane structure fails, lysosomal enzymes leak into the cytosol, and damage from oxygen-free radicals will occur. All of these processes will lead to irreversible loss of myocardial oxygen metabolism and failure of the respiratory enzymes in mitochondria. These events ultimately lead to myocyte necrosis. In patients with long-standing obstructive coronary artery disease or severe left ventricular hypertrophy due to aortic stenosis, it is common to find macroscopic scars throughout the left ventricular myocardium, with unexpected silent myocardial infarction a common pathologic feature in these circumstances. Indeed, 20 to 30 percent of all myocardial infarcts found in unselected populations occur without chest pain. Therefore, when patients are first seen with acute ischemia on the basis of coronary artery disease or left ventricular hypertrophy, or both, previous scarring and damage are common accompanying features, providing evidence that transient myocardial ischemia can exact permanent damage.

UNSTABLE CORONARY ARTERY DISEASE

Patients with unstable coronary artery disease can present with new-onset angina, angina at rest, or the acceleration of existing symptoms. These symptoms indicate the increased risk of myocardial infarction and sudden coronary death. Angina pectoris is not universal and ischemia may cause episodic sweating, epigastric distress, intermittent dizziness, palpitations, or unexplained bouts of shortness of breath. These angina equivalents are less specific but important clues in all patients who have risk factors or known coronary disease or both.

One illustrative example is the 65-year-old woman who is hypertensive and smokes. She now experiences episodic shortness of breath with sweating and the exercise stress test shows evidence of severe ischemia. A full history is vital, with an immediate search for evidence of anginal chest pain, previous diagnosis of coronary artery disease, cardiac medications, a family history of coronary artery disease, a history of myocardial infarction, or prior cardiac surgery. In the physical examination evidence of hyperlipidemia, tachycardia, an atrial fourth sound, a dyskinetic left ventricular apex, mitral regurgitation, pulmonary edema, or peripheral signs of occlusive atherosclerosis should be sought. The patient may be distressed and sweating, with a characteristic gesture of the hand pressed on the precordium or the throat. The physical examination should purposefully exclude aortic stenosis, severe left ventricular hypertrophy, gastrointestional bleeding, anemia, evidence of drug abuse, and cardiac arrhythmia, particularly tachyarrhythmias.

A 12-lead electrocardiogram (ECG) may show arrhythmia, planar ST-segment depression in two or more leads, ST-segment elevation, Q waves indicating prior myocardial infarction, or, occasionally, less specific signs such as symmetrical T-wave inversion, particularly across the precordium. The coincidence between transient ECG signs and symptoms that suggest myocardial ischemia is invaluable evidence and immediately establishes a provisionary diagnosis that should trigger admission and careful monitoring. After recording heart rate, blood pressure, and ventricular rate on the ECG, other tests might include cardiac enzymes, a chest x-ray if there are signs of cardiomegaly or heart failure, and a hematocrit. At this stage, the physician must decide if the clinical signs indicate ischemia on the basis of coronary artery disease, thus establishing a provisionary diagnosis.

PATHOPHYSIOLOGY

When the presentation of coronary artery disease is acute or unstable, or both, as was described previously, it is almost always the clinical manifestation of underlying stenosis of one or more epicardial coronary arteries. The occurrence of ischemia from moment to moment depends on the balance between coronary blood supply and the myocardial demands for oxygen. There is a growing appreciation that the supply—that is, the atherosclerotic coronary lesions—actively and intermittently interfere with coronary blood flow and thereby play a crucial role in causing the ischemic syndrome. Monitoring of regional coronary blood flow, radio isotope studies, and angiographic studies have all demonstrated that the vasomotion of these epicardial coronary artery lesions is abnormal, with loss of vasodilator responses and inappropriate constriction. In addition, angiographic studies, angioscopic studies in the coronary arteries, and pathologic evidence have also shown that these patients frequently have erosions or fissuring, or both, in an atherosclerotic plaque complicated by local thrombus formation (Fig. 18-1).

MANAGEMENT

Clinical management should be individualized and based on the coincidental problems of *coronary stenosis, disturbed vasomotion, and thrombus formation*. Immediate management should consist of explanation and reassurance, and sublingual nitroglycerin for symptoms or signs of ischemia on the electrocardiogram. Sublingual tablets of 0.3 or 0.4 mg are usual, with care to avoid a greater than 20-mm Hg decrease in systolic blood pressure. Oxygen by nasal prongs may be necessary to maintain an optimal arterial oxygen saturation.

The therapies that will be described are in order of application and should all be titrated individually against the patient's symptoms, electrocardiographic signs of ischemia, heart rate, and blood pressure. Any evidence of intracardiac conduction disturbances, cardiomegaly, or heart failure will modify the use of these drugs. Medications include sublingual nitroglycerin, intravenous morphine in l-mg increments every three minutes, intravenous nitroglycerin given at 10 to 200 μg per minute, and sublingual nifedipine (10 mg). Oral beta-blockers (propranolol, 20 mg, or metoprolol, 50 mg) or intravenous beta-blockers (propranolol, l-mg increments, or metoprolol, 5-mg increments, every five minutes) can be used. The importance of individual dose titration against each patient's symptoms, heart rate, blood pressure, and the other signs listed cannot be overemphasized. If contraindica-

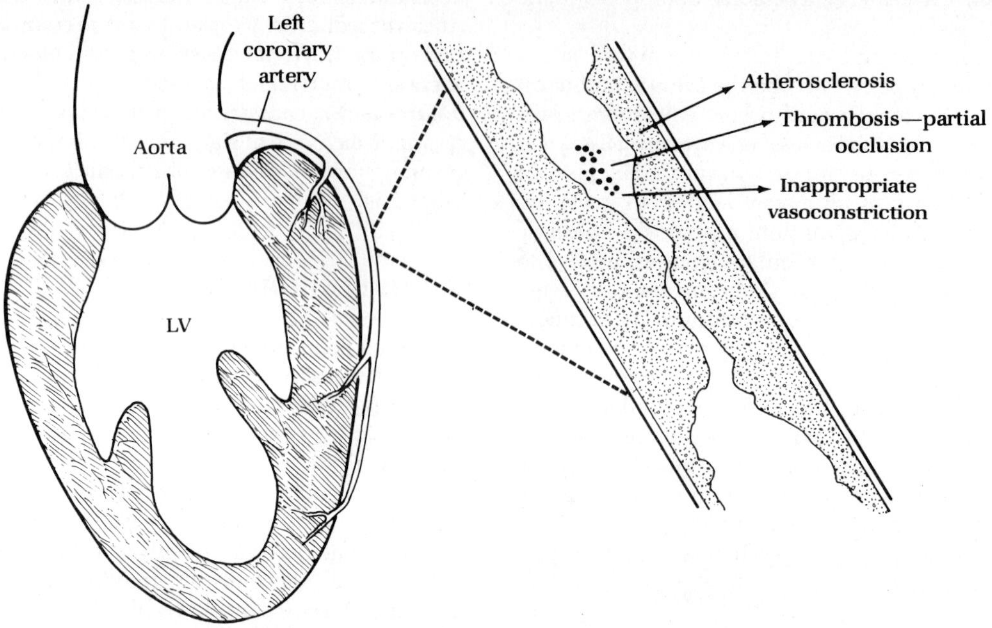

Fig. 18-1. Major pathology associated with the clinical presentations of coronary artery disease (i.e., angina, myocardial infarction, and left ventricular damage). There is a growing appreciation that these clinical syndromes are due to problems arising from the cell biology of atherosclerotic lesions. The major features of these problems seem to be inappropriate growth leading to stenosis; inappropriate constriction, particularly at the site of stenosis; and a tendency to vascular thrombosis. These underlying pathogenic mechanisms likely explain the acute clinical presentations of unstable angina and myocardial infarction.

tions do not exist, heparin or aspirin have been shown to decrease the occurrence of myocardial infarction and death in these circumstances. Heparin is given intravenously as 5,000- to 10,000-unit boluses, then 500 to 1,000 units per hour according to coagulation studies. Aspirin is given as one adult tablet (325 mg) daily. Further management may include sedation, increasing doses of the drug regimens just listed, insertion of a flow-directed balloon catheter to measure and maintain the pulmonary capillary wedge pressure at 5 to 20 mm Hg, and timely referral to cardiology services for consideration of intraaortic balloon counterpulsation or urgent coronary arteriography.

Unstable or accelerating ischemia that is refractory to medical therapy indicates the serious risk of myocardial infarction or death. Timely diagnosis is important, and the use of aspirin or heparin is the only therapy known to reduce these risks. Urgent cardiac catheterization is reserved for patients with recurrent angina and ischemia on medical therapy. Balloon angioplasty can be used if ischemia is uncontrollable and the coronary anatomy is suitable. Coronary surgery is reserved for recurrent ischemia in patients with left main-stem stenosis or severe three-vessel coronary artery disease. The emergency department physician needs to recognize the syndrome, admit the patient to the hospital, and refer the patient to cardiology services so that the management can be intensified in accordance with the presentation and progress in each individual case.

VENTRICULAR HYPERTROPHY

Patients who are first seen with anginal chest pain may show severe left ventricular hypertrophy with widespread ST-segment and T-wave changes on the 12-lead electrocardiogram (strain pattern or myocardial ischemia, or both). These patients frequently also show symptoms of worsening left ventricular failure, such as shortness of breath, orthopnea, and paroxysmal nocturnal dyspnea. They may have a history of hypertension, renal disease, or aortic stenosis. A complete physical examination may reveal tachycardia, hypertension, an atrial fourth sound, and physical signs of left ventricular failure (raised venous pressure and a gallop rhythm); it may also show cardiomegaly, pulmonary congestion or edema, and physical signs of aortic stenosis. This presentation carries a significantly increased risk of worsening congestive heart failure, arrhythmias such as ventricular tachycardia or fibrillation, and sudden death. The thickened left ventricle results in high wall tension and an abnormally high resistance to effective subendocardial myocardial blood flow. Myocardial demand is increased and coronary stenoses are poorly tolerated in these circumstances. Myocardial function can be further impaired by the drugs that are used to treat hypertension, the numerous biochemical disturbances that are caused by renal disease, or the fixed impedance to left ventricular outflow imposed by aortic stenosis. Since left ventricular hypertrophy and important atherosclerotic stenoses of the large coronary arteries frequently coexist, in initial management it should probably be assumed that coronary disease is present until proved otherwise.

A complete physical examination should focus on heart rate, blood pressure, the degree of congestive heart failure and left ventricular failure, adequate blood oxygenation, a search for aortic stenosis, and an assessment at the bedside of cardiac and urine output. The initial tests should include the 12-lead electrocardiogram, blood plasma levels of cardiac enzymes, electrolytes, renal function, arterial oxygen saturation, and acid-base balance.

The immediate management must focus on the relief of ischemia, with oxygen delivery by nasal prongs and sedation using intravenous morphine in 1-mg increments. The use of sublingual or intravenous nitroglycerin must carefully avoid rapid or excessive changes in aortic blood pressure ($\geq$ 20 mm Hg), which can lead to confusion, transient ischemic attacks, strokes, or worsening of myocardial ischemia and renal function. Sublingual and intravenous nitroglycerin should not be used in patients who have severe aortic stenosis. When present, heart failure is difficult to treat because myocardial compliance is poor, left ventricular volume may be small, and the cardiac output is highly sensitive to ventricular filling (preload). In addition to oxygen, morphine, and nitroglycerin (if no aortic stenosis is present), a diuretic (furosemide starting at 10 mg intravenously) can be given if the venous pressure is raised with cardiomegaly or pulmonary congestion, or both.

When dyspnea and fatigue are obvious, the respiratory rate exceeds 25 cycles per minute, and the oxygen saturation and blood gas analysis indicate respiratory failure, emergency endotracheal intubation with assisted ventilation may be necessary and life-saving. If heart rate and blood pressure are abnormally raised with no signs of left ventricular failure or conduction disturbances on the 12-lead electrocardiogram, intravenous beta-blockers (propranolol in 1-mg increments) can be used. Monitoring of heart rate, blood pressure, symptoms and signs of ischemia, and intracardiac conduction on the electrocardiogram is essential. Once again, all therapies must be individually titrated to avoid the problems of bradycardia, hypotension, and worsening of left ventricular failure.

A provisionary diagnosis of myocardial ischemia with left ventricular hypertrophy due to hypertension, renal disease, or aortic stenosis requires emergency admission and intensive monitoring. If heart failure accompanies the ischemia and left ventricular hypertrophy, or if a diagnosis of aortic stenosis is made at the bedside, the patient needs cardiology services. If angina, shortness of breath, electrocardiographic signs of ischemia, or physical signs of heart failure do not respond promptly, the patient needs referral to cardiology services in the emergency department to prevent or arrest the progressive deterioration of cardiac output, blood pressure, and coronary blood flow. Persistent ischemia indicates the need for consideration of intraaortic balloon-pump counterpulsation, temporary endotracheal intubation, and emergency cardiac catheterization. The importance of timely referral to cardiology services with consultation in the emergency department cannot be overemphsized.

MYOCARDIAL ISCHEMIA AND INFARCTION

In patients who are first seen with unstable angina as described previously, the pathophysiology (atherosclerotic stenosis with thrombosis) merges by small degrees into the occlusive thrombus that occurs in acute myocardial infarction. Therefore, when patients manifest recurring pain at rest and/or transient ST-segment depression or elevation despite the initiation of medical therapy, the syndromes of unstable angina and myocardial infarction merge and cannot be distinguished (Fig. 18-2). The following symptoms and clinical signs must be taken as alarms that indicate impending myocardial infarction: recurring anginal chest pain with ST-segment elevation, recurring chest pain that lasts longer than 10 minutes and responds poorly to nitroglycerin or the therapeutic measures listed previously, or persistent ST-segment depression or T-wave inversion in two or more leads that remains after chest pain and will not reverse with the specific therapy listed previously. If the initial treatment for unstable angina does not produce relief of symptoms and abolish signs of myocardial ischemia on the electrocardiogram, the physician must recognize the transition to myocardial infarction. The initiation of thrombolytic therapy and timely referral to a coronary care unit and cardiology services are discussed in Chapter 19.

ABUSE OF DRUGS

The increasing abuse of cocaine taken by nasal or intravenous routes, or by inhalation or smoking, will increase the release of and block the re-uptake of catecholamines, result-

Fig. 18-2. These ECG samples are taken from a calibrated tape during continuous monitoring of the electrocardiogram in an ambulant patient with coronary artery disease. The samples show normal complex at the outset and then episodes of typical square wave ST-segment depression indicating transient ischemia occurring throughout the day and during normal daily activities. The example shows that transient ischemia episodes occur in patients while at rest and active outside of the hospital and generally indicate an increased risk of adverse coronary events.

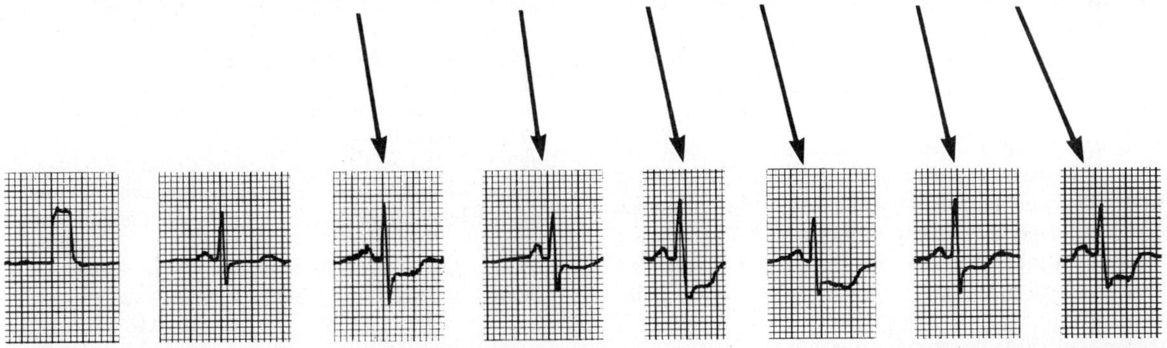

ing in excessive increases in heart rate, blood pressure, and myocardial contractility. A clinical syndrome is now recognized in drug abusers that occurs minutes to hours after cocaine abuse and consists of diaphoresis, agitation, hypertension, tachycardia, chest pain, and electrocardiographic signs of myocardial ischemia with ST-segment depression or elevation, or both. Early coronary arteriography and studies of ventricular function have demonstrated spasm and/or thrombosis of large epicardial coronary arteries or depressd ventricular function, or both. This clinical situation can lead to acute myocardial infarction, malignant arrhythmias, and sudden cardiac death.

Management must start with obtaining a record of drug abuse. The physical examination should include a search for signs of intravenous drug use and sympathetic stimulation (sweating, tachycardia, hypertension, and agitation). A 12-lead electrocardiogram should be performed to look for evidence of ischemia in ST-segment depression or elevation.

Immediate management should consist of monitoring the electrocardiogram, heart rate, and blood pressure. Intravenous nitroglycerin, propranolol, phentolamine, or labetalol have all been used to reverse the coronary spasm and sympathetic stimulation associated with this syndrome. If ST-segment elevation is present and persists with a clinical history of less than six hours, thrombolytic therapy must be considered for acute myocardial infarction. The immediate aims of therapy are reversal of the coronary constriction and thrombosis, followed by cessation of the drug abuse. Descriptive clinical reports have demonstrated the successful treatment of myocardial ischemia using this regimen.

MYOCARDIAL ISCHEMIA COMPLICATING ACUTE STRESS

Middle-aged and elderly patients who are first seen in the emergency department with a wide variety of urgent medical problems frequently have known or as yet undiagnosed underlying obstructive coronary artery disease in addition. Myocardial ischemia and infarction can occur unexpectedly and complicate the clinical management of a number of unrelated medical conditions. Typical examples include the elderly diabetic who is seen initially with severe infection or ketoacidosis, as well as the patient who suffers a gastrointestinal bleed or a severe motor accident. The management of these conditions may suddenly be complicated by chest pain, the unexpected onset of left ventricular failure, mitral regurgitation, pulmonary edema, unexpected hypotension, or arrhythmias. In all of these circumstances, it is important to realize that coronary artery disease can manifest itself under stress and requires management as outlined previously.

A number of miscellaneous and usually rare conditions must also be considered as clinical problems. Patients with a pheochromocytoma can first be seen with tachycardia and hypertension caused by excess catecholamines, which can lead to and cause myocardial ischemia; myocardial infarction; arrhythmias; and sudden cardiac death. Patients who have recently received thrombolytic therapy in the first six hours of a myocardial infarction are particularly susceptible to coronary reocclusion, with recurrent ischemia, chest pain, and electrocardiographic signs of recurring ischemia and myocardial infarction. Finally, patients with a personality disorder (Munchausen's syndrome), who seek medical attention, clinical testing, and usually analgesic narcotics, can be seen initially with typical anginal chest pain, and then go on to manipulate the available staff and facilities, describing false symptoms.

EMERGENCY CARE AND MYOCARDIAL ISCHEMIA

Obstructive coronary artery disease is generally a condition found in middle-aged and elderly people and can present with obvious chest pain and electrocardiographic signs or without any angina but with unexpected left ventricular failure, mitral regurgitation, or pulmonary edema with or without arrhythmias. In its unstable forms it is a dangerous but reversible condition that gives warning of myocardial infarction and death. The emergency department staff and facilities must be prepared by considering the following guidelines:

1. The history is essential and should quickly try to capture certain essential features, such as known coronary artery disease, a history of myocardial infarction, or drug abuse.
2. The physical examination must follow in order to assess cardiac rhythm, severity of left ventricular failure, onset of myocardial infarction, or mitral regurgitation.
3. The 12-lead electrocardiogram and electrocardiographic monitoring with careful interpretation must be immediately available.
4. Full equipment for cardiopulmonary resuscitation must be on hand and constantly maintained.
5. Simple tests such as blood gases, cardiac enzymes, electrolytes, and acid-base balance should be available.
6. Written guidelines should be discussed for the timely referral to and collaboration with specialty cardiology services, which are essential if the patient needs intraaortic balloon counterpulsation, thrombolytic therapy, cardiac catheterization, coronary angioplasty, or even cardiac surgery.

SELECTED READING

Ambrose, JA, et al. Angiographic morphology and the pathogenesis of unstable angina pectoris. *J Am Coll Cardiol* 5:608, 1985.

Braunwald, E, and Sobel, BE. Coronary Blood Flow and Myocardial Ischemia in Heart Disease. In E Braunwald (ed), *Heart Disease: A Textbook of Cardiovascular Medicine* (3rd ed). Philadelphia: Saunders, 1988.

Ross, R. The Pathogenesis of Atherosclerosis in Heart Disease. In E Braunwald (ed), *Textbook of Cardiovascular Medicine* (3rd ed). Philadelphia: Saunders, 1988.

Rutherford, JD, Braunwald, E, and Cohn, PF. Chronic Ischemic Heart Disease in Heart Disease. In E Braunwald (ed), *Textbook of Cardiovascular Medicine* (3rd ed). Philadelphia: Saunders, 1988.

Theroux, P, et al. Aspirin, heparin, or both to treat acute unstable angina. *N Engl J Med* 319:1105, 1988.

19. Acute Myocardial Infarction

Joseph R. Benotti

Over the past 30 years, the treatment of myocardial infarction has undergone major change. Indeed, since the first edition of *Emergency Medicine* was published, significant change has evolved in the emergency department treatment of myocardial infarction. With each decade the role of the emergency physician in the diagnosis and early management of acute myocardial infarction has assumed greater importance in terms of diagnosis, patient stabilization, and outcome.

Before the mid-1960s, acute myocardial infarction, commonly known as "coronary thrombosis," was considered a static and completed event at the time the patient was first seen. Treatment was dictated by the pathologic observation that the segment of myocardium undergoing ischemic necrosis required four to six weeks to evolve to a mature scar composed of fibrous tissue. Accordingly, treatment was entirely supportive and the mainstay was prolonged bed rest. The myriad of complications consequent to bed rest (thromboembolism, pneumonia, and so forth), especially in elderly patients, as well as those more specific for myocardial infarction, were treated in a supportive fashion. The emergency physician, other than having the first opportunity to diagnose myocardial infarction, had little to contribute to overall management and care, and the quality of emergency care did not materially affect outcome. Indeed, in-hospital mortality for acute myocardial infarction ranged between 20 and 30 percent.

With development of electrical defibrillation, synchronized cardioversion for ventricular and atrial tachyarrhythmias, continuous electrocardiographic (ECG) monitoring, and the induction of effective, rapid-acting, and relatively safe antiarrhythmic therapy (xylocaine and procainamide) came the realization in the late 1960s that sudden cardiac death in the early stages of acute myocardial infarction was a primary electrical event (ventricular tachycardia–ventricular fibrillation). Accordingly, the concept of the coronary care unit evolved. The standard of care dictated that the patient be rapidly triaged to a specially equipped in-hospital care area as soon as the diagnosis of acute myocardial infarction was entertained. Here the cardiac rhythm was continuously electrocardiographically monitored by nursing personnel skilled in the immediate diagnosis and treatment of malignant cardiac arrhythmias. Accordingly, it became incumbent on the physician in the emergency department to improve his or her skills in the electrocardiographic and clinical diagnosis of myocardial infarction and in the emergency management of malignant ventricular arrhythmias.

The decade of the 1970s was characterized by greater understanding of the prognostic determinates of myocardial infarction. At the same time, medical and surgical therapies evolved for complications of myocardial infarction, including ongoing myocardial ischemia, cardiogenic shock, acute mitral insufficiency, ventricular septal rupture, and left ventricular aneurysm. Concomitantly, more effective and definitive management of conditions that might mimic myocardial infarction (i.e., aortic dissection, esophageal rupture, pulmonary embolism, and so forth) was developed. It became important for the physician in the emergency department to be skilled in the differential diagnosis of acute myocardial infarction so that specific therapies for these other conditions could be made rapidly available. The emergency physician also became more proficient in the pharmacologic management of hemodynamic instability consequent to acute myocardial infarction.

Since the first edition of this textbook was published, therapeutic strategies have emerged to rapidly restore coronary blood flow after acute coronary thrombosis and to reduce infarct size both by expeditious reperfusion and by protection of the ischemic myocardium. The success and safety of these interventions depend on the rapidity with which the patient is seen at the hospital following the onset of infarction, the alacrity and accuracy with which the diagnosis is made, and the promptness with which the indications and contraindications to alternative therapeutic reperfusion strategies (pharmacologic thrombolysis, balloon angioplasty, or coronary artery revascularization surgery) are considered. Accordingly, the importance of the physician in not only the prompt diagnosis of myocardial infarction but also its initial management cannot be overemphasized.

PATHOPHYSIOLOGY

Myocardial infarction is defined as the irreversible loss (death) of myocardial tissue consequent to an acute severe and protracted deprivation of its blood supply. After 15 minutes of coronary artery ligation followed by reperfusion in experimental preparations, evidence of ischemic myocardial injury is seen. This injury is totally reversible with reperfusion (release of the arterial ligature). As the period of coronary occlusion increases, the relative extent of myocyte recovery after reperfusion is diminished. Beyond four to six hours of total coronary occlusion followed by reperfusion, little or no recovery of myocardial function is observed.

Over the past decade, it has become clear that the in-hospital and long-term prognosis after acute myocardial infarction is determined by the cumulative amount of ventricular damage. With more extensive cumulative irreversible injury from previous and current myocardial infarction, the risk of death becomes greater. It has also been unequivocally demonstrated that in over 80 percent of patients who are seen within the first few hours of acute transmural myocardial infarction, total coronary artery occlusion is the primary cause. It results from a fibrin-platelet thrombosis in the artery supplying the infarcted myocardial segment. The underlying propensity to acute thrombotic occlusion usually results from an underlying atherosclerotic lesion of the vessel. A secondary loss of the endothelial integrity results in acute thrombosis. This occurs, in part, from intimal disruption with the loss of endothelial anticoagulant function. Exposure of subendothelial collagen elicits platelet adhesion and aggregation, fibrin activation by circulating procoagulants, and thrombus formation.

The success of therapeutic medical strategies that have evolved for myocardial infarction relate to enzymatic thrombolysis, pharmacologic inhibition of platelet function and reduction in myocardial oxygen demand to preserve cellular structural integrity during the critical interval of acute ischemia. Thrombolytic agents digest the fibrin components of the culprit coronary artery thrombosis. This relieves the acute obstruction, restores arterial patency, and improves myocardial oxygenation to salvage ischemic yet viable myocardium downstream to the site of vessel occlusion. Aspirin reduces platelet adhesiveness to reduce the incidence of post-infarction ischemic events. Beta-blockers reduce myocardial oxygen demand to preserve cell viability and reduce the size of the myocardial infarction. These measures have dramatically reduced the in-hospital and one-year mortality following myocardial infarction. The establishment of these pathologic concepts since the first edition of *Emergency Medicine* has placed a great deal of responsibility on the emergency physician to promptly diagnose and treat myocardial infarction. It is incumbent that this diagnosis be made accurately and with alacrity; that the patient be promptly screened for contraindications to thrombolytic agents, aspirin, and beta-blockers; and that these drugs be administered promptly. Therapy should usually commence before the patient leaves the emergency department for the coronary care unit. There is generally only time for phone consultation to the cardiologist or internist before undertaking these more specific therapies. Time is insufficient to permit certain confirmation or exclusion of the diagnosis of myocardial infarction by serum enzyme analyses before institution of thrombolytic treatment, a very expensive and potentially hazardous therapy.

DIAGNOSIS

Presentation and History

Patients with myocardial infarction usually have initial symptoms of chest pain of a squeezing, oppressive nature. It is usually more intense and prolonged than the pain that is characteristic of angina pectoris and persists despite administration of nitroglycerin. The pain may radiate to the arm, neck, or jaw. It may be localized to the epigastric area and perhaps raise suspicion of a gastrointestinal problem. In the patient with one or more risk factors for coronary disease—that is, high blood pressure, a family history of coronary disease, diabetes mellitus, a history of cigarette smoking, or elevation in the serum cholesterol—any new discomfort experienced between the forehead and the umbilicus could raise the question of acute myocardial ischemia. Under appropriate circumstances this would mandate emergency department evaluation, including electrocardiography.

Patients with acute myocardial infarction may only have dyspnea initially. Elderly patients may have dyspnea, diaphoresis, or lightheadedness. These complaints reflect one or more of the following: pulmonary congestion, compensation by the sympathetic nervous system in an effort to compensate for the acute circulatory embarrassment, or moderate arterial hypoperfusion due to low cardiac output secondary to the primary myocardial insult or the complicating arrhythmia, or both.

Physical Examination

The physical examination may reveal pallor and acrocyanosis, which reflect inadequate cutaneous circulation with intense compensatory reflex vasoconstriction mediated by the sympathetic nervous system. Blood pressure should be measured in both upper extremities. Any difference in simultaneously recorded upper-extremity arterial pressures points to arterial obstruction, and this in turn points to acute aortic dissection rather than acute myocardial infarction as the cause of the patient's chest pain. The blood pressure may be elevated or diminished depending on the size of the myocardial infarction; a large zone of myocardial necroses results in a reduced cardiac output, more intense reflex activation of the sympathetic nervous system, and a greater degree of hypotension. A high level of circulating catecholamines evokes tachycardia, an elevated diastolic blood pressure, and a narrowed arterial pulse pressure. Diaphoresis may be present consequent to sympathetic overactivity. The pulse may be rapid and thready, reflective of catecholamine excess and low stroke output in conjunction with the acute myocardial insult. Auscultation of the chest may reveal rales and pulmonary congestion. Arterial hypoxemia may result in central cyanosis.

The cardiac examination may be unrevealing if the zone of infarction is relatively small or if the patient is in the very early stages of a large infarction. A fourth heart sound may be heard, reflecting a reduction in ventricular compliance. With more severe and extensive myocardial infarction, a third heart sound may be present. This indicates more severe systolic ventricular failure with impending clinical congestive heart failure or, perhaps, cardiogenic shock. A systolic murmur indicative of mitral insufficiency resulting from papillary muscle dysfunction, or a left-to-right ventricular shunt resulting from ventricular septal rupture, may be evident.

Laboratory Evaluation and Electrocardiogram

Blood is immediately obtained for a complete blood count, electrolytes, blood urea nitrogen, and serum creatinine; tests for myocardial enzymes (creatinine phosphokinase [CPK], total isozyme and myocardial fraction, lactic dehydrogenase [LDH], and serum glutamic oxaloacetic transaminase [SGOT]) should also be performed. A free-running intravenous (IV) line through a large-bore plastic cannula is immediately established to maintain a reliable intravascular access, should the rapid administration of antiarrhythmics or pressor agents, or both, become necessary.

All patients with chest pain or any clinical presentation compatible with myocardial infarction should immediately have a 12-lead electrocardiogram performed in the emergency department. The diagnosis of Q-wave myocardial infarction is suggested by Q waves and ST-segment elevation greater than 1 mm in two or more adjacent leads, reflecting the distribution of a single coronary artery. There are usually reciprocal leads that demonstrate depression in the ST segments. Anterior-wall myocardial infarction is suggested by Q waves and ST-segment elevation followed by T-wave inversion in the precordial leads, with reciprocal ST-segment depression in the inferior leads. It usually reflects coronary occlusion in the distribution of the left anterior descending artery. Inferior myocardial infarction is diagnosed by the presence of Q waves and ST-segment elevation in leads II, III, and F, with reciprocal ST-segment depression across the precordium. It usually results from acute thrombotic occlusion of the circumflex or right coronary artery. Lateral-wall myocardial infarction is diagnosed by Q waves and ST-segment elevation in leads 1, AVL, V_5, and V_6. It usually results from occlusion of the obtuse marginal branch of the circumflex vessel or the first diagonal branch of the left anterior descending artery. ST segment shifts or T-wave inversion, or both, in similar lead distributions in the absence of evolving Q waves indicate non–Q-wave infarction in the myocardial distribution of the respective coronary artery.

Early in the course of a myocardial infarction the T waves may become tall and peaked, resembling those seen in hyperkalemia (Fig. 19-1). These hyperacute T waves are usually a very transient phenomenon, rarely lasting more than a few hours, and are probably seen only several times a year in a busy emergency department. More commonly, patients present with one of three ECG patterns: subendocardial ischemia (Fig. 19-2), intramural infarction (Fig. 19-3), or transmural infarction (Fig. 19-4A). In subendocardial infarction, which is usually seen in older patients with rather large hemodynamically compromising infarcts, there are widespread ST depressions. In an intramural infarct, there are localized T-wave inversions without QRS abnormalities. In transmural infarction, we see the evolution of classic ST elevation (Fig. 19-5A), T-wave inversion, and Q-wave development (Fig. 19-5B). The differentiation between acute transmural infarction and acute pericarditis (Fig. 19-5) by ECG may be difficult.

It must be emphasized that the emergency department diagnosis of myocardial infarction must be reliably established on the basis of the patient's overall clinical presentation and the electrocardiographic findings. The emergency physician cannot generally rely on the rapid performance of serum enzyme analyses to confirm or refute the presence of acute myocardial necrosis. The total CPK may not rise significantly for five to seven hours after the onset of the acute thrombotic coronary artery occlusion responsible for myocyte necrosis (Fig. 19-6). This interval is required for the intracellular myocardial enzymes to permeate the deteriorating myocyte membrane and ultimately return to the circulation through venules and lymphatics. Though this ultimately results in a reliable and clinically meaningful elevation of the serum enzyme concentration, the time course is insufficiently rapid to allow enzyme analyses to be useful for the prospective diagnosis of myocardial infarction. The additional turnaround time for performance of the enzyme assays preclude this information from being prospectively useful in establishing the diagnosis of myocardial infarction with its protean implications; the need for coronary care unit triage; and consideration of acute revascularization strategies including thrombolytic therapy.

TREATMENT

Oxygen

Oxygen at two to four liters per minute via nasal cannula is administered to correct the mild arterial hypoxia that is al-

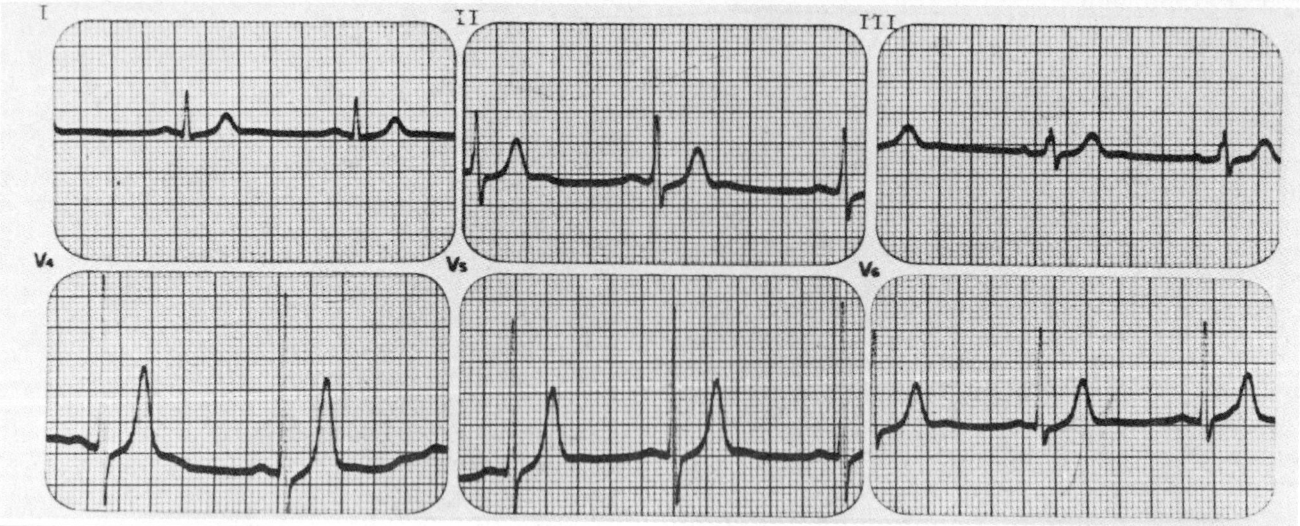

Fig. 19-1. Leads I, II, III, V_4, V_5, V_6 are shown. Tall, peaked, symmetrical (hyperacute) T waves, best seen in leads V_4 and V_5, can occasionally be the earliest sign of myocardial infarction.

most always present in patients with acute myocardial infarction. This results from ventilation-perfusion imbalance consequent to the elevation in mean left atrial and pulmonary artery wedge pressure, which is associated with systolic and diastolic left ventricular dysfunction and is characteristic of acute myocardial infarction.

Intravenous Access

Placement of an 18-gauge, intravenous plastic cannula into a reliable vein in the upper extremity should be rapidly accomplished. Through this procedure blood specimens for diagnostic evaluation are obtained. These should include a complete blood count, platelet count, prothrombin time, partial thrombin time, blood urea nitrogen, creatinine, glucose, and electrolytes, as well as cardiac enzymes. Access is maintained with a freely running IV line of D_5W at 10 to 20 ml per hour. If hypotension is a problem, the patient is placed in Trendelenburg's position; normal saline, one liter, should be administered at 250 to 500 ml per hour until the blood pressure rises, or until the specific cause of the hypotension can be elucidated and more specific treatment instituted. In more severely ill patients with evidence of congestive heart failure or shock, this frequently requires bedside right-heart catheterization with a flow-directed balloon-tipped catheter, performed in the coronary care unit.

Reliable vascular access is required for administration of antiarrhythmic drugs, opiate analgesic agents, and/or vasopressors should the need arise. It should be noted that drugs with potent alpha-adrenergic–stimulating properties such as dopamine or norepinephrine (indicated when arterial pressure falls below 90 mm Hg systolic) should not be administered through a peripheral IV line. Should infiltration occur, the intense arterial constriction resulting from the potent

Fig. 19-2. Leads I, II, III, V_4, V_5, V_6 are shown. There is subendocardial ischemia, with 1 mm ST-segment depression in lead I and 2-4 mm ST-segment depression in leads V_4–V_6. The persistence of these ST-segment depressions would differentiate infarction from angina.

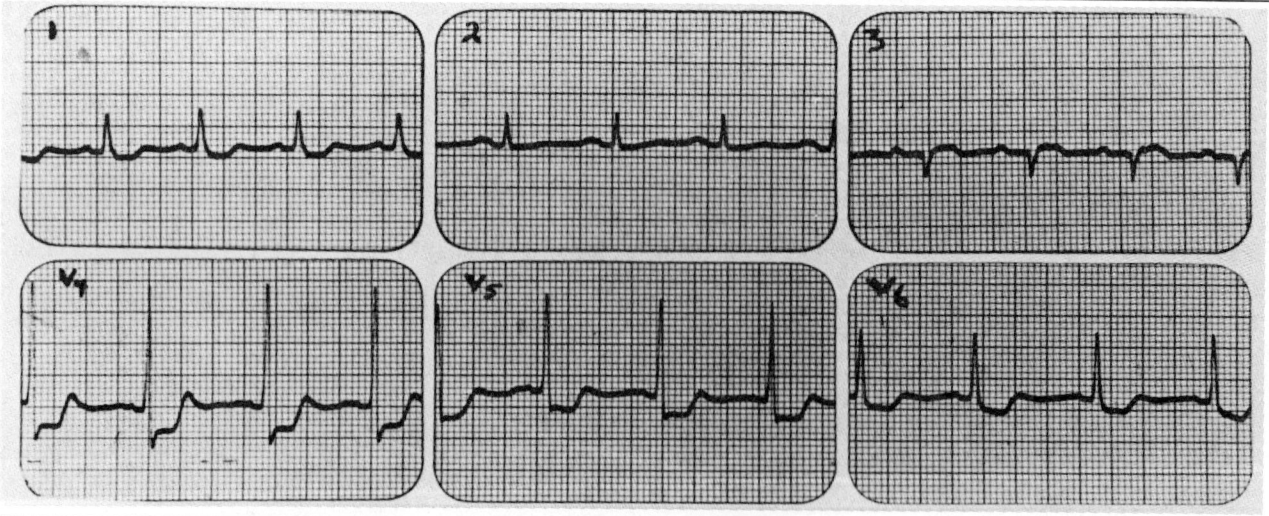

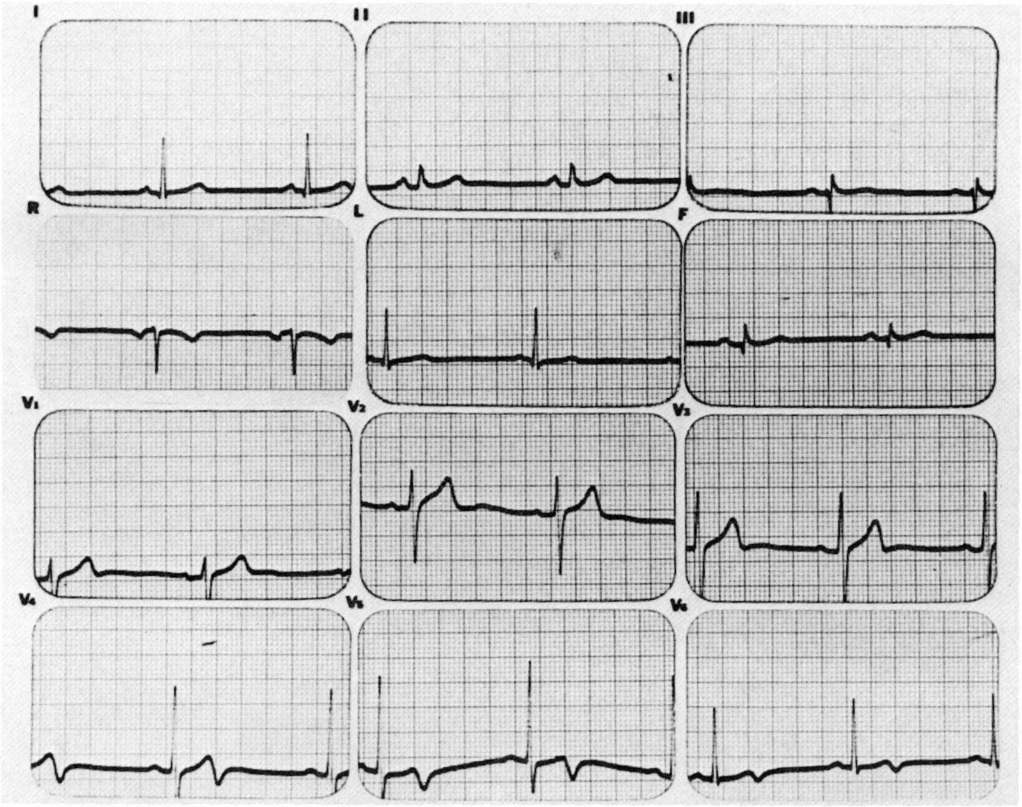

Fig. 19-3. Twelve-lead electrocardiogram demonstrates biphasic T waves in V_4–V_6 in a patient who has sustained an intramural infarction. There are no pathological Q waves and no loss of R waves. Therefore, no electrocardiographic evidence exists for transmural infarction.

alpha-adrenergic action of these agents may produce skin necrosis. Should infiltration of a peripheral IV line through which a potent alpha-adrenergic agent is being administered occur, immediate subcutaneous regional infiltration with a parenteral alpha-blocking agent such as phentolamine is indicated to reverse vasconstriction and prevent cutaneous ischemic injury.

Monitoring

The patient should be connected immediately to a portable ECG monitor capable of continuous oscilloscopic display of the ECG. Ideally, this should also have the capability of hard copy generation to facilitate rapid detection, diagnosis, and treatment of potentially life-threatening arrhythmias.

Patient Positions

It is important to position the patient comfortably with the head and thorax elevated approximately 45 degrees above the horizontal plane. This positioning will offset the gravitational propensity for development of pulmonary congestion.

Pain Relief

In the patient who lacks unequivocal ECG changes diagnostic of myocardial ischemia (ST-segment depression and T-wave inversion), it is reasonable to first attempt analgesia with sublingual nitroglycerin, 0.15 to 0.30 mg. This can be repeated once or twice over the next three to six minutes. If this treatment offers prompt relief, the clinical implication is that the patient is indeed afflicted with acute myocardial ischemia that has not as yet evolved into myocardial infarction. If sublingual nitroglycerin fails to relieve the pain, or if an obvious current of injury or an evolving transmural infarction pattern (Q waves and elevation of the ST segments), or both, are seen on the 12-lead ECG, it is prudent to administer morphine sulfate, 2 to 3 mg intravenously every 5 to 10 minutes, titrated to achieve satisfactory pain relief. If the systolic blood pressure drops below 100 mm Hg, the patient should be placed in Trendelenburg's position and a few hundred milliliters crystalloid should be rapidly administered to correct the hypotension. When using morphine or other narcotic analgesics, it is important to avoid respiratory depression due to hypoventilation (arterial carbon dioxide tension exceeding 45 mm Hg). However, in the patient with acute pulmonary edema, should a modest dose of morphine as just outlined result in respiratory depression or excessive obtundation, it is prudent to immediately intubate the trachea and ventilate the patient rather than to pharmacologically reverse the excessive narcotic effect with naloxone.

Relief of Myocardial Ischemia

In the patient with chest pain, ECG changes suggestive of evolving Q-wave infarction, and a systolic blood pressure exceeding 110 mm Hg, it is appropriate to start intravenous nitroglycerin at 5 to 10 μg per minute, slowly titrated up-

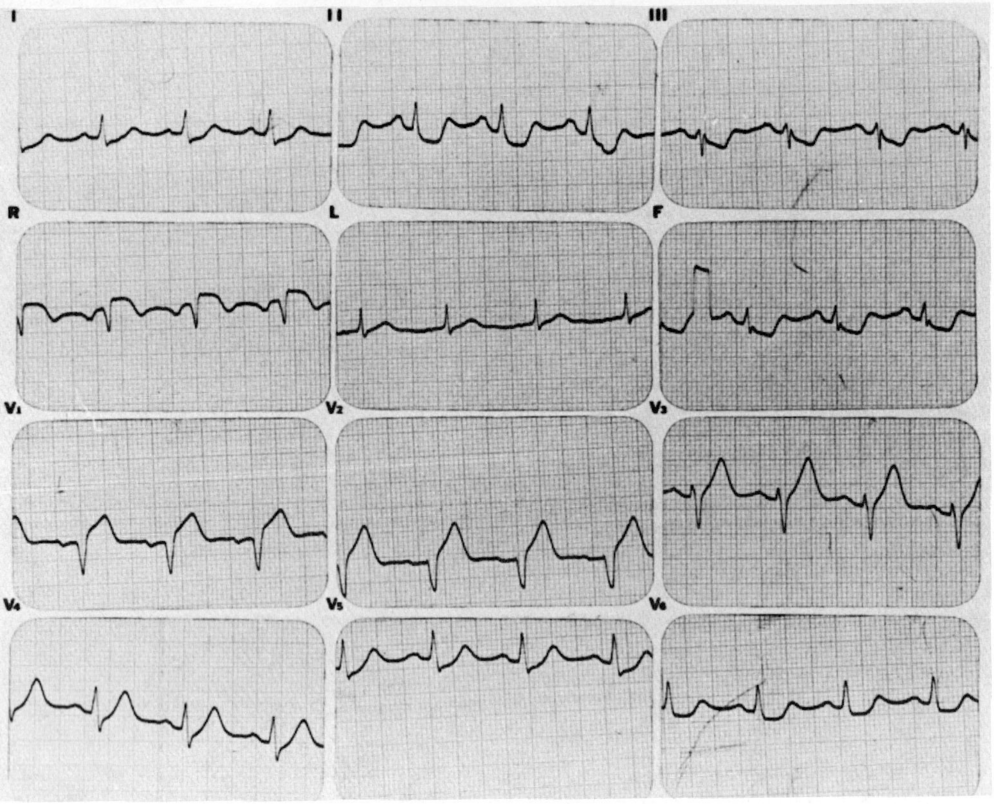

A

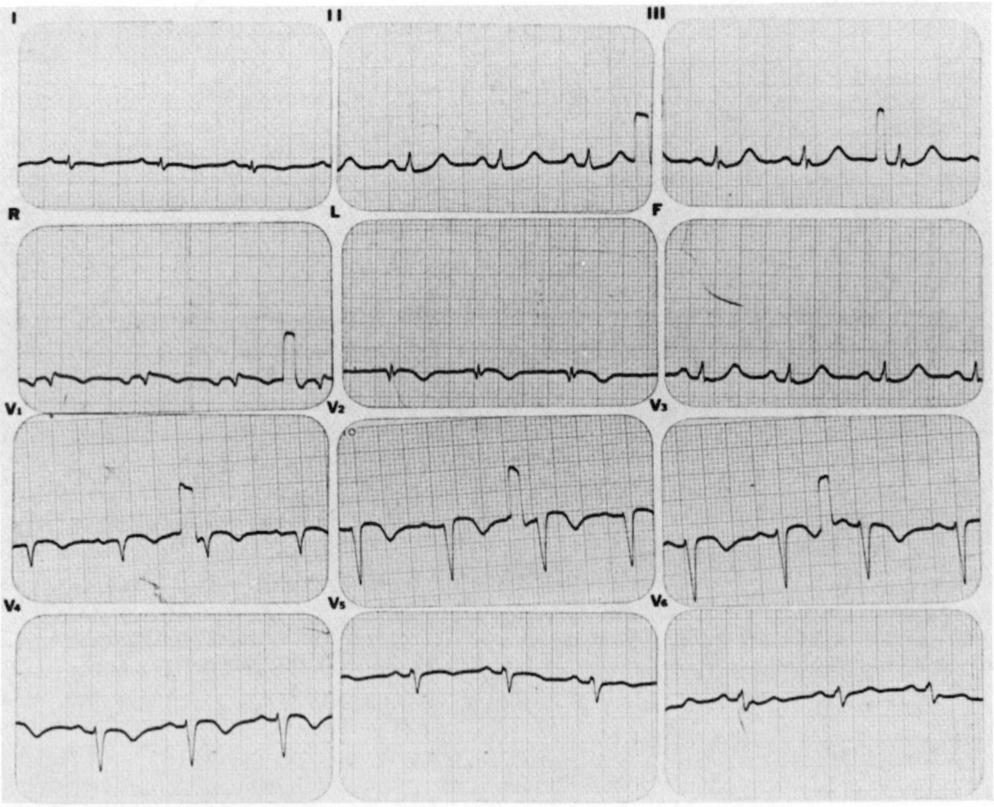

B

Fig. 19-4. A. Twelve-lead electrocardiogram from a 67-year-old woman demonstrates acute transmural anteroseptal infarction with ST-segment elevation in V_1, V_2. There is reciprocal ST-segment depression inferiorly (II, III, AVF) and laterally (V_6). (Tracing kindly supplied by Dr. L. Frederick Kaplan, Leonard Morse Hospital, Natick, MA). B. Twelve-lead electrocardiogram demonstrates evolution of transmural infarction in the same patient. This tracing was taken two days later. Note development of Q waves and the new loss of R waves in V_1, V_2. T-wave inversion has developed in leads V_1–V_4. The reciprocal ST-segment depression inferolaterally has resolved.

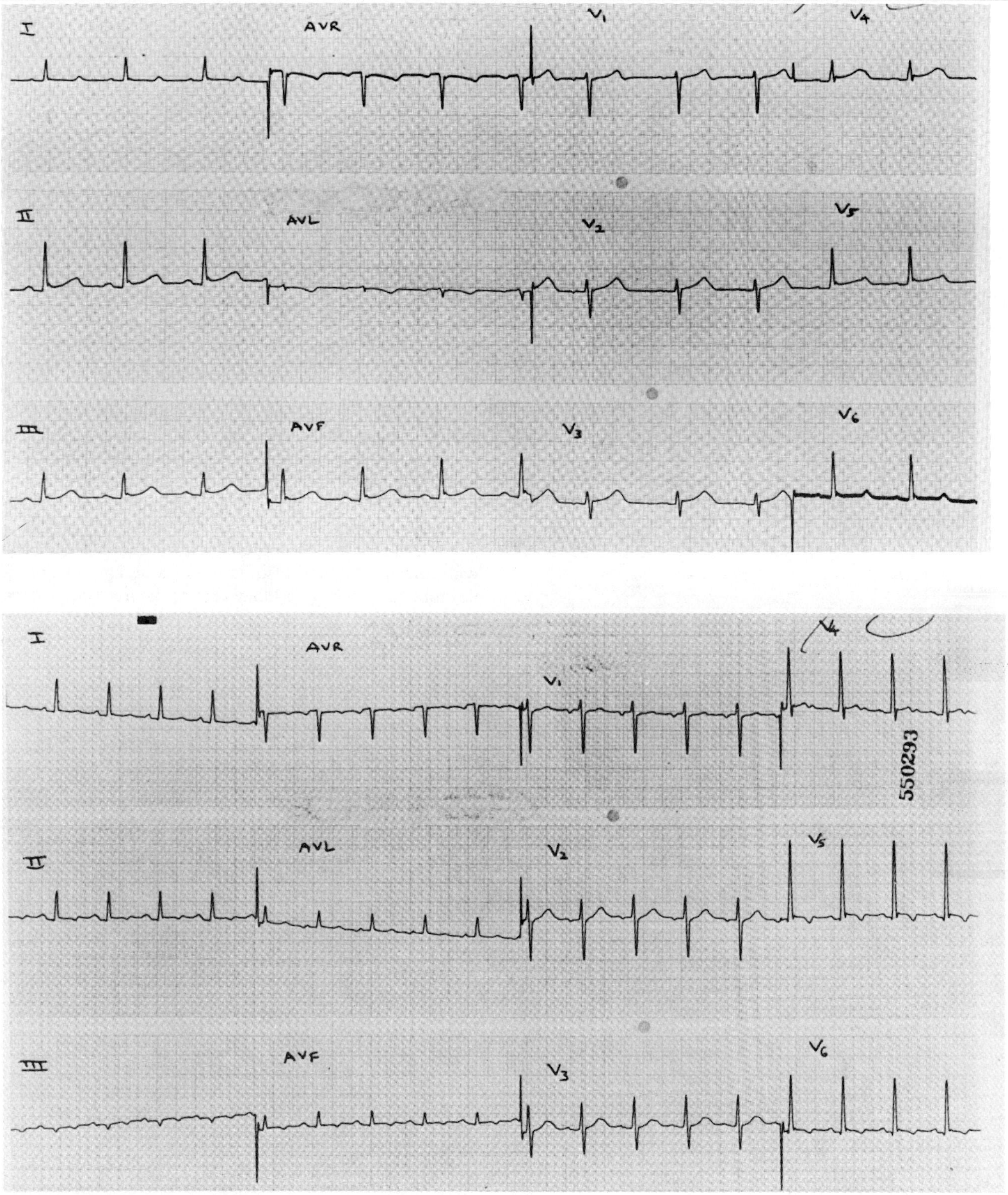

Fig. 19-5. A. Twelve-lead electrocardiogram demonstrates acute pericarditis in a 57-year-old man after aortic valve replacement. There is ST-segment elevation in leads I, II, III, AVF, V_2–V_6 with reciprocal ST-segment depression in endocardial lead aVr. Leads II, III, AVF have PR segments that suggest slight (0.5 mm) downward sloping depression. B. Twelve-lead electrocardiogram demonstrates evolution of acute pericarditis in same patient four days later. The inferolateral (II, III, AVF, V_4–V_6) T waves have inverted and the ST segments have returned toward normal.

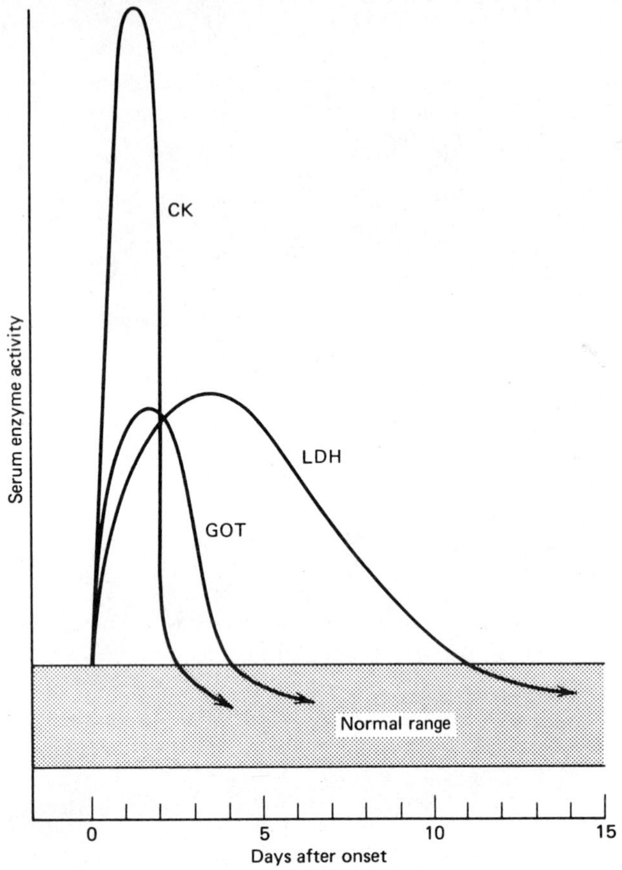

Fig. 19-6. Time course of release of cardiac enzymes during acute myocardial infarction. Creatine phosphokinase (CK) is released first, followed by glutamic-oxaloacetic transaminase (GOT) and lactic dehydrogenase (LDH).

ward by 5 to 10 μg per minute every 5 to 10 minutes. The end point is to reduce the systolic blood pressure no more than 10 to 15 mm Hg while not allowing it to fall below 105 to 115 mm Hg systolic. Nitroglycerin reduces the myocardial demand for oxygen, improves collateral flow into the area of ischemia-infarction, relieves pulmonary congestion, and may reduce infarct size. In the patient with acute myocardial infarction and hypertension, the addition of nitroprusside may also be required to reduce the systolic blood pressure below 130 to 140 mm Hg. It is important to institute intravenous nitroglycerin only in patients with clear-cut ECG changes suggestive of subendocardial ischemia or injury (ST-segment depression or T-wave inversion, or both) or in patients with a transmural injury current on the ECG (ST-segment elevation).

Antiarrhythmia Therapy

In the patient with an appropriate clinical story and unequivocal ECG evidence of transmural myocardial infarction with or without the presence of ventricular premature beats, intravenous lidocaine is indicated. It is administered intravenously as a slow bolus to a total dose of 1 to 2 mg/kg. A continuous lidocaine infusion at 2 mg per minute is started immediately. Such prophylactic treatment has been shown to reduce the incidence of primary ventricular fibrillation during the first two or three days after myocardial infarction.

Thrombolytic Therapy

Several thrombolytic agents have been shown to lyse coronary artery thrombi and restore coronary arterial patency. This was first demonstrated with agents administered via the intracoronary route and then by the intravenous route. The therapeutic rationale is based on the fact that acute coronary thrombosis is the proximate cause of myocardial infarction. Rapid pharmacologic dissolution of the thrombus through intravenous administration of a thrombolytic agent restores coronary-artery perfusion, lessens ventricular damage, and improves survival.

The most important determinant of prognosis after myocardial infarction is the cumulative extent of ventricular damage. This can be lessened and prognosis improved with the prompt intravenous administration of thrombolytic agents. It appears that the size of the myocardial infarction can be reduced and prognosis improved in direct proportion to the rapidity with which the coronary artery thrombus can be dissolved and coronary artery perfusion be reestablished through prompt administration of thrombolytic agents. Administration of aspirin and acute intravenous beta-blockade with metoprolol are also important in conjunction with thrombolytic therapy, as they reduce the frequency of recurrent myocardial ischemia after infarction.

Intravenously administered streptokinase (SK) and tissue plasminogen activator made from recombinant deoxyribonucleic acid (DNA) technology (rt-PA) have been approved as thrombolytic agents useful in the treatment of patients with acute, evolving, transmural myocardial infarction. The rationale is that either of these drugs rapidly lyses the coronary thrombi responsible for myocardial infarction in 60 to 90 percent of patients when they are administered rapidly (within four hours) after the onset of myocardial infarction (as measured by the elapsed time since the patient's first symptoms of chest pain). This restores coronary artery reperfusion to the infarct zone, reduces the size of the resultant myocardial infarction, and enhances hospital and one-year survival.

Thrombolytic therapy also may reduce the likelihood of structural complications following myocardial infarction (septal rupture, ventricular perforation, papillary muscle infarction, and rupture). To guarantee maximum therapeutic benefit, thrombolytic therapy should be administered within four to six hours of acute myocardial infarction onset to prevent myocardial necrosis. However, even when streptokinase has been administered up to 24 hours after chest-pain onset, patients seem to derive benefit. This may be because reperfusion, even though late, attenuates subepicardial structural myocardial injury to reduce the propensity for late infarct expansion with development of a late reentrant ventricular arrhythmia.

Previously, streptokinase administered directly into the occluded culprit coronary artery had been approved by the Food and Drug Administration as an effective agent to dissolve the coronary thrombus. However, intracoronary thrombolytic therapy for acute myocardial infarction is impractical and expensive. Less than 20 percent of hospitals in the United States have catheterization facilities, and only a fraction of these are staffed for round-the-clock operation. There is also an obligatory delay of one to three hours between the emergency department diagnosis of myocardial infarction and the administration of a thrombolytic agent via a catheter positioned in the coronary artery.

It is very important to underscore the overwhelming importance of expeditious emergency department triage and early clinical assessment in patients with chest pain. This must be conducted in a very thorough but rapid fashion. It includes obtaining vital signs, excluding the presence of active bleeding or other contraindications to thrombolytic therapy, determining the adequacy of overall cardiovascular compensation, performing a 12-lead ECG that is immediately interpreted by a capable physician, administering oxygen via nasal cannula, and establishing at least two reliable IV lines (no smaller than an 18-gauge catheter or plastic cannula). No unnecessary venous or arterial punctures should be performed and arterial puncture for the performance of blood gases should not be done routinely. Baseline diagnostic blood hematologic and chemistry studies should be obtained and ordered as outlined previously. It is important to obtain a red top tube so that the patient's blood can be typed and screened by the blood bank.

A rapid history and physical examination should be completed to determine if the patient has an overall clinical picture compatible with myocardial infarction. Administration of sublingual nitroglycerin is reasonable to rule out reversible myocardial ischemia (angina) or coronary spasm, as outlined previously. It is important that all of this be performed over a very abbreviated time frame to confirm the diagnosis and identify the presence of any absolute or relative contraindications to thrombolytic agents.

The two agents presently approved as thrombolytic agents in the treatment of myocardial infarction are SK and t-PA. The advantages of SK include cost, since it is approximately one-tenth as expensive as t-PA. Disadvantages include the behavior of SK as a nonspecific fibrinolytic agent. It depletes the circulating blood of fibrin and a number of other vital coagulation factors to introduce a lytic state (circulating fibrinogen concentration below 100 mg% or 50 percent of lower-limit-normal fibrinogen concentration), which can increase the risk of bleeding. Streptokinase, as a bacterial protein, is antigenic. It can cause fevers, chills, urticaria, or bronchospasm. Because of its nonspecific proteolytic effects, SK can produce a number of vasoactive peptides that cause hypotension during and shortly after its administration. However, this condition usually responds promptly to fluid or pressor administration. Streptokinase is most effective only within the first three hours of coronary thrombosis. Its efficacy as a thrombolytic agent for coronary artery clots older than two to three hours is clearly reduced relative to tPA.

A major advantage of t-PA is that it is nonallergenic. It also appears to be somewhat selective, preferentially activating plasminogen already bound to fibrin thrombi. As it is relatively inactive against circulating procoagulants, t-PA does not usually produce a systemic lytic state. However, the incidence of significant bleeding (requiring transfusion) with t-PA or SK is similar (<5 percent). Indeed, the risk of serious intracranial hemorrhage (approximately 0.5 percent) may be higher with t-PA than with streptokinase according to some studies.

When SK and t-PA were directly compared, it was shown that in patients who received either thrombolytic agent at a mean time of 4.5 hours after the onset of myocardial infarction, t-PA was nearly twice as effective as SK in recanalizing totally occluded coronary arteries. In several investigations in which SK was administered earlier (within two to three hours of infarct onset) and the patients underwent coronary angiography a few hours later, patency of the infarct-related artery was established in 70 to 90 percent of patients. No direct comparative study of infarct artery patency or reperfusion rates, mortality, or ventricular function in patients with myocardial infarction treated with either SK or t-PA in a controlled blinded fashion has as yet been published. However, t-PA appears to be a more effective thrombolytic agent.

Streptokinase is administered intravenously as 1.5 million units over 60 minutes. Tissue plasminogen activator is administered as a 10-mg slow IV bolus over one minute, 50 mg intravenously over the first hour, and 20 mg intravenously over the second and third hours. A total of 100 mg is given over three hours.

Eligibility criteria for thrombolytic treatment of myocardial infarction include:

I. Patient history consistent with acute myocardial infarction
   A. Prolonged (greater than 30 minutes) ischemic-type pain unrelieved with sublingual nitroglycerin
   B. Electrocardiographic evidence of evolving transmural myocardial infarction
      1. At least 1-mm ST-segment elevation in at least two or more inferior leads (II, III, AVF) or I and AVL
      2. At least 1- to 2-mm ST-segment elevation in at least two contiguous precordial leads (V_1–V_6)

II. Onset of pain less than four to six hours before initiation of thrombolytic agents

III. No contraindications to thrombolytic therapy

Absolute contraindications to thrombolytic treatment include any past history of stroke (cerebrovascular accident), symptoms compatible with transient ischemic attacks, or active bleeding. Major relative contraindications include pregnancy or recent delivery, recent puncture of a noncompressible artery or vein (especially the subclavian or internal jugular vein), prolonged cardiopulmonary resuscitation (more than one minute), history of recent gastrointestinal bleeding, malignant long-standing hypertension, recent severe trauma, surgery within the previous two weeks, and primary or metastatic cancer. Where there is an absolute contraindication to thrombolytic therapy, alternative reperfusion strategies include immediate coronary arteriography with intracoronary administration of a thrombolytic agent, percutaneous transluminal coronary angioplasty, or coronary-artery revascularization surgery.

Minor and relative contraindications to thrombolytic therapy include age exceeding 75 years, nonmalignant hypertension (systolic blood pressure greater than 110 mm Hg), diabetic retinopathy, left bundle branch block, bleeding disorder, active menstruation, endocarditis, concomitant anticoagulation therapy, recent minor trauma, or other advanced illnesses. The following conditions are not contraindications to thrombolytic therapy: hypotension, cardiogenic shock, previous myocardial infarction, Q waves on the electrocardiogram, heart block, or history of previous bypass surgery.

In the patient with myocardial infarction, lidocaine should be started at a 1- to 2-mg/kg IV loading dose, followed by an IV infusion at 2 mg per minute. In patients undergoing thrombolytic therapy, lidocaine may prevent the accelerated idioventricular rhythm or frequent premature ventricular contractions that commonly occur with reperfusion.

The patient with myocardial infarction should be heparinized after receiving thrombolytic therapy. This is accomplished by administering 100 units/kg as an IV loading dose shortly after the administration of t-PA. The bolus dose is followed by infusion of heparin at 20 units/kg per hour by continuous IV infusion through a constant-rate infusion pump. The goal is to prolong the partial thromboplastin time to 2 to 2½ times over control. This should be checked approximately four to six hours after IV heparin is instituted and four to six hours after upward or downward adjustment in the maintenance heparin dose. Heparin should not be administered for several hours after administration of SK until the thrombin time has returned to approximately two times that of control (usually 12–24 hours after SK administration).

Treatment with aspirin, 325 mg per day, in conjunction with thrombolytic therapy reduces the incidence of recurrent ischemic events. Likewise, rapid intravenous beta-blockade with metoprolol, administered slowly as an intravenous bolus over 1 minute (5 mg per dose, up to three doses, or a total of 15 mg), has been shown to reduce the likelihood of recurrent myocardial ischemic events after myocardial infarction. Contraindications to beta-blockade include symptomatic bradycardia, heart block (unless a pacemaker is in place), insulin-dependent diabetes with a history of insulin reaction, active asthma, or severe congestive heart failure with a third heart sound present.

The patient with acute myocardial infarction manifested by acute pulmonary edema should receive intravenous morphine (2–4 mg); oxygen should be administered by nasal cannula or face mask, and intravenous nitroglycerin or nitroprussides should be given to lower the blood pressure if it is above 120 mm Hg. The patient should also undergo diuresis (furosemide, 10–20 mg intravenously, titrated to induce diuresis in excess of 150 ml per hour for three to four hours). Careful attention must be paid to blood gas and acid-base derangements. Supplemental oxygen for arterial hypoxemia, mechanical ventilation for carbon dioxide retention with respiratory acidosis, and judicious sodium bicarbonate administration for metabolic acidosis ($pH < 7.2$) as a consequence of shock and organ hypoperfusion with lactic acidoses may be indicated. The serum potassium should be maintained in excess of 4.2 mEq per liter with supplemental potassium.

With the development of fibrinolytic treatment therapy for acute myocardial infarction, the emergency department physician has assumed preeminence in the management of patients with syndromes of acute myocardial ischemia. Rapid diagnosis with administration of a thrombolytic agent for acute myocardial infarction increases the patient's likelihood of survival and presence of ventricular function, and may improve the patient's quality of life. Conversely, inaccuracies in diagnosis or administration of thrombolytic agents where contraindicated (patients with active bleeding or cerebrovascular disease) may result in life-threatening hemorrhage. With thrombolytic therapy the realization that "time is muscle" has placed a great deal of responsibility and medicolegal culpability directly on the emergency physician for rapid diagnosis of acute myocardial infarction and the decision to either treat with or withhold a thrombolytic agent. Rapid identification of patients with myocardial infarction and screening for contraindications to thrombolytic treatment are vital. Rapid diagnosis of other life-threatening conditions mimicking myocardial infarction, for which specific and potentially life-saving therapy must be quickly instituted, is equally important.

TRANSFER OF THE PATIENT

As soon as the patient with acute myocardial infarction is somewhat stabilized with respect to control of arterial pressure, pain, and arrhythmia, he or she should be rapidly transferred from the emergency department to the coronary care unit. Transfer should always be undertaken with the following:

1. Continuous oscilloscopic monitoring of the electrocardiogram with immediate access to a defibrillator
2. Oxygen by nasal cannula
3. At least two large-bore, free-running IV lines; through one lidocaine is administered at 2 mg per minute for prophylaxis against ventricular fibrillation; through the other line nitroglycerin is administered at 50 to 200 μg per minute, titrated to lower blood pressure to 110 to 120 mm Hg systolic in order to reduce infarct size
4. A physician or paramedical personnel trained in advanced cardiac life support to accompany the patient; there should be immediate access to the drugs and standard resuscitative equipment available on a standard advanced cardiac life support code cart

PROGNOSIS

The mortality from myocardial infarction has been reduced to between 5 and 10 percent with the advent of thrombolytic therapy, beta-blockade, aspirin, and anticoagulation. These measures have been developed and recorded into direct clinical practice and evolved since the publication of the first edition of *Emergency Medicine*. Diagnostic factors that favorably affect hospital survival of the patient with an acute myocardial infarct include younger age, male sex, infarct location in the inferior or posterior distribution, first myocardial infarction, good preservation of overall left-ventricular performance (ejection fraction 0.55 or better after infarction), freedom from ventricular ectopic activity after the first 72 hours following myocardial infarction, prompt receptors of an intravenous thrombolytic agent, and treatment with a beta-blocker. Factors associated with a less favorable prognosis include older age, female sex, infarct location in the anterior wall of the left ventricle, history of previous myocardial infarction, congestive heart failure due to significant systolic left-ventricular dysfunction (ejection fraction under 0.45), and ventricular ectopic activity (more than one premature ventricular beat per minute) in the late hospital phase of recovery from myocardial infarction (after the first three to five days after infarction). Current revascularization strategies including thrombolytic therapy in the majority of patients and mechanical revascularization (by angioplasty or coronary bypass surgery in carefully selected patients) have improved hospital survival to approximately 95 percent.

Any further reduction in myocardial infarct mortality is predicated on patient education. This includes measures to alter lifestyle in order to reduce one's risk for development of coronary artery disease. Patients must also be educated to minimize delay in seeking medical attention should symptoms compatible with acute and unrelenting myocardial ischemia develop. Infarct mortality should decline with education of the public as to the importance of immediate presentation to a hospital emergency department (rather than placing a call to one's primary physician and awaiting its return) whenever symptoms suggestive of myocardial ischemia occur.

SELECTED READING

Alpert, JS, and Francis, GS. *Manual of Coronary Care* (4th ed). Boston: Little, Brown, 1987.

Gruppo Italiano per lo Studio della Streptochinasi nell-Infarcto Miocardio (GISSI). Effectiveness of intravenous thrombolytic treatment in acute myocardial infarction. *Lancet* 1:397, 1986.

ISAM Study Group. A prospective trial of intravenous streptokinase in acute myocardial infarction (ISAM). *N Engl J Med* 314:1465, 1986.

Johns, JA, Gold, HK, and Leinbad, RC. Acute Myocardial Infarction. In KA Engle et al. (eds), *The Practice of Cardiology*. Boston/Toronto: Little, Brown, 1989. Pp 403-454.

Pasternack, RC, Braunwald, E, and Alpert, JS. Acute Myocardial Infarction. In E Braunwald et al. (eds), *Harrison's Principles of Internal Medicine* (11th ed). New York: McGraw-Hill, 1987. Pp 982–992.

Pasternack, RC, Braunwald, E, and Sobel, BE. Acute Myocardial Infarction. In E Braunwald (ed), *Heart Disease: A Textbook of Cardiovascular Medicine* (3rd ed). Philadelphia: Saunders, 1988. Pp 1222-1313.

TIMI Study Group. The Thrombolysis in Myocardial Infarction (TIMI) Trial: Phase I findings. *N Engl J Med* 312:932, 1985.

20. Cardiac Arrhythmias

Charles I. Haffajee

The purpose of this chapter is to provide a practical present-day approach to both cardiac bradyarrhythmias and tachyarrhythmias. As with most practical subjects in medicine, such information may be out of date by the time a textbook such as this is published. It is also important to recognize that cardiac arrhythmias rarely occur in isolation and often accompany heart disease, which should be addressed simultaneously with the specific arrhythmia therapy.

Several questions need to be entertained when confronting a patient with an arrhythmia in the emergency or acute care situation: (1) How and why did it take place? (2) What company does the arrhythmia keep? (3) Is there a history or suggestion of an acute myocardial infarction? (4) Should any specific tests beyond an electrocardiogram (ECG) and chest x-ray be performed before acute intervention for the arrhythmia? (5) After termination of the arrhythmia, what steps should be taken to diagnose the underlying cause and to prevent recurrences?

In the diagnosis and treatment of arrhythmias, an understanding of the fundamental mechanisms of arrhythmogenesis is helpful. A knowledge of the normal cardiac conduction system will aid in understanding how deviations from this result in arrhythmogenesis.

BASIC ANATOMY AND ELECTROPHYSIOLOGY OF THE CONDUCTION AND IMPULSE FORMING SYSTEM

A simple overview of the heart reveals that it is composed of atrial and ventricular muscle fibers, blood vessels, and specialized electrical tissues that generate and conduct impulses. These specialized electrical cells are responsible for the appropriate sequence and rate of contraction of the heart that is synchronized to the cardiac output.

The physiologic pacemaker is the sinus node located at the junction of the superior vena cava and right atrium; its impulses are generated spontaneously and are influenced by physiologic, pathologic, and pharmacologic states. The normal heart rate is 60 to 100 beats per minute (bpm). The formed impulse leaves the sinus node, then traverses the atrium through three specialized atrial internodal tracts into the atrioventricular (AV) node, which is an elongated structure just below the septal leaflet of the tricuspid valve near the ostium of the coronary sinus. The AV nodal tissue penetrates the interventricular septum as the His-Purkinje network and then divides into a discrete right bundle branch and more distal left bundle branch of specialized electrical tissue. Both bundles spread to the endocardial septal surfaces and the left bundle divides further into anterior and posterior bundles. Numerous ramifications of these bundles spread and link throughout the right and left ventricles, allowing an electrical impulse to spread very rapidly from the

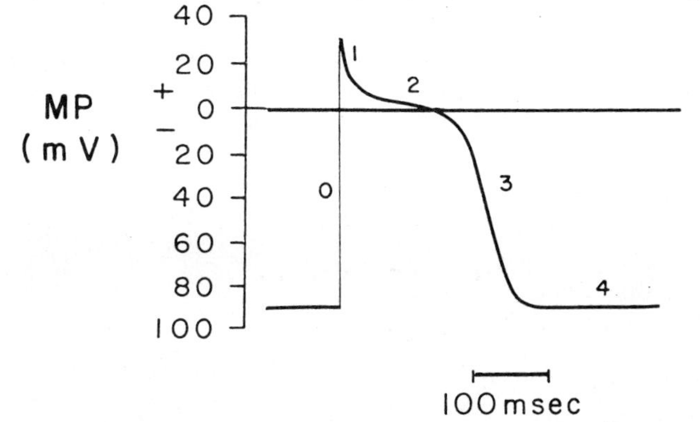

Fig. 20-1. An action potential with its four phases. (MP = membrane potential.)

AV node throughout the ventricles so as to result in an almost instantaneous depolarization of the entire ventricular muscle mass of the heart.

The electrically active cells maintain an electrical potential across their cell membranes. Spontaneous or active discharge of these cells will result in an action potential that is depicted in Fig. 20-1. The action potential is divided into four phases. Two basic types of action potentials are generated by the heart cells. The automatic or spontaneous discharging cells (sinus and AV node tissue) have a gradually upsloping phase 4 that will result in spontaneous discharge when it reaches a critical threshold potential (−50 mV); this is then followed by a slower phase 0 and phase 1 with little overshoot. This is in contrast to cells that are actively depolarized, such as Purkinje fibers or muscle cells (atrial, ventricular), which have a stable resting phase-4 potential that requires an active process to lower its transmembrane potential (−90 mV) so as to discharge or contract. These cells have a rapid upstroke to phase 0 and phase 1 (depression phase) with overshoot that is followed by slower phase 2 and phase 3, which constitute repolarization (see Fig. 20-1). This is characteristic of the nonautomatic tissues in the heart.

The different phases of the action potential are the result of active and passive exchanges of ions through pores across the cell membranes. The inside of the cells at rest are relatively negative (−90 to −60 mV) during phase 4 of the action potential or resting potential. During this phase, either by spontaneous or by an active process, sodium ions enter the inside of the cell and potassium ions leave the cell, causing transmembrane potential to reach a critical level that results in discharge or the rapid phase 0 of the action potential, which corresponds to the QRS of the ECG. In pacemaker cells this is due to influx of calcium rather than sodium through slower calcium channels. Phase 1 then ensues, a brief, initial rapid depolarization phase that is followed by the slower phase 2 and the more rapid phase 3 repolarization phases (corresponding to the QT interval on the ECG). Phase 2 is due to slow inward movement of calcium ions with opposing outward flow of potassium. In contrast, during phase 3 there is unopposed outward flow of potassium from the cell. During the early portion of phase 4 (resting) action potential, sodium, potassium, and calcium ions are returned to their original transmembrane gradient levels.

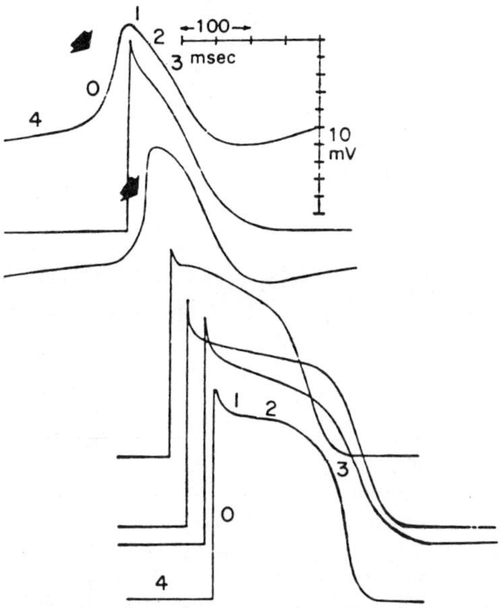

Fig. 20-2. The four phases of the action potential for the sinus node, AV node, His-Purkinje system, and ventricular muscle.

Once a pacing impulse is generated in the pacemaker tissue of the heart, it is transmitted in an orderly sequence throughout the specialized tissues of the heart. The different action potentials generated throughout the heart are depicted in Fig. 20-2.

There are three accepted "mechanisms" of arrhythmogenesis: automaticity, reentry (circus movement), and triggered automaticity. Under normal conditions the "automatic" electrical tissues such as sinus and AV nodes discharge spontaneously, and the faster-discharging sinus node prevails, resulting in the normal sinus rhythm of the heart (Fig. 20-3). From a knowledge of the sinus node action potential, it can be deduced that a drug such as verapamil that blocks or slows calcium entry into cells will slow the sinus node (and AV node) discharge rates (Fig. 20-3B). This can also occur under pathologic states and may then result in the slower subsidiary pacemaker in the heart becoming the dominant rhythm (junction rhythms) if the sinus node is selectively affected. Occasionally, the subsidiary pacemakers or Purkinje fibers become augmented and assume a dominant rhythm, which is referred to as *triggered automaticity* (Fig. 20-3C). This can result from acute ischemia, digitalis toxicity, hypocalcemia, or other electrolyte disturbances. This type of rhythm is due to "after-depolarizations" during phase 3 and phase 4 of the action potential.

The most common mechanism for arrhythmogenesis is reentry (Fig. 20-4). This occurs in abnormal cardiac tissue (e.g., infarct-related scars), in atrial disturbances, in the presence of functional dual pathways in AV node, and in the presence of accessory AV connections (Wolff-Parkinson-White [WPW] syndrome). Since an impulse can travel in either direction in electrical tissue, block or delay in one direction in an area can allow for retrograde penetration of the area by a propagated impulse from adjacent tissue. If an imbalance between refractoriness and conduction exists such that the "head" of an impulse can penetrate the "excit-

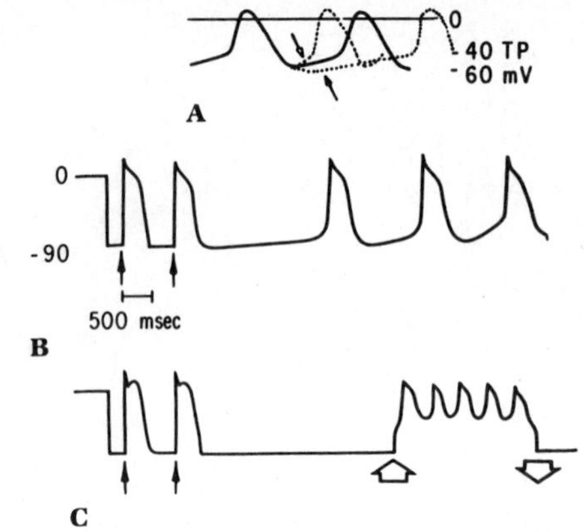

Fig. 20-3. Normal automaticity. A. A sinus node action potential. Spontaneous depolarization (phase 4) can cause automatic discharge or firing (normal automaticity). Change in the phase-4 slope, as depicted by arrows, can slow (*solid lines*) or increase (*open lines*) spontaneous automaticity. B. Action potentials of His-Purkinje fibers. The arrows show electrical stimulation; the three subsequent action potentials are generated spontaneously. C. Presence of "after-potentials" during phase 3 or 4 of the action potential, resulting in automatic firing of ventricular muscle (triggered automaticity). (TP = transmembrane potential.)

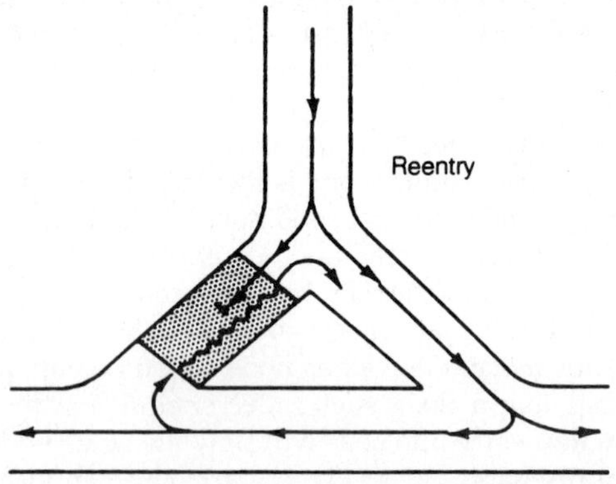

Fig. 20-4. Schematic model of reentry in an area of damaged ventricular muscle. Conduction in one limb is blocked antegradely and slow conduction occurs retrogradely in this limb after normal conduction in the opposite limb. This circuit then perpetuates itself (circus movement) with a shorter circuit time than sinus cycle length and takes over the rhythm of the heart.

able gap" between its head and the "tail" of refractoriness, then a reciprocating circuit can be established, resulting in reentrant, or circus-movement, tachycardia.

This mechanism may be the most common cause for clinical tachyarrhythmias. These arrhythmias can be initiated and terminated by timed extrasystoles or burst pacing. In contrast, arrhythmias with automaticity as their mechanism can be suppressed but not interrupted by overdrive pacing.

A *tachycardia* is said to exist if the heart rate exceeds 100 bpm. *Bradycardia* is usually defined as heart rate below 60 bpm.

MANIFESTATION OF ARRHYTHMIAS

Arrhythmias produce symptoms that depend on a variety of factors in any given patient. Some of the factors that determine arrhythmia manifestation are rate of arrhythmia, type of arrhythmia, underlying ventricular function, and level of ischemia that the arrhythmia produces or exacerbates. The clinical manifestations may be:

1. Palpitations
2. Presyncopal feelings, dizziness, weakness, lightheadedness
3. Syncope
4. Heart failure
5. Angina or chest pain
6. Sudden cardiac death

The normal heart can tolerate a wide range of heart rates even in the absence of atrioventricular synchrony without decompensation. It is not uncommon for normal hearts at rest to tolerate rates of 30 bpm or 250 bpm. However, when physical demand is increased, symptoms of low cardiac output may supervene in patients with normal hearts and earlier in patients with preexistent ventricular dysfunction when significant bradycardia or tachycardia occurs.

Tachycardia tends to shorten diastole so as to compromise ventricular filling. If atrial contraction is lost due to its absence (e.g., atrial fibrillation), dissociation (e.g., ventricular tachycardia), or improper timing (e.g., supraventricular tachycardia), then further compromise in ventricular filling can ensue, resulting in a drop in blood pressure, cardiac output, and coronary perfusion. Patients with certain diseases such as acute myocardial infarction, angina, or ventricular noncompliance (aortic stenosis, hypertension, or hypertrophic cardiomyopathy) are very dependent on the presence of appropriate atrial contraction. Similarly, bradycardia can compromise cardiac output as a result of the loss of atrial contraction, improper timing of atrial systole (AV dissociation), or marked sinus bradycardia, though it may be tolerated longer than most tachycardias.

Thus, it is important to assess both the arrhythmia and its tolerance by the patient to determine the urgency for intervention. For example, a patient with mitral stenosis who develops atrial fibrillation (Afib) and rapid ventricular response can be managed by measures such as digitalis therapy, beta-blockers, or calcium channel blockers to slow or moderate the ventricular response. On the other hand, the acute onset of Afib in patients with aortic stenosis or hypertrophic cardiomyopathy is best managed by urgent synchronized cardioversion (100–200 joules).

GENERAL PRINCIPLES IN MANAGEMENT OF ARRHYTHMIAS

The history, physical examination, ECG, and occasionally ancillary tests may have to be carefully analyzed and integrated to arrive at a working diagnosis for arrhythmias. The speed at which a diagnosis needs to be made may well depend on the patient's tolerance of the arrhythmia. However, a diagnosis should always be made, and both acute and preventive therapy are only successful and appropriate when the diagnosis of the arrhythmia and the underlying causative disease are known.

History

Underlying heart disease, prior drug therapy, previous arrhythmia episodes, and response to therapies can all be ascertained directly from the patient or relatives. Drug intoxication (such as digitalis, tricyclics, antiarrhythmic agents, beta-blockers) has to be considered, in addition to hypokalemia or other electrolyte disturbances that can occur as a result of diuretics or severe weight-reducing diets. Excessive alcohol consumption, cocaine, or other cardiotoxic agents should also be considered. The duration of the arrhythmia and symptoms caused by the arrhythmia should then be assessed. Response of prior episodes to Valsalva maneuvers or drugs may help determine therapy. If chest pain is present, it is important to determine if it preceded the arrhythmia (as with acute myocardial infarction).

Physical Examination

The general appearance of the patient, state of circulatory perfusion, blood pressure, mental status, and temperature may aid in determining the effects of the arrhythmia. The 12-lead ECG of the arrhythmia will help in guiding therapy but often the desire for acute intervention may appear not to permit time for an ECG. This temptation must be resisted where possible since an accurate diagnosis of arrhythmia may not be possible in the absence of a 12-lead ECG during the arrhythmia. If hemodynamic collapse is not present, a full physical examination, 12-lead ECG, and rhythm strip can provide important clues.

During the neck-vein examination, an assessment of the level and wave form of the jugular veins can provide information on atrial activity, which may be difficult to assess even with a 12-lead ECG. Intermittent a waves (e.g., AV block) or absent a waves (e.g., Afib) may be noted or more a waves than v waves (2:1 AV block) may be seen. Large, intermittent cannon waves are diagnostic of heart block whereas rapid a waves following closely or coinciding with v waves are suggestive of AV nodal tachycardias.

Analysis of the heart sounds and murmurs may reveal evidence for valvular heart disease, Afib, or heart failure (gallops). Variability of heart sounds, with intermittent cannon waves, rapid heart rate, and intermittent gallop sounds, often suggests ventricular tachycardia, which frequently is difficult to diagnose from the ECG. Presence of valvular disease should be noted.

In the general examination it is important to search for other diseases with arrhythmia manifestations, such as thyrotoxicosis, pulmonary disease, sarcoid, and collagen-vascular diseases.

Electrocardiogram

A 12-lead ECG with a sufficient rhythm strip is critical for the diagnosis of the arrhythmia. The approach to the ECG must be systematic and reasonably rapid. The following questions should be asked:

1. What is the rate of the arrhythmia?
2. Are P waves visible? Are the P waves normal and what is their relationship to the QRS complex? If P waves are absent, are there atrial fibrillatory or flutter waves or is there atrial standstill or sinus arrest?
3. Is the QRS complex normal or wide (>0.12 seconds); what is the QRS relationship to P waves; is the QRS rate regular or irregular; if the QRS complex is wide, is it due to a bundle branch block or nonspecific conduction delay?
4. Is the QT interval abnormally long (>0.50 seconds); what is the shape of the T wave; is a T-U wave present?
5. Are there abnormal pauses? Is there sinus arrest, sinoatrial exit block, AV block, or compensatory pauses from premature beats?

Rate

Bradycardia is defined as heart rates below 60 bpm. However, most patients are rarely symptomatic from simple bradycardia unless it is below 40 bpm or associated with a drop in cardiac output, or both. This is more noticeable on physical exertion or if the patient has compromise of the ventricular function. If AV dissociation or block is present in addition to bradycardia, symptoms may appear earlier. Sinus bradycardia is present when there is a 1:1 P-to-QRS relationship. Junctional bradycardia is present when sinus P waves are not conducted and escape rates from the AV node or His-Purkinje system appear. Occasionally, sinus node disease is manifest as periodic sinus arrest or sinoatrial exit block when sudden absence of the PQRS complex(es) occurs.

Tachycardia is arbitrarily defined as heart rates greater than 100 bpm. Patients rarely show symptoms at such rates. However, if rates exceed 130 bpm, symptoms such as palpitations may start to appear. When rates exceed 170 bpm and if there is underlying ventricular dysfunction, hemodynamic decompensation occurs, which may lead to cardiovascular collapse, especially if the tachycardia is ventricular in origin. Since a normal AV node permits one-to-one conduction up to 200 bpm, tachycardias below 200 bpm can be either supraventricular or ventricular in origin. Thus, when rates exceed 200 bpm, the tachycardia is usually ventricular in origin even if the patient walks into the emergency department, since rate alone is not the determinant of cardiovascular decompensation. Ventricular tachycardia occurs more commonly in the older patient or if the patient has a history of previous myocardial infarction. On the other hand, when young patients have rates greater than 200 bpm, supraventricular tachycardia is the most likely cause. These tachycardias are due to either the presence of accessory AV connection of the Wolff-Parkinson-White syndrome or true AV nodal bypass tracts, such as those due to Mahaim or James fibers (Lown-Ganong-Levine syndrome). Occasional patients may have "short" or facilitated AV nodal conduction when the PR interval is short (<0.10 seconds) in the 12-lead sinus rhythm ECG. However, in these patients tachycardias at rates greater than 200 bpm can occur, during which the

Table 20-1. Causes of wide QRS complex tachycardias

Ventricular tachycardia
Supraventricular tachycardia (SVT)
SVT with rate-related functional bundle branch block (intermittent)
SVT with preexistent bundle branch block
SVT associated with preexcitation (e.g., Wolff-Parkinson-White) syndromes

Table 20-2. Helpful electrocardiographic differences between ventricular tachycardia and supraventricular tachycardia with wide QRS complexes (aberrancy)

Feature	SVT with aberrancy	VT
AV dissociation or VA block	No	Highly diagnostic (3 of 4 pt)
QRS duration > 0.14 sec	Rare except when RBBB present	Common
Positive QRS concordance in V_1–V_6 (QRS in same direction)	No, except when RBBB present	Diagnostic in absence of RBBB
Preexistent BBB	Yes, if BBB similar to sinus	Unhelpful
Triphasic RSR in V_6 with LBBB	No	Yes
Triphasic RSR in V_1 with RBBB	Yes	Less likely
Response to carotid sinus massage	Can slow or convert tachycardia	Usually no response

Key: SVT = supraventricular tachycardia; VT = ventricular tachycardia; AV = atrioventricular; VA = ventricular atrial block; RBBB = right bundle branch block; LBBB = left bundle branch block.

QRS complexes are narrow and similar to sinus rhythm QRS complexes.

QRS Complex

The QRS width is an indirect measurement of the time taken for an impulse to travel from the AV node to the ventricle. This is normally less than 0.12 seconds. However, the rate can be altered by ventricular disease, disease affecting the major electrical bundles that transmit the impulse from the AV node, or drugs that alter conduction velocity. These alterations reflect in the QRS width and become more apparent at faster heart rates. Recent additions to antiarrhythmic agents such as the class IC agents (flecainide, encainide, and propafenone) prolong the QRS and make an accurate diagnosis of a tachycardia difficult. Supraventricular tachycardias with aberrancy (usually right bundle branch block) result in a wide QRS complex that may mimic ventricular tachycardia. It is important to distinguish between these tachycardias. Several indirect criteria can be employed to help separate the two using a 12-lead ECG. The probability of being correct may not be better than 60 to 70 percent. The major reasons for this are that several mechanisms can cause QRS widening: Impulse may start in the ventricular muscle (area of slow conduction) and may not have direct access to the conduction system (fast conduction); the conduction system may be diseased or affected by drugs such that conduction is slowed, especially at faster rates; and there may be permanent disease of a major conduction bundle in the His-Purkinje ventricular axis, resulting in aberrancy of the right or left bundle branch block type.

Knowledge of some helpful features will aid in separating ventricular tachycardia from supraventricular tachycardia with aberrancy. Most of these differences have been accurately observed during the study of these arrhythmias in the electrophysiology laboratory. A knowledge of the underlying heart disease will also aid in arriving at a correct diagnosis together with the ECG differences. Table 20-1 enumerates causes of wide QRS complex tachycardias and Table 20-2 depicts helpful ECG differences between ventricular tachycardias and supraventricular tachycardias with aberrancy (and QRS complexes).

DIAGNOSIS AND MANAGEMENT OF THE DIFFERENT ARRHYTHMIAS

Based on the preceding discussion, the 12-lead ECG of the arrhythmia, the history, and the company (underlying ventricular function) it keeps will allow for a specific diagnosis. Therapy for the arrhythmia revolves around the degree of hemodynamic decompensation and may vary from immediate cardiopulmonary resuscitation to withdrawing offending agents and correcting abnormalities such as hypokalemia, ischemia, other electrolyte disturbances, and heart failure. When possible, the 12-lead ECG and rhythm strip should always be obtained before intervention for the arrhythmia as it will permit a more accurate diagnosis.

The ECG should be approached in a systematic manner that includes the rate (P and QRS), QRS regularity, P-QRS relationship, QRS width and bundle branch configuration, and AV conduction status. The schema in Figs. 20-5 and 20-6 provide such a preliminary approach to arrhythmia diagnosis.

Tachycardias

Narrow QRS Regular Tachycardias

Of the tachycardias (heart rates > 100 bpm) that will be encountered in the emergency department setting, narrow QRS regular tachycardias are among the most common. By definition the width of the QRS of these tachycardias is less than 0.14 seconds and invariably the rhythm originates at or above the AV node region; they are lumped together as "supraventricular tachycardias." They include sinus tachycardia, atrioventricular reentry tachycardia, atrioventricular reciprocating (orthodromic) tachycardia associated with preexcitation syndromes (WPW syndrome), paroxysmal atrial (intraatrial reentry or focal) tachycardia, and atrial flutter with fixed AV nodal block (1:1, 2:1, or 3:1).

SINUS TACHYCARDIAS. Sinus tachycardias are usually physiologic and a function of other systemic abnormalities or heart failure. Rarely, a true, paroxysmal, reentrant sinus tachycardia is present that has the sudden onset-offset characteristics of paroxysmal tachycardias. The P wave always precedes the QRS complex in a fixed 1:1 relationship and

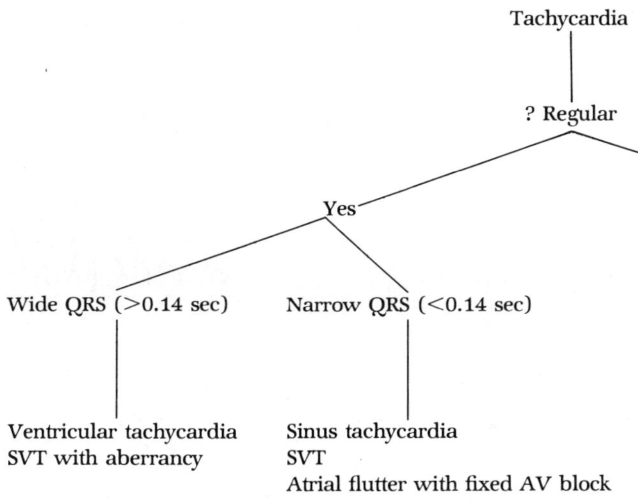

Fig. 20-5. Guide to diagnosis of tachycardias. (SVT = supraventricular tachycardia.)

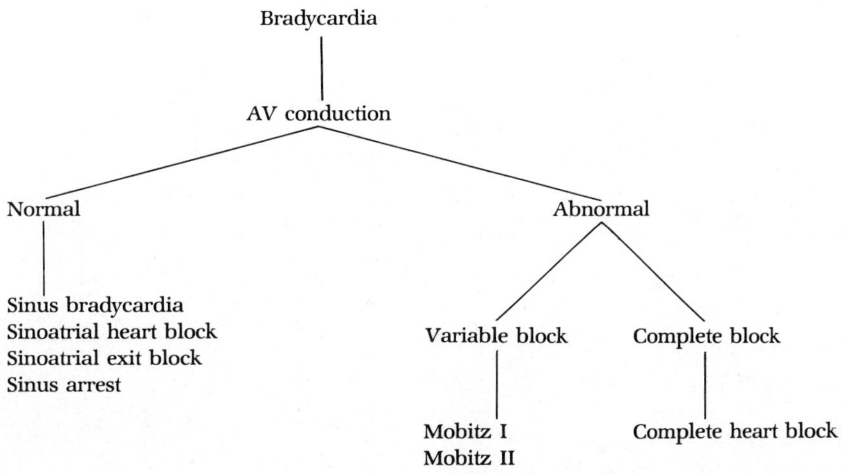

Fig. 20-6. Guide to diagnosis of bradycardias.

the PR interval is similar to that of sinus rhythm. Physiologic sinus tachycardia has gradual acceleration and rate variations and is unresponsive to carotid sinus massage. The P-wave axis is normal and usually upright in leads II, III, and aVF, with a P-wave axis around +60 degrees.

A careful search for causative disease such as thyrotoxicosis, fever, pneumonia, sepsis, acute abdomen, shock, heart failure, hypovolemia, anemia, pulmonary embolism, or anxiety should be made. When none of these causes can be identified and the patient has a history of paroxysmal tachycardia with sudden onset-offset, then beta-blockers (intravenous propranolol, 0.1 mg/kg; intravenous esmolol, 0.5 mg/kg; or oral beta-blockers) or calcium channel blockers (intravenous verapamil, 5-mg boluses every five minutes up to 20 mg; oral diltiazem, 60 mg three times a day; or verapamil, 80 mg three times a day) can be given for termination and prophylaxis.

AV NODAL REENTRY TACHYCARDIAS. Atrioventricular nodal reentry tachycardias are due to an imbalance in conduction and refractoriness of two functional pathways with different conduction velocities and refractoriness in the AV node region (Fig. 20-7). The classic rhythm strip shows that the P waves are buried in the QRS and thus are rarely identified on the ECG in this usually narrow QRS tachycardia (Fig. 20-8). The rate of the tachycardia varies between 140 and 180 bpm, which is a function of the circuit time of the AV node. This is the most common cause of narrow QRS tachycardias, with a 1:1 P-QRS relationship. This tachycardia has abrupt onset and offset, and measures to slow or block AV nodal conduction will result in termination.

Valsalva maneuvers, especially in the standing position, or carotid sinus pressure often result in termination and, when possible, should be instituted before drug or electrical therapy. If these measures fail, drugs that slow AV nodal conduction can be employed. The most effective is intravenous verapamil (5–20 mg in 5-mg boluses every two to five minutes) or oral verapamil (80–160 mg three times a day). Intravenous beta-blockers (propranolol, 2–10 mg or 0.1 mg/kg given at a rate of 1 mg per minute, or a 0.5-mg/kg infu-

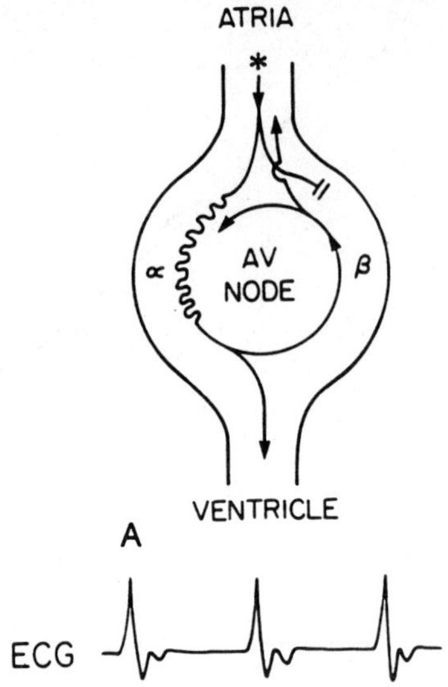

Fig. 20-7. Schematic model of AV nodal tachycardia (supraventricular tachycardia).

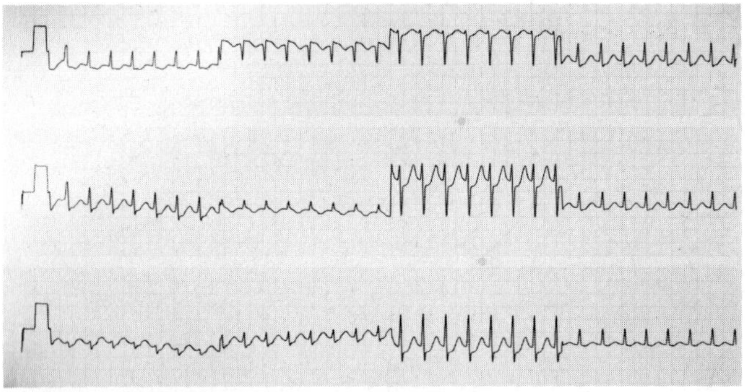

Fig. 20-8. Twelve-lead ECG showing a narrow, QRS regular tachycardia with no visible P waves. This is an example of AV nodal reentry tachycardia.

sion of esmolol) are also reasonably effective. If advanced ventricular dysfunction precludes the use of verapamil or beta-blockers, 0.5 mg intravenous digoxin can be given. It may take 20 minutes to 2 hours before full effect. On the other hand, if there is significant heart failure, hemodynamic decompensation, or hypotension, synchronized cardioversion with 20 to 100 joules will nearly always convert this rhythm and should be the treatment of choice. This can be performed with the patient under sedation with intravenous diazepam or midazolam (Versed). If these measures fail and if the diagnosis is in doubt, a temporary venous pacing electrode may be advanced to the right atrial level with ECG guidance. This is obtained by connecting the external pin of the electrode via alligator clips to the V_1 lead of the ECG machine. Once atrial activity is identified and if there is a 1 : 1 relationship to the QRS complex, overdrive pacing at rates faster than the atrial rate will often interrupt the tachycardia. After conversion a 12-lead ECG in sinus rhythm should be obtained to search for predisposing conditions such as preexcitation (WPW syndrome, where the PR interval will

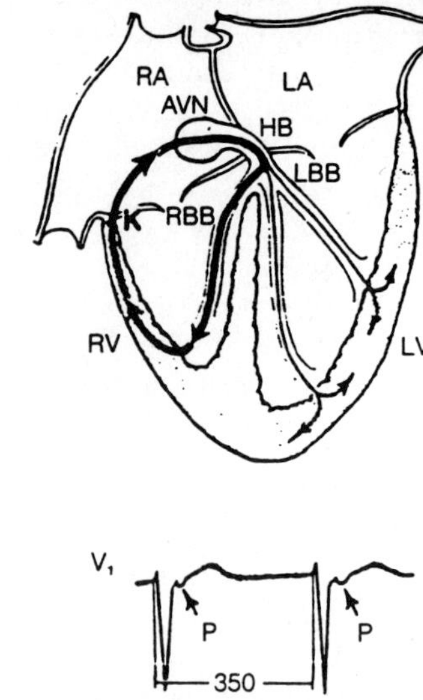

Fig. 20-9. Schematic model of AV reentrant reciprocating tachycardia (Wolff-Parkinson-White syndrome). (RA = right atrium; LA = left atrium; AVN = AV node; RBB = right bundle branch; LBB = left bundle branch; RV = right ventricle; LV = left ventricle; HB = His bundle.)

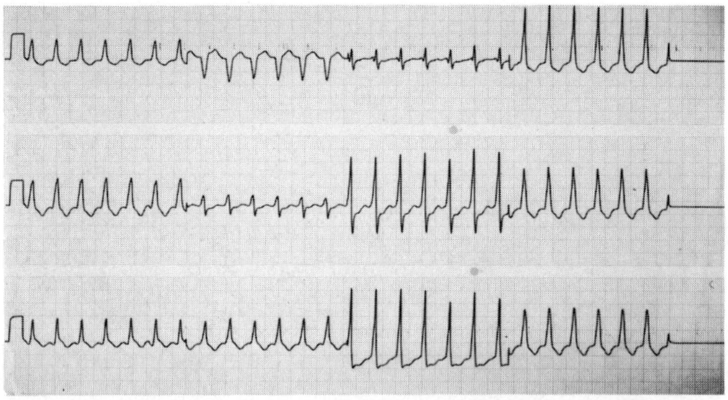

Fig. 20-10. Example of AV reciprocating tachycardia in a patient with Wolff-Parkinson-White syndrome. The P waves can be seen to follow the QRS complex and the RP interval is greater than 70 msec.

be very short—<0.10—with a delta wave inscription on the QRS) or acute myocardial infarction.

ATRIOVENTRICULAR RECIPROCATING (ORTHODROMIC) TACHYCARDIAS. These are frequently confused with and often cannot be separated from AV nodal reentry tachycardias. This tachycardia depends on the AV nodal conduction for its maintenance and its rate since the maximal 1 : 1 AV nodal conduction time usually determines the rate (Fig. 20-9).

The rate of this tachycardia varies from 160 to 200 bpm and there is a 1 : 1 P-QRS relationship. The P waves follow the QRS complex and the RP interval is usually greater than 70 msec and less than the PR interval (Fig. 20-10). The P waves are usually seen in the QT segment and are often inverted in ECG leads II, III, and aVF as the atrium is retrogradely depolarized (see Fig. 20-9).

Interruption of this tachycardia is similar to that of AV

nodal reentrant tachycardia, described in the preceding section. However, one should be cautious since degeneration to atrial fibrillation can occur, especially when intravenous verapamil or digoxin is used. If the rhythm degenerates into Afib or atrial flutter, rapid ventricular rates can occur in WPW syndrome patients. Thus, if verapamil or digoxin is used intravenously, facilities for immediate cardioversion should be available if this occurs.

Perhaps the safest and often the most effective agent for these reciprocating tachycardias associated with the WPW syndrome is intravenous procainamide since this agent will slow or block retrograde conduction over the accessory tract. Additionally, procainamide slows conduction and increases refractoriness in the atrium and AV node. Procainamide should be given intravenously at 10 to 15 mg/kg over 30 minutes. Beta-blockers are also safe and often effective both for termination and prevention of these tachycardias.

Long-term prophylaxis can be achieved by oral class IA antiarrhythmic agents (quinidine, disopyramide, or procainamide) or the newer class IC agents (flecainide, encainide) and beta-blockers singly or in combination with class IA agents. Oral verapamil and digoxin should be avoided, as was discussed earlier, unless the patient does not have evidence for antegrade conduction (absence of delta wave on the ECG or from results of prior electrophysiologic evaluation).

ATRIAL FLUTTER. The classic atrial flutter rhythm most often is characterized by a heart rate of about 150 bpm, which represents an atrial flutter rate of 300 bpm with 2:1 AV block. The atrial flutter rate can vary between 260 and 320 bpm in the absence of specific antiarrhythmic therapy (Fig. 20-11). This arrhythmia invariably accompanies or is due to underlying heart disease and is one of the more difficult tachycardias to prevent and interrupt with antiarrhythmic drugs.

After diagnosis, controlling the ventricular rate by drugs that slow AV nodal conduction, such as digoxin, beta-blockers, verapamil, or diltiazem, is the initial treatment. However, if sinus rhythm is important because of poor hemodynamics or if the ventricular rate is difficult to control and drugs such as beta-blockers or verapamil are contraindicated, low-energy synchronized cardioversion (40–100 joules) is very effective. In situations in which an atrial pacing electrode is indicated either for tachycardia diagnosis or prophylactic pacing, atrial overdrive pacing at rates 25 to 50 bpm in excess of the atrial flutter rate (e.g., 325–400 bpm) at high pacing energies may revert the rhythm to sinus. Class IA agents (e.g., quinidine) may convert atrial flutter to sinus rhythm. We often use procainamide intravenously (10 mg/kg) over 30 to 60 minutes for conversion, and oral quinidine gluconate (Quinaglute, 324–488 mg three times a day) or procainamide hydrochloride (Procan SR, 1,000 mg every six hours) for prophylaxis. It is not unusual for atrial flutter to convert to Afib with these agents and then to go on to revert to sinus rhythm. If Afib persists the ventricular rate tends to be slower and easier to modulate. Carotid sinus pressure not uncommonly, especially in digitalized patients, increases AV block and slows the ventricular rate, which will expose the classic sawtooth flutter waves. Any narrow QRS rhythm at 150 bpm should be considered to represent atrial flutter with 2:1 AV block until it can be proved to be otherwise.

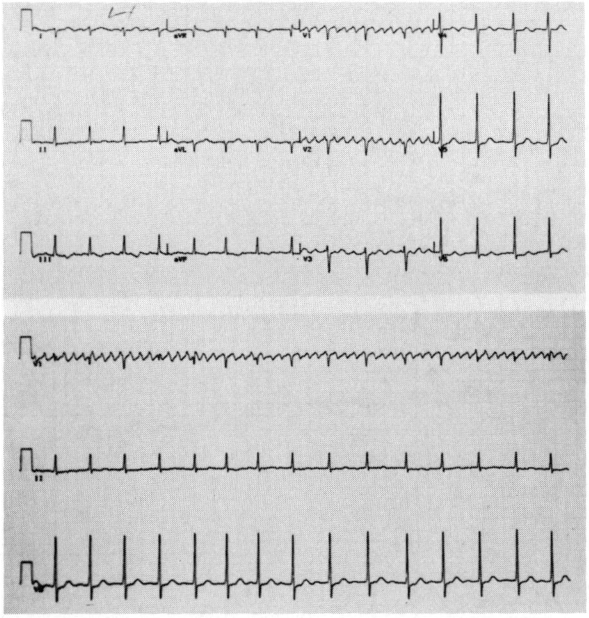

Fig. 20-11. Atrial flutter. The sawtooth flutter waves can be clearly seen.

Wide QRS Regular Tachycardias

These tachycardias should be considered to represent ventricular tachycardia (VT), especially in patients with significant ventricular dysfunction or previous myocardial infarction. The main differential diagnosis is supraventricular tachycardia (SVT) with aberrancy. The principles for distinguishing between the two have been outlined in preceding sections in this chapter (see Table 20-2) and the treatment of SVT with aberrancy is the same as that for narrow QRS-SVT.

Ventricular tachycardia is relatively common and diagnosable by careful analysis of the 12-lead ECG and rhythm strip. The QRS complexes are nearly always wide (>0.14 seconds); AV dissociation is present so that the slower atrial rate, if identified, appears to "march" through the tachycardia independent of the QRS complexes (Fig. 20-12). If the initiating beat of the VT is seen, then it is often a late-cycle ventricular premature beat (VPB), whose shape may differ from that of the tachycardia QRS complexes (Fig. 20-13). The rate can vary from 100 to 300 bpm and the patient's tolerance will depend on the rate, underlying left ventricular dysfunction, level of ischemia, or valvular dysfunction. Hemodynamic deterioration will very quickly lead to cardiac arrest, with or without the rhythm accelerating and degenerating into VT. Ventricular fibrillation is almost always associated with heart disease and thus occurs in older patients, most commonly with a history of a remote myocardial infarction or presence of an acute myocardial infarction or congestive cardiomyopathy. Rarely, VT can occur in the absence of heart disease; in this case it is paroxysmal and usually well tolerated.

Treatment depends on the hemodynamic impact of the VT in the patient. If no marked decompensation or hypotension is present, replacing K^+ if it is less than 4.0 mEq per liter is useful, and conversion may be achieved with lidocaine (5 mg/kg) over 20 minutes, given as 100- to 50-mg boluses every 5 to 10 minutes. If VT is terminated prevention can be

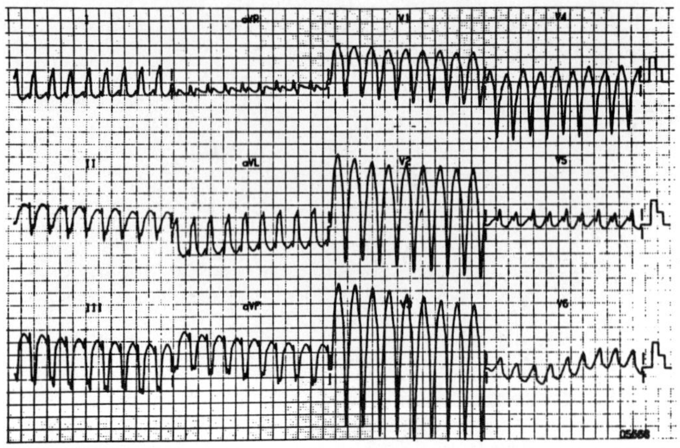

Fig. 20-12. Twelve-lead ECG of ventricular tachycardia.

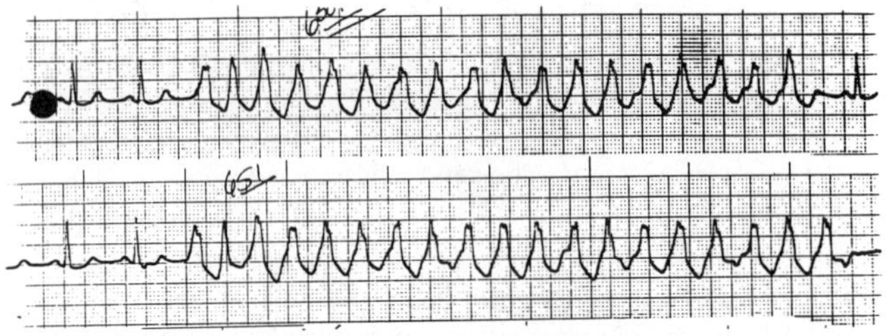

Fig. 20-13. Example of self-limited run of ventricular tachycardia. The initiating beat is seen as a late-cycle, wide QRS complex that differs from the QRS complexes in the salvo of tachycardia.

achieved by intravenous infusion of lidocaine at 2 to 5 mg per minute. Lidocaine is most effective in the setting of ischemia or acute myocardial infarction. Chronic VT is less likely to respond to lidocaine and more often responds to intravenous procainamide (10–15 mg/kg) given as an infusion over 30 minutes. Prevention of recurrence can be achieved by maintenance infusion of procainamide at 1 to 5 mg per minute. VT is nearly always slowed even if it is not terminated with procainamide, which results in less hemodynamic compromise. However, if the QRS complex widens and exceeds 0.20 seconds or if the blood pressure falls to less than 80 mm Hg during procainamide administration, it should be discontinued or the dose decreased. If these agents fail and the patient's blood pressure is adequate, bretylium can be administered intravenously. However, this ganglion blocker will nearly always decrease the blood pressure and should be used with great caution. We recommend using it as a slow infusion after a 400-mg bolus. The dose generally employed is 400 mg every six to eight hours for VT prevention.

If hemodynamic deterioration occurs or decompensation accompanies VT, immediate cardioversion is indicated, which can be effected by a direct current (DC) synchronized shock using 50 to 100 joules. For moribund patients or those with polymorphic VT, immediate defibrillation with 200 to 400 joules should be carried out. Synchronization should not be attempted for polymorphic VT.

Cardioversion is also the preferred treatment if a patient is in heart failure or is experiencing angina. After cardioversion or defibrillation, prevention of VT recurrence is necessary while the cause for VT is being determined. Lidocaine or procainamide infusion as described previously is often effective for prevention even if it did not terminate the VT.

In patients with recurrent well-tolerated VT, overdrive pacing may be very effective; this can be achieved at the bedside by floating a transvenous pacing electrode into the right ventricle with ECG or x-ray guidance. An ECG from the pacing electrode when it is in the right atrium will also help in confirming the VT diagnosis, as described in preceding sections. Overdrive pacing is performed by pacing at a rate that is 25 percent faster than the VT rate. Overdrive pacing for 5 to 10 beat bursts is ample and when longer bursts, especially at rates greater than 220 bpm, are employed, VF may be produced. Thus, an external cardioverter-defibrillator must always be available when overdrive ventricular pacing is attempted.

With all arrhythmias, but even more so with VT, underlying causes must be identified and measures instituted to prevent recurrences. Eliminating triggers such as low K^+, acidosis, ischemia, or drug toxicity is also important for VT prevention. The serum K^+ in patients with VT should be kept in the range of 4.0 to 5.0 mEq per liter.

Ventricular Fibrillation

Ventricular fibrillation (VF) and ventricular flutter are now considered to be variations of the same rhythm and treatment is identical. The treatment for VF is immediate defibrillation with 200 to 400 joules. When it occurs in the ischemic or acute myocardial infarction setting, it can recur; thus, lidocaine or procainamide infusions should be instituted in an attempt to prevent recurrences.

Irregular Narrow or Wide QRS Complex Tachycardias

Such tachycardias are invariably Afib (Fig. 20-14). Aberrant conduction due to fixed or rate-related bundle branch block will cause irregular, wide QRS complexes (Fig. 20-15). Generally, the baseline of the ECG between QRS complexes will reveal fine, rapid, irregular f waves. However, in chronic Afib these fibrillatory waves may be very fine and almost unapparent, thus making the diagnosis difficult. This rhythm often slows with carotid sinus pressure because of increase in AV block.

Atrial fibrillation invariably occurs in paroxysms initially and becomes chronic with time, especially if the underlying disease, such as advanced mitral valve disease or ischemic cardiomyopathy, is not corrected. Other causes, such as hypertension, cardiomyopathy (especially alcoholic), thyrotoxicosis, lung disease, pneumonia, pericarditis, and sick sinus syndrome, should be considered. In the United States, chronic hypertension and ischemic heart disease are by far the most common causes of Afib.

Atrial fibrillation with aberrancy is important to recognize as it mimics VT (see Fig. 20-15). Figure 20-15 demonstrates Afib with left bundle branch block, which resembles VT, especially when the ventricular rate is fast and more regular. The more common type is Afib with intermittent right bundle branch block (RBBB). This is usually seen in the short R-R cycles following a long R-R cycle and is referred to as *Ashman's phenomenon* (Fig. 20-16). Salvos of

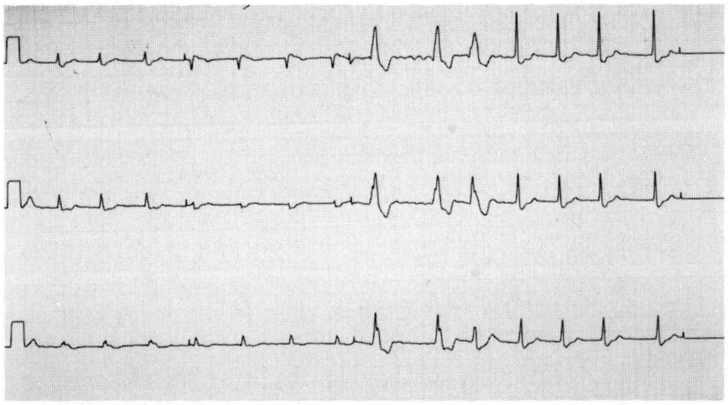

Fig. 20-14. Atrial fibrillation with occasional aberrant QRS complexes.

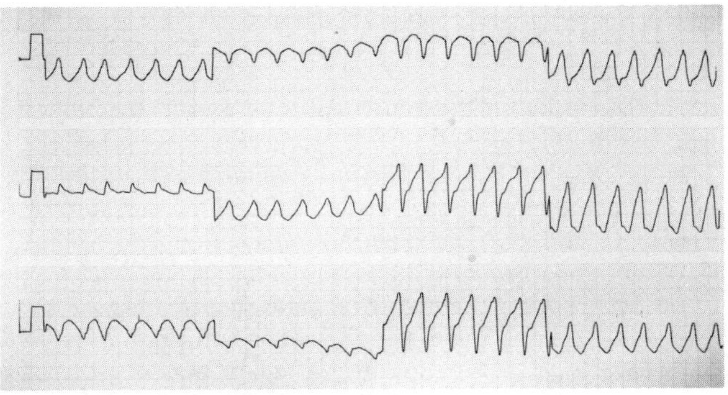

Fig. 20-15. Left bundle branch block–QRS complexes during atrial fibrillation that mimic ventricular tachycardia.

the RBBB-QRS complexes in Afib can look just like short paroxysmal runs of VT.

The treatment of Afib with aberrancy revolves around both ventricular rate control and reversion to sinus rhythm. Drugs that slow the AV node, such as digoxin (0.25 mg IV every two to four hours) or intravenous verapamil (2.5- to 5.0-mg bolus), or slow esmolol infusion (0.5 mg/kg) will achieve rapid ventricular rate control. Subsequent oral therapy with digoxin, 0.25 mg daily; verapamil, 80 mg three times a day; or beta-blocker (e.g., propranolol, 20 mg four times a day) will maintain ventricular rate control. In patients with congestive heart failure, verapamil or beta-blockers should be avoided or used with extreme caution for fear of exacerbating heart failure.

Conversion of Afib is usually not achieved by the drugs used to slow ventricular rate and more often requires class IA antiarrhythmics such as procainamide (1,000–1,500 mg IV over 20–30 minutes), oral quinidine (400 mg every six hours), or procainamide hydrochloride (Procan SR, 1 gm every six hours). If the ventricular rate is fast and difficult to control or if there is severe hemodynamic compromise or worsening angina, immediate synchronized cardioversion with 100 to 400 joules is the treatment of choice. This is especially so, irrespective of ventricular rate, in patients with stiff and noncompliant left ventricles (aortic stenosis, hyper-

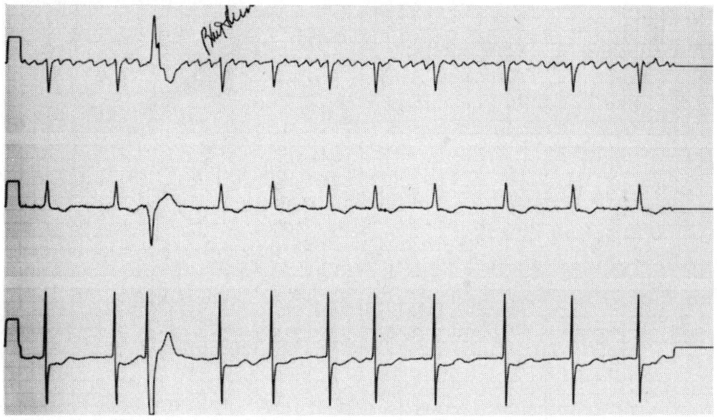

Fig. 20-16. Atrial fibrillation with intermittent right bundle branch block–QRS complexes due to Ashman's phenomenon. This mimics ventricular extrasystoles.

trophic cardiomyopathy, or acute myocardial infarction), when proper atrioventricular synchrony and atrial contraction are very important.

Prevention of Afib is achieved by controlling or eliminating the cause, where possible, and use of agents such as quinidine or procainamide. Long-term anticoagulation should be considered in those patients with recurrent Afib associated with an enlarged left atrium in whom anticoagulants are not contraindicated.

Multifocal Atrial Tachycardias

Multifocal atrial tachycardias usually occur in patients with chronic pulmonary disease and are characterized by irregular QRS complexes associated with varying P-wave morphologies of more than three configurations (Fig. 20-17). When associated with variable AV block, multifocal atrial tachycardia can be confused with Afib.

Treatment is directed at the cause (lung disease) and at improving hypoxia. A major mistake is to give these patients digoxin, which only sensitizes the atria and produces more atrial ectopy. This rhythm portends a poor long-term prognosis in patients with lung disease.

Paroxysmal Atrial Tachycardias with Variable AV Block

When the atrial rate is faster than the maximum permissible AV nodal conduction, varying degrees of AV block will result, with periodic absences of QRS complexes; this may take place in a Wenckebach manner. It occurs when the atrial rate exceeds 200 bpm or when drugs, such as digoxin, beta-blockers, or verapamil, which slow AV node rather than interrupt or convert the tachycardia, are employed. The diagnosis depends on recognition of atrial activity (P rate) and is usually due to intraatrial reentry or a rapidly discharging ectopic focus (Fig. 20-18).

Treatment is directed toward slowing AV nodal conduction and converting the arrhythmia at the atrial level, and is similar to that for Afib (quinidine, procainamide, and the newer class IC agents, such as flecainide and encainide). Occasionally, this rhythm is due to digitalis toxicity and should be suspected whenever a patient is receiving digoxin

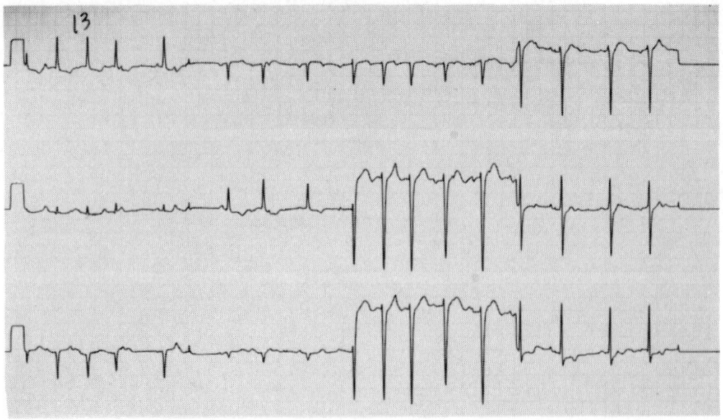

Fig. 20-17. Multifocal atrial tachycardia that reveals at least three different P-wave morphologies.

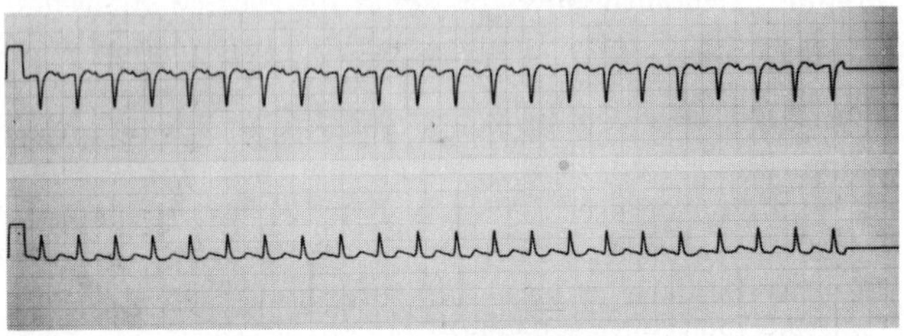

Fig. 20-18. Paroxysmal atrial tachycardia (ectopic). The ectopic P waves are visible with a long PR interval.

and ventricular rate is slow and very regular due to high grade AV block.

Bradycardias

The various bradycardias (rate < 60 bpm) are approached in the same manner as tachycardias: according to the setting in which they appear, P and QRS rates, and the P-QRS relationship. These arrhythmias result from sinus and AV node abnormalities and are apt to occur if the blood supply to the sinus or AV node is interrupted (e.g., in acute inferior myocardial infarction). They can also occur when there is infiltration of these structures (e.g., in sarcoid, collagen-vascular diseases, tumors, and amyloid).

Sinus Bradycardia

When the sinus rate is less than 60 bpm and there is a 1:1 P-QRS relationship, sinus bradycardia is present. The hemodynamic disturbance that this creates will depend on underlying ventricular function, cardiac output demand, and bradycardia rate.

This rhythm is relatively common today as a result of the widespread use of beta-blockers and calcium channel blockers such as verapamil and diltiazem; it is also common in well-trained athletes or joggers, in whom it is considered nonpathologic or physiologic. It can also be seen in patients during sleep or heightened vagal tone and in hypothyroidism.

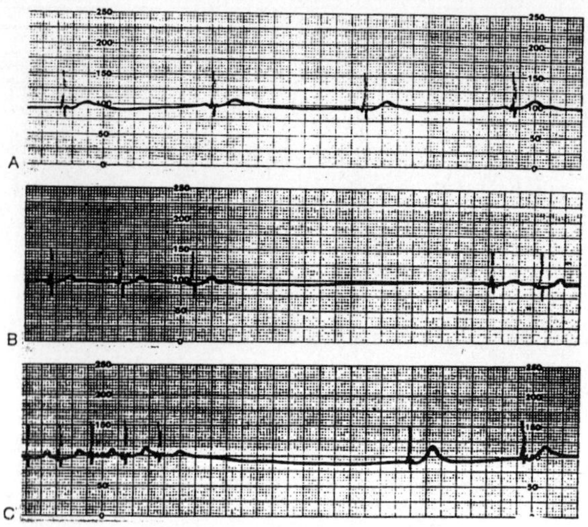

Fig. 20-19. Sinoatrial block. Sudden cessation of sinus rhythm with prolonged asystolic pause can be seen.

Pathologic sinus bradycardia is usually seen in the presence of acute inferior myocardial infarction, sick sinus syndrome, or end-stage cardiac failure.

When sinus bradycardia requires treatment, withdrawal of bradycardia-producing drugs with the use of intravenous atropine, 0.03 mg/kg (1–2 mg), is often sufficient. In patients with beta-blocker overdosage, or when atropine does not reverse the decompensating bradycardia, intravenous infusion of isoproterenol, 1–2 μg per minute, or, rarely, temporary pacing is indicated. Correction of diseases that lead to bradycardia (e.g., hypothyroidism) may be necessary.

Sinoatrial Exit Block

Sinoatrial exit block (Fig. 20-19) is characterized by sudden cessation of sinus rhythm that results in long pauses or cardiac standstill until the sinus resumes or junctional escape beats emerge. It is sometimes accompanied by sinus bradycardia and is then likely to be due to sick sinus syndrome. It is difficult to be certain whether this rhythm represents sinus arrest or sinoatrial exit block unless P waves are absent in a fixed periodic pattern so that a 2:1 or 3:1 exit block can be deduced.

Treatment of this rhythm is similar to treatment for sinus bradycardia. However, sinoatrial exit block is more resistant and occasionally will require temporary, followed by permanent, pacing.

Atrioventricular Block

Atrioventricular block is due to an abnormal AV node, which can show varying degrees of block from one-degree AV block (PR interval > 0.20 seconds) to Mobitz I (increasing PR intervals until a QRS complex is dropped), Mobitz II (sudden dropped QRS complexes preceded by a P wave), and complete heart block (failure of P waves to be conducted to the ventricle).

THERAPY FOR MOBITZ I ATRIOVENTRICULAR BLOCK. If a long PR is seen that progresses through varying PR inter-

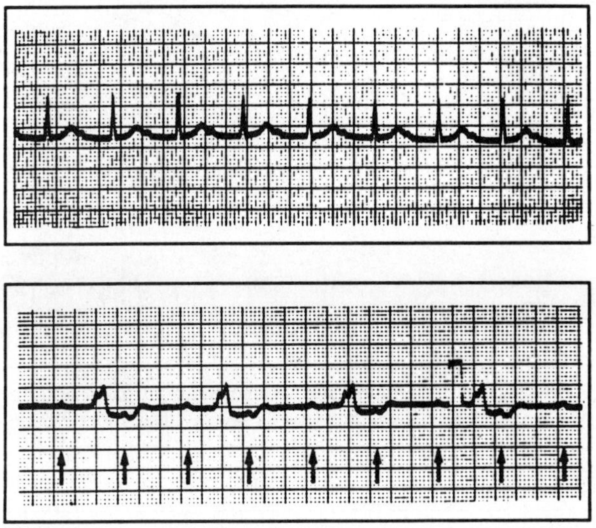

Fig. 20-20. Displays Mobitz I AV Wenckebach block that progresses to Mobitz I complete heart block.

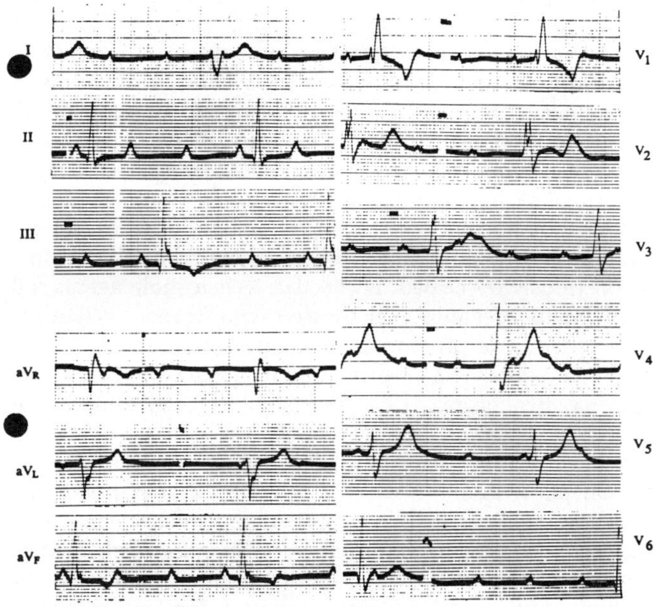

Fig. 20-21. Complete AV block (Mobitz II).

vals (Mobitz I) to complete heart block, then the block is at the AV node level and is often responsive to agents that facilitate AV nodal conduction, such as atropine (0.03 mg/kg or 1–2 mg IV) or infused isoproterenol (1–2 μg per minute). Treatment is indicated if symptoms such as dizziness, weakness, congestive heart failure, or syncope are present. This is usually the case when complete heart block occurs. Complete AV block of the Mobitz I type is characterized by an atrial rate that is faster, and is usually associated with narrow QRS complexes due to an escape (junctional) rhythm that is between 50 and 60 bpm (Fig. 20-20). When drugs do not accelerate the rhythm or improve AV nodal conduction, temporary pacing can be employed either by external transthoracic or temporary transvenous pacing. Drugs that cause AV nodal block, such as digoxin, beta-blockers, and calcium channel blockers (verapamil, diltiazem), should be discontinued. This type of AV nodal block is most often seen during an acute inferior myocardial infarction or digoxin toxicity. It can rarely be due to hypervagotonia.

THERAPY FOR MOBITZ II AV BLOCK. Mobitz II AV block (Fig. 20-21) is due to His-Purkinje conduction disease or advanced bifascicular bundle (right and left) disease. This rhythm is characterized by a slow escape rhythm (30–40 bpm) with wide QRS complexes, is rarely due to drugs, and is usually pathologic. Mobitz II AV block rarely responds to atropine but can be accelerated by isoproterenol infusion. However, since it may accompany acute anterior myocardial infarction, isoproterenol should be avoided, as it can extend myocardial infarction by increasing the oxygen demands via production of an uncontrollable increase in heart rate and an increase in contractility. Temporary external or transvenous pacing is usually the treatment of choice. When acute myocardial infarction is not present, idiopathic or degenerative AV block is the cause. Generally, these patients are compensated and will exhibit cannon waves in the neck, variable heart sounds, and a wide pulse pressure with a high systolic pressure. Their bradycardia symptoms occur when an increase in cardiac output is needed (e.g., during exercise), so that they should be hospitalized and investigated; temporary as opposed to permanent pacing is rarely necessary. Table 20-3 delineates the differences between Mobitz I and II complete heart block.

Table 20-3. Helpful differences in the electrocardiogram between Mobitz I and II block

Feature	Mobitz I	Mobitz II
PR interval	Progressive increases and periodicity present	Constant; may be increased or normal
QRS complexes of conducted beats	Usually normal	Generally broad and complete bundle branch block or hemiblock is present
Ventricular rate	Variable or 40–60 bpm when complete AV block	Slow, usually 30–40 bpm; occasionally asystole or <20 bpm
Response to drug (atropine/isoproterenol)	Improved conduction; speeding up of the escape rate	Little or no response
Underlying conditions	Digoxin toxicity; inferior myocardial infarction; excess beta-blockers; excess calcium channel blockers	Idiopathic/degenerative; acute anterior myocardial infarction
Site of block	AV node	His-Purkinje system

Arrhythmias in Special Situations

Acute Myocardial Infarction

Virtually all (approximately 90 percent) of patients with acute myocardial infarction (MI) exhibit an arrhythmia in the first 24 hours. The most common are VPBs. These rarely need treatment unless they cause salvos of unsustained VT (>120 bpm) or sustained ventricular tachycardia. Occasionally, early "R-on-T" VPBs trigger ventricular fibrillation and if they occur frequently, these VPBs should be suppressed. Intravenous lidocaine over 20 minutes, given as an initial bolus of 100 mg and then 50-mg boluses every 5 to 10 minutes (total of 5–10 mg/kg), is often successful for VT. This is followed by lidocaine infusion (1–4 mg per minute). If lidocaine fails, procainamide alone or in addition to lidocaine, as previously described, is effective. When these agents fail intravenous bretylium can be used with caution. When active ischemia is present, intravenous beta-blockers (metoprolol, 7.5–10.0 mg, or propranolol, 1 mg/kg) may be very effective. Synchronized cardioversion (50–100 joules) will convert resistant or decompensating VT.

Sudden VF or VT leading to VF occurs in 5 to 10 percent of patients with acute MI, especially in the first four hours after the attack. This may represent reperfusion, since it is seen more commonly in patients receiving thrombolytic therapy (streptokinase or t-PA). Ventricular fibrillation is treated by immediate cardiopulmonary resuscitation and defibrillation with 200 to 400 joules DC shock. In resistant VF cases, defibrillation can be attempted after "priming" with intravenous procainamide (500–1,000 mg) or intravenous bretylium (400 mg). Evidence suggests that priming with epinephrine may also increase the likelihood of successful defibrillation.

Bradycardias are common, especially in inferior myocardial infarction, and are usually due to increased vagal tone, which can be exacerbated by sublingual nitroglycerin. Unless they are symptomatic these patients should be observed. Symptoms will be due to hypotension (blood pressure < 90 mm Hg) or aggravation of ischemia. Intravenous atropine (0.03 mg/kg or 1–2 mg) is usually effective. Other bradycardias such as AV block are rare and are treated as described previously if hemodynamic decompensation occurs.

Sinus tachycardia is common in extensive MI (especially anterior) and is probably a result of the reflex augmentation of the sympathetic system, caused by a low cardiac output. Treatment is directed at pump dysfunction if possible.

Accelerated idioventricular rhythm is frequent and when it is greater than 100 bpm, it is considered VT and is treated as such. However, when the rate is less than 100 bpm, this rate is similar to the sinus rate and will appear to compete with sinus rhythm. It appears in salvos at a rate slightly faster than sinus rate and the QRS complexes are wide (>0.14 seconds) with no associated P waves. This rhythm rarely requires treatment. If suppression is required, increasing the sinus rate with atropine, 1 to 2 mg intravenously, is successful. Rarely, pacing or isoproterenol infusion (1–2 μg per minute) may be needed.

Wolff-Parkinson-White Syndrome

Wolff-Parkinson-White syndrome invariably has initial symptoms of supraventricular arrhythmias in young adults. If a delta wave is present on the ECG during sinus rhythm, the QRS is wide and represents fusion of excitation of the ventricle by both antegrade conduction over the accessory tract and over the normal AV node (Fig. 20-22). The degree of "preexcitation" represents the accessibility of the accessory tract to sinus impulse and its conduction-refractoriness properties. The presence of a delta wave implies that during atrial fibrillation or flutter, rapid conduction up to 300 bpm can occur into the ventricle if the accessory tract has a short refractory period. Thus, when Afib develops in patients with WPW syndrome, the tachycardia may show both narrow and wide QRS complexes unless the refractory period of the accessory tract is very short. In such a case wide QRS complexes will predominate and mimic VT. In some cases this rhythm will degenerate into VF and sudden cardiac death can occur (Fig. 20-23).

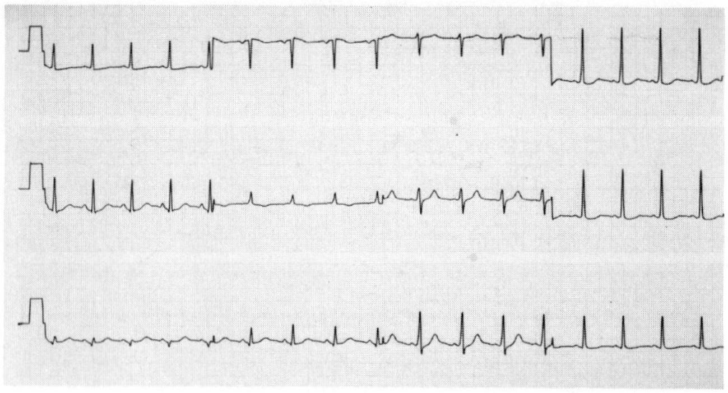

Fig. 20-22. Electrocardiogram of patient with left paraseptal accessory tract (WPW). A delta wave is seen with a short PR interval.

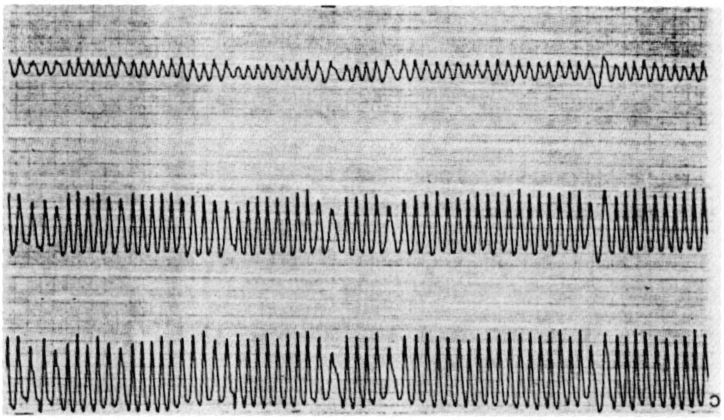

Fig. 20-23. Atrial fibrillation degenerating into VF as a result of rapid conduction over the accessory tract in a patient with WPW syndrome.

Treatment depends on the ventricular rate and hemodynamic decompensation. If symptomatic hypotension or hemodynamic decompensation is present, synchronized cardioversion with 100 to 200 joules is the preferred treatment. If only mild decompensation is present, intravenous procainamide (1,000–1,500 mg over 20–30 minutes) is very effective. It will slow or block conduction, resulting in slower and narrower QRS complexes, representing predominant AV nodal conduction. Procainamide will also result in conversion to sinus rhythm in a significant number of patients. Digoxin and verapamil are absolute contraindications for this rhythm since they can shorten the refractory period of the accessory tract either directly (digoxin) or indirectly (verapamil) as a result of the reflex augmentation of the

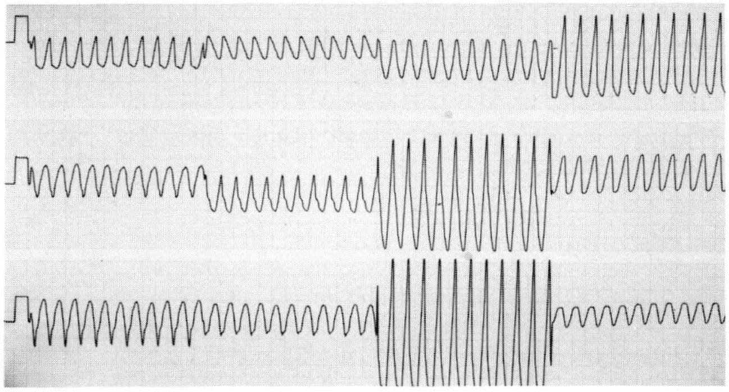

Fig. 20-24. Rare antidromic reciprocating atrioventricular tachycardia in a patient with WPW syndrome.

sympathetic system. In addition these drugs can slow AV node conduction and, hence, may facilitate accessory tract conduction further.

The most common tachycardia that patients with WPW experience is the narrow QRS tachycardia (AV reciprocating tachycardia; see Fig. 20-10), which has been described together with its treatment in a preceding section of this chapter. The rare antidromic SVT, during which conduction occurs down (antegrade) over the accessory tract into the ventricle and retrogradely through the AV node, will mimic VT. Recognition of P waves preceding the QRS complexes may aid in diagnosis (Fig. 20-24). Digoxin and verapamil should be avoided for this arrhythmia and procainamide or beta-blockers (IV propranolol or esmolol), or both, are the preferred treatments to slow or block accessory tract and AV nodal conduction. Low-energy (50–100 joules) cardioversion is also effective and should be used if the patient is decompensating.

Pacemaker-Related Arrhythmias

These arrhythmias are either due to appropriate or inappropriate pacemaker function or to lead malfunction. A variety of newer pacemakers are available whose characteristics and programmed mode need to be known before one can troubleshoot the arrhythmia in relation to the pacemaker. Single- (atrial or ventricular) and dual-chamber pacemakers are now available, and rate-adaptive (responsive) pacemakers have also become available that automatically increase pacing rate in response to a sensor such as activity or minute ventilation.

If there is a pacemaker spike (artifact) without capture of the paced chamber (atrium or ventricle), then pacer or lead malfunction is present (Fig. 20-25). However, in certain dual-chamber pacemakers with "safety pace" features, both atrial and ventricular spikes can fall immediately (in the refractory zone) after an intrinsic nonsensed P wave and a conducted native QRS, respectively. This is an idiosyncrasy that needs to be recognized; it is a "pseudomalfunction" due to atrial malsensing and may require reprogramming of the pacer. Failure to sense intrinsic complexes will result in a pacer output stimulus at the escape rate of the pacemaker (demand rate) irrespective of the underlying rhythm. Most pacemaker troubleshooting should be left to the pacemaker technician/physician, who can diagnose, and program out of, the problem if possible.

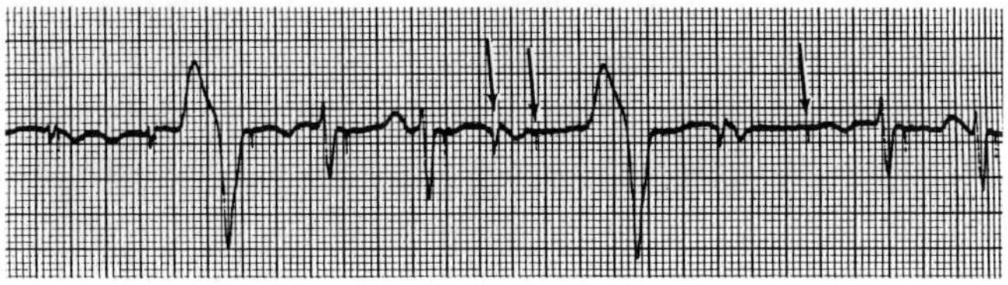

Fig. 20-25. Electrocardiogram showing pacer artifacts (stimuli) marching through the intrinsic rhythm at a rate faster than intrinsic rhythm. In a VVI pacemaker this is due to failure to sense and pace the ventricle.

Proarrhythmia Due to Antiarrhythmic Agents

Proarrhythmia due to antiarrhythmic agents is being seen increasingly often but is not correctly diagnosed. The tendency is to increase the dose or add another antiarrhythmic agent to patients who exhibit proarrhythmia. This is the result of misinterpreting the arrhythmia as being due to drug inefficacy or inadequate dosing. Electrolyte disturbances, especially hypokalemia, can precipitate ventricular proarrhythmia. Proarrhythmia should be considered if there is an increase in numbers of ectopic beats, there is precipitation of unsustained salvos or of a sustained tachycardia, it becomes more difficult to convert or cardiovert sustained tachycardias, or there is precipitation of polymorphic VT/VF (torsade de pointes).

An increase in ectopic beats is commonly seen with digitalis toxicity, especially if ventricular bigeminy occurs. Hypokalemia ($K^+ < 3.0$ mEq per liter) can also result in increased ventricular ectopic beats. If undiagnosed and uncorrected, the hypokalemia can lead to VT or VF.

The newer class IC antiarrhythmic agents such as flecainide and encainide are particularly prone to exacerbating or producing sustained VT, with very wide complexes that resemble ventricular flutter, can be very difficult to cardiovert, and can become incessant until the drugs are withdrawn and excreted. These drugs have long half-lives and thus can pose a problem. Patients with poor left ventricular function (ejection fraction < 30 percent) and with a history of VT are most likely to experience this type of proarrhythmia.

The most common and most easily recognized proarrhythmia is torsade de pointes (polymorphic VT/VF). This arrhythmia invariably occurs in the setting of class IA agents (quinidine, procainamide, disopyramide) in association with sinus bradycardia, long QT (increased QTc), and late-cycle ventricular extrasystoles (Fig. 20-26). Initially, they occur in self-limited bursts with near syncope, and if they are unsuspected or mistakenly diagnosed as being due to inadequate dosing, the patient may be given more of the offending class IA agent, resulting in sustained VT/VF and cardiac arrest from which the patient may be difficult to resuscitate. Hypokalemia and acute ischemic disease can cause this arrhythmia as well, and it rarely occurs with other antiarrhythmic agents (lidocaine, amiodarone, mexiletine) and tricyclic antidepressants.

Treatment of proarrhythmia includes withdrawal of the offending drug, elevating serum K^+ to levels greater than 4.5 mEq per liter, using empiric IV bicarbonate and magnesium sulfate (1–2 gm), and correcting other metabolic derangements (e.g., acidosis, renal failure). Overdrive pacing may

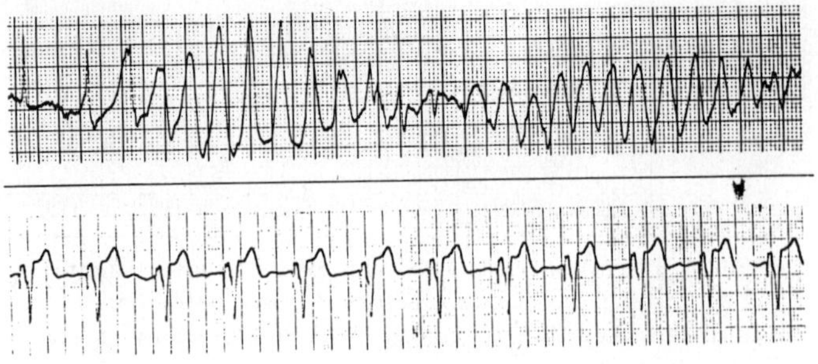

Fig. 20-26. Classic torsade de pointes (polymorphic VT/VF) due to quinidine (class IA antiarrhythmic agent). Pacing can be used to suppress this arrhythmia, as shown in lower tracing.

help in some patients, as will diphenylhydantoin (250–500 mg every four to six hours IV) and lidocaine, 1 mg/kg IV bolus followed by further boluses up to a total of 5 mg/kg.

SELECTED READING

General Principles and Mechanisms

Cranefield, PF, Wit, AL, and Hoffman, BF. Genesis of cardiac arrhythmias. *Circulation* 47:190, 1973.

Pick, A, and Langendorf, R. Differentiation of supraventricular and ventricular tachycardia. *Prog Cardiovasc Dis* 2:391, 1960.

Zipes, DP. Genesis of Cardiac Arrhythmias. In E Braunwald (ed), *Heart Disease. A Textbook of Cardiovascular Medicine* (3rd ed). Philadelphia: Saunders, 1988.

Zipes, DP. Specific Arrhythmias: Diagnosis and Treatment. In E Braunwald (ed), *Heart Disease: A Textbook of Cardiovascular Medicine* (3rd ed). Philadelphia: Saunders, 1988.

Tachyarrhythmias: Supraventricular

Akhtar, M. Electrophysiologic basis for wide QRS complex tachycardia. *PACE* 6:81, 1983.

Akhtar, M. Atrioventricular nodal reentry tachycardia. *Med Clin North Am* 68:819, 1984.

Benditt, DG, et al. Atrial flutter, atrial fibrillation and other primary atrial tachycardias. *Med Clin North Am* 68:895, 1984.

Donges, J, et al. Value of preexisting bundle branch block in the ECG differentiation of supraventricular from ventricular origin of wide QRS tachycardia. *Am J Cardiol* 55:717, 1985.

Gulamhussein, S, et al. ECG criteria for differentiating aberrancy and ventricular extrasystole in chronic atrial fibrillation. Validation by intracardiac recordings. *J Electrocardiol* 18:41, 1985.

Rinkenberger, RL, et al. Effects of intravenous and chronic oral verapamil administration in patients with supraventricular tachyarrhythmias. *Circulation* 62:996, 1980.

Sung, RJ, Elser, B, and McAllister, RG. Intravenous verapamil for termination of supraventricular tachycardias. Intracardiac studies correlated with plasma verapamil concentrations. *Ann Intern Med* 93:682, 1980.

Wellens, HJJ, et al. The value of the ECG in the differential diagnosis of a tachycardia with a wide QRS complex. *Am J Med* 64:27, 1978.

Wu, D. Dual AV nodal pathways. A reappraisal. *PACE* 5:72, 1982.

Tachyarrhythmias: Ventricular

Josephson, ME, et al. Recurrent sustained ventricular tachycardia: Mechanisms. *Circulation* 57:431, 1978.

Reiter, M, Smith, W, and Gallagher, J. Clinical spectrum of ventricular tachycardia with left bundle branch block. *Am J Cardiol* 51:113, 1983.

Bradycardias

Kerr, CR, et al. Sinus node dysfunction. *Cardiol Clin* 1:187, 1983.

Langendorf, R, and Pick, A. Atrioventricular block, type II (Mobitz). Its nature and clinical significance. *Circulation* 38:819, 1968.

Rosenqvist, M, Vallin, H, and Edhag, O. Clinical and electrophysiologic course of sinus node disease. Five-year followup study. *Am Heart J* 109:513, 1985.

Zipes, DP. Second degree AV block. *Circulation* 60:465, 1979.

Arrhythmias in Myocardial Infarction

Campbell, RWF, Murray, A, and Julian, DG. Relation of ventricular arrhythmias to ventricular fibrillation. *Br Heart J* 43:109, 1980.

El Sharief, N, et al. Electrocardiographic antecedents of primary ventricular fibrillation. Value of the R-on-T phenomenon in myocardial infarction. *Br Heart J* 38:415, 1976.

Ewy, GA. Ventricular fibrillation masquerading as asystole. *Ann Emerg Med* 13:811, 1984.

Josephson, ME. Treatment of ventricular arrhythmias after myocardial infarction. *Circulation* 74:653, 1986.

Lie, KJ. Lidocaine and prevention of ventricular fibrillation complicating acute myocardial infarction. *Int J Cardiol* 7:321, 1985.

Norris, RM, et al. Prevention of ventricular fibrillation during acute myocardial infarction by intravenous propranolol. *Lancet* 2:883, 1984.

Surawicz, B. Ventricular fibrillation. *J Am Coll Cardiol* 5 (Suppl 6):43B, 1985.

Wald, RW, et al. Management of intractable ventricular arrhythmias after myocardial infarction. *Am J Cardiol* 44:329, 1979.

Arrythmias in White-Parkinson-Wolff Syndrome

Benditt, DG, Pritchett, ELC, and Gallagher, JJ. Spectrum of regular tachycardias with wide QRS complexes in patients with accessory atrioventricular pathways. *Am J Cardiol* 42:828, 1978.

Gallagher, JJ, et al. The preexcitation syndromes. *Prog Cardiovasc Dis* 2:285, 1978.

Klein, GJ, et al. Ventricular fibrillation in WPW syndrome. *N Engl J Med* 301:1080, 1979.

Pryskowsky, EN, et al. Preexcitation syndromes. Mechanism and management. *Med Clin North Am* 68:831, 1984.

Wellens, HJJ, and Durrer, D. Effect of procainamide, quinidine and ajmaline in the WPW syndrome. *Circulation* 50:114, 1974.

Pacemakers

Haffajee, CI. Temporary cardiac pacing modes, evaluation of function, equipment and troubleshooting. *Cardiol Clin* 3:575, 1985.

Rosenthal, E, et al. Transcutaneous pacing for cardiac emergencies. *PACE* 11:2160, 1988.

Waldo, A, et al. Temporary cardiac pacing. Applications and techniques in the treatment of cardiac arrhythmias. *Prog Cardiovasc Dis* 23:457, 1981.

21. Congestive Heart Failure

John Gaca
Joseph Alpert

Congestive heart failure (CHF) is not a distinct pathophysiologic disorder but a syndrome arising from one or more causes—common, uncommon, or precipitating. The approach to the patient with heart failure in the emergency department should reflect current understanding of the diverse pathophysiologic natures of heart failure. In that way, optimal modalities of treatment, based on sound working hypotheses, can be chosen.

DEFINITION AND PATHOPHYSIOLOGY

The syndrome of CHF can be described as the inability of the heart to deliver blood in sufficient amounts to satisfy the oxidative needs of peripheral tissues despite an adequate intravascular volume. Conceptually and clinically, it is useful to think of heart failure in terms of:

1. Locus of dysfunction—right, left, or biventricular
2. Forward or backward ventricular failure
3. Phase of the cardiac cycle—systolic or diastolic dysfunction

Appreciation of the primary locus of dysfunction and the predominant direction of failure will help establish the etiologic differential. Although systolic and diastolic function are usually abnormal at the same time, they may occasionally be discordant. Therapy will then differ.

With left ventricular failure, the major abnormalities are a rise in pulmonary venous pressure (backward failure) and reduced forward output into the aorta (forward failure). "Pure" right ventricular failure results in abnormal elevation of systemic venous pressure (backward failure) and reduction of flow into the pulmonary arterial tree (forward failure). Although helpful conceptually, "pure" forms of isolated right or left ventricular failure do not exist since the two ventricles are arranged in series. Indeed, the most common cause of right ventricular failure is left ventricular failure. Backward heart failure is accompanied by a decrease in cardiac output—that is, by some of the features of forward failure. Backward failure of the right heart results in distended neck veins, peripheral edema, and, eventually, anasarca. Left ventricular backward failure results in dyspnea, pulmonary edema, and rales. Forward failure initially results in fatigue, weak pulse, and cool extremities.

The concept of diastolic dysfunction, as opposed to systolic dysfunction, is a relatively recent idea. Implicit in the concept of heart failure is the notion of the heart's inability to maintain its pumping function. There are parameters to evaluate myocardial contractility such as the rate of the development of pressure within the ventricle during isovolumic contraction (dP/dt) and the velocity of muscle fiber circumferential shortening (V_{cf}). These are used to evaluate alterations in systolic or contractile function.

There is evidence that clinical heart failure can be produced by different but interdependent mechanisms that control myocardial relaxation. The heart, unlike mechanical pumps, must structurally relax to receive incoming blood as well as eject a portion of the blood it receives. Ischemic or hypertrophied myocardium develops abnormalities in the rate of relaxation, which results in higher diastolic pressures for a given volume than in the normal heart. These pressure elevations are reflected back to the systemic or pulmonary venous systems. The modality of treatment of CHF will depend on whether the failure is secondary to the more common systolic dysfunction (a dilated ventricle with poor contractility) or diastolic dysfunction (normal or intact systolic function and probably normal ventricular size).

In the case of the former, the options for drug treatments include diuretics, vasodilators, and inotropic agents. In diastolic dysfunction with a nondilated ventricle, inotropic agents are not helpful and the response to vasodilators is less helpful.

CAUSES OF HEART FAILURE

The major pathophysiologic processes that result in congestive heart failure are:

1. Pressure overload
2. Volume overload
3. Loss of myocardial muscle
4. Diminished contractility
5. Restricted filling (Table 21-1)

Pressure overload is commonly seen in hypertension, either systemic or pulmonary, and in outflow obstruction such as aortic or pulmonic valve stenosis. Volume overload occurs with valvular regurgitant lesions and with some forms of congenital heart disease such as patent ductus arteriosus in which the left ventricle is volume overloaded by the low pressure "sump" created by the communication between the aorta and the main pulmonary artery. Pressure or volume overload eventually results in alterations in contractility and the syndrome of CHF.

Loss of myocardial muscle is seen in coronary artery disease, the most common cause of heart failure in developed countries. The cumulative insult of one or more infarctions decreases the pumping ability of the heart and, in effect, places both a volume and pressure burden on the remaining residual normal myocardium. Diminished contractility is seen in prolonged volume or pressure overload, or both, as well as in dilated cardiomyopathy of whatever etiology—idiopathic, alcoholic, viral, drug-induced, and so on. Restricted filling causing heart failure is seen in the aforementioned diastolic dysfunction of the hypertrophied stiff ventricle as well as in the extramyocardial pathologic processes of constrictive pericarditis and cardiac tamponade.

The common causes of heart failure in developed countries are, in decreasing frequency:

1. Coronary artery disease
2. Systemic hypertension

Table 21-1. Major pathophysiologic processes causing congestive heart failure

Pressure overload
Volume overload
Loss of myocardial muscle
Diminished contractility
Restricted filling

Table 21-2. Common causes of heart failure in the United States

Coronary artery disease
Systemic arterial hypertension
Valvular heart disease
Cardiomyopathy
Congenital heart disease

3. Valvular heart disease
4. Cardiomyopathy
5. Congenital heart disease (Table 21-2)

In the approach to the emergency department patient presenting with acute CHF, it is important to seek the underlying cause and the possible precipitating causes. Distinguishing worsening of the intrinsic heart failure and the imposition of a precipitating cause is important in directing therapy.

Common precipitating causes include:

1. Change or reduction of therapy
2. Cardiac arrhythmias
3. Cardiac or extracardiac infection
4. Pulmonary embolism
5. Physical or environmental stress
6. An additional form of heart disease
7. Noncardiac illness (Table 21-3)

Change or reduction of therapy includes dietary indiscretion such as increased salt or volume intake. Recent change in medical therapy or patient noncompliance is included in this category. Arrhythmias such as supraventricular and ventricular tachycardias and bradycardias as well as some forms of heart block can aggravate and cause heart failure. By decreasing diastolic filling time, supraventricular arrhythmias can cause elevation in atrial pressure. Pulmonary edema and systemic venous hypertension result. Ventricular tachycardia results in both shortened diastolic filling as well as atrioventricular dyssynchrony. The lack of coordinated atrial contraction followed by ventricular contraction results in a lowered forward output, intermittent ventriculoatrial valvular regurgitation, and atrial hypertension. Dyssynchronous atrioventricular activation leads to elevated systemic and pulmonary venous pressures. Cardiac infection such as endocarditis or myocarditis can aggravate or cause CHF.

The valvular regurgitant lesion of endocarditis imposes an acute volume overload that is poorly tolerated by even normal hearts. The increasing demands that sepsis places on the heart are poorly tolerated in individuals with limited ventricular reserve. Pulmonary embolism, if large enough, can im-

Table 21-3. Common precipitating factors of congestive heart failure

Change or reduction in therapy
Cardiac arrhythmias
Cardiac or extracardiac infection
Pulmonary embolism
Physical or environmental stress
An additional form of heart disease
Noncardiac illness

pose an acute pressure overload on the right heart, resulting in acute right heart failure and shock. With less extensive embolism, the resulting hypoxemia can cause a marginal left ventricle to fail.

Physical or environmental stress can aggravate an otherwise compensated state of CHF. With exercise, cardiac output fails to increase appropriately, and right and left ventricular filling pressures increase inappropriately for a given level of effort. Extremes of temperature—cold causing peripheral vasoconstriction and increased "afterload" and heat resulting in the need for increased skin blood flow—may impose an inappropriate circulatory load or demand on an initially abnormal, albeit compensated, heart. Some forms of noncardiac illness can precipitate heart failure. Acute renal failure and hepatic cirrhosis can result in volume overload. Anemia increases the need for more cardiac output secondary to the reduced oxygen-carrying capacity of a given volume of blood. Hyperthyroidism and the attendant increased total body metabolism result in the need for greater cardiac output. Arteriovenous fistulae cause shunting of blood to the venous system bypassing the capillaries. Volume overload of the ventricle follows.

HEART FAILURE AND THE CIRCULATORY SYSTEM

Although heart failure seemingly has myriad underlying and precipitating causes and the recognition of these causes is critical in the overall therapeutic approach, the syndrome of acute CHF is a final common pathway. This pathway is the expression of the interaction of the cause(s) of heart failure with the body's "normal" compensatory mechanisms in response to decreased stroke volume. These "normal" mechanisms may ultimately lead to a depression of cardiac output and a vicious cycle of progressive decompensation, disabling symptoms, and organ dysfunction.

To understand how an otherwise normal compensatory system could prove to be deleterious in heart failure and to prevent this from occurring, a review of the dynamics of the cardiovascular system in the normal and the abnormal state is necessary.

The four major factors that regulate cardiovascular performance are:

1. Myocardial contractility
2. Left ventricular preload
3. Afterload or aortic outflow impedance
4. Heart rate and rhythm

Myocardial contractility can be described as the force with which the heart beats. It is related to the rate of intraventricular pressure development and the rate of muscle fiber shortening. Preload is the force that stretches the muscle fiber to its precontraction length. The Frank Starling relationship shows that an increase in muscle fiber length within a physiologic range increases the number of filament interactions during contraction, allowing the heart a greater contractile force. This leads to an increase in stroke volume. Afterload is the tension the heart must develop to overcome forces opposing left ventricular ejection. These encompass resistance to blood flow in the aortic root area and beyond. Heart rate and rhythm determine the efficiency of myocardial contraction.

The cardiovascular system in the face of a declining stroke volume responds in a compensatory fashion as though volume depletion is the cause.

The sympathetic nervous system and the renin-angiotensin system are activated. There is a general rise in plasma catecholamines, particularly norepinephrine. Increased myocardial contractility, increased heart rate, and heightened vasoconstriction occur. The increased production of angiotensin II causes additional vasoconstriction and reduces sodium excretion via aldosterone production.

In the normal heart facing the consequences of hemorrhage, such adaptive mechanisms are life preserving. From a teleologic standpoint, the evolution of such compensatory adaptations undoubtedly helped prehistoric people in their adverse, predator-infested environment.

When the failing heart diminishes its stroke volume, the same sequence occurs: increased catecholamine production, sodium and water retention, and systemic vasoconstriction. However, the catecholamines usually have an inadequate inotropic effect since patients with chronic CHF have decreased numbers of beta-adrenergic receptors in the ventricular myocardium. The increased heart rate and increased systemic vascular resistance further impair the capability of the compromised left ventricle to eject blood. Myocardial work and oxygen demand are increased. Sodium and water retention further complicate the situation by increasing preload.

The clinical picture of cardiac failure is a result of the interactions among ventricular systolic and diastolic dysfunction and the peripheral response. Acute CHF presenting to the emergency department needs both emergent as well as subsequent definitive management.

Emergent intervention involves reversal of the overshooting "compensatory" dynamic cardiovascular changes. This encompasses altering, in a selective and controlled manner, one or more parameters of cardiac function—myocardial oxygenation and work, the contractile state, preload, and afterload. More definitive therapy involves reversing possible precipitating causes and rectifying, if possible, the underlying causes of heart failure.

EMERGENT ASSESSMENT AND MANAGEMENT

The approach to acute CHF in the emergency department involves a rapid assessment, improving tissue oxygenation, optimizing the patient's position, reversing acidosis, decreasing the work of breathing, treating arrhythmias, and producing a diuresis.

Evidence of Left Ventricular Failure

If the patient is able to provide a history, symptoms of progressive dyspnea and fatigue may be obtained. Dyspnea on exertion, the earliest symptom, is usually followed by orthopnea and paroxysmal nocturnal dyspnea. Pulmonary congestion secondary to an increase in the diastolic pressure in the left atrium and left ventricle produces the symptoms of left ventricular failure. The pathophysiologic mechanisms of orthopnea and paroxysmal nocturnal dyspnea are similar. When a patient moves from an erect to a supine position, blood that has been sequestered in the large venous reservoir in the legs returns to the central circulation and the pulmonary vessels. Pulmonary vascular pressure increases, fluid accumulates in the pulmonary interstitial spaces, breathing becomes more difficult, and the oxygen level in the blood decreases.

Extremely severe pulmonary congestion results in pulmonary edema, which is discussed in Chap. 11. Symptoms of pulmonary edema include severe dyspnea at rest and a cough productive of frothy sputum. Arterial hypoxemia, the result of ventilation/perfusion mismatches in a congested lung, further depresses left ventricular function, and hypoxemia combined with decreased cardiac output causes extreme fatigue.

Physical examination provides useful clues. The pulse pressure may be approximated by palpation of the carotid or brachial artery, which roughly indicates stroke volume. The small pulse of the low output state such as severe left ventricular dysfunction or mitral stenosis differs from the large pulse pressure of high output failure—that is, aortic insufficiency and mitral regurgitation. A slowly rising low-amplitude aortic pulse is characteristic of aortic stenosis. An S_3 (ventricular) gallop sound indicates rapid filling of a stiff, noncompliant ventricle and may signal left ventricular failure. An S_4 (atrial) gallop can occur in association with hypertension, aortic stenosis, cardiomyopathy, or coronary disease. Rales, indicating accumulation of fluid in the pulmonary interstitium, can be heard at the lung bases soon after the left ventricle begins to fail. As the decompensation worsens and pulmonary edema becomes more severe, rales are apparent over an increasing area of the lung fields.

The lungs' ability to supply the body with oxygen decreases, hypoxia increases, and tachypnea results. Some patients develop significant wheezing.

Dyspnea, on exertion or at rest, and orthopnea with arterial hypoxemia also frequently accompany chronic obstructive pulmonary disease (COPD). Therefore, the first question that must be answered by the physician evaluating the dyspneic patient is whether the dyspnea is secondary to cardiac or pulmonary dysfunction. A checklist such as the one in Table 21-4 is often useful in helping the physician distinguish one etiology from the other, but at times the differentiation cannot be made until the patient is admitted to the intensive care unit and the pulmonary wedge pressure is measured with a Swan-Ganz catheter.

Evidence of Right Ventricular Failure

The symptoms and signs of right ventricular failure are due to systemic venous congestion. Peripheral edema and fatigue are usually the earliest symptoms. Once venous congestion stretches the hepatic capsule, pain is felt in the right upper quadrant. Anorexia, nausea, and malabsorption, secondary to splanchnic venous congestion, eventually develop.

When the right ventricle fails, the patient's neck veins are usually distended, the liver is frequently enlarged and tender, hepatojugular reflux may be noted, and peripheral edema is often apparent. Ascites occurs only rarely, most commonly in patients with chronic right ventricular failure.

In either type of failure, careful auscultation for the characteristic murmurs of valvular stenosis or regurgitation should be performed.

Table 21-4. Differentiation of pulmonary and cardiac dyspnea

	Pulmonary	Cardiac
History	Industrial exposure; extensive tobacco use; recurrent respiratory infections; previous abnormal pulmonary function tests; daily cough-producing sputum, perhaps purulent	Previous angina, myocardial infarction, or rheumatic fever; previous evidence of abnormal cardiac function such as an abnormal ECG, presence of a murmur, or cardiomegaly seen on film
Physical examination	Increased respiratory rate; increased thoracic AP diameter; clubbing; localized rales; rhonchi; evidence of consolidation	Increased respiratory rate; S_3 and S_4 gallops; diffuse or symmetrical rales; murmur
ECG	Low voltage; poor R-wave progression; RVH	Old or recent MI; LVH except in mitral stenosis where RVH may be present
Chest film	Increased pulmonary volume with large AP diameter and flattened diaphragms; localized consolidation; small heart; normal pulmonary vasculature	Normal pulmonary volume and diaphragm; cardiomegaly; pulmonary vascular redistribution; Kerley B lines; interstitial or alveolar edema
Pulmonary capillary wedge pressure	Normal (< 12 mm Hg)	Elevated (usually > 20 mm Hg)
Pulmonary function tests	Markedly abnormal (restrictive or obstructive pattern)	Normal or mild abnormalities

LABORATORY TESTING

Routine laboratory testing, although helpful in assessing the patient's general condition, does not contribute much to the diagnosis of CHF. The electrocardiogram is usually abnormal and might provide clues as to etiology, including evidence of hypertrophy, new ischemic changes, or the presence of arrhythmias or heart block.

Radiographic Signs of Left and Right Ventricular Failure

The earliest roentgenographic sign of left ventricular failure is a "redistribution" of pulmonary venous flow; that is, more blood than normal flows through the vessels in the upper lobes of the lung and less flows through vessels in the lower lobes. As pulmonary venous pressure rises, pulmonary congestion worsens and the chest film reveals Kerley B lines and fluid in the major and minor fissures of the right lung, which are signs of fluid accumulation in the pulmonary interstices.

The marginal contours of the pulmonary vessels, normally sharply defined, gradually fade and a perihilar haze develops. Fluffy alveolar infiltrates and pleural effusion eventually appear. This results in the classic "butterfly" x-ray pattern.

Radiographic evidence of heart failure usually does not appear until 12 hours after the left ventricle begins to fail; signs of pulmonary congestion rarely disappear until approximately 1 to 2 days after the condition has resolved, even though hemodynamic evidence of resolution is observed earlier. The physician must keep these radiologic "phase lags" in mind when planning therapeutic strategy (see Chap. 11).

The evidence of right ventricular failure on chest films may be subtle. In fact, nothing abnormal may be evident except a distended azygous vein; the right ventricle is not always enlarged. Abdominal films may reveal hepatic and splenic enlargement.

Echocardiography in the Emergency Assessment of Acute Congestive Heart Failure

The determination of ventricular size and contractility can be easily accomplished through the use of M-mode, two-dimensional, and Doppler echocardiography. Echocardiography is more useful than the electrocardiogram or chest film for determining chamber size and ventricular function. It is virtually indispensable in the absence of very clear-cut clinical findings. It may detect causes of acute CHF that may, eventually, be surgically correctable—mitral or aortic stenosis or regurgitation. Echocardiography is quite helpful in demonstrating obstructive hypertrophic cardiomyopathy, pericardial constriction, and cardiac tamponade. Focal wall motion abnormalities seen in coronary artery diseases are delineated. The echocardiographic device is easily portable, and its use should be immediately available to the emergency physician for the rapid assessment of CHF.

MANAGEMENT

Providing Tissue Oxygenation

The crucial first step in the management of acute CHF is the administration of 30 to 40 percent oxygen by face mask. This will increase tissue oxygenation. In patients suspected of COPD, the amount should be 24 percent to avoid CO_2 narcosis. Adequacy of oxygenation should be confirmed with arterial blood gases. In those patients with respiratory insufficiency, intubation and artificial ventilation should be performed immediately.

Patient Position

The upright position of 90 degrees will result in some preload reduction by venous pooling. Vital capacity will increase.

Reversing Acidosis

There is some lactic acidosis in almost all patients with acute CHF; this will contribute to hypotension and arrhythmogenesis. The hazards of bicarbonate administration—rebound alkalosis and acute volume load of a hypertonic solution—often outweigh the benefits. Improvement of tissue oxygenation and cardiac performance with therapy usually reverses this form of acidosis. However, in the pulseless patient or in those with a pH of less than 7.0 or a bicarbonate less than 10 mmol/liter, exogenous bicarbonate therapy is indicated.

Decreasing the Work of Breathing

Intravenous morphine sulfate results in some increase in systemic venous capacitance, dilation of resistance vessels, and reduction in the work of breathing via its central sedative effect. It is best to give morphine sulfate as an intravenous push starting at 3 to 5 mg and repeated every 10 to 15 minutes until the respiratory rate is less than 20 breaths/minute. The phosphodiesterase inhibitor aminophylline can bronchodilate, increase myocardial contractility, and induce a diuresis. The usual intravenous bolus is 4 to 6 mg/kg over 20 minutes. The maintenance dose is 0.7 to 1.0 mg/kg/hour. This agent is particularly useful in patients with pulmonary edema, induced bronchospasm, or cor pulmonale. Caution should be exercised in patients with passive congestion of the liver since aminophylline is degraded by the liver; toxicity may result if doses are not reduced.

Treating Arrhythmias

Atrial fibrillation with a rapid ventricular response is a definite indication for digoxin. Cardioversion is indicated for any tachyarrhythmia causing hemodynamic embarrassment or unstable angina. If possible, prior to cardioversion, the parameters of pH, potassium, and PaO_2 should be normalized. Verapamil and beta-blockers should be used with caution owing to their negative inotropy.

Producing a Diuresis

In acute CHF, diuretic therapy is designed to reduce left ventricular preload. The diuretic of choice is furosemide, which both induces a diuresis and causes an immediate venodilation. In some situations, it may be wise to withhold or reduce the dose of furosemide; severe aortic stenosis and hypertrophic obstructive cardiomyopathy depend on a high preload to maintain forward output. Also, in the setting of acute infarction, there is usually a normal blood volume. Overdiuresis may result in hypotension. Inotropic therapy in the setting of infarction may be more appropriate.

The initial dose is an intravenous push of 20 to 40 mg of furosemide. If no effect is seen in 15 to 20 minutes, a second dose that is 3 to 4 times the initial dose may be used.

Subsequent Therapy in the Hospital or Outpatient Department

Once the emergent management has been undertaken, the phase of more definitive therapy is begun and long-term goals are formulated. Again, it is imperative that the patient's particular pathophysiology dictate the treatment. Specifically, an inadequate preload secondary to the restricted filling of constrictive pericarditis or cardiac tamponade requires pericardiectomy or evacuation, respectively; preload in these circumstances should be augmented until definitive management is performed.

Malignant hypertension is treated with a rapidly acting vasodilator such as nitroprusside; nifedipine can be used until the nitroprusside solution is prepared for intravenous usage. Severe aortic stenosis is transiently improved with urgent medical therapy, but aortic valvuloplasty or aortic valve replacement is ultimately necessary. In the setting of acute infarction, which is now known to be the result of acute intracoronary thrombosis, thrombolytic therapy should be used. This will depend on the time of the patient's presentation; the period of greatest efficacy of the thrombolytic agent is usually within 4 to 6 hours from the onset of pain. Contraindications to the use of thrombolysis include recent surgery or trauma, severe hypertension, bleeding disorders, and evidence of occult bleeding (positive guaiac).

The precipitating factors previously outlined should be sought and corrected.

The in-hospital management of CHF involves the use of certain invasive and noninvasive diagnostic procedures, diuretics, digitalis, vasodilators, and positive inotropic agents, and reversing correctable underlying and precipitating causes. Although diastolic dysfunction may play an important contributory role, CHF is usually related to a marked impairment in systolic performance, which is usually caused by an ischemic or cardiomyopathic process.

Diastolic dysfunction should be kept in mind, however, particularly when otherwise appropriate therapy for CHF fails or even results in deterioration (diuretics or arterial vasodilators in hypertrophic obstructive cardiomyopathy, diuretics in tamponade).

Noninvasive and Invasive Diagnostic Procedures for the In-Hospital Management of Left and Right Ventricular Failure

One of the most reliable ways to confirm a diagnosis of left ventricular failure is to determine the patient's *pulmonary venous pressure,* which reflects the filling pressure of the left ventricle. This is most easily done indirectly by measuring the *pulmonary capillary wedge pressure (PCWP),* which correlates with pulmonary venous pressure in most patients. The PCWP is determined with a Swan-Ganz balloon flotation catheter. A value greater than 12 to 15 mm Hg implies that the patient's left ventricle has failed. Insertion of this catheter is usually not performed in the emergency department, since it can be a time-consuming procedure requiring careful monitoring and possibly fluoroscopy. Placement is done in the intensive care unit (see Procedure 16).

Central venous pressure (CVP), an accurate reflection of right atrial or right ventricular filling pressure, should be measured in patients with suspected right ventricular failure. A value greater than 8 mm Hg confirms the diagnosis of right ventricular failure. Note that the CVP may be normal even when the PCWP is markedly elevated; CVP thus provides no information about left ventricular function.

The use of M-mode, two-dimensional, and Doppler echocardiography was described earlier.

Diuretics

Diuretics remain the mainstay of therapy for CHF, regardless of other drug therapy that may be used. These drugs promote the renal excretion of salt and water and may be particularly useful in preventing the sodium and water retention that may follow the administration of direct-acting vasodilator drugs. Although diuretics reduce the ventricular filling pressures and alleviate congestive symptoms, they do not increase cardiac output.

Diuretics are divided into three classes:

1. *Distal tubular diuretics,* which inhibit distal tubular sodium and water reabsorption
2. *Loop diuretics,* which primarily inhibit chloride absorption in the ascending Henle's loop
3. *Potassium-sparing diuretics,* which antagonize the effect of aldosterone on the distal renal tubule

Distal Tubular Diuretics

Distal tubular diuretics—the thiazide diuretics chlorothiazide, hydrochlorothiazide, and chlorthalidone—inhibit the active absorption of sodium and water in the distal tubule. The resultant obligatory increased delivery distally increases the availability at the site of aldosterone activity, where tubular sodium is more avidly exchanged for intracellular potassium. In conjunction with secondary aldosteronism resulting from diuretic-induced sodium and water depletion, this results in total body potassium depletion.

The distal tubular diuretics also cause an increase in the level of serum calcium and urate, as well as a tendency for glucose intolerance. The usual dose is 500 mg of chlorothiazide per day or 50 to 100 mg of hydrochlorothiazide per day.

Total body potassium depletion and clinically significant hypokalemia are particular problems in patients with heart failure who receive digoxin, because the patient's sensitivity to intoxication by digitalis is inversely proportional to the total body content of potassium and the serum potassium level. Because of its long duration of action, chlorthalidone is more problematic in this regard.

Loop Diuretics

Furosemide and ethacrynic acid inhibit chloride reabsorption in the ascending Henle's loop. They are potent diuretics that promote profound natriuresis and kaliuresis; the logical

Table 21-5. Most commonly used diuretics for left or right ventricular failure

Preparation	Mechanism	Usual Dosage	Onset of action	Duration of action
Hydrochlorothiazide (Esidrix)	Inhibits sodium reabsorption in the distal tubules	50 mg 1–2 times a day	2 hr	12 hr or longer
Furosemide (Lasix)	Inhibits sodium reabsorption in the loop of Henle	20–120 mg 1 time a day	Oral: 1 hr; IV: 5 min	Oral: 6 hr IV: 2 hr
Ethacrynic acid (Edecrin)	Inhibits sodium reabsorption in the loop of Henle	50–100 mg 1 time a day	Oral: 30 min IV: 15 min	Oral: 6–8 hr IV: 3 hr
Spironolactone (Aldactone)	Competitively inhibits renal tubular effects of aldosterone	25 mg 4 times a day	Gradually over 1–2 days	2–3 days after therapy ceases
Triamterene (Dyrenium)	Inhibits sodium reabsorption associated with potassium secretion	100 mg 1–3 times a day	2 hr	12–16 hr

extension of this is that there is greater risk of excessive intravascular volume depletion, prerenal azotemia, and hypotension.

Like the thiazides, the loop diuretics cause hypokalemia, metabolic alkalosis, hyperuricemia, and glucose intolerance. Unlike the distal tubular diuretics, loop diuretics promote calcium excretion.

In patients with decompensated CHF, furosemide is administered 20 to 40 mg intravenously, ethacrynic acid at 15 to 30 mg intravenously. For chronic treatment, a single morning dose of 20 to 160 mg of furosemide is usually enough.

Bumetanide is a new potent loop diuretic that is very effective in mobilizing edema fluid. The usual intravenous dose is 0.5–1.0 mg given over 1 to 2 minutes.

Aldosterone Antagonists

Spironolactone is a competitive antagonist of aldosterone; this antagonism results in inability of the distal tubule to reabsorb salt and water, with less potassium excretion. Triamterene has virtually the same ability but does so in a noncompetitive antagonistic manner.

Both of these agents are weak diuretics whose major clinical utility is minimizing potassium loss caused by the other forms of diuretics. Hyperkalemia is the major risk in the use of aldosterone antagonists. Table 21-5 lists commonly used diuretics and dosages.

Digitalis

Digoxin probably produces an inotropic effect by indirectly increasing intracellular calcium concentration. It binds to the myocardial muscle cell's sodium-potassium-ATPase membrane transport system and inhibits it. This increases intracellular sodium, which may lead to an increased intracellular calcium concentration through a sodium-calcium exchange mechanism. The increased calcium concentration at the contractile site promotes increased myocardial contractility.

Patients with CHF who will benefit from digitalis are those with:

1. Cardiac dilatation
2. Presence of an S_3 gallop
3. Chronic CHF
4. Atrial fibrillation
5. Elevated PCWP
6. Decreased ventricular ejection fraction

Digoxin has a low therapeutic ratio; its therapeutic serum level is 1 to 2 ng/ml. The risk of toxicity increases as the level exceeds 2.3 ng/ml. Digoxin metabolism relies on renal elimination; therefore, the daily dose should be adjusted downward if the glomerular filtration rate (GFR) falls.

The oral loading dose for a normal-sized adult is approximately 1.5 mg over 24 hours; the loading dose is 1 mg if given intravenously in the same time period. Maintenance dose is 0.25 to 0.375 mg per day. Toxic manifestations include adverse central nervous system (CNS) effects, nausea, vomiting, lassitude, and visual disturbances. The toxic cardiac effects of digoxin are a direct result of its electrophysiologic properties: depression of atrioventricular (AV) nodal conduction and acceleration of the rate of diastolic depolarization in subsidiary pacemakers. Hence, any combination of ectopic atrial, nodal, or ventricular beats or tachycardias in conjunction with AV nodal block may be a sign of digoxin toxicity (Table 21-6).

Regardless of the etiology of heart failure, systolic dysfunction should be documented as the cause of the CHF syndrome; digoxin has been shown to have little or no utility when diastolic dysfunction is the cause of failure.

Vasodilators

Vasodilators have an indirect effect on ventricular function. Arterial vasodilators reduce afterload by relaxing vascular smooth muscle. In acute CHF with an elevated left ventricular end-diastolic volume, this allows greater shortening of myocardial muscle fibers and facilitates increased ventricular emptying and ejection of a greater stroke volume. Venodilators increase capacitance of the venous system and, thus, reduce preload. This results in lower left ventricular end-diastolic volume and pressure. "Balanced" vasodilators work on both the arterial and venous systems.

Arterial Vasodilators

Arterial vasodilators include hydralazine, nifedipine, diltiazem, minoxidil, and diazoxide. Hydralazine is an arterial smooth muscle dilator that reduces resistance to left ventricular ejection. However, it does not affect left ventricular end-diastolic filling pressure since it does not venodilate. The

Table 21-6. Extracardiac manifestations of digitalis preparations

Gastrointestinal
Anorexia
Nausea
Vomiting
Diarrhea
Abdominal discomfort
Central nervous system
Headache
Drowsiness
Malaise
Nightmares
Disorientation
Delirium
Blurred vision
Altered color vision
White halos around dark objects
Diplopia
Scotomas
Optic neuritis
Hematologic
Thrombocytopenia
Eosinophilia
Skin
Rashes
Gynecomastia

intravenous preparation works rapidly in the acute setting. The starting dose is 20 mg. The oral dose is 50 to 150 mg/day as a tid dose. Exceeding this produces a lupus-like syndrome.

Combination therapy of hydralazine with a nitrate preparation, which, in effect, creates a "balanced" agent, has been shown to *prolong* life in patients with chronic CHF.

New drugs for treating *acute* CHF are the calcium channel blockers, nifedipine and diltiazem. They inhibit calcium ion influx in smooth muscle cells, and this results in relaxation of vascular tone. As a result, nifedipine and diltiazem reduce aortic outflow impedance. This allows for better ventricular emptying. They also cause coronary arterial vasodilatation, which increases myocardial oxygen supply.

Although nifedipine is an oral agent, the capsule can be punctured and swallowed for faster effect. The initial dose is 10 mg, and this may be repeated every 8 hours. Diltiazem is an oral agent; the dose is 30 to 60 mg every 6 hours.

Note: Caution should be exercised in the use of calcium channel blockers for *chronic* CHF. Nifedipine may increase digoxin levels by 50 percent. Both these agents have a slight negative inotropic effect. In the case of predominant diastolic dysfunction, they are more appropriate, since they may increase ventricular compliance. In patients with severe systolic dysfunction, calcium channel blockers may actually worsen heart failure.

Minoxidil and diazoxide have little use in the management of either acute or chronic CHF. Although minoxidil is a potent, direct-acting, smooth muscle relaxant that significantly reduces systemic vascular resistance, it also stimulates the renin-angiotensin system. Diazoxide's potency in reducing blood pressure renders it an agent for malignant hypertension. It has a rapid onset of action and long duration of action. It has some efficacy in *severe* CHF.

Venous Vasodilators

The primary agents in this class are the nitrates. Although it is now clear that nitrates affect both the systemic and myocardial vasculature, their most pronounced effect is to dilate the systemic venous vessels with consequent preload reduction but little change in cardiac output. For acute and chronic CHF, there are a variety of preparations. Sublingual nitroglycerin provides an immediate but short duration of action (5–30 minutes) at doses of 0.3 to 0.6 mg. Isosorbide dinitrate, on the other hand, has a longer duration of action (2–4 hours), and the chewable and sublingual forms have a fairly rapid onset (2 minutes) at doses of 5 mg.

Tolerance to these agents may develop with repeated, frequent dosage. An 8- to 10-hour "nitrate-free" interval is probably indicated each day.

"Balanced" Vasodilators

"Balanced" vasodilators include sodium nitroprusside and captopril. Another member, prazosin, has the problem of the rapid development of tolerance. Sodium nitroprusside is a potent vasodilator that produces both arterial and venous vasodilatation, reducing preload and afterload. It has no direct effect on the myocardium. In patients with acute CHF, these reductions translate into decreases in left ventricular end-diastolic and systemic arterial blood pressure without a significant rise in heart rate. In this setting, nitroprusside increases the left ventricular ejection fraction, decreases myocardial oxygen consumption, and increases cardiac output.

The initial dose is 0.5 μg/kg/minute; this can be titrated upward until the desired effect is achieved, systemic blood pressure falls below 100 mm Hg, or a dose of 10 μg/kg/minute is reached. Its use is largely restricted to severe acute CHF managed in the intensive care unit with systemic and pulmonary arterial pressure monitoring. Prolonged infusions can produce pulmonary shunting and cerebral and thyroid toxicity.

Captopril and enalapril have the same balanced effects as sodium nitroprusside, but their primary mechanism differs. They are angiotensin-converting enzyme (ACE) inhibitors that reduce the production of angiotensin II, the potent vasoconstrictor. ACE inhibitors interrupt one of the body's major pathologic responses to decreased cardiac output in patients with CHF. In so doing, they cause regionalized peripheral vasodilatation, reduced aldosterone synthesis, and decreased plasma levels of catecholamines. The net effect is a significant rise in cardiac output for most of these patients, coupled with a decrease in sodium and fluid retention, and a rise in renal blood flow and urinary output.

Captopril and enalapril are oral agents. Captopril is given in ascending doses up to 50 mg tid; enalapril's maximum dose is 20 mg bid. Higher doses cause no further beneficial effects. Both are excellent drugs for the management of chronic CHF.

Positive Inotropic Agents

This class of agents is largely reserved for those patients with severe CHF who manifest decompensation despite diuretic, digitalis, and vasodilator therapy. They are largely recommended for short-term therapy in these relatively refractory patients. There is no evidence of long-term benefit as seen by a reduction in mortality such as exists with the vasodilators.

The goal with these agents is to get the severely failing and refractory ventricle to a better position on the Starling function curve, thereby improving overall cardiovascular hemodynamics with the hope that the patients will become less refractory to the aforementioned therapy.

Dopamine is a catecholamine that enhances myocardial contractility via stimulation of myocardial beta receptors. It can restore systemic arterial blood pressure and improve cardiac output. At intravenous infusion rates of 1 to 2 μg/kg/minute, dopamine dilates renal arteries and increases urinary output. At 2 to 5 μg/kg/minute, there is a further increase in cardiac output and heart rate. Above this level, there is alpha receptor stimulation and vasoconstriction. The greatest utility of dopamine is in patients with severe left ventricular failure from acute myocardial infarction.

Dobutamine is a potent catecholamine that stimulates both $beta_1$ and $beta_2$ receptors, with more selectivity for the former. Dobutamine improves inotropy in a fashion similar to dopamine but without alpha receptor stimulation. Because it also affects both types of beta receptors, dobutamine induces an effect akin to that achieved with combined dopamine and sodium nitroprusside: increased myocardial contractility and increased arterial blood pressure from $beta_1$ stimulation and a simultaneous reduction in resistance owing to activation of $beta_2$ receptors in peripheral vessels. The average rate of infusion is 12 to 15 μg/kg/minute.

Dobutamine is most useful for short-term inotropic therapy in patients with acute CHF that is accompanied by hypotension and is refractory to treatment with digoxin and furosemide. Its use should be accompanied by arterial and pulmonary arterial monitoring.

There are several new positive inotropic agents that are bipyridine derivatives. The prototype is amrinone. Its mode of action is complex but includes phosphodiesterase inhibition and alteration in calcium transport. The inhibition results in higher intracellular levels of cyclic AMP and increased calcium availability. Amrinone also reduces vascular tone, resulting in vasodilatation—hence, the term *cardiotonic vasodilators*. To date, only intravenous amrinone is available for short-term use. The dose is 0.75 mg/kg as a bolus injected over 2 to 3 minutes; a hemodynamic benefit within 10 to 15 minutes that lasts for 1 to 2 hours can be expected. The maintenance infusion is 5–10 μg/kg/minute.

CONCLUSION

In the evaluation of CHF, acute or chronic, or both, the physician can supplement a careful and critical clinical evaluation with newer techniques of evaluating ventricular structure and function. By focusing on the specific pathophysiologic derangements, therapy can be tailored for the best possible benefit. Older traditional modalities of therapy can now be supplemented with appropriately chosen vasodilators and newer inotropic agents.

SELECTED READING

Alpert, JS, and Rippe, JM (eds). Heart Failure. In *Manual of Cardiovascular Diagnosis and Therapy* (3rd ed). Boston: Little, Brown, 1988.

Benotti, J. Therapy for heart failure: Current status. *Int Med* 7:51, 1986.

Braunwald, E. Clinical Manifestations of Heart Failure. In E Braunwald (ed), *Heart Disease.* Philadelphia: Saunders, 1988.

Bristow, M, and Mazzullo, J. A new look at therapy for acute congestive heart failure. *Emerg Med Rep* 5:181, 1984.

Katz, A. A physiologic approach to the treatment of heart failure. *Hosp Pract* 22:48, 1987.

Mallis, G. Management of congestive heart failure. *Cardiol Board Rev* 2:16, 1985.

Parmley, W. Pathophysiology of congestive heart failure. *Am J Cardiol* 55:9A, 1985.

Parmley, W. Medical treatment of congestive heart failure: Where are we now? *Circulation* 75(suppl):IV–4, 1987.

Schofield, PM. Use of vasodilators in the management of chronic heart failure. *Cardiovasc Rev and Rep* 8:48, 1989.

Smith, TW, Braunwald, E, and Kelly, RA. Management of Heart Failure. In E. Braunwald (ed), *Heart Disease.* Philadelphia: Saunders, 1988. Chap 17.

22. Congenital Heart Disease in the Adult

Michael S. Weinstock
Andrew E. Sama

In ever increasing numbers, patients with congenital heart disease are surviving well into adulthood. It is estimated that more than 500,000 patients with functionally important cardiac malformations fall into this category. The patient who presents to the emergency department with signs and symptoms referable to the cardiovascular system can sometimes challenge the most astute clinician. Emergency physicians need to understand the natural history, pathophysiology, anatomy, and clinical presentation of corrected and uncorrected congenital heart disease.

Palliative or corrective surgical procedures have been developed for most congenital cardiac anomalies, which continue to result in increasing numbers of patients who are born with congenital heart disease and survive into adulthood. When emergency physicians are faced with an acute presentation, the diagnosis of congenital heart disease may not initially be considered. However, as Perloff and colleagues wrote, "the anatomic principles are sound and the clinical manifestations are readily understood when information is handled within the framework of an orderly classification" (Table 22-1).

The patient who survives into adulthood after palliative or corrective surgery may have important residua (Table 22-2), which should be considered when evaluating someone with congenital heart disease. In addition, there are many possible causes of abnormal diastolic or systolic ventricular function and dysrhythmia in patients after corrective surgery for congenital heart disease (Table 22-3).

There are a group of patients who present to the emergency physician with undetected congenital heart disease. Explanations for this phenomenon reflect the subtle or silent nature of some congenital heart lesions and also point to the inadequate access to health care in underserved areas. There are textbooks devoted to the study of congenital heart disease; however, this chapter will focus on the more common lesions encountered in the daily practice of emergency medicine.

MITRAL VALVE PROLAPSE

Mitral valve prolapse syndrome was not elucidated until the 1960s, when Barlow and colleagues demonstrated that midsystolic clicks and late systolic murmurs were associated with prolapse of the mitral valve and mitral regurgitation. Initially, this condition was thought to be benign, but now, after intense study, it has been found to be ubiquitous and quite variable. The mitral valve prolapse syndrome may be found in 5 to 10 percent of the population, making it one of the most common cardiac valvular abnormalities. As a result

Table 22-1. A clinical classification of congenital heart disease

GENERAL

Innocent or normal murmurs
The cardiac malpositions
Congenitally corrected transposition of the great arteries
Congenital complete heart block

ACYANOTIC WITHOUT A SHUNT

Malformations Originating in the Left Side of the Heart (from most proximal to most distal)

1. Obstruction to left atrial inflow
   a. Pulmonary vein stenosis
   b. Mitral stenosis
   c. Cor triatriatum
2. Mitral regurgitation
   a. Endocardial cushion defect
   b. Congenitally corrected transposition of the great arteries
   c. Anomalous origin of the left coronary artery from the pulmonary trunk
   d. Miscellaneous (congenital perforations, accessory commissures with anomalous chordal insertion, congenitally short or absent chordae, cleft posterior leaflet, and so on)
3. Primary dilated endocardial fibroelastosis
4. Aortic stenosis
   a. Discrete subvalvular
   b. Valvular
   c. Supravalvular
5. Aortic valve regurgitation
6. Coarctation of the aorta

Malformations Originating in the Right Side of the Heart (from most proximal to most distal)

1. Acyanotic Ebstein's anomaly of the tricuspid valve
2. Pulmonic stenosis
   a. Subinfundibular
   b. Infundibular
   c. Valvular
   d. Supravalvular (stenosis of pulmonary artery and its branches)
3. Congenital pulmonary valve regurgitation
4. Idiopathic dilatation of the pulmonary trunk
5. Primary pulmonary hypertension

ACYANOTIC WITH A SHUNT (LEFT TO RIGHT)

Shunt at Atrial Level

1. Atrial septal defect
   a. Ostium secundum
   b. Ostium primum
   c. Sinus venosus
2. Partial anomalous pulmonary venous connection
3. Atrial septal defect with mitral stenosis (Lutembacher's syndrome)

Shunt at Ventricular Level

1. Ventricular septal defect
   a. Inlet septum
   b. Trabecular septum
   c. Perimembranous septum
   d. Infundibular septum
2. Ventricular septal defect with aortic regurgitation
3. Ventricular septal defect with left ventricular to right atrial shunt

Shunt Between Aortic Root and Right Side of Heart

1. Coronary arteriovenous fistula
2. Ruptured sinus of Valsalva aneurysm
3. Anomolous origin of left coronary artery from pulmonary trunk

Table 22-1. (Continued)

Shunt at Aortopulmonary Level

1. Aortopulmonary window
2. Patent ductus arteriosus

Shunts at More than One Level

Complete common atrioventricular canal

CYANOTIC

Increased Pulmonary Arterial Blood Flow

1. Complete transposition of the great arteries
2. Taussig-Bing anomaly
3. Truncus arteriosus
4. Total anomalous pulmonary venous connection
5. Univentricular heart with low pulmonary vascular resistance and no pulmonic stenosis
6. Common atrium
7. Fallot's tetralogy with pulmonary atresia and increased collateral arterial flow
8. Tricuspid atresia with nonrestrictive ventricular septal defect

Normal or Decreased Pulmonary Arterial Blood Flow

1. Dominant left ventricle
   a. Tricuspid atresia
   b. Pulmonary atresia with intact ventricular septum
   c. Ebstein's anomaly of the tricuspid valve
   d. Single morphologic left ventricle with pulmonic stenosis
   e. Congenital vena caval to left atrial communication
2. Dominant right ventricle
   a. No Pulmonary hypertension
      (1) Pulmonic stenosis or atresia with ventricular septal defect (Fallot's tetralogy)
      (2) Pulmonic stenosis with intact ventricular septum and right to left interatrial shunt
      (3) Pulmonic stenosis with complete transposition of the great arteries
      (4) Double outlet right ventricle with pulmonic stenosis
   b. Pulmonary hypertension
      (1) Atrial septal defect with reversed shunt
      (2) Ventricular septal defect with reversed shunt (Eisenmenger's complex)
      (3) Patent ductus arteriosus or aortopulmonary window with reversed shunt
      (4) Double outlet right ventricle with high pulmonary vascular resistance
      (5) Complete transposition of the great arteries with high pulmonary vascular resistance
      (6) Total anomalous pulmonary venous connection with high pulmonary vascular resistance
      (7) Hypoplastic left side of heart (aortic atresia, mitral atresia)
3. Normal or nearly normal ventricles
   a. Pulmonary arteriovenous fistula
   b. Vena caval to left atrial communication

Source: J. K. Perloff. *The Clinical Recognition of Congenital Heart Disease* (3rd ed.). Philadelphia: Saunders, 1987.

Table 22-2. Residua, sequelae, and late complications after surgery for congenital heart disease

Preoperative diagnosis	Residua, sequelae, and complications
VSD	Open VSD with CHF; elevated Rp; AV block; ventricular dysfunction
Endocardial cushion defect	Mitral, tricuspid regurgitation; elevated Rp; residual shunt; AV block; atrial dysrhythmia
Coarctation of the aorta	Residual or recurrent coarctation; aneurysm; aortic regurgitation
Aortic stenosis	Residual or recurrent stenosis; aortic regurgitation; ventricular dysfunction; altered ventricular distensibility
Transposition of the great arteries (atrial repair)	Atrial dysrhythmia and conduction disturbances; ventricular dysfunction; caval obstruction; pulmonary venous obstruction; increased Rp; residual shunt; pulmonary stenosis; tricuspid regurgitation
Tetralogy of Fallot	Ventricular dysrhythmia; AV block; aneurysm of RV outflow tract; VSD; residual or recurrent stenosis; pulmonary regurgitation; ventricular dysfunction; tricuspid regurgitation; increased Rp (usually in patients with prior shunt procedure)
Pulmonary atresia plus ventricular septal defect, truncus arteriosus, transposition post-Rastelli repair	All of those listed for tetralogy plus conduit stenosis

Key: VSD = ventricular septal defect; CHF = congestive heart failure; Rp = pulmonary vascular resistance; AV = atrioventricular; RV = right ventricular.
Source: T. P. Graham. Assessing the results of surgery for congenital heart disease—a continuing process. *Circulation* 65:1049, 1982. By permission of the American Heart Association, Inc.

Table 22-3. Possible causes for abnormal diastolic or systolic ventricular function and dysrhythmia in patients after surgery for congenital heart disease

I. Secondary to the defect or defects
  A. Hemodynamic overload—chronic hypertrophy—? fibrosis
  B. Intermittent myocardial oxygen supply–demand imbalance—? fibrosis
    1. ↑ O_2 demands— ↑ wall tension, ↑ heart rate and ↑ catecholamine stimulus during stress
    2. ↓ O_2 supply— ↑ wall tension; cyanotic patient— ↓ O_2 content, polycythemia— ↑ viscosity— ↑ coronary vascular resistance
  C. Residual shunts, obstructive lesions, valvular insufficiency
II. Complications of treatment
  A. ? Inadequate myocardial protection during operative interventions—ischemia → fibrosis
  B. ? Inadequate myocardial protection during low output states: e.g., severe congestive heart failure pre- or postoperatively with low coronary perfusion pressure
  C. Intraoperative coronary air embolus and myocardial ischemia
  D. Altered coronary supply: tetralogy with injured or transected coronary artery, ? post-Jatene arterial switch for transposition
  E. Ventricular scar from repair
  F. Atrioventricular block and ventricular pacing
III. Acquired disease
  A. Coronary artery disease
  B. Myocardial disease: myocarditis, endocarditis with valvular or myocardial damage, cardiomyopathy
  C. Hypertensive cardiovascular disease

Source: T. P. Graham. Assessing the results of surgery for congenital heart disease—a continuing process. *Circulation* 65:1049, 1982. By permission of the American Heart Association, Inc.

of multiple manifestations of this abnormality, Perloff and colleagues proposed guidelines for the diagnosis of mitral valve prolapse (Table 22-4).

Mitral valve prolapse has been associated with various forms of congenital heart disease and connective tissue disorders as well as acquired heart disease. Although not classically considered a form of congenital heart disease, it appears to have a strong hereditary component transmitted as an autosomal dominant trait.

Anatomy and Physiology

The connective tissue in most cases of mitral valve prolapse is congenitally defective, leading to mitral valvular dysfunction later in life. These abnormal valves may or may not contain excessive amounts of acid mucopolysaccharide material, but electron microscopy reveals alteration in collagen fibers in the leaflets and chordae tendinae. Anatomic findings associated with mitral valve prolapse include redundancy and myxomatous degeneration of the leaflets, dilatation and sometimes calcification of the mitral annulus, thinning and lengthening of the chordal structures, focal thickening of the mural left ventricular endocardium behind the posterior mitral leaflet, and fibrinous deposits on the atrial surface of the prolapsed portion of the mitral leaflet. This abnormal valvular structure causes abnormal and destructive stresses on the mitral valve during systole and diastole. Mitral valve prolapse is now the most common cause of pure isolated severe mitral regurgitation requiring mitral valve replacement.

Clinical Features

Physical examination may reveal a click, a late systolic murmur, or a holosystolic murmur. Provocative maneuvers or pharmacologic interventions that change left ventricular volume will alter the appreciation of the click and murmur. Decreases in left ventricular volume will result in earlier

Table 22-4. Diagnostic criteria and nonspecific findings in mitral valve prolapse

MAJOR CRITERIA
Auscultation
  Mid to late systolic clicks and late systolic murmur or whoop alone or in combination at the cardiac apex
Two-dimensional echocardiogram
  Marked superior systolic displacement of mitral leaflets with coaptation point at or superior to annular plane
  Mild to moderate superior systolic displacement of mitral leaflets with:
    Chordal rupture
    Doppler mitral regurgitation
    Annular dilatation
Echocardiogram plus auscultation
  Mild to moderate superior systolic displacement of mitral leaflets with:
    Prominent mid to late systolic clicks at the cardiac apex
    Apical late systolic or holosystolic murmur in the young
    Late systolic "whoop"

MINOR CRITERIA
Auscultation
  Loud first heart sound with an apical holosystolic murmur
Two-dimensional echocardiogram
  Isolated mild to moderate superior systolic displacement of the posterior mitral leaflet
  Moderate superior systolic displacement of both mitral leaflets
Echocardiogram plus history
  Mild to moderate superior systolic displacement of mitral leaflets with:
    Focal neurologic attacks or amaurosis fugax in the young
    First-degree relatives with major criteria

NONSPECIFIC FINDINGS
Symptoms
  "Atypical" chest pain, dyspnea, fatigue, lassitude, giddiness, dizziness, syncope
  Psychologic disturbances
Physical appearance
  Thoracic bony abnormalities
  Hypomastia
Electrocardiogram
  T-wave inversions in inferior limb leads or lateral precordial leads
  Premature ventricular beats at rest, on exercise, or on ambulatory ECG
  Supraventricular tachycardia
X-ray
  Scoliosis, pectus excavatum or carinatum, or loss of thoracic kyphosis
Two-dimensional echocardiogram
  Mild superior systolic displacement of anterior or anterior and posterior mitral leaflet

Source: J. K. Perloff, J. S. Child, and J. E. Edwards. New guidelines for the clinical diagnosis of mitral valve prolapse. *Am. J. Cardiol.* 57:1124, 1986.

prolapse of the valve during systole, causing the click and the onset of the murmur to drift closer to S_1.

Increases in left ventricular volume will cause both the click and onset of the murmur to be delayed and sometimes disappear. Electrocardiographic evaluation is generally normal, but there is an association with a myriad of atrial and ventricular tachy- and bradyarrhythmias. Paroxysmal supraventricular tachycardia is the most common tachyarrhythmia in patients with mitral valve prolapse syndrome. This may be related to the increased evidence of accessory atrioventricular (AV) bypass tracts. Inferolateral T-wave inversions (I, II, AVF, and V4-6) and prolongation of the Q-T interval are also common repolarization abnormalities.

Chest radiography in mitral valve prolapse is frequently unrevealing as opposed to echocardiography, which is most helpful in making the diagnosis. Two-dimensional and M-mode echocardiography frequently illustrate the dynamic anatomic abnormality and can be used to evaluate the mitral regurgitation. In patients with atypical chest pain and frequently in elderly patients with coexistent coronary artery disease, exercise thallium 201 scintigraphy as well as cardiac catheterization may be necessary to make a definitive diagnosis.

The majority of patients with mitral valve prolapse, who are asymptomatic, have minor physical findings and may go decades without diagnosis. Variability is the hallmark of this syndrome and is found when evaluating patients who are symptomatic. Asymptomatic patients without arrhythmias, ST segment changes, or serious mitral regurgitation should be reassured and have follow-up examination every 2 to 4 years. Endocarditis prophylaxis should be recommended liberally for all patients subjected to instrumentation of the upper respiratory tract and genitourinary tract.

Management

Symptomatic patients with mitral valve prolapse syndrome always pose a difficult problem for the clinician. Acute presentations of mitral regurgitation require immediate evaluation for infective endocarditis, spontaneous rupture of chordae tendineae, and myocardial infarction. Cerebral embolic events are treated with platelet aggregation inhibitor therapy (typically aspirin alone or with dipyridamole) after ruling out infective endocarditis.

Patients with mitral regurgitation unresponsive to medical therapy may require mitral valve replacement. Calcification of the mitral annulus alone rarely requires annuloplasty.

Those with palpitations, syncope, chest pain, and fatigue may benefit from ambulatory electrocardiographic (ECG) monitoring so that those with documented symptomatic arrhythmias may be treated. Typical anginal chest pains should be evaluated with treadmill exercise testing or cardiac catheterization, or both. Beta-blocker therapy may be beneficial for the treatment of fatigue and atypical chest pain, although reassurance may be all that is necessary.

An uncommon complication of mitral valve prolapse is sudden cardiac death that appears to be caused by ventricular fibrillation. The propensity for this occurrence is poorly understood, and postmortem findings in these cases reveal valvular abnormalities varying from mild to severe. Mitral valve replacement for refractory life-threatening arrythmias has been suggested.

CONGENITAL LEFT VENTRICULAR OUTFLOW TRACT ABNORMALITIES

Congenital obstruction to the left outflow tract can occur at the valvular, subvalvular, or supravalvular positions. The clinician's role in evaluating patients with outflow tract obstruction is in identifying and recognizing important signs and symptoms requiring further study. The bicuspid aortic valve is the most common congenital malformation of the heart, with a prevalence rate estimated at between 0.7 and 20 percent of the U.S. population. By age 45, approximately 50 percent of all bicuspid valves show some degree of stenosis.

Anatomy and Pathophysiology

Both supravalvular and subvalvular aortic stenosis are uncommon in adults. Discrete subaortic stenosis is usually tubular (fibromuscular) or the localized fibromembranous type. Supravalvular stenosis is usually found either as an hourglass deformity with segmental narrowing of the ascending aorta or the less common hypoplastic form, with the entire aorta being narrowed.

Many patients, when seen as adults, will have undergone a surgical procedure in childhood to palliate their congenital outflow tract obstruction. The complication of infective endocarditis is everpresent with congenital abnormalities of the aortic valve; all these patients should receive antibiotic prophylaxis.

Clinical Manifestations

Careful attention to history taking is important in identifying the "asymptomatic patient" with aortic stenosis. Subtle changes in exercise tolerance, fatigue, or dyspnea may be pointing to well-compensated heart failure. The major symptoms of congenital valve outflow tract obstruction in the adult includes angina pectoris, syncope (typically exertional or postexertional), and congestive heart failure (CHF).

The physical examination in patients with aortic stenosis is frequently accompanied by a loud harsh systolic murmur heard best at right upper sternal edge radiating to the carotids and may be associated with a palpable thrill. The carotid pulse may exhibit a delayed upstroke and a systolic shudder, and the precordial apical impulse may be sustained. Patients with unusual chest wall anatomy or elderly patients with underlying chronic lung disease may not have characteristic physical findings consistent with aortic stenosis.

Chest radiographs of patients with aortic stenosis are frequently normal but may show calcification of the aortic valve, left ventricular enlargement, or poststenotic dilatation of the ascending aorta. The ECG variably reveals left ventricular hypertrophy with a "strain" pattern but alone is a poor indicator of the severity of valvular obstruction. Noninvasive evaluation of congenital left ventricular (LV) outflow tract obstruction is most often done by echocardiography. M-mode, two-dimensional, and Doppler echocardiography can be helpful in defining the location and extent of obstruction. Despite advances in noninvasive quantitation of aortic stenosis, cardiac catheterization remains the definitive procedure for diagnosis.

Management

The reported incidence rate of sudden death from aortic stenosis has varied from 1 to 19 percent, with an accepted average incidence of 7.5 percent. Adults with congenital bicuspid aortic valves that are stenotic usually present for evaluation of a murmur or symptoms of angina, CHF, syncope, or presyncope. Generally, valve replacement is not considered until the development of symptoms occur, after which time average life expectancy is 5 years. Once symptoms are present, there is little role for medical management; cardiac catheterization with aortic valve replacement as indicated is the preferred management. These patients often require urgent or emergent evaluation of their symptoms.

It is preferable to intervene with aortic valve replacement when myocardial performance is good, with the hope of left ventricular hypertrophic changes being reversible. Aortic valve replacement carries an early mortality rate of 1.5 to 5 percent. Postoperative mortality is highest in the first 2 years after surgery, with the leading mode of late mortality being sudden death. In younger patients with congenital valvular aortic stenosis, valvulotomy or percutaneous balloon valvuloplasty may be the procedure of choice.

VENTRICULAR SEPTAL DEFECT

Ventricular septal defect (VSD) represents the third most common type of congenital heart disease found in the adult population (Mark). The second most common lesions are patent ductus arteriosus and atrial septal defect (Keith, et al.).

In looking at the natural history of VSD, it can be noted that spontaneous closure occurs in about one-third of all cases in early life, and in those individuals with a small VSD, there is generally a favorable course. An unknown number of adults who have VSD and are free of symptoms may go unrecognized and therefore escape medical statistics. In the adult population, there are two main complications that lead to death: (1) acquired aortic regurgitation and (2) bacterial endocarditis. The latter is, for the most part, preventable with antibiotics and can be reduced to a minimum with periodic indicated use of antibiotics. Acquired aortic regurgitation can be the direct result of endocarditis. Corone and coworkers reported aortic regurgitation in 6.3 percent of the 790 patients studied in their series.

Pathophysiology

The significant consequences of VSD relate to the pathophysiology determined by the size of the defect. Large VSDs can eventually result in equilibration of systolic pressure in both ventricles with acquired pulmonary vascular hypertension. In combination, these two factors result in the Eisenmenger's syndrome, which is the reversal in the direction of the shunt resulting in arterial desaturation.

Clinical Features

Although several sophisticated modalities are now readily accessible to the clinician for evaluation of cardiac disease, the emergency physician must still utilize the time honored diagnostic armamentarium of a good history, ECG, and cardiac x-rays.

In the adult patient with a small VSD, symptoms are few and the specific signs usually consist of a forceful apical impulse on inspection, a sometimes palpable thrill over the precordium, and a prominent high-frequency holosystolic murmur obscuring the first and second heart sounds. In the case of large septal defects that have gone on to produce Eisenmenger's syndrome, the striking diagnostic feature is the loudness and narrow splitting of the second heart sound; this is secondary to the pressure in the pulmonary artery being equal to that of the aorta. When the shunt reverses and becomes right to left, cyanosis appears as well as the associated plethora of polycythemia. These patients may present in cardiac failure.

Those adults with uncomplicated VSD have normal ECGs. If there is systemic pressure overload of the right ventricle, the ECG reflects a right axis deviation and may demonstrate right ventricular hypertrophy.

Chest x-rays are normal in individuals with small defects. However, pulmonary vascular markings associated with pulmonary arterial and left atrial and left ventricular enlargement are common with large defects and associated Eisenmenger's syndrome.

Most clinicians encounter adult patients who have undergone corrective surgery for their VSD many years prior to their presentation to the emergency department. It is important to note that most of these individuals still have soft systolic murmurs that may be accompanied by a thrill leading the physician to believe that there is a residual VSD. However, on these individuals, the chest x-ray and ECG should appear normal.

Management

In the emergency department, it is the complications of VSD that the clinician must initially manage. Infective endocarditis must be considered in the individual who presents with a cardiac murmur or history of VSD and febrile tendencies. Recent dental manipulation or other types of invasive procedures should be illicited in the history, if available. Those individuals with known VSD undergoing any invasive procedure or dental extractions should be given prophylactic antibiotics in therapeutic doses immediately before and a dose 4 hours after the procedure. If the diagnosis of infective endocarditis is contemplated, appropriate blood cultures and indicated antibiotics should be instituted along with hospitalization.

Additional complications of cerebral abscess and thrombosis can occur in those adults with Eisenmenger's syndrome. Thrombosis is more likely to occur in the young adult who is polycythemic. If the patient presents with cardiac failure, it should be addressed with immediate intervention and appropriate therapy, along with hospitalization.

The treatment of choice is surgical intervention and correction of the VSD in early childhood. This clearly reduces the morbidity and mortality associated with VSDs, especially those that present as large shunts.

HYPERTROPHIC CARDIOMYOPATHY

Hypertrophic cardiomyopathy (HCM) is a primary disease of the cardiac muscle characterized by inappropriate myocardial hypertrophy. It usually involves the left ventricle with an asymmetric interventricular septal thickening as compared to the left ventricular free wall. These findings must occur in a nondilated heart and in the absence of other hypertrophic cardiac disease in order for the diagnosis to be made. The basic defect resulting in hypertrophy in HCM is unknown, although there are data that suggest that the disease is inherited and in some cases HLA-linked. The disease appears to be transmitted as an autosomal dominant trait with a high degree of penetrance, although occasional cases probably represent new mutations.

The natural history of this disease has been altered with the use of beta-blockers, calcium channel blockers, amiodarone, and septal myotomy-myectomy, all making the clinical course of a given patient unpredictable.

In patients with HCM who are not treated surgically, the premature cardiac death rate is approximately 3 percent per year, with about 87 percent of all cardiac deaths being sudden and unexpected.

The study by Maron, et al. concluded that HCM was the leading cause of sudden cardiac death in young competitive athletes. The importance of early recognition of this disorder is clear, and the advent of echocardiography as a diagnostic tool has enhanced our appreciation of this disease.

Anatomy and Pathophysiology

The hallmark pathologic features of HCM are greater thickening of the interventricular septum than the left ventricular free wall with small or normal-sized left and right ventricular cavities. There is fibrous plaque on the mural endocardium of the outflow tract of the septum, a thickened mitral valve, and dilated atria. The intramural coronary arteries are abnormal and one sees myocardial fiber disarray and myocardial fibrosis microscopically. The most distinctive and controversial physiologic feature of HCM is the dynamic pressure gradient sometimes found in the subaortic region of the outflow tract.

Initially this was thought to be secondary to muscular sphincter action in the subaortic region, but now it is thought to be related to systolic anterior motion (SAM) of the mitral valve against the septum, causing further impingement of an already narrowed outflow tract. Pathophysiologically HCM is characterized by diastolic dysfunction. The left ventricle is abnormally stiff, causing impaired diastolic ventricular filling resulting in elevated LV end diastolic pressure.

Clinical Features

The most common complaint of symptomatic patients with HCM is dyspnea thought to be secondary to elevated LV end diastolic pressure reflected in elevated left atrial and pulmonary venous pressure. Angina pectoris, fatigue, and syncope are common with palpitations, overt CHF, paroxysmal nocturnal dyspnea, and dizziness, found less often. Physical exertion will often worsen symptoms. Examination often reveals a LV lift, a loud fourth heart sound, and an apical precordial impulse that is hyperdynamic and laterally displaced with a systolic thrill. The carotid pulse rises quickly, then declines in midsystole with the development of a gradient. The jugular venous pulse may show a prominent a-wave if right ventricular (RV) compliance is reduced secondary to interventricular septal hypertrophy. The systolic murmur is usually harsh and crescendo-decrescendo in quality and starts after S1. It is heard best between left sternal border and the apex. Dynamic auscultation may be useful when one suspects the murmur may be secondary to HCM. The murmur is decreased by increasing LV volume. Squatting and standing have opposite hemodynamic effects. Squatting results in increased venous return and an increase in aortic pressure, which increases LV volume and diminishes the murmur (standing has opposite effects and accentuates the murmur). The dynamic nature of this LV outflow tract obstruction differentiates it from other forms of fixed obstruction.

The ECG is usually abnormal, showing ST-segment and T-wave abnormalities, left ventricular hypertrophy, abnormal Q-waves in the inferior leads, left axis deviation, and P-wave abnormalities (usually left atrial enlargement). Ventricular arrhythmias are more common than supraventricular arrhythmias on continuous ambulatory ECG monitoring. Chest radiography findings are variable with heart size (left ventricle) being normal to enlarged and left atrial size frequently enlarged; calcification of the mitral valve annulus is also seen. The most useful noninvasive diagnostic instrument for studying HCM is echocardiography. The findings of a thickened septum (1.3 to 1.5 times the thickness of the left ventricular posterior wall) and narrowed LV outflow tract are helpful criteria for diagnosis. Patients with pressure gradients usually show systolic anterior motion (SAM) of the anterior leaflet of the mitral valve. Radionuclide imaging and cardiac catheterization are also used in the assessment of HCM. In patients over 45 years of age, obstructive coronary artery disease is frequently found at catheterization, but symptoms of angina pectoris have been reported in patients with hypertrophic cardiomyopathy and normal coronary arteriograms.

Management

Improvements in symptoms of patients with HCM have been noted when pharmacologic or surgical manipulation results in increased ventricular volume, systemic arterial pressure, size of the LV outflow tract or ventricular compliance, and decreases in ventricular contractility. Beta-blockers, calcium channel blockers, and surgical myotomy-myectomy have been used to effect these changes with some success. Symptomatic arrhythmias (ventricular and supraventricular) may be ameliorated with amiodarone, since conventional antiarrhythmics do not appear to control these arrhythmias effectively (Fig. 22-1). Atrial fibrillation and other symptomatic supraventricular tachyarrhythmias should be rapidly cardioverted in patients with HCM, since loss of the atrial kick may cause serious hemodynamic decompensation.

Patients presenting emergently with angina pectoris, syncope, pulmonary vascular congestion, or poorly controlled arrhythmias with known or suspected HCM should be hospitalized for careful evaluation and cardiac monitoring. Unfortunately, few clinical parameters are useful in predicting sudden death in patients with this disease. Predisposition to sudden death appears to be related to youthful age, familial predilection for premature death, and serious ventricular arrhythmias found in ambulatory ECG. It is recommended that patients with HCM not engage in competitive athletics or strenuous physical exertion because of the high incidence of

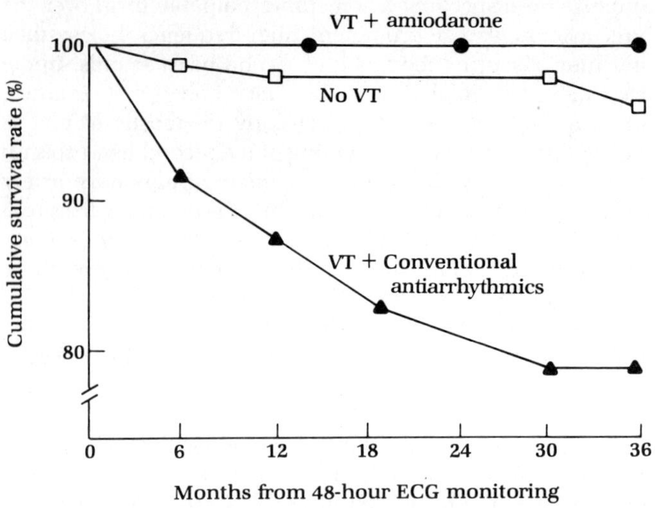

Fig. 22-1. Survival in patients with hypertrophic cardiomyopathy and ventricular tachycardia (VT) on 48-hour ambulatory electrocardiogram. Comparison of 21 patients with VT treated with amiodarone (circles), 24 patients with VT treated with conventional antiarrhythmic agents (triangles), and 123 patients without VT. (From W.J. McKenna, et al. Improved survival with amiodarone in patients with hypertrophic cardiomyopathy and ventricular tachycardia. *Br. Heart J.* 53:412, 1985.)

sudden cardiac death in this group of individuals. Endocarditis does occur with increased frequency in this patient population, and antibiotic prophylaxis is recommended. Anticoagulation should be considered in patients with chronic atrial fibrillation and no contraindications to its use.

COARCTATION OF THE AORTA

In adults, coarctation of the aorta is usually discovered during the medical evaluation for the etiology of hypertension. It is one of the surgically correctable causes of hypertension.

Anatomy and Physiology

The lesion consists of a congenital narrowing of the thoracic aorta beyond the origin of the left subclavian artery. There is usually an abnormal ridge of posterior aortic wall media protruding into the aortic lumen opposite the insertion of the ligamention arterosis. The left subclavian artery is often dilated, as is the descending thoracic aorta just distal to the sight of coarctation.

Coarctation is frequently associated with other congenital cardiac malformations including bicuspid aortic valve, patent ductus arteriosus, VSD, and mitral valve abnormalities. Arterial collateral circulation develops between the proximal high-pressure zone and the distal low-pressure area.

Extensive investigation as to mechanism of hypertension and relative roles of mechanical effects in the operation in the renin-angiotensin system still remains unclear. Even in those patients with surgically corrected coarctation, hypertension can persist. Persistent systemic hypertension associated with coarctation regardless of etiology results in premature arteriosclerotic cardiovascular disease.

Clinical Features

Patients who seek emergent care usually have symptoms associated with LV failure, endarteritis, aortic rupture, dissection, or cerebral hemorrhage. The most common nonemergent complaints are vague headaches, intermittent claudication, and leg fatigue. Individuals who have Turner's syndrome should be specifically evaluated for coarctation of the aorta since it is common to that disorder.

Systolic blood pressure is elevated disproportionately to the diastolic pressure, with a resulting wide pulse pressure. In most cases, there is a marked difference in the systolic pressure of the upper and lower extremities, and significantly diminished and delayed femoral pulses are diagnostic. The patient will commonly have a thrill in the suprasternal notch on precordial examination. There is an ejection-type murmur that can best be heard in the posterior thorax between the scapula. Chest roentgenography can be normal or may demonstrate cardiomegaly in a dilated ascending aorta. The characteristic "3" sign is produced by the dilated left subclavian artery, which produces a concave shadow proximal to the coarctate segment. Rib notching can be observed along the costal grooves. Erosion is caused by the dilated collateral intercostal arteries. The ECG is nonspecific for coarctation and may be within normal limits.

Management

Surgical correction of the coarctation is definitive therapy for the anatomic lesion; however, it may not necessarily correct the associated hypertension for reasons outlined previously. It is not always clear when the timing for surgery is most appropriate. For adults, correction consists of the resection of the coarcted segment and interposition of a graft between the proximal and distal ends. Balloon dilation angioplasty is primarily used for treating recurrent narrowing after repair in infancy.

As noted previously, the emergent care required by patients with coarctation of the aorta is directed at the complication of long-standing disease. The treatment of infectious endarteritis should begin as soon as the disorder is recognized. Cerebral vascular accidents secondary to rupture of berry aneurysm or dissection of the aorta require immediate stabilization and consultation with a neurosurgeon or thoracic surgeon, respectively. CHF should be treated accordingly.

ATRIAL SEPTAL DEFECTS

Atrial septal defects (ASDs) originate at specific sites anatomically and are referred to by their embryologic origins. ASDs account for 7 percent of all congenital heart disease and for 30 percent of congenital heart disease in adults, in whom it is second only to bicuspid aortic valve in frequency of occurrence. The most frequent type of ASD is the ostium secundum defect, followed by ostium primum defects, then sinus venosus defects (Fig. 22-2).

Anatomy and Pathophysiology

As a result of minimal or absent symptoms, subtle physical findings, and failure to suspect atrial lesions, ASDs may be difficult to diagnose. As age increases, progressive increases in symptoms, heart size, atrial arrhythmias, pulmonary arterial pressure, and systemic desaturation will frequently lead to diagnostic testing.

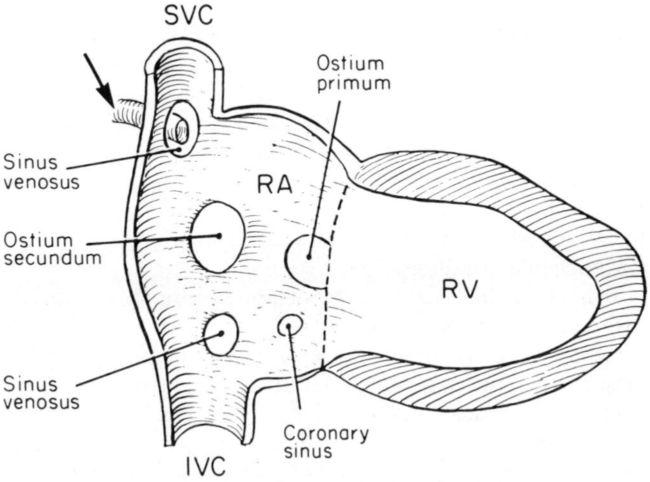

Fig. 22-2. The locations of ostium secundum and ostium primum atrial septal defects, sinus venosus defects of the superior vena caval (SVC) and inferior vena caval (IVC) types, and a coronary sinus defect. Unmarked arrow identifies the right superior pulmonary vein. (RV = right ventricle.) (From J.K. Perloff. *The Clinical Recognition of Congenital Heart Disease* [3rd ed.]. Philadelphia: Saunders, 1987.)

Patients with symptoms may present with palpitations, atrial arrhythmias, dyspnea, fatigue, respiratory illness, and chest pain. The severity and frequency of symptoms increase with age (especially in patients older than 40 years). The left to right shunting in ASD depends on the size of the defect, relative RV and LV compliances, and the ratio of pulmonary to systemic vascular resistance. Right to left shunting across the ASD may occur with severe obstructive pulmonary vascular disease or in sinus venosus defects.

Clinical Features

Physical examination may reveal a prominent V-wave in the jugular venosus pulse, a prominent first heart sound, fixed splitting of the second heart sound (with large ASD and left to right shunting), as well as a right-sided S4 gallop. The typical murmur heard is a pulmonic systolic murmur beginning shortly after the first heart sound.

Occasionally, with right to left shunting, clubbing and cyanosis may be present, and, if pulmonary vascular obstruction develops, one may appreciate a loud palpable pulmonary component of the second heart sound with a short pulmonic systolic murmur and tricuspid regurgitation. Chest radiography may be normal and may reveal cardiomegaly or increased pulmonary vascular markings, or both. The ECG shows sinus rhythm in most young patients, but as patients reach the fourth decade with ostium secundum defects, there is an increase in the incidence of atrial arrhythmias, especially atrial fibrillation. Other ECG findings include atrial flutter, supraventricular tachycardia, complete heart block, and incomplete or complete right bundle branch block (RBBB).

Management

The key noninvasive tool for evaluation of ASDs is echocardiography. Two-dimensional echocardiography is satisfactory for visualization in most uncomplicated ASDs. Doppler examination yields information regarding the volume and direction of flow through the defect. Cardiac catheterization may be avoided at times but is necessary in patients suspected of having ASDs who present with severe pulmonary hypertension, right heart failure, or uncharacteristic echocardiographic findings.

It is clear that with time, worsening symptoms, cardiomegaly, rhythm disturbances, and pulmonary vascular obstruction develop with most ASDs. Routine early surgical closure in all uncomplicated ASDs is strongly recommended, since spontaneous closure is uncommon in adults. Antimicrobial prophylaxis before or after repair of ostium secundum defects is usually unnecessary unless other valvular lesions that accompany the ASD require prophylaxis. Pregnancy should be avoided in patients with marked pulmonary hypertension, and cyanosis in patients with ASD is an absolute contraindication to the use of oral contraceptives owing to the risk of thromboembolism.

Other less common congenital atrial abnormalities may be present in adulthood. Patent foramen ovale abnormalities persistent into adulthood are significant as potential routes for paradoxical embolization. Interatrial septal aneurysms (often having mitral valve prolapse as an associated finding) may cause right atrial outflow obstruction or left atrial thrombus, producing peripheral embolization. Cor triatriatum (a membrane separating the atrium into two components) may present with dyspnea; pulmonary infections or exercise intolerance occasionally requires surgical intervention. Partial anomalous pulmonary venous connection often associated with an ASD of the sinus venosus type may also require surgical intervention if the pulmonary to systemic blood flow ratio exceeds 1.5:1.0.

Emergency evaluation of patients with congenital ASDs is usually the result of respiratory symptoms, symptomatic arrhythmias, chest pain, or palpitations. Those patients with sustained arrhythmias, pulmonary insufficiency, and chest pain frequently require hospital admission for emergency treatment and further cardiologic evaluation.

PATENT DUCTUS ARTERIOSUS

Patent ductus arteriosus (PDA) is rarely found in adults. Failure to close during infancy results in a persistent communication between the systemic and pulmonary vascular beds. When discovered late in adulthood, it may result in irreversible pulmonary hypertension, CHF, and premature death. Those patients reaching adulthood with PDA who receive medical therapy or no treatment have a decreased long-term life expectancy. PDA occurs more commonly as an isolated anomaly. When it occurs in association with other defects, it often represents a physiologic compensatory channel. The initial clinical presentation to the emergency specialist is, in part, the result of complications from a longstanding undiscovered PDA. CHF, pulmonary hypertension, or infected endocarditis are the most common late-stage complications and manifestations of a patent ductus.

Anatomy and Physiology

In the full-term neonate, if the ductus fails to close spontaneously within the first 2 months of life, persistent patency can be expected. In the adult, PDA is variable as to its length and diameter of the lumen and anatomically extends from the aortic isthmus near the origin of the left subclavian artery to the left pulmonary artery just distal to the pulmonary branch bifurcation. Occasionally, the PDA can be opened at one end and closed at the other.

The pathophysiologic consequences depend on the size of the shunt and ratio of the pulmonary-to-systemic vascular resistance. With a large shunt, blood continually flows to the lungs throughout the cardiac cycle, presenting systemic pressures to the pulmonary artery. This increase in pulmonary flow leads to engorgement and enlargement of the pulmonary artery, the left atrium, and the left ventricle and, eventually, to development of CHF. Bidirectional or reversed shunting through the ductus may develop if pulmonary artery hypertension and pulmonary vascular obstructive disease is present. Symptoms are frequently absent in adults with PDA until ventricular decompensation occurs.

Clinical Features

The most common symptom in adults with PDA is dyspnea on exertion. Atypical chest pain, angina pectoris, palpitations, coughing, and hemoptysis occasionally occur.

The classic auscultatory finding of a continuous "machinery"-type murmur is heard loudest in the second left interspace at the intraclavicular or left upper sternal border. It is associated with a wide arterial pulse pressure, bounding peripheral pulses, and a hyperdynamic LV apical impulse.

If pulmonary vascular resistance is high, the left to right shunt is diminished and the typical machinery murmur becomes a rough systolic murmur. Cardiomegaly on chest x-ray examination is a common finding, especially in patients with a moderate to large shunt. Enlargement of the pulmonary trunk is common, and enlargement of the left atrium can be observed on barium swallow.

If the shunt is small, the ECG may be normal. If the shunt is moderate to large, a LV hypertrophy or diastolic overload pattern is noted.

Management

The emergency physician is presented with complications of PDA that require interventional therapy. Attention to adequate oxygenation, treatment of CHF, and recognition of infective endocarditis are paramount.

Surgery in children for closure of PDA is the mainstay of interventional therapy and represents one of the simplest of cardiovascular procedures performed. In the adult patient, ligation or division of the PDA may present a number of difficulties.

PULMONIC STENOSIS

Pulmonic stenosis (PS) has an unclear etiology, and its cause is believed to be multifactorial. Repeated occurrences of PS in siblings have been noted. The natural course of uncorrected PS in the adult is unclear, and there is a paucity of cases in patients older than 35 years, implying a poor prognosis if uncorrected. A study by Johnson, et al. noted that in 5- to 24-year follow-up studies, there were no deaths in a group of patients with mild and moderate PS who did not undergo surgical correction.

Anatomy and Pathophysiology

There are three anatomic types of stenosis recognized: (1) at the level of the valve, 80 percent; (2) below the valve, 15 percent; and (3) above the valve, 5 percent of the cases. Acquired pulmonic stenosis is extremely rare and may result from rheumatic fever. The more common valvular PS is due to partial fusion and variable thickening of a tricuspid or, less commonly, a bicuspid pulmonary valve.

Regardless of the level of obstruction, RV systolic pressure overload and hypertrophy are nearly universal findings in PS. In cases in which there is severe PS, there may be right to left shunting across a patent foramen ovale leading to systemic arterial oxygen desaturation.

Clinical Features

Most patients, even those with significant obstruction, will deny symptoms. Those individuals with severe stenosis will complain of fatigue and dyspnea, especially on exertion. There are several prominent signs that may direct the clinician to the diagnosis. With a RV outlet obstruction, the RV wall hypertrophies with a decrease in compliance and distensibility. This increases impedance to right atrial emptying during atrial systole, and what the physician notes on physical findings is the resultant giant jugular A-wave.

On palpation of the thorax, a systolic thrill can be appreciated along the upper portion of the left sternal border in those patients with moderate to severe PS. Auscultative findings are typical, and the predominant finding is a systolic ejection murmur. It is heard loudest in the second left intercostal space parasternally and transmits to the clavicle.

The ECG can be normal or may demonstrate only a right ventricular conductive abnormality. In severe stenosis, right axis deviation, RV hypertrophy with strain, and right atrial enlargement are often present.

Management

Patients with mild stenosis do not require surgery. Those individuals with isolated severe or moderately severe valvular PS should undergo valvulotomy, which can be done with little risk. Mild pulmonic regurgitation is common after valvulotomy. In 1982, Karr and coworkers reported successful treatment of valvular PS by balloon valvuloplasty.

TETRALOGY OF FALLOT

Only 10 percent of patients who do not undergo surgical intervention for tetralogy of Fallot survive beyond 21 years of age (Holladay and Mulder). In rare cases, unusual longevity without surgical intervention is possible and is related to

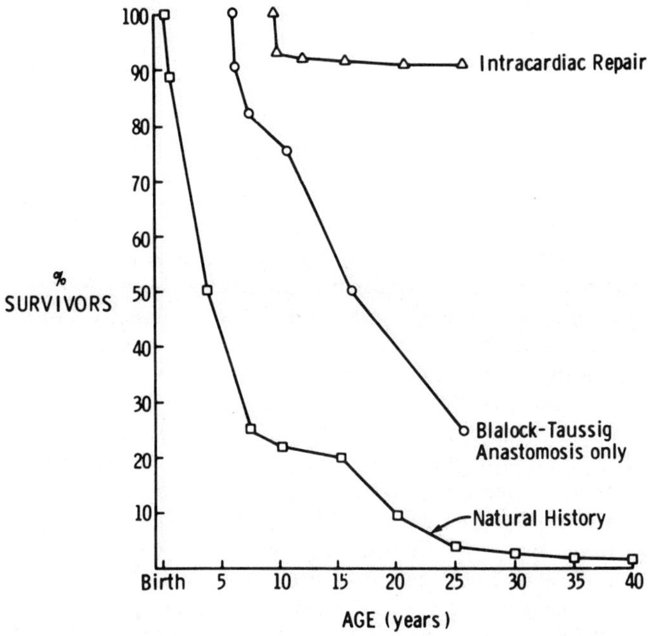

Fig. 22-3. Natural and surgically modified survival in patients with tetralogy of Fallot. The percentage of survivors at the end of each interval is graphed for each of 3 courses. The natural history data were combined from 6 authors, while the estimated survival following a single Blalock-Taussig anastomosis combined 2 studies, and the data following intracardiac repair (with or without prior operation) are ours combined with one other study. The curves representing survival following operation are constructed with the following assumptions: (1) the beginning point is the mean age at operation; (2) the initial vertical decrease corresponds to 30-day mortality; and (3) no patient died before operation. (From Roberts, William C., Congenital heart disease in adults. *Cardiovascular Clinics* Oct. 1, Albert N. Brest, M.D., Editor-in-Chief. F.A. Davis Company, Philadelphia, © 1979.)

large pulmonary blood flow resulting in only mild arterial desaturation. About 11 percent of all children with congenital heart disease are diagnosed as having tetralogy of Fallot. It is estimated that 87 percent of this group of patients will survive into adulthood. The reason for this survival rate is that most of these individuals have undergone some type of palliative surgery. The natural history of the disease is significantly modified, depending on the type of surgical intervention, as noted in Fig. 22-3.

In the clinical setting, the physician can usually assume that the adult patient with tetralogy of Fallot has had some palliative procedure and should make every attempt to ellicit what operation was performed and when. Keep in mind the predominant nonsurgical causes of death, which are paroxysmal hypoxemic spells, cerebrovascular accidents (CVAs) and brain abscess, infectious endocarditis, pneumonia, and CHF.

Anatomy and Pathophysiology

A large VSD associated with infundibular or valvular PS, RV hypertrophy, and an overriding aorta describe the classic and anatomic presentation of tetralogy of Fallot. Right to left shunting through the VSD is usual, and the pathophysiology is determined by the severity of the PS and the size of the VSD.

Clinical Features

The patient who has had a mild obstruction to the outflow tract of the RV is usually acyanotic with a predominant left to right shunt. Infants and children who present with cyanotic congenital heart disease have associated severe obstruction to the right outflow tract and undergo early palliative or total surgical repair. The palliative procedure most commonly encountered in the adult patient today is the Blalock-Taussig anastomosis. Other procedures that have been popular include the Potts anastomosis, the Waterston-Cooley anastomosis, and the Brock procedure.

In 18 percent of those adults who have had total correction, follow-up studies indicate that these individuals have unlimited exercise tolerance. Poor exercise tolerance generally implies a residual or RV hypertension.

Congestive heart failure is unusual in patients with tetralogy of Fallot; however, exertional dyspnea and poor exercise tolerance are described in unoperated adults with tetralogy of Fallot who survive into the third decade of life. Table 22-5 summarizes the prevalent signs of 147 adult patients older than 18 years who have not undergone total correction.

Most patients have a crescendo-decrescendo murmur at the left intercostal border postoperatively. The murmur becomes louder as the RV to pulmonary artery gradient increases.

The ECG is characterized by a right axis deviation, RV hypertrophy, and, in 80 to 95 percent of corrected patients, associated complete RBBB. On roentgenography, the boot-shaped heart described in children is less typical in the adult. Pulmonary vascularity is essentially normal in those individuals who are acyanotic.

Table 22-5. Signs of tetralogy of Fallot in adults

	Patients	
Signs	No.	%
Underdeveloped	17	11.6
Acyanotic	8	5.5
Congestive cardiac failure	23	15.6
Systemic hypertension (diastolic blood pressure > 90 mm Hg)	14	9.5
Parasternal lift	53	36.1
Systolic thrill in pulmonary area	79	53.7
Ejection click	50	34.0
Pulmonary component		
Not heard	119	81.0
Soft	25	17.0
Normal	3	2.0
Systolic murmur		
Short ejection	61	41.5
Long ejection	83	56.5
No murmur	3	2.0
Continuous murmur	24	16.3
Pulmonary regurgitant murmur	4	2.6
Aortic regurgitant murmur	10	6.7

Source: K. A. Abraham, et al. Tetralogy of Fallot in adults: A report of 147 patients. *Am. J. Med.* 66:811, 1979.

Management

The definitive management is total correction and should be performed early in life whenever possible. The emergency physician will be faced with managing the complications of uncorrected and corrected tetralogy of Fallot. The initial management of cerebral abscess, infective endocarditis, and cerebrovascular accidents are the most commonly encountered complications.

Polycythemia secondary to chronic arterial desaturation increases the risk of intravascular thrombosis, thrombotic emboli, infective endocarditis, brain abscess, and acute gouty arthritis. Phlebotomy can be dangerous in patients with tetralogy of Fallot and should be used only to relieve symptoms or to correct a bleeding disorder.

TRANSPOSITION OF THE GREAT ARTERIES

Transposition of the great arteries (TGA) refers to ventriculoarterial discordance; each great artery has an inappropriate ventricular relationship. The anatomic findings in complete transposition are normal atrial and ventricular relationships, with the aorta arising from the RV and the pulmonary artery arising from the LV (Fig. 22-4). This abnormality results in two parallel circulations, which is incompatible with life unless there is some communication between the two circulations.

Malposition of the great arteries or corrected TGA is defined by abnormal anatomic relationships (anteroposterior or lateral) of the great arteries to each other and to the ventricles, with each great artery arising from the "correct" ventricle. This transposition is "corrected" because the ventricles are inverted (RV on the left and LV on the right), there is AV discordance, and the great arteries are transposed (Fig. 22-5).

Clinical Features

Adults with TGA are cyanotic on physical examination. There is usually a hyperdynamic precordium, a single second heart sound, and a systolic murmur, none of which are diagnostic. Chest radiography is not specific in making the diagnosis of TGA. The ECG usually shows right axis deviation, right atrial enlargement, and RV hypertrophy. Two-dimensional echocardiography has revolutionized the evaluation of these patients and can provide essential information helping to guide patient management. The bi-plane angiocardiogram at cardiac catheterization remains the standard for diagnosis. Patients with complete TGA who survive into adulthood either have a VSD or single ventricle and achieve adulthood secondary to PS, limiting pulmonary blood flow. Those individuals with congenitally corrected TGA as an isolated defect may have no symptoms and no functional abnormality. Their clinical course is variable, depending on the nature and severity of associated congenital cardiac abnormalities.

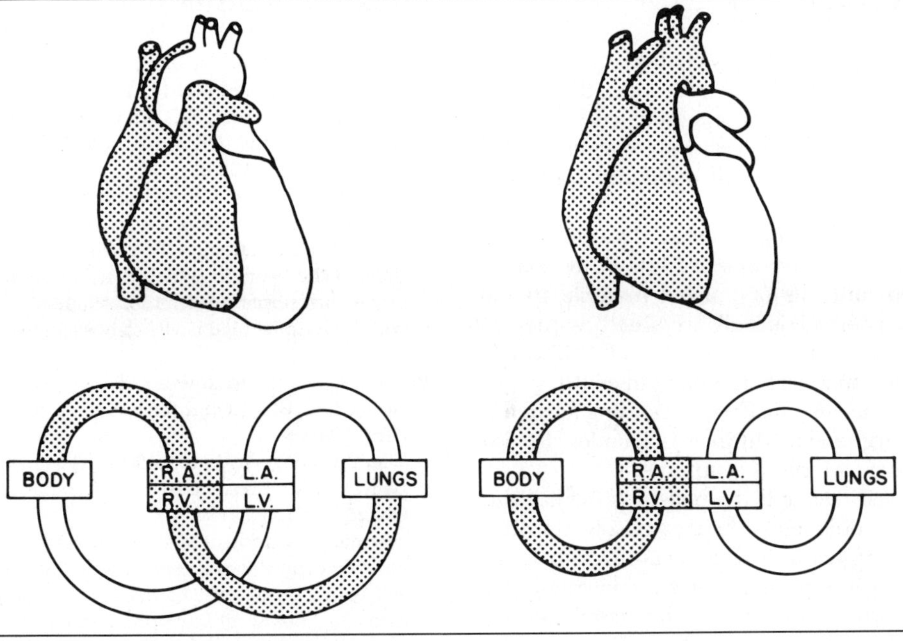

Fig. 22-4. Schematic diagram of blood flow in complete TGA as contrasted to normal. (From Roberts, William C., Congenital heart disease in adults. *Cardiovascular Clinics* Oct. 1, Albert N. Brest, M.D., Editor-in-Chief. F.A. Davis Company, Philadelphia, © 1979.)

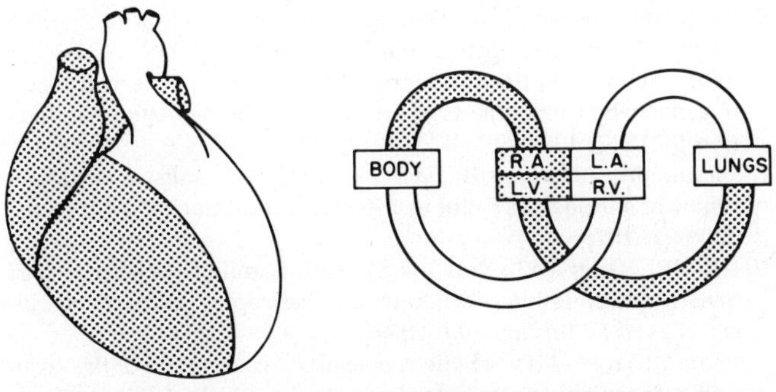

Fig. 22-5. Schematic diagram of blood flow in corrected TGA. (From Roberts, William C., Congenital heart disease in adults. *Cardiovascular Clinics* Oct. 1, Albert N. Brest, M.D., Editor-in-Chief. F.A. Davis Company, Philadelphia, © 1979.)

Management

A number of palliative and corrective surgical procedures have been developed that have allowed increasing numbers of patients with TGA to survive into adulthood. These patients may present acutely with arrhythmias, complications of pulmonary vascular hypertension and polycythemia, and, eventually, systemic congestion. Treatment is usually limited to management of these complications, which include bleeding, vascular thrombosis, skin changes, and infection. Careful attention must be paid to patients with febrile or diarrheal illnesses. When changes in intravascular volume occur, it may cause a dangerous rise in the hematocrit, which may require hydration and phlebotomy.

CONGENITAL HEART BLOCK

Congenital complete heart block is usually discovered in early childhood because of a persistent slow heart rate in an otherwise healthy child. Today, with constant fetal monitoring, the slow regular fetal heartbeat of congenital heart block is recognized before the onset of labor.

Most adults maintain clinical stability because of hemodynamic adjustments at rest and exercise. The presence of stable excelerated junctional pacemaker allows for this hemodynamic homeostasis under different physiological conditions.

Clinical Features

The general physical appearance of individuals with congenital complete heart block is normal and provides no initial insight in the assessment of the disorder. A slow arterial pulse is noted; however, the resting rate is generally greater than that found in acquired complete heart block. It is important to evaluate the jugular venous pulse since a distant A-wave is a prominent feature and, when timed with the carotid pulse, is found to be asynchronous. The definitive diagnosis is made by ECG. The P-wave and the QRS complex are completely independent with no relationships. The chest films in congenital complete heart block are usually normal.

Management

The clinician is usually faced with evaluating and treating the complications of congenital complete heart block, which include malignant ventricular tachyarrhythmias, Stokes-Adams attacks, and decreased cardiac output. Antiarrhythmic therapy or permanent pacing, or both, is the indicated therapy for persistent or potentially dangerous signs and symptoms.

MARFAN'S SYNDROME

Marfan's syndrome is characterized by changes in three connective system tissues. The extremities are long, the lens of the eye is dislocated, the ascending aorta is often dilated, and one or both of the left cardiac valves are regurgitant. The disease is inherited as an autosomal dominant trait with variable expression.

The most common fatal lesion is aortic dissection. Histologic study of the aorta shows massive loss of the elastic fibers with increased amounts of mucoid material in the media. Dissection is characteristically confined to the ascending aorta in Marfan's syndrome; however, the descending thoracic and abdominal aorta are often involved.

The major consequence of a fusiform ascending aorta aneurysm is aortic regurgitation. Mitral regurgitation is also frequent in patients with Marfan's syndrome.

The diagnosis is easily made if the patient presents with the Marfan habitus, ectopic lentis, kyphoscoliosis, and aneurysm of the ascending aorta. The echocardiogram is diagnostic in establishing the presence of an aneurysm, and the slit-lamp examination will delineate the ectopic lenses. There is no established treatment.

CYANOTIC CONGENITAL HEART DISEASE

Cyanotic congenital heart disease is rarely encountered uncorrected in older adult patients. Almost all such patients have undergone some palliative or corrective surgery in order to ensure survival to adulthood. The emergency specialist will encounter the complication of the corrected lesions or the end-stage of long-standing disease. The treatment is directed at the stabilization of the individual, along with the maintenance of adequate oxygenation and hemodynamic homeostasis.

CONGENITAL PULMONARY AV FISTULAS

Pulmonary AV fistulas are anomalous connections between the pulmonary artery and pulmonary veins, usually replacing the normal capillary bed. The pathophysiologic significance of these fistulas is a right to left shunt, with the size of the shunt usually dictating the cardiac manifestations of this derangement.

Patients with pulmonary AV fistulas frequently go unrecognized until adulthood. Currently, symptoms include hemoptysis, dyspnea, fatigue, and, rarely, cardiac failure. Asymptomatic pulmonary AV fistulas usually come to light because of the accidental discovery of abnormal shadows on the chest x-ray or because of cyanosis or telangectasias.

Physical examination is frequently normal, but occasionally a murmur may be heard over the fistula. Complications of pulmonary AV fistulas include rupture with hemoptysis or hemothorax, paradoxical embolism, infectious endarteritis, and cerebral abscess. Surgery can be performed for a singular pulmonary AV fistula that is symptomatic, but frequently congenital pulmonary AV fistulas are multiple. Catheter embolization may be most helpful in obliterating some of these lesions.

SELECTED READING

Abraham, KA, et al. Tetralogy of Fallot in adults: A report of 147 patients. *Am J Med* 66:811, 1979.

Anderson, RH, Lenox, CC, and Zuberbahler, JR. Morphology of ventricular septal defect associated with coarctation of aorta. Br Heart J 50:176, 1983.

Beckers, J, et al. HLA complex and hypertrophic cardiomyopathy in a European population. *Eur Heart J* 6:963, 1985.

Blalock, A, and Taussig, HB. The surgical treatment of malformations of the heart in which there is pulmonic stenosis or patent ductus arteriosus. *JAMA* 128:189, 1945.

Borow, KM. Congenital aortic stenosis in the adult. *J Cardiovas Med* 8:1163, 1983.

Borow, KM, and Braunwald, E. Congenital Heart Disease in the Adult. In E Braunwald (ed), *Heart Disease.* Philadelphia: Saunders, 1988.

Bowie, EA. Longevity in tetralogy and trilogy of Fallot. Discussion of patients and presentation of two further cases. *Am Heart J* 62:125, 1961.

Braverman, IB, and Gibson, S. The outlook for children with congenital aortic stenosis. *Am Heart J* 53:478, 1957.

Braunwald, E. *Heart Disease: A Textbook of Cardiovascular Medicine.* Vol. 2. Philadelphia: Saunders, 1988.

Campbell, M. Late results of operations for Fallot's tetralogy. *Br Med J* 2:1175, 1958.

Campbell, M, and Thorne, MG. Congenital heart block. *Br Heart J* 18:90, 1956.

Campbell, N. National history of patent ductus arteriosus. *Br Heart J* 30:4, 1968.

Canedo, MI, Frank, MJ, and Abdulla, AM. Rhythm disturbances in hypertrophic cardiomyopathy. Prevalence relation to symptoms and management. *Am J Cardiol* 45:848, 1980.

Cassels, DE. *Absence, Complications and Premature Closure of the Ductus Arteriosus.* Springfield, IL: Thomas, 1973.

Ciro, E, Nichols, PF, III, and Maron, BH. Heterogeneous expression of genetically transmitted hypertrophic cardiomyopathy. *Circulation* 67:1227, 1983.

Clapman, JA, Ankeney, JL, and Liebman, J. Results of complete repair of tetralogy of Fallot in 156 consecutive patients. *Am J Surg* 130:601, 1975.

Clark, CE, Henry, WL, and Epstein, SE. Familial prevalence and genetic transmission of idiopathic hypertrophic subaortic stenosis. *N Engl J Med* 259:709, 1973.

Clarkson, PM, et al. Prosthetic repair of the coarctation of the aorta with particular reference to dacron onlay patch grafts and later aneurysm formation. *Am J Cardiol* 56:342, 1985.

Cokkinos, DV, Krajcer, Z, and Leachman, RD. Coronary artery disease in hypertrophic cardiomyopathy. *Am J Cardiol* 55:1437, 1985.

Colucci, WS, et al. Hypertrophic obstructive cardiomyopathy due to Fabry's disease. *N Engl J Med* 307:926, 1982.

Corne, RA, and Mathewson, FAL. Congenital complete atrioventricular heart block. A 25-year follow-up study. *Am J Cardiol* 29:412, 1972.

Corone, P, et al. Natural history of ventricular septal defect. A study involving seven hundred and ninety cases. *Circulation* 55:908, 1977.

Davidson, GK, et al. Pulmonic stenosis with intact ventricular septum: Surgical considerations and results of operation. *J Thorac Cardiovasc Surg* 61:228, 1971.

Delman, AJ, and Stein E. Mitral Valve Prolapse. In *Dynamic Cardiac Auscultation and Phonocardiography.* Philadelphia: Saunders, 1979.

Dines, DE, Seward, JB, and Bernatz, PE. Pulmonary arteriovenous fistulas. *Mayo Clin Proc* 58:176, 1983.

Downing, DF. Congenital aortic stenosis: Clinical aspects and surgical treatment. *Circulation* 14:188, 1956.

Dunn, HP. Antenatal diagnosis of congenital heart block. *J Obstet Gynaecol Br Emp* 67:1006, 1960.

Ehlers, KH, and Engle, MA. Familial congenital heart disease. 1. Genetic and environmental factors. *Circulation* 34:503, 1966.

Ellison, RC, et al. Indirect assessment of severity in pulmonary stenosis. *Circulation* 56 (suppl): 114, 1977.

Engle, A, Kline, SA, and Borer, JS. Ventricular Septal Defect. In WC Roberts (ed), *Adult Congenital Heart Disease.* Philadelphia: Davis, 1987.

Engle, MA, Ito, T, and Goldberg, HP. The fate of the patient with pulmonic stenosis. *Circulation* 30:554, 1964.

Fairley, GH, and Goodwin, JF. Patent ductus arteriosus in adult life. *Br J Dis Chest* 53:263, 1959.

Feldman, T, and Borow, KM. Adults with pulmonic stenosis: Management. *Cardiovasc Med* 9:711, 1984.

Fenoglio, JJ, et al. Congenital bicuspid aortic valve after age 20. *Am J Cardiol* 39:164, 1977.

Fiorito, S, et al. HLA-DR3 antigen linkage in patients with hypertrophic obstructive cardiomyopathy. *Am Heart J* 111:91, 1986.

Fisher, RG, et al. Patent ductus arteriosus in adults—long-term followings: Nonsurgical versus surgical treatment. *J Am Coll Cardiol* 8:280, 1986.

Friedman, WF. Congenital Aortic Valve Disease: Natural History, Indications and Results of Surgery. In H Goldberg and D Morse (eds), *Important Topics in Congenital, Valvular and Coronary Artery Disease.* Mt Kisco, NY: Futura, 1975.

Gardin, JM, et al. HLA linkage vs association in hypertrophic cardiomyopathy. Evidence for the absence of an association in a heterogeneous caucasian population. *Chest* 81:466, 1982.

Garson, A, Jr, McNamara, DG, and Cooley, DA. Tetralogy of Fallot in adults. *Cardiovasc Clin* 10:344, 1979.

Garson, A, Jr, McNamara, DG, and Cooley, DA. Tetralogy of Fallot. In WC Roberts (ed), *Adult Congenital Heart Disease.* Philadelphia: Davis, 1987.

Graham, TP. Assessing the results of surgery for congenital heart disease—a continuing process. *Circulation* 65:1049, 1982.

Hall, RJ, et al. Massive pulmonary arteriovenous fistula in the newborn; a correctable form of "cyanotic heart disease"; an additional cause of cyanosis with axis deviation. *Circulation* 31:762, 1965.

Hardarson, T, et al. Prognosis and mortality of hypertrophic obstructive cardiomyopathy. *Lancet* 2:1462, 1973.

Haugland, H, et al. Hypertrophic cardiomyopathy in three generations of a large Norwegian family. A clinical, echocardiographic and genetic study. *Br Heart J* 55:168, 1986.

Higgins, CB, and Mulder, DG. Tetralogy of Fallot in the adult. *Am J Med* 29:837, 1972.

Hodgson, CH, et al. Hereditary hemorrhagic telangiectasia and pulmonary arteriovenous fistula; survey of a large family. *New Engl J Med* 261:625, 1959.

Holladay, WE, and Witham, AC. The tetralogy of Fallot. *Arch Intern Med* 100:400, 1957.

Huhta, JC, et al. Survival in atrioventricular discordance. *Pediatr Cardiol* 6:57, 1985.

Ikeda, M, and Huosawa, K. Tetralogy of Fallot. *Circulation* 37 (suppl V):21, 1968.

James, FN, Kaplan, S, and Chou, TL. Unexpected cardiac arrest in patients after surgical correction of tetralogy of Fallot. *Circulation* 52:691, 1975.

Joffe, HS. Effect of age on pressure-flow dynamics in secundum atrial septal defect. *Br Heart J* 51:469, 1984.

John, S, et al. The adult ductus. *J Thorac Cardiovasc Surg* 82:314, 1981.

Johnson, LW, et al. Pulmonic stenosis in the adult: Long-term follow-up results. *N Engl J Med* 287:1159, 1972.

Kaplan, S, Adolph, RJ, and Murphy, DJ. Pulmonic Stenosis. In WC Roberts (ed), *Adult Congenital Heart Disease.* Philadelphia: Davis, 1987.

Karr, JS, et al. Percutaneous balloon valvuloplasty: A new method for treatment of congenital pulmonary valve stenosis. *N Engl J Med* 307:540, 1982.

Keith, JD, et al. Ventricular septal defect. Incidents, morbidity and mortality in various age groups. *Br Heart J* 33:81, 1971.

Kidd, L, and Humphries, JO. Complete and congenital corrected transposition of the great arteries. In WC Roberts (ed), *Adult Congenital Heart Disease.* Philadelphia: Davis, 1987.

Kinsly, RH, et al. Pulmonary arterial hypertension after repair of tetralogy of Fallot. *J Thorac Cardiovasc Surg* 64:110, 1974.

Levine, RA, and Weyman, AE. Dynamic subaortic obstruction in hypertrophic cardiomyopathy: Criteria and controversy. *J Am Coll Cardiol* 6:16, 1985.

Lock, J, Keane, J, and Fellows K. The use of catheter intervention procedure for congenital heart disease. *J Am Coll Cardiol* 7:1420, 1986.

McAnulty, JH, Metcalfe, J, and Ueland, K. General guidelines in the management of cardiac disease. *Clin Obstet Gynecol* 24:773, 1981.

McKusick, VA. *Heritable Disorders of Connective Tissue* (4th ed.). St Louis: Mosby, 1972.

McManus, BM. Patent Ductus Arteriosus. In WC Roberts (ed.), *Adult Congenital Heart Disease.* Philadelphia: Davis, 1977. Pp. 455–476.

McManus, BM, et al. Eisenmenger's ductus arteriosus with prolonged survival. *Am J Cardiol* 54:462, 1984.

McReynolds, RA, and Roberts, WC. The intramural coronary arteries in hypertrophic cardiomyopathy (abstract). *Am J Cardiol* 35:120, 1975.

Malcolm, AD. Mitral valve prolapse associated with other disorders. Causal coincidence, common link or fundamental genetic disturbance. *Br Heart J* 53:353, 1985.

Mark YD. Congenital heart disease in the adult. *Am J Cardiol* 15:293, 1965.

Maron, BJ, et al. Hypertrophic cardiomyopathy. Interrelations of clinical manifestations, pathophysiology and therapy. *N Engl J Med* 316:780, 1987.

Maron, BJ, et al. "Malignant" hypertrophic cardiomyopathy: Identification of a subgroup of families with unusually frequent premature deaths. *Am J Cardiol* 41:1133, 1978.

Maron, BJ, et al. Patterns of inheritance in hypertrophic cardiomyopathy: Assessment by M-mode and two-dimensional echocardiography. *Am J Cardiol* 53:1087, 1984.

Maron, BJ, and Roberts, WC. Hypertrophic cardiomyopathy and cardiac muscle cell disorganization revisited: Relation between the two and significance. *Am Heart J* 102:95, 1981.

Maron, BJ, et al. Sudden death in young athletes. *Circulation* 62:218, 1980.

Maron, BJ, et al. Prognostic significance of 24-hour ambulatory electrocardiographic monitoring in patients with hypertrophic cardiomyopathy: A prospective study. *Am J Cardiol* 48:252, 1981.

Maron, BJ, et al. The intramural coronary arteries in hypertrophic cardiomyopathy. *J Am Coll Cardiol* 8:545, 1986.

Marquis, RM, et al. Patent ductus arteriosus with left to right shunt in the older patient. *Br Heart J* 48:469, 1982.

Mitchell, SC, Korones, SB, and Berends, HW. Congenital heart disease in fifty-six thousand, one-hundred and nine births. Incidents and natural history. *Circulation* 43:323, 1971.

Morrow, AG, Goldblatt, A, and Braunwald, E. Congenital aortic stenosis II. Surgical treatment and the results of operation. *Circulation* 27:426, 1963.

Moyer, JH, Glantz, G, and Brest, AN. Pulmonary arteriovenous fistulas. *Am J Med* 32:417, 1962.

Nishimura, RA, Giuliani, ER, and Brandenburg, RO. Hypertrophic cardiomyopathy. *Cardiovasc Rev Reports* 4:931, 1983.

Ongley, PA, et al. Aortic stenosis in infants and children. *Pediatrics* 21:207, 1958.

Pader, E. The familial incidence of mitral valve prolapse. A report of three generations in one family. *NY State J Med* 84:395, 1984.

Perloff, JK. Congenital Complete Heart Block. In *The Clinical Recognition of Congenital Heart Disease* (3rd ed.). Philadelphia: Saunders, 1987. Pp 49–61.

Perloff, JK, Child, JS, and Edwards, JE. New guidelines for the clinical diagnosis of mitral valve prolapse. *Am J Cardiol* 57:1124, 1986.

Perloff, JK. Patent Ductus Arteriosus. In *The Clinical Recognition of Congenital Heart Disease* (3rd ed). Philadelphia: Saunders, 1987. Pp. 467–497.

Pollick, C, et al. Muscular subaortic stenosis: The temporal relationship between systolic anterior motion of the anterior mitral leaflet and the pressure gradient. *Circulation* 66:1087, 1982.

Pollick, C, Rakowski, H, and Wigle, ED. Muscular subaortic stenosis: The quantitative relationship between systolic anterior motion and the pressure gradient. *Circulation* 69:43, 1984.

Prevention of Bacterial Endocarditis. A statement prepared by the Committee on Rheumatic Fever and Bacterial Endocarditis of the Council on Cardiovascular Disease in the Young. *Circulation* 70:1123A, 1984.

Przybojewski, JZ, Blake, RS, DeWitt Lubbe, JJ. Rupture of sinus of valsalva aneurysm into both right atrium and right ventricle. *S Afr Med* 63:616, 1983.

Reid, JM, Coleman, EN, and Doig, W. Complete congenital heart block—report of 35 cases. *Br Heart J* 48:236, 1982.

Roberts, WC. *Adult Congenital Heart Disease.* Philadelphia: Davis, 1987.

Roberts, WC. Left Ventricular Outflow Tract Obstruction and Aortic Regurgitation. In JE Edwards, M Lev, and MR Abell (eds), *The Heart.* Baltimore: Williams & Wilkins, 1974.

Roberts, WC. The congenitally abnormal bicuspid aortic valve—a study of 85 autopsy cases. *Am J Cardiol* 26:72, 1970.

Roberts, WC, and Ferrans, VJ. Pathologic anatomy of the cardiomyopathies. Idiopathic dilated and hypertrophic types, infiltrative types and endomyocardial disease with and without eosinophilia. *Human Pathol* 6:287, 1975.

Roberts, WC, and Honig, HS. The spectrum of cardiovascular disease in the Marfan syndrome. A clinicomorphologic study of 18 necropsy patients and comparison to 151 previously reported necropsy patients. *Am Heart J* 104:115, 1982.

Ruzzello, W, et al. Hemodynamic evaluation of 221 patients after mitrocardium repair of tetralogy of Fallot. *Am J Cardiol* 34:565, 1974.

Segal, BL, and Likoff, W. Late systolic murmur of mitral regurgitation. *Am Heart J* 66:443, 1964.

Serfas, D, and Borow, KM. Coarctation of the aorta: Anatomy, pathophysiology and history. *J Cardiovasc Med* 8:575, 1983.

Shah, PM, et al. The natural (and unnatural) course of hypertrophic obstructive cardiomyopathy. A multi-center study. *Circ Res* 34–35 (suppl II):II–179, 1973.

Smallborn, JF, Anderson, RH, and Mocartney, FJ. Morphological characterization of ventricular septal defects associated with coarctation of aorta by cross-sectional echocardiography. *Br Heart J* 49:485, 1983.

Sperling, DR, et al. Percutaneous transluminal angioplasty of congenital coarctation of the aorta. *Am J Cardiol* 51:562, 1983.

Standefer, JE, Tabakin, BS, and Hanson, JS. Pulmonary arteriovenous fistulas. Case report with cineangiographic studies. *Am Rev Respir Dis* 89:95, 1964.

Stringer, CJ, et al. Pulmonary arteriovenous fistula. *Am J Surg* 89:1054, 1955.

Taruz, M, DeGrovechy, J, and Schweisquth, O. Genetic and nongenetic factors in the etiology of congenital heart disease: A study of 1188 cases. *Am J Hum Genet* 9:17, 1957.

Thompson, WM, Cartaya, AL, Vanhoutte, JJ, et al. Tetralogy of Fallot. *J Okla State Med Assoc* 69:434, 1976.

Timber, J, et al. The natural history of isolated pulmonary stenosis. *Br Heart J* 27:151, 1965.

Warkamy, J. *Congenital Malformations.* Chicago: Year Book, 1971.

Watson, GH. Pulmonary stenosis, café-au-lait spots and dull intelligence. *Arch Dis Child* 42:303, 1967.

Weidman, WH, DuShane, JW, and Ellison, RC. Clinical course in adults with ventricular septal defect. *Circulation* 55:178, 1977.

23. Acquired Heart and Pericardial Disease

Richard Clinton Becker
Joel M. Gore

The sudden onset of symptoms, including chest pain, dyspnea, light-headedness, and syncope, may herald an acute cardiac process. The clinical presentations of acute myocardial infarction, myocardial ischemia, pulmonary embolism, and ventricular dysrhythmias are well known and the topic of other chapters in this text. The general clinical presentation of acquired diseases involving the heart and pericardium is important to recognize since the prompt institution of appropriate therapy can be lifesaving. Indeed, the majority of these conditions represent true medical emergencies.

ACUTE PERICARDIAL DISORDERS

The pericardium encloses the heart and great vessels. It consists of a fibroserous sac with an inner layer (visceral pericardium) and an outer layer (parietal pericardium), which is attached to the vertebral column, sternum, diaphragm, and costal cartilages. A small physiologic effusion commonly exists (15–25 ml) with constituents similar to serum, suggesting a transudative mechanism of formation (Fig. 23-1).

The pericardium has three main physiologic functions:

- Ligamentous
  - Limitation of cardiac displacement by attachments to adjacent structures
- Membranous
  - Reduction of external friction from heart movement
  - Barrier to inflammatory processes from contiguous structures
  - Buttressing of thinner portions of the myocardium (atria, right ventricle)
- Mechanical
  - Limitation of excessive acute dilation
  - Protection against ventriculoatrial regurgitation
  - Maintain cardiac output in response to venous inflow (preload)
  - Maintain normal ventricular compliance (volume–elasticity relationship)

Disease processes involving the pericardium may be divided into the following three categories:

- Inflammatory
- Constrictive
- Effusive
  - With tamponade
  - Without tamponade

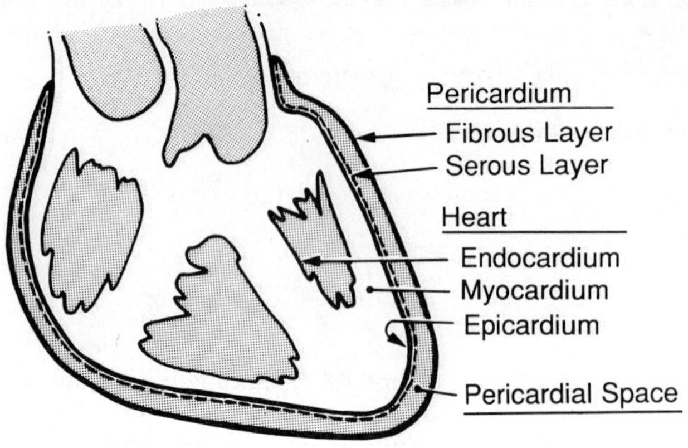

Fig. 23-1. Diagrammatic representation of the pericardium, showing its fibrous (parietal) and serous (visceral) layers. The pericardial space is exaggerated.

Table 23-1. Pericardial disorders—initial clinical presentation

Pericardial disorder	Symptom onset	Clinical signs/symptoms
Inflammatory pericarditis	Acute/subacute	Chest pain Viral prodrome Fever Friction rub
Constrictive pericarditis	Subacute/chronic	Jugular venous distention Peripheral edema Ascites Underlying disease state (frequent)
Effusive pericarditis with tamponade	Acute/subacute	Tachycardia Hypotension Narrow pulse pressure Pulsus paradoxus Jugular venous distention Tachypnea Distant heart sounds

Each category represents a specific pathoanatomic process with well-recognized clinical signs and symptoms (Table 23-1).

Inflammatory (Acute) Pericarditis

The incidence of pericarditis, as assessed in several autopsy series, ranges from 2 to 6 percent. However, clinically diagnosed acute pericarditis occurs in approximately 1 of every 1000 hospital admissions. All types of acute pericarditis are more common in men than in women and more common in adults than in children.

Pathophysiology

The pathologic changes found in acute pericarditis are those of acute inflammation, including polymorphonuclear leukocytes, increased vascularity, and fibrin. The inflammatory process frequently involves the superficial myocardium (epicardium). The exudation of fluid from the visceral pericardium is a response to injury.

Although there are many causes of acute pericarditis, the classification is based on a number of basic disease processes, which include infectious, immune/collagen vascular, metabolic, traumatic/iatrogenic, neoplastic, and idiopathic (Table 23-2).

Clinical Manifestations

Acute pericarditis is characterized by sharp and persistent substernal or precordial chest pain. Its onset is sudden or rapidly progressive and is frequently exacerbated by movement, coughing, lying supine, swallowing, or deep inspiration and is lessened by sitting upright and leaning forward. The pain of acute pericarditis may radiate, most commonly to the left trapezius ridge; however, radiation to the right trapezius ridge, and rarely down the arms, may also occur. Depending on the underlying etiology, other clinical manifestations may also be present.

The sine qua non of acute pericarditis is the pericardial friction rub. It is best heard along the left sternal border between the third and fourth intercostal space with the patient leaning forward in full expiration. Although variable, three components, representing atrial systole, ventricular systole, and ventricular diastole, are characteristically heard. Less commonly, two components are appreciated, and, rarely, only a single sound is present. Tachypnea of mild to moderate severity is frequently encountered in patients with acute pericarditis, reflecting a response to pain with inspiration. Therefore, respirations are characteristically shallow and splinted. Patients with infectious pericarditis and bacteremia may present in shock as may those with a large pericardial effusion causing cardiac tamponade.

Laboratory Findings

The electrocardiographic (ECG) findings of acute pericarditis are a manifestation of concomitant inflammation of the contiguous epicardium. While not diagnostic, the ECG supplements the history and physical examination. In the early stages of acute pericarditis, concave upward ST-segment elevation occurs in most leads, with the exception of aVR, in which ST-segment depression is seen. Lead V_1 may have a depressed or isoelectric ST segment. P-R segment–depression frequently accompanies ST-segment elevation and is both a sensitive and specific ECG marker of acute pericarditis (Fig. 23-2). Later in the process, the ST segments return toward normal, and concomitant diffuse T-wave flattening or T-wave inversion may occur. With time, the ECG usually reverts to normal. Occasionally, ECG changes may appear in only a few leads, suggesting a focal process. Unlike acute myocardial infarction, reciprocal ECG changes are not observed in acute pericarditis.

Arrhythmias of either atrial or ventricular origin, more frequently the former, have been observed in patients with acute pericarditis. Evidence to date suggests that underlying heart disease, particularly coronary artery disease, may explain the frequency of arrhythmias more than pericardial disease itself.

There are no radiographic findings that characteristically occur in the setting of acute pericarditis. In fact, the chest x-ray may be entirely normal. Depending on the underlying

Table 23-2. Etiology of acute pericarditis

Idiopathic
Infectious
Bacterial
Viral
Mycotic
Rickettsial
Parasitic
Spirochetal
Mycoplasma
Immune/collagen vascular
Rheumatoid arthritis
Systemic lupus erythematosus
Scleroderma
Sjögren's syndrome
Mixed connective tissue disease (MCTD)
Reiter's syndrome
Ankylosing spondylitis
Wegener's granulomatosis
Polymyositis (dermatomyositis)
Behçet's syndrome
Inflammatory bowel disease
Whipple's disease
Drug reactions (procainamide, hydralazine, isoniazid, methylsergide)
Serum sickness
Kawasaki's disease
Rheumatic fever
Metabolic disorders
Uremia (acute, chronic)
Myxedema
Gout
Cholesterol pericarditis
Diseases of contiguous structures
Myocardial infarction (acute)
Myocardial infarction (chronic; Dressler's syndrome)
Aortic dissection
Pneumonia
Pleuritis
Pulmonary embolism
Endocarditis
Neoplastic
Primary—mesothelioma
Secondary—metastatic
Traumatic
Penetrating chest injury
Esophageal perforation
Cardiac surgery
Cardiac catheterization
Radiation injury
Other
Pancreatitis
Sarcoidosis
Fabry's disease
Fat embolism

etiology, abnormalities of the cardiac silhouette, mediastinum, lung fields, great vessels, and bone structures may be present. If a moderate to large pericardial effusion accompanies acute pericarditis, an enlarged globular heart is observed.

An echocardiogram performed in the setting of acute pericarditis often demonstrates a pericardial effusion of variable size. Potential etiologies may be determined through evaluation of myocardial function, focal wall motion, valvular appearance and structure, chamber size, and the pericardial surface itself.

Leukocytosis with or without a left shift is frequently seen. In cases of acute viral pericarditis, a predominance of lymphocytes or, at times, a mild to moderate leukopenia may be observed. The sedimentation rate is increased. In the setting of acute transmural myocardial infarction with accompanying pericarditis, creatine kinase (CK) and its MB fraction are elevated. In addition, a small rise in CK-MB may at times be seen without myocardial infarction, suggesting epicardial extension of the inflammatory process.

Based on the history, physical findings, and overall clinical setting, more extensive diagnostic testing may be indicated to define the underlying cause of acute pericarditis. These include tuberculosis screening, blood cultures to rule out asssociated infective endocarditis/bacteremia; viral cultures of the urine, throat, and feces; acute/convalescent viral titers of the blood; an ASO titer in cases of suspected rheumatic fever; cold agglutinins to rule out mycoplasma; a heterophile antibody to rule out infectious mononucleosis; thyroid (T_4, TSH) studies; and an antinuclear antibody (ANA) when considering a diagnosis of a collagen vascular disease.

Differential Diagnosis

The most common disorders that must be considered in the differential diagnosis of acute pericarditis are

Acute myocardial infarction
Pneumonia
Aortic dissection (thoracic)
Pneumothorax
Musculoskeletal (chest wall) pain

Acute myocardial infarction is characterized by a gradual onset of chest, arm, neck, or back pain, which is pressure-like or squeezing in quality. Unlike acute pericarditis, the pain of acute myocardial infarction is not positional, nor is it influenced by coughing, inspiration, or swallowing. The ECG findings are those of "convex-upward" ST-segment elevation, frequently *with* reciprocal changes, which help differentiate it from the "concave-upward" ST-segment elevation *without* reciprocal changes of acute pericarditis.

Pneumonia is characterized by cough, fever, and nonspecific constitutional symptoms. The chest x-ray may be diagnostic. The ECG may reveal nonspecific ST–T-wave changes. Pleuritic involvement when present makes clinical differentiation from acute pericarditis difficult. Indeed, acute pleuropericarditis may be seen in viral and bacterial infections, trauma, and immune/collagen vascular disorders.

Dissection of the thoracic aorta presents with the sudden onset of back pain, which may radiate to the shoulders or through to the anterior chest. Pulse deficits, neurologic events, and rapid hemodynamic compromise are not uncommon. Hypertension is frequently observed. A widened mediastinum is seen frequently on chest x-ray.

Acute pneumothorax—spontaneous, traumatic, or iatrogenic—is characterized by sudden dyspnea. Breath sounds may be diminished or absent in the involved lung field(s). The diagnosis is secured by a chest x-ray revealing absent lung markings with or without mediastinal shift.

Musculoskeletal chest pain is a common phenomenon

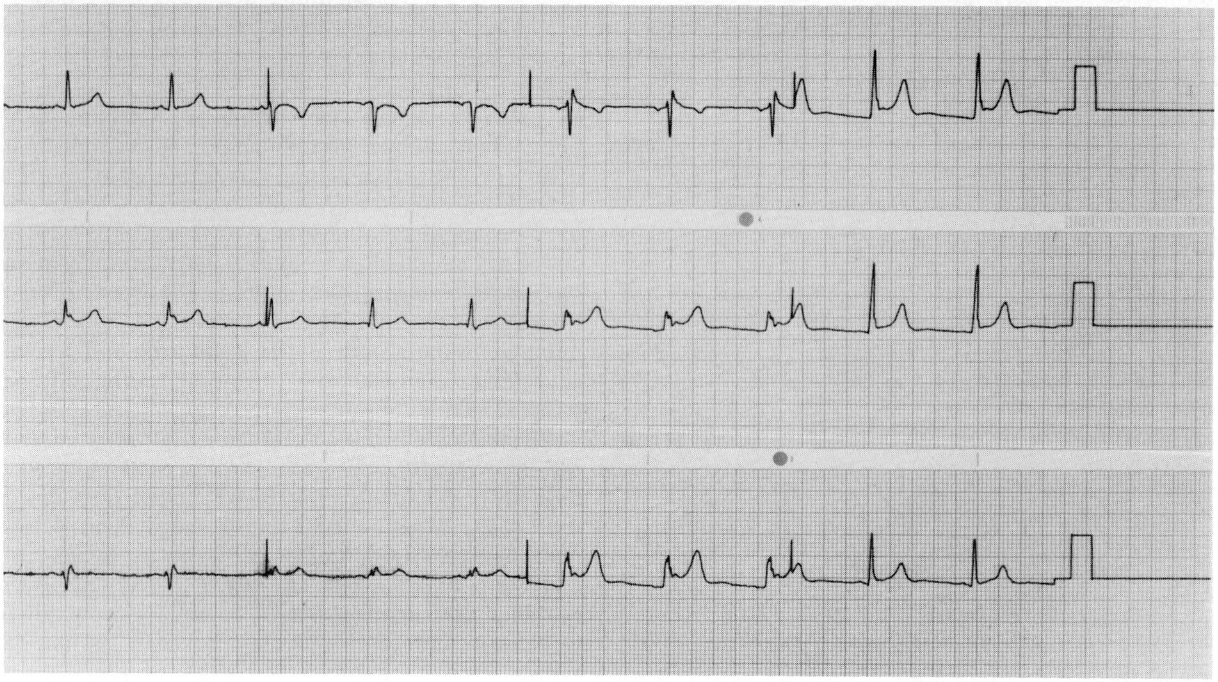

Fig. 23-2. Admitting ECG of a 34-year-old man with chest pain and a low-grade fever. Diffuse, concave-upward ST-segment elevation and P-R segment–depression are present, consistent with acute pericarditis.

that at times may be difficult to distinguish from true cardiac disease, particularly when they occur concomitantly. However, musculoskeletal pain tends to be well localized, sharp, and reproducible with manual compression. ECG changes are not present.

Management

The emergency department treatment of acute pericarditis is dictated by the patient's clinical condition and the underlying etiology. If acute pericarditis results in cardiac tamponade, urgent or emergent pericardial drainage may be indicated (see Procedure 21). Patients with either acute or chronic renal failure may require initiation or intensification of dialysis, respectively. For the majority of patients with acute pericarditis, emergent therapy is not indicated and a nonsteroidal anti-inflammatory agent given over a 7- to 14-day period results in a marked reduction in symptoms. Corticosteroids should be reserved for patients with refractory or chronic recurrent pericarditis and, when used, should be tapered slowly to prevent a rapid recurrence of symptoms. Azathioprine has also been used in this setting, as has surgical pericardiectomy.

Constrictive Pericarditis

Constrictive pericarditis is a disorder of the pericardium that typically follows a case of acute idiopathic or viral pericarditis, although a broad range of etiologies have been described (Table 23-3). It is far more common in adults than in children.

Table 23-3. Etiology of constrictive pericarditis

Idiopathic
Infections (viral, tubercular, fungal, parasitic)
Neoplastic (lymphoma, leukemia, primary [mesothelioma]); metastatic (lung, breast, other)
Trauma (blunt, penetrating)
Postcardiac surgery
Irradiation
Connective tissue disease (systemic lupus erythematosus, rheumatoid arthritis)
Other: rheumatic heart disease, renal failure, atrial septal defect

Pathophysiology

Constrictive pericarditis is present when a thickened and fibrotic pericardium restricts diastolic filling of the heart. A symmetric constricting effect from uniform scarring of the pericardium reduces filling of all cardiac chambers equally. However, systolic function on rare occasions may be affected.

Clinical Manifestations

Pericardial constriction is, in the majority of cases, a chronic process; therefore, the evolution of symptoms is slow and progressive. Patients complain of fatigue, weakness, weight loss, dyspnea on exertion, orthopnea, abdominal distention, and peripheral swelling. Presenting symptoms may suggest renal, hepatic, or myocardial disease. Rarely, symptom onset is rapidly progressive, particularly following cardiac surgery or acute inflammatory pericarditis.

Patients frequently appear chronically ill with muscle wasting and cachexia. The jugular veins are distended with a further increase during inspiration (Kussmaul's sign). The systemic blood pressure is normal or low, and, rarely, pulsus paradoxus is appreciated. The liver may be distended and tender. Ascites and peripheral edema are observed in a majority of cases. Basilar rales may or may not be present, and the heart sounds are either normal or soft. An early diastolic filling sound (pericardial knock) is frequently audible; however, it may be absent in subacute cases in which the pericardium is less rigid.

Laboratory Findings
The ECG in constrictive pericarditis reveals nonspecific findings. In long-standing cases, atrial fibrillation is common. The QRS voltage is frequently low in the limb and precordial leads. Diffuse T-wave flattening or shallow T-wave inversion may be seen.

Intrapericardial calcification is a radiographic finding that supports the diagnosis of pericardial constriction. However, it is present in less than 50 percent of cases. Moreover, pericardial calcification may be present without constriction. An enlargement of the cardiac silhouette is present in many patients; however, prominence of the pulmonary vasculature or interstitial edema are not common findings. More than half of the patients with pericardial constriction have a right-sided pleural effusion. Straightening of the left heart border, elevation of the left mainstem bronchus, and a "double density," each suggesting left atrial enlargement, may also be seen.

The echocardiogram, although not specific, frequently provides useful information, particularly in ruling out processes that may mimic pericardial constriction such as infiltrative (restrictive) cardiomyopathies and chronic cor pulmonale. Occasionally, a thickened pericardium may support the diagnosis of constriction; however, the pericardial thickness as assessed echocardiographically is frequently a function of instrument gain setting and, moreover, correlates poorly with thickness documented at surgery or necropsy. A number of echocardiographic findings have been described in patients with pericardial constriction, including left ventricular posterior wall flattening, paradoxical septal motion, early diastolic septal notching, and atrial systolic notching.

Newer methods of cardiac imaging such as computed tomography (CT) scanning and magnetic resonance imaging (MRI) are effective in documenting abnormal pericardial thickness. They may also be used to distinguish restrictive cardiomyopathy from pericardial constriction.

The thickened pericardium impairs diastolic filling of all cardiac chambers equally; therefore, diastolic pressure is elevated and nearly equal in the right ventricle, left ventricle, right atrium, and left atrium. Ventricular pressure tracings reveal the characteristic "square root" sign. The right atrial "a" and "v" waves are usually equal with rapid "x" and "y" descents, suggesting unimpeded early diastolic filling and a sudden pressure plateau as filling terminates abruptly (Fig. 23-3). The pulmonary artery pressure is normal or mildly elevated with a narrow pulmonary artery pulse pressure. The cardiac index is low-normal or mildly decreased.

As pericardial constriction commonly presents in a subacute or chronic fashion, echocardiographic and hemodynamic evaluation may not be required emergently. However, in cases in which hemodynamic compromise is present, these diagnostic studies may be important supplements to a chest x-ray, ECG, and arterial blood gas analysis.

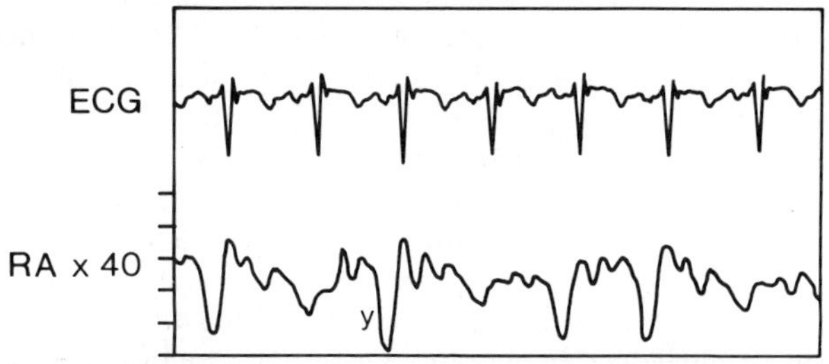

Fig. 23-3. Right atrial pressure tracing in a patient with constrictive pericarditis. Note the prominent "y" descent corresponding to early diastole.

Table 23-4. Restrictive cardiomyopathies

Amyloid
Hemochromatosis
Postirradiation fibrosis
Carcinoid
Doxorubicin cardiotoxicity
Scleroderma
Infiltrating tumor (primary, metastatic)
Pseudoxanthoma elasticum
Endocardial fibrosis (idiopathic)
Eosinophilic endomyocardial disease

Differential Diagnosis
Restrictive cardiomyopathy is by far the most common disorder in the differential diagnosis of pericardial constriction (Table 23-4). Others include:

Superior vena cava (SVC) syndrome
Hepatic cirrhosis
Chronic/subacute renal failure
Chronic cor pulmonale

In differentiating myocardial restriction from pericardial constriction, the following points must be considered: In *myocardial restriction*, (1) echocardiography may reveal an infiltrative process and abnormal left ventricular systolic function; (2) there is a disproportionate elevation in left ventricular end-diastolic pressure (LVEDP) or pulmonary wedge pressure (PWP), or both, particularly following fluid administration and exercise; (3) the cardiac index is moderately reduced and the pulmonary artery systolic pressure is frequently greater than 50 mm Hg; and (4) on physical examination, a third heart sound and murmurs of mitral and tricuspid insufficiency are commonly appreciated.

Management
Chronic constrictive pericarditis rarely requires emergent therapy. However, with constrictive-effusive processes, pericardial drainage may be indicated to improve overall cardiac function and raise systemic blood pressure. Digitalis

is useful in the setting of atrial fibrillation to control ventricular response and thus allow adequate diastolic filling time. Direct current (DC) cardioversion should be used if atrial fibrillation is accompanied by hemodynamic instability. Because constriction is primarily a disorder of diastolic function, adequate preload is essential. Therefore, volume support may be required initially to maintain an adequate cardiac output. Vigorous diuresis despite the external appearance of fluid overload or the use of potent venodilators such as nitroglycerin should be avoided. The only definitive therapy for pericardial constriction is surgical pericardiectomy.

Pericardial Effusion

A pericardial effusion is most commonly the result of inflammation from acute pericarditis; however, a number of clinical entities have been associated with the development of an excess in pericardial fluid (Table 23-5). As with acute pericarditis and pericardial constriction, pericardial effusions are more common in adults than in children.

Pathophysiology
Although a pericardial effusion may develop silently, if sufficient fluid accumulates and intrapericardial pressure increases, cardiac compression (tamponade) may develop. Overall, the development of increased pericardial pressure depends on (1) the absolute volume of fluid, (2) the rate of fluid accumulation, and (3) the mechanical characteristics of the pericardium. If fluid accumulates slowly, the pericardial space may accommodate 1 to 2 liters without a significant increase in intrapericardial pressure. However, the normal pericardium can allow no more than 100 to 200 ml of fluid acutely before there is a marked increase in intrapericardial pressure. With a noncompliant pericardium, smaller fluid volumes would be expected to cause an increased intrapericardial pressure.

As intrapericardial pressure increases, the transmural distending pressure within the cardiac chambers declines, preventing adequate filling, and, ultimately, a decrease in stroke volume and cardiac output.

Clinical Manifestations
The acute form of tamponade, as described by Beck in 1935, characterized by the classic triad of hypotension, jugular venous distention, and a small, quiet heart, is seen most frequently in cardiac trauma. Nontraumatic tamponade (subacute) may take days or weeks to evolve.

With rapidly developing tamponade, cyanosis, diaphoresis, restlessness, and hemodynamic collapse (shock) may quickly ensue (Table 23-6). Large effusions developing slowly are associated with nonspecific precordial discomfort and symptoms caused by pressure on adjacent mediastinal structures, resulting in hoarseness, coughing, tachypnea, and dysphagia.

In acute tamponade, the patient appears cool and clammy with marked diaphoresis, tachycardia, and hypoperfusion (shock). In subacute cases, the blood pressure is low-normal or low with a narrow pulse pressure and an inspiratory decline in systolic pressure of greater than 10 mm Hg (pulsus paradoxus). In addition, there is moderate jugular venous distention, distant heart sounds, and clear lung fields.

Table 23-5. Pericardial effusion

Idiopathic
Infectious (viral, bacteria, protozoal, tubercular)
Malignancy (primary, metastatic)
Connective tissue disease
Uremia
Trauma (blunt, penetrating)
Cardiac rupture (post-myocardial infarction)
Aortic dissection
Aortic aneurysm rupture
Post-cardiac surgery (post-pericardiotomy syndrome)
Complication of heart catheterization or pacemaker insertion
Postirradiation
Myxedema

Table 23-6. Clinical findings in acute cardiac tamponade

Hypotension
Narrow pulse pressure
Dyspnea, orthopnea
Tachycardia
Pulsus paradoxus
Jugular venous distention
Distant heart sounds
Shock

Laboratory Findings
The ECG may be normal, have nonspecific ST–T-wave changes, or have findings that reflect an underlying cardiac process such as acute pericarditis or myocardial infarction. With moderate to large effusions, QRS complex and T-wave amplitudes are decreased, while P-wave voltage is frequently preserved. Although not a frequent ECG finding, electrical alternans is considered specific for the presence of a large pericardial effusion.

The size and configuration of the cardiac silhouette depend on the compliance of the pericardium and the rate of fluid accumulation in the pericardial space. With large subacute or chronic effusions, the cardiac silhouette is enlarged and globular in appearance. A change in the cardiac silhouette from a previous chest x-ray may be informative. The absence of pulmonary vascular prominence aids in the exclusion of congestive heart failure.

The two-dimensional echocardiogram is the noninvasive diagnostic modality of choice in the evaluation of a pericardial effusion. It may be obtained in the emergency department, when the clinical status dictates, to confirm the presence of a pericardial effusion. With moderate to large effusions, an anterior and posterior echo-free space is seen (Fig. 23-4A and B). The swinging motion of the heart may cause pseudoprolapse of the mitral and tricuspid valves in systole. An inspiratory increase in right ventricular dimension and superior vena caval blood flow velocity, as assessed by Doppler examination, may be observed. Echocardiographic findings that correlate with hemodynamically significant pericardial effusions (tamponade) include right ventricular diastolic collapse, right atrial diastolic collapse, "plethora" of the inferior vena cava, and collapse of the

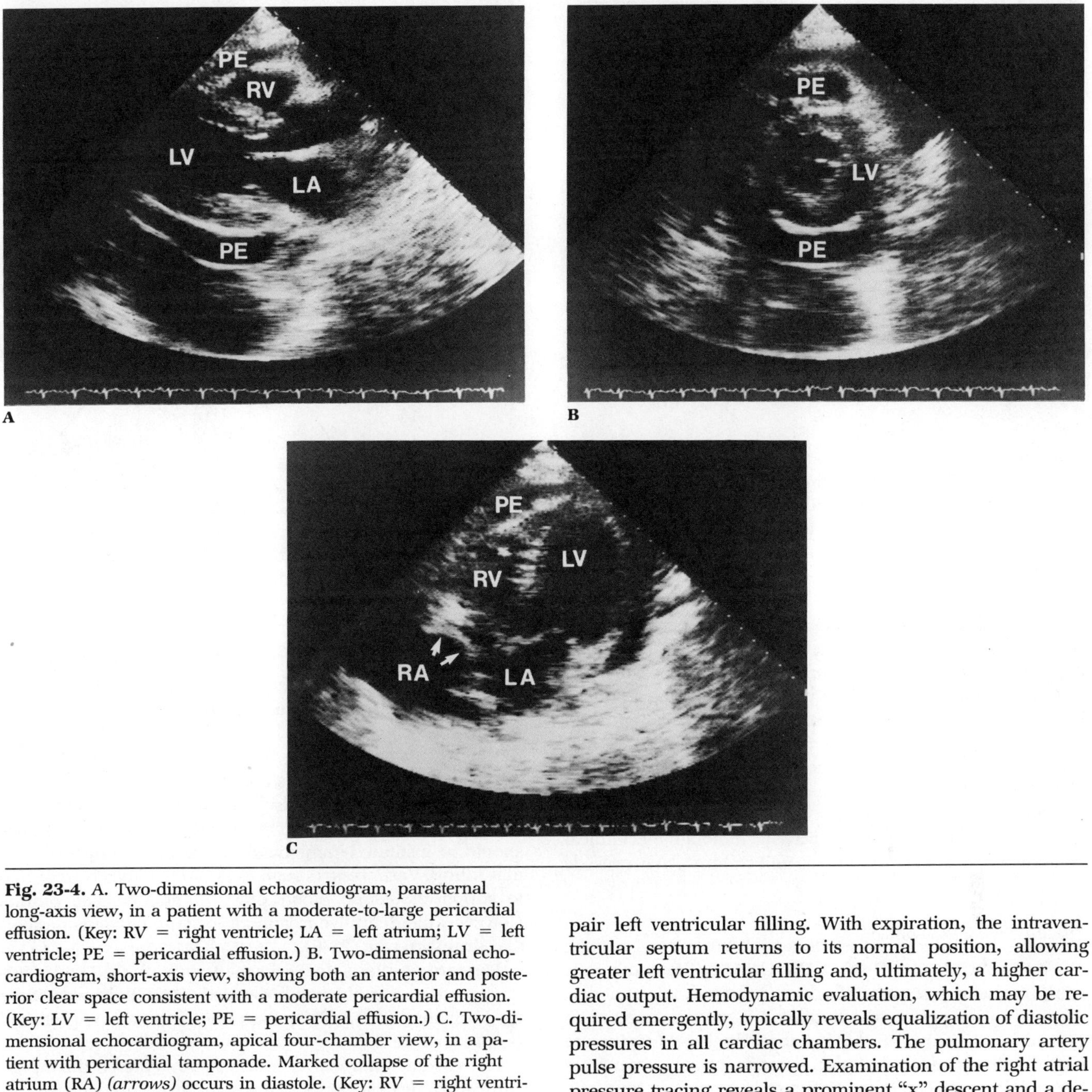

Fig. 23-4. A. Two-dimensional echocardiogram, parasternal long-axis view, in a patient with a moderate-to-large pericardial effusion. (Key: RV = right ventricle; LA = left atrium; LV = left ventricle; PE = pericardial effusion.) B. Two-dimensional echocardiogram, short-axis view, showing both an anterior and posterior clear space consistent with a moderate pericardial effusion. (Key: LV = left ventricle; PE = pericardial effusion.) C. Two-dimensional echocardiogram, apical four-chamber view, in a patient with pericardial tamponade. Marked collapse of the right atrium (RA) *(arrows)* occurs in diastole. (Key: RV = right ventricle; LV = left ventricle; PE = pericardial effusion.)

superior vena cava. The duration of chamber or vessel collapse correlates with the severity of hemodynamic compromise (Fig. 23-4C). The echocardiogram may also be useful in identifying localized hematomas causing atrial or ventricular compression.

As fluid accumulates, intrapericardial pressure rises and pericardial compliance declines. Pericardial compliance ultimately becomes dependent on the phase of the respiratory cycle, decreasing with expiration and increasing with inspiration. Therefore, venous return increases with inspiration and almost ceases with expiration. With an increase in venous return, right ventricular volume increases, causing a leftward shift of the intraventricular septum sufficient to impair left ventricular filling. With expiration, the intraventricular septum returns to its normal position, allowing greater left ventricular filling and, ultimately, a higher cardiac output. Hemodynamic evaluation, which may be required emergently, typically reveals equalization of diastolic pressures in all cardiac chambers. The pulmonary artery pulse pressure is narrowed. Examination of the right atrial pressure tracing reveals a prominent "x" descent and a decreased or absent "y" descent (Fig. 23-5).

Differential Diagnosis

Disorders that should be considered in the differential diagnosis of pericardial effusion with tamponade include:

- Right ventricular infarction
- Constrictive pericarditis (including constrictive-effusive pericarditis)
- Pulmonary embolism
- Tension pneumopericardium
  - Penetrating trauma
  - Mechanical ventilation
  - Gastric/esophageal rupture
  - Gas-producing mediastinal infection

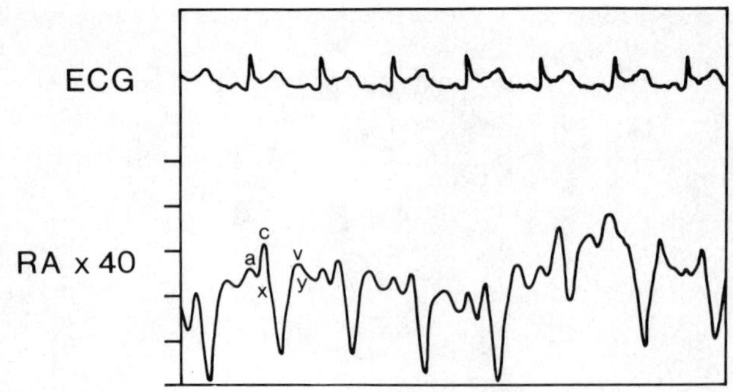

Fig. 23-5. Right atrial pressure tracing in a 63-year-old woman with a recent myocardial infarction and recurrent chest pain accompanied by hypotension. The "y" descent is obliterated; as intrapericardial pressure is maximum during diastole, rapid ventricular filling cannot occur. Pericardial tamponade.

Right ventricular infarction occurs in the setting of an acute inferior myocardial infarction and, like pericardial tamponade, limits ventricular filling and compromises overall cardiac output. The ECG typically reveals ST-segment elevation, with or without Q waves, in leads II, III, and aVF. ST-segment elevation is also seen in "right-sided" chest leads, particularly RV_4.

Constrictive pericarditis has previously been discussed and, as outlined, may cause acute symptom onset when an effusive component to the inflammatory process occurs.

Acute pulmonary embolism with cor pulmonale and cardiogenic shock may clinically mimic pericardial tamponade; however, profound hypoxia is more common in the former than in the latter. In addition, an ECG may reveal evidence of right ventricular strain or the classic "SI, QIII, TIII" pattern.

Tension pneumopericardium is seen most commonly in the setting of penetrating chest trauma, although mechanical ventilation, particularly in infants and children, may precede its development.

Special Considerations

LOW-PRESSURE CARDIAC TAMPONADE. Hemodynamic compromise may occasionally develop despite only a moderate amount of pericardial fluid and a modest increase in pericardial pressure. In this instance, the jugular veins are slightly distended, and close inspection reveals absence of the "x" descent. The blood pressure is normal or low, and pulsus paradoxus may be minimal or absent. In fact, the overall symptom profile may be unimpressive and the diagnosis of tamponade made only after hemodynamic improvement is obtained following the removal of pericardial fluid. Low-pressure tamponade occurs in states characterized by decreased central blood volume, either from dehydration or blood loss.

ATYPICAL TAMPONADE. Fluid within the pericardial space or mediastinum may be localized and cause regional compression of a cardiac chamber. This occurs most frequently following chest trauma or open heart surgery and usually involves the right atrium or right ventricle, although selective compression of any chamber or a combination of chambers may occur. Two-dimensional echocardiography is useful in identifying and localizing compressive fluid collections. Surgical drainage is usually required.

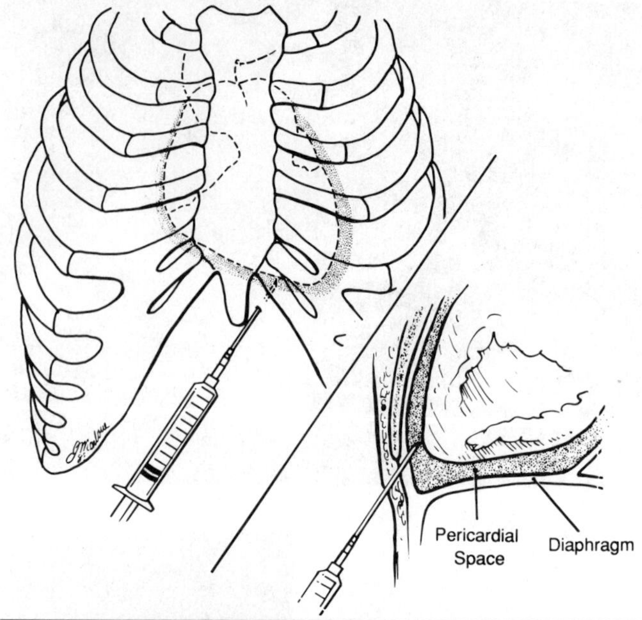

Fig. 23-6. Pericardiocentesis. Following anesthesia of the skin and subcutaneous tissues, an 18-gauge needle attached to a syringe is introduced to the left of the xiphoid process at a 30-degree angle to the frontal plane and advanced toward the left shoulder. Free aspiration of fluid confirms entry into the pericardial space.

Management

Acute cardiac tamponade is a medical emergency that must be treated swiftly and precisely. Rapid intravenous fluid administration, with either crystalloid or colloid solutions, should be instituted immediately to ensure adequate ventricular filling. Vasopressors such as dopamine may be required to support systemic blood pressure and cardiac output. However, the definitive treatment for tamponade is pericardial drainage (Fig. 23-6).

Pericardiocentesis is performed with the patient positioned supine and the trunk elevated 15 to 30 degrees above the horizontal plane. The subxiphoid approach is preferred (see Procedure 20).

If a cardiac chamber is inadvertently entered during attempted pericardiocentesis, the right atrial pressure should be monitored frequently thereafter. If right atrial pressure rises precipitously, hemorrhagic tamponade is likely, and provision for immediate pericardiocentesis followed by surgical pericardial exploration and drainage is indicated. Other complications of periocardiocentesis include:

Coronary artery laceration
Supraventricular arrhythmias
Ventricular arrhythmias (including ventricular tachycardia/fibrillation)
Pneumothorax
Hepatic laceration

Surgical drainage of the pericardium is preferred over blind pericardiocentesis in cases of traumatic tamponade and hemopericardium from leaking ventricular or aortic aneurysms, and with large purulent effusions.

ACUTE AORTIC INSUFFICIENCY

Acute aortic insufficiency (AI) is a unique clinical entity with specific clinical manifestations that differentiate it from the chronic form. Although the hemodynamic consequences of severe AI are consistent, the etiology and clinical manifestations vary.

The most common cause of acute severe AI is infective endocarditis caused by gram-positive bacteria, particularly *Staphylococcus aureus* and *Enterococci* (Table 23-7). Infective endocarditis often occurs on a functionally normal bicuspid aortic valve. Acute AI with refractory congestive heart failure resulting from destruction of one or more aortic valve leaflets is the most common cause of death in infective endocarditis.

Dissection of the ascending thoracic aorta may cause acute AI. The dissection may extend antegrade around the aortic arch, retrograde toward the aortic valve ring, or both. Dissection usually manifests itself as severe chest pain of abrupt onset. Occasionally, there is evidence of upper extremity or cerebral ischemia resulting from involvement of the aortic arch vessels. Dissection may disrupt one or more aortic cusps at their commissural attachments or dilate the aortic annulus, resulting in acute AI. Dissection may also compromise the coronary ostia, leading to acute myocardial infarction. In addition, hemopericardium and fatal pericardial tamponade may ensue if the dissection extends through the outer aortic media into the pericardium as it reflects about the origin of the aorta and main pulmonary artery.

The presence of acute AI complicating aortic dissection may at times be overshadowed by other presenting clinical manifestations, including stroke, upper extremity vascular compromise, chest pain, or tamponade. However, approximately two-thirds of patients requiring surgery for aortic dissection require concomitant replacement or resuspension of the aortic valve because of acute AI.

Aortic insufficiency is the valvular lesion most commonly found in patients surviving closed chest trauma. In this setting, autopsy or surgical aortic valve specimens demonstrate leaflet tears, avulsion of commissural attachments, and transmural tears in the proximal ascending aorta. The clinician must be aware that the occurrence of an AI murmur or clinical evidence of cardiac decompensation may be delayed for several days following closed chest trauma. The severity of AI may vary from mild to severe. In addition to trauma, aortic valve rupture has been reported following severe muscular strain, including snow shoveling and during childbirth.

Table 23-7. Etiology of acute aortic insufficiency

Infective endocarditis
Dissection of ascending aorta
Traumatic rupture
Inflammatory disease
Systemic lupus erythematosus
Aortitis
Ankylosing spondylitis
Takayasu's arteritis
Behçet's syndrome
"Spontaneous"
Prosthetic valve dysfunction (acute)
Sinus of Valsalva aneurysm rupture

There are several reports of acute AI complicating systemic lupus erythematosus, resulting from perforation of one or more aortic valve cusps weakened by localized fibrinoid necrosis. A number of other systemic disorders have also been associated with the development of AI, including ankylosing spondylitis, Whipple's disease, giant cell arteritis, Takayasu's disease, and Behçet's syndrome.

Severe AI following spontaneous rupture or prolapse of one or more aortic valve cusps has been described. AI resulting from rupture or prolapse of a myxomatous aortic valve, occurring either in the setting of Marfan's syndrome or an acquired degenerative process, has been reported. Spontaneous rupture of a bicuspid aortic valve causing acute severe AI has also been reported.

Sudden partial or complete dehiscence of a prosthetic valve sewing ring from the aortic annulus may precipitate acute, severe AI. This is a complication of emergency aortic valve replacement for acute bacterial endocarditis, when the prosthetic valve must be implanted into an infected annulus. Prosthetic valves may also develop pannus ingrowth, thrombus formation, or a vegetation, thus impeding proper seating of the ball or poppet with subsequent aortic insufficiency. Porcine bioprostheses can undergo spontaneous degeneration after several years, leading to acute AI.

Pathophysiology

The hemodynamic response that evolves in the setting of acute AI is determined by the volume of regurgitant blood and the rapidity with which it develops. A previously normal left ventricle suddenly faced with sudden, severe AI is not able to adequately compensate. With acute volume overload, left ventricular diastolic pressure increases precipitously with a concomitant relative decrease in stroke volume.

As effective forward stroke volume declines, there is an increase in heart rate via reflex sympathetic stimulation. In addition, total peripheral resistance increases to maintain perfusion pressure within vital organs. Since there is an insufficient increase in total left ventricular stroke volume, left ventricular and aortic systolic blood pressures are normal or low, in contrast to the marked elevations seen in chronic AI. Aortic diastolic pressure cannot decline below LVEDP. Therefore, in acute severe AI, the arterial pulse pressure is usually normal.

Clinical Manifestations

As previously mentioned, acute severe AI is most commonly the result of infective endocarditis; thus, most patients are acutely ill with symptoms of both systemic infection and hemodynamic compromise. The patient presents with symptoms suggestive of severe left-sided heart failure (dyspnea, orthopnea, paroxysmal nocturnal dyspnea, fatigue, exhaustion), the onset of which can frequently be specified (Table 23-8). Heart failure is usually progressive, intractable, and rapidly fatal unless definitive therapy is undertaken. Unlike chronic AI, the rapid progression of acute severe AI seldom

Table 23-8. Clinical manifestations of acute aortic insufficiency

Dyspnea
Orthopnea
Tachycardia
Hypotension
Pulsus alternans
Pulmonary rales
Cardiac ascultation
Midsystolic flow murmur
Variable second heart sound
Short diastolic murmur
Austin Flint murmur
S3 gallop

Table 23-9. Treatment of acute aortic insufficiency

Supplemental oxygen—intubation if needed
Treatment of pulmonary edema
Intravenous diuretics
Morphine sulfate
Potassium/magnesium supplementation as needed
Vasodilator therapy—nitroprusside
Inotropic therapy—dobutamine, dopamine
Valve replacement

allows time for significant renal retention of salt and water. Thus, few patients demonstrate symptoms related to systemic venous congestion such as edema, increasing abdominal girth, or weight gain.

Patients appear acutely ill with evidence of low cardiac output and pulmonary congestion. The distal extremities are pale and cool, and there may be acrocyanosis. Tachycardia is usually observed, and its absence should raise a question as to whether the AI is acute or severe. Pulsus alternans secondary to acute left ventricular failure may be appreciated. However, in contrast to chronic AI, Corrigan's (water-hammer) pulse and Quincke's pulse (alternating flushing and blanching of nailbed capillaries) are absent.

As left atrial and pulmonary capillary wedge pressures rise, pulmonary artery pressure also rises. A sustained elevation in pulmonary artery pressure can lead to right ventricular heart failure and subsequent elevation of the jugular venous pressure. The apical impulse is neither hyperdynamic nor displaced as the velocity of ventricular contraction is not augmented and the end-diastolic dimension is not significantly increased.

The auscultatory findings of acute severe AI are subtle and easily missed. The heart rate is rapid and the first heart sound (S1) is usually diminished or absent. A midsystolic flow murmur resulting from augmented total systolic flow across the incompetent aortic valve is heard. The quality of the second heart sound can be variable. It may be preserved if the aortic leaflets remain intact or soft to absent if they are flail. A decrease in the intensity of the aortic valve closure sound (S2–A2) contributes to the difficulty in separating diastole from systole in patients with acute AI. The diastolic murmur begins with the aortic S2 and is usually short in duration, since the totally incompetent valve allows equalization of aortic and left ventricular pressures early in diastole. The murmur may be surprisingly soft in intensity. A flail cusp may produce a low, musical (single frequency) diastolic murmur. An Austin Flint murmur (owing to antegrade flow across a mitral valve moving toward the closed position in late diastole) is often heard in severe AI. Antegrade diastolic flow velocity across the mitral valve is increased because of the shortened period during which the mitral valve is open. A third heart sound (S3) is common. It reflects rapid, early diastolic filling of the left ventricle, antegrade from the left atrium and retrograde from the aorta. Inrushing of blood causes abrupt distention of a poorly compliant ventricle, giving rise to the S3. A fourth heart sound (S4) is usually absent.

Laboratory Findings

Aside from sinus tachycardia, the ECG in acute AI commonly demonstrates nonspecific ST- and T-wave changes. If the acute AI is due to infective endocarditis, ECG findings of atrioventricular block may be present.

The chest x-ray shows little or no evidence of cardiac enlargement. In contrast to the normal cardiac silhouette, the lung fields demonstrate venous redistribution and interstitial edema. The aortic root and transverse aortic shadows are normal except in cases involving dissection of the thoracic aorta, where enlargement is typically observed.

Echocardiography, either by a transthoracic or transesophageal technique, is extremely important in evaluating patients with acute severe AI. Echocardiography often provides vital information concerning the severity of regurgitation, the status of other heart valves, and the presence of preexisting heart disease. Valuable information may be acquired concerning potential causes of AI, such as infective endocarditis and aortic dissection. In circumstances in which a high-quality echocardiogram is obtained and interpreted by an experienced cardiologist as being consistent with severe AI, cardiac catheterization may not be required to confirm the diagnosis. However, cardiac catheterization, left ventriculography, and coronary angiography are usually indicated for patients with clinical or echocardiographic evidence (or both) of preexisting heart disease.

Management

The treatment of patients with acute severe AI includes general supportive measures, as well as pharmacologic (medical) and surgical management (Table 23-9). These measures should be carried out simultaneously. Supplemental oxygen is invariably required, and intubation with assisted mechanical ventilation should be performed if tissue hypoperfusion or profound hypoxemia occurs. Pulmonary edema should be treated with inotropic agents, intravenous diuretics, and afterload reduction. Nitroprusside therapy may result in substantial clinical improvement. This pharmacologic agent primarily reduces the impedance to left ventricular ejection (afterload). If the cardiac index does not rise above 2.0 liter/minute/m^2 in response to nitroprusside, a sympathomimetic agent (dobutamine) should be added to increase cardiac output as well as coronary and cerebral perfusion. Intra-aortic balloon counterpulsation is contraindicated in patients with acute AI.

Pulmonary artery catheterization and intra-arterial cannulation should be utilized to monitor hemodynamic parameters and systemic blood pressure, respectively, in patients requiring vigorous medical support. However, patients in cardiogenic shock are unlikely to benefit substantially from medical therapy alone; therefore, early valve replacement should be undertaken.

ACUTE MITRAL REGURGITATION

Acute mitral regurgitation (MR) is a well-known clinical syndrome with characteristic physical and hemodynamic findings. Acute MR results from sudden disruption or dysfunction of the mitral valve apparatus, which includes the valve leaflets, chordae tendineae, papillary muscles, and attachments of the papillary muscles to the left ventricular wall.

The most convenient way to classify acute MR is to divide it according to the anatomic site of dysfunction or disruption (Table 23-10). The mitral valve is composed of two leaflets, designated as anterior and posterior. The anterior leaflet is adjacent to and continuous with the ascending aorta and aortic valve. The posterior leaflet is an extension of the lateral and posterior atrial walls. The leaflets are attached to the papillary muscles by multiple branches of collagenous strands known as the chordae tendineae. As the papillary muscles do not correspond exactly to the mitral leaflets, they are designated according to their anatomic positions as anterolateral and posteromedial. Because they are located at the most distal reaches of the coronary artery circulation, the papillary muscles are vulnerable to ischemia, particularly the posteromedial muscle, which typically derives its blood flow exclusively from the posterior descending coronary artery.

Leaflet disruption, a common cause of regurgitation in chronic MR, is an unusual cause of acute MR. However, infectious endocarditis, atrial myxoma, and chest trauma (blunt or penetrating) may cause sufficient leaflet damage to cause acute MR. Although a common finding in chronic MR, dilation of the mitral valve annulus is an extremely rare cause of acute MR. Rupture of one or more chordae tendineae is a common cause of acute MR, particularly in connective tissue disorders such as Marfan's syndrome, mitral valve prolapse, and multivalvular myxomatous degeneration. Pregnancy, infective endocarditis, congenital aortic valve disease with aortic regurgitation, acute rheumatic valvulitis, and systemic lupus erythematosus can also be complicated by chordal rupture. In cases of acute MR without a clear underlying cause, a classification of "spontaneous" has been given.

Acute MR owing to an abnormality within the papillary muscle results from one of three potential causes: (1) altered contraction of one or both papillary muscles, (2) rupture of all or part of a papillary muscle, or (3) altered left ventricular geometry. Papillary muscle dysfunction secondary to ischemia is a common cause of acute MR. Rupture of one head of a papillary muscle is hemodynamically equivalent to the rupture of several chordae tendineae, whereas rupture of an entire papillary trunk is a catastrophic event resulting in rapid hemodynamic collapse. A patient with a prosthetic mitral valve presenting with acute pulmonary edema may have prosthetic valve dysfunction and severe MR.

Table 23-10. Etiology of acute mitral regurgitation

Valve leaflet failure
Infectious endocarditis
Atrial myxoma
Trauma
Prosthetic valve dysfunction
Annulus failure
Dilation
Chordae tendineae/papillary muscle failure
Chordae tendineae rupture
Connective tissue disease (Marfan's syndrome, mitral valve prolapse)
Acute rheumatic fever
Spontaneous
Papillary muscle
Altered contraction secondary to ischemia
Rupture
Altered left ventricular geometry

Pathophysiology

The hemodynamic profile of acute MR is the result of a sudden and profound reduction in left ventricular afterload causing blood to flow into the low pressure left atrium. Up to 50 percent of left ventricular volume can be ejected into the left atrium prior to aortic valve opening. The rapid development of left atrial volume overload does not allow compensatory dilatation. Therefore, left atrial pressure increases rapidly, causing pulmonary venous hypertension, often with large "V" waves being seen on the pulmonary artery and pulmonary capillary pressure tracings. The volume of regurgitant flow is determined by two factors: the systolic pressure gradient between the left ventricle and left atrium, and the size of the regurgitant orifice. Systemic vasodilators and intraaortic balloon pumps reduce regurgitant volume by reducing the pressure gradient between the left ventricle and left atrium. Left ventricular function carries considerable prognostic significance. Initially, patients with acute MR have increased ejection fractions. An ejection fraction less than 40 percent in the setting of acute MR suggests such severe left ventricular dysfunction that mitral valve replacement may not result in significant symptomatic improvement.

Clinical Manifestations

Patients with acute MR can frequently pinpoint the time of symptom onset. The patient may give a history of chest trauma or symptoms suggestive of infective endocarditis. There may be a history of rheumatic fever or a long-standing heart murmur. In essence, the symptoms of acute MR are those of acute pulmonary edema.

On physical examination, the patient with acute MR appears acutely ill with tachypnea, tachycardia, and hypotension. Examination of the lungs reveals diffuse rales. Cardiac examination reveals a diminished or absent S1, and S2 may be widely split, reflecting early closure of the aortic valve. A prominent S3 is common. The systolic murmur of acute MR may vary in timing, location, intensity, duration, and auscul-

Table 23-11. Clinical presentation of acute mitral regurgitation

Abrupt onset
Tachypnea, tachycardia, and hypotension
Pulmonary rales
Cardiac examination
Diminished S1
Widely split S2
S3
Holosystolic murmur (variable intensity)
± Low-pitched diastolic murmur

tatory characteristics. A low-pitched diastolic murmur may be present, representing increased flow across the mitral valve during diastole (Table 23-11).

Laboratory Findings

The ECG findings in acute MR are not specific; however, occasionally, an underlying cause such as acute myocardial infarction may be identified. Sinus tachycardia is typically observed. The characteristic chest x-ray finding is interstitial edema with a normal-sized cardiac silhouette. Echocardiography can clarify potential underlying causes and rule out conditions that may mimic acute MR. Doppler echocardiography can detect both the presence and severity of MR. Left heart catheterization is frequently required prior to surgical correction to assess the severity of regurgitation, identify coexisting valvular lesions, assess left ventricular function, and determine the presence of coexisting coronary artery disease.

Differential Diagnosis

The murmur of acute MR may be difficult to distinguish from decompensated chronic MR, aortic stenosis, hypertrophic obstructive cardiomyopathy, or acute rupture of the interventricular septum. The ECG, echocardiographic, and chest x-ray findings assist in the differential diagnosis. A systematic approach to the diagnosis should reliably distinguish acute MR from other conditions.

Management

The medical management of acute MR should be regarded as a temporizing measure pending definitive surgical repair. The mainstays of medical therapy for acute MR are vasodilating drugs such as nitroprusside and the intra-aortic balloon pump. Nitroprusside infusion should be titrated to maintain the systemic systolic pressure in the 90 to 100 mm Hg range. As mentioned, surgery is the treatment of choice for acute MR.

CARDIAC RUPTURE

Cardiac rupture, although typically an acute catastrophic event, may at times be subacute; therefore, the diagnosis and surgical treatment of both cardiac tamponade and the underlying myocardial tear can be undertaken. Cardiac rupture is observed in three clinical settings. The most common is acute cardiac rupture, with sudden death occurring 3 to 5 days after an acute myocardial infarction. Cardiac rupture may also present with gradual leakage of blood into the pericardium and the development of clinically apparent tamponade. Perhaps as many as 15 to 35 percent of patients with myocardial rupture suffer from the subacute form, which is associated with a favorable prognosis if recognized and promptly treated.

Cardiac rupture may also result from blunt trauma or from overzealous cardiac resuscitation; however, it is most common following acute myocardial infarction, being observed in 10 percent of acutely infarcted hearts at autopsy. Rupture of the free wall follows transmural infarction. It is most common following large infarcts and first infarcts and in elderly hypertensive women. Its occurrence is increased with the use of corticosteroids and other anti-inflammatory drugs. There is no evidence that immobilization decreases the incidence of rupture or that anticoagulants or thrombolytic therapy increase the frequency.

Cardiac rupture and tamponade should be suspected in patients with myocardial infarction who develop hypotension, distended neck veins, and cardiogenic shock. Large ventricular tears will produce cardiac tamponade with electromechanical dissociation and death, but, with small tears, blood can distend the pericardium, gradually producing subacute tamponade. Small leaks can also be contained locally by the adherent pericardium producing false "pseudo" aneurysms without tamponade.

Prompt diagnosis is essential, since emergency surgical repair provides the only chance for survival following myocardial rupture. The echocardiogram is usually accurate in detecting or ruling out pericardial fluid. If there is a strong suspicion of rupture and tamponade and the echocardiogram shows no fluid or is technically inadequate, a pericardiocentesis should be attempted. It is questionable that afterload reduction or replacement of blood volume is of benefit; however, rapid initiation of intra-aortic balloon counterpulsation may be of use while awaiting surgery. Emergency surgery is usually limited to closure of the ventricular tear.

SELECTED READING

Boltwood, CM, JR, and Shah, PM. The pericardium in health and disease. *Curr Prob Cardiol* 9:1, 1984.

Fowler, NO, and Manitsas, GT. Infectious pericarditis. *Prog Cardiovasc Dis* 26:323, 1973.

Soffer, A. Electrocardiographic abnormalities in acute, convalescent, and recurrent stages of idiopathic pericarditis. *Am Heart J* 60:729, 1960.

Spodick, DH. Arrhythmias during acute pericarditis: A prospective study of 100 consecutive cases. *JAMA* 235:35, 1976.

Frame, JR, Lucas, SK, Pederson, JA, and Elkins, RC. Surgical treatment of pericarditis in the dialysis patient. *Am J Surg* 146:800, 1983.

Morask, RE, and Bousumros, G. Constrictive pericarditis due to chronic uremia. *N Engl J Med* 281:542, 1969.

Voelkel, AG, et al. Echocardiographic features of constrictive pericarditis. *Circulation* 58:871, 1978.

Shabetal, R. The pathophysiology of constrictive pericarditis. In PS Reddy, DF Leon, and JA Shaver (eds.), *Pericardial Disease*. New York: Raven, 1982. Pp. 267–274.

Glantz, SA, and Parmley, WW. Factors which effect the diastolic pressure-volume curve. *Circ Res* 42:171, 1978.

Beck, CS. Two cardiac compression triads. *JAMA* 104:714, 1935.
Kronzon, I, Cohen, ML, and Winer, HE. Diastolic atrial compression: A sensitive echocardiographic sign of cardiac tamponade. *J Am Coll Cardiol* 2:770, 1983.
Reddy, PS, et al. Cardiac tamponade: Hemodynamic observations in man. *Circulation* 58:265, 1978.
Shabetal, R, Fouilles, NO, and Gurrsoth, WG. The hemodynamics of cardiac tamponade and constrictive pericarditis. *Am J Cardiol* 26:480, 1970.
Perloff, JK. Acute severe aortic regurgitation—recognition and management. *J Cardiovasc Med* 3:209, 1983.
Weinstein, L, and Robin, RH. Infective endocarditis. *Prog Cardiovasc Dis* 16:239, 1973.
Braniff, BA, Shumway, NE, and Harrison, DC. Valve replacement in active bacterial endocarditis. *N Engl J Med* 276:1464, 1967.
Dalen, JE, et al. Dissection of the thoracic aorta—medical or surgical therapy? *Am J Cardiol* 34:803, 1974.
Dajee, H, Hurley, EJ, and Szarnick, RJ. Cardiac valve replacement in systemic lupus erythematosus. A review. *J Thorac Cardiovasc Surg* 85(5):718, 1983.
Olinger, GN, Korns, ME, and Bonchek, LI. Acute aortic valvular insufficiency due to isolated myxomatous degeneration. *Ann Intern Med* 88:807, 1978.
Becker, AE, and Curren, DR. Spontaneous rupture of bicuspid aortic valve, an unusual cause of aortic insufficiency. *Chest* 72:361, 1977.
Gore, JM, et al. Acute spontaneous failure of a porcine aortic valve. *Arch Intern Med* 142:1553, 1982.
Roberts, WC, Braunwald, E, and Morrow, AG. Acute severe mitral regurgitation secondary to ruptured chordae tendineae. *Circulation* 33:58, 1966.
Perloff, JK, and Roberts, RC. The mitral apparatus: Functional anatomy of mitral regurgitation. *Circulation* 46:227, 1972.
McLaughlin, JS, et al. Mitral valve disease from blunt trauma. *J Thorac Cardiovasc Surg* 48:261, 1974.
Felner, JM, et al. Ventricular septal rupture and mitral regurgitation in a patient with an acute myocardial infarction. *Chest* 75:614, 1979.
Voyce, SJ, et al. Accurate patient diagnosis of acute porcine valve failure. *Arch Intern Med* 147:585, 1987.
Braunwald, E. Mitral regurgitation: Physiological, clinical and surgical considerations. *N Engl J Med* 281:425, 1969.
Mann, JM, and Roberts, WC. Rupture of the left ventricular free wall during acute myocardial infarction: Analysis of 138 necropsy patients and comparison with 50 necropsy patients with acute myocardial infarction without rupture. *Am J Cardiol* 62:847, 1988.
Fox, AC. Infarction and rupture of the heart. *N Engl J Med* 309:551, 1983.

D. Hypertension

24. Principles of Circulation and Regulation of Blood Pressure

Lala Mathers Dunbar

Achieving the hemodynamic effects required to manage the hypertensive emergency is facilitated by understanding the physical laws of fluid dynamics that are applicable to the circulatory system and by appreciating the mechanisms of the three primary control systems that act to change resistance in the system of vessels or change the volume of blood pumped, or both.

Since appropriate intervention, differential diagnosis, and management of *urgent* and *emergent* hypertension are discussed in Chap. 25, this discussion will be limited to an overview of the components of the circulatory system, with an emphasis on the most promising areas for management of hypertension, which are the control mechanisms.

In dealing with the intricacies of the circulation, one should not overlook that, in simple terms, the purpose of the system is that of pickup and delivery—an elaborate, dynamic transportation system composed of vessels that act as conduits for the blood, powered by the pumping action of the heart. The blood receives nutrients, oxygen, and various metabolites and transports these to the tissues where they are utilized, and simultaneously removes by-products of metabolism from the tissues for disposal.

COMPONENTS OF THE HEMODYNAMIC MECHANISM

The Circulatory System

The hemodynamic mechanism is composed of two main divisions: the systemic and the pulmonary circulation, which meet and interchange at the heart (Fig. 24-1). The two main divisions differ markedly in the quantity of blood they contain. The systemic accounts for 84 percent by volume, composed in turn of 64 percent—veins, 15 percent—arteries, and 5 percent—capillaries. The pulmonary vessels by contrast account for 9 percent and the heart for 7 percent of the circulatory volume.

The Vessels

The systemic and pulmonary divisions each have an arterial and venous side, which are connected through low-resistance capillary beds in the tissues that they nourish. Blood entering the major arteries flows through a series of progressively smaller vessels to the thin-walled capillaries, which are permeable to small molecules and thus allow exchange to occur between the plasma and interstitial fluid in the case of systemic circulation, and the plasma and alveoli in the case of pulmonary circulation.

The driving force for fluid to leave the capillaries and move into the interstitial space is the hydrostatic pressure

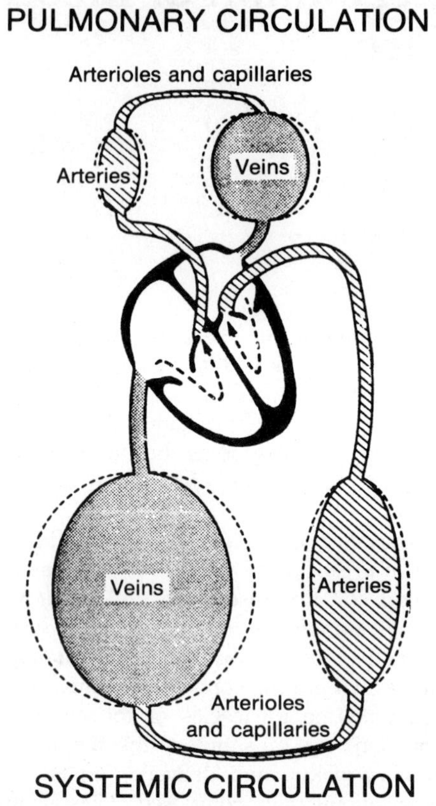

Fig. 24-1. A schematic diagram of the circulatory system reflecting relative volumes and distensibility of the pulmonary and systemic circulation. (From A.C. Guyton. *Textbook of Medical Physiology* [4th ed.]. Philadelphia: Saunders, 1971. P. 204.)

generated by the pumping action of the heart, which, with each beat, transfers a small but approximately equal volume of blood under pressure into the pulmonary artery and aorta from the right and left ventricle, respectively.

Those elements of blood that are too large to leave the vessel create an opposing force, the oncotic pressure, which on the distal end of the capillaries exceeds the hydrostatic pressure and thus attracts fluids back into the vessels to restore plasma volume and be returned to the heart via the venous circulation. Relaxation of the ventricles during diastolic filling creates the low pressure that promotes return of venous blood to the heart. In this capillary exchange, there is usually a small net flow of fluid to the interstitial space, which returns to the central circulation via the lymphatics.

The walls of blood vessels, unlike rigid tubes, have elasticity that allows distention and recoil—that is, volume changes—in response to changes in pressure. The fractional increase in volume per millimeter rise in pressure is the vascular distensibility. The total volume change per unit pressure change is the capacitance, or vascular compliance.

The distensibility of the veins is approximately 8 times that of the corresponding arteries, and, as just noted, the basic volume of the venous system is about 3 times as great. Compliance, which equals distensity times volume, is thus 8 times 3, or 24 times as great on the venous side. This large volume change in response to small pressure changes allows the venous circulation to act as a reservoir for large volumes of blood that can be redistributed to the central circulation when physiologic demand occurs.

On the arterial side, distensibility of the major vessels in response to the pressure rise during systolic ejection serves to buffer the force and thus lower the height of the systolic pressure. Loss of this elasticity in atherosclerotic vascular disease and aging leads to the higher systolic pressures seen in these states.

The vessel walls contain smooth muscle layers that play a major role in resistance through changes in diameter mediated by neural, humoral, and local mechanisms.

Symphathetic fibers enervate virtually all the vessels except the capillaries, precapilllary sphincters, and metarterioles. The arterioles and, to a lesser degree, the venules are particularly richly enervated and thus play a major role in vascular resistance mediated by neural mechanisms. Local stimuli play a greater role in regulation of blood flow in local tissues controlled by the metarterioles and precapillary sphincters.

The Pumps

In addition to the tubular arterial and venous circuity that contain the blood while in transit from the pulmonary to systemic systems and back again, the hemodynamic mechanism relies on two systems of pumps to provide impetus to flow of blood. The major pump is the contraction of the heart, which provides the motive force for the arterial flow by ejecting a bolus of blood into the pulmonary artery and aorta from the right and left ventricles.

The venous pumps consist of the contractions of the musculature through which the veins pass on their way back to the heart, aided by a system of one-way valves that facilitate forward flow in the lower pressure areas. The effect of this system is to increase the gradient between the two ends of the venous circuitry by lowering the volume in the dependent portion of the system. Recent findings indicate the muscles of the abdominal area can dramatically affect this process.

The Fluid

The physical properties of blood are important to the overall hemodynamic mechanism, with viscosity being a primary determinant of flow. The role of the blood stream as a conveyor of vasoactive substances to tissue areas not reached by the neurologic circuitry is also an essential element in control.

Control Mechanisms

Superimposed on the anatomic systems are a variety of physiologic control mechanisms that change the size/diameter of vessels, the capacity of the system, and other critical variables within seconds, minutes, or days.

This complex and exquisitely sensitive control system that regulates the circulatory system is composed of (1) neural mechanisms, specifically the autonomic nervous system; (2) humoral and locally synthesized vasoactive substances, and (3) factors that affect the volume of blood and extracellular fluid. The time frame of response and the long-term effects on blood pressure of the various control centers is variable (Fig. 24-2).

Hypertension arises more often from abnormalities of

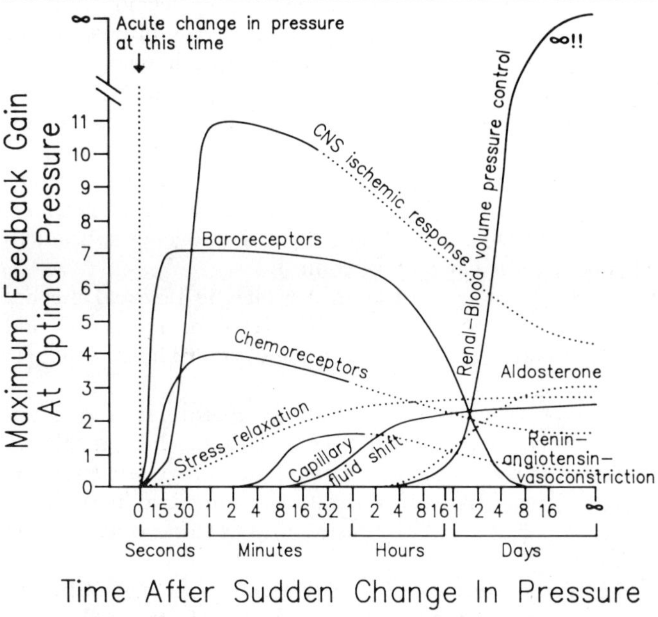

Fig. 24-2. The response of various arterial pressure control systems to an abrupt change in pressure expressed as feedback gain as a function of time. Note that the nervous system responses act most rapidly, with other systems adding in to provide long-term control. (From A.C. Guyton. *Arterial Pressure and Hypertension.* Philadelphia: Saunders, 1980.)

these long-term pressure regulator mechanisms than from the rapid control systems.

THE DYNAMICS OF BLOOD FLOW

Fluid Mechanics

The dynamics of blood flow and blood pressure throughout the vascular system follows certain general principles of fluid mechanics. One of these principles relates to rate of flow. It states that flow of a liquid is directly proportional to the pressure difference (ΔP) between the two ends of a vessel and inversely proportional to the resistance (R) to flow encountered by the liquid.

$$(1)\ \text{Flow (Q)} = \Delta\ \text{pressure} \times \frac{1}{\text{resistance}} \quad \text{or } \Delta P = Q \times R$$

The quantity of blood that will flow through a vessel in a given time may also be expressed as a product of velocity of flow (v) $\times$ cross-sectional area, expressed by the equation

$$(2)\ Q = v\,(\pi r^2)$$

Factors that affect velocity of flow are the pressure gradient, viscosity, and length of the vessel according to the equation:

$$(3)\ \text{Velocity} = \frac{\Delta P \times r^2}{8 \times \text{viscosity} \times \text{length}}$$

Substituting this value for velocity in equations (2) and (1), we have that

$$\text{flow (Q)} = \Delta P \times \left[\frac{\pi r^4}{8 \times \text{viscosity} \times \text{length}}\right] = \Delta P \times \frac{1}{R}$$

Resistance then equals

$$\frac{8 \times \text{viscosity} \times \text{length}}{\pi r^4}$$

From this it is important to note that flow is directly proportional and resistance indirectly proportional to the fourth power of the radius. Thus, small changes in vessel diameter have a major effect on resistance, blood flow, and pressure.

There is a progressive increase in cross-sectional area from the aorta (2.5 cm^2) to the capillaries (2,500 cm^2). Since velocity of flow is inversly proportional to cross-sectional area, as the blood travels from the major arteries to the capillaries there is a decrease in velocity, which allows time for exchange to occur across the capillary walls. As noted, the overall cross-sectional area of the veins is greater than that of the arteries, such that the volume of the venous circulation is approximately 3 times that of the arterial circulation.

Factors Affecting Resistance

Two important physical characteristics of blood vessels that affect their radius and thus resistance are (1) the distensibility of the vessel walls, and (2) the presence of smooth muscle in the vessel walls, which can change the vessel diameter in response to various physiologic stimuli.

Since vascular length, blood volume, and viscosity do not change abruptly in normal circumstances, we are left to conclude that changes in vessel diameter are responsible for the abrupt variations in resistance that lead to changes in pressure.

An important fact to note is that the calculated peripheral resistance includes changes in flow characteristics that result from changes in shape of the red cells in the small vessels so that the effective viscosity is diminished by half during the transition from larger vessels to capillaries. Most resistance in the circulatory system, however, still occurs as the result of smooth muscle tone in the small vessels, especially the arterioles.

Blood Pressure

The methods of calculating blood pressure integrate the formulas associated with calculating pressure in stable fluid dynamics with additional variables associated with the cardiac cycle. A summary of these factors follows.

Blood pressure, as the name implies, is the force exerted by the blood against any unit area of the vessel wall at the moment measured. This is conventionally expressed in millimeters of mercury (mm Hg). The numerical value of the systemic arterial blood pressure is determined by the extent of filling—that is, the fullness of the arterial side of the systemic vessels and the intrinsic resistance of these vessels to this volume of blood. This value is constantly changing owing to the pulsatile nature of filling and runoff related to a cardiac cycle.

The peak blood pressure occurs during systole when a bolus of blood is ejected into the aorta from the left ventricle.

The low point of pressure in the major arteries, the "diastolic pressure," is the result of flow of blood out of the larger arteries into lower pressure areas of the circulation while the heart is being refilled. Systemic arterial pressure thus undulates between systolic and diastolic values.

The mean arterial pressure is the integrated average pressure in the arteries during the cardiac cycle, which can be estimated by the following equation:

$$\text{MAP} = \text{diastolic pressure} + \tfrac{1}{3}\,(\text{systolic} - \text{diastolic pressure})$$

The mean arterial pressure is usually lowest in infancy, with an average value of about 70 mm Hg, rising to an average value of 110 mm Hg in healthy older persons. This pressure reaches even higher values in persons with hypertension and atherosclerosis.

Determinants of Blood Pressure

The total blood flow per unit time in the systemic circulation is the cardiac output. The pressure difference across the systemic circulation that promotes flow is the difference between the mean arterial pressure (MAP) on the upper end and the right atrial pressure (RAP) on the lower end—the latter being approximately zero. Substituting these values in equation, we have

$$\Delta P = \text{MAP} - 0 = \text{cardiac output} \times \text{resistance}$$

Pressure is thus a reflection of the cardiac output and peripheral resistance and will rise in response to an increase in output or any component that leads to a rise in resistance.

Blood pressure was defined earlier as the extent of filling of a vesssel and the intrinsic resistance to that filling. It seems logical therefore to include the residual volume of blood at end-diastole as another major determinant of pressure, although in the mathematic form, it is incorporated in the calculated resistance.

The most dramatic changes in peripheral resistance are effected by changes in the diameter of the vessels that may result from occlusive processes occurring over a period of months or years such as atherosclerotic vascular disease or through neural or hormonal signals acting within seconds. Modulating these changes in diameter has major importance in the selection of treatment for the emergent or urgent hypertensive patient.

THE PHYSIOLOGY OF CONTROL

The Major Control Mechanisms

The control mechanisms that regulate the hemodynamic mechanism are divided into three major systems.

1. The rapidly acting nervous system reflexes, which include the baroreceptors—sensitive to pressure changes; chemoreceptors—sensitive to hypoxia, hypercarbia, and acidosis; and the central nervous system (CNS) response, which causes intense sympathetic vasconstriction and increased vascular resistance in response to cerebral ischemia.
2. The hormonal and other humoral mechanisms for control of arterial pressure also provide rapid and moderately rapid responses. They are primarily adrenal release of epinephrine and norepinephrine, release of argenine vasopressin (AVP) from the pituitary and activation of the renin-angiotensin-aldosterone axis, with synthesis of angiotensin II as the early effect. Locally synthesized vasoactive substances also fall in this category of control.
3. The third area of control relates to physical mechanisms such as shifts of fluid between the interstitial and intravascular compartments in the capillary beds.

Changes in capacitance through stress-relaxation is another process of physical origin. This mechanism allows variation in size of blood vessels in the storage areas such as spleen, liver, veins, and lungs to accommodate increases of up to 30 percent and decreases of up to 15 percent in blood volume.

The responsiveness of a given tissue is controlled by the presence of substance-specific receptors in the cell membranes of that tissue. In the case of vascular smooth muscle enervated by adrenergic fibers, norepinephrine released by the nerve endings interacts with postsynaptic receptors of the cell to cause vasoconstriction. In the vessels of skeletal muscles, receptors are present that mediate an opposite effect—vasodilation to increase blood supply to that tissue in response to sympathetic stimulation. In cardiac muscle, receptors for adrenergic stimuli cause an increase in rate and contractility, whereas vagally mediated stimulation with release of acetylcholine (parasympathetic stimulation) slows heart rate. Some receptors are localized to nerve endings, whereas others are accessible to circulating or locally synthesized vasoactive substances.

As proposed by Page, hypertension is a disease of regulation that occurs when vascular resistance is not controlled effectively; therefore, a more extensive look at the specifics of regulation is necessary.

Specific Effects of Regulatory Systems

The Sympathetic Nervous System

The sympathetic nervous system activity establishes the basal tone of vascular smooth muscle and is a major effector of changes. A principal mechanism for modulation of sympathetic activity is through stimulation of the baroreceptors present in the internal carotid artery, carotid sinus, and aortic arch. The baroreceptors respond to pressure changes through stretch of the splayed sensory nerve endings, which alter the rate of impulse formation in response to changes in pressure. Signals are transmitted to the tractus solitarius of the medulla where they are relayed to the vasoconstrictor and vagal centers. A rising pressure results in increased vagal and decreased sympathetic outflow to decrease heart rate and contractility and relax vascular smooth muscle.

A decrease in arterial pressure conversely causes an increase in sympathetic stimulation. The effects of this are (1) an increase in rate and contractility in the heart, thereby to increase cardiac output; (2) vasoconstriction of the arterial resistance vessels, to increase afterload; (3) venous constriction, which effects an increase in blood pressure by translocation of blood from the venous storage vessels to the central circulation, thereby increasing preload; (4) stimulation of renin release to produce angiotension II—a powerful vasoconstrictor; and (5) stimulation of the posterior pituitary to release AVP—also a potent vasconstrictor.

The Chemoreceptor Response

The chemoreceptors are small bodies located at the bifurcation of the common carotids and adjacent to the aorta that are sensitive to decreased O_2 and increased CO_2 and H^+, which results from decreased perfusion of these bodies. These receptors are activated by severe decreases in blood pressure but act through mechanisms similar to those of the baroreceptors response.

The CNS Ischemic Response

The CNS ischemic response is a powerful vasoconstrictor response activated when blood flow to the vasomotor centers of the lower brain stem is diminished to a point of cerebral ischemia. It acts to rapidly increase sympathetic tone through direct stimulation of nerves. Its function is one of protection of blood flow to the CNS rather than as a modulator of normal pressures.

Renin-Angiotensin-Aldosterone System

Diminished blood pressure or renal perfusion, or both, activate the release of renin by the juxtaglomerular cells of the kidney.

Renin has an enzymatic role in conversion of circulating angiotensinogen to angiotensin I, which is further activated by a converting enzyme in the lungs to angiotensin II. This, in addition to being a powerful vasconstrictor with immediate effects on resistance and blood pressure, also stimulates release of aldosterone by the adrenal medulla.

Renin release is known to be regulated by a variety of mechanisms, including the beta-adrenergic system through direct effects or via renal nerve pathways and by prostaglandins, prostacyclin being a likely candidate in mediating this response.

The major effects of aldosterone are to cause Na^+ retention, K^+ excretion, and an associated retention of water. The overall long-term effect is to increase blood volume—ultimately increasing resistance and pressure.

Arginine Vasopressin

The release of AVP (also known as antidiuretic hormone) from the posterior pituitary also has both long- and short-term effects on blood pressure. As noted previously AVP is a powerful vasoconstrictor.

AVP is synthesized in supraoptic and paraventricular nuclei of the hypothalamus and stored in vesicles of the posterior pituitary from whence it is released in response to both osmotic and nonosmotic stimuli. A rise in serum osmolality triggers release to increase water retention by the kidney and thereby maintain fluid volume with its associated long-term effect on blood pressure. AVP also stimulates release of aldosterone, which acts synergistically to increase fluid volume through sodium retention. The release of AVP for its powerful vasoconstrictor action is important in the rapid response to a decreasing pressure. This nonosmotic release is triggered by sympathetic baroreceptor activity.

Atrial Natriuretic Factor

It has been recognized for some time that overfilling of the circulation stimulates diuresis. The mechanism of this effect has recently been elucidated through the identification of atrial natriuretic factor (ANF), a potent endogenous diuretic-like hormone. ANF has been identified in secretory granules that are particularly abundant in the muscle fibers of the atria of the heart, although they are also present in the ventricular muscle and in conduction tissue. The most important stimulant to release of ANF appears to be stretch of the cardiac muscle fibers. Thus, it is a sensitive mediator of volume status. Knowledge to date suggests that ANF acts as an inhibitor of the renin-angiotensin-aldosterone axis and an inhibitor of release of AVP.

Local Mechanisms of Control

The least understood mechanisms of blood pressure control are those that occur locally. Metabolites of arachidonic acid, collectively known as the prostanoids or eicosanoids, include several powerful vasoactive substances. Among these, thromboxane A_2 is a vasoconstrictor of smooth muscle, including arteries and bronchi as well as a platelet aggregant. Prostacyclin has an almost opposing effect in that it inhibits platelet aggregation, is a vasodilator, and stimulates renin release. Prostaglandin D_2, a major product of mast cells, is a vasodilator and bronchoconstrictor. Prostaglandin E_2 is a vasodilator that induces, in the kidney, diuresis and natriuresis. Although the overall importance in systemic blood pressure control is not clear, the vasodilator properties of PGE_2, and PGD_2, and prostacyclin and the vasoconstrictor properties of PGF and thromboxane A_2 undoubtedly play a role in perfusion of vascular beds.

Local control of vascular tone has also been shown to be mediated by substances synthesized by the vascular endothelium that diffuse to underlying smooth muscle cells. Chemical characterization of these substances is, to date, not well defined. Endothelium-derived relaxing factor (EDRF) may act through formation of nitrous oxide, although other potent vasodilators (e.g., prostacylin, leukotriene LTD_4, adenosine, ammonia) may also play a role in locally mediated vasodilation.

Endothelium-derived vasoconstrictor substances also exist and may include leukotriene LTC_4, thromboxane A_2, superoxide anions, and peptide endothelin. Studies to further characterize these substances and their mechanism of action are the subject of much current investigation.

SUMMARY

In summary, blood, like other fluids, is subject to the laws of fluid mechanics, in which pressure is a function of flow and resistance. The system in which the blood flows in humans is not, however, a rigid one, but rather is subject to constant change through the action of the various control mechanisms that respond to meet the physiologic needs. Through modulation of heart rate, stroke volume, and peripheral resistance, the blood pressure is normally maintained within normal limits while metabolic needs are met.

The assessment of the hypertensive patient is therefore a

search for malfunction in one or more of these regulatory systems.

The etiology of a large segment of hypertension, the so-called essential hypertensive patient, is still poorly defined. Evidence suggests that altered resistance is the likely unifying factor, but it is apparent that multifactorial reasons, including hereditary, hormonal, dietary, ethnic, and social factors, may each play a role. As an understanding of the local control mechanisms increases, so perhaps will our understanding of essential hypertension.

SELECTED READING

Guyton, AC. *Textbook of Medical Physiology* (7th ed.). Philadelphia: Saunders, 1986. Pp. 206–286, 410–436.

Schrier, RW. *Renal and Electrolyte Disorders* (3rd ed.). Boston: Little, Brown, 1986. Pp. 361–422.

Bailey, JM (ed.), *Prostaglandins, Leukotrienes and Lipoxins—Biochemistry, Mechanism of Action and Clinical Applications.* New York: Plenum, 1985.

Page, IH. The Mosaic Theory of Hypertension. In KD Bock and PT Cottier (eds.), *Essential Hypertension.* New York: Springer, 1960. P. 1.

Dustan, HP. Pathophysiology of Hypertension. In J Willis Hurst (ed.), *The Heart.* New York: McGraw-Hill, 1986. Pp. 1038–1047.

Feinmark, SJ. Cooperative synthesis of leukotrienes by leukocytes and vascular cells. *Ann NY Acad Sci* 524:122, 1988.

Morone, G, et al. Cardiovascular and metabolic effects of peptide leukotrienes in man. *Ann NY Acad Sci* 524:321, 1988.

Schrier, RW. Pathogenesis of sodium and water retention in high output and low output, cardiac failure, nephrotic syndrome, cirrhosis and pregnancy. *N Engl J Med* 319:1065–1072, 1127–1134, 1988.

Oates, JA, et al. Clinical implications of prostaglandin and thromboxane A_2 formation. *N Engl J Med* 319:689–698, 761–767, 1988.

Weinberger, MH. Sodium chloride and blood pressure. *N Engl J Med* 317:1086, 1987.

Laragh, JH. Atrial natriuretic hormone, the renin-aldosterone axis and blood pressure-electrolyte homeostasis. *N Engl J Med* 313: 1330, 1985.

Blaine, EH. Role of atriopeptin in blood pressure regulation. *Am J Med Sci* 295:293, 1988.

Rosenblatt, M, and Jacobs, JW. Atrial natriuretic factor. *Clin North Am* 16:1, 1987.

Vanhoutte, PM. The endothelium—modulator of vascular smooth-muscle tone. *N Engl J Med* 319:512, 1988.

25. Hypertension

Robert C. Goldszer
Harold S. Solomon
Norman K. Hollenberg

Hypertension, which ranges from a slight to an extreme elevation of blood pressure, is so common that an estimated 30 percent of visits to practitioners of adult medicine are for its treatment. Hypertensive emergencies, however, are rare; they occur in fewer than 1 percent of patients with high blood pressure. Although all hypertensive conditions require or benefit from treatment, two groups—emergent and urgent—must be distinguished because they are more effectively and more safely treated by different methods.

Truly emergent episodes of high blood pressure must be treated within minutes to prevent severe hemorrhagic or neurologic complications. Failure to act can result in rapid clinical deterioration and even death. Less immediately life threatening, but still serious, are urgent conditions for which treatment may be delayed without undue risk for a few hours or days. The distinction between these two classes of hypertension is important because rapidly acting antihypertensive drugs incur risk that must be weighed against potential benefit to the patient. In general, an emergent condition improves dramatically as the patient's blood pressure is reduced. An urgent condition, on the other hand, requires prompt attention, but its course is less threatening and somewhat less affected by a rapid lowering of blood pressure with parenteral medications. Tables 25-1 and 25-2 list emergent and urgent manifestations of hypertension.

The absolute level of blood pressure is only one indication of a hypertensive emergency and must always be interpreted in conjunction with other physical signs of accelerated disease and with the relevant history. Evidence of encephalopathy, signs and symptoms of cardiovascular complications, eclampsia, or the simultaneous ingestion of tyramine and monoamine oxidase (MAO) inhibitors coupled with an extreme elevation of blood pressure signal the need for immediate treatment.

Urgent conditions include those arising as hypertension progresses and damages small arteries and arterioles. Hemorrhages and infarctions in the eyes, kidneys, heart, or nervous system necessitate lowering the patient's blood pressure. Hospitalization with bed rest, observation, and oral rather than parenteral therapy are usually indicated. Postoperative patients who develop severe hypertension with bleeding and new patients, even if asymptomatic, whose diastolic blood pressure is above 130 mm Hg are also in need of urgent but not instant treatment.

INITIAL ASSESSMENT

Time is of the essence in hypertensive emergencies. Hence, eliciting a complete medical history should be waived in favor of obtaining a brief relevant history, including informa-

Table 25-1. Hypertensive emergencies

Malignant hypertension with or without encephalopathy
Acute complications of accelerated hypertension
Pulmonary edema
Cerebrovascular accident with hemorrhage or infarction
Aortic dissection
Hypertension with special causes
Eclampsia
Tyramine toxicity
Pheochromocytoma

Table 25-2. Urgent conditions associated with hypertension

Evidence of hemorrhage and exudates in eyegrounds
Myocardial infarction or severe angina
Occlusive stroke or transient ischemic attack
Renal failure or significant renal impairment
Burns, acute glomerulonephritis, or preeclampsia
Postoperative bleeding
New cardiovascular or neurologic symptoms in a previously hypertensive patient
Newly developed hypertension (diastolic blood pressure greater than 130 mm Hg)

tion about the current illness, medications the patient is taking, and prior adverse drug reactions. The goal is to identify a possible secondary cause of the hypertension. Except in rare cases, the patient's blood pressure should be lowered rapidly, but therapy depends to a large extent on the underlying condition. Table 25-3 outlines a suggested course of action.

An intravenous catheter should be inserted, and an electrocardiogram (ECG) should be obtained while the history is being taken and the patient is being examined. Blood should be drawn immediately for laboratory studies—a complete blood count (CBC) and measurement of blood urea nitrogen (BUN) and serum creatinine, electrolytes, and glucose. A urine specimen should also be sent to the laboratory for analysis. Therapy should not, however, be deferred until the results of any of these tests are known. Likewise, a posteroanterior x-ray film of the chest should be made but not at the expense of delaying therapy.

The patient's mental status and evidence of any neurologic changes are of paramount importance. Unfortunately, distinguishing immediately among hemorrhagic stroke, occlusive stroke, transient cerebral ischemia, eclampsia, and hypertensive encephalopathy is not always possible; yet therapy depends to some extent on the differential diagnosis. Lowering blood pressure too rapidly, for example, may exacerbate the symptoms of an occlusive stroke or a transient ischemic attack. A cardiovascular catastrophe is always a possible cause of severe hypertension if the patient complains of chest or back pain. Myocardial infarction or ischemia and dissecting aneurysm are the most important diagnoses to consider in the short term. Dissecting aneurysms, which are discussed in Chaps. 17 and 140, are exceedingly variable in their manner of presentation.

Therapy must often be determined from data gathered rapidly, and sometimes incompletely, at the bedside. Although incomplete, such information is sufficient to guide the initial therapy for most patients, and a more extensive evaluation can usually be safely postponed until a patient's condition has been stabilized. Unless a cause of the hypertensive emergency (e.g., eclampsia or ingestion of both tyramine and MAO inhibitors) is uncovered, however, a thorough evaluation of the patient is mandatory so that a secondary cause of hypertension can be confirmed, if present.

Table 25-3. Sequence of clinical events in hypertensive emergencies

Brief history emphasizing cardiovascular and neurologic systems and prior medications
Physical examination
Access to circulation
Electrocardiogram (ECG)
Determination of baseline CBC, BUN, creatinine, electrolytes, glucose levels; urinalysis
Parenteral therapy instituted with appropriate agent based on initial clinical evaluation
Chest film (posteroanterior, not portable anteroposterior)
Admission to intensive or coronary care unit
Reassessment and modification of therapy based on initial laboratory studies and clinical response; longer-acting agents or oral therapy begun
Further diagnostic evaluation considered

TREATMENT

General Considerations

Parenteral therapy should begin as soon as the physician has enough data to select an antihypertensive agent. The choice of medication depends on several factors, including the clinical setting in which the hypertension presents, the persistence and hemodynamic effects of the drugs available, and the availability of reliable monitoring and an experienced nursing staff. In general, a patient for whom the diagnosis cannot be established at bedside is more safely treated with a drug whose effects dissipate rapidly. If the agent worsens the patient's condition, the therapeutic strategy can then be rapidly altered. Agents such as reserpine and methyldopa, which may alter the level of consciousness, should be avoided. Patients hospitalized in facilities where they cannot be monitored minute by minute should be treated with agents such as diazoxide, intravenous methyldopa, or hydralazine, whose effects are more prolonged and do not require the constant attention that the more rapidly acting agents (nitroprusside, trimethaphan) do. Although parenteral therapy is mandatory for initial treatment of hypertensive emergencies, oral agents should be substituted as soon as possible.

Parenteral antihypertensives, listed in Table 25-4, are basically of two types: vasodilators and agents that act by interrupting the sympathetic nervous system at some level. All of them reduce either cardiac output or peripheral vascular resistance; some decrease both. These distinctions, which are discussed later in this chapter, are important. The dilators reduce peripheral resistance by dilating peripheral

Table 25-4. Hemodynamic effects of parenteral antihypertensives

Agent	Mechanism of action	Cardiac output	Total peripheral resistance	Venous return
Vasodilators				
Nitroprusside	Arteriolar and venous dilation	Decrease or unchanged	Decrease	Decrease
Diazoxide	Arteriolar dilation	Increase	Decrease	Increase
Hydralazine	Arteriolar dilation	Increase	Decrease	Increase
Enalapril	Arteriolar dilation	Increase	Decrease	Increase or unchanged
Nitroglycerine	Arteriolar dilation	Increase	Decrease	Increase or unchanged
Adrenergic inhibitors				
Trimethaphan	Autonomic blockade and arteriolar dilation	Decrease	Decrease	Decrease
Methyldopa	? Central depression ? False transmitter Direct Vasodilation	Decrease or unchanged	Decrease	Decrease
Phentolamine	Alpha inhibition	Increase	Decrease	Increase
Propranolol	Beta blockade	Decrease	Increase	Decrease
Labetalol	Alpha and beta blockade	Decrease	Decrease	Decrease

Table 25-5. Parenteral antihypertensives

Agent	Dose	Onset	Duration
Vasodilators			
Nitroprusside	0.5–10.0 μg/kg/min	<1 min	Minutes
Diazoxide	50–300 mg	1–2 min	4–18 hr
Nitroglycerine	5–100 μg/min	2–5 min	Minutes
Hydralazine	5–20 mg IV	10 min	2–6 hr
Enalapril	1.25 mg	10 min	2–4 hr
Adrenergic inhibitors			
Labetalol	20–80 mg	5–10 min	4–8 hr
Phentolamine	5–15 mg	1–2 min	1–2 hr
Trimethaphan	1–4 mg/min	1–5 min	Minutes
Methyldopa	250–500 mg	30–60 min	4–8 hr
Reserpine	0.5–5.0 mg IM	2–3 hr	4–8 hr

arterioles; they increase heart rate as well. Because nitroprusside acts both as a vasodilator and as a venodilator, it also reduces venous return; cardiac output therefore usually decreases. Diazoxide, hydralazine, and enalapril, which do not reduce venous return, cause increases in cardiac output. Of the agents acting on the sympathetic nervous system, trimethaphan, methyldopa, and labetalol decrease both peripheral resistance and cardiac output; phentolamine reduces peripheral resistance, and propranolol reduces cardiac output.

The most rapidly acting agents with broad application are nitroprusside, trimethaphan, diazoxide and labetalol. Hydralazine's onset of action is intermediate. Table 25-5 summarizes the route of administration, the usual adult dosage, and the approximate onset and duration of action of the parenteral medications.

Specific Medications

Vasodilators

SODIUM NITROPRUSSIDE. Sodium nitroprusside (Nipride), known as a parenteral antihypertensive agent since 1929, has gained widespread use since it became commercially available. Because it is consistently effective and because it combines several useful actions, the drug's popularity is warranted. Nitroprusside is particularly efficacious for treating hypertension complicated by left ventricular failure. By increasing venous capacitance, it permits blood to pool in the extremities; as a result, vascular resistance, cardiac output, and therefore blood pressure decrease. Nitroprusside is also effective for treating hypertensive encephalopathy or stroke because it does not affect the sensorium. It has an immediate onset of action and its effect dissipates very rapidly when the infusion is discontinued. As advantageous as these characteristics are, they are also responsible for the drug's major drawback—the necessity for constant supervision.

Prolonged administration of nitroprusside may result in thiocyanate toxicity, which is manifested by mental confusion and psychosis. In one study, however, continuous use for a mean period of 6 days produced no marked toxic reactions. Nevertheless, if nitroprusside is administered for longer than 72 hours, the patient's serum thiocyanate level should be measured every other day and the dosage reduced if the level exceeds 12 ml/dl. Other side effects—nausea, vomiting, apprehension, sweating, and muscle twitching—may occur acutely but can usually be reversed quite readily by reducing the infusion rate.

Nitroprusside is available in vials containing 50 mg of powder. Sterile 5% dextrose in water (D5W; 3 ml) should be instilled into the vial, then diluted in 500 ml of D5W to prepare a solution of 100 mg/ml. The usual adult dose averages 2 ml/minute (200 μg/min). The dosage should be adjusted as necessary to achieve the desired reduction of blood pressure. Both the bottle containing the solution and the intravenous tubing should be wrapped in aluminum foil to prevent light from altering the nitroprusside; once prepared, the solution, to which no other drugs should be added, should not be kept or used for longer than 4 hours.

DIAZOXIDE. Diazoxide (Hyperstat), a thiazide derivative that lowers blood pressure very rapidly, is effective for 4 to 12 hours. It acts directly by dilating resistance vessels, but because it does not affect capacitance vessels, its primary action does not interfere with reflex cardiac stimulation. Cardiac output and heart rate therefore increase as blood pressure decreases; because blood pressure is lowered, cardiac work and myocardial oxygen consumption decrease, despite increased cardiac output.

Relatively safe and effective, diazoxide is normally given for uncomplicated malignant hypertension, and it is also widely used to treat eclampsia. (However, it may produce fetal hyperglycemia.) The reflex increase in cardiac output, an effect of both diazoxide and hydralazine, contraindicates administering these drugs to patients with dissecting thoracic aneurysms; altered shear forces at the site of dissection can cause the aneurysm to extend even though blood pressure has been lowered.

Diazoxide is available in ampules containing 300 mg in a 20-ml solution. The dose can be repeated as often as necessary, usually 3 to 10 hours later. The ideal dose is 150 mg by intravenous bolus. If there is no response in 2 to 3 minutes, a second 150-mg bolus is given. If no response occurs after the second dose, switch to another antihypertensive agent.

NITROGLYCERINE. Nitroglycerine acts to dilate primarily the arteriolar beds. It is effective in the treatment of patients with coronary artery disease and hypertension and should be reserved for these patients. Vasodilation may result in increased cardiac output and reflex tachycardia. The usual dose is 5 to 100 μg/minute as a continuous intravenous infusion.

HYDRALAZINE. Hydralazine (Apresoline) has hemodynamic effects much like those of diazoxide; it dilates peripheral arterioles and increases cardiac output and heart rate. It can, however, precipitate or exacerbate angina pectoris in patients who present with coronary insufficiency unless it is administered with a drug (beta blocker) that interrupts the reflex cardiac stimulation.

Hydralazine has become popular for treating chronic congestive heart failure (CHF) because it reduces peripheral resistance, which is elevated in CHF, and thus allows cardiac output to increase. When administered to hypertensive patients, hydralazine has an effect that is immediate, peaks in 30 to 60 minutes, and persists for several hours.

Headache and tachycardia are common adverse reactions; coronary insufficiency is less frequent. Hydralazine, for the same reason as diazoxide, should not be given to a patient with a dissecting aneurysm.

Hydralazine is supplied in ampules of 20 mg in a 1-ml solution. An initial dose of 5 mg, given intramuscularly or intravenously, can be followed with additional doses of 5 to 20 mg as needed at 1- to 4-hour intervals.

ENALAPRIL. The angiotensin-converting enzyme inhibitor enalapril has recently been approved for intravenous use. This medication may be useful in patients with renal artery stenosis and renal insufficiency (high renin hypertensives). Because it has only recently been approved, there is minimal clinical experience. The recommended dose is 1.25 mg IV. One dose is given, and the patient is observed for 1 hour. If the blood pressure does not decrease, another 1.25 mg may be given. Patients should be started on oral therapy at the same time, if possible. If the blood pressure does not decrease after two doses, a different agent should be started. Possible side effects include headache, cough, and impaired renal function.

Sympathetic Blockers

TRIMETHAPHAN. A ganglionic blocker, trimethaphan (Arfonad) interrupts both sympathetic and parasympathetic functioning and also has a direct vasodilator action that is unrelated to ganglionic blockade. The drug, which dilates both capacitance and resistance vessels, reduces cardiac output. Like nitroprusside, it acts rapidly, its effects dissipate within a minute, and its administration requires constant supervision. Because it dilates capacitance vessels, trimethaphan has an orthostatic effect; elevating the head of a patient's bed therefore enhances the agent's antihypertensive effect. If trimethaphan is chosen as the initial therapeutic agent, longer-acting drugs should also be given as part of the early treatment regimen because tachyphylaxis to trimethaphan occurs after it has been used for 24 hours.

Because trimethaphan reduces cardiac output and consequently shear forces in the aorta, it is an agent of choice for the initial treatment of hypertension associated with dissecting aneurysms of the thoracic aorta. It is also useful for treating most other forms of hypertensive emergency; however, this drug may cause ileus, urinary retention, and blurred vision because of its parasympatholytic effect.

Trimethaphan is marketed in vials containing 500 mg in a 10-ml solution. One ampule added to 500 ml of D5W yields a concentration of 1 mg/ml. An intravenous infusion of 3 to 4 mg/minute (50–60 drops/min) should be adjusted to achieve the desired blood pressure response.

LABETALOL. Labetalol hydrochloride is a combined alpha- and beta-blocking agent. Its pharmacology is complex, with beta-adrenergic blockade being the major effect, with associated significant $alpha_1$-receptor blockade in the peripheral vasculature. After its administration, there is a decrease in peripheral resistance without a significant reduction in heart rate or cardiac output. Labetalol is effective in the upright or supine position. Intravenous labetalol has been used in patients with severe hypertension associated with coronary ischemia, renal insufficiency, acute dissection of the aorta, preclampsia, and hypertension in the setting of clonidine withdrawal.

Toxicities include those of other beta-blocking agents; thus, labetalol should not be used in patients with bronchospasm, bradycardia, or severe CHF. As with other intravenous antihypertensive agents, orthostatic hypotension may occur.

Patients receiving labetalol intravenously should be kept in the supine position to prevent orthostatic hypotension. It is given in an initial dosage of 20 mg by slow IV injection. Additional dosages are given at 10-minute intervals (20–80 mg) to maintain blood pressure control or until a total of 300 mg total dosage. Oral therapy can be initiated to maintain blood pressure.

METHYLDOPA. Methyldopa (Aldomet) has proved to have an antihypertensive effect that is still poorly understood. The formation peripherally of α-methylnorepinephrine from α-methyldopa led to the belief that the effect was due to the formation of a "false neurochemical transmitter." But methyldopa also has a prominent central effect, and it remains unclear whether the drug's antihypertensive property results from central inhibition of sympathetic activity, from action as a peripheral false transmitter, or even from direct vasodilation. Changes in blood pressure vary greatly from patient to patient; some patients respond dramatically within 2 hours, whereas others do not respond at all. Methyldopa is now often chosen as an agent with moderate rate of onset and duration of action.

Methyldopa is particularly appropriate for patients with renal insufficiency. Its primary metabolic product, α-methylnorepinephrine, which normally would be cleared by the kidney, is itself an effective antihypertensive. The drug thus works well if renal clearance is diminished and seemingly has little adverse effect on renal functioning.

Methyldopa does cause somnolence; therefore, it is relatively undesirable for treating patients with neurologic symptoms.

Methyldopa comes in 5-ml vials containing 250 mg. The dose should be added to 100 ml of D5W and administered in an intravenous drip over a 30-minute period. The usual dose for adults is 250 mg, but up to 3 gm may be administered at one time if necessary to reduce blood pressure to the desired level. If there is no effect on blood pressure 2 hours after an initial 250-mg dose, 500 to 750 mg should be given. The maintenance dose can be repeated every 6 hours.

PHENTOLAMINE. Phentolamine (Regitine), a competitive antagonist of norepinephrine, has very limited usefulness; in fact, it is effective only if a patient has pheochromocytoma or hypertension induced by the simultaneous ingestion of tyramine and MAO inhibitors. Phentolamine should be given in the operating room if pheochromocytoma is unexpectedly found during surgery and is associated with acute severe hypertension.

Phentolamine is supplied in vials containing 5 mg of powder, and each is accompanied with an ampule of 1 ml of sterile water. The 5 mg of the drug should be diluted in the 1 ml of sterile water to prepare a 5 mg/ml solution, which should be administered intravenously as a bolus. A dose of 5 mg usually effectively reduces blood pressure in 5 to 10 minutes, but up to 15 mg (3 ml) may be given. The dose may be repeated as often as necessary.

PROPRANOLOL. Propranolol (Inderal) is a competitive, beta-adrenergic inhibitor that has little antihypertensive effect when given intravenously. Although intravenous propranolol decreases cardiac output, the effect is offset by a reflex increase in peripheral vascular resistance, which is mediated by alpha-adrenergic responses. Consequently, arterial pressure decreases only slightly.

Propranolol is effective, however, for patients with dissecting thoracic aneurysm, which requires that myocardial contractility be decreased. The drug also partially interrupts the reflex tachycardia produced by diazoxide, hydralazine, and nitroprusside. A patient with pheochromocytoma who is given an alpha blocker (phentolamine, dibenzyline) may also require propranolol to block the beta-adrenergic effects of the catecholamine excess, especially if an arrhythmia occurs. Unless such a patient is first given adequate doses of alpha blockers, propranolol, because of its beta blockade, causes a dramatic increase in alpha activity and an increase in blood pressure.

Propranolol is supplied in 1-ml ampules containing 1 mg. The usual dose is 1 mg administered at a rate of 1 mg every 1 to 5 minutes by slow intravenous infusion. Careful monitoring of heart rate and blood pressure is mandatory. The dosage interval is determined by the heart rate response and can be as often as every 5 minutes. The total dosage should not exceed 0.1 mg/kg in a 4-hour period.

RESERPINE. Reserpine (Serpasil) depletes catecholamines in the central nervous system and in peripheral areas. Its effect begins 1 to 3 hours after administration, and hypotension occasionally complicates its use. Because the usual large parenteral doses commonly cause somnolence, reserpine should not be used to treat patients presenting with neurologic symptoms. Since diazoxide, nitroprusside, and methyldopa have become available, reserpine is used much less frequently than it was in the past.

Reserpine is supplied in ampules containing 5 mg in a 2-ml ampule. A test dose of 0.5 mg (0.2 ml) intramuscularly should be given intially and followed 30 minutes later with 5 mg (2 ml) intramuscularly if the test dose is effective and tolerated. If the 5-mg dose produces no response within a few hours, larger doses will not be particularly effective; the drug should therefore be discontinued.

Diuretics

Much has been written about the benefits of intravenously administering potent diuretics, such as furosemide or ethacrynic acid, to patients being treated with diazoxide. But all antihypertensive drugs, not just diazoxide, may cause sodium retention as a consequence of blood pressure reduction, a fact that the physician must keep in mind during any hypertensive emergency. Intravenous diuretics need not, however, be given the instant that the administration of antihypertensive drugs is begun; the physician can await the BUN and creatinine determination and the results of the urinalysis to select a diuretic and dosage.

Management of Excessive Hypotensive Effect

Occasionally, a patient reacts to antihypertensive therapy with too great a reduction in blood pressure. If rapidly acting agents (trimethaphan, nitroprusside) have been used, the hypotension does not require any therapy other than discontinuing the antihypertensive agent. But because the effects of longer-acting drugs cannot be stopped quickly, plasma expanders may be necessary; indeed, they may be lifesaving.

The most common reason for hypotension is a slight,

Table 25-6. Selection of parenteral antihypertensive agents

	Setting							
Agent	Acute pulmonary edema	Enceph-alopathy	Dissecting aneurysm; other chest pain	Cerebral vascular accident: thrombosis and hemorrhage	Malignant hypertension, including renal causes	Pheochro-mocytoma	MAO inhibitors and tryamine	Toxemia or eclampsia
Vasodilators								
Nitroprusside	1	2	3	1	1	2	2	1
Diazoxide	2	1	X	2	2	2	2	2
Hydralazine	3	3	X	2	3	3	3	2
Enalapril	2	2	X	2	2	2	2	X
Agents acting on sympa-thetic nervous system								
Trimethaphan	2	2	1	1	1	2	2	X
Labetalol	3	2	2	2	2	2	2	1
Methyldopa	3	X	2	3	3	3	3	3
Phentolamine	0	0	0	0	0	1	1	0
Propranolol	0	0	2	0	0	2	2	0

Key: X = usually contraindicated; 0 = not useful; 1 = usual first choice in acute setting; 2 = frequently useful in acute setting; 3 = occasionally useful in acute setting, frequently useful for long-term therapy.

preexisting volume deficit that becomes apparent when an agent that inhibits the sympathetic activity is administered. If hypotension persists once adequate volume has been restored, pressors may be required. Norepinephrine (Levophed) rather than sympathomimetics (ephedrine, mephentermine, amphetamine derivatives) should then be used because the sympathomimetics may be ineffective if a patient has been treated with catecholamine-depleting agents (reserpine, guanethidine).

CLINICAL SETTINGS

Probably the most important factor for the physician to consider when deciding which drug to use is the clinical setting in which the hypertensive emergency presents. Table 25-6 summarizes the relative usefulness of drugs for various conditions. Although guidelines can be given, no hard and fast rules can be made; each patient must be evaluated and treated individually.

Malignant Hypertension

Diagnosis and Prognosis

The most common hypertensive emergency is the syndrome of malignant hypertension. Blood pressure is dramatically elevated; evidence of papilledema, hemorrhages, and exudates appear in the patient's retinas; and spastic arteriolar changes can be observed. The condition may present alone or it may coexist with other clinical problems. An increasing number of patients with mild or moderate hypertension are being adequately treated, and consequently the de novo appearance of malignant hypertension as an outgrowth of progressive, untreated essential hypertension seems to be decreasing. Today, malignant hypertension occurs more often as a complication of another disease, such as renal failure or renal artery stenosis. The appearance of malignant hypertension in patients older than 60 years who have never been known to be hypertensive before is almost invariably a result of atherosclerotic renal artery disease in either or both renal arteries.

Antihypertensive drugs have greatly improved the survival rate of patients with malignant hypertension. Most studies conducted before the agents were available reported a 95 percent 1-year mortality rate if the condition was untreated. Vigorous therapy can now achieve a 50 percent 5-year survival rate. Cautious optimism is nevertheless the wisest attitude for a physician to adopt when discussing prognosis with a patient and family.

Therapy

If a patient with malignant hypertension presents with failing vision, left ventricular failure, or headache or any other neurologic symptom, parenteral treatment is mandatory. Although bed rest and oral therapy are at times permissible for patients who do not demonstrate these symptoms, treatment usually begins with parenteral agents. Nitroprusside is usually the agent of choice, but trimethaphan, labetalol, enalapril, or intravenous methyldopa may be used; the selection of the drug ultimately depends on the desired rate of blood pressure reduction (Table 25-7).

Because malignant hypertension is so often a complication of progressive renal disease, the patient's renal functioning must also be considered before a therapeutic decision is made. Severe renal insufficiency may require early dialysis to relieve fluid overload or the signs and symptoms of uremia. Many patients with mild or moderate renal insufficiency, on the other hand, experience a temporary worsening of renal function after blood pressure is reduced, but the condition usually improves. Acute renal failure, frequently with oli-

Table 25-7. Oral agents for rapid control of blood pressure

Agent	Dose
Captopril	6.25–25.0 mg tid
Labetalol	100–600 mg bid
Nifedipine	10–20 mg qid
Clonidine	0.1–0.2 mg/hr × 5 hr

guria, may accompany malignant hypertension. Minoxidil, a drug that often has intolerable long-term side effects, has been effective for treating rare patients with severe uncontrollable hypertension and end-stage renal disease when other therapies have been ineffective.

A few patients require surprisingly small doses of antihypertensive medications after the initial malignant phase is treated, but careful outpatient follow-up is mandatory. Because malignant hypertension can complicate every known form of high blood pressure, a complete diagnostic evaluation should be performed as soon as possible.

Acute Pulmonary Edema

Diagnosis

Hypertensive patients who develop acute pulmonary edema often improve greatly if arterial blood pressure and thus the afterload on the heart are reduced. Decreasing systemic vascular resistance, which is elevated in all but a few patients with hypertension and CHF, results in an increase in cardiac output and a decrease in cardiac work. The agents of choice in this setting are nitroprusside, nitroglycerine, and trimethaphan. They decrease peripheral vascular resistance and affect the capacitance vessels in such a way that venous return decreases. The myocardium consequently works against less resistance, and the reduction of venous return reverses the pulmonary edema.

The cause of acute pulmonary edema in the presence of hypertension is extremely important, because, if the patient has suffered an acute myocardial infarction or has a history of coronary artery disease, special caution is required when dilators are used to reduce blood pressure. Although nitroprusside has been reported to be beneficial in treating acute myocardial infarction and cardiogenic shock, too rapid or too great a reduction of pressure with vasodilators may reduce coronary artery perfusion and increase myocardial ischemia.

Therapy

Opiates, intravenous diuretics, oxygen, and rotating tourniquets are all effective for treating CHF while blood pressure is being reduced with dilators. Digitalis should be administered to any patient for whom it has not been previously prescribed, but its effect may be minimal if blood pressure is extremely high.

Some physicians would include diazoxide as an agent of choice for treating hypertension associated with pulmonary edema. However, because coronary insufficiency may underlie the condition and because the unpredictable lowering of pressure with diazoxide may result in adverse consequence, we elect to use nitroprusside first and nitroglycerine or trimethaphan only if nitroprusside is ineffective.

Hypertensive Encephalopathy

Hypertensive encephalopathy, the most serious complication of accelerated hypertension, mandates the immediate lowering of blood pressure. Although blood pressure is virtually always greater than 250/130 mm Hg, papilledema is not always present. On the other hand, some physicians have reported that hypertensive encephalopathy may develop at even lower blood pressure levels in patients with acute glomerulonephritis or eclampsia.

Diagnosis

Acute, although generally reversible, neurologic signs and symptoms may result from severe hypertension. Headache, photophobia, somnolence, vomiting, visual impairment, and other transient focal neurologic disturbances (e.g., seizures) are among the manifestations of this type of encephalopathy. Because visual disturbances are the most frequent presenting symptom, it is not surprising that an ophthalmologist or an optometrist is often the first to make to diagnosis.

Hypertensive encephalopathy must be differentiated from other syndromes of hypertension and neurologic dysfunction, including cerebral hemorrhage, occlusive stroke, rapidly growing brain tumors, pseudotumor cerebri, cerebral torulosis, and acute lead encephalopathy. Improvement of neurologic abnormalities when a patient's blood pressure is lowered is the hallmark of hypertensive encephalopathy. Spinal fluid proteins are elevated, and the spinal fluid is often mildly xanthochromic; superficial hemorrhages, multiple small thrombi, edema, and necrotizing arteritis in the brain are seen during autopsy of a patient who has died from this condition.

Therapy

Nitroprusside or diazoxide are the drugs of choice if the diagnosis of hypertensive encephalopathy is certain. If another neurologic diagnosis (such as stroke) that could be worsened by lowering the patient's blood pressure is a possibility, one of the more rapidly dissipating agents, nitroprusside or trimethaphan, should be used. These two drugs are preferable if the diagnosis has not been established beyond doubt because their effects are short-lived and thus can be controlled by discontinuing or reducing the dosage if the patient's neurologic status deteriorates as blood pressure decreases. The effects of diazoxide, on the other hand, persist for 4 to 12 hours and cannot be easily counteracted. Neither reserpine, which induces obtundation and may lower the patient's seizure threshold, nor methyldopa, which causes drowsiness and thus may obscure neurologic findings, should be given.

While efforts are made to lower blood pressure, precautions should be taken to prevent seizures and to control them and protect the patient if they do occur. Patients at risk for seizures should be restrained in the lateral recumbent, not the supine, position; side rails of the bed should be padded, suction should be available, and intravenous diazepam (Valium) should be at the bedside.

Cerebral Vascular Accident

The differential diagnosis to be considered is the same as that for hypertensive encephalopathy. If hemorrhage is suspected, a neurologist should be consulted and surgery considered. If cerebral thrombosis is likely, blood pressure should cautiously be reduced to the lowest level possible without precipitating or aggravating neurologic symptoms. The agent of choice in this setting is trimethaphan or nitroprusside, again because the effect of each dissipates rapidly.

Dissecting Aortic Aneurysm

Diagnosis
Any patient who presents with acute chest pain, back pain, or midline abdominal pain and with hypertension may be suffering a dissection of thoracic aorta; care must therefore be taken to establish or rule out the diagnosis (see Chap. 17). Dissection should be considered if chest pain is atypical for coronary pain, is absolutely midline, radiates to the back or abdomen, or is described as "tearing" or "burning." The ECG of a patient with chest pain and dissection may demonstrate left ventricular hypertrophy (LVH) without myocardial infarction or ischemia. A posterior anterior film of the chest usually reveals a widened mediastinum. Neurologic symptoms suggesting an occluded carotid or vertebral artery, especially if evidence of vascular obstruction elsewhere is also found, are another indication of dissection. In addition, if a murmur of aortic insufficiency is heard or if clinical signs of pericardial tamponade present, dissection is highly likely.

Therapy
Today, antihypertensive drugs are generally the preferred mode of therapy for dissection during its acute phase because medical management results in a better survival rate than does surgical intervention. The goal of therapy is to lower both blood pressure and the rate at which the left ventricle generates pressure in order to lessen the shear forces at the site of dissection and prevent it from extending. Trimethaphan is the parenteral drug of choice. Oral propranolol or labetalol may be given at the same time, and diuretics should be administered simultaneously. Because the renal arteries may be included in the area of dissection, urinary output must be carefully monitored. Only after the patient's condition has been stabilized and blood pressure lowered should angiography and surgery be considered.

Severe Preeclampsia or Eclampsia

Diagnosis
The presence of hypertension, seizures, and proteinuria in the third trimester of pregnancy constitutes a severe form of hypertension, eclampsia. It is important to remember that this syndrome can occur with blood pressure elevation that would be modest in a nonpregnant patient, from 150/100 upward. Ultimately, interrupting the pregnancy reverses the syndrome. Secondary forms of hypertension such as pheochromocytoma, or renal artery stenosis, should be considered.

Therapy
Reducing blood pressure and interrupting the pregnancy are mandatory for a pregnant patient with severe hypertension and seizures (eclampsia). Although magnesium sulfate, administered intramuscularly, has been popular with obstetricians for many years, diazoxide has been used with increasing frequency as its effectiveness has become apparent. Diazoxide can cause hyperglycemia in the fetus, but this condition does not seem to pose clinical problems. Intravenous labetalol is an effective and safe agent for severe hypertension during pregnancy. Trimethaphan should not be used because ganglionic blockade results in fetal ileus and stops labor; reserpine should also be avoided because it increases the likelihood of seizures.

Pheochromocytoma

Diagnosis
Patients with pheochromocytoma, a rare cause of hypertensive crisis, may present with characteristic episodic symptoms referable to the sympathetic nervous system (sweating, syncope, headaches, palpitation), or they may present with relatively sustained or episodic hypertension. Any patient with severe hypertension may therefore have a pheochromocytoma, but the diagnosis is more likely if the patient has a history of hyperparathyroidism, medullary carcinoma of the thyroid, or pheochromocytoma. Evidence of neurofibromatosis or the other phakomatoses also suggests that the hypertension is due to pheochromocytoma.

Therapy
In the past, the administration of 5 mg of phentolamine intravenously before any other drug was given was recommended as a diagnostic test. Pheochromocytoma could be confirmed if the patient's systolic blood pressure fell more than 35 mm Hg or diastolic more than 25 mm Hg. (Such changes suggest a catecholamine excess.) This procedure was necessary because the antihypertensive agents made it impossible to determine levels of catecholamine metabolites in the urine accurately and thus made pheochromocytoma difficult to diagnose if treatment had already been initiated. However, more recently developed laboratory methods allow catecholamines, metanephrines, and vanillylmandelic acid (VMA) to be measured after most drugs have been administered, and the precaution is no longer essential.

A patient with a pheochromocytoma responds to antihypertensive drugs as other hypertensive patients do, and nitroprusside, trimethaphan, or diazoxide can confer benefits. These agents may produce tachycardia and signs of a beta-adrenergic excess, conditions that necessitate the addition of propranolol to the therapeutic regimen. Propranolol, however, is contraindicated as a first agent because it can exacerbate alpha-adrenergic reflex effects (hypertension) in a patient with pheochromocytoma and actually cause an increase in pressure.

Tyramine Ingestion by Patients on Monoamine Oxidase Inhibitors

Hypertensive crises may occur in patients who are taking MAO inhibitors, such as pargyline (Eutonyl), tranylcypromine (Parnate), isocarboxazid (Marplan), and phenelzine (Nardil), although use of these drugs is becoming increasingly rare. A dramatic outpouring of catecholamines is triggered by the ingestion of sympathomimetic agents such as ephidrine, amphetamines, tyramine, phenylephrine, and foods and beverages containing tyramine (e.g., Chianti wine, certain beers, unpasteurized cheeses, pickled herring). The treatment of hypertension in this setting is the same as that for pheochromocytoma.

Many patients will present with severe hypertension without evidence of acute end-organ damage. These patients are classified as hypertensive urgencies. They require repeated monitoring at frequent intervals and rapidly acting oral medications. Depending on the monitoring capabilities, the patient may be managed in the office, clinic, or emergency room or as an inpatient. These patients do not have evidence of cerebral, cardiac, vascular, or renal dysfunction. The medications that are useful for these patients are shown in Table 25-7.

Captopril, nifedipine, labetalol, or clonidine have been given in frequent dosages to decrease blood pressure. Nifedipine and clonidine can be given hourly until blood pressure decreases. Captopril and labetalol should be given every 2 hours for severe hypertension. Patients with severe hypertension will frequently also benefit from diuretic therapy.

SELECTED READING

The 1988 Report of the Joint National Committee on Detection, Evaluation, and Treatment of High Blood Pressure. *Arch Intern Med* 148:1023, 1988.

Ram, CVS, and Hyman, D. Hypertensive crisis. *J Intensive Care Med* 2:151, 1987.

DeQuattro, V. Treating hypertensive crisis: Which drug for which patient? *J Crit Illness* 7:24, 1987.

Ramos, O. Malignant hypertension: The Brazilian experience. *Kid Intl* 25:209, 1984.

Grubb, BP, Sirio, C, and Zelis, R. Intravenous labetalol in acute aortic dissection. *J.A.M.A.* 258:78, 1987.

Koch-Weser, J. Hypertensive emergencies. *N Engl J Med* 290:211, 1974.

Cohn, JN, and Burke, LP. Nitroprusside. *Ann Intern Med* 91:752, 1979.

Koch-Weser, J. Diazoxide. *N Engl J Med* 294:1271, 1976.

E. Shock

26. Shock: General Considerations of Pathophysiology and Management

Arthur E. Baue

DEFINITIONS OF SHOCK

Support of the circulation has been a major achievement of modern medicine. For many years, traumatic or wound shock was thought to be a mysterious process produced by toxins, humors, or the neuroendocrine system. As recently as the beginning of World War II, shock, or inadequate circulation, was a common cause of death in otherwise normal individuals after injury. The recognition that with injury or with an operation there was loss of blood and also extracellular fluid volume, which produced hypovolemia and reduced blood flow to tissues, allowed the treatment of traumatic shock by replacement of such losses. The association of circulatory failure with infection, cardiac disease, and central nervous system injury led to treatment of these problems as well. How simple these definitions and concepts seem now in retrospect, but how difficult was the recognition of them earlier. In spite of this, shock or circulatory failure remains a major problem in the resuscitation, treatment, and survival of injured and operated patients. The severity and duration of shock after injury are major risk factors for the development of infection, multiple organ failure, and death in such patients.

The word *shock* was first used as a medical term in 1743 in an English translation by Clarke of the French surgeon Henri Francois Le Dran's *A Treatise of Reflections Drawn from Experience with Gunshot Wounds* (Clarke, 1743, Le Dran, 1737). Use of the word *shock* has been criticized for its lack of specificity. It is no more exact than *fever,* but it does describe a clinical abnormality that requires immediate attention in order to improve blood flow. It is thus a valuable word for the surgeon because injury, whether accidental or produced by an operation, so frequently results in abnormalities of the circulation. However, an all-encompassing definition of shock, wherein it becomes the final common pathway of many disease processes, is meaningless. The definitions historically reflect the emphasis and understanding of the time. Thus, Samuel Gross in 1872 described shock as "a manifestation of the rude unhinging of the machinery of life," and John Collins Warren said that it was "a momentary pause in the act of death." Blalock, after extensive studies, wrote, "Shock is a peripheral circulatory failure resulting from a discrepancy in the size of the vascular bed and the volume of the intravascular fluid." This concept of an inadequate circulating blood volume was further emphasized in 1942 by Wiggers, who said, "Shock is a syndrome resulting from a depression of many functions but in which reduction of the effective circulating blood volume is of basic importance and in which impairment of the circulation steadily progresses until it eventuates in a state of irreversible circulatory failure." The emphasis at the time was on blood volume, as the concept of hypovolemia after injury was being discovered. Harkins put this in pathophysiologic terms, describing shock as a "progressive vasoconstrictive oligemic anoxia." A more broad definition was given by Simeone a few years ago when he defined shock as "a clinical condition characterized by signs and symptoms which arise when the cardiac output is insufficient to fill the arterial tree with blood under sufficient pressure to provide organs and tissues with adequate blood flow." Of importance, then, are blood volume, the vascular system, the heart, and the distribution of blood flow, each of which can be abnormal.

Shock is not just a transient decrease in blood pressure as in syncope or hypotension alone, since controlled hypotension produced by ganglionic blockade during anesthesia may allow normal nutrient blood flow to tissues. It is also an acute generalized problem of the entire individual, even though it may produce failure of single organ systems such as the kidney. The circulation conducts its affairs at the capillary level. The common thread in all forms of shock is an inadequate circulation with diminished blood flow to tissues, resulting in cell ischemia and hypoxia and their sequelae. The final result was described by Haldane, who said, "Anoxia not only stops the machine but wrecks the machinery."

HISTORICAL NOTES

Recognition of a depression of vital processes after injury goes back to antiquity. The writings of Hippocrates, the Old Testament, and Homer clearly recognized the problem of blood loss after injury. As with other knowledge in the arts and sciences, the fundamental importance of hypovolemia after injury and operation was forgotten for centuries, and in the Renaissance, the problems with injury were ascribed to mystical relationships. Even though Ambrose Paré wrote in the sixteenth century that "the cause of swooning that happens to those that are wounded is . . . bleeding," he and others practiced bloodletting in injured patients. Paré wrote that phlebotomy is "required in great wounds where there is fear of deflexion, pain, delirium, raving and unquietness." Also, Le Dran in his description of shock wrote that "this coldness may likewise be occasioned by loss of blood." Clarke in his translation of Le Dran's treatise used the word *shock* to convey the impression of a blow or jolt (a *comonotio*), commotion, or concussion with an injury leading to progressive deterioration, loss of consciousness, and death. Le Dran had used the word *secousse,* or *saisissement.* The word *shock* was next used by John Latta in 1795 to describe the clinical picture after injury. Thomas Latta first used saline in 1831 for the treatment of hypovolemic shock due to cholera. In spite of this, shock was treated by strychnine and stimulants as late as the Boer War (1899–1902). Often the injury or insult seemed small in relationship to the profound effect (shock) on the patient. Sir Astly Cooper, in his *Commentary on War Injuries,* described the enigma of soldiers dying without significant blood loss, severe pain, or gross injury. The best clinical description of this dilemma was provided by John Collins Warren in 1895 when he wrote:

> A patient is brought into the hospital with a compound comminuted fracture or with a dislocation of the hip joint added to other injuries, where the bleeding has been slight. As the litter is gently deposited on the floor he makes no effort to move or look about him. He lies staring at the surgeon with an expression of complete indifference as to his condition. There is no movement of the muscles of the face; the eyes, which are deeply sunken in their sockets, have a weird, uncanny look. The features are pinched and the face shrunken. A cold, clammy sweat exudes from the pores of the skin, which has an appearance of profound anemia. The lips are bloodless and the fingers and nails are blue. The pulse is almost imperceptible; a weak, thread-like stream may, however, be detected in the radial artery. The thermometer, placed in the rectum, registers 96° or 97°F. The muscles are not paralyzed anywhere, but the patient seems disinclined to make any muscular effort. Even respiratory movements seem for the time to be reduced to a minimum. Occasionally the patient may feebly throw about one of his limbs and give vent to a hoarse, weak groan. There is no insensibility (coma is not observed in cases of shock), but he is strangely apathetic, and seems to realize but imperfectly the full meaning of the questions put to him. It is of no use to attempt an operation until appropriate remedies have brought about a reaction. The pulse, however, does not respond; it grows feebler and finally disappears, and "this momentary pause in the act of death" is soon followed by the grim reality. A postmortem examination reveals no visible changes in the internal organs.

Early studies of the circulation and its control during the beginnings of experimental physiology by Claude Bernard, Brown-Sequard, and Charcot led to the concept that shock was the result of inhibition of the vasomotor center, producing weakening of the heartbeat and peripheral pooling of blood. In 1889, George W. Crile, who worked originally with Victor Horseley in London, published a series of pioneering experimental studies of shock. He defined the importance of venous pressures and failure of venous return in hemorrhagic shock, of fluid loss in shock, and of saline therapy. Nine years later, Yendel Henderson wrote that "venous pressure is, so to speak, the fulcrum of circulation. Shock, as physicians use the word, is due to failure of the fulcrum."

The first systematic observations of clinical shock came during World War I when Cannon and Bayliss led a team of physiologists and clinicians who provided descriptions and measurements on the battlefield. Cannon defined hypotension and shock in terms of a fall in blood volume, reduction in alkali reserve, accumulation of fixed acids, loss of vasomotor tone, cardiac failure, and stagnation in venous reservoirs. Keith used dye dilution methods to show that the severity of shock correlated with reductions in blood volume. Archibald and McLean recognized the differences between blood flow and blood pressure in shock, emphasizing the importance of decreased blood flow. However, shock from injury without external blood loss, with crush injury, and in patients who did not respond to blood, gum acacia, or saline solutions was a problem. This was not understood as hypovolemia per se but rather as a problem of blood vessels holding fluid in the circulation and was called *wound shock* or *secondary shock.* Toxins were sought as an explanation, and, from the work of Dale and Richards at the time, histamine was implicated in producing *traumatic toxemia.*

In 1930, Blalock and Parsons, and Phemister, each working independently, documented that shock after trauma was due to blood and plasma loss in and around the wounds and not due to a toxin. Blalock further documented the importance of blood transfusion for such injuries and showed that histamine was not a factor. In spite of this, until the middle of World War II, the definition of shock by the National Research Conference was "the clinical condition characterized by progressive reduction in the circulatory blood volume due to increased capillary permeability." During World War II, further contributions were made by trauma research units, such as the one headed by Henry K. Beecher in the Mediterranean theater. Their studies indicated that the major cause of shock was hemorrhage and fluid loss leading to metabolic acidosis. Cournand and Richard first measured cardiac output in patients in shock in 1943. Surgical research units during the Korean War documented the importance of triage and early resuscitation and evaluation. Posttraumatic renal insufficiency was described when fluid resuscitation was not as rapid or extensive as required for renal function. During the Vietnamese conflict, shock and renal failure were no longer major clinical problems, but infection and posttraumatic pulmonary insufficiency were identified as frequent limitations for survival after injury. With further progress, the major limitations after injury and operations have now become head injury, infection, and multiple organ failure. The development of knowledge about septic and cardiogenic shock will be described later.

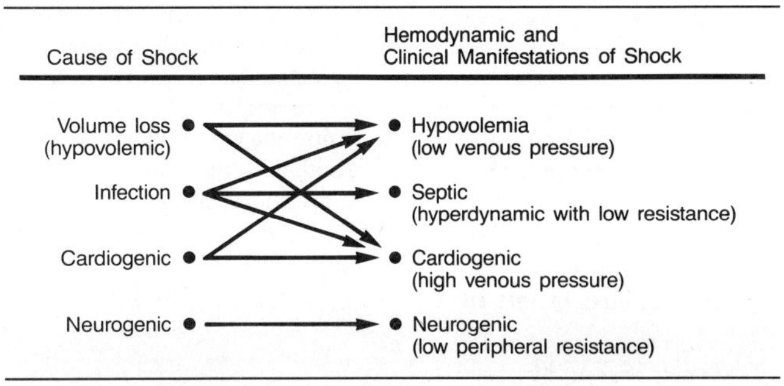

Fig. 26-1. Differences between the cause of shock and the hemodynamic and clinical manifestations of shock. Both are important.

Table 26-1. Causes of hypovolemic shock

Etiology	Type of fluid lost	Location of loss
Bleeding	Blood	External loss—blood, perspiration, vomitus, stool, fistulas
Soft tissue injury—blood and fluid loss—traumatic or wound shock	Plasma	
	Extracellular fluid (salt and water loss or deficiency)	
Burns		Internal loss
Intestinal obstruction	Gastric contents—succus entericus, colonic loss	Traumatic—hematoma, sequestration in wounds, body cavities, or bowel
Perforated ulcer		
Crush injury		
Dehydration from fever and perspiration	Exudate	
	Water	
		Obstructive—intestine, etc.
Gastrointestinal fistulas, diarrhea		Inflammatory—exudative

CLASSIFICATION

The causes of shock may be classified into four general categories, based on which circulatory component is abnormal (Fig. 26-1). Thus, an inadequate blood volume is called *hypovolemic shock.* If the heart is unable to provide an adequate cardiac output, it is called *cardiogenic shock.* Inability of the nervous system to maintain vascular resistance is called *neurogenic shock.* The inability of the circulation to meet the need for increased blood flow required by infection is called *septic shock.* This is similar to the original classification by Blalock in 1934 of hematogenic or oligemic shock, cardiogenic shock, neurogenic shock, and vasogenic shock. The vasogenic category of decreased vascular resistance and increased vascular capacity producing circulatory failure is accurate conceptually because it is the fourth component of the circulation, which can be abnormal—that is, the size of the vascular system, along with the pump, blood volume, and neurogenic control. This category resembles the early picture of septic shock with a hyperdynamic circulation but is not a characteristic clinical or etiologic entity. Therefore, it is preferable to eliminate it as a separate category and use the designation septic shock. There are many other problems that, although associated with hypotension or circulatory failure, are not considered primary circulatory problems. These include various types of organ failure such as adrenocortical insufficiency or hepatic failure, injuries such as traumatic tension pneumothorax, flail chest and vena caval obstruction or compression, and problems such as electrolyte abnormalities and increased intracranial pressure.

Hypovolemic shock may be classified according to the type of fluid lost, such as blood alone from a bleeding duodenal ulcer, loss of fluid with a high protein content, such as with a burn or perforated ulcer, extracellular fluid loss with intestinal obstruction, and water loss from fever and hyperventilation. Synonyms for hypovolemic shock include oligemic or hemorrhagic shock, traumatic shock, wound shock, and burn shock. The location of the loss and the disease or injury producing the loss may also be part of such categorization (Table 26-1).

Cardiogenic shock is classified according to the primary problems of the heart or myocardium (intrinsic) and problems extrinsic to the heart that interfere with its ability to provide adequate blood flow (Table 26-2). Although valvular heart disease, cardiomyopathies, and other forms of congestive heart failure (CHF) may eventually produce acute circulatory failure, they are not usually considered forms of shock.

Septic shock may be produced by any type of infection. The complex demands of an infection of the circulation fall into two categories: an increase in circulation required by fever and infection, and alterations in the circulation, heart, and vascular bed produced by the infection or its metabolic products (Table 26-3).

Vasogenic or *neurogenic shock* is primarily a problem of loss of vascular tone or resistance of both the peripheral arterial system and the venous capacitance system. It may result from injuries to the central nervous system or spinal

Table 26-2. Causes of cardiogenic shock

Intrinsic	Extrinsic to the heart
Myocardial infarction—aneurysm of the left ventricle Myocardial failure due to ventricular ischemia, depression from sepsis, pulmonary failure, or late hypovolemia Myocardial contusion Arrhythmias Drugs, including anesthetic agents	Pulmonary embolism Cardiac tamponade Respiratory failure and pulmonary hypertension High levels of PEEP

cord or be caused by agents that block vasoactive functions, such as spinal anesthesia, or by syncope.

Generally these four categories or etiologies of shock produce characteristic hemodynamic pictures that can be distinguished from each other (Figs. 26-2, 26-3, and 26-4). All, of course, have manifestations of inadequate peripheral tissue and organ perfusion differing in an inadequate filling pressure for the heart with hypovolemia, a high filling pressure with cardiogenic shock, and a hyperdynamic—albeit inadequate—circulation with early septic shock. However, clinical manifestations are frequently not so neatly categorized, and an abnormality may not occur in pure form. Clinical characteristics are determined not only by the etiology of the abnormality but also by the condition of the patient at the time shock develops and the stage of disease or injury. It is necessary, therefore, to recognize not only the etiology of shock but also the exact hemodynamic manifestations in the patient. This is particularly important because hypovolemia

Table 26-3. Causes of septic shock, bacteremia, or septicemia from any gram-negative or -positive organism or fungi

Peritonitis
Extensive abscesses
Genitourinary infection or instrumentation
Septic abortion
Intravenous catheters
Pulmonary or other infections
Toxic shock syndrome

or an inadequate vascular volume frequently occurs, no matter what the cause of shock. Increasing the vascular volume by fluid infusion could be helpful in many patients with shock from other causes. Thus, an elderly person with severe coronary artery disease who has gastrointestinal bleeding and develops circulatory failure would be said to have hypovolemic shock based on the etiology of the problem. However, because of coronary artery disease, myocardial blood flow may be decreased and produce ventricular failure. In such a patient, the hemodynamic manifestations may be those of cardiogenic shock with a high central venous pressure. On the other hand, a patient who develops circulatory failure due to an acute myocardial infarction may have previously received diuretic therapy and have decreased total body water and blood volume. Such a patient may initially have the hemodynamic manifestations of hypovolemic shock, with decreased central venous pressure. The same thing may be true with a patient who develops sepsis. Sepsis often produces peripheral vasodilation and a hyperdynamic circulation with a high cardiac output, but central venous pressure may be extremely low, indicating the need for volume replacement, and, therefore, the hemodynamic picture of hypovolemic shock (see Fig. 26-1).

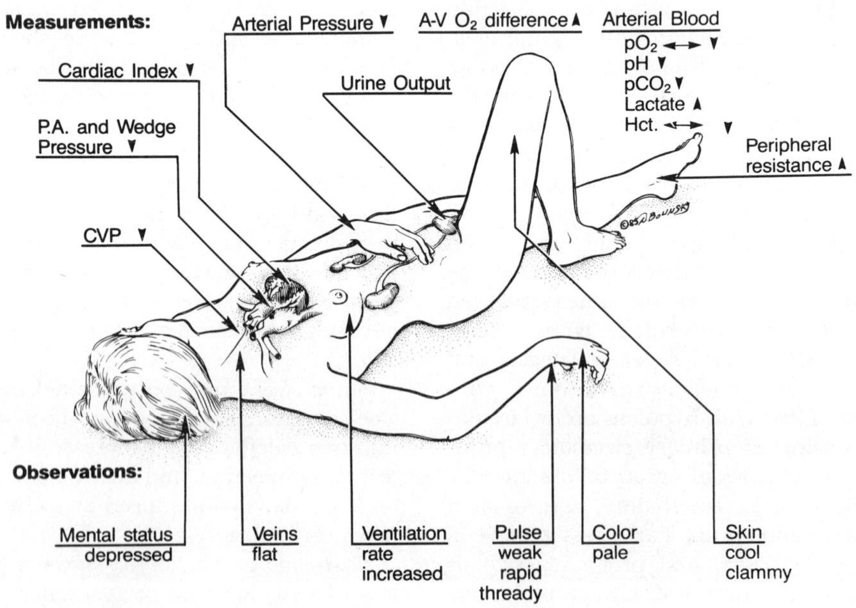

Fig. 26-2. The hemodynamic and clinical manifestations of hypovolemic shock are illustrated.

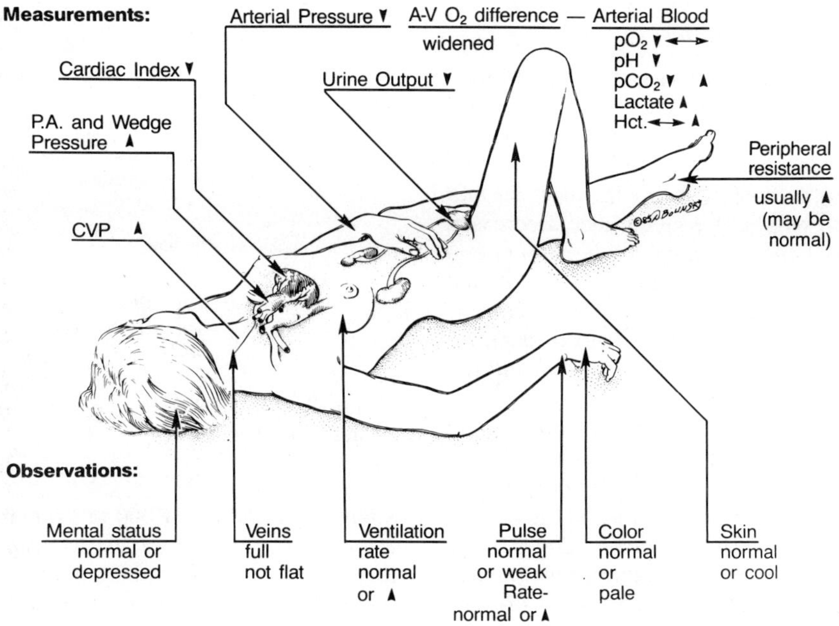

Fig. 26-3. The hemodynamic and clinical manifestations of cardiogenic shock are illustrated.

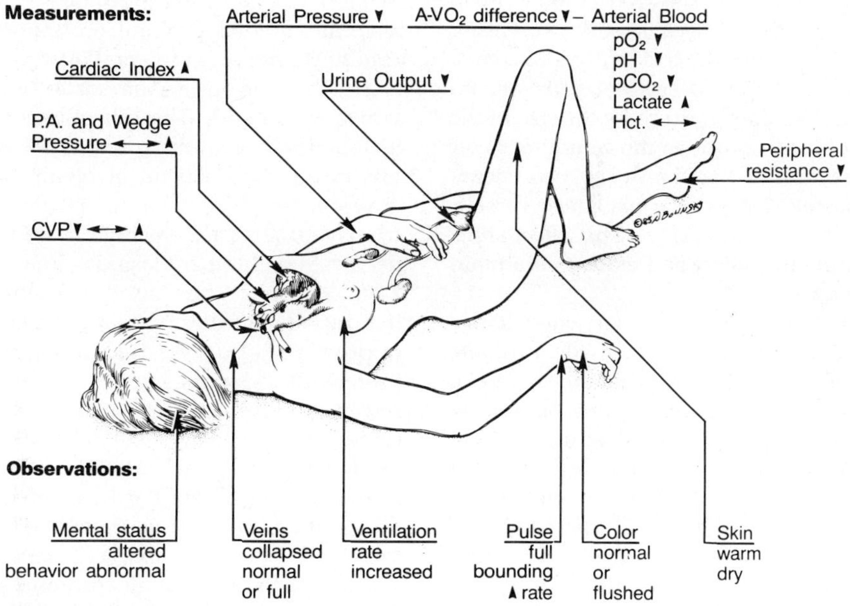

Fig. 26-4. The hemodynamic and clinical manifestations of hyperdynamic septic shock are illustrated. The sites for venous access and arterial puncture are illustrated.

PATHOPHYSIOLOGY OF CIRCULATORY INADEQUACY

Adaptation of the Vascular System

All forms of shock have similar characteristics when blood flow to organs and tissues is reduced. Therefore, the altered physiology produced by a failing circulation can be described for all types, using hypovolemic shock as an example, while recognizing certain differences with sepsis and cardiac problems, which will be described later. Decreased blood flow brings about a complex homeostatic response to try to protect the individual and maintain perfusion of vital organs. Thus, whether the decrease in blood flow (cardiac output) is due to decreased venous return (blood loss), increased circulatory demand (sepis), or myocardial failure, the compensatory mechanisms will be similar.

With an altered circulation, due to either blood or fluid loss or decrease in cardiac output, two things happen: First, there is compensation for this alteration by the cardiovascular system by transcapillary refilling and by endocrine changes; second, there are the effects of such changes in the circulation, including those on organ function, metabolism, microcirculation, and cellular alterations. With loss of circulating volume, the major responses are to decrease the size of the vascular bed, maintain circulation to the heart and brain, and mobilize body fluids to replace the loss.

When blood volume is lost, venous return to the heart is decreased and cardiac output is lessened. The medullary vasomotor center, aortic arch, and carotid baroreceptors sense the change in pressure and flow. This produces arteriovenous constriction, increased heart rate, and an inotropic effect on the ventricles due to sympathetic nervous system stimulation and decreased vagal tone. Arterial vasoconstriction has the effect of maintaining central arterial blood pressure and redistributing flow to vital organs while decreasing flow to organs and tissues that may be less in need. Since the arterial system is a small part of the overall vascular system, arterial vasoconstriction does little to decrease the size of the vascular bed or to shift blood volume to the central circulation. The decrease in volume of the circulatory bed occurs primarily through vasoconstriction of capacitance vessels, which are primarily in the venous system. This effect shifts more blood to the central circulation and tends to maintain venous pressure and return.

The splanchnic bed in humans is the primary capacitance region, and 500 to 1,000 ml of blood may be made available by venoconstriction in this area. Depending on the volume of loss, the initial compensatory mechanisms may be able to maintain a reasonable blood pressure, cardiac output, and venous return. Thus, loss of 350 (as would be given in a blood donation) up to 500 ml of blood may produce no particular hemodynamic effect, especially if the patient remains recumbent. However, syncope may occur even after giving a unit of blood as a blood donor. Thus, donors are given juice to drink and kept recumbent for a period of time until the circulation adjusts to this modest loss. A feeling of lightheadedness, syncope, or postural hypotension may occur if an individual sits up rapidly in such a circumstance. If an individual loses 1,000 ml of blood over a period of minutes, the effect may be profound. If the loss occurs slowly over hours, compensatory mechanisms may allow replenishment, with only evidence of postural hypotension. However, a fairly rapid loss of 1,000 to 1,500 ml of blood will produce evidence of circulatory inadequacy with hypotension, reduced organ flow, and beginning signs of shock. Losses larger than this, however, produce severe shock and will not allow survival unless treatment is provided.

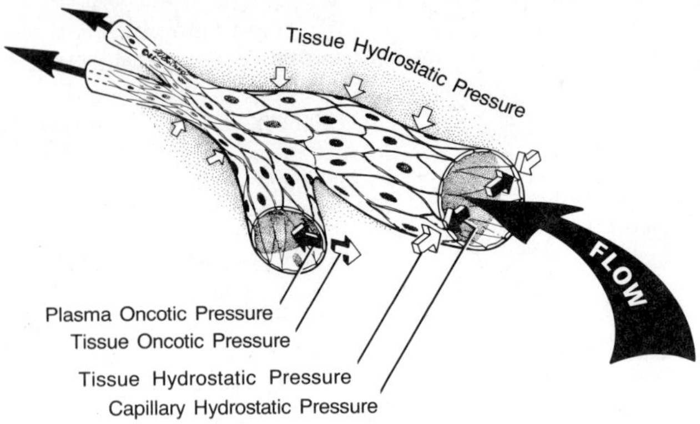

Fig. 26-5. The relationships of hydrostatic and oncotic pressure as described by Starling. These relationships allow for capillary refilling after hemorrhage.

Homeostatic mechanisms do compensate for moderate blood or extracellular fluid loss. After circulatory adjustments to maximize central blood flow and pressure to vital organs for survival, mechanisms to refill the circulation begin to function. The circulatory or cardiovascular compensatory mechanisms also contribute to this powerful mechanism. Volume is restored to the circulation by two mechanisms: transcapillary refilling of the circulation from extravascular extracellular fluid, and restoration of protein to the circulation for oncotic pressure. The first phase of restoration of fluid volume occurs because of Starling forces resulting from a fall in capillary hydrostatic pressure due to arteriolar vasoconstriction intracellular space into the capillaries (Fig. 26-5). This phenomenon has been studied by Skillman, Moore, and coworkers, who found that after the loss of 500 to 1,000 ml of blood by slow protein into the plasma, this plasma volume refilling in the capillary bed is usually quite rapid—as high as 2 ml per minute—and then decreases with time. Plasma volume is restored to normal in 24 to 48 hours. They found that albumin enters the circulation rapidly, at rates up to 4 gm per hour initially. Synthesis of protein is also increased, along with a decreased rate of protein degradation. The return of protein to the circulation seems to depend on interstitial volume and pressure as a driving force. The net result of this is a decrease in interstitial fluid, which is then restored only by autoingestion or by intravenous injection. Participation of cells and cell water in this phenomenon has been studied by Gann and colleagues, who believe that an extracellular increase in solute with shock, particularly by glucose and perhaps other osmotic-reactive solutes, draws water out of cells into the interstitial space. A number of factors may be necessary for this, including solute in the splanchnic bed, glucose, cortisol, and perhaps epinephrine, along with adequate nutrition and prior hydration.

If an individual before injury or operation suffers from malnutrition or dehydration, compensation may not be possible. In severe or late hypovolemic shock with decompensation, there may be a number of other factors involved, including impaired vasomotor activity, alteration in interstitial macromolecules and collagen, which may take up or bind fluids, and also the matter of cell swelling. With cell ischemia, sodium is taken up into the cell and potassium is lost. There is increased hydration of cells, resulting in a further decrease in extracellular fluid volume. In severe late shock, epinephrine, norepinephrine, and angiotensin may be deleterious by preventing capillary refilling and increasing capillary fluid loss by high venous pressures.

Neuroendocrine Compensation

The metabolic and neuroendocrine response to injury is an important part of the stress reaction and teleologically provides a better opportunity for the biologic organism to survive under adverse circumstances or when injured. Shock, blood loss, and inadequate circulation all represent powerful forces to initiate these changes. Thus, the responses brought about by hemorrhage and blood volume loss or shock are similar to those occurring in patients with the stress of an injury. With starvation, bed rest, and a general anesthetic alone, the neuroendocrine response is minimal. With modest hemorrhage, there is initial increased secretion of renin, aldosterone, antidiuretic hormone, and erythropoietin, with renal conservation of sodium and water. With more severe injury or hemorrhage, there is an increase in adrenocorticotropic hormone (ACTH) secretion. Sympathetic activity is increased as an early response to hypovolemia, as is an increase in epinephrine from the adrenal medulla when blood pressure and blood flow decrease. Additional stimuli include acidosis and hypercapnia. The effects of the catecholamines on the circulation are well known.

Other effects include the production of hypoglycemia due to glycogen breakdown from the liver, stimulation of glucagon production, innervation of insulin production and of its peripheral actions, and stimulation of ACTH. Decreased renal blood flow and pulse pressure stimulate the juxtaglomerular apparatus to produce renin, which stimulates the production of angiotensin. Angiotensin contributes its vasoconstrictor effect and stimulates the production of aldosterone. From the anterior pituitary, ACTH is released and further increases aldosterone production, along with cortisol. The posterior pituitary secretes vasopressin or antidiuretic hormone (ADH), with its dual effect on the circulation and water retention by the kidney.

The hypothalamus is activated, with production of beta-endorphin, which increases vasopressin release and may have a morphine-like effect throughout the body. The role, if any, of the other hypothalamic hormones, such as somatostatin, thyrotropin-releasing factor, beta-lipoprotein, and other pituitary hormones, such as prolactin, growth hormone, and thyroid-stimulating hormone (TSH), is not known. The gastrointestinal and metabolic hormones play a role after injury, but no specific activities of pancreatic polypeptide, vasoactive intestinal peptide, or secretin are recognized. The decrease in insulin and depression of its peripheral effects by epinephrine may be responsible for the diabetic-type picture seen in the injured and shocked patient. Glucagon would also contribute to this.

Precise alterations and effects of the cellular or tissue mediators and hormones such as the prostaglandin and kinin-kallikrein systems are not clear in humans. It seems likely that these may have an effect and may be an important factor in the later deterioration seen in prolonged and severe shock. Studies in experimental animals given some of these agents while blocking the effects of others suggest that they play a role.

Pathophysiology of Decreased Blood Flow—Changes in Organ Function with Decreased Blood Flow

Compensation for decreased vascular volume or for a decrease in cardiac output provides readjustment of the circulation, decreasing flow to those areas that can tolerate ischemia for brief periods of time. These include the skin, muscle, the splanchnic bed, and the kidneys, where decreased flow also serves the purpose of fluid conservation. Compensation for a severe decrease in vascular volume when carried out over a period of time will eventually result in alterations in organ function. There is no particular stage or combination of hemodynamic variables in which shock is said to be present. It certainly indicates an inadequate circulation with blood pressure, cardiac output, and blood flow to organs diminished so that compensation is either impossible or the compensation itself becomes deleterious.

The Kidney

As blood flow to the kidney is decreased, there is an alteration in the intrarenal distribution of flow from the cortex to the medulla. This distribution is probably affected by aldosterone. Along with this, there is decreased renal function, with a depression in glomerular filtration rate and oliguria. Medullary sodium is decreased, and there is loss of the medullar hyperosmolar zone and of the countercurrent concentrating system. If decreased blood flow continues and is associated with other changes such as the need for the kidney to handle large amounts of pigment (e.g., hemoglobin or myoglobin), eventually tubular necrosis and acute renal failure may occur. If the injury is severe, total renal shutdown with anuria and rapid development of azotemia, hyperkalemia, and acidosis may develop. However, if the injury is not severe enough to produce oliguric or anuric renal failure, there may be what is called *high output renal failure.* This is a less severe injury that may be more difficult to recognize because urine output may be normal or high in spite of inability to excrete waste products, along with a progressive rise in blood urea nitrogen (BUN) and creatinine.

Effects on the Heart

With hypovolemia and decreased cardiac output, the central circulation is initially maintained, and coronary blood flow may be adequate, particularly if there is no occlusive disease of the coronary arteries. However, with further decreases in cardiac output, coronary flow may not keep pace. This may then contribute to a further decrease in cardiac output. Myocardial oxygen extraction is normally high, so that increasing oxygen extraction is of modest benefit unless blood flow can be maintained or increased. Even though the coronary circulation has the ability of autoregulation and dilates as cardiac output decreases, this may not be possible if the decrease in cardiac output is extensive or if the patient has significant coronary artery disease. Electrocardiographic (ECG) changes or myocardial ischemia, premature ventricular contractions, or other arrhythmias may be seen. The ischemic heart produces lactate rather than using it for metabolic needs. There is also altered utilization of free fatty acids. In any form of shock, if cardiac output is depressed or if other changes take place, the myocardium may be affected. Myocardial depression is said to occur in late or severe septic shock and in other forms of circulatory failure. Thus, no matter what the etiology of the shock, a careful search for adequacy of ventricular performance is necessary. In any form of circulatory failure, there may ultimately be depression of the myocardium, which would be expressed clinically by low cardiac output and a high and rising venous pressure. Whether such changes in late shock in humans are due to toxic factors depressing the myocardium or are simply the late result of a prolonged decrease blood flow has not been determined.

The Liver

Although decreased splanchnic blood flow, including flow to the liver, occurs with any form of circulatory failure, the immediate acute manifestations of hepatic ischemia are difficult to recognize or describe. It is known that there is decreased ability to metabolize lactate and perhaps to detoxify other substances. Synthetic activities of the liver are probably depressed, such as the production of albumin and other acute-phase proteins. With severe shock, there may be elevation of certain enzymes, suggesting hepatic injury, and alterations in Bromsulphalein (BSP) retention or an abnormal cephalin floculation test, and so on. However, the effects of ischemia on the liver may not be evident until later, when bilirubin is elevated and other aspects of hepatic function are altered. Depression of the reticuloendothelial system, and particularly the Kupffer's cells in the liver, could be important. Much more study is required, especially in humans, as to the acute effects of hepatic ischemia with shock or circulatory failure.

The Brain

Although blood flow to the brain is maintained at the expense of many other organ systems, with circulatory failure there is often alteration in the sensorium, a distressed mental state, apathy, diminished responsiveness, fatigue, anxiety, and other factors. Electroencephalographic (EEG) activity may be depressed if circulatory failure and hypotension are severe. However, even with severe hypotension, an individual may be in contact and be lucid mentally.

The Gastrointestinal Tract

The gastrointestinal tract has decreased activity with shock. With decreased blood to the gastric mucosa, it is more susceptible to injury. This, along with hydrochloric acid in the stomach, contributes eventually to stress ulceration and bleeding.

The Lung

A decrease in blood flow produces hyperventilation. This is a central effect related to increased PCO_2 in the respiratory center of the medulla rather than a direct effect on the lung. This initial hyperventilation may produce respiratory alkalosis and contribute to a further decrease in cerebral blood flow due to the fall in arterial PCO_2. Later in shock, increased ventilation occurs due to metabolic acidosis from increased lactate production. Decreased blood flow to the lung may contribute to hypoxia and carbon dioxide retention. Pulmonary problems are frequent after injury and shock, with the development of posttraumatic pulmonary insufficiency and the need for ventilatory support. The lung itself is quite resistant to ischemia, and it is unlikely that hypovolemic or hemorrhagic shock per se produces significant damage to the lung. Not only does the lung receive whatever cardiac output there is that passes through it albeit with shunting, but the lung is exposed to whatever oxygen is breathed.

Studies during the Vietnam conflict indicated that hemorrhagic shock was not associated with a high incidence of pulmonary complications. Pulmonary changes, however, occurred with severe tissue injuries, particularly crush injuries and injuries of the extremities, thorax, and abdomen, and there was a high incidence of pulmonary dysfunction and failure with sepsis. Thus, the term *posttraumatic pulmonary insufficiency* is more for appropriate pulmonary failure occurring after shock and injury rather than *shock lung.* There are many factors involved in the production of pulmonary problems with injuries, shock being only one of them and probably not a major one. However, shock and decreased blood flow may make the lung more vulnerable to fluid overload and increase the likelihood of later pulmonary capillary permeability alterations.

Coagulation System

In injured and operated patients, particularly with shock, coagulation changes are frequent. With massive injuries, soft tissue injuries, and external and internal bleeding, clotting of blood in the pleural and peritoneal cavities, soft tissues, and retroperitoneal spaces are indeed problems. Probably trauma shock and blood loss activate the clotting cascade and thrombolytic activity. The possibility of intravascular coagulation is present. Available evidence suggests, however, that coagulation changes are not important factors with hypovolemic shock. With tissue injury, multiple operations, and multiple transfusions, abnormalities of coagulation are frequent. Even then, however, the coagulation change seems to follow the severity of the injury, and it is unclear how much that contributes to the problem, its severity, and its outcome.

The Immune System

Both components of host defense, the nonspecific immune system with neutrophils, macrophages, opsonins and complement, and the specific system of lymphocytes and antibodies, are depressed with circulatory failure. There is decreased capacity for phagocytosis by white blood cells and macrophages of the reticuloendothelial system. With some injuries, there are also circulating immunosuppressive factors that may be related to activation of suppressor T cells. It is clear that the patient in or after a period of shock has increased susceptibility to infection.

Metabolic Alterations

Although certain specific metabolic abnormalities occur with shock per se, it may be difficult to differentiate them from metabolic alterations that occur with injury and with stress. The cardiovascular and endocrine responses to shock along with decreased tissue blood flow produce characteristic metabolic changes.

Some changes are adaptive to provide energy during stress. Others are the direct effect of anoxia and ischemia. Hyperglycemia occurs early in shock in spite of increased glucose utilization. Epinephrine seems to be the major factor in glycogenolysis, in early hyperglycemia, and muscle glycogen breakdown into lactate. Both pyruvate and lactate increase in early shock, followed later by an increase in lactate production, leading to metabolic acidosis. With shock, there is decreased oxygen consumption, increased oxygen extraction, and an oxygen debt. Much of the increased lactate produced in shock has been thought to be due to anaerobic glycolysis, which occurs when cellular hypoxia forces a shift from the aerobic Krebs cycle–electron transport system. Certainly this is part of it, but there are also other mechanisms. In experimental animals, epinephrine induces muscle glycogenolysis. Some lactate production is also due to hyperventilation unrelated to hypoxia. Also, elevations of lactate have not correlated with lack of oxygen or decreased production of CO_2 or in patients with ultimate mortality. Thus, the high lactate in shock may indicate not only tissue and cell hypoxia but also decreased ability of the liver to clear organic acids and altered substrate metabolism produced by epinephrine.

In shock, protein synthesis is also decreased, and circulating amino acid levels increase, particularly alanine. Increased rates of urea production indicate greater breakdown of amino acids. The release of amino acid from muscle may result from pyruvate accepting the amino groups through glycolysis. Alanine so produced would then be available to the liver for gluconeogenesis.

In humans, free fatty acids increase when there has been modest blood loss, but when shock occurs, fat mobilization shuts off. With glycogenolysis, there is also a tendency toward hyperkalemia and decreased serum sodium. Evidence of adrenal activation is also present, with eosinopenia, lymphocytopenia, and reduced platelets. Other changes, if they occur, would indicate impaired organ function due to decreased blood flow to the liver, kidneys, muscle, and other organs.

The metabolic response to injury that may occur if shock is not severe and tissue injury is predominant, as with a major operation along with shock, produces a mobilization of carbohydrate reserves, increased breakdown of protein, and bypassing of fat stores. The excessive catabolism and alteration in glucose metabolism can be reproduced experimentally in humans by the simultaneous infusion of cortisol, epinephrine, and glucagon, with interleukin-1 as a major determinant of the degree of catabolism. During and after injury and shock, patients will have a diabetic glucose tolerance curve particularly due to increased glycolysis, reduced insulin secretion, and perhaps some tissue insulin resistance. Later in shock, particularly that due to sepsis, hypoglycemia may be present; this is probably related to the failure of glucose production by the liver and severe and prolonged decrease in blood flow.

Alterations in the Microcirculation with Shock

The central element of the vasculature is the microcirculation. Alterations in the microcirculation, particularly in humans, are not well understood. The microvasculature is thought of by definition as all vessels of 100 μ or less in size. This segment of the circulation thus consists of precapillary arterioles, capillaries, and venules. Once decreased blood flow occurs, not only is there a shutdown of many capillaries with lack of perfusion of those regions of the circulation, but cell swelling and permeability changes in the microcirculation that may produce problems later. Clearly, the objective of treatment of shock is improvement in blood flow to this segment of the vascular bed to improve cell nutrition.

In a normal capillary bed, there is an ebb and flow of circulation so that capillaries open and close periodically. Blood is a viscid fluid due to the presence of red cells and proteins, especially fibrinogen and globulins, and this quality becomes important in the microcirculation, when flow may be slow or halted temporarily. Thus, blood is thought to have a non-Newtonian behavior. It was observed many years ago that during shock, blood flow in capillary beds decreases, and Rouleaux of red cells form. Capillaries become plugged with such cell aggregates. This was called *sludging of blood* and was thought by some to be a pathologic event in itself, impairing the microcirculation with shock. Another explanation was that this is simply a transient phenomenon with low blood flow, which is reversed as soon as blood flow is improved. Most observations of the microcirculation suggest that capillaries open up and the red cell aggregates disappear if the blood flow is improved, no matter what is used to improve the flow. This suggests that sludging is a nonspecific event.

There have been a number of substances that have been targeted as specific agents to improve microcirculatory blood flow. Low-molecular-weight dextran (average molecular weight 40,000) was thought to be such an antisludging agent. Its effect, however, does not appear to be specific, and after considerable initial enthusiasm, it is no longer used for this purpose. It seems most likely that anything that decreases hematocrit by hemodilution increases blood flow. Lactated Ringer's solution and saline are as effective as dextran in decreasing the cell aggregates and improving capillary blood flow.

Another alteration that may occur in the microcirculation is that of increased capillary permeability. In some types of shock, such as septic shock, there may be a change in capillary permeability, particularly in the lung, producing pulmonary failure. In any form of shock with prolonged decrease in blood flow, there may also be a reversal of capillary fluid exchange, with loss of fluid from the capillaries rather than capillary refilling. Some possible explanations for such changes include an alteration in interstitial collagen and other macromolecules to form a gel and trap water and sodium; a movement of water and sodium into the cells, as suggested by Shires and colleagues and by our work; a failure of capillary refilling with major hemorrhage; or persistence of increased postcapillary resistance. Late alterations in capillary membrane permeability could also be a factor.

Thus, the microcirculation is important. There may be changes in late shock that are not reversed as rapidly. It may also be that specific agents to improve microcirculatory flow may have certain advantages after prolonged ischemia. The exact place, however, for such agents and what they might be has yet to be established, at least for clinical use.

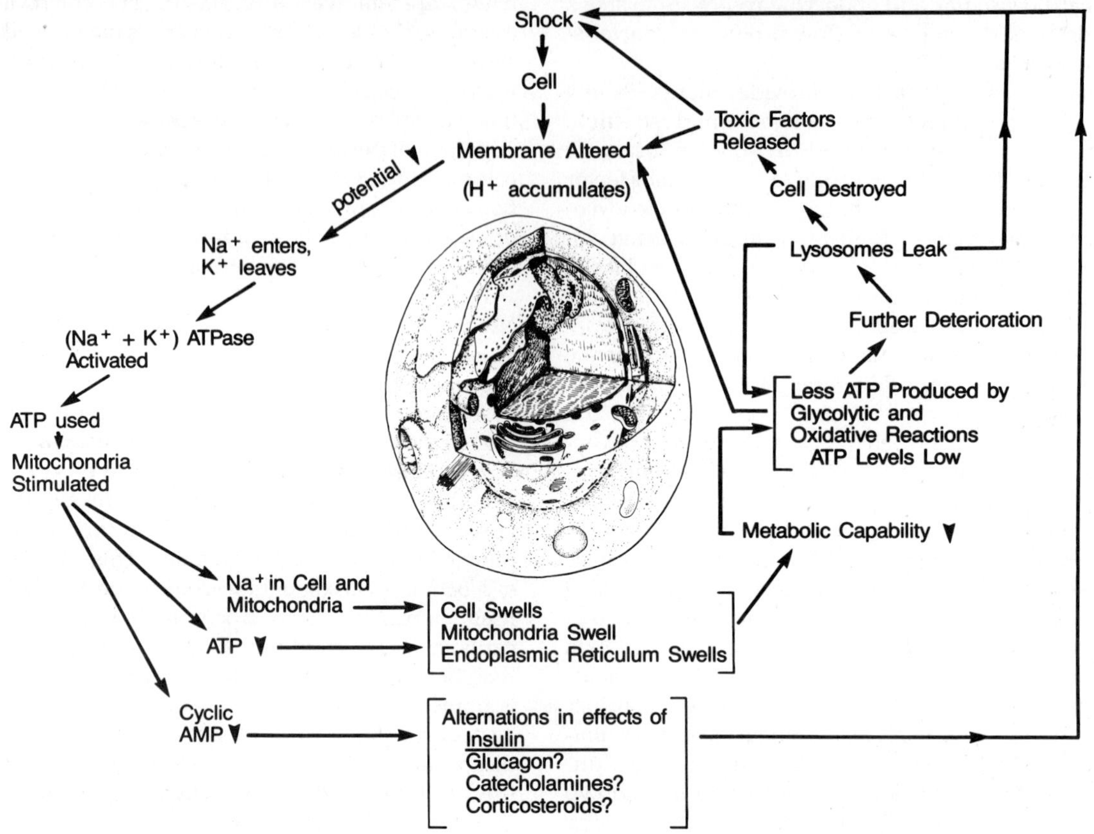

Fig. 26-6. Progressive changes in cell function occur with decreased blood flow, ischemia, and shock. This eventually results in cell destruction.

Progressive Abnormalities in Cell Function with Shock

With severe or prolonged shock in humans, organ malfunction becomes evident even if successful resuscitation of the circulation can be carried out. The effects of ischemia on the kidney, liver, lung, myocardium, and perhaps on other systems is evident clinically, particularly with single- or multiple-organ failure after severe injury along with shock. Organ injury must begin with progressive cell injury. It is well established that this occurs with shock and ischemia. The evidence for progressive cellular alterations with shock comes from studies, primarily in experimental animals, although there is sufficient clinical correlation of evidence to indicate the importance of these phenomena. The altered hepatic function seen in patients after injury is clearly due to ischemic damage to hepatocytes. Shires and coworkers have demonstrated the changes in muscle membrane potential and decreased functional extracellular fluid in patients with severe shock. The tissue, organ, and cell swelling that occur after injury or with ischemia are easily recognized. The major recent advance in cardiac surgery, using cold chemical cardioplegia intraoperatively for myocardial preservation, is an example of the use of this experimental information for practical clinical purposes. The same is true in the preservation of organs to be used for transplantation.

Extensive studies in our laboratory, with contributions from many other laboratories, have provided a sequence of events beginning with decreased blood flow or ischemia and leading to progressive cell injury and cell destruction. These changes are shown in Fig. 26-6. The initial change with ischemia seems to be an intracellular one, with increases in lactate and hydrogen ions, so that intracellular acidosis becomes a major factor. Cell membrane changes soon follow, with alterations in membrane transport and function. Later, membrane potential decreases and sodium enters and potassium leaves the cells. The Na–K adenosine triphosphatase (ATPase) enzyme system is activated. Metabolic capability of the cell is altered so that ATP is used but not replenished. Mitochondria, although stimulated, are unable to keep up with the energy needs, and ATP and cyclic adenosine monophosphate levels decrease. An important factor in the membrane change is an alteration in calcium regulation, and nuclear and protein synthetic activities are depressed. Cell swelling occurs as progressive deterioration in the metabolic systems of the cell takes place. Lysosomes eventually leak, mitochondria are disrupted, and the cell is gradually destroyed. There are many clinical examples of such altered cell and organ functions with ischemia and shock. They seem to play a critical role in the development of multiple systems or organ failure after injury. Treatment requires rapid restoration of adequate blood flow by initially providing fluid volume for what has been lost. Additional benefit may be achieved by biochemical support of these cell abnormalities; examples of such approaches will be discussed later.

EVALUATION, INITIAL RESUSCITATION, AND MONITORING

Rapid assessment of the status of the circulation and of the entire patient is required to determine not only the magnitude and urgency of the problem but also the etiology and hemodynamic manifestations or picture presented by the patient. This is followed by insertion of venous and arterial conduits for therapy and monitoring and institution of other methods of support as required. The manifestations of shock vary with the severity, the stage, and the cause of the problem. In early circulatory failure, there may be very different clinical characteristics produced by the various causes of shock. In late shock or the terminal stages, the clinical picture is similar no matter what the etiology. Patients may exhibit evidence of decreased blood flow to all organs and tissues, along with evidence of sympathoadrenal stimulation.

Beecher and coworkers defined three grades of shock in severely wounded soldiers. *Slight shock* was defined as normal or even slightly increased blood pressure and normal pulse but cool and pale skin. There is blanching of the skin and nails with pressure and a somewhat distressed mental state. *Moderate shock* was defined as a reduction in blood volume of 20 to 40 percent, a decrease in pulse volume, an increase in pulse rate, and a thready pulse, with cool and pale skin, prolonged blanching, thirst, and apathy. *Severe shock* was defined as a blood volume decrease of 40 percent or more and a blood pressure that is not recordable, with a pulse that is weak or imperceptible. The skin is cold, ashen, and cyanotic. There is sluggish capillary filling. The patient is either apathetic, stuporous, or comatose. If the patient is awake, there may be severe thirst. As shock progresses, the patient will appear fatigued and anxious. There may be restlessness progressing to unresponsiveness. If the patient is not recumbent, there may be faintness and vertigo. Postural hypotension may be demonstrable. Sweating may be present, with a clammy feeling of the skin. A decrease in blood pressure and blood flow will produce hyperventilation and tachycardia. Veins in the neck and extremities will be collapsed. There will be muscle weakness. Body temperature will be somewhat reduced. Some of the central nervous system depression with shock may be due to reduced blood flow and endorphin secretion from the hypothalamus. The response of an otherwise normal individual to injury will also be affected by sympathoadrenal, hypothalamic, and hypophyseal responses to the injury and the stress or alarm reaction.

The previous description is that of a patient with injury or operation or an illness in which there has been a loss of blood or extracellular fluid volume and body water; this is hypovolemic shock. In other forms of shock, such as cardiogenic or septic shock, the clinical appearance of the patient may be similar in the late phases. However, in the early stage of cardiogenic shock, the patient will have other manifestations, including neck vein distention, and may have more difficulty breathing and perhaps less anxiety than is produced by an injury. The clinical picture of a patient developing early septic shock will depend on the insult. Often there will have been a shaking chill with temperature elevation. The patient will be warm and dry, with a bounding pulse and evidence of a hyperdynamic circulation with a high cardiac output. The prodrome of septic shock has been described by McLean and includes hyperventilation and respiratory alkalosis, along with mental aberrations in a patient with sepsis. This prodrome may occur before the blood pressure begins to fall and before there is other evidence of circulatory failure. Sepsis is associated with a hyperdynamic circulation (increased cardiac output), and, if septic shock occurs, the circulation may continue to be hyperdynamic in the early phases, particularly if the patient has an adequate extracellular and vascular volume. When an inadequate blood volume or myocardial problems occur, the patient in early septic shock may have an immediate hypodynamic circulation with low cardiac output—the constricted state of hypovolemic or cardiogenic shock. In all forms of shock, the final or terminal phase is similar: cold, hypotensive, decreased organ function, and apathy progressing to coma.

After rapid initial assessment of the circulation and of the entire patient, the ABCs of resuscitation are required, with the establishment of an *a*irway if necessary, support of *b*reathing, and *c*irculatory support. If spontaneous ventilation is not adequate or may be a problem, insertion of an orotracheal or nasotracheal tube may be necessary. (An emergency tracheostomy is seldom if ever necessary in such a circumstance.) After establishment of an airway, inadequate ventilation must be supported by a volume-cycled ventilatory system. Finally, the circulation must be supported rapidly by intravenous fluid infusions, followed by other therapy determined by the type of shock that seems to be present. Giving intravenous fluids rapidly is often of help in all patients unless there is overt evidence of circulatory overload, suggesting a primary myocardial problem.

Percutaneous insertion of catheters into several major veins allows the safest and best access to the circulation for rapid infusion of fluids, blood, and drugs. Peripheral veins may be collapsed and difficult to cannulate; therefore, in patients with severe shock, central venous catheters can be lifesaving (Fig. 26-7). Insertion of catheters into the subclavian veins or internal jugular veins can be carried out safely and quickly by trained personnel. The veins in the upper extremities should be used first, considering the antecubital, cephalic, subclavian, or jugular veins, depending on availability. However, if there is evidence of chest injury, particularly with the possibility of either subclavian or jugular vein injury, the veins of the lower extremities should be used. In patients with abdominal injury, the possibility of inferior vena caval or iliac vein injury must be considered, and cutdowns or venous access in other locations may be necessary. Several large bore 14- or 15-gauge catheters should be inserted. Initial blood samples are obtained for determination of the patient's blood type and crossmatching for blood and other basic studies, including a hematocrit, hemoglobin, white blood count, electrolytes, BUN, creatinine, and blood sugar. Fluids are then given with an initial bolus infusion of 500 to 1,000 ml of lactated Ringer's solution over 10 to 15 minutes unless venous pressure is noticeably elevated.

After instituting serial and frequent measurements of blood pressure, heart rate, and rhythm; providing venous access and rapid fluid infusion; and inserting a Foley catheter to begin monitoring urine output, venous filling and venous pressure must be assessed. Although the initial judgment may be made by the appearance of the patient and

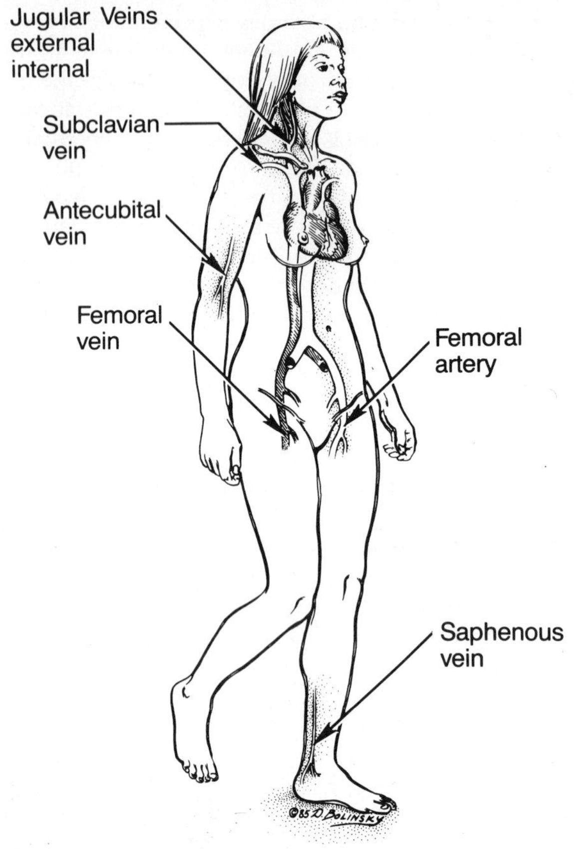

Fig. 26-7. Venous and arterial access points are illustrated.

status of venous filling, particularly with injury and hypovolemic shock, direct measurement of central venous or atrial filling pressure can be helpful if the problem is severe or unclear. Percutaneous insertion of a catheter through the subclavian vein into the right atrium will allow measurement of central venous pressure (CVP) or right atrial pressure. However, central venous pressure is affected not only by intrathoracic and intrapericardial pressures but also by venomotor tone. Therefore, a single measurement is not as helpful as are serial measurements and the response of central venous pressure to volume replacement. A low central venous pressure (below 5 cm H_2O) indicates an inadequate vascular volume. However, a normal ventral venous pressure is difficult to evaluate. Thus, it is more important to determine the response of central venous pressure to fluids than to rely on the initial measurement.

If the patient does not respond rapidly to the initial therapy, an indwelling arterial catheter for continuous blood pressure monitoring can be helpful. This also allows for obtaining blood samples to measure blood gas tensions and pH. Before the radial artery is cannulated percutaneously, the patency of the ulnar artery should be determined by digital occlusion of the radial artery. Arterial pH and PCO_2 measurements will help determine whether the metabolic acidosis of decreased perfusion has been corrected. The persistence of metabolic acidosis in a patient who does not have diabetes indicates an inadequate circulation, regardless of the blood pressure. With pelvic injuries and urethral bleeding, a cystourethrogram may be necessary to determine that the urethra has not been injured prior to the insertion of a catheter. Monitoring of the circulation then allows assessment of the major circulatory components: arterial pressure, venous return, atrial (and ventricular) filling pressures, and heart rate and rhythm. Peripheral perfusion is judged by urine output and appearance of the patient and skin temperature (Table 26-4).

Further measurement and monitoring may be helpful, particularly by insertion of a Swan-Ganz catheter. A Swan-Ganz catheter that provides the capability of measuring cardiac output by the thermodilution technique should be used. This allows measurement of pulmonary artery pressure (PAP) and (with peripheral placement and inflation of the balloon) pulmonary artery wedge pressure (PAWP) as well as cardiac output. PAWP is a direct reflection of left atrial pressure and is indicative of left ventricular filling pressure.

There are circumstances where measurement of left atrial pressure (from pulmonary capillary wedge pressure [PCWP]) and central venous pressure are both necessary. With infection, ventilatory failure, and pulmonary embolism, pulmonary artery and right atrial pressures may be high. With cardiac disease, myocardial infarction, and long-standing shock, left-sided pressures may be higher than suspected. The PAWP often more accurately reflects the effect of volume infusion than does right atrial pressure. In addition, serial measurements of cardiac output will allow appropriate adjustments of therapy, particularly with more accurate volume replacement and the use of inotropic agents if they become necessary.

Full monitoring, which should be carried out for any patient who does not respond to initial resuscitation and therapy, is illustrated in Fig. 26-8. Some of these measurements are critical and necessary in all patients. Others are necessary only in those patients who do not respond rapidly to treatment. There are a number of automated data processing systems now available, one of which has been described by Delguercio and colleagues as the automated physiologic profile. Using a minicomputer or a calculator as described by Barash is known as the hemodynamic tracking profile. Measurement of blood volume by isotopic dilution techniques or by indicator dye dilution is no longer done because the blood volume gives no indication of the adequacy of the circulation. It is a static measurement that does not describe the size of the vascular bed that the volume measured must fill. Arterial blood lactate determinations are made in some centers. They have some prognostic significance for predicting the severity of the metabolic abnormality of shock; however, such measurements are not useful in therapy.

Other adjunctive measurements may be helpful, such as oxygen administered by mask or nasal catheter. A nasogastric tube emptying the stomach may prevent aspiration and allow initiation of a program to prevent stress ulceration and bleeding. Close observation and communication with the patient by the surgeon is required. The most important thing in the treatment of shock is continuous observation and adjustment of therapy. It is not possible to write orders and leave for several hours. The patient must be observed minute by minute for circulatory improvement and alteration of therapy, depending on their hemodynamic picture.

Table 26-4. Monitoring of cardiovascular renal function during shock

Measurement	Normal values	Derived variables	Importance of measurement
Observation of patient	Appearance and sense of well-being	—	—
Heart rate	70–80/min	—	Critical
ECG-monitor	Normal sinus rhythm normal tracing	—	Important
12-lead ECG	No ischemia or strain	—	Critical for cardiac problems
Arterial pressure	95–140/70–90 mm Hg	Pulse pressure 40 mm Hg	Critical
Intermittent		Mean pressure 80–105	
Continuous			Critical for major problems
Postural change in blood pressure	Decrease in pressure with upright posture suggests hypovolemia	—	—
Central venous (right atrial pressure)	5 ± 2 cm saline	—	Critical if shock does not respond immediately
Pulmonary artery pressure	20–30/7–12 mm Hg	Mean posteroanterior pressure 10–16	Can be helpful
Pulmonary artery wedge pressure	5 ± 2 cm saline	—	Very important (reflects lateroanterior pressure)
Cardiac output	4–6.5 liters/min	Cardiac index—cardiac output/m^2 (body surface area) allows calculation of stroke index, systemic and pulmonary vascular resistance, left and right ventricular work index	Very important
Blood volume	3 liters/m^2 (8.5–9.0% body weight)	—	Little or no help in treating patients (may mislead)
Arterial blood samples			
PO_2	85–100 mm Hg (at sea level)	—	Important if ventilation is a problem
PCO_2	39–41 mm Hg	—	Important if ventilation is a problem
pH	7.39–7.41	—	Important if ventilation is a problem
O_2 content	17–20 ml/100 ml	—	Limited value
Lactate	—	—	Little help
Mixed venous O_2 content	14 ± 1.0 ml/100 ml	—	Limited value
Venous blood			
Hematocrit	38–42	—	Important
Hemoglobin	14 ± 1 gm/100 ml	—	Important
Creatinine	0.7–1.5 mg/100 ml	—	—
Osmolality	285–295 mOsm/kg water	—	Important to monitor renal function
Urine			
Volume	50 ml/hr optimal	—	Critical
Specific gravity	1.005–1.030	—	Helpful
Sodium	<20 mEq/liter with injury or operation	—	Helpful
Creatinine	75 mg/100 ml	Urine/plasma creatinine ratio >20	Helpful
Osmolality	900–1330 mOsm/kg water	Urine/plasma ratio—osmolality >3–4.7	

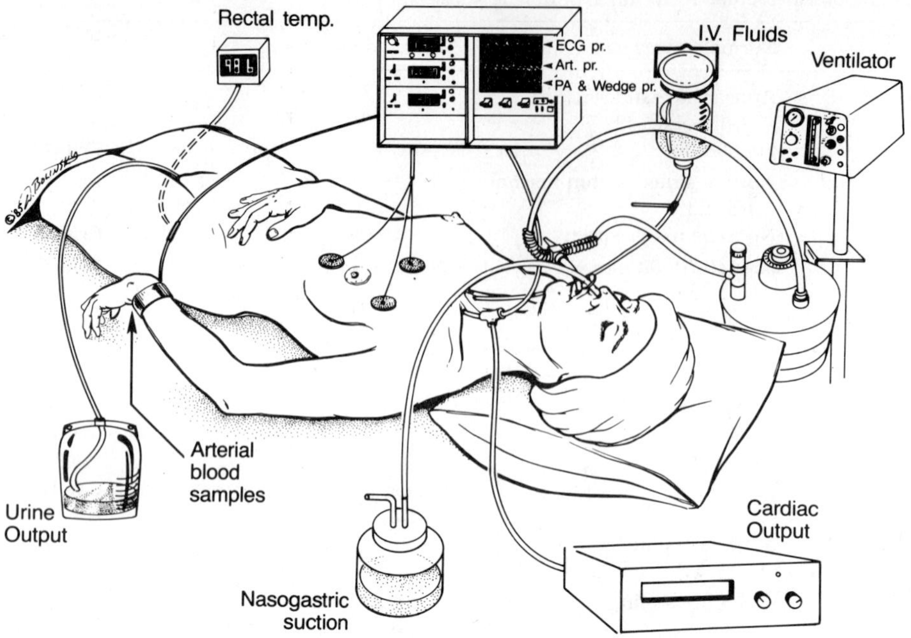

Fig. 26-8. Monitoring and care of the severely injured patient usually require measures illustrated.

THE CULMINATION OF PROLONGED SHOCK—MULTIPLE ORGAN FAILURE

With rapid resuscitation of injured patients, careful support of operated patients, postinjury and postoperative monitoring, and the careful treatment of shock, most patients should get along satisfactorily. Support of the circulation is usually possible to improve blood pressure and flow to some reasonable extent. Such support, however, may not allow optimal perfusion of various organs, and the ultimate effect may be individual and multiple organ failure. Thus, in severely injured patients, patients developing complications after major operations or those that develop severe sepsis, the circulation may be supported only to have the progressive development of pulmonary failure, renal failure, alterations in hepatic function, inability of the gastrointestinal tract to work satisfactorily, and other problems. This has resulted in a syndrome called *multiple organ failure,* which has increasingly been recognized. It is still the major cause of death in patients who survive initially after an injury but later develop complications, particularly infection.

HYPOVOLEMIC SHOCK

ETIOLOGY

Inadequate circulating blood volume is the most common cause of circulatory failure in surgical and injured patients. This may be due to an overt and readily determined cause, such as blood loss with injury, or to a more obscure cause, such as restriction of extracellular fluid volume due to sodium restriction and diuretics for hypertension. Anything that results in the loss of body water, if extensive, may produce hypovolemic shock (see Table 26-1).

With an operation, blood loss in the operating room can be measured by the weight of sponges used and the volume of blood suctioned from the operative field or site of injury. With injury, however, blood loss may not be measurable, and estimates must be made of the amount of loss and the amount of replacement that is necessary to restore the circulation to normal. It is recognized that with a fracture of the femoral shaft, there is considerable muscle injury, and that blood loss into the thigh can be as much as several liters. A severe soft tissue injury of the thigh with a femoral fracture may be sufficient in itself to produce hypovolemic shock. Fractures of the pelvis and lumbar spine with retroperitoneal hemorrhage may produce extensive blood loss in the muscles, subcutaneous tissue, and retroperitoneal region. With injury, there is also fluid loss of extracellular fluid into the site of injury (the swelling and bruises of an injury due to blood and fluids in the tissues).

Blood loss after operation can be estimated only if it comes out through drains and is collected. In addition, there is extracellular fluid lost in the area of the wound or injury. This has been called "the third space" or sequestration of extracellular fluid volume in the site of injury. After a simple elective cholecystectomy where measured blood loss may be as low as 200 ml, there may be 500 to 1,000 ml of extracellular fluid sequestered in the incision and the site of the injury. With an operation of greater magnitude, such as resection of an abdominal aortic aneurysm, extracellular fluid sequestration in the bowel wall, the peritoneal cavity, and the retroperitoneal space, may be up to 5 to 6 liters. Thus, third-space sequestration may, in itself, be sufficient to produce shock. With burn injury, there is considerable loss of fluid into the site of injury. As fluid is given to such patients, swelling of the burned region produces the massive edema characteristic of an extensive body burn. The magnitude of fluid loss is related to the extent of burn, leading to various formulae for the treatment of these patients. Intestinal obstruction produces extracellular fluid volume loss and eventual circulatory failure due to fluid in the lumen of the obstructed bowel (which may be vomited), swelling of the bowel wall, and transudate into the peritoneal cavity. A perforated ulcer releasing gastric and duodenal contents into the peritoneal cavity produces an acid burn with considerable fluid sequestered in the peritoneal cavity and eventual shock on that basis. Crush injury and other forms of injury can result in appreciable volume loss. Losses from the gastrointestinal tract by means of fistulas, vomiting, or diarrhea, will cause electrolyte and fluid deficiencies that may result in shock.

Vigorous preparation of the colon for an operation on the large bowel can produce desalting water loss and be the setting for circulatory failure, as can the extensive use of diuretics, salt restriction, and dehydration from perspiration and high environmental temperatures. Recognition of the etiology or etiologies involved in producing a volume deficit is important. However, it is almost never possible to have an exact documentation of the amount lost. This estimate must be made in two ways: (1) *The severity of the shock* will provide some initial estimate of the circulatory deficit and the amount required to replace the deficit. Rough estimates of the severity of shock and volume loss were described earlier. Three hundred to 500 ml of blood loss may produce little circulatory inadequacy and allow for compensation. Loss of blood volume of 500 to 1,000 ml or a comparable amount of extracellular fluid volume will result in modest hypotension. Rapid loss of more than 1,000 ml of blood or 3 to 4 liters of extracellular fluid will lead to significant shock, hypotension, and the characteristic hemodynamic picture of hypovolemic shock. (2) *The response to fluids* given intravenously is the ultimate measure of what has been lost and what is needed. Thus, blood or fluids must be given to provide adequate circulation. The amounts required for replacement may exceed the amount lost originally, particularly if the patient has been in shock for a period of time.

PATHOPHYSIOLOGY

Although the critical problem in producing hypovolemic shock is an inadequate circulating vascular volume, an exact definition or measurement of the blood volume is not helpful. Measurement of blood volume can be accomplished by several dilution methods: (1) using albumin tagged with radioactive iodine to measure the plasma volume, (2) using a dye, T-1824, for measurement of plasma volume; and (3) various tags, such as radioactive chromates on red cells, to measure red cell volume. Measurement of plasma volume and hematocrit provide a reasonable approximation of total blood volume. A measurement of blood volume, however, is a static measurement and does not describe the size of the vascular bed in which that volume must circulate. Blood volumes were once measured frequently and extensively in intensive care units until it was found that such measurements were not particularly helpful. It did not matter if the measured blood volume was high or low. The important factors were the characteristics of the circulation. Thus, the actual blood volume measurement gave way to the concept of an adequate *functioning* vascular volume. This can be determined only by filling the circulation by volume replacement until venous pressure begins to increase and the arterial circulation and organ function return toward normal. If a patient is hypotensive with a low filling pressure of the atria, he or she requires volume replacement regardless of what the measured blood volume would be. Similarly, if filling pressures are high, there is a cardiac problem regardless of the blood volume measurement or the extent of fluid loss.

Maintenance of vascular volume also requires adequate total body water and extracellular fluid volume. The size of the extracellular fluid volume is determined in good part by the primary extracellular cation, sodium. Thus, if total body sodium is decreased by sodium restriction or by diuresis, extracellular fluid and vascular volume will be reduced accordingly.

Alteration in cell and organ function, metabolic changes, and other processes that take place with hypovolemic shock are described earlier in this chapter.

HEMODYNAMIC CHARACTERISTICS

The primary distinguishing hemodynamic characteristic of hypovolemic shock is a reduced filling pressure for the ventricles that does not allow an adequate cardiac output and arterial circulation. In an otherwise normal individual, the filling pressures of the right and left ventricles will be low (below 5–6 cm H_2O). The level of an accurately measured right atrial pressure or left atrial pressure as measured by PCWP is a reasonable reflection of the extent of hypovolemia. With modest hypovolemia, central venous pressures may be normal. If, however, the patient has heart disease, such as mitral stenosis, pulmonary hypertension, or right ventricular failure, or has secondary myocardial depression from drugs, prolonged hypovolemia, or other problems, the central venous pressure may be normal or high in spite of the presence of hypovolemia. Thus, the importance of venous pressure is not the absolute or initial measurement, but rather what happens to venous pressure as treatment is initiated and circulatory volume is replenished.

Also included in the hemodynamic characteristics is the fact that the patient's skin will be cool, clammy, and pale and ventilatory rate will often be increased (see Fig. 26-2). The patient's mental status may be altered, varying from decreased awareness to decreased responsiveness. Peripheral veins will either be flat, nondistended, or invisible. Arterial pressure will be decreased and heart rate increased, whereas urine output is decreased. Peripheral vascular resistance will be increased as cardiac index is decreased. The arterial-venous oxygen difference will be increased. Arterial blood PO_2 may be normal or decreased, and pH will be lower. PCO_2 is diminished as a compensation for metabolic acodisis. Lactate levels rise, and hematocrit, although initially normal, will decrease as hemodilution occurs. If shock continues or becomes more severe, decreased organ function may be manifest, particularly initially with the kidney. In a patient with coronary artery disease and hypovolemic shock, ischemic changes may be seen on electrocardiography. Arrhythmias may also be evident. Progressive alterations in other organs and metabolic events will occur as described earlier.

TREATMENT

In any patient with hypotension or an inadequate arterial circulation, a volume deficit should be considered to be the most likely possible cause, and initial resuscitation and treatment should be started with volume replacement. Unless there is evidence of cardiac failure, such as distended neck veins, elevated venous pressure, tachypnea, moist rales at the lung bases, or other signs of cardiac problems, it is safest and best to assume that the patient may be hypovolemic, and an initial test infusion of a fluid should be given. An algorithm for therapy is provided in Fig. 26-9.

Generally speaking, hypovolemic shock is best treated by providing volume replacement of the type of fluid that has been lost. However, if hypotension is present, the response of the patient to an initial infusion of 500 to 1,000 ml of lactated Ringer's solution over a period of 15 minutes will provide information about the etiology of the problem and to the need for fluids. Fluids should be given in the amount and with the rapidity needed to support the arterial circulation. If hypotension is severe, with arterial blood pressure reduced 90/60 to 80/50, rapid resuscitation and fluid replacement is critical. With hypotension to this degree, it will probably take at least 2 to 3 liters of crystalloid solution to begin to correct the problem.

Crystalloid Solutions

Lactated Ringer's solution is the best initial fluid for resuscitation. Compared to isotonic saline, it has the advantage of not producing a dilutional decrease in pH. Although lactate levels will be elevated in shock, infused lactate will be rapidly metabolized and will not add to the lactic acidosis if the circulation is improved. Isotonic saline solution is, however, almost as effective and can be quite helpful. If Ringer's lactate solution is to be given initially for resuscitation when there has been evidence of blood loss, it will require approximately 2.5 to 3 times as much volume of Ringer's lactate as lost blood. Studies by Moyer and Butcher indicated that when blood is removed from a normal individual in modest amounts, a volume of Ringer's lactate solution equal to the plasma volume and 4 times the red cell volume removed will maintain a normal circulating blood volume.

Other crystalloid solutions that have been considered are 5 percent dextrose and saline with two ampules (90 milliequivalents) of sodium bicarbonate added; hypertonic saline, or sodium lactate solutions; and Hartman's solutions. At the present time, these have no specific advantages over the use of lactated Ringer's solution.

Colloid Solutions

A number of colloid solutions have been used in the treatment of shock. In most circumstances, they are no longer believed to be necessary. Plasma was the initial colloid to be used in resuscitation of the injured in World War II. It is no longer used, primarily because of the continued risk of transmission of hepatitis. Serum albumin has also been used; however, it is rapidly metabolized and expensive and has no particular advantage. Dextran solutions have been studied extensively and also have been used clinically. Clinical dextran, with a molecular weight of about 70,000 (which approximates albumin), has been available as a resuscitative fluid to provide colloid osmotic pressure. If used in modest amounts—up to 2 liters—it can be helpful in supporting the circulation. If used in larger amounts, however, it dilutes coagulation factors and may lead to increased blood loss, particularly in injured patients. This effect seems to be through increased capillary blood flow, by hemodilution, and also a dilutional decrease in circulating coagulation factors. Hydroxyethyl starch has also been used for such purposes, especially to provide colloid osmotic pressure after cardiac operations where hemodilution has been carried out. Low-molecular-weight dextran, which was once proposed as a solution to help improve the microcirculation and decrease sludging, is no longer used for that purpose. It is ineffective as a colloid osmotic agent because its molecular weight is only 40,000, and it is rapidly lost from the circulation. It also appears that it has no special advantages over any other solution that produces hemodilution in promoting blood flow in the microcirculation. Other plasma protein preparations have no particular advantage. Although it is recognized that colloid osmotic pressure is an effective and important part of the circulation, replacement of colloids and increasing colloid osmotic pressure do not seem important factors in resuscitation of the injured and in the treatment of hypovolemic shock. Thus, there is no reason to use any of these colloid solutions. In initial resuscitation, Ringer's lactated solution will be equally effective if not better provided that red cell volume is maintained at a reasonable level for transport of oxygen.

Other solutions include stroma-free hemoglobin solution, which is now being evaluated experimentally. At the present time, it is not generally available nor is it sufficiently safe and useful to be recommended.

Blood and Red Blood Cells

When blood loss is not excessive, volume replacement with Ringer's lactate solution may be adequate as long as hemodilution does not result in a hematocrit below 25 percent. The breaking point at which a reduction in hematocrit results in adequate transport of oxygen to the tissues is between 25 and 30 percent. Hemodilution to some modest extent may be helpful in improving microcirculatory flow. Cardiac output must increase, however, to compensate for a reduction in hematocrit and oxygen-carrying capacity. At a hematocrit of 25 percent, an increase in cardiac output can no longer compensate for the decreased oxygen-carrying capacity, and tissue hypoxia will result. Thus, if blood loss is 500 to 1,000 ml, total resuscitation with Ringer's lactate solution may be possible. If, however, it is more extensive, or if hematocrit becomes reduced, red cells must be given. This can be accomplished by giving fresh blood, packed red cells, whole banked blood, or reconstituted frozen red cells. Many surgeons believe that there is some advantage to giving fresh, warm, blood that is adequately typed and crossmatched and given immediately to the recipient. It has not been possible,

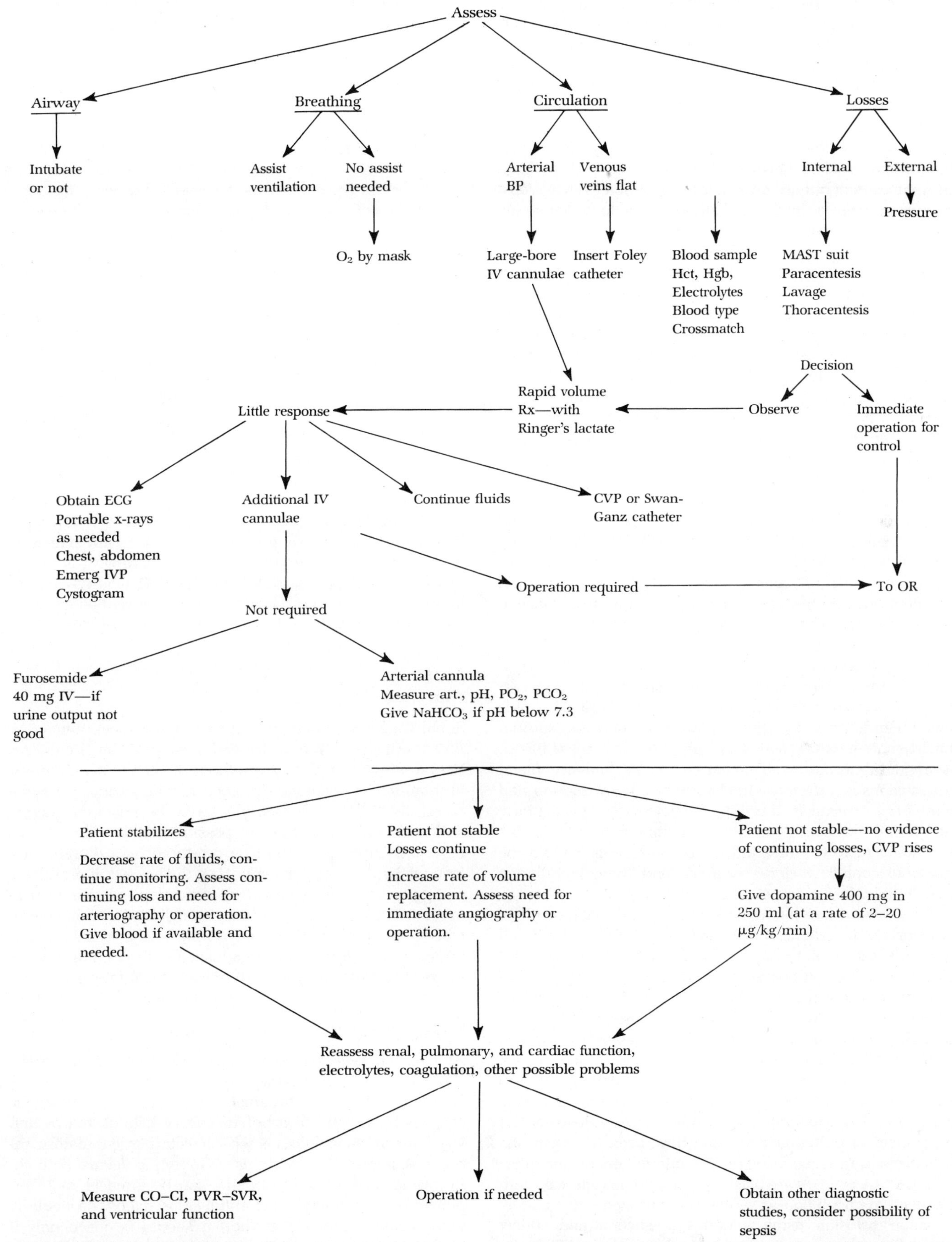

Fig. 26-9. Therapy for hypovolemic shock.

however, to document specific advantages of this approach, and it is difficult and expensive to carry out. Thus, whole banked blood, stored for up to 3 weeks to a month, has been available. More recently, it has been thought that components of whole blood can be used to better advantage, allowing the use of other parts of the blood for more specific purposes. As a result, packed red cells have been provided for use for blood loss along with other fluids, such as Ringer's lactate solution. Reconstituted frozen red cells are used in some centers but are not generally available. When transfusions are given in modest amounts—3 to 4 liters—no problems should be expected with properly typed and crossmatched blood if either whole banked blood or packed red cells are given. If, however, blood transfusions must be given in larger volumes or more rapidly, a number of problems may be produced. Banked blood or packed red cells are cold and should be warmed before being infused. Central hypothermia can occur with rapid, massive transfusions of cold blood, producing cardiac irritability and ventricular fibrillation. If blood is stored for a prolonged period of time, there is a progressive rise in serum postassium as red cells are broken down. The high potassium could be a problem with massive rapid transfusions. In addition, red cells stored for a length of time have a decrease in 2,3-diphosphoglycerate, shifting the oxyhemoglobin desaturation curve so that oxygen is not unloaded in the peripheral circulation and made available as easily to the tissues. The anticoagulant used in banked blood, whether it be acid, citrate, dextrose (ACD) or citrate, phosphate, dextrose (CPD) may produce a problem in decreasing the serum calcium to abnormal levels. This probably occurs only in patients with significant liver disease, where the citrate cannot be metabolized. In addition, blood stored in a blood bank becomes progressively more acidotic, and pH can be significantly lowered. Thus, in patients requiring multiple blood transfusions, it is recommended that the blood be warmed and that sodium bicarbonate be given with 1 to 2 ampules per unit of blood. A major abnormality in patients receiving massive blood transfusions is a decrease in clotting factors by dilution and loss from excessive bleeding. Platelets are particularly deficient in banked blood. When clotting abnormalities occur with massive transfusion, measurements should be made to replace factors required, and the possibility of platelet transfusions must be considered.

Blood stored in a blood bank accumulates small particles or debris of platelet and white cell aggregates and red cell ghosts. These are not caught in the standard filtration sets for blood, and they embolize to the pulmonary capillary bed during transfusion. If a patient receives 10 or fewer transfusions, such particles seem to be of little consequence and are probably broken up in the lungs. With massive transfusions, these microaggregates could produce a problem. However, this has not been well documented in patients. Microfilters to remove these particles are available and are helpful during extracorporeal circulation for cardiac surgery. However, no differences in pulmonary function have been demonstrated in patients transfused through such microfilters during operations. If microfilters are used, they should not interfere with the need to give blood as rapidly as is needed.

Autotransfusion using a device to suction and collect blood from the operating field can be lifesaving. This requires the use of filters in the system and is worthwhile only when a large amount of blood may be lost quickly. The use of stroma-free hemoglobin to replace red blood cells is not yet ready for clinical use.

Position

The patient in shock should be kept supine and horizontal. Elevation of the legs has the effect of a single-unit blood transfusion and can be done during initial resuscitation. The Trendelenburg position was developed, however, for exposure of the pelvic organs during operation—not for the treatment of shock. The head-down position may compromise ventilation and provide a false gravitational stimulus to the baroreceptors.

Oxygen

Since one of the problems with shock is decreased oxygen delivery to tissues, it may be thought that supplemental oxygen would be useful. However, if the patient's lungs are normal and the patient is breathing adequately, arterial blood oxygenation should be normal. Since there may be some small advantage in increasing the oxygen dissolved in arterial blood, increasing alveolar PaO_2 oxygen by mask with an FIO_2 of 50 percent should be given to all patients in shock. If alveolar ventilation is inadequate or there is arterial hypoxemia, assisted ventilation is needed. In any patient in shock who does not respond to initial therapy, it is best to measure blood gas tensions, including PaO_2, $PaCO_2$, and pH to determine whether the patient requires ventilatory assistance. This is particularly true with septic shock where ventilatory failure is frequent.

Diuretics

Renal function should be restored in the shock patient by fluids, transfusions, and drugs that support the circulation. However, along with these methods of treatment, an ampule of mannitol, an osmotic diuretic, may be given, or a small dose (10–20 mg) of furosemide (Lasix) to assist in beginning a diuresis and to decrease any possibility of developing renal failure. A diuresis will not be produced by a diuretic in a severely hypovolemic patient. Also, the hazard of producing or aggrevating hypovolemia by a diuretic must be kept in mind. With injury, myoglobin, hemoglobin, and other proteins from injured tissue may contribute to renal tubular injury, so that flushing these substances through and out of the renal tubules may help to prevent renal failure.

Buffering Agents

Although it is recognized that shock produces metabolic (lactic) acidosis, the best way to correct this is to improve the circulation. In certain circumstances, correction of metabolic acidosis by sodium bicarbonate can be helpful, but by and large, metabolic acidosis is self-correcting by circulatory improvement provided by fluids or inotropic agents, or both. Intravenous sodium bicarbonate can be given (1 to 2 ampules) as an adjunct during initial resuscitation, particularly with cardiac arrest. After that, it should be given only if blood pH measurements indicate significant acidosis. Even then, such continuing metabolic acidosis indicates the need for greater improvement in the circulation and not just administration of a buffering agent. The lactate in Ringer's solution does not contribute to the lactic acidosis, since it is not an acid and is metabolized rapidly by the liver.

Vasoactive Agents

Vasoconstrictor agents (drugs with strong alpha-adrenergic action) have little, if any, place in the initial therapy of hypovolemic shock. These drugs include norepinephrine (Levophed), phenylephrine (Neo-Synephrine), metaraminol (Aramine), and other agents. The only role for a vasoconstrictor agent is in a patient whose blood pressure is so low that cardiorespiratory arrest is imminent or has occurred. Then, an initial increase in central perfusion pressure to the heart and brain by the use of one of these agents for a short time along with volume replacement may be necessary. Otherwise, vasoactive agents should be used only if volume replacement does not correct the problem or if there is a problem with myocardial depression and cardiogenic shock. In such a circumstance, as indicated earlier, dopamine is the initial drug of choice. Isoproterenol (Isuprel) can also be quite useful in certain circumstances. It is a pure beta-stimulating agent with a positive inotropic and chronotropic effect and produces peripheral vasodilation in certain vascular beds. Isoproterenol can be given at a rate of 1 to 2 μg/minute with several milligrams mixed in 500 ml of intravenous fluid. Since isoproterenol has a potent chronotropic effect, caution must be taken that heart rate is not increased beyond an effective level (130–140 per minute). Digitalis is not as helpful in an emergency situation. Even the rapidly acting digitalis preparations (digoxin, ouabain, deslanoside) take a half hour or so for the initial effect, and they cannot be controlled minute-to-minute, as can an intravenously infused inotropic agent. If a patient responds to an intravenous inotropic infusion, digitalization can be done slowly to supplement or take the place of the other drug. Epinephrine and dobutamine (Dobutrex) may be helpful. Other inotropic agents such as amrinone (Inocor) have had insufficient use in the treatment of shock in surgical patients to recommend their use at the present time. Such agents, however, may be used if the response to dopamine, isoproterenol, epinephrine, and digitalis are not effective. Pure vasodilator drugs such as alpha-adrenergic blocking agents (phenoxybenzamine) or ganglionic blocking agents (trimethapan camsylate) are dangerous in treating shock and should not be used.

Antibiotics

Although shock contributes to the later development of infection by interference with host resistance, there is no specific need for antibiotics in the initial therapy of shock. Antibiotic therapy should be based on the injuries or the operative procedures performed rather than on shock per se. However, with injury, there is ample evidence that a broad-spectrum antibiotic given as rapidly as possible after the time of wounding and continued for the next 2 days will decrease the possibility of wound infection if such a patient requires operative treatment. Antibiotics given 4 to 6 hours after tissue contamination, however, have been shown experimentally to be of no value.

Hypertonic Solutions

Hypertonic solutions, particularly hypertonic saline or hypertonic Ringer's solution, have been used in the treatment of burn shock and are effective in maintaining the circulation with a much smaller volume than with an isotonic solution. In burn patients, the burn swelling was also greatly reduced. Hypertonic solutions such as mannitol have been used by Leaf and others to improve reflow to ischemic organs. Hypertonic mannitol has also been used to improve glomerular filtration rates in injured patients and to improve the ventilation perfusion coordination in patients with adult respiratory distress syndrome. Such hypertonic solutions may be beneficial in shock patients, particularly in late shock, to utilize the increased cell water for resuscitation or to reduce cell flowing. However, evidence for use of such solutions in patients with shock in general is not available.

Organ Preservation by Cooling

The use of cold chemical cardioplegia in cardiac surgery has amply demonstrated how cooling can be helpful in preserving organ function during a period of ischemia. In injured patients in shock, cooling of intraperitoneal organs during exploration has been suggested as an acid. This may be particularly important for the liver if interruption of the hepatic circulation is necessary during repair of injury, or for the kidney as well.

Substrates for Cell Metabolism

Considerable research has been done on the use of substrates to maintain cell and organ function after periods of ischemia or with shock. It has been recognized for a long period of time that an organ, such as the heart, will tolerate a period of ischemia, such as during a cardiac operation, for a longer period of time if substrate nutritional support has been provided before the period of ischemia. In animal studies, giving substrate after the insult is helpful in certain circumstances, particularly with low blood flow, circulatory failure, or shock. Substrates that have been used include inosine, adenosine, creatine phosphate, allopurinol, other kreb cycle intermediates, nicotinamide, and, more recently, the use of high-energy phosphate compounds such as ATP complexed with magnesium chloride. Studies are now beginning in humans on the efficacy of such approaches, and evidence should be forthcoming on whether any of these substrates are of value in the treatment of patients.

Continuing Management

After initial resuscitation and treatment of the patient in shock, continuing care must be provided to maintain an excellent circulation, correct the underlying abnormalities, treat the injury, and allow the patient to recovery satisfactorily. Two problems can occur during this period: One is overtreatment with excessive volume replacement. Rapid successful resuscitation supporting the circulation and providing for renal function may jeopardize the lungs and contribute to the development of posttraumatic pulmonary insufficiency. Thus, during resuscitation, pulmonary function must be monitored by arterial blood gases, by listening to the lungs, and by monitoring atrial pressures. Interstitial edema of the lungs can occur, of course, with little initial change. After initial resuscitation, if the circulation is functioning normally and renal function is good, consideration may have to be given to decreasing extracellular fluid volume if the lungs seem to be in jeopardy. The other difficulty encountered is unresponsiveness to treatment. The most common problem is that of an unrecognized volume deficit or continuing losses of blood volume and inadequate replacement of losses. Other problems must be considered such as myocardial failure, sepsis, peripheral pooling of blood flow, inadequate ventilation with hypoxia, carbon dioxide retention, persistent metabolic acidosis, hyponatremia, hyperkalemia, hypocalcemia, and renal failure. Other injuries can be involved in producing the problem, such as pneumothorax, hemothorax, cardiac tamponade, gastrointestinal perforation, or increased intracranial pressure. The term *irreversible shock* has been used for such difficult problems. This is an inappropriate term, however, because no patient should be considered to be in irreversible shock while he or she is still alive. Even though there are patients who do not respond satisfactorily to treatment, diagnosis and treatment must continue with the hope that the process can be reversed to provide survival for the patient.

SEPTIC SHOCK

Circulatory failure occurring with infection was described by Laennec in 1831. Boise, in 1897, drew a clear distinction between shock due to hemorrhage and that owing to sepsis. Blood stream invasion by gram-negative organisms, particularly after urinary tract instrumentation, was recognized early in this century but was not a frequent occurrence. It remained for Waisbren in 1951 to provide a clear description of the hypotension and shock-like appearance that occurred with sepsis. He described two distinct clinical pictures with gram-negative bacteremia in particular. In one picture, the patient appeared toxic, the other picture was of a patient in a shock-like state. In the same year, Borden and Hall described fulminating circulatory failure after transfusion of blood contaminated with gram-negative bacilli. In recent years, the focus of attention has been septic shock occurring with gram-negative infection because it has been the most frequent and devastating problem. It is important to recognize, however, that shock from infection may occur with any infecting agent, including viruses, rickettsiae, parasites, fungi, and gram-positive bacteria. It is now recognized that the hemodynamic picture and characteristics of septic shock are the same regardless of the type of infecting organism. Despite the availability of new information and the further development of new and perhaps better antimicrobial agents, septic shock remains a serious problem with a high mortality rate. Gram-negative bacteremia remains the most common problem in part because of the widespread use of antibiotics, the occurrence of nosocomial or hospital-acquired infections, the emergence of resistant strains of organisms, more extensive and complicated operations on the elderly or poor risk patients, and lowered resistance from trauma, chronic disease, steroid therapy, anticancer drugs, and immunosuppressive agents. The performance of procedures such as urethral catheterization by unskilled personnel remains a problem in certain areas.

ETIOLOGY

The setting for occurrence of septic shock is that of a hospitalized patient who has had an injury, an operation, or an underlying disease process that makes the patient susceptible to the growth of organisms, blood stream invasion, and septicemia. The urinary tract is a frequent site of infection, with many cases preceded by instrumentation such as catheterization of the bladder, cystoscopy, or passage of a sound, or by operations on the urogenital system. Recognition of this as a source of gram-negative septicemia and careful techniques for these procedures have decreased the frequency of this problem. The incidence of hospital-acquired urinary tract infections has been decreased by the routine use of closed systems when catheter drainage of the bladder is necessary. The respiratory tract is also a frequent source of such infections, often with an endotracheal tube in place or with a tracheostomy. The gastrointestinal tract may be involved when there has been an injury, perforation, anastomoses, or other contamination of the peritoneal cavity either by operation or injury. The biliary tract and the development of cholangitis can produce septic shock or it can develop from the skin with burns. A number of cases result from prolonged use of intravenous infusion sites. This has increased with the use of indwelling catheters in the central circulation for total intravenous nutrition, for chemotherapeutic agents, for prolonged antibiotic therapy, and for other purposes. Septic abortions and postpartum infections account for a number of such problems. Recognition of many of these sites of invasive infection has decreased both the frequency and the severity of septic shock from such problems. Predisposing factors include advancing age, diabetes mellitus, cirrhosis, leukemia, lymphoma, disseminated carcinoma, chemotherapy, transplantation with its associated immunosuppressive therapy, and a variety of surgical procedures and injuries that may lead to peritoneal contamination and areas of infection or abscess.

It is now increasingly recognized that injury and operation produce immunosuppression. Shock is known to decrease the capability of neutrophils and both lung and liver macrophages. Protein calorie malnutrition and prolonged catabolism with starvation are known to alter immunoglobin production and also depressed T- and B-cell function. Such deficiencies are associated with decreased reactivity to skin test antigens, producing partial or complete anergy. Steroid secretion with injury and anesthetic agents also alters or depresses host resistance. Finally, it has been recognized that there are circulating immunosuppressive factors with injury, particularly when there is tissue necrosis. This probably occurs through suppressor T-cell activation, which greatly alters the immune response. Thus, it is clear that injury and operation depress host resistance and increase the possibility of invasive infection, even in a previously normal individual.

The most frequent single organism producing septic shock has been *Escherichia coli,* followed by *Aerobacter aerogenes, Pseudomonas aeruginosa,* and *Klebsiella pneumoniae.* Bacteroides and proteus organisms have also been implicated. Organisms that are not thought to be pathogens may, in immunosuppressed patients, produce shock with infection. *Staphylococcus aureus* and other gram-positive organisms can also produce septicemia with shock, as can pneumococcal and streptococcal infections. The widespread use of antibiotics, however, particularly in injured and operated patients, has decreased the incidence of these infections because of their general sensitivity to most broad-spectrum antibiotics. Fungus infections, particularly those caused by *Candida albicans,* which occur in patients on broad-spectrum antibiotics and with immunosuppression, can be lethal. Because of the frequency of occurrence and the devastating effect, however, gram-negative organisms have been emphasized because of their associated problem.

PATHOPHYSIOLOGY—THE RESPONSE TO INFECTION

Infection requires an increased circulation that must be provided locally at the site of the infectious process and generally to the entire organism. If the circulation of the individual can keep up with the demands of the septic process, a hyperdynamic but adequate circulation results. If, however, the individual's circulation cannot keep up with the demands, either because of lack of volume, excessive vasodilation, effects on the heart or other toxic factors, circulatory failure and septic shock will ensue. A characteristic sequence of alterations in the circulation, organ function, and metabolism occurs if a septic process is not controlled, either by drainage, antibiotics, or both. The term *septic* is used generically to indicate a focus of infection that has a systemic effect such as generalized peritonitis, an abscess within the peritoneal cavity, a hepatic abscess, empyema of the lung, pulmonary infection, severe cellulitis, tissue ischemia with infection, or any other process with necrosis and invasion by pathogenic organisms. The similarity of circulatory response to sepsis and to that of the stable cirrhotic patients has been pointed out by John Siegel and others. The septic process elevates temperature and increases metabolic demands. The mediators of the increased need for circulation and the various toxic factors may be complex but certainly are not mysterious. The first indication of an exogenous product with pyrogenic activity clearly distinct from endotoxin was provided by Beeson in 1948. This material was called endogenous pyrogen and could be obtained from granulocytes. Injection of this material produced a number of different activities, including the release from bone marrow of neutrophils, granulopoiesis, synthesis of acute-phase proteins, and flux of amino acids from the muscle to the liver. Owing to its source and the multiplicity of host alterations produced, the active material was called *leukocyte endogenous mediator.* Initially, there was some question as to whether endogenous pyrogen and leukocyte endogenous mediator were the same. Gradually, evidence was produced that they were the same or related proteins. In addition, it was determined that monocytes produced a larger quantity of endogenous pyrogen than did neutrophils. Activation then of neutrophils or monocytes by bacteria, viruses, endotoxin, and other stimuli resulted in neutrophil release, granulopoiesis, lactoferrin production, stimulation of the reticuloendothelial system, and lowering of plasma iron. There is also increased iron storage in the liver, increased acute-phase protein synthesis, and increased release of amino acids from muscle, and a lymphokine was produced in lymphocytes that stimulated lymphocytes. Then it was found that the lymphocyte activating factor also seemed to be identical with endogenous pyrogen, stimulating mitogenic activity for T cells. This lymphocyte activating factor, a peptide of macrophage origin that stimulates T-lymphocyte proliferation and thus enhances immune responses, has now been called *interleukin-1 (IL-1).* The mitogenic action of IL-1 on T cells is probably mediated by the lymphocyte product or lymphokine called *interleukin-2 (IL-2).* There is now evidence indicating both functionally and biochemically that endogenous pyrogen, leukocyte endogenous mediator lymphocyte activating factor, and IL-1 are identical.

Early studies demonstrated that this material stimulated the uptake of amino acids by the liver and that this factor is totally unrelated to any hormonal effects. There is increased synthesis of RNA, preceded by enhanced hepatic production of a number of the acute-phase globulins. This effect appears to be direct without mediation by other hormones and is independent of cyclic adenosine monophosphate (AMP). More recently, it has been demonstrated that highly purified leukocyte pyrogen, or IL-1, when incubated with muscles, stimulates net protein degradation and proteolysis increases, but the rate of muscle protein synthesis does not change. This material also stimulated muscle synthesis of prostaglandin E_2, which promotes protein breakdown in muscle. Indomethacin prevented prostaglandin E_2 synthesis and abolished the increase in proteolysis. Thus, Baracos and coworkers concluded that human leukocyte pyrogen can act on skeletal muscle to stimulate intralysosomal proteolysis by increasing the production of prostaglandin E_2. Clowes and colleagues developed a rat muscle in vitro bioassay for proteolytic activity and found that the plasma of patients with trauma or sepsis had greatly increased proteolytic activity and that the rate of amino acid release from the legs of patients correlated with the bioactivity of the plasma in this proteolytic system. These investigators then found that the plasma factor that induced proteolysis seemed to be a peptide, probably containing sialic acid, with a chain of 32 amino acids and a molecular weight of approximately 4200 daltons. They also found that peritoneal or thoracic effusions associated with inflammation and extracts of human macrophages, as well as white cells and buffy coats, markedly increased proteolytic activity in their assay system.

More recently, Loda and associates pointed out that IL-1 has not been demonstrated in human blood. Their group did, however, find the small 4,000-dalton peptide, which they called a *proteolysis-inducing factor (PIF).* They concluded from their study that this proteolysis-inducing factor, not IL-1, is present in human plasma and that both are produced by active beta macrophages. The PIF seems to be the stable circulating cleavage product of IL-1, inducing not only muscle proteolysis but also hepatic protein synthesis. It is believed that IL-1 is the autacoid and that the proteolysis-inducing factor is the circulating hormone responsible for the acute-phase response. Luger and a group from Vienna recently found that the ability of cells from patients to produce IL-1 was markedly decreased in those who eventually died of sepsis, suggesting a metabolic inability to produce this material in the end stages. This may be consistent with an overall problem of decreased protein synthesis and energy utilization on a cellular and subcellular basis as a terminal event. Blackburn and colleagues have found that endogenous pyrogen obtained from the leukocytes of patients with protein malnutrition produced an attenuated fever and little change in plasma iron concentration. This defect was corrected after 7 days of nutritional support. Thus, the synthesis of endogenous pyrogen by human peripheral leukocytes may be sensitive to the availability of key substrates and of malnutrition. Survival and recovery from the septic process would then seem to require macrophage activation with a subsequent release of IL-1 or its breakdown active form and, in turn, the response of hepatocytes to this agent to produce acute-phase protein.

One aspect of the value of temperature elevation and of fever with sepsis comes from the demonstration by Duff and Durum that the T-cell proliferative response to IL-1 and to the lymphokine IL-2 was greatly increased at 39°C compared to 37°C. Thus, the immune response may be helped by temperature elevation.

Cachectin is a monokine polypeptide (subunit size, 17 kilodaltons) produced primarily by macrophages, which has many varied and profound effects on biologic organisms. It is now believed to be the major or proximate mediator of endotoxin. It has been isolated, characterized, and produced for study and has been found to be identical to another substance called tumor necrosis factor (TNF).

The discovery of TNF was the result of earlier work in which a factor that produced hemorrhagic necrosis of tumors in patients with infections was sought. Lipopolysaccharide (endotoxin) would induce this substance. The early researchers were also looking for a substance that would explain the cachexia occurring with neoplasms and infections. Trypanosome infection in rabbits produced profound wasting and lipemia, which led to studies of endotoxin injection and identification of the mediator that was called cachectin. It was then purified by Beutler and coworkers. Thus, two lines of research—one on tumor necrosis and the other on cachexia—converged with the discovery of cachectin/TNF.

Recombinant human cachectin/TNF, as a potential antineoplastic agent, has been injected in patients with tumors as part of a clinical trial. It produced a rise in C-reactive protein, a reduction in serum zinc, afflux of amino acids (alanine, glutamine) from skeletal muscle, and a decrease in arterial levels of alanine, glutamine, and total amino acids. This reaction is similar to the effect of IL-1. Cortisol levels also rose with the injections.

Although endotoxin is the major stimulus for cachectin production, virus particles and other biologic agents will induce it. Other infectious agents may also stimulate its production.

The functions and beneficial effects of cachectin are many. It activates neutrophils, stimulating their adhesion to endothelial surfaces and enhancing their phagocytic activity with degranulation or superoxide production. Cachectin also stimulates IL-1 production as well as the stress hormones epinephrine, norepinephrine, dopamine, cortisol, and glucagon.

Metabolic effects include loss of triglycerides from fat and decreased uptake and storage of fat. Lipoprotein lipase is suppressed. TNF increases peripheral muscle proteolysis when injected in rats by activation of the hypothalamic-adrenal stress response. It also produces liver hypertrophy, thus mediating interorgan substrate flux. Cachectin and IL-1 are also both endogenous pyrogens and therefore have other similar effects. Antiviral effects have been described, as have other protective effects against inflammation.

Activation of cachectin by endotoxin injection in vivo or injection of larger amounts of cachectin in animals, however, produces severe toxic reactions and death. The effects are the same as those ascribed to endotoxin injections. In dogs, cachectin injection produced hypotension, shock, and death within three hours, with pulmonary interstitial inflammation, intravascular thrombosis, hemorrhagic necrosis, and adrenal and renal tubular necrosis. Stress hormones were increased with hyperglycemia, and there were direct effects on muscle. When a sublethal infusion of TNF was given to dogs, Evans and coworkers found that there was a decrease in arterial blood pressure, pulmonary artery pressure, CVP, and PCWP with an increase in urine output, pyrexia, tachycardia, hypermetabolism, and increased hormone concentrations. These hemodynamic effects could be blocked and other septic like responses attenuated by pretreatment with ibuprofen indicating that TNF works in part through cyclooxygenase pathways. In rats, many of the deleterious effects of endotoxin were produced by injecting human cachectin. Smaller doses produced mild effects, and the animal recovered. Schirmer and coworkers found that a low dose of recombinant human TNF produced a hyperdynamic septiclike picture in rats, but hepatic flow was reduced at any dose. In baboons, Tracy and coworkers found that passive immunization with a monoclonal anti-TNF Fab (fragments of antibodies) protected against *E. coli* infusions that were otherwise fatal.

Cachectin levels can be measured in animals given endotoxin. The lethal effect of endotoxin can be eliminated in animals passively immunized by specific polyclonal antiserum to cachectin. The febrile effect, however, remains. In addition, a high dose of cachectin could overcome the protection of the immunization. Mice of the C3HHEJ strain are resistant to endotoxin and are unable to produce cachectin.

The host response to cachectin production probably involves other secondary mediators and complex interactions with interleukins, interferons, prostaglandins, leukotrienes, complement activation, and platelet activating factor.

The toxic effects seem to be an exaggeration of the normal responses to cachectin, which should be protective. Vascular effects with endothelial damage, permeability increase, fluid loss, induction of coagulation, vascular obstruction, and hemorrhagic necrosis are prominent. Obviously, a biologic organism cannot be prepared for the sudden injection of a large dose of endotoxin or cachectin. Much remains to be learned about these monokines and their effects and relationships.

There are several potential therapeutic relationships of cachectin. First, it has been understood for a long time that cortisol antagonizes the effects of endotoxin if given *before* the infectious insult or endotoxin injection. Now it is recognized that cortisol will completely inhibit cachectin biosynthesis. This occurs only if it is given before macrophage activation. It is ineffective after activation. This explains in biochemical terms why steroids are not effective after septic shock has occurred.

Michie and coworkers gave a bolus infusion of *E. coli* endotoxin to normal healthy male volunteers and found a response of TNF that increased to peak at 90 minutes and returned to normal by 4 hours. Temperature and heart rate also increased, as did ACTH and epinephrine. The white blood cell count increased after the infusion. Gamma-interferon was not detectable. The volunteers had symptoms of chills, headaches, myalgia, and nausea with the fever and tachycardia. Blood pressure did not decrease. Ibuprofen given before the endotoxin infusion did not alter the TNF levels but did eliminate the symptoms and attenuate the fever, tachycardia, and stress hormone responses. Thus, the responses to TNF seem to be mediated through a cyclooxygenase pathway. A similar experiment in humans has been reported by Fromm and coworkers. Michie and coworkers have also given TNF to a number of tumor-bearing patients and found that IL-1 levels did not change. They noted physiologic and metabolic changes that were the same as those found with endotoxin infusions and suggest that TNF may be the primary afferent signal that initiates many metabolic responses with sepsis. Waage and coworkers have now found TNF in 10 of 11 patients who died of meningococcal disease but in only 8 of 68 who survived.

In another study of TNF infusion for 5 days, Michie and coworkers found that it was associated with anorexia, fluid retention, acute phase responses, and negative nitrogen balance. However, the negative nitrogen balance was due to anorexia and not to hypermetabolism or increased tissue breakdown. Thus, TNF is not the entire answer.

Cachectin (TNF) was measured in monocytes from trauma and burned patients and was found to be elevated. The levels were highest in those patients who became septic and in those who ultimately died. This occurred in spite of high levels of PGE_2, which should be immunosuppressive.

Thus cachectin (TNF) can produce severe problems and death in experimental animals and a septiclike state in humans. Cerami and Beutler have indicated, however, that this cannot be the whole story. The high degree of conservation of the gene in mammals led them to hypothesize that the gene and TNF play an important role in host defense. In fact, they suggest some potential therapeutic benefits of its use.

An antibody to cachectin in humans could be deleterious with injury—unless the injured person receives a bolus injection of endotoxin. These questions and complexities have been reviewed in an editorial by Elizabeth Ziegler that accompanies Michie's 1988 study.

The severe proteolysis and excessive gluconeogenesis typical of accidental trauma with infection suggests an energy fuel deficit in skeletal muscle perhaps due to insulin resistance or insufficient perfusion with diminished blood flow with sepsis; glucose metabolism is altered, with hyperglycemia, progressive insulin resistance and increased gluconeogenesis, which is not suppressed by glucose administration; and lactate and pyruvate levels increase without a change in the lactate-pyruvate ratio. Fat metabolism is altered, with increased free fatty acids for the levels of glucose. Ketone bodies are present. There is rising beta-hydroxybutyric acid concentration and decreased acetoacetate. Triglyceride levels are high, and there is decreased utilization of fats. In protein metabolism, there seems to be increased peripheral utilization of the branched-chain amino acids in muscle. As branched-chain amino acids are used, nitrogen is transferred to alanine and glutamine, which is then released from the muscle. Branched-chain and glutamate circulating levels are low. Other amino acids released from muscle are used for systemic metabolism and go to the liver. Proline and the aromatic amino acid levels are high. This seems to indicate a peripheral energy deficit—most likely in the muscle. Terminally, the branched-chain amino acids that initially were low now increase. Glutamine, ornithine, ammonia, proline, and the aromatic amino acids increase even higher. This seems to be due to multiple metabolic blocks. This end stage with a rise in all amino acids, branched chain, and so on, suggests that nothing can be metabolized and a secondary hepatocellular defect occurs. Whether this is due to some specific factor from the septic process or to the overwhelming challenge of alterations in protein provided is not known.

The major acute-phase proteins are all synthesized in the liver by hepatocytes that have been activated. The acute-phase proteins include C-reactive protein, fibrinogens, ceruloplasmin, $alpha_1$-antitrypsin, transferrin, albumin, and $alpha_1$-macroglobulin. Siegel and colleagues recently demonstrated that in nonseptic traumatized patients and in septic traumatized patients, C-reactive protein, fibrinogen, ceruloplasmin, and $alpha_1$-antitrypsin levels rose in the initial 5 days postinjury, whereas transferrin, albumin, and $alpha_1$-macroglobulin levels fell.

$Alpha_2$-macroglobulin is also produced by lymphocytes and fibroblasts. There is evidence that IL-1 or related leukocytic endogenous mediator (LEM) can initiate synthesis of many if not all acute-phase proteins. Inflammatory stimuli have been shown to increase acute-phase protein production, and albumin synthesis is decreased. In patients who become septic, there is a further increase in C-reactive protein and greater decreases in albumin and transferrin. This could occur in the hepatocyte-ribosomal complex and is consistent with the alterations induced by sepsis. The reprioritization of acute-phase proteins shown by Siegel and colleagues support their theory that the primary shift from glucose to essential amino acids for substrate fuel oxidation and accompanying increased aversion to ureagenesis of amino acids essential for protein synthesis may be important factors in influencing the septic pattern.

The relatively simple phenomenon of the local response to infection helps in understanding these changes. The throbbing pain, heat, redness, and swelling described originally by Galen is a result of local release of substances producing vasodilatation and increased blood flow to the area with altered capillary permeability, exudation, and swelling. Heat is produced by increased blood supply and pain from the edema and release of vasodilating peptides. These local effects may be due to the effects of the bacterial organism itself, from endotoxin (a high-molecular-weight phospholipid polysaccharide protein complex found in the wall of gram-negative organisms), or from exotoxins produced by gram-positive organisms. Interaction with white blood cells and macrophages liberates several materials, including, in particular, IL-1. These materials alter the temperature control center in the midbrain and produce other effects on the individual. With the increase in temperature, the initial hemodynamic event is a fall in peripheral vascular resistance. This may be brought about by release of vasodilating substances, by the increased temperature, and by altered neurogenic control. An increase in cardiac output is required. Chills and fever increase heat production with increased skin blood flow to regulate heat production and heat loss. Catecholamine output and protein catabolism begin. There is increased oxygen consumption. However, measurement of oxygen consumption in patients with sepsis and in animal models have shown that for every 1°C rise in temperature, the oxygen consumption increases only 12 percent. Thus, the increase in cardiac output with infection is far in excess of the increase in oxygen consumption. Thus, the increased cardiac output is only partially related to the increase in metabolism and oxygen demand. The initial decrease in total peripheral resistance could be mediated by such endogenous substances as histamines, beta-endorphin from the hypothalamus, changes in components of the complement system, particularly C-3 and C-3 proactivator, and stimulation of the kallikrein system, particularly bradykinin production.

With septic shock, there is an increase in mixed venous oxygen content returning to the heart, in contrast to all other forms of shock, where there is increased extraction of oxygen in the peripheral circulation. This increase in venous oxygen content could be due to several possible mechanisms. First, it could be due to an overall increase in peripheral blood flow but whether high peripheral blood alone can reduce oxygen extraction is not known. Second, there is the possibility of opening of arteriovenous shunts due to high blood flow or diversion of blood from certain capillary beds. Third, there may be a direct cytotoxic effect on cells of the various organs, decreasing their capability to utilize oxygen or decreasing the ability of oxygen to get from the capillary bed into cells and into mitochondria. Perhaps all these factors play a role to some extent. There is no clear-cut evidence as yet for any single explanation. There has been some evidence for inability of cells to function and utilize oxygen with severe infection. However, the major mechanism for this increase in venous oxygen content seems to be increased blood flow with vasodilatation rather than the other mechanisms. The hemodynamic situation does behave somewhat like an atrioventricular (AV) shunt and establishes a new steady-state equilibrium with a very high blood flow and low resistance system. The fact that total body oxygen consumption is not greatly increased suggests that this may not be peripheral oxygen insufficiency.

If at this point of adaptation the circulation can meet the needs of the patient and of the septic process, stability will be maintained with the hyperdynamic state. If, however, the disease process continues and further septicemia or other changes ensue, the hyperdynamic phase will slowly progress to a hypodynamic situation. Initially, cardiac output and blood pressure will fall, and, as this happens, peripheral vascular resistance will increase to compensate, leading to a hypodynamic cold hypotensive state of late shock similar to all other types of shock. An increase in venous capacitance could be one of the factors with infection that initiates this deteriorating state of affairs. As the hyperdynamic process continues, cardiac fatigue may occur, and there is increasing evidence of toxic effects on the myocardium. What these toxic factors are is not known. There have been several myocardial depressive factors identified. Thus, eventually, cardiogenic shock may develop and may be a major limiting factor. Decreases in left ventricular function have been described in patients with septic shock. This depressed ventricular function may persist for 2 to 4 days. If the patient survives, eventually the left ventricular ejection fraction returns toward normal.

The various toxins produced by bacteria or within bacteria have been studied extensively. The various exotoxins of gram-positive organisms have profound effects. Purification of endotoxin from the cell walls of gram-negative organisms has stimulated extensive study, and this material has been implicated in the production of septic shock in humans when caused by gram-negative organisms. This high-molecular-weight phospholipid-polysaccharide-protein complex causes shock and death when injected into a number of animals. This has been a very convenient model for research, but endotoxin injection in animals has different effects than septic shock in humans. Ollodart and colleagues injected *E. coli* endotoxin in human volunteers, half of whom had no response; the other half had shaking chills, fever, a fall in white count, and some vasoconstriction. Smith and Grohlman demonstrated peripheral vasodilatation and rising cardiac output in humans after the injection of endotoxin. Waisbren pointed out some differences in the effects of endotoxin injection in animals and humans, suggesting that in humans there may be a hypersensitivity, an allergic reaction, or an accelerated type of Shwartzman reaction. This may be a better explanation for what occurs in gram-negative shock in humans. An immune mechanism has been suggested by others. As an example, the California hagfish shows no tissue response to injected antigen and is completely resistant to the lethal effects of endotoxin. It has now been evident in strains of mice that are resistant to endotoxin that the morbidity and mortality from experimental sepsis such as with cecal ligation and puncture is much less. This provides further evidence for the importance of endotoxin in gram-negative infection. There have also been studies indicating improved survival of patients when anti-endotoxin has been given. There are also clinically relevant models of peritonitis, abscesses, or injection by *E. coli* organisms. These have established that with localized infection there is increased blood flow to the area of sepsis, but this is only a small fraction of the total increase in cardiac output of the septic animal. Much of the increased blood flow seems to go to abdominal viscera, the splanchnic circulation, and the kidneys. The heart is affected after prolonged experimental sepsis, and the septic animals are very sensitive to the small changes in vascular volume. Further evidence has been provided of the narrow arterial venous oxygen difference in sepsis. Experimentally, it is due to higher blood flow rather than a direct cytotoxic effect. Skeletal muscle capillary blood flow has also increased in septic patients acting functionally like an AV shunt.

The effects of infection on other organs may result in multiple organ failure. In recent years, the identification of single- and multiple-organ failure in patients has led to study and identification of the profound effects of systemic infection on the entire individual and on other organs remote from the site of the infection. The development of multiple or sequential organ or system failure has as its most common feature a septic process. Thus, the development of respiratory failure, renal failure, hepatic failure with an elevated bilirubin, eventual failure of the myocardium, alterations in coagulation, demands on metabolism and gastrointestinal failure all may result from infection in which the circulation is supported so that shock in itself is not evident but damage to other organs develops. There have been a number of hypotheses as to how a septic process, an abscess, peritonitis, or other problems may produce remote organ failure. An infectious process such as peritonitis is often associated with respiratory failure and increased pulmonary vascular resistance as a characteristic of severe septic shock. The development of respiratory failure, the need for ventilatory assistance, or deterioration in ventilatory function may be the initial sign of occult infection. The reason why a septic process such as peritonitis produces ventilatory failure or is related to it is not completely clear. There is considerable experimental evidence that various factors such as a polypeptide toxin from the septic process, immune complexes, aggregation of white blood cells with superoxide production, complement activation, platelet and fibrin debris, kallikrein and kinin activation, and prostaglandin effects through arachidonic acid and lipoxygenases may all damage the capillary endothelium. Such a pulmonary capillary microcirculatory injury would produce an increase in permeability, interstitial edema, loss of protein, and finally the development of the full syndrome of posttraumatic pulmonary insufficiency or adult respiratory distress syndrome.

The kidneys may fail due to remote infection. The mechanism for such renal damage is still unclear. Circulating factors from an infection may produce direct damage or may alter renal and intrarenal blood flow. With the hyperdynamic septic state in humans, renal blood flow is increased, and there may be high normal levels of urine production. There is some suggestion, however, of a juxtaglomerular apparatus injury or injury to tubules in this region due to immune complexes, complement activation, or other factors. This injury may then produce polyuria inappropriate for the level of renal blood flow and filtration. The kidney would then be susceptible to a decrease in blood flow. If the high urine output is interpreted as excess fluid volume being given, a reduction in fluid administration could further decrease renal blood flow and produce acute renal failure. Either high-output renal failure or anuric or oliguric failure could develop.

It is now recognized that posttraumatic hepatic failure also occurs and that the liver is altered by the septic process. Whether this is a direct toxic effect due to decreased blood flow or abnormal intrahepatic distribution of blood flow is not known. If a septic process continues even though the circulation seems adequate, there is often a rise in bilirubin to high levels of 6 to 8 mg/dl with clinical evidence of jaundice. The liver may be enlarged and tender. There is a decrease in liver synthetic and detoxifying activities, which may progress to the full picture of hepatic failure.

Severe or late septic shock is frequently associated with myocardial depression, reduction of ejection fraction, and decreased contractility. Whether this is due to production of some toxic factor damaging the myocardium per se or from "fatigue" of the myocardium from a prolonged hyperdynamic circulation is not well understood.

Coagulation abnormalities are frequent, particularly those of alterations in circulating clotting factors. Circulating fibrinogen degradation products may be identified. However, overt abnormalities in coagulation with evidence of abnormal bleeding are less frequent. There may occasionally be disseminated intravascular coagulation (DIC), which occurs particularly with septic abortions and other overwhelming events. Changes in prothrombin time, fibrinogen levels, platelet count, and detection of fibrin split products may be found in a number of patients with sepsis, but they become severe and have clinical importance in only a few instances. Whether or not such microscopic intravascular coagulation plays a role in the development of multiple organ failure is not understood. There is experimental evidence for the deposition of fibrin within the microcirculation. Whether this is a primary or secondary effect has not been established.

The demands of an infectious process over a number of days or weeks on the metabolism of an individual can be overwhelming. This has been called a form of *autocannibalism* by Cerra and colleagues. A final event in such a patient may be exhaustion of the metabolic processes of skeletal muscle and of the liver that are called on to provide the protein for glucose production and for continuation of defense against the septic process. Detailed studies of the metabolic effects of sepsis with multiple systems organ failure in patients have been described in a series of papers by Borders, Cerra, and their group. They have defined a peripheral metabolic defect that reduces oxidative metabolism of conventional energetic fuels, including glucose, fatty acids, and triglycerides. The catabolism of essential branched-chain aminoacids is enhanced. Along with this, there is reduced hepatic protein synthesis and increased albumin catabolism. This produces what has been called an autocannibalism of skeletal muscle with ultimate death of such a patient due to metabolic exhaustion.

Thus, there may be a number of components of septic shock:

1. Loss of vascular and extracellular fluid volume in the area of infection, such as in peritonitis or in a large abscess, may produce a volume deficit and hypovolemia.
2. With a high temperature and increased blood flow, there is peripheral vasodilatation and extremely low resistance.
3. Cellular and circulatory abnormalities are produced by endotoxins, exotoxins, leukocyte mediators, prostaglandins, kallikreins and kinins, and other toxic factors.
4. The heart, adrenals, lungs, and other organs are eventually affected and may become significant factors in perpetuating or intensifying the original disease process.

CLINICAL PICTURE AND HEMODYNAMIC CHARACTERISTICS

A septicemic episode usually begins with chills, followed by elevation of the temperature above 101°F, with the temperature often going to 103° to 104°F. Initially, the circulation may be stable, particularly if the patient is otherwise in reasonable condition. A prodrome suggesting the development of septic shock has been suggested by MacLean and others. This includes the triad of mental confusion or aberrations, hyperventilation, and metabolic alkalosis. This is one of the best indicators of the potential development of septic shock at a time before blood pressure has been decreased. The most likely explanation for this prodrome is that there is a reduction in central nervous system (CNS) blood flow, even though blood pressure still remains normal in such patients. A reduction in CNS blood flow results in mental changes and produces hyperventilation with consequent reduction in PCO_2 and respiratory alkalosis.

If shock develops, it may occur slowly or it may develop rapidly. During the initial period, the patient will be warm and dry, despite the development of hypotension and reduction in cardiac output. Vasodilation or arteriovenous shunting, or both, with warm dry extremities is typical of early septic shock, with the classic picture of shock with vasoconstriction and hypotension seen only later in the course. Heart rate may be slow rather than fast, and vomiting and diarrhea may occur initially with blood in the stool later, depending on the infection. It is apparent now that the clinical picture of septic shock is determined in good part by the condition of the individual and his or her response to the infection at the time that the septic process occurs. Thus, fever and sepsis require an increased circulation. There is a demand for a higher cardiac output, and the patient is warm and dilated and has a hyperdynamic circulation. If the circulation can respond because the patient has adequate cardiac function and adequate vascular volume, cardiac output increases, with bounding pulses and increased peripheral blood flow (even though blood pressure may be low). If, however, the circulation cannot meet this need or demand because of either decreased circulating vascular volume or decreased cardiac reserve or excessive vasodilation, further circulatory inadequacy will develop with further reduction in blood pressure. At this point, the patient may have the hemodynamic manifestations of either:

1. Hypovolemic shock due to inadequate vascular volume
2. Cardiogenic shock due to exceeding the capabilities of cardiac reserve
3. A distributive problem with excess vasodilation in which cardiac output cannot maintain flow

If circulatory inadequacy is prolonged and progressive, this will eventually lead to attempts at compensation and then a cold, constricted, and hypodynamic circulation prior to death. Thus, the two varieties—cold, clammy hypodynamic hypotensive and the hyperdynamic, warm, dilated but hypotensive picture—are not different responses to infection but rather are determined by the condition of the patient at the time septicemia occurs or the stage of septic shock.

Thus, septic shock requires a higher cardiac output, there is a change in peripheral arterial resistance with a dilated circulation, and there is a change in venous capacitance and peripheral AV shunting. Thus, septic shock may have the hemodynamic and clinical manifestations of hypovolemia with low venous or filling pressures, of cardiogenic shock with a high venous pressure and inadequate ventricular contractile function, and simply a septic picture with a hyperdynamic circulation and extremely low peripheral vascular resistance.

Initially in the septic patient, cardiac index is increased; PAWP and PCWP may be the same (low or increased); central venous pressure may be low, normal, or increased; arterial pressure is decreased with a widened pulse pressure; urine output is increased; the $AV\text{-}O_2$ difference is decreased; and mixed venous oxygen content is increased. Arterial blood PO_2 may be decreased or normal; pH will be decreased with metabolic acidosis; PCO_2 will be decreased; lactate in the arterial blood will be increased; and hematocrit may be normal. Peripheral resistance will be decreased initially, particularly total peripheral resistance. However, pulmonary vascular resistance may be increased, particularly if ventilatory failure is developing.

Observation of the patient will show that mental status is altered. Behavior may be abnormal. Veins may be collapsed—normal or full. Ventilatory rate is increased. Pulses will be full and bounding with an increased rate. Color of the patient may be normal or flushed, and the skin initially will be warm and dry. The decrease in AV oxygen difference indicates less oxygen being taken up in the periphery of the body. Whether this is due to AV shunting or decreased utilization of oxygen by the tissues has not been determined completely.

The white blood cell count may be 15,000 to 20,000 or higher, but leukopenia may occur, particularly early in shock or with severe septic shock. There are no other characteristic laboratory findings other than progressive development of circulatory failure and its attendant features.

In summary, with sepsis, cardiac output is increased, oxygen consumption is increased, $AV\text{-}O_2$ difference is decreased, total peripheral resistance is decreased, pulmonary vascular resistance is often increased, and oxygen delivery is increased; however, oxygen consumption either is the same or is decreased. Eventually left ventricular ejection fraction and also right ventricular ejection fraction are decreased as progressive cardiac failure occurs. Seigel and colleagues have described the entire spectrum of clinical severity in patients with trauma and sepsis as being in four pathophysiologic states. In state A, there is a normal stress response that may be seen in compensated sepsis or after trauma or injury that is characterized by an increase in heart rate and cardiac index with an improvement in contractility of the heart and an increase in oxygen consumption without any overt metabolic abnormality. The B state represents increasing stages of severity and deterioration from the septic process. In the B state, there is a hyperdynamic cardiovascular pattern that fails to supply peripheral needs adequately with reduced oxygen extraction, narrow $AV\text{-}O_2$ difference, and metabolic acidosis. The C state represents further deterioration with respiratory decompensation on top of the unbalanced septic process with profound metabolic and respiratory acidosis occurring. This is characteristic of profound septic shock with hypotension in spite of normal or increased cardiac output and a further fall in arterial vascular tone. The final state is the D state or cardiogenic state, a pattern of primary myocardial rather than primary peripheral failure. There is a fall in cardiac output, a decline in myocardial contractility, prolonged mixing time, and a widening of the $AV\text{-}O_2$ difference.

Extensive studies of patients with septic shock in intensive care units have now provided considerable information. Wiles and coworkers found that there was no difference in any physiologic variable between infection and septic shock produced by either gram-positive or gram-negative organisms or by fungi. There were also no differences between any specific organisms. After volume loading, all their patients exhibited a hyperdynamic cardiovascular response with abnormally decreased vascular tone. Some degree of myocardial depression was seen in all forms of bacterial and fungal septicemia. Heart rate was the primary variable producing the increased cardiac output in their patients. This study emphasizes that the primary defect with sepsis is decreased total peripheral resistance that is out of proportion to changes in cardiac output. This can be called a *vascular tone abnormality*. Vincent and colleagues found that in patients who developed circulatory shock from purulent peritonitis, surviving patients had lower initial plasma and total blood volumes, and they improved with fluid replacement. Patients who died, however, failed to respond to infusion of equivalent volumes of fluid and had increases in both right- and left-sided cardiac filling pressures indicative of biventricular failure. This is further evidence that when myocardial depression occurs, the outlook is worse. Increased evidence for profound myocardial depression both of the right and left ventricle in septic patients has been found. In patients who survive, this gradually improves over a period of days. Whether this is a specific toxic effect or a general effect of the hyperdynamic circulation is not known. At the present time, there are no specific ways to combat this problem other than by inotropic agents.

Patients who do poorly are those who have lower white blood counts, right ventricular failure, no hypovolemia or response to fluid replacement, cardiac output that cannot increase, myocardial depression, and no response to digitalis, dopamine, and steroids. These findings of course are also characteristic of a much more severe septic process.

TREATMENT

Early recognition and treatment of sepsis and septicemia by appropriate antibiotics, drainage, and circulatory support before shock develops is the best way to prevent the deleterious effects of septic shock. The decreasing mortality rate from sepsis is described primarily to the prevention of development of septic shock. The ineffectivensss of prevention with prophylactic antibiotics, however, must be recognized. The treatment of infection in patients requires support of the circulation in addition to the usual treatment of the infection. If this is done effectively, many patients will not develop septic shock.

When mental confusion occurs with hyperventilation and there is respiratory alkalosis, one can predict the development of septic shock. The hyperventilation is probably due to decreased brain stem blood flow as cardiac output cannot keep up with the demand. If the patient is treated vigorously for sepsis at this time and the circulation is supported, septic shock may be avoided. The problems of severe overwhelming infection and mortality from infection in surgical patients still continues; however, we should now be able to prevent classic septic shock more frequently. The problem now is that of development of organ failure rather than septic shock per se. The reasons for the development of organ failure may be decreased blood flow in spite of what seems to be a generalized hyperdynamic circulation. Blood flow to organs such as the liver and the kidneys, the coronary circulation, and other areas may not be adequate, or intraorgan distribution of flow may result in organ malfunction and damage. At the present time, the measurement of organ flow, particularly the distribution of flow in patients is difficult if not impossible; thus, maintenance of the hyperdynamic circulation with infection is imperative.

The patient with sepsis and a failing circulation should be observed by careful and continuous arterial and central venous pressure monitoring, urine output measurement, ECG monitoring, and other observations as previously described for hypovolemic shock. Body temperature, arterial blood gas tensions, pH, and physical signs must also be observed (Fig. 26-10).

Of critical initial importance is the obtaining of cultures, both aerobic and anaerobic, of blood and other septic sites. Although identification of the causative organism may take hours or days, the prompt institution of cultures may be a critical factor in eventual outcome. At the same time, appropriate antibiotic sensitivities should be ordered with the results obtained as soon as possible. In certain infections, there are rapid staining or culturing techniques. Gram's stains may be helpful in getting some idea about the type of organism. This may be particularly true for clostridial infections and others in which Gram's stain may provide some morphologic evidence for the type of organism.

Following this, treatment consists of four separate but related and simultaneous approaches: (1) support of the circulation, (2) treatment of the infection by antibiotics, (3) treatment of the infection by operation, and (4) the use of adjunctive measures.

Support of the Circulation

Frequently, patients with sepsis have reduced vascular or extracellular fluid volumes. Thus, volume replacement by Ringer's solution or other solutions may allow cardiac output and cardiac index to increase to meet the circulatory demands, and a stable circulation and organ function can be obtained. If volume replacement alone with elevation of central venous pressures to high normal levels solves the problem, some would believe that the patient did not truly have septic shock. However, others have provided evidence that responses to volume replacement are compatible with increased chances of survival. Patients who do not respond to volume replacement will then have evidence of myocardial depression, and they do not fair as well. If, with volume replacement, central venous pressure, right atrial pressure, and left atrial pressures or PAWP and PCWP increase to high normal levels or even to abnormal levels, the circulatory problem is myocardial depression or inadequacy. An inotropic agent must be used. For this purpose, either dopamine, isoproterenol, or epinephrine can be given. If there is a satisfactory response with reasonable arterial pressure, a fall in venous pressure, and increase in urine output and an otherwise adequate circulation, this agent can be continued or digitalis can be given for more long-term support of the myocardium. If, however, the response is not satisfactory and the circulation remains inadequate, other agents should be tried such as one of the new inotropic agents, amrinone. An extremely high cardiac output and cardiac index may be necessary in some patients if there is a defect in peripheral resistance. If peripheral resistance is extremely low and the circulation is very hyperdynamic, possible benefit from mild vasoconstriction such as with phenylephrine (Neo-Synephrine) must be determined. More potent vasoconstric-

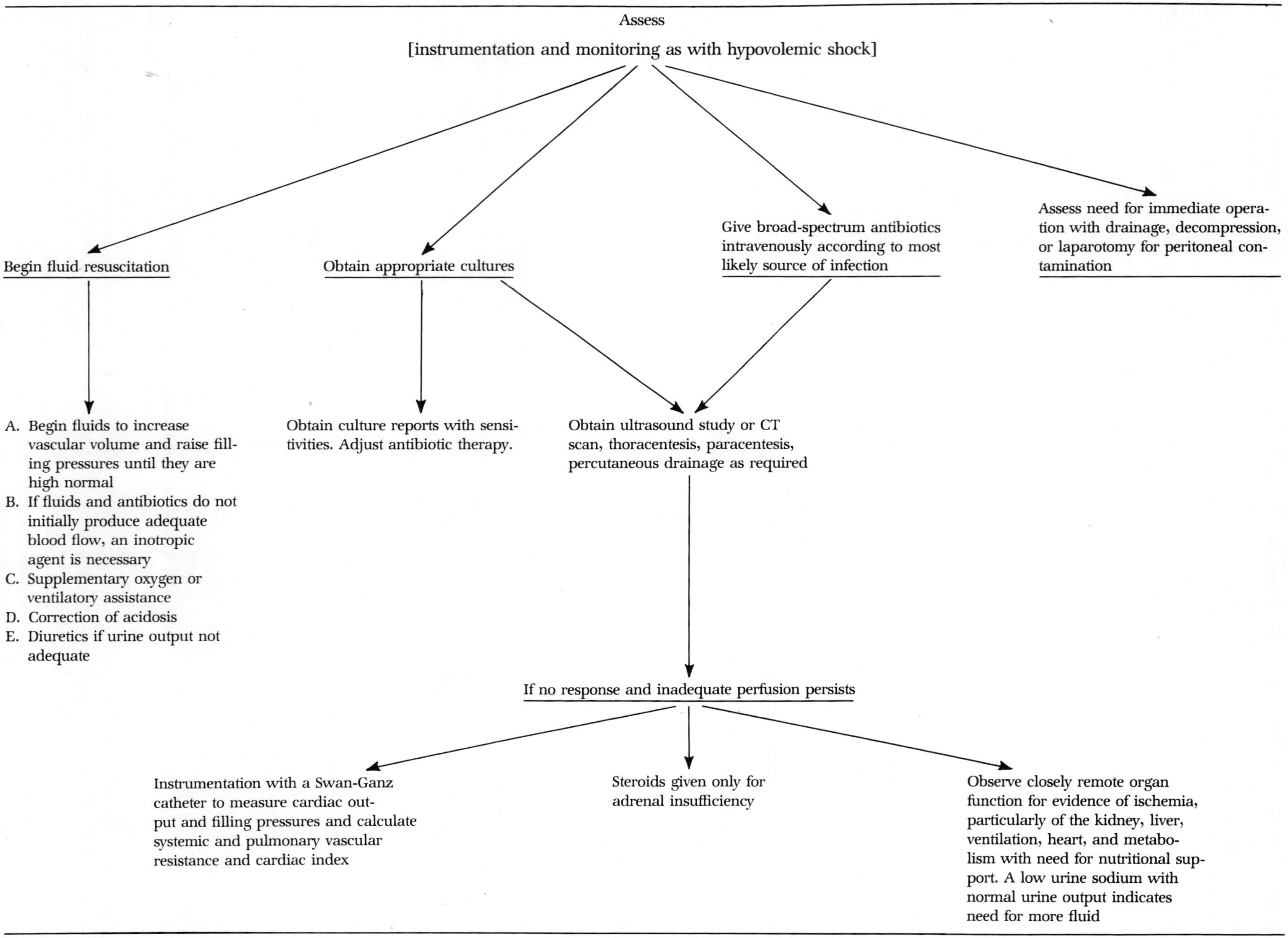

Fig. 26-10. Therapy for septic shock.

tor agents, however, will often produce further evidence of myocardial failure by increasing the afterload. An algorithim for the treatment of septic shock is shown in Fig. 26-10.

Antibiotics

After prevention, the next most important factor in successful treatment of sepsis and septic shock is selection of an appropriate antibiotic for the patient who is desperately ill. If antibiotics are selected and given initially for the organisms present and they are sensitive to those antibiotics, it is more likely that the patient will survive. Altemeier and colleagues and others established that the selection of the most appropriate antibiotic for a patient with sepsis is the most important determinant in final morbidity and mortality. The antibiotics must be given intravenously and a broad-spectrum antibiotic or combination of antibiotics in large dosages is critical. Whether the agent is bactericidal or bacteriostatic does not seem to be as important as selection of an antibiotic for the organism that seems most likely. For this purpose, the site of the infection, whether it be the urinary tract, biliary tract, peritoneal cavity, lungs, or elsewhere, may be helpful in predicting the most likely organisms. Gram's stain can be useful. The local record of experience in the hospital and susceptibility in that institution of various organisms to antibiotics should be used. In general, it is recommended that treatment be started with an aminoglycoside such as gentamycin. If the infection is a gram-positive one and the organisms are known to be cocci, a large dose of intravenous penicillin should also be used. With peritonitis or abdominal wall infections with necrotizing fasciitis and other infections where anaerobes may be active or where there is a mixed infection, including aerobes and anaerobes, a combination of gentamycin, 5 mg/kg; clindamycin, 600 mg a day; and 20,000,000 units of pencillin is recommended. For a potential clostridial infection, a large dose of intravenous penicillin should be given. With enteric infections or nosocomial infections, penicillinase-resistant agents should be used such as oxacillin or a cephalosporin such as cefoxitin, cefamandole, or cefazolin. This should be combined with aminoglycosides such as gentamycin or tobramycin. Clindamycin instead of a cephalosporin has been used for anaerobic infections along with an aminoglycoside. If patients are neutropenic or if a *Pseudomonas* infection is suspected, carbenicillin or ticarcillin should be used along with an aminoglycoside.

Specific treatment for *Pseudomonas* species now consists of an antipseudomonal aminoglycoside such as tobramycin or gentamycin and an antipseudomonal penicillin such as ticarcillin or piperacillin.

Some investigators believe that if only *Enterobacteriaceae* such as *E. coli* or *Klebsiella* are found, a third-generation cephalosporin such as cefotaxime or ceftizoxime is appropriate.

After initial antibiotic therapy is begun, it must be adjusted according to the response of the patient and the organisms cultured and sensitivities obtained.

Operative Therapy of the Infection

The old adage that the sun should not set on underdrained pus or on contaminated body cavities is still true. Prevention of septic shock by prompt exploration of patients with peritonitis, acute abdominal processes, or abscesses is of critical importance. The clinician must continue to evaluate the patient to determine the possibility of a localized infection that can be drained. A subphrenic abscess, an hepatic abscess, an intraloop abscess within the peritoneal cavity, a pelvic abscess, or an empyema or necrotizing fasciitis as well as other infections must be treated early and adequately. Retroperitoneal infection, particularly that associated with pancreatitis, pancreatic abscesses, or other areas of accumulation, requires early and complete drainage. The documentation that remote organ failure may be produced by an intraperitoneal septic process requiring surgical intervention has provided further evidence for this concept. It should now be possible to treat septic shock adequately by support of the circulation, maintenance of blood flow, and initial treatment of the septic process. The final outcome will depend on the ability of the surgeon and the patient to control the septic process by getting rid of the infection or the contamination.

Initial diagnostic studies that may be helpful in localizing a septic process include ultrasound and computed tomography (CT) scans. Percutaneous drainage may help initially. Patients with closed space infections such as cholangitis must be operated on promptly. If there is peritoneal contamination from wounds of the colon, anastomotic breakdown, or other factors, the continuing peritoneal contamination must be eliminated by exteriorization of the leak, by sealing of the hole such as by repair of a perforated ulcer, or by other procedures. If this is done before organ failure occurs, the process could be reversed, particularly if a single definitive drainage procedure or elimination of a source of contamination can be achieved. If, however, there is a generalized process, multiple procedures may be necessary. A number of approaches have been recommended for this, including radical peritoneal debridement, the insertion of catheters for continuous irrigation of the peritoneal cavity after the exploration, leaving the incision open for continuous irrigation of the peritoneal cavity with an open wound, or repeated exploration on a regular basis such as every other day to further debride, irrigate, and clean the peritoneal cavity. All these procedures may occasionally be helpful. It is unlikely that any single approach will take care of all problems or be necessary in all patients.

Adjunctive Measures

Included here are various approaches to modulate or support, or both, various aspects of body functions that can be helpful in the outcome of a severe infection with septic shock. These include evaluation of host resistance and attempts to support it, nutritional support, steroids, and the use of oxygen and other measures for specific organ support.

Steroids

The use of massive or pharmacologic doses of steroids has become common practice in the treatment of patients with septic shock, but it is also an area of great controversy. The use of large doses of steroids is not based on the development of adrenal insufficiency but rather on the pharmacologic effects of these agents. An initial suggestion of help in the treatment of patients with septic shock came from a report from Altemeier and Cole in 1958 when hydrocortisone seemed helpful in three patients with septic shock. There is little, if any, clinical or laboratory evidence of adrenal insufficiency in most septic patients, and there has been no improvement with physiologic doses of corticosteroids. One report indicated that some patients with sepsis and septic shock may not mount an adrenal response appropriate for the situation; therefore, relative adrenal insufficiency may be present. Because of such possibilities, it is generally believed that patients who do not respond to initial therapy should be given a pharmacologic dose of steroids to be sure that adrenal insufficiency is not developing.

There has been a great deal of experimentation, particularly in animals using steroids for endotoxic shock or for *E. coli* septicemia. When steroids have been given before the insult, such as before the injection of gram-negative organisms or of endotoxin, there has been a protective effect. If, however, the steroids are given a half hour to an hour after the injection of organisms or endotoxin, there has been little or no effect. Attempts to study the mechanisms for such a protective effect have not led to specific information. It has been thought that pharmacologic doses of steroids help to stabilize cell and lysosomal membranes. There is a decrease in vasoconstriction, alteration in the deleterious effects of endotoxin, and improvements in cell function with steroids. Several prospective randomized trials have been carried out that suggest that steroids, when given early in septic shock, may be helpful. In one report, patients given steroids improved hemodynamically, but there was no increase in survival. Whether these results would have been improved if the steroids had been given earlier is not known. Part of the controversy is that early in septic shock, when some investigators have recommended that steroids be given, they are probably not necessary and the patient will respond satisfactorily to the usual forms of resuscitation and treatment, whereas late in septic shock, the problem is complex and may also be irreversible. In reported series, it is often extremely difficult to separate out the effects of steroids and other treatment programs being carried out simultaneously. At the present time, it is fair to say that if a patient does not respond quickly to support of the circulation by fluids, inotropic agents, and other measures along with antibiotics and appropriate drainage, a trial of pharmacologic doses of steroids can be tried for several reasons.

1. Adrenal exhaustion can occur late in sepsis. Although it is best to try to document this, treatment should not be withheld.
2. If a patient does not respond to the usual treatment of septic shock, the addition of pharmacologic doses of steroids might be helpful. Since the evidence for this is minimal, steroids are best avoided at present.

There are few problems associated with the injection, for example, of 250 mg to 1 gm of methylprednisolone sodium succinate as a bolus injection to be repeated in 6 to 12 hours if the patient improves or survives and then stopped. Prolonged use of steroids in injured patients has been associated with increased respiratory infections, decreased host resistance, and, perhaps, increased morbidity and mortality.

Nutritional Support

The severe catabolism of infection results in metabolic depletion and cell and organ failure based on this metabolic failure. Thus, nutritional support is important to provide adequate calories and protein. Caloric needs may be way beyond those ordinarily required. The severely septic patient may require as many as 3,000 to 4,000 calories a day. There is some evidence to suggest that branched chain amino acids or short-chain carnitine independent fatty acid such as acetoacetate or butyrate may be helpful. It is unlikely, however, that adequate protein calorie nutrition can in itself alter the course of sepsis and septic shock. It seems, however, to be an important adjunct in the support of such patients.

Host Resistance

Depressed host resistance and increased susceptibility to infection in patients with injury and operation has been well documented. Protein calorie malnutrition in itself depresses host resistance, particularly T- and B-cell function, and many such patients are anergic to nonspecific skin test antigens. If nutrition can be restored and anergy can be eliminated, such patients have increased capability to survive. Support of the immune system, however, has not been possible as yet, although there are studies underway, particularly in experimental animals to evaluate nonspecific immunostimulation. Immune support by giving gamma globulin or by anti-A factors against endotoxin may have some immediate potential use. Nonspecific immune stimulation by using *Corynebacterium parvum,* levamisole, or muramyl peptide and other factors are being evaluated. There is no practical and sound approach as yet.

Finally, the treatment and support of organ function, maintaining good renal function, pulmonary function, and perfusion of vital organs is important in preventing the devastating effects of sepsis and septic shock.

Antibodies

Antibodies and antiserum prepared against the endotoxin core, to exotoxin A, and lipopolysaccharide show some promise in initial trials. Such approaches could be extremely worthwhile.

CARDIOGENIC SHOCK

ETIOLOGY

Failure of the heart to be able to provide an adequate circulation may be due to problems intrinsic to the heart itself or may be related to things outside the heart. Specific intrinsic cardiac problems are those of myocardial infarction, ventricular ischemia, myocardial contusion, arrhythmias, and drug depression of the myocardium. More frequently, however, in surgical patients, the problem is a nonspecific one in which there is myocardial failure due to depression of the myocardium. Whether this is caused by disease-related suppression of the myocardium from sepsis or general illness or is due to nonspecific stress is not known. It has been recognized, however, that after severe injury with significant infection or septicemia or in diseases that produce tissue necrosis such as with pancreatitis, the heart may quickly become the limiting factor in the circulation. This may occur in individuals who are young and otherwise normal prior to the injury or the septic episode. Thus, the definition of cardiogenic shock must be a broad one to include any circumstance in which the arterial circulation and perfusion of vital organs is less than adequate due to inability of the ventricles to pump the blood returning to them and provide an adequate cardiac output. There may be a specific extrinsic or intrinsic problem (see Table 26-2). In addition, the failure may initially be due to failure of the right ventricle as a primary problem or to a primary left ventricular problem. Right ventricular failure by ventricular distention and shift of the septum may decrease the filling capacity of the left ventricle and produce what seems to be left ventricular failure as well. The definition of shock following myocardial infarction was developed only in later years by Fishberg and associates in 1934. Classifications of circulatory failure in 1935 by Harrison and in 1940 by Blalock included for the first time the term *cardiogenic shock*. When cardiac output could first be measured in 1941, Grisham and Master found that cardiac output was reduced after myocardial infarction in humans. Freis in 1952 described the hemodynamic abnormalities of cardiogenic shock developing after a myocardial infarction. It is estimated that infarction of more than 40 percent of the left ventricle must occur before severe and progressive cardiogenic shock develops. Since that time, Wiggers, Guyton and Crowell, Siegel and DelGuercio, and others have described the importance and problems of the heart in all forms of shock.

Extrinsic problems include those that increase afterload, including pulmonary embolism or high levels of positive end-expiratory pressure (PEEP). Respiratory failure and pulmonary hypertension can also produce right ventricular failure. Cardiac tamponade, on the other hand, restricts the ability of the ventricles to fill, producing another type of cardiogenic shock.

PATHOPHYSIOLOGY

Cardiogenic shock may be produced by an abnormality of any of three of the determinants of cardiac output. The first determinant of cardiac output, preload, or filling pressure of the ventricles during diastole if inadequate is by definition hypovolemia and should be corrected by volume expansion. A high volume or high preload, on the other hand, would produce CHF rather than output failure initially. The Frank Starling relationship is that increased ventricular filling pressure produces an increase in the length of myocardial fibers at the end of diastole. This alteration increases the force of ventricular contraction, which then increases cardiac output. However, if the optimal length of stretch of the fibers is exceeded, contractions cannot increase and myocardial failure results. This is the so-called descending limb of the Starling curve. Also, decreased ventricular filling by pericardial tamponade, which compresses the ventricles and does not allow them to fill, or PEEP, which decreases blood return to the thorax, will produce a form of extrinsic cardiogenic shock that is, in actual fact, a preload problem. The measurements needed to determine preload are the atrial pressures that are an indication of ventricular filling pressures. Although ventricular end-diastolic pressure is the most important measurement, it is impractical to measure other than during cardiac catheterization. Also, if ventricular function is depressed by injury, by operation, by infection, or by other factors, a higher atrial pressure or preload may be necessary to obtain optimal ventricular muscle stretch and force of contraction. For this reason, a trial of increase in preload is always necessary, even with an acute myocardial infarction. Pulmonary edema should not occur until a wedge pressure of 20 to 25 cm of water is reached unless colloid osmotic pressure has been reduced.

The second determinant of cardiac output, contractility, reflects the health and vigor of the myocardium and can be effected by a number of primary and secondary problems. Its exact definition is the rate of myocardial fiber shortening independent of the initial length or afterload. Alterations in contractility are the most common problems producing cardiogenic shock. This can occur because of myocardial necrosis after myocardial infarction, ischemia, anoxia, or depression of function by drugs or disease and with such problems as peritonitis or severe injury. A commonly used measure to document such an abnormality is the ventricular function curve. Sarnoff and colleagues developed a family of ventricular function curves with changes in stroke work of the left ventricle plotted over a range of end-diastolic volumes or pressures, or both. Thus, the relationship of ventricular stroke work to a certain end-diastolic volume is the measure of contractility. To get an exact measurement of this, one would have to hold the other variables—preload, afterload, and heart rate—as constants. Obviously, in the clinical situation, this is impossible. Thus, an approximation of contractility is generally used, such as measurement of a left ventricular stroke work and the filling pressure (PCWP) or left atrial pressure. Such points can then be plotted and can be compared with those obtained from normal individuals. This allows a comparison of whether contractility at a particular time is in the normal range or is low. If the circulation is inadequate and filling pressures are high and contractility is low by ventricular function curve measurement, an inotropic agent is necessary and the measurements can be repeated to determine whether there is improvement. A ventricular function curve can also be constructed using the shape of an indicator dilution curve in relating this to ventricular work. Ventricular work is the product of stroke volume and arterial pressure. Ventricular contractility can also be expressed in terms of the ejection fraction and other measures. The ejection fraction is an important measurement. This can be measured in a number of ways, none of which is easily carried out in patients, particularly those in an intensive care unit, emergency room, or operating room. Contrast angiography, echocardiography, and, more recently, gaited blood pool imaging with a scintillation camera will allow accurate measurement of ejection fraction. Acute changes in ejection fraction are most diagnostic of rapidly changing ventricular events and capabilities. The *Vmax* is defined as the velocity of maximal shortening of the myocardial muscle; however, it is not independent of afterload and preload. VCF is a velocity of circumferential muscle fiber shortening that can be analyzed from an ECG. Other measures of myocardial capability, such as the dP/dt-, can be helpful. This is the first derivative of the maximal rate of pressure rise in the left ventricle divided by the intraventricular pressure at that point. This is a good measure of contractility but requires a catheter tip pressure transducer in the left ventricle, which is not suitable for intensive care monitoring. Ventricular function curves can also be developed for the right ventricle and can occasionally be important. The original concept of ventricular function curves, particularly the Frank Starling mechanism, related stroke work to diastolic volume. Since diastolic volume cannot be measured easily, the wedge or filling pressure has been substituted for this. This produces a problem, however, in interpretation of ventricular contractility because it does not consider ventricular compliance and how the situation or problems of one ventricle can affect the other. Thus, with respiratory failure, reduced cardiac blood flow to the right ventricle, or pulmonary hypertension, the failure of one ventricle can affect the other by septal shift and other changes in relationship.

The changes in contractility that occur with acute myocardial infarction with various forms of myocardiopathy, with ventricular scarring, and with aneurysms are fairly well understood. Of particular importance, however, for surgical patients is the nonspecific depression of myocardial function that occurs with a number of problems of acute illness. Depression of the ventricles may occur with pancreatitis, peritonitis, septic abortion, severe multisystem injury, prolonged illness, and other problems of infection. A number of factors have been implicated in the production of such changes in the myocardium. Lefer and others have identified a myocardial depressant factor with experimental pancreatitis and with other problems such as experimental burns. There have been a number of hypotheses and considerable evidence in experimental animals indicating that with late hemorrhagic shock, gram-negative septicemia, and other problems that a circulatory substance is produced that depresses the myocardium. There is considerable difference of opinion, however, as to the nature and significance of such substances. Lysosomal enzymes from ischemic cell, materials produced by macrophages or leukocytes, and plasma kinins such as bradykinin, endotoxin, and other substances may be implicated. It has not been possible to identify exact etiologic agents in humans. Of particular importance is the fact that at the present time nothing can be done to reverse these agents other than to treat the septic or necrotic process. It is most important to remember, however, that myocardial depression may occur or develop in many seriously ill patients, even those who are young and in otherwise good health with previously normal hearts. This must be treated appropriately by support of ventricular function.

Problems of heart rate can produce cardiogenic shock if heart rate is above 150 to 160 beats/minute. Diastolic filling time may be too short to allow satisfactory stroke volume and cardiac output. Thus, uncontrolled atrial fibrillation with a rapid ventricular response or ventricular tachycardia can be a life-threatening problem requiring immediate therapy. Bradycardia with a heart rate of below 40 to 50 beats/minute may also be associated with an inadequate cardiac output. This may be due to complete heart block or to drug toxicity or other problems.

The fourth component of determination of cardiac output is that of afterload. Problems of afterload may occur both with high or low peripheral or pulmonary vascular resistance. Low afterload or decreased resistance is characteristic of neurogenic shock and of septic shock. It has been determined that certain patients with acute myocardial infarction have a lower peripheral vascular resistance than would be predicted from the decrease in cardiac output. Thus, hypotension could be the result. Such happenings indicate the importance of measuring not only cardiac output and cardiac index but also peripheral vascular resistance. Decreases in afterload, however, do not, as far as is known, produce cardiogenic problems. An acute increase in afterload, however, can quickly result in ventricular dilatation and failure. This may occur with spontaneous aortic dissection, with crossclamping of the aorta during the treatment of aneurysms, or for other hypertensive problems. Adjustment of afterload in such circumstances may be a critical factor in preserving myocardial function. If the ventricles are depressed or damaged, even normal resistance may not be tolerated. In such circumstances, a reduction in afterload may be necessary in order to maintain adequate ventricular performance. With ventricular injury, it may be necessary to provide a higher preload and lower afterload to maintain a satisfactory cardiac output. With pulmonary embolism, the major problem for the right ventricle is increased afterload.

Shock produced by cardiogenic problems will initiate a chain of events to compensate for decreased blood flow and pressure similar to those of hypovolemic shock. Eventually, the effects on organ function metabolism, particularly on cellular events, will be similar to those described previously.

HEMODYNAMIC CHARACTERISTICS

The measurements and observations found in a patient with cardiogenic shock are shown in Fig. 26-3. The patient may have normal or depressed mental status. Veins in the neck and extremities, if the extremities are below the level of the right atrium, will be full and not flat. Ventilatory rate may be normal or increased. Pulse is normal or may be weak. The heart rate may be normal or increased. Color may be normal or pale, and the skin may be cool or normal in temperature. Central venous pressure or right atrial pressure will be elevated as will be PAWP unless the failure is limited to the right ventricle initially. Cardiac index, arterial pressure, and urine output will be decreased. The AV-O_2 difference will be widened, and arterial blood PO_2 may be low or normal, and pH will be decreased with the development of metabolic acidosis. PCO_2 may be increased or decreased. Lactate levels in the blood will be increased, and hematocrit will be unchanged. Peripheral resistance, if measured, may be normal or increased.

It is also necessary to remember that a patient with a primary myocardial problem may have the manifestations of other forms of shock. For example, if a patient who has been on digitalis and diuretics and on a salt-restricted diet develops an acute myocardial infarction and shock, the etiologic diagnosis is cardiogenic shock. However, the patient may actually be volume deficient and may respond to intravenous fluids to support the circulation and cardiac output. In the same way, an elderly patient with coronary artery disease and gastrointestinal bleeding would by definition have hypovolemic shock but may in actual fact have the hemodynamic manifestations of cardiogenic shock (see Fig. 26-1). The major differential feature between cardiogenic shock and other circulatory problems is the high filling pressures of the left or right ventricles, or both. Septic shock may eventually result in cardiogenic shock as circulatory and myocardial depression occur. Thus, the clinical features of cardiogenic shock are similar to those of hypovolemia with the exception of increased venous pressure. This major differential point is critical in treatment. A cardiogenic problem may also be associated with or produce pulmonary problems leading to CHF or pulmonary edema with dyspnea, rales, and x-ray findings of pulmonary congestion.

TREATMENT

Appropriate therapy for cardiogenic shock requires an exact definition of the problem. The finding of a high or rising venous pressure in the face of an inadequate arterial circulation or inadequate peripheral perfusion indicates that the heart is the problem no matter what the original etiology of the patient's illness. This determination must be made by initial monitoring and measurements of cardiovascular function. Since so many problems in surgical patients are those of hypovolemia, it is critical to be sure that the patient does not have a volume deficit or to determine whether the patient will improve if vascular volume is increased by fluid administration. Even though a patient has had an acute myocardial infarction, it is necessary to determine whether hypotension, if present, will respond to a careful infusion of intravenous fluids such as Ringer's lactate solution. A patient with an acute myocardial problem may, because of prior diuresis and salt restriction, have a low vascular and extracellular fluid volume. It is also important to determine whether or not there is a mechanical problem such as a pulmonary embolus producing right ventricular failure or pericardial tamponade producing inability for ventricular filling and thus a preload problem. Thus, the checklist of diagnostic possibilities must be considered; however, treatment must be based on an exact determination of whether the problem is that of preload, altered contractility, an afterload problem, or heart rate. Other diagnostic studies will be necessary, including a 12-lead ECG, chest x-ray, ventilation/perfusion lung scan, pulmonary arteriography, or other diagnostic procedures (Fig. 26-11).

If the problem is bradycardia, an infusion of isoproterenol should be started. This is the most rapid and expeditious way to increase heart rate to a reasonable level. Following this, consideration must be given as to whether a temporary and then permanent pacemaker will be needed. For tachyarrhythmias, initial therapy may be by intravenous lidocaine, calcium channel–blocking agents, propranolol, cardioversion, or digitalis.

The combination of muffled or distant heart sounds, rising or high venous pressure, an enlarged heart to percussion, and pulsus paradoxus indicates pericardial tamponade. An ultrasound study of the heart should provide this diagnosis, or a diagnostic-therapeutic pericardiocentesis can be carried out.

If the problem seems to be that of a pulmonary embolus with increased afterload on the right ventricle confirmed by ventilation/perfusion lung scan or pulmonary arteriogram, or both, a number of measures must be carried out. Supplementary oxygen, ventilatory assistance, intravenous heparin, and an inotropic agent may be helpful. Consideration, however, must be given to percutaneous catheter embolectomy or an open pulmonary embolectomy if the patient does not respond.

With decreased ventricular capability or an alteration in contractility for whatever reason, infusion of an inotropic agent is necessary beginning with dopamine, epinephrine, or isoproterenol. Although digitalis may be used, rapid-acting digitalis preparation still requires 20 minutes for initial effect and a number of hours for maximum effect. The intravenously infused inotropic agents will provide an immediate effect on the myocardium and can also be titrated minute by minute depending on changing circulatory circumstances.

A most difficult problem in the evaluation and treatment is the balance between producing an inotropic effect on the ventricle to improve contractility and the need to decrease afterload on the left ventricle. A depressed ventricle after a myocardial infarction or after a cardiac surgical procedure may be unable to work effectively against a normal peripheral vascular resistance. In such a circumstance, an attempt at afterload reduction can be carried out. This requires frequent measurement of cardiac output, however, to determine a satisfactory effect. Afterload reduction can be carried out by the use of nitroglycerin paste and by the intravenous infusion of sodium nitroprusside. Another method for afterload reduction is the use of an intra-aortic balloon pump, which is frequently used before, during, and after cardiac surgical procedures.

Along with the specific therapy of a cardiogenic problem, other adjuncts should be used. If urine output does not respond quickly, a diuretic should be given, either furosemide or ethacrynic acid. Supplemental oxygen or ventricular assistance along with correction of acidosis may be helpful. If the patient responds initially to an inotropic agent, a rapidly acting digitalis preparation may be helpful in order to wean the patient from the intravenous inotrope. If the patient does not respond, the possibility of coronary arteriography, cardiac catheterization, and an emergency operative procedure should be considered.

Vasoactive Drugs

The vasoactive agents are those that affect the sympathetic nervous system receptors or effect blood vessels directly. The classification provided by Ahlquist is most useful in discussing the effects and usefulness of such drugs. Alpha receptors are those in the peripheral circulation that when stimulated produce vasoconstriction. Pure alpha-stimulating drugs, therefore, are vasoconstrictor agents that increase vascular resistance and tend to elevate blood pressure. These include methoxamine hydrochloride (Vasoxyl) and angiotensin (Hypertensin). These drugs can be extremely helpful in circumstances in which peripheral vascular resistance is decreased, such as in several forms of neurogenic or spinal shock or with a spinal anesthetic where peripheral vascular resistance is lowered. They have little place in the therapy of other forms of shock and are to be avoided in general because they will simply increase resistance and not improve organ or microcirculatory blood flow.

There are strong alpha-stimulating drugs that have some

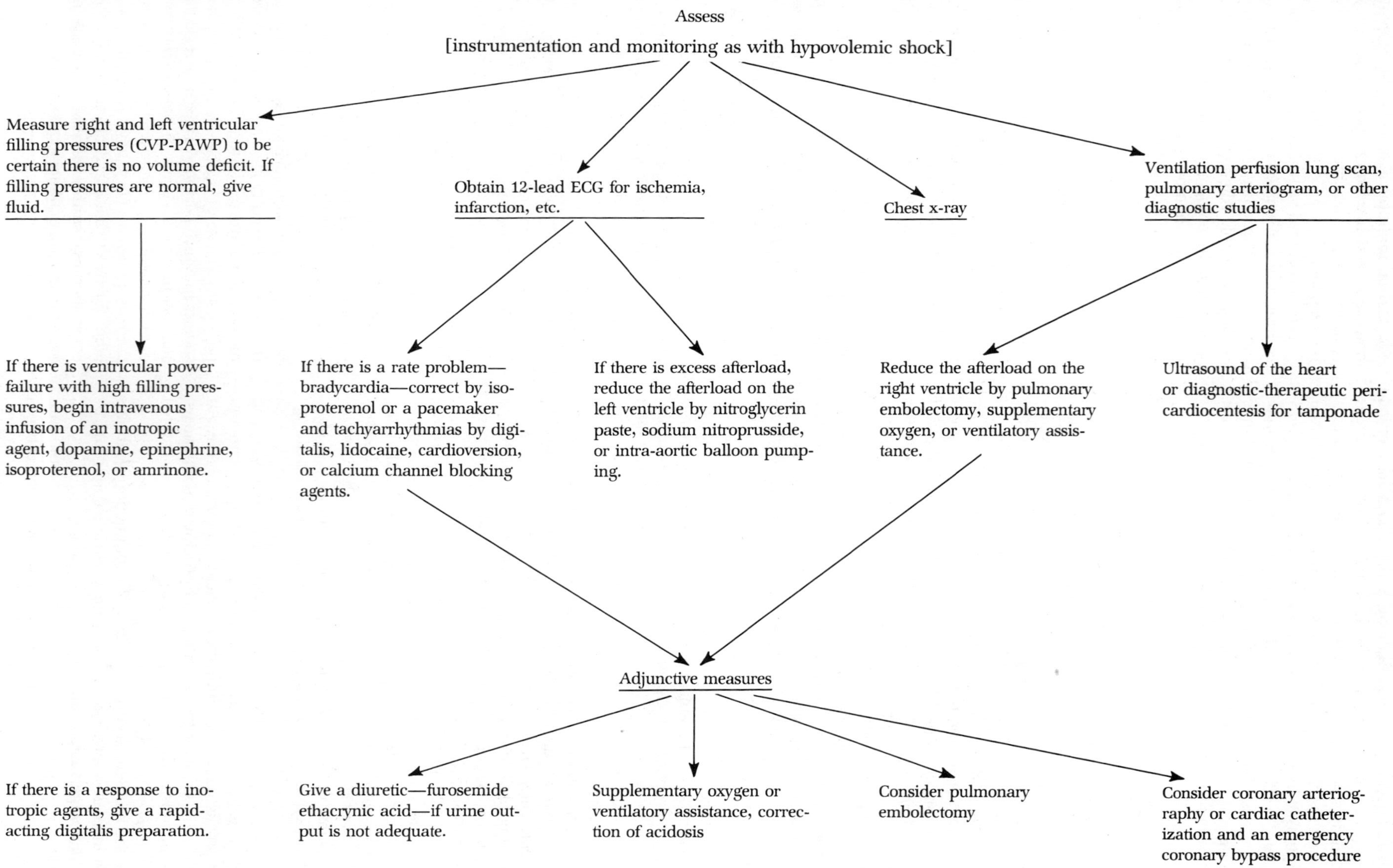

Fig. 26-11. Therapy for cardiogenic shock.

effect on the heart. The cardiac receptors are all beta receptors, and stimulation of these beta receptors in the myocardium produces an increased force of contraction (inotropic effect) and often an increase in heart rate—also a chronotropic effect. Such agents include phenylephrine (Neo-Synephrine). This drug has a very slight cardiac effect. It can be useful in circumstances in which slight or modest increase in peripheral vascular resistance would be helpful. The vasodilated septic patient may benefit from such a drug. Phenylephrine is a gentle vasoconstrictive agent that does not produce great problems or decreased flow to vital organs as do some of the more potent agents. Strong alpha drugs are metaraminol (Aramine), which has some beta cardiac effect and mephentermine (Wyamine), which also has some beta cardiac effect. At the present time, these agents are not particularly useful in the treatment of any of the various forms of shock.

Beta receptors in the peripheral circulation produce vasodilatation. Some vascular beds are more responsive than others. The splanchnic circulation and the skin have particularly active beta receptor systems. A pure beta-stimulating drug is isoproterenol hydrochloride (Isuprel). This agent produces some peripheral vasodilatation so that peripheral vascular resistance is decreased. However, isoproterenol also has a strong beta effect on the heart, increasing both contractility and heart rate. Isoproterenol can be effective for the immediate treatment of bradycardia and for any problem where an inotropic effect is needed with a decrease in peripheral vascular resistance. This agent can be particularly helpful for the sluggish ventricle in patients with diseases such as mitral valve disease, and with other problems. The increased heart rate produced by isoproterenol also increases myocardial oxygen consumption. This has been considered a hazard by some investigators. Therefore, it should be used carefully in patients with acute myocardial ischemia.

A number of drugs have a mixed alpha and beta effect. These include epinephrine (Adrenaline), dopamine (Inotropin), dobutamine (Dobutrex), and norepinephrine (Levarterenol, Levophed). These drugs can be particularly useful. Dopamine is the inotropic agent most commonly used in most circumstances. It stimulates dopaminergic receptors in the kidney. At a low dose, dopamine will improve renal blood flow and not alter peripheral vascular resistance. At a higher dose, however, it vasoconstricts and increases peripheral vascular resistance. Dopamine has a potent inotropic effect as well. Dobutamine is similar to dopamine but has less of a chronotropic effect and can be helpful in certain circumstances. Norepinephrine has such strong alpha or vasoconstricting effects that it is not considered a useful drug under most circumstances for surgical patients. It can be helpful, however, with a sudden cardiac arrest where peripheral vascular resistance disappears and both an alpha and beta effect may be helpful in restoring cardiovascular function.

There are blocking agents for both alpha- and beta-stimulating drugs. Alpha-adrenergic blocking agents include phenoxybenzamine hydrochloride (Dibenzyline), phentolamine (Regitine), and thymoxamine, which is a competitive blocker. The alpha-adrenergic blocking agents can be helpful in the preparation of a patient with a pheochromocytoma for operation and for other acute hypertensive events. However, they are not recommended for the therapy of shock. The beta-adrenergic blocking agents include propranolol (Inderal). Propranolol can be helpful for certain arrhythmias and for the chronic treatment and prevention of angina pectoris. There is no particular use or place for it in the treatment of cardiogenic shock per se.

Other circulatory agents can be helpful. The digitalis or digitalis-like compounds are helpful when a prolonged increase in contractility is needed. In acute situations with shock, however, it is better to use an agent that acts more rapidly and that can be easily titrated intravenously. Following this, digitalis can be given and the intravenous agent discontinued. It takes some time for even the rapid-acting digitalis drugs to have an effect. They also have a narrow therapeutic-toxic ratio. If the degree of circulatory depression is not acute, digoxin is the most appropriate drug. Digoxin or Lanoxin may have an initial effect in 5 to 30 minutes. Its maximum effect occurs in 1.5 to 3 hours. For rapid intravenous therapy, 0.5 to 0.7 mg can be given intravenously initially, followed by 0.5 mg in 0.5 hour to 4 hours, followed by 0.3 to 0.5 mg in 2 to 4 hours for a total digitalizing dose of 1.5 mg. Digitoxin has an initial effect in 30 to 120 minutes, with a maximum effect in 4 to 8 hours. Ouabain has a similar action to digoxin, as does deslanoside (Cedilanid-D). A new digitalis-like drug that has a different mechanism is amrinone, which has been found to be a very useful agent and is undergoing extensive clinical trial. It may be helpful as an inotropic agent in certain patients with cardiogenic shock.

Afterload reduction can be carried out by nitroglycerin paste as a 2 percent ointment on a section of 2.5 to 5 cm of skin. Sodium nitroprusside (Nipride) can be given as 50 mg in 500 ml of solution with 0.1 to 3 μg/kg/minute.

Anti-arrhythmic drugs can be classified according to those that interfere with depolarization of the muscle, those that have an antisympathetic activity, and those that prolong the action potential and the calcium channel–blocking agents. Those drugs that interfere with depolarization of the muscle include lidocaine, which can be given as a 1 to 2 mg/kg bolus intravenously followed by 20 to 50 μg/kg/minute as a continuous infusion. Procainamide can be given as 100 mg intravenously in 1 minute repeated every 5 minutes as needed. For ventricular tachycardia, diphenylhydantoin can be given as is procainamide. Quinidine, however, which is in the same class of agent, is best given orally. The class II or antisympathetic blocking or interfering agents include propranolol (Inderal), which is given as 0.5 to 0.1 mg intravenously every 3 to 5 minutes as needed. Bretylium is in the same group and can be given as 5 mg/kg intramuscularly or 5 to 10 mg/kg intravenously over 10 to 20 minutes. An example of a class III agent that prolongs the action potential is amiodorone. The class IV calcium channel blockers are exemplified by verapamil, which is given as a 10-mg intravenous bolus for control of ventricular arrhythmias.

Inotropic Agents

The most useful inotropic agent at the present time and one that is used most commonly is dopamine, which is given in a dose of 400 mg in 250 ml with a rate of 2 to 20 μg/kg/minute.

The lowest dose possible to achieve a maximum inotropic effect should be given so that peripheral vascular resistance is not increased. Epinephrine is given as 5 mg in 250 ml. A dose of 0.003 to 0.1 μg/kg/minute can be quite helpful in providing an inotropic effect. It has been used primarily by cardiac surgeons because of its potent effects on the ventricles. It does increase ventricular irritability and must be used with great caution if there are frequent premature ventricular contractions. Isoproterenol, described previously, can also be helpful as an inotropic agent. Glucagon has an inotropic effect but is weak and has many side effects. It has been useful when propranolol overdoses occur. Amrinone may also be of benefit.

Vasoconstrictor Agents

There is little place for these agents in most forms of shock, particularly in cardiogenic shock. Such a drug may be necessary when peripheral resistance is low for a very brief period of time to increase blood pressure above dangerous levels, or in an emergency situation while resuscitation and diagnosis can be carried out. If a mild increase in resistance with minimal side effects is desired, the drug of choice is Neo-Synephrine. In contrast to norepinephrine, Neo-Synephrine can be infused for a number of days with little organ or tissue ischemia.

Vasodilating Agents

There was a time when catecholamine effects and persistent vasoconstriction were thought to be part of the progressive pathophysiology of shock. Indeed, this may be a significant problem. However, reduced blood flow is the problem rather than increased resistance, and there is little to be accomplished by decreasing resistance unless one improves flow. Thus, unless afterload reduction is necessary to aid ventricular function, nothing will be accomplished by vasodilatation. Afterload reduction should be carried out by rapidly acting compounds such as sodium nitroprusside or nitroglycerin paste rather than the alpha blocking agents. Alpha blocking agents have no place at the present time in the treatment of clinical shock.

Combinations of Drugs

For the treatment of cardiogenic shock, there is no agent that is uniformly successful; thus, trial and error will have to be used, and in certain circumstances, combinations of drugs have made a difference. Dopamine and sodium nitroprusside have been used together to get a maximum inotropic effect but to decrease afterload on the ventricle. The same effects, however, can be achieved by using isoproterenol alone. Some investigators have used the alpha blocking agent phentolamine along with norepinephrine to obtain the inotropic effects of norepinephrine but to decrease its strong alpha vasoconstrictive activity. The catecholamines all produce ventricular irritability through an excitatory effect increasing automaticity. Thus, they must be used with caution. We have found that if isoproterenol produces ventricular premature beats or incipient ventricular tachycardia, the addition of 20 to 40 mEq of potassium to the infusion will often eliminate this problem.

PREVENTION

Many patients with cardiovascular disease, prior myocardial infarction, or arrhythmias require operations or sustain injury. In such surgical patients with urgent problems or even those requiring elective operations, study and support of the patient's circulation and cardiac reserve may prevent the development of cardiovascular decompensation. Control of hypertension by reduction in afterload; improvement in ventricular performance, if marginal, by elective digitalization; reduction in high preload of CHF; control of or maintenance of normal rate and rhythm; and careful maintenance of oxygenation during the operation may allow the patient to survive with a very limited cardiovascular system or previous myocardial infarction. Prospective consideration of these factors can be lifesaving. A patient with marginal cardiovascular status can be admitted to a surgical intensive care unit preoperatively with measurement of cardiovascular parameters and fine-tuning to provide maximum performance during and after a necessary operation.

NEUROGENIC SHOCK

ETIOLOGY

Neurogenic shock has also been called *vasogenic shock* or *vasomotor collapse.* Syncope is a form of this problem. It may also occur with spinal anesthesia, spinal cord injury (also called spinal shock), or anaphylactic shock. Any factor that causes decreased peripheral vascular resistance could result in hypotension and decreased blood flow. Thus, a decrease in peripheral vascular resistance can occur from a number of insults. It can be a sudden and brief transient episode, such as syncope. It can result from a CNS injury, such as spinal shock, or from the effects of an anesthetic agent, particularly a spinal anesthetic, which causes decreased vascular tone from the level of the anesthetic downward.

Decreased vascular resistance is also characteristic of early septic shock, as the patient's temperature is elevated with the infection. Vasodilatation occurs to attempt to increase heat loss and control the pyrogenic effect. Thus, this may resemble vasomotor collapse or vasogenic shock. The setting and the circumstances, however, are usually quite different. The septic patient with hypotension owing to excessive vasodilatation will certainly be warm and dry; temperature, however, will be elevated; pulse will be bounding, but usually will be associated with tachycardia. The patient will appear quite ill. In patients with acute myocardial infarction, there have also been circumstances described in which peripheral vascular constriction does not occur as cardiac output falls owing to the myocardial infarction. Thus, there may be a mismatch between cardiac output and the peripheral circulation's response to it. This has been the rationale for the use of mild vasoconstrictors in some patients with early or mild cardiogenic shock. Here again, this situation would be associated with acute changes of chest pain or ECG changes indicating something more than simply a vasogenic problem.

PATHOPHYSIOLOGY

A decrease in peripheral vascular resistance may not produce overt changes in a patient's hemodynamic status if there are adjustments elsewhere. Also, a modest decrease in blood pressure is well tolerated if it occurs with vasodilatation. Most anesthetic agents are associated with some decrease in blood pressure. However, any alteration in cardiac output is probably due to a direct cardiac depressant effect.

At one time, ganglionic blocking agents were used to decrease peripheral resistance and blood flow, particularly with certain neurosurgical operations. An extremely low mean arterial blood pressure is well tolerated as long as cardiac output is normal. With CNS injury, particularly to the spinal cord, reduced vascular tone from lost sympathetic innervation may lower blood pressure. If the individual cannot compensate for this, reduced tissue blood flow may occur as cardiac output falls. If neurogenic shock persists and is associated with a significant decrease in cardiac output, the manifestations of this would be a reduction of blood flow to tissues and organs with a response similar to that of hypovolemia or cardiogenic shock. Because of the low pressure, capillary refilling may occur; vasoconstriction would occur where it was possible to vasoconstrict the circulation and where vasomotor tone had not been eliminated. In most circumstances, however, the situation does not deteriorate to that point.

HEMODYNAMIC CHARACTERISTICS

By definition, in neurogenic shock, the blood pressure will be reduced. Usually, however, the heart rate is slow and the patient is warm and dry. Thus, the characteristic picture of neurogenic shock is quite different from that of other types of shock. Initially, the pulse may be steady, although slow; if blood flow decreases, tachycardia may eventually occur along with other changes suggestive of a prolonged decrease in blood flow. This would occur, of course, only if vascular volume and cardiac status were inadequate to deal with the loss of vasomotor tone.

TREATMENT

With mild forms of neurogenic shock such as syncope, placing the patient in a supine position with legs elevated for a short period of time will probably be sufficient. If the decrease in resistance is excessive, such as with spinal shock or with a spinal anesthetic, a mild vasoconstrictor agent would be helpful. Vasoxyl is effective in this regard because it has a safe and mild alpha-adrenergic stimulating effect to increase peripheral vascular resistance without altering blood flow to vital organs. If neurogenic shock, such as with spinal cord injury, occurs with severe generalized trauma, careful monitoring, resuscitation, and treatment are required. Blood and fluid loss, along with decreased vascular resistance and tone, may produce a complicated situation. In most such circumstances, increased vascular volume or overexpansion is much more appropriate than is the use of vasoconstrictor agents. In addition to Vasoxyl, Neo-Synephrine, or phenylephrine, may also be used safely and appropriately to produce a mild increase in peripheral vascular resistance without a reduction in blood flow to vital organs such as the kidneys and the myocardium.

Different problems such as acute gastric dilatation have been described as producing a form of neurogenic shock. Acute gastric dilatation, of course, requires the insertion of a nasogastric tube on an emergent basis and decompression of the stomach. Acute gastric dilatation can occur after injury and with air swallowing, such as with some forms of hysteria.

SELECTED READING

General and Culmination of Shock

Barash, PG, et al. The hemodynamic tracking system. An aid to data management and cardiovascular decision making. *Anesth Analg* 59:169, 1980.

Baue, AE. Shock and Cardiac Arrest. In JD Hardy (ed.), *Hardy's Textbook of Surgery*. Philadelphia: Lippincott. 1983. P. 33.

Baue, AE. Metabolic abnormalities of shock. *Surg Clin North Am* 56:1059, 1976.

Baue, AE, and Chaudry, IH. Prevention of multiple systems failure. *Surg Clin North Am* 60:1167, 1980.

Baue, AE. Multiple, progressive, or sequential systems failure. A syndrome of the 1970s. *Arch Surg* 110:779, 1975.

Beecher, HK, et al. The internal state of the severely wounded man on entry to the most forward hospital. *Surgery* 22:672, 1947.

Blalock, A. Experimental Shock: Cause of low blood pressure produced by muscle injury. *Arch Surg* 22:959, 1930.

Blalock, A. Acute circulatory failure as exemplified by shock and hemorrhage. *Surg Gynecol Obstet* 58:551, 1934.

Boucher, CA, et al. Determination of cardiac risks by Dipyridamole-Thallium imaging before peripheral vascular surgery. *New Engl J Med* 312:389, 1985.

Cannon, WB. *Traumatic Shock*. New York: Appleton, 1923.

Chaudry, IH, Clemens, MG, and Baue, AE. Alterations in cell function with ischemia and shock and their correction. *Arch Surg* 116:1309, 1981.

Clarke, J. Translation from the French original of HF LeDran. *A Treatise, or Reflections Drawn from Practice on Gun-Shot Wounds*. London, 1743.

Cooper, Sir A. *A Dictionary of Practical Surgery* (7th ed). London: Longmans, 1938.

Cournand, A, et al. Studies of circulation in clinical shock. *Surgery* 13:964, 1943.

Crile, GW. *An Experimental Research into Surgical Shock*. Philadelphia: Lippincott, 1889.

Crowell, JW, and Guyton, AC. Evidence favoring a cardiac mechanism in irreversible hemorrhagic shock. *Am J Physiol* 201:893, 1961.

Daniel, AM, et al. The metabolic utilization of protein and muscle glycogen in experimental shock. *J Surg Res* 26:663, 1979.

DelGuercio, LRM, and Cohn, JD. Monitoring operative risk in the elderly. *JAMA* 243:1350, 1980.

Drucker, WR, Chadwick, CDJ, and Gann, DS. Transcapillary refill in hemorrhage and shock. *Arch Surg* 116:1344, 1981.

Eiseman, B, Beart, R, and Norton, L. Multiple organ failure. *Surg Gynecol Obstet* 144:323, 1977.

Gann, DS, et al. Role of solute and the early restitution of blood volume after hemorrhage. *Surgery* 94:439, 1983.

Harkins, HN, and Long, CNH. Metabolic changes in shock after burns. *Am J Physiol* 144:661, 1945.

Hippokrates: Corpus hippocraticum. Epidemien, Buch I-III nach W. Capelle. Hippokrates, 5 auserlesene Schriften. Fischer, Frankfort, 1955.

Kreis, DJ, Jr, and Baue, AE. *Clinical Management of Shock.* Baltimore: University Park Press, 1984.

LeDran, HF. Traite ou reflexions tirees de la practique sur les playes d'armes a feu. Paris: C. Osmont, 1737.

Liddell, MJ, et al. The role of stress hormones in the catabolic metabolism of shock. *Surg Gynecol Obstet* 149:822, 1979.

Moore, FD. The effects of hemorrhage on body composition. *N Engl J Med* 273:567, 1965.

Moore, FD, and Ball, MR. The metabolic response to injury. Springfield, IL: Thomas, 1952.

Parsons, E, and Phemister, DB. Hemorrhage and "shock" in traumatized limbs: An experimental study. *Surg Gynecol Obstet* 51:196, 1930.

Polk, HC, Jr, and Shields, CL. Remote organ failure: A valid sign of occult intraabdominal infection. *Surgery* 81:310, 1977.

Shires, GT, et al. Alterations in cellular membrane function during hemorrhagic shock in primates. *Ann Surg* 176:288, 1972.

Skillman, JJ, Awwad, HK, and Moore, FD. Plasma protein kinetics of the early transcapillary refill after hemorrhage in man. *Surg Gynecol Obstet* 125:983, 1967.

Swan, HJC, et al. Catheterization of the heart in man with use of a flow directed balloon-tipped catheter. *N Engl J Med* 283:447, 1970.

Warren, JC. *Surgical Pathology and Therapeutics.* Philadelphia: Saunders, 1895.

Wiggers, CJ. *Physiology of Shock.* Cambridge, MA: Harvard University Press, 1950.

Hypovolemic Shock

Monafo, WW, Chuntrasakul, C, and Ayvazian, VH. Hypertonic sodium solutions in the treatment of burn shock. *Am J Surg* 126:778, 1973.

Moss, GS, et al. Colloid or crystalloid in the resuscitation of hemorrhagic shock: A controlled clinical trial. *Surgery* 89:434, 1981.

Moyer, CA, and Butcher, HR. *Burns, Shock and Plasma Volume Regulation.* St. Louis: Mosby, 1967.

Septic Shock

Albrecht, M, and Clowes, GHA. The increase of circulatory requirements in the presence of inflammation. *Surgery* 56:158, 1964.

Altemeier, WA. Bodily response to infectious agents. *JAMA* 202: 1085, 1967.

Altemeier, WA, and Cole, WR. Nature and treatment of septic shock. *Arch Surg* 77:498, 1958.

Baracos, V, et al. Stimulation of muscle protein degradation and prostaglandin E_2 release by leukocytic pyrogen (interleukin-1). *N Engl J Med* 308:353, 1983.

Baue, AE. The treatment of septic shock, a problem intensified by advancing science. *Surgery* 63:850, 1969.

Beeson, PB. Temperature—elevating effect of a substance obtained from polymorphonuclear leukocytes. *J Clin Invest* 27:524, 1948.

Beutler, B, and Cerami, A. Cachectin: More than a tumor necrosis factor. *N Engl J Med* 316:379, 1987.

Beutler, B, Milsark, IW, and Cerami, AC. Passive immunization against cachectin/tumor necrosis factor protects mice from lethal effect of endotoxin. *Science* 229:869, 1985.

Beutler, B, et al. Control of cachectin (tumor necrosis factor) synthesis: Mechanisms of endotoxin resistance. *Science* 232:977, 1986.

Beutler, BA, Milsark, IW, and Cerami A. Cachectin/tumor necrosis factor: Production, distribution, and metabolic fate in vivo. *J Immunol* 135:3972, 1985.

Beutler, B, et al. Purification of cachectin, a lipoprotein lipase-suppressing hormone secreted by endotoxin-induced RAW 264.7 cells. *J Exp Med* 161:984, 1985.

Boise, E. The differential diagnosis of shock, hemorrhage and sepsis. *Trans Am Assoc Obstet* 9:433, 1897.

Borden, CW, and Hall, WH. Fatal transfusion reactions from massive bacterial contamination of blood. *N Engl J Med* 245:760, 1951.

Burke, JF, Pontoppidan, H, and Welch, CE. High output respiratory failure: An important cause of death ascribed to peritonitis or ileus. *Ann Surg* 158:581, 1963.

Cerami, A, and Beutler, B. The role of cachectin/TNF in endotoxic shock and cachexia. *Immunol Today* 9:28, 1988.

Cerra, FB, et al. Septic autocannibalism—a failure of exogenous nutritional support. *Ann Surg* 192:570, 1980.

Clowes, GHA, Jr, et al. Muscle proteolysis induced by a circulation peptide in patients with sepsis or trauma. *N Engl J Med* 308:545, 1983.

Clowes, GHA, et al. The significance of altered protein metabolism regulated by proteolysis inducing factor, the circulating cleavage product of interleukin-I. *Ann Surg* 302:446, 1985.

Clowes, GHA, Jr, Vucinic, N, and Weidner, N. Circulatory and metabolic alterations associated with survival or death in peritonitis. *Ann Surg* 163:866, 1966.

Clowes, GHA, Jr, et al. Observations on the pathogenesis of the pneumonitis associated with severe infections in other parts of the body. *Ann Surg* 167:630, 1968.

Coley, WB. The treatment of malignant tumors by repeated inoculations of erysipelas: With a report of ten original cases. *Am J Med Sci* 105:487, 1893.

Demaria, EJ, et al. Septic complications of corticosteroid administration after central nervous system trauma. *Ann Surg* 302:248, 1985.

Dinarello, CA, et al. Tumor necrosis factor (cachectin) is an endogenous pyrogen and induces production of interleukin 1. *N Engl J Med* 163:1433, 1986.

Duff, GW, and Durum, SK. Fever and immunoregulation: Hyperthermia, interleukins I and II, and T-cell proliferation. *Yale J Biol Med* 55:437, 1982.

Evans, DA, et al. The effects of tumor necrosis factor and their selective inhibition by Ibuprofen. *Ann Surg* 209:312, 1989.

Fromm, RE, et al. Serum tumor necrosis factor response in humans receiving endotoxin. *Clin Res* 36:372A, 1988.

Hess, ML, Hastillo, A, and Greenfield, LJ. Spectrum of cardiovascular function during gram-negative sepsis. *Prog Cardiovasc Dis* 23:279, 1981.

Hoffman, MJ, et al. Unsuspected right ventricular dysfunction in shock and sepsis. *Ann Surg* 198:307, 1983.

Hoffman-Goetz, L, et al. Febrile and plasma iron responses of rabbits injected with endogenous pyrogen for malnourished patients. *Am J Clin Nutr* 34:1109, 1981.

Kawakami, M, et al. Lipoprotein lipase suppression in 3T3-L1 cells by an endotoxin-induced mediator from exudate cells. *Proc Natl Acad Sci USA* 79:912, 1982.

Laennec, RTH. *Traite de L'auscultation Mediate et des Maladies des Poumons et du Coeur.* Paris: JS Chaude, 1831.

Loda, M, et al. Induction of hepatic protein synthesis by a peptide in blood plasma of patients with sepsis and trauma. *Surgery* 96:204, 1984.

MacLean, LD, et al. Treatment of shock based on physiologic principles. *Surg Gynecol Obstet* 120:1, 1965.

MacLean, LD, et al. Patterns of septic shock in man: A detailed study of 56 patients. *Ann Surg* 166:543, 1967.

McMenamy, RH, et al. Multiple organ failure. I. The basal state. *J Trauma* 21:99, 1981.

Mealy, K, et al. Are the catabolic effects of tumor necrosis factor mediated by glucocorticoids? *Arch Surg* 125:42, 1990.

Michie, HR, et al. Detection of circulating tumor necrosis factor after endotoxin administration. *N Engl J Med* 318:1481, 1988.

Michie, HR, et al. Chronic TNF infusion causes anorexia but not accelerated nitrogen loss. *Ann Surg* 209:19, 1989.

Michie, HR, et al. Tumor necrosis factor and endotoxin induce similar metabolic responses in human beings. *Surgery* 104:280, 1988.
Ollodart, RM, Hawthorne, I, and Attar, S. Studies in experimental endotoxemia in man. *Am J Surg* 113:599, 1967.
O'Malley, WE, Achinstein, B, and Shear, MJ. Action of bacterial polysaccharide on tumors. II. Damage of sarcoma 37 by serum of mice treated with Serratia marcescens polysaccharide, and induced tolerance. *J National Cancer Institute* 29:1169, 1962.
Parker, MM, et al. Profound but reversible myocardial depression in patients with septic shock. *Ann Intern Med* 100:483, 1984.
Pollack, M, and Young, LS. Protective activity of antibodies to exotoxin A and lipopolysaccharide at the onset of *Pseudomonas aeruginosa* septicemia in man. *J Clin Invest* 63:276, 1979.
Pontoppidan, H, Geffin, B, and Laver, MB. Respiratory Failure in Septic Shock. In SG Hershey, LRM DelGuercio, and R McConn (eds.), *Septic Shock in Man.* Boston: Little, Brown, 1971. P. 37.
Rouzer, CA, and Cerami, A. Hypertriglyceridemia associated with Trypanosoma brucei brucei infection in rabbits: Role of defective triglyceride removal. *Mol Biochem Parasitol* 2:31, 1980.
Ruggerio, V, et al. Induction of the synthesis of tumor necrosis factor receptors by interferon-psi. *J Immunol* 136:2445, 1986.
Schirmer, WJ, Schirmer, JM, and Fry, DE. Recombinant human tumor necrosis factor produces hemodynamic changes characteristic of sepsis and endotoxemia. *Arch Surg* 124:445, 1989.
Schumer, W. Steroids in the treatment of clinical septic shock. *Ann Surg* 184:333, 1976.
Sibbald, WJ, et al. Variations in adrenocortical responsiveness during severe bacterial infections. *Ann Surg* 186:29, 1977.
Siegel, JH, et al. Physiological and metabolic correlations in human sepsis. *Surgery* 86:163, 1979.
Siegel, JH, Greenspan, M, and DelGuercio, LRM. Abnormal vascular tone, defective oxygen transport and myocardial failure in human septic shock. *Ann Surg* 165:504, 1967.
Sprung, CL, et al. The effects of high-dose corticosteroids in patients with septic shock. A prospective control study. *N Engl J Med* 311:1137, 1984.
Takayama, T, et al. Elevated tumor necrosis factor (TNF) production concomitant to elevated PGE_2 production by trauma patients' monocytes. *Arch Surg* 125:29, 1990.
Tracey, KJ, et al. Shock and tissue injury induced by recombinant human cachectin. *Science* 234:470, 1986.
Tracey, KJ, et al. Anti-cachectin/TNF monoclonal antibodies prevent shock during lethal bacteraemia. *Nature* 330:662, 1987.
Tracey, KJ, et al. Cachectin/tumor necrosis factor induces lethal shock and stress hormone responses in the dog. *Surg Gynecol Obstet* 164:415, 1987.
Vincent, JL, et al. Circulatory shock associated with purulent peritonitis. *Am J Surg* 142:262, 1981.
Waage, A, Halstensen, A, and Espevik, T. Association between tumour necrosis factor in serum and fatal outcome in patients with meningococcal disease. *Lancet* 1:355, 1987.
Waisbren, BA. Bacteremia due to gram-negative bacilli other than the *Salmonella;* a clinical and therapeutic study. *Arch Intern Med* 88:467, 1951.
Warren, RS, et al. The acute metabolic effects of tumor necrosis factor administration in man. *Arch Surg* 122:396, 1987.
Wiles, JB, et al. The systemic septic response: Does the organism matter? *Crit Care Med* 8:55, 1980.
Ziegler, EJ. Tumor necrosis factor in humans. *N Engl J Med* 318:1533, 1988.
Ziegler, EJ, et al. Treatment of gram-negative bacteremia in shock with human antiserum to a mutant *Escherichia coli. N Engl J Med* 307:1225, 1982.

Cardiogenic Shock

Braunwald, E. On the difference between the heart's output and its contractile state. *Circulation* 43:171, 1971.
Freis, ED, et al. Hemodynamic alterations in acute myocardial infarction. I. Cardiac output, mean arterial pressure, total peripheral resistance, "central" and total blood volumes, venous pressure and average circulation time. *J Clin Invest* 31:131, 1952.
Sarnoff, SJ, et al. Homeometric auto-regulation in the heart. *Circ Res* 8:1077, 1960.

F. Acute Alteration in Function of the Central Nervous System

27. Physiology of Consciousness

Gregory L. Henry

From the time of the earliest recorded Greek philosophers up to and including the present day, the origins and definitions of consciousness have been debated. Leaving aside the more metaphysical concepts of social and political consciousness over which there is never any general consensus, this discussion will turn toward the concepts involved in physiologic consciousness and their implications in both health and disease.

ANATOMY AND PHYSIOLOGY OF CONSCIOUSNESS

Physiologic consciousness, like truth and beauty, is a concept much better understood at a visceral level than articulated in a simple definition. For our purposes, it is reasonable to think of consciousness as a state in which an individual is aware at a cognitive level of self and environmental factors. Being aware at the cognitive level means that a person has the ability to process environmental stimuli and make selected decisions as to responses to those stimuli. Whether the patient who is totally devoid of the mechanisms of sensory input and totally devoid of motor pathways for response is actually conscious is a philosophical debate that we shall leave for others.

Consciousness requires both the machinery able to perceive an environmental stimulus and a sufficient central nervous system (CNS) computer that can process such a stimulus. Thus, the body must have the machinery necessary to perceive an environmental change and cause arousal of the CNS. It then must have a sufficient central computer that can not only process sensory stimuli but also present the higher intellectual functions with a picture of what such stimuli mean. The CNS must finally be able to sort out various options and respond to an incoming stimulus.

The actual physiologic machinery involved in consciousness includes not only the cerebral hemispheres but the reticular activating formation system that carries arousal pathways within the brain. Extensive research in mammals has identified tracks that run through the upper spinal cord and brain stem and connect in regions of the thalamus that provide the arousal mechanism.

From a conceptual standpoint, the entire peripheral nervous system, which carries information into the CNS, should be viewed as the initial gateway into the system. The reticular activating formation may be thought of as the center where stimuli are processed; if a sufficient stimulus is perceived, information is sent to the brain to cause arousal and wakefulness. The reticular activating formation therefore acts as a filter or sieve that brings the brain to a full state of alertness when it perceives a threat or stimulation sufficient enough to require the brain's attention. The reticular activating formation makes no responses in and of itself but merely prepares the brain to be ready to analyze incoming information. Once higher centers in the thalamic nuclei and cerebral cortices have been properly put on alert, they take over the role of analysis of incoming stimuli and selection of proper response.

Transections of the upper cervical cord do not affect consciousness. Lesions within the brain stem, however, that can be anatomically placed in regions in the high pericollicular region definitely impair consciousness. Lesions that lie centrally to the mesencephalon may also affect reticular activating formation tracks and can produce profound unconsciousness that can be documented by electroencephalic (EEG) changes.

Conversely, stimulation of these various tracks in properly prepared animals produces marked wakefulness and appropriate EEG changes exactly analogous to those seen in humans. Although there is some debate as to the exact location and numbers of various tracks involved in consciousness, it is well understood that central brain stem structures, including the dorsomedial pontine tegmentum, are intimately involved.

It is interesting to note that when cerebral trauma is induced in various experimental animals, glucose uptake is decreased within the brain everywhere except in the regions associated with the reticular activating formation. Biochemical means using injections of various substances into the brain stem as well as traumatic means have been tried, and all produce similar alterations of consciousness. It is interesting to note that experimentation using injections of cholinergics can produce cerebral depression that is reversed by injection of atropine. This gives some credence to the idea that cholinergic neurotransmission in this area is necessary for normal wakefulness. The degree to which this indicates a role for the autonomic nervous system and wakefulness is still an area of much debate.

Comparing animal data from lesions that cause consciousness or unconsciousness with human pathologic materials confirms the fact that rostral brain stem structures are required for consciousness. The neuropathology on patients with hemorrhages or infarcts involving the brain stem regions can be correlated to their physical findings and, again, reproduce the idea that brain stem activation is required for consciousness. It is important to note that limited lesions or lesions that are unilateral in nature can be perfectly compatible with an alert patient. Thus, as long as one half of the brain stem is providing arousal to the brain, normal wakefulness can be maintained.

The reticular activating formation and the various tracks that comprise it are believed to synapse and relay their stimulation through the hypothalamus and the thalamus. Lesions that depress the hypothalamus—such as third ventricular tumors, various infections, and various forms of hydrocephalus—can cause marked alterations in consciousness that would not be present if such lesions exist in the cerebral hemispheres. Students of neurophysiology have long been aware of the various hyperactivity syndromes that can be produced by stimulation of hypothalamic nuclei. There is well-documented pathologic evidence that unilateral thalamic infarcts leave the consciousness unaltered, whereas bilateral thalamic infarcts can produce profound unconsciousness. It is clear, therefore, that along with a reticular activating formation that carries the arousal mechanism, at least a partially intact hypothalamus and thalamus are required to maintain normal consciousness.

The integrity of brain stem structures and deep gray matter must, however, be viewed as the inarticulate warning signals that are sent forth from the body to be processed by central neuromechanisms. For even with an intact sensory apparatus, reticular activating formation, and thalamic structures, consciousness still depends on cerebral interpretation, integration, and action. Physical destruction of the cerebral hemispheres bilaterally causes a loss of consciousness.

Unilateral lesions in the hemispheres rarely affect consciousness unless they have created edema or other intracranial pressure situations in which both hemispheres or the brain stem structures are compromised. Indeed, neurosurgical experience and literature clearly document the fact that whole cerebral hemispheres can be removed without interfering with consciousness. Such radical surgery does affect the various focal outputs of the nervous systems but allows the central mechanisms to maintain wakefulness.

The dominant hemisphere seems to have considerably more influence on consciousness than the nondominant hemisphere, but data on this hypothesis are somewhat circumspect at this time. It is difficult on an experimental basis to isolate the various hemispheres completely owing to crossed information through the corpus callosum and the arterial network. Amytal studies seem to indicate, however, that the dominant hemisphere plays a larger role in what we externally view as consciousness than does the nondominant hemisphere. Since much neurologic disease involves all areas of the brain, combinations of lesions involving the cerebral cortex, thalamic structures, and the reticular activating formation, any of which may not be enough to cause unconsciousness, can in combination with other lesions produce severe alterations in consciousness.

An operational model of consciousness can now be constructed from our anatomic and physiologic base. It is important when constructing such a model to remember that the nervous system is programmed to respond at multiple levels, and merely producing a response to a stimulus does not indicate consciousness. A patient can be severely comatose, and yet withdrawal or at least motor movement to a painful stimulus can be elicited. This is handled at a spinal cord and brain stem level. The organism at that point may not have any cognitive understanding of a stress being placed against the body, nor does it have choices in the type of response it will produce.

For example, in a person whom we will describe as having normal consciousness, the following actions take place. A person is reading as another person enters the room. The auditory excitement pathways or the visual excitatory mechanisms, or both, send messages through their respective cranial nerve pathways to alert the CNS of an approaching change in the environment. On a reflex basis, the eyes will pick up a stimulus and will track to that object. Information necessary to cause such tracking will be processed first in eye tracking areas located in the occipital cortex. This information is then sent to anterior eye poles that transmit information down the brain stem to the cranial nerves involved in moving the eyes.

Simultaneously, the visual image is transmitted from the

calcarine cortex to secondary association areas in which the brain is cognitively processing the visual image against known patterns. The two halves of the brain will talk to each other through the corpus callosum so that information concerning the new environmental stimulus is shared by both halves of the cerebral cortex. The brain can then make a reasoned decision as to whether further actions (i.e., an acknowledgement of the other person, an immediate exit) are required.

In the sleeping individual, all systems are activated except the formal processing mechanisms. During sleep, sound activation or arousal by some other stimuli causes information to be immediately transmitted through the reticular activating formation in which some currently unknown mechanism causes the return of alertness. This turns on the processing mechanism to allow new information to be utilized for the benefit of the individual.

THE PATHOPHYSIOLOGY OF ALTERED CONSCIOUSNESS

Using our anatomic, physiologic, and functional models of consciousness, the factors that cause alteration in consciousness can be rather simply understood. Although specific etiologies will be covered in Chap. 28, it is good to divide alterations of consciousness into their two major broad categories: structural lesions and metabolic lesions.

Structural lesions of the apparatus required to maintain consciousness can readily be understood. Strokes, tumors, and certain forms of trauma cause direct injury to the machinery necessary to process information. It is important to note that, in order for unconsciousness to be produced by a structural mechanism, both hemispheres or the brain stem must be involved. Isolated lesions of one hemisphere or half the brain stem do not produce unconsciousness.

By far the most common causes for alterations of consciousness are metabolic. The neuromechanisms require a continuous supply of both glucose and oxygen to maintain their activity. Anything that interferes with the normal supply of glucose or oxygen can cause alterations of consciousness that may vary from minimal to profound coma. The central neurologic structures are extremely susceptible to not only a lack of nutrients but also the presence of depressant chemicals. Drugs that can suppress the nervous system usually do so in a nonselective, diffuse manner, affecting all areas of the nervous system. The principle overriding difference between structural and metabolic causes of coma is the presence of focal findings. It is relatively rare for simple metabolic disease to produce localized or focal neurologic deficits. In contradistinction to this, structural lesions, particularly those of a rapidly progressing nature or of sudden onset, almost always produce asymmetric findings on neurologic examination. Alterations of consciousness that have occurred on a rapid basis and that have focal neurologic findings should be considered structural problems until proved otherwise when evaluating the patient.

Structural lesions causing alterations of consciousness can be in multiple areas. Supratentorial lesions generally produce unconsciousness by putting pressure downward on the brain stem. Both central herniation, where pressure is applied in a rostral-caudal manner in a relatively symmetric way, and in uncal herniation, in which the temporal lobe compresses the midbrain, are possible mechanisms for supratentorial interference of consciousness.

Subtentorial lesions—hematomas, tumors, infarcts, and direct trauma—can produce unconsciousness in multiple ways. An intrinsic brain stem process, such as a tumor or a sudden bleed, may destroy the ascending reticular formation fibers. Another possible mechanism is that extrinsic disease, such as a tumor or hematoma in the posterior fossa, may compress the midbrain and cause unconsciousness by compromising the blood flow to these vital structures. In certain cases, a brain stem may actually herniate downward through the foramen magnum, causing circulatory compromise to brain stem structures.

Metabolic lesions, although occurring at the biochemical level, can be of multiple varieties. The subarachnoid hemorrhage, although usually resulting from the bleeding from a structural lesion, causes its associated loss of consciousness owing to arterial spasm and relative brain ischemia. Anoxia, renal failure, liver disease, electrolyte imbalances, alterations of temperature, variances in serum osmolality, and epileptic seizures, as well as ingested drugs and toxins, can all contribute to alterations of consciousness.

BRAIN DEATH VERSUS THE PERSISTENT VEGETATIVE STATE

Even the most profoundly comatose patient with no cortical activity will, after several weeks of intensive care, seemingly have some signs of wakefulness. These patients may actually open their eyes, have some blinking movements, and have primitive responses to stimuli. Such patients are still unconscious and will have profound abnormalities on EEG, as well as total lack of ability to function at other than a brain stem level. These patients are, however, not officially brain dead. The various criteria will still show that the patient will not have an isoelectic EEG and still has primitive brain stem functions. Such patients can, however, be considered to have irreversible cortical death, of which there are no reported improvements. A patient who has a normal body temperature and no sedative drugs in his or her system and is not in circulatory shock can be considered to have irreversibility of cortical brain death. If there are abnormal oculocephalic responses, apnea without assisted ventilations, or no discernible motor posturings, the patient can be considered to have irreversibility of their comatose state.

In conclusion, consciousness can be viewed as a complex interaction in which stimulation from the environment evokes decision making and action by an individual. For this system to function correctly, an intact brain stem, thalamus, and cortical structures are required. This delicate and sophisticated machinery can be affected by both structural and metabolic disease processes that will be covered more fully in Chap. 28.

SELECTED READING

Albert ML, et al. Cerebral dominance for consciousness. *Arch Neurol* 33:453, 1976.

Ames, A, III, Gurian BS. Effects of glucose and oxygen deprivation on function of isolated mammalian retina. *J Neurophysiol* 26:617, 1963.

Arduini, A, and Arduini MG. Effects of drugs and metabolic alterations on brainstem arousal mechanisms. *J Pharmacol Exp Ther* 110:76, 1954.

Bates, D, et al. A perspective study of nontraumatic coma: Methods and results in 310 patients. *Ann Neurol* 2:211, 1977.

Beecher, HK. After the "definition of irreversible coma." *N Engl J Med* 281:1010, 1967.

Brendler, SJ, and Selverstone B. Recovery from decerebration. *Brain* 93:381, 1970.

Chapman, LF, and Wolff, HJ. The cerebral hemispheres in the highest integrative functions of man. *Arch Neurol* 1:357, 1959.

Gelenberg AJ. The catatonic syndrome. *Lancet* 1:1339, 1976.

Ingvar DH, and Sourander P. Destruction of the reticular core of the brainstem. A patho-anatomical follow-up of a case of coma of three years duration. *Arch Neurol* 23:1, 1970.

Jefferson, M. Altered consciousness associated with brainstem lesions. *Brain* 75:55, 1952.

Levy, DE, Knill-Jones, PR, and Plum, F. The vegatative state and its prognosis following nontraumatic coma. *Ann NY Acad Sci* 315:293, 1978.

Plum, F, and Posner, JB. *A Diagnosis of Stupor and Coma* (3rd ed.). Philadelphia: Davis, 1980.

28. Coma: Assessment and Initial Management

Gregory L. Henry

The arrival of a comatose patient in the emergency department can bring fear and dread to an emergency physician who is not well schooled in this most dramatic of neurologic alterations. Although initially perplexing, the case of the comatose patient, if viewed and examined in a logical manner, can result in a rapid and specific diagnosis and treatment plan. The central nervous system expresses its general health through the individual's level of consciousness. A change in mental status is often the first sign of a severe pathologic process. Coma, although the most obvious and distressing change in mental status, is only the end point of a continuum that may begin with very minimal alterations of mental status. Any process that can cause minor alterations of mental status can cause coma. It is only a matter of degree or the time at which the process is observed that truly delineates one presentation from another.

DEFINITIONS

Definitions and strict terminology with regard to alterations of mental status vary widely, and there is no one acceptable system. When in doubt, it is always wiser for the examining physician to describe those physical findings that he or she has observed and the actual performance level of the patient than to worry about whether the term *stuporous* or *lethargic* should be used. Nonspecific terms are often misleading and are of little value to future examiners. Specific comments on the patient's ability to perform certain mental functions, however, are reproducible and give an excellent base for future examinations.

In general terms, *consciousness* can be defined as the awareness of self and the environment. Implicit in this very simple definition is the individual's ability to process sensory input and make reasonable choices and his or her response to such environmental stimuli. Patients with alterations of mental status can be divided into those who appear asleep and those who appear awake but are unresponsive. In the group of patients who appear asleep, the most common alteration seen is sleep itself.

Sleep can be defined as a state of nonpathologic decreased mental status from which the patient can be easily aroused to full consciousness. *Lethargy*, also a common finding in patients seen in the emergency department, is that state in which the patient appears wakeful but has depressed awareness of self and the environment globally.

Stupor is a state of unresponsiveness from which the patient can only be aroused with vigorous stimuli. The stuporous patient, however, does not return to a normal baseline awareness of self or environment as does the sleeping patient. The comatose patient is in a state of unresponsiveness and is unarousable to both verbal and physical stimuli, to a level at which he or she can make no meaningful response. Finally, *psychogenic coma* is a state of unresponsiveness, either voluntary or involuntary, from which the patient cannot be brought to give a reasonable cortical response to noxious, verbal, or physical stimuli. Patients in this state do, however, have normal physiologic testing and electroencephalographic (EEG) responses.

COMA-LIKE STATES

The group of disorders in which the patient appears awake but is unresponsive is a truly eclectic one. The *abulic state,* also known as *akinetic mutism* or *coma vigil,* is one in which the patient is awake with open eyes but is extremely slow to respond to any questions asked. The patient's frontal lobe function is depressed from any number of possible disease entities so that the patient is unable to make any meaningful response in a normal time frame. Such patients may have meaningful response, but because of huge delays in their ability to process information and answer questions, they are frequently misdiagnosed during initial evaluations.

In the *locked-in syndrome,* also referred to as the *Count of Monte Cristo syndrome* or the *Messr. Notier de Villefort syndrome,* the patient appears motionless, but the eyes are half open. Such patients are suffering from the destruction of the ventral pontine motor tracks. The only motor function that these patients maintain is an ability to look upward due to maintenance of the third-nerve tracks for vertical eye movement. It is important to ask such patients to look up. If the patient can look up but not move the eyes from side to side, the diagnosis of locked-in syndrome is secured.

All severely comatose patients who survive eventually enter a state known as *persistent vegetative state.* In this state, the patient has no true cortical output. He or she can open and close the eyes and make some motor motions; however, above a simple reflex level, information is not processed and the patient is cortically brain dead.

Psychogenic unresponsiveness, the catatonic state, is still seen in severely disturbed psychiatric patients. At this level of unresponsiveness, the patient appears awake and may maintain normal motor posturing and neurologic testing, but for voluntary or involuntary reasons, he or she is not able to communicate with the examiner in any way.

Confusional patients can present a difficult diagnostic dilemma in the emergency department. Such patients may have normal alertness or even a state of hyperalertness. Their principal problem is that they have an abnormal thought content and are unable to integrate sensory information into any meaningful pattern or give appropriate responses. The disorders in which confusion is paramount early on may be mistaken for an agitated depression of mental status and, indeed, the disease entities can initially overlap. The hallmark of the acute confusional state is a global confusion, inability to appropriately process stimuli, and inability to make meaningful responses, in the presence of an unaltered energy and output of neurologic activity. Such findings are found early in many toxic ingestions, metabolic encephalopathy, and central nervous system infections.

CAUSES

The specific causes of coma and the various alterations of consciousness can basically be divided into two groups (Table 28-1). The first group includes those lesions that are caused by structural damage to the nervous system proper. Direct trauma, mass lesions, tumors, and cerebrovascular accidents of all types fit well within this category. The second major category, which represents by far the largest cause of altered mental status, is the toxic-metabolic group. This group includes alterations in the supply of nutrients to the brain, as well as those toxic substances, whether endogenous or exogenous, that affect the nervous system tissue. Environmental factors, such as temperature and state of hydration, are also part of the toxic-metabolic group.

Although the causes of altered mental status are numerous (see Table 28-1), the two major groups can usually be divided on the basis of focal neurologic findings. Learning the two mnemonics "TIPS" and the vowels "aeiou," is a simple way to remember the various categories into which all comatose patients must fall (Table 28-2).

COMA FROM TRAUMA OR PRIMARY CENTRAL NERVOUS SYSTEM DISEASE

Structural lesions that lie wholly or partially above the tentorium cerebelli can seriously alter mental status, either through their causing increased intracranial pressure, thus decreasing cerebral blood flow, or by pressure that is exerted downward, causing various forms of brainstem compression. Such brainstem compression can be of the uncal herniation or central herniation type. Expanding supratentorial lesions can also affect consciousness if they become large enough to compress both cerebral hemispheres simultaneously. A supratentorial lesion causing uncal herniation should always be considered when a patient with altered mental status has a complete third-nerve palsy, decreasing mental status, and contralateral weakness.

Trauma

Subdural Hematoma

Subdural hematomas can be extremely confusing in both their onset and presentation. In older patients, victims of moderate to severe trauma, alcoholics, and patients receiving anticoagulants, subdural hematomas must always be considered when altered mental status is present. Even if focal neurologic findings are not found on examination, this does not rule out the possibility of a unilateral subdural hematoma. The presence of bilateral subdural hematomas should be considered in the elderly with rapid, nonfocal, decreased mental status. Subdural hematomas can compress supratentorial structures bilaterally and thus can present symptoms similar to those seen with dementia or progressive encephalopathy. Although past trauma is a useful diagnostic indicator, it is not part of the history of all patients with a subdural hematoma. Particularly in elderly patients in whom the bridging veins are long and tenuous between the cortex and the dural sinuses, minor amounts of trauma too insignificant to be remembered can cause slow subdural

Table 28-1. Causes of coma

I. Coma from trauma or primary central nervous system (CNS) disease
  A. Trauma
    1. Subdural hematoma
    2. Epidural hematoma
    3. Laceration or traumatic intracerebral hemorrhage
    4. Contusion
    5. Concussion
  B. Vascular disease
    1. Intracranial hemorrhage
      a. "Hypertensive" intraparenchymal hemorrhages
        (1) Cerebellar
        (2) Thalamic, pontine, putaminal, lobar
      b. Intraparenchymal hemorrhage from ruptured aneurysm
      c. Other causes of intraparenchymal hemorrhage—arteriovenous malformation rupture, bleeding dyscrasias
    2. Subarachnoid hemorrhage
      a. Aneurysm
      b. Arteriovenous malformation
    3. Infarction
      a. Thrombotic
      b. Embolic
        (1) Cardiac source
        (2) Other vascular source
      c. Vasculitis
  C. Infections
    1. Meningitis
    2. Encephalitis
    3. Abscess
  D. Neoplasms
    1. Metastatic
    2. Primary CNS
    3. Paraneoplastic effects
  E. Seizures
    1. Status epilepticus
    2. Postictal state

II. Coma from causes affecting the brain diffusely
  A. Hypoxic encephalopathies
    1. Severe congestive heart failure
    2. Severe obstructive pulmonary disease
    3. Severe anemia
  B. Hypertensive encephalopathy
  C. Metabolic encephalopathies
    1. Cardiac or pulmonary arrest, hypotension
    2. Hypoglycemia
    3. Diabetic ketoacidosis
    4. Nonketotic hyperosmolar coma
    5. Hepatic encephalopathy
    6. Uremia
    7. Hyponatremia
    8. Myxedema
    9. Hypercalcemia
    10. Hypocalcemia
    11. Reye's syndrome
  D. Toxins/drug reactions
    1. Carbon monoxide
    2. Alcohols
    3. CNS sedatives—barbiturates, opiates, tricyclics, phenothiazines
    4. Other toxins—heavy metals, aspirin, acetaminophen, hallucinogens
    5. Neuroleptic malignant syndrome
  E. Environmental causes
    1. Heat stroke
    2. Hypothermia
  F. Deficiency states
    1. Thiamine deficiency—Wernicke's encephalopathy

Table 28-2. Causes of altered mental status

TIPS		Vowels	
T	Trauma, temperature changes	a	Alcohol and ingested drugs and toxins
I	Infection (neurologic and systemic)	e	Endocrine, all types exocrine, liver, electrolytes
P	Psychiatric and porphyria	i	Insulin: diabetes mellitus
S	Space-occupying lesions, stroke, subarachnoid hemorrhage, shock	o	Oxygen and opiates
		u	Uremia, renal causes including hypertensive problems

Source: G.L. Henry and N. Little. *Neurologic Emergencies: A Symptom-Oriented Approach.* New York: McGraw-Hill, 1985.

bleeding. With chronic subdural hematomas, symptoms can fluctuate mildly from day to day as a result of hemostatic and oncotic forces within the hematoma itself. If a subdural hematoma is suspected, skull x-rays, EEGs, and laboratory tests are of little or no value. Computed tomographic (CT) scanning or angiography is needed if the strong possibility of a subdural hematoma exists.

Acute Epidural Hematomas

Acute epidural hemorrhage is the result of arterial bleeding and is most commonly associated with fractures of the basilar skull that cross the middle meningeal groove, causing tears in the middle meningeal artery. Unlike subdural bleeding, which is venous, epidural bleeding is arterial and therefore rapidly progressive. The patient with a suspected epidural hematoma must be treated quickly and aggressively if the patient is to be salvaged. The patient with a major head trauma who has a short lucid interval and then goes downhill quickly should be strongly suspected of having an epidural hematoma.

Intracerebral Lacerations and Traumatic Intracerebral Hemorrhage

Direct injury to the brain can cause alteration of mental status. The open laceration represents an immediate threat from exsanguination but is usually not a problem from compression. Open brain injury always represents the possibility of infection, as well as the direct physical damage to the underlying tissue.

An intracerebral hematoma represents a difficult diagnostic and therapeutic dilemma to both the emergency physician and the neurosurgeon. The decision as to management will depend on the size of the intracerebral hemorrhage, the structures involved, and the immediate clinical condition of the patient. Considerable thought must be given to the cost-benefit analysis to each intracerebral hemorrhage and whether the risks and complications of surgery outweigh the benefits of a conservative approach.

Cerebrovascular Accidents

It is rare that thrombotic or embolic cerebrovascular events are associated with coma or even significant decreases in mental status. Intracerebral hemorrhages, however, are commonly associated with unconsciousness. Bleeding can be from a ruptured artery, aneurysm, or arteriovenous malformation. When a bleed is the result of a hypertensive crisis, exact location of the bleeding site will usually not be obvious. In patients who are deteriorating rapidly in their mental status because of such severe hypertension, it is advisable to stabilize the patient's blood pressure before attempting to localize the bleeding site with ancillary studies. It is neither necessary nor advisable to drop such a patient's blood pressure into the normal range. The diastolic blood pressure should be brought down to the range of 110 mm Hg.

The intraventricular hemorrhage is a particular subset of cerebrovascular accident. Patients who suffer intraventricular hemorrhage are usually profoundly comatose and have an extremely poor prognosis. Death usually occurs rapidly after pontine level findings appear.

Traumatic Posterior Fossa Hemorrhage
Bleeding below the tentorium cerebelli into the posterior fossa can occur in severe trauma without destruction of the brainstem proper. A hematoma in the posterior fossa can compress the brainstem and should be considered immediately life-threatening. It is impossible to tell this type of hematoma from several other posterior fossa lesions based on physical examination findings alone. Since it represents a potentially treatable surgical lesion, it must be considered as a possibility in trauma cases.

Basilar Artery Occlusion
The brainstem receives its arterial supply through the basilar artery. The reticular activating formation receives its blood supply through the paramedian branches of this single basilar artery. Anything that interferes with the blood supply to the vertebral-basilar system can cause alterations of consciousness. Posterior circulation transient ischemic attacks are often characterized as drop attacks during which there may be a total loss of muscular tone and, depending on which fibers are involved, a loss of consciousness as well. Problems involving the posterior circulation are extremely difficult to manage but must be separated from more treatable entities.

Acute Cerebellar Hemorrhage
The symptoms of head pain and the sudden onset of vertigo with conjugate deviation of the eyes toward the side of positive cerebellar findings strongly suggest an acute cerebellar hemorrhage. Bleeding into the cerebellum is usually the result of a nontraumatic rupture of an arteriovenous malformation or hypertension. The cerebellar hemorrhage is the most treatable of all the intraparenchymal hemorrhages; if it is relieved promptly, a reasonable return of neurologic function is possible. Since the cerebellum and the brainstem essentially occupy the same space, any lesion that involves the cerebellum will in short order involve the brainstem proper.

Pontine Hemorrhage
Bleeding into the substance of the pons is a devastating neurologic event that can rapidly produce coma. It is often difficult to differentiate acute pontine hemorrhage from acute cerebellar hemorrhage. Both lesions are associated with sudden decreases in consciousness, ataxia, breathing disorders, pinpoint pupils, absent or abnormal oculovestibular reflexes, and meningismus. Although there are some reports of successful drainage of intrapontine hematomas, prognosis remains grave. Rapid diagnosis is important to separate this problem from the acute cerebellar hemorrhage, which is potentially a surgically treatable disease.

Brainstem tumors are an exceedingly rare cause of coma. Parenchymal lesions of the brainstem, including angiomas, gliomas, and ependymomas, can cause brainstem compression syndromes. These lesions, however, are usually slow growing and will be associated with positive neurologic findings over a long period of time before causing any changes in mental status. Other posterior fossa tumors, such as meningiomas and acoustic neuromas, usually show positive cranial nerve findings before any significant alteration of mental status is seen, and should not generally be confused with the acute causes of coma.

Subarachnoid Hemorrhage
Subarachnoid hemorrhage is the only intracranial hemorrhage that is usually not focal in nature. Bleeding into the subarachnoid space quickly spreads throughout the cerebrospinal fluid. The resultant vasospasm, which causes decreased bleeding, can also cause decreased mental status as a result of a reduced cerebral blood flow. In all patients who experience headache with decreasing mental status, subarachnoid hemorrhage should be a prime diagnostic consideration.

Infections of the Central Nervous System

Central nervous system infections, as well as generalized septicemia, can cause alterations of mental status by their direct actions on the nervous system and through changes induced throughout the body. Bacterial and viral meningitis, as well as encephalitis, may be seen early in the disease course, with marked confusion that progresses to delirium and finally to lethargy and coma.

Cerebral Neoplasms

It is unusual for coma or even stupor to be the presenting sign in patients with a neoplasm within the supratentorial region. Such patients may have a seizure disorder followed by a prolonged postictal state; during investigation the tumor is discovered. Bleeding into a tumor itself can cause symptoms that are indistinguishable from those of other types of cerebrovascular accidents. The slow encroachment of a supratentorial tumor produces brain swelling, which, over a period of time, can dull mental status but rarely causes an acute alteration of consciousness.

Tumors in the lateral or third ventricles can obstruct outflow of cerebral fluid, causing acute downward pressure and displacement of the brainstem. In rare instances, neoplasm is directly infiltrated to destroy the cerebral connections for the reticular activating formation, causing irreversible coma.

Carcinoma

Cancers of various types can cause severe depression of mental status and coma from multiple mechanisms. Hyponatremia as a direct result of inappropriate antidiuretic hormone (ADH) secretion from cancers involving the lung, pancreas, and prostate is well recognized as causing severe alterations of mental status. Metabolic alkalosis in association with Cushing's syndrome may become severe enough to alter mental status. The leukoencephalopathies seen with lymphomas can significantly affect mental status. Both hypercalcemia and hypocalcemia, although not usual causes of coma, can definitely cause alterations of mental status.

Seizures

A patient who has had a seizure may be seen in the emergency department in a postictal state that resembles coma. It is important to remember that all seizures are not simple epilepsy. If the underlying disease is truly idiopathic epilepsy, the patient generally has a rapid return to normal mental status without residual focal neurologic deficits. Seizures with residual deficits or those lasting more than 15 minutes should be suspected of being structural in nature. It is important to check for underlying causes of seizures, such as encephalitis, metabolic abnormalities, structural lesions, and trauma.

COMA FROM TOXIC-METABOLIC CAUSES

Oxygen Deprivation

The cerebral tissues require a constant stream of oxygen for the patient to remain conscious. When any portion of the cardiorespiratory system is so altered as to prevent the orderly supply of oxygen, coma can result. If sudden in onset, severe anemia that decreases the total delivered oxygen to the brain can cause profound changes of mental status and coma. Low cardiac output due to dysrhythmias or loss of myocardial contractility can also cause decreased cerebral perfusion and therefore decreased oxygen delivery. Antihypertensive medications in the elderly can cause altered mental status by also reducing total cerebral blood flow. Rapid increases in carbon dioxide from pulmonary disease or hypoventilation also correlate closely with depression of mental status.

Hypertensive and Hypotensive Encephalopathies

Alterations of blood pressure on both ends of the scale can cause severe alteration of mental status and coma. The cause of alteration of mental status in hypotension is an inadequate cerebral perfusion and decreased supply of oxygen nutrients. The specific cause for hypotension in the altered mental state should always be sought and should not be assumed to be on a neurogenic basis.

Hypertensive encephalopathy that results in severe altered mental status is a relatively rare condition. Patients with extremely high blood pressure can exhibit disorientation as well as head pain, and if the condition persists, end-organ damage can affect mental status. In patients with significant severe hypertension and altered mental status, the possibility of cerebrovascular accident must also be considered.

Glucose Metabolism

In multiple series, the most common cause of altered mental status seen in the emergency department has been glucose metabolism. Both hyperglycemia and hypoglycemia can cause alterations of mental status. Patients with diabetes are at high risk for altered mental status not only because of glucose but also because of infection and other metabolic derangements. Hyperglycemic patients also suffer changes in mental status secondary to the alterations of the serum osmolality caused by poor control of blood sugar. Hypoglycemia is seen not only in diabetics but also in patients with pancreatic tumors and retroperitoneal sarcomas, in patients with chronic alcoholism accompanied by liver disease, and in patients who have had drug overdoses.

Hepatic Encephalopathies: Cirrhosis

Cirrhosis can contribute to cellular changes within the brain. Rapid elevations of serum ammonia levels can also contribute to changes in mental status. Patients with advanced liver disease frequently have decreased ability to store glycogen and are thus predisposed to hypoglycemia as well.

Reye's Syndrome

Reye's syndrome should be considered a cause of altered mental status in children. It is a multisystem disease that occurs principally in children under the age of 12. Reye's syndrome is associated with viral infections, such as influenza B and chickenpox. The clinical course includes the abrupt onset of vomiting some 7 to 10 days after the initial viral illness. Within 24 to 48 hours, the patient's condition usually progresses to agitation, lethargy, and finally coma. No prominent focal neurologic signs are seen. Tremendous controversy exists as to whether any specific therapy for Reye's syndrome is effective. However, the clinical stages of the disease determine the need for aggressive control of intracranial pressure, which is thought by some to influence the disease outcome. Laboratory findings in Reye's syndrome can be deceptive early in its course. Patients usually have elevated levels of serum glutamic oxaloacetic transaminase (SGOT) and serum glutamic pyruvic transaminase (SGPT) with normal alkaline phosphates. Blood ammonia levels are usually elevated. Any child with severe alteration of mental status and vomiting and an elevated SGOT twice the normal level should be considered to have early Reye's syndrome and be hospitalized for possible control of intracranial pressure.

Uremia

Uremic patients do not undergo actual pathologic changes in the brain cells but experience alterations of mental status based on rising levels of the blood urea nitrogen (BUN) that severely alter serum osmolality. Although the cerebral water content may adjust to gradual changes in BUN, rapid rises in nitrogenous wastes will usually produce depression of mental status and even coma.

Electrolytes

Alteration of serum electrolytes can influence mental status through changes in osmolality. Multiple mechanisms appear to exist by which alterations in serum osmolality can affect neuronal functioning. Hypoosmolality can result from the hyponatremia seen with dialysis or dysequilibrium syndrome, or during correction of diabetic ketoacidosis. Hyponatremia can also result from many disorders, such as congestive heart failure, inappropriate ADH, renal failure, and adrenocortical disease. Hyperosmolality, either from hypernatremia or diabetic hyperosmolar nonketogenic states, causes shifts of fluids and affects membrane potentials and cortical functioning.

Endocrine Disorders

Shifts in serum sodium cause changes in serum osmolality that can affect the central nervous system and produce changes in intracellular water. Extreme hypothyroidism can likewise cause metabolic shifts that result in depressed mental status or even coma. Hyperthyroidism, on the other hand, usually causes an agitated tremulous state. Coma is not usually seen in the hyperthyroid patient until the disease is so severe that thyroid storm occurs or the patient suffers a cerebrovascular accident.

Cofactor Disorders

Lack of specific metabolic cofactors, such as cobalt, manganese, zinc, and thiamine, has been reported to cause coma. Although most of these cofactors are exceedingly rare, thiamine deficiency is well noted in patients with alcoholism and in other persons with severe nutritional deprivation. Wernicke's encephalopathy due to carbohydrate overload and lack of thiamine can cause multiple neurologic deficits, some of which are nonreversible if not treated in a timely manner.

Poisons and Toxins

The most widely used drug of abuse, and still the most common metabolic poison, is ethyl alcohol. The effects of alcohol, although usually short lived, can be profound in causing mental status changes and even coma. Ethyl alcohol is particularly dangerous in young children with poorly developed glycogen storage capabilities, in whom it can produce profound hypoglycemia.

Barbiturates, on the other hand, can cause alteration of mental status over extremely long periods of time, depending on the specific agent ingested. Cases of barbiturate coma that last weeks and are followed by a return to normal mental status have been reported. Severe metabolic acidosis with drugs such as methyl alcohol, ethylene glycol, and paraldehyde can also be seen in patients who abuse drugs.

Environmental Causes: Temperature Regulation

Both hypothermia and hyperthermia are well-recognized causes of coma. Hypothermia below 32°C core body temperature can depress neurologic functioning enough to cause coma. Hypothermia can be the result of underlying diseases such as myxedema or hypoadrenalism, or ingested drugs and toxins.

Hyperthermia with core body temperatures above the level of 42°C can also depress mental status to the point of coma. Patients with severe hyperthermia or hypothermia frequently have underlying neurovascular disease and are often left with severe neurologic residuals.

Subdural Empyema

Empyemas of the subdural space are a rare cause of coma but are extremely lethal. They are usually related to recent surgeries involving the paranasal sinus structures. A subdural empyema can also be seen in conjunction with acute meningitis when *Streptococcus* is the principal causative organism. Meningitis itself is not associated with focal neurologic signs. However, if a patient has symptoms of meningitis plus focal findings, a subdural empyema or brain abscess should be considered.

Viral Infections

Although viral infections should be considered a part of the toxic-metabolic group of causes of coma, certain infections can have focal findings that are confusing in the early presentation. Herpes simplex encephalitis, although a diffuse disease, tends to have a particular affinity for the temporal lobes. Patients can have temporal lobe symptoms and appear to have a focal neurologic process when, indeed, a diffuse viral infection is present. The focality of herpes simplex encephalitis is added to further by the fact that the CT scan is often positive for the temporal lobe areas involved.

In the majority of emergency settings, toxic and metabolic factors are the most common causes for alteration of mental status. When ingestion of drugs and alcohol is included in this group, they become by far the leading cause of stupor and coma. Although intrinsic brain cell diseases can have symptoms similar to the toxic-metabolic conditions, they are usually slow in onset, cause deterioration over long periods of time, and are not often confused with the treatable causes of delirium, encephalopathy, or coma.

GENERAL APPROACH TO THE PATIENT WITH ALTERED MENTAL STATUS

When dealing with a patient in stupor or coma, the usual clinical approach (i.e., careful history followed by physical examination, studies, and treatment) must be abandoned. Since severe alteration of mental status is of such major importance and constitutes potentially immediate serious damage to the patient, an action-oriented approach is required (Table 28-3). As for all critically ill patients in emergency medicine, the ABC_3 approach should be activated immediately. *Airway* management is paramount. Patients who do not have an adequate gag reflex require intubation by one

Table 28-3. General approach to the patient with altered mental status

- Airway established
- Breathing checked (including auscultation to rule out pneumothorax)
- Cardiac output assessed
- Cervical spine immobilization
- Obvious hemorrhage compressed
- Intravenous (IV) line started
- Vital signs (full set)
- Thiamine, 100 mg IV
- Glucose, 50 ml, 50% IV
- Naloxone, two ampules IV, repeated if no response
- The stable patient historical features obtained, including the rate of onset, drugs, trauma, fever, prior episodes
- General physical examination: signs of trauma, i.e., Battle's sign, hemotympanium, scalp hematomas and lacerations, subcutaneous emphysema of the chest, etc.
- Obvious lesions of the abdomen, lesions of the pelvis, and long-bone injuries
- Skin: needle marks, cyanosis, pallor, rashes, dehydration
- Breath and odors: alcohol, acetone, fecal material, fetor hepaticus
- Cardiac examination: rhythm, signs of decreased output
- Abdominal findings: organomegaly, ascites, bruits, flank ecchymoses (Grey Turner's sign); rectal and pelvic examination as time permits
- Neurological examination (general)
  - Observation
  - Respiratory pattern
    - Normal
    - Cheyne-Stokes
    - Hyperventilation
    - Apneustic breathing
    - Ataxic breathing
    - Agonal breathing
    - Autisms
      - Yawning
      - Coughing
      - Hiccupping
      - Vomiting
- Neurological examination (specific)
  - Mental status
    - Responds to voice
    - Responds to touch
    - Responds to noxious stimuli
  - Cranial nerves
    - Visual threat
    - Inspection of fundi for papilledema and hemorrhages
  - Pupils
    - Size
    - Reactions—direct and consensual
  - Extraocular movements
    - Oculovestibular testing
    - Oculocephalic testing (if appropriate)
  - Corneal reflex
  - Facial asymmetry
  - Motor system
    - Posturing
    - Ability of the limbs to move
    - Stimuli
  - Decerebration, decortication, or true abduction by high-level centers
  - Pathologic reflexes
- X-rays and laboratory studies (the need for all x-ray and laboratory studies are relative; their use will be guided by the initial examination and the patient's initial response to therapy)
- Complete blood count
- BUN
- Electrolytes
- Glucose
- Calcium
- Toxic screen for drugs
- Arterial blood gases
- Cervical spine x-rays
- CT scan
- Lumbar puncture
- Electrocardiogram

Source: Modified from G.L. Henry and N. Little. *Neurologic Emergencies: A Symptom-Oriented Approach.* New York: McGraw-Hill, 1985.

of the standard approaches, not only to support their respirations, which may be quickly diminishing, but to prevent aspiration, which in many series has been found to be an important cause of death in patients with altered mental status. Regurgitation and aspiration take place so quickly that a "wait and see" attitude is fraught with disaster.

After an appropriate airway has been established, ventilation *(breathing)* should be of concern. The emergency physician should note not only the volume of air being exchanged but also the respiratory pattern of the patient. This should be recorded and will subsequently be integrated with other neurologic data in establishing the cause of the patient's coma. Assuring adequate ventilation helps to provide adequate oxygenation to the patient during the evaluation phase, and mild hyperventilation helps to lower the carbon dioxide pressure and decrease intracranial pressure.

Concomitant with airway control and ventilatory support, the patient's *cervical spine* should be protected in all cases in which trauma is a possibility. If cervical spine fractures are suspected or the mechanism of coma is unknown, the neck should be stabilized while an airway is secured. Either endotracheal intubation with continuous monitoring of the head position or nasotracheal intubation in breathing patients is an excellent form of airway control that should minimize cervical spine movement. In patients who have had severe midfacial and oral trauma and in whom the standard approaches to airway control are contraindicated, a cricothyrotomy or tracheostomy may be necessary.

Another one of the three *Cs* of initial approach is *cardiac status.* Just as patients with inadequate ventilation require support, patients with inadequate cardiac output also require support. It is useless to begin a detailed neurologic evaluation and search for a correctable intracranial cause if the patient does not have adequate cardiac output. Once cardiac stability has been established and the immediate life-threatening arrhythmias have been eliminated, a more careful evaluation of the patient's cardiovascular system can be carried out.

The last of the three initial *Cs* of initial resuscitation is *control* of obvious hemorrhage. Again, detailed evaluation of the nervous system should come after obvious arterial and venous bleeding has been compressed. Although detailed wound management is not required early on, the patient should not be allowed to exsanguinate while being evaluated or awaiting studies. All obvious hemorrhage should be stopped before detailed physical and neurologic examination has begun. Early signs of shock include apprehension and confusion. As shock deepens, mental status quickly deteriorates and thus the patient in hemorrhagic shock can be lethargic or comatose.

Initial treatment should be essentially simultaneous with the performance of the initial *ABCs*. An intravenous line should be inserted and blood removed for further laboratory analysis. It has become standard that thiamine, 100 mg; glucose, 25 gm; and naloxone, 2 mg, are given intravenously on an empiric basis. It is of the utmost importance that nutritionally deficient patients, such as alcoholics, patients receiving cancer chemotherapy, and the very elderly who may have improper diets, receive thiamine before glucose administration. Thiamine is given to facilitate carbohydrate metabolism through its effect on two carbon transfers. An excessive glucose load in the face of inadequate thiamine can precipitate Wernicke's syndrome. In the awake patient, Wernicke's syndrome will be characterized by abnormal eye movements and incoordination. In the comatose patient, the earliest findings may be sixth-nerve palsies, which can be confused with increasing intracranial pressure. Any debilitated or alcoholic patient with a sudden onset of sixth-nerve palsies should have Wernicke's syndrome included as a prominent part of the differential diagnosis.

The administration of glucose, usually as a 50% solution, has also become standard. There are some minor theoretical arguments against giving glucose load until the patient's serum sodium is known, but these are of no clinical significance. No good experimental data suggest that comatose patients should not immediately receive glucose. For patients who are comatose because of hyperglycemia, the recommended dose of glucose is inconsequential. For patients who are hypoglycemic, however, immediate administration of the glucose can be brain-saving, if not lifesaving. Glucose also increases the serum osmotic load and is therefore potentially beneficial in reducing increased intracranial pressure in patients who have mass lesions.

Naloxone is an effective antagonist of opiates in synthetic narcotics such as propoxyphene and pentazocine. Generally, 2 mg naloxone is given intravenously, followed by 2 mg more if no response is seen. No dose-related adverse effects of naloxone have been reported, although the possibility of an acute opiate withdrawal syndrome increases along with each dose of naloxone. Unlike its predecessor, nalorphine, naloxone does not produce respiratory depression. It should be noted that a very large dose of naloxone may be required to overcome the endorphin receptor effects of synthetic narcotics. Any patient who can be aroused with naloxone may become combative and disoriented. Proper precautions should be taken, therefore, before its administration.

Obtaining the History

The patient is often an unreliable or impossible source of history in the face of altered mental status. Medical information can be obtained from the patient's personal effects, such as medical alert tags, information in his or her wallet or purse, or medication containers. Friends and family accompanying the patient should be queried to provide further history, or family members can be contacted by phone. Such sources may be able to describe previous episodes or events that led up to the current problem. Specific questions about abnormal motor movements, food or drug ingestions, trauma, and underlying disease entities should be asked. It is important to provide reassurance that the medical history obtained remains part of the medical record and will not be capriciously or arbitrarily given to law enforcement officials without due process.

General Physical Examination

Vital Signs

Complete vital signs should be taken and repeated at regular intervals (see Table 28-3). The patient should be monitored for dysrhythmias, which should be treated as clinically indicated. As mentioned earlier, both the patient's respiratory rate and rhythm should be carefully observed to be integrated into the total neurologic picture. Initial tachypnea should be considered a sign of inadequate oxygenation, at least early on, and treatment should err on the side of improving oxygenation as opposed to assuming that the tachypnea is triggered by a central neurologic event. Oxygenation and ventilation should be properly corrected, followed by reevaluation of the patient's mental status.

Both hypertension and hypotension should be considered to have nonneurologic causes until proved otherwise. Although systemic hypertension can be caused by an elevation in intracranial pressure, it should not initially be ascribed to a neurologic mass lesion. Hypotension, likewise, should always be considered to be on a hypovolemic or distributive shock basis, rather than from a neurogenic cause when initially noted. Correction of hypotension through proper fluid administration and other support measures should be vigorously instituted. Alterations of mental status are difficult to evaluate in patients in profound shock, and their mental status should always be reviewed after restoration of normal tissue profusion.

Knowledge of the patient's rectal temperature is important in looking for both hyperthermia and hypothermia. Extremes at either end of the scale can in and of themselves cause alteration of mental status from mild lethargy to coma.

Head and Neck Region

As the patient is examined, signs of trauma should be carefully sought. These signs, such as hematomas in the region of the mastoid processes (Battle's sign), raccoon eyes, and local tenderness or crepitus all suggest severe trauma and should be specifically sought. Blood behind the tympanic membranes should be considered a sign of a basilar skull fracture until proved otherwise. Careful palpation of the head may reveal cephalohematomas that are not visible at first glance. Palpation of the neck, although often advocated, is generally nonproductive in the comatose patient. It is best to assume that a cervical spine injury is present and to immobilize the neck until the necessary x-rays are performed. Even without specific signs of trauma to the head and neck region, areas of multiple trauma on the rest of the body in a comatose patient should suggest trauma to the central nervous system.

Skin

Needle tracks suggest intravenous (IV) drug use. Cyanosis can suggest hypoxemia, polycythemia, or abnormal hemoglobin. Pallor can likewise be an early indication that the patient has inadequate oxygen-carrying capacity as a result of blood loss with resultant anemia. Carbon monoxide poisoning, in rare cases, can produce a cherry-red glow of the mucous membranes. Other more generalized skin findings, such as multiple abscesses, cellulitis, uremic frost, or icterus, can point to underlying conditions that are affecting the patient's mental state.

The odor of alcohol on the breath should not be equated with alcohol as the cause of the patient's deteriorated mental status. Alcoholics and individuals under the influence of alcohol are certainly susceptible to trauma, hypoglycemia, and all the other usual causes of coma; however, to assume that altered mental status is the result of alcohol alone ignores other potential disease processes. The fruity fragrance of acetone or the distinct odor of an infection should be evident to the experienced examiner with developed olfactory skills. Fetor hepaticus indicates advanced liver disease. A feculent smell suggests bowel obstruction. Cyanide has the distinctive odor of bitter almonds.

Cardiac Examination

The presence of tachyarrhythmias or bradyarrhythmias can alter mental status through the mechanism of decreased cardiac output. Endocarditis or various dysrhythmias can produce mural thrombi that can be dislodged, causing cerebral emboli that can, in unusual cases, affect the level of alertness. In cases of severe myocardial infarction, cardiac output can be reduced enough to cause depressed consciousness.

Abdominal Examination

The presence of organomegaly, pulsatile masses, ascites, and bruits should be sought. Such conditions can indicate intraabdominal pathology associated with alterations of mental status. Hepatomegaly and ascites can be associated with severe hepatic failure and the resultant hepatic encephalopathy. The presence of an intraabdominal aortic aneurysm is consistent with advanced vascular disease, and in the presence of shock, can show the origins of the patient's inadequate cerebral perfusion. In cases in which the cause of the patient's coma is still unknown, a rectal examination should be performed to detect bleeding, masses, infection, or foreign bodies.

General Neurologic Examination

Observation

The first part of the neurologic examination should be observation (see Table 28-3). The patient should be carefully observed for involuntary movements or abnormal posturing, or both. The patient who is agitated and yet has decreased mental status may have a toxic encephalopathy. Tonic contractions can be due to tetanus, strychnine poisoning, dystonic reactions, or decerebration. Seizures should be observed to see if they are focal or generalized in nature.

Respiratory Pattern

Both the rate and pattern of respiration should be noted since it can indicate the level of neurologic injury in the patient (Fig. 28-1). An awake patient at rest generally breathes 14 to 18 times per minute and has occasional sighing or deeper respirations as demanded by carbon dioxide levels. When the cortex is no longer functioning, the nervous system is relying on diencephalic control of breathing. Cheyne-Stokes respirations then occur. This type of breathing is characterized by periodic, regularly increasing breaths alternating with short periods of apnea. The breathing crescendos to a peak and then ceases or decrescendos suddenly. The apneic phase is usually short. The most frequent cause for a Cheyne-Stokes respiration pattern is bilateral involvement of the hemispheres through metabolic disease or structural disease of the cerebral hemispheres and basal ganglia. The principal mechanism underlying Cheyne-Stokes respirations has to do with loss of forebrain control of ventilatory stimulation.

Hyperventilation in the stuporous or comatose patient can stem from a variety of causes. Attempts to correct hypoxia or compensate for metabolic acidosis, as well as brain injury itself, are possible explanations for hyperventilation. Central neurogenic hyperventilation is seen in midbrain lesions with the impairment of those areas that normally monitor ventilatory patterns. When hyperventilation is caused by central nervous system disease, it indicates upper brainstem damage.

Apneustic breathing is characterized by a prolonged pause at the end of inspiration with breath-holding. It is seen with lesions in and about the brainstem at the level of the fifth cranial nerve. Cluster breathing is breathing in short bursts and is almost always associated with lesions at the level of the pons. Ataxic breathing, irregular breathing without pattern or regularity, is a forerunner of agonal respirations and death.

Autisms

Autisms are involuntary neurologic acts carried out for the maintenance and protection of the body. Yawning, although its mechanism is not well understood, frequently accompanies expanding lesions of the posterior fossa. Other autisms, such as vomiting, coughing, and hiccupping, have neurogenic centers involved in their control. In the face of altered mental status, hiccupping, coughing, and vomiting can be indications of lesions that involve brainstem centers.

Specific Neurologic Examination

Mental Status

The most sensitive early indicator of nervous system disease is alteration of mental status (see Table 28-3). It is the first function to be affected in a variety of lesions. The ability to respond to voice and follow commands should be recorded. If the patient cannot respond to voice but responds to firm but gentle touch, the manner of response must be assessed. Response to noxious stimuli is recorded.

Since early changes in mental status are subtle, the examination and recording of that examination must be equally refined. In the patient who has mild decrease in mental status, it is best to chart orientation and recall of specific facts to help establish a baseline for future questioning. Subtle changes, such as perseveration of words, lack of orientation to place, or even out-of-proportion anxiety, can lead one to suspect early cortical compression or swelling.

There is no need to inflict pain on a patient suspected of feigning coma, since other more humane techniques are available to detect functional disease. In the patient in whom

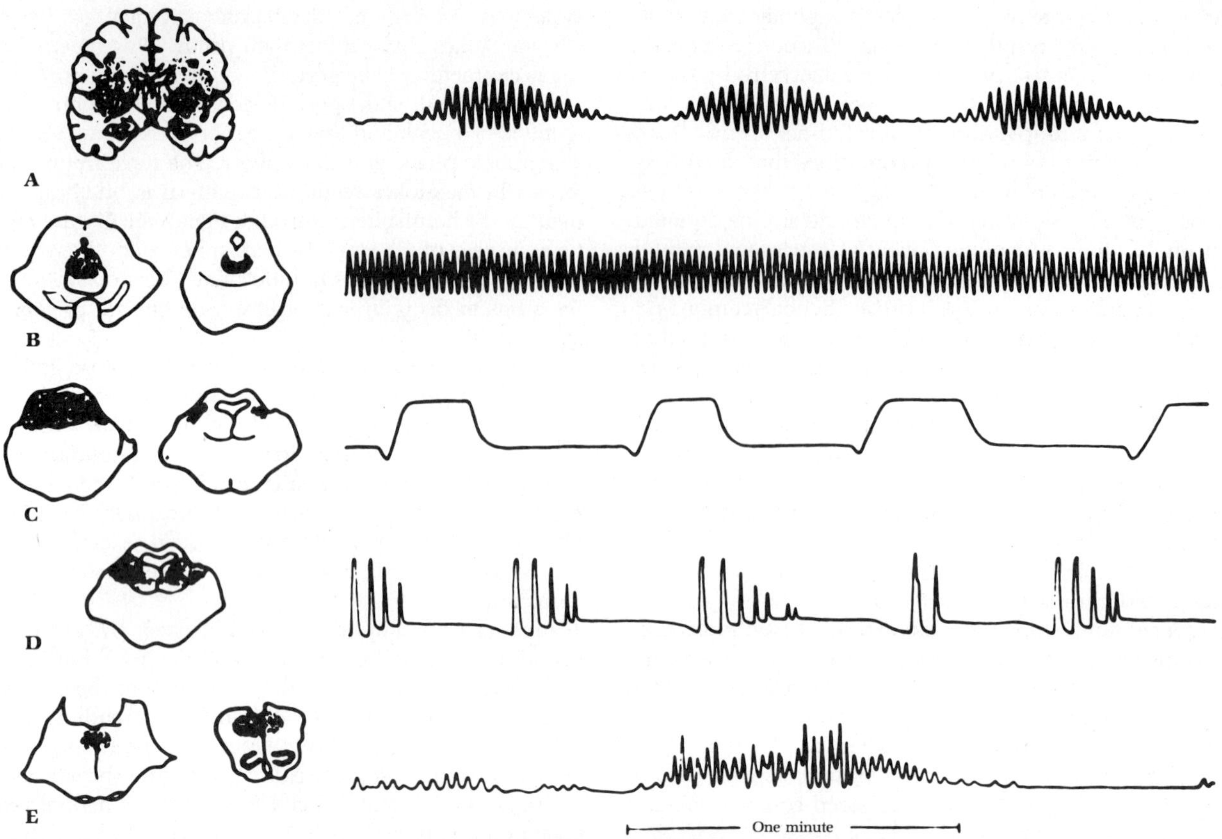

Fig. 28-1. Abnormal respiratory patterns associated with pathologic lesions *(shaded areas)* at various levels of the brain. Tracings by chest-abdomen pneumograph inspiration read up. A. Cheyne-Stokes respiration. B. Central neurogenic hyperventilation. C. Apneusis. D. Cluster breathing. E. Ataxic breathing. (From F. Plum and J. Posner. *Diagnosis of Stupor and Coma* [2nd ed.]. Philadelphia: Davis, 1972. P. 26.)

the psychogenic cause for altered mental status is suspected, relatively painless techniques can be employed to establish the diagnosis of psychogenic coma. One common technique is to gently lift the eyelids. It is almost impossible for a patient to fake the lack of resistance to eyelid-opening and the slow fall of the eyelids seen in a truly comatose patient. Any patient who vigorously fights the opening of the eyes is not comatose. Even with gentle eye-opening, most patients will have a response to protect the eyes.

Another useful technique is ocular tracking. When open, the eyes of an awake patient will track to themselves if placed in front of a mirror. When the examiner holds a mirror slightly to the side and in front of a patient and the eyes are opened, they will look toward the eyes in the mirror. This ocular tracking is a very difficult response for a patient to suppress.

In cases in which it is difficult to discern the exact cause of the coma, cold caloric testing, as mentioned in the next section, will provide a definitive separation between pyschogenic and organic causes of coma.

Motor Examination

The most important part of the motor examination—observation—should be completed early on in the evaluation of the comatose patient. Spontaneous motor movements and general posturing should be noted. Spontaneous motor movements are generally a good sign. The ability of the muscles to move without external stimuli indicates that the patient is sending some cortical instructions or some movement instructions down the motor pathways. Any patient who can follow a command or move a body part and can manage, showing high-level motor-system function, is not comatose.

The response to stimuli helps isolate the level at which the nervous system is functioning. Abduction of the limb or movements toward the site of the noxious stimuli show motor-system involvement at least at a diencephalic level. Decorticate posturing is hyperextension of the legs and flexion of the arms and elbows, with hands coming in toward the center of the body. Such posturing can occur with lesions of the internal capsule to the upper midbrain, which interfere with corticospinal pathways.

Decerebrate rigidity, in which the teeth are clenched and the arms and legs are extended, is seen in only a few situations. It is usually caused by severe disease involving the central midbrain, leaving the lower brainstem below the lesion intact. Posterior fossa lesions that cause pressure against the brainstem can likewise result in this type of posturing. Decerebrate posturing can also accompany post-anoxic cerebral demyelination.

Total paralysis in the comatose patient with no posturing despite the application of nocuous stimuli should be considered a grave finding, indicating that no protective brainstem mechanisms are functioning. It can be seen in severe, deep metabolic or toxic comas, but is more likely to occur in

Table 28-4. Drugs and toxins capable of producing constriction and dilatation of pupils

Constriction		Dilatation		
Parasympathetic stimulators (cholinergics)	Sympathetic inhibitors (antiadrenergics)	Parasympathetic inhibitors (anticholinergics)		Sympathetic stimulators (adrenergics)
Acetylcholine	Guanethedine	Botulinus toxin	Imipramine (Tofranil)	Cocaine
Nicotine	Bretylium	Hemicholine	Doxepin (Sinequan)	Paradrine
Tetraethyl ammonium	Reserpine	Pentolinium	Diphenhydramine (Benadryl)	Ephedrine
Bromide	Alpha-methyl dopa (Aldomet)	Atropine-like drugs	Desipramine (Pertofrane)	Adrenaline
Physostigmine	Monoamine oxidase inhibitors	Scopolamine	Meprobamate and benactyzine (Deprol)	Phenylephrine (Neo-synephrine)
Neostigmine	Phenoxybenzamine (Dibenzyline)	Homatropine	Teldrin	Tyramine
Pyrophosphates	Phentolamine (Regitine)	Eucatropine	Sominex	
Carbachol (Doryl)	Tolazoline (Priscoline)	Tropicamide (Mydriacyl)	Compoz	
Mecholyl		Cyclopentolate (Cyclogyl)	Cope	
Pilocarpine		Methantheline (Banthine)	Toadstool toxin	
Lesions of third nerves		Dicyclomine (Bentyl)	Jimson weed	
Midbrain lesions		Isopropamide (Darbid)	Wild sage	

Source: G.L. Henry and N. Little. *Neurologic Emergencies: A Symptom-Oriented Approach.* New York: McGraw-Hill, 1985.

structural lesions that affect the brainstem nuclei. To be certain that no movement is possible, stimuli must be given both above and below the foramen magnum. Patients with cervical spine injuries may only be able to grimace the facial musculature if their motor tracks have been severed in the cervical cord region.

Eyes

Visual threat is an unreliable test in unresponsive patients. This reaction can be suppressed in certain individuals voluntarily, and the actual movement of air against the cornea can produce a blink response even in patients who have no vision. Lack of response to visual threat is not certain evidence for coma, and response is not evidence for wakefulness.

The ocular fundi can give the examiner the only opportunity to view an extension of the brain. Evidence of papilledema, subhyoid hemorrhages, and spontaneous venous pulsations should be sought. Spontaneous venous pulsations in erect patients indicate normal intracranial pressure. This is often difficult to assess with comatose patients, however, since they are generally recumbent. If spontaneous venous pulsations are seen when the patient is in the recumbent position, they clearly indicate that the possibility of increased intracranial pressure is remote.

Pupils

The size, shape, and reactivity, both direct and concentric, of the pupils should be recorded. The pupillary pathways are relatively resistant to metabolic insult. They receive their parasympathetic supply from the thalamic pretectal region and their sympathetic supply from the superior cervical ganglion, which courses along the carotid artery.

Pupillary findings must be interpreted along with the entire neurologic examination. As a general rule, hemispheric disease has very little influence on pupillary function. Usually, patients who are comatose from metabolic involvement of the cerebral hemispheres will have small to midrange pupils that are reactive to light. Structural lesions involving the diencephalon can cause small but reactive pupils. Pupillary size and reactivity can be altered by eye trauma, ocular drugs, or previous surgery (Table 28-4). Such common causes for pupillary asymmetry should be sought.

A unilateral fixed and dilated pupil should not necessarily be equated with an intracranial mass lesion. It can be the result of a cycloplegic agent instilled into one eye. An expanding aneurysm that compresses the third cranial nerve can cause an ipsilateral fixed and dilated pupil, but does not usually affect mental status. The general rule is that if a patient is alert, a dilated pupil is most likely not the result of increasing intracranial pressure. The mechanism for the fixed and dilated pupil seen with severe head injury is herniation of the uncus of the temporal lobe through the tentorial notch, which compresses the third cranial nerve. No patient with this degree of increased intracranial pressure will exhibit normal mental status (Fig. 28-2).

Lesions that involve the midbrain tectal regions can cause midsized to large pupils that may respond poorly to light. Pontine lesions frequently cause fixed pinpoint pupils that are not affected by naloxone. Anoxia, atropine, and cycloplegic agents can all cause dilated pupils. Pinpoint pupils, which are reversible with naloxone, are the result of the effects of narcotics. Certain narcotics, however, such as propoxyphene, can leave the pupils intact and reactive. One cannot rule out a narcotic overdose strictly on the basis of pupillary size and reactivity (Table 28-5).

Ocular Movements

In the awake patient, eye movements are directed by both anterior frontal lobe and posterior occipital lobe control centers, which are connected to the pontine gaze centers. These gaze centers lie adjacent to the sixth cranial nerves and in turn direct eye movements by way of the medial longitudinal fasciculus (MLF). The MLF, which turns from the upper cervical spine through the area of the third cranial nerve, is the principal interconnection for all conjugate eye movements. Because it extends over the entire length of the brainstem itself, testing the MLF is the single best method for judging intactness of the brainstem.

When freed from cortical control mechanisms, most comatose patients will exhibit roving eye movements, assuming that the brainstem is intact. Eye movements can be dysconjugate or conjugate, but as long as both eyes cross the midline, there is no evidence of damage at the brainstem level.

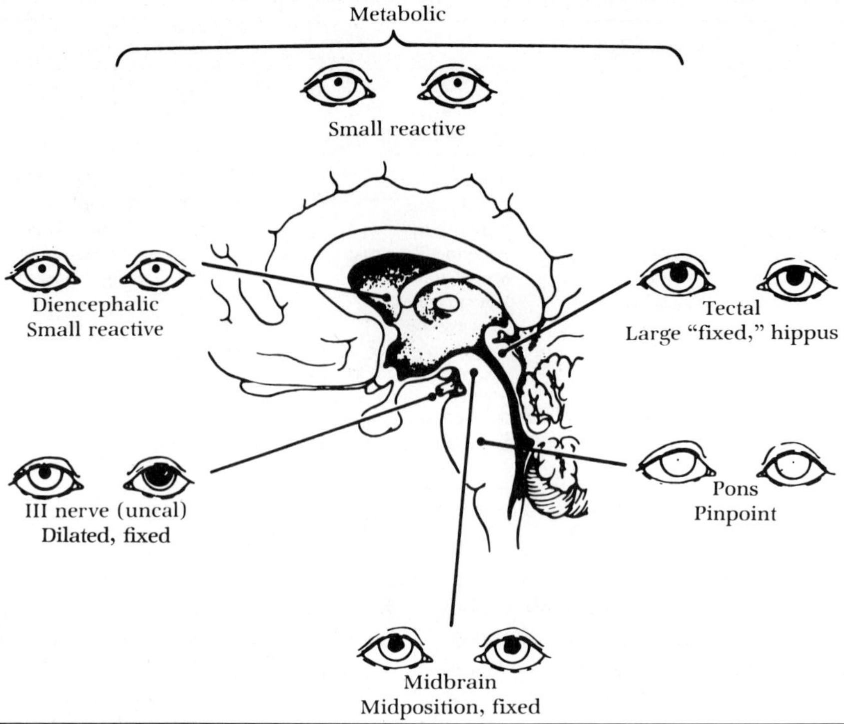

Fig. 28-2. Pupils in comatose patients. (From F. Plum and J. Posner. *Diagnosis of Stupor and Coma* [2nd ed.]. Philadelphia: Davis, 1972. P. 36.)

A general rule regarding cortical injuries is that the eyes will turn toward a dead or nonfunctioning hemisphere and away from an irritative one. For example, during a seizure the eyes will look away from the side of excess activity or seizure focus. The eyes may be abnormally deviated in a comatose patient because of injury involving cortical or pontine gaze centers.

To decide whether the cause of coma is a cortical or brainstem lesion, oculocephalic mechanisms can be tested. The presence of oculocephalic reflexes depends on whether the MLF receives constant information as to the position of the patient's head through the output of the semicircular canals. Without cortical influences, an intact brainstem maintains the eyes forward or upward when the patient is supine. This is the basis of the "doll's eye maneuver," the involuntary movement of the eyes upward and downward on passive flexion and extension of the head. In a comatose patient in whom a cervical spine injury is suspected, the performance of this test is contraindicated.

Oculovestibular testing, commonly referred to as "caloric testing," is a more sophisticated method to test the integrity of the brainstem (Table 28-6). To perform the test, the examiner injects 50 ml ice-cold water against the tympanic membrane. Countercurrent flow is set up in the semicircular canals and the information is transmitted to the pontine gaze centers near the ipsilateral sixth-nerve nucleus. The altered endolymphatic flow allows centers to believe that the head has been rapidly turned in the opposite direction. Only four clinical responses are possible: bilateral nystagmus, bilateral fixed conjugate gaze, no response whatsoever, and unilateral eye deviation. If caloric stimulation of the eye produces

Table 28-5. Summary of pupillary findings

Pupil size	Interpretations
Midposition 3- to 5-ml nonreactive pupils	Midbrain damage, drugs
Normal-sized reactive pupils	Metabolic abnormality; toxins, drugs; normal
Unilaterally dilated and unreactive to light or pilocarpine pupil without other third-nerve finding	Topical chemical in the eye, local eye trauma
Unilaterally dilated and unreactive pupil in a comatose patient with complete motor third-nerve findings	Uncal herniation: compression of the third nerve, expanding posterior communicating artery aneurysm; ruptured
Unilaterally dilated and unreactive pupil with third-nerve motor findings in awake patient	Compression of the third nerve by posterior communicating artery aneurysm
Bilaterally small and poorly reactive pupils	Pontine lesion, infarct, hemorrhage
Small pupils bilaterally reactive to naloxone (Narcan)	Systemic chemical, i.e., narcotics; alteration of pupil
Bilaterally dilated pupils, unresponsive to pilocarpine	Severe anoxia; topically instilled drugs, i.e., atropine; eye trauma
Dilatation of the pupils bilaterally with painful stimulus below the level of the neck (ciliospinal reflex)	Indicates connection between brainstem and spinal cord

Source: G.L. Henry and N. Little. *Neurologic Emergencies: A Symptom-Oriented Approach.* New York: McGraw-Hill, 1985.

Table 28-6. Caloric testing

Ice-water effect	Interpretation
Both eyes deviate and good nystagmus is produced	Patient is not comatose
Both eyes deviate toward cold water, bilateral, no fast phase	Coma but intact brainstem function
No eye movement despite cold stimuli to both sides; indirectly	Brainstem: complete structural damage, metabolic paralysis, hypothermia
Movement of eye ipsilateral to side stimulant but not opposite eye	Internuclear ophthalmoplegia, structural lesion of brainstem

Source: G.L. Henry and N. Little. *Neurologic Emergencies: A Symptom-Oriented Approach.* New York: McGraw-Hill, 1985.

prominent nystagmus of both eyes, the cerebral cortex, the corticobulbar tracts, the MLF, and the brainstem are working. All forms of nystagmus are based on a slow deviation component that results from brainstem-directed eye movements, with a correcting response directed by the cortex. Any patient who is able to produce nystagmus is not truly comatose.

If both eyes move conjugately toward the side irrigated with the cold water and if they remain deviated without nystagmus, then the midbrain and its brainstem reflexes are intact, but there is no checking or monitoring correction component from the cortex. This indicates that the brainstem mechanisms on the side tested are working and that information has been carried to the opposite side of the brainstem to move the contralateral eye. When the cold water is instilled in the opposite ear and both eyes again move conjugately toward the side of the cold irrigation, there is further confirmatory evidence that the entire brainstem reflex mechanism is intact and that, although cortical control is not present, no brainstem failure has occurred.

If cold-water irrigation of both ears done sequentially produces no eye movement of any kind, the brainstem is structurally or physiologically functionless. This brainstem failure can represent total destruction of the brainstem or severe physical or chemical suppression. Deep hypothermia and certain drugs, such as barbiturates and glutethimide (Doriden), can totally suppress the brainstem reflexes without structurally damaging the tracks or nuclei. Therefore, lack of any response to caloric stimulation does not necessarily prove irreversible disease. It does indicate, however, that the brainstem nuclei are not working. In a patient who is normothermic and has no drugs in the bloodstream, absent caloric responses mean brain death.

If one ear is irrigated and the ipsilateral eye moves to that side but the contralateral eye does not move, internuclear ophthalmoplegia is present. This means that the sixth cranial nerve on the side tested is functioning, but it is unable to transmit information to the opposite side of the brainstem. The opposite third cranial nerve, which would cause the conjugate medial movement of the contralateral eye, has not been stimulated. Such a finding almost always indicates severe structural damage or compression of the brainstem.

The corneal reflex may also be a useful test in examining comatose patients. The sensory portion of the corneal reflex is mediated through the fifth cranial nerve. Its efferent motor reaction is produced through the seventh cranial nerve. One must look for both the direct and the concentric response to determine if the reflex is working properly.

Sensory Examination

The sensory examination of the comatose patient essentially parallels the motor examination. The sensory or afferent fibers and the motor or efferent fibers are tested concomitantly.

Reflex Status

Reflexes in comatose patients can be sensitive but not very specific. An upgoing toe can indicate lesions along the corticospinal tract all the way from the cortex down to the motor neuron in the spinal cord. The importance of reflex testing in the comatose patient, as in the awake patient, lies in determining the general level of lesion. Reflexes must be compared for symmetry side to side and top to bottom. Abdominal reflexes are of extremely low value and not worth testing in comatose patients.

Table 28-7. Rostrocaudal brainstem deterioration secondary to expanding right supratentorial mass

Anatomic level	Consciousness	Respiration	Pupils	Oculovestibular	Motor
Upper diencephalon	Drowsy (dull)	Eupnea with yawns and sighs	Small, reactive	Depression of ocular checking and fast component of nystagmus	Left hemiparesis, bilateral paratonia
Lower diencephalon	Coma	Cheyne-Stokes (CSR)	Small, reactive	Loss of above	Left hemiparesis, decorticate
Mesencephalon	Coma	CSR; central neurogenic hyperventilation (CNH)	Midposition fixed (MPF)	Dysconjugate response (loss of medial rectus function on horizontal gaze)	Decerebrate
Upper pons	Coma	CNH, ataxic	MPF	As above	Weak decerebrate
Lower pons	Coma	Ataxic, eupnea	MPF	None	Flaccid, areflexic
Medulla	Coma	Apnea	MPF	None	Same

Source: G.L. Henry and N. Little. *Neurologic Emergencies: A Symptom-Oriented Approach.* New York: McGraw-Hill, 1985.

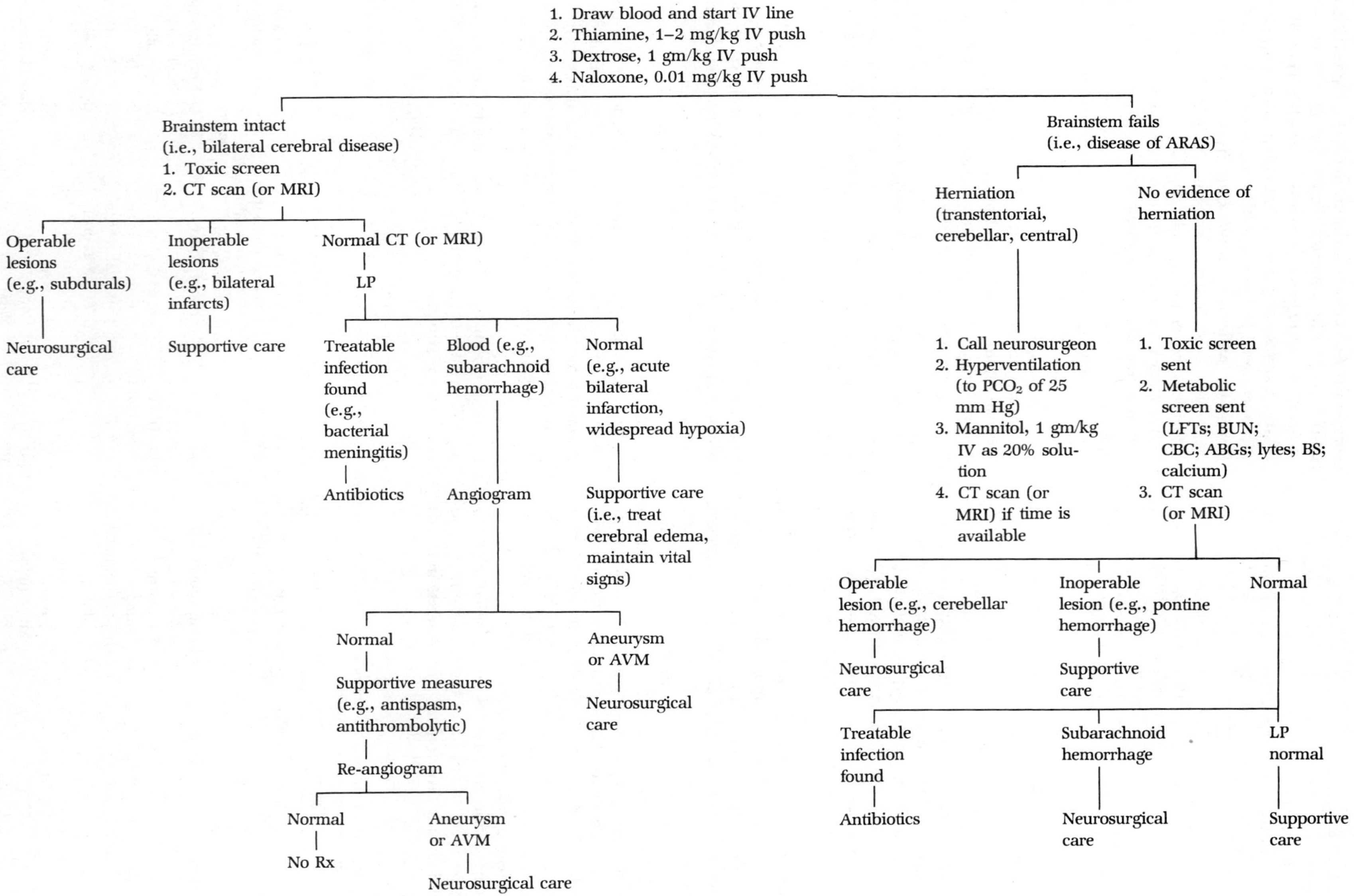

Fig. 28-3. Diagnosis and treatment protocol in the comatose patient. (CBC = complete blood count; LP = lumbar puncture; AVM = arteriovenous malformation; ARA = anterior reticular activating system; LFT = liver function tests; BS = blood sugar.) (From M.A. Samuels. *Manual of Neurologic Therapeutics.* Boston: Little, Brown, 1982. P. 13.)

Examination Summary

The neurologic examination of the patient with altered mental status has only a few areas of vital importance. Correct assessment of the level of mental status is paramount. Examinations of respiratory pattern, extraocular movements, pupils, and motor function need to be simultaneously integrated to determine the level of neurologic function. These various levels should be internally consistent. The principal goal of the neurologic examination is to distinguish structural localized lesions from diffuse metabolic ones (Table 28-7).

MANAGEMENT

Integration of laboratory and x-ray evaluation into the management of the patient is important. The selection of laboratory and radiographic testing is guided by the initial history and initial physical evaluation. Support therapy for the comatose patient must be performed first, however, as indicated in the "initial approach" section; then an orderly approach to the laboratory testing can follow. A complete blood count, serum osmolality, serum glucose, electrolytes, BUN, and blood gases can all be of significance in determining a metabolic cause of coma. Toxic drug screening should be ordered for those patients who have a nonfocal cause for coma and in whom no other discernible laboratory abnormalities are found. Toxic screens usually take several hours to complete, however, and basic decisions must be made before results are obtained. The indication for an emergency lumbar puncture is a strong suspicion of a nonfocal infection of the central nervous system in the patient without focal neurologic findings. The lumbar puncture is contraindicated in the presence of a mass lesion or focal findings. Except for the immediate evaluation of what appears to be nonfocal meningitis, the lumbar puncture can be postponed until a CT scan is performed. In cases in which meningitis is suspected, antibiotic therapy should be started even before the lumbar puncture if there is any delay in obtaining CT scanning when focal findings are present.

The most important plain-film radiologic study is of the cervical spine to rule out fracture or dislocation. A cross-table lateral view followed by anterior, posterior, and odontoid views are the minimum views needed. Even if the cervical spine films are found to be normal, the neck should remain immobilized if cervical cord injury is suspected.

The CT scan has become the definitive test in the management of focal neurologic disease. In coma patients, the CT scan can detect not only intracranial lesions but also fractures of the skull as well. It can detect amounts of blood as minute as 5 ml. Cervical spine films should be performed before a CT scan, as it is virtually impossible to position the patient in the scanner without some manipulation of the neck. If an emergency department does not have access within its hospital for CT scanning, it should have transfer arrangements available to obtain the study when focal neurologic disease entities are suspected (Fig. 28-3).

The most important function of the emergency department evaluation of the comatose patient is separation of structural, potentially surgically treatable disease from metabolic disease, followed by initiation of appropriate therapy. Fig. 28-3 provides a basis for immediate stabilization, generic treatment, and general physical and neurological examination. It then represents an algorithm for the management of comatose patients after initial treatment has been performed and the data have been obtained.

An example for the use of the diagnostic and treatment algorithm is the patient who is seen in a comatose state with a dilated, fixed right pupil and the right eye looking downward and outward. No history is obtainable, as the patient was found alone. The algorithm indicates that blood be drawn for analysis and an IV line started. Thiamine, glucose, and naloxone (Narcan) should be administered immediately. In the case of our patient, no result is obtained. Since the physical examination shows a brainstem alteration (i.e., potential herniation), the next actions should include notification of members of the neurosurgical department, basic support for the patient, and performance of a CT scan. In the case of our patient, a subarachnoid hemorrhage was noted on CT scan and the patient was immediately transferred to the neurosurgical department for angiography and possible operation.

It is important to note that had the CT scan been negative, a lumbar puncture would have been required to make the diagnosis. There is no reason to perform a spinal tap on any focal finding in the emergency department before CT scanning is obtained.

Stupor and coma are radical changes from the normal state of the nervous system and require definitive action to be taken in a timely manner. Rapid assessment and application of the correct testing techniques should allow the emergency physician to arrive at a diagnosis swiftly. Rapid performance of CT scanning and neurosurgical evaluation should never be contingent on the return of preliminary laboratory tests or any other unnecessary delays. There is no reason to ever delay CT scanning in the comatose patient (e.g., to obtain plain skull x-rays). When cortical and brainstem failure is the result of compressive structural disease, only rapid diagnosis and action will maintain any chance of the patient having reasonable functional capacity.

SELECTED READING

Adams, HD. Aneurysmal subarchnoid hemorrhage. *Mod Concepts Cardiovasc Dis* 50:49, 1981.

Adams, RD, and Foley, JM. The neurological disorder associated with liver disease. *Res Publ Assoc Res Nerv Ment Dis* 32:198, 1953.

American College of Surgeons. Advanced Trauma Life Support Program, 1980.

Ames, A III, and Gurian, BS. Effects of glucose and oxygen deprivation on function of isolated mammalian retina. *J Neurophysiol* 26:617, 1963.

Anderson, A, and Arduini, M. Effects of drugs and metabolic alterations on brain stem arousal mechanism. *J Pharmacol Exp Ther* 110:76, 1954.

Arief, AI, Llach, R, and Massry SG. Neurological manifestations and morbidity of hyponatremia: Correlation with brain water and electrolytes. *Medicine* 55:121, 1976.

Barr, M. *The Human Nervous System* (2nd ed). New York: Harper & Row, 1972.

Beecher, HK. After the "definition of irreversible coma." *N Engl J Med* 281:1010, 1967.

Bickerstaff, ER. Impairment of consciousness in migraine. *Lancet* 2:1057, 1961.

Bird, TD, and Plum, F. Recovery from barbiturate overdose and with a prolonged isoelectric electroencephalogram. *Neurology* 18:456, 1968.

Brennen, RW, and Ergland, RM. Acute cerebellar hemorrhage. Analysis of clinical findings and outcome in 12 cases. *Neurology* 27:527, 1977.

Brown, HW, and Plum, F. The neurologic basis of Cheyne-Stokes respiration. *Am J Med* 30:849, 1961.

Bull, JM, et al. Whole body hyperthermia: A phase I trail of a potential adjuvant to chemotherapy. *Ann Intern Med* 90:317, 1979.

Byrnes, D. Head injury and the dilated pupil. *Am Surg* 45:139, 1979.

Charness, MD, and Diamond, I. Alcohol and the Nervous System. In SH Appel (ed), *Current Neurology* (vol 5). New York: Wiley, 1984. Pp 383–422.

Cogan, DG. *Neurology of the Ocular Muscles.* Springfield, IL: Thomas, 1966.

Daroff, RB, and Hoyt, WF. Supranuclear Disorders of Ocular Control Systems in Man: Clinical, Anatomical and Physiological Correlations. In P Bachy-Rita, CC Collins, and JE Hyde (eds), *The Control of Eye Movements.* New York: Academic, 1971.

Davis, RA, et al. Decerebrate rigidity in humans. *Neurosurgery* 10:635, 1982.

DeCampo, J, et al. How useful is the skull x-ray in trauma? *Med J Aust* 2:553, 1980.

DeJong, R. *The Neurological Examination* (4th ed). New York: Harper & Row, 1979.

Feldman, MH. Physiological observations in a chronic case of locked-in syndrome. *Neurology* 21:459, 1971.

Feldman, MH. The decerebrate state in the primate. I. Studies in monkeys. *Arch Neurol* 25:501, 1971.

Finney, LA, and Walker, AG. *Transtentorial Hematuria.* Springfield, IL: Thomas, 1962.

Fischer, CM. Some neuro-ophthalmological observations. *J Neurol Neurosurg Psychiatry* 30:383, 1967.

Fischer, CM. The neurological examination of the comatose patient. *Acta Neurol Scand* 45 (Suppl 36):1, 1969.

Fishbeck, K, and Simon, RP. Neurologic manifestations of accidental hypothermia. *Ann Neurol* 10:384, 1981.

Glenberg, AJ. The catatonic syndrome. *Lancet* 1:1339, 1976.

Higashi, K, et al. Five-year follow-up study of patients with persistent vegetative state. *J Neurol Neurosurg Psychiatry* 44:552, 1981.

Jameson, KG, and Yelland, JD. Extradural hematoma. Report of 167 cases. *J Neurosurg* 29:13, 1968.

Jefferson, G. The tentorial pressure cone. *Arch Neurol Psychiatry* 40:857, 1968.

Jennett, B, et al. Prognosis of patients with severe head injury. *Neurosurgery* 4:283, 1979.

Lange, RI, and Hecht, HH. The mechanism of Cheyne-Stokes respiration. *J Clin Invest* 41:42, 1962.

Levin, BE. The clinical significance of spontaneous pulsations of the retinal vein. *Arch Neurol* 33:356, 1976.

Levy, DE, et al. Prognosis in the non-traumatic coma. *Ann Intern Med* 94:293, 1981.

MacCuish, AC, Munro, JF, and Duncan, LJP. Treatment of hypoglycemic coma with glucagon, intravenous dextrose and mannitol infusion in 100 diabetics. *Lancet* 2:946, 1970.

McKissock, W, Richardson, A, and Walsh, L. Spontaneous cerebellar hemorrhage: A study of 34 consecutive cases treated surgically. *Brain* 83:1, 1960.

Maragos, GD. The unconscious child. *Pediatrics* 7:142, 1978.

Messert, B, et al. Central pontine myelinolysis. *Neurology* 29:147, 1979.

Moore, RA, et al. Naloxone: Underdosage after narcotic poisoning. *Am J Dis Child* 134:156, 1980.

Neslon, JR. The minimal ice water caloric test. *Neurology* 19:577, 1969.

Plum, F. Neurological integration of behavioral and metabolic control of breathing. In R Porter (ed), *Breathing: Hering-Breuer Centenay Symposium.* London: J & A Churchill, 1970. Pp 159–75.

Plum, F. Mechanisms of "central" hyperventilation. *Ann Neurol* 11:636, 1982.

Plum, F, and Alvord, EC. Apneustic breathing in man. *Arch Neurol* 10:101, 1964.

Plum, F, and Posner, J. *The Diagnosis of Stupor and Coma* (2nd ed). Philadelphia: Davis, 1972.

Plum, F, and Posner, JB. *The Diagnosis of Stupor and Coma* (3rd ed). Philadelphia: Davis, 1980.

Plum, F, and Swenson, AG. Central neurogenic hyperventilation in man. *Arch Neurol Psychiatry* 81:535, 1959.

Rawlinson, WS, and Kelloway, CH. Studies of injury by heat. 2. The liberation of enzymes from the liver. *Aust J Exp Biol Med Sci* 22:69, 1944.

Samek, D. Coefficient of glucose consumption of the brain in hyperthermia. *Acta Physiol Pol* 17:740, 1966.

Samuels, M, et al. *Manual of Neurologic Therapeutics* (2nd ed). Boston: Little, Brown, 1982.

Shaffer, MA. Limitation of the cross-table lateral view in detecting cervical spine injuries: A retrospective analysis. *Ann Emerg Med* 10:508, 1981.

Swanson, PD. Neurological Manifestations of Hypernatremia. In PJ Vinken, GW Bruyn, and HL Klawans (eds), *Handbook of Clinical Neurology* (vol 28). Amsterdam: North Holland, 1976. Pp 443–461.

Tyler, HR. Neurologic disorders in renal failure. *Am J Med* 44:734, 1968.

Vicario, S, et al. Emergency presentation of subdural hematoma. *Ann Emerg Med* 11:45, 1982.

29. The Confusional-Delirious States

Maurice Victor

The inclusion of a chapter on the confusional states in a textbook of emergency medicine hardly requires justification. A significant proportion of patients who are seen in an emergency ward are mentally confused, a state that invariably signifies the presence of serious underlying neurologic or psychiatric disease, systemic infection, metabolic derangement, alcohol abuse, or drug intoxication. Moreover, the underlying disorder may be life-threatening and represent a clinical emergency in the true sense of the word. In this situation, the physician must be able to assess, quickly and accurately, the cognitive and behavioral functions of the patient. Without such data, errors will be made in evaluating the patient's history, in diagnosing the disease from which he or she suffers, and in initiating an appropriate therapeutic program.

DEFINITION OF TERMS

Defining the acute confusional states is difficult, mainly because the terms used to describe them have been given so many different meanings, both in medical and nonmedical writings. The difficulty is compounded by the fact that the pathophysiology of most confusional states is not understood, with the result that the definitions depend mainly on their clinical relationships, with all the imprecision that this entails. The following definitions would probably not satisfy most behavioral psychologists and psychiatrists. Nevertheless, we have found them to be highly practical in categorizing the clinical problems and initiating appropriate investigative and therapeutic measures.

We use the term *confusion* in only a general sense, to denote *any* state in which the patient cannot think with customary speed, clarity, and coherence. Disorientation, inattentiveness, an inability to register immediate events and recall them later, and a general diminution of all mental activity are its most conspicuous characteristics. Logical thinking, speaking, and the performance of even simple tasks are interrupted or suspended by the intrusion of irrelevant thoughts. Reduced perceptiveness with visual and auditory illusions and even hallucinations and paranoid delusions (i.e., a psychosis) are variable features.

These psychologic disturbances can be observed in several different clinical contexts. A confusional state is an essential element in delirium (described later), in which case it depends mainly on a disorder of perception and is associated with agitation and tremor. A confusional state can appear at a certain stage in the evolution and devolution of diseases that lead to drowsiness, stupor, and coma, in which instance it must be aligned with disorders of consciousness. Also, confusion is a characteristic feature of the more chronic syndrome of dementia, in which deterioration of memory, other intellectual functions, and perhaps language facility, has already occurred. Intense emotional and affective disturbances, either hypomania or a retarded depression, can interfere with attentiveness and coherence of thinking. Finally, confusion can occur in association with focal cerebral lesions, particularly of the nondominant parietal lobe. Then, instead of tremor, asterixis, and myoclonia—the generalized motor abnormalities that characterize confusional states of toxic-metabolic origin—there may be a contralateral neglect of self and environment and motor-sensory defects.

The many mental and behavioral aberrations that are observed in confused patients and their occurrence in various combinations and clinical contexts make it unlikely that they all derive from a single psychological abnormality, such as a disturbance of attention. Phenomena as diverse as drowsiness and stupor, hallucinations and delusions, disorders of perception and registration, impersistence and perseveration, and so forth, cannot logically be reduced to a disturbance of one psychological or physiologic mechanism. More likely, a number of separable disorders of function are involved, all acute and usually reversible. We refer to all of them as the *confusional states,* for want of a better term.

In our nomenclature, the term *delirium* is used to denote a special type of confusional state. In addition to many of the negative features of the confusional states, mentioned previously, delirium is distinguished by a prominent disorder of perception (misinterpretations and misidentifications), terrifying hallucinations and vivid dreams, a kaleidoscopic array of strange and absurd fantasies and delusions, inability to sleep, tendency to convulse, and intense emotional disturbances. These "positive" aspects of disordered consciousness are sometimes designated by the term *oneirism* or *oneiric consciousness* (from the Greek *oneiros,* "dream"). The *twilight state* is probably a related disorder, but the clinical descriptions have been so divergent and imprecise that this term now has little useful meaning. Delirium is also distinguished by a state of heightened alertness, that is, an increased readiness to respond to stimuli, and by marked overactivity of psychomotor and autonomic nervous system functions. Implicit also in the term *delirium* are its nonmedical connotations—intense agitation, frenzied excitement, and trembling.

This distinction between delirium and other acute confusional states is not universally accepted. Some authors attach no particular significance to the autonomic and psychomotor overactivity and the oneiric or dreamlike features of delirium, or to the underactivity and somnolence that characterize other types of confusional states. All such states are lumped together under the headings of toxic psychosis, infective-exhaustive psychosis, febrile delirium, exogenous reaction type of psychosis, acute organic reaction, or symptomatic psychosis, with the implications that they are all induced by toxic or metabolic disturbances of the brain. We believe that delirium should be set apart from other confusional states, because in most cases the two conditions are descriptively different and have different clinical and etiologic connotations, as will be indicated later. Nevertheless, implicit in both is the idea of an acute, transient, completely reversible disorder.

Also to be considered here is an impairment or loss of memory (amnesia), a symptom that is often included in descriptions of delirium and confusion. However, if the term *amnesia* or *amnesic state* is to have any clinical meaning, it should be used in a much more restricted manner, that is, to refer to both a loss of past memories and an inability to form new ones (i.e., to learn), despite an alert state of mind. The definition also presupposes that the patient can grasp the problem at hand, can comprehend and use language normally, and is sufficiently motivated and cooperative to take part in the testing of mental function. The failure in the amnesic state is essentially one of retention and recall. Undoubtedly, the drowsy, acutely confused, or delirious patient is often unable to retain information from one moment to the next and, on recovery, may remember little or nothing of what had happened during the illness. In these latter situations, however, the failure is not one of retention, but one in which information and events seem never to have been adequately perceived and registered in the first place. Finally, the amnesic state can be partial (selective)—for example, for words, visual images of faces, patterns, objects, colors, or motor skills. Then it is referred to as a form of aphasia, agnosia, or apraxia.

The term *dementia* literally means a loss or dissolution of the mind, and more particularly of the intellectual and cognitive functions, again without disturbance of consciousness or perception. The term implies a gradual deterioration of memory and other intellectual functions due to chronic progressive degenerative disease of the brain. Such a definition, however, is too narrow, since the term covers a number of closely related syndromes that are characterized not only by deterioration of intellectual functions (i.e., the capacity to remember, think logically and abstractly, calculate, make appropriate deductions from given premises, and so forth) but also by certain behavioral abnormalities and changes in personality. We propose that there are several states of dementia of multiple causes and mechanisms and that a diffuse degeneration of neurons is only one of the causes. Therefore, it is more correct to speak of the *dementias* or the *dementing diseases.*

Although the dementias are usually chronic in nature, they are not always so and can pose serious problems for the emergency physician. Many elderly patients in whom a medical or surgical illness or drug toxicity develops are seen in the emergency ward in a state of acute mental confusion. Often this state is caused by a preexisting mild or early dementing disease, which may not have been obvious to the family before the onset of the complicating illness. We refer to this type of confusional state as a *beclouded dementia.*

OBSERVABLE ASPECTS OF BEHAVIOR AND THEIR RELATION TO CONFUSION, DELIRIUM, AMNESIA, AND DEMENTIA

The components of mentation and behavior that lend themselves to bedside examination are (1) the processes of sensation and perception; (2) the capacity for memorizing; (3) the ability to think and reason; (4) temperament, mood, and emotion; (5) initiative, impulse, and drive; and (6) insight. Behavioral psychologists speak of (1) as sensorial, (2) and (3) as cognitive, (4) as affective, and (5) as conative or volitional. Insight (6) includes the introspective observations made by the patient concerning his or her normal or disordered functioning. Each of these components has its objective side, expressed in behavioral responses that are produced by certain stimuli, and its subjective side, expressed in what the patient thinks and feels in response to the stimuli.

Disturbances of Perception

Perception—that is, the processes used in acquiring through the senses a knowledge of the "world about" or of one's own body—involves a number of psychologic mechanisms in addition to a simple awareness of the stimulus. Most important, it requires the *maintenance of attention,* the selective focusing on a stimulus, the elimination of extraneous stimuli, and the identification of the stimulus by recognizing its relationship to remembered experience. With cerebral disease there is a reduction in the number of perceptions in a given period of time and failure to synthesize and relate them to the ongoing activities of the mind; always there is inattention or fluctuations of attention, distraction (pertinent and irrelevant stimuli have equal value), and impaired ability to persist in an assigned task. Qualitative sensorial changes also appear, causing misinterpretation of sounds and objects (illusions) and misidentification of persons. These changes, at least in part, form the basis of hallucinatory experience in which the patient reports and reacts to stimuli not evident to the examiner. There is also an inability to perceive simultaneously all elements of a complex of stimuli. These major disturbances in the perceptual sphere, sometimes called "clouding of the sensorium," are most prominent in deliria and other acute confusional states, but a quantitative deficiency may also become evident in the advanced stages of dementia.

Disturbances of Memory

Memory—that is, the retention of learned information and experiences—is involved in all mental activities. It can be subdivided arbitrarily into several parts, namely, registration, which includes all that was mentioned previously under "perception"; mnemonic integration and retention; recall; and reproduction. As was indicated previously, severe disturbances of perception and attention can be attended by a complete failure of learning and, consequently, of memory, because the material to be learned was never registered and assimilated ("imprinted") in the first place. In Korsakoff's amnesic syndrome, newly presented material appears to be temporarily registered but cannot be retained for more than a few minutes, and there is always an associated defect in the recall and reproduction of memories that had been formed some days, weeks, or even years before the onset of the illness *(retrograde amnesia).* Intact retention (especially of proper names) with failure of recall is a common normal phenomenon, sometimes referred to as the "tip of the tongue" syndrome or "benign forgetfulness." A severe disorder of recall, extending to all events of past life and even personal identity, is usually due to hysteria or malingering. Proof that the processes of registration and retention are intact under the latter circumstances comes from hypnosis and suggestion, and from questioning the patient under barbiturate narcosis, whereby the lost items are fully recalled and reproduced. Since some aspect of memory is involved to some extent in all mental processes, it becomes the most testable component of mentation and behavior.

Disturbances of Thinking

Thinking, which is central to practically all intellectual activity, remains the most elusive of all mental operations. If by thinking one means the capacity to solve problems and to reason and form sound judgments (the usual definition), then the working units of this type of mental activity are mainly words and numbers. The substitution of words and numbers for the objects that they represent (symbolization) is a fundamental part of the process. The formation of these symbols into ideas or concepts and the arrangement of new and remembered ideas into certain orders or relationships, according to the rules of logic, constitute other intricate parts of thought. One test of logical thinking is problem-solving—the capacity to formulate a problem into several hypotheses, to analyze critically the evidence for and against each hypothesis, and to make a correct choice. In a general way one can examine thinking for speed and efficiency, ideational content, coherence and logical relationships of ideas, quantity and quality of associations with a given idea, and the propriety of the feeling and behavior engendered by an idea.

Information concerning the thought processes and associative functions is best obtained by engaging the patient in conversation and analyzing his or her spontaneous speech. If the patient is taciturn or mute, one may have to depend on the responses to direct questions or on written material (i.e., letters, and so forth). One should note the prevailing trends of the patient's thoughts; whether the ideas are to the point, reasonable, and coherent, or whether they are vague, circumstantial, tangential, and irrelevant; and whether the thought processes are shallow and fragmented. Fragmentation of thought processes and their disruption by repetition and perseveration are spoken of as an *incoherence of thinking,* which characterizes deliria and other confusional states as well as dementia and schizophrenia. The patient may be excessively critical, rationalizing, and hairsplitting; this type of thinking is often manifest in depressive psychosis. Derangement of thinking can also take the form of a flight of ideas; the patient moves nimbly from one thought to another, and associations are numerous and loosely linked. This is a common feature of hypomanic or manic states. The opposite condition, poverty of ideas, is characteristic both of depression, in which it is combined with gloomy thoughts, and of dementing diseases, in which it is part of a general reduction in intellectual activity. Thinking can be distorted in such a way that patients fail to check their ideas against reality. When a false belief is maintained in spite of convincing evidence to the contrary, the patient is said to have a delusion. Delusions are particularly common in manic-depressive and schizophrenic states. Ideas may seem to the patient to have been implanted in his or her mind by some outside agency, such as radio, television, or atomic energy. These reflect the "passivity feeling" characteristic of schizophrenic psychosis. Gaps in thinking or condensations of logical associations also typify the latter disease.

Disturbances of Emotion, Mood, and Affect

Disturbances in the emotional life of the individual are difficult to judge. To begin with, marked individual differences in basic temperament are observed in the normal population; some persons are cheerful, gregarious, optimistic, and free from worry throughout life, whereas others are just the opposite. Also, it should be noted that certain strong emotional states, such as fear and anxiety, are common (and normal) reactions to life situations and may be accompanied by derangements of visceral function. If these reactions are clearly disproportionate to the stimulus and persistent, they are usually manifestations of an anxiety neurosis or depression. In depression, all stimuli tend to enhance the somber mood of unhappiness. Emotional responses that are excessively labile and poorly controlled or uninhibited are common manifestations of cerebral diseases that involve the corticopontine and corticobulbar pathways (pseudobulbar palsy). All emotional expression may be lacking, as in apathetic states or severe depressions, or the patient may be a victim of every trivial problem in daily life (i.e., unable to control worries). Finally, the emotional responses may be inappropriate to the stimulus (e.g., a depressing or morbid thought may seem amusing and be attended by a smile or arouse no emotional reaction), as appears to be the case in schizophrenia.

Temperament, mood, and other emotional experiences just described are evaluated by the appearance of the patient and by verbalized accounts of his or her feelings. For these purposes some psychiatrists divide emotionality into mood and feeling (affect). *Mood* refers to the prevailing emotional state of the individual without reference to the impinging stimuli; it can be cheerful or melancholic. Language (e.g., the adjectives used) and facial expressions, attitudes, postures, and speed of movement most reliably betray the patient's mood. By contrast, *feelings* (or *affect*) are said to be emotional experiences evoked by particular stimuli.

Disturbances in Impulse (Conation)

Impulse, the basic biologic urge, drive, or purpose by which every organism is directed to attain its objectives, is another important and observable, though somewhat neglected, dimension of behavior. Again, wide normal variations are seen in strength of impulse and these individual differences are present throughout life. One of the most conspicuous pathologic deviations is a constitutional weakness of impulse in certain neurotic persons. Moreover, with many types of cerebral disease (particularly those involving the medial-orbital parts of the frontal lobes), a reduction in impulse is coupled with an indifference or lack of concern about the consequences of actions; in such cases all other measurable aspects of psychic function may be normal. Pathologic lack of impulse, or *abulia*, can reach an extreme degree, to the point of mutism and immobility, a state that Cairns originally referred to as *akinetic mutism*. *Psychomotor retardation* is a lesser degree of the same state and is a feature of both cerebral disease and depression.

Loss of Insight

Insight, the state of being fully aware of the nature and degree of one's deficits, becomes manifestly impaired or abolished in patients with all types of cerebral disease that cause complex disorders of behavior. The patient with such a disorder does not seek advice or help for the illness; instead, the family usually brings the individual to the physician. It is a clinical truism that diseases producing complex neurologic abnormalities not only evoke observable changes in mentation and behavior but also alter or reduce the patient's awareness of the significance and severity of the abnormalities.

APPROACH TO THE PATIENT WITH A CONFUSIONAL STATE, DELIRIUM, DEMENTIA, OR AN AMNESIC SYNDROME

Confronted by a patient with one of these disorders, the physician must adopt an examination technique designed to expose the perceptual and intellectual defect. Abnormalities of posture, movement, sensation, and reflexes cannot be relied on for a full demonstration of the neurologic deficit, for the association and limbic areas of the brain can be severely damaged without displaying neurologic signs of this type.

Three sources of data are required for the recognition and diagnosis of these mental disorders: a reliable history of the illness; findings on mental examination (i.e., so-called mental status), as well as on the rest of the neurologic examination; and special ancillary examinations, such as skull films, lumbar puncture, electroencephalogram (EEG), computed tomography (CT) or magnetic resonance imaging (MRI) of the brain, and sometimes angiography.

The history must always be supplemented by information obtained from a person other than the patient. Through lack of insight, patients are often unaware of their illness; indeed, they may be ignorant even of their chief complaint. The person(s) accompanying the patient must not be allowed to leave the emergency ward before being interviewed.

The mental status evaluation need not be lengthy or elaborate, but it must be systematic. At a minimum it should provide answers to the following questions:

1. Insight (patient's replies to questions about the chief complaint): What is your difficulty? Are you ill? When did your illness begin?
2. Orientation
   a. Knowledge of personal identity and present situation: What is your name? Your occupation? Where do you live? Are you married? What are you doing now?
   b. Place: What is the name of the place where you are now? How did you get here? What floor is it on? Where is the bathroom?
   c. Time: What is the date today? What day of the week is it? What is the time of day? When was the last holiday?
3. Memory
   a. Remote: Tell me the names of your children and their birth dates. When were you married? What was your mother's maiden name? What was the name of your first school teacher? What jobs have you held?
   b. Recent past: Tell me about your recent illness (compare with previous statements). What did you have for breakfast today? What is my name? When did you see me for the first time? What were the headlines in the newspaper today? Give the patient a set of three or four items or a simple story, oral or written, and ask him or her to recall it after three to five minutes.
   c. Immediate recall (short-term memory): Repeat these numbers after me (give a series of up to eight digits at the speed of one per second). Then give the patient a

series of three to five numbers and ask him or her to repeat them in reverse order.

d. Visual span: Show patients a picture of several objects; ask them to name what they have seen and note any inaccuracies.

4. General information: Ask about the names of presidents, well-known historic dates, the names of large rivers or cities, and so forth.
5. Capacity for sustained mental activity.
   a. Calculation: Test the ability to do simple arithmetic. Serial subtraction of 7s or 3s from 100 is a good test of calculation as well as of concentration.
   b. Abstract thinking: Test the patient's ability to detect similarities and differences between classes of objects, or to explain a proverb or a fable.
6. General behavior: Attitudes, bearing, attentiveness, manner of dress, and so forth.
   a. Content of thought: What ideas occupy the patient's thoughts? Does the patient believe that his or her thoughts and actions are being controlled or broadcasted to others? Are there hallucinations or delusions, or both? Is there a press of speech or lack of speech?
   b. Mood: Does the patient appear cheerful or sad? How does he feel? Is he nervous, worried, or apprehensive? What feeling is revealed through speech, attitude, facial expression?
7. Special tests of localized cerebral functions: Grasping, sucking, tests of aphasia, praxis with both hands, corticosensory function, visual field defects, drawing a clock face, map of the United States or Europe, floor plan of the patient's house, and so forth.

It will be recognized that many of these questions are selected items from the various subtests of the Wechsler Adult Intelligence Scale (WAIS). Using the full form of the test, the discrepancy between the vocabulary, picture-completion, and object-assembly tests as a group (these correlate well with premorbid intelligence and are relatively resistant to dementing brain disease) and arithmetic, block design, digit-span, and digit symbol tests provide an index of deterioration. The Wechsler Memory Scale is a reliable method for quantitating the degree of impairment of retentive memory. Characteristically, in patients with Korsakoff's amnesic syndrome, a striking discrepancy is seen between performance on the WAIS and on the Wechsler Memory Scale.

COMMON SYNDROMES

Delirium

Clinical Features

The clinical features of delirium are most perfectly depicted in the alcoholic patient. The symptoms usually develop over a period of two or three days. The first indications of the approaching attack are difficulty in concentrating, restless irritability, tremulousness, insomnia, and poor appetite. One or several generalized convulsions precede the delirium in almost 30 percent of the cases. The patient's rest becomes troubled by unpleasant or terrifying dreams or by illusions and hallucinations. There may be momentary disorientation or an occasional inappropriate remark.

These initial symptoms give way to a clinical picture that, in severe cases, is one of the most colorful and dramatic in medicine. The patient is inattentive, restless, and agitated. He or she may talk incessantly and incoherently, and look distressed and perplexed; the facial expression is in keeping with vague notions of being annoyed or threatened. From the patient's manner and speech content, it is evident that he or she misinterprets the meaning of ordinary objects and ambient sounds and has vivid visual, auditory, and tactile hallucinations, often of a most unpleasant type. At first the patient can be brought momentarily in touch with reality and may answer questions correctly, but almost at once there is a relapse into the preoccupied, confused state. He or she gives wrong answers and is incapable of self-orientation or rational thought. Before long the patient is unable to shake off the hallucinations even for a second and does not recognize family or physician. Coarse tremor and jactitations are usually present. Sleep is impossible or occurs only in brief naps. The countenance is flushed, the pupils are dilated, and the conjunctivae are injected; the pulse is rapid and the temperature may be raised. There is much sweating, and the urine is scanty and of high specific gravity. In particular, the signs of overactivity of the autonomic nervous system distinguish delirium from other confusional states.

In most cases the symptoms abate after two or three days, although in some patients they can persist for weeks. The most certain indication of the end of the attack is the occurrence of sound sleep and of lucid intervals of increasing length. Recovery is usually complete.

Delirium can differ greatly in degree, not only from patient to patient but in the same patient from day to day and even hour to hour. The entire syndrome may be observed in one patient and only one or two components in another. In its mildest form, as so often occurs in febrile diseases (particularly in young children and the elderly), it consists of an occasional wandering of the mind and incoherence of verbal expression, interrupted by periods of lucidity. This form, lacking motor and autonomic overactivity, is sometimes referred to as a *quiet delirium* (or *hypokinetic delirium*) and is difficult to distinguish from other confusional states. The most severe form, best exemplified by delirium tremens, ends in death in 5 to 10 percent of patients.

Morbid Anatomy and Pathophysiology

The brains of patients who died in delirium tremens have shown no pathologic changes of significance. A number of diseases, however, such as focal embolic encephalomalacia, viral encephalitis, or trauma, can cause delirium and also give rise to focal lesions in the brain. The topography of these lesions is of interest; they tend to be localized in the high midbrain and subthalamus, and in the temporal lobes, where they involve the reticular activating and limbic systems.

Electrical stimulation of the human cortex during surgical exploration has demonstrated the importance of the temporal lobe in producing visual, auditory, and olfactory hallucinations. With subthalamic and midbrain lesions, there may be visual hallucinations that are pleasant, animated, and accompanied by good insight (the peduncular hallucinosis of Lhermitte).

The EEG in delirium may show nonfocal slow activity in the five- to seven-per-second range, a state that rapidly returns to normal as the delirium clears. In other cases only low-voltage, fast activity in the beta range is seen, and milder degrees of delirium may show no abnormality at all.

An analysis of the several conditions conducive to delirium suggests at least three different physiologic mechanisms. (1) The withdrawal of alcohol, barbiturates, or other (benzodiazepine) sedative drugs, after a period of chronic intoxication, is the most common cause of delirium. These drugs have a strong depressant effect on certain areas of the central nervous system; presumably, the release and overactivity of these parts, after withdrawal of the drug, are the basis of the delirium. (2) In the case of bacterial infections and poisoning by certain drugs, such as atropine and scopolamine, the delirious state is probably due to the direct action of the toxin or chemical agent on these same parts of the brain. (3) Destructive lesions, such as those of the temporal lobes in trauma or herpes simplex encephalitis, can cause delirium by disturbing the function of these particular areas.

Acute Confusional States Associated with Reduced Alertness and Psychomotor Activity

Clinical Features

Characteristically, all mental functions are reduced to some degree, but alertness (readiness of response), attentiveness, and the ability to grasp all elements of the immediate situation suffer most. In mildest form, the patient may pass for normal, and only the failure to recollect and reproduce events of the past few hours or days reveals the inadequacy of mental function. The more obviously confused patient spends much time in idleness and what he or she does may be inappropriate. Only the more automatic acts and verbal responses are properly performed, but these may permit the examiner to obtain from the patient a number of relevant replies to questions about age, occupation, and residence. Reactions are slow and indecisive, and it is difficult for the patient to sustain a conversation. The patient may fall asleep during the interview and if left alone sleeps more hours each day than is natural. Responses tend to be abrupt, brief, and mechanical. Disturbances of perception are frequent, resulting in the misinterpretation of voices, common objects, and the actions of other persons. Often one cannot discern whether the patient is hallucinating (i.e., hearing and seeing things that do not exist), or merely misinterpreting stimuli in the environment. Inadequate perception and forgetfulness result in a constant state of bewilderment. Failing to recognize the surroundings and having lost all sense of time, the patient repeats the same question and makes the same remarks over and over again. Irritability may or may not be present. Some patients are suspicious, demanding, and aggressive; in fact, a paranoid trend may be the most pronounced and troublesome feature of the illness.

As the confusion deepens, conversation becomes more difficult, and at a certain stage the patient no longer notices or responds to much of what is occurring. Questions may be answered with a single word or a short phrase spoken in a soft tremulous voice or whisper, or the patient may be mute. In the most advanced stages, confusion gives way to stupor and finally to coma. As the patient's condition improves, there may again be a stage of stupor and confusion, occurring in the reverse order. All this informs us that at least one category of confusion is a manifestation of the disease processes, which, in their severest form, cause coma.

In typical cases, this type of confusional state is readily distinguished from delirium; in others, with more than the usual degrees of irritability and restlessness, one cannot fail to notice the resemblance of one to the other. Similarly, when a delirium is complicated by an illness that superimposes stupor (e.g., delirium tremens with pneumonia, meningitis, or hepatic encephalopathy), it may be difficult to distinguish the delirium from other confusional states.

When the clouding of consciousness is minimal and the confusion is of insidious onset and several weeks' duration, it can mimic dementia. Lipowski has called this state "reversible dementia," claiming it to be intermediate between delirium and dementia and still potentially reversible. We classify it as a protracted confusional state.

Morbid Anatomy and Pathophysiology

Confusional states are so diverse and are associated with such a wide variety of diseases that one would not expect a common anatomic or pathophysiologic basis. Occurrence may be more frequent with lesions of the right (nondominant) hemisphere, especially its posterior parts. Large vascular and other acute lesions of the parietal lobe tend to render patients underactive, apathetic, and unaware of their neurologic disabilities; disorientation and inattentiveness are often associated. Only if the lesion is large enough to cause a hemiplegia, hemisensory disorder, or homonymous hemianopia will the focal nature of the lesion be appreciated.

As was discussed in Chap. 27, the basis of the confusional state is most often an acute metabolic disease, and the pathologic changes, if detectable (many are not visible by light microscopy), are bilateral and diffuse. Hypoxia, hyperglycemia, uremia, metabolic acidosis or alkalosis, hepatic stupor, hyponatremia, and certain drug intoxications are the commonly recognized causes, readily corroborated by appropriate examinations of blood, urine, and cerebrospinal fluid (CSF). Clues to these biochemical derangements are often provided by alterations of respiration and the presence of asterixis, myoclonus, and tremor, with preserved pupillary reflexes. Correction of the biochemical abnormalities can result in rapid improvement in the patient's condition.

Classification of Delirium and Acute Confusional States

I. Delirium
   A. In a medical or surgical illness (no focal or lateralizing neurologic signs; CSF usually clear)
      1. Postoperative and postconcussive states
      2. Pneumonia
      3. Typhoid fever
      4. Septicemia, particularly erysipelas and other streptococcal infections
      5. Rheumatic fever
      6. Thyrotoxicosis and adrenocorticotropic hormone or corticosteroid intoxication
   B. In neurologic disease that causes focal or lateralizing signs or changes in the CSF
      1. Vascular, neoplastic, or traumatic lesions, particu-

larly those involving the temporal lobes and high brainstem
2. Acute bacterial and tuberculous meningitis
3. Subarachnoid hemorrhage
4. Viral encephalitis or meningoencephalitis, particularly herpes simplex encephalitis

C. Drug withdrawal syndromes, exogenous intoxications, and postseizure state (signs of other medical, surgical, and neurologic illnesses are absent or coincidental)
1. Withdrawal of alcohol (delirium tremens), barbiturates, and nonbarbiturate sedative drugs, after chronic intoxication
2. Drug intoxications: amphetamine, camphor, caffeine, ergot, scopolamine, atropine, and so forth
3. Postconvulsive delirium

II. Acute confusional states associated with psychomotor underactivity

A. Associated with a medical or surgical disease (no focal or lateralizing neurologic signs; CSF clear)
1. Metabolic disorders: hepatic stupor, uremia, hypoxia, hypercapnia, hypoglycemia, porphyria, electrolyte imbalance
2. Infective fevers
3. Congestive heart failure
4. Postoperative and posttraumatic states

B. Associated with drug intoxication (no focal or lateralizing signs; CSF clear): opiates, barbiturates, other sedatives, trihexyphenidyl (Artane), and so forth

C. Associated with diseases of the nervous system (the focal or lateralizing neurologic signs and CSF changes are more common in these conditions than in delirium)
1. Cerebrovascular disease, tumor, abscess
2. Subdural hematoma
3. Meningitis
4. Encephalitis
5. Senile or other brain disease in combination with infective fevers, drug reactions, heart failure, or other medical or surgical disease (beclouded dementia)

Management of the Delirious and Confused Patient

The primary effort is directed to the recognition and control of the underlying medical disease. Other important objectives are to quiet the patient and protect him or her against injury. A nurse, an attendant, or a member of the family should be with the patient at all times, if this can be arranged. Depending on the degree of the patient's activity, a locked room, screened windows, and a low bed should be provided. It is preferable that the patient be allowed to walk about the room than be tied into bed, which may provoke a struggle to the point of exhaustion and collapse. If less active, the patient can be kept in bed by padded wrist restraints, a restraining sheet, or a net thrown over the bed. The patient should be permitted to sit up or walk part of the day, unless this is contraindicated by the primary disease.

Any drug that could possibly be responsible for the acute confusional state or delirium should be discontinued, unless withdrawal effects are believed to underlie the illness. In the latter circumstances, chlordiazepoxide, chlorpromazine, and diazepam are the drugs favored by most physicians, but the older sedatives, paraldehyde and chloral hydrate, are equally safe and effective if given in full doses. Whichever drug is chosen, it should be given until natural sleep is restored. In the case of severe delirium, drugs must be used with caution. One should not attempt to suppress agitation completely; to accomplish this may require that very high doses be given and vital functions may then be dangerously impaired. The purpose of sedation is to blunt the agitation so that the patient does not become exhausted and nursing care is facilitated.

A fluid intake and output chart should be kept, and any fluid and electrolyte deficit should be corrected. The pulse and blood pressure should be recorded at frequent intervals in anticipation of circulatory collapse. Transfusions of whole blood and administration of vasopressor drugs may be lifesaving if shock develops.

Finally, the physician should be aware of the many small therapeutic measures that can allay fear and suspicion and reduce the tendency to hallucinations. The room should be kept dimly lit at night and if possible the patient should not be moved from one room to another. Every procedure should be explained in detail, even such simple ones as the taking of blood pressure or temperature. The presence of a member of the family may enable the patient to maintain contact with reality.

Most delirious patients recover if they receive competent medical and nursing care. The family should be reassured on this point and must also understand that the abnormal behavior and irrational actions of the patient are not willful but rather symptomatic of a brain disease. Once recovered, the patient will be at least partly amnesic for the period of confusion, a gap that can only be filled by information provided by the physician and family.

Dementia

The term *dementia* and the concept of the dementias or the dementing diseases have already been defined. Another concept that requires qualification is that of dementia as a global loss, in which all intellectual functions are affected more or less equally. When the dementias are carefully analyzed, they are found to include several separable though related functions, such as memory, verbal facility, and the ability to deal with mathematical symbols, to perceive visuospatial relationships, and to think abstractly and solve problems. Each of these functions (except thinking) has a definable anatomy in the cerebrum and can therefore be affected individually by a disease. For example, retentive memory depends on the integrity of neural mechanisms in the inferomedial parts of the temporal lobes (usually bilateral), and the language mechanisms lie in the parasylvian region of the left (dominant) hemisphere. It comes as no surprise, therefore, that the dementing illnesses can affect certain intellectual functions predominantly or in various combinations and sequences.

Another point of importance is that most dementing diseases appear during the senium and many others during late adult life. In 17 series, comprising 15,000 persons over the age of 60 years, the mean incidence of moderate to severe dementia was found to be 4.8 percent. In 1983, according to Terry and Katzman, about 1.3 million persons in the United

States had severe dementia, and an additional 2.8 million had mild to moderate intellectual impairment. Since the elderly population in the Western world is increasing, both in percentage of the population and in absolute numbers, the magnitude of the medical problems they will present is alarming. Finally, it needs to be emphasized that the dementias of the elderly are to be regarded not merely as the inevitable consequences of growing old, but as age-linked diseases, some 15 percent of which are treatable.

Clinical Features

Clinical features are observed most commonly and prototypically in patients with Alzheimer's disease. The earliest signs of dementia can be so subtle as to escape the notice of even the most discerning physician. Often an observant relative or an employer of the patient is the first to become aware of a certain lack of initiative, irritability, loss of interest, forgetfulness, and inability to perform up to the usual standard. Later the patient may become easily distracted, inattentive, and unable to think with accustomed clarity. Reduced general comprehension; perseveration in speech, action, and thought; and defective memory, especially for recent events, become prominent. Changes in mood are frequent, taking the form more often of apathy than of depression or elation. Excessive lability of mood may be observed—for example, easy fluctuation from laughter to tears on slight provocation. Lapses in social graces, conduct, and judgment occur early in some cases and late in others. Paranoid ideas, delusions, and sometimes hallucinations develop. Early in the disease the patient may be aware of his or her declining capacities and become depressed, but as the condition progresses, insight is invariably lost.

Later almost all intellectual faculties are lost. Dysarthria, aphasia, sphincteric incontinence, reduced responsivity, and finally mutism are added to the clinical picture. Also, in the late stages, a secondary physical deterioration takes place. Food intake, which may be increased in the beginning of the illness, is usually limited in the end, with resulting emaciation. Locomotion fails and voluntary movements become poorly coordinated. Degenerative diseases can terminate in virtually complete decortication. The patient is unaware of what is happening but lies with eyes open. He or she no longer responds to spoken commands and does not speak. The patient has no interest in food or drink, though they are swallowed if placed in the mouth. The facial and limb muscles are stiff, with increased tendon reflexes and occasionally with Babinski signs. Grasping, sucking, and sphincteric incontinence are prominent. Finally, the patient dies of pneumonia or some other intercurrent infection. This whole process can evolve over a period of months or years, usually the latter.

Morbid Anatomy and Pathophysiology

Dementia is usually related to obvious structural disease of the cerebrum and the diencephalon. In some of these diseases, such as Alzheimer's and Pick's disease, the main process appears to be a degeneration and loss of nerve cells in the association areas of the cerebral cortex, with secondary changes in the cerebral white matter. Very rarely, a degeneration of neurons confined to the thalamus can also cause dementia. In other diseases, such as Huntington chorea and certain of the spinocerebellar and cerebral-basal ganglionic degenerations, dementia is associated with a loss of neurons in the putamen and caudate nuclei. Arteriosclerotic vascular disease can result in multiple foci of infarction, which can include the motor, sensory, or visual projection areas, as well as the association areas. This condition, which takes many forms, is called *multiinfarct dementia* in the relatively rare instances in which mental deterioration dominates the clinical picture. Trauma can cause contusions of cerebral convolutions, particularly of the inferior and anterior parts of the frontal and temporal lobes, as well as necroses and hemorrhages in the high midbrain; the latter lesions are responsible for protracted stupor and coma. Most traumatic lesions that produce dementia are extensive and the frontal lobes are affected more often than other parts of the cerebrum.

One of several other mechanisms may be operative in the pathogenesis of dementia. Chronic increased intracranial pressure or chronic hydrocephalus (with large ventricles the pressure may not exceed 180 mm Hg), regardless of cause, is often associated with a general impairment of mental function. Compression of cerebral white matter is the main factor. The compression of one or both of the cerebral hemispheres by chronic subdural hematomas can cause a widespread disturbance of cortical function. A diffuse inflammatory process is the basis for dementia in syphilis and in certain viral infections such as acquired immunodeficiency syndrome (AIDS) and herpes simplex encephalitis. Lastly, several toxic and metabolic diseases (e.g., bromism, hepatic encephalopathy) can interfere with nervous function over a period of time and create a clinical picture similar, if not identical, to that of dementia.

Bedside Classification

I. Diseases in which dementia is usually the only evidence of neurologic or medical disease
   A. Alzheimer's disease
   B. Pick's disease
II. Diseases in which dementia is associated with other neurologic signs but not with other obvious medical disease
   A. Invariably associated with other neurologic signs
      1. Huntington's chorea (choreoathetosis)
      2. Leukodystrophies: Schilder's disease, adrenoleukodystrophy, metachromatic leukodystrophy and related demyelinative diseases (spastic weakness, pseudobulbar palsy, blindness, deafness)
      3. Lipofuscinosis and other lipid storage diseases (myoclonic seizures, blindness, spasticity, cerebellar ataxia)
      4. Myoclonic epilepsy (diffuse myoclonus, generalized seizures, cerebellar ataxia)
      5. Creutzfeldt-Jakob disease (diffuse myoclonus and cerebellar ataxia)
      6. Cerebrocerebellar degeneration (Cerebellar ataxia of olivopontocerebellar type and others)
      7. Cerebral-basal ganglionic degenerations (apraxia-rigidity) and supranuclear palsy (paralysis of vertical gaze, neck dystonia)
      8. Dementia with spastic paraplegia
      9. Basal ganglia calcification (idiopathic and hypoparathyroidism)

10. Hallervorden-Spatz disease (pyramidal and extrapyramidal signs)
11. Dementia with Parkinson's disease (tremor, rigidity, bradykinesia)

B. Often associated with other neurologic signs
1. Cerebral arteriosclerosis and ischemic infarction
2. Brain tumor
3. Brain trauma (cerebral contusions, midbrain hemorrhages, chronic subdural hematoma)
4. Normal-pressure hydrocephalus (always with ataxia of gait and often with sphincteric incontinence)
5. Marchiafava-Bignami disease (apraxia and other frontal lobe signs)
6. AIDS

III. Diseases in which dementia is usually associated with clinical and laboratory signs of other medical disease
A. Hypothyroidism
B. Cushing's disease

Problems in Diagnosis

A common error is to assume that mental function is normal if patients complain only of nervousness, fatigue, insomnia, or vague somatic symptoms, and to label them as psychoneurotic. This will be avoided if one keeps in mind that psychoneuroses rarely begin in middle or late adult life. A practical rule is to assume that all mental illnesses beginning during this period are due either to structural disease of the brain or to a depressive psychosis.

A mild aphasia must not be mistaken for dementia. Aphasic patients may be anxious and appear uncertain of themselves, and their speech may be incoherent. Careful attention to the language performance will lead to the correct diagnosis in most instances, and further observation will disclose that their behavior, except that which is related to the language disorder, is within normal limits.

Depressed patients present another type of problem. They may complain of being forgetful or being unable to concentrate. Careful examination, however, will show that they can remember details of their history and that no qualitative change in cognitive function has occurred. Their difficulty is either a lack of energy and interest or an anxiety that prevents the focusing of attention on anything except their own problems. During mental tests their performance may be impaired by their emotional state in much the same way as that of a worried student during examinations. When patients are calmed by reassurance and given more time in the performance of tests, mental function improves, indicating that intellectual deterioration has not occurred. Hypomanic patients may fail in tests of intellectual function because they are restless and distracted. As was indicated previously, demented patients rarely complain of mental deterioration and those who admit to poor memory do not realize the degree of their disability. The physician must never rely on the patient's statements of the efficiency of mental function and must always evaluate a poor performance on tests in the light of the patient's emotional state and motivation at the time the test is given. An especially difficult problem is posed by the mildly demented patient who is also depressed and whose CT scan shows some degree of ventricular enlargement, raising the question of normal-pressure hydrocephalus. Sometimes the contribution of depression can only be ascertained by an empiric trial of antidepressant drugs.

Certain metabolic or endocrine disorders, such as those seen with prolonged corticosteroid therapy, hypothyroidism, Cushing's disease, Addison's disease, or a postpartum mental disturbance, can create difficulties in diagnosis because of the wide variety of symptoms by which they manifest themselves. Some such patients appear to be suffering from a dementia, others from an acute confusional psychosis; if mood change or delusions predominate, a manic-depressive pyschosis or schizophrenia is suggested. In all these metabolic and endocrine disorders, some degree of clouding of the sensorium can usually be recognized, and these findings alone should be enough to exclude schizophrenia and manic-depressive pyschosis. The acute onset of mental symptoms should always suggest a confusional psychosis or delirium; inasmuch as these conditions are generally reversible, they must be distinguished from the dementing diseases.

Once it has been concluded that the patient suffers from a dementing disease, it needs to be determined, by careful physical examination, whether other signs of neurologic or medical disease are present. This enables the physician to place the case in one of the three categories of the bedside classification (see previous section). Skull films, EEG, lumbar puncture, and CT scans or MRI should be carried out in most cases. Usually these procedures necessitate admission to a hospital. The final step is to determine, from the total clinical picture, the particular disease within any one category. This task can sometimes be difficult. If the dementia is of recent onset, complicated by the use of drugs or associated with temporal lobe seizures or an endocrine disease (beclouded dementia, see the following section), a period of observation may be required before the diagnosis can be settled. Finally, it is important to keep in mind that the correct diagnosis of treatable forms of mental disease (e.g., general paresis, subdural hematoma, brain tumor, chronic drug intoxication, normal-pressure hydrocephalus, pellagra and other deficiency states, and hypothyroidism) is of greater practical importance than the diagnosis of the untreatable ones.

Obviously, not all of these diseases are of equal importance as causes of dementia, and some are rare. In a series of 84 demented patients (<65 years of age) who were admitted to a British neurologic center, 58 percent had brain atrophy, probably of the Alzheimer type, 10 percent had multiinfarct dementia, and nearly 10 percent had tumors. Normal-pressure hydrocephalus, Creutzfeldt-Jakob disease, Huntington chorea, posttraumatic sequelae, and alcoholism accounted for the remainder. In an older population (>65 years) the incidence of brain atrophy was found in approximately 80 percent and multiinfarct dementia in 15 percent.

Beclouded Dementia

It has already been mentioned that in certain clinical circumstances, a patient with a mild or inconspicuous dementing disease can suddenly become severely confused. Characteristically, this occurs when an early form of Alzheimer's disease is complicated by a medical illness, surgical operation, or the excessive use of drugs, and attests to the precarious state of cerebral compensation. Other cerebral diseases (vascular, neoplastic, demyelinative) can have the same effect. *Beclouded dementia,* as we have chosen to designate this state, is arguably the most common type of confusional state observed in hospital practice.

All the clinical features that one observes in the acute confusional states may be present. The severity varies greatly. The confusion may be reflected only in the patient's inability to relate sequentially the history of the illness, or it can be so severe that the patient is virtually *non compos mentis.*

Almost any complicating illness can bring out the confusion, but it is particularly frequent with febrile illnesses; with posttraumatic and postoperative states, notably after concussive brain injuries and surgical procedures that require covering of the eyes; with congestive heart failure; with chronic obstructive respiratory disease (hypercapnia) and other metabolic or electrolyte disturbances; with severe anemia, especially pernicious anemia; and after the injudicious administration of medication. Often it is difficult to determine which of several possible factors is responsible for the confusion, and there may be more than one. In a cardiac patient with a confusional psychosis, for example, low-grade fever, a marginally reduced cerebral blood flow, intoxication with one or more drugs, impaired renal function, and water and electrolyte imbalance may all be present. When patients with beclouded dementia recover from their medical or surgical illnesses, they usually return to their premorbid state, though their shortcomings, now drawn to the attention of the family and physician, may be more obvious than before.

The Amnesic Syndrome: Amnesic (Amnestic) Confabulatory Syndrome and Korsakoff's Psychosis

The amnesic syndrome, the amnesic (amnestic) confabulatory syndrome, and Korsakoff's psychosis are terms used interchangeably to designate a unique but common disorder of cognitive function, in which memory is deranged out of all proportion to other components of mentation and behavior. It possesses two salient features that can vary in severity but are always conjoined: an impaired ability to recall events and other information that had been well established before the onset of the illness *(retrograde amnesia),* and an impaired ability to acquire new information—i.e., to learn or to form new memories *(anterograde amnesia).* Other cognitive functions (particularly the capacity for concentration, spatial organization, and visual and verbal abstraction), which depend little or not at all on memory, are also impaired, but to a relatively minor degree. The patient tends to lack initiative and spontaneity and is usually complacent and apathetic. Ability to repeat a series of numbers or a spoken sentence *(immediate memory)* is intact. Recent memories are affected more than remote ones (Ribot's law) but this varies in degree with the nature and severity of the disease. *Confabulation,* the fabrication of ready answers or the recital of fictitious experiences, is variably present. It is observed mainly in the acute phase of the illness.

The definition of Korsakoff's psychosis is also predicated on the intactness of certain aspects of behavior and mental function. The patient should be alert, attentive, responsive, and capable of understanding the written and spoken word, of making appropriate deductions from given premises, and of solving such problems as can be concluded within his or her forward memory span. These "negative" features are of particular importance because they help distinguish Korsakoff's psychosis from a number of other disorders in which the basic defect is not in retentive memory but in some other psychological mechanism—for example, in attention and perception (as in the delirious, confused, or stuporous patient), in recall (as in the hysterical patient), or in volition (as in the abulic patient with frontal lobe disease).

Pathologic Anatomy

The anatomic structures of particular importance in memory function are the diencephalon (more specifically the medial nuclei of the thalamus) and the inferomedial portions of the temporal lobes, particularly the hippocampal formations. Bilaterally placed lesions in either of these regions derange memory and learning out of all proportion to other cognitive functions, and even a unilateral lesion in the dominant thalamus or hippocampus produces a lesser degree of the same effect. It appears that the aforementioned anatomic structures are involved in all forms of learning and integration of newly formed memories and that they form a tenuous but vital link between the high brainstem reticular formation (the integrity of which is necessary to maintain an alert state of mind, a prerequisite for any learning) and the cerebral cortex, which is the locus for special memories (i.e., for words, geometric figures, numbers, and so forth).

Classification of Diseases Characterized by an Amnesic Syndrome

I. Amnesic syndrome of sudden onset, usually with gradual but incomplete recovery
   A. Bilateral or unilateral (dominant) hippocampal infarction due to atherosclerotic-thrombotic or embolic occlusion of the posterior cerebral arteries or their inferior temporal branches
   B. Trauma to the diencephalic or inferomedial temporal regions
   C. Spontaneous subarachnoid hemorrhage
   D. Carbon monoxide poisoning and other hypoxic states (rare)
II. Amnesia of sudden onset and brief duration with full recovery
   A. Temporal lobe seizures
   B. Postconcussive states
   C. Transient global amnesia
III. Amnesic syndrome of subacute onset with varying degrees of recovery, usually leaving permanent residua
   A. Wernicke-Korsakoff disease
   B. Herpes simplex encephalitis
   C. Tuberculous and other forms of meningitis characterized by a granulomatous exudate at the base of the brain
IV. Slowly progressive amnesic states
   A. Tumors involving the walls of the third ventricle and temporal lobes
   B. Alzheimer's disease and other degenerative disorders (early stage only)

Some of these amnesic syndromes are unique and some demand early recognition if therapy is to be effective. For example, in *transient global amnesia,* so named by Fisher and Adams, an elderly person (usually over 50 years) will suddenly become bewildered, being uncertain of his or her whereabouts, the time of day, and what he or she is doing. If told, the patient quickly forgets and asks the same questions repeatedly. In contrast to the patient with a temporal lobe seizure, the patient with transient global amnesia is in contact with the environment and can reply to complex questions, read, calculate, and perform routine tasks. Memory is also impaired for events that occurred hours or days before the attack began. During the episode of amnesia, pallor, convulsive phenomena, or altered consciousness are not evident. Within several hours (five to seven hours as a rule) the patient makes a complete recovery but is left with a gap in memory for the period of the attack and a short period before its onset. During the attack, the EEG may disclose minor changes in the temporal regions. An ischemic attack due to occlusive disease of the temporal branches of the posterior cerebral arteries is one postulated cause. Most patients have only a single attack and no treatment is necessary. Second, third, or several attacks can occur, however, and nothing is known about how to prevent them.

Herpes simplex encephalitis is a common cause of an amnesic state, because of its localization to the inferomedial parts of the temporal lobes. An acute confusional state marks the onset of the illness. Early diagnosis, using lumbar puncture and CT or MRI, and treatment with antiviral agent acyclovir, are mandatory if a fatal outcome or a crippling dementia is to be avoided. In some patients with carcinomatosis, a limbic encephalitis of unknown cause has been found. Some gliomas infiltrate the temporal lobes, fornices, and thalamus over a period of weeks to months, resulting in a characteristic amnesic syndrome.

Perhaps the most important member of this group, from the point of view of the emergency physician, is the Wernicke-Korsakoff syndrome. The occurrence of this disorder represents a genuine neurologic emergency. It is observed mainly but not exclusively in severe alcoholics and is due to a deficiency of thiamine. The syndrome has an acute onset, with ocular palsies, nystagmus, ataxia of stance and gait, and a drowsy-apathetic-confusional state, occurring singly or more often in some combination. The ocular palsies are remarkably sensitive to the administration of thiamine and can be ablated by a meal or two before admission. The nystagmus and ataxia can be overlooked unless they are carefully sought. The failure to recognize the confusional state for what it is—that is, an acute thiamine deficiency—can result in irreparable damage to the mind (Korsakoff's amnesic state). Even in the absence of ocular and ataxic signs, it is good practice to administer large doses of thiamine (50 mg intravenously and 50 mg intramuscularly daily until the patient takes a normal diet) to all confused alcoholics and to all nutritionally depleted patients who are receiving hyperalimentation or intravenous glucose solutions. The administration of thiamine at the first hint of the disease, when only ocular and ataxic signs are present, will prevent the occurrence of the amnesic state. The acute confusional state also responds to the administration of thiamine, and early diencephalic lesions (which cause Korsakoff's amnesic state) can be reduced, reversed, or arrested.

SELECTED READING

Adams, RD, and Victor M. *Principles of Neurology* (4th ed). New York: McGraw-Hill, 1989.

Benson, DF, and Blumer, D (eds). *Psychiatric Aspects of Neurologic Disease* (vol 2). New York: Grune & Stratton, 1982.

Engel, GL, and Romano, J. Delirium, a syndrome of cerebral insufficiency. *J Chronic Dis* 9:260, 1959.

Fisher, CM, and Adams, RD. Transient global amnesia. *Acta Neurol Scand* 40 (Suppl 9):1, 1964.

Lishman, WA. *Organic Psychiatry: The Psychological Consequences of Cerebral Disorders.* Oxford: Blackwell, 1978.

Lipowski, ZJ. *Delirium: Acute Brain Failure in Man.* Springfield, IL: Thomas, 1980.

Mori, E, and Yamadori, A. Acute confusional state and acute agitated delirium. *Arch Neurol* 44:1139, 1987.

Terry, RD, and Katzman R. Senile dementia of the Alzheimer type. *Ann Neurol* 14:497, 1983.

Tomlinson, BE. The Pathology of Dementia. In CE Wells (ed), *Dementia.* Philadelphia: Davis, 1977. Pp 113–153.

Victor, M, Adams, RD, and Collins, GH. *The Wernicke-Korsakoff Syndrome and Related Neurologic Disorders Due to Alcoholism and Malnutrition.* Philadelphia: Davis, 1989.

Wang, HS. Dementia in Old Age. In LW Smith and M Kinsbourne (eds), *Aging and Dementia.* New York: Spectrum, 1977. Pp 1–4.

Wells, CE. *Dementia* (2nd ed). Philadelphia: Davis, 1977.

Wells, CE. Treatable Forms of Dementia. In KJ Isselbacher et al (eds), *Update II: Harrison's Principles of Internal Medicine.* New York: McGraw-Hill, 1981. Pp 221–238.

30. Syncope

Daniel J. Shea

Syncope is a common presenting complaint of emergency department patients and is estimated to account for approximately 3 percent of emergency department visits and 1 percent of hospital admissions. Institutionalized elderly patients have an annual incidence of syncope of approximately 6 percent, and from 5 to 20 percent of adults will experience at least one episode of syncope by age 75. Although syncope is more common in the elderly, an incidence of up to 47 percent has been demonstrated in college students and Air Force personnel.

Syncope is defined as a transient loss of consciousness and motor tone secondary to a reversible disturbance in cerebral function, from which the patient recovers spontaneously without any therapeutic intervention. Presyncope represents a milder form of the same disorder. The causes of syncope are numerous and varied, ranging from a simple, benign "faint" to a life-threatening arrhythmia or subarachnoid bleed. In some cases it can be a harbinger of sudden death. Syncope, even when the cause is benign, can lead to serious injury. Patients with recurrent syncope may become chronically anxious and restrict their activities as a result.

A gold standard for the precise definition of syncope has yet to be developed. This makes it difficult to compare statistical information from different studies since the inclusionary criteria vary widely. The most common causes of syncope in any particular study depend heavily on patient age, diagnostic criteria, and the setting of the study (emergency department, hospital, or office).

Even after extensive evaluation, the specific cause of syncope remains undiagnosed in up to 47 percent of patients. When a cause can be clearly identified, it can be diagnosed by history and physical examination alone approximately 72 to 89 percent of the time. Further evaluation at the time of recurrence only occasionally provides a diagnosis when the cause was unclear at the time of the initial evaluation.

Since syncope is transient and episodic by definition, its cause is often not evident at the time of examination. The episodes usually do not occur in the presence of the physician and often fail to recur while the patient is being monitored. In addition, many of the abnormalities found during evaluation are commonly present in age- and comorbidity-matched patients without syncope and may be difficult to relate to the syncopal episode without a direct temporal relationship.

The evaluation of syncope should ideally be focused and cost effective. However, it is essential for the evaluating physician to recognize those patients at increased risk for sudden death and, after an appropriate initial evaluation, to assure that they are admitted to the hospital or referred for timely and suitable outpatient evaluation and treatment.

Table 30-1. Disorders potentially confused with syncope

Dizziness (light-headedness)
Vertigo
Loss of consciousness secondary to trauma, alcohol intoxication, or other causes
Generalized seizures
Complex-partial or psychomotor seizures
Hypoglycemia
Functional disorders
Drop attacks
Narcolepsy

PATHOPHYSIOLOGY

Syncope is the end result of a transient, diffuse reduction in cerebral blood flow, which can be caused by a number of aberrant physiologic mechanisms. True loss of consciousness requires bilateral cerebral hemisphere dysfunction, suppression of the reticular activating system, or both. For this reason, isolated, focal neurologic defects do not result in syncope.

The metabolic energy requirements of the brain are high, accounting for approximately 20 percent of the basal oxygen consumption in a normal adult. Even at rest the average adult brain (1,500 gm) consumes approximately 120 calories per minute and has a storage capacity of only about 300 calories. Energy requirements are supplied almost exclusively by oxygenation of glucose, which must be continuously supplied because of the brain's poor energy reserves. Changes on an electroencephalogram (EEG) have been demonstrated within a few seconds after oxygen deprivation to the brain.

Because of the brain's high energy requirements, dependence on glucose for metabolism, and lack of energy storage capabilities, a sudden, significant reduction in blood flow requires only about 10 to 15 seconds to cause syncope in normal adults. This response can be enhanced by preexisting hypoxemia or hypoglycemia. In normal adults, an acute reduction in cerebral blood flow of 60 percent or more is required to cause syncope. This critical level corresponds to a mean arterial blood pressure of approximately 25 mm Hg.

The autonomic nervous system plays a major role in the pathophysiology of syncope by influencing cardiac output through both heart rate and force of contraction and controlling the diameter of both capacitance (preload) and resistance (afterload) vessels. The mechanisms of the various specific causes of syncope are discussed in the following section.

DIFFERENTIAL DIAGNOSIS

Disorders Potentially Confused with Syncope

A number of disorders may be falsely diagnosed and treated as syncope unless a careful evaluation is performed (Table 30-1). True syncope must be distinguished by history from isolated dizziness or vertigo and from loss of consciousness secondary to other causes, such as trauma, alcohol intoxication, or drug overdose.

Generalized seizures can initially present as unexplained syncope. A careful history is often sufficient to make the diagnosis. Generalized seizures usually involve a prolonged postictal phase, commonly present on arrival in the emergency department, as opposed to the more rapid recovery in patients with syncope. The aura that precedes seizures can be distinguished from the typical premonitory symptoms that precede vasovagal syncope or the lack of warning associated with cardiovascular syncope. A witness may describe tonic-clonic movements. Evidence of tongue-biting, incontinence, a Babinski sign, or all three, may be noted on examination, lending weight to the diagnosis of seizure rather than syncope. Todd's paralysis, a hemiplegia or monoplegia that lasts from minutes to days, is occasionally present after seizures.

A more difficult problem is seen in patients with complex-partial or psychomotor seizures, who may have loss of consciousness without tonic-clonic movements. Difficult cases may require an EEG to make the final diagnosis. The presence of tonic-clonic movements, however, does not always indicate a true seizure. Cardiac syncope with hypoxemia can result in a short burst of seizure activity. Even vasovagal syncope can involve a few tonic-clonic movements when the period of cerebral hypoxia is prolonged (such as when the patient is prevented from assuming a supine position). Care must be taken to avoid diagnosing a seizure disorder in a patient who suffered a "simple faint," thus committing that patient to an expensive evaluation or prolonged and unnecessary treatment.

Hypoglycemia does not cause sudden loss of consciousness with rapid recovery and can usually be distinguished from true syncope. Testing for levels of serum glucose in an alert patient who has recovered from a syncopal episode is rarely, if ever, revealing.

Functional disorders can mimic syncope, but the episode is typically prolonged and often accompanied by bizarre movements and unusual responses to stimuli. The changes in heart rate, blood pressure, and skin color (pallor) typical of syncope are absent. Patients with these disorders frequently demonstrate conjugate gaze toward the floor, as if to avoid eye contact with the examiner. Turning the patient's head to the other side will result in conjugate gaze toward the floor in the opposite direction, a response not seen in true coma.

Drop attacks (a sudden, unexpected fall often following head-turning) are occasionally seen in elderly individuals. Since these patients vigorously deny loss of consciousness, drop attacks are not considered syncopal episodes.

Narcolepsy is an uncommon disorder in which patients, usually young, experience an uncontrollable desire to sleep when they are relaxed, often with inappropriate timing. They may be difficult to arouse from this sleep for a period of time. These patients frequently suffer from cataplexy (an abrupt loss of muscle tone following an emotional stimulus) as well.

Causes

For practical purposes, the various causes of syncope can be divided into two general categories: cardiovascular (heart and great vessels) and noncardiovascular (Table 30-2).

Table 30-2. Known causes of syncope

Cardiovascular
Ventricular tachyarrhythmias
Supraventricular tachyarrhythmias
Stokes-Adams syndrome
Severe bradycardia of any cause
Acute myocardial infarction
Artificial pacemaker failure
Sudden, severe obstruction to blood flow through the heart or great vessels
Dissection of a thoracic aortic aneurysm
Leakage or rupture of an abdominal aortic aneurysm
Congenital heart disease
Noncardiovascular
Vasovagal (vasodepressor) syncope
Orthostatic hypotension
Medication induced (see Table 30-3)
Carotid sinus hypersensitivity
Situational syncope (cough, laugh, deglutition, micturition, defecation)
Postprandial syncope
Hyperventilation
Subclavian steal syndrome
Vertebrobasilar insufficiency
Hypertensive encephalopathy
Takayasu's disease (pulseless disease)

Cardiovascular Causes

Cardiovascular causes of syncope include any arrhythmia that is significant and prolonged enough to reduce blood flow, including an absolute or relative bradycardia. Ventricular tachyarrhythmias, especially runs of ventricular tachycardia, cause syncope much more commonly than do supraventricular tachyarrhythmias. Supraventricular tachyarrhythmias are more likely to cause syncope in patients with valvular heart disease, especially those with aortic or subaortic stenosis who may decompensate after loss of atrial contraction and subsequently reduced diastolic filling of the ventricle. Arrhythmias should be strongly suspected in all elderly patients, whenever syncope occurs in the reclining position and whenever the prodromal period is very brief or absent.

Severe bradycardia for any reason can cause syncope secondary to reduced cardiac output, especially in hemodynamically compromised patients. Stokes-Adams syndrome refers to a high-degree heart block with resultant syncope, although the term is commonly used to describe syncope associated with any acute rhythm disturbance or heart block.

Syncope is an early symptom in up to seven percent of patients with an acute myocardial infarction (MI). This can be the result of a transient heart block, an arrhythmia, or a transient reduction in inotropy during the early stages of the MI. It can also be vasovagel in nature, secondary to severe pain or fear induced by the chest pain.

Artificial pacemaker malfunction, including battery failure, electrode displacement, and fracture of the wire secondary to trauma can cause syncope. Unexplained syncope in a pacemaker patient mandates admission for monitoring and further evaluation.

Other cardiac causes of syncope include any sudden, severe obstruction to blood flow through the heart or great vessels, such as a massive pulmonary embolism with acute cor pulmonale. Either aortic stenosis or hypertrophic cardiomyopathy (subaortic stenosis) restricts flow through the heart chronically, but the patient is usually able to compensate up to a certain point. Any further reduction in flow, such as from loss of atrial contraction or peripheral vasodilatation, can result in syncope. Cardiac tamponade is another cause of decreased cardiac output, and any additional stress that reduces output further can induce syncope. An atrial myxoma can be a rare cause of syncope if its position results in a sudden, transient reduction in blood flow through the heart.

Syncope can occur in patients with aortic dissections or leaking abdominal aortic aneurysms. Although a history of pain is normally present, patients with leaking abdominal aortic aneurysms may experience syncope without any other significant symptoms, including abdominal pain. A high index of suspicion is essential to make the proper diagnosis and initiate proper treatment immediately.

Various types of congenital heart disease, including tetralogy of Fallot, predispose a patient to syncope and should be considered in children who have a syncopal episode and in young patients who experience exertional syncope.

Noncardiovascular Causes

Noncardiovascular causes of syncope are many and varied. Vasomotor instability for any reason can transiently reduce systemic vascular resistance or venous return, or both, resulting in decreased cerebral blood flow.

Vasovagal (vasodepressor) syncope is common in young, healthy patients but should be diagnosed with caution in older adults. Definitive diagnosis requires the history of a precipitating factor, such as fear, excitement, pain, fright, or apprehension, and typical premonitory symptoms, such as nausea, diaphoresis, and light-headedness. Dilated pupils may be noted just before the syncopal episode if it is witnessed. There is often a history of standing erect or being immobile for a prolonged period of time before the episode, frequently in a warm environment. Exacerbating factors include hunger, fatigue, crowding (especially in a hot room), alcohol, certain medications, and anxiety.

Vasovagal syncope begins with a decrease in arterial blood pressure that is not accompanied by a compensatory increase in cardiac output. Heart rate changes are variable at this early stage, which is followed by a sudden bradycardia, a drop in blood pressure, and a decrease in peripheral vascular resistance. At this point skeletal muscle blood flow is increased, with a concomitant decrease in cutaneous and central (renal, mesenteric, and cerebral) blood flow. As a result of these factors, if the process is not aborted in time, pallor and typical premonitory symptoms develop, followed shortly by syncope.

The precise pathophysiology of vasovagal syncope is not entirely understood, although overall it seems to be secondary to a general reduction of sympathetic tone accompanied by a relative increase in vagal tone. It is clear that the bradycardia is not solely responsible since atropine has been shown to reverse the bradycardia but not the other features of this disorder. Pooling of blood in the lower extremities, long a favored explanation for vasovagal symptoms, now appears to only partially account for the syndrome.

Central venous pressure is consistently low to unobtainable during vasovagal syncope. This seems to correspond to

Table 30-3. Medications that cause or predispose to syncope

Prazosin (first-dose effect)
Quinidine (torsade de pointes)
Digitalis
Toxicity from any antiarrhythmic medication
Beta-blockers
Calcium channel blockers
Diuretics
Nitrates
Any antihypertensives, vasodilating agents, antianginal agents
Tranquilizers
Antidepressants
Sedatives (including alcohol)
Lithium toxicity
Ganglionic blockers

pooling of blood in a dilated central venous reservoir. Ventricular function during vasovagal reactions may also be impaired, although the evidence for this is inconclusive.

The lack of compensatory rise in cardiac output and heart rate is possibly due to diminished venous return secondary to a blunted rise in plasma renin, causing a loss of renin-angiotensin–controlled vasoconstriction. Oliguria has been noted after vasovagal syncope, unlike other forms of syncope, secondary to increased secretion of antidiuretic hormone, indicating that posterior pituitary hormones may play a role in some of the clinical features of vasovagal syncope, such as nausea and pallor.

One theory on the inciting mechanism for vasovagal syncope is that it may represent an enhanced baroreceptor response to a sudden increase in carotid sinus blood pressure secondary to one of the previously mentioned stimuli. Stimulation of intracardiac receptors has also been postulated to play a role, but there is no definitive evidence for this theory.

Orthostatic hypotension can cause syncope and is usually seen after a change from the supine position to sitting or standing. It may be caused by volume depletion, decreased cardiac output, decreased peripheral resistance, or the Shy-Drager syndrome (multiple central nervous system defects associated with idiopathic orthostatic hypotension). Premonitory symptoms, as with vasovagal syncope, are common. Definitive diagnosis requires a symptomatic, orthostatic decrease in systolic blood pressure of at least 25 mm Hg or a symptomatic decrease in standing systolic blood pressure to less than 90 mm Hg. Blood pressure and heart rate should be measured immediately after standing and five minutes later. Patients who cannot stand may have their upright pressure measured while sitting with the legs dangling. A rise in the heart rate with standing is often a more sensitive indicator of early orthostatic changes, especially in children. However, this response may not be present in patients who are taking beta-blockers.

Medications can cause syncope directly or indirectly (Table 30-3). There are several different mechanisms through which a variety of medications can lead to syncope in susceptible patients, including orthostatic hypotension, cardiac arrhythmias, and anaphylactic reactions.

Prazosin often causes syncope when it is first taken, a side effect commonly known as the "first-dose effect." This phenomenon is probably secondary to a combination of vasodilation from the medication and chronic intravascular volume depletion. Patients should be instructed to take their first dose at night while supine and diuretics should be discontinued for at least 48 hours before starting prazosin.

Quinidine-induced syncope is related to transient episodes of rapid polymorphic ventricular tachycardia (torsade de pointes) or, occasionally, ventricular fibrillation. Digitalis toxicity can produce any arrhythmia, including complete heart block. Toxicity from any antiarrhythmic agent and from tricyclic antidepressants can result in arrhythmias that lead to syncope.

Diuretics can cause volume depletion, leading to orthostatic hypotension, and can exacerbate digitalis toxicity through induction of hypokalemia. Tranquilizers, ganglionic blockers, nitrates, and other vasodilators can also contribute to orthostatic hypotension. Medications such as sedatives, tranquilizers, and antidepressants can predispose a patient to development of syncope after the addition of a usually benign stress to his or her system.

Carotid sinus hypersensitivity can be cardioinhibitory, vasodepressor, or a combination of both in nature. The cardioinhibitory (vagal) type causes syncope by means of significant bradycardia or a short (up to five seconds) episode of asystole and responds to atropine. The vasodepressor type, which is less common, produces syncope through a drop in systolic blood pressure of up to 50 mm Hg.

Situational syncope results from normal physiologic functions (including coughing, laughing, swallowing, urinating, and defecating) that cause decreased cerebral blood flow under certain conditions in predisposed patients. In some cases, these functions produce an additional stress in a hemodynamically compromised patient. Frequently, however, the mechanism is not clear.

Defecation syncope might be secondary to a decreased venous return and bradycardia from the Valsalva maneuver often associated with defecation. Urination in the presence of prostatic hypertrophy can require a Valsalva maneuver as well, resulting in micturition syncope for the same reasons. Micturition syncope might also be related to increased vagal tone as a result of a combination of sleeping and a full bladder, accompanied by incomplete compensatory vasoconstriction with standing and a sudden decompensation after micturition. This condition can be exacerbated by alcohol, fatigue, and hunger.

The mechanism of cough syncope remains unknown but is thought to be related to sudden posttussive rises in intracranial pressure, possibly causing a cerebral "concussion" or a regional decrease in blood flow secondary to the sudden rise in intracranial pressure. Intrathoracic and intracranial pressures can rise to as high as 300 mm Hg after paroxysms of coughing in patients predisposed to this condition. Other proposed mechanisms include a sudden decrease in cerebral blood flow due to the excessive Valsalva maneuver (increased intrathoracic pressure causing decreased venous return to the heart) associated with coughing in these patients, who tend to be short, heavy-set, barrel-chested, middle-aged male smokers who often have chronic lung disease. The mechanism of laugh syncope is also unknown, but is most likely similar to that of cough syncope.

Deglutition (swallow) syncope can be secondary to a combination of increased vagal tone in response to swallowing in the face of cardiac conduction abnormalities. It may be seen with glossopharyngeal neuralgia or tumor invasion of the glossopharyngeal nerve, resulting in an increase in vagal tone secondary to the pain produced by swallowing. Deglution syncope is frequently associated with esophageal disorders, incuding tumors, spasm, and diverticula, but is also seen in patients with no discernable underlying abnormality. Recurrent deglutition syncope may require a permanent pacemaker for control.

Postprandial syncope is seen in some elderly patients in whom heavy meals induce a postprandial drop in blood pressure, predisposing them to syncope. Possible mechanisms include a blunted baroreceptor response, exaggerated vagal tone, and pooling of splanchnic blood.

Hyperventilation, through a reduction in the arterial carbon dioxide pressure, causes cerebral vasoconstriction and hypoxia, along with a decrease in peripheral vascular resistance. Early symptoms include light-headedness and paresthesias of the lips, hands, and feet. With continued hyperventilation, tightening of the facial muscles and carpal-pedal spasm can develop, sometimes followed by syncope.

The *subclavian steal syndrome* occasionally causes syncope. This syndrome involves a stenosis of the subclavian artery in an area proximal to the vertebral artery, resulting in a diversion of blood flow from the vertebrobasilar circulation to the ipsilateral arm with vigorous exercise of that extremity. The diagnosis is suggested by a difference in the systolic blood pressure of more than 20 mm Hg between the upper extremities and symptoms of vertebrobasilar ischemia on exercise of the affected upper extremity.

Vertebrobasilar artery insufficiency is an uncommon cause of syncope. In this case the syncope is always accompanied by diplopia, vertigo, dysarthria, hemiparesis, or other symptoms suggesting brainstem ischemia. Other focal cerebrovascular diseases, including transient ischemic attacks (TIA) and strokes, do not cause true syncope.

Other unusual causes of syncope include *hypertensive encephalopathy* (probably secondary to diffuse spasm of the cerebral arterioles) and *Takayasu's disease* (arteritis of the aorta and large arteries that can affect the carotid circulation).

Table 30-4. Basic evaluation of syncope

History

Each patient should be questioned concerning the following factors:

- Was there truly loss of consciousness?
- Rapidity of onset and recovery
- Duration of the syncopal episode
- Presence or absence of prodromal symptoms or an aura
- Symptoms before, during, and after the syncopal episode (palpitations, chest pain, apprehension, vertigo, diplopia, dysarthria, focal neurologic signs, incontinence, tongue-biting, postictal phase)
- Environment (temperature, crowding, and so forth) and position at the time of syncope
- Actions just before syncope (rising from bed, exertion, micturition, emotional upset, turning of head, and so forth)
- Was any trauma associated with the syncopal episode or before it?
- Symptoms of hyperventilation (paresthesias of lips, hands, or feet)
- Postsyncopal residua
- Account of eyewitness (if available)
- Past medical history (including any prior episodes of syncope and any predisposing factors)
- Medication history (especially any recent changes in medication)

Physical examination

Routine

- Complete vital signs
  - Orthostatic blood pressure and heart rate measurements in stable patients
  - Blood pressure in both upper extremities
- Palpation of carotid, femoral, and peripheral pulses for quality, rate, regularity, and symmetry
- Auscultation of the heart for murmurs, prominent pulmonary component of the second heart sound, other abnormal sounds, rate, and regularity
- Auscultation of the lungs
- Abdominal examination for tenderness, masses, organomegaly, and bruits
- Rectal examination for occult blood
- Neurologic examination for focal neurologic defects, peripheral neuropathy, and evidence of seizures
- Mental status examination
- General inspection for signs of trauma

When indicated

- Blood pressure in lower extremities
- Auscultation for carotid artery bruits
- Inspection of the neck for cannon a waves
- Carotid sinus massage
- Hyperventilation to reproduce symptoms
- Exercise of the upper extremities

EVALUATION

Because of syncope's frequency as a presenting symptom and its myriad causes, there should be a goal-directed, individualized evaluation of each case rather than a "routine" syncope work-up applied indiscriminately to all patients.

History

A thorough and accurate history is of paramount importance. Careful questioning of the patient or a witness, or both, often leads to the correct diagnosis or significantly limits the possibilities. The following aspects of the history are essential and should be obtained in each patient who experiences a syncopal episode (Table 30-4).

The first objective of the history is to determine whether there was an actual loss of consciousness as opposed to dizziness or vertigo without true syncope. The distinction should be clear in most cases, but some patients are uncertain whether loss of consciousness actually occurred. The physician should not accept a statement such as, "I fainted," at face value. Since near-syncope does not involve full loss of consciousness, it may be difficult to distinguish from the other conditions.

The rapidity of onset and recovery should be ascertained, as well as the duration of the syncopal episode. Very sudden onset of syncope can be seen with ventricular arrhythmias, seizures, and carotid sinus hypersensitivity. The latter is also associated with turning of the head before syncope, especially in elderly patients who are wearing stiff collars. A rapid recovery suggests a ventricular tachyarrhythmia while a slower recovery points to a vasovagal episode. An extended period of unconsiousness or prolonged recovery might be secondary to a persistent bradycardia, hypovolemia, or shock. A prolonged recovery from syncope must be distinguished from a postictal phase or Todd's paralysis.

Prodromal symptoms such as diaphoresis, blurred vision, and nausea suggest vasovagal syncope, especially when combined with a precipitating factor (fright, hunger, stress) and an upright posture at the time of the episode. An aura is often noted before a seizure.

The patient should be questioned concerning symptoms and circumstances before, during, and after the syncopal episode. If palpitations preceded the syncopal episode, an arrhythmia should be considered as the cause. Chest pain suggests an acute MI and respiratory distress or apprehension may indicate a pulmonary embolism as the cause of syncope. Symptoms associated with seizures include tonic-clonic movements, tongue-biting, and incontinence.

The environment and the patient's position and actions just before the onset of syncope are often enlightening. Vasovagal syncope is commonly seen in the setting of a warm, crowded room, and the patient is usually standing, often for a prolonged period of time, before the syncopal episode. Syncope shortly after rising from a supine or sitting position suggests orthostatic hypotension, especially when the patient is receiving a predisposing medication or has some other condition that can lead to an orthostatic drop in blood pressure. The patient should be questioned as to any activity before the syncopal episode, normal or otherwise, including micturition, defecation, coughing, laughing, eating, or exertion. Syncope following exertion frequently indicates a serious cause and may be seen in patients with critical aortic stenosis, hypertrophic cardiomyopathy, and pulmonary hypertension.

Trauma can be a cause of syncope or a result of it. The patient should be questioned carefully in this regard and any injuries sustained at the time of syncope need to be evaluated carefully. A history of trauma preceding the syncope should also be obtained. A chronic subdural hematoma should be considered in any patient with a history of recent head trauma, especially in alcoholic patients, in patients receiving anticoagulants, or in individuals with bleeding disorders.

Hyperventilation can lead to syncope and is usually associated with dysesthesias of the lips, hands, and feet as well as shortness of breath. The patient may not be aware of having hyperventilated, even when questioned directly in this regard. Postsyncopal residua can indicate a stroke or TIA (focal neurologic deficits), migraine syncope (headache), or seizure (Todd's paralysis).

The description of an eyewitness can be invaluable and can, at times, provide more objective and complete data than the patient's own account. Even when the syncopal episode was not witnessed directly, additional information provided by family members or other parties familiar with the patient can provide valuable insight into the underlying problem and is always worth seeking.

A thorough medical history should be obtained, concentrating on possible contributory factors such as cardiovascular, cerebrovascular, and pulmonary disease; hypertension; diabetes mellitus; anemia; gastrointestinal or excessive vaginal bleeding; peptic ulcer disease; seizures; renal disease; deep venous thrombosis; embolic disease; aortic aneurysm; dehydration; and recent surgery. A careful medication history is mandatory and any recent changes in medication should be diligently noted.

Physical Examination

Routine Physical Examination

As the first step in the physical examination, one must obtain careful vital signs, including orthostatic blood pressure and heart rate measurements in stable patients, excluding those who are hypotensive while supine (see Table 30-4). A drop in systolic blood pressure of more than 25 mm Hg, or of more than 10 mm Hg when the supine systolic blood pressure is 90 or less, is considered positive. Blood pressure should also be checked in both arms since a significant difference can indicate subclavian steal syndrome.

Carotid, femoral, and peripheral pulses should be palpated for quality, rate, regularity, and symmetry. Persistently weak or absent pulses can be associated with shock. Lack of radial pulses suggests Takayasu's (pulseless) disease. Bradycardia can indicate sinus node dysfunction, vasovagal syncope, or carotid sinus hypersensitivity.

The heart and lungs should be auscultated carefully, listening for murmurs, rubs, gallops, clicks, muffled heart sounds (cardiac tamponade), heart rate, and rhythm. The murmur of aortic stenosis or hypertrophic cardiomyopathy (which increases with the Valsalva maneuver) should be sought in patients with exertional syncope. An increased pulmonary component of the second sound suggests pulmonary vascular hypertension or pulmonary embolism. An irregular rhythm mandates appropriate monitoring and a 12-lead electrocardiogram (ECG).

The abdomen should be palpated carefully for pulsatile and stationary masses, hepatomegaly, splenomegaly, and tenderness. The abdomen should be auscultated for the presence of bruits. A rectal examination should be performed to check for occult bleeding unless the history clearly indicates another cause.

It is essential to perform a careful neurologic examination, searching for evidence of seizures, stroke, TIA, or peripheral neuropathy. Focal neurologic defects can indicate intracranial disorders. A mental status examination and an inspection for signs of trauma are also part of the routine examination.

Additional Physical Examination

When indicated based on history, the following aspects of the examination should also be performed (see Table 30-4). Lower-extremity blood pressure readings may be useful in some patients. A significant difference between upper- and lower-extremity measurements raises the possibility of a dissecting aortic aneurysm or coarctation of the aorta. The carotid artery should be auscultated for bruits whenever carotid sinus hypersensitivity, a stroke, or TIA is suspected. When a Stokes-Adams attack is considered, the neck should be inspected for cannon a waves.

When hyperventilation is a likely cause of syncope, it is helpful to have the patient purposely hyperventilate in order to determine if the symptoms can be reproduced in this manner, thus making the diagnosis. Exercise of the upper extremities is useful to diagnose the subclavian steal syndrome since it will often reproduce the symptoms. Also, a supraclavicular bruit or thrill should be checked for when this condition is suspected.

Carotid sinus massage (CSM) can be helpful in selected patients whose histories suggest carotid sinus hypersensitivity. It is generally a safe procedure. However, serious complications (e.g., stroke) can arise, making it contraindicated in patients with carotid artery bruits or known carotid artery disease. It is relatively contraindicated in elderly patients with hypertension and atherosclerosic heart disease. Even when properly performed on appropriate patients, CSM can result in bradycardia or hypotension, or both. Therefore, the patient should be tested in the supine position, on cardiac and blood pressure monitors, with an intravenous line in place and with atropine and pressor agents readily available.

To perform CSM, the first side should be massaged for 10 to 20 seconds, with only light pressure applied in the beginning. If there is no response, the other side should be massaged; this process can be repeated. An abnormal response is a drop in systolic or diastolic blood pressure of at least 50 mm Hg or asystole for at least 3 seconds. Detection of carotid sinus hypersensitivity does not establish it as the definitive cause of syncope since it can be found in up to 10 percent of normal elderly patients.

Basic Laboratory and Diagnostic Testing

When a cause for a patient's syncope is diagnosed, approximately 72 to 89 percent of the time it is based primarily on history and physical examination. When the diagnosis is clear and certain with a high degree of confidence (e.g., vasovagal syncope or hyperventilation), no further testing is required. The threshold for obtaining laboratory studies should be lower with elderly patients, who are more likely to have a cause that can be diagnosed by laboratory studies, especially ECG.

If the diagnosis is uncertain after the initial evaluation, a complete blood count (CBC), basic chemistry screen (serum electrolytes, serum glucose, blood urea nitrogen, and creatinine), and ECG should generally be performed (Table 30-5). A creatine phosphokinase isoenzyme level should be obtained if there is any suspicion of an acute MI. An arterial blood gas may be useful in some cases (e.g., suspicion of a pulmonary embolism or of hyperventilation that is not clearly evident on examination). A chest x-ray is indicated if there is any suspicion of a cardiac or pulmonary cause (such as a dissecting aortic aneurysm). Whenever an irregularity of the heart rate is noted on physical examination or there is any suspicion of a cardiovascular cause for the syncope (which includes all elderly patients), the patient should be placed on a continuous cardiac monitor while he or she is in the emergency department.

A routine ECG will specifically diagnose the cause of syncope in only three to six percent of patients. Definitive diagnosis requires evidence of a symptomatic bradyarrhythmia or tachyarrhythmia, an acute MI, or symptomatic pacemaker malfunction. Other abnormalities found on a routine ECG, while not specifically diagnosing the cause of syncope, can indicate the presence of structural heart disease and the need for further evaluation. Structural heart disease is suggested by any heart block, ventricular hypertrophy, significant atrial or ventricular arrhythmias, and preexcitation syndromes (such as Wolff-Parkinson-White syndrome). Of course, all of these abnormalities are commonly present in patients without syncope and, conversely, a patient with structural heart disease can have a normal ECG.

Table 30-5. Basic laboratory and diagnostic tests for syncope

Routine*
Complete blood count
Basic serum chemistry screen (electrolytes, glucose, blood urea nitrogen, and creatinine)
Electrocardiogram
Continuous cardiac monitoring while in the emergency department
When indicated
Chest x-ray
Arterial blood gas
Creatine phosphokinase isoenzyme level
Ventilation-perfusion lung scan
Hepatic and renal chemistries
Alcohol level
Toxicology screen
Blood for type and cross-match

*In some cases it is appropriate not to order any tests (e.g., clear-cut vasovagal syncope in a young patient) or to order one or two specific tests (e.g., complete blood count).

A CBC and basic chemistry screen are not likely to provide a specific cause for the syncopal episode, but an abnormal result may indicate a contributing factor. For example, anemia suggests gastrointestinal bleeding or a leaking abdominal aortic aneurysm. Significant hyponatremia suggests the possibility of a seizure rather than true syncope.

Further Testing

Testing beyond the basic evaluation just outlined becomes expensive and the invasive procedures carry an inherent risk. It also has a low likelihood of producing a diagnosis in patients without structural heart disease. Since many episodes of syncope are isolated single events, extensive evaluation is usually reserved for patients with recurrent syncope unless a specific problem is noted on initial evaluation that indicates the need for further testing. The overall recurrence rate in patients with unexplained syncope has been shown to be as low as 13 percent over 2.5 years.

Young patients (under 30 years old) do not usually require extensive testing. In these patients, the cause of syncope is likely to be benign, unifactorial, and clearly evident on initial evaluation. In addition, young patients with unexplained syncope have an excellent prognosis and low incidence of recurrence, mainly because of the infrequent presence of structural heart disease.

In spite of these admonitions, additional testing is advisable for a distinct subgroup of patients who experience syncope. This subgroup includes patients with recurrent syncope (regardless of age), heart block, arrhythmia, or evidence of structural heart disease (even if the syncope is not clearly secondary to a cardiac cause). Also included are patients who suffered significant morbidity, such as a fractured hip, as a result of the syncopal episode. Elderly pa-

Table 30-6. Additional tests for further evaluation of syncope

24-hour ambulatory (Holter) monitoring
Electrophysiologic studies
Exercise tolerance testing
Echocardiography
Computed axial tomography
Electroencephalography

tients with recurrent syncope after correction of any metabolic abnormalities found on previous evaluations or after empiric medication adjustments should also be evaluated carefully and thoroughly. The following tests may be of benefit in the further evaluation and management of selected patients (Table 30-6).

24-Hour Ambulatory (Holter) Monitoring
Holter monitoring should be the first step in patients who are undergoing further evaluation on an outpatient basis for syncope of uncertain cause. An accurate and complete diary of symptoms is essential to determine the temporal relationship of the syncope to arrhythmias, making patient cooperation and understanding a prerequisite for proper interpretation.

The ideal duration of monitoring is still unknown. In general, all patients with recurrent syncope of uncertain cause, or with recurrent syncope, risk factors for coronary artery disease, and a normal resting ECG, should undergo Holter monitoring for 24 hours. Patients with a high probability of a cardiac cause should be monitored for an additional 24 to 48 hours if the initial 24-hour monitor is negative. In some cases monitoring for several weeks may be necessary, with the patient initiating a recording whenever he or she shows symptoms.

Holter monitor results must be interpreted with care. Asymptomatic arrhythmias are common in patients with and without syncope. Only symptomatic arrhythmias can be considered diagnostic and a basis for treatment. However, a Finnish study demonstrated that asymptomatic pauses of greater than 2.5 seconds are more likely to predict a cardiac cause of syncope than asymptomatic short bursts of ventricular tachycardia.

The actual diagnostic yield with Holter monitoring is fairly low. In one study, only 1 percent of approximately 1,500 patients had syncope during 24-hour ambulatory monitoring. Another 16 percent experienced presyncopal symptoms, but the symptoms could be related to an arrhythmia in only 1.5 percent. A typical episode of syncope during documented normal sinus rhythm is useful in that it eliminates arrhythmias as a cause of that patient's syncopal episodes.

Patients with negative results on Holter monitoring who have no evidence of structural heart disease and a single episode of syncope do not require any further evaluation. Those with recurrent syncope or evidence of structural heart disease, or both, should undergo additional testing.

Electrophysiologic Studies
Electrophysiologic studies (EPS) involve catheterization of the heart with intracardiac leads for determination of baseline rhythm as well as response to ventricular and supraventricular stimulation and to various antiarrhythmic agents. EPS is useful primarily in patients with recurrent syncope and known heart disease. The diagnostic yield of EPS depends on patient selection and is high when the test is reserved for patients with known structural heart disease. EPS has a yield of up to 68 percent in patients with heart disease, as compared to 10 to 15 percent in those without heart disease. The overall diagnostic yield in patients with recurrent syncope is approximately 50 to 60 percent.

The risks associated with EPS have an occurrence rate of approximately 0.1 percent and include bleeding, perforation of major vessels or the myocardium, infection, phlebitis, pneumothorax, arrhythmias, MI, and death. The majority of complications are related to the catheterization procedure itself rather than to the induction of arrhythmias. As with Holter monitoring, EPS results must be interpreted carefully. EPS is capable of inducing false-positive results, as well as yielding false negatives. Patients with negative results on EPS have a good prognosis, a recurrence rate of only 5 percent, and no need for prophylactic treatment.

Exercise Tolerance Testing
Exercise tolerance testing (ETT) may be helpful in patients at high risk for structural heart disease in whom a Holter monitor shows normal results. Patients with a normal resting ECG, negative Holter monitor, and normal ETT do not usually require EPS.

Echocardiography
Two-dimensional echocardiography is useful for diagnosing valvular heart disease, subaortic stenosis, ventricular hypertrophy, atrial myxoma, congenital heart disease, and ventricular aneurysms. It does not usually produce a specific diagnosis for the syncopal episode but does aid in the selection of patients for EPS.

Computed Axial Tomography
Computed axial tomography (CT) scanning has a low yield in diagnosing the cause of syncope. It should be reserved for patients with focal abnormalities noted on neurologic examination and for those with a significant head injury resulting from the syncopal episode (i.e., suspicion for a subdural hematoma). In addition, CT scanning may be useful when there is suspicion of a leaking abdominal aortic aneurysm or of a subcapsular splenic or hepatic hematoma in patients who experience a syncopal episode several days after abdominal trauma. If CT scanning is not readily available, ultrasound should be considered for some of these indications.

Electroencephalography
Electroencephalography is a low-yield procedure that should be limited to patients in whom the suspicion for seizures is high. These patients include those with a history of seizures, evidence of metabolic acidosis on initial evaluation, and recurrent syncope of uncertain cause.

THE ELDERLY

Syncope is more frequent in the elderly than in younger patients, and is often multifactorial, whereas a single cause is more common in younger patients. A number of age- and disease-related factors may work in a synergistic manner to decrease cerebral blood flow and set the stage for syncope. Syncope in an elderly person is more likely to have a serious and recurrent cause, such as an arrhythmia. It is also more likely to result in a serious injury because of age-related factors (arthritis, poor balance) that result in a harder fall and osteoporotic bones that are more prone to fracture. For these reasons, syncope, especially when recurrent, can create a fearful patient who restricts his or her activity significantly, leading to further physical and emotional disability.

A number of conditions predispose the elderly to syncope. Elderly patients often receive medication regimens that, alone or in combination, can lead to syncope. When medical care is fragmented among several different physicians, the chances of a drug interaction leading to syncope or other complications are more likely.

Age-related changes can also contribute to syncope. These include the presence of cardiovascular and cerebrovascular disorders, anemia, chronic dehydration, a lower resting cerebral blood flow, and a diminished capacity to compensate in response to sudden hypotension or vasodilation. Under these conditions, the addition of a factor that decreases cerebral blood flow to a normally insignificant degree can result in a syncopal episode. These usually trivial factors include several normal daily functions, such as eating, urinating, defecating, taking a hot bath, and even rising from a sitting or supine position.

Falls in the elderly are common and occur for a number of reasons, including syncope. However, an injury related to the fall may be the chief complaint and the syncopal episode may not be mentioned by the patient unless he or she is questioned carefully concerning the circumstances that led to the fall. For this reason, it is essential to obtain a thorough and accurate history, including a medication history, from any elderly person who falls and from any available witnesses.

MANAGEMENT

Upon discharge, patients should be advised to avoid potentially dangerous activities (driving, climbing, swimming, using power tools, and so forth) for at least several days in case of a recurrence. Any treatment should be specific and aimed at a demonstrable cause of the syncope.

Young patients with vasovagal syncope need only be advised to rest and to avoid prolonged standing or sudden positional changes until they feel better. When appropriate, increased fluid intake should be advised. Patients should be further instructed to lie down or sit with the head lowered between the knees at the onset of any future premonitory symptoms and to avoid precipitating conditions whenever possible.

Patients with situational syncope (micturition, defecation, cough) should be instructed to avoid precipitating factors (i.e., sit while urinating, use stool softeners). Patients with cough syncope should be advised to quit smoking and to avoid hard coughing. Those with a chronic cough that does not respond to direct measures such as cessation of smoking require a more extensive evaluation (including pulmonary function tests) to determine a specific cause and treatment for the cough.

Any identifiable contributing or precipitating factor should be corrected, including arrhythmias, volume depletion, and metabolic abnormalities. Medication adjustment should be undertaken whenever appropriate. Patients with quinidine-induced syncope require admission for monitoring, discontinuation of quinidine, and specific antiarrhythmic treatment as indicated. Syncope secondary to digitalis toxicity also mandates inpatient treatment and monitoring.

Patients with vasodepressor-type carotid sinus hypersensitivity may avoid syncope by wearing soft, loose collars and not turning the head too far in either direction. A permanent pacemaker is the preferred treatment for documented, isolated, cardioinhibitory-type carotid sinus hypersensitivity.

Elderly patients often have multiple medical problems and may be receiving numerous medications, any one of which could be the cause of the syncopal episode. Treatment should be aimed at a specific cause whenever possible. However, the inciting event may be difficult or impossible to determine and may in fact be a combination of several factors or medications. When the cause is uncertain, and a cardiovascular cause is not strongly suspected, empiric medication adjustment may be beneficial. Any metabolic abnormalities noted on the initial, basic laboratory evaluation should also be corrected. The patient should be warned to avoid precipitating events and should continue to be evaluated carefully for recurrence of symptoms. The treatments of various other cardiovascular and neurologic causes of syncope are discussed in detail in other chapters.

DISPOSITION

Prognosis

The majority of patients with syncope have an excellent prognosis and it is important to provide reassurance whenever appropriate. Patient age under 30 years old and a noncardiovascular cause of the syncope are major factors associated with a good prognosis. Recurrence of vasodepressor and situational (e.g., micturition) syncope can often be prevented by avoidance of certain environmental factors or minor behavioral changes, or both.

Patients with syncope of cardiovascular origin have a high rate of mortality, in the range of 18 to 33 percent, with approximately 80 percent of the deaths occurring suddenly. Patients with syncope of noncardiovascular origin (including an uncertain cause after full evaluation) have a low mortality, in the 6 to 12 percent range. This rate does not differ significantly from the mortality in comorbidity and age-matched control subjects without syncope.

During 26 years of the Framingham Study, three percent of the patients reported at least one syncopal episode. Nonrecurrent syncope was not associated with any increased incidence of stroke, TIA, MI, or cardiovascular mortality.

Recurrence in patients with a noncardiovascular or unclear cause of syncope is not associated with an increased rate of mortality. In fact, frequently recurring syncope may indicate a benign process and lower mortality, since the more serious causes of syncope will often manifest themselves or result in sudden death rather than lead to multiple recurrences.

Elderly patients who suffer a significant injury, such as a fractured hip, as a result of a syncopal episode have an increased rate of morbidity and mortality. In addition, frequent falls secondary to syncope, even with only minor injuries, can cause an elderly person to severely restrict his or her activities and become dependent because of the constant fear of falling.

Inpatient Versus Outpatient Evaluation

The decision to admit a patient for further evaluation should be based on whether the syncopal episode is isolated or recurrent, the age of the patient, the likelihood of a cardiovascular cause, and the severity of the episode, with any resultant injuries (significant head trauma, fractured hip) taken into account. Any patient in whom a cardiovascular cause of syncope is likely should be admitted to the hospital for monitoring and further evaluation. Patients with known structural heart disease, recurrent syncope, or age over 70 years should also be admitted when the cause of the syncope is uncertain, as should any patients with significant injuries as a result of the syncope. Outpatient evaluation is appropriate and safe for most others.

Branch divided patients into three categories: (1) Low-risk patients are those less than 30 years old with a history that suggests vasovagal syncope. These patients require only careful follow-up study. (2) High-risk patients are those with a history that strongly suggests syncope of cardiovascular origin. These patients should be hospitalized for cardiac monitoring and should be considered for EPS. (3) Intermediate-risk patients are those who do not fall into either of these categories. They require a basic evaluation and an individualized decision, based on clinical judgment, in regard to follow-up study and further evaluation as an outpatient versus admission for monitoring and more extensive testing.

Patients who are discharged from the hospital or emergency department with the cause of syncope still uncertain should continue to be evaluated carefully because up to 25 percent will experience a recurrent episode within a year. Repeat evaluation will demonstrate a specific cause in 2 to 5 percent of these patients.

SELECTED READING

General

Branch, WT. Approach to syncope. *J Gen Intern Med* 1:49, 1986.

Day, SC, et al. Evaluation and outcome of emergency room patients with transient loss of consciousness. *Am J Med* 73:15, 1982.

Henry, GL, and Little, N. *Neurologic Emergencies: A Symptom Oriented Approach.* New York: McGraw-Hill, 1985. Pp 250–260.

Linzer, M. Syncope. *South Med J* 80:545, 1987.

Martin, GJ, et al. Prospective evaluation of syncope. *Ann Emerg Med* 13:499, 1984.

Ormerod, AD. Syncope. *Br Med J* 288:1219, 1984.

Schultz, K. Vertigo and Syncope. In P Rosen (ed), *Emergency Medicine: Concepts and Clinical Practice* (2nd ed). St. Louis: Mosby, 1988.

Sobel, BE, and Roberts, R. Hypotension and Syncope. In E Braunwald (ed), *Heart Disease* (2nd ed). Philadelphia: Saunders, 1984.

Specific Causes of Syncope

Baron, SB, and Huang, SK. Cough syncope presenting as Mobitz type II atrioventricular block—an electrophysiologic correlation. *PACE* 10:65, 1987.

Glick, G, and Yu, PN. Hemodynamic changes during spontaneous vasovagal reactions. *Am J Med* 34:42, 1963.

Goldstein, DS, et al. Circulatory control mechanisms in vasodepressor syncope. *Am Heart J* 104:1071, 1982.

Haldane, JH. Micturition syncope: Two case reports and a review of the literature. *Can Med Assoc J* 101:712, 1969.

Kadish, AH, Wechsler, L, and Marchlinski, FE. Swallowing syncope: Observations in the absence of conduction system or esophageal disease. *Am J Med* 81:1098, 1986.

Kapoor, WN, Peterson, J, and Karpf, M. Defecation syncope. *Arch Intern Med* 146:2377, 1986.

Leung, FW, and Oill, PA. Ticket for admission: Unexplained syncopal attacks in patients with cardiac pacemaker. *Ann Emerg Med* 9:527, 1980.

Lipitz, LA, et al. Cardiovascular and norepinephrine responses after meal consumption in elderly (older than 75 years) persons with postprandial hypotension and syncope. *Am J Cardiol* 58:810, 1986.

McIntosh, HD, Estes, EH, and Warren, JV. The mechanism of cough syncope. *Am Heart J* 52:70, 1956.

Schellack, J, et al. The carotid sinus syndrome: A frequently overlooked cause of syncope in the elderly. *J Vasc Surg* 4:376, 1986.

Thomas, JE, et al. Orthostatic hypotension. *Mayo Clin Proc* 56:117, 1981.

Zangerle, KF, and Wolford, R. Syncope and conduction disturbances following sublingual nifedipine for hypertension. *Ann Emerg Med* 14:1005, 1985.

Ziegler, MG, Lake, CR, and Kopin, IJ. The sympathetic-nervous-system defect in primary orthostatic hypotension. *N Engl J Med* 296:293, 1977.

Syncope in the Elderly

Kapoor, W, et al. Syncope in the elderly. *Am J Med* 80:419, 1986.

Whiteside-Yim, C. Syncope in the elderly: A clinical approach. *Geriatrics* 42:37, 1987.

Diagnostic Testing

DiMarco, JP. Electrophysiologic studies in patients with unexplained syncope. *Circulation* 75 (Suppl III):III-140, 1987.

Gibson, TC, and Heitzman, MR. Diagnostic efficacy of 24-hour electrocardiographic monitoring for syncope. *Am J Cardiol* 53:1013, 1984.

Kapoor, WN, et al. Prolonged electrocardiographic monitoring in patients with syncope. *Am J Med* 82:20, 1987.

Krol, RB, et al. Electrophysiologic testing in patients with unexplained syncope: Clinical and noninvasive predictors of outcome. *J Am Coll Cardiol* 10:358, 1987.

Morady, F. The evaluation of syncope with electrophysiologic studies. *Cardiol Clin* 4:515, 1986.

Reiffel, JA, et al. Electrophysiologic testing in patients with recurrent syncope: Are results predicted by prior ambulatory monitoring? *Am Heart J* 110:1146, 1985.

Miscellaneous

Kapoor, WN, et al. Diagnostic and prognostic implications of recurrences in patients with syncope. *Am J Med* 83:700, 1987.

Kramer, MR, Drori, Y, and Lev, B. Sudden death in young soldiers: High incidence of syncope prior to death. *Chest* 93:345, 1988.

Rosenberg, ML. The eyes in hysterical states of unconsciousness. *J Clin Neuro Ophthalmol* 2:259, 1982.

G. Disorders of Thermoregulation

31. Mechanisms of Thermoregulation

John D. Patrick

A consequence of the complexity of the human organism is the need for maintenance of effective body temperature within a relatively narrow range (Fig. 31-1). If body temperature varies from this ideal range, the complex cascade of chemical reactions that enables us to function as living organisms becomes more disorganized; at further extremes, this disruption is enough to cause death. This chapter discusses the intricate mechanisms we have evolved in becoming homeotherms, creatures who maintain constant core body temperatures despite the wide temperature variations found in the environment.

TEMPERATURE AND ITS MEASUREMENT

The "set point" at which homeotherms maintain internal temperature is not arbitrary but is defined by the biophysiology of life on our planet. Evolution has selected for an ability to maintain the temperature at which the complex proteins, lipids, and carbohydrates on which animal life is based can best maintain cellular structural integrity and chemical efficiency. This is well illustrated by the fact that the set point for nearly all active homeotherms lies in the relatively narrow range of 39 ± 3°C. Extremes of heat can cause errors in protein synthesis, cellular metabolism, and protein denaturation. Extremes of cold retard the rate of chemical reaction in the cell to such an extent that metabolism approaches zero, while the formation of ice crystals and modification of lipid structure as temperatures dip into the freezing range can irreversibly damage individual cells.

In humans, the normal core temperature varies with time of day, emotional state, bodily activity, age, and, in women, the menstrual cycle. The average oral temperature is between 36.5°C and 37.5°C (97.7°F and 99.5°F), and 0.6°C or 1°F higher when measured rectally; the axillary temperature is generally about 0.7°C lower than oral. Since oral temperatures can vary significantly with respiratory rate, time of equilibration, prior oral intake, and location of the probe tip in the oropharynx, and axillary temperatures are often insensitive detectors of fever, rectal temperatures are generally believed to be the most accurate of the three in approximating core temperature. However, even rectal temperatures vary, sometimes significantly, with thermometer tip location and equilibration time. Electronic thermometers that measure infrared radiation from the tympanic membrane have recently become available. Benzinger and Taylor found that the temperature of the tympanic membrane closely approximates that of the hypothalamus, so this may be the method of external temperature measurement that most accurately reflects the true set point.

The core temperature in humans is generally maintained within 1.0°C of baseline despite wide variations in environ-

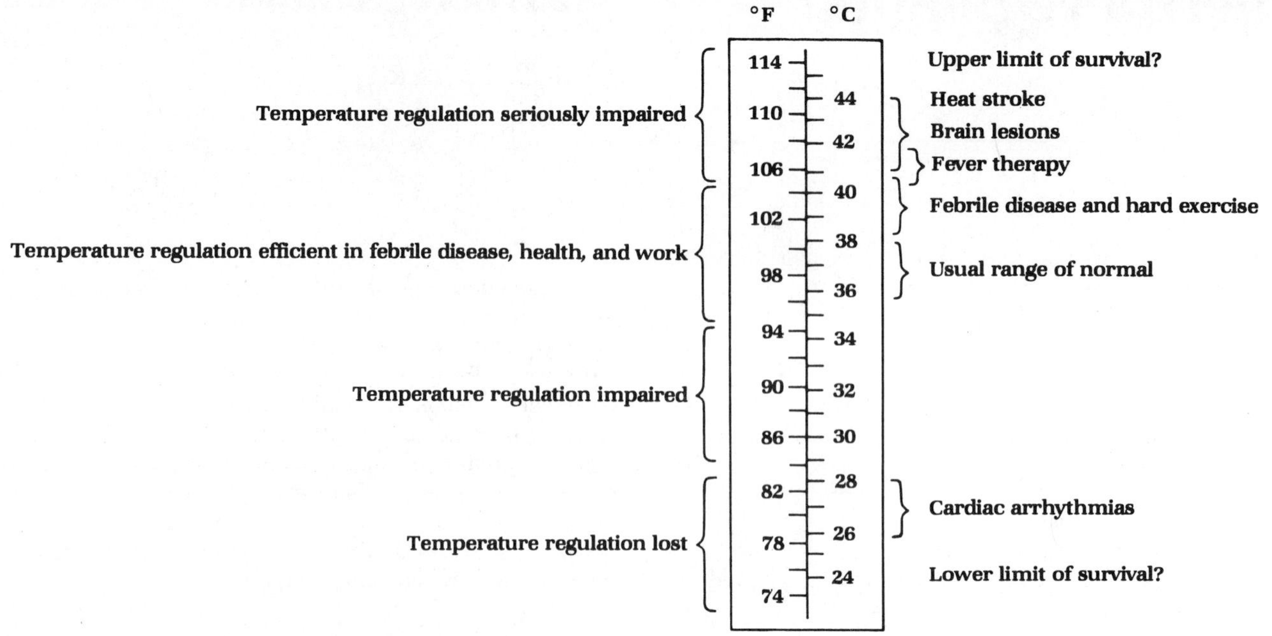

Fig. 31-1. The range of effective human body temperature. (From E.F. DuBois. *Fever and the Regulation of Body Temperature.* Springfield, IL: Thomas, 1948. Courtesy of Charles C Thomas, Publisher, Springfield, Illinois.)

mental temperature. The temperature of the body's surface, on the other hand, varies widely with environmental extremes, tending to approach the temperature of the environment in the more distal extremities. There is a normal diurnal variation of core temperature of up to 1.5°C, with the temperature falling lower during sleep as a result of decreased muscular activity and less perfect autoregulation. Profound emotional stimulation can raise the body temperature by as much as 2°C, probably secondary to a centrally mediated increase in metabolic activity. During sustained extremes of exertion such as long-distance running, the temperature can rise to as high as 40 to 41°C (104–106°F), depending on environmental conditions.

Neonatal temperature control is imperfect, with wider swings in temperature with variations in environment or activity. The temperature in infants is generally 0.5 to 1.0°C higher than in adults and gradually approaches the adult normal temperature with increasing age. The elderly often have a slightly reduced core temperature as well as a diminished ability to compensate for environmental changes. Average female temperature is at a nadir during menstruation and tends to peak at about the time of ovulation.

MECHANISMS OF HEAT GAIN

Like all vertebrates, humans have a water-based biochemistry that depends on the oxidation of foodstuffs as an energy source. Since, even under optimal conditions, these reactions are only about 40 percent efficient (and because thermodynamic principles prevent a closed system maintained at uniform temperature from converting the remaining 60 percent of the stored energy into useful work), the remainder of the stored energy is released as "waste" heat. The production of this thermal energy, along with that produced by the sum of all the other chemical reactions intrinsic to our cellular function, is called *thermogenesis.* Thermogenesis is responsible for the approximately 75 kcal per hour of heat generated by a typical 70-kg man at rest, enough to raise body temperature by 1°C per hour. Exercise, by increasing the rate of chemical reaction in muscle, can dramatically increase the production of heat, to as many as 10 to 16 times the basal level with extremes of exertion. At rest, then, metabolically active organs such as the heart, liver, and kidneys produce most of the body's heat. With exertion, skeletal muscle becomes the primary source; this is the reason why shivering has an important compensatory function in cold environments.

In many animals (especially those awakening from hibernation) and in human neonates, a specific tissue called "brown fat" can increase heat production by, in effect, reducing the efficiency of the cellular machinery. Under central nervous system control, sympathetic stimulation of brown fat causes mitochondria there to become more permeable to adenosine diphosphate. This in turn reduces the efficiency of oxidative phosphorylation of glucose, thereby increasing heat production. The significance of this mechanism in adult human thermogenesis is not clear but is probably minimal.

Besides altering their rate of metabolic activity, humans can also, under certain circumstances, take up thermal energy from the environment. Human skin acts like a classic black body for thermal radiation and will absorb nearly all such radiation that lands on the skin's surface and is not reflected by clothing. If air temperature (or whatever other medium is in contact with the skin, such as water) is warmer than the skin itself, heat will be transferred from the environment. The very significant role of behavioral change (such as moving closer to a heat source, changing clothes, or taking a warm bath) in effective heat gain is primarily manifested through this mechanism, since in most societies today individuals find it easier to move to a warmer environment than to perform sustained physical exertion.

MECHANISMS OF HEAT LOSS

When the temperature of the environment is cooler than that of the body, thermodynamic principles mandate heat loss to the environment. This takes place in several ways; the primary mechanism of heat loss at moderate temperatures is radiation. About 60 percent of the total heat loss at rest and at room temperature is through radiation in the infrared spectrum from the body to its surroundings.

A second method of heat loss involves the transfer of the kinetic energy of molecular motion in the skin to the molecules of the immediate environment in the process known as *conduction.* Since energy also moves from the air to the skin, the net transfer of energy occurs in the direction of thermodynamic equilibrium so that heat loss will take place if the skin is warmer than the microenvironment. Under perfectly static conditions, heat loss by this mechanism would be limited since the air immediately surrounding the body is quickly warmed to skin temperature, a condition where no net transfer of heat can occur. Since these conditions are essentially never seen in nature, unheated air is generally exchanged with the air warmed by the skin in amounts that vary with ambient wind or air current speed and our own motion. This heat loss through warmed air exchange is called *convection* and is responsible for about 5 to 10 percent of heat loss at rest in quiet air with light clothing. Clothes trap warmed air near the skin, and normal indoor apparel reduces heat loss by some 50 percent compared to that lost when one is nude. Specially designed winter clothing can further reduce the loss to less than 10 percent than when nude by decreasing convection and increasing infrared reflection back to the skin. Since the specific heat of water is far greater than that of air, water immersion can increase the rates of conduction and convection by a factor of 20 or more. This is the reason hypothermia can occur much more rapidly in water than in air at the same temperature. Likewise, the insulating value of clothing is almost entirely lost when it is wet, since it will transfer heat so much more readily to the environment.

Heat cannot be lost to the environment through conduction, convection, or radiation if the ambient temperature is warmer than the body temperature. Under these circumstances, the only way the body can dispose of the heat generated by normal metabolism is through evaporation; any conditions that prevent effective evaporation, such as extreme humidity, profound dehydration, or sweat gland dysfunction or absence, can be rapidly fatal. Water's unusually high heat of vaporization makes evaporation a particularly effective means of heat loss; up to 0.58 kilocalorie of heat is lost for each gram of evaporated water. Unacclimatized individuals can produce a maximum of about 700 ml sweat per hour, more than enough to offset basal heat production if it is all lost to evaporation. After several weeks of exposure to high temperatures, acclimatized individuals can excrete as much as 1.5 to 3.0 liters per hour of sweat, potentially 10 to 15 times the amount necessary to carry away the heat of basal metabolism. Acclimatization also causes a decrease in the concentration of sodium chloride in sweat, probably mediated through increased aldosterone secretion. Insensible water losses through evaporation from the skin and respiratory tract generally amount to an additional 600 to 700 ml per day.

The quantity of sweat produced is rarely lost entirely to evaporation, however; much is often absorbed by clothing or simply rolls off the body, and the amount lost to the environment varies directly with the ambient humidity. A person immersed in water or in air that is fully saturated with water may be unable to lose any sweat through evaporation. Since strenuous exercise can increase basal heat production by a factor of 10 to 15, it is impossible for even a trained acclimatized individual to maintain temperature homeostasis with vigorous exertion in a climate with ambient temperatures above body temperature. Untrained individuals in humid environments may develop hyperthermia at temperatures considerably lower than 37°C.

BODY TEMPERATURE CONTROL

The efficiency of human thermoregulatory mechanisms is such that a nude human can maintain a core body temperature of 36 to 38°C in dry air at an air temperature of anywhere between 60 and 130°F. To do so requires a control center and a system of sensors and temperature regulation mechanisms all connected through the nervous system. The area where temperature information seems to be integrated and acted on is the hypothalamus. Careful thermal probe experiments have shown that large numbers of heat-sensitive neurons are present in the preoptic area of the anterior hypothalamus; destruction of these neurons in animals causes a steady increase in temperature that can culminate in death from hyperthermia. In humans, careful warming of the same area with thermal microprobes increases the neuronal firing rate and initiates cooling by stimulating sweating and peripheral vasodilatation. Cold-sensitive neurons have been found in the posterior hypothalamus and midbrain; their destruction in animals abolishes the normal response to cold.

The hypothalamus receives afferent impulses from other temperature-sensitive receptors in the skin, spinal cord, abdominal viscera, and great veins. Cold receptors outnumber warm receptors in these peripheral locations, a sensible arrangement since it is likely that they are primarily responsible for preventing hypothermia. The signals from all these receptors appear to be processed in the posterior hypothalamus, where appropriate adjustments in the temperature-regulating systems can then be signaled.

The set point at which core temperature is maintained is determined by hypothalamic integration of input from all the temperature sensors and can be altered by levels of some neurotransmitters, prostaglandins, interleukin-1, and tumor necrosis factor. Exercise itself can cause an acute increase in the set point, while regular training can cause an adaptive decrease in core temperature when at rest, both through as yet unknown mechanisms.

Individuals with high spinal cord injuries that interrupt sympathetic discharge lose the ability to coordinate central hypothalamic temperature control with sweating and vasodilatation. Autonomic temperature regulation is then very

Table 31-1. Human responses to cold

Peripheral vasoconstriction
Piloerection (ineffective in humans)
Increases in basal metabolic rate via increased secretion of catecholamines and thyroxine
Shivering
Thermogenesis in brown fat (significant only in neonates)
Behavioral changes—increased activity, warmer clothing or environment, and so forth

Table 31-2. Human responses to heat

If environment is cooler than body temperature:
Radiation of infrared to the environment
Conduction
Convection
Vasodilation (with increased losses through above mechanisms)
Behavioral changes—decreased activity, cooler clothing or environment, fans, and so forth
If environment is warmer than body temperature:
Evaporation through sweating and other insensible water losses
Behavioral changes

poor, and temperature control in these persons must rely almost entirely on their conscious perception of temperature in order to effect appropriate behavioral changes.

It is interesting to note and of some clinical significance that the central nervous system gives temperature regulation priority over vasomotor regulation. This may become important in the treatment of shock and near-shock states; if a hypovolemic patient who is in shock is kept too warm, sweating and vasodilatation may persist until complete circulatory collapse occurs.

THE HUMAN RESPONSE TO COLD

When the hypothalamus senses that temperatures are too cold, a complex series of events is triggered (Table 31-1). Stimulation of the sympathetic nervous system causes vasoconstriction of the blood vessels in the skin throughout the body. The small-vessel anatomy of the body is designed to very efficiently reduce heat loss by using countercurrent heat exchange. Immediately adjacent to the skin's surface is an extensive venous and capillary bed that is relatively unprotected by the insulating properties of the comparatively avascular subcutaneous fat. Buried deeper beneath the skin is a second and larger-caliber venous system that more closely parallels the skin's arterial blood supply. In the vasodilated state, numerous arteriovenous shunts open and increase blood flow to the skin's superficial venous plexus and capillary beds by a factor of as high as 15 to 20, causing large amounts of heat loss through radiation and conduction; returning blood remains cool as it does not pass close to the deep arteries. Arteriolar vasoconstriction preferentially routes blood through the deeper system, significantly reducing heat loss through the skin and allowing rewarming of the returning blood by the adjacent arteries (the countercurrent heat exchange) before it reaches the core.

Sympathetic stimulation also causes piloerection, a somewhat vestigial reflex intended to reduce conductive heat loss from the skin by increasing the amount of air trapped and held motionless over the skin's surface. Clothing has essentially supplanted piloerection as a mechanism for heat retention, and the human body's relative hairlessness makes it ineffective in any case.

Both epinephrine and norepinephrine are released in increased amounts with cold exposure; they act directly on cells to increase chemical thermogenesis by both increasing the metabolic rate and reducing metabolic efficiency. The brown fat of neonates may contribute significantly to heat production after sympathetic stimulation. Cooling also causes the hypothalamus to release increased amounts of thyrotropin releasing hormone, which in turn stimulates secretion of thyroid-stimulating hormone, then of thyroxine, which in turn further increases metabolic rate and heat production.

The primary motor area for shivering is a small area in the posterior hypothalamus, which triggers shivering when core temperature falls fractionally below a critical value. Maximal shivering can increase heat production by some four to five times normal. Unacclimatized naked humans will begin to shiver when the generalized skin temperature drops below about 33°C (91°F) or the air temperature below 27°C (81°F). Some adaptation to cold can take place by improving the usual generalized vasoconstriction in a process called *insulative hypothermic acclimatization*. The Australian aborigine, for instance, can sleep nearly naked in temperatures as low as 4°C (39°F) and with a skin temperature down to 27°C (81°F) without shivering.

Finally, efferents to the cortex from the hypothalamus allow humans to become consciously aware that they are "cold." This sensation in turn causes behavioral changes that are probably the most potent means of heat conservation, such as putting on more clothes, becoming more active, or seeking a warmer environment.

There are also some local skin temperature reflexes that cause the localized vasoconstriction and suppression of sweating seen with cold application to a limited area of the skin. These reflexes are caused by direct effects of the cold on the vascular tree locally and to some extent by spinal cord reflexes.

THE HUMAN RESPONSE TO HEAT

Evolution in a warmer climate combined with a limited tolerance for high temperatures have forced humans to develop efficient heat elimination reserves (Table 31-2). If they fail, death generally occurs at or above temperatures of 48°C (118°F). In very warm climates, the body faces the task of losing excess heat against a temperature gradient, requiring some type of heat pump mechanism. In humans, evaporation of sweat serves this purpose; many animals that lack sweat glands use panting as an alternative means of evaporative heat loss.

When ambient temperature increases beyond a certain point or enough extra heat is generated by exertion, passive heat loss via conduction, convection, and radiation may not be enough to maintain hypothalamic temperature at the set point, and immediate measures to increase cooling begin.

There is a generalized cutaneous vasodilatation, increasing passive heat loss to the environment. The drop in peripheral vascular resistance caused by this vasodilatation can cause nearly a quadrupling of cardiac output in order to maintain blood pressure. Thus, orthostatic syncope is much more common in hot environments, and very warm conditions can provoke ischemia in patients with heart disease.

Sweating begins and will progressively increase if hypothalamic temperature does not drop back toward normal. Epinephrine and thyroxine secretion are decreased in order to reduce metabolic heat production. Adrenocorticoid secretion is increased, preserving salt and water necessary for sweating. Efferents from the hypothalamus to the cortex generate a subjective sensation of warmth. Subsequent changes in behavior such as disrobing or moving to a cooler location can play a significant role in furthering heat loss.

A recently discovered class of proteins called *heat-shock proteins* may play some role on a more basic level in helping to protect against thermal injury. Heat-shock proteins are cytosolic proteins that seem to be involved in protein transport across endoplasmic reticulum and mitochondrial membranes as well as in protein folding and assembly. Some authors believe that this last function may help to renature proteins that have been denatured by heat and to help prevent such denaturation from occurring.

SELECTED READING

Thermophysiology

Benzinger, TH. Heat regulation: Homeostasis of central temperature in man. *Physiol Rev* 49:671, 1969.

Benzinger, TH, and Taylor, GW. Cranial Measurements of Internal Temperature in Man. In CM Herzfeld (ed), *Temperature: Its Measurement and Control in Science and Industry.* Vol 3. New York: Reinhold, 1963.

Cossins, AR, and Bowler, K. *Temperature Biology of Animals.* New York: Chapman & Hall, 1987.

Hales, JRS (ed). *Thermal Physiology.* New York: Raven, 1984.

Mitchell, D. Physical basis of thermoregulation. *Int Rev Physiol* 15:1, 1977.

Robertshaw, D (ed). *International Review of Physiology III* (vol 20). Baltimore: University Park Press, 1979.

Swan, H. *Thermoregulation and Bioenergetics.* New York: American Elsevier, 1974.

Temperature and Its Measurement

Baker, NC, et al. The effect of type of thermometer and length of time inserted on oral temperature measurements of afebrile subjects. *Nurs Res* 33:109, 1984.

Edwards, RJ, Belyavin, AJ, and Harrison, MH. Core temperature measurement in man. *Aviat Space Environ Med* 49:1289, 1978.

Ilsley, AH, Rutten, AJ, and Runciman, WB. An evaluation of body temperature measurement. *Anaesth Intensive Care* 11:31, 1983.

Tandberg, D, and Sklar, D. Effect of tachypnea on the estimation of body temperature by an oral thermometer. *N Engl J Med* 308:945, 1983.

Togawa, T. Body temperature measurement. *Clin Phys Physiol Meas* 6:83, 1985.

Temperature Control

Bruck, K, and Olschewski, H. Body temperature related factors diminishing the drive to exercise. *Can J Physiol Pharmacol* 65:1274, 1987.

Cabanac, M. Temperature regulation. *Ann Rev Physiol* 37:415, 1975.

Heller, HC, et al. The thermostat of vertebrate animals. *Sci Am* 239:102, 1978.

Keele, CA, Neil, E, and Joels, N (eds). Regulation of Body Temperature in Man. In *Samson Wright's Applied Physiology* (13th ed). New York: Oxford, 1982.

Pelham, H. News and views: Heat-shock proteins: Coming in from the cold. *Nature* 332:776, 1988.

32. Fever

Eric W. Schmidt

Descriptions of fever have filled all known historic medical literature. Our predecessors were fascinated with fever as a primary and sometimes sacred process. This view held until the germ theory of medicine started late in the nineteenth century. Despite the mystical history of the febrile process, the daily challenge to emergency medicine is to distinguish life-threatening febrile diseases from self-limited illnesses.

PATHOPHYSIOLOGY

Fever is defined as a temperature of 38°C (101°F) or greater, or greater than 2°C above baseline temperature in certain disease states (e.g., renal failure). The human body closely maintains a normal temperature of 36 to 38°C. There is a normal circadian variation of up to 2°C, peaking at about 6:00 A.M. For unknown reasons this may be reversed in elderly patients, with peak temperatures in the evening.

Thermostasis is regulated by the pituitary-hypothalamic axis. Fever is considered an elevation in the thermal set point, as opposed to heat production or dissipation failure with a normal set point, as discussed in Chapter 33.

The search for humoral pyrogens initially focused on bacterial toxins and then leukocyte products, leading finally to interleukin-1. Interleukin-1 is a 15,000-mW monokine liberated by monocyte stimulation. It increases circulatory acute-phase reactants, granulopoiesis, leukotaxis, and T-cell proliferation. Centrally, interleukin-1, and perhaps other peptides, act as calcium-dependent thermostimulators, increasing neuronal prostaglandins, predominantly of the PGE series. These prostaglandins then increase neuronal cyclic adenosine monophosphate (cAMP). This acts in the hypothalamic axis to increase heat production or decrease dissipation, or both, increasing the set point. Sympathomimetics can directly stimulate neuronal cAMP.

Monocytes can be stimulated to produce interleukin-1 by a myriad of acute and chronic processes (Table 32-1). Any infecting organism from viral to parasitic can induce inflammation and therefore fever. Any inflammatory process, such as the collagen-vascular diseases, antigen-antibody complexes, or complement activation, can be pyrogenic. "Tumor fever," especially from solid or hemopoietic neoplasms, is a well-documented phenomenon.

Drugs can produce fever directly or via allergic reactions. Traumatized, burned, or otherwise necrotic tissue can also be pyrogenic, as with stroke and pulmonary emboli. In addition, in endocrinopathies or rare inherited conditions, fever may be the first symptom.

Whether fever has a positive or negative effect has long been argued and probably depends on the underlying disease state. The metabolic rate increases approximately seven percent for each 1°C, potentially taxing the metabolic reserves of the chronically ill or traumatized patient. Some

Table 32-1. Causes of fever

Infectious
Viral
Mycoplasmal
Chlamydial
Bacterial
Fungal/yeast
Protozoan
Neoplasms
Connective tissue diseases
Rheumatoid arthritis
Systemic lupus erythematosus
Vasculitides
Granulomatous diseases
Sarcoid
Crohn's disease
Endocrine disorders
Hyperthyroidism
Drug reactions
Allergic
Direct
Aspirin
Bleomycin
Neuroleptics (phenothiazines)
Stimulants
Trauma
Tissue damage
Burns
Miscellaneous
Pulmonary embolus
Familial fever
Fabry's disease
Factitious fever

viral infections proceed more rapidly at elevated temperatures. Leukocytes and lymphocytes are, however, most active at temperatures between 38 and 40°C. Isothermic organisms (e.g., reptiles) have a markedly decreased survival when blocked from their normal heat-seeking behavior after bacterial inoculation. Studies in homeothermic organisms are less clear.

Very young or old patients may not mount a febrile response. With young patients this may be due to an immature immune system, and the physical examination may not allow a reliable diagnosis (see Chap. 160). Older patients with severe diseases may not be febrile. Studies in animals suggest that this may be due to poor nutritional status rather than to senescence of the immune system.

Antipyretics have long been the cornerstone of symptomatic therapy for fever. Acetaminophen and its more toxic congeners act centrally as prostaglandin inhibitors, sharing the same mechanism of action as salicylate and the other nonsteroidal antiinflammatory drugs (NSAIDs). Both classes of drugs block the interleukin-1–stimulated, prostaglandin-mediated increase in cAMP.

Neither class of drugs has ever been shown to be more efficacious, and both require similar dosages of 10 to 15 mg/kg every four hours. Combining doses of acetaminophen and salicylate does not cause a greater decrease in absolute temperature but does prolong the effect, providing about six hours of defervescence. Rapid or marked response to antipyretics should not cause the emergency physician to assume a benign process, as studies have shown response to be a poor predictor of disease severity. Salicylate should be avoided in young patients with influenza or primary varicella because of its rare association with Reye's syndrome.

Table 32-2. Characteristics of a compromised host

Extremes of age
Malnutrition
Chronic ethanol consumption
Malignancy (especially after chemotherapy)
Steroid therapy
Immunodeficiency syndromes
Splenectomized patients
Diabetes
Severe coronary disease
Renal failure
Chronic obstructive pulmonary disease
Sickle cell disease

EVALUATION OF THE FEBRILE PATIENT

Prolonged evaluation in the emergency department rarely occurs. Definitive diagnosis may take up to several weeks, pending cultures, scans, and biopsies. It is contingent on the emergency physician to correctly identify three groups of patients: (1) patients with a toxic presentation or underlying conditions that predispose them to rapid decompensation, (2) patients who have nontoxic presentations but require initiation of expedient therapy, and (3) nontoxic patients in whom nonspecific therapy may confuse or delay definitive diagnosis and treatment.

History

As with all complaints, obtaining the history is of paramount importance. Finding out the duration and spectrum of symptoms begins with the search, along with awareness of recent travel and concomitant household or community infections. Any underlying or past illness can limit the patient's ability to tolerate the stress of a febrile process (e.g., chronic obstructive pulmonary disease and coronary artery disease), and may suggest a source of the fever (Table 32-2). The alcoholic, elderly, or debilitated patient may have a blunted febrile response as a result of malnutrition.

Acquired, congenital, or iatrogenic immunodeficiency syndromes predispose the patient to a fulminant course from otherwise trivial disease and present the emergency physician with a spectrum of pathogens that until recently were considered rare. This is of special concern, as patients with previously undetected human immunodeficiency virus, especially heterosexuals without classic risk factors, have unusual febrile illnesses. Sickle cell disease or splenectomized patients are at increased risk for infections with encapsulated organisms.

NSAID therapy or acetaminophen use can alter the initial presentation. Use of beta-blockers will blunt the tachycardia that is present in many severe cases. Patients with fever will frequently have taken antibiotics. Studies of urine samples have shown traces of antibiotics even in patients who deny self-treatment.

A history of possible illicit drug ingestion should be sought. Stimulants are directly pyrogenic. Any febrile intravenous drug abusers, especially those with a heart murmur or hematuria, should be considered to have bacterial endocarditis until this has been proved otherwise.

Classic teaching has been that the pattern of the fever is suggestive of etiology. However, this pattern is of little, if any, predictive value.

Physical Examination

The clinical appearance of the patient in the eyes of an experienced clinician is the best predictive factor, especially in children (see Chap. 160). Pallor, lethargy, depressed level of consciousness, or responsiveness should be noted.

The posterior lingual sulcus is the warmest part of the mouth, with variations of oral temperature up to 1.6°C depending on the placement of the probe. Tachypnea directly correlates with decreased oral readings.

Rectal temperature is the most consistent, simple temperature measurement. It is slightly less than central venous temperature and between 0.5 and 0.8°C higher than oral temperature. Rectal probe monitoring may be necessary in hyperthermic and hypothermic states.

Axillary temperatures are at best a crude and now obsolete method of temperature measurement with the advent of reliable infrared tympanic thermometers. Antipyretics administered early or active cooling measures are indicated in patients with temperatures that exceed 40°C (see Chap. 33).

Tachypnea may represent a pulmonary cause or diabetic ketoacidosis (DKA). If not marked, tachypnea and tachycardia may be due to the increase in metabolic rate associated with fever. On average the heart rate increases only 10 to 20 beats per minute per degree centigrade. Rates beyond this suggest dehydration or septic vasodilatation, and orthostatic changes should be sought with initiation of fluid replacement as needed.

Any remarkable muscle rigidity in the febrile patient suggests neuroleptic malignant syndrome or malignant hyperthermia. Neuroleptic malignant syndrome is a potentially life-threatening side effect of the major tranquilizers and responds to dantrolene and bromocriptine. Malignant hyperthermia involves uncontrolled muscle contraction. It is usually familial and precipitated by anesthesia or other drug stimulants. Malignant hyperthermia may not respond to active cooling, and dantrolene therapy may be diagnostic and lifesaving.

The physical examination should then proceed with the physician seeking any focality, noting rashes, bulging fontanels, tympanic membrane or pharyngeal inflammation, nuchal rigidity, adenopathy, and splenomegaly; carefully auscultating the lung fields; documenting any murmurs; and performing an abdominal examination, including a rectal examination.

LABORATORY EXAMINATION

Many emergency department patients require laboratory evaluation. These tests are expensive and are not routinely indicated in the nontoxic, noncompromised patient with a relatively short illness and an obvious site of infection.

Gram's Stain

Gram's stain is the most useful study for the emergency physician. It is rapid, requires no special equipment, and is easily performed in the department. A good sample should contain a large number of leukocytes with less than five epithelial cells per high-power field. A good sputum sample will easily direct therapy in a pulmonary process. Lancet-shaped gram-positive diplococci suggest pneumococcus. Predominant gram-positive flora without obvious pneumococcal morphology should lead to antistaphylococcal coverage. Pleomorphic gram-negative rods suggest *Haemophilus* influenza. A mixed flora without a great number of epithelial cells suggests aspiration pneumonitis. A good sputum sample without obvious flora suggests a nonbacterial process and should lead the clinician to consider a viral, mycoplasmal, *Legionella,* or tuberculosis pneumonitis. The urine may be gram stained in urinary tract infections though it may be safe to assume a gram-negative rod infection.

Cerebrospinal fluid gram-staining is still one of the cornerstones of treating the patient with suspected meningitis. Some authors note a higher sensitivity when they use acridine orange staining. This technique requires a fluorescent microscope and does not differentiate gram-positive from gram-negative organisms.

Counterimmunoelectrophoresis may be giving way to the newer, faster, and more sensitive latex agglutination techniques. These two processes are the only methods of definitive diagnosis in the emergency department.

Complete Blood Cell Count

The complete blood cell count has long been relied on as indicating severe infectious processes. The clinician should be aware that the white blood cell count may be elevated, usually without a left shift, in trauma and hyperadrenergic states. DKA and corticosteroids elevate the total white count and also cause a left shift. Toxic granulation is found in vasculitis and neoplastic disease and is absent in up to 25 percent of patients with positive blood cultures. Many studies show the lack of sensitivity of the absolute white count, total leukocytes, or the presence of a left shift as reliable predictors of infection. In patients up to the age of one year, a normal white cell count can be as high as 15,000. Several studies suggest that a total white count of greater than 15,000 with or without a left shift, in combination with an erythrocyte sedimentation rate greater than 30 mm per hour, is a good predictor of a significant infectious process.

DISPOSITION

The challenge for the emergency physician is to rely on history and physical examination to identify the toxic or possi-

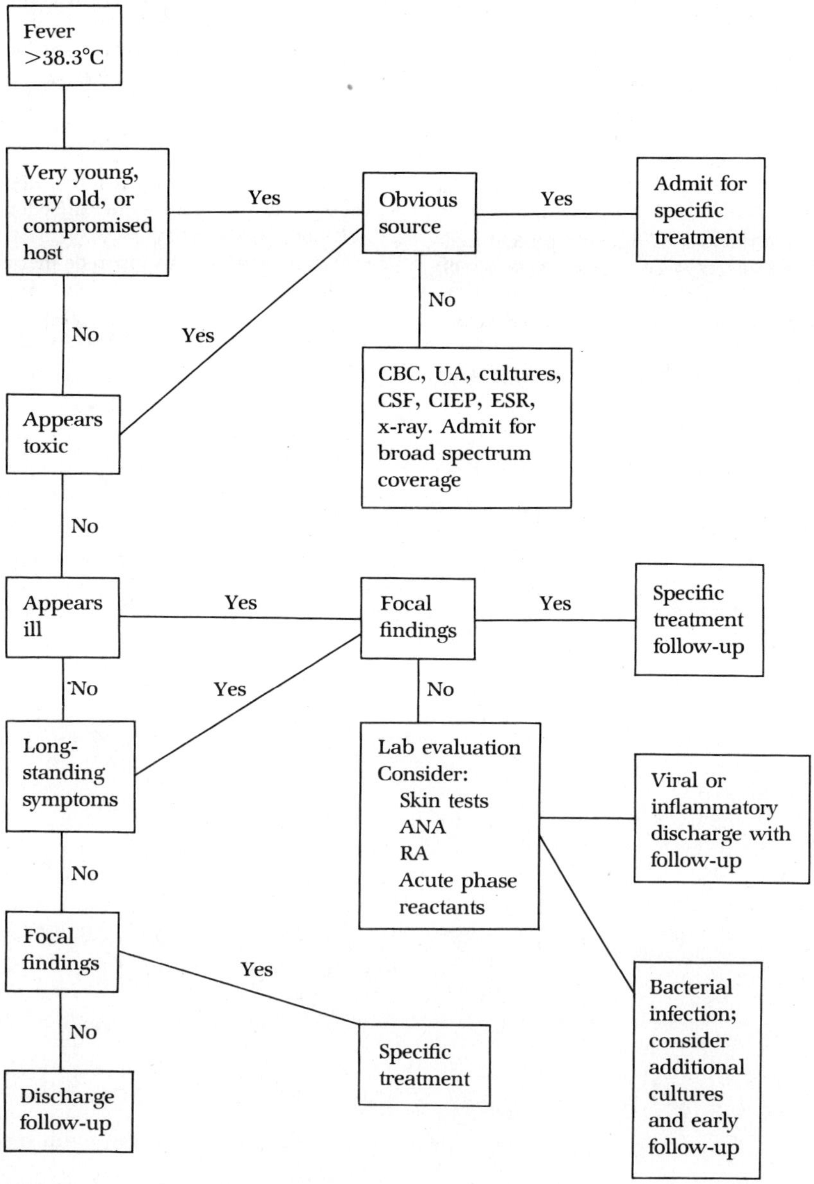

Fig. 32-1. Approach to the management of fever. (CBC = complete blood count; UA = urinalysis; CSF = cerebrospinal fluid; CIEP = counterimmunoelectrophoresis; ESR = erythrocyte sedimentation rate; RA = rheumatoid factor.)

bly compromised patient who needs aggressive therapy (Fig. 32-1). It is important to repeat the history and the physical examination if the source of the fever is not obvious. Many patients will remember additional historical information and the clinical examination findings may change. If the patient is compromised or appears toxic, he or she should be admitted to the hospital. Admission should also be considered if the patient will not be able to return if signs of worsening symptoms occur or cannot reliably fill and take prescribed medication. These patients include the elderly who live alone and young patients, when the clinician believes that the parents will not be able to treat them at home. Once the decision to admit has been made, therapy should be initiated in the department. Frequently, long delays in therapy occur if the patient waits to get to the hospital floor for initial treatment. For the adult patient with no obvious source of fever, broad-spectrum coverage should include a third-generation cephalosporin, a semisynthetic penicillin, and an aminoglycoside.

For patients who do not require admission, expectant therapy with clear instructions and follow-up evaluation is adequate. In the adult patient, antibiotics should not be initiated unless a site of infection is identified. Family and patient education should include instruction on what each medication is for, along with its common side effects. Symptomatic relief, including over-the-counter remedies, should be discussed. Timely return to the department or regular physician should be encouraged if the patient's condition is not improving as expected, or certainly if it is getting worse. The patient who returns to the department should lower the clinician's threshold for evaluation. A frequent trap occurs when the clinician does not consider causes other than those identified on the previous encounter.

SELECTED READING

Baker, MD, Fosarelli, PD, and Carpenter, RO. Childhood fever: Correlation of diagnosis with temperature response to acetaminophen. *Pediatrics* 80:315, 1987.

Barriere, SL. Therapy of choice for the empiric treatment of the febrile neutropenic patient. *Drug Intell Clin Pharm* 20:767, 1986.

Bernheim, HA, Block, LH, and Atkins, E. Fever: Pathogenesis, pathophysiology and purpose. *Ann Intern Med* 91:261, 1979.

Bradley, SF, Kluger, MJ, and Kauffman, CA. Age and protein malnutrition: Effects on the febrile response. *Gerontology* 33:99, 1987.

Cooper, KE. The neurobiology of fever: Thoughts on recent developments. *Ann Rev Neurosci* 10:297, 1987.

Dinarello, CA, and Wolff, SM. Pathogenesis of fever in man. *N Engl J Med* 298:607, 1978.

Dinarello, CA, and Wolff, SM. Molecular basis of fever in humans. *Am J Med* 72:799, 1982.

McCarthy, PL, et al. Observation, history, and physical examination in diagnosis of serious illnesses in febrile children ≤ 24 months. *J Pediatr* 110:26, 1987.

Nolan, SM, and Fitzgerald, FT. Fever of unknown origin. *Postgrad Med* 81:190, 1987.

Norman, DC, Yamamura, RH, and Yoshikawa, TT. Fever response in old and young mice after injection of interleukin 1. *J Gerontol* 43:M80, 1988.

Steele, RW, et al. Oral antipyretic therapy. *Am J Dis Child* 123:204, 1972.

33. Heat Illness

Harvey Louzon

The spectrum of heat illness is wide and ranges from such minor syndromes as heat cramps and heat exhaustion to the life-threatening syndrome of heat stroke. The precise incidence of heat-related deaths is unknown, but estimates of 100 to 400 cases a year in the United States have been made. The incidence of the minor syndrome of heat illness are undocumented but can reliably be estimated to be many times higher. With the increasing popularity of competitive running and other athletic activities, these problems are likely to be encountered with even greater frequency in the future.

Our discussion of heat illness is prefaced by a review of thermoregulation and the process of acclimatization. This is followed by a description of the individual clinical syndromes, their pathophysiology and treatment, and a brief discussion of the differential diagnosis, prognosis, long-term sequelae, and prevention of heat illness.

THERMOREGULATION

Body temperature represents the balance between heat gain and heat loss, the former being of either endogenous (metabolism, exercise) or exogenous (environmental) origin. Endogenous heat production, a normal by-product of the metabolism of foodstuffs, amounts to approximately 75 kcal per hour. Absorbed radiant solar energy can add an additional 150 kcal per hour of heat load. Heat can also be transferred to the body when environmental temperature exceeds skin temperature. Finally, exertion can increase endogenous heat production to the range of 300 to 900 kcal per hour. At ambient temperatures below 32°C (89.6°F), convection and radiation contribute to maintain a normal body temperature. As environmental temperature increases and approaches body temperature, sweating becomes an increasingly important mechanism in the defense of normothermia. The evaporation of 1.7 ml sweat will dissipate 1 kcal heat energy, and since sweating rates can approach 1.5 liters per hour, this mechanism theoretically can dissipate 900 kcal per hour of heat (and twice this amount in acclimatized humans). However, sweating is only approximately 80 percent effective as some of it is lost by dripping and not evaporation. Thus, in practice only about 650 kcal per hour can be lost by the evaporation of sweat. As ambient humidity increases sweating becomes less effective. The importance of these compensatory mechanisms is underscored by the fact that in the absence of heat dissipation, body temperature can rise 1.1°C per hour (2°F per hour) under basal resting conditions. Even when compensatory mechanisms are intact, as in well-acclimatized athletes, core body temperatures of up to 42°C (107.6°F) have been recorded after strenuous exertion. Measurements of muscle and hepatic venous blood may be 1 to 2°C (1.8–3.6°F) higher than core temperature as measured by a rectal probe. This rise in core body temperature increases basal metabolic rate by 13 percent for each 1°C (1.8°F) rise in temperature, thus initiating a vicious cycle. Although high temperature and humidity impair the body's ability to dissipate a heat load, heat stroke has been described at ambient temperatures as low as 16°C (60.8°F) in the setting of marked elevations of endogenous heat production.

Adequate cardiac reserve plays a central role in maintaining a normal body temperature under diverse environmental conditions. Heat stress promotes cutaneous vasodilation, with a corresponding increase in cardiac output of up to 17 to 20 liters per minute. Splanchnic vasoconstriction diverts blood flow to muscle and skin. Rates of sweating can increase to 1.5 liters per hour in unacclimatized and 3.0 liters per hour in acclimatized subjects. Renal blood flow and, to a lesser degree, glomerular filtration rate fall and thus filtration fraction increases.

ACCLIMATIZATION

The process of acclimatization involves a complex interplay of metabolic, hormonal, and cardiovascular adjustments. Exertion in a warm environment for 1 to 2 weeks is necessary for this to occur. An increase in metabolic efficiency occurs wherein a given level of exertion results in lower endogenous heat production. Aldosterone secretion rises, lowering sweat and urine sodium concentrations and raising potassium excretion. Potassium deficits in the range of 400 to 500 mEq occur during this process. Sweating rates may increase from 1.5 to 3.0 liters per hour. Maximal cardiac output rises and is attained at a lower heart rate and with an increase in stroke volume. Although plasma volume increases initially, this increase is not maintained for a long period of time.

CLINICAL SYNDROMES

Heat Edema

Heat edema is an uncommon phenomenon that is typically observed in unacclimatized individuals. It is characteristically dependent in distribution, occurring soon after a move to a warm environment, and resolves within a week during the normal process of acclimatization. A transient gain in weight is also occasionally noted. Its etiology is unclear but may be related to the normal vasodilation that occurs on exposure to heat. The few published clinical studies on this phenomenon have demonstrated transient hyponatremia and hypervolemia, which have been attributed to the normal rise in antidiuretic hormone in the early days of exposure to a heat stress.

Heat Tetany

Heat tetany is characterized by classic carpopedal spasms when individuals are exposed to a source of heat stress. Additionally, it can be associated with numbness of the hands, feet, and lips, and a positive Chvostek's sign may be noted on physical examination. The normal process of hyperventilation observed when subjects are exposed to heat stress induces a rapid fall in arterial carbon dioxide tension and rise in pH. Although total serum calcium concentrations are normal, this may be associated with a fall in serum ionized calcium. Whatever the precise mechanisms involved, however, the carpopedal spasms resolve promptly after removal of the subject from the source of heat.

Heat Syncope

Heat syncope is a not uncommon syndrome observed in poorly acclimatized individuals. Its pathophysiology is unclear, but peripheral vasodilation induced by heat, with resultant venous pooling and hypotension, has been implicated in its development. Consciousness should return promptly after assumption of the recumbent position. Since syncope can also be a feature of heat stroke, if its cause is unclear or consciousness does not return promptly, a rectal temperature should be obtained to rule out the latter syndrome.

Heat Cramps

Heat cramps typically occur at variable periods after exertion in well-acclimatized individuals. Their onset is often delayed by several hours. Heavily exercised muscle groups are most commonly affected. Thus, there is a predilection for the lower extremities, but any area including the abdominal musculature can be involved. Heat cramps are believed to result from relative sodium depletion, which can occur when sodium deficits incurred through sweating are replaced by hypotonic solutions. The presence of sodium is believed essential to the calcium-dependent relaxation phase of skeletal muscle contraction.

Short-lived, painful muscular contractions are observed. Edema or muscle tenderness would indicate the presence of exertional rhabdomyolysis, which is associated with marked elevation of serum creatine kinase (CK), myoglobinuria, and occasionally acute renal failure. Heat cramps should also be distinguished from carpopedal spasms secondary to hyperventilation induced by heat stress.

Laboratory findings in heat cramps may disclose hyponatremia, hypophosphatemia, and hypomagnesemia. Treatment consists of sodium replacement in the form of an oral, balanced electrolyte solution. Salt tablets, which can cause gastric irritation or hyperosmolarity and actually increase the likelihood of more severe heat syndromes, should be avoided. If oral intake is precluded, intravenously administered normal saline or lactated Ringer's solution can be used.

Heat Exhaustion

Heat exhaustion is seen in individuals who engage in work or athletic activities in the setting of high environmental temperatures and humidity. It has been repeatedly demonstrated that workers in a hot environment consistently underestimate their fluid requirements and thus develop an extracellular fluid (ECF) deficit up to two percent of their body weight.

Heat exhaustion is characterized by symptoms of nausea, vomiting, dizziness, and headache. Hyperventilation and piloerection over the chest and upper arms are also seen. Occasionally, mild personality changes, impaired judgment,

Table 33-1. Causes of heat illness

Increased endogenous heat production
Hard work or exercise
Neuroleptic malignant syndrome
Malignant hyperthermia
Phencyclidine or amphetamine ingestion
Decreased heat dissipation
Cardiovascular disease
Dehydration
Lack of acclimatization
Scleroderma, cystic fibrosis
Anticholinergic drugs
Previous heat stroke
Miscellaneous
Cerebrovascular accidents
Ethanol (via vasodilation)
Extremes of age
Intercurrent medical illness

Table 33-2. Role of drugs in causing heat illness

Increases endogenous heat production
Amphetamines
Phencyclidine
Cocaine
Thyroid hormone
Impairs heat dissipation
Anticholinergics
Antihistamines
Phenothiazines
Cyclic antidepressants
Impairs thermoregulation
Phenothiazines (central effect)
Ethanol (via vasodilation)
Impairs cardiovascular compensation
Diuretics
Beta-blockers

and syncope occur. Body temperature may be mildly to markedly elevated. Many cases of severe heat exhaustion should more properly be considered as true heat stroke. Indeed a continuum exists in the physiologic derangements and clinical presentation of patients with heat exhaustion and those with heat stroke.

Volume depletion, orthostatic symptoms, and occasionally syncope are observed. This syndrome can be associated with either predominant salt depletion or predominant water depletion, although this distinction is of questionable clinical significance. The latter syndrome occurs in individuals whose access to water is limited. The former occurs when an unacclimatized individual replaces losses due to sweating with hypotonic solutions. Thus, serum sodium concentrations are variable. Hemoconcentration and respiratory alkalosis are usually observed.

Treatment consists of intravenous (IV) rehydration with isotonic solutions and rest in a cool environment. If body temperature is elevated to the range compatible with heat stroke, active cooling measures as described later should be instituted.

Heat Stroke

Heat stroke, the most severe manifestation of heat illness, occurs in both exertional and nonexertional (classic) varieties. This clinical dichotomy reflects the physiologic observation, noted previously, that hyperthermia can arise from increased endogenous heat production (exertional heat stroke), an impairment of heat dissipation (classic heat stroke), or a combination of both (Table 33-1).

Exertional heat stroke has most consistently been observed in military recruits, miners, and marathon runners. Among military recruits it is usually seen during the first few weeks of basic training before the full benefits of acclimatization have occurred. High motivation combined with fatigue and relative dehydration are often-cited contributory factors in this group. Classic heat stroke is seen typically in an urban environment during prolonged heat waves in elderly individuals (80 percent are over 65 years of age) and is of multifactorial etiology.

The use of drugs that can impair heat dissipation and an inadequate cardiovascular response to heat stress are two of the more common likely mechanisms in this group. Drugs can impair thermoregulation in several ways (Table 33-2). Phenothiazines and butyerophenones can directly disrupt hypothalamic thermoregulation. Drugs can interfere peripherally with the sympathetic cholinergic control of sweating; the anticholinergics, cyclic antidepressants, and antihistamines are in this category. Less commonly, drugs that increase endogenous heat production, such as amphetamines and phencyclidine (PCP), have been implicated. Ethanol, by promoting cutaneous vasodilation, can predispose to heat illness. Finally, diuretics and beta-blockers, by blunting the cardiovascular response to a heat stress, can play a contributory role. Patients with scleroderma and other diffuse dermatologic disorders may have an impaired ability to sweat. Patients with cystic fibrosis, which is characterized by sweat gland dysfunction and an increased concentration of sweat chloride and sodium, have an increased susceptibility to heat stroke. Finally, diabetes, obesity, cerebrovascular accidents (CVA), and other chronic disorders have been implicated in heat stroke. Heat stroke, by causing sweat gland necrosis, has itself been associated with an increased susceptibility for recurrence. The urban preponderance of classic heat stroke has been ascribed to an attenuation of the normal diurnal drop in nighttime temperatures observed in big cities. Heat stroke has also been described in subjects exposed to high radiant heat loads, a condition that can occur in boiler rooms or enclosed automobiles in the midday sun.

Pathophysiology

Physiologic alterations in heat stroke include an increase in heart rate and respiratory rate and a variable fall in blood pressure. Cardiac output is usually markedly elevated in the setting of cutaneous vasodilation but can fall with myocardial damage. Central venous pressure and pulmonary vascular resistance are usually elevated. Cutaneous and muscle blood flow are increased in proportion to the elevated temperature but splanchnic and renal blood flow are reduced.

Pathologic findings in cases of fatal heat stroke have disclosed abnormalities in virtually every organ system. Above

42°C (107.6°F), the so-called "critical thermal maximum temperature," oxidative phosphorylation is uncoupled, cellular membrane integrity is compromised, and critical enzymes are denatured. Skeletal muscle fibers display cytolysis. Sweat glands show subcellular disorganization and luminal obstruction. Petechial and macroscopic hemorrhages have been observed in numerous organs, including the heart, where lesions have had a peculiar predisposition for the left side of the interventricular septum. Renal tubular necrosis and pigmented casts are seen in kidney specimens. The gastrointestinal tract is the site of mucosal erosions and hemorrhage. Liver specimens may show cholestasis and centrolobular necrosis. Pancreatic hemorrhage is seen in the setting of a generalized bleeding diathesis, but pancreatitis has not been described. Cerebral edema and petechial brain hemorrhages, particularly in the walls of the third ventricle and floor of the fourth ventricle, are an almost invariable finding in fatal cases. The Purkinje cells of the cerebellar cortex appear to be peculiarly vulnerable to hyperthermia. The pancreas, adrenal glands, and hypothalamus are relatively spared. Microscopic evidence of diffuse vascular endothelial cell damage and intravascular thrombosis has been noted.

Clinical Presentation

Clinically, the presence of severe hyperthermia (temperature greater than 40.6°C, 105°F) and profound central nervous system (CNS) dysfunction (obtundation, coma, seizures, and so forth) are essential for diagnosis. The presence of anhidrosis, considered in the past to be an invariable feature of heat stroke, is now known to be an inconstant finding. Sweating is maintained approximately 50 percent of the time in the exertional variety and somewhat less often in the classic cases. The cause of sweat gland failure in some cases of heat stroke has been the object of some controversy. Ultimately, it may merely be the result of the microscopic changes in sweat gland morphology noted previously.

Onset during exertion is often abrupt although premonitory symptoms, including a sensation of impending doom, can occur. Prodromal symptoms, as have been described for heat exhaustion, are sometimes seen.

Central nervous system abnormalities are varied. Mental status changes, ranging from delirium, psychosis, and obtundation to profound coma, are observed. If loss of consciousness is seen, it may or may not be followed by a lucid interval. Pupils may be fixed and dilated. Occasionally, papilledema is seen. Focal neurologic findings and seizures have been described. Extensor plantar responses, decerebrate posturing, oculogyric crises, opisthotonus, and hemiplegia are sometimes seen. Hyperventilation and tachycardia are common. Hypotension can occur and be secondary to peripheral vasodilation, high-output cardiac failure, volume contraction, or, less commonly, a low-output state secondary to direct myocardial damage. Various ventricular and supraventricular arrythmias can occur. Acute tubular necrosis, most common in the setting of exertional heat stroke, may be secondary to hypotension, volume contraction, and myoglobinuria. Renal failure can also be caused by hyperuricemia and disseminated intravascular coagulation (DIC). Gatrointestinal bleeding secondary to gastric and intestinal erosions is common. Hepatic necrosis manifested by right upper quadrant tenderness, hepatomegaly, and jaundice may be seen several days into the illness. In fatal cases a bleeding diathesis may ensue, characterized by coagulation factor and platelet inactivation. Endothelial cell damage may promote platelet adhesion and initiate the clotting mechanism. Frank DIC may supervene and result in conjunctival petechiae, visceral hemorrhages, and renal failure. Thermal injury to pulmonary vascular endothelium can cause cor pulmonale and congestive heart failure.

Laboratory Findings

Laboratory findings reflect visceral organ damage. Serum sodium can be normal, high, or low depending on the relative losses of salt and water. Hypocalcemia secondary to calcium deposition in injured skeletal muscle can occur. Secondary hyperparathyroidism can cause hypercalcemia in the convalescent phase. Hypokalemia and hypophosphatemia may be secondary to respiratory alkalosis, although hyperkalemia can occur if rhabdomyolysis and renal failure supervene. Hypomagnesemia results from sweat and urinary losses. Often a lactic acidosis is observed, particularly in exertional heat stroke. Serum glutamic oxaloacetic transaminase (SGOT), serum glutamic pyruvic transaminase, (SGPT), lactic dehydrogenase (LDH), and CK levels are elevated to a variable degree, reflecting skeletal muscle and liver injury. These enzyme levels typically peak several days into the illness. A leukocytosis with a leukocyte count of up to 30,000 to 50,000, in part reflecting catecholamine release and hemoconcentration secondary to volume contraction, is seen. Fibrinogen and prothrombin depletion, thrombocytopenia, and prolongation of prothrombin and partial thromboplastin times may be seen in the setting of DIC. Serum glucose may be low secondary to increased metabolism and liver glycogen depletion. Occasionally, hyperglycemia has been described. Hyperuricemia from skeletal muscle damage can cause renal failure. Elevations of blood urea nitrogen and serum creatinine are common. The latter is sometimes disproportionately elevated because of rhabdomyolysis. Cerebrospinal fluid can be completely normal or demonstrate an elevation of protein, xanthochromia, and a lymphocytic pleocytosis. Urinalysis commonly shows pyuria, proteinuria, hematuria, and granular casts. Metabolic (lactic) acidosis, respiratory alkalosis, or a combination of both may be seen. Since oxygen and carbon dioxide are more soluble at lower temperatures, arterial blood gases may disclose a low oxygen tension (PO_2), carbon dioxide tension (PCO_2), and elevated pH if uncorrected for body temperature. Electrocardiographic abnormalities are common and include sinus tachycardia, T-wave and ST-segment changes, and transient bundle branch blocks. Supraventricular arrhythmias can occur.

Treatment

The goals of treatment are twofold: management of hyperthermia itself (Table 33-3) and treatment of any complications (Table 33-4). Maintenance of airway, breathing, and circulation, as usual, takes precedence over more specific interventions. Comatose patients, in general, will require endotracheal intubation. Measured PO_2 and PCO_2 will be 7.2 percent and 4.4 percent lower, respectively, for each degree above 37°C (98.6°F) as compared to in vivo values at the elevated body temperature. The relevance of these changes to clinical management, however, is unclear at this time. Body temperature should be continuously measured with

Table 33-3. Initial treatment of heat stroke

Intubation of patient if comatose
Disrobing of patient
Rest in a cool air-conditioned environment
Immediate cooling using evaporative technique, possibly augmented by ice packs over axilla, groin, and neck
Establishment of intravenous line
Cardiac monitoring
Foley catheterization
Baseline blood work, including complete blood count with platelets, blood urea nitrogen, creatinine, liver and cardiac enzymes, coagulation profile, and glucose
Continuous monitoring of rectal temperature

a high rectal thermistor probe and not a standard clinical thermometer, which may only register to 42.5°C (108.5°F). An indwelling urethral catheter is useful for monitoring urine output and gauging the adequacy of fluid replacement.

Various methods for reducing body temperature have been suggested. The ice-water bath is a time-tested and reliable method of lowering body temperature. However, immersing a comatose or seizing patient in ice water in the emergency department setting is awkward, dangerous, and unnecessary. Moreover, cold water will promote shivering, which itself will increase body temperature, and cause cutaneous vasoconstriction, which will impair heat loss. Thus, ice-water immersion has largely been supplanted by the method of evaporative cooling. In this technique the patient's body is kept continually moist with a spray bottle of tepid water, and air is circulated with the aid of fans to promote evaporation. Alternatively the patient's body is covered with cool wet sheets and air is circulated as above. The rate of cooling can be augmented by applying ice packs to the axilla, groin, and neck areas. The goal should be a reduction in core temperature to 39°C (102.2°F) within no more than 30 to 60 minutes. Active cooling measures should be stopped at this point, as further spontaneous lowering of body temperature is expected and hypothermia can otherwise result. Shivering, if it occurs, can be controlled with chlorpromazine, 25 to 50 mg IV. A rebound increase in temperature should be anticipated within three to six hours and treated if it develops.

Other techniques that can be used to lower body temperature, but are rarely necessary, include chilled IV solutions, iced gastric lavage, and cold enemas. Cold peritoneal lavage and hemodialysis have also been used successfully.

Coma should reverse promptly with cooling and, if not, other causes of altered mental status, such as hypoglycemia, should be considered. Occasionally, return of consciousness is delayed for hours to days and may be a bad prognostic sign.

Hypotension generally responds to cooling measures alone, as vasoconstriction occurs in the setting of high-output heart failure. If not, cautious fluid administration is indicated. Many reports have now documented that actual fluid deficits are modest and average only 1.2 to 1.4 liters in the first four to six hours of treatment. Overly vigorous fluid administration during this time can result in pulmonary edema. Specific fluid composition depends on determination of serum electrolytes. If hypotension is a manifestation of a low cardiac output state, the use of IV isoproterenol beginning at 1 μg per minute may help restore blood pressure. Agents with alpha agonist activity, such as levarterenol or high-dose (>10 μg per minute) dopamine, should be avoided, as they tend to promote cutaneous vasoconstriction and can impair heat dissipation.

Table 33-4. Treatment of complications of heat stroke

Complication	Treatment
Coma	Reverses with cooling
Hypotension	Cooling and cautious fluid administration; if low-output state, isoproterenol, 1 μg/min IV, titrated upwards to blood pressure
Seizures	Diazepam, 5–10 mg IV
Shivering	Chlorpromazine, 25–50 mg IV
Pigmenturia	Urinary alkalinization, diuretics, and mannitol
Acidosis	Bicarbonate (controversial)

Seizures are common, particularly during the cooling process. They are usually short-lived, however, and respond to IV diazepam. It is important that both seizures and shivering be controlled since they substantially increase endogenous heat production.

Controversy exists regarding the aggressiveness with which metabolic acidosis should be corrected. It should be kept in mind that the measured pH will be artifactually high if not corrected for body temperature. To make this correction 0.015 pH units should be subtracted for each degree above 37°C (98.6°F). Often, surprisingly large amounts of sodium bicarbonate are needed to correct the (predominant) lactic acidosis.

If pigmenturia is observed a trial of mannitol, diuretics, and urinary alkalinization can be tried to forestall renal failure. Acute tubular necrosis (ATN), if it develops, will resolve in time, but dialysis may be necessary for the usual medical indications. DIC has been variably treated with heparin or plasma and platelet transfusions, or both. Liver failure, renal failure, and DIC generally are complications observed during hospitalization but are rarely problems in the emergency department.

Steroids have not been found to be of value in heat stroke, and antibiotics should be reserved for specific infectious complications. Antipyretics, such as aspirin or aceteminophen, which work by lowering the body's thermoregulatory set point, are ineffective.

Diagnosis

Differential diagnosis includes thyroid storm, meningitis, encephalitis, CVA, anticholinergic poisoning, and, rarely (in tropical settings), cerebral falciparum malaria. Thyroid storm may be accompanied by goiter and exophthalmos, but in any case initial management of the hyperthermic state should proceed as discussed previously. Meningitis is usually accompanied by nuchal rigidity, but this finding may be lost when coma supervenes, and the occasional finding of a cerebrospinal fluid (CSF) lymphocytic pleocytosis in hyperthermia can further complicate the diagnosis. Encephalitis is typically associated with a normal CSF and may provide some diagnostic confusion, particularly if key historical information about the illness is not available. Cerebrovascular accidents can result in hyperthermia if the hypothalamic thermoregulatory center is disrupted; computed tomographic scanning may be needed to make this distinction. Blood smears examined by an experienced pathologist will almost invariably disclose malarial parasites if they are present.

Malignant hyperthermia is a syndrome observed in genetically susceptible individuals in whom muscular rigidity, rhabdomyolysis, and hyperthermia develop when they are exposed to inhalational anesthetics and depolarizing neuromuscular blocking agents. Cases precipitated by physical or emotional stress have also been described. The neuroleptic malignant syndrome has similar clinical features but is seen as a complication of phenothiazine use. Dantrolene, 2 mg/kg IV, has been used to treat both disorders, which should be suspected whenever muscular rigidity is observed in the setting of hyperthermia and CNS dysfunction.

Prognosis

Many features of the initial presentation of heat stroke have been proposed as predictive of outcome. The extent of hyperthermia and length of time in coma are two often-mentioned variables. SGOT levels greater than 1,000 within 24 hours of presentation correlate with visceral organ damage and death. Lactic acidosis, in classic heat stroke, of greater than 3.3 mEq per liter has a similar poor prognosis, although lactic acidosis in exertional heat stroke is often profound and does not appear to correlate with outcome.

Overall mortality reported in the literature has ranged from 5 to 80 percent. Early deaths probably occur from CNS injury. After three to four days, mortality occurs from a generalized bleeding diathesis. Late deaths follow liver or kidney failure or vascular thrombosis.

Long-Term Sequelae

The two most common complications observed after heat stroke are persistent cerebellar deficits and impaired thermoregulation. The latter can predispose to recurrent heat illness after exposure to even moderate heat stress. Hepatic injury, although at times considerable, does not appear to impair long-term liver function in survivors. Renal function also tends to return to normal in patients who sustain ATN, although several cases of chronic interstitial nephritis have been described.

Prevention

Athletic activities should be canceled or postponed during periods of high environmental heat and humidity. The degree of heat stress is best assessed by determination of the wet-bulb globe temperature (WBGT). This index takes into consideration the effects of dry-air temperature, humidity, and radiant solar energy. A WBGT index of greater than 28 to 30°C (82.4–86°F) should prompt cancellation of athletic events. The wearing of light-colored absorbent clothing is advisable but may not be possible in some settings, such as football games, where bulky uniforms may be necessary to avoid injuries.

Adequate intake of fluids is critical, both before and during exertion. As was noted previously, athletes and manual laborers consistently underestimate their fluid requirements even when water is freely available. Five hundred ml of fluids should be ingested before activities and 200 to 300 ml should be ingested every 20 minutes during exertion. The precise composition of the fluid ingested is not important. Water or any of a number of commercially available weak eletrolyte solutions, with or without added glucose, is acceptable.

Finally, sufficient time should be allotted for the normal process of acclimatization to occur. One to two hours of exertion a day for at least 1 to 2 weeks in a warm environment are necessary before more strenuous activities should be undertaken. Also, the avoidance of exertion during times of excessive fatigue, stress, or intercurrent medical illnesses, particularly those that predispose to dehydration, is advisable. Realization of these simple facts has resulted in a reduced incidence of heat stroke among military recruits.

SELECTED READING

Clark, WG, and Lipton, JM. Drug-related heat stroke. *Pharmacol Ther* 26:345, 1984.

Clowes, GHA, and O'Donnell, TF. Heat stroke. *N Engl J Med* 291:564, 1974.

Costrini, AM, et al. Cardiovascular and metabolic manifestations of heat stroke and severe heat exhaustion. *Am J Med* 66:296, 1979.

Gold, J. Development of heat pyrexia. *JAMA* 173:1175, 1960.

Graham, BS, et al. Nonexertional heat stroke: Physiologic management and cooling in 14 patients. *Arch Intern Med* 146:87, 1986.

Gronert, GA, Thompson, RL, and Onofrio, BM. Human malignant hyperthermia: Awake episodes and correction by dantrolene. *Anesth Analg* 59:377, 1980.

Iampietro, PF. Heat-induced tetany. *Fed Proc* 22:884, 1973.

Irwin, GE, Simon, JE. Neuroleptic malignant syndrome. *J Emerg Med* 1:207, 1984.

Kew, MC, Bershas, I, and Sefteh, H. The diagnostic and prognostic significance of the serum enzyme changes in heat stroke. *Trans R Soc Trop Med Hyg* 63:325, 1971.

Knochel, JP. Environmental heat illness: An eclectic review. *Arch Intern Med* 137:841, 1974.

Knochel, JP, and Caskey, JH. The mechanism of hypophosphatemia in acute heat stroke. *JAMA* 238:425, 1977.

May, DC, et al. Neuroleptic malignant syndrome: Response to dantrolene sodium. *Ann Intern Med* 98:183, 1983.

O'Donnell, T, and Glower, G. The circulatory abnormalities of heat stroke. *N Engl J Med* 287:734, 1972.

Saxton, CR. Treatment of heat stroke at Parkland Memorial Hospital. *West J Med* 133:447, 1980.

Schiff, HB, MacSearraigh, EJM, and Kallmeyer, JC. Myoglobinuria rhabdomyolysis, and marathon running. *Q J Med* 188:463, 1978.

Schrier, RW, et al. Renal, metabolic and circulatory responses to heat and exercise. *Ann Intern Med* 73:213, 1970.

Shapiro, Y, et al. Heat intolerance in former heat stroke patients. *Ann Intern Med* 90:913, 1979.

Shibolet, S, Lancaster, M, and Danon, Y. Heat stroke: A review. *Aviat Space Environ Med* 47:200, 1976.

Simon, HB. Extreme pyrexia. *JAMA* 236:2419, 1976.

Sitprija, V. Heat oedema: A clinical study. *Postgrad Med J* 55:728, 1979.

Smego, R, and Durack, D. The neuroleptic malignant syndrome. *Arch Intern Med* 142:1183, 1982.

Stine, R. Heat illness. *JACEP* 8:154, 1979.

Talbott, JH, and Michelsen, J. Heat cramps: A clinical and chemical study. *J Clin Invest* 12:533, 1931.

Weiner, JS, and Khogali, M. A physiological body-cooling unit for treatment of heat stroke. *Lancet* 1:507, 1980.

Wyndham, CH. Heat stroke and hyperthermia in marathon runners. *Ann NY Acad Sci* 301:128, 1977.

34. Hypothermia

Paul N. Seward
Mel Robinson

Hypothermia is said to exist when the patient's core temperature is 95°F or below. (All temperatures in this chapter are given as Fahrenheit; for centigrade/Fahrenheit conversion see Table 34-1.) A large number of factors have been found to predispose individuals to hypothermia. However, both etiologically and practically, hypothermia is most clearly related to problems in one of three areas: increased heat loss, the failure of heat production, or the failure of thermoregulation.

The category of *increasing heat loss* can in turn be divided into the broad areas of physiologic and environmental factors. Physiologic factors that predispose to an increase in the loss of heat into the environment include, first and foremost, anything that increases the body surface area or the permeability of that surface to heat loss. Thus, something as simple as the ratio of body mass to body surface area predisposes infants and small children to become more readily hypothermic than adults. Similarly, burns and major trauma, with violation of the integument, are commonly associated with hypothermia, and the degree of hypothermia is well correlated with ultimate morbidity and mortality. Similarly, significant degrees of exfoliative dermatitis or other chronic problems on the skin surface will predispose the patient to heat loss.

Drugs and intoxicants can likewise predispose to heat loss by increasing peripheral vasodilatation or blunting the vasoconstrictive response to cold stress. By far the most important of these is alcohol, which produces vasodilatation, reduces shivering, blunts the sensation of cold, limits mobility, and produces the impaired judgment that can lead to exposure situations and associated trauma in the first place. To a lesser degree, barbiturates and other intoxicants have been shown to do the same.

Environmental factors include, first and foremost, immersion injury. Because of the excellence of water as a conductor of heat and the fact that water at a temperature comfortable for swimming is well below body temperature, hypothermia is a nearly universal complication of immersion injury. Moreover, even as immersion injury predisposes to hypothermia, the blunting of judgment and consciousness caused by hypothermia can lead to drowning, even in the case of otherwise competent swimmers. In situations of extreme cold, the act of attempting to swim to shore, by increasing the conduction of heat into moving water, can hasten the loss of consciousness and increase the likelihood of subsequent drowning.

Rapid hypothermia, by decreasing cerebral metabolism and blood flow, can exert a protective effect on the individual with submersion injury, particularly cerebral asphyxia. Thus, a number of reports exist of patients who, despite submersion in ice water for times extending to nearly an hour, have complete neurologic recovery. However, at

Table 34-1. Centigrade/Fahrenheit conversion

°C	°F
40	104.0
39	102.2
38	100.4
37	98.6
36	96.8
35	95.0
34	93.2
33	91.4
32	89.6
31	87.8
30	86.0
29	84.2
28	82.4
27	80.6
26	78.8
25	77.0
24	75.2
23	73.4
22	71.6
21	69.8
20	68.0

warmer water temperatures, the degree of hypothermia is likely to be correlated less with a protective effect of decreased body temperature than with the duration of submersion and thus an increased risk of adverse outcome.

Hypothermia can also occur from nonimmersion exposure injury. This is particularly common in outdoor exposure during conditions of extremely cold weather. In these cases, the onset of hypothermia is uniformly slow, and the degree of hypothermia is therefore strongly correlated with the length of exposure and thus an adverse outcome. Moreover, nonimmersion exposure hypothermia is also much more likely to be associated with peripheral frostbite injury, which also will correspond closely to the length of exposure and the degree of hypothermia.

The common underlying problem in *failure of heat production* is inability to produce heat, due either to a lack of substrate or a failure of endocrine regulation. These underlying issues, rather than age itself, has led in some series to an association of hypothermia with the extremes of age. Failure of heat production can occur with malnutrition, as well as inactivity, or endocrinologic failure due to hypothyroidism, hypopituitarism, or hypoadrenalism.

Patients with neurologic impairment or patients who are receiving medications such as phenothiazines, which directly impair thermoregulation, will have even greater difficulties with cold stress since they have *limitation of thermoregulation.* Moreover, any of a variety of serious underlying illnesses can incidentally affect thermoregulation and heat production as a part of a more general homeostatic impairment. The obvious examples of sepsis, diabetic ketoacidosis, or severe cardiopulmonary disease readily come to mind.

It is important to remember also that these situations are not mutually exclusive. On the contrary, many of them are likely to coexist in the same individuals and thus complement and reinforce one another. Thus, the exposed alcoholic patient may also be malnourished; the elderly person on limited income may be unable to purchase sufficient nourishment or to adequately heat the home; infants in deprived circumstances may at once be undernourished, exposed, and relatively immobile. All of these individuals may have concomitant relative or absolute endocrine deficiencies, take medications that diminish thermoregulation, or have underlying diseases such as diabetes, which can produce substrate problems, a predisposition to infection, and concomitant vascular disease.

Climate as an exogenous factor is worthy of some independent mention. On the one hand its importance to the problems of environmental heat loss is obvious: People will lose consciousness and drown much faster in water that is 35°F than in water that is 80°F. Being stranded in one's car in winter or lost on a camping trip is obviously a different risk when the weather is below zero than on a mild summer afternoon. However, severe cold injury can occur in all climates and all seasons and does not require exposure to extremes of cold. A room at a temperature of 77°F would feel uncomfortably warm to most of us, yet humans cooled to that temperature have rarely survived. Moreover, whereas hypothermia in the snowbound individual is expected and will be looked for, hypothermia in normal inhabitants of nursing homes may be missed, despite its documented frequency.

Mortality from hypothermia ranges from 10 to 80 percent and is related to core temperature if it is 78°F or below; there is little or no association between temperature and mortality above this range. Mortality is very closely associated, however, with underlying illness as an inciting cause. Finally, in addition to central hypothermia, localized injury to tissue (frostbite) accounts for many cases of serious morbidity.

PATHOPHYSIOLOGY

When the core temperature of the body begins to drop, a number of physiologic responses occur. The hypothalamic "thermostat" senses blood-cooling and immediately initiates sympathetic neurogenic signals, which cause increased muscle tone and metabolic rate. When muscle tone reaches a certain level, shivering begins. These factors combine to increase heat production by about four times the normal rate. Sympathetic impulses also create intense cutaneous vasoconstriction, thereby pooling cold blood at the surface and extremities, maximizing core temperature. Situations that create heat loss through convection and conduction greatly accelerate the development of hypothermia. High winds and wet clothes intensify body heat loss in this way. The most profound effects occur during immersion in cold water. In this environment rapid heat loss is intensified by any movement. Death can occur in as little as 15 minutes.

Core body temperature begins to drop when homeostatic mechanisms are no longer able to compensate for environmental cold. Virtually every organ system is affected by hypothermia. Physiologic responses occur in two phases. Between 90 and 95°F organ systems exhibit an "excitation" phase in which responses are geared to generate and retain heat. When core body temperature drops below 90°F, excitation gives way to slowing of organ system function. The following organ system effects are seen in hypothermia:

1. *Cardiovascular.* Blood pressure, heart rate, and cardiac output initially rise and then fall at temperatures below

90°F. Dysrhythmias and conduction delays frequently occur at core body temperatures below 86°F. Sinus bradycardia and atrial fibrillation with a slow ventricular response are commonly encountered. On occasion, the bradycardia is so profound as to resemble asystole, though with warming a rhythm can return. In addition, pulse and blood pressure may be difficult to determine at these temperatures. The risk of spontaneous ventricular fibrillation progressively increases as core temperature drops below 82°F, most likely because of an increase in the degree of nonuniform recovery of excitability in ventricular muscle. Also, at this temperature and below, manipulation that transmits physical force to the myocardium can produce fibrillation. The Osborne wave (J wave) is a characteristic conduction abnormality that often appears on the electrocardiogram (ECG) tracing when core temperature nears 86°F. Intravascular volume decreases as a result of plasma shift to the extracellular space and renal losses.

2. *Central nervous system.* At core temperatures below 90°F, a progressively decreasing level of consciousness is seen. Confusion and incoordination give way to unconsciousness at temperatures below 86°F. Pupils may be dilated and unresponsive.

3. *Metabolic.* The metabolic requirements of all tissues, including the brain, are decreased with profound hypothermia. An initial alkalosis gives way to a lactic acidosis produced by shivering and poor tissue perfusion at lower temperatures. Hypothermia also causes a leftward shift of the oxyhemoglobin dissociation curve, impairing oxygen release at tissues. Hyperglycemia proportional to the temperature is common.

4. *Local cold injury.* Vasoconstriction causes a profound drop in tissue temperatures (especially in extremities). Hemoconcentration and sludging of vascular elements can lead to thrombosis. Coagulopathy can occur if sufficient amounts of tissue thromboplastins are released. Finally, actual ice crystallization occurs when tissue temperature nears the freezing point of water. Rhabdomyolysis can occur in immobilized hypothermic patients.

5. *Renal.* Hypothermic patients have impaired ability to concentrate urine, which induces a diuresis. Acute tubular necrosis can occur in severe hypothermia secondary to renal hypoperfusion and myoglobinuria.

6. *Pancreas.* The pancreas seems particularly subject to cold injury with subsequent pancreatitis. Temporary or permanent alterations in glucose metabolism are common.

7. *Pulmonary.* Progressive hypothermia blunts the cough reflex and produces bradypnea. Respiratory arrest commonly occurs at core temperatures below 77°F.

PRESENTATION

Common signs and symptoms of progressive hypothermia are as follows:

1. *Mild (90–95°F).* In neonates, the presentation may be atypical, with decreased activity and feeding as early signs of hypothermia. In older patients, shivering is often present. However, slurred speech, mild incoordination, and poor judgment may be the only manifestations. In the elderly, these symptoms may be mistaken for cerebrovascular insufficiency. Moreover, in patients who are already impaired in their mental function, this may be regarded as merely a variation on a normal state. Similarly, in active individuals who are suffering from acute exposure hypothermia, though shivering is often present, findings may be mistaken for the fatigue associated with exertion.

2. *Moderate (82–90°F).* Progressive deterioration of mental status occurs in this range. Unconsciousness is likely at core temperatures less than 86°F. The skin becomes cyanotic and edematous. Shivering is replaced by muscle rigidity. Respiratory drive and cardiac output decrease. Osborne waves and bradydysrhythmias appear on the ECG.

3. *Severe (<82°F).* Patients are usually comatose and areflexic with dilated unresponsive pupils. Ventricular dysrhythmias and respiratory arrest may occur at core temperatures below 82°F.

DIAGNOSIS

The diagnosis of hypothermia is made on the basis of the core temperature. However, a number of pitfalls lie in the way of that determination. First among these is an index of suspicion, particularly when evaluating the comatose, hypotensive patient. Particularly in cases of chronic hypothermia in the elderly or in intoxicated patients with minimal apparent exposure, the possibility of obtaining the temperature inadequately or ignoring an apparently mistaken result while busy with other problems is a real danger.

Second, core temperature, when sought, must be measured correctly. Ideally, an esophageal probe is used, as this will most closely approximate the temperature of the heart and great vessels. This is practical, however, only in the comatose, intubated patient. For other patients, in settings in which this technology is both familiar and available, tympanic temperature is closely correlated with core temperature. For all other circumstances a rectal probe is an acceptable alternative. When this is used, however, it must be remembered that rectal and true mediastinal core temperatures can differ substantially during periods of rapid rewarming. If there is any clinical suspicion of hypothermia, under no circumstances should oral thermometers or those that do not register temperatures less than 95°F be used.

Finally, a diagnosis of hypothermia immediately mandates the constant monitoring of core temperature with equipment capable of detecting and continuously displaying temperature below 95°F, until such time as it has returned to a normal and stable level.

PREHOSPITAL CARE

Mild to Moderate Hypothermia

First aid for patients with hypothermia consists of extrication to a warm environment and removal of wet clothing. If the patient is conscious and alert, warm fluids can be administered orally.

Local tissue injury occurs most commonly to ears, nose, fingers, toes, hands, and feet. Proper first aid for local tissue injury (frostbite) includes the following:

1. Constricting or wet garments should be removed and affected parts wrapped with warm, dry material.

2. Affected parts should not be rubbed or exposed to dry heat.
3. Rapid rewarming should be accomplished by immersion of the affected parts in water warmed to 104 to 108°F for 20 to 40 minutes or until a flush has returned to the most distal tip of the thawed part. Care must be taken to avoid injury of frozen tissue against the water container. Rewarming should not be accomplished if there is any possibility of refreezing because extensive tissue damage will result.
4. A loose padded dressing should be applied.

Transport for hospital evaluation is required for all patients suspected of being hypothermic.

Severe Hypothermia: The Comatose Patient

In most cases paramedical personnel will not be equipped to measure core temperature in the field. Because of this, a carefully directed, rapidly performed history combined with such clinical assessments of temperature as can be readily performed are critical. Wet clothing must be removed and replaced with dry blankets or other insulating material. A basic airway should be provided and high-flow oxygen administered. If it is possible to warm the inspired gas to a temperature of 104 to 108°F safely, this should be done. However, as hot gases can be hazardous, unfamiliarity with equipment or technique is a contraindication to this procedure. An intravenous line of normal saline or Ringer's lactate should be started if possible. Naloxone, thiamine, and 50% dextrose in standard doses are indicated for comatose patients.

BASIC AND ADVANCED LIFE SUPPORT IN THE PROFOUNDLY HYPOTHERMIC PATIENT

In arrested hypothermic patients, two difficulties exist: first, determining the appropriateness of the initiation of basic life support (BLS) and advanced life support (ALS) procedures in the first place, and second, changes in responsiveness to therapy. Patients whose core temperature is below 82°F may appear similar not merely to patients in cardiac arrest but also to individuals after prolonged death, and both prehospital care and emergency department personnel may be reluctant to institute resuscitative measures. In this quandary, two apparently contradictory principles should govern: *First, do no harm.* This principle most particularly applies to the danger of producing ventricular fibrillation with presumptively therapeutic manipulations such as intubation, chest compression, or central venous cannulation. In a more general way it also applies to the risks of overly aggressive resuscitation and rapid transport to the safety of the paramedics and to the emotional well-being of the patient's family. The other principle states that *no patient is dead until he or she is warm and dead.* This principle applies to the potential reversibility with prompt resuscitation of what in normothermic patients would be irreversible physiologic derangements in circulation and central nervous system activity.

Because of these concerns, the caretaker first responsible for the profoundly hypothermic patient may experience a great deal of uncertainty regarding the appropriateness of initiating BLS and ALS procedures. On the one hand the apparent danger is present of producing irreversible nonperfusing dysrhythmias by the irritation of chest compressions, in patients who may in fact have undetectable but life-sustaining cardiorespiratory function. Also, there is a natural reluctance to begin resuscitation, with its real emotional and financial costs, in patients who have already been irreversibly dead for some time. On the other hand, there may be good reason to institute such procedures with some hope of success in hypothermic patients with what would otherwise be the most profound appearance of death. In short, in the profoundly hypothermic, apparently dead patient, there seem to be powerful reasons both to limit the vigor of resuscitation and to pursue resuscitation with greater than normal fervor.

This is a controversy that has not been entirely resolved. However, it is also one in which awareness of the question and attention to the issues involved are likely to be more helpful than any specific protocol. A practical approach includes:

1. *Intubation.* While this should be performed gently, the indications for performing this procedure are the same as for patients who are not hypothermic. Moreover, the dangers of intubation alone may have previously been overstated, as a substantial number of series have now been reported of the intubation of patients with temperatures below 90°F without complications.

2. *Institution of resuscitation.* If doubt exists, the patient still deserves the benefit of that uncertainty. Thus, despite appearances, resuscitation should be instituted in patients known or suspected of having exposure hypothermia unless "do not resuscitate" status is documented and verified, obviously lethal injuries are present, chest wall depression is impossible, any signs of life are present, or resuscitators are endangered by evacuation delays.

3. *Pulselessness and the institution of chest compressions.* If monitoring is unavailable, a longer time should be taken to determine pulselessness (up to one minute) before one decides whether the pulse is absent. Otherwise cardiopulmonary resuscitation (CPR) under the same guidelines as in other advanced cardiac life support (ACLS) situations. If monitoring is available, CPR should be instituted for ventricular fibrillation but withheld for other pulseless rhythms, such as atrial fibrillation, bradycardias, junctional rhythms, and so forth, as these are usually adequately managed with rewarming. In all cases, appropriate ventilation should be performed, either with bag and mask or with careful intubation, and the patient should be transported rapidly.

4. *Medications and other ACLS procedures.* The principal difference in ACLS in profoundly hypothermic patients is the relative unresponsiveness to medication or defibrillation in these patients. If there is uncertainty about the patient's true temperature, pharmacotherapy and defibrillation guided by ACLS protocols should be attempted. Defibrillation at two to four joules per kilogram should be tried. However, response is unusual if the temperature is less than 86°F, and, as such, failure to respond to such therapy should

not be considered an indication to discontinue resuscitation. Moreover, if initial therapy with medication or defibrillation is not successful, and strong suspicion of profound hypothermia exists, excessive repetition of cardiac drugs should be avoided, as they are unlikely to be effective. Instead, the next step should be rapid transport to an environment where rewarming can take place. In addition, bretylium has been recommended both for the prevention and treatment of ventricular fibrillation in the profoundly hypothermic patient and has been associated with successful defibrillation when electrical defibrillation has failed.

5. *Continued resuscitation* until the patient is rewarmed.

MANAGEMENT IN THE EMERGENCY DEPARTMENT

Proper emergency department management of hypothermic patients requires a high index of suspicion and early measurement of core temperature. Patients with core temperatures greater than 90°F are invariably conscious with spontaneous cardiac activity unless other severe underlying problems are present. Passive rewarming with warm blankets is usually the only therapy required.

Patients with initial core temperatures less than 90°F usually require more extensive treatment. If intubation is believed to be necessary, adequate preoxygenation should precede insertion of an endotracheal tube, and the procedure should be performed as gently as possible. The inspired gases should be warmed to 104 to 108°F.

Peripheral vascular access should be obtained and, as the vast majority of hypothermic patients will be hypovolemic, appropriate warmed crystalloid solutions should be administered. If they have not been given in the field, glucose, naloxone, and thiamine should be administered as well. A Foley catheter should be inserted to monitor urinary output. Insertion of a nasogastric tube and central venous pressure line should be deferred until a core temperature of 86°F is obtained in order to prevent ventricular fibrillation. Once these priorities have been addressed, rewarming procedures should be instituted.

Rewarming

Various rewarming methods have been advocated for profoundly hypothermic patients. On the one hand, in neonates with hypothermia, rapid external rewarming has been suggested to decrease mortality substantially, and active external rewarming has been used successfully in many patients without complications. On the other hand, active external rewarming with heating blankets or total body immersion has been implicated as a cause of core temperature afterdrop in older patients. This phenomenon results when external rewarming causes peripheral vasodilatation. The result is sudden hypovolemia and a bolus of cold acidotic blood to the core, which can produce fatal cardiac dysrhythmias.

For this reason, active core rewarming is probably preferred for the severely hypothermic patient and can be accomplished by the following techniques:

1. Delivery of humidified oxygen warmed to 104 to 108°F. The respiratory therapy department should be able to provide this technology readily in any emergency department in which even a small number of hypothermic patients are seen. Of particular importance is the ability to ensure that the temperature of the inspired gases does not exceed the prescribed limits in order to avoid the possibility of upper-airway injury.

2. Warmed intravenous (IV) fluids at 104 to 108°F. Crystalloid solutions can be readily warmed in a microwave oven in a matter of seconds, with close monitoring of the temperatures involved. Studies have failed to show evidence of toxic contamination from the plastic bags or tubing used with such procedures. In addition, most facilities have water baths that are used to heat blood to body temperature for exchange transfusion or the transfusion of the trauma patient. These can be readily adapted for the warming of IV fluids.

3. Peritoneal dialysis with K^+ free dialysate heated to 104 to 108°F (similar microwaving of fluids can be used for this technique as well). If dialysate is unavailable, normal saline can be used. However, regardless of what is used, close monitoring of serum electrolytes must be performed throughout the procedure, and the potential complications of emergency peritoneal lavage in the emergency department must be weighed against the risks of prolonged hypothermia.

4. Hemodialysis, cardiopulmonary bypass, or mediastinal lavage can be used in desperate situations. If blood or blood products are used, microwave rewarming is contraindicated and warm water baths for warming are mandatory.

Aggressive resuscitation must continue until a core temperature of at least 86°F is reached. At this point, standard ACLS drug protocols should be followed in an attempt to restore a viable cardiac rhythm.

Finally, it is interesting to note that in a growing number of studies on the use of microwave radiation in the rapid rewarming of artificially chilled laboratory animals, no apparent morbidity has been found, and the technique has been performed in one-fourth to one-third the time required for other methods. As yet these techniques are not applicable to humans.

Laboratory Evaluation

Initial laboratory studies should include an ECG, electrolytes, blood sugar, amylase, renal and liver function studies, complete blood cell count and coagulation studies, and urinalysis. An important question in the interpretation of blood gases lies in the fact that the pH of blood in a sealed container will rise by a factor of approximately 0.008 units for every drop of 1°F (Table 34-2). Therefore, if blood is taken from a patient whose core temperature is 77°F, a pH reading of 7.4 will represent an actual pH of 7.58. Therefore, it has long been advocated that such readings be corrected for this temperature change and that the calculated rather than the measured reading be reported (Figs. 34-1 and 34-2).

More recently, a number of authors have advocated that blood gas determinations not be corrected. They suggest that change in pH with temperature is paralleled by physiologic changes that render an alkaline environment physiologic. In essence, therefore, for any temperature, the pH that should

Table 34-2. Normal arterial pH/temperature relationship

°C	pH	°F	pH
37	7.40	98.6	7.40
36	7.41	97.6	7.41
35	7.43	96.6	7.42
34	7.44	95.6	7.42
33	7.46	94.6	7.43
32	7.47	93.6	7.44
31	7.49	92.6	7.45
30	7.50	91.6	7.46
29	7.52	90.6	7.47
28	7.53	89.6	7.47
27	7.55	88.6	7.48
26	7.56	87.6	7.49
25	7.58	86.6	7.50
		85.6	7.51
		84.6	7.51
		83.6	7.52
		82.6	7.53
		81.6	7.54
		80.6	7.55
		79.6	7.56
		78.6	7.56
		77.6	7.57
		76.6	7.58
		75.6	7.59
		74.6	7.60

be considered "normal" is that which will be read as normal at 98.6°F. The authors base this on a number of contentions. First, at lower temperatures, the metabolic production of carbon dioxide (CO_2) is decreased while its solubility is increased. Thus, the maintenance of CO_2 balance with bicarbonate will be constant at lower levels of CO_2. Second, it has been pointed out that in various tissues in the body, physiologic temperatures may differ considerably and pH differs accordingly. However, these differences obviously do not alter normal function. Finally, the change in pH with temperature parallels the temperature-dependent change in the pH of neutrality of water, which also increases at a rate of approximately 0.017 units for each degree of temperature loss.

On a practical level, in a patient with a core temperature of 26°F, one may be presented with an uncorrected blood gas result of 7.22. A number of responses to this are possible. On a basic level, one might say that such a patient is moderately acidotic. A more sophisticated response would be to recognize that at that core temperature, such a reading represents a true tissue pH of 7.4 and is thus physiologic. However, the most correct interpretation would be to realize that a normal pH for tissues at that temperature is 7.56 and that the patient is therefore moderately acidotic physiologically.

While these concepts may appear complex, their implications are simple. First, it is important to know whether the determinations received have been corrected by one's laboratory or not. Secondly, as it is likely that corrected values are being received, the uncorrected values should be obtained as well. Thirdly, in considering the use of alkalinization, either with metabolic acid or hyperventilation, calculations should be based on the uncorrected value.

DISPOSITION AND PROGNOSIS

All patients with core hypothermia should be admitted for 24 to 48 hours of observation. Patients with core temperatures of less than 90°F should be admitted to the intensive care unit for continuous cardiac monitoring until rewarming is accomplished. Underlying problems are frequently discovered during the observation period.

Complications that may need to be addressed after the first hour of care include metabolic abnormalities; gastrointestinal bleeding; acute tubular necrosis and renal failure; pulmonary problems including pneumonia and pulmonary edema; pancreatitis; thrombosis and coagulopathy; and cardiac dysrhythmias and electrolyte abnormalities. Management of these problems should be addressed in the customary way as they become manifest.

The management of frostbite deserves some special mention. First, the extent of local tissue injury may be difficult to appreciate acutely in patients with cold injury. Initial management is as previously discussed. However, if the patient

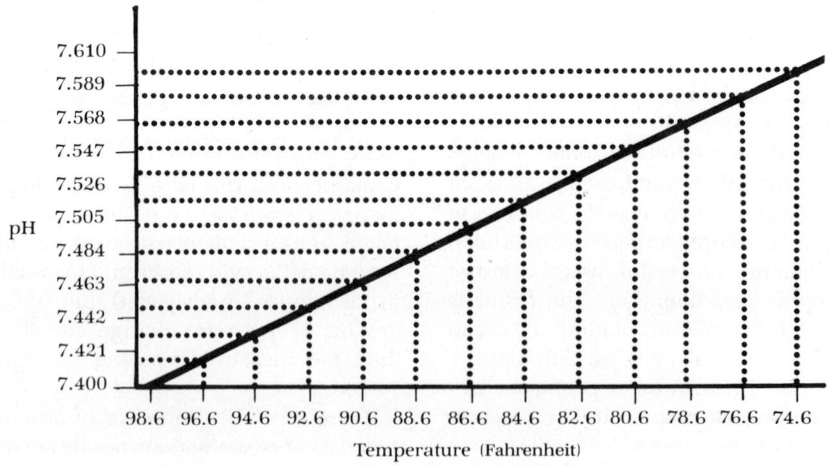

Fig. 34-1. Change in normal arterial pH with cooling (Fahrenheit).

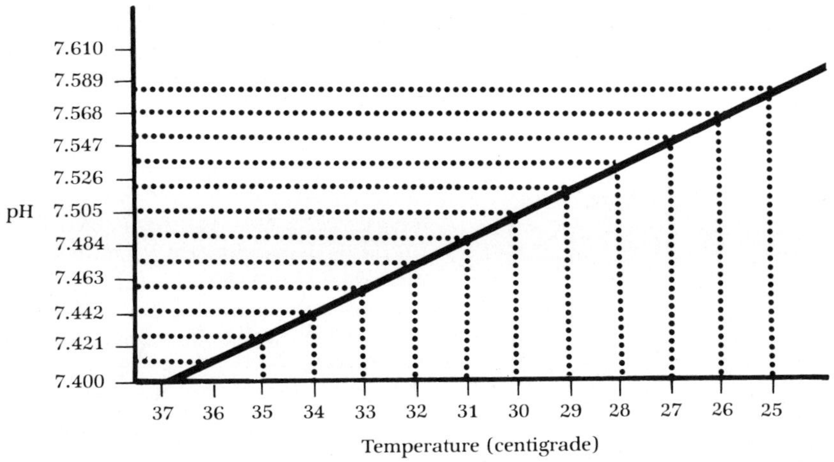

Fig. 34-2. Change in normal arterial pH with cooling (centigrade).

has an associated profound hypothermic injury, peripheral rewarming can be deferred until central rewarming has been accomplished. Thereafter care should be directed toward minimizing the possibility of infection or trauma. In a manner analogous to that used with burn injury, whirlpool bath débridement, protective isolation techniques, and physical therapy are all essential parts of management. Progressive necrosis occurs over 24 to 48 hours and ultimate demarcation of tissue loss can take weeks. Hyperemia and burning suggest superficial injury. Blister formation and paresthesias imply at least second-degree injury. Edema, ulceration, and anesthesia suggest full-thickness injury with involvement of subcutaneous tissues. Surgical amputation should be deferred as long as possible, as subsequent clarity of demarcation can minimize the amount of tissue that must be removed. Medical therapy to reduce coagulation and improve perfusion has been tried with mixed results. Finally, patients with frostbite have an increased susceptibility to subsequent frostbite and should be appropriately cautious about subsequent exposure to cold. See Chap. 76 for discussion of frostbite.

SELECTED READING

Danzel, DF, et al. Multicenter hypothermia survey. *AEM* 16:1042, 1987.

Han, J, and Moe, G. Nonuniform recovery of excitability in ventricular muscle. *Circ Res* 14:44, 1964.

Jurkovich, GJ, et al. Hypothermia in trauma victims: An ominous predictor of survival. *J Trauma* 27:1019, 1987.

Luna, GK, et al. Incidence and effect of hypothermia in seriously injured patients. *J Trauma* 27:1014, 1987.

Miller, J, Danzel, D, and Thomas, D. Urban accidental hypothermia: 135 cases. *AEM* 9:456, 1980.

Nugent, S, and Rogers, M. Resuscitation and intensive care monitoring following immersion hypothermia. *J Trauma* 20:9, 1980.

Olsen, RG, and David, TD. Hypothermia and electromagnetic rewarming in the rhesus monkey. *Aviat Space Environ Med* 55: 1103, 1984.

Ornato, J. Special resuscitation situations: Near drowning, traumatic injury, electric shock and hypothermia. *Circulation* 74 (Suppl IV):23, 1986.

Pickering, B, Bristow, G, and Craig, D. Core rewarming by peritoneal irrigation in accidental hypothermia with cardiac arrest. *Anesth Analg* 56:574, 1977.

Rahn, H, Reeves, R, and Howell, B. Hydrogen ion regulation, temperature, and evolution. *Am Rev Respr Dis* 112:165, 1975.

Ream, A, Reitz, B, and Silverberg, G. Temperature correction of pCO_2 and pH in estimating acid base status. *Anesthesiology* 56:41, 1982.

Reuler, J. Hypothermia: Pathophysiology, clinical settings and management. *AEM* 89:519, 1978.

State of Alaska. Hypothermia and cold water near drowning guidelines. EMS Section, Department of Public Health, Alaska, April 1982.

White, D. Hypothermia: The Bellevue experience. *AEM* 11:417, 1982.

White, F. A comparative physicological approach to hypothermia. *J Thorac Cardiol Surg* 82:821, 1981.

White, JD, et al. Comparison of rewarming by radio wave, regional hyperthermia and warm humidified inhalation. *Ann Emerg Med* 16:1, 1987.

Wong, K. Physiology and pharmacology of hypothermia. *West J Med* 138:227, 1983.

Zell, S, and Kurtz, K. Severe exposure hypothermia: A resuscitation protocol. *Ann Emerg Med* 14:339, 1985.

H. Alterations in Renal Function and Electrolyte Balance

35. Renal Physiology: Regulation of Volume, Potassium, Tonicity, and Acid-Base Status

David M. Poppel

PRINCIPLES OF RENAL PHYSIOLOGY

As an excretory organ, the kidney is responsible for maintenance of balance between intake and output of fluids, minerals, and nutrients, which by their metabolism form potentially toxic waste products. Excess or deficient excretion can cause serious acute and chronic physiologic disturbances, many of which are encountered in the emergency department. Additionally, the kidney plays important roles in chronic control of blood pressure, red-cell mass, and bone metabolism.

The excretory functions of the kidney demand considerable expenditure of physiologic resources. To process body wastes adequately, the kidney receives about 20 percent of the cardiac output, which, on the basis of flow per weight, far exceeds the flow to most other organs, including the heart and exercising muscle. The metabolic energy used to power the many epithelial transporters that process the plasma filtrate, generated in the glomerulus, is considerable and makes the kidney particularly vulnerable to hemodynamic or ischemic insults.

Waste excretion is achieved by a filtration-reabsorption process whereby, despite the large volume of blood that is filtered (approximately 180 liters per day in adults), only modest amounts of fluid are actually excreted to eliminate the waste water and excess solutes necessary to balance intake with output. Multiple passive and active mechanisms are responsible for returning the bulk of the filtered load to the systemic circulation.

The Nephron

The nephron is the basic unit responsible for filtration and reabsorption. Each kidney contains approximately 1.0 to 1.2 million nephrons. The glomerulus, a system of capillaries interposed between an afferent and efferent arteriole, is the site of filtration where a portion of plasma water and dissolved small solutes leaves the circulating blood and enters a series of tubules, which constitute the remainder of the nephron (Fig. 35-1). The tubules are lined by a single-cell-layer epithelium with variable luminal surface morphology and intrinsic cellular functions that give each nephron segment unique capacities to alter the character of the plasma filtrate, forming a urine that will suit the body's excretory needs. The tubules are in turn surrounded by the peritubular capillaries (Fig. 35-2), derived from the glomerular efferent arteriole. The juxtamedullary nephrons deep in the cortex, which send long loops of Henle into the inner medulla, are

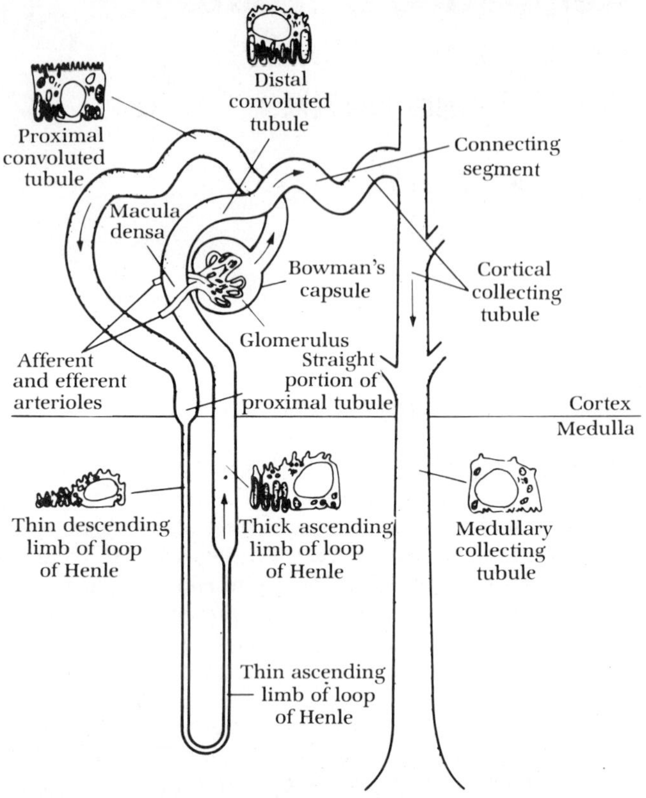

Fig. 35-1. Components of the nephron. Systemic blood, derived from the renal artery, enters the glomerulus via the afferent arteriole and leaves via the efferent arteriole. An ultrafiltrate of plasma crosses the glomerular capillary wall into Bowman's capsule and subsequently flows along the proximal tubule, into the loop of Henle, distal tubule, and collecting tubules. During passage through the tubules, reabsorption and secretion alter the character of the filtrate. (From B. D. Rose. *Clinical Physiology of Acid-Base and Electrolyte Disorders* [3rd ed.]. New York: McGraw-Hill, 1989. Reproduced with permission.)

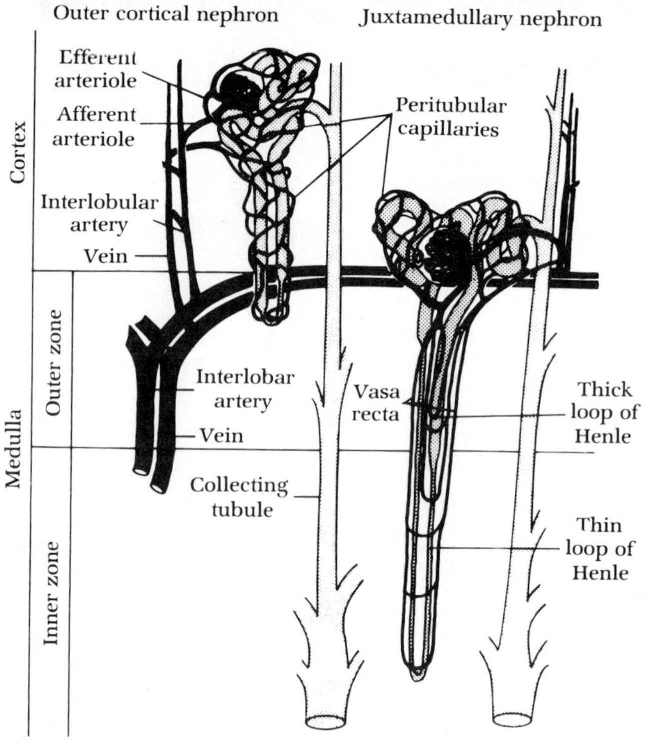

Fig. 35-2. The renal capillary circulation. Efferent arterioles form the peritubular capillaries that surround the tubular system of the nephron. Those accompanying the long loops of Henle, derived from juxtamedullary nephrons, are known as the vasa recta and are critical components in maintenance of the hypertonicity of the medullary interstitium. (From B. D. Rose. *Clinical Physiology of Acid-Base and Electrolyte Disorders* [3rd ed.]. New York: McGraw-Hill, 1989. Reproduced with permission.)

surrounded by the vasa recta, which are long hairpin capillary loops responsible, as are all peritubular capillaries, for clearing reabsorbed fluid and solutes back to the systemic circulation (see later in text).

A tubular epithelial cell can be thought of as having an apical or luminal surface, facing the tubular lumen, and an opposite, basolateral surface, facing the renal interstitium and peritubular capillaries. The arrangement and activity of solute transporters on one or both of these surfaces provide a vector for the movement of solutes and fluids across these cells. For example, basolateral sodium–potassium–adenosine triphosphatase (Na-K-ATPase) pumps actively transport sodium from tubular cells into the peritubular interstitium, and by lowering intracellular sodium concentration, maintain a gradient for sodium entry into the cell from the tubular lumen. Active transport processes are thus responsible for creation of gradients that promote passive transport as well (Fig. 35-3).

The Glomerulus

The separation of a glomerular filtrate from plasma is achieved across the glomerular capillary endothelium, the underlying glomerular basement membrane, and the visceral epithelial layer, which constitutes one of the borders of Bowman's space, the initial part of the tubular system (Fig. 35-4). This filtration barrier allows unrestricted movement of water and small solutes—for example, sodium, chloride, potassium, bicarbonate, urea, and glucose—while restricting movement of larger molecules, such as albumin and other plasma proteins. In addition to size, molecular charge affects filtration, as anions are more restricted from traversing the glomerular wall, given the negative charge that predominates on the basement membrane.

As is true of other capillary systems, fluid movement across the glomerular wall is controlled by Starling's forces, the balance between the hydrostatic pressure (P) and oncotic pressure (π) on either side of the capillary wall. Higher glomerular capillary hydrostatic pressure (P_{GC}) and lower plasma oncotic pressure (π_P) favor filtration, whereas similar changes in Bowman's space (BS) retard filtration. This balance is modulated by the permeability characteristics of the capillary wall–basement membrane, such that

$$GFR = Kf[(P_{GC} - P_{BS}) - (\pi_p - \pi_{BS})]$$

where Kf is the ultrafiltration coefficient (permeability) of the membrane and GFR is glomerular filtration rate. Kf is affected by structural changes in the glomeruli induced by diseases such as inflammatory nephritides but also can be

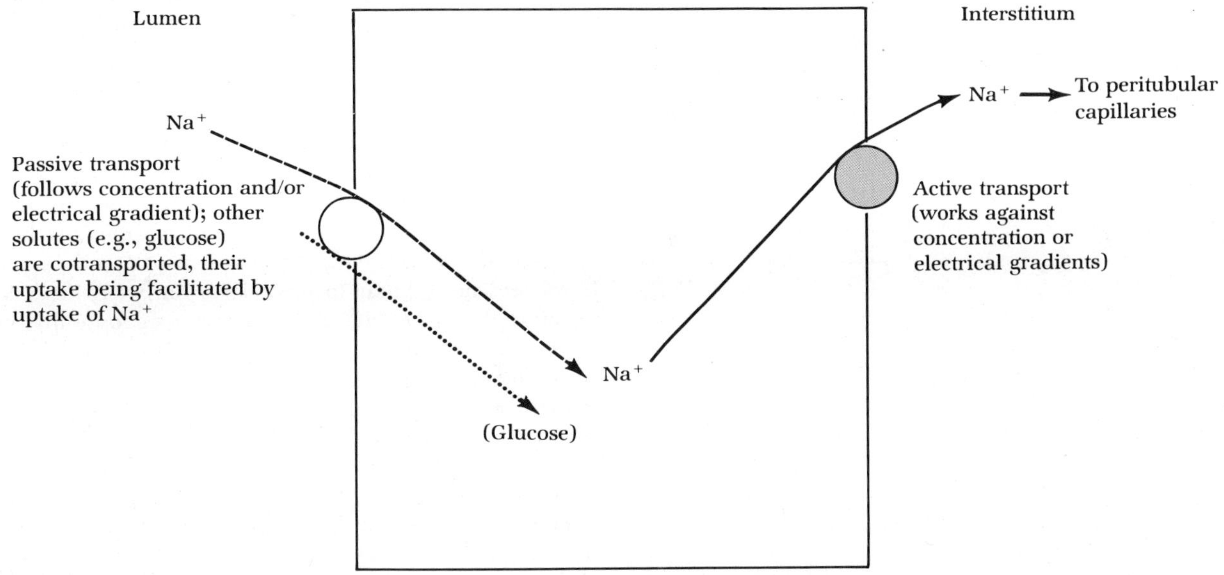

Fig. 35-3. Transepithelial gradients. This generalized schematic represents transporter-mediated movement of solutes from one side of the tubular epithelium to the other—in this case reabsorption of sodium from the lumen through the cell into the peritubular interstitium, where it can be taken up by peritubular capillaries. The active pump on the basolateral cell membrane creates a gradient for passive movement across the luminal membrane.

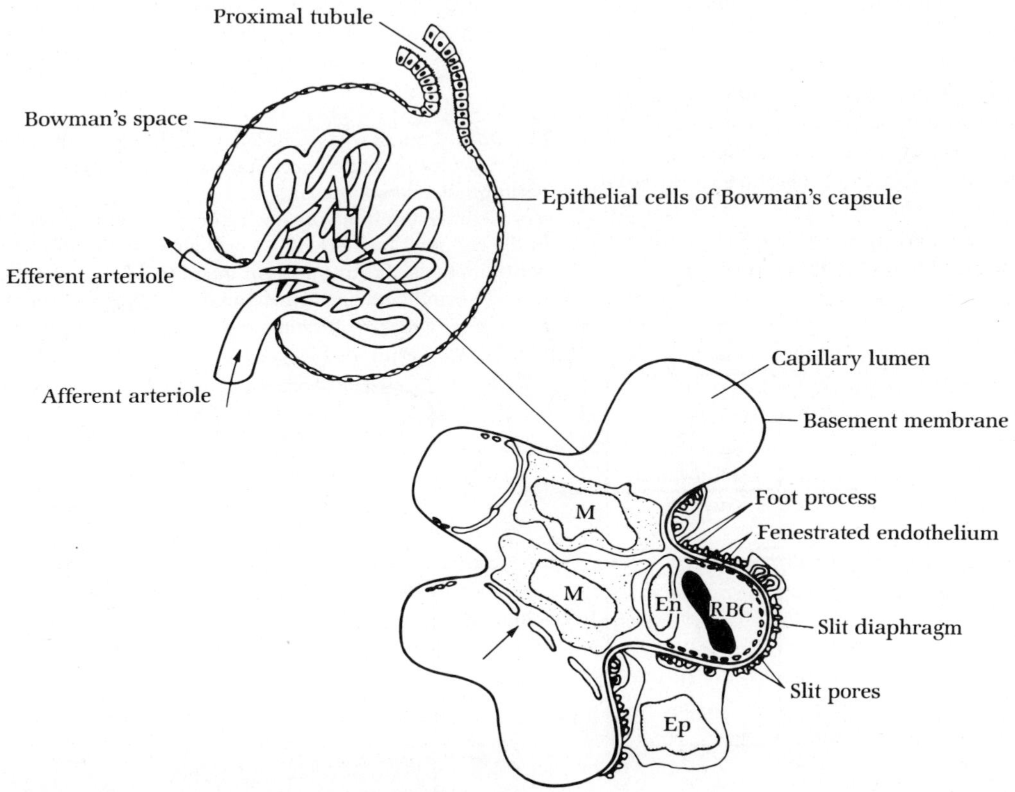

Fig. 35-4. Anatomy of the glomerulus. This schematic magnifies the glomerular capillary tuft, supported by the mesangial cells (M). The fenestrated endothelium (En), basement membrane, and visceral epithelial cell (Ep), with their foot processes, constitute the filtration barrier across which plasma filtrate enters Bowman's space. (RBC = red blood cell.) (From B. D. Rose. *Clinical Physiology of Acid-Base and Electrolyte Disorders* [3rd ed.]. New York: McGraw-Hill, 1989. Reproduced with permission.)

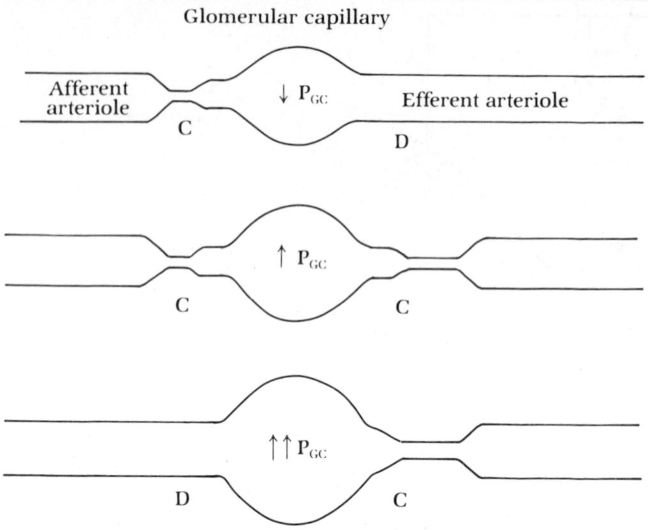

Fig. 35-5. Relationship of intraglomerular hydrostatic pressure to arteriolar tone. Efferent arteriolar constriction raises pressure within the glomerular capillary. The increase can be augmented by dilatation of the afferent arteriole. In states of generalized arteriolar constrictions, such as shock, or impaired renal arterial inflow due to renal artery stenosis, maintenance of intraglomerular hydrostatic pressure favoring filtration may depend on intense efferent arteriolar constriction and can be abolished by prostaglandin and angiotensin converting enzyme inhibitors. (C = constriction; D = dilatation.)

altered functionally by hormones such as prostaglandins and angiotensin II, which alter glomerular capillary surface area via changes in conformation of mesangial cells.

Glomerular capillary hydrostatic pressure, the major force that drives glomerular filtration, depends on cardiac output and the resistance to capillary blood flow offered by the renal arteries and particularly the preglomerular afferent and postglomerular efferent arterioles. Intraglomerular hydrostatic pressure is maximized by afferent arteriolar dilatation and efferent arteriolar constriction, resulting in increased flow into the capillary and retarded outflow (Fig. 35-5).

The Tubule

As the ultrafiltrate of plasma generated at the glomerulus moves from Bowman's space through the remainder of the nephron, its composition is changed considerably by reabsorption and secretion. Both active and passive mechanisms remove or add solutes and water. Alterations in luminal permeability affect fluid movement across the tubular epithelium, and peritubular factors, particularly Starling's forces affecting the postglomerular capillaries surrounding the tubules, influence the reuptake of filtered fluid and solute into the systemic circulation (Fig. 35-6).

Each nephron segment has specific capacities for reabsorption and secretion. The proximal tubule reabsorbs the bulk (70%) of filtered sodium chloride and water isosmotically. In addition, large amounts of potassium, calcium, phosphorus, magnesium, bicarbonate, amino acids, and urea are reclaimed in this nephron segment via several active and passive transport systems. A degree of secretion of protons and organic acids and bases also occurs proximally.

In the loop of Henle, an additional 20 percent of the filtered load of sodium chloride is reabsorbed, mainly in the thick ascending limb (TALH) via active transporters. This region of the nephron is also important in the regulation of serum tonicity, in that the differential permeabilities and transport activities of the descending and ascending limbs of the loop, as well as their hairpin configuration, create a steep osmotic gradient between the cortical and medullary interstitia. This countercurrent multiplier effect occurs in the 30 to 40 percent of nephrons that originate in the juxtamedullary region and send long loops into the inner medulla.

Fig. 35-6. Function of peritubular capillaries. This schematic depicts the factors that control uptake of solute and water from the peritubular interstitium into the peritubular capillaries. Solute enters the interstitium across the tubular cells via transporters located in the cell wall (see Fig. 35-3) or between cells through "leaky" tight junctions. Starling's forces then control uptake into the capillaries. Normal values for interstitial pressures are not known.

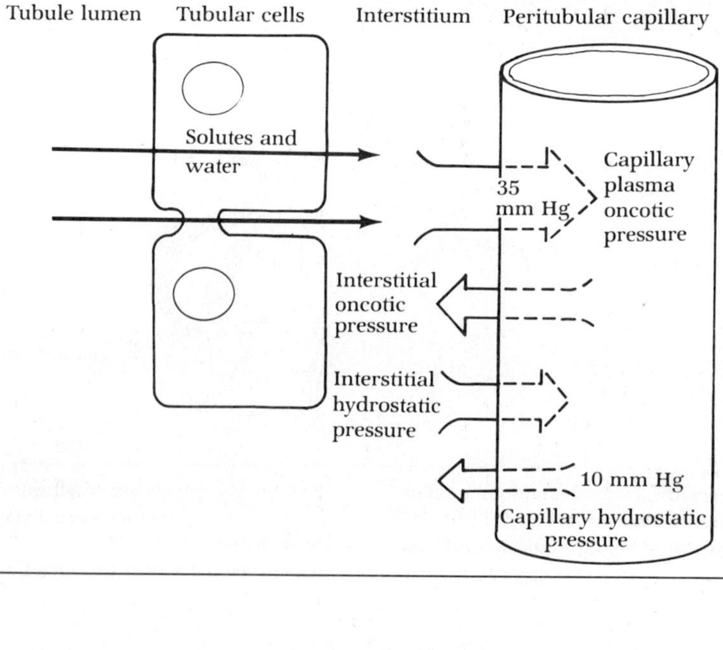

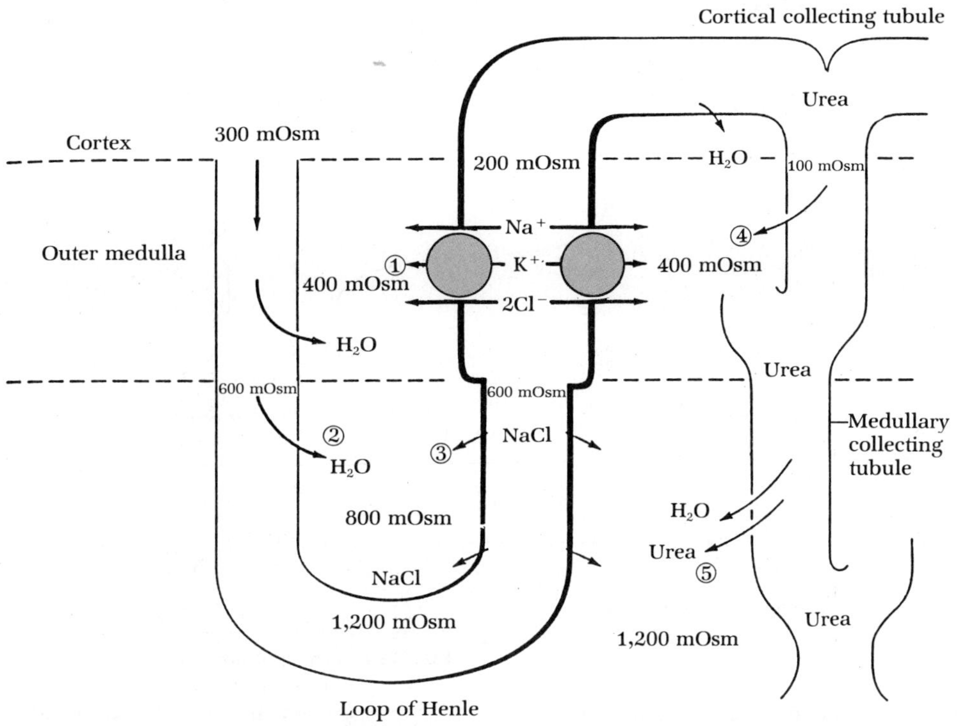

Fig. 35-7. Counter-current multiplier. Active transport of sodium chloride out of the thick ascending limb of Henle's loop (1) creates a small gradient between the tubular lumen and surrounding interstitium. Passive water movement following the concentration gradient out of the descending limb (2) increases the tonicity of tubular fluid descending toward the tip of the loop. In the water-impermeable thin ascending limb, sodium chloride passively follows a concentration gradient from the luminal fluid (3), made progressively more concentrated by repetitions of steps (1) and (2) as the modest transverse gradient across the tubular wall is multiplied into a steep axial gradient by the countercurrent flow between the limbs of the loop. Water reabsorption from the water-permeable cortical collecting tubule (4) raises urea concentration in the tubule and promotes urea movement from the medullary collecting tubule into the interstitium, enhancing interstitial tonicity (5). The tonicities in the schematic represent the approximate maximal values created by the countercurrent multiplier. (Modified from B. D. Rose. *Clinical Physiology of Acid-Base and Electrolyte Disorders* [3rd ed.]. New York: McGraw-Hill, 1989.)

Active sodium chloride reabsorption in the TALH increases the tonicity of the interstitium, generating an osmotic and concentration gradient that promotes passive movement of water and solutes from the descending and thin ascending limbs of the loop, respectively (Fig. 35-7). Even though the gradient from tubular lumen to interstitium is limited at any level of the renal medulla, the hairpin configuration, with fluid in adjacent tubular segments flowing in opposite directions, allows a substantial increase in osmolarity to occur at the bend of the loop, as fluid leaving the descending limb becomes progressively hypertonic secondary to water moving into the hypertonic interstitium. In addition, urea, passively leaving the collecting tubule, contributes equally to the creation of medullary tonicity, which can reach 900 to 1,200 mOsm/kg, and provides a steep gradient across the lining of the collecting tubule. In the presence of ADH, this gradient promotes urinary concentration (see later in text). The tonicity of the medullary interstitium is protected from dilution as water entering the interstitium is carried away by the vasa recta (see Fig. 35-2).

Finally, the distal and collecting tubules, responsible for regulated absorption and secretion of water, potassium, calcium, and protons, provide the final pathway to conserve or eliminate water and these physiologically important solutes. Details of these mechanisms are discussed later in this chapter.

Sodium reabsorption occurs along the entire nephron, with the majority in the proximal tubule (50–70% of filtered load) and Henle's loop (25–30%). Distal tubular and collecting duct reabsorption, though of lesser magnitude, provides the critical final control. Sodium is reabsorbed isotonically in the proximal tubule, about two-thirds of this via an active process driven by basolateral membrane Na-K-ATPase pumping sodium out of the cell into the peritubular interstitium (Fig. 35-8). This lowers intracellular sodium concentration and facilitates sodium uptake from the luminal fluid via cotransporters on the luminal membrane that "absorb" sodium in conjunction with bicarbonate, glucose, amino acids, phosphate, and other organic acids. In later segments of the proximal tubule, coupled countertransport of sodium and hydrogen is the primary active mechanism for sodium reabsorption. Passive reabsorption also occurs as sodium follows the electrical gradient, in part created by chloride reabsorption down a concentration gradient generated by greater reabsorption of bicarbonate proximally. Passive sodium chloride reabsorption probably occurs through the "leaky" paracellular pathways, which are more permeable to chloride than other anions (see Figs. 35-6 and 35-8).

The epithelium of the descending limb of Henle's loop is impermeable to sodium, but this is not so in the ascending

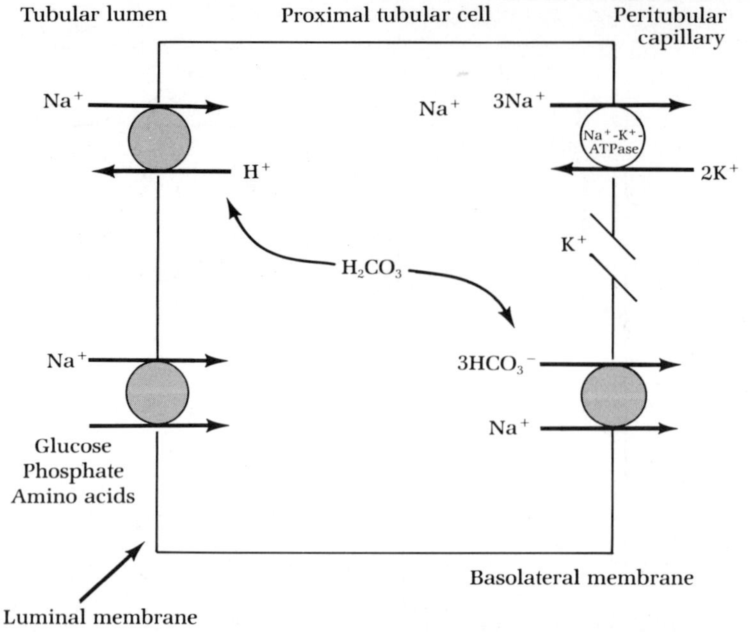

Fig. 35-8. Proximal tubular transporters. Active excretion of sodium out of cells via Na-K-ATPase in the basolateral membrane creates a gradient that favors uptake of sodium into the cell across the luminal membrane. Various cotransporters couple sodium uptake with that of glucose, phosphate, and amino acids such that their reabsorption across the luminal membrane is essentially powered by basolateral Na-K-ATPase. Antiporters that exchange sodium for hydrogen also exist. Note also the tendency for potassium to leak down its concentration gradient into the interstitium, where it can be removed by peritubular capillaries and returned to the circulation.

limb, where sodium moves passively along gradients set up by active chloride reabsorption. As this segment is impermeable to water, the fluid in the tubular lumen is made dilute and the medullary interstitium is made concentrated (see Fig. 35-7). Significant active reabsorption of sodium occurs in the thick ascending limb of the loop via sodium chloride–potassium cotransporters (Fig. 35-9), as well as sodium-hydrogen and chloride-bicarbonate antiporters. Active sodium reabsorption continues in the distal convoluted tubule via several recently described mechanisms (Fig. 35-10).

Final adjustment of sodium excretion occurs in the collecting duct, where prominent roles are played by aldosterone and natriuretic peptides. The mechanisms of these actions are discussed in the following section.

Renal Handling of Potassium

Potassium is freely filtered at the glomerulus, and 90 to 95 percent is reabsorbed before the filtrate reaches the early distal tubule. The proximal convoluted tubule accounts for 50 to 70 percent of reabsorption, mainly coupled to sodium and water (see Fig. 35-8), and 20 to 40 percent is reabsorbed in the thick ascending limb of Henle's loop.

Both secretory and reabsorptive capacities are present in the distal tubule, which generally receives less than 10 percent of filtered potassium but is responsible for the major adjustments in potassium excretion, largely affected by the principal cells. Na-K-ATPase in the basolateral cell membrane loads these cells with potassium, which then diffuses passively across the luminal membrane down its concentration or electrical gradient, or both (Fig. 35-11). Principal cells adapt to chronic potassium loading by increasing the surface area of the basolateral membrane, which increases Na-K-ATPase activity. The latter is controlled by aldosterone.

Though the distal nephron usually exhibits net potassium secretion, the capacity to reabsorb potassium persists and at times affects net absorption. The luminal surface of intercalated cells, a subpopulation of cells in the collecting tubule, demonstrates amplification of surface area in states of potassium depletion, presumably facilitating increased potassium reabsorption, by K-Cl coupled transporters, or possibly luminal Na-K-ATPase.

Renal Mechanisms of Acid-Base Homeostasis

The kidney is also critical in regulating acid-base balance, since it is responsible both for reclamation of the large amount of bicarbonate filtered at the glomerulus, as well as excretion of organic acids and protons and regeneration of new buffer in the process. Details of these mechanisms are described in Chap. 38.

In essence, reclamation of the huge amount of bicarbonate filtered daily (approximately 25 mEq per liter $\times$ 180 liters per day $\rightarrow$ 4,500 mEq) is achieved in the proximal tubule, where carbonic acid is formed in a reaction between water and carbon dioxide, catalyzed by intracellular carbonic anhydrase. The acid dissociates into a proton and bicarbonate, and the proton enters the tubular lumen via coupled transport in exchange for reabsorbed sodium and combines with filtered bicarbonate, which will eventually dissociate into water and carbon dioxide and be excreted. The bicarbonate generated in the cell enters the peritubular interstitium and ultimately returns to the circulation by uptake into peritubular capillaries via coupled transport with sodium. Thus, a

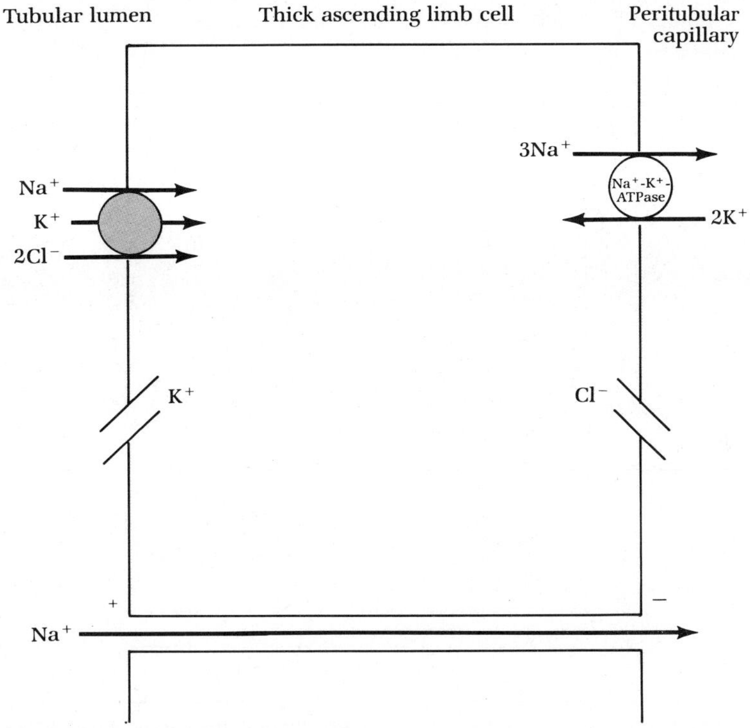

Fig. 35-9. Transporters in the thick ascending limb of the loop of Henle. Energy for luminal cotransport of Na-K-2Cl is indirectly provided by basolateral Na-K-ATPase activity. Note that back leak of potassium into the lumen creates a lumen-positive setting that favors the occurrence of sodium movement passively via paracellular pathways. (From B. D. Rose. *Clinical Physiology of Acid-Base and Electrolyte Disorders* [3rd ed.]. New York: McGraw-Hill, 1989. Reproduced with permission.)

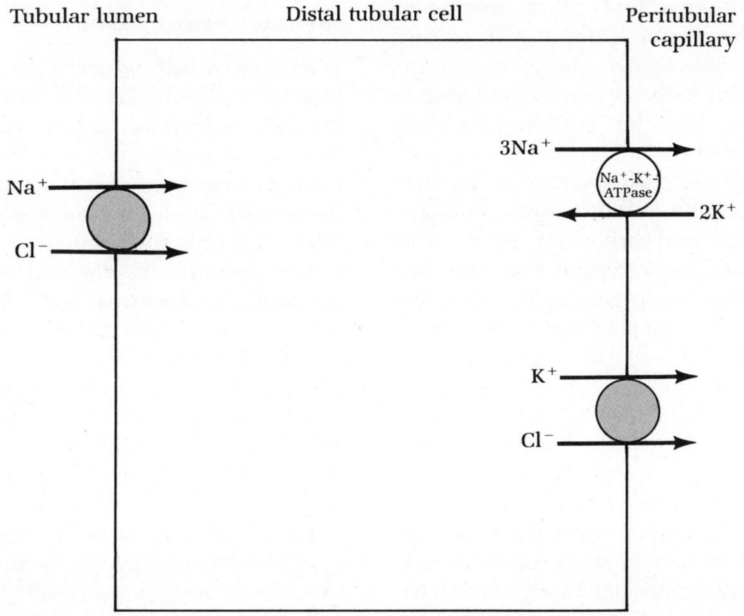

Fig. 35-10. Transport in the distal convoluted tubule. The active transport generated by basolateral membrane Na-K-ATPase creates an intracellular milieu favorable to both luminal sodium chloride cotransport into the cell and basolateral KCl cotransport out of the cell into the interstitium. (From B. D. Rose. *Clinical Physiology of Acid-Base and Electrolyte Disorders* [3rd ed.]. New York: McGraw-Hill, 1989. Reproduced with permission.)

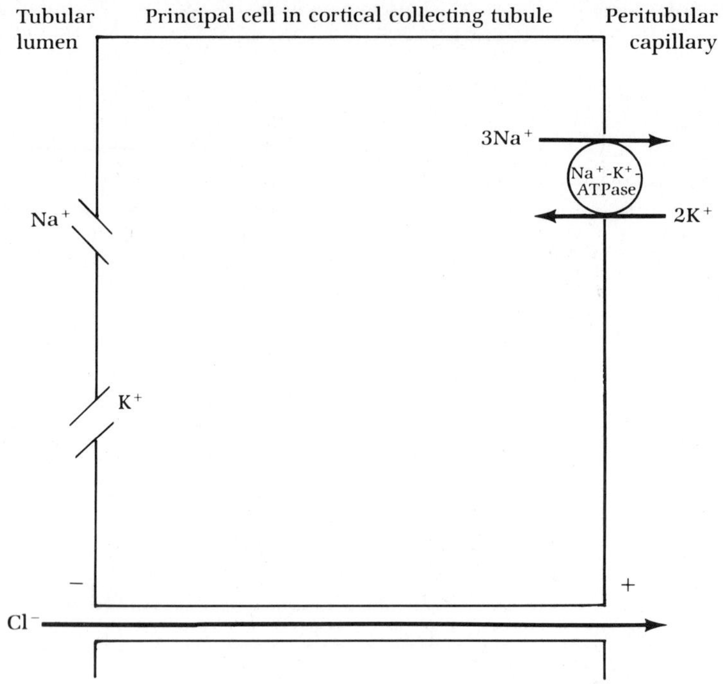

Fig. 35-11. Potassium secretion. Principal cells in the cortical collecting tubules secrete potassium down a concentration gradient created by basolateral Na-K-ATPase activity. In addition, the uptake of sodium from the lumen down its concentration gradient (also created by Na-K-ATPase activity) creates an electronegative lumen, and both potassium secretion across the luminal membrane and chloride reabsorption via paracellular pathways are favored. Aldosterone stimulates these processes in a variety of ways (see text). (From B. D. Rose. *Clinical Physiology of Acid-Base and Electrolyte Disorders* [3rd ed.]. New York: McGraw-Hill, 1989. Reproduced with permission.)

molecule of bicarbonate is reclaimed to compensate for the one that is filtered (Fig. 35-12).

In the collecting tubule, carbonic acid is formed in a similar fashion, and protons are excreted, though not via countertransport with sodium, but rather via a voltage-dependent process in which protons follow the electrical gradient into the tubular lumen, made electronegative by independent sodium uptake into the cells. In the lumen the proton can combine with weak acids, primarily HPO_4^2 (so-called titratable acid) and the base ammonia (NH_3), forming ions that cannot back leak out of the tubular lumen; thus, protons are excreted without loss of bicarbonate (Fig. 35-13). In fact, the bicarbonate generated intracellularly by breakdown of carbonic acid is free to return to the systemic circulation as regenerated buffer, repleting base lost buffering the daily acid load produced by normal metabolism (approximately 70–100 mEq). Regulation of hydrogen excretion by changes in circulating volume, aldosterone, and serum potassium concentrations, as well as dissolved carbon dioxide and arterial pH, allows adjustment of acid secretion to compensate for processes that tend to disturb acid-base balance. Further discussion of renal mechanisms of acid-base homeostasis can be found in Chap. 38.

VOLUME REGULATION

Control of body fluid volume is primarily affected by renal handling of sodium and its accompanying anions, as these constitute greater than 90 percent of the solutes in extracellular fluid. A complex array of monitoring and effector mechanisms influence sodium balance and, thus, volume status, a system largely separate from, and more complex than, that regulating body fluid tonicity, the osmoreceptor–pituitary–antidiuretic hormone–renal axis, which is discussed later in this chapter.

Afferent (Sensor) Limb

Mechanisms exist whereby the level of extracellular and intravascular fluid volume is assayed to provide signals affecting sodium balance. Volume receptors have been described in both the high-pressure, arterial side of the circulation and the low-pressure, venous capacitance side. In some manner, these integrate a message that defines effective circulatory volume, a ratio of volume to capacity.

Low-pressure receptors have been described in the atria and intrathoracic great veins, in which acute volume alterations induce compensatory changes in renal salt excretion. Volume expansion leads to natriuresis, partly by local release of atrial natriuretic peptide as well as inhibition of antidiuretic hormone (ADH) release, promoting excretion of solute and water. Chronic changes, however, can decrease the sensitivity of volume receptors and blunt signals for natriuresis, possibly playing a role in the maintenance of salt retention, as in congestive heart failure.

Arterial baroreceptors in the carotid sinuses and aortic arch sense changes in blood pressure or wall tension and induce change in sympathetic nervous system activity that affects renal salt excretion. Given a sufficiently large decrement in pressure or volume, these baroreceptors also stimulate ADH release.

Finally, *an intrarenal baroreceptor,* the juxtaglomerular

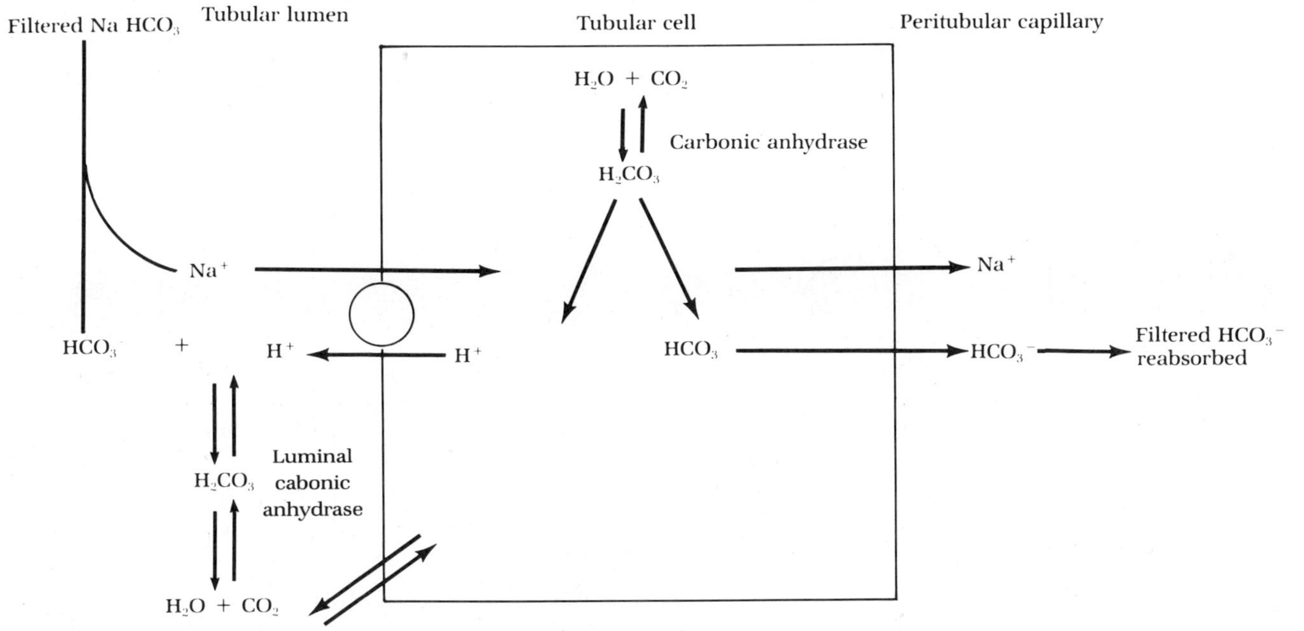

Fig. 35-12. Bicarbonate reabsorption. Intracellular carbonic acid (H_2CO_3), formed from CO_2 and H_2O, dissociates into H_2 and bicarbonate (HCO_3^-). The latter returns to the peritubular capillary across the peritubular membrane, while the former is secreted into the lumen via Na-H antiporters. The secreted H^+ combines with HCO_3^- in the filtrate, forming H_2CO_3, which then dissociates into H_2O and CO_2. The net effect is HCO_3 reabsorption, though the HCO_3 returning to the systemic circulation is not the same molecule as that which had been filtered in the glomerulus.

apparatus, appears to play a role in volume regulation (Fig. 35-14). Juxtaglomerular cells, specialized cells in the walls of the afferent arteriole, release renin in response to decreased pressure in the arteriole. In addition, stretch receptors in this region of the arteriole may have a role in regulation of sympathetic nervous system activity, and the composition of the fluid that reaches the adjacent macula densa segment of the distal tubule likewise affects renin release. Renin is a proteolytic enzyme that releases the decapeptide angiotensin I from renin substrate. Subsequent catalysis of angiotensin I by converting enzyme yields angiotensin II, a potent vasoconstrictor and antinatriuretic hormone that both affects tubular reabsorption directly and stimulates adrenal secretion of another antinatriuretic hormone, aldosterone.

Efferent (Effector) Limb

Early descriptions of the mechanisms that control renal sodium excretion postulated effects of filtered sodium load, a function of GFR; aldosterone; and a nebulous "third factor" to account for inconsistencies and inadequacies of the other two factors in explaining all observed phenomena. The nature of this third factor has more recently been elucidated, at least in part. It is more likely a multiplicity of factors, both humoral and nonhumoral, the most important of which are: natriuretic hormones, prostanoids, angiotensin II, the sympathetic nervous system, and physical factors—that is, Starling's forces operating on the postglomerular-peritubular capillaries.

Autoregulation and Other Glomerular Mechanisms of Volume Regulation

Though it appears that the filtered load of sodium should play a role in regulating sodium excretion, several factors moderate this effect. Renal autoregulation tends to maintain GFR at a relatively constant level over a wide range of renal perfusion pressures. In conditions of elevated pressure secondary to expansion of circulating volume, the expected natriuresis may be blunted. The filtered load of sodium may not increase proportional to the expanded plasma volume, as intrinsic afferent arteriolar constriction dampens the transmission of increased systemic perfusion pressure to the glomerular capillary.

Differential responses of afferent and efferent arterioles are critical for protection of renal function during periods of hemodynamic stress (e.g., hypotension-hypovolemia), in which the generalized response is vasoconstriction, largely induced by angiotensin II and catecholamines. The renal circulation, among others, is potentially compromised in this setting, but GFR tends to be preserved by preferential constriction of the efferent arteriole and opposition of afferent arteriolar constriction by locally produced prostaglandins, endothelial-derived relaxant factors, and possibly kinins, stimulated by angiotensin II and norepinephrine (see Fig. 35-5). The preservation of intraglomerular capillary hydrostatic pressure assures ongoing filtration. Profound states of vascular collapse or prostaglandin synthesis and converting enzyme inhibitors can overwhelm or block these protective mechanisms and compromise renal function.

Glomerular filtration rate is also affected by glomerular capillary surface area and permeability, which can be decreased by angiotensin II–induced contraction of the glomerular mesangium (see Fig. 35-4), the cells that support glomerular capillaries. By inducing arteriolar constriction,

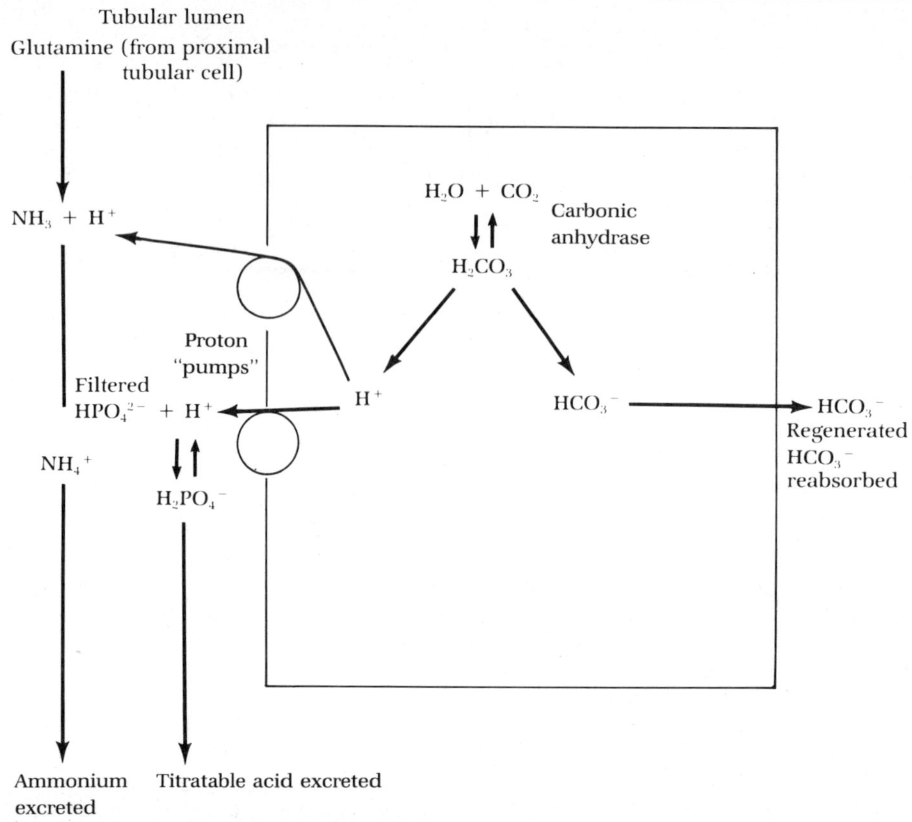

Fig. 35-13. Bicarbonate regeneration. In distal tubular cells, H_2O and CO_2 combine in a reaction catalyzed by carbonic anhydrase and form H_2CO_3. The bicarbonate is reabsorbed in the peritubular capillary and returned to the systemic circulation, while the hydrogen ion is secreted into the lumen. In the lumen, it can combine with NH_3 to form ammonium ions that cannot be reabsorbed back into the tubular cell, or the hydrogen ion can combine with urinary HPO_4^{2-} to form H_2PO_4 ion, which likewise cannot return through the tubular cell. Thus, a hydrogen ion is excreted and not buffered by filtered bicarbonate. Therefore, the bicarbonate returning to the circulation is new bicarbonate—that is, it has been generated to replace bicarbonate that was previously lost in the act of buffering the acid load produced by normal metabolism. Several types of proton "pumps" are located on the luminal cell surface.

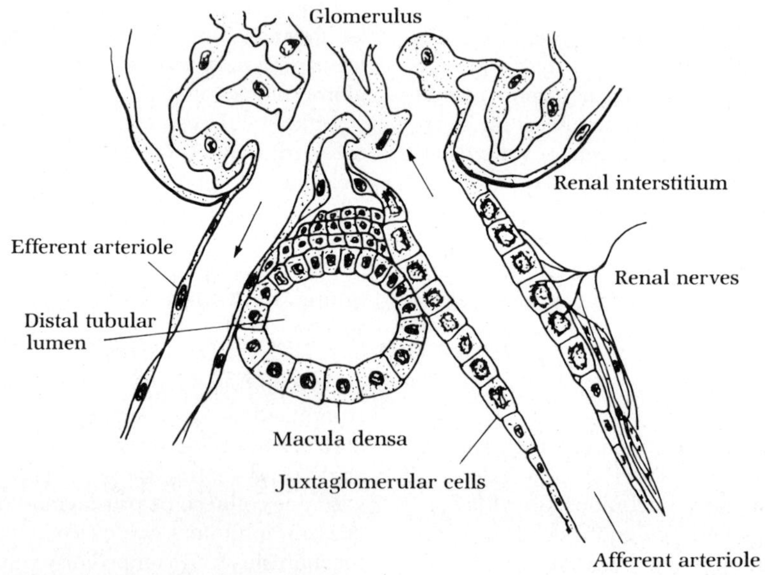

Fig. 35-14. Juxtaglomerular apparatus. Specialized cells in the wall of the afferent arterioles secrete renin in response to decreased perfusion pressure. Stretch receptors also influence the sympathetic nervous system at well as renin release. Finally, specialized cells in the macula densa of the distal tubule likewise influence renin release, possibly as a result of sampling the composition of tubular fluid. Renin subsequently promotes synthesis of the vasoconstrictor and antinatriuretic peptide angiotensin II, as well as the antinatriuretic hormone aldosterone. (From B. D. Rose. *Clinical Physiology of Acid-Base and Electrolyte Disorders* [3rd ed.]. New York: McGraw-Hill, 1989. Reproduced with permission.)

angiotensin II also causes renal plasma flow to fall and increases the *filtration fraction*, which is the percentage of renal blood flow filtered into Bowman's space. As more fluid leaves the capillaries and enters Bowman's space, the oncotic pressure of capillary blood is increased and hydrostatic pressure is lowered. Both factors tend to increase sodium reabsorption by decreasing the rate of sodium back leak into the tubular lumen and enhancing the return of sodium to the systemic circulation via uptake into the postglomerular capillaries (see Fig. 35-6).

Increases in GFR that increase delivery to the distal nephron can, via *tubuloglomerular feedback*, dampen the rise in GFR by unclear mechanisms related to the response of the macula densa to changes in distal tubular flow, which appear to induce afferent arteriolar constriction and alter capillary permeability. In addition, the largely unexplained phenomenon of *glomerulotubular balance* dampens the effect of changes of filtered load on sodium excretion, since the percentage of solute reabsorbed is kept constant, as are the quantity and composition of fluid delivered to the distal nephron. In summary, autoregulation, tubuloglomerular feedback, and glomerulotubular balance all prevent distal delivery from overwhelming the somewhat limited reabsorptive capacities of the collecting tubules, preserving for this region of the nephron the ability to make small but important adjustments in excretion to balance changes in fluid and solute intake.

Aldosterone

Aldosterone, a steroid hormone synthesized in the adrenal zona glomerulosa, is stimulated by hyperkalemia or angiotensin II, which, in turn, is stimulated by hypovolemia-induced renin release. Its principal effects are to increase reabsorption of sodium and chloride and secretion of potassium and hydrogen. When aldosterone binds to and enters epithelial cells lining the renal tubules, it binds to specific cytoplasmic receptors. The hormone-receptor complex moves into the nucleus and initiates ribonucleic acid transcription and protein synthesis by binding to an intranuclear receptor. The newly synthesized proteins mediate in some manner aldosterone's physiologic effects to increase sodium reabsorption and potassium secretion, possibly by increasing the quantity of basolateral membrane Na-K-ATPase or increasing its activity, or both, and perhaps altering membrane phospholipids and luminal membrane permeability. This sequence is blocked by the diuretic spironolactone, which competitively binds to the cell membrane receptor for aldosterone.

Aldosterone is not the major acute regulator of sodium excretion, as evidenced by the acute onset of natriuresis with salt loading and the significant lag time that is required for aldosterone to affect protein synthesis. Also, patients with hyperaldosteronism, or those who are receiving fixed doses of exogenous mineralocorticoids with aldosteronelike activity, "escape" from progressive sodium retention and maintain a new, steady state of sodium balance.

Atrial Natriuretic Peptide

Considerable attention has focused on various natriuretic hormones. In response to maneuvers that increase atrial pressure, such as volume expansion or balloon dilatation, a peptide hormone has been noted to be released from granules stored in the atria. This atrial natriuretic peptide (ANP), or factor ANF, has been shown to be a vasodilator, both directly and possibly by decreasing angiotensin II levels and effect. This vasodilatation, which in the renal circulation primarily affects afferent arterioles, is somewhat dependent on the state of preexisting vasoconstriction. In fact, when prior vasodilatation predominates, ANP can cause mild constriction. ANP also inhibits aldosterone release from the adrenal gland and ADH release from the pituitary and impairs angiotensin II–induced thirst. Afferent arteriolar dilatation causes an increased filtration fraction, increasing proximal sodium reabsorption, but this is offset by the increased filtered load of sodium that is in part passed through to the loop and distal nephrons. ANP has little effect on loop function, but in the cortical and medullary collecting ducts, it impairs the response to ADH, thus promoting a water diuresis, and decreases sodium transport in the medullary collecting duct, possibly via decreased aldosterone levels and direct effects on tubular function. Finally, increased medullary blood flow caused by ANP can "wash out" interstitial tonicity, contributing to increased free water clearance. Thus, ANP can induce both a natriuresis and a diuresis. The true physiologic significance of ANP vis-à-vis other regulators of volume balance is not as yet clear.

Other Natriuretic Mediators

Other hormonal mediators of sodium excretion have been proposed—for example, an endogenous "ouabainlike" hormone that inhibits basolateral Na-K-ATPase. Angiotensin II plays a role by virtue of its promotion of aldosterone synthesis, constrictor effects on systemic and intrarenal arteriolar tone, and, possibly, a direct effect on proximal tubular function. Prostaglandins, because of their vasodilatory properties, can modulate the antinatriuretic effects of angiotensin II. Other mediators of renal salt handling include the sympathetic nervous system and the several "physical" factors that influence Starling's forces in the postglomerular-peritubular capillaries (see previous section). Adrenergic activation affects both systemic and renal hemodynamics, and, in general, has antinatriuretic effects.

When renal function is normal, the capacity to reabsorb sodium and thus preserve or expand body fluid volume is remarkably effective, as daily excretion of sodium can be reduced to less than 5 mEq, or about $^2/_{10}$ of 1 percent of the daily filtered sodium load. Sodium excretion during natriuresis can increase by more than 100-fold. This range of response allows maintenance of normal body fluid volume under widely varied challenges. On the other hand, impaired ability to conserve sodium can contribute to states of marked volume depletion, while inappropriate avidity for sodium leads to edema.

Regulation of Potassium Balance

Both hormonal and nonhormonal factors regulate renal transport activities that contribute to potassium balance (Table 35-1). Aldosterone plays a dominant role, increasing the activity of basolateral cell membrane Na-K-ATPase, luminal membrane potassium conductance, and sodium reabsorption across the luminal membrane, which in turn increases luminal electronegativity and favors potassium crossing the

Table 35-1. Renal mechanisms of potassium homeostasis

Hormonal
Aldosterone
Glucocorticoids
ADH
Catecholamines
Insulin?
Nonhormonal
Distal tubule flow
Distal tubule sodium concentration/delivery
Distal tubule lumen electronegativity
Nature of anion in distal lumen
Magnesium
Serum potassium concentration
pH
Drugs
Diuretics
Sodium penicillin derivatives
Gentamicin
Old tetracycline
Amphotericin B
Rifampin
Polymyxin B
Cis-platinum
L-dopa
Lithium
Toluene
Thallium
Carbenoxolone

membrane into the tubular lumen. Acute increases in potassium excretion initially can be opposed by decreased delivery of filtrate to the distal nephron secondary to aldosterone's antinatriuretic effect, but net secretion will ensue once aldosterone-induced volume expansion restores adequate distal sodium and volume delivery. In fact, any state of increased distal delivery—for example, volume loading, or diuretics in patients with secondary hyperaldosteronism, as in congestive heart failure—will augment the kaliuretic effect of aldosterone.

Glucocorticoids augment potassium secretion through hemodynamic changes, resulting in increased GFR and urine flow rate, though evidence suggests a direct effect on Na-K-ATPase. Antidiuretic hormone exerts both direct and indirect effects, which tend to oppose each other, but generally net secretion results. Insulin or catecholamines, which enhance extrarenal cellular uptake, can also impair potassium secretion by direct inhibitory effect on collecting tubule secretory cells.

Potassium secretion varies directly with changes in distal tubule luminal flow rate. Distal delivery of sodium and luminal sodium concentration influence potassium secretion, primarily because of the generation of luminal electronegativity from sodium reabsorption. When luminal concentration of sodium falls below 30 mM, potassium secretion is limited. This can occur during water diuresis, marked sodium depletion, or mineralocorticoid excess. If chloride concentration falls below 10 mM, sodium/potassium chloride–coupled reabsorption in the TALH is decreased and potassium excretion is increased. In addition, if less permeable anions such as bicarbonate or certain drugs—for example, sodium penicillin derivatives—replace chloride, luminal electronegativity is increased and potassium secretion is augmented. Magnesium depletion is often associated with potassium depletion, and correction of potassium deficits can be difficult without prior magnesium repletion.

Acid-base status affects renal handling of potassium by several mechanisms. First, extracellular pH influences intracellular potassium concentration by shifting potassium into cells during alkalosis and out of cells during acidosis. Thus, in alkalosis, distal tubule cells are "loaded" and the gradient for efflux to the lumen is increased. In addition, because of the increase in luminal bicarbonate, the electrical gradient also favors potassium secretion. Acute acidosis causes opposite effects, though chronic acidosis can augment potassium secretion by decreasing proximal sodium reabsorption, increasing distal flow.

Finally, many drugs affect excretion of potassium. Diuretics, in general, cause increased potassium secretion by several mechanisms: increased distal urine and sodium delivery, stimulation of aldosterone secretion secondary to volume depletion, and increased delivery of nonabsorbable anions such as bicarbonate during diuretic-induced alkalosis. Loop diuretics directly block potassium reabsorption in the TALH, and thiazide diuretics block reabsorption in the distal tubule. Osmotic diuretics increase potassium secretion primarily by increased distal fluid delivery. Potassium-sparing diuretics induce less diuresis-natriuresis and therefore less volume contraction and alkalosis. In addition, they interfere directly with tubular transport of potassium. Amiloride blocks sodium conductance channels of distal tubule luminal membrane, resulting in decreased generation of luminal electronegativity. Triamterene may work in a similar way. Spironolactone competitively blocks aldosterone's effect, and therefore its action depends on ambient aldosterone levels.

Other medications that augment potassium secretion are listed in Table 35-1. Antibiotics, such as carbenicillin, which present both a large sodium load and nonreabsorbable anion to the distal tubule, cause potassium wasting. Gentamicin and several other antibiotics increase potassium secretion by unknown mechanisms. Amphotericin B increases potassium permeability across the distal tubule luminal membrane, and outdated tetracycline induces a proximal renal tubular acidosis with potassium wasting. Cis-platinum increases sodium permeability in the collecting duct, increasing luminal electronegativity while also causing magnesium depletion. Carbenoxolone and excessive ingestion of licorice and certain chewing tobaccos can induce potassium wasting by aldosteronelike action. Finally, lithium can cause increased renal potassium losses.

REGULATION OF OSMOLAR HOMEOSTASIS

Osmolality of solutions is determined by the presence of solutes in solution. As cell membranes are usually permeable to water and less so to the passive movements of certain solutes, the osmolality created by these solutes determines the distribution of body water among the several fluid compartments kept separate by cellular membranes. Changes in osmolar gradients across membranes will induce water movement from compartments with lower osmolality, and therefore more water relative to solute, to those of higher osmolality or tonicity, and result in dehydration and overhydration of the respective compartments. The relative volume changes that result, particularly in cells of the central nervous system (CNS), can induce clinically significant syndromes. As sodium salts, primarily sodium chloride and sodium bicarbonate, constitute the major osmotically active particles in extracellular fluid, and as water movement across cell membranes maintains osmotic equality between extracellular and intracellular fluids, the concentration of sodium in serum is proportional to serum osmolality and reflects osmolality within cells as well. Hypernatremia reflects hyperosmolality and hyponatremia usually indicates hypoosmolality.

Control of serum tonicity depends on components of the CNS, the kidney, and a peptide hormone, vasopressin or ADH. Osmoreceptors in the brain control release of ADH by the posterior pituitary, and ADH affects retention of free water by the kidney. The system forms a feedback loop that normally maintains serum sodium concentration and, thus, tonicity, within close limits of 135 to 145 mEq Na per liter or 280 to 295 mOsm per liter.

Antidiuretic Hormone

In the presence of ADH, renal conservation of free water is maximized, producing a concentrated urine while lowering plasma osmolality. The dilute urine produced in the absence of ADH eliminates free water from the body and elevates plasma osmolality.

Antidiuretic hormone (or arginine vasopressin) secretion is very low or even nondetectable when plasma osmolality is less than 280 mOsm/kg, but as osmolality increases over 280, ADH secretion rises in a linear manner. Areas of the anterior hypothalamus monitor plasma osmolality and induce ADH secretion from the posterior pituitary by neural impulses, causing exocytosis of ADH that was previously synthesized in the hypothalamic neurons and transported to the pituitary for storage. Antidiuretic hormone, only slightly protein bound, is rapidly cleared from the blood with a half-life of 10 to 25 minutes.

Control of ADH Release

OSMOTICALLY ACTIVE SOLUTES. Only osmotically active solutes—that is, those that generate a transmembrane osmotic gradient—induce ADH release. Sodium chloride and solutes, such as mannitol, which are limited to the extracellular space, act as "effective" osmols, whereas urea is only about 25 percent as "effective" and glucose, though it induces an osmotic gradient, is actually not very effective. Although the osmotic threshold does not usually change with advancing age, older patients tend to secrete greater amounts of ADH for a given osmotic stimulus. Pregnancy causes a resetting of the osmostat, with plasma osmolality running 2 to 4 percent less than normal throughout gestation.

BLOOD PRESSURE AND VASCULAR VOLUME. Also important in regulation of ADH secretion are blood pressure and vascular volume; a fall of sufficient magnitude in either induces ADH release. Stretch receptors in the left atrium and baroreceptors in the aortic arch and carotid sinuses detect volume and blood-pressure changes, respectively, and send impulses to the CNS via vagal and glossopharyngeal nerves. Though relatively small changes in osmolality (e.g., 2%) induce maximum osmotically stimulated increases in ADH secretion, greater degrees of change in volume or pressure (e.g., 10–15%) are required to elicit a response. However, once ADH secretion is induced by these nonosmotic stimuli, there is an exponential, not linear, rise in secretion, and the significantly higher level of ADH required for pressor effects is achieved.

THIRST. An important but less well-understood mediator of osmolar homeostasis is thirst, which most normal individuals rarely experience at full intensity, as both anticipatory and habitual drinking satisfy most requirements for water intake. The thirst "centers," located close to, but not identical with, the hypothalamic centers that regulate ADH release, also respond to osmotic and hemodynamic stimuli, though the thresholds are greater; for example, thirst is "turned on" when serum osmolality exceeds approximately 290 mOsm/kg, a level at which maximal antidiuresis from ADH is already in effect. This response is also governed only by osmotically active solutes—for example, sodium and mannitol, not glucose or urea. The renin–angiotensin II system also stimulates thirst, though the importance of its role in most physiologic states is unclear.

OTHER FACTORS. ADH secretion can be influenced by several other factors, such as nausea, with or without emesis. This may be the major mechanism by which opiates induce ADH release. Hypoxia can cause ADH release by a similar mechanism or secondary to its hypotensive effect. Glucopenia induces moderate increases in ADH release, possibly via alterations in CNS metabolism, rather than by induction of an osmotic gradient. Other potential stimuli for ADH release are norepinephrine and angiotensin II, which directly affect ADH release but indirectly depress release secondary to increased blood pressure; cholinergic agonists, which stimulate ADH release; and prostaglandins, as well as other drugs that promote ADH release or potentiate its action (see Table 36-4).

Mechanism of ADH Action

In the absence of ADH, the cells of the collecting ducts are water impermeable, and the filtrate remains dilute through its passage to the lower urinary tract; urine with osmolality as low as 50 mOsm/kg, or specific gravity of approximately 1.003, is produced. In this way, the normal kidney is capable of excreting 15 to 20 liters of free water each day.

The presence of ADH allows reabsorption of free water into the medullary interstitium surrounding collecting tubules, producing urine with a concentration of up to 1,200 mOsm/kg or specific gravity of about 1.030. The capacity of the kidney to greatly alter the filtrate made dilute more proximally depends on both ADH and the hypertonicity of the medullary interstitium, which is created and maintained by active sodium chloride reabsorption from Henle's loop and passive urea movement from collecting tubules. The vasa recta clear the reabsorbed water and contribute to maintenance of medullary tonicity (see previous discussion).

The mechanism by which ADH exerts its influence on cells of the collecting duct has been explored in considerable detail. Basically, ADH binds to a receptor on the basolateral membrane of these cells and activates adenylate cyclase, which produces intracellular cyclic adenosine monophosphate (cAMP); this in turn activates a protein, ultimately causing formation and insertion of intramembranous particle aggregates in the apical luminal membrane. These aggregates may function as channels for water movement.

Several physiologic factors affect ADH action at the cellular level. Prostaglandins antagonize ADH action, possibly via a direct effect on adenylate cyclase, but also by impairing sodium chloride reabsorption in the TALH and urea reabsorption from the inner medullary collecting duct, and promoting washout of the medullary gradient secondary to increased medullary blood flow. Kinins may have similar effects. Adrenal steroids decrease phosphodiesterase activity and thus augment the effect of ADH via increasing levels of cyclic AMP. Alpha catecholamines interfere with adenylate cyclase stimulation and can affect ADH release. Beta catecholamines can have opposite effects. Hypokalemia impairs the response of the collecting tubule to ADH, as does hypercalcemia. Both electrolyte disturbances also induce thirst and cause a decrease in medullary tonicity. A wide variety of drugs influence the action of ADH on the collecting tubule (see Table 36-4). Some of these, as well as other drugs (e.g., lithium), can also stimulate ADH release or thirst.

Factors Other than Antidiuretic Hormone that Affect Urinary Concentration

Decreased filtered load or increased proximal sodium and water reabsorption impair free water clearance secondary to decreasing distal fluid delivery, thus limiting the amount of free water that can be excreted. In addition, sluggish flow in the collecting tubule allows prolonged exposure of tubular fluid to the concentration gradient with hypertonic medullary interstitium, producing a greater degree of free water reabsorption. Thus, any state of volume depletion can promote urinary concentration even in the absence of ADH. Accelerated filtration rates in states of volume excess have opposite effects.

Diuretics also affect urinary concentration. Thiazides impair sodium reabsorption in the cortical diluting segment, limiting the extent to which the urine can be made dilute. Loop diuretics do the same, but this effect is countered by their action in the TALH, where inhibition of sodium chloride reabsorption limits the creation of a hypertonic medullary interstitium. In fact, urine from a patient who is receiving loop diuretics tends toward osmolality equal to plasma. Diuretic-induced volume depletion can limit free water excretion as noted previously.

SELECTED READING

Brenner, BM, and Rector, FC. *The Kidney* (3rd ed). Philadelphia: Saunders, 1986.

Maxwell, MH, Kleeman, CR, and Narins, RG. *Clinical Disorders of Fluid and Electrolyte Metabolism* (4th ed). New York: McGraw-Hill, 1987.

Rose, BD. *Clinical Physiology of Acid-Base and Electrolyte Disorders* (3rd ed). New York: McGraw-Hill, 1989.

Schrier, RW, and Gottschalk, CW (eds). *Diseases of the Kidney* (4th ed). Boston: Little, Brown, 1988.

36. Disorders of Water Balance and Osmolality: Hypernatremia and Hyponatremia

David M. Poppel

The physician who is evaluating a patient with an abnormal serum sodium concentration must remain aware of the following dictum: Abnormalities of serum sodium concentration are secondary to abnormalities of water balance, not primarily sodium balance. Regulation of serum sodium concentration preserves body fluid osmolality compatible with normal cellular functions. As water is able to move freely across most cell membranes, following its concentration gradient, the concentration of impermeable solutes on either side of cell membranes will influence the relative water volume in both the intra- and extracellular compartments. As sodium and the most common associated anions, chloride and bicarbonate, are the principal solutes in the extracellular space, their concentrations also reflect the concentration of solutes (primarily potassium, chloride, and proteins) inside cells. The ratio of solute to solvent (tonicity or osmolality) influences not only the distribution of body water across cell membranes but also creates the basic physical/chemical milieu for all extra- and intracellular processes. Thus, abnormalities of the serum sodium concentration, as they reflect abnormalities of extra- and intracellular osmolality or tonicity, can lead to pathologic processes secondary to water movement across cell membranes, or impaired biochemical activities, or both.

HYPERNATREMIA

In a survey of hospital admissions, it was found that approximately 1 percent of the patients demonstrated hypernatremia, though only one-third of them were hypernatremic on admission. Most patients were elderly and likely to reside in nursing homes.

Pathophysiology

As described in Chap. 35, urinary concentration depends on the ability to form and maintain a markedly hypertonic medullary interstitium. The presence of antidiuretic hormone (ADH) at the collecting tubules allows concentration of the dilute tubular fluid formed in more proximal parts of the nephron (thick ascending limb of Henle's loop, or TALH, and distal convoluted tubules). This process is impaired by any of the following:

1. Impaired solute reabsorption into the medullary interstitium (e.g., use of loop diuretics)
2. Accelerated urinary losses of the solute delivered to the

reabsorptive segment of Henle's loop (e.g., diuretics, including the osmotic diuresis associated with glycosuria or the obligate solute diuresis in hyperalimentation or renal failure)

3. Accelerated vascular losses of interstitial solute by vasa recta, so-called medullary washout (see Chap. 35)
4. Absence of ADH or impaired alteration of tubular water permeability in response to ADH (e.g., central or nephrogenic diabetes insipidus)
5. Alterations of normal tubular epithelial architecture (e.g., chronic renal failure, sickle cell disease, analgesic abuse, or obstruction)

Hypernatremia is always associated with increased plasma tonicity. However, the reverse is not always true: Hyperosmolality can exist without hypernatremia. The usual cause of this is the presence of solutes such as urea, ethanol, or methanol. Hypertonicity (generally associated with hypernatremia) can be caused by pure water loss, hypotonic fluid loss, or gain of impermeant solutes (e.g., hypertonic sodium chloride, sodium bicarbonate, or mannitol).

Causes

Only some of the disorders listed in Table 36-1 are likely to be seen in the outpatient setting. Many will more likely develop in the hospital.

Central diabetes insipidus secondary to operation or trauma often shows a triphasic pattern of transient polyuria due to functional suppression of ADH release, followed, after four to five days, by excess ADH release, and finally by diabetes insipidus, as ADH stores are exhausted. Central diabetes insipidus often has an abrupt onset and presents with polyuria and polydipsia, but not always hypernatremia, which can be prevented by adequate intake of water. It is important to realize in any case of hypernatremia that urine osmolality need not always be extremely low, as volume depletion, if it occurs, can cause some degree of urinary concentration by mechanisms independent of ADH (see Chap. 35).

Polyuria and polydipsia can occur despite an intact hypothalamic pituitary axis with adequate release of ADH if the response of the distal collecting duct to ADH is impaired. A common cause of this is lithium, which can produce a type of nephrogenic diabetes insipidus even with normal therapeutic levels of this commonly used drug. In addition, the effect of lithium on the tubular cell may be evident for long periods or even indefinitely after the drug has been discontinued. Lithium enters the collecting tubule cell and impedes the ability of ADH to stimulate formation of cyclic adenosine monophosphate, which, as a secondary messenger, ultimately promotes the insertion of water channels into the luminal membrane of the cell. Profound hypokalemia and hypercalcemia also impair cellular response to ADH.

Structural abnormalities of the medullary region can induce functional defects in distal tubular cells as well as diminish the number of such tubules. Disorders that primarily affect the medullary region—for example, obstruction, sickle cell disease, or medullary cystic disease—are the most common causes of this phenomenon. In addition, loop and osmotic diuretics impair the response to ADH by diminishing the tonicity of the medullary interstitium, thus limiting the capacity to concentrate urine.

Table 36-1. Causes of hypernatremia

I. Pure water loss
   A. Central diabetes insipidus
      - Posthypophysectomy
      - Trauma
      - Tumors
      - Granulomas
      - Infections
      - Vascular (cerebrovascular accident, aneurysm, Sheehan's syndrome)
      - Autoimmune (idiopathic)
      - Clonidine
   B. Nephrogenic diabetes insipidus ("true NDI" due to abnormal response of collecting duct to ADH in presence of normal medullary hypertonicity)
      - Familial (usually fully penetrant in men, partially in women)
      - Lithium
      - Demeclocycline
      - Colchicine
      - Methoxyflurane
      - Hypokalemia
      - Hypercalcemia
   C. Renal concentrating defects secondary to abnormal anatomy or solute delivery, or both
      - Acute or chronic renal failure
      - Polycystic kidney disease
      - Obstruction
      - Infection
      - Allergic interstitial nephritis
      - Sarcoidosis
      - Sjögren's disease
      - Myeloma
      - Amyloidosis
      - Sickle cell disease
      - Osmotic diuresis
      - Prolonged diuretic use
   D. Increased insensible water loss
      - Fever
      - High environmental temperatures
      - Thyrotoxicosis
      - Burns or exfoliative dermatitis
      - Hyperventilation
   E. Impaired thirst (primary hypodipsia)

II. Hypotonic fluid losses
   - Vomiting, nasogastric suction, diarrhea
   - Diuretics and osmotic diuresis
   - Skin losses
   - Peritonitis or peritoneal dialysis

III. Solute gain
   - Hypertonic sodium chloride or sodium bicarbonate
   - Dialysis malfunction
   - Incorrect infant-formula dilution

As the solute content of sweat is low, skin losses via excessive sweating primarily eliminate water from the body, and if these losses are not replaced by water intake, hypernatremia can result. Fever, burns, or exfoliative dermatitis and high environmental temperatures are potential causes of such a problem and can be compounded by inadequate access to or ability to ingest water. Other forms of body fluid loss—for example, gastrointestinal (GI) or renal secondary to diuretics, will usually be hypotonic (that is, contain some salt) but at osmolalities below that of plasma. Such losses thus reduce body water content to a greater degree than solute content and hypernatremia results if repletion of water is insufficient.

Clinical Presentation and Evaluation

The emergency department physician should be alert to the possibility of hypernatremia in any patient who is receiving diuretics, manifests polyuria or urinary tract obstruction, or has a history of interstitial renal disease, febrile illness, or use of certain drugs (e.g., lithium). As hypernatremia is unlikely to develop in patients with intact thirst mechanisms and adequate access and ability to obtain drinking water, it should be expected in infants and debilitated or restrained patients or those with impaired mental status. One should suspect hypernatremia especially in the elderly, particularly patients in nursing homes or other institutional settings, and especially when increased insensible water losses, as in febrile states, occur.

Signs and symptoms of hypertonicity depend primarily on the speed with which osmolar changes develop. Slow increases in extracellular (ECF) tonicity allow cells, especially those of the central nervous system (CNS), to generate "idiogenic osmols," such as various proteins and phosphates that retard cellular water loss and prevent cell shrinkage. Rapid changes in cell volume that result from rapid osmolar shifts can cause rupture of cerebral blood vessels, as cells shrink away from the rigid skull wall.

Signs and symptoms will also depend on the cause of hypernatremia, as conditions in which hypotonic fluid losses occur will produce greater changes in ECF volume compared with pure water losses, in which only one-third of the fluid loss comes from the ECF, and of this, only one-fourth from the intravascular space. Signs and symptoms of volume depletion (hypotension, orthostatic changes in blood pressure and pulse, and decreased skin turgor) are more likely with hypotonic fluid loss, in which some degree of salt loss occurs.

Hypernatremic patients often complain of thirst, and dry mucous membranes and decreased sweating may be noted. Neurologic symptoms can range from lethargy and confusion to seizure, coma, and death. Patients will have the signs and symptoms of the various disorders underlying their hypernatremic states—for example, fever, CNS lesions, and intrinsic renal diseases.

History

Often, the underlying cause will be apparent from the history, if the physician pays particular attention to the following: any history of CNS surgery or trauma; family history (e.g., nephrogenic diabetes insipidus); drug use (especially lithium, demeclocycline, colchicine, or diuretics); renal and genitourinary diseases such as interstitial nephritides, urinary tract infections, and/or obstruction; excess GI or renal fluid losses; fever; signs and symptoms of CNS lesions; or conditions associated with hypokalemia or hypercalcemia.

Physical Examination

Physical examination should concentrate on determination of volume status to assess whether water loss has been coincident with some salt loss (e.g., diarrhea or osmotic diuresis), or occurred mainly as free water losses (e.g., central and nephrogenic diabetes insipidus or skin losses). Supine, sitting, and, if possible, standing blood pressure and pulse should be obtained and compared for any significant orthostatic drop in the former or rise in the latter. Comparison with the patient's baseline blood pressure measurements, if known, can confirm relative hypotension in a previously hypertensive patient. Central venous pressure should be estimated by evaluation of the internal or, if necessary, the external jugular venous pulse. Normally, this pulse can be seen approximately 3 cm above the level of the sternal angle. This will be noted when the patient is approximately 30 to 45 degrees above the supine position. If it is necessary for the patient to lie flatter in order for the jugular venous pulse to be seen, its position is likely to be closer to or perhaps even below the level of the sternal angle, indicating a low central venous pressure and an element of volume depletion. In patients with significant volume depletion, the jugular venous pulse may not be apparent even with the patient completely flat. Skin turgor should be assessed as a reflection of interstitial fluid status. Areas such as the thighs, which tend to maintain stable tone and skin elasticity even in the elderly, should be pinched and stretched, while the physician watches for the ability of the tissue to quickly recover from such manipulations. Tenting or delay in recovery indicates decreased interstitial fluid and a volume (salt and water) deficit.

Uncommonly, patients show signs of volume excess, as in primary hyperaldosteronism or Cushing's syndrome, or exposure to hypertonic salt-containing solutions, such as sodium bicarbonate, sodium chloride tablets, or hypertonic dialysis fluid. Edema and elevated venous pressures may be noted. Determination of volume status is important, not only to aid in discovering the cause of hypernatremia but also in guiding therapy, as some patients require salt as well as water repletion; uncommonly, diuresis may be necessary in the patient with volume overload and hypernatremia.

Laboratory Examination

The presence of hypernatremia will be obvious from serum electrolyte determinations. Laboratory results can be helpful in demonstrating hypokalemia, hypercalcemia, glycosuria, pyuria, renal insufficiency, and anemia (raising the possibility of such conditions as myeloma or sickle cell disease).

Assessment of urinary sodium and osmolality can be helpful as well. An osmolar gap between the calculated serum osmolality

$$\left(2 \times \text{serum sodium concentration} + \frac{\text{serum glucose}}{18} + \frac{\text{blood urea nitrogen}}{2.8}\right)$$

and the measured osmolality of greater than 10 mOsm should raise the suspicion of ethanol, ethylene glycol, or methanol ingestion. Ethanol ingestion can be confirmed by serum ethanol levels, and this level can be correlated with the osmolar gap, as each 100 mg% ethanol raises serum osmolality by 22 mOsm per liter. Ethylene glycol and methanol ingestion should be suspected when the serum anion gap is elevated, particularly since signs and symptoms of these ingestions may not be present early on in the emergency department; however, the presence of calcium oxalate crystals may be noted secondary to the oxalate load due to metabolism of ethylene glycol, and early findings of optic disk changes with hyperemia may be noted in methanol ingestion. The levels of these poisons can be estimated from the osmolar gap, as each 100 mg% methanol produces 31 mOsm per liter and each 100 mg% ethylene glycol produces 16 mOsm per liter.

Urinary osmolality varies in hypernatremia and can help to identify the underlying cause. When renal water losses are responsible for hypernatremia, urine will be quite dilute, usually less than 300 mOsm/kg in complete central or nephrogenic diabetes insipidus, whereas values of 300 to 800 mOsm/kg may be seen in partial diabetes insipidus or with osmotic diuresis in which an osmolar load, such as urea, necessitates relatively salt-free urinary water losses. When the renal concentrating capacity is well preserved—for example, with a urinary osmolality greater than 800 mOsm/kg—nonrenal sources of water loss are likely, such as insensible or GI losses. Less commonly, such a situation is seen with sodium overload—for example, intravenous fluids or salt tablets, or the unusual condition of primary hypodipsia, in which patients lack the normal thirst response to serum tonicity and tolerate hypernatremia.

In the polyuric patient without marked urinary dilution—that is, urinary osmolality greater than 300 mOsm/kg—assessing for glycosuria, marked azotemia, or the presence of other osmotically active species, such as mannitol, can indicate the cause of polyuria. The response to ADH can be very helpful in differentiating among the causes of relatively pure water loss, but such testing cannot be performed in the emergency department. Measurements of urinary sodium and fractional excretion of sodium

$$\left(\frac{\text{Urinary sodium}}{\text{Plasma sodium}} \times \frac{\text{plasma creatinine}}{\text{urinary creatinine}} \times 100\%\right),$$

can be very helpful in corroborating clinical assessment of volume status or aid in cases in which the history and physical examination are not satisfactory. A low urinary sodium (less than 20 mEq per liter) or fractional excretion of sodium (less than 1%) indicates a volume deficit due to extrarenal causes. The urinary sodium or fractional excretion of sodium will exceed these values when little if any volume has been lost or if salt excess has led to hypernatremia.

Treatment

Hypernatremia of any cause indicates a deficit in body water content, and appropriate therapy will include measures to replete this deficit and, as needed, to match continued losses of free water. Specific therapy of underlying disorders may not be possible within the confines of the emergency department, and a full diagnostic evaluation often requires hospitalization.

As usual, stabilization of vital signs is the first order of business, and evaluation of a patient's hemodynamic status will be the first step in determining appropriate replacement therapy for hypernatremic patients (Table 36-2). Those with evidence of a volume deficit (flat neck veins, orthostatic blood pressure changes, tachycardia, decreased skin turgor) will require both salt and water repletion. It may be easier to consider their deficit as having a free-water component (see the following paragraph for calculation of free water deficit) and an isotonic fluid component, to be replaced by normal saline, which will not contribute directly to correction of hypertonicity.

Table 36-2. Treatment of hypernatremia

1. Assess patient for hemodynamic stability and treat hypotension with volume replacement (normal saline and/or colloid) and/or pressors as needed. Lesser degrees of hypovolemia may require some replacement with normal saline (or hypotonic saline, which allows coincident correction of free water replacement deficits).
2. Estimate extent of free water deficit (see text).
3. Estimate ongoing free water losses—e.g., sweat, hypotonic urinary and GI losses.
4. Administer one-half of estimated free water deficit over 12–24 hr along with amount needed to cover ongoing losses, given as D_5W IV.* (In conditions that require simultaneous volume repletion, D_5 ½ NS can be used, remembering that each liter contains 500 ml free water and 500 ml normal saline. Quarter-normal saline can also be considered in such situations.)
5. Recheck clinical condition and serum electrolytes within first 12–24 hours to assess adequacy of therapy and need for further replacement.
6. In the unusual situation of hypernatremia and volume overload, free water replacement remains necessary, but salt excess can be eliminated by use of loop diuretic (furosemide or bumetanide). Dialysis may be indicated in cases with severely impaired renal function.
7. Address the underlying illness that is precipitating hypernatremia.

Key: NS = normal saline.
*Patients who are able to take fluids by mouth can be encouraged to drink water or juices, and these quantities should be figured into calculations of replacement needs.

The free water deficit can be estimated by the following calculation:

Free water deficit (in liters)

$$= [(\text{WT})\,(0.6)] \times \frac{\text{patient's serum sodium}}{140} - [(\text{WT})\,(0.6)],$$

where WT is the patient's lean body weight in kg and (WT × 0.6) equals total body water in liters. This calculation indicates the approximate amount of free water needed to return the patient's sodium to 140 mEq per liter. Total body sodium content will remain the same, but weight will increase as water is added to cause dilution of serum hypertonicity. It is important to remember three points: (1) First, this is only an approximation, providing a working definition of the deficit and permitting initial plans for repletion. Frequent follow-up assessments of the patient's clinical status and electrolytes are mandatory to allow any necessary alteration in therapy. (2) This quantity represents the free water deficit at one point in time. Continuing GI, urinary, and skin losses must also be matched by free water intake, in addition to that required for repletion of the deficit. In general, insensible losses represent 30 to 50 ml per hour. (3) It is rarely necessary, and certainly rarely appropriate, to correct free water deficits abruptly. Generally, one-half of the deficit should be replaced over the first 12 to 24 hours and the other half over the next 24 to 48 hours. As an example, a 70-kg patient with a serum sodium of 160 mEq per liter has a free water deficit of $[(70)\ (0.6)] \times 160/140 - [(70)\ (0.6)] =$ approximately 6 liters. This patient should receive 3 liters D_5W over 12 to 24 hours, with electrolytes reassessed periodically to assure the need for an additional 3 liters D_5W over the subsequent 24 hours. If the patient is experiencing continued loss of free water—for example, dilute urine or sweat—even more free water will be required. Extensive deficits, such as in the previous example, usually require a considerable component of intravenous replacement, though more trivial deficits can be repleted orally by encouraging ingestion of water, soda, juices, and the like in patients who are capable of such intake.

Free water replacement contributes minimally to repletion of volume deficits, as only one-third of the free water administered will remain in the ECF, and of this, only one-fourth in the plasma space. Therefore, in a patient with evidence of volume deficit due to hypotonic fluid losses, efforts to restore volume will require adequate replacement of the salt deficit. Solutions such as "half-" or "quarter-" normal saline can be useful. In patients with any hemodynamic compromise, priority must be given to restoration of volume with normal saline or colloid, as these will remain entirely within the ECF space. The rare patient with hypernatremia secondary to solute gain—for example, hypertonic salt solutions received in illegal abortions, after cardiac arrest, or dialysis malfunctions—will show evidence of ECF volume expansion (e.g., edema). The free water "deficit" can be repleted slowly as previously described, but there is also a role for loop diuretics to remove excess salt. In cases of impaired renal function, dialysis may be necessary.

Additional therapy that can be initiated in the emergency department is correction of any apparent underlying cause for impaired urinary concentrating capacity—for example, hypokalemia, hypercalcemia, urinary tract obstruction, and infection. However, as fluid replacement often requires considerable time, as does thorough evaluation of underlying illnesses, only initial stabilization and therapy will be accomplished by the emergency department physician, who should also coordinate appropriate plans for admission to the hospital.

Disposition

Patients with mild hypernatremia secondary to medications (e.g., diuretics or lithium) or known renal diseases such as certain tubulointerstitial diseases (sarcoid, Sjögren's disease, sickle cell disease, analgesic nephropathy, and polycystic kidneys) may only require water replacement and adjustment of medications. Elderly, debilitated patients who have become dehydrated secondary to febrile illnesses or other fluid losses may respond to rehydration and be released, provided their conditions are clinically stable, their underlying illness is resolving, and their adequate follow-up care (e.g., attention to continued fluid requirement and further medical evaluation) can be assured.

It is critical that the physician in the emergency department make thorough arrangements for continuing outpatient care and appropriate medical follow-up evaluation for all patients discharged from the emergency department after therapy for disturbances of water balance. This includes careful and well-understood instructions to patients and family. Most patients can be treated by their primary care physician without immediate referral to subspecialists. Hypernatremic patients with continuing febrile illness, urinary tract obstruction, or significant polyuria will need to be further treated and evaluated in the hospital. The full evaluation of polyuria, including deliberate dehydration and vasopressin challenge, can only be accomplished in a controlled setting. A description of these tests is beyond the scope of this chapter.

The physician responsible for arranging admission for patients with hypernatremia should make certain that appropriate fluid and electrolyte replacement therapy, initiated in the emergency department, will continue until another physician becomes responsible, and should see that necessary follow-up laboratory results are checked to reduce the possibility of inadequate correction or over-correction. It is always helpful to obtain urine for urinalysis, urine sodium, and osmolality in the emergency department and to obtain serum for serum osmolality determinations. Other studies should be obtained as appropriate (e.g., cultures and x-rays) and therapy, such as antibiotics, should be initiated as indicated.

HYPONATREMIA

Hyponatremia is probably the most common electrolyte abnormality seen in hospitals, and one-third of cases are present on admission. The possibility of hyponatremia is suggested by patients who are either volume depleted or have edematous disorders, are receiving diuretics or are taking drugs associated with increased ADH activity (see Table 36-4), or have neurologic or pulmonary processes, associated with increased ADH levels (see later in text).

Pathophysiology

The capacity to produce dilute urine and thus eliminate excess water and avoid plasma dilution (i.e., hyponatremia) also depends on solute reabsorption in the TALH, as well as in the diluting segment of the cortical and medullary collecting ducts. This dilute urine must be protected from reequilibration with the hypertonic medullary interstitium by maintenance of water impermeability in the medullary collecting duct. Thus, ADH must not be present. In addition, quantitative aspects of free water clearance are affected by the rate of flow to the diluting segment, as it is only that volume, and no more, that can be diuresed. Any process that decreases distal delivery decreases the amount of dilute urine excreted and predisposes to conditions in which free water intake can exceed output.

In summary, urinary dilution depends on (1) adequate delivery of urine to the diluting segment, which can be limited by a state of proximal sodium avidity—for example, volume depletion and congestive heart failure; (2) adequate function of the diluting segment, potentially limited by diuretics, particularly thiazides; and (3) absence of ADH,

Table 36-3. Causes of hyponatremia

- I. In the setting of *hypovolemia* (deficit in total body sodium greater than deficit in total body water)
  - A. Extrarenal losses
    - Gastrointestinal—e.g., vomiting, diarrhea, cathartics
    - Third spacing—e.g., pancreatitis, peritonitis, ileus
  - B. Renal losses
    - Diuretics and osmotic diuresis
    - Adrenal insufficiency
    - Salt-losing nephritides
    - Renal tubular acidoses (bicarbonaturia)
    - Ketonuria
- II. *Hypervolemia* (salt-retaining disorders with decreased circulating plasma volume)
  - Congestive heart failure
  - Cirrhosis
  - Nephrotic syndrome
  - Renal failure
- III. In setting of clinically *normal ECF volume*
  - Hypothyroidism
  - Adrenal insufficiency
  - Renal failure
  - Drugs (see Table 36-4)
  - SIADH (see Table 36-5)

Table 36-4. Antidiuretic drugs

Vasopressin
Oxytocin
d-Desamino-arginine vasopressin (dDAVP)
Vincristine
Carbamazepine
Psychotropic drugs
Opiates
Isoproterenol
Nicotine
Chlorpropamide
Other sulfonylureas
Salicylate
Nonsteroidal antiinflammatory drugs
Clofibrate
Cyclophosphamide
Colchicine

which, if present secondary to "appropriate" secretion under nonosmotic volume stimuli or "inappropriately" due to a variety of nonphysiologic stimuli, will allow reconcentration of dilute tubular fluid by water movement back into the hypertonic medullary interstitium (see Chap. 35).

A low serum sodium level can occur, along with low, high, or normal plasma osmolality. Only the first of these conditions constitutes true hyponatremia related to free water excess. In pseudohyponatremia, a low serum sodium concentration is associated with normal osmolality and occurs in conditions that lower the percentage of plasma volume in the aqueous phase. The actual concentration of sodium in the aqueous phase remains normal, but, as this phase constitutes a reduced portion of plasma, the autoanalyzer perceives a decrease in sodium concentration with respect to the entire plasma sample. The freezing point depression, as a true measure of osmolality, remains normal. If an increased osmolar gap (greater than 10 mOsm) occurs between calculated and measured osmolality, one must suspect pseudohyponatremia or the presence of ethanol, methanol, or ethylene glycol. Pseudohyponatremia occurs in hyperlipemic and hyperproteinemic states. No primary therapy is required, as the solute concentration of serum is normal.

Hyponatremia can also exist in states of hyperosmolality, particularly hyperglycemia, in which movement of water out of cells dilutes sodium concentration of the extracellular fluid. Generally, serum sodium concentration will fall by 1.6 mEq per liter for every 100 mg% elevation of blood glucose greater than 100 mg%. Other osmotically active agents (e.g., mannitol and glycerol) will induce a similar condition. Therapy should be directed at the primary disorder (e.g., hyperglycemia).

Causes

A review of the pathogenetic mechanisms responsible for hyponatremia (see Chap. 35) reveals the relationship of plasma volume status to the ability to excrete free water. Table 36-3 lists common causes of hyponatremia. States of both true volume depletion and volume overload (e.g., congestive heart failure or cirrhosis) often induce hyponatremia. A dissociation between ADH release and serum tonicity occurs when ADH release is induced by nonosmotic stimuli. Antidiuretic hormone retains the vasopressor action for which the hormone is used exclusively in more primitive organisms, and its release can be provoked by signals from volume receptors, sensing inadequate filling of the vascular space. Thus, in both conditions of true volume deficit (e.g., after gastrointestinal fluid losses) or with total body volume excess associated with inadequate intravascular filling (e.g., congestive heart failure, ascites, or nephrosis), ADH may be called on as a vasopressor and coincidentally as an antidiuretic hormone to affect both vascular capacitance and fluid retention. These same conditions will also limit the capacity to excrete free water secondary to sodium avidity: Flow to the diluting segment of the nephron and beyond is diminished, and there is an often coexistent alteration in diluting segment function induced by diuretics used in edematous disorders. A common scenario is the patient who, despite an episode of gastroenteritis with vomiting and diarrhea, dutifully continues taking prescribed thiazide diuretics used for treatment of hypertension or heart failure.

In the patient who appears by examination to be normovolemic and whose laboratory assessment (e.g., urinary sodium > 20) confirms this, the syndrome of inappropriate ADH secretion (SIADH) can be considered, once other causes of impaired urinary dilution (e.g., hypothyroidism or adrenal or renal insufficiency) have been ruled out. SIADH is likely to be somewhat chronic and associated with certain drugs (Table 36-4), CNS or pulmonary diseases, or various malignancies (Table 36-5). Chlorpropamide is a common cause of SIADH related to drugs, potentiating the effects of ADH on the collecting tubule and also possibly stimulating sodium chloride reabsorption in the TALH, thus augmenting medullary interstitial tonicity.

As renal prostaglandins antagonize ADH action, nonsteroidal antiinflammatory drugs can potentiate the effect of

Table 36-5. Causes of SIADH*

Carcinoma
Bronchogenic
Duodenal
Pancreatic
Thymoma
Lymphoma
Ewing's sarcoma
Mesothelioma
Bladder
Prostate
Pulmonary
Pneumonia
Abscess
Tuberculosis
Aspergillosis
Positive pressure breathing
Asthma
Pneumothorax
Cystic fibrosis
Central nervous system
Encephalitis
Meningitis
Trauma
Abscess
Delirium tremens
Peripheral neuropathy
Guillain-Barré
Acute intermittent porphyria
Subarachnoid hemorrhage
Subdural hemorrhage
Acute psychosis
Cavernous sinus thrombosis
Hydrocephalus
Shy-Drager syndrome
Rocky Mountain spotted fever
Multiple sclerosis
Stress

*See Table 36-4 for drugs that can stimulate ADH release or augment its effect.

ADH by limiting prostaglandin synthesis, though these drugs are rarely sufficient to cause hyponatremia alone. When they are used in the setting of congestive heart failure or volume deficits, the likelihood of worsening hyponatremia is high.

Pulmonary diseases of virtually any type (e.g., infection, obstruction, bronchospasm, or ventilator dependency) can induce ADH release unrelated to either serum tonicity or volume. The mechanism is not clear but may relate to hypoxia or to alterations in pulmonary venous return, with consequent activation of volume receptors or feedback from stretch receptors to the CNS that "inappropriately" signal for pituitary release of ADH.

Central nervous system processes from trauma to infection, vascular events, or even stress, psychosis, or vomiting can induce ADH release via stimulation of hypothalamic output through the pituitary gland. Finally, certain tumors (e.g., oat cell carcinoma of the lung) can produce ADH ectopically, unaffected by the usual stimuli. In many patients in whom no cause for SIADH is found after thorough evaluation, long-term follow-up study may demonstrate an occult malignancy.

Presentation and Evaluation

Hyponatremic patients often develop signs and symptoms of underlying conditions—for example, volume depletion secondary to GI or renal losses, edematous disorders, endocrine abnormalities, or CNS, pulmonary, or malignant conditions that can induce SIADH. The signs and symptoms that are related to hyponatremia are modulated not only by the absolute level of serum sodium but also by the rate of change. Central nervous system findings can include lethargy, apathy, disorientation, agitation, seizures, coma, and death. Muscle cramps, depressed and pathologic reflexes, anorexia, and pseudobulbar palsy can be seen.

History

Evaluation of the hyponatremic patient starts with critical assessment of the state of total body sodium—that is, total body volume and ECF volume status. In taking the history, the physician should concentrate on evidence for GI, third-space, and renal fluid losses (e.g., due to diuretics or renal tubular acidosis) and a history of renal insufficiency, edematous disorders, thyroid and adrenal diseases, and pulmonary and CNS disorders. He or she should also take a careful drug history (see Table 36-4).

Physical Examination

Critical to the evaluation and treatment of hyponatremia is a careful assessment of volume status (see Table 36-3). As was detailed in the discussion of hypernatremia, documentation of orthostatic blood pressure and pulse changes, character of neck vein distention, and skin turgor should be obtained. Evidence of congestive heart failure (e.g., rales, gallop rhythm, edema) or liver disease (e.g., hepatomegaly, telangiectasia, or ascites) should be sought.

Laboratory Examination

PLASMA OSMOLALITY. Laboratory test results can help by first ruling out hyponatremia associated with normal or high plasma tonicity—that is, lipid and protein excess in the former and hyperglycemia in the latter (see previous discussion).

URINE OSMOLALITY. Determinations of urinary sodium and osmolality are very useful and should always be obtained unless the cause of hyponatremia is completely obvious from the history and physical examination. Maximal urinary dilution (osmolality < 100 mOsm per liter) is the normal response to serum hypotonicity, and any value higher than that, even if it remains lower than plasma tonicity, represents an inadequate diluting capacity. This will generally be secondary to either (1) impaired delivery to the diluting segment of the nephron as in states of decreased glomerular filtration rate and increased proximal sodium reabsorption, (2) impaired function of the diluting segment due to thiazide diuretics, or (3) the presence of ADH, "appropriately" in response to diminished plasma volume or "inappropriately" due to drugs, CNS processes, ectopic ADH release, and so forth (see Table 36-5). Urinary osmolality by itself cannot separate these disorders. Hyponatremia in the presence of dilute urine (osmolality < 100 mOsm per liter) implies polydipsia or a reset osmostat—that is, normal mechanisms for control of serum tonicity operating to maintain an abnormal level of osmolality.

URINE SODIUM CONCENTRATION. A low urinary sodium value (<20 mEq per liter) or fractional excretion of less than 1 percent suggests states of volume depletion or edematous disorders with inadequate effective plasma volume, conditions that should also be obvious from physical examination. The two exceptions to this are states of volume depletion secondary to renal salt losses (diuretics, osmotic diuresis, mineralocorticoid deficiency, and salt-losing nephritides) or volume overload secondary to acute and chronic renal failure. Patients who appear normovolemic, have a urinary sodium value greater than 20 mEq per liter, and have no evidence for renal, thyroid, or cortisol deficiency may have SIADH (see Table 36-5).

Treatment

Only hyponatremia associated with hypoosmolality requires treatment to correct the abnormality of water balance (Table 36-6). Hyponatremia seen with hyperlipidemia or elevated plasma protein does not reflect a true abnormality of serum tonicity and, in fact, the sodium concentration of the aqueous phase of plasma is normal. Treatment of hyperglycemia will "cure" the associated hyponatremia by inducing fluid shifts back into cells without any adjustment in total body water balance. Such patients should be observed for signs of ECF volume collapse secondary to these fluid shifts and may require volume replacement to maintain blood pressure as hyperglycemia is corrected.

In treating hypoosmolar hyponatremia, the initial step is clinical evaluation of volume status—that is, total body sodium content (see previous discussion). Correction of hyponatremia in patients who are volume depleted will follow correction of volume deficit with normal saline or colloid, as nonosmotic stimuli to ADH release are eliminated and flow to the urinary diluting segment improves, thus augmenting capacity to excrete free water. Generally, no other therapy is required except, possibly, repletion of the potassium losses that often accompany volume-depleted states (see Chap. 37) and discontinuation or adjustment of medications such as thiazide diuretics that may have contributed to the underlying condition. Persistent causes of fluid loss must be investigated and corrected.

Patients with edematous disorders require therapy for the underlying process. For example, inotropes and vasodilators may be required for congestive heart failure (CHF), and the patient may benefit from free water restrictions (e.g., 1.0–1.5 liters per day). Converting enzyme inhibitors (CEI) may be particularly useful in CHF through a variety of mechanisms, as angiotensin II may play a role in the development of hyponatremia, possibly by augmenting ADH release and thirst, independent of changes in renal hemodynamics. The effects of CEI on ADH may be via a direct pathway as well as by increasing prostaglandins that can impair the effect of ADH. Furosemide, which also causes an increase in prostaglandin levels, may be necessary to augment the effect of CEI.

Hyponatremia in the clinically normovolemic patient requires consideration of the underlying cause. If corticoid or thyroxine deficiencies can be implicated, hormone replacement therapy will generally suffice to reverse the defect of water excretion, though these diagnoses cannot always be made in the emergency department. Likewise, discontinuation of drugs that augment ADH effect is the primary means of treating drug-related ADH excess (see Table 36-4).

In the meantime, severe or symptomatic hyponatremia requires correction. Fluid restriction should be a component of the therapeutic regimen, but will not have an impact on serum tonicity until several days have passed and insensible and urinary losses of free water exceed free water ingestion even if restricted. This modality is thus not part of the physician's primary therapy in the emergency department. The administration of saline solutions may be indicated in the emergency department, however, not only to correct volume deficits and the consequent deficit in free water clearance, but also to "salt load" the patient who has a relative deficit of salt with respect to water and ongoing salt losses seen in SIADH. Often, normal saline will not suffice in a patient with SIADH as urinary osmolalities are generally fixed above the osmolality of normal saline (300 mOsm per liter). The os-

Table 36-6. Treatment of hyponatremia

1. Rule out pseudohyponatremia (hyperlipidemia/hypertriglyceridemia, hyperproteinemia) or hyponatremia in hypertonic states (e.g., hyperglycemia).
2. Assess volume status and treat hemodynamic instability with volume repletion (normal saline or colloid) and/or pressors.
3. In volume-depleted patients, correct volume deficit with normal saline. Check for and correct other electrolyte abnormalities (e.g., hypokalemia). Investigate and treat underlying problem (e.g., vomiting, diarrhea, diuretic use).
4. In volume-overloaded patients, treat underlying disorders (e.g., congestive heart failure (CHF) with inotropes and/or vasodilators), and restrict daily free water intake (1,000–1,500 ml/day). Long-term therapy of CHF with converting enzyme inhibitors and furosemide can be considered in certain patients.
5. In normovolemic patients, rule out underlying renal, adrenal, and thyroid disease and assess for drugs or other conditions that promote ADH release or action; then treat accordingly.
   A. In patients without symptoms of hyponatremia and/or serum sodium greater than 120 mEq per liter, fluid restriction should be started.
   B. In severely hyponatremic patients (<110 mEq per liter), particularly in the setting of symptoms related to hyponatremia (mental status changes, seizures), more acute correction to moderate levels of hyponatremia is indicated. This usually requires hypertonic (3%) saline. To estimate volume of 3% saline, calculate:

   $$(120 - \text{patient's serum sodium concentration}) \times (\text{TBW})$$

   where TBW = total body water = patient's lean body weight in kg × (0.6). This gives the number of mEq required to correct the patient to a serum sodium of 120 mEq per liter. Dividing by 513 mEq Na per liter gives the amount of 3% saline to use in liters.

   Rate of correction should be 0.5–1.0 mEq per liter per hour; therefore, administer appropriate volume of 3% saline over

   $$\frac{(120 - \text{patient's serum sodium concentration})}{0.5\text{–}1.0} \text{ hours}$$

   (see text)

   Use furosemide as needed to avoid volume overload.
6. *Closely* follow clinical status and repeat electrolytes.

motic load of normal saline can thus be excreted in a more concentrated form, and a portion of the administered volume will be retained as free water and worsen the hyponatremic state.

When immediate correction of hyponatremia is deemed necessary, hypertonic saline, usually 3% (513 mEq Na per liter), can be used, possibly with a diuretic to avoid volume overload. The salt "deficit" vis-à-vis the actual surfeit of free water can be estimated by multiplying total body water (total lean body weight × 0.6) by the difference between a "normal" serum sodium value and the patient's actual value. For example, in a 70-kg individual with a serum sodium value of 110, the sodium "deficit" equals (70) × (0.6) × (140 − 110) = 1,360 mEq. *There is, however, a critical error in the clinical use of this calculation.* There is *never* a need to correct the patient to a "normal" value of serum sodium, and, in fact, correction to values above 130, particularly when done abruptly, can be associated with significant morbidity and mortality. In this example, a more appropriate calculation would have been to determine the salt load needed to bring the serum sodium to 120 to 130 mEq per liter, a deficit of 420 to 840 mEq sodium. This would require the administration of 800 to 1,600 ml of 3% saline.

The speed with which such corrections can be made safely has been the subject of much debate. First, it is important that significant hyponatremia by itself not be considered an indication to rapidly correct serum sodium toward normal. Many patients, particularly if hyponatremia has developed slowly, can be well compensated and show few, if any, signs of neuromuscular or CNS abnormalities. In these patients, aggressive therapy is not indicated. Rather, reliance should be on volume repletion and control of edematous disorders, or fluid restriction as appropriate for hypo-, hyper-, and normovolemic states, respectively (see previous discussion).

The issue of rate of correction must be considered in the patient who manifests signs, particularly CNS signs, of hyponatremia (confusion, lethargy, seizure, coma). Even patients with a sodium value of 110 to 120 mEq per liter, or possibly even lower, who do not manifest symptoms can be treated conservatively. Generally, patients with a serum sodium of at least 120 mEq per liter will not be at risk for CNS abnormalities, and this level should serve as a target for correcting lower levels associated with symptoms. Most authorities agree that correction much above this level is not only unnecessary but can be the cause of severe neurologic abnormalities that have been seen in association with hyponatremia and its treatment.

The rate of correction remains a point of controversy. Some believe that profound hyponatremia, especially in patients otherwise debilitated by chronic alcoholism or cachexia, is itself associated with demyelinating lesions of the CNS, particularly central pontine myelinolysis, and advocate correction to serum sodium levels of 120 to 130 relatively "rapidly" (i.e., at 2 mEq per liter per hour), possibly limiting total change in sodium to 20 mEq per liter if starting at a serum sodium below 105 mEq/kg. Other authorities believe that rapid correction by itself can cause demyelinating syndromes and recommend correction at 0.5 mEq per liter per hour. In the previous example of correcting a serum sodium of 110 to 120 via administration of 800 ml 3% saline, the rate of administration could be 40 to 160 ml per hour.

Perhaps the major risk in choosing a more rapid correction is that the hospitalized patient will be affected by other maneuvers to correct hyponatremia beyond volume and salt repletion—that is, control of excessive fluid intake and discontinuation of diuretics and other medications. These factors can accelerate the rate of correction independently and create the potential to overshoot target levels. As there is no need to achieve a normal serum sodium level, this should be avoided. It is thus advisable to choose a more modest rate of correction (e.g., 0.5–1.0 mEq per liter per hour), and follow the patient clinically, frequently reassessing serum electrolytes to adjust therapy.

Many patients have several coincident causes for hyponatremia, such as fluid losses from vomiting or poor intake in an elderly patient with pneumonia who has been taking diuretics. The initial evaluation, including laboratory findings, may point to hypovolemia, but correction of this may not correct hyponatremia secondary to inappropriate release of ADH that persists despite turning off the volume-related signal. After the acute treatment of symptomatic hyponatremia has stabilized the patient's condition, ongoing SIADH may require therapy (e.g., with demeclocycline) to block ADH's chronic effect on the kidney. This treatment is usually not initiated in the emergency department.

Disposition

Many, if not all, patients with significant disturbances of serum sodium will require hospitalization for further correction of electrolyte abnormalities, as well as evaluation and treatment of underlying illnesses. In the patients with mild, asymptomatic hyponatremia secondary to volume depletion, if ongoing fluid losses are not anticipated, the volume deficit can be corrected in the emergency department and the patients discharged if their conditions are stable. Edematous patients who are not seriously ill and are only mildly hyponatremic and without symptoms may only need conservative therapy of the underlying illness (e.g., CHF) and close outpatient follow-up study. Drugs implicated in hyponatremia (e.g., thiazide diuretics, chlorpropamide, or carbamazepine) can be discontinued or replaced. Concurrent electrolyte disorders such as hypokalemia can also be corrected before the patient is released from the emergency department.

Hyponatremic patients with symptoms, significant ongoing fluid losses, severe CHF, cirrhosis, renal failure, or SIADH will require hospital admission. More sophisticated tests of renal capacity for free water excretion, such as the water load test, can only be performed in a supervised setting.

SELECTED READING

Anderson, R J, et al. Hyponatremia: A prospective analysis of its epidemiology and the pathogenetic role of vasopressin. *Ann Intern Med* 102:164, 1985.

Arieff, A I. Hyponatremia, convulsions, respiratory arrest and permanent brain damage after elective surgery in healthy women. *N Engl J Med* 314:1529, 1986.

Ayus, J C, et al. Treatment of symptomatic hyponatremia and its relation to brain damage: A prospective study. *N Engl J Med* 317:1190, 1987.

Berl, T. Treating hyponatremia: Damned if we do and damned if we don't. *Kidney Int* 37:1006, 1990.

Cluitman, F H M, and Meinders, A E. Management of severe hyponatremia: Rapid or slow correction? *Am J Med* 88:161, 1990.

DeFronzo, R A, and Thier, S O. Pathophysiologic approach to hyponatremia. *Arch Intern Med* 140:897, 1980.

Hayes, R M, et al. Effect of antidiuretic hormone on the collecting duct. *Kidney Int* 31:530, 1987.

Jamison, R L, and Oliver, R E. Disorders of urinary concentration and dilution. *Am J Med* 72:308, 1982.

Miller, M, and Moses, A M. Drug induced states of impaired water excretion. *Kidney Int* 10:96, 1976.

Robertson, G L, et al. Neurogenic disorders of osmoregulation. *Am J Med* 72:339, 1982.

Robertson, G L, et al. Differential diagnosis of polyuria. *Ann Rev Med* 39:425, 1988.

Rose, B D. New approach to disturbances in the plasma sodium concentration. *Am J Med* 81:1033, 1986.

Weisberg, L S. Pseudohyponatremia: A reappraisal. *Am J Med* 86: 315, 1988.

37. Disorders of Potassium Metabolism

David M. Poppel

PRINCIPLES OF NORMAL POTASSIUM BALANCE

Tight control of potassium concentration in extracellular fluid (ECF) is critical for maintenance of normal cellular metabolism. The steep concentration gradient between intracellular (140–150 per liter) and extracellular (3.5–5.0 mEq per liter) concentrations of potassium, largely responsible for control of neuromuscular excitability and cardiac rhythmicity, can be markedly affected by small changes in ECF potassium concentration. Intracellular potassium is important as a major intracellular osmol and contributes to maintenance of cell volume and regulation of intracellular pH, enzyme functions, and synthetic processes.

Both extrarenal and renal mechanisms control ECF or serum potassium concentration. Extrarenal factors regulate internal disposition of potassium, particularly in response to acute loads, while renal mechanisms maintain long-term balance between input and output. The average diet provides 70 to 100 mEq potassium each day, which equals or exceeds the entire amount of potassium in the extracellular fluid (only about 2% of total body potassium). Since it takes several hours for complete renal excretion of a potassium load, acute internal disposition of a potassium load is crucial. Given sufficient time, wide variations of renal excretory capacity are possible, and as little as 5 mEq, or as much as 1,000 mEq, can be excreted per day to accommodate variations in intake. The kidney thus exerts the dominant role in chronic maintenance of potassium homeostasis.

Both internal and external balance can be up- or down-regulated in settings of chronic excess or deficiency, and a person's "tolerance" to an acute perturbation can be improved. Numerous therapeutic interventions, in particular medications, also affect potassium homeostasis.

Extrarenal Mechanisms of Potassium Homeostasis (Internal Balance)

Several hormonal and nonhormonal factors affect the distribution of potassium across cell membranes and facilitate rapid disposition of a potassium load into a large intracellular "sink" (Table 37-1). The two major hormonal regulators of cellular potassium uptake are catecholamines with beta-2 agonist action and insulin. Epinephrine infusion causes an early, transient rise of plasma potassium as a result of alpha agonist–mediated potassium release from hepatocytes, but the predominant effect is beta-2–mediated cellular uptake. Insulin-stimulated cellular uptake of potassium is independent of its mediation of glucose uptake, and even basal levels of insulin are important in tonic regulation of extracellular potassium concentration. Both insulin and epinephrine ap-

Table 37-1. Extrarenal mechanisms of potassium homeostasis

Hormonal	Nonhormonal
Insulin	Cellular integrity
Catecholamines	ECF tonicity
Aldosterone	pH
Glucagon?	Drugs
Thyroxine?	
Growth hormone?	
Increase cellular uptake or decrease leak	Decrease cellular uptake or increase leak
Insulin/glucose	Digitalis
Beta-2 agonists	Beta-2 antagonists
Alpha antagonists	Alpha agonists
Barium	Nonsteroidals
Thiazides	Converting enzyme inhibitors
Vitamin B_{12} therapy	Succinylcholine
Refeeding	
Arginine HCl	

Table 37-2. Conditions that predispose to hypokalemia and hyperkalemia

Conditions that predispose to hypokalemia
Dietary insufficiencies/alcoholism
Hypertension ← aldosterone excess
Edematous disorders ← diuretics
Diabetes/diabetic ketoacidosis
Any significant loss of fluids (vomiting, diarrhea, sweat, urine)
Drugs, especially diuretics (see Table 37-3)
Conditions that predispose to hyperkalemia
Hypertension
Salt substitutes
Potassium-sparing diuretics
KCl supplements
Beta-blockers
Renal insufficiency
Trauma
Acidoses (acute)
Diabetes
Insulin deficiency/DKA
Renal insufficiency
Low renin-aldosterone
Renal failure/transplants
Drugs, especially potassium-sparing diuretics, nonsteroidal antiinflammatory drugs, converting enzyme inhibitors (see Table 37-7)

pear to activate sodium–potassium–adenosine triphosphatase (Na-K-ATPase), though via different mechanisms. Insulin also stimulates sodium-hydrogen exchange, which can augment potassium influx. The physiologic importance of alpha agonist inhibition of cellular uptake is less clear. Though elevation of serum potassium induces the synthesis and release of aldosterone, acute effects of aldosterone on transcellular potassium distribution may be limited.

The principal nonhormonal regulators of transcellular potassium distribution are ECF tonicity and pH (see Table 37-1). In addition, a variety of medications or an interruption of cellular integrity by trauma, necrosis, or cell lysis cause leakage of potassium into the ECF. Exercise, particularly in the nonconditioned patient, can raise ECF potassium concentration. Elevation of ECF tonicity, as in hyperglycemia, causes cellular dehydration, increasing intracellular potassium concentration and the gradient for potassium efflux.

Acidemia induces exchange of intracellular potassium for extracellular hydrogen ions, and alkalemia tends to cause opposite shifts. The impact of acidemia is more pronounced than that of alkalemia, while metabolic disorders cause greater changes than respiratory disturbances by virtue of the considerable extracellular buffering that is present in the latter. Greater shifts of potassium out of cells occur with mineral acidoses (normal anion gap) because the accompanying anions (chloride, phosphate, sulfate) are less permeable than anions of organic acids (lactate, ketoacids), which are transported with their proton into cells, maintaining electroneutrality without obligating outward movement of potassium. By rough approximation, a fall in pH by 0.1 units can induce a rise of the serum potassium by 1.5 mEq per liter in mineral acidoses and 0.66 mEq per liter in organic acidoses.

The most important drugs to affect transcellular potassium concentration are insulin, beta-2 and alpha agonists and antagonists (see previous discussion), digitalis, and inhibitors of prostaglandin and angiotensin II synthesis. Beta-blocker inhibition of cellular uptake may be especially important when in the presence of additional factors or drugs, or both, that impair potassium disposition or excretion, such as in diabetic patients with renal failure, elevated ECF tonicity, or acidemia. Digitalis inhibits Na-K-ATPase activity, which impairs cellular uptake, but significant elevation of serum potassium concentration occurs only in serious overdose. Other, less common, drug effects are listed in Table 37-1.

Renal Mechanisms of Potassium Homeostasis (External Balance)

Renal excretion or conservation of potassium is affected mainly by aldosterone, distal tubule luminal flow rate, the make up of distal tubule luminal content, and the integrity of distal tubular cells and their function. The mechanisms are explained in greater detail in Chap. 35.

HYPOKALEMIA

By understanding the mechanisms that protect the concentration of potassium in the ECF, the emergency medicine physician should be able to recognize situations in which hypo- or hyperkalemia is likely to occur. Once they are identified, the clinician can rationally proceed with treatment.

The physician should anticipate the possibility of abnormal serum potassium levels in evaluating patients with a variety of chronic diseases or acute illnesses and in those who use certain drugs (Table 37-2). Serum levels should always be checked in these settings.

Causes

The causes of hypokalemia can be divided into three categories: inadequate intake, abnormal transcellular distribution, and increased output (Table 37-3). It is unusual for *inadequate intake* to cause hypokalemia without simultaneous increase in potassium excretion, but patients with alcohol-

Table 37-3. Causes of hypokalemia

Inadequate intake
High-carbohydrate diet
Alcoholism
Anorexia nervosa
Abnormal transcellular distribution
Alkalosis
Insulin/glucose infusion
Mineralocorticoids
Beta-2 agonists
Barium poisoning
Vitamin B_{12} therapy for pernicious anemia
Refeeding/hyperalimentation
Familial hypokalemic periodic paralysis
Increased output
Renal excretion
Diuretics
Other medications (see Table 37-1)
Aldosterone excess
Primary hyperaldosteronism
Adrenogenital syndromes
Cushing's syndrome
Accelerated, malignant, and renovascular hypertension
Renin-producing tumors
Vasculitis
Edematous states
Pseudohyperaldosteronism
Licorice gluttony/certain chewing tobaccos
Carbenoxolone
Exogenous mineralocorticoids
Renal disease
Renal tubular acidosis (types I and II)
Fanconi's syndrome
Bartter's syndrome
Liddle's syndrome
Other
Magnesium depletion
Hypercalcemia
Diabetic ketoacidosis
Leukemia
Metabolic alkalosis of extrarenal origin
Gastrointestinal losses
Vomiting/lavage
Lower gastrointestinal losses
Skin losses

ism or anorexia nervosa may develop profound deficits of total body potassium over time.

Abnormalities of transcellular distribution do not reflect deficits in total body potassium stores and thus need not be corrected by repletion. Rather, the underlying disturbances, such as alkalosis and mineralocorticoid excess, should be reversed.

Renal loss of potassium is the major cause of hypokalemia. Even hypokalemia in patients with upper gastrointestinal (GI) fluid loss is due mainly to increased renal excretion. Gastric juice contains little potassium (< 10 mEq per liter), but metabolic alkalosis, generated by upper GI acid loss, and volume depletion–induced hyperaldosteronism promote renal potassium wasting. In contrast, lower GI loss can induce hypokalemia directly, as the potassium concentration of this fluid is significant (approximately 90 mEq per liter). This occurs in numerous settings, such as diarrhea of any cause, Zollinger-Ellison syndrome, pancreatic cholera, jejunoileal bypass, laxative and enema abuse, malabsorption syndromes, fistulas, villous adenoma, congenital chloride diarrhea, ureterosigmoidostomy, and obstructed or long ileal loops. The mechanism by which various drugs, such as diuretics, mineralocorticoids, beta-2 agonists, and others, induce potassium wasting has been described in Chap. 35.

Hypokalemia can occur in any condition associated with an excess in aldosterone. Only a small percentage of patients with Cushing's syndrome will have significant hypokalemia, usually due to adrenocorticotropic hormone–producing tumors or increased levels of deoxycorticosterone. Increased aldosterone is seen in any state of hyperreninism, such as renovascular hypertension or accelerated/malignant hypertension, juxtaglomerular cell tumors, Wilms' tumor and hypernephroma, vasculitis, and, more commonly, edematous disorders. Marked potassium-wasting in the latter can occur in patients who are being treated concomitantly with diuretics that intensify the effects of aldosterone. Exogenous mineralocorticoids (e.g., 9-fluoroprednisolone nasal spray) and mineralocorticoidlike substances (licorice, certain chewing tobaccos, carbenoxolone) cause pseudohyperaldosteronism.

Both proximal (type II) and distal (type I) renal tubular acidoses (RTA) lead to potassium-wasting. The former causes proximal bicarbonate-wasting with increased distal flow of nonreabsorbable anions and secondary hyperaldosteronism due to volume depletion. The latter is due to failure of distal proton pumps associated with abnormal ion permeability, as well as decreased proximal sodium reabsorption secondary to chronic metabolic acidosis. Fanconi's syndrome of multiple defects in proximal reabsorption behaves like a type II RTA. Bartter's syndrome, a rare and not well-understood disorder, probably of tubular function, is also associated with potassium-wasting, as is Liddle's syndrome. Functional abnormalities of potassium-handling with potassium-wasting are seen in states of hypomagnesemia and hypercalcemia, though the cause is not clear.

Diabetic ketoacidosis (DKA) is commonly associated with severe potassium depletion (up to 10 mEq/kg), though serum levels can be normal or elevated due to the effects of hypertonicity, metabolic acidosis, insulin and catecholamine deficiencies, and abnormal cellular metabolism. Potassium losses are largely due to osmotic diuresis and the delivery of poorly reabsorbable ketoacid anions to the distal tubule. Patients with leukemia, with or without lysozymuria, may have renal potassium-wasting of unclear cause, as well as gastrointestinal losses, abnormal dietary intake, and use of kaliuretic drugs.

Clinical Presentation

Patients with hypokalemia often have signs and symptoms of their underlying illness, in many cases associated with volume depletion or states of effective circulating volume deficiency (congestive heart failure, ascites), hypertensive states, or ketoacidosis. Other signs and symptoms that may be seen in the emergency department and are referable to hypokalemia are (1) tetany, (2) weakness, (3) ileus, (4) orthostatic hypotension, (5) rhabdomyolysis, (6) encephalopathy in patients with liver disease, (7) polyuria and polydipsia, and (8) edema (Table 37-4).

Table 37-4. Effects of hypokalemia

Systemic acid-base effects
Metabolic alkalosis
Enhanced ammonia synthesis (can aggravate hepatic encephalopathy)
Impaired endogenous acid production
Carbohydrate intolerance due to decreased insulin release and hepatic and skeletal muscle glycogen synthesis and storage
Growth retardation due to decreased growth hormone release, altered protein synthesis, negative nitrogen balance
Abnormal muscle resting potential, decreased muscle blood flow and depletion of energy stores, weakness, fatigue, myalgias, restless legs, tetany, paralysis; when extreme can cause cell necrosis
Impaired smooth-muscle function with decreased gastrointestinal and bladder motility, decreased vascular resistance, and pressor response to angiotensin II
Increased cardiac automaticity, decreased conduction velocity, and refractory period; ECG may show increased Q-wave duration, decreased voltage, wide T waves with flattening and appearance of U waves, ST segment depression (see Fig. 37-1)
Renal effects
Tubular cell vacuolization and interstitial nephritis and fibrosis
Decreased glomerular filtration rate and renal blood flow
Impaired concentrating ability via insensitivity to antidiuretic hormone, decreased interstitial tonicity, and primary polydipsia
Mild sodium retention
Abnormal response to parathyroid hormone with phosphate wasting
Decreased aldosterone secretion

Evaluation

A diagnosis of hypokalemia is not difficult to make by routine laboratory testing. The diagnostic challenge is obtaining the test at appropriate times (see previous discussion) and defining the cause, allowing directed acute therapy and follow-up care. As in any diagnostic evaluation, a thorough history and physical examination are critical and often define the problem, making more elaborate evaluation unnecessary. Certain routine laboratory tests can clarify more difficult presentations.

Before any thorough examination is performed, the ABCs of emergency department care must be assured. Initial efforts should be directed toward stabilization of vital signs and attention to any severe symptoms. In critical settings it is helpful to set aside serum for evaluation as initial stabilization is under way. Disorders of potassium homeostasis will often be seen in settings in which urgent control of volume depletion or overload, hypo- and hypertension, arrhythmias, and related profound metabolic abnormalities is required. Limited history and physical examination will assist in this phase.

After initial stabilization, a more thorough history and physical examination can be pursued. In all cases careful attention should be directed toward drug use—in particular, diuretics, insulin, mineralocorticoids, antibiotics, and chemotherapy. Dietary history may also be important, particularly salt substitutes and low-salt diets, alcoholism, and anorexia nervosa. The patient should be assessed for past and present history of hypertension, diabetes, edematous disorders, renal disease, malignancy, and surgery. Evaluation of the patient's recent history may reveal gastrointestinal fluid losses or trauma. The electrocardiogram (ECG) should be assessed for flattened T waves, the presence of U waves, ST segment depression, and increased atrial and ventricular ectopy, particularly in patients who are receiving digitalis (Fig. 37-1).

In the emergency department setting, further evaluation of hypokalemia could start with determination of urinary electrolytes (Table 37-5). Urinary potassium greater than 20 mEq per liter indicates renal losses, whereas values less than 20 mEq per liter generally indicate extrarenal losses, especially if adequate urine flow is present (normovolemia on

Fig. 37-1. Altered cardiac conduction. In hypokalemia, the T wave is flattened and the U wave is prominent. In hyperkalemia, the ECG changes do not always correspond to the serum potassium values given, but the progression from minor to severe changes correlates to some degree with the potassium level. With a potassium concentration of less than 6.5 mEq per liter, the early ECG abnormality is peaking or tenting of the T waves. The next change, shown with a level of potassium concentration greater than 6.5, includes flattening of the P wave, prolongation of the PR interval, and widening of the QRS complex, with development of a deep S wave. With severe hyperkalemia (>8.0 mEq per liter), a sine wave pattern develops and ventricular fibrillation or cardiac arrest is imminent.
(From R.W. Schrier [ed.]. *Manual of Nephrology: Diagnosis and Therapy* [3rd ed.]. Boston: Little, Brown, 1990.)

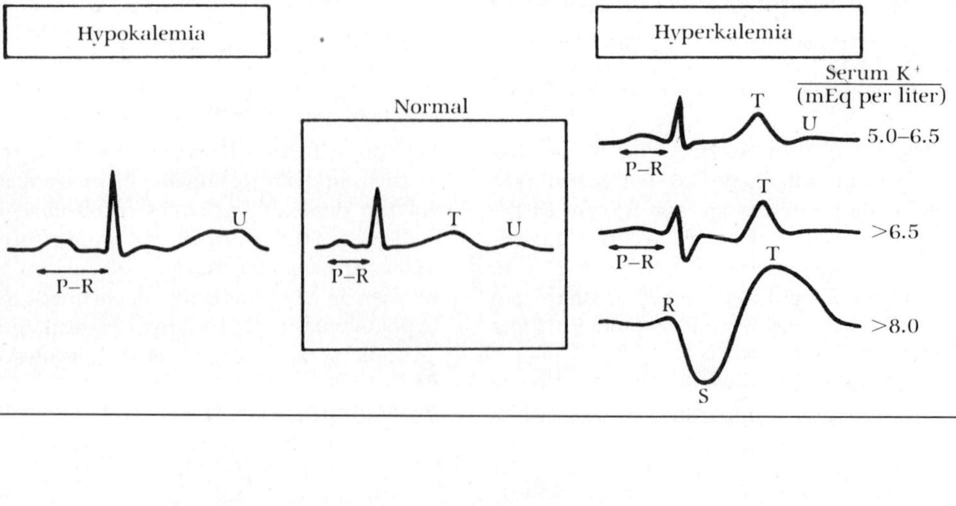

Table 37-5. Evaluation of hypokalemia

1. History and physical examination may suggest poor intake, upper or lower GI losses, or use of medication associated with hypokalemia, either by renal potassium losses or shifting potassium into cells, or states associated with hyperaldosteronism (hypertension, edematous disorders); see Table 37-3
2. Check serum bicarbonate level, pH, glucose, complete blood count; possibly magnesium
3. If unable to define cause with the above:
   a. Check urine potassium:
      Renal losses if >20mEq per liter
      Extrarenal losses if <20 mEq per liter
   b. If renal losses probable, check arterial pH:

Acidemia	=	DKA, RTA, carbonic anhydrase inhibitors, ureterosigmoidostomy
Alkalemia*	=	Diuretics, hyperaldosteronism (any cause) Nonreabsorbable anions, including bicarbonate due to upper GI loss–induced alkalosis
Normal	=	Suspect osmotic diuresis (postobstruction, recovery phase of acute renal failure)

   If extrarenal losses:

Acidemia	=	Lower GI losses
Alkalemia	=	Upper GI losses, some laxatives
Normal	=	Inadequate intake Skin losses

*Urinary chloride determination can assist in defining among these causes:

Urinary Cl < 10 mEq/day	=	Upper GI losses Volume depletion due to prior diuretic use
> 10 mEq/day	=	Mineralocorticoid excess if hypertensive Diuretics

examination or urinary sodium > 100 mEq per day). Renal losses can be further divided by either arterial pH or the presence or absence of hypertension, or both. The latter may ultimately require assessment of the renin-aldosterone axis. Patients with acidemia (pH < 7.36) may be hypokalemic because of DKA or distal RTA, while alkalotic patients (pH > 7.43), lose potassium either as a result of diuretics, excess mineralocorticoid or mineralocorticoidlike substances, vomiting with subsequent bicarbonaturia, or other nonreabsorbable anions (e.g., carbenicillin). Patients with normal pH may have experienced osmotic diuresis.

In patients with suspected extrarenal losses and nondiagnostic history, acidemia indicates the probability of lower GI fluid loss and alkalemia points toward vomiting. Laxative abuse and villous adenomas can manifest variable pH.

Therapy

Three principles should guide therapy for hypokalemia. First, the emergency department physician must decide whether or not potassium repletion should be undertaken emergently; this, of course, depends on the patient's clinical condition. The presence of significant cardiac or neuromuscular abnormalities, or both (see previous discussion), demands urgent attention. Conditions associated with profound deficits, such as DKA, likewise warrant aggressive intervention. Potassium replacement in these settings should generally be via intravenous (IV) administration (see guidelines in Table 37-6), whereas oral therapy is preferred in nonemergent settings.

Table 37-6. Guidelines for treatment of hypokalemia

1. Deficits may be large (100–200 mEq for each 1 mEq fall of serum potassium in mild deficits; 200–400 per 1 mEq fall below 3 mEq per liter)
2. Oral therapy preferred; IV administration to reverse acute cardiac or neuromuscular abnormalities
3. IV replacement generally at no more than 10 mEq/hr (maximum 40 mEq per liter fluid); in severe cases, up to 40 mEq/hr, via large, peripheral vein in ICU with careful monitoring
4. Chronic therapy with oral supplements as needed, usually 40–120 mEq/day; follow levels until stable
5. May need to correct any magnesium deficits
6. Usually use KCl, but consider K citrate or K acetate in acidosis and KPO_4 in DKA
7. Issue adequate instructions to patient discharged from emergency department about medications and arrange appropriate follow-up

The second principle is quantitation of potassium deficits. Given the large intracellular store of potassium, low serum levels likely reflect considerable deficits in total body potassium. Estimates vary, but a fall in serum potassium from about 4 to 3 mEq per liter is associated with a minimum of 100 to 200 mEq deficit, while every decrement of 1 mEq thereafter indicates an additional 200 to 400 mEq deficit. Therapy should be monitored to avoid any overshoot and development of hyperkalemia as deficits are repleted.

The third principle of therapy is safety. Not only the magnitude of replacement but the route and speed of replacement are important (see Table 37-6). In the most emergent settings (profound neuromuscular abnormalities and serious arrhythmias), rapid IV therapy may be needed but should be undertaken in a closely monitored setting as in an intensive care unit. A large, but not central, vein should be used and potassium administered at up to 40 mEq per hour, with ECG and serum levels followed closely. When IV therapy is indicated in a noncritical condition (profound deficits without severe acute clinical abnormalities), the rate should not exceed 10 mEq per hour and not more than 40 mEq should be put in a liter of IV fluids. Oral therapy, preferred whenever possible, can be tailored to replace estimated deficits and any anticipated ongoing losses, if the underlying cause of potassium loss cannot be eliminated—for example, diuretics or hyperaldosteronism of any cause. Doses can range from 40 to 120 mEq per day and a variety of preparations are available in tablet and liquid forms. Patient tolerance for taste and possible gastrointestinal side effects will determine the choice of preparation. Extreme caution is warranted when replacing potassium deficits in patients with evidence for existing or impending renal failure.

In most situations, potassium repletion with potassium chloride is appropriate. In conditions associated with metabolic alkalosis, potassium and chloride deficits generally coexist. However, in metabolic acidoses, a base may accompany potassium—for example, potassium bicarbonate, gluconate, acetate, or citrate. Several commercial preparations are available. In DKA, since considerable phosphate deficits are often seen potassium phosphate may be a better choice for repletion of at least part of the potassium deficit. Patients with coexisting magnesium deficits require magnesium repletion to allow maximum potassium conservation. These patients may also be hypocalcemic and overaggressive repletion of potassium can further lower serum calcium levels and precipitate tetany or seizures. Hypokalemia associated with abnormal transcellular distribution warrants only correction of the underlying abnormality, as no true deficit of potassium exists.

Disposition

Some patients with hypokalemia require hospital admission, though generally this decision is based on the nature and severity of the underlying illness. Severe nutritional deficits, volume deficits (especially if continuing losses are likely), severe hypertension, symptomatic edematous disorders, and DKA mandate consideration for admission. Patients who require large amounts of IV potassium or patients with ongoing neuromuscular and cardiac abnormalities need continued close monitoring. The emergency physician should make sure that appropriate initial orders are given for cardiac monitoring, volume and potassium repletion, and specific therapy, such as antihypertensive agents and insulin. Patients with less severe symptoms may need extended therapy in the emergency department before discharge, particularly if fluid repletion is necessary. The emergency physician must establish suitable end points for acute control of underlying illness, volume and potassium repletion, and control of other metabolic abnormalities. If these cannot be achieved completely in the emergency department in a timely manner, hospital admission is warranted.

Many patients with hypokalemia who can be discharged from the emergency department will require little, if any, follow-up study, provided the underlying process is self-limited. When this is not the case, or ongoing losses and need for repletion can be anticipated, arrangements for follow-up evaluation should be made. Patients should be seen by a physician within several days to several weeks, depending on the situation. Careful instruction about use of potassium supplements and other medications, as well as diet, are important. Unless particular care is taken, patients may leave the emergency department confused about changes necessary in medications they may have been taking chronically—for example, diuretics. Patients who appear to have previously undiagnosed states of aldosterone excess, renal and gastrointestinal disorders, and diabetes deserve particular care in arranging follow-up study, possibly with referral to appropriate subspecialists.

HYPERKALEMIA

Causes

The causes of hyperkalemia can be divided into three categories: increased intake, abnormal transcellular distribution, and decreased renal excretion (Table 37-7). Factitious hyperkalemia, though not common, should also be considered. This occurs when red blood cells lyse in vitro or with traumatic blood drawing. Also, white cells and platelets release potassium into the serum sample and, when present in unusually high numbers, can cause a rise in potassium. A simultaneous unclotted specimen normally has a plasma po-

Table 37-7. Causes of hyperkalemia

Factitious
Laboratory error
Pseudohyperkalemia
In vitro hemolysis
Thrombocytosis ($>10^6$)
Leukocytosis ($>10^5$)
Increased intake
Exogenous
Diet
Salt substitutes/low-sodium diet
Potassium penicillin
KCl supplements
Stored blood
Endogenous
Hemolysis
Gastrointestinal bleed
Catabolic states
Crush injury/rhabdomyolysis
Tumor lysis
Abnormal transcellular distribution
Acute acidemia
Hypertonicity
Insulin or aldosterone deficiency
Beta-2 antagonists/alpha agonist
Digitalis intoxication
Succinylcholine
Arginine HCl
Familial hyperkalemic periodic paralysis
Decreased renal excretion
Inadequate distal flow/sodium delivery
Renal failure: acute or severe chronic
Abnormalities of aldosterone axis
Aldosterone deficiency
Addison's disease
Bilateral adrenalectomy
Primary hypoaldosteronism (acquired idiopathic zona glomerulosa defect)
Enzyme deficiencies
Chronic heparin therapy
Acquired insensitivity to angiotensin II
Cyclosporine
Renin deficiency (hyporenin hypoaldosteronism)
Primary hyporeninism
Diabetic nephropathy
Tubulointerstitial diseases
Obstructive uropathy
Transplants
Angiotensinogen deficiency
Medications
Beta-blockers
Prostaglandin synthesis inhibitors
Converting enzyme inhibitors
Insensitivity of tubule to aldosterone (pseudohypoaldosteronism)
Classic type I of infancy
Type II
Chronic tubulointerstitial disorders
Spironolactone
High levels of antagonist, e.g., progesterone
Severe renal failure
Other
Amiloride/triamterene
Lithium

tassium value within 0.2 to 0.3 mEq per liter of the serum value. A greater difference suggests factitious hyperkalemia.

Excessive potassium intake will usually not cause hyperkalemia without a concomitant defect in renal excretion. Patients on low-salt diets, using salt substitutes or potassium supplements, are at risk. Medications such as potassium penicillin or stored blood provide exogenous potassium loads. Crush injuries, rhabdomyolysis, hemolysis, tumor lysis, or catabolic states can produce large endogenous loads.

Hyperkalemia due to *abnormal transcellular distribution* is not associated with true excesses in total body potassium. Acute acidemia shifts potassium from cells in exchange for hydrogen and transiently decreases potassium excretion by the kidney. This is seen primarily in metabolic acidoses, especially hyperchloremic (normal anion gap) acidoses (see previous discussion). Hypertonicity, insulin or aldosterone deficiency, beta-blockers, severe digitalis overdose, and succinylcholine cause hyperkalemia by the mechanisms described previously.

Decreased renal excretion is the most significant cause of elevated serum potassium. Impaired distal delivery and abnormalities of the aldosterone axis (synthesis or end-organ effect) are the major renal causes of impaired excretion. Any state of diminished glomerular filtration rate (GFR) or distal urine flow rate, or both, especially when acute, can cause hyperkalemia. Generally, in chronic renal failure, renal adaptation prevents hyperkalemia until GFR has fallen below 20 ml per minute. Increased gastrointestinal losses can also blunt the tendency toward hyperkalemia. In certain patients with chronic renal failure (e.g., diabetics, who may have a significant component of tubulointerstitial disease), hyperkalemia develops, with less profound decreases in GFR.

The aldosterone axis is impaired by deficiencies of hormone production, as in Addison's disease; after bilateral adrenalectomies; and in acquired zona glomerulosa defects. Deficiency in 21 hydroxylase activity decreases both aldosterone and glucocorticoid synthesis, whereas deficiency of corticosterone methyl oxidase impairs aldosterone synthesis alone, as does functional inhibition of 18 hydroxylase activity by chronic heparin therapy.

Aldosterone synthesis can also be limited by deficiencies in renin synthesis. Hyporenin-hypoaldosteronism, often associated with hyperkalemic RTA, can be a primary disorder or secondary to chronic renal diseases—for example, diabetic nephropathy, tubulointerstitial diseases (e.g., analgesia abuse, sickle cell disease, gout), chronic hypertension and glomerulonephritis, obstructive uropathy, or renal allografts. Patients are often elderly and often diabetic, with mild to moderate chronic renal insufficiency. Their low baseline renins also show impaired response to stimulation, and they may have impaired adrenal response to hyperkalemia caused by adrenal atrophy.

Production of renin or angiotensin II, or both, is affected by several drugs. Beta-blockers inhibit renin release, as do prostaglandin synthesis inhibitors, which also impair insulin release, decrease GFR via decreasing vasodilators, and can induce acute renal failure. Angiotensin converting enzyme inhibitors, especially in the setting of low GFR or beta-blockade, or both, can cause hyperkalemia by inhibiting conversion of angiotensin I to angiotensin II, resulting in inadequate aldosterone synthesis.

Table 37-8. Algorithm for evaluation of hyperkalemia

1. History and physical examination may suggest excess ingestion or endogenous load (hemolysis, trauma, etc.), medication, or diseases associated with hyperkalemia, either by impaired renal excretion or shifting of potassium out of cells, in particular diabetes and renal insufficiency (see Tables 37-1 and 37-2)
2. Check serum bicarbonate, pH, glucose, BUN, creatinine, and ECG
3. Rule out factitious hyperkalemia, if a possibility, with plasma level
4. Further evaluation, if above not definitive, is generally pursued outside the emergency department

Finally, in pseudohypoaldosteronism both renin and aldosterone levels are elevated, but the distal tubule exhibits insensitivity to aldosterone. Classic (type I) pseudohypoaldosteronism occurs in infants, and a selective defect of tubule function, possibly increased absorption of chloride, occurs in type II pseudohypoaldosteronism in adults. Chronic tubulointerstitial diseases, obstruction, and transplants, as well as cyclosporine, can cause hyperkalemia as a result of aldosterone insensitivity. Spironolactone specifically inhibits aldosterone effects at the tubule, as do high levels of antagonists, such as progesterone, seen in 21-beta-OHase deficiency. Other potassium-sparing diuretics (amiloride and triamterene) can cause hyperkalemia, and it is important to remember that potassium supplements are often given to patients who are receiving diuretics, both kaliuretic and potassium-sparing. Both cases (especially, but not exclusively, the latter) can lead to hyperkalemia.

Evaluation

Hyperkalemic patients may primarly show manifestations of the underlying illness, such as acute or end-stage chronic renal failure, trauma, sepsis, acidosis, Addison's disease, or chronic tubulointerstitial renal diseases. Specific manifestations of hyperkalemia can include weakness or paralysis; ECG abnormalities such as tall, peaked T waves; wide QRS complexes; ventricular arrhythmias; or cardiac arrest (see Fig. 37-1). Though many patients who come to the emergency department with these conditions or signs and symptoms will certainly have their electrolytes evaluated, concern about possible hyperkalemia (see Table 37-2) should prompt the emergency physician to check serum levels in any ill patient with a known history of chronic renal disease, diabetes, hypotension, or accelerated hypertension and other severe illnesses.

In the emergency department, it should be possible to attribute hyperkalemia to one of the following causes: (1) factitious hyperkalemia, (2) acidosis, (3) excessive intake, (4) inadequate distal nephron delivery, (5) drugs, or (6) renal failure (Table 37-8). After a thorough history and physical examination have been performed, arterial pH, serum bicarbonate, blood urea nitrogen (BUN), creatinine, and glucose determinations will be helpful. Given sufficient concern for factitious hyperkalemia, a plasma potassium can be checked. An ECG should be obtained promptly in any case of significant hyperkalemia. A history of daily urine output greater than 800 ml makes inadequate delivery an unlikely cause. If doubt still remains as to specific cause, evaluation of the renin-aldosterone axis, tubular secretory capacity, and extrarenal uptake of potassium may be necessary but are beyond the scope of an emergency department evaluation, though an index of aldosterone action can be obtained by solving the equation,

$$\frac{\text{Urine potassium}}{\text{Plasma potassium}} \times \frac{\text{plasma osmolality}}{\text{urine osmolarity}}$$

Values below 6.0 indicate impaired aldosterone response to hyperkalemia (low level or tubular insensitivity).

Therapy

The urgency of treating hyperkalemia depends on the presence of signs and symptoms of cardiac or neuromuscular toxicity—for example, ECG abnormalities, paresthesias, weakness, or paralysis (see previous discussion). Acute therapy is needed for levels greater than 6.0 in most cases, even without signs or symptoms, though some patients with mild chronic hyperkalemia (e.g., patients with chronic renal failure) may be tolerant of such levels. There are several categories of acute therapy (Table 37-9) and selection among these depends on the clinical condition.

Direct antagonism of the membrane effect of hyperkalemia with calcium gluconate is necessary when serious abnormalities are seen in the ECG (widening QRS complexes, loss of P waves, presence of sine waves, conduction defects, and arrhythmias) or when significant neuromuscular symptoms (tetany, paralysis) occur. In most cases, acute control of hyperkalemia can be achieved by shifting potassium into cells, though this does not eliminate excess potassium from the body. Glucose and insulin should be used acutely in most cases. Glucose should not be given without insulin, as patients may have undiagnosed diabetes and develop hyperglycemia, which can worsen hyperkalemia. Likewise, insulin should not be used without concomitant glucose infusion to avoid hypoglycemia.

Evidence suggests that beta-2–specific agonists, such as albuterol, can be effective in lowering serum potassium acutely. Administration of bicarbonate can exacerbate volume overload in patients with congestive heart failure, but if tolerated, will help shift potassium into cells.

Even in the acute setting, measures to eliminate potassium excess should be initiated. Diuretics can accomplish this if GFR is adequate, but often the physician must rely on the gut. Acutely, cation exchange resin, sodium polystyrene sulfonate (Kayexalate), should be used with a cathartic (sorbitol) to assure rapid movement through the GI tract. As cation exchange occurs in the colon, Kayexalate enemas may be necessary if upper gastrointestinal motility is inadequate to deliver an oral dose to the colon. In cases of critically elevated potassium, the physician should avoid the tendency to undertreat with insufficient amounts of exchange resins. Doses can be repeated hourly if necessary while potassium levels are followed. Kayexalate also removes magnesium and calcium and presents a sodium load that can compromise patients with congestive heart failure. Dialysis, especially hemodialysis, can effectively remove potassium if other means fail, but availability of this technique and creation of acute vascular access cause delays. Chronic therapy should be initiated in the emergency department in appropriate cases (see the following section).

Table 37-9. Guidelines for treatment of hyperkalemia

Acute therapy

I. Direct antagonism of membrane effect
- A. Calcium (raises threshold potential)
  - 10–20 ml 10% calcium gluconate IV
    - Onset: immediate
    - Duration: 30–60 min
    - Repeat: after 5–10 min if no effect and as needed as effect wanes
    - Caution: patient on digitalis, infuse slowly in 100-ml D_5W over 20–30 min
- B. Hypertonic saline: 50–100 ml
  - (Rarely used, mainly in patients with coexisting severe hyponatremia, which can exacerbate potassium's membrane effect)

II. Redistribution of potassium into cells
- A. Bicarbonate
  - 50 mEq (1 ampule $NaHCO_3$) over 5 min
    - Onset: 5–10 min
    - Duration: 2 hr
    - Repeat: as needed (avoid alkalosis)
    - Caution: patients with hypocalcemia, volume overload
- B. Insulin (regular)
  - 10–20 units with 1 ampule D50 (or 500 ml D10 over 1 hr)
    - Onset: 30 min
    - Duration: 4–6 hr
- C. Albuterol, recently described for use in patients in renal failure
  - Further evaluation necessary before it can be recommended for routine use (0.5 mg in 100 ml D_5W IV over 15 min or 10–20 mg nebulized inhalation treatment)

III. Removal of potassium from body
- A. Diuretics (loop, thiazide)
- B. Sodium polystyrene sulfonate (Kayexalate; 1 gm removes 0.5–1.0 mEq potassium, in exchange for 2–3 mEq sodium)
  - 25–50 gm in 15 ml 70% sorbitol
  - or
  - 50 gm in 200 ml D_5W per rectum as 30–60 min retention enema
  - Repeat every 1–4 hr as needed
- C. Dialysis (particularly hemodialysis)

Chronic Therapy

1. Low-potassium diet (<60 mEq/day)
2. Avoid or adjust beta-blockers, nonsteroidal antiinflammatory drugs, converting enzyme inhibitors, heparin, potassium-sparing diuretics
3. Control blood sugar
4. Avoid volume contraction
5. $NaHCO_3$ or $CaCO_3$
6. Thiazides
7. Kayexalate (no sorbitol for chronic therapy, unless significant constipation occurs)
8. Fludrocortisone acetate (Florinef) if mineralocorticoid deficient, or possibly hyporeninism

Disposition

Disposition largely depends on the nature of the underlying illness, which will often mandate hospital admission—for example, trauma, severe hemolytic anemia, undiagnosed renal disease, sepsis, and other catabolic states. Patients with known chronic renal diseases, who may have a degree of tolerance for hyperkalemia, may not require admission unless it is indicated by other acute problems. Adequate chronic therapy and appropriate follow-up examination are necessary, however. Hyperkalemia can complicate episodes of acute renal failure due to volume depletion, and effective emergency volume resuscitation may obviate any further treatment. Some patients may only require adjustment of medications, eliminating or changing doses of drugs such as beta-blockers, nonsteroidal inflammatory drugs, and converting enzyme inhibitors. The physician should make sure that patients who need hospitalization will have appropriate monitoring and follow-up laboratory examinations.

Patients who are discharged should be instructed about medications, sources of potassium in the diet, and maintenance of adequate hydration and blood sugar control when appropriate. Use of diuretics or cation binding resins requires explanation and any patient so treated needs immediate and close outpatient follow-up study. Generally, all patients who demonstrate hyperkalemia in the emergency department, regardless of underlying cause, should have follow-up examination with a physician within several days to weeks depending on the situation. Some will require further evaluation—for example, specialized workup of the renin-aldosterone axis, renal secretory capacity, or other aspects of renal function. Referral to a nephrologist may be appropriate. In general, obtaining serum levels of renin and aldosterone in the acute setting is not helpful, as interpretation of results is best accomplished in controlled settings.

SELECTED READING

Brown, R S. Extrarenal potassium homeostasis. *Kidney Int* 30:116, 1986.

DeFronzo, R A. Hyperkalemic States. In, M H Maxwell, C R Kleeman, and R G Narins (eds), *Clinical Disorders of Fluid and Electrolyte Metabolism* (4th ed). McGraw-Hill, 1987.

DeFronzo, R A, et al. Clinical disorders of hyperkalemia. *Ann Rev Med* 33:521, 1982.

Field, M J, and Giebisch, G J. Hormonal control of renal potassium excretion. *Kidney Int* 27:379, 1985.

Gabow, P A, and Peterson, L N. Disorders of Potassium Metabolism. In R W Schrier, *Renal and Electrolyte Disorders* (3rd ed). Boston: Little, Brown, 1986.

Gennari, F J, and Cohen, J J. The role of the kidney in potassium homeostasis: Lessons from acid base disturbances. *Kidney Int* 8:1, 1975.

Ponce, S P, et al. Drug induced hyperkalemia. *Medicine* 64:357, 1985.

Raymond, K H, and Kunau, R T, Jr. Hypokalemic States. In M H Maxwell, C R Kleeman, and R G Narins (eds.), *Clinical Disorders of Fluid and Electrolyte Metabolism* (4th ed). New York: McGraw-Hill, 1987.

Wright, F S. Renal potassium handling. *Semin Nephrol* 7:174, 1987.

38. Acid-Base Disorders

Sharon Silbiger
Jeffrey Stoff

The importance of recognizing and understanding acid-base abnormalities in the emergency department cannot be overstated. Certain medical situations warrant immediate intervention whereas a "wait and watch" posture suffices in others. At times, the acid-base abnormality is an expected companion to an obvious medical problem, but at other times it may be the only clue to the existence of an otherwise occult and serious illness. The correct diagnosis and intervention depend on the physician's understanding of the principles of acid-base physiology and their impact on health and disease.

PATHOPHYSIOLOGY

An understanding of acid-base physiology begins with the Bronsted-Lowry definition of acids and bases. Acids are defined as "proton donors" and bases as "proton acceptors." Strong acids are substances with a weak affinity for a proton or a propensity to "donate" a proton, while weak acids are defined as substances with a strong affinity for a proton and a low propensity to "donate" a proton.

Acids and bases in equilibrium follow the law of mass action, first described by Guldberg and Waage:

$$K' = [A^-]\,[H^+]/[HA] \qquad (1)$$

where [HA] is the concentration of acid, $[A^-]$ the concentration of base, $[H^+]$ the hydrogen ion concentration, and K' the apparent dissociation constant of the acid. Under a given set of circumstances (specifically temperature and pressure), the K' of a particular acid is a constant—that is, the acid and base pair is in equilibrium. Strong acids have a large dissociation constant K' and weak acids a small constant. From the law of mass action, we can derive the commonly used Henderson-Hasselbach equation. Solving for $[H^+]$ in equation 1:

$$[H^+] = K'\,[HA]/[A^-].$$

As defined by Sorensen in 1909, $pH = -\log [H^+]$; therefore:

$$-\log [H^+] = -\log K' - \log [HA]/[A^-]$$

Since $-\log K' = pK'$, the Henderson-Hasselbach equation becomes:

$$pH = pK' + \log [A^-]/[HA] \qquad (2)$$

As defined by this equation, the pH of a solution depends on the pK' and the ratio of the base $[A^-]$ and its corresponding acid [HA]. The Henderson-Hasselbach equation is commonly used to describe the carbonic acid–bicarbonate pair, which is the major acid-base pair that determines the serum pH in humans.

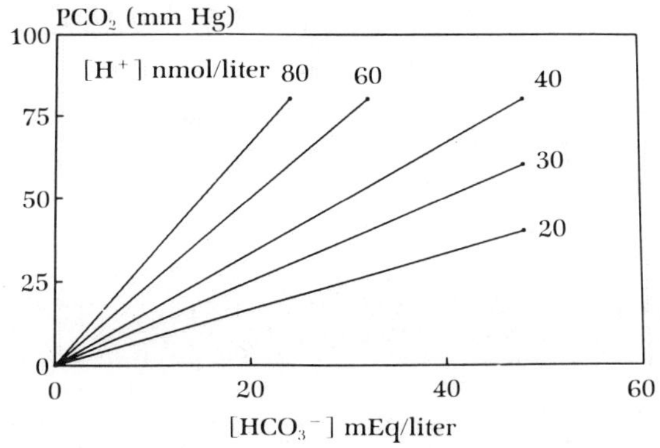

Fig. 38-1. Nomogram depicting the relationship between the [HCO_3^-], the PCO_2, and the arterial [H^+].

Table 38-1. pH corresponding to [H^+]

pH	[H^+] (nmole/liter)
7.8	16
7.7	20
7.6	25
7.5	32
7.4	40
7.3	50
7.2	63
7.1	79
7.0	100
6.9	126
6.8	158

Since the pK′ of this bicarbonate–carbonic acid pair at 37°C is 6.1, the Henderson-Hasselbach equation becomes:

$$pH = 6.1 + \log [HCO_3^-]/[H_2CO_3] \quad (3)$$

where [HCO_3^-] represents the concentration of bicarbonate and [H_2CO_3] the concentration of carbonic acid. Since [H_2CO_3] is approximately equal to CO_2 (dissolved) and CO_2 (dissolved) is approximately equal to $\alpha \times PCO_2$, the equation becomes:

$$pH = 6.1 + \log [HCO_3^-]/\alpha PCO_2 \quad (4)$$

where α = the solubility coefficient at 37°C = 0.03 and PCO_2 = the partial pressure of CO_2. The pH depends on the pK′ (6.1) and the ratio of [HCO_3^-] to PCO_2 (the base:acid ratio). As depicted graphically in Fig. 38-1, the [H^+] or pH remains stable over a wide range of [HCO_3^-] and PCO_2 values, if the ratio of these two components is constant.

The logarithmic functions of the Henderson-Hasselbach equation are cumbersome for a clinician to use. This relationship can be further modified to its nonlogarithmic form:

$$[H^+] = 24PCO_2/[HCO_3^-] \quad (5)$$

This equation is sufficiently accurate over a pH range from 7.2 to 7.6 units, where there is linearity in the relationship between the pH and the [H^+]. Table 38-1 provides a range of pH values and the corresponding [H^+]. Conversion of pH to [H^+] is necessary if equation 5 is to be used. The [HCO_3^-] (mEq/liter) can be obtained from a mixed venous blood sample and the PCO_2 (mm Hg) and pH from an arterial blood gas determination. Measurement of any two of these variables permits calculation of the third.

Biologic pH Maintenance

Normal serum pH is maintained between 7.36 and 7.44 pH units. Within this range, many cellular processes are optimized. Changes in pH (or [H^+]) are sensed by central nervous system (CNS) receptors in the medulla oblongata and in the arterial circulation by the carotid body. Within these tight limits, pH is maintained by a sophisticated system of "buffering." A buffer is an acid-base pair that resists changes in pH with the addition of hydrogen ion (H^+) or hydroxyl ion (OH^-) over a certain pH range. The buffering systems of the body are in continuous operation, minimizing changes in blood pH from the daily addition of approximately 50,000 mmole carbon dioxide and 50 to 100 mEq nonvolatile acids. These strong acids (sulfuric, phosphoric, and other organic acids) are generated from the metabolism of fats, carbohydrates, and amino acids.

The importance of this buffering system is apparent when one calculates the pH change that would result if 1 mmole daily acid production went unbuffered in 10 liters of body water:

$$[H^+] = 1 \text{ mmole/10 liters} = 0.1 \text{ mmole/liter} = \text{pH of } 4.0$$

When acid production or the delivery of exogenous acids exceeds daily excretion, buffer systems maintain the pH within the "normal" range. There are three major buffering spaces: the extracellular space, the intracellular space, and bone.

The extracellular buffering system consists mainly of the bicarbonate–carbonic acid buffering pair and, to a lesser degree, inorganic phosphates and proteins. The effect of extracellular buffering on an acid load is virtually instantaneous. Using the bicarbonate–carbonic acid pair, the acid (H^+) is buffered as follows:

$$H^+ + HCO_3^- \longleftrightarrow H_2CO_3 \longleftrightarrow H_2O + CO_2$$

The intracellular system consists mainly of protein buffers such as hemoglobin (Hb^-) as in the red blood cell. Inorganic and organic phosphates also play a small role. Several hours are required for intracellular buffers to reach equilibrium with extracellular buffers.

$$H^+ + HCO_3^- + Hb^- \longleftrightarrow H^+Hb^- + HCO_3^-$$

Between the extracellular and intracellular compartments, the exchange of H^+ for sodium (Na^+) and potassium (K^+) also occurs. In situations of low pH or high [H^+] due mainly to inorganic acid addition into the extracellular space, H^+ is transported into cells in exchange for intracellular Na^+, K^+, or both. These H^+ ions are buffered by intracellular mechanisms. In clinical situations, it is not uncommon for the serum potassium level to rise as a consequence of this pro-

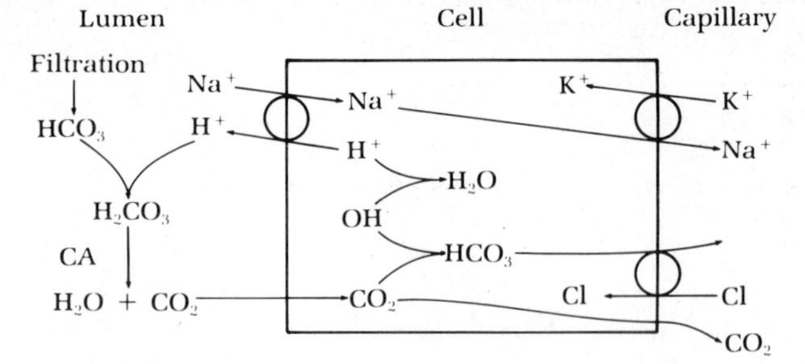

Fig. 38-2. Ion transport occurring between lumen and capillary across a renal tubular cell. (CA = carbonic anhydrase.)

cess. It is estimated that a decrease of 0.1 pH units results in a rise in the $[K^+]$ of 0.6–0.8 mEq/liter.

The third major buffering space is that of bone, which constitutes a large reservoir of bicarbonate. The bicarbonate in bone is able to buffer a large amount of both acute and chronic acid loads.

$$H^+HCO_3^- \longleftrightarrow H_2CO_3 \longleftrightarrow H_2O + CO_2$$

Although the low pK′ of the bicarbonate–carbonic acid buffer pair of 6.1 is not optimal for efficient buffering at physiologic pH (7.4), it is still principally responsible for the maintenance of serum pH at this level. The effectiveness of this system resides in the uniqueness of the buffer pair. Unlike other buffer pairs, in which the sum of the components of the system is fixed, the bicarbonate–carbonic acid buffer system is "open ended." The dissolved CO_2 is in equilibrium with an infinite gaseous reservoir (PCO_2), which can be excreted or retained by the lungs.

The pulmonary and renal systems are the major organ systems responsible for pH maintenance in humans. The lung controls PCO_2 through ventilation, and the kidney maintains serum $[HCO_3^-]$ through bicarbonate reabsorption and hydrogen ion secretion.

Pulmonary Mechanisms of Acid-Base Balance

Low pH stimulates the respiratory center in the medulla oblongata and causes an increase both in respiratory rate and tidal volume. There is a subsequent fall in PCO_2 and therefore an increase in pH (equation 4). Conversely, elevated pH causes a lowering of the respiratory rate, an increase in PCO_2, and subsequent drop in pH toward normal.

Rapid changes in arterial pH can induce equally rapid changes in the respiratory rate. This change in respiratory rate and concomitant change in PCO_2 are considered the normal respiratory compensation for a metabolic derangement in the pH.

Renal Mechanisms of Acid-Base Balance

Through the processes of bicarbonate reabsorption and hydrogen ion secretion, the kidney can restore the principal buffer base bicarbonate and stabilize systemic pH.

BICARBONATE REABSORPTION. The proximal tubule reclaims as much as 90 percent of the daily filtered load of bicarbonate. It does so via a complex system of ion transport between the tubular lumen, the proximal tubular cell, and the peritubular capillary (Fig. 38-2).

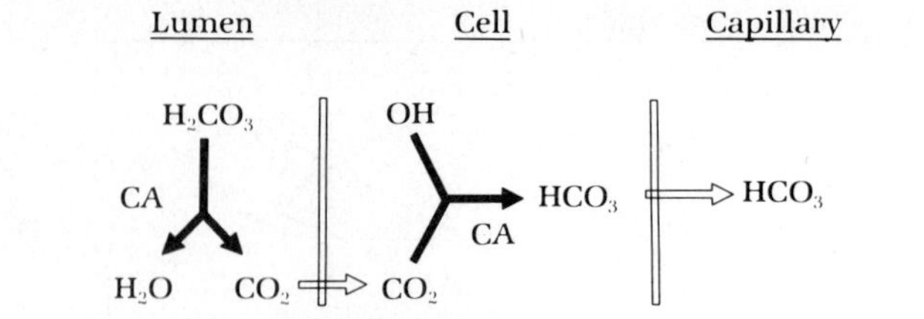

Fig. 38-3. Mechanism of bicarbonate reclamation by the renal tubule. (CA = carbonic anhydrase.)

Bicarbonate is reabsorbed by an indirect process through which intracellular hydrogen ions are exchanged for filtered sodium ions. Hydrogen ion in the tubular lumen combines with filtered bicarbonate to form H_2CO_3, which is hydrolyzed to $CO_2 + H_2O$ in the presence of carbonic anhydrase localized to the luminal brush border (Fig. 38-3).

As depicted in Fig. 38-2, the reabsorption of bicarbonate depends on the transport of other ions and the secretion of hydrogen ions via sodium-hydrogen exchange at the luminal membrane and via bicarbonate-chloride exchange at the basolateral membrane. Several factors promote proximal tubular bicarbonate reabsorption, including elevated PCO_2, hypokalemia, and extracellular fluid volume contraction. The distal tubule also reabsorbs bicarbonate (although less than 20% of the filtered load is reabsorbed here), and actively secretes hydrogen ions.

HYDROGEN ION SECRETION. There are two major mechanisms for hydrogen ion secretion into the distal tubule: titratable acidity and ammonium (NH_4^+) formation. Titratable acidity is the process whereby hydrogen ions combine with urinary buffers (mainly HPO_4^{2-}) and are excreted as depicted by the following:

$$H^+ + HPO_4^{2-} \longleftrightarrow H_2PO_4^-$$

This mechanism accounts for approximately one percent of the total hydrogen ion secreted by the kidney. Using this process, 10 to 40 mEq hydrogen ion can be buffered and eliminated daily. This process is limited by the filtration and reabsorption of phosphate and other urinary buffers.

The second mechanism by which hydrogen ions are excreted involves the combination of hydrogen ion with ammonia (NH_3) to form ammonium (NH_4^+).

$$H^+ + NH_3 \longleftrightarrow NH_4^+$$

Ammonia, produced by the proximal tubule, diffuses into the tubular lumen and combines with hydrogen ion secreted by the distal nephron. The NH_4^+ ion formed is trapped in the lumen and excreted principally as the ammonium salt of chloride or sulfate. Under normal circumstances, this process also accounts for approximately one percent of the hydrogen ion titrated (30–50 mEq per day). Whereas titratable acidity has a fixed nature, the renal proximal tubule cell has the capacity to increase NH_3 production in the presence of metabolic acidosis and hypokalemia and thereby increase H^+ elimination. This process requires deamination and deamidation of glutamine by proximal tubular cells to produce NH_3.

Table 38-2. Physical signs in acidemia and alkalemia

Signs	Mechanisms
Severe acidemia (pH < 7.2) Kussmaul's respiration Hypotension Pulmonary edema Arrhythmia (ventricular fibrillation)	Depressed myocardial contractility, decreased peripheral resistance and tissue hypoxia
Severe alkalemia (pH > 7.55) CNS changes Paresthesias Carpopedal spasm Angina	Vasoconstriction of the cerebral vasculature, coronary vasospasm, and leftward shift of the oxygen-hemoglobin dissociation curve

Failure to completely reabsorb bicarbonate or maximally secrete hydrogen ion results in renal tubular acidosis. The renal response to perturbations in systemic pH requires several days to exert a maximal effect. These alterations in the absorptive and secretory processes of the kidney in response to changes in arterial pH due to respiratory disturbances are termed *normal metabolic compensations.* The degree of metabolic compensation depends on the severity and the duration of the respiratory abnormality.

DIAGNOSIS

The first step in diagnosing acid-base disturbances in the emergency department is having sufficient clinical suspicion to warrant pursuit of appropriate laboratory tests. As in other medical conditions, clinical suspicion can be aroused by a complete history and physical examination of the patient. The importance of these two factors should not be minimized. For example, the physician should suspect a potential metabolic acidosis in a patient who admits to a toxic ingestion of antifreeze or metabolic alkalosis in an individual with a history of protracted vomiting. With respect to the physical examination, acidemia and alkalemia predispose to certain physical findings, which, although not specific for these acid-base disorders, may be helpful in diagnosis.

Table 38-2 lists some of these findings. Kussmaul's respiration, hemodynamic instability, and arrhythmias may be seen in severe acidemia (pH < 7.2), while central nervous system findings and neuromuscular and cardiac irregularities may be seen in severe alkalemia (pH > 7.55).

After an adequate history is taken, physical examination is performed, and acute intervention directed toward stabilizing the patient's condition is accomplished, pursuit of certain laboratory tests is invaluable in deciphering the acid-base disorder in a given situation. The basic laboratory tests necessary for adequate assessment of acid-base balance are arterial blood gas determination (ABG) and serum electrolyte values.

Arterial blood gas sampling provides information regarding the arterial pH, PCO_2, and partial pressure of oxygen (PO_2). The pH and PCO_2 are two components of the modified Henderson-Hasselbach equation, where $[H^+] = 24 \times PCO_2/[HCO_3^-]$ (see equation 5). It is possible to calculate the serum bicarbonate concentration from the PCO_2 and pH. The bicarbonate concentration reported on an arterial blood gas specimen is a calculated value using the Henderson-Hasselbach equation.

Serum electrolytes provide direct information regarding the venous blood concentrations of sodium $[Na^+]$, potassium $[K^+]$, chloride $[Cl^-]$, and bicarbonate $[HCO_3^-]$. Abnormalities in one or several of these parameters provide clues to the underlying disease process.

The combination of an arterial blood gas determination and serum electrolytes provides sufficient laboratory information to determine the acid-base derangement. Additional tests such as urinary pH measurement and urinary electrolytes may be required to further define the specific etiology of the abnormality.

Before delineating a stepwise approach to the diagnosis of acid-base disorders, certain definitions should be noted. The suffix "osis" denotes the presence of an abnormal acid-base process. For example, *acidosis* means that a process is under way that increases the amount of acid (H^+) in the body. Several processes may be operant simultaneously, producing additive or neutralizing effects. Thus, there may be no net increase in hydrogen ion (or decrease in pH). Acidosis therefore does not necessarily imply that the measured arterial pH will be low.

The suffix "emia" refers to the state of acid-base balance in the blood. For example, *acidemia* means that the arterial pH is low or that the $[H^+]$ is increased. It does not define which acid-base processes are present that result in a low arterial pH. Acidemia is defined as an arterial pH less than 7.36 and alkalemia as an arterial pH greater than 7.44 pH units. Metabolic processes involve the accumulation or loss of bicarbonate ion, and respiratory processes are associated with an increase or decrease in the PCO_2.

The following steps should be consistently followed when acid-base disorders are analyzed:

1. *Obtain history and perform physical examination.*
2. *Obtain arterial blood gas and serum electrolyte values.*
3. *Determine "internal consistency" of laboratory values.* The modified Henderson-Hasselbach equation shows that the hydrogen ion concentration equals $24 \times PCO_2$ divided by the bicarbonate concentration (see equation 5). The hydrogen ion concentration (or pH) and the PCO_2 are obtained from an arterial blood gas specimen, and the bicarbonate concentration from the venous serum sample. Regardless of the acid-base abnormality, the $[H^+]$, PCO_2, and $[HCO_3^-]$ can be substituted into equation 5 to determine internal consistency of these parameters. If this equation does not hold true, then the arterial blood gases and electrolytes do not provide accurate information for determination of the patient's acid-base status. This commonly occurs when the arterial blood gas and electrolytes are not obtained simultaneously. If the values are inconsistent—that is, the $[H^+] \neq 24PCO_2/[HCO_3^-]$ based on the laboratory values—a new complement of serum electrolytes and arterial blood gas determinations should be obtained to provide accurate information. It is suggested that these laboratory tests be drawn as simultaneously as possible. If the values are internally consistent, one should proceed to the following step.

Table 38-3. Simple acid-base disorders

Primary abnormality	pH	$[HCO_3^-]$ (mEq/liter)	PCO_2 (mm Hg)
Metabolic acidosis	<7.36	<24	<40
Respiratory acidosis		>24	>40
Metabolic alkalosis	>7.44	>24	>40
Respiratory alkalosis		<24	<40

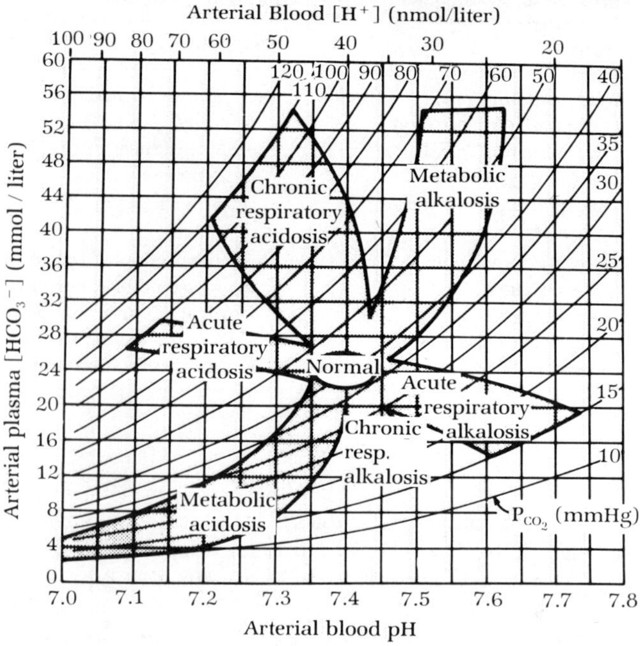

Fig. 38-4. Acid-base nomogram. The 95 percent confidence limits of the normal respiratory and metabolic compensations for primary acid-base disturbances are shown. (From B.M. Brenner and F.C. Rector, Jr. [eds.]. *The Kidney* [3rd ed]. Philadelphia: Saunders, 1986.)

Table 38-4. Respiratory and metabolic compensations for primary acid-base disorders

A. Expected respiratory response to metabolic derangements
 I. Metabolic acidosis
  1. $PCO_2 = 1.5\ ([HCO_3^-]) + 8 \pm 2$
  2. $\Delta\ PCO_2 = 1.2\ (\Delta\ [HCO_3^-])$
  3. $PCO_2 \approx$ last 2 digits of the arterial pH
 II. Metabolic alkalosis
  1. $\Delta\ PCO_2 = 0.6\ (\Delta\ [HCO_3^-])$

B. Expected metabolic response to respiratory derangements
 I. Respiratory acidosis
  1. Acute respiratory acidosis
   a. $\Delta\ [HCO_3^-] = 0.1\ (\Delta\ PCO_2)$
  2. Chronic respiratory acidosis
   a. $\Delta\ [HCO_3^-] = 0.35\ (\Delta\ PCO_2)$
 II. Respiratory alkalosis
  1. Acute respiratory alkalosis
   a. $\Delta\ [HCO_3^-] = 0.2\ (\Delta\ PCO_2)$
  2. Chronic respiratory alkalosis
   a. $\Delta\ [HCO_3^-] = 0.5\ (\Delta\ PCO_2)$

4. *Check arterial pH.* If the arterial pH is less than 7.36, the patient has acidemia; if it is greater than 7.44, the patient has alkalemia. A normal pH does not exclude the presence of acid-base abnormalities; for example, acidosis can be present without acidemia.

5. *Check serum bicarbonate concentration and PCO_2 values.* The bicarbonate concentration and PCO_2 values help determine the type of acid-base abnormality present. For example, an arterial pH of less than 7.36 (acidemia) and a low serum bicarbonate concentration (< 24 mEq/liter) indicate a metabolic acidosis. If the arterial pH is less than 7.36 and the PCO_2 is greater than 40 mm Hg, a respiratory acidosis is present. Table 38-3 lists the four types of simple acid-base disorders and the expected values of pH, PCO_2, and $[HCO_3^-]$ in each.

6. *Evaluate compensatory response.* During primary respiratory acid-base abnormalities (increases or decreases in PCO_2), expected metabolic or renal mechanisms are activated that normalize arterial pH. In contrast, during primary metabolic abnormalities (increases or decreases in $[HCO_3^-]$), respiratory or pulmonary mechanisms are activated to compensate. For a given primary metabolic or primary respiratory process, the magnitude of the compensatory change can be calculated and should move in the same direction as the primary process. For example, in metabolic acidosis, a fall in the serum bicarbonate concentration is compensated for by a fall in PCO_2, which minimizes the decline in arterial pH (see equation 5). Thus, in "simple" acid-base disorders, compensation tends to return the serum pH toward normal. If the direction of the compensatory change is in a direction opposite to the primary abnormality, then a second primary abnormality exists in the compensatory system. For example, a patient with an arterial pH of 7.0, a serum $[HCO_3^-]$ of less than 24 mEq/liter, and a PCO_2 of greater than 45 mm Hg has both a primary metabolic acidosis and a primary respiratory acidosis. This is called a "mixed acid-base disturbance."

The expected change in the compensatory component depends on the primary process and can be interpolated from a metabolic acid-base map (Fig. 38-4) or calculated from formulas listed in Table 38-4. The specific formulas listed can be used to calculate "appropriate compensation" as follows: When a patient arrives in the emergency department in septic shock, it is likely that metabolic acidosis secondary to lactic acid accumulation is present. This is confirmed by a low serum pH and $[HCO_3^-]$. In this hypothetical case the $[HCO_3^-]$ is 16 mEq/liter. Using the appropriate formula the expected compensatory change in PCO_2 is calculated in this situation:

In metabolic acidosis: $PCO_2 = 1.5\ ([HCO_3^-]) + 8 \pm 2$

Therefore: $PCO_2 = 1.5\ (16\ \text{mEq/liter}) + 8 \pm 2$

$PCO_2 = 30 - 34$ mm Hg

If the actual PCO_2 (ABG) is within this range, a simple metabolic acidosis with appropriate respiratory compensation exists. If the actual PCO_2 is less than 30 mm Hg, a superimposed respiratory alkalosis is present, and if it is

Table 38-5. Metabolic acidosis with elevated anion gap

Ketoacidosis
Diabetic
Alcoholic
Starvation
Glycogenesis I, defects in gluconeogenesis
Lactic acidosis
Infection
Ischemia
Seizures
Strenuous exercise
Hepatic necrosis
Tumors
Poisoning (see below)
Short bowel syndrome
Renal failure
Ingestions/exposures
Salicylates
Carbon monoxide, cyanide, iron, isonicotinic acid hydrazide, strychnine, phenformin (lactic)
Methanol
Ethylene glycol
Hydrofluoric acid

Table 38-6. Metabolic acidosis with normal anion gap

Gastrointestinal loss of bicarbonate
Diarrhea
Laxatives
Pancreatic drainage
Chloride containing anion-exchange resins
Magnesium chloride, calcium chloride
Ureteral diversions (ileal-bladder, ileal-ureter, uretero-sigmoidostomy, obstructed ileal loop conduit)
Renal
Renal tubular acidosis
Early renal failure
Interstitial renal disease
Hyperparathyroidism
Ingestions/intoxications
Ammonium chloride
Hyperalimentation
Carbonic anhydrase inhibitors (acetazolamide)
Miscellaneous
Posthypocapneic
Recovery from diabetic ketoacidosis
Diuretic-phase acute tubular necrosis
"Expansion" acidosis

greater than 34 mm Hg, a superimposed respiratory acidosis exists. The latter two conditions are examples of mixed acid-base disorders. It is necessary to recognize (by pH, PCO_2, $[HCO_3^-]$, and clinical scenario) at least one of the acid-base disorders operating in a patient at a given time so the appropriate formula in Table 38-4 can be used.

The map in Fig. 38-4 was constructed based on studies measuring the metabolic or respiratory response in volunteers to alterations in acid-base balance. Based on these results, "confidence bands" were established. Acid-base disorders whose values place them within the confidence bands of a particular disorder are "simple" acid-base disorders, as those listed in Table 38-3. "Mixed acid-base disturbances" are defined as those situations in which the values fall outside of these confidence bands.

7. *Determine the unmeasured anion gap.* The anion gap (AG) is helpful in differentiating between the various types of metabolic acidosis. It is defined as the difference between the sodium concentration $[Na^+]$ and the sum of the chloride concentration $[Cl^-]$ and the bicarbonate concentration $[HCO_3^-]$.

$$AG = [Na^+] - ([Cl^-] + [HCO_3^-]) \qquad (6)$$

The normal anion gap is between 8 and 12 mEq/liter when the serum albumin is normal. These 8 to 12 mEq/liter are attributed to unmeasured extracellular anions, such as phosphate, sulfate, organic anions, and negatively charged serum proteins. Elevations in the calculated anion gap occur when there is an accumulation of these anions—for example, ketones, lactate, or sulfate.

MANAGEMENT

Management of acid-base disturbances is ultimately directed toward the diagnosis and treatment of the underlying medical disorder. However, since extremes in the serum pH can have profound life-threatening effects, emergent treatment directed solely at moving the arterial pH from the "dangerous" zone into the "safe" zone may be required. It should be remembered that even if therapy is instituted to change the arterial pH, the underlying pathophysiologic conditions must be recognized and specific treatment instituted. Treatment should be accompanied by frequent measurements of serum electrolytes and arterial blood gas values to assess the patient's status and the response to therapy. Specific treatment modalities are discussed in their respective sections.

Metabolic Acidosis

Metabolic acidosis is the result of accumulation of $[H^+]$ ions in the extracellular space. Certain types of metabolic acidoses are accompanied by the accumulation of "unmeasured" anions and therefore tend to increase the anion gap. The calculation of the anion gap in metabolic acidosis can help determine the etiology of the acid-base imbalance and is a useful initial step in limiting the diagnostic options (Tables 38-5, 38-6).

It is helpful in the management and treatment of metabolic acidosis to estimate the amount of bicarbonate required to return the serum $[HCO_3^-]$ to normal (24 mEq/liter). This calculation is based on the volume of distribution of the HCO_3^- ion, which can be estimated as approximately 0.5 × body weight (kg). This calculation assumes a steady state and does not account for ongoing HCO_3^- ion losses.

$$HCO_3^- \text{ "deficit" (mEq)} = 0.5 \text{ (or} \sim 0.7 \text{ in severe metabolic acidosis)} \times \text{body weight (kg)} \times (\text{normal } [HCO_3^-] - \text{actual } [HCO_3^-]) \qquad (7)$$

For example, to calculate the amount of bicarbonate required to restore a normal serum $[HCO_3^-]$ (24 mEq/liter) in a 70-kg man whose $[HCO_3^-]$ is 14 mEq/liter, the amount of HCO_3^- required is:

$$0.5 \times 70 \text{ kg} \times (24 \text{ mEq/liter} - 14 \text{ mEq/liter}) = 350 \text{ mEq}$$

In practical terms, less bicarbonate is usually administered to partially correct the serum [HCO_3^-], since complete normalization is unnecessary. When using bicarbonate therapy in metabolic acidosis, it is important to carefully assess the arterial pH during administration since measurement of serum [HCO_3^-] alone fails to reflect persistent ventilatory compensation and can lead to overshoot treatment and alkalemia. Bicarbonate therapy is justified in certain clinical situations, but it is controversial or contraindicated in others. Bicarbonate is usually administered as sodium bicarbonate ($NaHCO_3$). A solution of $NaHCO_3$ nearly isotonic to plasma can be achieved by the addition of three ampules of $NaHCO_3$ to one liter of dextrose in water (D_5W).

In most medical centers, one ampule (50 ml) of $NaHCO_3$ contains 44.6 mEq sodium (Na^+) and 44.6 mEq bicarbonate (HCO_3^-). Therefore, administration of bicarbonate necessitates administration of sodium. Sodium bicarbonate therapy therefore may be detrimental in situations associated with volume overload, congestive heart failure, renal failure, or liver failure.

The expected respiratory compensation for a metabolic acidosis can be calculated using any of the following formulas.

1. $PCO_2 = 1.5\,[HCO_3^-] + 8 \pm 2$
2. $\Delta\ PCO_2 = 1.2\ (\Delta\ [HCO_3^-])$
3. $PCO_2 \approx$ last 2 digits of the arterial pH

Elevated Anion Gap Metabolic Acidosis

There are several different types of elevated anion gap metabolic acidosis (see Table 38-5). Those commonly encountered in the emergency department include diabetic and alcoholic ketoacidosis, lactic acidosis secondary to infection or ischemia, severe renal failure, and toxic ingestion of salicylates, methanol, or ethylene glycol.

DIABETIC KETOACIDOSIS. In the presence of insufficient insulin to meet metabolic demands, fatty acids are mobilized and used for energy in place of glucose. The end products of fatty acid metabolism include acetoacetic and beta-hydroxybutyric acids. Acetoacetic acid is decarboxylated to acetone, which is a ketone. The anion gap is elevated in diabetic ketoacidosis (DKA) due to the accumulation of these anions. The serum and urine tests for ketones using the nitroprusside reaction react with acetoacetic acid and acetone but not with beta-hydroxybutyrate.

In DKA, volume depletion due to osmotic diuresis and poor oral intake is often present. The physical examination may reveal orthostatic hypotension, tachycardia, poor skin turgor, dry mucous membranes, and a fruity odor to the patient's breath. Abdominal complaints are frequently present. Aside from the expected elevation in blood sugar, serum electrolytes reveal a low serum [HCO_3^-] and an elevated anion gap. The arterial blood gas confirms the presence of a metabolic acidosis. The urine and serum tests for ketones show positive results.

Intravenous fluids, insulin therapy, and potassium repletion are the mainstays of treatment for DKA. In the presence of insulin, accumulated ketoacids and lactic acid are converted by the liver and peripheral tissues to bicarbonate, helping to restore normal acid-base balance.

Bicarbonate therapy in the treatment of DKA remains controversial. Concerns include impaired tissue oxygen delivery, possible paradoxical cerebrospinal fluid (CSF) acidosis, and worsening hypokalemia. Since therapy with insulin and intravenous hydration allows for metabolism of ketones and lactate into bicarbonate, treatment with $NaHCO_3$ may actually overcorrect the acidosis and cause an overshoot metabolic alkalosis. In DKA, consideration should be given to a potentially beneficial role of $NaHCO_3$ when severe hyperkalemia is present (>6 mEq/liter) or when the serum pH is less than 7.00.

Close monitoring of laboratory data should begin early in treatment, with hourly assessment of electrolytes and acid-base status. Since beta-hydroxybutyrate is converted to acetoacetate during treatment, conventional serum or urine tests for ketones will continue to detect ketones even during the reparative process. Therefore, reliance on serum or urine ketone tests to assess the success of early therapy in DKA is inappropriate. Further information regarding DKA is found in Chap. 114 of this text.

ALCOHOLIC KETOACIDOSIS. The consumption of large amounts of alcohol without adequate nutritional intake can precipitate alcoholic ketoacidosis. Alcohol is metabolized to acetaldehyde and then to both acetoacetic and acetic acid. Fasting decreases insulin levels, which further exacerbates the accumulation of acetoacetic acid and beta-hydroxybutyric acid. Increased glucagon release also promotes hepatic acetoacetic acid production. Acetoacetic acid is then decarboxylated to acetic acid and converted to beta-hydroxybutyric acid. Since beta-hydroxybutyric acid is not detected by the commonly used urine and serum tests for ketones, the presence of a large amount of this ketoacid may be unnoticed. An elevated anion gap metabolic acidosis in the presence of a low blood glucose (25% of patients) may be the only clue to the diagnosis of alcoholic ketoacidosis.

Serum electrolytes show a depressed [HCO_3^-] with an elevated anion gap. The arterial blood gas determination confirms the diagnosis of metabolic acidosis. A coexistent metabolic or respiratory alkalosis may be present. As was mentioned previously, blood glucose concentration may be depressed. The urine and serum screens for ketones are usually positive.

Treatment of alcoholic ketoacidosis is geared toward repletion of volume and glucose deficits. Glucose treatment alone appears to reduce the levels of ketones and the ratio of beta-hydroxybutyrate to acetoacetate. The requirement for bicarbonate administration is controversial. Patients have been successfully managed with and without its use. When considering bicarbonate therapy in this disturbance, its potential adverse effects should be recognized. These include volume overload, hypokalemia, and paradoxical CSF acidosis. Most reports support the use of bicarbonate in alcoholic ketoacidosis to maintain a serum pH greater than 7.10. Information regarding alcoholic ketoacidosis is also found in Chap. 114.

LACTIC ACIDOSIS. Lactate is produced as well as used by most tissues of the body, with the liver accounting for 25 percent of its metabolic clearance. Lactic acidosis occurs when excess lactate is produced, lactate is not effectively utilized, or a combination of both of these processes is present. A number of pathologic processes can result in lactic acid accumulation (see Table 38-5). Lactic acidosis should be suspected when an elevated anion gap acidosis is detected in the presence of infection, ischemia (shock, hypovolemia), seizures, fulminant hepatic necrosis, or certain toxic ingestions.

The history and physical examination will reflect the underlying process. Serum electrolytes show an elevated anion gap acidosis and a decrease in [HCO_3^-] roughly equivalent to the increase in serum lactate level. The normal resting lactate level is approximately 1 mEq/liter and can rise to more than 5 mEq/liter in severe lactic acidosis.

As is the case for other acid-base disorders, treatment of lactic acidosis requires therapy aimed at the underlying cause. Controversy surrounds the utility of bicarbonate administration in this disorder. Information as to the effect of bicarbonate administration on tissue oxygen delivery, CSF pH, and increase in lactic acid production points toward a detrimental effect of bicarbonate administration. However, supporters of bicarbonate treatment cite the paucity of clinical applicability of this evidence and the life-threatening potential of severe acidemia. At present, it is reasonable to weigh the beneficial and possibly detrimental outcomes of bicarbonate administration in individual clinical situations. Most clinicians advocate the use of bicarbonate for a serum pH less than 7.10 in order to mitigate the cardiac and hemodynamic toxicities of such severe acidemia. A multicenter trial is under way to assess the efficacy of the drug dichloroacetate in the treatment of lactic acidosis. Dichloroacetate appears to increase tissue oxygenation and decrease circulating lactate concentrations. Uncontrolled trials appear to show some beneficial effect of dichloroacetate on the very high mortality associated with severe lactic acidosis. Routine therapy with this agent is not recommended at this time. Lactic acidosis is also discussed in Chap. 114.

RENAL FAILURE. Acid-base balance is well maintained until the glomerular filtration rate is decreased below approximately 10 ml per minute. At this point the kidney is unable to adequately excrete acid or regenerate bicarbonate because of the reduction in nephron mass. The anion gap is elevated, primarily due to the retention of sulfates and phosphates.

In uremia, the history may be one of fatigue, malaise, difficulty in sleeping, poor appetite, and muscle cramps. Urine output may be diminished. The physical examination may reveal grayish skin color in whites, uremic fetor, and asterixis. If the serum calcium is depressed, Chvostek's and Trousseau's signs may be present. Serum electrolytes reveal an elevated anion gap acidosis. Blood urea nitrogen and creatinine levels are elevated. Commonly, an elevated phosphate and a low hematocrit are seen. The increased anion gap acidosis of chronic renal failure rarely requires emergent intervention. Since chronic acidosis has long-term deleterious effects, particularly on bone, oral bicarbonate therapy may be indicated. If the renal failure is very severe, signs and symptoms of uremia may be present and dialysis therapy should be initiated. In this situation dialysis will provide bicarbonate or bicarbonate equivalents in the form of acetate. Renal failure is also discussed in Chap. 39 of this text.

TOXIC INGESTION WITH AN ELEVATED ANION GAP (SALICYLATES). An elevated anion gap acidosis is commonly seen in toxic salicylate ingestion. Since salicylates stimulate the respiratory center, respiratory alkalosis may also be present. The unmeasured anions from salicylate ingestion include both ketones and lactate.

History may reveal a large intake of aspirin or other salicylate-containing compounds. The physical examination may be unremarkable or may be significant only for tachypnea. At times, symptoms may include tinnitus, vomiting, diarrhea, and confusion. Serum electrolytes and the arterial blood gas determination commonly show an elevated anion gap metabolic acidosis with a respiratory alkalosis. The salicylate level is elevated. Symptoms are commonly seen with plasma levels above 40 mg/100 ml and toxicity at levels greater than 50 mg/100 ml.

The goals of treatment of salicylate intoxication are to decrease gastrointestinal absorption and increase renal salicylate excretion. The former is achieved by gastric lavage and the latter by alkalinization of the urine and initiation of an alkaline diuresis. An alkaline diuresis can usually be effected by providing an isotonic solution of sodium bicarbonate (three ampules, 50 ml each, of $NaHCO_3$ per liter of D_5W), given at 200 to 300 ml per hour intravenously. Because of the marked kaliuresis associated with this therapy, potassium should be supplemented. The urine pH should be maintained above 7 pH units. The average adult without cardiac, hepatic, renal, or pulmonary disease tolerates this regimen well. A loop diuretic may be required to avoid positive fluid balance.

Volume status, electrolyte and acid-base status, urinary pH, and serum salicylate levels should be assessed frequently. The intravenous hydration prescription should be modified as necessary based on the results of electrolyte, acid-base, and clinical status. In patients who are unable to tolerate large amounts of intravenous (IV) fluids, maintaining a urinary pH above 7.0 without a brisk diuresis may be beneficial in clearing salicylates. This still requires the administration of $NaHCO_3$, which may be detrimental in individuals with borderline cardiopulmonary status. If urinary alkalinization cannot be achieved or renal failure is present, and salicylate levels continue to rise to greater than 90 mg/100 ml despite appropriate alkalinization, hemodialysis should be considered. Further discussion of salicylate intoxication is found in Chap. 156.

TOXIC INGESTION WITH AN ELEVATED ANION GAP AND ELEVATED OSMOLAR GAP. Normal plasma osmolality is regulated between 285 and 295 mOsm/liter. The main components that contribute to the plasma osmolality are sodium (Na^+), glucose, and urea (blood urea nitrogen). An estimate of plasma osmolality (Posm) is calculated as follows:

$$\text{Posm} = 2\,[Na^+] + \frac{[\text{glucose}]}{18} + \frac{[\text{urea}]}{2.8} \qquad (8)$$

Since this formula does not account for other plasma osmols, the "true" or measured Posm is 5 to 10 mOsm/liter higher than the calculated osmolality (equation 8). When the difference between these two values exceeds 10 mOsm/liter, an "osmolar gap" exists. This should alert the physician to the possibility of a toxic ingestion. Ethanol, methanol, and ethylene glycol can significantly elevate the osmolar gap. Under certain situations the osmolar gap may be normal (<10 mOsm/liter) despite ethanol, methanol, or ethylene glycol ingestion. This occurs when the plasma osmolality is measured by the vapor pressure method. Ethanol, methanol, and other alcohols evaporate with this method and therefore are not measured. The osmolar gap can also be elevated by hyperlipidemia and ketone body accumulation (diabetic ketoacidosis), as well as by chronic renal failure.

Methanol intoxication. Methanol ingestion is a serious and potentially life-threatening condition. Intake of as little as 100 to 250 ml is usually fatal. Hepatic metabolism of methanol by alcohol dehydrogenase yields formic acid. Formic acid interferes with normal oxidative metabolism and causes the accumulation of other organic acids, especially lactic acid. The accumulation of lactate and formate accounts for the elevation in the anion gap.

A wide spectrum of presentations follows methanol ingestion, depending on the amount imbibed and the length of time between ingestion and medical attention. Patients may complain of abdominal pain, headache, and feelings of inebriation followed by visual disturbances. With more severe ingestions confusion, obtundation, coma, or cardiovascular collapse can develop. Within 12 to 20 hours after ingestion, pupillary dilation, loss of pupillary reflexes, and edematous optic disks may be seen. Laboratory tests reveal an elevated anion gap acidosis with an elevated osmolar gap, reflecting an increased methanol level. Treatment of methanol intoxication includes reduction of the gastrointestinal absorption (lavage), plasma volume expansion, and infusion of ethanol to inhibit hepatic methanol metabolism. Bicarbonate administration is used to treat the accompanying severe acidosis. Hemodialysis is required in severe cases (methanol levels of 50–100 mg/100 ml) to remove methanol and its toxic metabolite, formic acid, as well as to correct the acidosis. The severity of the acidosis and the extent of the anion gap are related to the elevated serum formic acid concentration. Therefore, inhibition of methanol metabolism (by ethanol) and extracorporeal removal (by hemodialysis) reduce the extent of the acidosis. The diagnosis and treatment of methanol intoxication are discussed further in Chap. 156.

Ethylene glycol intoxication. Ethylene glycol, a major constituent of antifreeze, is an extremely dangerous intoxicant. It is also present in some lacquers and detergents. Ingestion of 60 ml can be lethal. As in the case of methanol breakdown, initial metabolism of ethylene glycol by hepatic alcohol dehydrogenase forms glycolate and glycoxalate. Further metabolism yields oxalic, formic, beta-hydroxy, and beta-keto acids. Glycolic and lactic acids appear to be the major contributors to the acidosis.

Vomiting and lethargy with eventual obtundation and coma are commonly seen. The severity of the medical condition depends on the amount of ethylene glycol ingested and the elapsed time after ingestion. Serum electrolytes and arterial blood gas determinations confirm the presence of an elevated anion gap acidosis. An osmolar gap of greater than 10 mOsm/liter will likely be present. Urinalysis may show the presence of oxalate crystals. Blood urea nitrogen and creatinine levels may be elevated secondary to oxalate deposition in the renal tubules. A serum ethylene glycol level will be elevated and hypocalcemia may also be present.

As in the case of methanol ingestion, initial therapy is aimed at reduction of absorption (lavage/charcoal). Since there is no evidence that the anion metabolites in ethylene glycol intoxication are further metabolized to bicarbonate, bicarbonate therapy is recommended for severe acidosis. To decrease the metabolism of ethylene glycol, ethanol is infused to competitively inhibit the enzyme alcohol dehydrogenase. Some studies advocate the use of 4-methylpyrazole, an alcohol dehydrogenase inhibitor, in place of ethanol, to produce more effective enzyme inhibition.

Toxic acids can be converted to nontoxic metabolites by administration of thiamine (glycolic acid → alpha-hydroxy or beta-hydroxy ketoadipate) and pyridoxine (glyoxalate → glycine), which act as cofactors in these reactions. Since thiamine and pyridoxine are relatively safe to administer, they should be provided in the treatment of this intoxication.

Hemodialysis is the adjuvant treatment of choice in ethylene glycol ingestion when associated with an elevated anion gap metabolic acidosis. This procedure removes both ethylene glycol and glycolic acid. Dialysis can be provided using a bicarbonate-based bath, and ethanol can be added to the dialysate (100 mg/100 ml) to prevent reduction in the serum level during the dialysis treatment. An in-depth discussion of ethylene glycol intoxication can be found in Chap. 156.

Normal Anion Gap Metabolic Acidosis

Table 38-6 lists conditions commonly associated with a normal anion gap metabolic acidosis. In the emergency department, a normal anion gap acidosis is frequently caused by diarrhea. It is important, however, for the emergency department physician to recognize other causes of this acid-base abnormality as well.

GASTROINTESTINAL LOSS OF BICARBONATE. Ileal and cecal fluids contain large amounts of bicarbonate (approximately 20–30 mEq/liter), and therefore diseases that provoke a large daily stool output can affect the serum bicarbonate concentration. Viral, bacterial, and drug-induced diarrhea as well as primary diseases of the gastrointestinal (GI) tract such as colitis and sprue can have this effect. As would be expected, excessive laxative use also promotes large GI bicarbonate losses. Pancreatic fluid contains an even greater concentration of bicarbonate (approximately 90 mEq/liter), and diseases that promote large amounts of pancreatic drainage can also cause a normal anion gap metabolic acidosis. Certain urinary tract diversion procedures place a loop of bowel in contact with the ureter or bladder. Urine generally has a low bicarbonate concentration; however, if urine is in prolonged contact with bowel mucosa, bicarbonate exchanges for urinary chloride, and bicarbonate may be lost through the urine. Other factors that explain this normal anion gap acidosis include intestinal absorption of ammonium chloride and renal tubular damage.

The history is indispensable in eliciting a gastrointestinal etiology of a normal anion gap acidosis. Physical examination findings will depend on the degree of volume contraction and the underlying disease process.

Laboratory tests will confirm a normal anion gap acidosis if volume contraction is absent or mild. The serum chloride level is usually elevated. If volume contraction is severe, a superimposed metabolic alkalosis may be present. In the case of large stool losses, the urinary pH will be low (<5.5). Serum potassium levels may be normal or low. Urinary

Table 38-7. Causes of hypokalemic or normokalemic distal renal tubular acidosis

A. Hereditary
  1. Fructose intolerance (with nephrocalcinosis)
  2. Galactosemia
  3. Elliptocytosis
  4. Fabry's disease
  5. Ehlers-Danlos syndrome

B. Acquired
  1. Metabolic
    a. Hyperparathyroidism (with nephrocalcinosis)
    b. Hyperthyroidism (with nephrocalcinosis)
  2. Hypergammaglobulinemic states
    a. Systemic lupus erythematosus
    b. Sjögren's syndrome
    c. Cryoglobulinemia
    d. Sarcoidosis
    e. Tuberculosis
    f. Hodgkin's disease
    g. Idiopathic hypergammaglobulinemia
  3. Other
    a. Renal transplantation
    b. Hepatic cirrhosis

C. Drug induced
  1. Amphotericin B
  2. Vitamin D (with nephrocalcinosis)
  3. Lithium carbonate
  4. Toluene

D. Miscellaneous
  1. Medullary sponge kidney

drainage from urinary diversion through a bowel loop may show a high urinary pH.

Therapy in these disorders is aimed at correcting the underlying disturbance as well as reestablishing euvolemia and acid-base balance. Treatment of the latter two situations involves IV or oral hydration if volume depletion exists, and supplementation with bicarbonate and potassium to correct the acid-base and electrolyte disturbances. If volume depletion and acidemia coexist, a solution of $NaHCO_3$ in D_5W can be used for rehydration and correction of the acidemia. The serum $[Cl^-]$ in these disorders is usually elevated, and therefore chloride administration as part of the therapeutic protocol is not indicated. The concentration of $NaHCO_3$ in D_5W will depend on the serum electrolyte values, volume status, and stool and urinary losses of electrolytes. The amount of electrolytes required to correct the electrolyte disturbances can be estimated by knowing the stool electrolyte composition and replacing it either orally or intravenously. Since most types of acute diarrhea are short lived, therapy can be terminated when the underlying disorder resolves.

The situation is somewhat different in regard to the acidosis caused by urinary diversion procedures. This acidosis is usually chronic and therefore long-term treatment with bicarbonate or citrate and electrolytes may be required.

RENAL CAUSES. Normal anion gap metabolic acidosis can result from renal tubular dysfunction (e.g., renal tubular acidosis), early renal insufficiency, or interstitial renal disease. Renal tubular acidosis (RTA) generally results from either defective hydrogen ion secretion (distal RTA, type I), bicarbonate wasting (proximal RTA, type II), or abnormalities in the renin-aldosterone axis (type IV). The multiple causes of classic types I and II RTA are listed in Tables 38-7 and 38-8, respectively. Although types I and II are the results of derangements in the function of different portions of the renal tubule, the serum electrolyte values associated with these disorders are similar (normal or $\downarrow [K^+]$, $\downarrow [HCO_3^-]$, $\uparrow [Cl^-]$. On the other hand, type IV RTA results in different electrolyte perturbations ($\downarrow [Na^+]$, $\uparrow [K^+]$, $\uparrow [Cl^-]$, $\downarrow [HCO_3^-]$). Other causes of hyperkalemic RTA include hypoaldosteronism, sickle cell nephropathy, and obstructive uropathy.

Table 38-8. Causes of proximal renal tubular acidosis

A. Associated with multiple proximal tubular defects
  1. Hereditary
    a. Wilson's disease
    b. Cystinosis
    c. Tyrosinosis
    d. Lowe's syndrome
  2. Acquired
    a. Hyperparathyroidism
    b. Vitamin D deficiency
    c. Nephrotic syndrome
    d. Amyloidosis
    e. Multiple myeloma
    f. Sjögren's syndrome
  3. Drugs/ingestions
    a. Outdated tetracycline
    b. 6-Mercaptopurine
    c. Heavy metals (lead, cadmium, copper, mercury)
  4. Miscellaneous
    a. Medullary cystic disease

B. Bicarbonate wasting solely
  1. Drugs
    a. Sulfonamides
    b. Acetazolamide

A normal anion gap hyperchloremic metabolic acidosis may be seen with moderate renal insufficiency of any etiology and particularly in renal diseases that affect the medullary interstitium. This is commonly due to proximal tubular chloride reabsorption secondary to volume depletion.

Instituting therapy aimed at correcting the acidosis secondary to RTA or mild renal failure is rarely an emergency. Therapy usually consists of bicarbonate treatment and management of other electrolyte imbalances. Long-term management of these disorders should be provided in consultation with a physician who is well versed in this area.

DRUG/CHEMICAL INGESTION. Although rare, certain exposures may be associated with a normal anion gap metabolic acidosis. In the acute emergency department setting, it is important for the physician to be aware of the ingestion of carbonic anhydrase inhibitors. The most widely used of these agents is acetazolamide, commonly prescribed for the treatment of open-angle glaucoma. As was discussed in the pathophysiology section of this chapter, carbonic anhydrase, an enzyme present in the proximal renal epithelium, plays a role in the reabsorption of carbon dioxide and the subsequent generation of HCO_3^-. Blockade of this enzyme's activity results in bicarbonate loss from the proximal renal tubule and a normal anion gap metabolic acidosis. Although this acidosis is typically mild, it can be more severe in elderly or

Table 38-9. Causes of respiratory acidosis

Central depression in ventilation	
	CNS lesion
	O_2 treatment in chronic CO_2 retention
	Cardiac arrest
	Drugs (narcotics, sedatives, anesthesia)
Musculoskeletal	
	Crush injury of chest wall, flail chest
	Kyphoscoliosis
	Muscle weakness (Guillain-Barré, myasthenia gravis, polio, amyotrophic lateral sclerosis, familial periodic paralysis, hypokalemia)
	Pickwickian syndrome
Intrinsic lung disease/conditions affecting lungs	
	Chronic obstructive pulmonary disease
	Pneumonia
	Pulmonary edema
	Pneumothorax
	Pleural effusion
	Bronchospasm (asthma)
Anatomic obstruction	
	Foreign-body aspiration
	Laryngospasm
Miscellaneous	
	Mechanical ventilation

diabetic patients or in those with underlying renal insufficiency.

A history of acetazolamide ingestion or of glaucoma is invaluable in establishing this compound as the cause of the acid-base imbalance. As expected, the serum bicarbonate concentration is depressed and the serum chloride concentration is elevated. If the serum bicarbonate has not reached its new steady-state value and acetazolamide has recently been ingested, the urinary pH may be elevated, despite the systemic acidosis.

If the metabolic acidosis is severe, replacement with sodium bicarbonate is acceptable. Long-term decisions with regard to continuation or discontinuation of the therapy should be made with the patient's primary outpatient physician.

Respiratory Acidosis

Respiratory acidosis is characterized by an elevation in the partial pressure of carbon dioxide (PCO_2). A variety of clinical and physiologic conditions are associated with respiratory acidosis. A comprehensive list is provided in Table 38-9. Respiratory acidosis can be acute (of relatively short duration) or chronic (of longer duration). The degree of metabolic compensation (i.e., an increase in the serum $[HCO_3^-]$) depends on the duration of the underlying respiratory acidosis. The metabolic compensation for chronic respiratory acidosis is greater than for acute respiratory acidosis.

The expected metabolic compensation can be estimated using the following formulas:

Acute respiratory acidosis:

$$\Delta [HCO_3^-] = 0.1 (\Delta PCO_2)$$

Chronic respiratory acidosis:

$$\Delta [HCO_3^-] = 0.35 (\Delta PCO_2)$$

Physical signs and symptoms depend on the severity of the respiratory acidosis. Extreme elevation in the PCO_2 can manifest itself in a constellation of neurologic symptoms, referred to as "CO_2 narcosis." Early on, nondescript symptoms such as weakness and headache predominate. However, with prolonged extreme respiratory acidosis, delirium, somnolence, asterixis, myoclonus, combativeness, and seizures may be seen. Physical examination findings may include papilledema from elevated cerebrospinal fluid pressure.

As expected, admission of narcotic/sedative intake, symptoms of pneumonia or pulmonary edema, or the presence of overt musculoskeletal abnormalities will point toward a cause of this acid-base disturbance. In uncomplicated respiratory acidosis, serum electrolytes will reveal an elevated $[HCO_3^-]$ (compensation for the PCO_2). The ABG will disclose elevation in the PCO_2 and a low serum pH.

Treatment of respiratory acidosis depends on the underlying disease, the severity of the PCO_2 and pH changes, the chronicity, and the likelihood of speedy reversal with treatment. For example, in acute respiratory acidosis due to laryngospasm, relief of the airway obstruction in a conscious patient should quickly reverse the acidosis. However, if this patient has had a cardiopulmonary arrest due to hypoxemia and no spontaneous respiration exists, relief of the obstruction alone is insufficient in reestablishing normal acid-base balance. In this situation, it is necessary to provide artificial ventilation to the patient. Another situation commonly encountered is that of chronic respiratory acidosis in an individual with chronic obstructive pulmonary disease. Renal mechanisms have been maximally employed to compensate for the chronic CO_2 elevation. Attempts to significantly reduce the PCO_2 to a level below the patient's chronic baseline value would not be beneficial to long-range acid-base balance. The PCO_2 would be reduced but the elevation in the serum $[HCO_3^-]$ would persist for at least several days, resulting in alkalemia. Since underlying physiologic mechanisms maintaining hypercapnia in this patient are still operating, the PCO_2 would return to its baseline value after the acute intervention had been withdrawn.

Metabolic Alkalosis

Severe alkalosis, like severe acidosis, can be life threatening. Symptoms and signs can include mental status changes ranging from mild confusion to obtundation. Neuromuscular manifestations may also be evident and present as cramping, paresthesias, or frank tetany. As in the case of acidemia, cardiac arrhythmias can be provoked or aggravated by the presence of alkalemia (see Table 38-2).

Metabolic alkalosis is caused by either H^+ loss or HCO_3^- addition to the extracellular compartment. The net result of either of these perturbations is an increase in the serum $[HCO_3^-]$. Since the normally functioning kidney is able to excrete amounts of bicarbonate greatly in excess of the quantity it normally excretes, the maintenance of metabolic alkalosis requires factors in addition to an elevated serum $[HCO_3^-]$. Potassium and chloride depletion with associated reduction in glomerular filtration rate aids in maintaining

Table 38-10. Causes of metabolic alkalosis

A. H^+ loss
  1. Gastrointestinal
    a. Gastric HCl (vomiting, nasogastric suction)
    b. Stool losses (in congenital chloridorrhea, villous adenoma)
  2. Urinary
    a. Diuretics
    b. Nonreabsorbable anions (e.g., carbenicillin)
    c. Mineralocorticoid excess
      Primary: 1. Primary hyperaldosteronism
        2. Cushing's syndrome
        3. Adrenogenital syndromes
      Secondary: 1. Volume contraction
        2. Renal artery stenosis
        3. Magnesium depletion
        4. Bartter's syndrome
      Other: licorice ingestion (glycyrrhizic acid)
    d. Posthypercapnia
    e. Hypoparathyroidism

B. HCO_3^- addition
  1. Alkali therapy
  2. Massive blood transfusions
  3. Milk-alkali syndrome

C. Miscellaneous
  1. Contraction alkalosis

the elevated serum [HCO_3^-] of metabolic alkalosis. Since the kidney is maintaining the metabolic alkalosis, one often sees a "paradoxically acid" urine. Knowledge of the association between these electrolyte disturbances and metabolic alkalosis will help the clinician in diagnosis and subsequent therapy.

As in other acid-base disorders, therapy in metabolic alkalosis is aimed at correcting the underlying disease state. At times, however, specific treatment of the alkalosis is required.

In metabolic alkalosis, the excess amount of bicarbonate present can be calculated using a mildly modified version of the formula that is used to calculate bicarbonate "deficit" in metabolic acidosis. In this case:

$$\text{Bicarbonate "excess" (mEq)} = 0.4 \times \text{body weight (kg)} \times (\text{actual } [HCO_3^-] - \text{"normal" } [HCO_3^-]) \quad (9)$$

That is, if it were possible to remove a certain amount of total body bicarbonate, the acid-base disorder would be corrected.

There are two approaches to correcting this HCO_3^- "excess": (1) therapy directed at the initiating factors and perpetuators of the metabolic alkalosis, or (2) providing sufficient H^+ to titrate the excess HCO_3^-. The latter method is usually reserved for cases of severe alkalemia (pH > 7.55–7.60), which are associated with a high mortality rate; cases in which physical signs and symptoms of alkalemia are prominent; in certain cases of renal or hepatic failure; and in situations in which correction of the underlying disorder cannot be accomplished. Hydrochloric acid is delivered in a concentration range between 0.05 and 0.2N via a central vein. Care must be taken when administering this compound since it is very corrosive to subcutaneous tissues. A 0.15N hydrochloric acid solution can be prepared by mixing 150 ml of 1N HCl and 850 ml of dextrose in water (D_5W) in a glass container. This contains 150 mEq of HCl per liter. Solutions of this concentration can be given at flow rates up to 125 ml per hour. Flow rates should be determined by the patient's clinical status and the severity of the acid-base imbalance. Theoretically, in pure metabolic alkalosis with no evidence of ongoing HCl acid losses, the mEqs of bicarbonate "excess" calculated from the formula should equal the mEqs of H^+ ion needed to titrate this bicarbonate. As with other severe acid-base disorders, the acute goal is not to reestablish a "normal pH," [HCO_3^-], and PCO_2 but to prevent dangerous extremes in these values.

Table 38-11. Saline responsive and saline unresponsive metabolic alkalosis

Saline responsive (U_{Cl} < 10 mEq/liter)
  Gastric HCl losses (vomiting, nasogastric suction)
  Stool losses (congenital chloridorrhea, villous adenoma)
  Diuretics (late)
  Posthypercapnia

Saline unresponsive (U_{Cl} > 20 mEq/liter)
  Mineralocorticoid/mineralocorticoid-like excess
  Primary hyperaldosteronism
  Cushing's syndrome
  Adrenogenital syndromes
  Bartter's syndrome
  Renal artery stenosis
  Licorice ingestion

Key: U_{Cl} = urinary [Cl^-].

Occasionally, the carbonic anhydrase inhibitor acetazolamide can be used to reduce the serum [HCO_3^-]. When using this drug, care should be taken to avoid dehydration and hypokalemia.

The expected respiratory compensation for a given primary increase in the serum [HCO_3^-] can be calculated using the following formula:

$$\Delta PCO_2 = 0.6 (\Delta [HCO_3^-])$$

That is, for every 10 mEq/liter rise in the serum [HCO_3^-], the PCO_2 is expected to increase by 6 mm Hg. In an adult with adequate pulmonary function and no other acid-base abnormalities, the PCO_2 rarely increases beyond 60 mm Hg as compensation for metabolic alkalosis. The anion gap (see the section on diagnosis) may be elevated due to organic anion synthesis.

Table 38-10 lists the common causes of metabolic alkalosis. This list is divided into two categories: those associated with H^+ loss and those associated with HCO_3^- addition to the extracellular compartment. Table 38-11 further divides these causes into those associated with a low urinary [Cl^-] (saline responsive) and those associated with a high urinary [Cl^-] (saline resistant). This differentiation will become more important when specific treatment is discussed.

H^+ Loss

GASTROINTESTINAL HCL LOSS. The pH and quantity of gastric fluid lost through either vomiting or nasogastric suction will determine net H^+ loss. For example, one liter of gastric fluid of pH 2.0 contains more H^+ content than one liter of fluid of pH 4.0. For each mEq of H^+ lost through this route, 1 mEq HCO_3^- is added to the extracellular space. Normally, H^+ secreted by the stomach stimulates the duodenum to secrete HCO_3^-. If H^+ is lost before it enters the duodenum, HCO_3^- is not secreted and the serum [HCO_3^-] increases.

A history of excessive vomiting or nasogastric suction is indispensable in making this diagnosis. Physical examination will depend on the extent of fluid losses (volume status) and the cause of the vomiting (e.g., gastric outlet obstruction, gastroenteritis).

Serum electrolytes reveal an elevated [HCO_3^-] with a low serum [Cl^-]. Commonly, the serum [K^+] is also depressed. An arterial blood gas determination confirms the presence of a metabolic alkalosis (PCO_2 increased). The urinary chloride concentration is commonly less than 10 mEq/liter.

At this point mention should be made of the rare condition of congenital chloridorrhea, in which an acid stool is produced. As would be expected, massive stool losses in this condition can also produce a picture of metabolic alkalosis.

URINARY LOSSES of H^+. Under this category two major causes will be discussed, the metabolic alkalosis caused by diuretic use and that caused by mineralocorticoid excess.

Diuretics. Metabolic alkalosis secondary to diuretic use is most often seen with administration of the loop (e.g., furosemide) or thiazide class agents. Diuretics cause metabolic alkalosis in two ways: through volume contraction and by augmenting distal sodium delivery. Chloride losses also stimulate aldosterone secretion and further distal renal tubular H^+ secretion. The result is an elevation in the serum [HCO_3^-] and metabolic alkalosis.

A history of diuretic ingestion is helpful in this situation. If diuretic use is seriously suspected and the patient is unable or unwilling to acknowledge diuretic use, urine toxicology screens may be informative.

Electrolytes reveal an elevated serum [HCO_3^-], which may be associated with a depressed serum [Cl^-], [Na^+], and [K^+]. Arterial blood gas values confirm the presence of a metabolic alkalosis (increased PCO_2). Early in diuretic use, urinary [Cl^-] will be elevated ($>$20 mEq/liter) but later, in the face of volume contraction, is commonly less than 10 mEq per liter.

Mineralocorticoid excess. Mineralocorticoids have specific effects on the renal tubule. They promote Na^+ reabsorption distally and augment H^+ and K^+ secretion. Metabolic alkalosis occurs as the result of these tubular actions. The alkalosis is often sustained by hypokalemia and may be potentiated by enhanced distal Na^+ delivery (as with diuretics) or by the presence of a nonreabsorbable anion presented with Na^+ (as with carbenicillin). Mineralocorticoid excess can be primary, as in primary hyperaldosteronism or Cushing's syndrome, or secondary to elevated renin, as in volume contraction or renal artery stenosis.

In both primary and secondary causes of mineralocorticoid excess, electrolytes reveal an elevated serum [HCO_3^-] and hypokalemia. Hypernatremia may also be present. The urinary [Cl^-] is frequently greater than 20 mEq/liter.

HCO_3^- Addition

Alkali therapy, massive blood transfusions, and milk-alkali syndrome can also cause metabolic alkalosis. Elevations in serum [HCO_3^-] due to excess therapy with $NaHCO_3$, particularly in the situation of resolving acidosis (e.g., DKA, cardiac arrest), are commonly seen. Blood used in transfusions contains citrate (16.8 mEq/unit), which is converted to bicarbonate in the body. By this mechanism, massive blood transfusions can cause metabolic alkalosis. Ingestion of large amounts of calcium carbonate–containing antacids can result in accumulation of HCO_3^-, which is generated from CO_3^{2-} in the serum. This situation is called the *milk-alkali syndrome.*

Electrolytes and ABG are similar to those seen in other types of metabolic alkalosis. In the milk-alkali syndrome, serum [Ca^{2+}] is elevated.

Contraction Alkalosis

With extracellular fluid loss, the remaining extracellular volume is said to "contract" around the fixed amount of bicarbonate, resulting in a higher [HCO_3^-] in this compartment. Part of the etiology of diuretic-induced metabolic alkalosis can be attributed to this effect. Large extracellular fluid loss is required to engender a significant increase in the serum [HCO_3^-] by this mechanism.

Table 38-11 divides the common causes of metabolic alkalosis into characteristics that directly affect therapy. Treatment of disorders listed in the "saline responsive" category focuses on repletion of chloride. This is provided by NaCl solutions. When euvolemia is reestablished, normal renal mechanisms will act to excrete the excess serum bicarbonate. This action can be detected by a rising urinary pH. Hypokalemia, if present, should also be corrected to reduce stimuli acting to maintain the alkalosis. When treating the alkalosis secondary to gastric HCl acid loss, prevention of vomiting or cessation of nasogastric suction is an important treatment goal. If gastric acid loss cannot be controlled adequately, treatment with an H_2-receptor antagonist (cimetidine, ranitidine) will diminish the [H^+] of the gastric fluid and reduce the cumulative gastrointestinal acid losses. Efficacy of treatment can be determined by measuring the gastric fluid pH.

Saline-unresponsive alkaloses are more difficult to treat. Therapy in this group of disorders is directed toward removal of the cause of mineralocorticoid excess—for example, adrenal adenoma resection in primary hyperaldosteronism or renal artery dilatation in renal artery stenosis. Electrolyte disturbances should also be corrected since, as in saline-responsive alkalosis, they act to maintain the metabolic alkalosis.

Respiratory Alkalosis

When the PCO_2 is reduced (hypocapnia) due to an increase in tidal volume or respiratory rate, alkalosis ensues. Neurologic symptoms and signs due to respiratory alkalosis are more commonly seen than with metabolic alkalosis since CO_2 easily traverses the blood-brain barrier while HCO_3^- does not. The symptoms are identical to those caused by hypocalcemia and include lightheadedness, paresthesias, cramps, and carpopedal spasm.

Respiratory alkalosis may be of short duration, as in acute respiratory alkalosis, or of a persistent nature, as in chronic respiratory alkalosis. The metabolic compensation for acute respiratory alkalosis occurs within 10 minutes of onset and principally involves transcellular shifts of H^+ ions. The H^+ ions then buffer extracellular HCO_3^- ions, resulting in a return toward pH 7.4. This mechanism would be inadequate

Table 38-12. Causes of respiratory alkalosis

CNS disorders
Cerebrovascular accident
Diseases of the medulla
Tumor
Infection
Anxiety, pain, psychosis
Hypoxemia
Cardiac: congestive heart failure, congenital heart disease (right-to-left shunts)
Pulmonary: interstitial disease, $\dot{V}/\dot{Q}$ mismatch (e.g., pulmonary embolus)
High altitude
Metabolic/endocrinologic
Anemia
Thyrotoxicosis
Pregnancy
Fever
Drugs
Salicylates
Progesterone
Xanthines
Nicotine
Infection
Gram-negative sepsis
Liver disease
Mechanical ventilation

to compensate for hypocapnia of long duration. Renal mechanisms that act to diminish H^+ ion secretion are therefore called into play in chronic respiratory alkalosis. These renal mechanisms are very effective in stabilizing the serum pH within the normal range.

The expected metabolic compensations for acute and chronic respiratory alkalosis are listed below.

ACUTE RESPIRATORY ALKALOSIS:

$$\Delta\ [HCO_3^-] = 0.2\ (\Delta\ PCO_2)$$

That is, for every 10-mm Hg fall in PCO_2, the serum $[HCO_3^-]$ is expected to fall by 2 mEq/liter.

CHRONIC RESPIRATORY ALKALOSIS:

$$\Delta\ [HCO_3^-] = 0.5\ (\Delta\ PCO_2)$$

That is, for each 10-mm Hg fall in PCO_2, the serum $[HCO_3^-]$ is expected to fall by 5 mEq/liter.

Table 38-12 provides a list of clinical situations associated with respiratory alkalosis. Certain stimuli result in an acute alkalosis, while others have a long-term effect and result in chronic respiratory alkalosis. Recognizing the underlying stimuli for respiratory alkalosis in emergency department patients is important, since, as will be discussed later, therapy should be aimed at the underlying cause of the acid-base abnormality.

Acute Respiratory Alkalosis

Acute respiratory alkalosis is commonly seen in conditions associated with pain, acute congestive heart failure, salicylate intoxication, and acute cerebrovascular accidents. With reasonable attention to the history and physical examination, these causes become evident.

Tachypnea is a frequent finding. Laboratory values reveal a depressed serum $[HCO_3^-]$ in the electrolyte screen and an arterial blood gas that confirms the presence of alkalemia (serum pH $>$ 7.44) and a reduced PCO_2. The serum phosphate level may be depressed.

Chronic Respiratory Alkalosis

Chronic respiratory alkalosis is frequently seen in individuals with liver cirrhosis and in those residing at elevated altitudes. As in the case of acute respiratory alkalosis, the history and physical examination are indispensable in determining the cause of the acidosis. Depending on the cause, tachypnea may be undetectable. As seen in acute respiratory alkalosis, the serum $[HCO_3^-]$ is depressed. Commonly, in this condition mild hypokalemia secondary to shifts in H^+ and mild hyperchloremia due to Cl^- for HCO_3^- exchange can occur. Hypophosphatemia may be seen in this condition as well. The arterial blood gas shows a diminished PCO_2, but frequently a relatively "normal" serum pH, especially if the respiratory alkalosis is over two weeks in duration.

The presence of respiratory alkalosis prompts a search for the underlying cause. At times, the cause will be clinically apparent (as in pregnancy) but at other times more obscure (as in salicylate toxicity). Treatment of respiratory alkalosis is aimed at correction of the underlying cause. Rarely is the alkalemia severe but occasionally, for example, in states of extreme agitation, the degree of hypocapnia and alkalemia is indeed severe. In these situations, reduction of the respiratory rate by sedation or CO_2 rebreathing may be beneficial. Before any therapy directed at reducing the respiratory rate is begun, the physician should be convinced that the decreased PCO_2 is a primary process and not the expected respiratory compensation for an underlying metabolic acidosis. In that situation hypocapnia is not pathologic but is critical to the maintenance of an adequate serum pH.

Mixed Acid-Base Disorders

When more than one primary disturbance in acid-base balance is present at a given time, a "mixed" acid-base disorder is said to exist. A mixed disturbance should be suspected when, despite gross abnormalities in the serum $[HCO_3^-]$ and PCO_2, the pH is completely within the normal range. Other clues include a serum $[HCO_3^-]$ that is elevated with a PCO_2 that is low and a depressed serum $[HCO_3^-]$ in the presence of an elevated PCO_2.

The simplest way to approach this situation is illustrated in the following example: If the pH is greater than 7.44, assume that the individual has, at the minimum, an alkalosis. Check the serum $[HCO_3^-]$ and PCO_2. An elevated $[HCO_3^-]$ would imply a metabolic alkalosis. Calculate the appropriate compensatory elevation in PCO_2 from the formula discussed in the section on alkalosis: $\Delta\ PCO_2 = 0.6\ (\Delta\ [HCO_3^-])$. If the actual magnitude of the PCO_2 elevation is not what is expected from the formula—that is, the PCO_2 is lower or higher—a superimposed respiratory alkalosis or acidosis exists concomitantly with the metabolic alkalosis. The same rationale applies for assessing mixed acid-base problems that result in a low serum pH. Table 38-13 lists

Table 38-13. Examples of mixed acid-base disorders

Disorder	Cause
Metabolic acidosis and respiratory acidosis	Cardiogenic shock and respiratory arrest
Metabolic acidosis and respiratory alkalosis	Salicylate intoxication; sepsis and cirrhosis
Metabolic alkalosis and respiratory alkalosis	Fever and vomiting
Metabolic alkalosis and respiratory acidosis	Diuretic use in chronic obstructive pulmonary disease

some clinical situations commonly associated with mixed acid-base disturbances.

Recognition of complex acid-base disturbances is necessary to prevent misguided therapy. As with other acid-base disorders, treatment should be aimed at the underlying cause(s). Life-threatening extremes in pH due to mixed acid-base disturbances are approached as one would approach similar life-threatening extremes in pH due to simple acid-base disorders.

SELECTED READING

General Acid-Base Balance

Al-Awquati, Q. The cellular response to respiratory acid-base disorders. *Kidney Int* 28:845–855, 1985.

Bidani, A. Electrolyte and acid-base disorders. *Med Clin North Am* 70:1013–1036, 1986.

Emmett, M, and Narins, RG. Clinical use of the anion gap. *Medicine* 56:38–54, 1977.

Gennari, FJ. Serum osmolality. Uses and limitations. *N Engl J Med* 310:102–105, 1984.

Jehle, D, and Harchelroad, F. Bicarbonate. *Emerg Med Clin North Am* 4:145–173, 1986.

Kaehny, WD. Respiratory acid-base disorders. *Med Clin North Am* 67:915–928, 1983.

Koeppen, BM, and Steinmetz, PR. Basic mechanisms of urinary acidification. *Med Clin North Am* 67:753–770, 1983.

Narins, RG, and Emmett, M. Simple and mixed acid-base disorders: A practical approach. *Medicine* 59:161–187, 1980.

Oh, MS, and Carroll, HJ. The anion gap. *N Engl J Med* 297:814–817, 1977.

Schwartz, WB, and Cohen, JJ. The nature of the renal response to chronic disorders of acid-base equilibrium. *Am J Med* 64:417–428, 1978.

Ventriglia, WJ. Arterial blood gases. *Emerg Med Clin North Am* 4:235–251, 1986.

Acidosis

Elevated Anion Gap Metabolic Acidosis

KETOACIDOSIS

Adams, SL, Matthews, JJ, and Flaherty, JJ. Alcoholic ketoacidosis. *Ann Emerg Med* 16:90–97, 1987.

Felts, PW. Ketoacidosis. *Med Clin North Am* 64:831–843, 1983.

Keller, V. Diabetic ketoacidosis: Current views on pathogenesis and treatment. *Diabetelogia* 29:71–77, 1986.

Krane, EJ. Diabetic ketoacidosis. Biochemistry, physiology, treatment and prevention. *Pediatr Clin North Am* 34:935–960, 1987.

Morris, LR, Murphy, MB, and Kitabchi, AE. Bicarbonate therapy in severe diabetic ketoacidosis. *Ann Intern Med* 105:836–840, 1986.

LACTIC ACIDOSIS

Kreisberg, RA. Pathogenesis and management of lactic acidosis. *Annu Rev Med* 35:181–193, 1984.

Narins, RG, and Cohen, JJ. Bicarbonate therapy for organic acidosis: The case for its continued use. *Ann Intern Med* 106:615–618, 1987.

Stacpoole, PW. Lactic acidosis: The case against bicarbonate therapy. *Ann Intern Med* 105:276–279, 1986.

INTOXICATIONS

Gabow, PA. Ethylene glycol intoxication. *Am J Kidney Dis* 11: 277–279, 1988.

Gabow, PA, et al. Organic acids in ethylene glycol intoxication. *Ann Intern Med* 105:16–20, 1986.

Jacobsen, D, et al. Ethylene glycol intoxication: Evaluation of kinetics and crystalluria. *Am J Med* 84:145–152, 1988.

McMartin, KE, Ambre, JJ, and Tephly, TR. Methanol poisoning in human subjects. Role for formic acid accumulation in metabolic acidosis. *Am J Med* 68:414–418, 1980.

Osterloh, JD, et al. Serum formate concentrations in methanol intoxication as a criteria for hemodialysis. *Ann Intern Med* 104: 200–203, 1986.

Prescott, LF, et al. Diuresis or urinary alkalinization for salicylate poisoning. *Br Med J* 285:1383–1386, 1982.

RENAL FAILURE

Sabatini, S. The acidosis of chronic renal failure. *Med Clin North Am* 67:845–858, 1983.

Normal Anion Gap Metabolic Acidosis

Battle, D. Renal tubular acidosis. *Med Clin North Am* 67:859–878, 1983.

Krochel, JP. The syndrome of hyporeninemic hypoaldosteronism. *Annu Rev Med* 30:145–153, 1979.

Quintanilla, AP. Renal tubular acidosis. Mechanisms and management. *Postgrad Med* 67:60–73, 1980.

Sabatini, S. The acidosis of chronic renal failure. *Med Clin North Am* 67:845–858, 1983.

Stinebaugh, BJ, et al. Pathogenesis of distal renal tubular acidosis. *Kidney Int* 19:1–7, 1981.

Alkalosis

Cogan, MG, et al. Metabolic alkalosis. *Med Clin North Am* 67:903–914, 1983.

Duncan, DA. Use of intravenous hydrochloric acid for the treatment of metabolic alkalosis in renal or hepatic failure. *Intern Med Specialist* 5:56–63, 1984.

Kassirer, JP, et al. The critical role of chloride in the correction of hypokalemic alkalosis in man. *Am J Med* 38:172–189, 1965.

Kassirer, JP, et al. On the pathogenesis of metabolic alkalosis in hyperaldosteronism. *Am J Med* 49:306–315, 1970.

39. Acute and Chronic Renal Failure

David M. Clive
Linda Brown

Patients rarely come to physicians complaining of renal dysfunction. Whereas dyspnea can help the clinician focus attention on cardiac or respiratory problems, kidney failure has no localizing signs or symptoms. Back pain may occur in a few renal disorders but is unusual. Oliguria, on the other hand, occurs frequently in patients with acute and chronic renal disease, although it is rarely documented by patients themselves. Nausea, anorexia, malaise, weakness, and insomnia, among other symptoms, are common in renal failure but are nonspecific findings.

For these reasons, in the emergency department renal failure is usually discovered through laboratory tests. Elevated levels of urea nitrogen and creatinine in the blood are the most common clues to the presence of renal dysfunction.

The causes of renal failure are many and the pathophysiology is complex. A detailed analysis of these subjects would be inappropriate for this chapter. Rather, the sections that follow are intended to provide a foundation for understanding, diagnosing, and treating renal failure and its related complications.

Well-functioning kidneys are central to the maintenance of chemical stability in the body's internal milieu. Their homeostatic role comprises several key functions, which include excretion of metabolic wastes, excretion of water and electrolytes at a rate appropriate for their intake, and regulation of acid-base balance through normal hydrogen and bicarbonate ion metabolism. The kidneys also possess endocrine functions, specifically the synthesis of erythropoietin and renin, and the activation of vitamin D. In acute and chronic renal failure of any cause, any or all of these activities can be impaired.

ACUTE RENAL FAILURE

The term *acute renal failure* can be applied to anyone who sustains a marked diminution in renal function over a period of several days or less. Patients with acute renal failure generally have oliguria, azotemia, or both. It is important to realize that acute renal failure is not a specific diagnosis, but rather a syndrome that can be evoked by renal disorders of diverse causes. In discussing the various causes of acute renal failure, it is traditional, and very useful, to categorize them according to where they arise—in the renal circulation (prerenal acute renal failure), the renal parenchyma itself (intrinsic acute renal failure), or the collecting system and bladder (postrenal renal failure).

Prerenal Renal Failure

Prerenal azotemia is the most prevalent and usually the most easily reversed form of acute renal failure. Its most common

Table 39-1. Causes of prerenal azotemia

Hypovolemia
Hemorrhage, diarrhea, vomiting, perspiration, diuretic therapy, mineralocorticoid and glucocorticoid insufficiency, third-spacing, diabetes insipidus, osmotic diuresis
Hypotension
Hemodynamic abnormalities
Renal artery stenosis
Drugs (nonsteroidal antiinflammatory drugs, various antihypertensives)
Renovascular occlusion or spasm (e.g., scleroderma, hepatorenal syndrome)
Edematous disorders
Low cardiac output
Cirrhosis
Nephrotic syndrome (hypovolemia may play a role)

cause is hypovolemia. In prerenal azotemia, reduced blood flow to the kidneys results in a lowered glomerular filtration rate (GFR). A variety of disorders other than hypovolemia can also result in prerenal azotemia (Table 39-1). Cirrhosis and congestive heart failure are commonly associated with prerenal azotemia. In these conditions, plasma volume may be normal or expanded; however, the reduction in effective renal blood flow leads to prerenal azotemia and the sodium and water retention that accompany it.

Pathophysiology

When perfusion of the kidneys is compromised, the afferent glomerular arteriole dilates, maximizing the inflow of blood. This response occurs independent of any humoral or neural signal to the kidneys and is therefore termed *autoregulation of renal blood flow*. Constriction of the efferent arteriole also occurs in these circumstances, raising intracapillary pressures in the glomerulus and increasing the filtration fraction—that is, the portion of the renal blood flow that is removed as filtrate. This process, called *autoregulation of glomerular filtration*, maintains glomerular filtration at a rate as nearly normal as possible despite the decline in perfusion. When the reduction in blood flow outstrips the ability of these mechanisms to maintain normal renal hemodynamics, prerenal azotemia results.

In prerenal azotemia, the nephrons are morphologically and physiologically normal. The GFR is reduced solely through hemodynamic alterations and returns rapidly to normal when normal hemodynamics are restored.

The diagnosis of prerenal acute renal failure begins with examination of the patient for signs of volume depletion. Hypotension, orthostatic lability of the blood pressure, and poor skin turgor all suggest contraction of the extracellular compartment. Severe, protracted hypotension can also lead to intrinsic acute renal failure (see the section on acute tubular necrosis). This may confound the differentiation of prerenal from intrinsic acute renal failure.

Since congestive heart failure and cirrhosis can also be associated with prerenal renal failure, their stigmas should be sought on physical examination as well. Since prerenal renal failure is usually a hallmark of severe congestive heart failure and cirrhosis, the presence of rales, edema, or ascites will be evident.

The results of urinalysis in prerenal azotemia are nonspecific. However, urinary chemistries should reveal low sodium concentration and a fractional excretion of sodium of less than 1 percent.*

Flow through the renal tubules is reduced in "prerenal states," enhancing the reabsorption of water, sodium, and urea. Since creatinine is nonreabsorbable solute, the urea clearance is reduced disproportionately to the creatinine clearance, and the ratio of urea to creatinine in the serum rises, typically to greater than 1:20.

When prerenal azotemia due to hypovolemia is suspected, administration of isotonic saline is appropriate. The rate of volume repletion is determined by the severity of the deficit, which usually ranges from 100 to 500 ml per hour. Occasionally, a patient's state of fluid balance is not readily discernible by physical examination. In these settings, if prerenal azotemia is a concern, the clinician can elect to offer a "fluid challenge" of 500 to 1,000 ml isotonic saline over two to four hours while monitoring the patient's general condition and urine output. Prerenal azotemia in the setting of congestive heart failure or cirrhosis with ascites requires inpatient evaluation and treatment. Patients with these conditions are so finely balanced between vascular overload and underfill that, unless shock is present, they should only receive intravenous crystalloid in the most controlled and gradual fashion.

Intrinsic Acute Renal Failure

Inflammatory, ischemic, and toxic insults to the renal parenchyma can lead to abrupt onset of renal failure. The specific lesions are quite diverse in their pathophysiology and morphology.

Acute Tubular Necrosis

The syndrome known as *acute tubular necrosis* (ATN) is one of the most important causes of acute renal failure and the most prevalent form of intrinsic acute renal failure. Although ATN most commonly arises during hospitalization, patients are occasionally seen in the emergency department in the early phases of the disorder.

PATHOPHYSIOLOGY. In ATN, the predominant pathophysiologic alterations occur in the renal tubules. Thus, acid excretion, potassium secretion, urinary concentration, and sodium absorption are all impaired. Although the glomeruli appear relatively unaffected, the GFR is also reduced in this syndrome, reflecting changes in the ultrafiltration (K_f) of the glomerulus. The mechanism behind this phenomenon remains to be elucidated. One popular explanation is that impaired proximal tubular reabsorption leads to increased solute delivery to the distal nephron. The macula densa responds to the increased solute traffic by initiating localized

*The fractional excretion of sodium (FE_{Na}) represents the percent amount of filtered sodium that is excreted in the urine. A low FE_{Na} suggests avid sodium reabsorption from the nephrons and is the hallmark of prerenal physiology. In clinical practice, it is most common to calculate the FE_{Na} as follows:

$$FE_{Na} = \frac{\text{urine sodium} \times \text{plasma creatinine}}{\text{plasma sodium} \times \text{urine creatinine}} \times 100$$

Table 39-2. Causes of acute tubular necrosis

Ischemia
Toxins
Heavy metals (e.g., cisplatin, mercury salts)
Radiographic contrast agents
Antibiotics
Aminoglycosides
Amphotericin B
Tetracyclines
Nonsteroidal antiinflammatory agents
Other (e.g., carbon tetrachloride)
Sepsis (with endotoxemia)
Pigmenturia (myoglobinuria and hemoglobinuria)

activation of the renin-angiotensin system. This culminates in preglomerular vasoconstriction and mesangial cell contraction. Histopathologic examination of the kidney in ATN may reveal cell swelling and vacuole formation in the tubular epithelial cells, with occasional nuclear pyknosis. Disruption of the proximal tubular brush border and mitochondrial degeneration may be seen at the ultrastructural level. In most studies of renal morphology in human ATN, the degree of functional impairment is disproportionate to the visible extent of tissue damage.

The pathogenesis of ATN remains poorly understood. Several hypotheses have been advanced to explain the mechanism of renal failure in ATN, including intratubular *obstruction* by sloughed or damaged cells, disordered renal *vasomotor* response after the specific insult, and loss of epithelial integrity, leading to *back leak* of filtered wastes into the systemic circulation. A wide body of clinical and experimental literature exists to support or refute each of these constructs. The fact that a variety of disparate insults, both toxic and ischemic, can produce ATN (Table 39-2), plus subtle differences in presentation between patients (e.g., oliguria vs. nonoliguria, high vs. low fractional excretion of sodium) with ATN of differing causes, suggest that this syndrome probably represents a complex of distinct, if related, disorders.

COURSE. In the vast majority of patients, ATN is a self-limited process and will resolve within two to four weeks after the provoking insult. The course may be protracted in patients with particularly severe intercurrent illnesses or coexisting renal disease. It has been observed that oliguric patients have a more prolonged course and a higher likelihood of requiring interim dialysis than do nonoliguric patients with ATN.

DIAGNOSIS. The diagnosis of tubular necrosis in a patient with acute onset of renal failure rests largely on historical data. Was the patient predisposed to developing ATN as a result of a recent episode of hemodynamic instability, sepsis, or exposure to a nephrotoxic agent or radiographic contrast material? In most patients, such a history can be elicited. The physical examination is usually nonspecific, although it may be of use in ruling out hypovolemia or bladder outlet obstruction as the cause of renal failure. Eighty percent of patients will have the characteristic urinary sediment findings of brown granular casts and abundant renal tubular epithelial cells in the urine.

Urine chemistries are also useful, particularly in distinguishing between ATN and prerenal azotemia (see the section on prerenal renal failure). Typically, the fractional excretion of sodium is high in ATN, reflecting the impairment of the kidneys' ability to reabsorb sodium from the filtrate. In rare cases, however, particularly when ATN arises as a result of radiographic contrast exposure or in a patient with liver disease, the fractional excretion of sodium may be low. In these instances or in the event that a patient is believed to have an element of reversible prerenal renal failure in addition to ATN, observing the reponse to a cautious fluid challenge (e.g., 500 ml isotonic saline over two hours) may help to clarify the diagnosis.

MYOGLOBINURIC ATN: SPECIAL CONSIDERATIONS. It is particularly important for the emergency department physician to be familiar with myoglobinuric acute renal failure. In this disease, myoglobin released from damaged muscle cells is filtered and exerts toxic effects on tubular cells. This is a common complication in severe trauma. Rhabdomyolysis can also occur nontraumatically as a result of drug intoxication, hyperthermia, or infectious and inflammatory processes. The risk of developing frank renal failure in this setting is greatest when muscle injury has been sufficient to elevate the serum creatine phosphokinase to 10,000 IU/per liter or greater, and if volume depletion is present. The urine of patients with myoglobinuria is often reddish or brownish in color. The dipstick test for heme will be positive, regardless of the degree of hematuria. Acute renal failure is much rarer with hemoglobinuria than with myoglobinuria. Very large amounts of free hemoglobin must be present in the serum before the binding capacity of haptoglobin is saturated and hemoglobin can gain entry into the glomerular filtrate. Any pathologic process that produces massive intravascular hemolysis—for example, fresh-water drowning—must be considered a potential cause of hemoglobinuric acute renal failure.

TREATMENT. There is no specific therapy for ATN. Fluid and electrolyte problems should receive top therapeutic priority in a patient with suspected ATN.

Volume overload can be treated with diuretics; generally, the patient with ATN requires high-dose, intravenous loop diuretics. If this measure fails to provoke a diuresis, dialysis may be indicated. There is some evidence to suggest that osmotic or loop diuretics administered at the time of an ATN-provoking insult can protect the kidneys. These agents lower the metabolic oxygen requirements of the kidneys by interrupting nephronal transport processes, rendering tubular cells less vulnerable to toxic and ischemic injury. Diuretic protection is most easily practicable in patients in whom the time of the renal insult can be anticipated—for example, the patient about to undergo a radiographic contrast study. Prophylaxis is best afforded by administering intravenous fluids conjointly with diuretics to keep the urine flow rate at about 200 ml per hour or greater. *Volume restoration and forced diuresis are critical in preventing myoglobinuric renal failure in patients at risk.*

Hyperkalemia is the most serious of the electrolyte imbalances seen in acute renal failure and should be handled in the same manner as for patients who do not have kidney failure. Since total body potassium stores are usually more

Table 39-3. Acute interstitial nephritides that cause intrinsic acute renal failure

Drugs	Infections	Infiltration	Idiopathic
Common	Direct invasion	Lymphoma	Diagnosed by exclusion
Methicillin	*Staphylococcus*	Leukemia	
Ampicillin	Various gram-negative organisms	Sarcoidosis	
Penicillin	Brucellosis		
Sulfonamide	Indirect effects		
Rifampicin	*Streptococcus*		
Phenindione	*Pneumococcus*		
Uncommon	Typhoid		
Allopurinol	Diphtheria		
Diphenylhydantoin			
Cimetidine			
Thiazides			

Source: M.R. Rudnick, et al. The Differential Diagnosis of Acute Renal Failure. In B.M. Brenner and J.M. Lazarus (eds.), *Acute Renal Failure* (2nd ed.). Churchill Livingstone, New York, 1988. Pp. 177–232.

massively overloaded in hyperkalemic patients with renal failure than without, dialysis may be necessary for remediation. The technical aspects of dialysis, including its use in treating the uremic manifestations of acute and chronic renal failure, are discussed later in this chapter.

Acute Interstitial Nephritis

Acute interstitial nephritis (AIN) is an inflammatory disease of the renal tubules and surrounding interstitial tissue. In the majority of cases, the disease is triggered by exposure to a pharmacologic agent. The reaction is idiosyncratic and can be associated with allergic manifestations. Renal failure is common with this lesion and can last four to six weeks, although the disease is almost always reversible.

Allergic manifestations such as a rash, eosinophilia, fever, and excretion of polymorphonuclear leukocytes and eosinophils in the urine occur in as many as 75 percent of patients with AIN. Some patients have elevated immunoglobulin E (IgE) levels in the blood. Acute interstitial disease also occurs, albeit rarely, in association with bacterial and viral infections, or may be entirely idopathic (Table 39-3).

Histologically, the kidney shows a patchy or diffuse inflammatory cell infiltrate throughout the interstitium, which can be quite edematous. Neutrophils and eosinophils are occasionally identified within tubular lumens.

Withdrawal of any agents believed to be potentially responsible for the disorder is the mainstay of therapy in AIN. In patients with severe renal failure, attention to the fluid and electrolyte disturbances, as described in the section on ATN, is paramount. Interim dialysis may be indicated in such patients. It has been suggested, but never proved, that the use of high-dose daily corticosteroid therapy can shorten the course of AIN.

Other Causes

Numerous vascular and glomerular diseases can cause acute renal failure (Table 39-4). Differentiating among them usually requires special serologic tests or renal biopsy. In some diseases, such as idiopathic crescentic glomerulonephritis, the glomerulonephritides associated with collagen-vascular diseases, and Goodpasture's syndrome, a rapid diagnosis is essential in order that definitive therapy with steroids, cytotoxic drugs, or plasmapheresis can be instituted in time to salvage kidney function. In the emergency department, however, the initial management of the patient need not be directed at establishing a specific diagnosis but rather at correcting the life-threatening metabolic and chemical derangements of acute renal failure.

Table 39-4. Glomerular and vascular diseases that can cause acute renal failure

- Glomerular
  - All forms of idiopathic nephrotic syndrome
  - Glomerulonephritides
    - IgA nephropathy
    - Postinfectious glomerulonephritis
    - Idiopathic crescentic glomerulonephritis (including Goodpasture's syndrome)
    - Bacteremia-associated glomerulonephritis (endocarditis, shunt nephritis, abscess-related glomerulonephritis)
    - Membranoproliferative glomerulonephritis
- Vascular
  - Collagen-vascular diseases
    - Systemic lupus erythematosus
    - Hypersensitivity vasculitis
    - Essential mixed cryoglobulinemia
    - Polyarteritis nodosa and related syndromes
    - Hypocomplementemic vasculitis
    - Henoch-Schönlein purpura
    - Wegener's granulomatosis
    - Scleroderma
  - Atheroembolic disease
  - Renal artery thromboembolism
  - Aortic dissection
- Miscellaneous
  - Hemolytic-uremic syndromes
  - Preeclampsia

Table 39-5. Causes of postrenal acute renal failure

- Obstruction of the collecting system, ureters, or bladder outlet
  - Urolithiasis
  - Pelvic and retroperitoneal neoplasms
  - Blood clot
  - Retroperitoneal fibrosis
  - Sloughed renal papilla
  - Fungus ball
  - Prostatic hypertrophy
  - Neurogenic bladder
  - Urethral stricture or infection
  - Surgical ligation of ureters
- Renal tubular microobstruction
  - Crystal nephropathies
    - Uric acid (seen in association with tumor lysis and uricosuric drugs)
    - Oxalic acid
    - Drugs (sulfa, sulindac, methotrexate, acyclovir)
  - Pigmenturia
  - Myeloma cast nephropathy

Postrenal Renal Failure

Postrenal renal failure denotes renal failure due to obstruction of urinary outflow from the kidneys. Anatomically, there are two major categories of obstruction (Table 39-5). Diffuse microobstruction of the renal tubules can result from crystal deposition within the lumens. An example of this is the tumor lysis syndrome, in which intracellular products such as purine metabolites and phosphates are released from dying tumor cells, are filtered by nephrons in large amounts, and crystallize in the renal tubules. This situation, occasionally referred to as *blockade nephropathy*, can also be caused by several drugs. Macroscopic obstructions can occur anywhere from the renal pelvis to the bladder outlet and may be related to a variety of anatomic lesions.

In general, both kidneys must be obstructed to cause acute renal failure in a person with previously normal renal function. Therefore, azotemia is most likely to develop in an individual with two intact kidneys if the site of the obstructing lesion is the bladder outlet or, as occurs more rarely, if both ureters are simultaneously blocked.

Of all the forms of acute renal failure, obstructive uropathy is most likely to produce frank anuria. A popular misconception, however, is that patients with renal failure due to obstructive uropathy inevitably have a reduced urine output. In fact, obstruction impairs the ability of the renal collecting tubule to concentrate the urine, and, hence, patients in whom the obstruction is not complete may be polyuric. The other tubular functions are hindered in obstruction also, particularly urinary acidification, ammonia excretion, and potassium secretion. Most of the functional abnormalities are attributable to the direct effect of increased urinary pressures on nephron components. However, in experimental models of obstructive uropathy, other key pathogenetic events can be demonstrated, including enhanced local synthesis of the vasoconstrictive substance thromboxane A_2, which reduces renal blood flow, possibly resulting from infiltration of the renal interstitium by inflammatory cells.

Diagnosis of Obstructive Uropathy

Postrenal, like prerenal, causes should be considered at the time a patient is seen with acute renal failure, since corrective measures can be undertaken with rapid success. Bladder catheterization should be performed both as a diagnostic and therapeutic measure; a vigorous diuresis on insertion of a bladder catheter suggests bladder outlet obstruction. If no diuresis ensues, a more proximal site of obstruction—for example, in the ureters—is still possible. In this case, the catheter should be removed, and renal sonography performed to rule out the continued possibility of obstruction. If the sonogram reveals hydronephrosis, or if one still suspects an obstructive cause despite normal results on renal sonography, cystoscopy and retrograde pyelography are indicated.*

The diagnosis of acute renal failure due to intratubular crystal deposition is generally based on historical information. The patient will have oliguria and azotemia after administration of drugs known to precipitate in the renal tubules, or in the first several days after chemotherapy for lymphoproliferative or myeloproliferative disease.

*Although the renal sonogram has a greater than 90 percent sensitivity in detecting urinary obstruction, in some settings it may fail to yield a diagnosis. At times a functionally obstructed patient fails to demonstrate hydronephrosis because of coexistent volume depletion, encasement of the renal pelvis by fibrotic tissue, or extremely rapid onset of the obstruction. Furthermore, in some settings obstruction must be considered the cause of renal failure until proved otherwise—for example, in the patient with a known history of bilateral nephrolithiasis, retroperitoneal tumor, or a solitary functioning kidney. In such a setting, we recommend routine retrograde pyelography, unless specifically contraindicated.

Table 39-6. Causes of chronic renal failure

Cause	Percentage*
Diabetes mellitus	30
Glomerulonephritis	25
Hypertensive renal disease	15
Chronic interstitial nephritis	10
Hereditary, including polycystic kidney disease	7
Chronic obstructive uropathy	3
Other causes	10

*Percentages represent approximate prevalence among those with end-stage renal disease in the United States.

Treatment of Postrenal Renal Failure

Therapy of obstructive renal failure depends on the anatomic nature of the obstruction. Bladder outlet obstructions, of which prostatic hypertrophy is the most common, may be temporarily relieved in the emergency department by insertion of an indwelling bladder catheter. More proximal lesions, such as ureteral obstruction by tumor or stones, require urologic intervention.

There is no curative measure for the crystal blockade nephropathies. Hemodialysis may help the patient both by replacing renal excretory function, and by clearing the offending substance, particularly in the case of acute uric acid nephropathy. By far, the most prudent management is preventative. Patients at risk for crystal nephropathy should be hydrated and a diuresis should be maintained to keep the urine flow rate at or above 200 ml per hour. Patients at risk for uric acid nephropathy should be given an alkalinizing agent, such as sodium bicarbonate, and pretreated with allopurinol to mitigate purine degradation into uric acid.

CHRONIC RENAL FAILURE

In acute renal failure, the decline in renal function occurs over a period of days to weeks and can often be traced to a discrete illness or event. Most lesions that produce acute renal failure are reversible. On the other hand, in chronic renal disease, the decline in renal function is more apt to have an insidious onset and a slower course. Renal function is lost gradually; when the GFR is detectably reduced below expected levels, the patient is said to have *chronic renal insufficiency*. When further erosion of renal function leads to a GFR of less than 25 percent of normal, *chronic renal failure* is said to be present.

A number of the disease processes that cause acute renal failure can also produce irreversible chronic renal injury if resolution is incomplete. For example, uncorrected obstructive uropathy can cause permanent loss of functioning renal parenchyma. The most common causes of chronic renal failure, however, are renal parenchymal diseases (Table 39-6). Hypertension, chronic glomerulonephritis, and diabetes mellitus are the leading causes of end-stage renal disease in the United States.

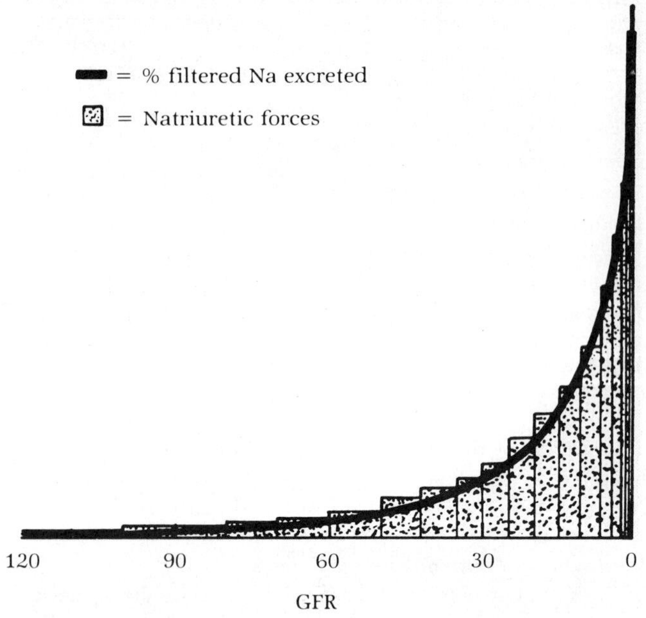

Fig. 39-1. As the GFR declines, the fractional excretion of sodium increases. The "natriuretic forces" act to maximize sodium excretion in a manner that offsets, in part, the reduction in filtered load. (From N.S. Bricker. On the pathogenesis of the uremic state. Reprinted, by permission of the New England Journal of Medicine 286:1097, 1972.)

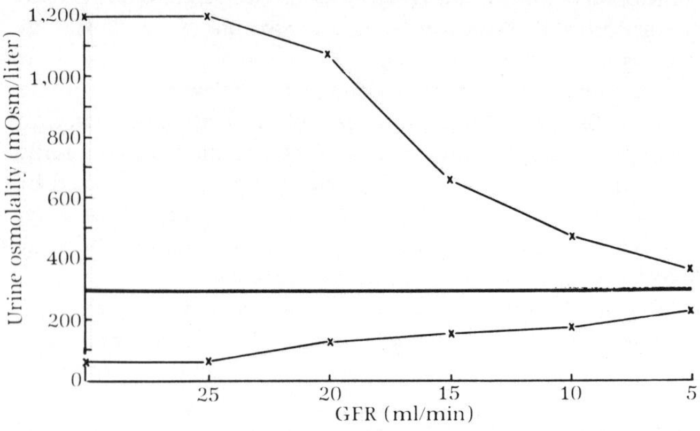

Fig. 39-2. Theoretical maximum and minimum urine osmolalities in moderate to advanced chronic renal failure. This diagram presupposes that each residual nephron is functionally intact and that daily solute excretion is fixed at 600 mOsm. The solute diuretic state effectively reduces maximal urinary concentration and dilution. The ability of the kidney both to maximally excrete and conserve electrolytes is also limited. (From N.S. Bricker, et al. Observations on the concentrating and diluting mechanisms of the diseased kidney. Reproduced from the *Journal of Clinical Investigation,* 1959, 38:516 by copyright permission of the American Society for Clinical Investigation.)

Close to 200,000 people in the United States currently have end-stage or near end-stage renal failure. The size of this population is a tribute to the increased availability over the past 20 years of superior dietary and pharmacologic management, particularly antihypertensive agents, and widespread dialysis and transplantation resources. In spite of these advances, such patients remain susceptible to a wide variety of complications with which the emergency department physician must be familiar.

Pathophysiology

A significant reduction in the number of functioning nephrons obviously limits the total excretory capacity of the kidney. In chronic renal failure, each surviving nephron is anatomically enlarged and physiologically adapted to expand its individual excretory contribution.

The glomerular adaptation is primarily hemodynamic. Micropuncture studies in rats with experimental forms of chronic renal failure reveal that afferent arteriolar blood flow is increased, culminating in extremely high blood pressure in the glomerular capillary. The resulting rise in the net filtration pressure maximizes the single nephron GFR. It is thought that the long-term effect of glomerular capillary hypertension is to shorten the life of the glomerulus itself, making this phenomenon potentially maladaptive.

Adaptive changes also occur in the tubules of remnant nephrons. In general, the fractional reabsorption of filtered solutes is reduced. In the case of sodium, as Bricker has shown, the fractional reabsorption of filtered sodium falls hyperbolically with the fall in GFR (Fig. 39-1). If this reduction in reabsorption of filtered sodium by the tubules did not accompany renal failure, the body would be much more vulnerable to sodium overload. The mechanism by which sodium reabsorption is inhibited in the remnant nephron is still unclear. It is possible that factors such as renal prostaglandins, atriopeptins, and changes in renal neural activity mediate the inhibition of tubular sodium transport that occurs in renal failure. Fractional potassium excretion per nephron also occurs and is in part mediated by aldosterone. The ability of surviving nephrons to maximize their contribution to the total excretory capacity of the kidney is often referred to as the *magnification phenomenon.* In some instances, the magnification is mediated by substances that engender deleterious effects to the body. In the syndrome of secondary hyperparathyroidism, for example, the high levels of parathormone serve to maximize the phosphaturic capacity of the reduced renal mass. Excretory capability is preserved at the expense of hyperparathyroid bone disease. This concept is often referred to as the *trade-off hypothesis.*

The flow rate in remnant tubules is high, owing to the large number of osmotically active particles being processed by these nephrons. This solute diuretic state enhances the fractional excretion of water and electrolytes relative to those in a normal nephron. For this reason, the surviving nephron cannot maximally conserve water or electrolytes. Thus, patients with chronic renal failure are more prone than normal individuals to dehydration or electrolyte depletion when dietary intake is inadequate or extrarenal losses are increased. Under usual circumstances, however, the reduction in the filtered load of these substances offsets impaired tubular conservation. Fluid overload and hyperkalemia are common complications of chronic renal failure.

Thus, the ability of the chronically failing kidney both to conserve or eliminate substances is restricted (Fig. 39-2). Dietary therapy must be aimed at adjusting intake of sodium, potassium, water, and protein to levels appropriate for the residual excretory capacity.

Metabolic Consequences of Renal Failure

Patients with renal failure are subject to two major categories of problems: metabolic abnormalities and fluid-electrolyte imbalances. The metabolic group of problems comprise the syndrome known as *uremia*. The chemical imbalances are discussed in depth in Chaps. 36, 37, and 38 and will be treated in more cursory fashion here. As a general rule, uremic manifestations are more common in patients with chronic renal failure, whereas the fluid and electrolyte disturbances are a greater concern in patients with acute renal failure, presumably because adaptive renal homeostatic mechanisms may not yet have developed in these patients. Both classes of morbidity are of major concern in both types of renal failure, however.

Uremia

The uremic syndrome represents tissue injury by endogenous toxins and waste products. Virtually every organ system can be affected. Although it has been recognized for centuries, the uremic syndrome remains poorly understood, mainly because the identities of the culpable uremic toxins are still largely controversial.

The symptoms of uremia do not appear until 85 to 90 percent of renal function is lost. Patients complain first of fatigue, lassitude, generalized weakness, anorexia, and bad taste in the mouth. As the condition continues and further kidney function is lost, the signs and symptoms become more dramatic. Mild glucose intolerance, a result of acquired insulin resistance, is often present. Hypertriglyceridemia may also be noted.

A number of cardiovascular abnormalities can occur. Hypertension is the most prevalent of these and is usually due to salt and water retention. More rarely, and depending on the nature of the underlying renal disease, vasoconstrictive hypertension related to inappropriate activation of the renin-angiotensin system may be seen. Congestive heart failure is also common and, like hypertension, usually reflects fluid overload. It has also been suggested that a uremic toxin may exert an antiinotropic effect, directly impairing myocardial performance. This hypothesis is based on the observation that isovolemic dialysis in some patients can improve cardiac function.

Pericarditis is one of the most urgent cardiovascular complications of uremia. Effusions are common and are generally small, although on occasion they may be of sufficient magnitude to cause tamponade. Uremic pericarditis probably represents the response of the pericardium to an offending uremic toxin. The pericardial fluid is typically hemorrhagic or serosanguinous. Uremic pericarditis is considered an indication for prompt initiation of dialysis therapy. Uremic pleuritis has been reported, although most pleural effusions in uremic patients signify fluid overload or infectious comorbidities.

Skeletal myopathy can occur in uremic patients. Although toxins may play a role in this disorder, uremic myopathy is more likely related to derangements in calcium-parathormone-vitamin D metabolism. The shoulder and pelvic girdle are most commonly involved.

Overt gout occurs less often than might otherwise be expected, despite the prevalence of hyperuricemia in uremic patients. Pseudogout (calcium pyrophosphate deposition disease) is not uncommon, particularly in patients with an elevated calcium-phosphate product. All patients with chronic renal failure have abnormal calcium and phosphorus metabolism. There are several reasons for this. With the decline in GFR, phosphate retention occurs. The excess phosphorus binds to soluble calcium in the plasma, forming insoluble complexes that precipitate. The resultant hypocalcemia provides a tonic stimulus for parathyroid hormone (PTH) release, which, in turn, raises the plasma calcium concentration via accretion of calcium from bone, and augmented calcium reabsorption from the renal tubules. Parathyroid hormone also directly enhances renal phosphate excretion, as was mentioned earlier in this chapter (magnification phenomenon). With GFRs of less than 30 ml per minute, the phosphaturic capacity of the kidney, even with maximal levels of PTH present, is exceeded, and frank hyperphosphatemia is seen.

Vitamin D is the other hormonal system that controls bone mineralization and calcium and phosphorus balance. Vitamin D requires biochemical activation in the renal tubules. With extensive renal parenchymal loss, insufficient vitamin D activation can occur. Furthermore, the 1-hydroxylase enzyme that catalyzes the activation step is inhibited by hyperphosphatemia. Experimental evidence suggests that uremia can induce end-organ resistance to vitamin D. The end result is acquired functional vitamin D deficiency.

The term *renal osteodystrophy* is used to denote the complex metabolic bone disease that occurs in patients with chronic renal failure. This represents a composite of several different lesions. One of these lesions is *osteomalacia*, the diffuse demineralization caused by vitamin D deficiency and, in some cases, aluminum overload. *Osteitis fibrosa* is the lesion attributable to hyperparathyroidism and consists of resorption and scarification of bone cortex.

Uremia is associated with a number of gastrointestinal complications. A bad taste in the mouth, fetid breath, and loss of taste for food (dysgeusia) are highly prevalent. Erosive peptic disease of the stomach and duodenum is common.

Anemia occurs in almost all uremic patients. There are several explanations for this, including marrow suppression by uremic toxin(s); shortened red-cell life span, possibly also related to toxins; failure of the diseased kidneys to manufacture erythropoietin; and increased blood loss due to repetitive venipuncture, hemodialysis, and occult gastrointestinal bleeding. The anemia typically has normocytic and normochromic features, similar to those seen in many forms of chronic disease. There is a loose correlation between the degree of anemia and the severity of renal functional impairment; in most patients with end-stage renal failure, the hematocrit eventually stabilizes in the 15 to 25 percent range. The recent availability of recombinant human erythropoietin for therapeutic use promises to eliminate the widespread need for frequent transfusions in patients with advanced renal failure.

Thrombocytopenia is occasionally observed but is not significant. Far more important from a hemostatic standpoint are qualitative abnormalities of platelet function—that is, impaired adhesion and aggregation. These are likely related to circulating platelet inhibitors in uremic plasma. Platelet function can be normalized in most patients with dialysis.

Uremic toxins also inhibit host defenses, including both the inflammatory and immunologic response. Humoral immunity is less affected than cellular immunity.

The neurologic manifestations of uremia can involve both the central and peripheral nervous systems. The primary central nervous system disorder comprises an encephalopathy indistinguishable from other metabolic and toxic encephalopathies. Although this disorder may be seen in simple uremia, the presence of biochemical and vascular abnormalities such as acidosis, hypoxia, hyper- or hypoosmolality, and severe hypertension may play additive roles. The signs of uremic encephalopathy are nonspecific and include clouded consciousness, reduced attention span, memory lapses, irritability, and disturbed sleep pattern. Asterixis is frequently demonstrable. Left untreated, uremic encephalopathy eventuates in seizures, coma, and death.

Peripheral neuropathy is extremely common. Characteristically, uremia produces a distal, sensorimotor, symmetric polyneuropathy. Nerve conduction studies are very often abnormal in patients with advanced renal disease and no symptoms of neuropathy. The earliest clinical finding is reduced vibratory sensation in the distal lower extremities. With progression of the disorder, patients become aware of weakness, numbness, and even pain in the affected distributions. As with so many other components of the uremic syndrome, the identities of the specific toxins responsible for uremic neuropathy remain unknown.

Autonomic nervous system abnormalities frequently occur in uremia and can lead to impotence, orthostatic hypotension, and dysfunction of the sweat glands. These problems are most severe in diabetic patients, since diabetes itself contributes to autonomic dysfunction.

Dermatologic disorders seen in uremic patients include nail changes, hair loss, and a pale and sallow complexion resulting from a combination of anemia and retained pigmented wastes. Ecchymoses are common due to tissue fragility and the bleeding diathesis. Pruritus is a particularly common and unpleasant symptom that may relate to cutaneous neuropathy, intradermal calcium and phosphorus deposition, and other waste products that accumulate in these tissues.

Therapy

The definitive therapy for renal failure or *renal replacement therapy* includes dialysis and transplantation. These are modalities that need not be employed until late in the course of chronic renal disease. Transplantation is never an emergency procedure. Acute dialysis may, on occasion, be initiated in the emergency department but only when a delay is anticipated in relocating the patient to a more permanent hospital site.

In both acute and chronic renal failure, optimal management comprises a preventative approach. Measures must be taken to adjust the dietary intake of fluid and electrolytes to a level commensurate with residual renal function. Reducing protein intake (0.5–1.0 gm/kg body weight per day) has several beneficial effects, including reduction of substrate from which nitrogenous wastes are generated and amelioration of the workload on hyperfiltering remnant glomeruli. The predialytic management of patients with progressive renal failure requires the expertise of nephrologic and dietary consultants. With careful management, critical complications are rare in these patients. In the following paragraphs, the major emergencies are considered.

Managing Fluid Imbalances in Patients with Renal Failure

As has already been discussed, the patient with failing kidneys is prone to both hypervolemia and hypovolemia. *Hypovolemia* is important to recognize since it is common, readily reversible, and can exacerbate renal failure in patients with intrinsic renal disease by adding a prerenal component. A volume-depleted patient with acute or chronic parenchymal renal disease will often have substantial amelioration of uremic symptoms with fluid repletion.

Fluid deficits in patients with renal failure should always be treated with isotonic fluid unless hypernatremia is present. Isotonic fluids are more effective in restoring extracellular volume than are hypotonic solutions and will not cause hyponatremia. Clinically assessing the magnitude of a volume deficit can be difficult. An adult patient with hypotension, postural blood pressure change, and grossly reduced tissue turgor clearly needs to receive several liters of fluid. Frequently, however, a patient who could benefit from a liter or two of saline replacement may not display these obvious signs of fluid depletion. In such cases, and barring any overt signs of fluid overload, we generally administer a liter of normal saline over two to four hours, reassessing the patient hourly. Before the patient is discharged, the causes of hypovolemia should be identified and corrected. Typically, these include supervening acute illnesses, overly aggressive use of diuretics, inadequate intake, or enhanced insensible fluid loss, as is common during summer months.

Hypervolemia in patients with renal failure results from failure to restrict sodium intake adequately, which can be iatrogenic or related to poor patient compliance with dietary restrictions. Pulmonary vascular congestion and pulmonary edema are the only manifestations of hypervolemia that need emergent treatment. Depending on the extent of the patient's renal failure, this can be accomplished with an appropriately high dose of a loop diuretic (e.g., furosemide, $\leq$ 200 mg intravenously, or bumetanide, $\leq$ 5 mg intravenously), perhaps in conjunction with a thiazide. Topical, oral, or intravenous nitrates can help "buy time" while waiting for a therapeutic diuresis to occur. Patients in whom these measures fail, and patients who are already receiving maintenance dialysis therapy will require emergency dialysis or ultrafiltration to correct fluid overload.

Electrolyte Abnormalities in Patients with Renal Failure

Most of these are discussed in depth in Chap. 37. This section is limited to special considerations for patients with renal dysfunction.

HYPERKALEMIA. Hyperkalemia is the most immediately life-threatening electrolyte disturbance and a major cause of death in patients with acute renal failure. Although hyperkalemia is occasionally seen in patients with chronic renal disease, it is less common than in acute renal failure, since the adaptive changes that occur in remnant nephrons increase their ability to secrete potassium. As a rule, patients with chronic renal failure do not require dietary potassium restriction until the GFR falls below 15 ml per minute.

Hyperkalemia that arises in a previously stable, normokalemic patient with chronic renal failure should alert the clinician to the possibility of an unrecognized potassium load, either exogenous (dietary noncompliance or medication error) or endogenous (gastrointestinal hemorrhage, increased tissue catabolism). Medications that predispose to hyperkalemia should be avoided or used with great caution in these patients. Such agents include potassium supplements, converting enzyme inhibitors, and potassium-sparing diuretics.

The treatment of hyperkalemia in patients with acute or chronic renal failure is as outlined in Chap. 37. Two of these modalities, orally or rectally administered sodium polystyrene sulfonate resin (Kayexolate) and intravenous sodium bicarbonate, commit the patient to a considerable sodium load. If the patient is volume depleted when first seen, this is not a problem, and, in fact, fluid repletion with isotonic saline is also recommended. However, acute dialysis is generally necessary in a volume-overloaded, hyperkalemic patient with renal failure.

HYPONATREMIA. The ability to excrete free water is impaired in anyone with a reduced GFR. For this reason, patients with acute or chronic renal failure are maintained on daily fluid restrictions of one to two liters per day. Failure to comply with these restrictions can lead to the development of dilutional hyponatremia. The serum sodium level in this setting rarely falls below 120 mEq per liter, although this degree of hyponatremia can precipitate the appearance of uremic symptoms in a previously well-compensated patient. Fluid restriction is usually sufficient to correct the problem over several days. Patients who have neurologic symptoms at presentation should receive hypertonic (3%) saline according to the formula mentioned in Chap. 36, unless they are volume overloaded. In this latter instance, patients should be dialyzed against a high-sodium dialysate. Hyponatremia in volume-depleted patients is known as *hypotonic dehydration* and can occur whenever salt loss exceeds water loss in magnitude. Restoration of the extracellular volume with isotonic saline rapidly corrects this disorder. Care should be taken to avoid correcting the fluid deficit too rapidly lest hypervolemia result. It has been suggested that raising the serum by more than 2 mEq per liter per hour can have adverse neurologic consequences.

HYPOCALCEMIA. The causes of hypocalcemia in renal failure have already been discussed. It is rare that hypocalcemia of sufficient magnitude to cause symptoms such as tetany, muscle fibrillation, hypotension, or seizures arises in uncomplicated renal failure. Almost invariably, the hypocalcemia is accompanied by hyperphosphatemia. It has generally been taught that raising the "calcium-phosphorous product" by supplementing calcium can lead to precipitation of calcium salts in soft tissues. It is therefore preferable to avoid administration of calcium supplements. Any situation serious enough to warrant immediate calcium supplementation should be treated with calcium gluconate IV solution; our practice is to administer the equivalent of 200 mg of elemental calcium in 5% dextrose in water over the first 20 minutes. Additional supplementation may be given more slowly over the ensuing 1 to 3 hours until satisfactory control of hypocalcemic symptoms is achieved. For the reasons previously cited, the therapeutic end point should be elimination of hypocalcemic symptoms, not normalization of the serum calcium level.

The use of oral phosphate binders, by helping to lower the serum phosphorus level, may aid in raising the serum calcium. This maneuver acts slowly and is not useful in the emergency setting. Oral phosphate binders should be included in the maintenance regimen of most patients with chronic renal failure and dialysis. Likewise, vitamin D supplementation has no role in the emergent management of hypocalcemia.

HYPERMAGNESEMIA. The kidney is the main organ of magnesium homeostasis, and predictably magnesium retention can occur in the setting of chronic renal failure, particularly if the patient has been ingesting magnesium-containing antacids. Mild hypermagnesemia (3–4 mEq per liter) is rarely symptomatic. As the magnesium level rises, lethargy and weakness ensue, and very high levels (>10 mEq per liter) can produce fatal respiratory, cardiac, and cerebral depression. In severe cases of hypermagnesemia, dialysis is indicated.

METABOLIC ACIDOSIS. The treatment of metabolic acidosis is outlined in Chap. 38. This is by far the most common acid-base abnormality in acute or chronic renal failure.

By itself, renal failure rarely produces acidosis of sufficient proportion to require emergency treatment. The finding of a serum bicarbonate level less than 15 mEq per liter or a significant fall in the serum bicarbonate from previously stable levels, should prompt an investigation to rule out the coexistence of another cause of acidosis—for example, ketoacidosis or lactic acidosis.

Treatment of metabolic acidosis is a controversial topic. Our approach is as follows: (1) Ascertain that the disorder is attributable to renal failure alone—that is, rule out lactic acidosis, ketoacidosis, and toxic ingestion. If these are present, treat their underlying cause as recommended in Chap. 38. (2) Check the arterial blood gas profile to establish that hypocarbia reflects a true metabolic acidosis as opposed to another acid-base disturbance such as a compensated respiratory alkalosis or a mixed disturbance. (3) If renal failure is believed to be the sole cause of the acidosis, supplement with sodium bicarbonate only as needed to maintain the arterial pH at or greater than 7.20 or the serum bicarbonate concentration at or greater than 15 mEq per liter. Dialysis is rarely needed in the treatment of metabolic acidosis and it is not very effective as a sole modality. In severe metabolic acidosis, dialysis is best viewed as an adjunct to bicarbonate supplementation.

Emergency Dialysis

Careful conservative management—that is, a cohesive dietary and medication regimen—of the patient with renal failure should make emergency dialysis a rare event. Periodically, however, situations arise in which acute dialysis is unavoidable. Any life-threatening fluid or electrolyte imbalance that cannot be treated by medical means is an indication for urgent dialysis. The same is true of drug intoxications, even in patients without renal disease, which produce potentially lethal manifestations and in which drug levels cannot be lowered by less aggressive modalities such as forced emesis, enteric charcoal, or specific medical antidotes.

Uremia is rarely an indication for urgent dialysis, since uremic manifestations usually evolve over a long enough period that they can be anticipated and dialysis can be initiated on an elective basis. Furthermore, uremic symptoms are rarely life threatening. However, there are two exceptions. Uremic pericarditis, evidenced by the development of a pericardial rub in a patient with renal failure, rarely, but occasionally, causes tamponade and is best treated with prompt and aggressive dialysis. The other urgent uremic indication for dialysis is severe encephalopathy as characterized by seizures or coma.

Dialysis treatments effect substance transfer through two means: *diffusion* of waste solutes down a concentration gradient from blood to dialysate and *ultrafiltration*, in which plasma water and the small, dissolved molecules it contains move across the dialysis membrane in response to a hydrostatic pressure gradient (hemodialysis) or fixed osmotic gradient (peritoneal dialysis). A detailed description of the technical aspects of peritoneal and hemodialysis would be impossible within the confines of this chapter. The emergency physician should be acquainted with some basic principles.

Hemodialysis

Although both peritoneal and hemodialysis are effective for engendering fluid and solute removal, hemodialysis is more rapid. It should therefore be considered the preferred modality for treating dire situations such as coma due to intoxication by a dialyzable drug, hypercalcemic coma, or hyperkalemia with electrocardiographic changes. Hemodialysis does have several drawbacks. Vascular access is needed; in patients who do not already have a working arteriovenous fistula for this purpose, temporary subclavian or femoral venous catheters have become the preferred substitute. They are usually easy to place and are of large enough caliber to afford satisfactory blood flow for hemodialysis.

Another drawback of hemodialysis is that it also requires systemic anticoagulation during the procedure, and therefore it may be contraindicated in patients with ongoing bleeding problems. Lastly, hemodialysis represents more of a cardiovascular stress than does peritoneal dialysis. Hypotension in hemodialysis is common and relates to several factors, including rapid osmolar and volume shifts and depression of myocardial performance by rapid transfer of acetate buffer from the dialysate. For this reason, peritoneal dialysis may be preferable for hypotensive patients and those with preexisting heart disease.

Peritoneal Dialysis

Hemodialysis is performed exclusively by specialized personnel. Peritoneal dialysis, on the other hand, should be within the technical repertoire of any physician who cares for critically ill patients. Access to the peritoneal cavity is afforded by a plastic catheter, either rigid or soft. Percutaneous placement of a rigid peritoneal dialysis catheter is a simple bedside technique (Fig. 39-3). The bladder must be emptied before insertion; this may involve catheterizing a debilitated or unconscious patient. The insertion site is usually in the midline, three fingerbreadths below the umbilicus. The abdominal wall is infiltrated with lidocaine and a

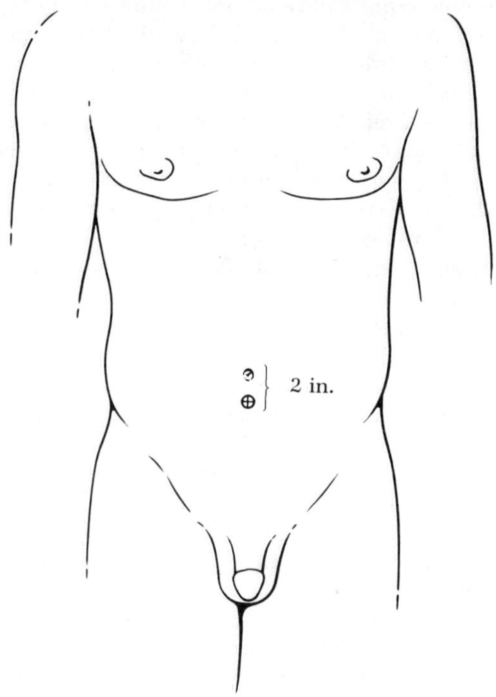

A

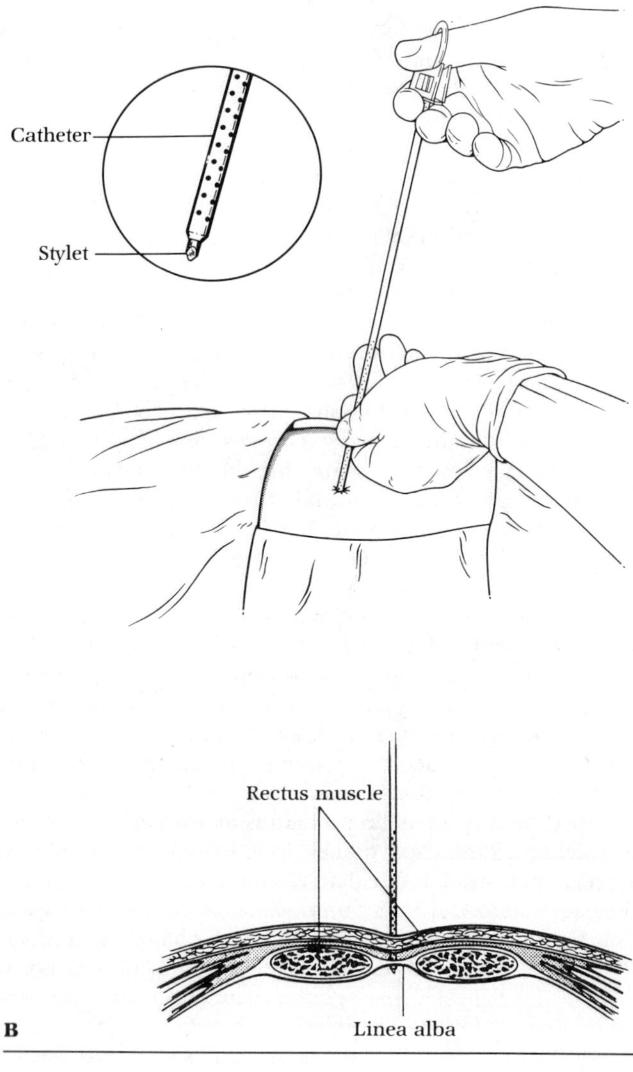

B

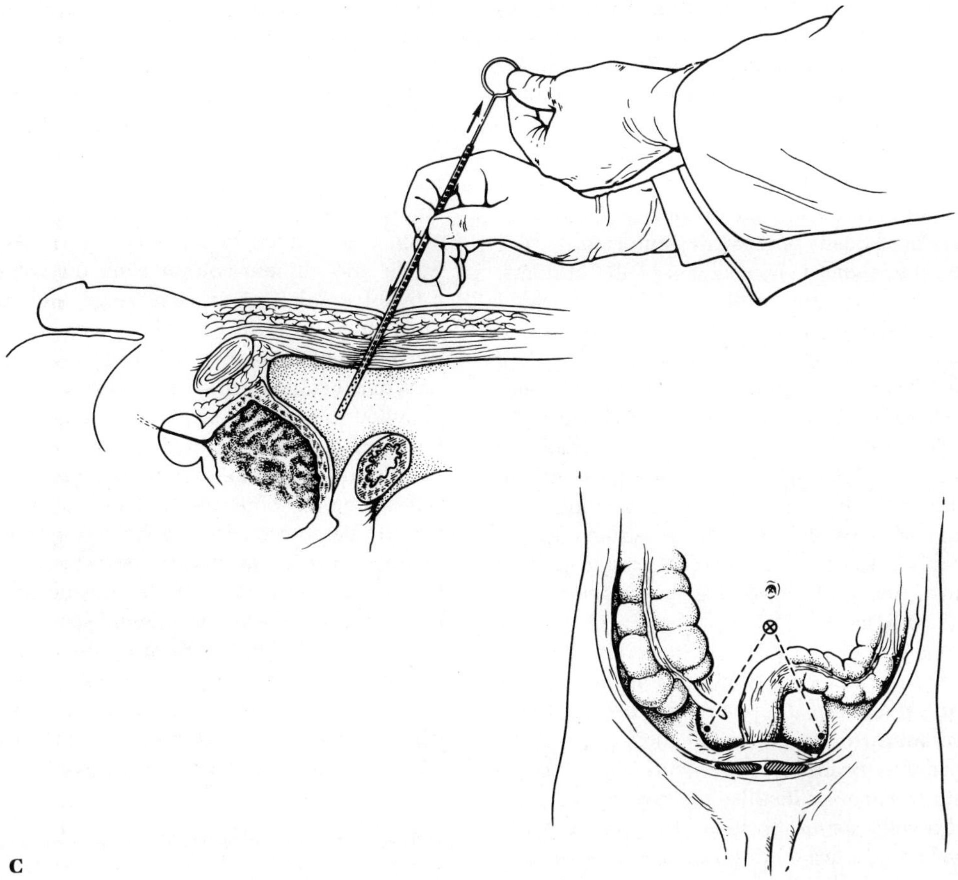

C

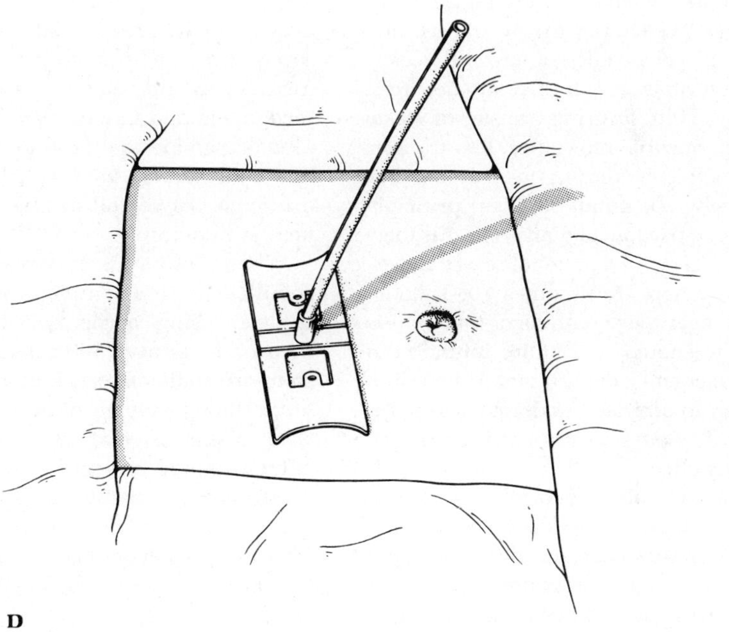

D

Fig. 39-3. Proper technique for bedside insertion of a rigid catheter for peritoneal dialysis. A. Step 1: Position. Infiltrate local anesthetic. B. Step 2: Place peritoneal dialysis catheter with stylet in incision. Insert dialysis catheter into peritoneal cavity. C. Step 3: Advance peritoneal dialysis catheter. D. Fix catheter position. (From T.J. Vander Salm, B.S. Cutler, and H.B. Wheeler. *Atlas of Bedside Procedures.* Boston: Little, Brown, 1979.)

small incision is made, through which the catheter is passed with a trochar in place. When the catheter enters the peritoneum, the physician will feel a distinct pop followed by a change in tissue resistance to further advancement of the catheter. At this point, the trochar is removed and the catheter tip advanced toward the left pelvic gutter.

The following conditions contraindicate percutaneous placement of a rigid peritoneal catheter: (1) bowel dilatation, (2) extensive abdominal surgery or history of abdominal adhesions, (3) significant hemostatic abnormality, (4) marked hepatosplenomegaly, (5) infections of the abdominal wall, and (6) vascular abnormalities of the abdominal wall, such as the dilated collateral vessels common in cirrhosis, which might be injured during placement. In some of these situations, operative placement of a soft, cuffed catheter may be feasible. These devices, of which the Tenckhoff catheter is the prototype, are better tolerated for long periods of time, more resistant to bacterial entry into the peritoneum, and thus preferable for patients in whom a longer course of dialysis is anticipated. The presence of an ostomy in the abdominal wall raises the risk of bacterial contamination and poses a relative contraindication to the placement of any peritoneal dialysis catheter.

Although peritoneal dialysis can be performed in ambulatory patients, emergent peritoneal dialysis is almost always performed with the patient in the recumbent position. The treatment can be initiated in the emergency department while the patient awaits transfer to the acute care floor or intensive care unit. Dialysate is instilled through the catheter and allowed to "dwell" for a specified period of time. A typical dialysis cycle might last 60 minutes. The first 10 minutes might elapse while dialysate is infused and be followed by a 30-minute dwell; the last 20 minutes would be spent draining the fluid to gravity. The shorter the dwell time, the more rapid the clearance of permeable solutes and water. Short dwells mean frequent replacement of dialysate; fresh dialysate maximizes the gradient, favoring transfer of waste solutes. For small, freely permeable molecules, this transfer occurs so rapidly as to eliminate the plasma-to-dialysate gradient within approximately 20 minutes. This principle should be used in prescribing peritoneal dialysis. If this therapy is indicated for the emergency treatment of severe hyperkalemia of fluid overload, short dwell times (0–1 hour) should be ordered. Rapid, aggressive dialysis of this kind is indicated for any patient ill enough to require initiation of peritoneal dialysis in the emergency department. When dialysis is undertaken electively to alleviate moderate symptoms of uremia, fewer cycles per 24 hours are required, and dwell times of 2 to 6 hours may suffice.

Ultrafiltration in peritoneal dialysis depends on the osmotic force generated by the high concentration of dextrose in the dialysate. The greater this concentration, the more fluid can be "pulled" per exchange. For example, with two liters of 1.5% dextrose dialysate solution dwelling in the peritoneum for one hour, 100 to 200 ml fluid will be removed. If the same volume of 4.25% dextrose dialysate is dwelled instead, over a liter of fluid can be removed in the same amount of time. Thus, when rapid ultrafiltration is necessary, a concentrated dialysate should be employed. Care must be taken, however, to avoid causing hypotension through overly zealous fluid removal. Vital signs are monitored closely during acute peritoneal dialysis treatments. Should a sudden drop in blood pressure occur, the system should be temporarily clamped and corrective measures, such as fluid repletion and Trendelenburg's positioning, undertaken.

Therapeutic success in peritoneal dialysis is best assured through meticulous technique. A flow chart must be kept, recording the progress of the dialysis (Fig. 39-4). This should include daily changes in body weight, and, for each exchange, the concentration of dialysate used, medications or electrolytes added to the dialysate, measurements of the influent and effluent volume with the calculated net fluid removal (or gain) for that exchange, and cumulative fluid balance since the start of dialysis therapy. The start times and durations of each run should also be noted.

When drainage of dialysate from the peritoneum is slow or when the volume of effluent fluid is consistently less than the original dwell volume, the source of the problem must be identified. Most commonly, sequestration of dialysate within the abdomen is the cause of the difficulty. This can usually be corrected by repositioning the patient during the drainage cycle. Rarely, the catheter itself will need repositioning, particularly if its fenestrations are occluded by an overlying bowel loop or omental sheet. Fibrin clots occasionally form in the abdomen or on the catheter itself. These can be cleared by irrigating the catheter with heparinized saline. Subsequent exchanges should be done with lightly heparinized dialysate (e.g., 500 units per liter dialysate) until whitish fibrin particles are no longer seen in the dialysate runoff.

Other Emergencies in Dialysis Patients

The most significant complication of both chronic ambulatory and acute peritoneal dialysis is infection in the peritoneal cavity. Although dialysis-related peritonitis is rarely as severe as that associated with surgical disorders of the abdomen, sepsis and death can occur in cases that are not rapidly recognized and treated. The hallmarks of developing peritonitis are abdominal pain and tenderness, fever, turbidity of dialysis drainage, and an excessive amount of fibrin in the drainage. Any or all of these may be present when the patient is first seen.

When peritonitis is suspected, the physician or nurse should remove a sample of the dialytic effluent through the catheter using sterile technique. A peritoneal fluid white blood cell count of 500 cells per mm^3 and a positive Gram's stain are confirmatory, and these studies should be obtained at the first suspicion of peritonitis even though the yield on Gram's stain is relatively low. In addition, a sample of the effluent should be sent for culture and sensitivity testing. The most common pathogens are coagulase-negative staphylococci, *Staphylococcus aureus*, and enteric gram-negative bacilli. Fungal peritonitis can also occur and is most common in diabetic patients who have been receiving peritoneal dialysis for longer periods of time. A polymicrobial infection, or the presence of feculent material in the dialysate effluent, should alert the clinician to the possibility of a complicated or surgical peritonitis.

If peritonitis is believed to be present, after samples of the initial dialysate runoff are sent for Gram's stain, cell count, and culture, three quick irrigating (zero dwell time) exchanges should be performed. This will clear fibrin and greatly reduce the patient's discomfort. Next, the patient

UNIVERSITY OF MASSACHUSETTS MEDICAL CENTER
PERITONEAL DIALYSIS TREATMENT RECORD

Total Number of Exchanges: ____________

Treatment Duration: ____________

Time On: ____________ Time Off: ____________

PRINT IN INK OR STAMP WITH PATIENT CARD.

Exchange Number	Solution Type		MEDICATION ADDED	NURSING NOTES	SOLUTION IN			SOLUTION OUT			Difference + or -	Cumulative Difference + or -
	1.5%	4.25%			Starting Time	Finish Time	Vol.	Starting Time	Finish Time	Vol.		

	TEMP.	BP Lying/Sitting	BP Standing	WEIGHT	WEIGHT + or -	BLOOD WORK
PRE - DIALYSIS						
POST - DIALYSIS						

MR DIAL 234 ED 11/80 GS 810767

Fig. 39-4. An example of a flow record for acute peritoneal dialysis.

should recommence dialysis exchanges in which broad-spectrum antibiotics providing staphylococcal and gram-negative coverage should be added to the dialysate in concentrations equal to plasma bactericidal levels (Table 39-7). In particularly ill patients, a systemic loading dose is also administered. The antibiotic regimen can be refined pending culture results. Treatment should be continued for at least seven days after the first negative repeat culture.

Hypotension complicates 25 percent of all hemodialysis treatments. As was already mentioned, it can have many causes. A patient seen in the emergency department with postural hypotension, dizziness, or severe weakness after a dialysis treatment will usually respond to the rapid administration of 500 to 1,000 ml isotonic saline. In milder cases, a cup of bouillon may suffice.

The neurologic problems associated with dialysis bear mentioning. The *dialysis disequilibrium syndrome* refers to a group of symptoms, including nausea, visual blurring, headache, restlessness, disorientation, tremor, seizures, and even coma, that occur after hemodialysis treatment. Its onset correlates with rapid lowering of the serum urea and other solutes, as might occur in a particularly intensive dialysis treatment or a patient's first treatment. It is theorized that the disequilibrium syndrome relates to a rise in cerebrospinal fluid (CSF) pressure resulting from the dialysis-induced osmotic gradient between the plasma and brain water. This gradient drives fluid into CSF.

The disequilibrium syndrome is usually self-limited in duration and severity. Patients rarely need seizure treatment or prophylaxis. Dizziness and headache often respond to the administration of 20 to 50 ml hypertonic saline. Patients with severe symptoms, such as seizures, obtundation, or coma, and long-term hemodialysis patients who experience disequilibrium-type symptoms for the first time, should undergo cranial computed tomography. Subdural hematoma occurs in approximately 3 percent of hemodialysis patients, probably as a result of repetitive anticoagulation, and must be ruled out with alacrity.

It is not uncommon for hemodialysis patients to be brought to the emergency department from the dialysis unit with complaints of chest pain. Coronary artery disease is a common comorbidity of end-stage renal failure, probably as a result of the abnormalities of lipid metabolism in these patients, the prevalence of hypertension, and the large number of patients with diabetes mellitus and atherosclerosis who are currently undergoing dialysis. The chemical and volume shifts of hemodialysis and the anemia of chronic renal failure pose additional stresses that can trigger symptoms of myocardial ischemia. In general, chest pain in dialysis patients should be handled as it would in any patient (see Chaps. 17 and 18). Special attention should be given to ensuring that the patient is euvolemic and that the hematocrit has not been allowed to drift too low.

Relatively few problems related to vascular access require emergent attention. Access infections can produce symptoms of cellulitis of the overlying skin or nonlocalized sepsis (e.g., fever rigors). Fistulas are less prone to infection than are shunts, grafts, and temporary venous catheters. When infections in fistulas do occur, they are especially likely to be free of localized signs. Infections in new access sites represent a potential emergency, since dissolution of the anastomotic suture ring can result in spontaneous hemorrhage. When access site infection is suspected, blood cultures should be obtained and an attempt to express material for culture from the access itself should be made. Broad-spectrum coverage, including an antistaphylococcal agent (we prefer vancomycin, 500–1,000 mg intravenously once a week) should then be instituted pending the culture results.

Rupture or leakage of access sites is a true emergency, since the resulting hemorrhage can be of massive proportions. This rare catastrophe generally results from trauma, infection, or the spontaneous rupture of an aneurysm or pseudoaneurysm. Acute management is identical to that for an arterial hemorrhage from a native vessel; the extremity should be tourniqueted, pressure should be applied to the bleeding site, the blood pressure should be maintained with fluids and transfusion, and the access site should be repaired or ligated as soon as possible.

Clotted access sites generally do not constitute emergency situations, although it is worth remembering that loss of an access site greatly complicates a dialysis patient's care and commits the patient to further surgery. Fistulas and grafts can often be thrombectomized successfully by a trained surgeon using a Fogarty catheter or similar device. The sooner the clot is recognized, the more likely the chance of successful thrombectomy. Sudden disappearance of a bruit and spontaneous collapse of the access vessel are the two most common presenting signs.

Emergencies in Renal Transplant Patients

Nephrologists widely regard renal transplantation as the most desirable mode of therapy for end-stage renal disease. An allograft kidney can provide its recipient with total replacement of renal excretory and endocrine function. Newer modifications of immunosuppressive medical regimens, particularly the advent of the agent cyclosporine A, have markedly improved graft survival and reduced the incidence of opportunistic infections. In spite of these developments, the two most important complaints that bring transplant patients to the emergency department remain infection and acute renal failure.

Infection

Renal transplant patients have an enhanced rate of viral, bacterial, and fungal infections. The incidence of specific types of infections has been shown to vary depending on the length of the posttransplant interval (Fig. 39-5). In the immediate postoperative period, bacterial infections such as wound infections, line sepsis, urinary tract infections, and other typical nosocomial infections prevail. Surveillance cultures are important during this time; once detected, infections are dealt with in the routine manner.

Viral infections, such as cytomegalovirus and hepatitis B and non-A, non-B, can occur in the three-week to two-month posttransplant period. Cytomegalovirus infection is a common problem in transplant recipients who were seronegative for the pathogen before transplant. The spectrum of illness can range from low-grade fever and malaise to major multisystem disease, including hepatitis, renal failure, pneumonia, and high fever. Care is usually supportive; antiviral agents have been utilized in particularly severe cases.

Opportunistic infections involving more exotic pathogens occur at a longer time interval from the time of transplant.

Table 39-7. Pharmacokinetics of antibiotics in CAPD patients and proposed regimens for the treatment of CAPD peritonitis

	Half-life			Dose (per 70-kg adult)[a]		
					Maintenance	
Antibiotic	Normal	ESRD	CAPD	Initial (mg/2-liter bag)	Intermittent mg/2-liter bag per dosing interval	Continuous (mg/2-liter bag)
Aminoglycosides						
Amikacin	1.6	39	40	500	150/d	12–15
Gentamicin	2.2	53	32	70–140	50/d	8–16
Netilmicin	2.1	42	18	70–140	60/d	8–16
Tobramycin	2.5	58	36	70–140	50/d	8–16
Cephalosporins						
First generation						
Cefazolin	2.2	28	30	500–1,000	1,000/d	250–500
Cefonicid	4.0	68	50	250	ND	50
Cephalothin	0.2	3.7	ND	1,000	ND	200
Cephradine	0.9	12	ND	500	ND	250
Cephalexin	0.8	19	9	1,000 PO	500/qid PO	NA
Second generation						
Cefamandole	1.0	10	8.0	1,000	1,000/d	500
Cefmenoxime	1.3	11.3	6.0	2,000	1,000/d	100
Cefotiam	1.0	7.0	8.0	1,000	1,000/d	50
Cefoxitin	0.8	20	15	1,000	ND	200
Cefuroxime	1.3	18	15	1,000	ND	150–400
Third generation						
Cefixime	3.2	11.5	15	400 PO	400/d PO	NA
Cefoperazone	1.8	2.3	2.2	2,000	ND	400–1,000
Cefotaxime	0.9	2.5	2.4	2,000	2,000/d	500
Cefsulodin	1.8	11	11	1,000	1,000/d	50
Ceftazidime	1.8	26	13	1,000	500/d	100–250
Ceftizoxime	1.6	28	11	1,000	1,000/d	250
Ceftriaxone	8.0	15	12	1,000	1,000/d	250–500
Moxalactam	2.2	20	16	1,000	1,000/d	350
Penicillins						
Azlocillin	0.9	5.1	ND	500	ND	500
Mezlocillin	1.0	4.3	ND	3,000 IV	3,000/bid IV	500
Piperacillin	1.2	3.9	ND	4,000 IV	4,000/bid IV	500
Ticarcillin	1.2	15	ND	1,000–2,000	2,000/bid	250
Quinolones						
Ciprofloxacin	4.0	8.0	10	750 PO	750/bid PO	50
Fleroxacin	13	27	27	800 PO	400/d PO	NA
Ofloxacin	7.0	30	25	400 PO	200/d PO	NA
Vancomycin and others						
Vancomycin	6.9	161	92	1,000–2,000	1–2,000/7 d	30–50
Teicoplanin	50	260	260	400	400/bid	40[b]
Aztreonam	2.0	7.0	7.1	1,000	ND	500
Clindamycin	2.8	2.8	ND	300	ND	300
Erythromycin	2.1	4.0	ND	ND	500/qid PO	150
Metronidazole	7.9	7.7	11	500 PO/IV	500/tid PO/IV	ND
Rifampin	4.0	8.0	ND	600 PO	600/d PO	NA
Antifungal agents						
Amphotericin	360	360	ND	NA	20–30/d IV	2–8
Flucytosine	4.2	115	ND	2,000–3,000 PO	1,000/d PO	NA
				200	400/d	100–200
Ketoconazole	2.0	1.8	2.4	400 PO	200–800/d PO	NA
Miconazole	24	25	ND	200	ND	100–200
Combinations						
Ampicillin	1.3	15	9.5	1,000–2,000	1,000/bid	100
Sulbactam	1.0	19	9.7	1,000–2,000	1,000/bid	100
Imipenem	0.9	3.0	3.3	500–1,000	500/bid	100–200
Cilistatin	0.8	15	9	500–1,000	500/bid	100–200
Sulfamethoxazole	10	13	14	1,600 PO	1,600/1–2 d PO	200–400
Trimethoprim	14	33	34	320 PO	320/1–2 d PO	40–80

[a] The route of administration is intraperitoneal unless otherwise specified. The phamacokinetic data and proposed dosage regimens presented here are based on published literature reviewed through January 1989. There is no evidence that mixing different antibiotics in dialysis fluid (except for aminoglycosides and penicillins) is deleterious for the drugs or patients. Do not use the same syringe to mix antibiotics.

[b] This is in each bag × 7 days, then in 2 bags/day × 7 days, and then in 1 bag/day × 7 days.

Key: CAPD = chronic ambulatory peritoneal dialysis; ESRD = creatinine clearance < 10 mL/min, patient not on dialysis; NA = not applicable; ND = no data; IV = intravenous; PO = oral; d = once a day; bid = twice a day; tid = three times a day; qid = four times a day.

Source: W.F. Keane, et al. Continuous ambulatory peritoneal dialysis treatment. Recommendations; 1989 update. Reprinted with permission from *Peritoneal Dialysis International* 9:247, 1989, Pergamon Press plc.

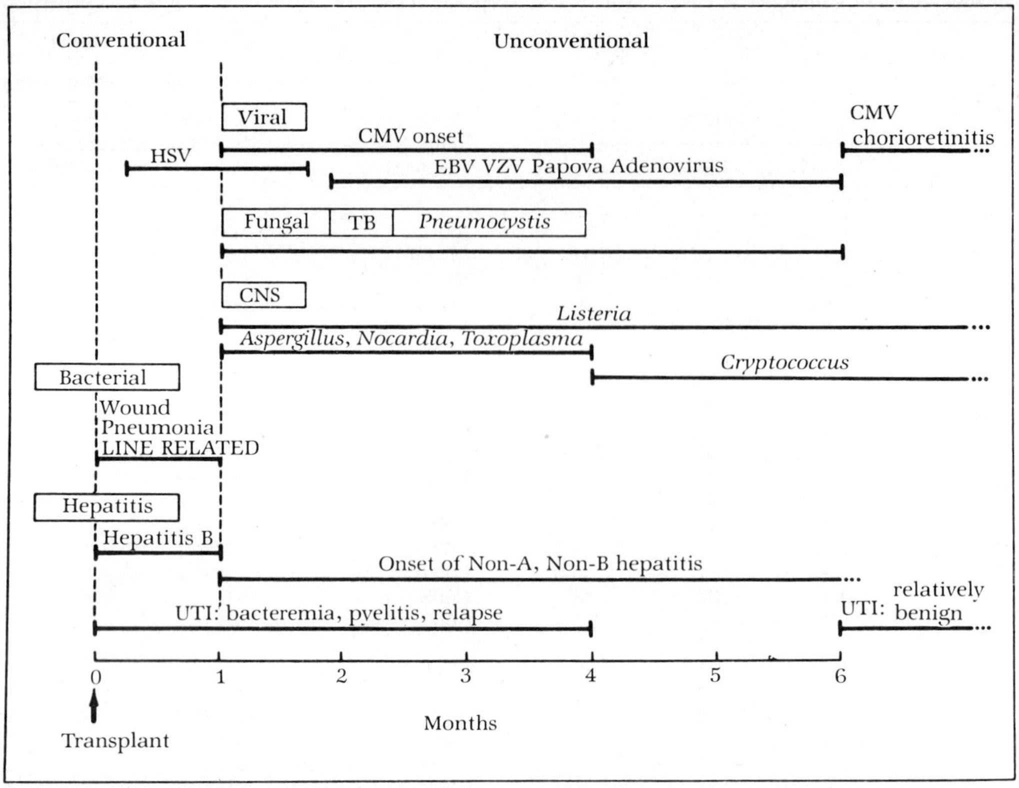

Fig. 39-5. The proclivity of the host for specific types of infectious changes with time after renal transplantation. (CMV = cytomegalovirus; EBV = Epstein-Barr virus; TB = tuberculosis; CNS = central nervous system; UTI = urinary tract infection; HSV = herpes simplex virus; VZV = varicella-zoster virus.) (From R. H. Rubin, et al. Infection in the renal transplant recipient. *Am. J. Med.* 70:405, 1981.)

Pneumonia caused by gram-negative organisms, *Legionella*, or even *Pneumocystis carinii* has been reported, although these causes became less common in the 1980s. The diagnostic evaluation of a transplant patient with fever, malaise, myalgias, or other symptoms suggestive of a possible occult infection should include a chest x-ray, urinalysis, sputum culture (if available), and blood cultures. It must be remembered that the immunosuppressed status of the transplant patient means that mild symptoms can belie the true seriousness of the infection.

Infections involving the head and central nervous system are also seen. Diabetic transplant patients may develop mucormycosis, a *Rhizopus* infection that arises in the nasal or oral mucosa and can rapidly spread to the orbits, sinuses, and, by direct extension, into the cavernous sinus and central nervous system. Worsening of glucose intolerance and a small lesion in the oropharynx or nares should alert the clinician to the possible presence of this illness, which can prove rapidly fatal. The occurrence of neurologic abnormalities or meningeal signs should prompt investigation to rule out possible meningitis or brain abscess. Brain abscesses due to *Listeria* have been well described in transplant recipients. Cryptococcal meningitis, although rare, also occurs with enhanced frequency in this population. *Cryptococcus* sometimes arises as a cutaneous, cellulitic lesion that may resemble a typical bacterial cellulitis. For this reason, cellulitic lesions in transplant patients should always be biopsied for culture as well as histopathologic examination.

Because serious infections in a transplant patient pose a potentially life-threatening problem, it is usually prudent to discontinue immunosuppressive medications until the infection is under control. Steroid doses should be temporarily increased, however, to cover the stress of severe infections.

Acute Renal Failure

An acute deterioration in function of the transplant kidney should be approached in a manner similar to that used for acute renal failure in native kidneys. The differential diagnosis should include prerenal, renal, and postrenal causes.

Volume depletion, perhaps a result of vomiting or diarrheal losses, can cause prerenal azotemia in patients with an intercurrent gastrointestinal illness. Overly aggressive diuretic or antihypertensive therapy can also result in a decline in transplant renal function. Converting enzyme inhibitors have been reported to cause acute transplant kidney failure, apparently by altering glomerular hemodynamics. Prerenal azotemia of the transplant, like that of native kidneys, is reversible on rehydration or cessation of the offending drug.

Intrinsic renal failure after transplantation carries a limited differential diagnosis. In the immediate postoperative stage, ATN is the most common cause. This is an unusual diagnosis, however, in the ambulatory patient seen in the emergency department with reduced renal function, unless a severe intercurrent illness has arisen accompanied by hypotension or sepsis. Reduction of transplant renal function, like native kidney disease, can occur in the absence of clinical signs or symptoms. Unless such a patient has fever, graft pain, or severe fluid overload, it is unlikely that he or she will seek urgent medical attention.

The differential diagnosis in acute intrinsic transplant kidney failure commonly reduces to cyclosporine nephrotoxicity versus acute rejection. It is notoriously difficult to differentiate clinically between these two entities. Biopsy of the transplant kidney is often necessary for this reason. Fever, graft tenderness, and sterile pyuria are suggestive of acute rejection. A sonogram may demonstrate swelling of the rejecting graft. Patients with these findings are to be admitted and treated aggressively for acute rejection, generally with high-dose intravenous methylprednisolone or, especially if rejection episodes have occurred previously, with alternative forms of therapy such as antilymphocyte globulin.

Cyclosporine nephrotoxicity has no specific clinical correlates and often forces a presumptive diagnosis that can be strengthened by the subsequent finding of a high serum cyclosporine level. It is now common to begin posttransplant cyclosporine therapy at high doses (10–15 mg/kg per day) and to taper the dose over a period of months to a low maintenance dose (3–5 mg/kg per day). In the absence of clinical signs of rejection, a patient who is receiving doses of cyclosporine that are still in the higher range can be treated with reduction of the dose and careful daily monitoring of the serum creatine. If improvement is noted, antirejection therapy can be begun, possibly after a confirmatory biopsy.

Recurrence of native renal disease in the transplant kidney occurs commonly, particularly in patients whose original renal disease was some form of progressive glomerulonephritis. Recurrent native disease rarely causes rapid diminution of graft function. A slow recapitulation of the course of the original illness, diagnostic features of which may be present on urinalysis, is more likely.

Postrenal or obstructive transplant renal failure is not common but is important to rule out, since it would generally require intervention. Ischemia of the distal portion of the graft ureter or anatomic obstruction at the transplant ureterovesicular junction (i.e., the ureteroneocystostomy) are the most common causes. The evaluation of any transplant patient with a sudden change in renal function should include a sonogram of the graft.

SELECTED READING

Ahmad, S, Blagg, CR, and Scribner, BH. Center and Home Chronic Hemodialysis. In RW Schrier and CW Gottschalk (eds), *Diseases of the Kidney* (4th ed). Boston: Little, Brown, 1988. P 3281.

Anderson, RJ, et al. Nonoliguric acute renal failure. *N Engl J Med* 296:1134, 1977.

Bricker, NS. On the pathogenesis of the uremic state. *N Engl J Med* 286:1097, 1972.

Bricker, NS, et al. Observations on the concentrating and diluting mechanisms of the diseased kidney. *J Clin Invest* 38:516, 1959.

Gloor, HJ, et al. Peritoneal access and related complications in continuous ambulatory peritoneal dialysis. *Am J Med* 74:593, 1983.

Manis T, and Friedman, EA. Dialytic therapy for irreversible uremia. *N Engl J Med* 301:1260, 1979.

Miller, TR, et al. Urinary diagnostic indices in acute renal failure. A prospective study. *Ann Intern Med* 89:47, 1978.

Morris, PJ. Renal Transplantation: Indications, Outcome, Complications, and Results. In RW Schrier and CW Gottschalk (eds), *Diseases of the Kidney* (4th ed). Boston: Little, Brown, 1988. P 3211.

Popovich RP, et al. Continuous ambulatory peritoneal dialysis. *Ann Intern Med* 88:449, 1978.

Rubin, RH, et al. Infection in the renal transplant recipient. *Ann J Med* 70:405, 1981.

Rudnick, MR, et al. The Differential Diagnosis of Acute Renal Failure. In BM Brenner and JM Lazarus (eds), *Acute Renal Failure* (2nd ed). New York: Churchill Livingstone, 1988. Pp 177–232.

Vas, SI (Principal Discussant). Microbiologic aspects of chronic ambulatory peritoneal dialysis. *Kidney Int* 23:83, 1983.

II. Acute Injuries

A. The Critically Injured Patient

40. Pathophysiology of Critical Injury

THE INJURY AND THE BODY'S INITIAL RESPONSES

Harold L. May

More than 62 million injuries occur each year in the United States, and of these, 96,000 were fatal in 1988 and 9.1 million were either temporarily or permanently disabling. Accidents are currently the fourth largest cause of death in the United States, exceeded only by cardiovascular disease, cancer, and cerebrovascular disease, but they are by far the leading cause of mortality in young people between the ages of 1 and 37 (Fig. 40-1). The pattern of accident fatalities in 1986 was similar to that of other recent years, showing a substantial increase in accident fatalities to persons between the ages of 14 and 21, then a gradual decrease from 21 to 48, and a relatively stable rate from age 48 to age 90.

Motor vehicle accidents, falls, drownings, and fires and burns are the leading causes of accidental death in the United States (Fig. 40-2). Motor vehicle accidents, the leading cause, show a sharp increase for persons aged 12 to 21 years, with peak incidence at age 21. (More than half of the motor vehicle accident fatalities of persons between the ages of 5 and 34 are alcohol related.) Falls, the second most common cause of accidental death, lead all other causes of accidental death in individuals aged 79 and over. Drowning follows as the third leading cause of accidental death, reaching its peak incidence in 1-year-olds. (In many parts of the country, including the South, Southwest, and California, drownings are the leading cause of accidental death in children under age 5.) The fourth leading cause of accidental death is fires and burns, which also peaks at the age of 1. One of the major causes of death between the ages of 15 and 24 is homicide, whether by firearms, stabbing, beating, or other means.

Deaths as a result of trauma tend to have a trimodal distribution (Fig. 40-3). The first peak of deaths occurs within seconds or minutes after the injury. Invariably, these deaths are a result of lacerations in the brain, brainstem, upper spinal cord, heart, aorta, or other large vessels. Few patients with such injuries can be saved. The second peak occurs within the first two hours of injury. These deaths are usually caused by subdural and epidural hematomas, hemopneumothorax, ruptured spleen, lacerations of the liver, fractured femur, or multiple injuries associated with significant blood loss. The third death peak occurs days or weeks after the injury, and these deaths are almost always a result of sepsis and multisystem organ failure.

Many of the deaths that occur in the latter two groups are unavoidable, regardless of the excellence of the care that is

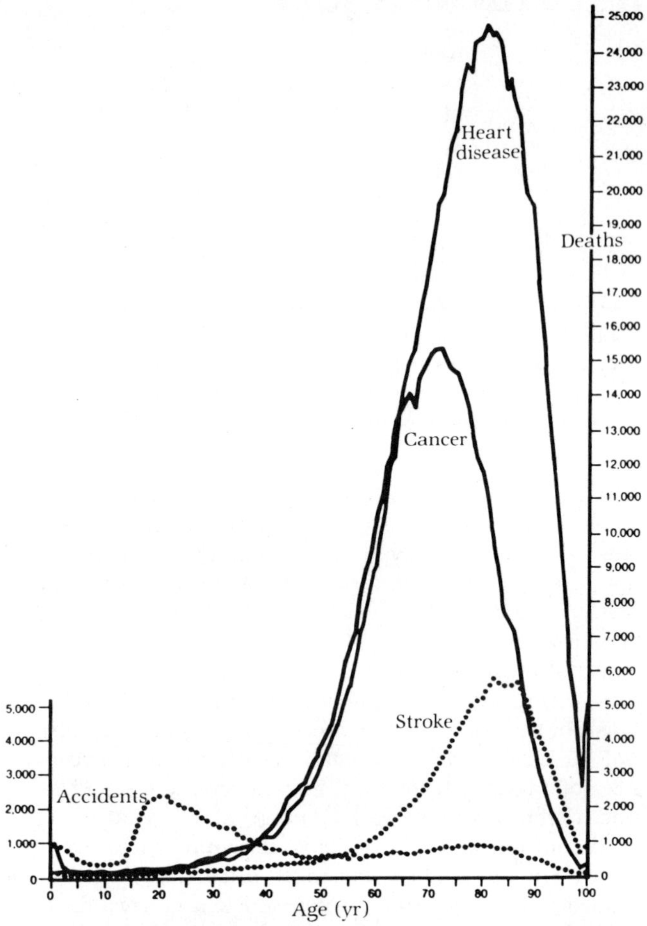

Fig. 40-1. Leading causes of death by age in 1986. (From National Safety Council, *Accident Facts,* 1989.)

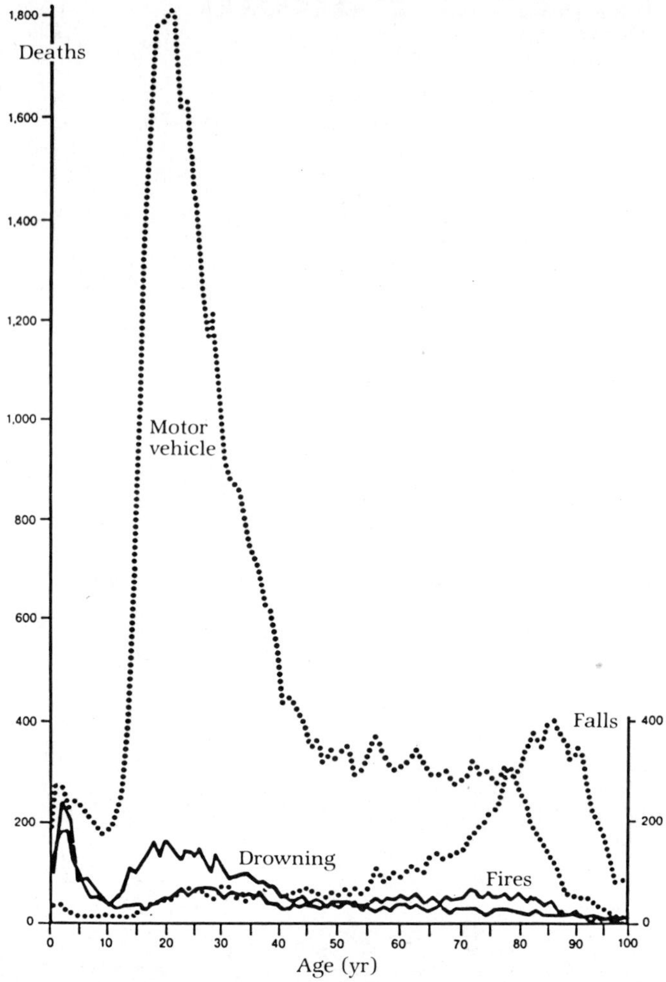

Fig. 40-2. Leading causes of accidental death by age in 1986. (From National Safety Council, *Accident Facts,* 1989.)

given, but the prevention of avoidable death and the minimizing of disability from injury did not become generally recognized as a major priority until 1966. In that year, a landmark white paper, "Accidental Death and Disability: The Neglected Disease of Modern Society," was published, identifying several problem areas: lack of public awareness, neglect of prehospital emergency medical services, lack of research, and inadequate medical facilities for care of the injured. Although many improvements in the care of the injured have occurred since that time, an effective trauma system that ensures prompt, definitive surgical treatment of severe injuries is available to only 25 percent of the population of the United States at this time.

THE INJURY

Improvement in care of the injured requires an understanding of the pathophysiology of the injury and of the body's response to it. Injury occurs only when the amount of energy that impacts on the body is more than it can absorb. Tissue damage must result. An overload of kinetic energy causes blunt or penetrating injury; thermal, electrical, chemical, and radiation energy cause other forms of tissue damage and body injury, either immediately or over a period of time.

Fig. 40-3. The trimodal distribution of death from trauma. (MOF = multisystem organ failure.) (This figure was prepared by Donald D. Trunkey, Chairman of the Department of Surgery, Oregon Health Sciences University, Portland, OR, and is used with his kind permission.)

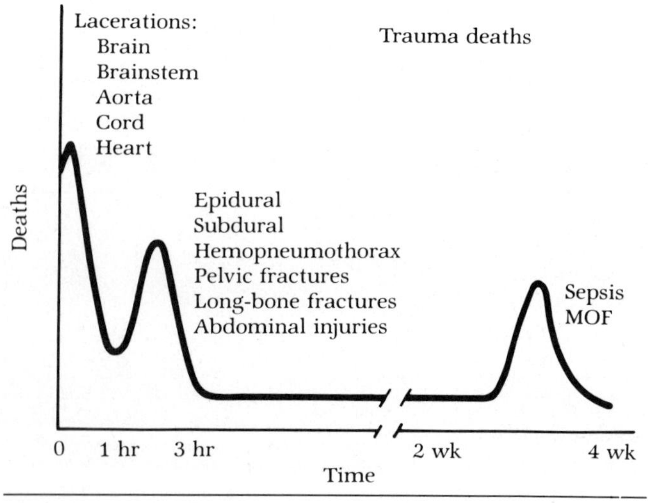

Blunt Injury

Injuring Forces

In 1942, DeHaven called attention to the magnitude of injuries suffered in collisions, reporting survival of individuals after free falls from heights that varied from 55 to 146 ft. In each case, in spite of the violent impact, survival was possible because the victim landed in a variant of the supine or prone position onto a yielding structure, such as a roof or soft earth, that allowed time for deceleration.

Typical of the reported cases was that of a woman who jumped from a 10-story window, falling 93 ft onto a garden where the earth had been freshly turned and striking the soft earth in a nearly supine position. The stopping distance was 6 in.

The magnitude of the energy exchange at the time of impact is expressed primarily in terms of kinetic energy, force, or gravitational (g) units.* Table 40-1 shows the velocity of a falling body at impact in relation to the distance fallen. Since the velocity of the 115-lb falling woman at the time of impact was 73 ft per second (50 mph), the kinetic energy of her body when it hit the ground was 9,516 ft-lb.

To stop a moving object, the opposing force that must be exerted times the distance over which it acts exactly equals the kinetic energy of the object. In other words, force (apparent weight at time of impact) × stopping distance = kinetic energy. The apparent weight of the woman's falling 115-lb body at the time of impact (and the force that had to be absorbed by her body) was 19,090 lb. Survival was possible because the apparent weight of almost 10 tons was distributed throughout her body rather than being concentrated in a small point of impact, and the stopping distance of 6 in., though small, moderated the forces of deceleration. In addition, the supine position limited the amount of stretching to which the supporting ligaments of her organs were subjected, thereby limiting the disruption of these supporting structures. The increase in the "apparent weight" of human organs during violent impact (Table 40-2) not only subjects them to unaccustomed forces but at some critical point causes rupture of their supporting structures.

Forces can cause injury directly by impact or indirectly by acceleration or deceleration. Deceleration or acceleration is best understood in terms of gravity units, the factor by which the weight of an object is apparently increased by a sudden velocity change. In the example, the g units of force of the woman's body at the time of impact were 166 g.

There are many kinds of force (e.g., gravity, the weight of any object, or atmospheric pressure, the weight of the air that is pressing on a specific area of a surface), but three basic types are recognized in terms of their effects: tensile, compressive, and shearing. These forces can act alone or in combination, or they can be coupled in ways that cause bending or torsion.

**Force* is a push or a pull.
Weight (the pull of gravity on a given mass) = mass × gravitational acceleration (32.2 ft/sec²).

$$\textit{Kinetic energy} = \frac{\text{mass} \times \text{velocity}^2}{2}$$

$$\textit{Kinetic energy}\ \text{(ft-lb)} = \frac{\text{weight (lb)} \times \text{velocity}^2\ \text{(ft/sec)}^2}{2 \times 32.2\ \text{ft/sec}^2}$$

$$g = \frac{\text{velocity}^2\ \text{(mph)}}{30 \times \text{stopping distance (ft)}}$$

In the metric system, kinetic energy is expressed in joules, weight in kilograms, and velocity in meters per second. Gravitational acceleration is 9.8 m/sec².

Table 40-1. Relation of distance fallen to velocity at impact

Duration of fall (sec)	Distance fallen (ft)	Velocity at impact (ft/sec)	(mph)
1	16.1	32.2	21.9
2	64.4	64.4	43.9
3	144.9	96.6	65.8
4	257.6	128.8	87.8
5	402.5	161.0	109.8
6	579.6	193.2	131.7

Source: A. Besson and F. Saegessor. *Color Atlas of Chest Trauma and Associated Injuries*. London: Wolfe Publications, 1983.

Table 40.2. "Apparent weight" of the organs of the human body during a violent impact

Actual organ weight (kg)	Apparent weight (kg)* 36 km/hr	72 km/hr	108 km/hr
Spleen (0.25)	2.5	10	22.5
Heart (0.35)	3.5	14	31.5
Encephalon (1.5)	15.0	60	135.0
Liver (1.8)	18.0	72	162.0
Blood (5.0)	50.0	200	450.0
Whole body (70)	700.0	2,800	6,300.0

*At 37 km/hr, the inertial weight of the body and its parts is increased 10-fold over resting weight; at 72 km/hr the increase is 40-fold; at 108 km/hr the increase is 90-fold.
Source: A. Besson and F. Saegessor. *Color Atlas of Chest Trauma and Associated Injuries*. London: Wolfe Publications, 1983.

The Body's Response to Injuring Forces: Stress and Strain

Newton's third law of motion—for every action there is always an opposed and equal reaction—helps to explain the difference between externally applied forces and the ones that occur in the body in response to them. Force applied to the human body (or any object) elicits two responses: stress and strain. *Stress* is the internal resistance to the deforming effect of an external force. *Strain,* the reciprocal of stress, is the deformity produced by the applied force. Stress and strain, like force, can be tensile, compressive, or shearing.

Mechanical stress in the body is probably best exemplified by the architecture of the weight-bearing portion of the skeletal system. The trabeculae of the upper femur (Fig. 40-4) are arranged in the familiar pattern of arching struts; these lines of stress within this part of the bone are the body's adaptation to the bearing of the weight (force) of the trunk when the person is in an upright position. Similarly, the trabecular pattern of the calcaneus (Fig. 40-5), reflects the stress that makes its weight-bearing function possible. Although stress cannot be seen directly and cannot be measured, it can be computed in terms of the magnitude of the applied force, divided by the cross-sectional area of the

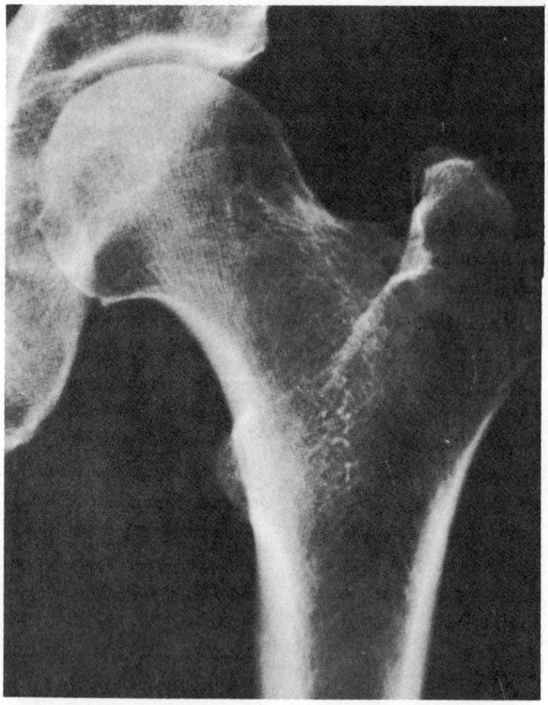

Fig. 40-4. Lines of stress in the femur from weight-bearing.

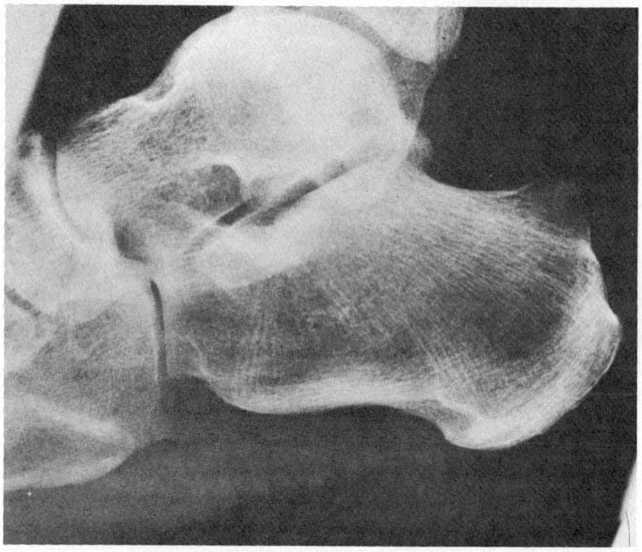

Fig. 40-5. Stress lines in the calcaneus and other bones of the foot.

distribution of the force. Its units, therefore, are those of pressure: pounds per square inch (psi).

Strain is the deformity produced by a given force; it is measured by the degree of lengthening, compression, or shearing. The characteristics of the tissues determine their responses. Highly elastic tissue can stretch enormously without breaking. Even normal bone possesses a small amount of elasticity. The distensibility of organs such as the colon and the bladder makes it possible for their walls to be stretched greatly without damage. Most of the body's structures can stand much greater loads than are required by ordinary activities, but all of the structures have a breaking point and any that are deformed beyond that point will break. Even before that point is reached, however, if some tissues are stretched beyond their normal limits of tolerance, they will be injured to some degree (strained) although not broken.

Table 40-3. Severity of injury of 57,597 victims of rural automobile accidents*

Severity of injury	Percent of injured occupants
Minor	52.0
Nondangerous	34.5
Dangerous	7.6
Fatal	5.9

*From study by Automotive Crash Injury Program of the Cornell Aeronautical Laboratory.
Source: E. S. Gurdjian, et al. (eds.). *Impact Injury and Crash Protection.* Springfield, IL: Thomas, 1970. P. 15.

Table 40-4. Number of body areas involved in 57,597 injured occupants of automobile accidents*

Number of body areas involved	Percent of injured occupants
One	30.0
Two	32.0
Three	23.4
Four	10.9
Five	3.2
Six	0.5

*From study by Automotive Crash Injury Program of the Cornell Aeronautical Laboratory.
Source: E. S. Gurdjian, et al. (eds.). *Impact Injury and Crash Protection.* Springfield, IL: Thomas, 1970. P. 14.

Injury Patterns

When blunt forces of great magnitude are absorbed by the body, it is not surprising that multiple injuries are frequently the result. Analysis of injury data for automobile occupants who were injured in rural automobile accidents revealed that 7.6 percent had serious injuries and 5.9 percent were fatally injured (Table 40-3). Only 30 percent of the injuries were limited to one body area; 62 percent involved at least two body areas and 38 percent involved more than two (Table 40-4). The data from this study and the evidence from many others confirm the observation that multiplicity of injury is a dominant feature for victims injured in automobile accidents. The head was the area that was most often involved, and the lower limbs were more commonly injured than the thorax or the abdomen (Table 40-5). Those injuries that were dangerous or fatal commonly included the head, neck, thorax, and abdomen in some combination. On the other hand, less dangerous injuries were generally not multiple and tended to involve the limbs rather than the other parts of the body.

For victims of blunt trauma treated in the Maryland Trauma Institute, 42 percent had central nervous system (CNS) injuries, 27 percent had thoracic injuries, 16 percent had abdominal injuries, and 65 percent had fractures (Table

Table 40-5. Body areas involved in 57,597 injured occupants of automobile accidents*

Body area involved	Percent of injured occupants
Head	70.8
Neck	10.8
Thorax	38.6
Abdomen	17.1
Upper limb	38.9
Lower limb	50.4

*From study by Automotive Crash Injury Program of the Cornell Aeronautical Laboratory.
Source: E. S. Gurdjian, et al. (eds.). *Impact Injury and Crash Protection.* Springfield, IL: Thomas, 1970. P. 14.

Table 40-6. Blunt trauma in 1,286 victims*

Body area	Number	Percent
CNS	540	42
Thorax	347	27
Abdomen	205	16
Fracture	835	65

*Maryland Trauma Institute figures.
Source: Adapted from W. Gill and W. B. Long. *Shock Trauma Manual.* Baltimore: Williams & Wilkins, 1979. Pp. 25–27.

40-6). Of those with abdominal injuries, 44 percent had CNS injuries and 41 percent had thoracic injury. Of those with thoracic injury, 56 percent required laparotomy. Simultaneous involvement of the thorax, CNS, and abdomen was present in 6 percent of the patients.

FACTORS THAT INFLUENCE THE BODY'S RESPONSE TO ANY INJURING FORCE. The injuring potential of a force is determined not only by the nature and magnitude of the force but also by the characteristics of the body tissues. The amount of energy absorbed by the body tissues is the primary determinant of the magnitude of the injury. Animal experiments have confirmed the common-sense observation that a force that seriously injures a small animal may not injure a large one. The magnitude of injuring force is measured against the individual's capacity to withstand it.

The area over which a force is concentrated is an important factor in determining the magnitude of an injury. If a force is distributed over a wide area, the body may be able to absorb it, since the number of pounds of force per square inch is thereby minimized. As the area of distribution becomes smaller, the amount of force that is concentrated over that area increases, sometimes exceeding the limits of tolerance of the underlying tissues, and injury results. The smaller the area becomes, the more the injuring force becomes penetrating instead of blunt. A relatively small amount of force can readily penetrate tissues if it is concentrated over a small enough area.

The location of impact of a blunt force helps to determine its injuring potential. Under most circumstances (especially if forces are distributed over a wide area) only a small percentage of the force is actually transmitted directly to vital structures such as the liver because much of the applied energy is absorbed by structures such as the rib cage and the abdominal parietes. However, relatively small blunt forces can produce severe injuries of solid abdominal viscera when the point of impact is the upper part of the abdomen since fluid-filled, sinusoidal, encapsulated structures such as the liver and spleen transmit applied hydrokinetic energy through their internal architecture to their capsules with bursting force if the pressure is great enough. Much greater force is needed to produce comparatively severe injuries in the lower abdomen because the abdominal parietes can absorb much of the force unless the visceral structures are distended at the time of impact (Mays). These issues are discussed in more detail later in relation to torso injuries.

The duration of action also influences the degree of injury. In general, the injury produced by a given force applied over a long period of time is much more severe than if that same force is applied briefly. On the other hand, when compressive force is applied slowly enough, it sometimes allows a turgid organ, such as the liver, to deform to a distorted shape without sustaining injury.

Safety equipment and protective clothing can often prevent or diminish the severity of an injury. According to National Highway Traffic Safety Administration studies, safety belts are 45 percent effective in preventing fatalities, 50 percent effective in preventing moderate to critical injuries, and 10 percent effective in preventing minor injuries.

Although the likelihood of fatality increases as the speed of the vehicle increases, most automobile accidents that produce fatal injuries occur at the speed of about 40 mph, as the consequence of delayed braking. As is true of the body in free fall, the critical variable is the stopping distance. If a vehicle that is traveling at a velocity of 40 mph stops in a distance of 2 ft (including the compressing deformation of the front of the vehicle), it is subjected to 26.7 g units. A passenger who is securely strapped in by lap and shoulder belts is subjected to approximately the same g forces. However, the unrestrained passenger continues forward at the moment of impact and will not stop until he or she is thrown out of the vehicle or hits the steering wheel, dashboard, windshield, or other obstruction—the second collision. Although the velocity at the time of the second collision is less than that of the automobile at the time of impact, if the structure is unyielding, such abrupt crashes are almost always fatal (Stapp).

Extensive studies in Australia revealed that the use of protective headgear reduced the risk of fatal injuries to motorcyclists to about one-third of the risk without the helmet. Not only does the helmet distribute the impact over a larger area, but it also protects the skull from deformity which would otherwise occur from a direct impact against an unyielding surface. Athletic equipment, such as shoulder pads, offer energy-absorbing protection, and even street clothing (especially heavy clothing) offers some degree of protection. Not surprisingly, leather clothing offers the highest degree of protection to the motorcyclist, who is subjected to great shearing forces when thrown off the vehicle. The tough hide of an animal absorbs shearing forces to which the motorcyclist's skin would otherwise have been subjected.

Mechanisms of Body Injury

There are three basic mechanisms for the production of blunt injury. It is commonly caused by direct impact, by

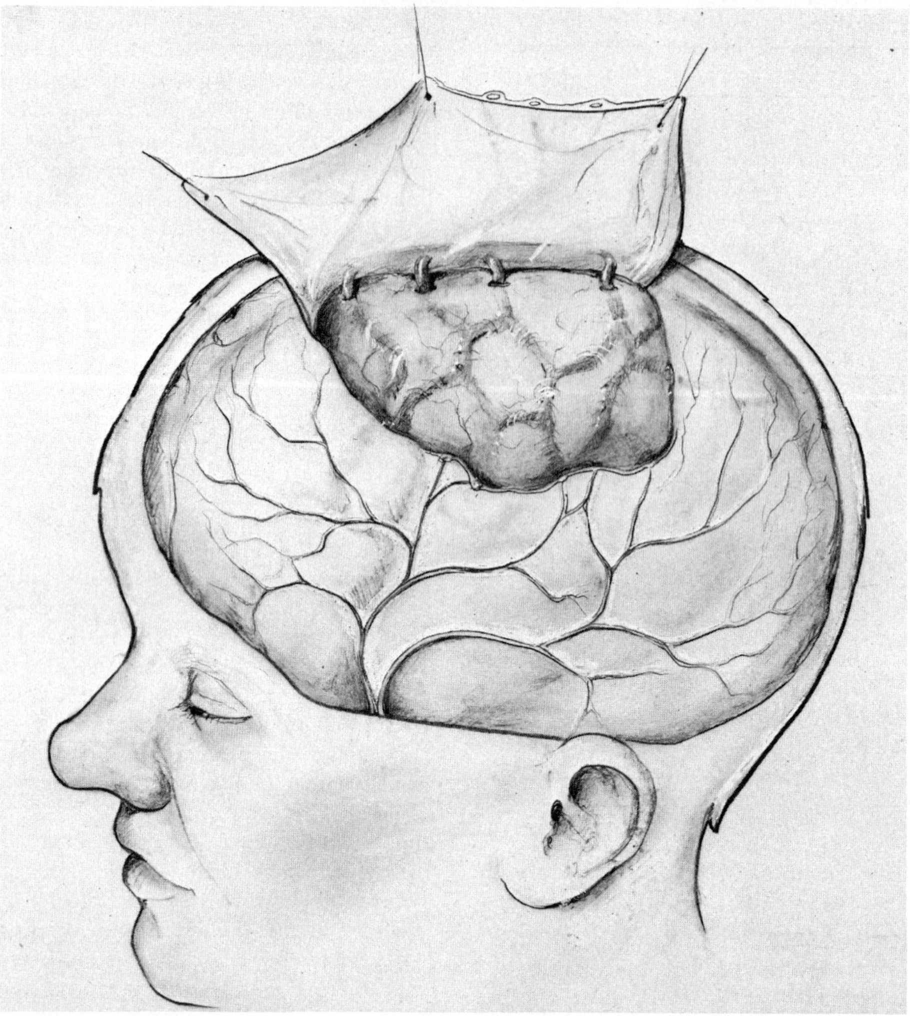

Fig. 40-6. The subdural bridging veins between the sagittal sinus and the cortical vessels are shown. These can shear at the time of violent deceleration, causing a subdural hematoma. The middle meningeal artery, which runs in the meningeal groove on the inner cortex of the temporal region, can be lacerated by a fracture of the overlying bone, leading to an epidural hematoma.

inertial forces, or by air- or liquid-transmitted blast waves that transmit pressure to large parts of the body or major segments of it (see Chap. 79). Exposure to a blasting force can involve all three types of force application. Crash injury involves forces of both the first and second type.

HEAD INJURY. A blunt injury to the head can result from a direct blow to the head or from violent acceleration or deceleration of the brain, associated with sudden hyperextension or hyperflexion of the neck. In fact, any impact to the head (except very slowly applied compression) involves acceleration or deceleration, whether the head is fixed or free. When deformation (compression, stretching, or shearing) occurs simultaneously or in succession during an impact to the head, the scalp is compressed, thereby absorbing a significant amount of force. The scalp is able to absorb up to 35 percent of a force so that in certain low-intensity impacts, the scalp and a thick head of hair may be effective in preventing an injury to underlying structures.

Violent acceleration or deceleration can cause injury because of differences in the rate of acceleration or deceleration of various parts of the intracranial contents. Cortical veins emptying into the superior sagittal sinus and other veins emptying into the sphenoid sinus can be torn and produce subdural hematomas as a result of relative movement of the brain in relation to the skull (Fig. 40-6). The base of the skull, which is irregular in the anterior and middle fossae, and the knife-like edge of the lesser wing of the sphenoid and the unbudging sharp border of the tentorium can produce tears and contusions of the brain as it moves in relation to these structures (Fig. 40-7).

Direct impact over the skull can cause a fracture that, in turn, may be responsible for injuring an underlying blood vessel such as the middle meningeal artery (see Fig. 40-6), thereby causing an epidural hematoma. If a large force is concentrated over a small area—for example, a blow from a hammer—a depressed fracture can result. The total energy that is required to cause a skull fracture ranges from 33 to 75 ft-lb, which is the amount of energy that is transmitted to the head when it strikes a hard flat surface after a free fall from a height of 5 ft. Striking the head at 50 mph against a surface that bends or dents 5 or 6 in. may expose it to less force than it receives when a person slips on the ice. Of patients with linear skull fractures, 78 to 80 percent are

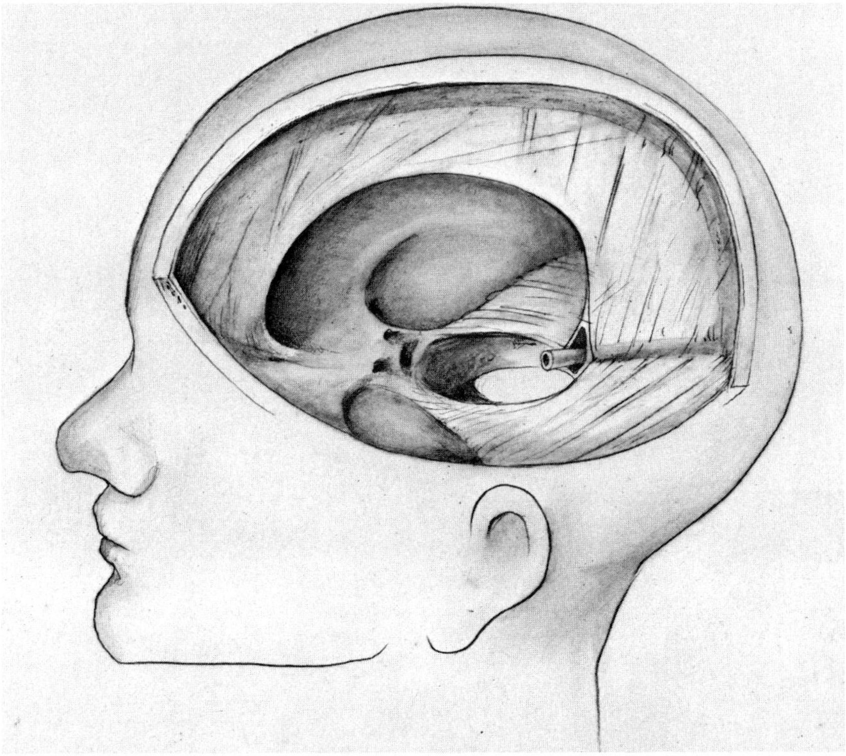

Fig. 40-7. The base of the skull, the edge of the lesser-wing sphenoid, and the unbudging edge of the tentorium are structures against which the decelerating or swelling brain can be injured.

rendered unconscious. The presence of a linear skull fracture can therefore usually be taken as an index of severity of a blow, representing an impact effect that is slightly stronger than the impact level that can cause a concussion (Gurdjian).

Ordinarily, a combination of forces is involved in producing a head injury. As is discussed in Chap. 54, the intracranial pressure changes that result from a head injury can secondarily produce movement and compression of portions of the brain, which can result in neurologic deficits and threaten life.

NECK INJURY. Although the neck is injured much less frequently than the head, blunt neck injury must be suspected whenever the head is injured. Direct force to the anterior part of the neck, such as that caused by the impact of a steering wheel during a collision, can compress and crush the larynx. Commonly, the forces responsible for blunt injury to the neck are indirect. Violent hyperextension or hyperflexion of the neck, associated with violent acceleration or deceleration of the head, can tear the supporting ligaments and protecting muscles and rupture intervertebral disks. If compressive force is great enough, fractures of the vertebrae can result and shear forces may lead to dislocation (see Chap. 55).

When indirect forces alone are involved, significant differences are found between the injuries sustained in a rear-end collision and those that result from front-end and side collisions. McNab and Hohl found that rear-end collisions were the most disabling. Their explanation is that hyperflexion, caused by front-end collision, has a built-in restraint when the chin strikes the chest, and, to a lesser extent, the lateral flexion is limited when the head strikes the shoulder. On the other hand, if a rear-end collision is forceful enough, the resulting hyperextension of the neck is stopped only when the head strikes the dorsal spine, causing movement well in excess of the range permitted by the anatomic structures.

TORSO INJURY. Direct impact to the chest wall produces injury primarily to the chest wall or to intrathoracic or upper-abdominal structures, depending on the force of impact. Since clothing often provides an effective cushion and protection for the skin, the skin is often unbruised and apparently undamaged in spite of severe underlying soft-tissue damage and intrathoracic injury.

The torso can be divided into three coronal zones (Fig. 40-8A). Zone 1 is the upper torso from clavicles to nipples, zone 2 is between the nipples and umbilicus, and zone 3 is the remaining torso, including the pelvis. It can also be divided sagittally into three zones (Fig. 40-8B), two lateral and one midline. Table 40-7 indicates the possible injuries that can result from blunt trauma to various zones of the torso. Because the heart, great vessels, and spinal cord occupy the midline zones, blunt trauma involving this zone is more likely to be lethal than trauma in the lateral zones.

Approximately 40 percent of victims of nonpenetrating thoracic trauma sustain fractures of the ribs, the most common of all chest injuries. Fractures of the ribs are more common in adults than in children because the cartilage in children is more resilient and can absorb an impact without breaking. The ribs of elderly individuals are brittle and can be broken even by minor trauma. The number of ribs frac-

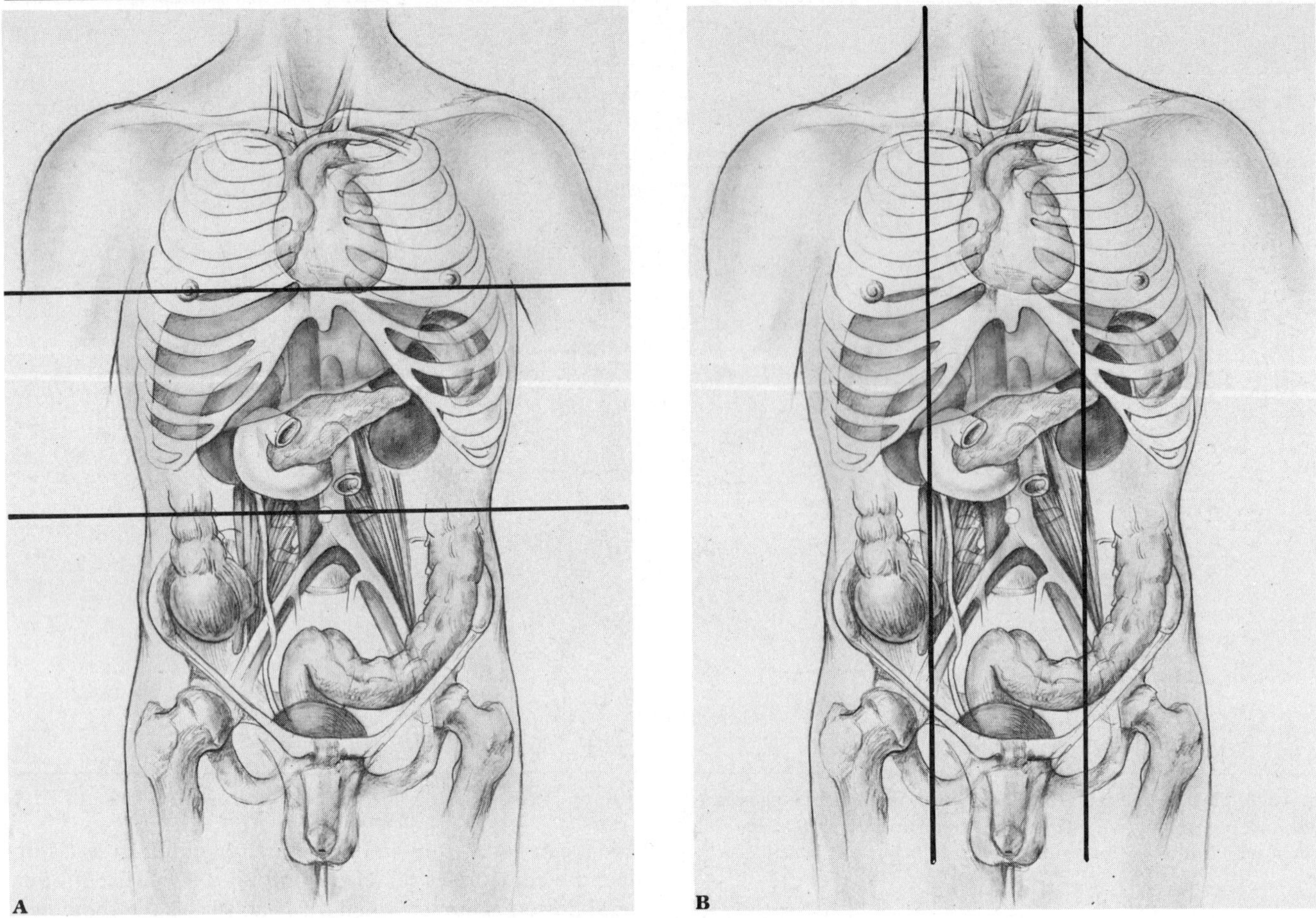

Fig. 40-8. The three coronal zones of the torso. Zone 1 is the upper torso from clavicles to nipples; zone 2 is between the nipples and umbilicus; zone 3 is the remaining torso. B. The three sagittal zones of the torso: one midline and two lateral.

tured, the degree of displacement of the rib fragments, and injury to the underlying lung depend on the force and direction of the impact and the area of its distribution. If the injuring force is applied over a wide area, especially in the anteroposterior projection, the ribs tend to buckle outward, breaking in midshaft position without injuring the pulmonary parenchyma. Direct impact over a limited area of the chest tends to drive the rib fragments inward (in the same way that a similar force can cause a depressed skull fracture) and can result in laceration of the pleura, pulmonary parenchyma, and intercostal vessels, producing pneumothorax, hemothorax, or both.

The sternum is seldom fractured in children and young adults because of the elasticity of the ribs and anterior costal cartilages. It has been demonstrated experimentally that the force of impact can press the sternum backward almost against the spinal column without breaking it. The fact that severe trauma is usually necessary to produce a sternal fracture explains the high incidence of serious associated injuries with such fractures. Blunt direct force readily produces pulmonary or myocardial contusion, and the blunt force can cause sharp intrathoracic damage if ribs are broken and sharp edges are forced backward, causing laceration of underlying structures.

Fractures of the first rib are uncommon. Because the first rib is small and protected by the shoulder girdle, fractures of this rib usually occur only if the impact force is tremendous. These fractures, almost always accompanied by fracture of the overlying clavicle, are frequently associated with injuries of the thoracic aorta or major bronchi; they are also associated with an increased incidence of disruption of the neurovascular structures to the upper extremities (Fig. 40-9).

Myocardial contusion following blunt trauma is usually the result of direct impact of an automobile steering wheel over the precordium, causing compression of the heart between the sternum and the vertebral column. This injury is most commonly associated with multiple rib or sternal fractures.

Mediastinal injuries rarely result from direct impact because the lungs presumably serve as protective cushions, somewhat like plastic air splints while they are momentarily at positive pressure. At time of impact, the sternum is forced posteriorly, displacing and twisting the heart to the left, while the mediastinal contents suddenly decelerate. The decelerating aorta is arrested sharply at points of attachment, such as the ligamentum arteriosum (Fig. 40-10). Although the factors responsible for the tearing or transection of the aorta have not been completely elucidated, it seems clear that an imbalance of forces of deceleration, compression, and restraint are involved. Torsion stress is critical at the

Table 40-7. Blunt injuries in torso trauma

Zone	Lateral	Midline	Lateral
Zone 1*	Lung Chest wall	Great vessels Heart Spinal cord	Lung Chest wall
	Majority managed nonoperatively	High morbidity and mortality	Mortality ranges from 15–40%
Zone 2*	Diaphragm Liver Colon Kidney Gallbladder	Liver Pancreas Duodenum Stomach Colon Aorta Cava	Diaphragm Spleen Kidney Colon
	Most require operative treatment	Almost all require surgery	Should have low mortality
Zone 3*	Colon Small bowel Pelvis	Small bowel Aorta Rectum Bladder Ureters Genitalia	Colon Small bowel Pelvis
	Most can be managed without operation	Potentially high mortality	Mortality should be low

*Zones of injuries in the torso with organs susceptible to injury and the probability of an organ injury requiring surgery.
Source: D. D. Trunkey. Torso trauma. *Curr. Probl. Surg.* 24:218, 1987.

base of the heart and shearing stress is critical at the ligamentum.

At the time of direct impact, compression and sudden increase in pressure in an enclosed system can cause further injury. Ordinarily, the airway is open, but the open system in the awake and aware subject is converted into a closed box by closure of the glottis at the moment of or just before impact. The increase in pressure can result in bursting phenomena, causing mediastinal, pleural, tracheal, bronchial, or intrapulmonary damage. When the force is removed, the distorted thorax springs back, creating an instant of increased negative intrathoracic pressure.

Zone 2 injuries are particularly common in steering column injuries in the unrestrained driver. Injury patterns associated with this zone include contusion or rupture of the myocardium, rupture of the liver, laceration of the spleen, and injuries to the pancreas and duodenum. The lower two ribs are mobile and yielding, and therefore they are the ones that are least often fractured. Because of their location, lower-rib fractures are often associated with injuries to the liver, spleen, and kidneys (Figs. 40-11, 40-12, and 40-13). Fractures of the left tenth rib also are sometimes associated with fractures of the spleen.

The mechanisms for diaphragmatic rupture remain conjectural, but it is believed that it is caused by a tremendously high gradient between intraperitoneal and intrathoracic pressure at the time of injury if the glottis is open when a severe crushing force is applied to the abdomen. At the time of impact with the glottis closed, the sudden rise in intrathoracic pressure is usually matched by a rise in intraabdominal pressure. This apparent neutralization of pressures probably accounts for the relative infrequency of diaphragmatic rupture associated with blunt injury to the torso (Blair).

The severity of abdominal injury is greatly influenced by the location of the impact. As was previously noted, although the turgid liver and spleen are somewhat protected by the rib cage, they are much more easily injured than are the lower abdominal organs. This observation is supported by the statistics in Table 40-8, Blaisdell's summary from the literature of the relative incidence of organ injury in blunt abdominal trauma. The hollow viscera can absorb a considerable amount of transmitted pressure unless they are distended.

Blunt force to the abdomen can cause injury by a variety of mechanisms, acting singly or in combination: direct compression of abdominal solid organs, direct or shearing force as midlying structures are caught between the abdominal wall and the vertebral column, shearing forces applied to relatively fixed supporting mesentery or vessels, rupture of hollow viscera when intraluminal pressure exceeds bursting wall tension, diaphragmatic rupture following sudden increase in intraabdominal pressure, and direct penetration of soft tissue by fragments of fractured bones, especially fractured pelvis. When a hollow viscus ruptures, the injury effect is compounded by the intense inflammation caused by spillage of sterile, but irritating, or bacteria-laden contents of the viscus into the body cavity.

Associations of injuries include pelvic fractures and rupture of structures of the urinary tract, concomitant hepatic and splenic injuries following steering wheel injuries to the torso, and ruptures of the small bowel and its mesentery with or without lumbar fracture in patients who were wearing seat belts at the time of the automobile accident.

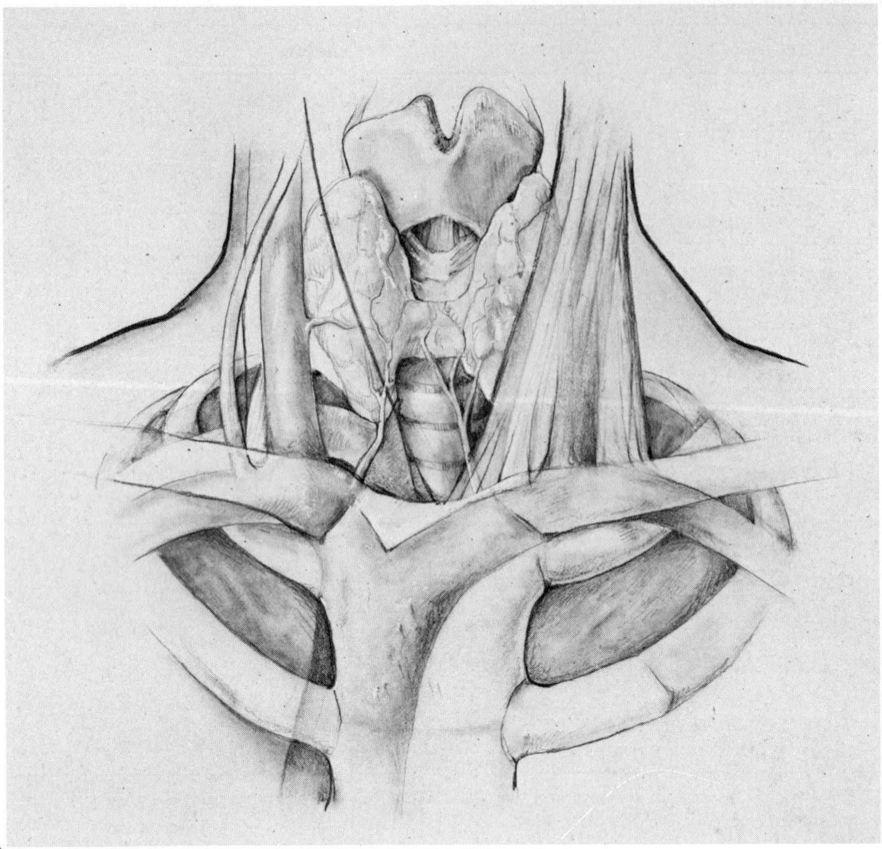

A

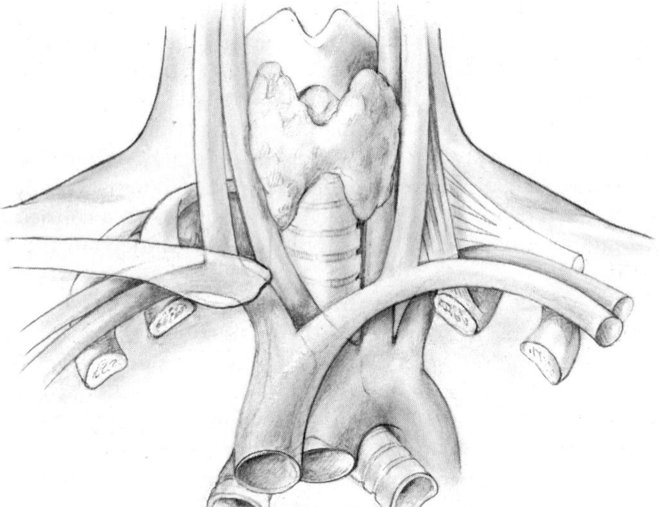

B

Fig. 40-9. A. The root of the neck showing the relations of the subclavian vessels, which lie immediately behind the clavicle, to the first rib, to which they are closely attached. The dome of the pleura rises just above the first rib. B. The structures of the brachial plexus are immediately lateral to the subclavian artery. The aortic arch arches close to the first rib.

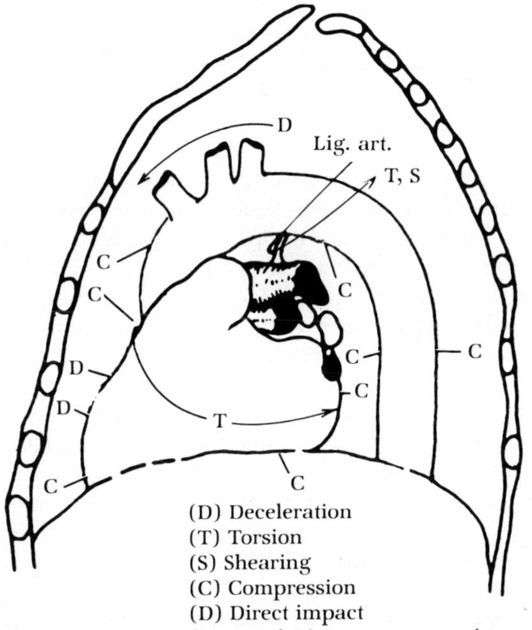

Fig. 40-10. Some of the forces involved in injury to the chest. (From E. Blair, C. Topulzu, and R. S. Deane. Major blunt chest trauma. *Curr. Probl. Surg.* May 1969, P. 2.)

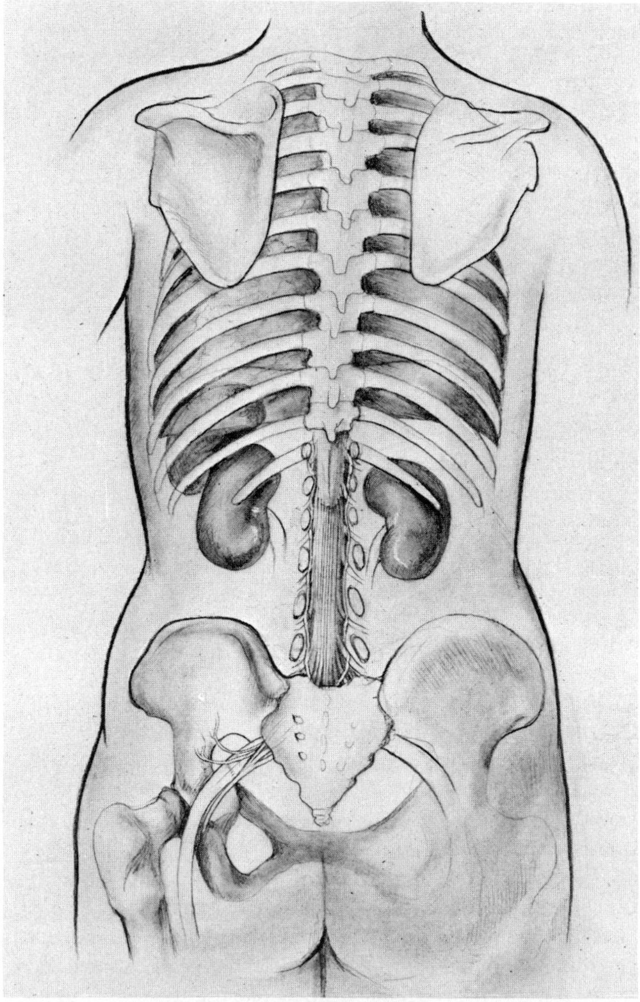

Fig. 40-11. The relations of the posterior structures of the torso.

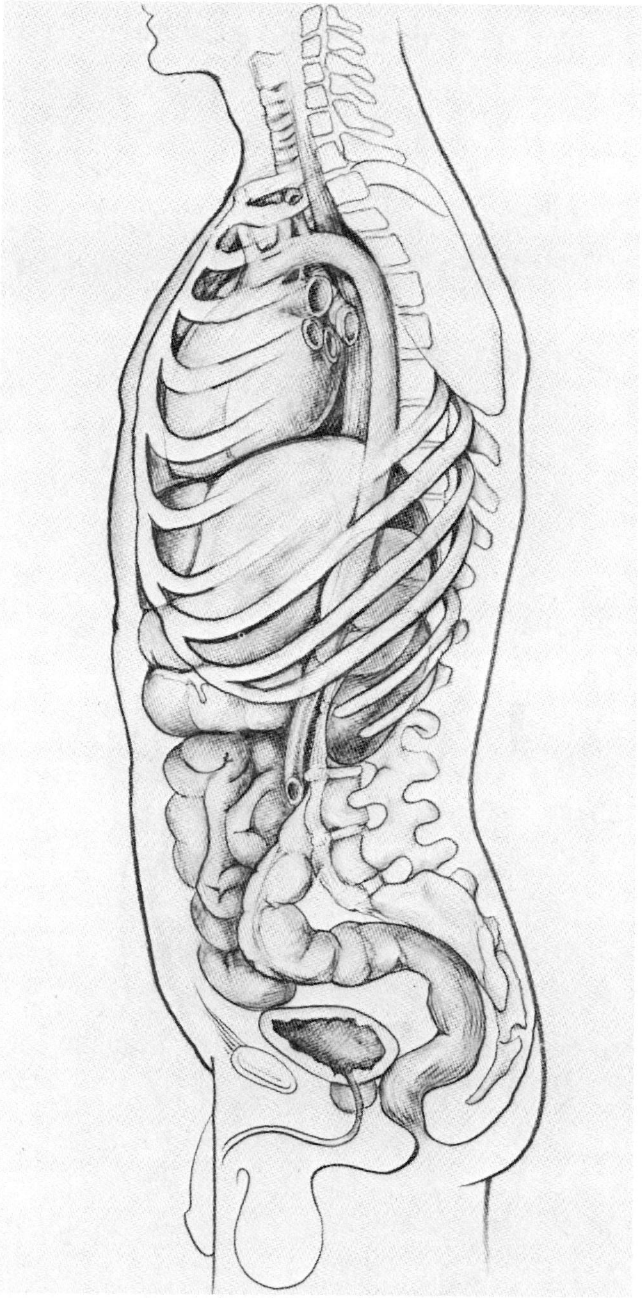

Fig. 40-12. The left lateral view of the torso showing the relationship of the ligamentum teres to the aorta and pulmonary artery and the relationship of the subclavian vessels to the first rib. Also shown are the relationships of the spleen and the left kidney to the lower left ribs.

The rigid, strong, bony ring of the pelvis cannot be fractured unless great force is applied to it, and bony displacement can occur only if the ring is disrupted in at least two places. Other portions of the pelvis—the obturator rings, sacrum, and coccyx—can be fractured from the application of much less force, such as occurs commonly from falls. Although the pelvis can absorb a tremendous amount of force that would otherwise cause injury to underlying soft tissue, once it is broken, it can become the wounding force for underlying pelvic vessels, urethra and bladder, vagina, and rectum and perianal structures. Fractures of the pelvic ring commonly occur from industrial accidents in which crushing forces are applied. In recent years, automobile accidents in which a pedestrian is struck from the side, is thrown sideways in a crashing vehicle, or has the heavy wheels of a vehicle run over the pelvis, have also become common causes of pelvic fractures.

INJURIES OF THE EXTREMITIES. If the applied force is great enough, bones of the extremities will be broken or dislocated, depending on the way the force is applied. Then the bones that protected the nearby soft tissues, including neurovascular structures, can damage them. Figures 40-14 and 40-15 identify some of the sites where neurovascular structures are particularly vulnerable and are sometimes injured by the displaced fragment of bone. The subclavian vein or artery or portions of the brachial plexus are sometimes injured by displaced fragments of a fractured clavicle or first rib. The axillary nerve, curving around the head of the humerus, can be injured by a dislocated head of the humerus. The radial nerve can be damaged as it curves behind and close to the midhumerus, or the ulnar nerve can be injured as it passes behind the medial epicondyle. The brachial artery can be damaged, especially in children, by

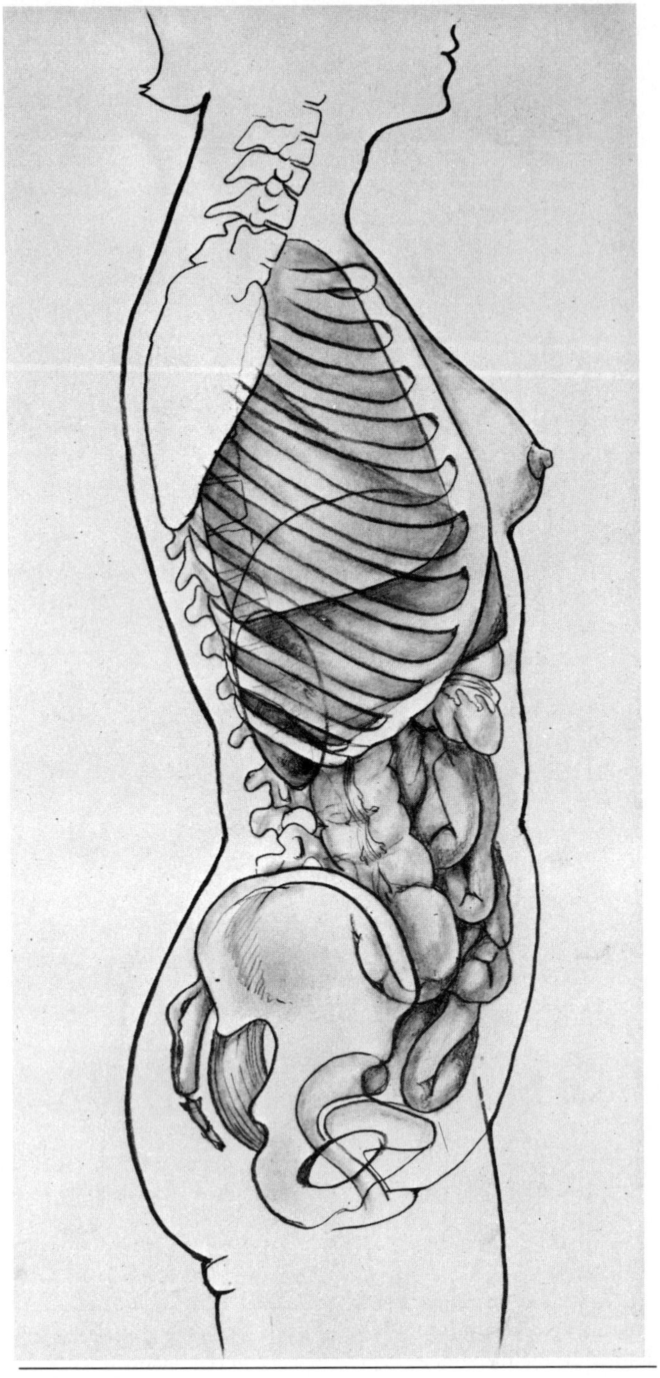

Fig. 40-13. Anatomic relationships for the right lateral aspect of the torso.

certain fractures or dislocations of the elbow, and the median or ulnar nerves can be injured by some fractures of the wrist.

The sciatic nerve, coursing behind the head of the femur, is sometimes injured by a posteriorly displaced femoral head. In much the same way that the brachial artery can be injured at the elbow, the popliteal artery can be compromised by a posteriorly displaced fracture at the knee. The common peroneal nerve, curving behind and around the head of the fibula, can be injured either by a bony injury at that point or by a tight-fitting cast.

Table 40-8. Blunt trauma: Relative incidence of organ injury

Organ	Percentage
Spleen	25
Liver	15
Retroperitoneal hematoma	13
Kidney	12
Small bowel	9
Bladder	6
Mesentery	5
Large bowel	4
Pancreas	3
Urethra	2
Diaphragm	2
Vascular	2
Stomach	1
Duodenum	1

Source: F. W. Blaisdell. General Assessment, Resuscitation, and Exploration of Penetrating and Blunt Abdominal Trauma. In F. W. Blaisdell and D. D. Trunkey (eds.), *Trauma Management*, vol 1—*Abdominal Trauma*. New York: Thieme-Stratton, 1982. P. 13.

Deep soft tissues of the extremities can be damaged by the primary injuring force or can be secondarily damaged, either by ischemia caused by compromise of the arterial supply or by compartment syndrome if venous drainage of the structures within the compartment is compromised, especially in the presence of a crush injury (see Chap. 73). Shearing force (applied, for example, when an extremity is caught in a roller or run over by a vehicle) can cause a degloving injury in which the skin and subcutaneous tissues are pushed ahead of the deeper tissues, tearing the skin's nutrient blood supply from the deeper muscular sources (see Chap. 67).

Penetrating Injury

The damage caused by penetrating injury from such objects as knives, impaling objects, or low-velocity missiles depends on the tissues that have been injured. Such secondary effects as infection depend on the nature of the weapon, the material that is carried into the body, and spillage of contents of any hollow viscus that has been injured. Table 40-9 indicates mortality for penetrating torso injuries, and Table 40-10 indicates relative incidence of organ injury resulting from penetrating injury to the abdomen. As is true of blunt trauma, mortality is highest for penetrating injury to midline structures, especially for zone 1 injuries. Mortality for lateral injuries of zone 1 is low unless systemic vessels are injured, because the pulmonary circulation is a low-pressure system. Zone 2 penetrating injuries almost invariably require exploration.

Gunshot Wounds

Classifying all gunshot injuries in a broad category of penetrating wounds is an oversimplification associated with the widely held belief that the seriousness of a bullet wound depends only on the structures that are directly in its path. A stab wound or an injury caused by a low-velocity missile

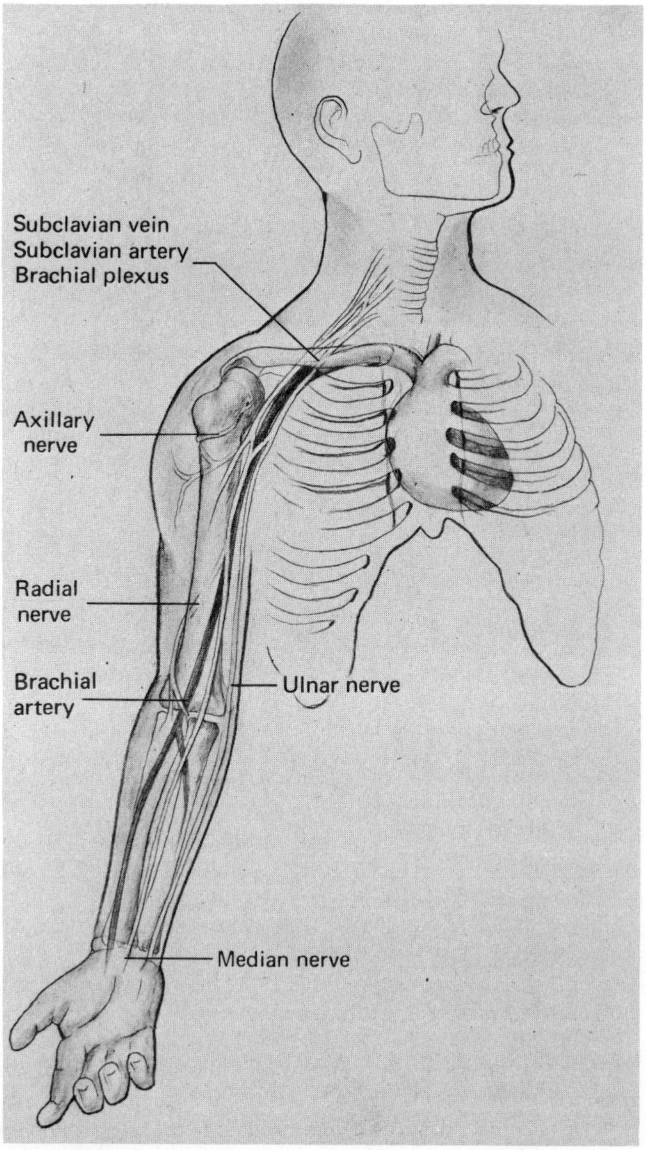

Fig. 40-14. Neurovascular structures that can be damaged by fracture or dislocation of overlying bony structures of the upper extremity.

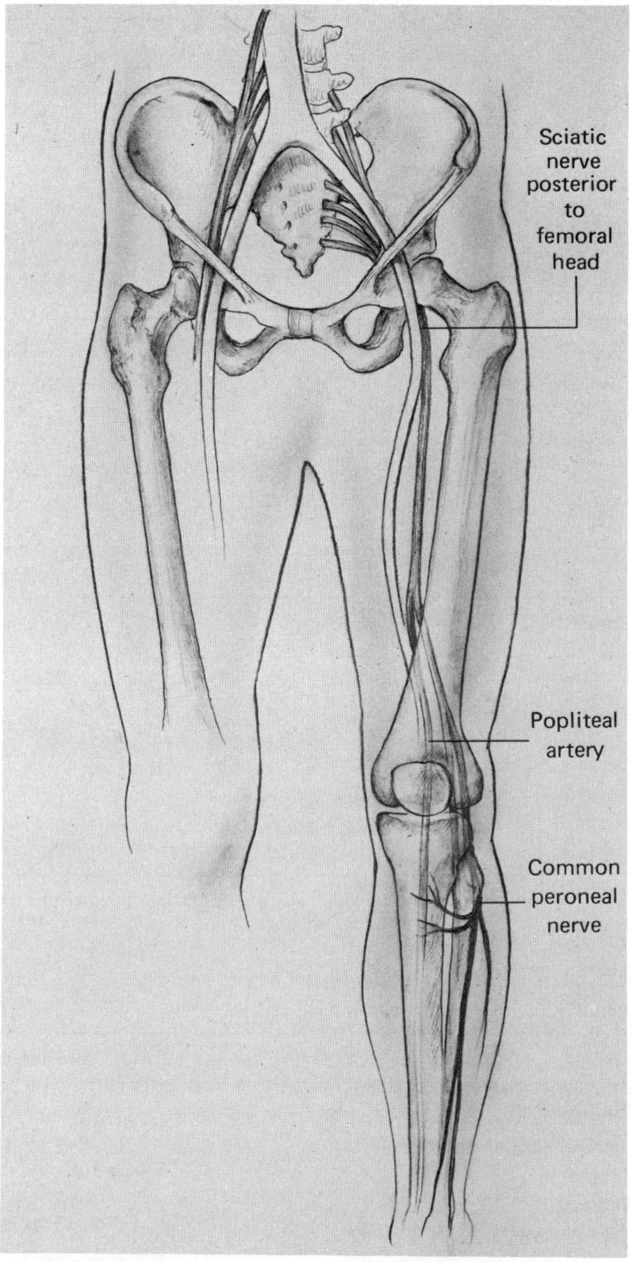

Fig. 40-15. Neurovascular structures that can be damaged from fracture or dislocation of overlying bony structures of the lower extremity.

can be rapidly lethal if a vital structure is injured. However, a wound caused by a high-velocity missile, such as a hunting or military rifle, can be lethal even if a vital structure has not been penetrated.

The three primary theories that have been used to explain the wounding mechanism of bullets are the kinetic energy, momentum, and power theories.* Most authorities now hold that the kinetic energy theory is most compatible with the experimental observation that the damage inflicted by a penetrating missile primarily depends on the kinetic energy that is absorbed by the tissue.

The main groups of weapons that commonly produce gunshot wounds are rifles, shotguns, and handguns. American rifles and handguns are designated by caliber, the ap-

*Kinetic energy $= \dfrac{\text{mass} \times \text{velocity}^2}{2}$

Momentum $=$ mass $\times$ velocity
Power $=$ mass $\times$ velocity^3

Since the weight of the bullet is usually expressed in grains and approximately 7,000 grains equals 1 lb, the kinetic energy of the bullet at the gun muzzle is approximated by the formula,

$$\text{Energy (ft-lb)} = \frac{\text{weight (grains)} \times \text{velocity}^2\ (\text{ft/sec})^2}{7{,}000\ (\text{grains/lb}) \times 64.4\ (\text{ft/sec}^2)}$$

$$= \frac{\text{weight (grains)} \times \text{velocity}^2\ (\text{ft/sec})}{453{,}600}$$

Table 40-9. Penetrating injuries in torso trauma

Zone	Lateral	Midline	Lateral
Zone 1*	Lung	Great vessels Heart Spinal cord	Lung
	Approximately 15% will require operation; great majority can be managed with tube thoracostomy	High mortality, almost all will require operation if patient makes it to the emergency department	Low mortality
Zone 2*	Diaphragm Liver Colon Kidney Gallbladder	Liver Pancreas Stomach Colon Duodenum Aorta Cava	Diaphragm Spleen Colon Kidney
	Almost all require operation	All require surgery, modest mortality	Mortality should be low
Zone 3*	Colon Small bowel Pelvis	Small bowel Aorta Rectum Bladder Ureters Genitalia	Colon Small bowel Pelvis
	Most will require operation	Almost all will require surgery, mortality can be modest	Mortality should be low

*Zones of injury in the torso with organs susceptible to injury and the probability of an organ injury requiring surgery.
Source: D. D. Trunkey. Torso trauma. *Curr. Probl. Surg.* 24:219, 1987.

Table 40-10. Penetrating trauma: Relative incidence of organ injury

Organ	Percentage
Small bowel	30
Mesentery and omentum	18
Liver	16
Colon	9
Diaphragm	8
Stomach	7
Spleen	6
Kidney	5
Major vascular	4
Pancreas	3
Duodenum	2
Bladder	1
Ureter	1

Source: F. W. Blaisdell. General Assessment, Resuscitation, and Exploration of Penetrating and Blunt Abdominal Trauma. In F. W. Blaisdell and D. D. Trunkey (eds.), *Trauma Management*, Vol. 1—*Abdominal Trauma*. New York: Thieme-Stratton, 1982. P. 11.

proximate diameter of the bullet in inches. European weapons are designated in millimeters.

RIFLES. Rifles, the most powerful of the weapon types, have been developed for military or for civilian use. Unfortunately, as new military weapons have been developed, the older models and modern semiautomatic assault rifles, which are copies of fully automatic military rifles, have become available and are being used in civilian shootings. Early military rifles were patterned after hunting rifles, using heavy bullets to maximize the knockdown capability, under the assumption that the momentum of the bullet was primarily responsible for its wounding capacity. However, the U.S. military M-16 rifle, used in Vietnam, was developed with the recognition of the fact that the velocity of a missile contributes more to its kinetic energy than does its mass. Its bullet is tiny (55 grains, or 3.6 gm), but its muzzle velocity is so high (approximately 3,250 ft/sec, or 991 m/sec), that its kinetic energy is 1.218 ft-lb. Table 40-11 indicates the relative contribution of the mass and velocity of a missile to its kinetic energy. By convention, bullet velocity is classified as low if it is under 1,000 ft/sec, medium if it is between 1,000 and 2,000 ft/sec, and high if it is above 2,000 ft/sec. The velocity of all bullets falls off with increasing distance, but the velocity retained by most hunting and military rifles at the range of 300 to 1,000 yd approximates the velocity of the handgun at close range.

Table 40-11. Representative ballistic data for hunting and military rifles

	Bullet		Velocity (ft/sec)				Energy (ft-lb)			
Cartridge	Weight (grains)	Type	Muzzle	100 ft	200 ft	300 ft	Muzzle	100 ft	200 ft	300 ft
22 Hornet	46	Hollow point	2,690	2,030	1,510	1,150	740	420	235	135
223 M-16 (US 5.56 mm)	55		3,200	2,630	2,120	1,700	1,218	837	541	330
243 Winchester	80	Hollow point	3,450	3.050	2,675	2,330	2,115	1,650	1,270	965
270 Winchester	100	Pointed soft point	3,480	3,070	2,690	2,340	2,690	2,090	1,600	1,216
30-06 Springfield	110	Pointed soft point	3,370	2,830	2,350	1,920	2,770	1,960	1,350	900
30 M-1 US	150		2,970	2,670	2,400	2,130	2,930	2,370	1,920	1,510
300 Winchester magnum	150	Plastic point Pointed core lok	3,400	3,050	2,730	2,430	3,850	3,100	2,480	1,970
458 Winchester magnum	510	Soft point	2,130	1,840	1,600	1,400	5,140	3,830	2,900	2,220
460 Weatherby magnum	500	Full metal jacket	2,700	2,416	2,154	1,912	8,095	6,482	5,153	4,060

Table 40-12. Comparison of different handgun calibers commonly used in shootings

Caliber (in. or mm)	Bullet (grains)	Velocity (ft/sec)	Energy (ft-lb)
0.25	45	815	66
0.22LR	36	1,080	93
0.32	60	970	125
0.38 special	148	710	166
0.380	85	1,000	189
0.38 +P	158	915	294
9 mm	95	1,355	387
0.45 automatic	200	917	421
0.357 magnum	125	1,450	583
0.44 magnum	180	1,610	1,045

Key: LR = long rifle; +P = power.
Source: Modified from E. Barach, M. Tomlanovich, and R. Nowak. Ballistics: A pathophysiologic examination of the wounding mechanisms of firearms: Part II. *J. Trauma* 26:374, 1986.

HANDGUNS. Table 40-12 compares the calibers of 10 different handguns that are frequently used in shootings. Most handgun injuries treated in urban emergency departments are caused by small, easily concealed weapons that deliver small-caliber, low-velocity bullets with such low kinetic energy that their range is short and the damage is usually limited to the tissue directly in the path of the bullet. Unfortunately, multiple woundings are increasing in urban hospitals because automatic weapons have become popular in the drug wars. Although the bullets of the popular MAC-10 0.22-caliber semiautomatic pistol are light and the muzzle velocity is low, the weapon is lethal because it is easily converted to fire like a machine gun so that multiple wounds are common. On the other hand, a single bullet from the 9-mm Uzi can cause much more damage because the bullet is heavier and has a higher muzzle velocity and therefore a higher kinetic energy. The 0.38 special + P, a popular bullet with police departments, also has added power that increases its velocity and its kinetic energy.

BULLETS AND THEIR WOUNDING FORCES. A "magnum" rifle or handgun (for example, the 0.357 magnum revolver or the 0.338 Winchester magnum rifle) uses the same diameter and weight and the same type of powder as a regular bullet, but the cartridge case is longer and holds more gunpowder, thereby increasing the velocity and kinetic energy of the weapon.

The most important determinant of the wounding capability of a bullet is the kinetic energy absorbed by the victim.* Although the impact velocity is the most important contributor to the kinetic energy, the composition and design of the bullet are almost as important in determining its wounding capability because they play an important role in determining how much of the kinetic energy of the bullet will be absorbed by the body. The bulk of most bullets consists of a lead alloy. Since lead's melting point is low, it is easily deformed when heated above its melting point. This fact

$$^{*}KE = \frac{m \times (V1^2 - V2^2)}{2\,g}$$

where m = mass, V1 = striking velocity, V2 = exit velocity, and g = gravitational acceleration.

Table 40-13. Relationship of specific gravity to wounding capacity

Tissue	Specific gravity	Severity of wound
Lung	0.4–0.5	Minimum
Fat	0.8	Moderate
Liver	0.01–1.02	Marked
Skin	1.09	Marked
Muscle	1.02–1.04	Marked
Bone	1.11	Extreme

Source: W. E. DeMuth, Jr. Bullet velocity and design as determinants of wounding capability: An experimental study. *J. Trauma* 6:226, © by Williams & Wilkins, 1966.

does not limit its use in handguns because their muzzle velocity is so slow that the bullet does not become distorted by frictional heat during its passage through the gun barrel; on the other hand, the portion of a high-velocity rifle bullet that comes in contact with the barrel must be covered with a jacket of metal that has a higher melting point than lead to prevent distortion produced by heat. Geneva Convention rules, established before World War I, required that military bullets must be full jacketed and nonexpanding, but hunting bullets are ordinarily soft-nosed so that they mushroom after entering the target, expanding to several times their original caliber and establishing a wide wound tract. Whereas some bullets are designed to expand, others are intended to disintegrate or to tumble once they have penetrated the target. Any of these actions increases their wounding power.

The damaging effect of moving bullets increases with the increase in the specific gravity of the tissues involved. This explains the seeming paradox that lung injury appears to be greater if a bullet strikes the thorax tangentially than if the bullet moves directly through lung tissue. Table 40-13 indicates the specific gravity of a number of tissues. In contrast to the high-velocity bullet that transverses human tissue in a straight line, a low-velocity missile often has its course changed as it encounters tissue of varying density so that its course within the body is not that of a straight line.

Low-velocity missiles inflict penetrating injuries that are similar to those produced by knives or other sharp pointed instruments. Since tissues are pushed aside, the damage that is inflicted is limited to a small radius from the center of the track; morbidity and mortality depend only on the structures that have been penetrated. However, when a bullet of similar caliber but high velocity penetrates, the tremendous amount of kinetic energy that is absorbed by the surrounding structures causes momentary acceleration of the tissues in a direction forward and laterally away from the bullet, thereby forming a temporary cavity around the bullet and its track. The cavity, resulting from the expending of an enormous explosive force during the passage of the bullet through the tissues, continues to enlarge to many times its diameter after the bullet passes. Since the cavity is initially at subatmospheric pressure, foreign materials and tissue fragments may be sucked into it; then within a few milliseconds the cavity begins to collapse under atmospheric pressure. The reforming and collapsing of the cavity continues until all imparted energy has been dissipated, alternately stretching and compressing the tissues and producing severe damage, sometimes at a great distance from the permanent wound track. The cavity temporarily formed is principally a function of the velocity of the bullet (DeMuth). Figure 40-16 illustrates variations of ballistic effects on animal tissue.

SHOTGUNS. Shotguns, which have unique wounding effects, are designated by the archaic system of gauge, indicating the number of lead balls of a specific diameter (made from one pound of lead) that would just fit the barrel of the gun. Thus, a 12-gauge shotgun accepts lead balls weighing one-twelfth of a pound, and a 16-gauge shotgun accepts a ball weighing one-sixteenth of a pound. As the gauge number decreases, the bore opening increases in size. Shotguns shoot multiple pellets instead of single bullets since they are used primarily for hunting birds and fast-moving animals. The pellets are held in a shotgun shell, along with powder in a metal base, with cardboard or plastic wads to separate the pellets from the powder. The tissue damage depends on the range. At close range, the amount of kinetic energy delivered to the tissues is overpowering (over 2,200 ft-lb). In addition, at close range, the wadding that accompanies the shotgun shell is delivered to the wound along with the total mass of the shot, adding considerably to the blast effect and driving the foreign body deeply into the body tissues, along with clothing and sometimes other foreign material.

The long-range shotgun injury is very different. At 40 yd approximately 200 to 300 pellets hit in a circle 30 in. in diameter. As the range from the target increases, fewer pellets will hit it and the kinetic energy at time of impact will decrease so that the seriousness of the injury depends only on the site of injury. These pellets do not hit the target at the same time; rather, the first pellet may strike a person in one position and the last pellet may strike the victim after he or she has changed from the earlier position (Mays).

INITIAL RESPONSES OF THE BODY TO INJURY

If critical injury does not cause immediate death, the body instantly begins to mobilize a highly organized series of cellular and neurohumoral responses in its effort to stop bleeding and to meet the energy requirements that will prolong survival. Immediate activation of clotting mechanisms to limit blood loss, shifting of body fluids from the extravascular compartment into the intravascular space to conserve blood volume, and redistributing blood flow to ensure perfusion of vital structures with enough oxygen and energy substrate to maintain life are the highest immediate priorities.

Early Local Responses

Depending on the nature of the trauma, some tissues are injured or destroyed directly; others are damaged subsequently and deteriorate because of hypoxia or damage from metabolic products of adjacent injured cells or from noxious effects of inflammatory cells that are recruited to defend the threatened tissues. Cellular injury releases metabolic products locally that greatly influence subsequent events.

Platelet Aggregation and Blood Clotting

Damage to a blood vessel disrupts its endothelium, exposing the underlying layer of collagen. Platelets adhere to the colla-

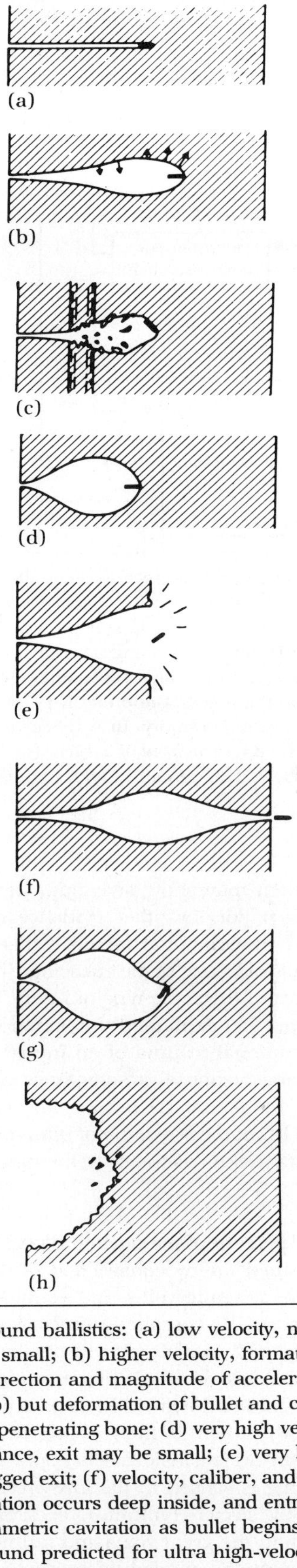

Fig. 40-16. Wound ballistics: (a) low velocity, no cavitation, entrance and exit small; (b) higher velocity, formation of cavity; arrows show direction and magnitude of acceleration of tissue; (c) velocity as in (b) but deformation of bullet and creation of secondary missiles on penetrating bone: (d) very high velocity, large cavity and small entrance, exit may be small; (e) very high velocity, thin target, large ragged exit; (f) velocity, caliber, and thickness of tissue such that cavitation occurs deep inside, and entrance and exit are small; (g) asymmetric cavitation as bullet begins to deform and tumble; (h) wound predicted for ultra high-velocity, small-caliber projectiles now under development, no exit wound, fragmentation of the bullet. (From K. G. Swan and R. C. Swan. *Gunshot Wounds, Pathophysiology and Management.* Chicago: Mosby-Year Book, 1980. P. 9.)

gen and stick to each other, forming clumps and secreting the contents of their granules. As discussed in Chap. 1, some of the secreted materials—serotonin, adenosine diphosphate (ADP), calcium, lysosomal enzymes, prostaglandins, thromboxane A_2 (TxA_2), and other eicosanoids—assist in producing local vasoconstriction, and some make the platelets sticky, thereby promoting further aggregation of platelets to form a temporary hemostatic plug. Stimulation of the coagulation cascade then causes the formation of fibrin, which consolidates and stabilizes the thrombus. Some of the compounds, such as TxA_2, are strong stimulators of platelet aggregation; others, such as prostacyclin, modulate the response in such a way that when an injury is minor, platelet thrombi form but parts break off to be washed away by the circulation. The size of the thrombus depends, at least in part, on the degree of injury; for the development of a large thrombus, severe damage or physical detachment of the endothelium must occur. Platelet-plug formation is especially important in capillary hemostasis, whereas vasoconstriction and fibrin formation seem to be more important in larger-vessel hemostasis.

Increase in Vascular Permeability

Tissue mast cells, found in cutaneous and mucosal surfaces and around venules, contain stored mediators of the inflammatory response—histamine, heparin, and chemotactic factors for neutrophils and eosinophils—and synthesize other mediators, including leukotrienes, in response to perturbation of cellular membranes. These mediators, along with others, participate in a biphasic inflammatory pattern of increased permeability of vessels 20 to 100 μ in diameter in response to injury. The immediate phase is transient, occurring within minutes after the injury and then disappearing. It is replaced by the delayed phase, which occurs over a 3- to 6-hour period as the vasopermeability factors induce a reversible opening of the junction between the endothelial cells by producing a contraction of the cells, thereby permitting passage of plasma solutes across the vascular barrier.

Depending on the local balance between the vasoconstricting and vasodilating agents that are secreted or synthesized in response to injury, local vasoconstriction or vasodilatation occurs in the injured area. The blood flow in the microvascular bed slows because of the increased viscosity of the packed red blood cells associated with loss of fluid from the vessels. These changes permit increased adherence of polymorphonuclear leukocytes to the endothelial lining and their diapedesis into the inflammatory focus. Neutrophils are present in large numbers within four hours after injury because of the chemotactic factors generated by blood clotting, injured tissues, complement (especially C5A), bacteria (if present), lymphocytes, and eicosanoids.

Blood sequestered in an injured area, together with decreased tissue perfusion brought about by local vascular injury, hypotension, and edema, leads to local acidosis because of anaerobic energy metabolism of the cells and consequent breakdown of the sodium-potassium pump, allowing sodium to enter the cells and potassium to move from cells into the interstitial compartment. In some cases, the early movement of sodium into the cells is accompanied by water, leading to swelling of the cells. For cells that are not irreversibly damaged by the initial trauma, the sodium-potassium fluid shifts are reversible early.

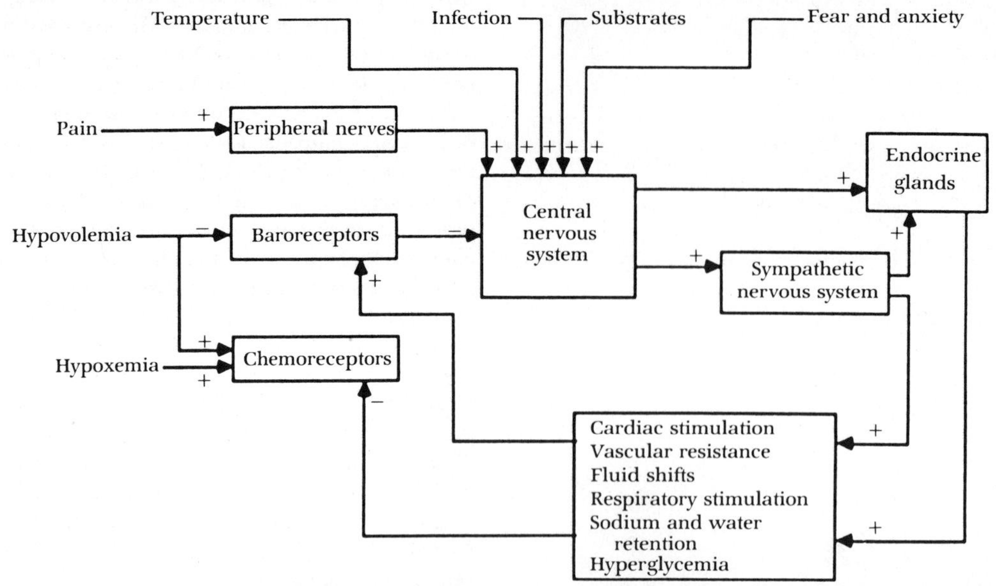

Fig. 40-17. Overview of the neuroendocrine reflexes induced by shock and injury. At least seven stimuli consequent to injury elicit neuroendocrine reflexes. These include hypovolemia; pain; changes in PO_2, PCO_2, or pH; infection; changes in substrate availability; and changes in temperature. The most common of these are hypovolemia and pain. (From D. S. Gann and J. F. Amaral. Endocrine and Metabolic Responses to Injury. In S. I. Schwartz, G. T. Shires, and F. C. Spencer [eds.], *Principles of Surgery* [5th ed.]. New York: McGraw-Hill, 1989. P. 4. Reproduced with permission.)

Stimuli and Early Systemic Neurohumoral Responses

Early local changes at the injury site are accompanied by systemic alterations as the neuroendocrine reflexes are activated by any or all of the following stimuli: (1) pain; (2) hypovolemia; (3) emotional response; (4) changes in the concentration of oxygen, carbon dioxide, or pH of tissues or blood; (5) alterations in the availability of glucose or other vital substrate; (6) changes in core or ambient temperature; and (7) sepsis (Fig. 40-17). The most critical are hypovolemia and pain.

Pain

Since the quickest route for signals to arrive at the central nervous system following stress is via the afferent sensory nerve pathways, it has long been postulated that pain may provide the initial afferent signal after injury. In a classic experiment, Egdahl and Hume showed that the outpouring of adrenocorticotropic hormone (ACTH) that followed the injury to the hind limb of a dog was eliminated if all nerves to the extremity were divided. This observation confirmed the fact that the afferent nerves from an injury site play a critical role in mobilizing the body's responses and explains the observation that paraplegic or quadriplegic patients fail to demonstrate an increase in ACTH after trauma to denervated areas. Pain impulses ascend in the spinothalamic tracts to the thalamus, but because of association of these pathways to the cortex and limbic system in the conscious patient pain commonly evokes strong emotional responses, including fear, anxiety, and possibly anger, which intensify the sympathetic outpouring that is stimulated by the pain. This pain-mediated response occurs before blood volume loss is sufficient to activate the autonomic system. The initial release of norepinephrine may be from the postganglionic sympathetic fibers in the wound. The release of both epinephrine and norepinephrine from the adrenal medulla occurs soon thereafter. The local pain is augmented by the local outpouring of prostaglandins, potassium, and histamine.

Emotion

The injured patient may show sweating, tremor, tachycardia, dry mouth, pallor, or other evidence of epinephrine release triggered by emotional factors. Some of the differences in the effects of injury in the conscious individual compared to the effect of the same type of injury in the anesthetized patient can be explained by emotional reactions. Although the emotional trauma of an injury usually stimulates the endocrine response, it sometimes can also inhibit it. Endorphins, which are released in the central nervous system, can also blunt the sensation of pain and the response of the sympathetic nervous system to the pain.

Hypovolemia

Loss of up to 10 percent of the normal blood volume can be readily compensated for by constriction of the capacitance vessels. Since the systemic veins and venules—the capacitance system—normally contain 14 times as much blood as does the capillary bed, loss of up to 10 percent of circulating blood volume from loss of whole blood or plasma and from sequestration of fluid in the interstitial space can be compensated for by an adjustment in the venous tone, accomplished primarily through an intrinsic mechanism. Further loss of circulating volume is sensed in the low-pressure portion of the circulation by stretch (volume) receptors in the atria and by receptors in the great veins and pulmonary vascular system, and later by the arterial baroreceptors in the aortic arch and the carotid bodies. As blood volume decreases, the tonic inhibitory influence that these receptors normally maintain over the medullary vasomotor center is reduced.

The resulting stimulation of the vasomotor center, the hypothalamus, and the anterior and posterior pituitary gland results in a rapid increase in the secretion of ACTH, vasopressin (antidiuretic hormone [ADH]), and growth hormone. Stimulation of the hypothalamus results in enhanced secretion of epinephrine and norepinephrine from the adrenal medulla, of norepinephrine from the autonomic nervous system, of renin from the kidney, and of glucagon from the pancreas.

This mobilization is the body's response to hypovolemia and its attempt to compensate for it initially and to correct it as rapidly as possible by initiating clotting in order to stop blood loss, by repleting blood volume through refilling of capillary beds from the surrounding interstitial spaces, by shunting blood to vital organs, and by minimizing the renal loss of body fluids and sodium.

PLASMA REFILLING. The body's attempt to restore blood volume occurs in two phases. The first phase depends at least in part on hydrostatic forces. The capillary hydrostatic pressure is reduced because of decreased systemic blood pressure, as well as because of the predominantly sympathetically induced precapillary vasoconstriction. Interstitial fluid, which is essentially protein free, moves into the capillaries. It was long thought that the hydrostatic pressure differential between the capillaries and the interstitial fluid was the predominant factor in replacement of fluid volume after hemorrhage, but during the past few years the importance of hyperglycemia, first described by Claude Bernard over 100 years ago, to the plasma refilling process has been recognized. Changes in both the capillary hydrostatic pressure and the plasma osmolality (because of hyperglycemia and increased levels of plasma phosphate, lactate, and pyruvate) are equally important in determining the rate of vascular fluid replacement early after relatively severe hemorrhage (i.e., the first 1 or 2 hours). Since the fluid that is absorbed into the capillaries is relatively protein-free, the hematocrit and plasma oncotic pressures decrease together as the interstitial fluid pressure decreases during this early phase of plasma refilling. A 20 to 50 percent restitution of plasma volume occurs in 2 to 6 hours before an equilibrium is achieved between capillaries and interstitial space, making further restitution of blood volume impossible without the addition of plasma protein.

The second phase of plasma refilling requires movement of plasma protein from the interstitium, either across the capillary membrane or through lymphatic channels. This, in turn, requires an increase in interstitial pressure, which occurs as a result of increased osmolality of the interstitial space. This produces an osmotic gradient between the cells and the surrounding interstitial space and leads to a loss of fluid from the cells to the interstitium. This second phase in the restitution of blood volume, which appears to be critical for cardiovascular stabilization after injury, depends on the metabolic effects of the hormones that are released after injury. Although this response depends critically on increased concentration of cortisol, there is evidence that glucagon, epinephrine, and growth hormone are also involved in this response. The restitution of blood volume is complete in 24 hours (Gann and Amaral). Although the nonglucose elements responsible for the increased concentration of solute have not been completely identified, the changes in concentration of amino acids, of free fatty acids, and sometimes of lactate are sufficiently large to account for at least a portion of the solute. The antianabolic actions of cortisol and glucagon, which impede the entry of amino acid into cells, lead to the catabolic effect, a major component of the metabolic response to injury. In one sense, the protein loss, fat mobilization, and hypoglycemia and carbohydrate depletion associated with injury may be viewed as late metabolic consequences of an initial attempt by the body to restore blood volume through this second phase of restitution. As little as 12 percent reduction in blood volume, which causes no change in blood pressure, is sufficient to initiate absorption of extracellular fluid.

SHUNTING OF BLOOD TO VITAL AREAS. The proportion of cardiac output available to an individual organ under normal circumstances depends on the perfusion pressure and the degree of smooth-muscle tone of the supplying vessels. For most of the body tissues, the pressure-flow relationship is passive; the lower the pressure, the lower the flow. However, in the heart, brain, and kidneys, the flow is maintained at an almost normal level, in spite of lowering of blood pressure to 90 mm Hg. Below this pressure, renal blood flow and glomerular filtration decrease to defend blood flow to the brain and heart. When a pressure of approximately 50 mm Hg is reached, the flow to the brain and heart decreases precipitously. This mechanism, autoregulation, is the body's compensation for reduced perfusion pressure to vital organs (see Chap. 35).

CONSERVATION OF RENAL WATER AND SALT LOSS. Through the action of ADH, aldosterone, renin, and angiotensin, the kidney participates in the body's defense of the blood volume by minimizing the renal loss of sodium and by decreasing (and sometimes stopping) the renal loss of water. The combined action of ADH and aldosterone is extremely effective in preventing renal sodium loss; if sodium is found in the urine of a severely injured patient, it can be assumed that either renal or adrenal failure has occurred. Injured patients continue to produce 800 to 1,200 mOsm solute per day. Since the normal kidney, maximally concentrating in the presence of ADH and aldosterone, can excrete 1 mOsm of solute per ml of urine, urine volume after a major injury should be in the range of 800 to 1,200 ml per day. If urine flow decreases much below 800 ml per day, decreased renal blood flow and glomerular filtration rate of renal failure have occurred.

UNDERPERFUSION. At the same time that the heart, brain, and kidneys are being protected, the splanchnic region and other parts of the body are being hypoperfused. The following mechanisms for the shock-induced pancreatic hypoperfusion have been noted by Lefer and others: passive decrease in vessel lumen diameter in response to a reduced perfusion pressure; vasoconstriction resulting from active increase in sympathetic tone to the splanchnic resistance vessels; release of humoral vasoconstrictor agents such as angiotensin II, TxA_2, and vasopressin; and physical obstruction of the microcirculatory vessels by the formation of microthrombi and platelet aggregation. The primary consequence of these events is reduced perfusion to the pancreas and, to a lesser extent, other splanchnic viscera.

As previously described, autoregulation can maintain the

glomerular filtration rate almost to a normal level in spite of lowering of systemic blood pressure to approximately 90 mm Hg. Unfortunately, any fall in blood pressure below that level decreases the ability of the kidneys to excrete waste products while still protecting extracellular fluid volume. Renal damage as a result of hypotension does not normally occur until arterial pressure falls below 60 mm Hg and activates the renin-angiotensin system. Then, as the body attempts to defend extracellular fluid volume, urine flow stops or decreases to a negligible volume. If abnormal pigments, such as hemoglobin or myoglobin, are present in the plasma, acute renal failure can result (see Chap. 39).

Hypoxia

Respiratory failure does not occur early in the injured patient unless an injury to the chest has been sustained or an injury to the head, neck, or abdomen has interfered with the mechanics of breathing. During the initial phase of the body's response to injury, the pain and emotional response stimulate the respiratory center, leading to an increased rate and depth of breathing. This hyperventilation response, which occurs even before hypoxia or metabolic acidosis has stimulated the center, produces respiratory alkalosis and, at the same time, increases the work of breathing. Between 1 and 2 percent of the total oxygen consumption of the body is normally used for ventilation, but the hyperventilation that occurs after injury (if the injury itself does not prevent it) increases the work of breathing. As ventilatory exchange increases to 15 liters per minute, up to five times as much oxygen is required for each additional liter of ventilation, reflecting the increased work of breathing, even in patients without chest injuries. As cardiac output decreases in patients who are in shock, the muscles of respiration receive inadequate circulation, further impairing their efficiency and resulting in a deterioration of ventilatory function. In the low-flow state in which there is a maximum extraction of oxgyen in the tissues, the low venous oxygen content exceeds the oxygen transport capability of the lungs. Cellular adenosine triphosphate (ATP) production in body tissues is severely curtailed in the absence of aerobic metabolism. Ultimately, the acidosis decreases the responsiveness of the body to sympathomimetic agents.

When hypoxia does occur, it is detected by the chemoreceptors of the medulla and of the carotid and aortic bodies (which are also sensitive to hypercarbia and to acidosis). Chemoreceptor activation stimulates an increased sympathetic output and the increased production of other hormones.

Temperature

The temperature of the environment in which an injury occurs or to which a victim is subjected after injury can have a profound effect on the body's response to it. Extremes of ambient temperature can directly trigger neuroendocrine responses or they can stimulate these reflexes indirectly through changes in the core temperature, sensed in the hypothalamus. Core temperature change can result not only from alterations in ambient temperature but also from the loss of the normal thermal insulating barrier (burns), from inadequate hepatic blood flow (hypovolemia) or substrate supply (starvation), or from inadequate peripheral vasconstriction or vasodilation (sepsis). Heat and cold by themselves can each produce changes in the output of many hormones, including ACTH, cortisol, aldosterone, ADH, epinephrine, norepinephrine, and thyroxine (Gann). A hot or cold environment produces striking changes in skin circulation, sometimes with associated fluid and electrolyte losses. Fever increases cardiac work and oxygen consumption, which are associated with increased catabolism and water and salt loss.

Substrates or Damaged Tissue

The primary substrate alteration that activates neuroendocrine reflexes is the change in the plasma glucose concentration. A decrease in this concentration, sensed by receptors in the hypothalamus and in the pancreas, stimulates the release of catecholamines, growth hormone, cortisol, ACTH, beta endorphin, and vasopressin through central pathways (hypothalamus and autonomic nervous system) and stimulates the release of glucagon, both by central (autonomic nervous system) and peripheral (direct pancreatic activation) pathways. In addition, the secretion of insulin is inhibited by central pathways (autonomic nervous system) and by the pancreas itself.

By mechanisms that are not completely understood, changes in the concentration of individual amino acids also produce alterations in the secretion of various hormones. Amino acids exert an important role in the neuroendocrine response as well, because they are the parent compound for a number of hormonal agents and neurotransmitters (Gann).

The damaged tissues of the wound elicit additional signals that profoundly affect the body's response to injury. Reporting in 1918 and 1919 on some of his studies of battlefield casualties, Walter Cannon observed that the degree of shock always appeared worse than the amount of measured or predicted blood loss. He postulated that a toxic material was given off by smashed and dying tissue and probably came from the wound. His observations are still valid. Products are released from damaged tissue, and inflammatory mediators—the eicosanoids, histamine, the kinins, serotonin, interleukin-1, tumor necrosis factor (TNF), and others—are activated as part of the body's response to injury. The inflammatory mediators, which combine local with systemic effects, are discussed in Chap. 1. If the body's defenses are overwhelmed, these mediators contribute to the development of multisystem organ failure, which is discussed in the second part of this chapter.

Infection

Infection does not always accompany injury, but it is often a major contributor to the body's response. As discussed in Chap. 1, it may stimulate the neuroendocrine system directly through the action of endotoxin or of cytokines, such as tumor necrosis factor or interleukin-1. It also may have indirect effects through secondary changes in blood volume, oxygen concentration, or pain.

Early Hormonal Responses to Injury

The body's response to injury is graded; the more severe the injury, the greater the response. The response will generally increase until a maximum level is reached; injury severity above this level will simply result in a maximum response (Wilmore). Physiologic reserve decreases as the extent of

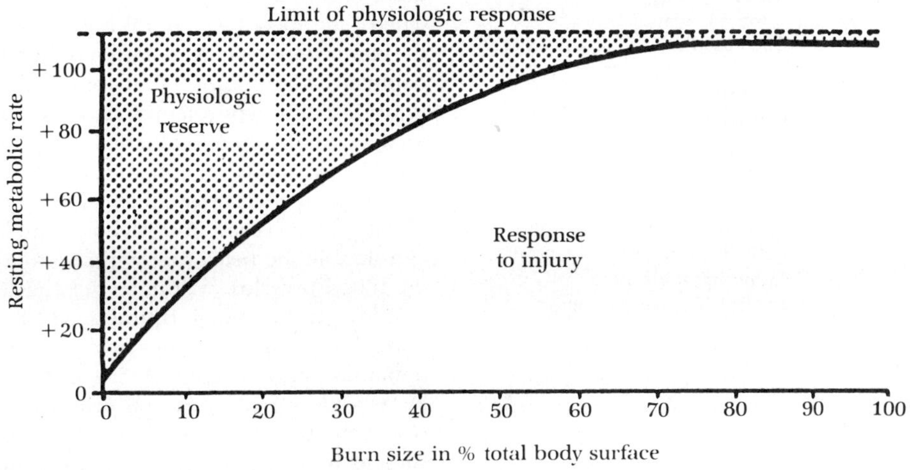

Fig. 40-18. The body's response to injury in relation to its physiologic reserve. The physiologic reserve diminishes as the extent of injury increases. (From D. W. Wilmore. The metabolic management of the critically ill. New York: Plenum, 1971.)

injury increases. Because patients with extensive injuries approach maximal responses, limited physiologic reserve is present to adjust to subsequent complications (Fig. 40-18). These patients are among the group in which multisystem organ failure is likely to develop (see the second section of this chapter).

The intensity of the initial hormonal responses to injury depends on the severity of the injury. These responses include the release of ACTH, cortisol, epinephrine, norepinephrine, glucagon, renin, angiotensin, aldosterone, and growth hormone (Table 40-14). They also include the suppression of other hormones such as insulin. As noted above, most injuries also recruit inflammatory mediators, with combined local and systemic effects (Table 40-15).

Corticotropin Releasing Factor, ACTH, and Cortisol

The mechanisms by which the body increases the level of circulating glucocorticoids in response to injury or other stress are essential for survival. In the injured patient, a number of stimuli, including pain, emotional stimuli, and pressure-sensitive baroreceptor signals, stimulate the paraventricular nuclei of the hypothalamus to produce corticotropin releasing factor, which, in turn, activates the anterior pituitary gland to synthesize ACTH and release it into the circulation. Cortisol, the most prominent glucocorticoid, is synthesized in cells of the adrenal cortex and secreted very rapidly into the circulation (within a minute or two) after the adrenal has been stimulated by ACTH. ACTH production can also be potentiated by angiotensin II, vasopressin, possibly oxytocin, and also possibly interleukin-1. ACTH release is inhibited by cortisol and by ACTH itself.

Cortisol has widespread effects on the metabolism and utilization of glucose, amino acids, and fatty acids. Along with the catecholamines and glucagon, it increases the availability of glucose during the early stages after injury in order to maintain hyperglycemia, or at least euglycemia, at that time. In the liver, it inhibits the action of insulin and enhances gluconeogenesis by a number of mechanisms, partly by potentiating the action of glucagon and epinephrine. It

Table 40-14. Some metabolic effects of hormones with generally increased secretion in trauma

Hormone	Proteolysis (in muscle)	Gluconeogenesis (in liver and kidney)	Glycolysis		Glycogenolysis		Lipolysis (adipose tissue, liver, muscle)	Insulin antagonism	Insulin secretion	Plasma sodium	Plasma potassium	Water retention
			Muscle	Adipose tissue	Liver	Muscle						
ACTH-cortisol	+ + +	+ + +	0	0	—	0	+ + +	+ +	+ +	+	0	0
Renin-aldosterone			—							+ + +	00	
Epinephrine Norepinephrine	+	+ +[a]	0	+ +	+	+ +	+ + + +[a]	+ + +	0	+	0	
ADH											+ + + +	
Growth hormone	0		0	+ +			+ +[a]	+ +	+ + +			
Glucagon	+	+ + +[a]	0		+ + + +[b]		+ +[a]		+ + +			

[a]Only in the presence of the adrenal corticosteroids.
[b]By stimulating catecholamine secretion.
Note: Lipolysis stimulates gluconeogenesis; + to + + + + = stimulates or increases; 0 or 00 = antagonizes or decreases.
Source: D. S. Gann. Endocrine and Metabolic Responses to Injury. In S. I. Schwartz (ed.), *Principles of Surgery* (3rd ed.). New York: McGraw-Hill, 1979. P. 17. Reproduced with permission.

Table 40-15. Neuroendocrine response

Increased release	Decreased release or unchanged
Epinephrine	Insulin
Norepinephrine	Estrogen
Dopamine	Testosterone
Glucagon	Thyroxine
Renin	T_3
Angiotensin	Thyroid-stimulating hormone
Vasopressin	Follicle-stimulating hormone
ACTH	Luteinizing hormone
Cortisol	Insulin-like growth factor
Aldosterone	
Beta endorphin	
Growth hormone	
Prolactin	
Somatostatin	
Eicosanoids	
Histamine	
Kinins	
Serotonin	
Interleukin-1	
TNF	

Source: D. S. Gann and J. F. Amaral. Endocrine and Metabolic Responses to Injury. In S. I. Schwartz, G. T. Shires, and F. C. Spencer (eds.), *Principles of Surgery* (5th ed.). New York: McGraw-Hill, 1989. Reproduced with permission.

also inhibits insulin-mediated glucose uptake in skeletal muscle tissue, and, in addition, it induces proteolysis in skeletal muscles by reducing the uptake and increasing the release of amino acids by these muscles. In adipose tissue, cortisol increases lipolysis through its potentiating action on other lipolytic hormones such as epinephrine and growth hormone and it also decreases glucose uptake in adipose tissue. Therefore, cortisol appears to exert an important role in maintaining at least euglycemia during stressful conditions by increasing the availability of gluconeogenic substrates to the liver.

The pattern of cortisol increase following injury closely parallels that observed for ACTH. In pure hypovolemia, if the blood volume is restored quickly, the plasma cortisol concentration returns rapidly to normal. Commonly, the cortisol level is elevated for a few days after hemorrhage and for less than one week following soft-tissue trauma. The plasma concentration of cortisol remains elevated for up to four weeks after thermal injury. Supervening infection, however, will prolong the increase in plasma cortisol in all these injuries (Gann).

Catecholamines

One of the most basic of all hormonal responses to stress is the elaboration of catecholamines—epinephrine and norepinephrine. Many stimuli that are present to some degree after injury—pain, hypovolemia, hypoglycemia, hypoxemia, fear, anxiety, infection, and others—reach the hypothalamus, are quickly integrated there, and then are released by nerve pathways to effect sympathetic control rapidly and intensely. The rapid increase in catecholamine secretion after injury can double the heart rate within 3 to 5 seconds and double the blood pressure within as little as 10 to 15 seconds.

Epinephrine, which is produced almost exclusively by the adrenal medulla, functions primarily as a hormone, whereas dopamine and norepinephrine, produced for the most part by nerve terminals, function primarily as neurotransmitters. Norepinephrine exerts direct effects on innervated tissue, such as blood vessels and visceral organs, as it is elaborated from nerve endings to these structures. Its effects depend on the localization of the nerve endings. If stimulation is sustained, some norepinephrine diffuses into the bloodstream and thereby may exert effects on distant organs. Catecholamines increase immediately after injury and achieve peak concentrations at about 24 to 48 hours after injury, from which time they decrease to baseline levels. The increase appears to be related to the severity of injury.

Epinephrine appears to exert a major role in stress-induced hyperglycemia by increasing glucose production in the liver and decreasing glucose uptake in peripheral tissues. It stimulates glycogenolysis in the liver and skeletal muscle. (This process in muscles leads to the formation of lactic acid.) In the liver it enhances gluconeogenesis, lipolysis, and ketogenesis. It stimulates lipolysis in adipose tissue, stimulates glycogenolysis, and inhibits insulin-stimulated glucose uptake in skeletal muscle. The correlation between plasma glucose concentrations after injury and plasma catecholamine concentrations is very strong.

Hemodynamic effects of catecholamines include venous and arterial vasoconstriction, mediated by α_1 receptors, and arterial vasodilation of other vessels, such as the coronary arteries and arteries to skeletal muscle, mediated by β_2 receptors. They also increase myocardial rate, contractility, and conductivity, under the mediation of β_1 receptors (Table 40-16).

Catecholamines also modulate the production of other hormones. In addition to inhibiting the insulin-mediated uptake of glucose by skeletal muscle, they also inhibit the secretion of insulin by the pancreas. Catecholamine stimulation of the pancreas results in increased secretion of glucagon. Catecholamines also increase the release of renin.

Table 40-16. Cardiovascular effects of adrenergic stimulation

Receptor site	Systemic arteries	Pulmonary arteries	Veins	Heart
$Alpha_1$	Constriction (+ + +)	Constriction (+)	Constriction (+ +)	0
$Beta_1$	0	Constriction (secondary to renin secretion in kidneys)	0	↑ Rate ↑ Contractility (+ + +) ↑ Conductivity (+ + +)
$Beta_2$	Dilatation (+ +)	Dilatation (+)	Dilatation (+ +)	0

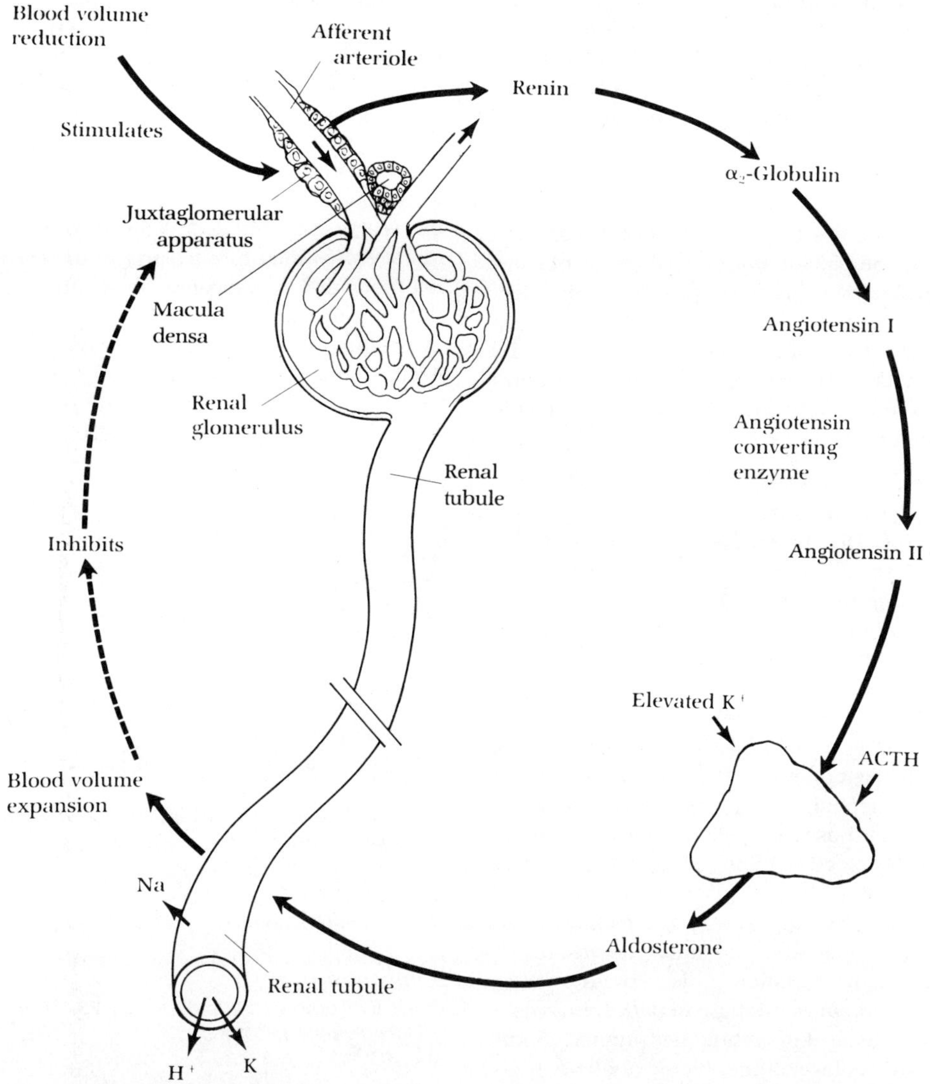

Fig. 40-19. Schematic diagram of the renin-aldosterone-angiotensin system. Renin is secreted in the cells of the juxtaglomerular apparatus in response to increased sympathetic stimulation of the juxtaglomerular arterioles, decreased renal arterial perfusion pressure, and/or decreased delivery of sodium to the macula densa. Aldosterone is secreted in the adrenal cortex in response to elevation in levels of ACTH, angiotensin II, and potassium.

Glucagon

Although Wilmore noted an immediate increase in plasma glucagon concentration that correlated with plasma glucose concentration after thermal injury, most studies of glucagon metabolism following nonthermal injury have reported no increase in plasma glucagon until 12 hours after injury (Gann and Amaral). Glucagon is released from the alpha islet cells of the pancreas and acts, along with insulin, to ensure a steady supply of substrate from the liver. It stimulates gluconeogenesis in the liver and facilitates hepatic amino acid extraction. When insulin production in the pancreas is stimulated, glucagon is suppressed, favoring anabolism and protein conservation, and when glucagon is elaborated relative to insulin, there is glycogenolysis and gluconeogenesis at the expense of protein biosynthesis.

Insulin

Although a primary effect of insulin is in the membrane transport and intracellular metabolism of glucose, it also plays an important role in the synthesis of protein and of fat. Under normal conditions, it is stored in the pancreas and released into the portal venous blood, exposing the liver to high insulin concentrations. Approximately 50 percent of the insulin is captured and degraded by the liver, while the remaining insulin exerts its effect on peripheral tissue, mainly skeletal muscle and adipose tissue. In early injury, insulin concentrations are low, even in the face of hyperglycemia, due to regulation of the endocrine pancreas by the sympathetic nervous system; in this case, insulin release is inhibited by alpha-adrenergic stimulation. Insulin inhibition accounts in part for the posttraumatic hyperglycemia and thus allows glucose to be utilized primarily by noninsulin-mediated tissue—that is, the brain and the peripheral nervous system (Gann and Amaral).

Growth Hormone

Tissue injury and hemorrhage are potent stimuli for the release of growth hormone from the anterior pituitary gland.

In the injured patient, stress and other hormones, such as vasopressin and ACTH, can stimulate its secretion, so it is not surprising that the secretion of growth hormone is increased in virtually all forms of injury. Its plasma concentration remains elevated for approximately 24 hours after injury and then returns to normal. Growth hormone increases plasma glucose concentration by an inhibition of glucose transport in liver and skeletal muscle. It increases plasma fatty acids and ketone bodies by stimulation of lipolysis in adipose tissue and by the potentiation of the actions of catecholamines on adipose tissue. As part of its catabolic effect on carbohydrate and lipid metabolism, it increases plasma ketone bodies by stimulation of ketogenesis in the liver. Its actions on protein metabolism are anabolic, as it promotes protein synthesis in the liver and in skeletal muscle after the acute phase of injury has passed (Gann and Amaral).

Vasopressin (Antidiuretic Hormone)

Antidiuretic hormone (ADH) is released from the posterior pituitary in response to an increase in plasma osmolality (mediated by the osmoreceptors of the hypothalamus) or to decreased blood volume (mediated by the low-pressure receptors in the left atrium, the great veins, and the pulmonary vessels). Pain, anxiety, and other emotions that are aroused from trauma can also stimulate its release. ADH increases the permeability of the cells of the distal tubules and collecting ducts of the kidneys so that water in the tubule enters the hypertonic interstitium (see Chap. 35). The urine becomes concentrated and its volume decreases as the body attempts to increase the blood volume and lower the osmolality of body fluids.

In addition to its osmoregulation function, vasopressin also has vasoactive and metabolic functions. Its vasoactive properties are important in regulation of blood pressure after hemorrhage because it mediates increase in peripheral vasoconstriction, especially in the splanchnic bed, under conditions of reduced intravascular volume. Its metabolic actions include the stimulation of hepatic glycogenolysis and gluconeogenesis.

Renin

Renin is secreted in the cells of the juxtaglomerular apparatus of the preglomerular afferent arteriole (Fig. 40-19). Its release can be triggered by at least three mechanisms: increased sympathetic stimulation of the juxtaglomerular arterioles, decreased renal arterial perfusion pressure, and decreased delivery of sodium to the macula densa of the distal tubule. The macula densa is a group of modified cells of the distal tubule immediately adjacent to the juxtaglomerular apparatus of the afferent arterioles. The renin acts as an enzyme in the liver to convert angiotensinogen, an α_2 globulin normally found in the plasma, into angiotensin I. Then most of the angiotensin I is converted in the lung or in the plasma to angiotensin II, the most powerful hypertensive agent known. (Its pressure activity is about 200 times that of norepinephrine.) It increases the contractility of the heart and constricts the veins, thereby reducing the capacity of the circulatory system; it also constricts arterioles, thus limiting the excretion of water and sodium by decreasing glomerular filtration. Angiotensin II is an important stimulus for aldosterone secretion by the adrenal cortex, and it also acts to increase the production of ACTH and of ADH from the pituitary gland (see Chap. 35).

Aldosterone

Aldosterone, secreted by the adrenal cortex in response to injury, acts in the early distal convoluted tubule to increase the reabsorption of sodium and of chloride, and in the late distal convoluted tubules and in the early collecting ducts to promote the reabsorption of sodium and the excretion of potassium and hydrogen ions (see Fig. 40-19). This is an important mechanism since it is the principal means of renal excretion of potassium and acid, which build up rapidly in the injured patient. Aldosterone is secreted in response to three factors: angiotensin II, ACTH, and potassium.

SELECTED READING

Epidemiology of Trauma and Mechanisms of Injury

Accidental Death and Disability: The Neglected Disease of Modern Society. Committee on Trauma and Committee on Shock, Division of Medical Sciences, National Academy of Sciences, National Research Council, 1966.

Baker, CC, et al. Epidemiology of trauma deaths. *Am J Surg* 140:144, 1980.

Injury in America: A Continuing Public Health Problem. Committee on Trauma Research, Commission of Life Sciences, National Research Council and the Institute of Medicine, National Academy Press, 1985.

National Safety Council. *Accident Facts,* 1989.

Blunt Injury

Blair, E, Topuzlo, C, and Deane, RS. Major blunt chest trauma. *Curr Probl Surg.* 1969.

Blaisdell, FW, and Trunkey, DD (eds). *Trauma Management Abdominal Trauma,* Vol 1. New York: Thieme-Stratton, 1982.

Brinkhouse, KM (ed). *Accident Pathology.* Proceedings of an International Conference, No. FH-11-6595, National Highway Safety Bureau, 1968.

DeHaven, H. Mechanical analysis of survival in falls from heights of fifty to one hundred and fifty feet. *War Med* 2:586, 1942.

Foley, RW, Harris, LS, and Pilcher, DB. Abdominal injuries in automobile accidents: Review of care of fatally injured patients. *J Trauma* 17:611, 1977.

Gurdjian, ES, et al (eds). *Impact Injury and Crash Protection.* Springfield, IL: Thomas, 1970.

Hohl, M. Soft tissue injuries of the neck. *Clin Orthop* 109:42, 1975.

Kulowski, J. *Crash Injuries.* Springfield, IL: Thomas, 1960.

Stapp, JP. Voluntary Human Tolerance Levels. In ES Gurdjian, et al (eds), *Impact Injury and Crash Protection.* Springfield, IL: Thomas, 1970. P. 308.

Trunkey, DD. Torso trauma. *Curr Prob Surg* 24:215, 1987.

Penetrating Injury

Barach, E, Tomlanovich, M, and Nowak, R. Ballistics: A pathophysiologic examination of the wounding mechanisms of firearms: I. *J Trauma* 26:255, 1986.

Barach, E, Tomlanovich, M, and Nowak, R. Ballistics: A pathophysiologic examination of the wounding mechanisms of firearms: II. *J Trauma* 26:374, 1986.

DeMuth, WE, Jr. Bullet velocity and design as determinants of wounding capability: An experimental study. *J Trauma* 6:222, 1966.

DeMuth, WE, Jr, and Smith, JM. High-velocity bullet wounds of muscle and bone: The basis of rational early treatment. *J Trauma* 6:744, 1966.

Mays, ET. *Clinical Evaluation of the Critically Injured.* Springfield, IL: Thomas, 1975.

Walt, AJ, and Grifka, TJ. Blunt Abdominal Injury: A Review of 307 Cases. In ES Gurdjian, et al (ed), *Impact Injury and Crash Protection.* Springfield, IL: Thomas, 1970. P 101.

The Body's Response to Injury: Stimuli and Initial Responses

Local Responses

Austin, KF. The heterogeneity of mast cell populations and products. *Hosp Pract* 19:135, 1984.

Cannon, WB. The course of events in secondary wound shock. *JAMA* 73:174, 1919.

Davis, JM, and Dineen, P. Chemoattractants in Trauma. In P Dineen and G Hildick-Smith (eds), *The Surgical Wound.* Philadelphia: Lea & Febiger, 1981. P. 26.

Lewis, RA, and Austin, KF. Mediation of local homeostasis and inflammation by leukotrienes and other mast-cell dependent compounds. *Nature* 293:103, 1981.

Moncada, S, and Vane, JR. Prostacyclin, Platelet Aggregation, and Thrombosis. In G deGaetano and S Garattini (eds), *Platelets: A Multidisciplinary Approach.* New York: Raven Press, 1978. P 239.

Weissman, G, Smolen, JE, and Korchak, MM. Release of inflammatory mediators from stimulated neutrophils. *N Engl J Med* 303:27, 1987.

Yurt, RW. Role of the Mast Cell in Traumas. In P Dineen and G Hildick-Smith (eds), *The Surgical Wound.* Philadelphia: Lea & Febiger, 1981. P. 37.

Systemic Responses

Chaudry, IH, and Baue, AE. Overview of hemorrhagic shock. In RA Cowley and BF Trump (eds), *Pathophysiology of Shock, Anoxia, and Ischemia.* Baltimore: Williams & Wilkins, 1982. P 203.

Cowley, RA, and Trump, BF (eds). *Pathophysiology of Shock, Anoxia, and Ischemia.* Baltimore: Williams & Wilkins, 1982.

Drucker, WR, Chadwick, CDJ, and Gann, DS. Transcapillary refill in hemorrhage and shock. *Arch Surg* 116:1344, 1981.

Egdahl, RH. Pituitary-adrenal response following trauma to the isolated leg. *Surgery* 46:9, 1959.

Gann, DS, and Amaral, JF. Endocrine and Metabolic Responses to Injury. In SI Schwartz, GT Shires, and FC Spencer (eds), *Principles of Surgery* (5th ed). New York: McGraw-Hill, 1989.

Lefer, AM. Vascular Mediators in Ischemia and Shock. In RA Cowley and BF Trump (eds), *Pathophysiology of Shock, Anoxia, and Ischemia.* Baltimore: Williams & Wilkins, 1982. P 165.

Mason, J, and Thurau, K. Physiological Mechanisms Responsible for the Adjustment of Renal Function During Acute Renal Failure. Sixth International Congress on Nephrology. Stuttgart: Symposium Verlag, 1975. P 100.

Pirkle, JC, and Gann, DS. Restitution of blood volume after hemorrhage: Role of the adrenal cortex. *Am J Physiol* 230:1683, 1976.

Powers, SR. Maintenance of renal function following massive trauma. *J Trauma* 10:554, 1979.

Trunkey, DD. Inflammation and trauma. *Arch Surg* 123:1517, 1988.

Wilmore, DW. Homeostasis: Bodily Changes in Trauma and Surgery. In DC Sabiston (ed), *Textbook of Surgery* (13th ed). Philadelphia: Saunders, 1986.

POSTTRAUMATIC MULTISYSTEM ORGAN FAILURE

Malcolm DeCamp, Jr.
Robert H. Demling

Multisystem organ failure (MSOF) is a syndrome of progressive, sequential failure of physiologic organ systems after a traumatic or septic insult. It affects a wide variety of critically injured or ill patients and represents a final common pathway for traumatic, surgical, and medical illness. In surgical units alone, MSOF is the most common cause of death, with a mortality rate well in excess of 60 percent. A better understanding of the syndrome of MSOF can assist the emergency physician in successfully resuscitating the critically ill patient, while minimizing the risk of subsequent dysfunction of organ systems.

The emergence of MSOF as a significant health problem is due in part to a more aggressive approach to resuscitation of traumatized patients and to an understanding of the need to volume-load the septic patient. These therapeutic maneuvers have significantly altered the causes of postresuscitation mortality. In the 1950s, renal failure was a common cause of death after successful initial therapy for trauma. With improved emergency medical transport systems and a better understanding of the need for rapid intravascular volume restoration, prolonged hypovolemic shock states were eliminated. In the 1960s, respiratory failure predominated as a frequent cause of death. Early hypoxemic demise was averted with the advent of mechanical ventilation, but the adult respiratory distress syndrome (ARDS) often developed. Mortality rates still approached 70 percent for what appeared to be single-organ failure. The cause of death in ARDS in these days was failure of gas exchange. Refinements in ventilator management, the evolution of positive end-expiratory pressure (PEEP), and an aggressive approach to invasive hemodynamic monitoring and cardiopulmonary support have markedly decreased the incidence of early posttraumatic pulmonary death.

Beginning in the 1970s, a more chronic form of ARDS evolved, characterized by increased protein permeability in the pulmonary microcirculation (and other systemic tissue beds). Associated with this capillary leak syndrome, in certain patients a hyperdynamic state developed that we recognize as sepsis, which is manifested by increased cardiac output and decreased systemic vascular resistance. In the late 1970s and on into the 1980s, clinicians and their basic science colleagues further defined the metabolic, endocrine, and immune responses of patients who appeared "septic." The MSOF victim then became broadly defined as the patient who, after a traumatic or septic insult, develops a hyperdynamic circulation, is hypermetabolic, and shows evidence of dysfunction in several physiologic organ systems.

Multisystem organ failure was first described as a discrete entity in 1973 by Tilney and associates. They discussed a series of patients who had sequential organ-system failure after suffering postoperative septic complications. The same course has unfortunately been recapitulated in series of patients after multiple trauma or severe burns. The system involved most prominently remains the lungs, followed closely

Table 40-17. Clinical presentation of multisystem organ failure

Stage 1 (sepsis syndrome)	Onset hours to days after insult
Cardiovascular	Hyperdynamic state Increased cardiac output Decreased systemic vascular resistance Risk of splanchnic hypoperfusion Increased fluid requirements (third space)
Respiratory	Early ARDS Tachypnea Metabolic alkalosis
Renal function	Possible oliguria No chemical abnormalities
Hepatic function	Increased acute-phase protein synthesis Fibronectin consumption No measured change in liver function tests
Gastrointestinal	Gastric ileus common No bleeding Potential for ongoing mucosal ischemia and gut leak, especially if not enterally fed
Central nervous system	No change
Metabolism	Increased oxygen consumption per minute ($\dot{V}O_2$) Hypermetabolism catabolism Mild glucose intolerance No lactic acidosis
Hematology	Probable leukocytosis Decreased red cell production
Stage 2 (early MSOF)	Onset 7–14 days after insult
Cardiovascular	Persistent hyperdynamic state O_2 consumption dependent on O_2 delivery
Respiratory	ARDS with need for PEEP and ventilatory support Increased shunt
Renal function	Mild increase in blood urea nitrogen (BUN) Decreased creatinine clearance even with normal creatinine
Hepatic function	Chemical jaundice Cholestasis if not fed enterally
Gastointestinal	Continued ileus Ongoing mucosal leak Possible early mucosal bleeding
Central nervous system	Lethargic or confused
Metabolism	Negative nitrogen balance Visceral and skeletal catabolism Glucose intolerance Mild to moderate lactic acidosis
Hematology	Anemia, thrombocytopenia Leukocytosis or leukopenia possible
Stage 3 (established MSOF)	Onset 2 weeks to months after insult
Cardiovascular	Unstable circulation Often requires fluid and inotropes Anasarca common
Respiratory	Progressive ARDS Early fibrosis, decreased compliance Nosocomial pneumonias
Renal function	Rising BUN and creatinine Oliguria common May need dialysis
Hepatic function	Clinically jaundiced Cholestasis Coagulopathy possible
Gastrointestinal	Stress ulceration and bleeding Persistent ileus Feeding intolerance
Central nervous system	Obtunded, may be comatose

Table 40-17 (continued)

Metabolism	Lactic acidosis Hyperglycemia Poor O_2 extraction
Hematology	Coagulopathy, disseminated intravascular coagulation (DIC) common
Stage 4 (preterminal MSOF)	Onset weeks to months after insult
Cardiovascular	Hypotensive; refractory to fluid, inotropes, and alpha-agonists
Respiratory	Persistent ARDS Pneumonias common Barotrauma
Renal function	Oliguric renal failure
Hepatic function	Hypometabolism Hypoglycemic as gluconeogenesis fails Encephalopathic
Gastrointestinal	Intermittent bleeding
Central nervous system	Coma
Metabolism	Severe lactic acidosis Falling oxygen consumption
Hematology	DIC

by the liver and gastrointestinal tract. The kidneys, bone marrow, central nervous system, heart, and endocrine and immune systems are also at risk.

The time course over which frank MSOF develops is often weeks to months after injury, with the emphasis on sequential rather than simultaneous dysfunction. Such a broad clinical entity can be viewed in stages, with stage 1 being indistinguishable from early sepsis without discrete organ failure. Stage 2 can be termed early MSOF, with multiple quantifiable defects in organ functions. Stage 3 is established MSOF, with obvious failure of physiologic systems, some approaching end stage. Stage 4 is a preterminal or moribund condition characterized by cardiovascular collapse and a refractory hypometabolic state. These stages can be reviewed in Table 40-17 and are discussed in greater detail later.

PATHOPHYSIOLOGY

Multisystem organ failure is characterized by a hyperdynamic, hypermetabolic state similar to that seen in sepsis. While invasive infection remains the most common initiating factor in the development of MSOF, it is not obligate. It is now clear that a septic state can be induced by any agent that activates the host inflammatory process. Bacteria, endotoxins, exotoxins, viruses, fungi, and necrotic tissue have all been found to produce a similar systemic response. Positive blood cultures in patients with established MSOF are present in only 50 percent of cases. The term *sepsis syndrome* has evolved to reflect the fact that ongoing infection, although frequently present, is not essential for initiating or perpetuating progressive organ failure. An endogenous, systemic host inflammatory response modulated by a cascade of soluble lipid and peptide mediators appears to be the pathway that links the sepsis syndrome with MSOF. Various autocrine, paracrine, and endocrine mediator loops are active in MSOF. The factors responsible are both lipid and protein in chemical composition and are derived from a wide range of tissues and cell types. Many of these mediators and their actions are discussed in detail in the first section of this chapter and can be reviewed in Table 40-18 and Fig. 40-20.

Table 40-18. Inflammatory mediators active in multisystem organ failure

Mediator	Symbol	Action
Complement	C_{5a}	Neutrophil chemotaxis
Oxygen radicals	H_2O_2 O_2^- $OH^{\cdot}$	Cell membrane disruption
Proteases		Denatures cellular proteins
Clotting factors	I–XII	Intravascular coagulation
Bradykinin		Local vasodilation
Serotonin		Local vasoconstriction
Eicosanoids		
Prostacyclin	PGI	Vasodilation
Prostaglandin E_2	PGE_2	Thermoregulation Immune modulation
Thromboxane	TxA_2 TxB_2	Vasoconstriction
Leukotriene B_4	LTB_4	Neutrophil chemotaxis
Peptidoleukotrienes	LTC_4 LTD_4	Vasoconstriction and bronchoconstriction
Platelet activating factors	PAF	Vasoactive, increased permeability
Interleukin-1	IL-1	Pyrogenic, neutrophil chemotaxis
Tumor necrosis factor	TNF	Permeability edema Neutrophil chemotaxis Tissue necrosis

Ischemia-Reperfusion Injury

Necrotic or injured tissues as a consequence of trauma or burns are obvious potent stimulators of an inflammatory response. The attendant hypovolemic state, with or without measured hypotension, that accompanies these injuries pre-

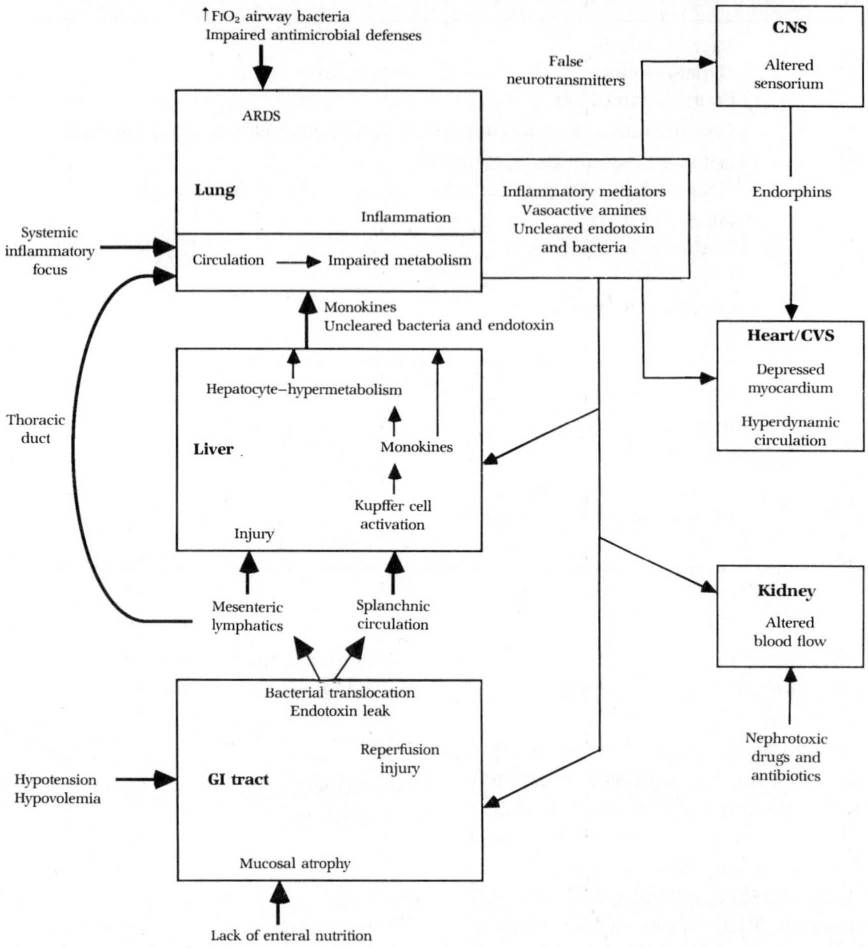

Fig. 40-20. Self-perpetuation process in MSOF. (FIO_2 = inspired oxygen concentration; CNS = central nervous system; CVS = cardiovascular system.)

pares the host for a second insult after adequate volume resuscitation. This insult is known as *reperfusion injury*. There is a growing body of literature documenting the detrimental effects that the products of reperfusion have on local organ function as well as the systemic consequences if these locally generated oxidants and mediators gain access to the circulation. After the volume resuscitation of a traumatized or burned patient, the early manifestations of the sepsis syndrome (from which MSOF evolves) can be blamed on reperfusion-generated mediators. Furthermore, the severity of this reperfusion injury is directly proportional to the volume of tissue that was rendered ischemic and the length of the ischemic interval. The evolution to MSOF over the ensuing days to weeks depends on the physician's ability to limit the reperfusion injury and control the host inflammatory response.

The principal mediators implicated in reperfusion injury include the prostanoids (thromboxanes) and oxygen radicals [hydrogen peroxide (H_2O_2), superoxide anion O_2^-, hydroxyl radical ($OH^{\bullet}$)]. After reperfusion, thromboxanes are generated from arachidonic acid liberated from cell membranes by the action of phospholipase A. These, in turn, cause local arteriolar constriction, resulting in decreased microvascular blood flow and further tissue injury. Also during ischemia, intracellular adenosine triphosphate (ATP) stores are consumed. If oxygen is restored early, the intracellular energy crisis is averted and normal cell function can resume. With prolonged ischemia, altered purine metabolism intervenes and a severe ATP deficit ensues. Residual ATP is broken down into xanthine and hypoxanthine. Concurrently in the anaerobic environment, xanthine dehydrogenase is converted to xanthine-hypoxanthine oxidase. On reperfusion, there is an influx of oxygen. In the presence of excess intracellular xanthine and hypoxanthine and catalyzed by xanthine oxidase, uric acid, O_2^- and H_2O_2 are generated. If local radical production exceeds local antioxidant defenses, then further cell damage occurs. The most common site of oxidant injury is the cell membrane where lipid peroxidation occurs. Circulating lipid peroxides have been detected after trauma and burns, underscoring the role that ischemia-reperfusion injury may play in system-wide dysfunction after injury. The process of oxygen radical–mediated reperfusion injury is schematically represented in Fig. 40-21.

SPECIFIC ORGAN FAILURE

Despite the obvious complexities of mediator-induced MSOF, most organ systems involved fail along well-defined pathways (Table 40-19). In most clinical series, the lungs

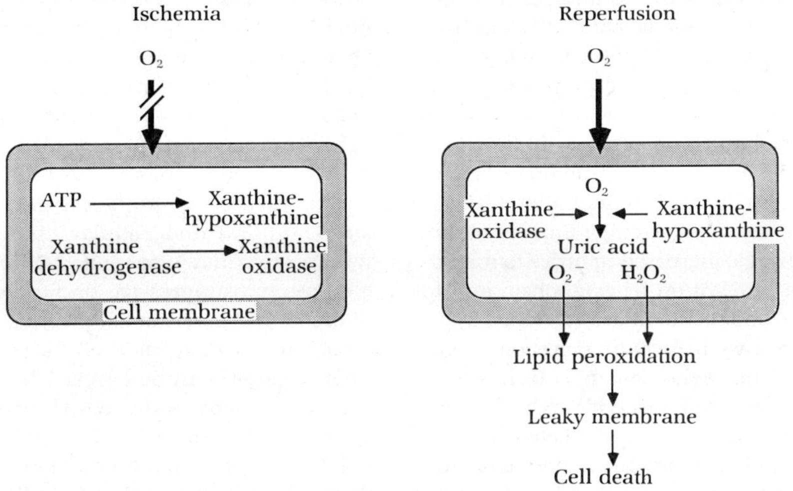

Fig. 40-21. Posttraumatic ischemia-reperfusion injury.

Table 40-19. Specific organ failure in multisystem organ failure

Organ	Pathophysiology	Result
Lung	↑ Permeability, $\dot{V}/Q$ mismatch	↓ Compliance, ↓ PO_2
	↓ Metabolism of vasoactive substances	Hemodynamic instability
	Antimicrobial dysfunction	Nosocomial pneumonia
Liver	Early increase	Hypermetabolism
Synthetic		↑ Acute-phase proteins
	Late decrease	Jaundice, coagulopathy
	↓ IgA	↑ Gut bacteria
	↓ Bile salts	↑ Gut endotoxin
Immunologic	Kupffer cell activation	Hepatocyte depression
		Monokine expression
		Peripheral catabolism
	↓ Fibronectin, ↓ phagocytosis	Bacteremia, endotoxemia
		Microvascular emboli
Gastrointestinal tract	Ischemia-reperfusion	↑ Luminal bacteria and endotoxin
	Antacids, antibiotics, ↓ IgA	Bacteria and endotoxin/leak
	Mucosal atrophy and permeability	Stress bleeding
Kidney	Hypovolemia	Azotemia, ± oliguria
	Altered blood flow away from cortex	
	Nephrotoxic drugs	
Heart	Circulating myocardial depressant factor	↓ Ejection fraction
Central nervous system	Circulating false neurotransmitters	Altered sensorium
	Endogenous opioid-mimetics	Labile hemodynamics
Immune system	↑ PGE_2 production and sensitivity	Immune suppression
	↓ Il-2 elaboration from T cells	

have been found to be the first organ to fail, strongly suggesting that the respiratory failure (ARDS) is a key component to subsequent organ injury. The pulmonary failure is characterized by increased permeability of the lung microvasculature to both protein and water, leading to decreased lung compliance, hypoxia, and ventilation-perfusion mismatch. With current ventilator techniques, life-threatening hypoxia and hypercapnia can usually be avoided. A defect in peripheral tissue oxygen extraction from hemoglobin becomes evident. This is a critical observation and is compelling circumstantial evidence linking ARDS with a systemic perfusion defect. The ARDS lung may also act as a source of inflammatory mediators, which in turn lead to distant organ injury, as an intense alveolar and interstitial macrophage and neutrophil infiltration are characteristically seen. Paradoxically, this inflammatory cell infiltrate is associated with an impairment in overall lung antimicrobial capability. This, in turn, makes nosocomial pneumonia a frequent complication, thus providing a continued inflammatory stimulus to drive the MSOF process forward. Finally, the lung fails metabolically, with impaired clearance of vasodilator prostanoids and bradykinin and with decreased production of angiotensin II secondary to angiotensin converting enzyme inhibition or destruction. In about 60 percent of patients with ARDS, at least early evidence of MSOF develops. Of patients dying with ARDS, 75 percent die from MSOF rather than primary pulmonary failure.

Failure of synthetic, metabolic, and phagocytic functions in the liver characterizes the hepatic manifestation of MSOF. The failure usually becomes clinically evident after ARDS is established though it can evolve concurrently. Early in MSOF or sepsis, hepatic metabolism is increased in order to metabolize the amino acid load brought on by catabolism and to provide sufficient glucose and acute-phase proteins. Concomitant with this is a decrease in hepatic secretion of immunoglobulin A (IgA) and bile salts, which in turn allows gut bacteria to proliferate and decreases endotoxin detoxification ability. Hepatic macrophages—Kupffer cells—are activated by uptake of circulating debris and endotoxin and secrete their own mediators, which exert local and distant effects. Later, as opsonic fibronectin levels fall, Kupffer cell phagocytosis fails, allowing more widespread circulation of endotoxin and other microaggregates and activation of distant mononuclear phagocyte populations.

The gastrointestinal tract may be the organ system that is most sensitive to the ravages of ischemia-reperfusion injury. Autoregulatory mechanisms, active after trauma, burns, or any form of hypovolemia, shunt blood flow away from splanchnic organs even after clinical signs of hemodynamic stability are restored early during resuscitation. Thus, the gut remains relatively ischemic for longer periods of time. As discussed earlier, this prolonged ischemia results in more reperfusion injury in the bowel wall. The consequences of such injury are the translocation of luminal bacteria and endotoxin into portal venous blood and mesenteric lymphatics. This process has been documented in several posttraumatic and burn animal models and can be reduced by limiting oxygen radical production with the use of a xanthine oxidase inhibitor.

The gastrointestinal tract may also be the principal reservoir of substances that perpetuate systemic inflammation and propel the host down the MSOF pathway. Broad-spectrum antibiotics, gastric antacids, and failed liver immunoglobulin and bile salt excretion allow for bacterial overgrowth. Stress and lack of enteral nutrients lead to further mucosal atrophy, which, in turn, allows bacteria and their cell-wall constituent endotoxins to continually translocate. This could explain the high incidence of the *sepsis syndrome* without a definable focus of infection. Unfortunately, failure of the gut mucosal barrier function is not clinically measurable. Later in the course of MSOF, gastrointestinal dysfunction is manifest as stress bleeding.

Renal failure often follows hepatic and pulmonary dysfunction even if adequate preload and inotropic support have been instituted. Its etiology is presumed to be secondary to inadequate local perfusion or failed autoregulation during the hyperdynamic state. Prostanoids have been implicated in the redistribution of renal blood flow away from the cortex. Other factors that contribute to azotemia include the use of nephrotoxic antibiotics, alpha-agonist agents, increased pigment loads as bilirubin increases, and the poorly understood hepatorenal syndrome.

The cardiovascular system is affected by the mismatch of circulating vasodilatory and vasoconstricting mediators, while the heart is directly impaired by an as yet poorly defined circulating peptide myocardial depressant factor. The central nervous system can be severely impaired by circulating false neurotransmitters, which are by-products of catabolism. Endorphins, which are endogenous, centrally active opioid-mimetics, can also contribute to both altered sensorium and hemodynamic instability.

Finally, there is ample evidence for a variety of defects in both humoral and cellular immune responses in patients with posttraumatic or septic MSOF. Prostaglandin E_2 (PGE_2) has immunosuppressive properties on the host. After traumatic or thermal insults, patients appear to have increased sensitivity to PGE_2 as well as increased PGE_2 production. This response can be blocked by cyclooxygenase inhibition (i.e., ibuprofen). A decreased production of the lymphokine interleukin-2 (IL-2) by T lymphocytes is also well documented after trauma. Interleukin-2 is important in cell-mediated immunity, natural killer cell activity, and for the elaboration of colony-stimulating factors necessary to stimulate neutrophil production. Interleukin-2 repletion in studies on animals appears to be beneficial in ameliorating their response to subsequent septic episodes.

CLINICAL PRESENTATION

Multisystem organ failure is a syndrome of sequential progression rather than simultaneous failure. Its true course can stretch from weeks to months. The clinical course can be arbitrarily divided into four stages, which define the degree of organ injury and underline the progressive nature of the disease (see Table 40-17). Stage 1 is really a prodrome and looks like early sepsis. Patients with stage 1 injury may show fever and leukocytosis and are usually hyperdynamic. If seen in the emergency department, they appear vasodilated with low to normal blood pressure and mild tachycardia. Aggressive institution of resuscitative and supportive measures at this time are crucial to limit the ischemic interval and prevent progression to full-blown MSOF.

In early MSOF (stage 2), multiple organ systems manifest clinically measurable signs of dysfunction. Its onset is insidious, arising several days to two weeks after the initial traumatic or septic event. Increased mixed venous oxygen tension in the face of increased tissue oxygen demands indicates the presence of a defect in peripheral oxygen extraction. The process is still reversible; however, mortality exceeds 50 percent if more than two systems are involved.

Over the next several weeks, MSOF becomes well established (stage 3), while the consequences of sustained hypermetabolism become more obvious. Hyperglycemia is seen until hepatic gluconeogenesis fails. Evidence of muscle mass wasting and impaired wound healing is seen. Patients remain hemodynamically labile. The low-pressure pulmonary edema indicative of ARDS gives way to fibrosis with worsening lung compliance. Recurrent nosocomial pneumonias are common and perpetuate the system-wide inflammatory state. The gastrointestinal tract, heretofore silent, begins to bleed intermittently, though its mucosal barrier function has been failing for weeks. Mortality approaches 100 percent when three or more systems are involved.

Stage 4 is a preterminal state marked by a hypodynamic circulation now refractory to inotropic or vasopressor sup-

Table 40-20. Therapeutic options in multisystem organ failure

Prevention
Aggressive fluid resuscitation
Early cardiopulmonary support
Invasive monitoring
Mechanical ventilation and PEEP
Inotropic support
Early excision of burn wounds
Early fracture fixation
Aggressive surveillance and treatment-drainage of infection
Aggressive and early nutritional support
Combination of enteral and parenteral routes
Attention to protein and caloric needs
Supportive care
Maximize oxygen delivery and consumption
PGE_1 and/or prostacyclin infusion
Red cell transfusions to increase O_2-carrying capacity
Optimize nutrition and modify the inflammatory response
Branched-chain enriched amino acid formulas
Preferred fuel in MSOF
Increase fish oils; decrease linoleic acid in lipid preparations
Stimulate wound healing and positive nitrogen balance
Recombinant growth hormone and other growth factors
Immune enhancement (experimental)
Replete IL-2
Replete fibronectin
Consider adjuvants (muramyl dipeptide)
Mediator-specific treatment
Prostanoids
Cyclooxygenase inhibitors (ibuprofen)
Thromboxane synthetase inhibitors
Lipoxygenase inhibitors
Leukotriene antagonists
Platelet-activating factor antagonists
Oxygen radicals
Scavengers (superoxide dismutase and/or catalase)
Antioxidant drugs (pentoxifylline)
Tumor necrosis factor antibodies
Endotoxin
Antilipid A antibodies to block endotoxin activity
Lipid X to block lipid A activity
Gut sterilization with nonabsorbable antibiotics

port. Metabolic pathways also fail. Cells are no longer able to use oxygen and the liver cannot generate sufficient glucose to sustain life. Irreversible lactic acidosis ensues leading to death.

TREATMENT AND PREVENTION

The self-perpetuating nature of MSOF, with its complex and intertwined physiology and mediator feedback loops, makes prevention of the syndrome a most attractive therapeutic strategy. It therefore falls to the emergency physician, in coordination with surgical and critical care colleagues, to identify traumatized or septic patients early in their course and to aggressively initiate appropriate care. The principles for preventing MSOF or interrupting its evolution are found in Table 40-20. They include vigorous volume resuscitation and early inotropic and respiratory support. The goal is rapid restoration of homeostasis in all organ systems, thereby limiting the reperfusion injury. Adequate end-organ perfusion, not just normal blood pressure, is necessary.

The second important concept is to rid the host of the focus of inflammation via débridement of necrotic tissue, drainage of pus, fracture fixation, and appropriate antibiotic therapy. Finally, early emphasis on nutrition, especially via the enteral route, is essential to prevent gut mucosal atrophy and leak of luminal bacteria and endotoxin. Gut sterilization with nonabsorbable antibiotics is currently under investigation in an effort to decrease the bacterial load available for translocation.

Once MSOF is established, the therapeutic options are reduced to surveillance for infection and multiorgan system support. Given the observed defect in oxygen extraction in established MSOF, several experimental strategies have evolved to increase oxygen delivery. Prostaglandin E_1 and prostacyclin have been used, with measurable improvement in specific organ function but no increase in patient survival. Red blood cell transfusions can also be helpful, as they increase oxygen-carrying capacity. If multiple, however, they are known to be immunosuppressive.

Other supportive options with measured salutary effects include fibronectin repletion with either a purified product of fibronectin-rich cryoprecipitate, the use of parenteral nutrition formulas enriched in branched-chain amino acids, and the use of recombinant growth factors to stimulate wound healing and restore positive nitrogen balance. All three approaches have met with success in animal and early clinical trials. Their widespread efficacy and effect on survival have yet to be determined.

There is currently an explosive investigative effort aimed at modifying the host inflammatory response to trauma and sepsis. Nutritional modifications, substituting larger amounts of omega-3 polyunsaturated fatty acids (fish oils), and decreasing the linoleic acid content of parenteral lipid formulations have the potential to decrease the amount of arachidonic acid metabolism and prostanoid expression on cellular stimulation.

Other investigators have targeted specific mediators implicated in the MSOF syndrome. Regimens involving ibuprofen to block cyclooxygenase have met with clinical success. Studies focusing on thromboxane synthetase inhibitors, lipoxygenase inhibitors, leukotriene antagonists, platelet-activating factor inhibitors, and endorphin antagonists all show some benefit. Similarly, oxygen radical scavengers have been helpful in animal models of endotoxin-induced MSOF, while pentoxifylline, an antioxidant, has proved helpful in some patients with ARDS.

Immunotherapy is also showing promise in the treatment of experimental MSOF. Monoclonal antibody to tumor necrosis factor has blocked the lethal response to endotoxin or bacteremia in animals. Antibody directed at the lipid A molecule common to many bacterial endotoxins has also been helpful, as has lipid X, which blocks lipid A binding and competitively inhibits endotoxin activity. Nonspecific immune enhancement with substances such as muramyl dipeptide has also protected animals from developing organ dysfunction after subsequent traumatic or septic insults. Corticosteroid therapy has been attempted in refractory cases with no statistically demonstrable survival benefit and multiple infectious and wound healing complications. Until these trials produce a therapy with obvious clinical efficacy, prevention of MSOF will continue to provide the largest impact on survival of the critically injured or ill patient.

SELECTED READING

Baue, AE. Multiple, progressive or sequential systems failure: A syndrome of the 1970s. *Arch Surg* 10:779, 1975.

Baue, AE, and Chaudry, IH. Prevention of multiple system failure. *Surg Clin North Am* 60:1167, 1980.

Bell, R, Coalson, J, and Smith, J. Multiple organ system failure and infection in adult respiratory distress syndrome. *Ann Intern Med* 99:293, 1983.

Beutler, B, Milsark, JA, and Cerami, AC. Passive immunization against cachectin/tumor necrosis factor prevents mice from lethal effect of endotoxin. *Science* 229:869, 1985.

Bihari, D, et al. The effects of vasodilation with prostacyclin on oxygen delivery and uptake in critically ill patients. *N Engl J Med* 317:397, 1987.

Border, JR, et al. The gut origin septic states in blunt multiple trauma (ISS-40) in the ICU. *Ann Surg* 206:427, 1987.

Burke, J, Quinby, W, and Bondoc, C. Primary excision and prompt grafting as routine therapy for the treatment of thermal burns in children. *Surg Clin North Am* 56:477, 1976.

Carrico, CJ, et al. Multiple organ failure syndrome. *Arch Surg* 121:196, 1986.

Cerra, F. Hypermetabolism, organ failure, and metabolic support. *Surgery* 101:1, 1987.

Cerra, FB, et al. Enteral feeding in sepsis: A prospective randomized, double-blind trial. *Surgery* 98:632, 1985.

Christou, NV, et al. Lymphoctye-macrophage interactions in the response to surgical infections. *Arch Surg* 122:239, 1987.

Clowes, G, George B, and Villar, C. Muscle proteolysis induced by a circulating peptide in patients with sepsis or trauma. *N Engl J Med* 308:545, 1983.

Danner, RL, Joiner, KA, and Parrillo, JE. Inhibition of endotoxin-induced priming of human neutrophils by lipid X and 3-Aza-lipid X. *J Clin Invest* 80:605, 1987.

DeCamp, MM, and Demling, RH. Posttraumatic multi-system organ failure. *J Am Med Assoc* 260:530, 1988.

Deitch, E, et al. Hemorrhagic shock-induced bacterial translocation is reduced by xanthine oxidase inhibition or inactivation. *Surgery* 104:191, 1988.

Demling, RH. The pathogenesis of respiratory failure after trauma and sepsis. *Surg Clin North Am* 60:1372, 1981.

Dinarello, C, and Mier, J. Lymphokines: Current concepts. *N Engl J Med* 317:940, 1987.

Dunn, DL, et al. Immunotherapy of gram-negative bacterial sepsis: A single murine monoclonal antibody provides cross-genera production. *Arch Surg* 121:58, 1986.

Eiseman, B, Beart, R, and Norton, L. Multiple organ failure. *Surg Gynecol Obstet* 144:323, 1977.

Ernster, L. Biochemistry of reoxygenation injury. *Crit Care Med* 16:947, 1988.

Faist, E, et al. Immunoprotective effects of cyclooxygenase inhibition in patients with major surgical procedures. *Surg Forum* 39:114, 1988.

Filkins, JP. Monokines and the metabolic pathophysiology of septic shock. *Fed Proc* 44:300, 1985.

Fisher, M, et al. Effect of dietary fish oil supplementation of polymorphonuclear leukocyte inflammatory potential. *Inflammation* 10:387, 1986.

Fry, DE. Multiple system organ failure. *Surg Clin North Am* 68:107, 1988.

Goris, R, et al. Multiple organ failure: Generalized auto destruction inflammation. *Arch Surg* 120:1109, 1985.

Granger, DN. Role of xanthine oxidase and granulocytes in ischemia-reperfusion injury. *Am J Physiol* 255:H1269, 1988.

Jansson, I, et al. Primary fracture immobilization as a method to prevent post traumatic pulmonary changes. *Acta Chir Scand* 148:329, 1982.

Jin, LJ, LaLonde, C, and Demling, RH. Lung dysfunction after thermal injury in relation to prostanoid and oxygen radical release. *J Appl Physiol* 61:103, 1986.

Kariman, K, and Burns, S. Regulation of tissue oxygen extraction is disturbed in adult respiratory distress syndrome. *Am Rev Respir Dis* 132:109, 1985.

Klausner, JM, et al. Post ischemic renal injury is mediated by neutrophils and leukotrienes. *Am J Physiol* 256:F794, 1989.

LaLonde, C, Demling, RH, and Pecquet, GM. Tissue inflammation without bacteria produces increased oxygen consumption and distant organ lipid peroxidation. *Surgery* 104:49, 1988.

Olson, NC, Grizzle, MK, and Anderson, DL. Effect of polyethylene glycol–superoxide dismutase and catalase on endotoxemia in pigs. *J Appl Physiol* 63:1526, 1987.

Parrillo, JE, et al. Profound but reversible myocardial depression in patients with septic shock. *Ann Intern Med* 100:483, 1984.

Polk, HC, and Shields, CL. Remote organ failure: A valid sign of occult intra-abdominal infection. *Surgery* 81:310, 1977.

Revhaug, A, et al. Inhibition of cyclo-oxygenase attenuates the metabolic response to endotoxin in humans. *Arch Surg* 123:162, 1988.

Rinaldo, J, and Rogers, R. Adult respiratory distress syndrome: Changing concepts of lung injury and repair. *N Engl J Med* 306:900, 1982.

Stoutenceck, C, et al. The effect of selective decontamination of the digestive tract on colonization and infection rate in multiple trauma patients. *Intensive Care Med* 10:185, 1984.

Tilney, NL, Bailey, GL, and Morgan, AP. Sequential system failure after rupture of abdominal aortic aneurysms: An unsolved problem in post operative care. *Ann Surg* 179:117, 1973.

Tracey, KJ, et al. Anti-cachectin/TNF monoclonal antibodies prevent septic shock during lethal bacteremia. *Nature* 330:662, 1987.

Watters, JM, et al. Both inflammatory and endocrine mediators stimulate host response to sepsis. *Arch Surg* 121:179, 1986.

Waymack, JP, et al. Effect of blood transfusions on immune function: III. Alterations in macrophage arachidonic acid metabolism. *Arch Surg* 122:56, 1987.

Wilmore, D, Aulick, L, and Mason, A. Influence of the burn wound on local and systemic response to injury. *Ann Surg* 186:444, 1977.

Ziegler, T, et al. Metabolic effects of recombinant human growth hormone in patients receiving parenteral nutrition. *Ann Surg* 208:6, 1988.

41. Stabilization and Transport of the Critically Injured Patient

Pradip Sahdev
Lenworth M. Jacobs

PRINCIPLES OF TRAUMA CARE IN THE FIELD

The goal of any advanced life support prehospital team responding to a call for a patient in extremis is to identify and correct life-threatening conditions and then to initiate transportation to an appropriate facility. There is a fundamental difference in the philosophy of management of trauma and medical patients. Definitive care for a trauma patient is in the hospital, whereas the cardiac patient can frequently be stabilized in the field before transfer to the hospital.

The severely traumatized patient who is in extremis requires basic interventions, such as securing the airway, ensuring ventilatory exchange, and controlling obvious external hemorrhage. Prolonged efforts at stabilization in the field are not indicated because the cause of instability in these patients cannot be definitely managed in the prehospital setting. This must await evaluation and treatment, often including surgical intervention, in the trauma center. It has been documented in several studies that the most important factor influencing survival in patients who sustain trauma is the duration of time that elapses between injury and the undertaking of definitive care. This finding formed the basis for the "scoop and run" philosophy. An exception to this is the situation in which arrival to a hospital is delayed beyond one-half hour because of prolonged extrication, traffic conditions, or long distances to the hospital. In these circumstances, intravenous lines and fluid resuscitation should be initiated. In the cardiac arrest situation from medical causes, this implies stabilization of the patient in the field with advanced cardiac life support (ACLS) before and during transport to the facility. This has improved survival of such patients. The time at which basic life support (BLS) and ACLS have been initiated has been shown to be of prime importance in survival.

Trunkey has shown that death in patients with major trauma has a trimodal distribution. The first peak occurs immediately or within a few minutes of injury and accounts for one-half of all trauma deaths. These deaths are almost invariably due to major brain injury, high spinal cord injury, or major cardiac or vascular disruption. As these patients are often found dead at the scene, or within minutes thereafter, no significant salvage can be expected from this group.

The second peak of trauma-induced fatalities occurs within two hours of the incident and results primarily from internal hemorrhage, respiratory compromise, or smaller injuries that lead to large cumulative fluid losses and hemodynamic instability. It is toward this group of potentially salvageable patients that major prehospital emphasis and subsequent rapid inhospital stabilization and definitive therapy need to be addressed. Nearly three percent of trauma patients fall within this group, and substantial reduction in mortality can be achieved by a comprehensive expeditious approach to their management. Finally, the third peak of trauma deaths occurs three to four weeks after the initial insult and is usually related to sepsis and multiple organ failure.

Fifty to sixty percent of early trauma deaths occur in the prehospital phase. Of the remaining deaths, 60 percent occur during the first four hours after arrival at the hospital. Establishing appropriate trauma systems that encompass all aspects of trauma care, including prehospital care, triage, and management in a definitive facility, will decrease the number of preventable deaths.

TRAUMA SYSTEMS

An organized response to trauma as a public-health problem first began in the United States in 1966. This resulted in Federal legislation in 1973 that mandated comprehensive emergency medical service (EMS) systems. Fifteen components were identified and implemented nationally during the 1970s. The military experience accumulated from Korea and Vietnam enhanced the philosophy that optimal care of the trauma victim was best served by rapid initial assessment, control of life-threatening conditions, and rapid transfer by helicopter, bypassing smaller units, to definitive-care hospitals.

In the civilian setting, improvement in morbidity and mortality of trauma victims by the deployment of a trauma system was reported by West and associates, when they showed an alarming incidence of "preventable" deaths before the institution of hospital categorization in Orange County, California. This finding has been replicated in other geographic sites.

A trauma system is composed of four primary components: access to care, prehospital care, hospital care, and rehabilitation. Access to the trauma system implies availability of a universal, free, and easily remembered emergency telephone number (911). This number must be directly linked to the dispatch of trained emergency response teams and must be widely disseminated so that no confusion or delay arises in activating the system. Prehospital care includes education and certification of primary responders, an organized rapid response to the incident, certified transport vehicles, protocols for medical management of the patient at the scene, and predetermined destination hospitals.

The American College of Surgeons Committee on Trauma has developed guidelines for categorization of hospitals into level I, II, and III trauma centers in order to provide optimal care for the trauma patient and to make the best possible use of community resources. The most significant ingredient for excellent care of the trauma patient by individuals and the hospital is a commitment to providing all available resources 24 hours a day. These resources, and hence the categorization of the hospital, are a direct reflection of the institution's commitment to care for the trauma patient.

A level I trauma center is one with maximal resources, personnel, and commitment in the care of trauma victims, as well as a commitment to education and research. Such an institution should treat 600 to 1,000 trauma victims a year. Physicians representing all the major subspecialties must be available 24 hours a day. All radiographic investigations, including computed tomographic (CT) scanning and angiography, and laboratory examinations relevant to the trauma victim should be available for immediate performance when the patient is received at the institution. The operating room and intensive care unit should be immediately available 24 hours a day. These hospitals are tertiary-care facilities and are able to manage the most severely injured trauma victims.

Level II facilities are similar to level I in their ability to provide optimal clinical care. The major difference is the absence of research in trauma-related topics.

Level III trauma centers are hospitals that have demonstrated a maximum commitment to trauma commensurate with available resources. Physicians who must be available 24 hours a day are a general surgeon, anesthesiologist, emergency physician, and internist. Capability to process all routine chemistries and routine x-rays should also exist. Additional capabilities are desirable but may not be present depending on the resources. Such centers are appropriate for the initial management of trauma victims who are too far from a level I or level II trauma center for primary triage and for definitive treatment for the less severely injured patients. These centers are usually located in rural areas.

PREHOSPITAL MANAGEMENT

Primary Survey

It is the responsibility of the first responding team to immediately recognize and treat life-threatening conditions. The initial rapid examination is popularly known as the *primary survey*. The objective is to open and control the airway, assure that ventilation is adequate, and control obvious hemmorrhage. A rapid neurologic examination is also included here.

Airway

Of prime importance in the trauma victim is the establishment of a patent airway to permit unimpeded ventilatory exchange. The airway is most often compromised due to secretions, blood, or alterations in consciousness. In the case of secretions, blood, or other foreign bodies, it is essential to clear the oropharynx. A jaw-thrust or chin-lift maneuver may be needed to open the airway. This is especially important in patients with altered mental status. Any persistent obstruction could be from a retained oropharyngeal foreign body (blood, teeth, dentures). A finger sweep should be performed to remove any obstruction. Suction is a useful adjunct for removing foreign bodies and clearing the airway. It is of prime importance that during attempts to secure a patent airway, the cervical spine is immobilized with one or more of the following: manual traction, a cervical collar, sandbags, or a spine board.

If the airway can be opened by these maneuvers, constant vigilance should be maintained to prevent secretions or blood from reobstructing it. If the patient is unconscious, a nasopharyngeal or oropharyngeal airway will prevent the tongue from being displaced posteriorly and the glottis from being closed. If the patient is awake, the gag reflex usually prevents such an airway from being employed. This is an indication that the patient can protect his or her own airway. It is important to remember that this is a changing situation and the patient may lose the gag reflex and the ability to protect the airway during extrication and transport to the trauma center. In cases in which the airway cannot be satisfactorily maintained by these methods, as well as in patients who either are not breathing spontaneously or who require hyperventilation or positive-pressure ventilation, urgent consideration of an alternate airway is needed.

OROTRACHEAL TUBE. In patients who have no evidence of cervical spine injury, an orotracheal tube should be inserted using an appropriate laryngoscope. The technique requires someone who has been trained to perform such intubations. It is often difficult to accomplish, especially in a patient who is inebriated or combative.

It is important to ensure the proper positioning of the tube by auscultation over both lung fields, at which time equal bilateral air entry should be heard. If air entry is heard only over one hemithorax, the tube may have been advanced too far distally in the trachea. It will be in the right main-stem bronchus and should be pulled back until adequate air entry is heard bilaterally. If the tube is accidentally placed into the esophagus, it must be promptly recognized, as this allows no ventilation and carries a potential for gastric distention. Vomiting may occur once the tube is withdrawn. Appropriate suction must therefore be available and vomiting anticipated. Two options are available if esophageal intubation occurs. A second endotracheal tube can be passed anterior to the first tube. In a difficult intubation with an anterior trachea, leaving a first tube in situ provides a guide for positioning the second tube. As this may be cumbersome, an alternate procedure is to remove the tube and press on the cricoid cartilage in order to obstruct the esophagus and prevent regurgitation.

NASOTRACHEAL TUBE. In patients with suspected cervical spine injury, movement of the neck must be avoided at all cost. Nasotracheal intubation, which is blind passage of an endotracheal tube through the nares and posterior oropharynx into the trachea, is the procedure of choice. This allows control of the airway without movement of the cervical spine. This technique requires considerable training and skill. However, once the practitioner has mastered the technique, it is extremely useful in both the prehospital and emergency department resuscitative arenas.

If in addition to possible cervical spine injury, the patient also has severe midfacial (Le Fort I, II, or III) fractures, passage of a nasotracheal tube is contraindicated. This is because of the association of basal skull fractures with major facial fractures and hence the possibility of inadvertently passing the tube into the cerebrum. The presence of cerebrospinal fluid rhinorrhea or otorrhea should alert the practitioner to the possibility of a fracture with a communication to the cerebrospinal space.

ESOPHAGEAL OBTURATOR AIRWAY. The esophageal obturator airway is designed for assisting ventilation when endotracheal or orotracheal intubation is not possible for technical reasons or because of lack of personnel trained in its performance. It consists of a curved, blind ending tube with a mask attached to its proximal end. It has a cuff at the distal end to obstruct the esophagus and holes placed more proximally in the tube to allow air to pass through the tube into the oropharynx and trachea.

The technique of using the tube is simple. It is passed blindly through the mouth and into the esophagus, where the cuff is inflated. This prevents gastric distention when the patient is ventilated with a bag-mask apparatus, as well as vomiting and aspiration. The mask is positioned snugly around the patient's nose and mouth to prevent air leaks. When air is passed via a bag-valve device through the tube, it escapes from the side holes situated in the oropharynx and then into the trachea.

This tube has many disadvantages, including injuries to the esophagus, accidental tracheal intubation with asphyxiation, and problems related to vomiting when the tube is subsequently removed to provide more definitive airway control. As training of paramedic and rescue personnel in nasotracheal and orotracheal intubation becomes more widespread, opportunities for using the esophageal obturator airway will decrease.

NEEDLE CRICOTHYROIDOTOMY. If both nasotracheal and orotracheal intubation are contraindicated or have failed in spite of repeated attempts, a needle cricothyroidotomy or a formal cricothyroidotomy should be considered. In performing the needle cricothyroidotomy, a No. 14 or No. 16 sheathed needle attached to a syringe is used to puncture the lower half of the cricothyroid membrane in the anterior midline of the neck. During this puncture, negative pressure should be applied to the syringe so that as soon as the trachea is entered, there is a free flow of air. Care should be exercised not to puncture the posterior tracheal wall. Once the trachea is entered, the sheath is advanced and the metal stylet is removed. The hub of the needle is attached to a Y connection. One end of the Y is connected to a 50-psi source of oxygen. The remaining limb of the Y should be intermittently occluded with the index finger, so that oxygen flows into the trachea for two to three seconds, and then released to allow spontaneous exhalation. Satisfactory oxygenation can be maintained in this way for up to 45 minutes.

SURGICAL CRICOTHYROIDOTOMY. A formal cricothyroidotomy can also be performed, but should only be done by persons trained in the technique. After the cricothyroid membrane has been palpated, a skin incision is made over its lower half and up to 0.5 to 1.0 cm on either side of the anterior midline of the neck. This is deepened through the subcutaneous tissue and the cricothyroid membrane. Once the trachea is entered, the back of the handle of the knife is passed into the opening in the membrane and rotated 90 degrees to enlarge the opening. A suitably sized endotracheal tube is then inserted through the opening.

It must be emphasized that even in an unconscious patient, an open airway can usually be maintained using the jaw-thrust or chin-lift maneuver. In an unconscious patient the use of an oropharyngeal or nasopharyngeal airway will aid in maintaining a patent airway. Elective nasotracheal or orotracheal intubation can then be performed as needed.

Cricothyroidotomies are only needed in cases of severe facial or laryngeal fractures, and in patients with extensive bleeding that is causing airway obstruction. Though a simple procedure under elective circumstances, it can be difficult to accomplish in a combative patient who has extensive injuries and hemorrhage. It should not be undertaken lightly and should be regarded as a procedure of last resort.

Breathing

Once airway patency has been assured, breathing must be evaluated to ensure an adequate ventilatory exchange. Inadequate ventilatory exchange may be obvious, as in cases in which there is no attempt at breathing, as noted by absence of chest and abdominal wall movements and of exhaled air. In other cases respiration may be shallow, slow, or rapid, and with or without the use of accessory muscles. Vigorous attempts at breathing, often with "air hunger," may signify ventilatory compromise. Any of these types of breathing may be accompanied by cyanosis and altered sensorium (lethargy in cases of carbon dioxide narcosis, or agitation in cases of hypoxia).

In any patient suspected of having sustained a traumatic injury, oxygen therapy should be initiated. This can be achieved by mask or via the endotracheal tube if the patient is intubated. In cases in which spontaneous ventilatory exchange is insufficient in spite of a patent airway, assisted ventilation is essential. This may take the form of a bag-valve-mask technique, usually for initial ventilation, or ventilation via the endotracheal tube using an Ambu bag or a portable ventilator.

An immediate examination of the ventilatory status of the patient includes palpation of the position of the trachea in the neck, palpation for any gross chest wall injuries, and auscultation of breath sounds. The three life-threatening conditions that should be specifically looked for and treated at this stage are tension pneumothorax, flail chest, and an open (sucking) chest wound.

TENSION PNEUMOTHORAX. A tension pneumothorax presents with tracheal deviation away from the side with the tension, decreased breath sounds, and hyperresonance on the side of the tension. Distended neck veins and hemodynamic compromise may also be seen. The tension pneumothorax is caused by a parenchymal lung injury that allows air to escape into the pleural cavity during inhalation. During expiration, the air in the pleural space remains trapped, causing collapse of the affected lung. With successive respirations, more and more air is trapped in the pleural cavity due to the valvelike behavior of the parenchymal injury, leading to progressive collapse of the affected lung, shift of the mediastinum toward the unaffected side, decrease in venous return, and resultant fall in cardiac output. This in turn results in systemic hypotension and hypoxemia. The diagnosis of tension pneumothorax is a surgical emergency and can be made clinically, without the need for a confirmatory chest x-ray.

Treatment of this condition relieves the pressure of the trapped air in the affected pleural cavity. Emergency treatment can be performed in different ways, with the exact option used to be defined by the local EMS treatment protocol.

The simplest technique is to insert a No. 16 or No. 14 angiocatheter into the chest wall, at a point just superior to the third rib margin in the anterior axillary line or just above the superior margin of the fifth rib in the lateral axillary line. The latter approach is more useful in muscular individuals, as they tend to have well-developed pectoralis muscles over the anterior chest. The angiocatheter should be attached via a three-way stopcock to a 50-cc syringe and advanced into the pleural space, with negative pressure applied on the syringe. Free aspiration of air signifies entrance into the pleural cavity, and the sheath of the needle should then be advanced and the stylet removed. The air is allowed to escape, and its exit with a hissing sound both confirms the diagnosis and treats the condition.

Additional air can be sucked out with the syringe, and the needle is then attached to an IV extension tubing. The end of the IV tubing should be submerged under water to form a seal that prevents air from reentering the pleural cavity. The disadvantage of this method (needle thoracostomy) is that the narrow diameter of the sheath allows for occlusion when the expanding lung occludes the tip, causing recurrence of the tension. Kinking and displacement are other frequent problems. A refinement of the technique consists of placing a finger condom or the finger of a glove over the end of the angiocatheter. As the air escapes, it distends the condom and confirms the diagnosis. The condom can then be incised to allow further release of the tension.

The McSwain dart can also be employed to decompress a tension pneumothorax. This device, a 16F catheter with expanding wings, is placed through the chest wall in a manner similar to that used for needle thoracostomy. Once in place, the trocar is removed and the wings automatically expand, securing the catheter in place. A one-way valve can be attached to the end of the catheter to prevent reentry of air into the pleural space. Finally, insertion of a chest tube into the pleural space is the definitive treatment for a tension pneumothorax or hemothorax.

FLAIL CHEST. The second condition that requires urgent recognition and appropriate therapy is a flailed chest. A flail of the chest wall is said to exist when part of the usually rigid chest wall is disrupted and moves paradoxically. It is also defined as the fracture of two or more contiguous ribs in two or more places. In general, the greater the number of fractured ribs involved in the flailed segment, the more significant the respiratory compromise. The force that broke the ribs and caused the flail segment is usually sufficient to cause an underlying pulmonary contusion and additional respiratory compromise.

The diagnosis is made by inspecting the chest for paradoxical movement of part of the chest wall and feeling for extensive bony and pneumocrepitus. Associated subcutaneous emphysema is diagnostic of an underlying pneumothorax.

Any patient with a suspected flail segment should be treated with supplemental oxygen and at times ventilatory assistance with the bag-valve-mask technique. For patients with a large flail and for those who show signs of respiratory decompensation, endotracheal intubation with positive-pressure ventilation should be initiated. High oxygen flow rates should be begun to suppress the respiratory drive. Analgesics should not be used without an appropriate physician's order, as they can induce changes in the patient's sensorium and clinical examination.

SUCKING CHEST WOUND. The third condition that can prove rapidly fatal and therefore needs to be recognized and treated expeditiously, is an open chest wound, or "sucking" wound of the chest. This is a through-and-through wound of the chest wall that permits air to pass to and from the pleural cavity to the atmosphere. This leads to a collapse of the ipsilateral lung, and pendular movement of the mediastinum, resulting in ineffectual ventilation. This in turn leads to rapid respiratory compromise.

Emergency treatment consists of covering the wound with Vaseline-covered gauze and taping it on three sides to the chest wall. This allows air to escape from the fourth untaped side and at the same time prevents reentry of air into the chest. A needle or tube thoracostomy may also be needed to permit full lung expansion.

Circulation

Next, a rapid assessment of the circulatory status with appropriate intervention needs to be undertaken. It should be again emphasized that prolonged efforts at cardiovascular stabilization are not justified in the field, and only those interventions should be undertaken that are essential to maintain patient viability en route to the hospital.

The multitrauma victim is at high risk for development of hypovolemic shock. This clinical presentation is usually associated with a loss of at least 30 percent of total blood volume. Lesser degrees of shock are seen with blood losses up to 20 percent of total blood volume (class I shock). This is characterized by normotension and tachycardia. Loss of 20 to 30 percent of blood volume is associated with narrowing of pulse pressure due to elevation of diastolic pressure, tachycardia, and delayed capillary refill (class II shock). Class I and II shock may be subtle in presentation and require careful assessment to identify. Class III shock occurs after loss of 30 to 40 percent of total blood volume and class IV shock after loss of greater than 40 percent of total blood volume. Symptoms include hypotension; cold, clammy skin; and cyanosis. Metabolic acidosis is also present, and blood transfusions are required to reverse these states of profound shock.

Treatment of shock in the prehospital setting includes administration of 10 liters of high-flow oxygen, positioning in the recumbent position, and application of the pneumatic antishock garment (PASG). Two large-bore (No. 14 or No. 16 gauge) intravenous lines should be started, one in either arm, if extrication and transport time of the patient are likely to be prolonged and if it does not delay transportation to the hospital. Any obvious bleeding point should be controlled, with direct pressure and/or dressings.

PNEUMATIC ANTISHOCK GARMENT. Pneumatic splinting of pelvic and long-bone lower-extremity fractures with the PASG is appropriate in the prehospital stabilization of trauma patients. Stabilization of fractures assists in decreasing blood loss and continuing soft-tissue injury. Splinting also decreases additional damage to arteries, nerves, and other soft tissues by movement of bony fragments.

The PASG exerts its primary effect by elevating peripheral vascular resistance, thus allowing better perfusion of vital structures (brain, heart, kidney) and stabilizing the blood pressure. Autotransfusion of blood on inflating the trousers occurs, but this is of small volume and is responsible for only a small part of the effect of this device.

The trousers are constructed in three compartments: one for the abdomen and one for each of the lower extremities. Each compartment usually has a pop-off valve activated at a predetermined pressure (104 mm Hg), which prevents excessive compartmental pressures. During inflation, the extremity sections are inflated first, then the abdominal section. Deflation should be performed in the hospital and in the reverse sequence. Indications for use are systolic blood pressure lower than 90 mm Hg, intraabdominal hemorrhage, pelvic fractures, lower-extremity long-bone fractures or soft-tissue hemorrhage, and neurogenic shock. An absolute contraindication to its use is pulmonary edema; care needs to be exercised in cases of pregnancy (to prevent harm to the fetus) and in cases of intrathoracic hemorrhage. Care needs also to be exercised in patients with head injury. The abdominal section should not be inflated in diaphragmatic rupture as abdominal contents are forced into the left hemithorax. This results in respiratory compromise.

TOURNIQUETS. Bleeding in the extremities is controlled by direct pressure over the bleeding point, as this causes minimal ischemia distal to the bleeding. Application of a tourniquet is controversial, and its use should be limited to situations in which point pressure is not effective—for example, in traumatic extremity amputation with excessive bleeding. Tourniquets should be applied only proximal to the elbow or knee to provide adequate vessel compression. The forearm and leg have two bones with interosseous vessels that are immune from tourniquet pressure. Thus, the hemorrhage is likely to continue if the tourniquet is inappropriately placed.

CARDIAC TAMPONADE. It is important during the primary survey to be able to differentiate hypotension secondary to hypovolemia from hypotension that results from cardiac tamponade, as the treatment for the two conditions is different. Most important in the diagnosis of cardiac tamponade is a high index of suspicion. Although it can occur secondary to blunt trauma, it is most often associated with penetrating injury in the chest or upper abdomen. Clinical diagnosis is based on a suspicion of the condition, along with the presence of an elevated jugular venous pulse, systolic hypotension, distant heart sounds (Beck's triad), and pulsus paradoxus. The absence of one or more signs does not, however, exclude the diagnosis.

Treatment in the field consists of application of PASG, establishment of adequate ventilation, and rapid transport to a hospital. Treatment in the emergency department consists of pericardiocentesis and thoracotomy for definitive treatment.

Neurologic Examination

It is important to perform a rapid neurologic examination on the patient at this time. This consists of assessment of pupil size and reaction to light and evaluation of patient responsiveness in terms of being awake, responding to vocal or painful stimuli, or being unconscious.

Secondary Survey

The secondary survey is a more detailed examination of the patient than the primary survey. An attempt is made to identify injuries and conditions that will require special treatment en route to the hospital. Only examinations that will assist in more effective management of the patient in the prehospital phase should be carried out here. Examinations and procedures that will not aid during transfer but will only add to the time spent in the field (e.g., endoscopic or rectal examinations), should not be done. A rapid and relatively complete "head-to-toe" examination should be performed, starting at the head.

Head Examination

The airway should be reexamined and any deficiencies noted should be corrected. The scalp and face are inspected and quickly palpated for any tenderness, swelling, or laceration. Open wounds are covered with sterile dressings, and bleeding is controlled with pressure dressings. Scalp wounds can bleed profusely in spite of dressings, and the best policy in this situation is to transport the patient to the hospital as soon as possible after dressings have been applied.

Neck Examination

The neck is gently and thoroughly examined, with inline traction to the head maintained if neck injury is suspected. Areas of bruising, swelling, and tenderness are looked for in all cases in which a cervical spine injury is suspected. Cervical spine immobilization on a short or long board and with or without inline traction and sandbags or other devices (e.g., foam pillows) to support the head should be used. A semi-rigid collar is appropriate. A useful adjunct is to immobilize the head to the spine board using tape before transfer.

In general, short boards are used for spinal immobilization during extrication, and long boards during transport. It is important to remember that a soft collar does not adequately immobilize the neck. If used, it must be accompanied by one of the aforementioned adjuncts.

Finally, wounds of the neck should be dressed and bleeding controlled with direct pressure or dressings. The dressings should not be circumferential.

Chest Examination

Next to be examined is the chest. The chest wall should be assessed for stability. Tracheal deviation should be identified and breath sounds auscultated. If a tension pneumothorax or sucking chest wound is present, it should be managed as discussed under the section on the primary survey. In the case of a flail chest, paradoxical motion of the flail section should be controlled by applying a towel or sandbag over the area and taping it to the chest. If possible, the patient should be made to lie on the side of the injury.

No prehospital treatment is usually required for fractured ribs, fractured sternum, pneumothorax, and hemothorax. Needle pericardiocentesis should not be performed in the field. It should only be attempted if the patient is in extremis, as potential complications from the procedure are serious.

Patients with multiple trauma should always be placed on a cardiac monitor, especially if chest injury is overt or suspected. This will identify arrhythmias and other electrocardiographic (ECG) changes resulting from myocardial contusion or underlying heart disease.

Abdominal Examination

Examination of the abdomen should be directed toward identifying wounds, gross intraabdominal hemorrhage, pelvic fractures, and pregnancy. Principles of treatment of abdominal wounds are the same as elsewhere. External hemorrhage is controlled by local pressure and clean, sterile pressure dressings placed over the wound. Impaled objects are secured in place with dressings unless the physician orders them removed. In case of evisceration, a sterile cloth should be placed over the eviscerated organ. The patient should then be transported immediately to the hospital.

If intraabdominal hemorrhage is suspected, and in the event of a pelvic fracture, PASG should be considered. In the latter case, the PASG acts by stabilizing the fracture fragments and diminishing further hemorrhage that can result from bony fragments lacerating the pelvic vasculature. The venous system is particularly at risk as the vessels are thin walled.

In the event that the patient is pregnant, the mother's life takes precedence over the unborn child's. This philosophy should dictate management at all times. Hence, if hemorrhagic control is indicated, the PASG should not be withheld on the basis of the patient's pregnancy alone.

Examination of Extremities

In the examination of the extremities, the focus should be on preserving the integrity of the vessels and nerves. Disruption of either major arteries or veins or damage to nerves could lead to significant compromise of the extremity, requiring operative intervention or subsequent amputation.

The extremity should be inspected and palpated for any evidence of long-bone fractures or joint dislocations. This includes inspection for obvious bony deformity and palpation to identify local tenderness and crepitus. Distal pulses should be palpated and neurologic function should be assessed. In cases in which the fracture is thought to be causing compression on the vessel with vascular compromise, traction in the long axis of the extremity should be applied to realign bony fragments. The suspected bony injuries should be splinted. This decreases pain, prevents further soft-tissue damage, and decreases blood loss.

Neurologic Examination

A rapid survey of the neurologic status of the patient should be performed. This is invaluable for comparison with later neurologic examinations. It also provides an objective criterion that can aid in the decision as to which hospital is most appropriate. This survey, also known as the mini-neurologic examination, consists of evaluating and grading eye-opening and best verbal and best motor responses, with the sum of the judged responses providing the Glasgow Coma Score. The actual values given to the responses noted are as listed in Table 41-1.

TRANSPORT TO HOSPITAL

Once the patient has been fully evaluated in the field, rapid transportation to the appropriate center is essential. Once the problems identified by the primary and secondary survey

Table 41-1. Glasgow Coma Scale*

Type of response	Score
Best eye response	
Spontaneous	4
To verbal command	3
To painful stimulus	2
No eye-opening	1
Best verbal response	
Full comprehension	5
Confused	4
Inappropriate words	3
Unintelligible sounds	2
No sounds	1
Best motor response	
Obeys commands	6
Controlled movements	5
Withdraws	4
Flexes	3
Extends	2
No response	1

*The Glasgow Coma score is obtained by adding the individual scores for each of the three parameters measured.

have been appropriately managed, the patient is secured on a long board. The cervical spine must be protected at all times. If the PASG has been applied prophylactically, it can be deflated and left in position if the patient is currently hemodynamically stable. The patient is loaded onto the stretcher for transfer to an appropriate facility.

The patient must be adequately monitored during transfer. Continuous cardiac monitoring is essential in patients suspected of having major trauma. The vital signs, respirations, and neurologic status should be reassessed every five minutes or less to evaluate the need for additional ventilatory support, treatment of arrhythmias, and possible additional fluid resuscitation in patients with intravenous access.

Additional monitoring of the respiratory and physiologic status of the patient can be performed using pulse oximetry and end-tidal carbon dioxide monitoring. The pulse oximeter noninvasively measures arterial oxygen saturation continuously. The device attaches to a finger or toe in adults and to a heel in infants and continuously displays arterial oxygen saturation. This saturation is a calculated value determined by measuring the differential absorption of two frequencies of light emitted by the device. The values obtained are accurate when the saturation is 70 percent or greater. Arterial saturations less than 70 percent, hypothermia, shock, arterial disease, and infusion of vasopressors decrease the accuracy of this device. Continuing improvements in its design are targeted at overcoming these problems.

End-tidal carbon dioxide ($PeCO_2$) refers to the partial pressure of carbon dioxide in expired air at the end of exhalation. This measurement can be obtained using a portable device with a sampling port attached to the endotracheal tube or tight-fitting face mask. Though interpretation of changes noted in $PeCO_2$ requires considerable experience, this measurement can provide important information regarding the state of oxygenation, metabolism, circulation, and ventilation when used in combination with pulse oximetry. Though experience with this device in the prehospital phase of the care of trauma patients is limited, its use in this setting appears promising.

If the secondary survey at the scene was incomplete, it should be concluded en route to the trauma center. The status of any injuries noted either in the field or en route should be frequently reassessed to identify deterioration.

Throughout the prehospital care of the patient, it is essential that the EMTs remain in voice contact with the designated physician. Standing orders and protocols can be used for certain situations in true emergencies. The details of the medical protocols should be established in writing for each emergency care system. Frequent evaluations and audits must be in place to review the quality of care being provided by the prehospital crew. Any violation detected must be thoroughly investigated.

In the event that a trauma victim is thought to be dead in the field, the order for nonresuscitation must be given by a physician, either by direct voice order or by the physician being present at the scene. This is an extremely important decision both medically and legally. It requires careful transmission of accurate information. The usual criteria are decapitation, hemicorporectomy, rigor mortis, putrefaction, and obvious extrusion of brain in an asystolic patient. Most communities will then require the coroner or medical examiner to pronounce the patient dead in the prehospital setting.

TRIAGE PARAMETERS

Triage of the multiply injured trauma victim becomes important when two or more hospitals, each with varying capacity to care for trauma victims, are present in a reasonable distance from the site of the accident. In many rural areas where only one hospital is located in the region, the patient must be taken there first for management. Once the patient has been evaluated and initial treatment begun at this hospital, triage to a definitive-care institution can be performed if indicated.

A problem can arise in the field if two or more hospitals are in reasonable distance of the accident. In these situations directly triaging patients to the hospital best equipped to deal with major trauma is appropriate (usually a level I or II trauma center). It has been demonstrated that up to 30 percent of the deaths that occur within four hours of injury can be prevented if the patient is initially evaluated and resuscitated in a trauma center.

Clearly, however, this does not mean that all trauma patients should be triaged to trauma centers. About 90 percent of injured patients can be adequately treated at the locally available hospital. Only the 10 percent of patients who are severely injured should be transferred to a trauma center. Selective triage is not only appropriate but essential; it prevents the overloading of major trauma centers with patients who would do equally well elsewhere and avoids an unnecessary increase in the cost of trauma care for the individual and the state.

If any major injury is suspected, even in a patient who appears well, triage to a more advanced trauma receiving facility is appropriate. A 50 percent over-triage rate is considered acceptable to avoid triaging patients with occult injuries to lower-level facilities, thereby jeopardizing the lives of these patients. Once the patient is received at a level I or II trauma center, a comprehensive multidisciplinary team will be engaged in his or her management. Numerous laboratory examinations and radiologic studies are routinely performed, often according to a predetermined protocol. This leads to an extremely low incidence of missed or inappropriately treated injuries.

Field triage involves an estimation of the severity of the injury (apparent and potential) incurred by the patient and subsequent transport to the available facility most likely to be able to take care of the patient without the need for subsequent interhospital transfer after stabilization. This decision depends on the actual or potential injuries received by the patient, the available resources to treat the patient, and time and distance factors.

The severity of injury sustained by the trauma victim can be judged in the field by the presence of obvious anatomic injuries, such as facial trauma or bony fractures, as well as alterations in physiologic functions, such as in pulse, blood pressure, and respiration. Unfortunately, some injuries, including some injuries to the chest, abdomen, brain, or spine, may not cause obvious changes on the physical examination. In such cases, a consideration of the mechanism of injury is important, as some mechanisms are more commonly associated with significant injuries than are others. Age and associated diseases, if known, can also influence triage to a higher-level facility. Figure 41-1 outlines the algorithm that can guide appropriate triage decisions.

It is important for prehospital personnel to confer with the online physician as to the appropriateness of triage to a trauma center, especially in cases where the extent of injuries is unclear. The triage decision may have to be altered en route as a result of previously unsuspected deterioration in the patient's condition or the development of a new finding on physical examination.

INTERHOSPITAL TRIAGE

Once the patient has been brought to a hospital, the physician performs a rapid primary and detailed secondary survey. The primary survey is similar to the one performed by the EMTs in the field but with more definitive treatment of the conditions needing attention—for example, establishment of large-bore intravenous lines for rapid fluid and blood administration in hypovolemic patients, tube thoracostomy for pneumothorax, and pericardiocentesis for pericardial tamponade. Hence, the airway, breathing, circulation, and rapid neurologic examination are performed by the receiving physician. Any change in status as compared to the patient's condition in the field is important in proper evaluation. An assessment of the appropriateness and effectiveness of measures taken in the field (e.g., endotracheal intubation) is undertaken immediately, and any deficiencies noted are rapidly addressed and corrected.

The secondary survey is much more detailed than the one performed in the field and consists of a rapid but detailed head-to-toe examination, following the dictum "finger or tube in every orifice." Included in this survey are examinations of the head and neck, chest, abdomen, pelvis, rectum, extremities, and spine, and a detailed neurologic examination; these have previously been described. It is important to establish a routine for examining all the organ systems in a systematic manner that is repeated in the same way for every patient. This complete comprehensive examination ensures that nothing significant is missed in any patient.

While the secondary survey is in progress, hematologic investigations should be obtained for each patient. These should include, but need not be limited to, hemoglobin, hematocrit, electrolytes, blood urea nitrogen, creatinine, glucose, liver function tests, creatine phosphokinase, amylase, lipase, alcohol level, and blood gases. A urine dipstick and urinalysis should also be routinely performed. X-rays should include lateral, anteroposterior, and odontoid views of the cervical spine (this *must* be inclusive of the C7–T1 interspace, in addition to all seven cervical vertebrae); an anteroposterior chest x-ray; and an x-ray of the pelvis. A 12-lead electrocardiogram completes the essential initial investigations in the stable patient. Additional blood work or further investigations (e.g., intravenous pyelography, head or abdominal CT, arteriograms, and so forth) may also be needed for full evaluation, or emergent peritoneal lavage may be chosen as the quickest way to exclude or confirm an intraabdominal problem, especially in hemodynamically unstable patients.

It must be appreciated that the extent of evaluation will depend on the actual or potential severity of injuries of the patient, the presence of injuries that require operative intervention, and the decision regarding treatment of the patient definitively at the present institution versus transfer to another hospital. In each of these situations, the number of the investigations can be modified to provide the best care for the patient. An extensive evaluation should never be allowed to hamper timely operative intervention or transfer in injured patients.

In cases in which it is determined that it is in the patient's best interest to effect a transfer, it is usually unwise to waste time in obtaining extensive studies to prove or rule out conditions that will be treated at the other institution. Such an example would be performing arteriography for suspected aortic rupture when the patient is being transferred to a trauma center for definitive treatment.

The majority of patients evaluated in a hospital will not need to be transferred. Guidelines as to the types of injuries that require higher-level trauma center care have been established by the American College of Surgeons Committee on Trauma. A listing of these is given in Table 41-2. The Committee also recommends an anatomic and physiologic categorization of trauma patients, as well as consideration of the mechanism of injury and the circumstances surrounding the event. Evaluation of these parameters should enable the treating physician to make appropriate triage decisions.

In the anatomic categorization, patients are grouped into categories based on the severity of injuries that are apparent on examination. Three categories have been proposed.

Category 1 includes patients who have the most severe injuries, which could rapidly prove fatal and require emergent management if the patient is to survive. Patients with chest or abdominal injuries with shock, severe head injury, or quadriplegia are included in this category. These patients are best treated at a level I or II trauma center.

Category 2 is made up of patients who have stable hemodynamic and respiratory status and no severe neurologic

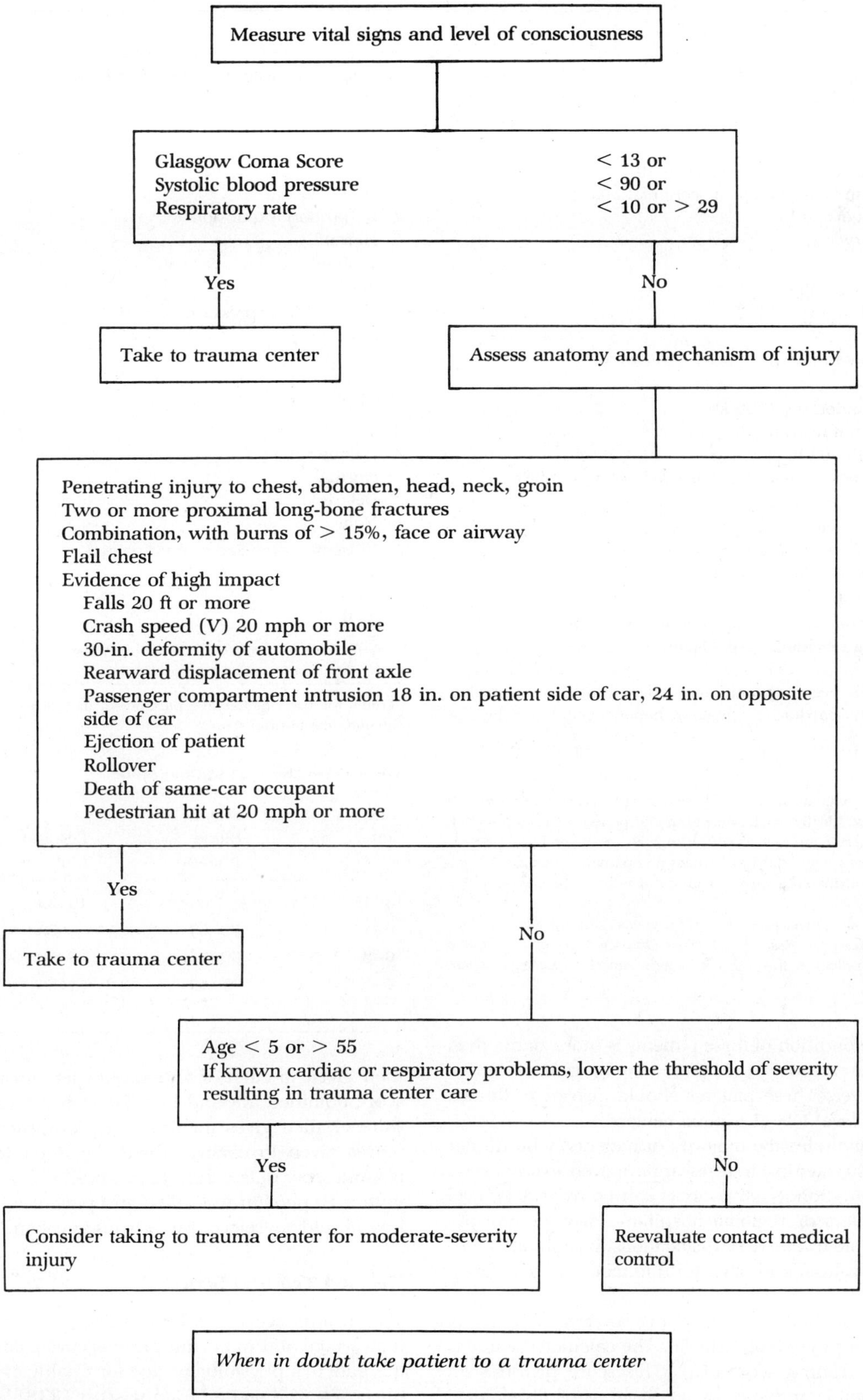

Fig. 41-1. Primary triage criteria for a level I trauma center. (Adapted from American College of Surgeons Committee on Trauma, *Hospital and Prehospital Resources for the Optimal Care of the Injured Patient* and Appendices A through J. Chicago: American College of Surgeons, 1987.)

Table 41-2. Interhospital triage criteria*

Central nervous system
Head injury
Penetrating injury
Depressed skull fracture
Open injury
Cerebrospinal fluid leak
Severe coma (Glasgow Coma Score < 10)
Deterioration in Glasgow Coma Score of 2 points or more
Lateralizing signs
Spinal cord injury
Chest
Wide superior mediastinum
Major chest-wall injury
Cardiac injury
Patients who may require protracted ventilation
Pelvis
Pelvic ring disruption with shock
More than five-unit transfusion
Evidence of continued hemorrhage
Compounded (open) pelvic injury or pelvic visceral injury
Multiple system injury
Severe face injury with head injury
Chest injury with head injury
Abdominal or pelvic injury with head injury
Burns with head injury
Secondary deterioration (late sequelae)
Patient requiring mechanical ventilation
Sepsis
Single or multiple organ system failure (deterioration in central nervous system, cardiac, pulmonary, hepatic, renal or coagulation systems)
Osteomyelitis

*This list identifies patients at a particularly high risk of dying from multiple and severe injuries. Ideally, such patients should be treated in a high-level trauma center where continued exposure to such problems by multidisciplinary team systems may afford the patient an optimal outcome. Such patients should be considered for transfer to high-level centers whenever possible.

Source: Adapted from American College of Surgeons Committee on Trauma, *Hospital and Prehospital Resources for the Optimal Care of the Injured Patient* and Appendices A through J. Chicago: American College of Surgeons, 1987.

injury. As the condition of these patients is more stable than that of those in category 1, the pace of management can be somewhat slower. These patients should also be evaluated and treated at level I or II trauma centers.

Category 3 includes the majority of patients, who do not have any life-threatening injuries apparent on examination and initial evaluation. Such patients can be treated at level III trauma centers or regional hospitals. They include patients with simple fractures or dislocations, lacerations without severe blood loss, and other mild to moderate soft-tissue trauma.

The second method of determining severity of injury is measurement of physiologic criteria. The calculated value is known as the trauma score (TS). This score provides an easily reproducible measure of the severity of physiologic derangement of trauma patients. It is useful in making triage decisions, in determining prognosis, and, in the research setting, for comparing patients with different injuries. To calculate the TS, a group of readily measured and quantifiable physiologic parameters are evaluated, and scores are then given to each of four parameters measured. The total score obtained after adding the scores of each separate parameter then gives the TS. The parameters tested and the scores given to each of them are listed in Table 41-3. A trauma score of less than 12 has been shown to be associated with a 10 percent mortality, and patients with a TS of 12 or less should be referred to a trauma center.

Table 41-3. Trauma score*

Parameter	Point value
1. Respiratory rate (breaths per minute)	
10–24	4
25–35	3
More than 35	2
1–9	1
None	0
2. Respiratory expansion	
Normal	1
Shallow	0
Retractive	0
3. Systolic blood pressure (mm Hg)	
90 or less	4
70–89	3
50–69	2
0–49	1
No pressure	0
4. Capillary return	
Normal	2
Delayed	1
None	0
5. Glasgow Coma Score (total points)	
14–15	5
11–13	4
8–10	3
5–7	2
3–4	1

*Points for each of the five parameters measured are added together to calculate the trauma score.

Table 41-4. Revised trauma score

Glasgow Coma Scale	Systolic blood pressure	Respiratory rate	Coded value
13–15	>89	10–29	4
9–12	76–89	>29	3
6–8	50–75	6–9	2
4–5	1–49	1–5	1
3	0	0	0

Revised Trauma Score

The trauma score has been revised to increase the ease of field triage and to permit more accurate characterization of the patient's physiologic state for quality of care assessment purposes. The revised trauma score (RTS) is computed from coded values (from 0 to 4) of the Glasgow Coma Scale, systolic blood pressure, and respiratory rate (Table 41-4). A score below 4 for any variable represents a probability of survival of 90 percent or less. The actual value of the revised trauma score is obtained by multiplying the coded values for each parameter by weighted constants. The sum of all the values so obtained is the RTS.

Application of the RTS is made easier in the field by elimination of the capillary return and respiratory expansion criteria measured in the (old) trauma score. Triage to a trauma center is presently advised if the sum of the three coded values is 11 or less (see Table 41-4).

Mechanism of Injury

In addition to the anatomic and physiologic categorizations, mechanism of injury is important to consider. Certain mechanisms of injury are more likely to cause significant injury than others. Patients injured as a result of such mechanisms should be evaluated with a low threshold for transfer to a more comprehensive center. The circumstances that precipitate or influence the injury—for example, alcohol or drug intoxication—are important, as such factors can induce an altered mental state and pain perception. This could mask significant physical findings.

If the physician is unsure of the severity of the patient's clinical status, it is safer to transfer the patient to a trauma center. Some of the injuries that should alert the physician to the need for transfer are listed in Table 41-2.

Duties of the Referring and Receiving Physicians

Once the decision to transfer the patient has been made, the responsibility for the initiation of the transfer lies with the referring physician. It is his or her responsibility to identify an institution that will be able to provide the level of care needed by the patient. This institution must not only be willing to accept the patient in transfer but must also be in a position to provide the required care as soon as the patient arrives. The referring physician must identify the physician at the receiving hospital who will be taking primary care of the patient. Direct communication with the receiving physician regarding the patient's history and examination in the field and in the emergency center is essential. Resuscitative measures undertaken, inclusive of the amount of blood and other fluids administered, and treatment and medications given, along with relevant laboratory values and x-ray findings, should also be communicated.

It is the responsibility of the receiving physician to communicate to the referring physician any additional investigations that may be needed before transfer and what therapies may be useful and should be available in the air ambulance. This is especially important if the patient's condition is unstable, in spite of initial resuscitation. It is also essential that adequately trained personnel accompany the patient en route, especially in cases of long transportation times. The patient's family must be informed of the arrangements made and adequate permission for transfer must be obtained from them before initiation of the transfer.

Table 41-5. Checklist of measures to be considered for interhospital transfer

Airway
- Nasal/oropharyngeal airway
- Nasotracheal tube
- Orotracheal tube
- Cricothyroidotomy

Breathing
- Oxygen: mode and rate of administration
- Mechanical ventilation
- Suctioning as needed
- Chest tubes

Circulation
- Control external bleeding
- Establish large-bore IV, internal jugular, subclavian, or cutdown lines
- Determine type of fluid to be given and rate of administration
- PASG

Nervous system
- Hyperventilation in head injuries
- Diuretics, e.g., mannitol load
- Cervical collar/thoracolumbar spine immobilization

Monitoring
- ECG
- Blood pressure, pulse, mental status monitoring every five minutes
- Continue adequate ventilatory and circulatory support monitoring
- Continuous oximetry
- End-tidal carbon dioxide
- Urinary catheter: record output
- Keep nasogastric tube to suction
- Maintain communications with both the receiving and referring physicians

Diagnostic studies (discussed in text)

Wounds
- Clean and dress
- Tetanus prophylaxis
- Antibiotics

Fractures
- Appropriate splinting
- PASG, especially for pelvic fractures
- Cervical and thoracolumbar spine immobilization

Record-keeping
- All appropriate prehospital and hospital records as discussed earlier must accompany the patient
- Accurate account of the treatment rendered and the response of the patient to treatment en route
- All orders from physicians and details of conversations with the receiving hospital should be recorded; this should include medication and therapeutic orders transmitted

DOCUMENTATION

Adequate written documentation must accompany the patient. Such a record must include a complete history and physical examination (including prehospital data), treatment rendered to the patient, results of laboratory tests, and reports of x-rays and ECGs, along with any other diagnostic study that was conducted. If a peritoneal lavage was performed, an aliquot of the effluent fluid should accompany the patient. Copies of all x-rays and ECGs should also accompany the patient. Additional information that needs to be specified and sent along with the patient includes details of the fluid administered by type and amount; identification of both referring and receiving physicians by name, phone number, and address; signed permission for transfer and, if applicable, for surgery, taken from the family before transfer; and a specific transfer form summarizing all pertinent data.

MANAGEMENT OF THE PATIENT EN ROUTE

The condition of most patients has been stabilized before transfer. However, it may be impossible to stabilize some patients without interventions (e.g., surgery) that are available only at the receiving hospital. Though such transfers pose additional risk to both patient and physician, transfer should be accomplished once the best stabilization possible has been attained. Some factors that require consideration before and during transfer are listed in Table 41-5.

SUMMARY

A comprehensive, well-thought-out assessment plan should be clearly in the mind of the medical professional who is responsible for the early management of the trauma patient. This minimizes errors and confusion, and maximizes the patient's chances of surviving a severe multitrauma injury.

SELECTED READING

American College of Surgeons Committee on Trauma. *Hospital and Prehospital Resources for the Optimal Care of the Injured Patient and Appendices A through J.* Chicago: American College of Surgeons, 1987.

American College of Surgeons Committee on Trauma. *Advanced Trauma Life Support Course: Student Manual.* Chicago: American College of Surgeons, 1985.

Biskell, WH, et al. Randomized trial of pneumatic antishock garments in the prehospital management of penetrating abdominal injuries. *Ann Emerg Med* 16:653, 1987.

Bivins, HG, et al. Blood volume displacement with inflation of antishock trousers. *Ann Emerg Med* 11:409, 1982.

Cales, RH. Advanced life support in prehospital trauma care: An intervention in search of an indication? *Ann Emerg Med* 17:651, 1988.

Carlson, WJ, Hunter, SW, and Bonnabeau, RC. Esophageal perforation with obturator airway. JAMA 241:1154, 1979.

Cohen, MH, and Jacobs, LM. Transcutaneous and transconjunctival oximetry. *Emerg Care Q* 3:72, 1987.

Cottington, EM, et al. The utility of physiological status, injury site, and injury mechanism in identifying patients with major trauma. *J Trauma* 28:305, 1988.

Crompton, RS, et al. Reduction of prehospital ambulance and community death rates by the community-wide emergency cardiac care system. *Am J Med* 58:151, 1975.

Gaffney, FA, Thal, ER, and Taylor, WF. Hemodynamic effects of medical antishock trousers. *J Trauma* 21:931, 1981.

Ivatury, RR, et al. Penetrating thoracic injuries: In-field stabilization vs prompt transport. *J Trauma* 27:1066, 1987.

Jacobs, L, et al. Endotracheal intubation in the pre-hospital phase of emergency medical care. *JAMA* 250:2175, 1983.

Jacobs, L, et al. Pre-hospital advanced life support: Benefits in trauma. *J Trauma* 24:1:8, 1984.

Jacobs, LM, Lydon, P, and Sinclair, A. The pneumatic antishock garment. *Med Instrum* 16:194, 1982.

Kilberg, L, et al. Effectiveness of implementing a trauma triage system on outcome: A prospective evaluation. *J Trauma* 28:1493, 1988.

Kissoon, N, et al. The child requiring transport: Lessons and implications for the pediatric emergency physician. *Paediatr Emerg Care* 4:1, 1988.

McSwain, NE. Pneumatic anti-shock garment: State of the art 1988. *Ann Emerg Med* 17:506, 1988.

Melton, JD. Noninvasive monitoring techniques. *Emerg Care Q* 3:63, 1987.

National Academy of Sciences/National Research Council: Committee on Trauma and Committee on Shock. *Accidental Death and Disability; The Neglected Disease of Modern Society.* Washington, DC, 1966.

Reed, J. Orotracheal and nasotracheal intubation. *Emerg Care Q* 3:1, 1987.

Reines, DH, et al. Is advanced life support appropriate for victims of motor vehicle accidents: The South Carolina Highway Trauma Project. *J Trauma* 28:563, 1988.

Rose, LB, and Press, E. Cardiac defibrillation by ambulance attendants. *JAMA* 219:63, 1972.

Rhodes, M, et al. Field triage for on-scene helicopter transport. *J Trauma* 29:963, 1986.

Trunkey, DD: Is ACLS necessary for pre-hospital trauma care? *J Trauma* 24:86, 1984.

West, JG, Trunkey, DD, and Lim, RC. Systems of trauma care; A study of two counties. *Arch Surg* 114:455, 1979.

Yealy, DM. Surgical methods of emergency airway control. *Emerg Care Q* 3:11, 1987.

Yelderman, M, and New, W. Evaluation of pulse oximetry. *Anesthesiology* 59:349, 1985.

42. Emergency Department Assessment and Management of the Critically Injured Patient

Marvin A. McMillen
John D. MacArthur

Far more remarkable than the surgeon's skill in repairing the traumatic insult is the organism's ability to tolerate the traumatic injury and compensate for it. Highly lethal injuries, such as penetrating wounds of the heart, aortic transection, and major hepatic or bowel disruption may present in a patient with sufficient physiologic reserve to be evaluated, diagnosed, and treated. The body's compensatory mechanisms are marvelous, but the compensation is of finite duration. Traumatologists refer to the "golden hour," before poor oxygenation, hypoperfusion, tissue anoxia, and acidosis overwhelm the patient and cause his or her demise. Most trauma patients who die after reaching the hospital alive have surgically treatable disease. It is the loss of their physiologic reserve that kills them. Rapidity of diagnosis and therapy and efficient prioritization are essential for preservation and support of this physiologic reserve. A clearly defined chain of command and a single decision maker are essential to this prioritization and the focus and efficiency of subsequent diagnosis and care.

The Committee on Trauma of the American College of Surgeons has recommended a standardized approach to the critically injured patient that is simple in concept yet elegant in its organization and flexibility. The care of the critically injured patient is divided into four distinct, although somewhat overlapping phases, including the initial survey, the resuscitation phase, the secondary survey, and the definitive care phase. The definitive care phase can be further divided into immediate and chronic. This concept was introduced in Chap. 41 regarding prehospital management. Although good paramedic systems can be relied on to have identified many of the problems prehospital, the entire drill should be repeated in initial evaluation in the emergency department. Close adherence to this schema is recommended, as this division keeps one from becoming so preoccupied by the obvious femoral triangle gunshot wound that the posterior chest gunshot wound is unappreciated.

THE EMERGENCY DEPARTMENT AND STAFF

The emergency department assessment and management of the critically injured patient necessitates that the emergency department caregivers and institution recognize their capabilities and limitations and identify where each patient fits into their system. The American College of Surgeons has created three levels of trauma care, and each emergency department and institution can be classified according to

Table 42-1. Injuries appropriate to each level of trauma center

Type of injury	Level III	Level II	Level I
Neurologic	Scalp laceration, concussion	Skull fracture (simple, compound, or depressed), thoracolumbar spine fracture with deficit, persistent central or peripheral neurologic deficit	Skull fracture (simple, compound, or depressed), intracranial injuries necessitating intracranial pressure monitoring
Head and neck	Lacerations	C-spine fracture; mandible and maxillofacial fracture, penetrating neck wounds	Major facial injury requiring reconstruction, major facial injury with polytrauma
Thoracic	Lacerations, rib fracture, simple hemopneumothorax	Flail chest, ventilation, management of pulmonary contusion, emergency thoracotomy and arterial-atrial-ventricular repair or emergency lobectomy	Aortic transection, injuries necessitating chest wall reconstruction
Cardiac	Cardiac contusion with injury current	Penetrating injury	Traumatic papillary muscle rupture
Abdominal	The decision to perform laparotomy is usually based on the presence of a positive abdominal tap, a positive abdominal CT scan, or an obvious penetrating injury. Organ injury—severity and complexity—is established at laparotomy and is often quite different or more complex than was established preoperatively. The trauma surgeon, even at a level I institution, who performs laparotomy must be prepared to deal with any visceral, hepatic, splenic, pancreatic, vascular, urologic, or gynecologic injury encountered. Most patients with abdominal injury are operated on first, then transferred according to their support needs.		
Orthopedic	All long bone fractures and dislocations (simple, compound, open, and comminuted)	Vertebral body fractures and dislocations, pelvic fractures	Fractures with associated neurovascular injuries, fractures requiring flaps for closure
Urologic	Renal contusion, emergency nephrectomy	Ureteric, bladder, or urethral injury	Renal devascularization, major penile injury, bladder injuries requiring reconstruction
Pediatric	Lacerations	Major neurologic trauma	Facial and genitourinary trauma
Burns	$<5\%$ BSA	$<10\%$ BSA	Facial or genital second-degree burn, $>25\%$ BSA; inhalation injury, electrical injury with burn

Key: BSA = body surface area.

where it fits in the schema. The resources that should be available in level I, II, and III centers are listed in Chap. 41. Hospital size is a surprisingly poor indicator of trauma care in the United States. Some very large centers are, in reality, level II centers, and some committed community hospitals provide excellent level I care. Some of the necessities for level I centers may seem self-evident (e.g., 24-hour presence of in-house emergency department physician and the capability to provide intubation/anesthesia in less than 15 minutes), but most Veterans Administration hospitals and a surprising number of highly specialized university facilities may not offer some of these services and should play a minimal role in the trauma network. Table 42-1 outlines the type of injuries that are appropriate to each level within the system. Table 42-2 is an outline of minimal logistic support for optimal trauma care.

PRIMARY SURVEY

The initial survey is carried out as soon as the patient arrives. It consists of evaluating five parameters: *a*irway, *b*reathing, *c*irculation, *d*isability, and *e*xposure, remembered by the mnemonic ABCDE.

Airway

Regardless of the catastrophic appearance of the patient's wounds, the first priority is maintenance of a patent, unobstructed airway, free of blood and secretions. The jaw thrust, chin lift, and finger sweep were described in Chap. 41. Most unconscious patients transported now arrive with an airway in place. It is important to identify the subgroup of patients with possible C-spine injury and ensure that no manipulation of the head and neck takes place until a C-spine film is obtained showing all seven cervical vertebrae. The conscious patient with a C-spine fracture usually has some component of neck pain; the unconscious patient must have a film taken before intubation. The tongue falls back against the posterior pharynx in most unconscious patients, and stertorous breathing is the rule, not the exception. An oral airway will be sufficient in 80 percent of these patients to allow adequate ventilation and can be carefully placed without manipulating the head or neck.

The therapeutic choices to maintain an adequate airway are:

No airway
Oral airway
Nasal airway

Table 42-2. Logistic support necessary for trauma care

	Level III	Level II	Level I
Operating room	Vital signs Accurate I & O	Invasive monitoring (Swan-Ganz and cardiac output)	Auto transfusion blood warmer
Anesthesia	Intubation Laparotomy <15 min	Intubation Laparotomy Thoracotomy <15 min	Intubation, laparotomy, thoracotomy, neurosurgical and cardiac anesthesia
Blood bank	Immediate 6 units O negative, TSUB in <30 min	Immediate 6 units TSUB in <15 min, platelets, factor concentrates, cryoprecipitate, and FFP in <1 hr	—
Radiology	Cervical spine, thoracic, abdominal, bone, and IVP	Immediate CT scan	Immediate CT Immediate angiography
Critical care	ECG monitor Accurate I & O	Ventilator Invasive monitoring Total parenteral nutrition Dialysis (peritoneal) Committed surgical nursing in-service program	ABS certified critical care surgeon Bronchoscopy Cardiac balloon assist Nutritional support

Key: I & O = intake and output; TSUB = type-specific uncrossed blood; FFP = fresh frozen plasma; IVP = intravenous pyelogram; CT = computed tomography; ABS = American Board of Surgery.

Nasotracheal intubation
Orotracheal intubation
Needle cricothyroidotomy
Surgical cricothyroidotomy
Surgical tracheostomy

The patient who is fully awake and alert, is able to cough and swallow, and has an intact gag reflex can be managed with no airway. In the unconscious patient without oral or maxillofacial injury, an oral airway may be used. If oral or maxillofacial trauma is present or if a semiconscious patient repeatedly gags on an oral airway, a nasal airway may be used. Orotracheal intubation with a 7.5- to 8-mm OD tube in men or a 7.0- to 7.5-mm OD tube in women should be established in any unconscious patient or any patient with facial injury or head and neck injury or who is at risk of aspiration from bleeding, secretions, or vomitus. Nasotracheal intubation with a tube 0.5 mm smaller is used in patients with suspected C-spine injury. Nasotracheal intubation is also better tolerated in conscious patients who require airway control. The disadvantages of nasotracheal intubation include the inability to perform bronchoscopy through the smaller tube and the increased incidence of purulent maxillary sinusitis. Needle cricothyroidotomy with a No. 10-, 12-, or 14-gauge needle and jet ventilation with 100 percent O_2 is advocated by some as a temporizing measure in the scenario of supraglottic airway compromise and the absence of surgical experience. It is a temporizing measure only and may be associated with massive subcutaneous emphysema if improperly performed. It is appropriate only if no skilled surgeon is immediately available to perform a cricothyroidotomy or tracheostomy. Under emergent conditions, conventional tracheostomy through the second tracheal ring may be associated with bleeding problems from the external jugular branches, thyroid ima artery, or the thyroid itself. In thick necked men, exposure may be poor and the tube may be inadvertently placed alongside or in front of the trachea. An extraluminal tube can lethally collapse the trachea with the first insufflation. Cricothyroidotomy has therefore been proposed as an alternative. The incision is above the thyroid, there is less bleeding, and the exposure is better. Emergency department surgical personnel should be familiar with both techniques and individualize the choice according to the availability of lights and equipment, their own experience, and the anatomy they encounter. An esophageal obturator should play no role in in-hospital management of airway problems.

Breathing

Once an adequate airway is achieved, the next priority is adequacy of ventilation. Either a 40 percent ventimask or 10 liters of O_2 via nasal prongs should be placed on all trauma patients until they are stable. One should quickly consider whether pain, secretions, vomitus, aspiration, bleeding, chest trauma, or neurologic trauma are impairing phrenic nerve signals, diaphragmatic excursion, chest wall expansion, or alveolar ventilation. If the answer to any of these considerations is "Yes," a nasotracheal, orotracheal, or surgical airway should be established and the patient ventilated with an FIO_2 of 100 percent, a tidal volume of 10 to 15 ml/kg, and a respiratory rate of 10 to 12 breaths per minute. A blood gas should be obtained immediately and again in 15 minutes by someone other than the primary physician evaluating the patient. If no one else is available, the blood gas should be delayed until after resuscitation is begun.

Circulation

With an airway in place and adequacy of ventilation established, one checks for the adequacy of the circulation. With

Table 42-3. Estimated blood volume lost*

Pulse lost	Systolic blood pressure	Blood volume lost (%)
Radial	80	20
Femoral	70	30
Carotid	60	40

*Note that the systolic blood pressure plus % blood volume lost equals 100 for radial, femoral, and carotid. This is a useful way of remembering this chart.

a clothed patient, blood pressure measurement may be awkward and unreliable, and a quick check of the radial, carotid, and femoral pulses should be carried out. The radial pulse is lost at a systolic pressure of 80 mm Hg, the femoral is lost at a systolic of 70, and the carotid disappears at a systolic of 60 mm Hg (Table 42-3). The patient with spinal cord injury may be hypotensive in the face of adequate perfusion; a quick check of the capillary refill of the thenar eminence or the nailbed should be done. Normal capillary refill is 2 seconds.

Disability

In the primary survey, one should note whether the patient is alert, responds to words or painful stimuli, or is unresponsive. The mnemonic of AVPU is useful to describe whether the patient is *a*lert, *v*ocally responsive, *p*ain responsive, or *u*nresponsive. Further neurologic evaluation is carried out in the secondary survey.

Exposure

Modesty has no place in the care of the critically injured patient; all the patient's clothes should be removed, and every inch of the skin and scalp should be inspected. This is particularly true with patients with penetrating trauma. Beware of the patient with an obvious and life-threatening injury (Table 42-4). Overlooked wounds above the hairline, of the back, and in the perineal area are common in the experience of every busy emergency department. The time to look for them is when the patient is first encountered—before resuscitation, the more detailed secondary survey, and the definitive care phase supervene. When a patient is deteriorating despite rapid and appropriate therapy, it is time for reexamination.

RESUSCITATION

The best monitor of adequate resuscitation and restoration of flow to critical organs is restored urine output. A urinary catheter should therefore be routinely placed in every critically injured patient. However, the presence of blood at the urethral meatus, a scrotal hematoma, or a nonpalpable or high-riding prostate on rectal examination suggests urethral transection. A Foley catheter should *not* be placed until a retrograde urethrogram has ensured urethral patency.

The focus of the resuscitation phase is (1) to rapidly establish two sites of large-bore venous access and (2) identify the presence of shock and then initiate its correction while trying to determine its cause (Table 42-5). Supplemental nasal or mask oxygen is placed on all trauma patients to ensure that the red cells that reach the tissue are fully saturated.

Table 42-4. Correctable life-threatening injuries identified in primary survey

Location	Type of injury
Neurologic	None
Head and neck	Airway obstruction or injury
Chest	Tension pneumothorax Open pneumothorax Flail chest Massive hemothorax Cardiac tamponade
Abdomen and extremity	Major vascular injury with pulsatile bleeding

Table 42-5. Shock nomogram

Establish venous access
Identify the presence of shock
Initiate resuscitation
Determine its magnitude
Calculate its correction
Determine its cause
Reevaluate

Two No. 12-, 14-, or 16-gauge intravenous cannulas should be placed in the antecubital veins or, if great vessel injury is suspected, in an antecubital vein and a saphenous or femoral vein. There is *no value* to central lines in terms of volume delivered, and their placement can waste considerable time. Electrocardiographic (ECG) monitoring should be established immediately on all major injury victims.

Major critical injury may produce shock either because of internal/external bleeding or because of the loss of plasma, salt, and water into contused tissue. Shock has classically been divided into a *compensated, decompensated,* and *irreversible* phase. In the compensated phase, cardiac output and tissue perfusion are maintained despite lost effective blood volume by increased heart rate and vasoconstriction. Clinically, patients are tachycardic and sweaty because of sympathetic nervous stimulation. In decompensated shock, increased heart rate and vasoconstriction are inadequate to sustain cardiac output in the face of lost blood volume, and blood pressure falls. In irreversible shock, cellular metabolism and injury have produced a state of refractory acidosis and tissue/cellular dysfunction that does not respond to restored effective blood volume, nor does blood pressure respond to either volume or pressors. Shock can be caused by hypovolemia (low effective blood volume), cardiac compromise (low cardiac output), sepsis, or spinal cord injury (loss of systemic vascular resistance).

In the majority of injured patients, the cause of shock will be hypovolemia, although a cardiac event may have precipitated the automobile accident, the gunshot patient may have cocaine-compromised cardiac function, or a spinal cord injury may complicate the resuscitation in a hypovolemic patient. Clinically, the patient may complain of thirst and be tachycardic and oliguric. The restoration of effective blood volume and critical organ perfusion is of primary importance. Calculation of the estimated loss of blood volume is extremely helpful in assessing the adequacy of volume

Table 42-6. Magnitude of hypovolemia in a 70-kg male

Hemorrhage	Blood volume loss	Heart rate	Systolic blood pressure	Urine output	Capillary refill	No. of units (volume lost)
Class I	(<15%)	<110	Maintained	Oliguric	Slow	3 (750)
Class II	(15–30%)	100–125	Maintained	Anuric	Slow	3–6 (750–1500)
Class III	(30–40%)	100–140	Decreased	Anuric	Slow	6–8 (1500–2000)
Class IV	(>40%)	125–160	Profoundly decreased	Anuric	Slow	>8 (>2000)
Death	(50–60%)					

replacement and evaluating whether losses are stable or continuing.

Blood volume is about 7 percent of lean body weight or 70 ml/kg; hence, in a 70-kg man, blood volume will be about 5 liters. Crystalloid resuscitation generally follows the "three-for-one" rule: If one has a 70-kg man with a palpable femoral pulse but no radial pulse, one can assume that the loss of effective blood volume has been on the order of 30 percent of 5 liters, or 1.5 liters (Table 42-6). Following the three-for-one rule, blood volume should be restored and critical organ perfusion well supported after 4.5 liters of normal saline or Ringer's lactate. Acidosis, hypothermia, neurologic injury, or sepsis may increase requirements, but if this volume has not resulted in restoration of blood pressure and capillary refill, continued loss from a missed injury or some metabolic, anatomic, or intercurrent compromise of cardiac output and critical organ perfusion should be suspected. The end point of resuscitation is not restoration of blood pressure but support of cellular oxidative metabolism. Capillary refill and a brisk urinary diuresis are better indicators of perfusion than is blood pressure. Young persons, in particular, are notorious for manifesting only mild tachycardia in the face of a 20 to 25 percent blood volume loss and then precipitously decompensating. Unexplained mental status changes may also herald severe injury and be the only sign of underresuscitation. Patients with hepatic or splenic injuries may initially be well resuscitated but "sag" over the next several hours as low pressure bleeding continues.

The pneumatic antishock garment (PASG) compresses the lower extremity, increases systemic vascular resistance, increases venous return, and may decrease blood loss in the lower extremity. It is usually placed in the field (see Chap. 41). Once in place, it should not be taken down until blood pressure is restored. (It should be left on all patients going to the operating room.) When the PASG is removed, one section should be removed at a time in a sequence proceeding from abdomen to distal extremity. Blood pressure should be rechecked after each deflation, and 5 or 10 minutes should be allowed to elapse before moving on to the next section.

Once resuscitation is initiated, the source of loss of blood volume must be vigorously sought. External signs of major blood loss are usually major injuries involving major vessels. (The absence of pulsatile bleeding in a major extremity injury does *not* rule out major vascular injury. Vascular spasm, hypotension, and tissue edema may combine to mask major vessel injury or even transection.) Direct pressure over a sterile dressing should be applied to obvious pulsatile bleeding. Tourniquets should generally be avoided. Internal cavities that permit occult major bleeding are the thorax, the intraperitoneal space, the retroperitoneal space (particularly in pelvic fractures), and the thigh (particularly in femur fractures). Evaluation of these cavities in confused or unconscious patients requires a chest x-ray, abdominal tap, pelvic film (if appropriate to the mechanism of injury), and clinical evaluation of the thigh.

EMERGENCY DEPARTMENT THORACOTOMY

The patient with life-threatening hypotension (systolic blood pressure <60) who does not respond to 4 to 5 liters of crystalloid resuscitation should be considered for immediate thoracotomy. Generally, these are patients with penetrating trauma in proximity to the heart. The role of emergency department thoracotomy for victims of blunt, decelerating, or automobile trauma has been carefully studied and found to be without value. Candidates for emergency thoracotomy generally fall into two distinct groups: Candidates in the first group have an obvious stab or gunshot wound to the heart and no vital signs and are either agonal or clinically dead. Candidates in the second group have a wound in proximity or a low-caliber gunshot wound whose path may cross the pericardium or great vessels and have poor vital signs or are deteriorating rapidly. The first group of patients must have thoracotomy performed in the emergency department. Despite the requisite speed, the ABC's must *not* be neglected. Successful repair of a right atrial laceration in an inadequately ventilated patient who cannot be given fluid, blood, and bicarbonate will still result in an unsatisfactory outcome. The second group of patients may be better served by a fast run down the hallway to the operating room. Better lighting, better exposure, a wider variety of instruments, and trained operating room personnel are extremely important factors in technical surgery that translate into lives saved. Furthermore, once the cardiac injury is controlled, immediate laparotomy may be indicated. An emergency department operating suite may be well equipped, but if a hospital performs one or two hundred cardiac operations per year and only one or two emergency thoracotomies per month, patients may be better off in the operating room. Obviously, an operating room that is located some distance from the emergency department is unacceptable for this strategy;

however, calling the full operating room staff to the emergency department for emergency thoracotomies is advisable.

There are two goals in emergency department thoracotomy. The first goal is to preserve brain perfusion by cross-clamping the aorta and decreasing the perfusion of the acidotic, vasodilated lower body. The second goal is to identify and resolve those lesions that are causing the life-threatening hypotension. These include right atrial, right ventricular, left atrial, and left ventricular lacerations and thoracic aortic injury. Central pulmonary artery and vein lesions are usually mortal, even when emergency department thoracotomy is performed under the best of circumstances by in-house cardiac surgeons. However, peripheral pulmonary lesions of lobar vessels may also result in exsanguinating bleeding. The bony thoracic cage greatly restricts the flexibility of incisions. Most surgeons are familiar with a median sternotomy learned from elective coronary artery or valve surgery. Although this is a good incision for anterior cardiac injury and an acceptable incision for anterior pulmonary injury, it is a poor incision for posterior thoracic injury. Neither bullets nor knives respect the restrictions of elective surgery, and the incision of greatest flexibility is indicated. This is the left thoracotomy with transverse sternotomy. The skin incision is made along the fourth rib and carried down to the anterior surface of the rib in one swipe. The chest is entered *above* the rib, avoiding the intercostal vessels. The pleura is entered, a rib spreader is placed, and the left chest is opened widely. The left hand is used to manually identify the aorta at the esophageal hiatus. (It may *not* be pulsating.) A large Cooley cross-clamp is placed. This should take less than 60 seconds. The sternum is then transected with a heavy scissors or rib cutter. The internal mammaries will be transected and will bleed. Clamps should be placed on them, but they should not be tied. The pericardium should be opened, usually transversely.

Trying to close holes in a beating heart is tricky. Right atrial, right ventricle, and left atrial holes are low pressure and can be occluded with gentle finger pressure. Left ventricular injury is harder to sew, and because of higher luminal pressures, it is easier to inadvertently injure a coronary artery. Left ventricular injury is also far more likely to be lethal at the scene and present to the morgue. Sutures, once placed, may easily pull through cardiac muscle; thus, sutures with pledgets are often used to prevent this from occurring. Once the cardiac injury has been repaired, the mammaries are tied off and the patient is transferred to the operating room for chest closure or abdominal procedure.

SECONDARY SURVEY AND DEFINITIVE CARE

History

In the confusion that often accompanies the critically injured patient to the emergency department, the history of the incident is often overlooked or reduced to "auto trauma" or "GSW abdomen." A good description of the mechanism of wounding is often critical in determining how high one's index of suspicion should be and how aggressive the workup should be. A 5-mile-an-hour fender bender in a parking lot would be unlikely to produce a torn thoracic aorta; however, running into a bridge abutment at 60 miles an hour on the interstate certainly could produce such an injury. Both patients may be awake, alert, and complaining primarily of a forehead scalp laceration, but the vigor with which one should pursue a "soft sign" such as the suggestion of a cap on the chest x-ray would be determined mostly by the likelihood that the mechanism of injury would produce the pathology with which one is concerned. Most ambulance crews and paramedics are quite good about observing and obtaining the information that the emergency department caregivers require. Like many of us, they are sometimes less efficient about writing it all down. Therefore, the history of the mechanism of injury should be obtained from these parties before they leave the hospital.

For automobile trauma, the history should include the following:

What kind of car?
What was the speed of the car at the time of the accident?
What type of stop—sudden, sliding, or roll-over?
What was the position in the car of the injured person(s)?
Were seatbelts used?
Was there a stellate window break, broken steering wheel, or broken dashboard?
Did seats break loose from their mooring?
Was the patient thrown from the car?
Was anyone dead at the scene?

Any patient with only abrasions and contusions who was involved in an accident where someone died should nevertheless be admitted for 24 hours of observation. The mechanism of the injury was clearly severe enough to produce major occult organ injury, and the pain of abrasions and contusions may mask the less intense pain of more severe visceral injury.

For penetrating trauma, the history should include the following:

How many assailants?
Was the patient shot, stabbed, beaten, or thrown from a height?

(Street gangs do not issue uniform armaments, and it is not uncommon for the injured to be stabbed, shot, and beaten.)

If the patient was shot, try to estimate the caliber and type of weapon and the distance at which the patient was shot. As discussed in Chap. 40, the amount of tissue injured is a function of the kinetic energy delivered to the tissues. "Saturday Night Specials" are handguns of small caliber (.22, .32, and 9 mm) with small bullets (less than 100 grains) and fairly slow muzzle velocities (800–1000 feet per second [fps]). Although they can certainly kill if they penetrate the brain or left ventricle, they do far less damage if they penetrate the liver than a .44 magnum with its 200-grain slug and 1800 fps muzzle velocity. Shotgun slugs have low muzzle velocities (800–1000 fps) but a weight of nearly 1000 grains. Hunting rifles often have low bullet weights but extremely high muzzle velocities of 2500 to 3000 fps. As a consequence, people with hunting rifle injuries to the chest and abdomen more commonly present to the pathologist than to the emergency department physician. Automatic weapons are becoming especially popular in settling disputes in the streetcorner pharmaceutics industry, and multiple woundings seem to be increasing in urban hospital settings. The MAC-10 .22 caliber is particularly popular. It has a low muzzle velocity and a light bullet. The Uzzi, on the other hand, has a substantial bullet weight and an intermediate muzzle velocity and can do considerably more damage. Many streetcorner warriors know the difference and can provide the necessary history.

If the patient was stabbed, the obvious most important question is, "How long was the knife?" If the patient is severely enough injured to be unable to answer this question, one can safely assume that the knife was long.

Trauma patients often lead disordered lives. It is not uncommon for injury to have multiple components. A patient encountered by one of the authors was caught with an extra ace in his hand during a poker game with his brothers-in-law. Their response was to shoot him in the chest, stab him in the abdomen, cut his throat, hang him out the fourth floor window by the neck, douse him with kerosene, start him on fire, and cut the rope. His admission diagnosis was "polytrauma, multiple mechanisms of injury." (He survived.) Prioritization and triage of such patients is often facilitated by identifying all the components of injury and writing down the plan in the first few minutes of evaluation, before the hard work and confusion begin.

It is also not uncommon for trauma patients to conceal other medically significant events from their treating physicians. Concurrent drug and alcohol abuse should be assumed until proved otherwise. Sixty to 80 percent of felons have measurable drug levels when arrested. Any wounded criminal perpetrator therefore has a two-thirds chance of having measurable drug levels. A toxicology screen and ethanol level should be routine in any critically injured patient. (Toxicology screens do not quantitate cocaine; they simply indicate its presence. Any young trauma patient who has an unexpected cardiac event should be considered for cardiac contusion, cardiac tamponade, and cocaine-related coronary vasospasm.) Drug and alcohol abuse are in no way limited to inner city hospitals, and alcohol and toxicology screens should still be routinely drawn in suburban and rural hospitals.

If the patient is not a streetcorner gladiator but an older solid citizen, an extremely brief but thorough history should be obtained:

What operations has he or she had?
What medicines does he or she take?

We have found it useful to rapidly ask the patient or available family: Have you ever been treated for allergy, anemia, bleeding trouble, bronchitis, cancer, "colon trouble" or colitis, diabetes, emphysema, "falling spells," goiter, gall bladder, high blood pressure, heart attack/heart failure, hepatitis/cirrhosis/jaundice, immune disorders (AIDS), kidney disease, prostate trouble, strokes, tuberculosis, "low thyroid," pancreatitis, ulcers, or venereal disease? This semialphabetical list covers most important common diseases, jogs the patient's or family's memory despite the pain of the injury or the confusion of the emergency department, yet spares a detailed, time-consuming and unnecessary description of each hospitalization.

Neurologic Assessment

During the secondary survey, evaluation for neurologic and orthopedic disability can be readily carried out in the first 5 minutes. As pain is a significant indicator of injury, the conscious patient should be asked to perform the maneuvers him- or herself. A conscious and oriented patient who can see, squint, look left and right, grimace, stick out his or her tongue, shrug, grasp one's hands, make a fist, flex his or her arms, raise his or her legs from the table, and bend his or her knees has just had most major neurologic and extremity trauma ruled out, although he or she may still have a torn thoracic aorta, ruptured spleen, or pelvic fracture. (His or her Glasgow Coma Score is 15.)

Evaluating disability as part of the primary survey in the patient who is unconscious is considerably more difficult. Doll's maneuver evaluates cranial nerves III, IV, V, VI, and VII but should not be performed on any patient suspected of cervical spine injury. The presence of a gag reflex indicates that cranial nerve IX is intact. The presence or absence of deep tendon reflexes neither rules in or out significant central nervous system (CNS) or spinal cord trauma. Normal tightness of the rectal sphincter, noted on rectal examination, is an indication of an intact cord and is of considerable value in the unconscious patient. Familiarity with the Glasgow Coma Scale (see Chap. 41) should be encouraged. It should be recorded as soon as possible after admission and periodically reevaluated until the patient is stable.

Head and Neck

Head and neck injuries provide some of the greatest diagnostic and therapeutic challenges in the management of critically injured patients. A bloody human face is a striking image that provokes an emotional response of urgency in an onlooker, patient, and caregiver, yet the scalp laceration that caused it is relatively benign, and it should assume an immediate, but not urgent, priority in trauma triage. On the other hand, an unstable C2 or C3 fracture may pass unnoticed until neck movement produces quadriplegia and death. The diagnostic challenge is to correlate the nature and mechanism of injury with those morbid or mortal injuries for which the patient is at risk and not to become preoccupied with disfiguring yet benign problems. The mortality of head and neck injury is primarily due to CNS injury or airway compromise. Whereas scalp lacerations are generally immediate but not urgent priorities, it is possible for an adult patient to exsanguinate from a severe scalp laceration alone (particularly an intoxicated patient who presents with three or four more critically injured friends).

The scalp should be inspected for lacerations, entrance wounds, or depressions. Palpation will often reveal abnormalities at first unimpressive on inspection. Extraocular movements should be tested on conscious patients. Although conjunctival hemorrhage may be dramatic, it is the anterior chamber bleeding (hyphema), the traumatic cataract, or the detached retina that is most vision threatening. Diplopia on upward gaze suggests a blow-out fracture of the orbital floor with entrapment. The zygomatic prominence is often contused in blunt facial trauma, but the loss of prominence should make one suspect zygomatic fracture. The nose should be palpated for fracture, and the nares should be inspected for bleeding. The upper dentition should be palpated and the maxilla evaluated for mobility. The mandible should be palpated along its contour for fracture. The mouth should be opened, and oral lacerations and missing dentition should be noted. (A common place to find broken teeth is in the right lower lobe bronchus.) The grimace, tongue, and gag should be evaluated in conscious or semiconscious patients. With extraocular movements, this evaluates cranial nerves III, IV, V, VI, VII, IX, and XI. The larynx should also be palpated for crepitus, and the carotid pulses should be evaluated (see Chap. 59). Although most important facial injuries can be identified and noted in the secondary survey, cardiothoracic, neurologic, and abdominal injuries are usually more immediately life threatening and thus take priority.

Chest Injuries

Chest injuries have a high mortality and account for one fourth of all deaths from trauma. But fewer than 15 percent of patients with significant injury limited to the chest who reach the emergency department and who are hemodynamically unstable or have significant impairment of oxygenation will require thoracotomy for correction of their pathology. The hemodynamic instability and ventilatory compromise of hemothorax and pneumothorax and the rapidity with which the patient may deteriorate pose a far greater threat to life than the underlying pathology that caused these problems (Table 42-7).

Table 42-7. Diagnoses sought in chest injury

Tracheal fracture
Bronchial disruption
Esophageal perforation
Diaphragmatic rupture
Myocardial contusion
Partial aortic tear
Pneumothorax
Hemothorax
Rib fracture

Evaluation

Evaluation of the patient with chest injury should consist of the simple triad of physical examination, chest x-ray, and arterial blood gas. The physical examination should be carefully repeated as resuscitation progresses and the situation becomes more controlled.

Physical Examination

In the conscious patient, one of the most reliable indicators of rib fracture is the patient's complaint of sharp, pleuritic pain. A moment's observation of chest excursion and inspection for contusion may provide valuable clues in the semiconscious patient. Crepitus and chest wall flail may be appreciable on palpation. In the adult, percussion is often a more reliable indicator of pneumothorax or hemothorax than is auscultation. The hypertympanic note of pneumothorax or the flat note of hemothorax may be more easily appreciated than breath sounds in a noisy emergency department. (The lateral borders of the pleural cavity may reach the level of the umbilicus, and the "intra-abdominal" portion of the lung is often unappreciated by physicians unaccustomed to thoracic anatomy.) Once the neck is cleared, the patient should be quickly rolled from side to side so that the back can be inspected.

Chest X-Ray

An anteroposterior (AP) supine chest film should be obtained on all hypotensive or unconscious patients. If chest injury has occurred, posteroanterior (PA) and lateral chest films are helpful. Because hemothorax and pneumothorax are the most life-threatening complications of severe chest injury, their diagnosis takes greatest precedence. A small hemothorax (>500 m) may not be appreciated on an AP supine chest film, but neither will this hemothorax be life threatening. Pneumothoraces are notoriously easy to miss, and sometimes the largest ones are the most difficult to identify (Fig. 42-1). First and second rib fractures have a high association with significant neurovascular or pulmonary injury. Whereas other rib fractures sustained in blunt trauma may be distractingly dramatic, their detailed enumeration adds little to the overall management of the patient, and detailed rib films *should not be done* in the unstable polytrauma patient. A high diaphragm is most commonly caused by a poor inspiration but may be helpful if lateralized to one side or the other as a sign of splinting, phrenic nerve or diaphragmatic rupture or injury, or subdiaphragmatic pathology.

Arterial Blood Gas

In the rapid secondary survey of the patient with a chest component to his or her injury, an arterial blood gas must be obtained. Because speed is critical, the femoral site is recommended. Hypovolemia, shivering, vasoconstriction, and combativeness all compromise brachial and radial sticks. Most traumatized patients are hyperventilating and are frequently alkalotic with PCO_2s of 28 to 32. Metabolic acidosis is *never* compensatory but is usually indicative of tissue acidosis from poor perfusion. A PO_2 of 75 to 150 on room air or 10 liters of O_2 is acceptable. A PO_2 of 60 to 75 mm is an indication for close observation, and any PO_2 of less than 55 mm Hg is a clear indication for intubation and mechanical ventilation.

It is impossible to overemphasize the speed with which the chest evaluation should be carried out. In a patient with a high likelihood of having a hemo-pneumothorax who is rapidly deteriorating hemodynamically without other obvious source, logistic delay in obtaining a chest x-ray should not delay the expedient placement of a chest tube. Patients do not die from unnecessary chest tubes placed by trained personnel; patients do die from delay in diagnosis of hemopneumothorax.

Abdominal Trauma

While it is always possible to find creative new ways of sustaining abdominal injury, the epidemiology and pathogenesis of injury tends to be fairly predictable: Children fall on handlebars or fire hydrants or are struck by baseball bats. Adults suddenly decelerate in their cars and are traumatically restrained by their seat belts or are thrown against

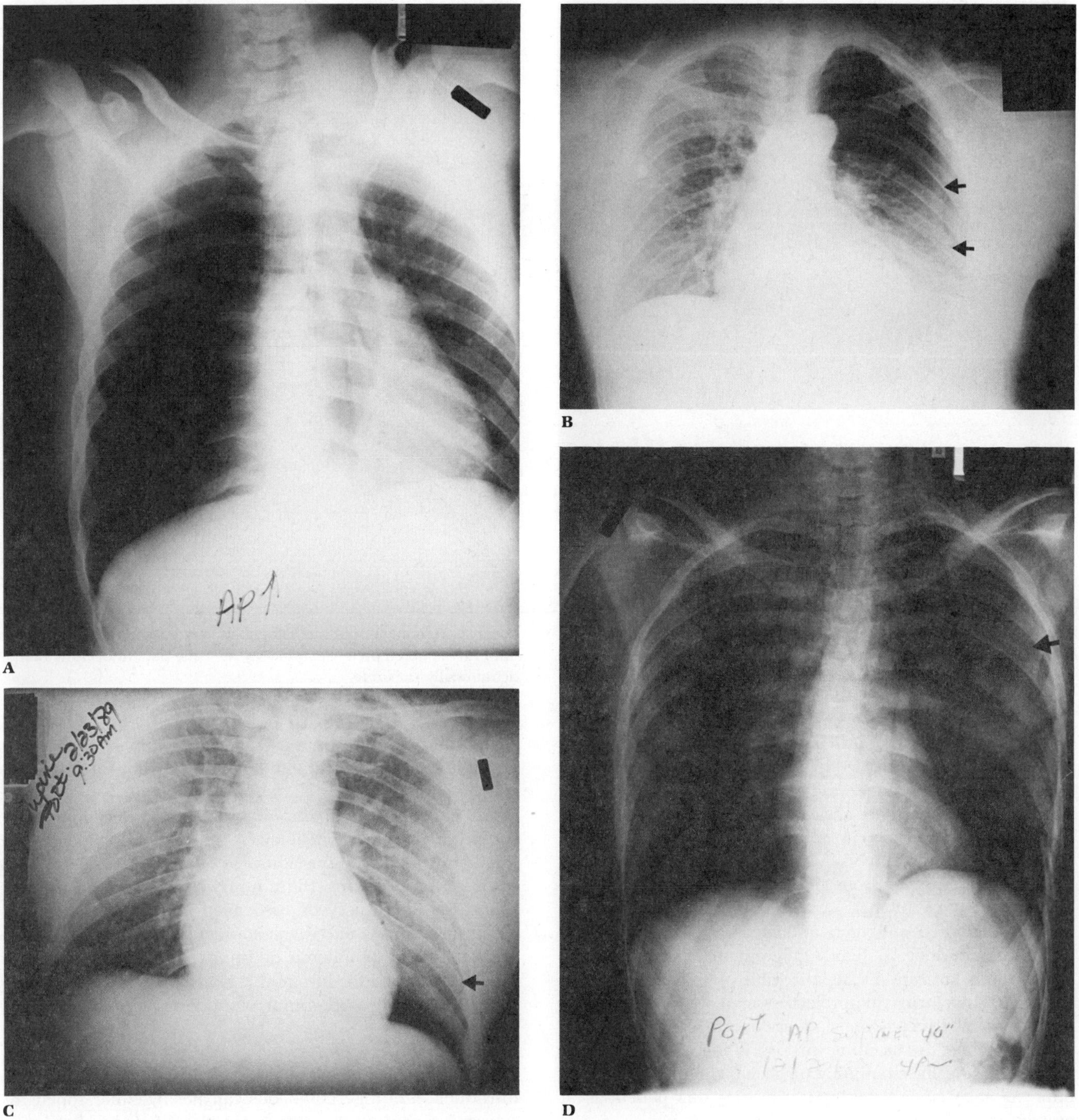

Fig. 42-1. A. Obvious right-sided tension pneumothorax in a patient with blunt trauma. B. Obvious left-sided pneumothorax with subcutaneous emphysema in a patient with an isolated stab wound above the left nipple in the anterior axillary line. C. Not so obvious pneumothorax in the same patient as in B in a supine film taken at the same time. This illustrates how easily large pneumothoraces can be missed and result in a later tension pneumothorax with hemodynamic instability after intubation and positive pressure ventilation while exploring the abdomen. D. Not so obvious pneumothorax in a young woman with blunt trauma after a motor vehicle accident. A seventh rib fracture and subcutaneous/mediastinal air are highly suggestive of the diagnosis.

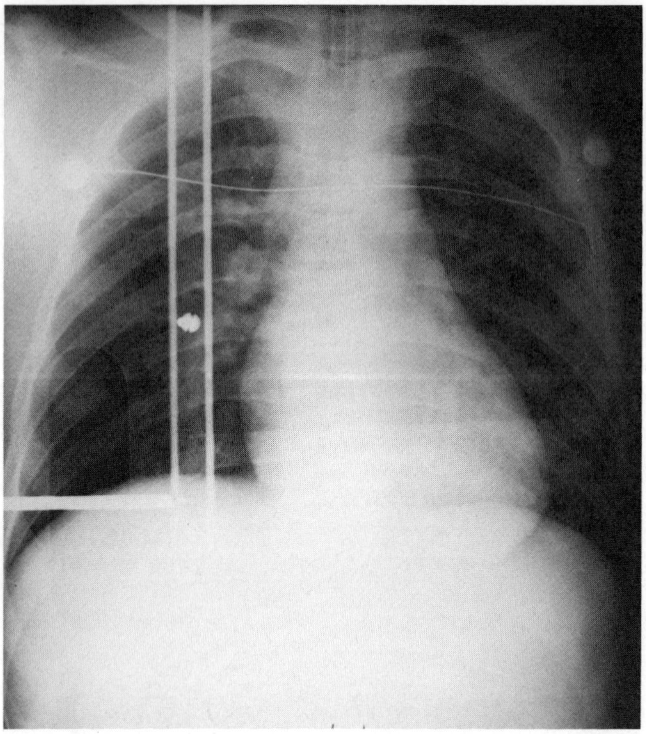

E

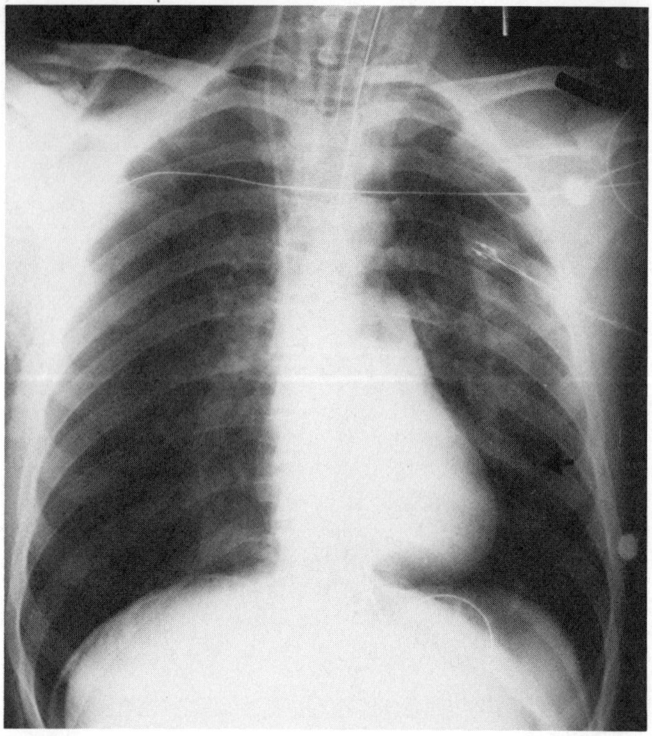

F

Fig. 42-1 (continued). E. Admission chest film on a patient with craniofacial, abdominal, and extremity blunt trauma after a motor vehicle accident. F. Left pneumothorax (and left pneumopericardium) on the same patient as in E after general anesthesia and positive pressure ventilation. Diagnosis was missed for over 9 hours until it was noted on a second x-ray after the patient became hemodynamically unstable.

the steering wheel or dashboard. Motorcyclists impact on the gas tank or are impaled by the handlebars or abrasively decelerate while dismounting at high speed. Persons fall from heights and sustain shearing injuries when their bony pelvis and retroperitoneum stop before their more mobile viscera.

Penetrating injuries from low-caliber, low-velocity weapons are a matter of luck. A .22 or 9-mm slug may pass through the bowel mesentery and succeed in missing vessel, viscera, and kidney. A slightly different angle with the same entry would lacerate the hepatic hilus and result in a fatal injury. High-velocity rifle projectiles create a large "cone of injury" on entering tissue and are more likely to present to the morgue. An accurate history is therefore extremely important, and the examining physician should try to determine as early as possible what injuries this patient is at greatest risk of having sustained.

While we divide the examination into thoracic and abdominal portions, it is quite often that the mechanism of wounding involves both cavities. In particular, with penetrating injury in the lower half of the chest or upper half of the abdomen, involvement of the other cavity should be rigorously sought. Abdominal examination should include observation; percussion; palpation and auscultation of the abdomen for contusion/laceration, organ size, or peritoneal tenderness; and notation of the presence or absence of bowel sounds. (Absent tenderness may *not* rule out perforation of a viscus and subsequent peritonitis.) A rectal and vaginal examination are part of any abdominal evaluation. Patients with penetrating wounds of the abdomen *must* be examined thoroughly. Blunt trauma presents a different set of diagnostic challenges and generally requires peritoneal lavage or computed tomography (CT) scanning or both.

All unconscious victims of blunt or deceleration injury should undergo peritoneal lavage, as should all patients with fluctuating levels of consciousness who are to undergo neurosurgical procedures. Blunt injury anywhere from the nipple to the knees may be associated with significant intra-abdominal injury, and even shoulder pain may suggest subdiaphragmatic hematoma or injury. CT scanning may be safely substituted for lavage if it is available within 15 minutes. Penetrating abdominal wounds require laparotomy, not lavage.

Peritoneal Lavage

Introduction of a percutaneous catheter by either "open" or "closed" technique permits evaluation of significant intra-abdominal bleeding. Gross blood on initial aspiration is an indication for laparotomy, as is a red cell count greater than 50,000 on the fluid return after 1 liter of normal saline lavage. Peritoneal lavage primarily detects injury to the large vascularized organs—liver and spleen—although it is usually also helpful with hollow viscus and pancreatic injury. Lavage amylase, as well as red cell count, may thus be a useful parameter to evaluate. A positive peritoneal lavage in patients with pelvic fracture is a special case. The large retroperitoneal hematoma is usually associated with a positive tap, yet these patients can be managed without laparotomy if CT scan confirms that liver, spleen, and other viscera are uninjured.

Computed Tomography
CT scan is often presented as an alternative to lavage. It is, in fact, complementary. CT scan may pick up a serious pancreatic injury that lavage may not, and the use of luminal contrast may also demonstrate duodenal hematomas and other significant abnormalities that lavage would miss. CT scanning may also allow the identification and follow-up of hepatic or splenic injuries that would give a positive lavage necessitating laparotomy, whereas scanning techniques may allow nonoperative care. The value of the CT enema in evaluating colorectal injury is still uncertain.

Extremity Soft Tissue Injury

Soft tissue injury is less dramatic than chest, abdominal, or orthopedic injury and less often the cause of hemodynamic instability. Yet soft tissue injury can be surprisingly morbid. Low-caliber bullet wounds, in particular, may cause significant injury to nerve, muscles, and vessels in an extremity with minimal apparent damage. A rapid mode of screening, a high index of suspicion, and an awareness of diagnostic and therapeutic pitfalls is therefore essential.

Muscle
Although striated muscle forms the bulk of tissue in an extremity, the muscles themselves are relatively tolerant of major blunt or penetrating injury. Debilitating injury most commonly occurs with denervation or ligamentous disruption and less commonly from injury to the muscle itself. Swelling is a common event with severe muscle contusion or blast, and it is often the major cause of morbid sequelae when it causes *compartment syndromes.* Compartment syndromes occur when extensive soft tissue injury causes swelling within the fascial compartment, inhibiting capillary blood flow, raising tissue pressure, and eventually compromising arterial blood flow. This will result in necrosis of the entire muscle group within the compartment and have a highly morbid outcome with significant disability. The most common loci of compartment syndromes are the anterior compartment of the lower leg, which contains the muscles involved in dorsiflexion of the foot, and the extensor compartment of the forearm, which contains the muscle involved in dorsiflexion of the hand. Compartment syndromes should be clinically suspected when the distal pulses disappear and paralysis of distal function develops (see Chap. 73).

Nerve
Penetrating injuries can often be managed with observation and antibiotics if one can ensure that no critical structures have been involved. Injury to small cutaneous nerve branches may produce significant anesthesia, but the results of nerve repair are so disappointing at this time that seldom is repair attempted for sensory branches only. Attempted repair is indicated for brachial plexus trunk, median, ulnar, femoral, and sciatic nerves. It is therefore essential that the primary caregiver include a brief evaluation of function in his or her secondary survey. Five-finger grasp, hand extension and flexion, forearm flexion, extension and pronation/supination, shrug, leg lifts, knee flexion and extension, foot dorsiflexion, and plantar flexion rule out major nerve injury and can be accomplished in less than 1 minute.

Table 42-8. Scenarios of major vascular injury

Penetrating wounds of the neck
Wrist and forearm lacerations
Deceleration injuries with aortic tears
Retrohepatic caval injuries
Aortoiliac penetrating injuries
Visceral artery transection
Femoral triangle injury
Popliteal disruption with fracture

Arterial, Venous, and Lymphatic Injury
The diagnosis of major arterial injury may be more occult then one would first suspect (Table 42-8). Soft young vessels may spasm down and retract into vascular sheaths where hematoma may partially tamponade them. Distal palpable pulses, particularly in the upper extremity, may be present despite proximal arterial interruption. Whereas missed venous injury may self-repair or occlude, missed major arterial injury either continues to bleed or forms expanding pseudoaneurysms. Fifteen percent of torn thoracic aortas reach the emergency department alive. Half remain stable for another 48 hours if the diagnosis is unsuspected. Injury to both artery and vein within a relatively intact vascular sheath may result in traumatic arteriovenous (AV) fistulae, as flow will be greatest into the area of lowest resistance. A "machinery murmur" is often present over these fistulae or in veins just cephalad. Proximity alone is an unreliable indicator of injury, as penetrating wounds at some distance may ricochet or disrupt vessels via the "cone of injury" of impact. A high index of suspicion and an awareness of the pitfalls are essential in the diagnosis and management of vascular injury.

While the techniques of vascular surgery have dramatically improved the results in repair of vascular injuries, the pathophysiology of traumatic and atherosclerotic ischemia are considerably different. Atherosclerotic limbs have time to develop collaterals; traumatized devascularized limbs do not. Tissue edema and prolonged hypotension in trauma patients may worsen reperfusion problems, and associated injuries may create instability, venous hypertension, or contamination. These problems combine to significantly decrease the warm ischemic time from the 4 to 8 hours often quoted in the treatment of atherosclerotic vascular lesions and increase the incidence of compartment syndromes and other morbid complications.

Diagnosis
Pulsatile bleeding, unilateral absence of distal pulses, and a unilateral pallid extremity are associated with major vascular injury nearly 100 percent of the time. But patients with combined systems injury often present hypotensive and vasoconstricted. Systolic blood pressure of less than 80 mm Hg is usually associated with loss of radial, dorsalis pedis, and posterior tibial artery pulses. During the resuscitation phase, the phenomena of *discriminant rewarming* should be watched for: As blood pressure and critical organ perfusion improves, one extremity warms up, the other does not.

Proximity of a bullet or stab entrance or exit wound to a vessel would *seem* a good indication for operative exploration. In fact, it is not. Of 143 patients with extremity injury in proximity to major vessels in one collected series, only 8 percent were found to have real injury. Furthermore, arterial injuries such as endothelial disruption occur where the media and adventitia remain in continuity. The luminal occlusion of flow may not be appreciated when vessels are examined extraluminally, yet it is the natural history of these injuries to progressively dissect and ultimately occlude the vessel.

Proximity is therefore an indication for arteriography rather than exploration in a hemodynamically stable patient. Logistic decision making (such as in a multiply injured patient) may necessitate delaying angiography for up to 24 hours, but it should nevertheless be performed. Although femoral and popliteal venous injury often accompany arterial injury, the value of venography is less well established. The patient who was hemodynamically unstable but is now resuscitated may have a significant decrease in his or her renal dye tolerance. Studies should therefore be limited to those absolutely essential to make the diagnosis. On-table occlusion arteriography or venography may give better definition with a lower dye load.

The care of the critically injured patient is a challenging unfolding of events. Adherence to an organized schema of evaluation and care is essential to keep from repeating the mistakes of the past. But there can be no substitute for careful, thoughtful, constant attention to detail and an assiduous effort to understand both the underlying pathophysiology and the body's attempt to compensate for and recover from it.

INITIAL LABORATORY TESTS, RADIOLOGIC EXAMINATION, AND OTHER STUDIES (TABLE 42-9)

Hematology

Although it is customary to obtain a complete blood count (CBC) and differential, prothrombin time (PT), and partial thromboplastin time (PTT) in most emergency departments as part of the initial blood work, these tests are seldom of significant value. The hematocrit reflects the percentage of blood that is red cell mass before resuscitation commences, just as the PT/PTT reflects plasma clotting before resuscitational dilution. But the initial hematocrit and postresuscitation hematocrits can be used to calculate the blood volume lost in the injury, and the coagulation studies are helpful in determining whether patients have concurrent hepatic disease or coagulation disorder, or are on anticoagulants.

Type and Cross, Type and Screen

Whereas the CBC and coagulation studies are of questionable value, the type and screen/cross is essential. Blood type can be obtained in 10 to 15 minutes, and six units of type-specific blood should be set up for any patient with a systolic blood pressure of less than 110 mm Hg or obvious pulsatile bleeding. Although fresh frozen plasma may not be of benefit for colloid support, it is essential for correction of coagulopathy associated with massive transfusion. It is type specific.

Table 42-9. Initial admission studies, polytrauma (blunt and penetrating)

1. Blood work (minimal)
   - Hemoglobin and K^+
   - Toxicology screen and blood alcohol
   - Type and screen/cross for 6 units packed cells
   - Arterial blood gas
2. Radiologic studies
   - Lateral cervical spine (if unconscious, blunt or deceleration trauma, facial injury, or neck pain)
   - AP chest
   - AP abdominal film
   - AP pelvis
   - AP view of any deformed extremity (*not* a complete study until resuscitation and stabilization are underway)
3. Urinalysis for blood, ketones, and glucose

Serum Electrolytes, BUN, and Glucose

Sodium, potassium, chloride, and bicarbonate together with blood urea nitrogen (BUN) (or creatinine) and glucose are part of most emergency departments' admission screen. Although they may suggest premorbid conditions such as diabetes, diuretic use, severe vomiting, or renal dysfunction, they are seldom of much real value in resuscitation or initial therapy.

Liver Function Tests

Both hepatocellular (SGOT and SGPT) and cholangiolar (alkaline phosphatase and gamma-glutamyl transferase) enzymes may become of value in the long-term care of the trauma patient, and there may be some value in knowing their initial levels. However, SGOT and SGPT also rise with skeletal muscle injury and are unlikely to be of any value acutely. An increased bilirubin is indicative of premorbid disease.

Calcium, Phosphorus, and Magnesium

Although massive resuscitation with blood products may slightly lower the plasma ionized calcium, the total body calcium pool is enormous and the deficit in ionized calcium is quickly made up from protein-bound calcium. Serum phosphate may be increased from skeletal muscle in scenarios of muscle crush injury and renal dysfunction. Deficiency of divalent anions or cations seldom becomes a major clinical problem, and changes in ECG Q-T interval may be more valuable in indicating problems than are serum levels.

Albumin, Prealbumin, Transferrin, Colloid Oncotic Pressure, and Cholesterol

Although an estimation of critical serum proteins is valuable in predicting the need for nutritional support in the recovery phase after trauma, the dilutional effect of resuscitation usually invalidates the results. Attempts to preserve a high colloid oncotic pressure to minimize adult respiratory distress syndrome (ARDS) have not been successful, and this parameter is of little use acutely.

Arterial Blood Gas

Once an airway has been established and ventilation ensured, an arterial blood gas (ABG) should be obtained on all patients who are unconscious, hypotensive, or chest-injured or have multiple long bone fractures. An adequate PO_2 (80–120) and the ensurance of adequate alveolar ventilation (PCO_2 of 38–42) should be noted. Despite the shortcomings of the "calculated" bicarbonate on most blood gas machines, it is a useful number to note, as many trauma patients may have a combination of respiratory acidosis from alveolar hypoventilation with metabolic acidosis from hypoperfusion and excess lactate production. These problems necessitate separate and distinct therapeutic maneuvers.

Radiologic Evaluation

In the multiply injured patient, diagnostic radiologic accuracy is sometimes sacrificed for speed. Single AP films of injured extremities in the initial survey will screen for major long bone injuries. Detailed studies can follow resuscitation and stabilization.

Unconscious or semiconscious victims of automobile deceleration injury should all have a lateral C-spine film, an AP chest film, an AP abdomen and pelvis film, and a single AP view of any contused, deformed, or crepitant extremity. Following resuscitation, stabilization, and initial evaluation of chest and abdomen, they should have a head CT with cuts at least 1 cm in thickness. Intravenous contrast is desirable but not essential.

CT scanning plays an increasing role in evaluation of the trauma patient. Its greatest value has been in identifying and following injuries that might give a positive lavage but at laparotomy are frequently found to have stopped bleeding. Thus, small hepatic lacerations and contained splenic injury can now sometimes be carefully followed nonoperatively by experienced surgical teams in hemodynamically stable patients without other significant organ injury. CT scanning has its greatest utility in the treatment of head injury, blunt abdominal trauma and automobile deceleration injury, and pelvic fractures.

Retrograde Transurethral Cystography

If a male trauma patient has blood at the urethral meatus, a hand injection of 50 ml of full-strength contrast retrograde through the urethra should be performed prior to Foley catheterization. Urethral injury occurs most commonly with falls and straddle injuries with resultant pelvic fractures. Evidence of urethral disruption contraindicates Foley catheterization and necessitates suprapubic cystotomy (see Chap. 136).

DISPOSITION

Trauma patients were formerly divided into those requiring hospitalization, those requiring operation, and those who could be discharged home. Contemporary trauma care is increasingly associated with delayed or serial operative care with intercurrent diagnostic studies and supportive critical care. Therefore, the secondary survey and definitive care may easily extend beyond the first few hours of the emergency department through the first few days of hospitalization. An attempt to predict the disposition of the patient is, however, appropriate within 6 to 8 hours of admission, to determine appropriate utilization of resources and required supportive care.

Table 42-10. Missed traumatic diagnosis

An unappreciated puncture or bullet wound (head and rectum)
Fractured pancreas (sepsis)
Duodenal laceration (sepsis)
Duodenal hematoma (bowel obstruction)
Missed enterotomy (on mesenteric border)
Renal artery disruption or ureteric injury

The Chronic Phase of Critical Injury

Advances in trauma care have allowed the salvage of many polytrauma patients previously considered unrecoverable, but this often requires an extensive and prolonged "team effort." Resolution of an epidural hematoma, repair of a ruptured spleen and hepatic lacerations, wiring of a facial fracture, open reduction and internal fixation of bilateral femur fractures, and treatment of hemopneumothorax may easily stretch out to 24 to 48 hours of very hard work under the best of circumstances. Superimposed problems of ventilatory insufficiency, hypothermia, coagulopathy, renal insufficiency, and electrolyte imbalance further complicate management. It is very easy to get intellectually and therapeutically "lost" in very complicated decision analysis. We therefore once or twice daily perform a system-by-system review of each decision point, reprioritizing and retriaging as we go. The purpose of the daily note is not to summarize data and laboratory work available elsewhere in the chart but to attempt to define the resolution or deterioration of both the initiating event and the body's response to it. Most young healthy trauma victims should be afebrile by the third postoperative day and ready for discharge by the tenth to fourteenth day. "Falling off the recovery curve" is an indication for careful attention to commonly missed traumatic diagnoses (Table 42-10).

Observation

Patients with single-system organ injury that is resolved within 6 hours of admission may nevertheless require 1 to 3 days of observation, particularly elderly patients with controlled intercurrent disease or the individual with contusions and abrasions who survived a mechanism of injury that killed several of his or her companions. Tissue swelling, muscle stiffness, pain, hypercoagulability, and tissue necrosis may not manifest until 24 to 48 hours postinjury, and significant physiologic deterioration may occur in the period of observation.

Close Observation

The difference between observation and close observation occurs when an injury that could rapidly deteriorate into a life-threatening situation is suspected but cannot be proved. For example, a patient with head injury may have minor abnormalities that are observed on neurologic examination and a skull fracture. But if no epidural is observed on CT scan, an abdominal tap is negative, and only a small duodenal hematoma was noted on abdominal CT scan, close observation is indicated. An elderly patient with four rib fractures may have acceptable ABGs but considerable pain with coughing and requires close observation. Patients requiring close observation are sometimes extremely challenging and require the greatest amount of insight and judgment.

Intensive Care Unit Monitoring
Intensive care unit (ICU) monitoring should not necessarily be reserved for the intubated, oliguric patient requiring pressors for hemodynamic support. If the injury suspected could lead to life-threatening hemodynamic or cardiopulmonary compromise in less than 1 hour, the patient should be in a surgical ICU. Any patient requiring nursing observation or evaluation at less than 3-hour intervals requires a special unit or ICU for his or her stay.

Invasive Radiologic Procedures
Although the new technologies of invasive radiology enhance diagnosis and may enhance therapy, it should *not* be assumed that "sparing a patient an operation" is necessarily desirable. Radiologic embolization of a spleen may control bleeding, but surgical splenorrhaphy may be immunologically more efficacious in preserving reticuloendothelial function. Whereas trauma surgeons are responsible for both the operative and nonoperative care of the patient, trauma radiologists have decided to be only proceduralists, with someone else delivering the routine patient care and observation. The decision to utilize an invasive radiologic technique should therefore be made by the surgeon, who is in the best position to determine that it may offer anatomic and physiologic advantages to the accepted surgical procedure.

Operation
General anesthesia is a cardiac depressant and results in loss of vasomotor tone that may be compensatory for hypovolemia. Appropriate resuscitation should therefore be achieved before entering the operating room suite, not therein. Triage decisions regarding concurrent neurologic, thoracic, abdominal, and extremity injuries should be made *before* the first procedure has been started, even though the findings of that procedure may alter the initial prioritization. All operated on patients with injury of more than two systems require postoperative care by a trauma team experienced and certified to expect, seek, present, and treat the expected systemic complications of major injury.

Although every trauma surgeon attempts to minimize the number of "unnecessary laparotomies" that he or she performs, no apologies should be offered or scornful glances cast when laparotomy reveals only a few hepatic capsular lacerations that gave a positive tap but have now stopped bleeding (Table 42-11). A knife wound that traverses skin, rectus fascia, and peritoneum may involve no visceral injury in 75 percent of patients, but if patients were observed for the 25 percent that would develop peritoneal signs, the one fourth that come to laparotomy would have a morbidity and mortality that far outstrip that of the "unnecessary laparotomies." A successful outcome of a past case in no way justifies a deviation from the established protocols of trauma management. A mode of management such as "close observation of penetrating abdominal injury" that may work well in a single anecdotal case may be unacceptable when repeated with a *large* population.

Table 42-11. Indications for operative exploration

	Penetrating injury	Blunt trauma
Neck	All or angiography, gastrograffin, swallow, and bronchoscopy	Expanding hematoma; evolving neurologic injuries; airway compromise
Chest	>300 ml/hr of blood loss	>300 ml/hr of blood loss
Abdomen	All	Positive tap (liver, spleen, and vessels); CT suggestive of bowel luminal injury; nonvisualizing kidneys on CT
Extremity	Proximity of injury to vessels, plus suspicious arteriogram	Loss of pulses; signs of compartment syndrome; major nerve deficit

After blood loss and hypoperfusion, the next great killer of the critically injured is sepsis. A well-resuscitated young patient with a missed colonic injury and gross peritoneal contamination may manifest little more than midrange fever (101°–102°) and leukocytosis for 48 to 96 hours, and then dramatically deteriorate into septic shock. While it takes several days for the pathophysiology of sepsis to develop its mortal course, the occult forms of injury leading to sepsis (such as a fractured pancreas or retroperitoneal duodenal leaks) should be high on one's diagnostic suspicions, vigorously sought in any patient with elevated temperature and white count on the fourth postinjury day, and aggressively treated.

The interplay between premorbid intercurrent medical conditions, severity of shock, and number and severity of injuries impacts greatly on subsequent surgical decision making. An ice pick injury of the left colon may be closed primarily with a few silk sutures. The same injury associated with multiple stabs, enterotomies, hypovolemia, and refractory tissue perfusion should probably best be managed with proximal colostomy or exteriorization. The wound has not changed, but the patient's ability to heal may have.

Interhospital Transfer
The management of the critically injured patient may initially appear to be straightforward. But as the definitive care phase evolves, competing diagnostic and therapeutic events may severely tax the judgment of the level II or III trauma surgeon as well as the logistics of his or her institution. A major goal of trauma networks is to achieve 250- to 300-mile transport in less than 4 hours. If one's emergency department is part of such a system, long-term management of any polytrauma patient (greater than three systems injured) should be weighed against the benefit of centralized referred care and rehabilitation. A polytrauma patient who should

be considered for transfer to a level I center is anyone in whom injuries to at least two major systems continues to require definitive care 8 hours beyond the primary survey and resuscitation phase. For example, a healthy 18-year-old man who has a mild concussion with no neurologic deficit, fractured ribs, a left-sided pneumothorax, and a ruptured spleen would have two out of three system injuries resolved with his neurologic examination, chest tube insertion, and resuscitation prior to his splenic repair or splenectomy. Care could be well delivered at most level III centers. However, if the physiologic burden of the injuries were unresolved 8 to 12 hours into the definitive care phase, with a level of consciousness still fluctuating and a pulmonary contusion resulting in very poor blood gases, transfer to a level II or I center should be seriously considered.

Deaths in the Emergency Department

Injured patients die; some die in the field, whereas others die in the emergency department. There are several important professional, interpersonal, legal, and institutional guidelines that should be observed when death occurs in the emergency department.

1. The staff did not shoot the patient. The motivation of almost all emergency department staff nationwide is remarkably positive. A bad outcome is usually the result of severe injury, loss of physiologic reserve from delay in transport, and inability to control blood loss and ensure the ABCs. When a bad outcome occurs, it is no one's *fault*, although systems failures may be the collective responsibility of the institution, its administration, and its caregivers. Therefore, systems analysis of bad outcomes is appropriate; finger pointing never is.

2. Document everything. Trauma sheets are extremely helpful in this regard because they graphically demonstrate what the institutional standard of care is and document that it is consistent with community standards of care. Brief annotations of deviation from expected recovery are also extremely helpful:

11:33 P.M. Still hypotensive after 4.5 liters saline. No external bleeding, Abd tap negative, CXR O.K., No evidence missed injury. Cardiac problem?

Even if the suppositions are wrong, they demonstrate that caregivers were aware that a bad outcome might be developing and were vigorously evaluating possibilities. The standard of care is not to always be right but to identify when things are not going well and vigorously attempt to identify the reason. Brief annotations are often extremely helpful.

If the family wants to see the patient after death, the body should be cleaned and the room should be straightened. However, the tubes, lines, clamps, or dressings should not be disturbed until the medical examiner has been contacted.

43. Pediatric Trauma

Ronald A. Dieckmann

EPIDEMIOLOGY

For almost 50 years, trauma has been the number one cause of death and disability in young Americans. Accidents cause more than one half of all deaths in children older than 1 month of age—surpassing the combined death rates for infections, heart disease, cancer, and congenital anomalies. The absolute dimensions are staggering: more than 15,000 children killed and 500,000 permanently crippled each year; approximately 21 million nonfatal injuries; more than 13.5 million hospital days, and $15 billion in yearly costs of acute and long-term care of children who are permanently or partially disabled. Despite an upsurge in interest in trauma care over the last decade, overall death rates remain stubbornly high, especially among the young. In addition to accidents, deliberate events—child abuse, assaults, and suicide—are now identified as significant components of childhood trauma.

Recent reports on pediatric emergency preparedness decry recalcitrant problems in trauma care:

- Inadequate training and equipping of emergency response personnel
- Lack of guidelines and clinical protocols for field care
- Lack of planned systems for transportation of trauma victims to specialized receiving hospitals for children
- Lack of clinical training for physicians in pediatric emergency care and pediatric trauma
- Failure to transfer unstable pediatric patients in a timely manner to centers capable of specialized critical care

Adult trauma center experiences over the last 15 years have yielded much cogent analysis of injury patterns and the cost-effectiveness of early definitive care provided within the first "golden hour."

The epidemiology of childhood injury, on the other hand, is not as well documented. Mortality from trauma appears to be higher for children than for adults, particularly in regions without pediatric trauma centers. Seidel's study revealed mortality rates of 12 percent in serious pediatric trauma cases compared to only 7 percent in adults. Romenofsky's review concluded that 53 percent of its childhood trauma deaths were potentially salvageable.

Special difficulties occur in caring for the young trauma victim that frequently delay early diagnosis, prolong field management, and complicate transport of the critically injured child. Furthermore, emergency department treatment is often inadequate, usually because of inappropriate resuscitative measures or because of long delays in arrival of the treating physician. Accordingly, the "platinum half-hour" has come to characterize the early phase of pediatric trauma care—where immediate actions and prospective organization are most likely to affect outcome.

SPECIAL CONSIDERATIONS IN PEDIATRIC TRAUMA

Most significant childhood trauma involves blunt force. Penetrating injury accounts for only about 10 percent of cases. Blunt injury from motor vehicle accidents constitutes 30 percent of total trauma deaths. Pedestrian deaths and falls pose major problems in urban areas, whereas bicycle accidents and child abuse are responsible for a smaller proportion of cases. (Burns and submersion injuries in children are discussed below.)

General Principles

Children are not small adults. Indeed, trauma in children distinguishes itself from adults in its patterns, anatomy, and pathophysiology.

Patterns of Injury in Children

1. The critical trauma victim is older than the critical medical patient. The peak age for significant injury is 8 years, with a range of 4 to 12 years. Serious medical conditions, in contrast, usually present in children younger than 2 years of age.
2. Multiple system involvement is common. The triad of pediatric blunt trauma is concurrent head, chest, and abdominal injuries.
3. Penetrating trauma is unusual. Impaled objects, gunshot wounds, and stabbings happen to children, but these injury patterns mostly occur in urban, adult victims.
4. Head trauma is the most frequent form of severe injury and usually determines prognosis. It is present in about 80 percent of critical cases and may camouflage associated injuries by distracting the examiner from less evident processes in the chest or abdomen.
5. Probability for death is highest when spinal, chest, or abdominal injury, respectively, is present. When such injuries are detected, a heightened sense of urgency is imperative.
6. The youngest occupant in a motor vehicle is the most likely to be injured.

Anatomic Differences

1. The tracheal orifice is tiny, allowing easy airway obstruction.
2. The tongue is large, and the larynx is more anterior, presenting unfamiliar landmarks during laryngoscopy and endotracheal intubation.
3. The head is larger and not as well supported; thus, head injury is frequent.
4. The scalp is well vascularized and may be the source of life-threatening hemorrhage.
5. In young children, the cranial vault can accommodate enough blood to cause shock.
6. Most cervical spinal injuries are partial or incomplete, and spinal fractures are unusual.
7. The chest wall is less muscularized and the mediastinum more flexible, thereby increasing vulnerability to internal thoracic injuries, especially pulmonary contusion and pneumothorax.
8. The abdomen is less protected by muscle, and the solid organs are less covered by the bony thorax, causing a higher incidence of liver, spleen, and kidney injury.
9. The pelvis is relatively small, so that pelvic fractures and urethral injuries are less frequent.
10. The axial skeleton is also more exposed, and fractures of long bones are common.

Table 43-1. Normal vital signs in children

Age	Mean wt in kg	Minimum systolic blood pressure	Normal heart rate	Normal respiratory rate
Premature	2.5	40	120–170	40–60
Term	3.5	50	100–170	40–60
3 mo	6	50	100–170	30–50
6 mo	8	60	100–170	30–50
1 yr	10	65	100–170	30–40
2 yr	13	65	100–160	20–30
4 yr	15	70	80–130	20
6 yr	20	75	70–115	16
8 yr	25	80	70–110	16
10 yr	30	85	60–105	16
12 yr	40	90	60–100	16

Physiologic Differences

1. Vital signs are age-related, difficult to obtain, and difficult to interpret. Table 43-1 lists normals by age and weight. (Rapid formula for blood pressure calculations: mean blood pressure = 80 + 2 times age in years.)
2. Blood volume is 7 to 8 percent of a child's body weight—about 20 percent higher than adults.
3. Hematocrits are lower.
4. Vigorous early hemodynamic compensation for hemorrhage maintains blood pressure, until 20 to 25 percent blood loss, at which point decompensation can occur abruptly and sometimes irreversibly. Blood pressure measurements in children are poor measures of volume status.
5. Surface is larger, in proportion to body mass, thereby increasing insensitive water loss and heat loss. Thermogenesis in the child derives from shivering and, in the infant, from brown fat metabolism—homeostatic processes that are readily overwhelmed by stress and environmental exposure. Hypothermia can drastically interfere with successful resuscitation by causing or complicating acidosis, hypoglycemia, and cardiopulmonary dysfunction.
6. Life-threatening injuries are often occult. Objective initial evaluation may evidence little cause for suspicion, yet profound and progressive internal injury may be present.
7. The effects of internal metabolic decompensation often outweigh the initial insult in determining patient outcome. Hypoxia and acidosis, regardless of precise origin, initiate a cascade of degenerative cellular events that ultimately cause organ failure. Treatment must be aimed first at reversing pathophysiology rather than at a specific diagnosis.

Emotional Development and the "Injured Family"

Finally, health care providers must be cognizant of the immature developmental stage and emotional profile of the injured child. Whenever possible, procedures must be explained, pain control optimized, and communication made supportive. Also, interaction with the "injured family" must seek understanding, confidence, and cooperation. A nurturant emotional support system for the child facilitates the physician's role in the delivery of care and safeguards the mental health of the child and family.

PLANNING FOR PEDIATRIC TRAUMA

Preparation is the primary ingredient for good pediatric trauma care. Prospective planning must include organizing field and hospital personnel, ensuring adequate training, and developing treatment protocols. All appropriate specialties must participate in both the planning process and the practical implementation of the "trauma plan" at the patient's bedside. Key specialists include emergency medicine, pediatrics, pediatric emergency medicine, surgery (pediatric, neurosurgery, and orthopedic), radiology, critical care, anesthesia, and laboratory medicine, as well as nursing and hospital administration. The "trauma plan" provides for a clear-cut, predetermined system and hospital commitment to coordinated delivery of care.

Planning for trauma involves personnel training and protocol development both in the prehospital and in-hospital settings. The emergency medical technician or paramedic rendering field trauma care needs directed education in pediatric emergency care, as well as proper equipment in the ambulance. Moreover, field practice must occur within a physician-directed system that provides both immediate online radio direction and retrospective case review. Treatment protocols and patient destination to appropriate receiving facilities must be carefully regulated. Short field times (under 10 minutes), rapid transport to definitive care, and minimal field interventions are imperative for optimal outcome. Airway management requires primary attention, and intravenous access should be attempted only en route to the hospital.

Eichelberger and others have described a hospital trauma plan that requires both a reliable method for mobilizing personnel and a scheme for task assignment and communication within the provider team. While the pediatric trauma center is the ideal model for coordinated "trauma team" functions, most hospitals do not have in-house multispecialty backup. Nonetheless, in every emergency department receiving trauma cases, optimal care involves the synchronized functioning of available call-in specialists with the emergency physician or pediatrician.

A coordinated response begins with notification of the members of the trauma team as soon as shock-trauma is recognized or suspected in the field. Tasks in the resuscitation are assigned by a single team captain and, whenever possible, should be determined prior to patient arrival. Ideally, team members should include at least three physicians: an anesthesiologist, a pediatrician or emergency specialist, and a pediatric surgeon. Ordinarily, the surgeon serves as captain. Interventions are guided by protocol, based on anatomic and physiologic criteria.

The resuscitation arena must also be strategically arranged. Proper-sized equipment, monitoring devices, and pediatric drugs and fluids must be immediately available (Fig. 43-1). Equipment operation, sequences of drug delivery, and a hospital scheme for rapid access to blood products—as well as task assignments and treatment protocols—should be rehearsed and routinely updated. Then, when a trauma victim arrives in the emergency department, a deliberate, orchestrated approach unfolds. At all times, a single physician leader must oversee the resuscitation process, give all orders, ensure clear communications among personnel, and expedite definitive disposition to the appropriate in-hospital area.

THE RESUSCITATION SEQUENCE

Exposure

When the traumatized child arrives in the emergency department, a crucial transformation occurs—the field "victim" is converted to a "patient."

1. The child is fully exposed. Overhead heating devices provide essential thermal regulation by maintaining a homeostatic ambient temperature (e.g., 90°F. in young children). This prevents dangerous hypothermia and minimizes insensible water loss.
2. The cervical spine remains immobilized, either by manual axial traction or by other means—towel rolls and tape across the forehead, or sandbags and tape. Rigid hard collars and soft cervical collars are inadequate forms of immobilization.
3. A cardiac monitor is applied.
4. One hundred percent oxygen is administered by mask in the shock patient, or by nasal cannula at 5 to 10 liters per minute in the stable, conscious patient.

History

Crucial information is obtained *rapidly* from field personnel by the physician as the patient is exposed and initial maneuvers are completed. A thorough history is delayed until after initial stabilization. Essential historical data includes:

Mechanism of injury
Status of the airway and respiratory effort
Vital signs and skin signs of perfusion
Gross neurologic status (Glasgow Coma Scale)
Response to field intervention

The Primary Survey

The physician's first examination evaluates only airway, cardiopulmonary function, and gross neurologic status and detects life-threatening problems. This initial "primary survey" takes about 2 to 3 minutes. A secondary, comprehensive, head-to-toe examination is performed after stabilization.

Airway

EVALUATION. Rule out airway obstruction and apnea.

1. Determine airway patency by inspecting pulmonary effort—the frequency, rhythm, effort, and symmetry of chest movement. Attach pulse oximeter.
2. Listen for normal air movement and for pathologic respi-

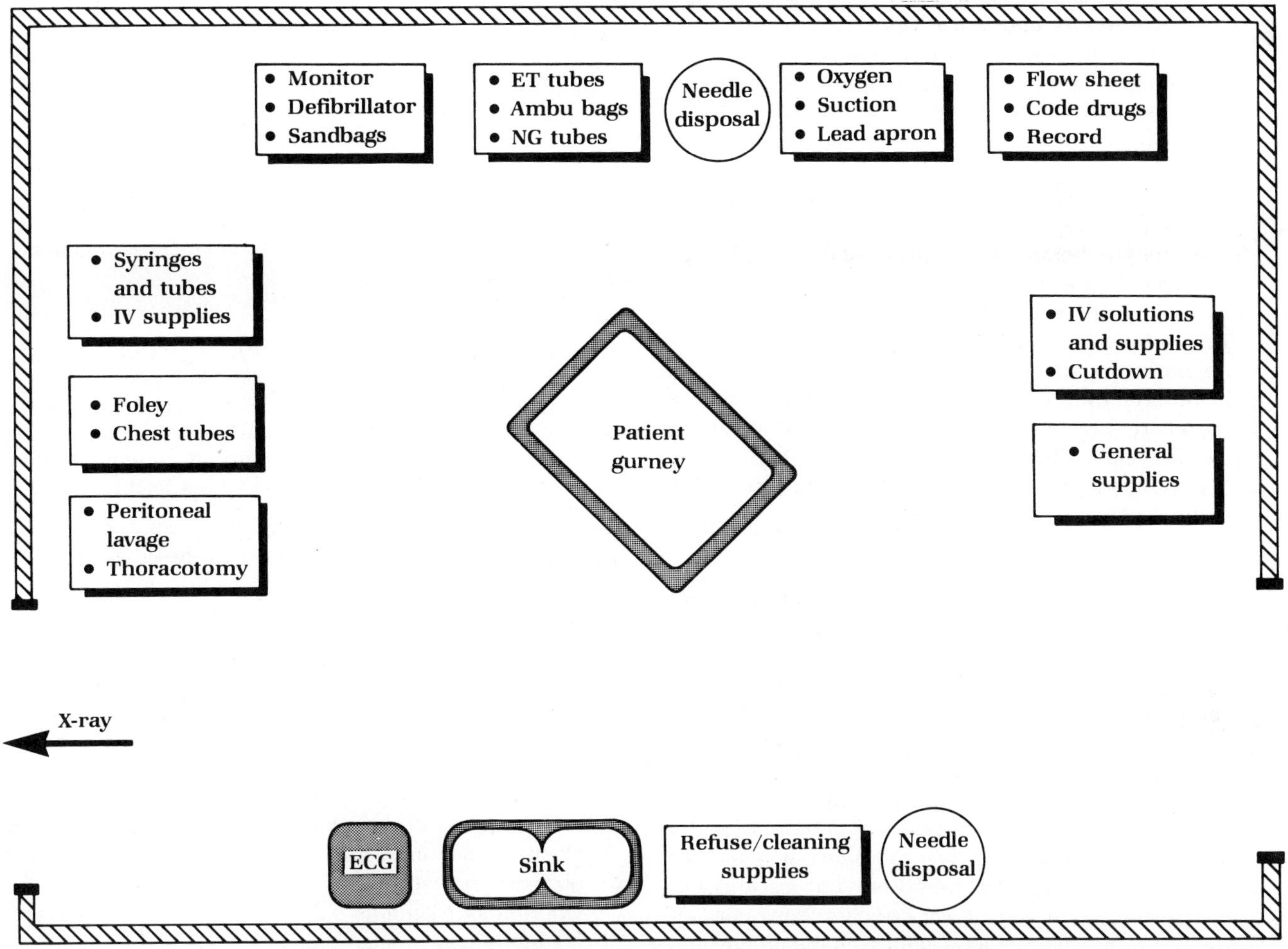

Fig. 43-1. Trauma room organization.

ratory sounds—grunting, gasping, stridor, and wheezing.

3. Evaluate the child's competency for airway protection, especially in high-risk circumstances such as head trauma, drug intoxication, or direct airway or chest injury.

MANAGEMENT

1. *Open the airway* with a chin lift, jaw thrust maneuver, lifting the tongue away from the posterior pharynx. If necessary, grip the tongue with a sponge or, where severe maceration is present, with a towel clip.
2. *Use copious but carefully applied suction* to evacuate blood, secretions, and foreign bodies. Suction is extremely useful, since small volumes in the wrong places can cause significant airway obstruction.
3. *If apnea or airway obstruction is present and bag-mask ventilation will not inflate the chest, do immediate orotracheal intubation* using the following technique:
   a. Assistant provides in-line, axial traction of the cervical spine.
   b. Select an appropriate endotracheal tube size, using wall chart (Table 43-2). Alternatively, choose an endotracheal tube that approximates the diameter of the child's fifth digit. In children younger than 6 years of age, use an uncuffed tube.
   c. After suctioning, visualize the vocal cords by direct laryngoscopy, preferably with a proper-sized, straight Miller laryngoscope blade. Check wall chart for size (see Table 43-2).
   d. Apply cricoid pressure. Insert endotracheal tube 2 cm

Table 43-2. Proper-sized pediatric equipment

Age	Endotracheal tube (mm)	Laryngoscope blade	Chest tube (Fr)	Nasogastric/ Foley (Fr)
Newborn	2.5–3	0–1	8–12	5
1 mo	3.5	1	12	8
6 mo	3.5	1	16	8
1 yr	4	1	20	8
2–3 yr	4.5	1	24	8
4–5 yr	5–6	2	28	10
6–8 yr	6–6.5	2	32	10
10–12 yr	7	2–3	32	12
14 yr	7.5	3	40	12

past cords; ensure correct placement by auscultating each hemithorax and epigastrum; then secure tube. Inadvertent dislodgment or right mainstream intubation can readily occur with neck flexion or extension.

e. Place nasogastric tube and evacuate stomach contents. Use orogastric tube when facial trauma or nasal blood or fluid is present.
f. In rare cases, where orotracheal intubation is impossible either because of obstruction in the mouth (e.g., tongue hematoma), uncontrollable oropharyngeal bleeding, or anatomic distortion, perform percutaneous needle cricothyroidotomy (see Procedure 7). This technique can provide adequate oxygenation and ventilation for about 30 minutes.
g. In children over 12 years of age, the standard incision cricothyroidotomy is preferred, using adult technique (see Procedure 7).
h. Maintain oxygen saturation on pulse oximeter greater than 92 percent.

CAVEATS

1. Do not manipulate the neck unnecessarily during airway management.
2. Do not delay orotracheal intubation when obstruction or apnea is present, even in the setting of possible cervical spine injury. The greater threat of life (hypoxia) must be managed first. Also, the unstable trauma patient is far more likely to suffer morbidity and mortality from ventilatory insufficiency than from spinal cord injury.
3. Avoid use of mechanical airway devices in the emergency department for unstable patients. They are not well tolerated in the conscious patient, and any unconscious patient requiring an airway device usually requires an endotracheal tube. Their greatest value is in the prehospital setting, where endotracheal intubation cannot be accomplished due to time, technical difficulty, or restrictions on paramedic scope of practice.
4. Nasotracheal intubation is quite difficult in the uncooperative young child in extremis. Bleeding from tonsillar and pharyngeal trauma is common, and esophageal intubation is frequent. Furthermore, there are no data to indicate reduction in cervical spine injury with this technique compared with orotracheal intubation using in-line traction. Both are risky.
5. Tracheostomy is contraindicated in the young child in the emergency department.

Breathing

EVALUATION. Rule out flail chest, open pneumothorax, closed tension pneumothorax, massive hemothorax, and pulmonary contusion.

1. If the airway does not require urgent management, continue with the primary assessment of breathing.
2. Look carefully at the chest wall for evidence of trauma (hematomas, ecchymoses, abrasions, penetrating wounds), splinting, and paradoxical movement.
3. Palpate the thorax to detect subcutaneous emphysema, rib instability, flail segments, or sucking wounds. Note the position of the trachea relative to the sternal notch.
4. Auscultate the hemithoraces, listening for quality and discrepancy in breath sounds.

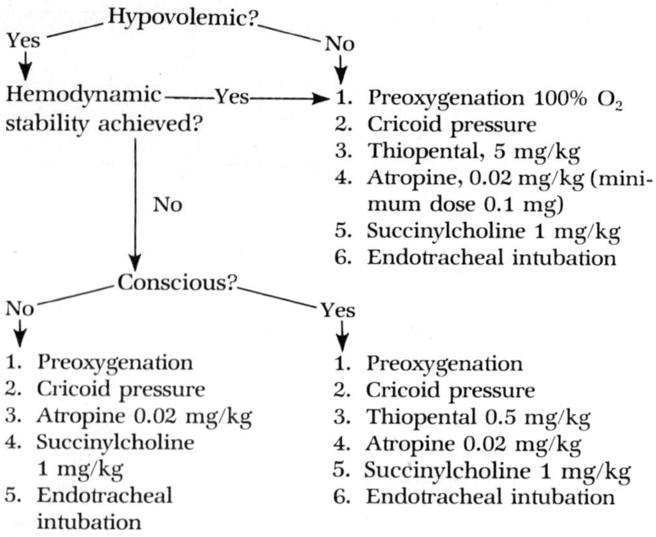

Fig. 43-2. Rapid induction anesthesia in pediatric trauma.

MANAGEMENT

1. If rapid assessment discloses clinical evidence for ventilating insufficiency (e.g., flail chest) and bag-valve-mask technique does not adequately inflate the chest, proceed to immediate endotracheal intubation, with in-line cervical traction.
2. Radiographic evaluation of the cervical spine and rapid-induction anesthesia should ordinarily precede orotracheal intubation in the perfusing patient without airway obstruction *who can be successfully ventilated by bag-valve-mask technique.* Figure 43-2 presents an algorithm for intubation in such patients.
3. If respiratory distress continues after endotracheal intubation, tube thoracostomy is required. If tube thoracostomy cannot be accomplished immediately, do needle thoracostomy first (see Procedure 41D).
4. When prepared, proceed to tube thoracostomy. A unilateral chest tube is placed when injuries appear one-sided. However, if one tube is ineffective or if physical findings are not lateralized, insert bilateral chest tubes (see Pediatric Procedure 41E).
5. When open pneumothorax (sucking chest wound) is diagnosed, cover the open site with petrolatum gauze to prevent further air entry and increased intrapleural tension. Insert chest tube through a surgical incision, as described previously, on the involved side.

CAVEATS

1. Rapid-induction anesthesia may precipitously decrease blood pressure in the traumatized child, especially in the presence of hypovolemia.
2. Chest auscultation is frequently unreliable. A difference in breath sounds *alone* should not indicate tube thoracostomy. In the patient who is not in respiratory distress, usually there is time to obtain a chest radiograph.
3. Needle or tube thoracostomy should not be delayed for chest radiography in an *unstable* patient in respiratory distress when clinical findings suggest significant pneumothorax or hemothorax (i.e., tracheal deviation, decreased breath sounds, subcutaneous emphysema,

jugular venous distention with hypotension). Immediate decompression may be lifesaving.

4. Tube thoracostomy can appropriately *precede* endotracheal intubation when clinical assessment suggests pneumothorax of hemothorax as the major problem. This sequence is especially appropriate for penetrating injuries.
5. Airway and breathing problems not requiring urgent intubation must be constantly reassessed while radiographs of the cervical spine and chest are obtained. Too often, however, endotracheal intubation is dangerously delayed.
6. Continued air leaks, after the thoracostomy tube is connected to water seal drainage and suction, may indicate tracheal or bronchial rupture.

Perfusion

EVALUATION. Rule out external or occult hemorrhage (especially abdominal), myocardial contusion, and pericardial tamponade.

1. After assessment of the airway and adequacy of breathing, the examiner turns to evaluation of the degrees of shock and requirements for fluids and blood products.
2. Inspect cardiac monitor for rate and rhythm.
3. Evaluate clinical indicators of perfusion in children:
   a. *Skin.* The earliest hemodynamic response to blood loss is peripheral vasoconstriction. Delayed capillary refill (>2 seconds) and pale color and cool, clammy skin in a properly warmed environment are sensitive and specific signs of hypovolemia. Since vasoconstriction occurs first in the lower extremities, check skin at the kneecaps.
   b. *Heart rate and respiratory rate.* Very sensitive but nonspecific indicators of hypovolemia.
   c. *Pulse pressure.* More sensitive and specific than blood pressure, but often the diastolic level is difficult to obtain without a Doppler device.
   d. *Blood pressure.* Extremely insensitive, although quite specific. Twenty-five percent blood loss can occur before hypotension appears in children. Also, it is difficult to obtain and interpret age-dependent vital signs in children.
   e. *Jugular venous distention.* This finding is useful only if positive. When shock is present along with external jugular venous distention, pericardial tamponade, tension pneumothorax, or myocardial contusion are likely causes.
   f. *Mental status.* Agitation or confusion may indicate hypoperfusion. However, since hypoxia or head trauma or both may also affect the level of consciousness, this sign is nonspecific.

MANAGEMENT. *Stop hemorrhage*

1. Stop external hemorrhage by direct pressure.
2. If clinical assessment indicates pericardial tamponade, do immediate pericardiocentesis (see Procedure 43).

Establish Intravascular Access

1. *Percutaneous approach.* Establish intravenous access, with at least two lines, preferably one above and one below the diaphragm. Access can be extremely difficult in the traumatized child in shock with low venous pressures and may pose a major obstacle to resuscitation. Percutaneous venous cannulation is especially difficult in children younger than 2 years of age.
2. *Surgical cutdown and intraosseous approach.* The following sequence is used to obtain vascular access in the hemodynamically unstable patient:
   a. In children older than 2 years, perform an immediate open surgical cutdown on the greater saphenous vein, at the ankle. The vein lies predictably above the tibia, one finger breadth anterior and one finger breadth proximal to the medial malleolus (see Procedure 9). In children, the saphenous vein may not require distal ligation. Appropriate catheters in children include a short 14-gauge over-the-needle catheter, or a No. 5 or No. 8 infant feeding catheter.
   b. A second line is started by percutaneous cannulation in high yield areas: the femoral area, the antecubital fossa, the external jugular, the fifth interdigital space. Guidewires, where available, can significantly improve success when cannulating large veins (e.g., femoral vein).
   c. If percutaneous cannulation is unsuccessful after 1 to 2 minutes, establish an intraosseous line in either the distal femur or proximal tibia. The intraosseous route accommodates moderate infusion rates (see Procedure 42D). If necessary, multiple intraosseous lines can be used. Volume administration is enhanced when pressure is applied to infusion apparatus.
   d. Alternative sites for open venous access when greater saphenous cutdown or percutaneous cannulation fail include cutdown at the basilic vein in the antecubital fossa or at the cephalic vein in the wrist. Cutdown on the greater saphenous vein at the fossa ovalis will usually be successful.
   e. In children younger than 2 years, in cases in which surgical cutdown is technically difficult even in experienced hands, attempt initial cutdown at the greater saphenous vein, at the fossa ovalis. A No. 5 feeding catheter is advanced directly into the femoral vein. A second line is established by the intraosseous route, usually in the femur.

Table 43-3. Fluid therapy in shock

Push 20 ml/kg of Ringer's lactate or normal saline.
Repeat 20 ml/kg of crystalloid, if no improvement.
10 ml/kg packed cells or whole blood; repeat, as needed.
Expedite operative management of hemorrhage.

Begin Fluid Therapy

1. Begin vigorous fluid therapy with two large lines in place (Table 43-3). Crystalloid solution—Ringer's lactate or normal saline—is quickly infused at 20 ml/kg. Colloid (e.g., albuminated saline) offers no clear advantage over crystalloid when administered to the same hemodynamic end point. Due to its primary distribution within the vascular space, colloid volume requirements are lower, usually about one-third those of crystalloid. The main deterrent to use of colloid is cost: It is 20 to 50 times as expensive as crystalloid.
2. If signs of hypoperfusion persist after 20 ml/kg, repeat with a second 20 ml/kg bolus.

Table 43-4. Initial treatment of pediatric dysrhythmias

Dysrhythmia	Treatment
Ventricular fibrillation	Defibrillate at 2 joules/kg Repeat at 4 joules/kg Lidocaine, 1 mg/kg, then 50 μg/kg/min
Ventricular tachycardia	Synchronized counterversion 1 joule/kg Repeat at 2 joules/kg Lidocaine, 1 mg/kg, then 50 μg/kg/min
Bradycardia	Atropine, 0.02 mg/kg (minimum dose, 0.1 mg) Dopamine, 5–10 μg/kg/min
Asystole	Epinephrine 0.01–0.2 mg/kg (Higher doses usually necessary)

3. If 40 ml/kg of crystalloid does not restore hemodynamic stability, blood component therapy is required.

Transfusion

1. In initial resuscitation, either type O negative (females) or O positive (males) packed red blood cells are mixed with normal saline and administered at 10 ml/kg aliquots. Fresh whole blood is best but is not usually available.
2. If blood loss is not immediately life threatening, use type-specific blood (10 minutes in most blood banks), or crossmatched blood (20–30 minutes).
3. Use blood warmer and micropore filters with blood products.
4. Fresh frozen plasma and platelets should be considered after 40–60 ml/kg of blood is given.
5. When stabilization requires blood product administration, definitive care often requires the operating theater.

Emphasize Monitoring and Early Surgical Consultation

1. Insert a urinary bladder catheter in all shock patients (see Table 43-2 for size) and follow urinary output—a highly sensitive indicator of perfusion and response to therapy. Establish output of at least 1 ml/kg/hr. Withhold urinary bladder catheter in the setting of clinical pelvic fracture, urethral blood, or perineal or scrotal hematoma.
2. Rarely, drug therapy or electrical therapy is required to manage cardiac rhythm disturbances causing or contributing to shock. Myocardial contusion will sometimes cause heart rate and rhythm abnormalities. Such disturbances include ventricular fibrillation, ventricular tachycardia, and bradycardia. Table 43-4 provides specific dose forms for such therapies.
3. Penetrating trauma arrests and shock that is refractory to blood component therapy are indications for emergency department open thoracotomy (see Chap. 42). Direct visualization of the major vascular structures may permit emergent repair, as well as evacuation of pericardial tamponade. Moreover, aortic crossclamping preserves cerebral and myocardial perfusion so that bleeding sites (often in the abdomen) can be controlled in the operating theater.
4. Early surgical consultation in shock is imperative since definitive management may require laparotomy or other operative intervention.

Table 43-5. Emergency department tubes for major trauma patients

Endotracheal tube
Nasogastric tube
Two large intravenous or intraosseous lines
Urinary bladder catheter
Rectal temperature probe

CAVEATS

1. After stabilization, titrate fluid, glucose, and electrolyte administration to accommodate maintenance requirements and ongoing losses. Do not overhydrate, since pulmonary edema may result.
2. Use a flow sheet to keep track of temperature, vital signs, input and output, and key laboratory data.
3. Do not delay administration of blood products when clinical signs of shock exist. This is a common error in preventable deaths.
4. Central venous lines are dangerous in pediatric trauma resuscitation. Complication rates are high among inexperienced practitioners. Guidewires may reduce complications.
5. Avoid use of military anti-shock trousers (MAST) in children. They may mask significant injury to the abdomen or lower extremities as well as compromise ventilation. Moreover, although the MAST may elevate blood pressure, available data do not show actual improvement in patient outcome. One possible role for the garment in children is pelvic fracture.
6. Constant reassessment is critical. Ensure that every major trauma patient is appropriately "packaged" in the emergency department (Table 43-5), with essential tubes.
7. In the hemodynamically stable patient, occult abdominal bleeding, especially from the spleen and liver, can be evaluated in the emergency department by peritoneal lavage (see Procedure 25). However, when available, computed tomography (CT) of the abdomen offers specific localization and quantification of hemorrhage.

Neurologic Status

EVALUATION. Rule out intracranial hemorrhage and spinal cord trauma.

Assess the initial level of consciousness based on the Glasgow Coma Scale (see Table 41-4).

MANAGEMENT

1. Early neurosurgical consultation is mandatory in the resuscitation of the head-injured patient.
2. Perform endotracheal intubation and hyperventilation early to decrease pCO_2 to the 25 mm Hg range.

3. Mannitol, 1.0 gm/kg, may be administered by rapid intravenous bolus for presumed intracranial hypertension in the comatose child who is hemodynamically stable.

CAVEATS

1. In the young child, intracranial hemorrhage alone can cause shock. This differs from the adult, in whom hypotension occurs either as a terminal event with brainstem failure or with "spinal shock"—diffuse loss of sympathetic tone from spinal cord injury. Spinal shock occurs rarely in children.

2. Do not use mannitol or furosemide for lowering intracranial pressure in children with hemodynamic instability. Central nervous system (CNS) salvageability depends on maintenance of minimal perfusion pressures.

CONSIDERATIONS AFTER RESUSCITATION

The Secondary Survey

When the primary survey discloses life-threatening injury, immediate emergency department interventions are instituted. Operative management is sometimes required to stop bleeding or remove intracranial blood in unstable patients. However, when emergency department maneuvers successfully stabilize the patient, a thorough secondary examination should be done. The components of the "secondary survey" include:

1. *Head, eyes, ears, nose, face, and cranial nerves.* Inspect the scalp and face for depressions, hematomas, or lacerations. Look for blood or cerebrospinal fluid in the ears or nose. Check pupils for size and reactivity and eyes for hyphema and oculocephalic and oculovestibular reflexes (doll's eyes). Delay doll's eyes maneuver if the child has potential cervical spine injury or when clinical clearance of the cervical spine is impossible because of young age or altered mental status.

2. *Cervical spine.* Search for stepoffs, hematomas, and tenderness.

3. *Chest.* Palpate the entire chest wall, sternum, and clavicles. Compress the ribs laterally and sternum anteroposteriorly. Carefully auscultate breath and heart sounds.

4. *Back.* Logroll the patient and inspect his or her entire back, including axillae. Palpate the spinous processes for alignment and stepoffs. Note abrasions, hematomas, and areas of tenderness. Repeat lung auscultation at lung bases.

5. *Abdomen.* Inspect for distention, ecchymoses, and penetration. Auscultate for bowel sounds and percuss for tenderness and the presence of fluid. Palpate for masses and tenderness. (Hemoperitoneum from organ rupture or vascular injury may have immediate clinical signs in only 40% of cases.) Rectal examination evaluates prostate, sphincter tone, and bulbocavernous reflex.

6. *Pelvis.* Inspect the urethral meatus for blood. Evaluate rock tenderness and pelvic bone stability.

7. *Musculoskeletal.* Search for deformities of long bones. Evaluate peripheral pulses.

8. *Neurologic.* Perform motor, sensory, and reflex examinations. Reevaluation is essential, seeking evidence of occult intracranial hemorrhage, contusion, or concussion, as well as partial or complete spinal cord lesions.

Trauma X-Rays in the Emergency Department

1. *Cervical spine.* Well-visualized, cross-table lateral, anteroposterior, and odontoid views are part of early evaluation of every trauma patient who is either young or has impaired sensorium. Children usually have high fractures (C1–C3), making all views necessary. Overall, cervical cord injury is uncommon in children, especially in those younger than 2 years of age. It may be present in the absence of any radiographic abnormalities.

2. *Chest x-ray.* This high yield study is imperative in all major trauma patients. If in-room x-ray is unavailable, a portable film is usually acceptable. Once detected, most serious trauma to the chest can be treated with tube thoracostomy alone (e.g., hemothorax, pneumothorax). If chest x-ray is negative in the patient who is in shock without major external bleeding sites, the abdomen is almost always the source of hemorrhage.

3. *Pelvis.* Fractures of the pelvis and, less commonly in children, urethral injury can be the source of significant blood loss.

4. *CT scan.* This procedure offers great sensitivity, especially in head (e.g., epidural, subdural hematoma) and abdominal injuries (e.g., liver, spleen). CT has high utility in the diagnosis of serious internal injury and is ordinarily obtained immediately after stabilization. Patients must have careful physician monitoring during the procedure. However, if the patient is hemodynamically unstable or has bilateral, fixed and dilated pupils, the need for immediate operative intervention usually precludes CT evaluation.

5. *Miscellaneous.* Extremity and facial x-rays, skull x-rays, intravenous pyelogram, angiography, and ultrasonography all have important roles in emergency department evaluation of selected trauma patients. Magnetic resonance imaging (MRI) may have a greater role in trauma diagnosis in the near future.

Use of the Clinical Laboratory

1. Routine laboratory tests include arterial blood gases (ABGs), complete blood count (CBC), platelets, electrolytes, glucose, calcium, type and crossmatch, amylase, BUN, creatinine, and coagulation studies. During resuscitation, these tests have secondary value to the clinical assessment, but they do provide essential information to postresuscitation care.

2. Serial hematocrits will often provide an important indicator of occult hemorrhage.

3. Urinalysis discloses the presence of gross or microscopic hematuria—markers for renal injury, a common complication of blunt trauma in children.

Pain Control

Analgesia must be used with great caution in the emergency department trauma patient because of the potential for dangerous cardiopulmonary or CNS depression. Even in the ostensibly stable patient, occult hemorrhage may be present. Furthermore, mental status provides a key clinical monitor of cardiovascular and CNS function. However, severe pain may significantly impede ventilation in the setting of rib fractures or occasionally preclude thorough clinical evaluation. In these circumstances or when trauma is clearly minor (e.g., isolated extremity injuries), low doses of a short-acting reversible agent such as morphine sulfate or meperidine may be given intravenously (see Chap. 48).

Disposition

For the seriously traumatized patient, the team captain, in collaboration with appropriate specialists, including an anesthesiologist, a pediatrician, a neurosurgeon, and an orthopedist, determines the disposition: immediate operative intervention, intensive care unit admission, or pediatric-surgical floor admission and observation.

In a facility without specialist pediatric anesthesia or pediatric surgical consultants, early transfers to a pediatric trauma center, adult trauma center, or pediatric intensive care unit should be considered. Patient outcome may be highly influenced by the availability of specialized care. Such transfer arrangements, as noted earlier, need to follow guidelines determined prospectively.

Patients with obvious clinical brain death may be candidates for organ procurement. Premortem consideration is mandatory for heart, heart-lung, liver and pancreas transplantation, and ideally for renal transplantation. Such considerations must occur within an appropriate ethical and legal milieu, after sensitive parental dialogue. Often, organ donation provides bereaved families with important elements of consolation and renewal in the face of overwhelming grief. The effect on organ recipients may be lifesaving.

Family Considerations

The physician must communicate clearly with the child and the child's family as soon as possible after initial disposition. The injured child is best translated to the "injured family." Disposition decisions, as well as progress reports, need to be presented frequently, carefully, and succinctly. Psychological support to the injured family is mandatory through the entire continuum of care—from emergency department, to operating room, to surgical floor, to rehabilitation.

SELECTED READING

American College of Surgeons, Committee on Trauma. Hospital and prehospital resources for optimal care of the injured patient. *Bull Am Coll Surg* 68:1, 1983.

Baker, SP, O'Neill, B, and Karpf, R. *The Injury Fact Book.* Lexington, MA: Lexington Books, 1984.

Bickel, WH, et al. Effect of anti-shock trousers in trauma score: A prospective analysis in the urban setting. *Ann Emerg Med* 14:208, 1985.

Brunette, DD, Fifield, G, and Ruiz, E. Use of pneumatic antishock trousers in the management of pediatric pelvic hemorrhage. *Pediatr Emerg Care* 3:86, 1987.

Committee on Trauma, American College of Surgeons. *Advanced Trauma Life Support Course Student Manual,* 1985.

Committee on Trauma Research, Commission on Life Sciences, National Research Council and the Institute of Medicine. *Injury in America: A Continuing Public Health Problem.* Washington, DC: National Academy Press, 1985.

Department of Transportation, National Highway Traffic Safety Administration. *National Training Course, Emergency Medical Technician/Paramedic Course Guide,* 1973.

Eichelberger, MR, and Pratsch, GL. *Pediatric Trauma Care.* Rockville: Aspen Publishers, Inc., 1988.

Eichelberger, MR, and Randolph, J. Pediatric trauma: An algorithm for diagnosis and therapy. *J Trauma* 23:91, 1983.

Eichelberger, MR, Stossel-Pratsch, G, and Mangubat, EA. A pediatric emergencies training program for emergency medical services. *Pediatr Emerg Care* 1:177, 1985.

Federle, MP, et al. Evaluation of abdominal trauma by computerized tomography. *Radiology* 138:637, 1981.

Haller, J, et al. Organization and function of a regional pediatric trauma center. *J Trauma* 23:691, 1983.

Holmes, MJ, and Teyes, HM. A critical review of pediatric trauma. *J Trauma* 24:253, 1984.

Iserson, KV, Criss, EA. Pediatric venous cutdowns: Utility in emergency situations. *Pediatr Emerg Care* 2:231, 1986.

King, D. Trauma in infancy and childhood: Initial evaluation and management. *Pediatr Clin North Am* 32:1299, 1985.

Mackensie, RC, Christensen, JM, and Lewis, FR. The prehospital use of counter pressure: Does MAST make a difference? *J Trauma* 24:882, 1984.

Mullner, R, and Goldberg, J. The Illinois trauma system: Changes in patient survival patterns following vehicular injuries. *JACEP* 6:393, 1977.

National Center for Health Statistics. *National Health Interview Survey.* Hyattsville, MD: National Center for Health Statistics, 1980.

National Safety Council. Accident Facts, 1984.

Pollack, MM, et al. Evaluation of Oregon Pediatric Critical Care Outcome by Hospital Resource Level. The National Conference on Pediatric Trauma. September 1987.

Ramenofsky, M, Luterman, A, and Quinlen, E. Maximal survival in pediatric trauma: The ideal system. *J Trauma* 24:818, 1984.

Robertson, LS. Present Status of Knowledge in Childhood Injury Prevention. In *Preventing Childhood Injuries.* Report of the Twelfth Ross Roundtable on Critical Approaches to Common Pediatric Problems. Columbus: Ross Laboratories, 1982.

Seidel, J, and Henderson, DP. *Prehospital Care of Pediatric Emergencies.* Los Angeles Pediatric Society, California Chapter 2, American Academy of Pediatrics, 1987.

Seidel, J, et al. Emergency medical services and the pediatric patient: Are the needs being met? *Pediatrics* 73:769, 1984.

Seidel, J, et al. Emergency medical services and the pediatric patient: Are the needs being met? II. Training and equipping emergency medical services providers for pediatric emergencies. *Pediatrics* 78:769, 1986.

Tolan, DA, Simon, RR, and Hoffman, JR. Cephalic vein cutdown at the wrist: Comparison to the standard saphenous vein ankle cutdown. *Ann Emerg Med* 17:38, 1988.

Weiskopf, RB, and Fairle, HB. Anesthesia. In DD Trunkey and FR Lewis (eds.), *Current Therapy of Trauma.* Toronto: B.C. Decker, 1986.

B. Control of Pain in the Emergency Department

44. Physiologic Mechanisms of Pain

Stephen T. Hickey
Paul M. Paris

Our ability to survive relies on the interpretation and integration of a continuous barrage of information from our environment. Whereas the primary senses are the major long-range warning systems, the skin is the most proximal monitor of danger from the external environment. Sensations via the skin provide crucial data alerting us to danger and protecting us from injury. How pain perception occurs is a complex question and not fully elucidated. In this chapter, we briefly review the history of pain theory and summarize current beliefs. Based on those theories, possible methods of improving pain management are discussed. It must be remembered that the pain experience consists of the actual noxious stimulus and, perhaps as important, the emotional and cognitive reaction to the stimulus. In this chapter, we are concerned only with the first component of the pain experience.

HISTORY

As outlined in the work of Fields and Pert, et al., the word *pain* is a derivation of the Greek and Latin words for punishment. The earliest interpretations of pain were that it represented punishment from offended gods and entered the body as demons. The earliest theories on the physiology of pain perception date from Aristotle, who believed that an excess of "vital heat" caused increased pain sensitivity through the blood to the heart. This concept of the heart as a sensory and feeling organ for the experience of pain persisted for centuries.

Adams and Victor report that by the nineteenth century, scientific data and theory began to supplant such ancient dogma. Magendie and Bell showed that the ventral roots of the spinal nerves were associated with motor function and the dorsal roots with sensory function. In 1840, Muller (Table 44-1) proposed that the central nervous system (CNS) received information about external objects and the body structures only by way of sensory nerves. He believed that sensory nerves for each of the five senses carried particular information specific for each sensation. This became known as the *specificity theory*, which stated that pain was a specific sensation independent of touch and other senses. Muller believed that the body's pain system had its own peripheral receptors (nociceptors) and its own central connections. Even though specific receptors for pain were not isolated, the specificity theory gained dominance and remained accepted until the 1920s.

Hughes, Crue, and Stimmel describe how in the 1920s, Wollard and Sinclair independently developed a pattern theory of pain. This theory stated that when a stimulus is ap-

Table 44-1. Theories of pain perception

Specificity theory (Muller): There exist specific receptors for pain.	
Pattern theory (Wollard and Sinclair): Multiple receptors form specific patterns of pain sensation.	
Gate theory (Melzack and Wall): Peripheral fibers carry pain information to spinal gate where it is modulated before being transmitted to the brain for perception.	

Source: P.M. Paris and R.D. Stewart (eds.). *Pain Management in Emergency Medicine.* East Norwalk, CT: Appleton & Lange, 1988.

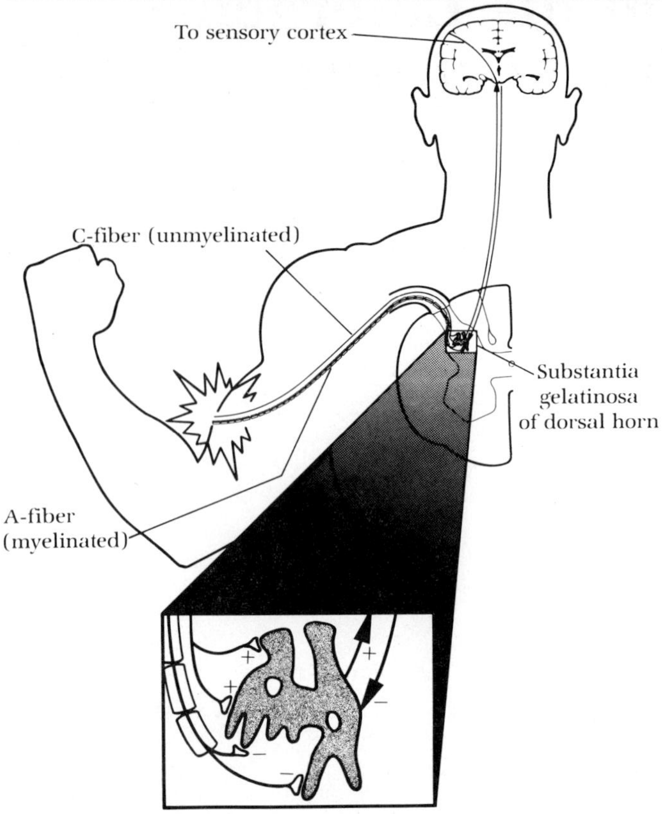

Fig. 44-1. An illustration of the gate control theory. The noxious stimuli originating in the arm are transmitted via large myelinated A fibers and small unmyelinated C fibers to the substantia gelatinosa of the dorsal horn of the spinal cord. These fibers synapse at a "T" (target) cell that controls the gate by the balance of input of the two types of fibers. C fibers open the gate and promote transmission of noxious stimuli to higher levels in the CNS, whereas the A fibers tend to close the gate and block further transmission. (From P.M. Paris and R.D. Stewart [eds.]. *Pain Management in Emergency Medicine.* East Norwalk, CT: Appleton & Lange, 1988.)

plied to the skin, it produces a nerve impulse pattern in a group of fibers rather than exciting a single specific receptor or fiber. As discussed by Levin, Mense, and Pasternak, this idea of a timing-spatial pattern rather than specific receptor stimulation was proposed to explain the differences in pain sensation and the source of it (i.e., mechanical, chemical, thermal). This was supported by the work of Adrian when the intensity theory was shown to be limited after his research showed intense cutaneous receptive discharge could occur without pain. Over the next 20 years, this spatiotemporal pattern continued in vogue as the first pain afferent fiber components and their characteristics were identified. Mayer states that in 1965, Melzack and Wall (Fig. 44-1) expanded this concept and proposed the gated theory of pain modulation. Briefly, they suggested that afferent impulses were perceived as pain only if permitted through the presynaptic "gates" before synapsing on the second-order neuron. Afferent fibers were presynaptically influenced by the substantia gelatinosa (SG), which in turn was modulated by descending central centers primarily related to the affective and memory component of pain. Furthermore, nociceptive input may be gated at segmental and superspinal levels prior to the cognitive pain experience.

Wall, Crue, Mayer, and others, in reviewing the gate theory, proposed that nerve impulses from the skin are relayed to three spinal cord areas: (1) SG, (2) the dorsal column, and (3) the transmission cells in the dorsal horn (T). It also stated that the SG functions as a gating mechanism that modifies the afferent impulses before they can influence the T cells. Stimulation of the dorsal column system was believed to influence supersegmental systems, which in turn also modified the gate control by way of descending fibers. The resulting modified impulses transmitted to T cells located also in the dorsal horn of the spinal cord would then signal the system responsible for pain perception to occur.

Whereas the relative concept of gated pain transmission remains intact, the specific gate control theory has undergone modification as more information and better experimental evidence have become available.

The elucidation of the exact mechanisms of pain transmission are complex and ongoing. More detailed information can be found in Wall, Field, Crue, and others, but briefly they outline the following: The gate control theory essentially proposes that sensory input from peripheral large and small nerve fibers is transmitted to T cells in the dorsal horn in the spinal cord. When the sensory input is from large, myelinated fibers (A-δ fibers), there is negative feedback to the T cells and the gate is affectively closed. When the sensory input is transmitted by small fibers (C-fibers), there is a positive feedback and the gate is open, allowing the painful sensory information to be relayed to the CNS. The final perception is thought to be the result of the number of nociceptive impulses reaching the gate through small unmyelinated fibers, compared to the number of inhibitory impulses reaching the gate through the large myelinated fibers. All of this is also subject to modulation from descending fiber pathways from the brain.

The gate theory has been shown to have a number of shortcomings that are related to the lack of anatomic and physiologic evidence for the "gate." The interaction of the SG with the large and small fibers as well as other laminae of rexed is not completely understood. Also, this theory does not explain certain clinical phenomena such as some peripheral neuropathies in which there is a selective loss of large myelinated A-δ fibers, leaving the predominance of C-fibers. Victor and Adams state that the gate theory would predict these to be painful neuropathies, but many are not. It could, however, explain the analgesia obtained from acupuncture, massage, and transcutaneous nerve stimulation activating the large A fibers and thereby increasing inhibitory tone. In summary, the neurogate is facilitated by small peripheral fiber input and inhibited by inputs originating in large pe-

Table 44-2. Comparison of sensory fibers

Fiber	Sensation	Dorsal horn termination	Ascending tract	Conduction rate (m/sec)	Size (μm)	Myelin
A-alpha	Light touch	Deep	Ipsilateral dorsal column	15–30	6–7	Heavy
A-beta						
A-delta	Sharp pricking	Superficial	Contralateral spinothalamic tract	5–30	1–5	Thin
C	Long-lasting burning	Superficial	Contralateral spinothalamic tract	5–2	3–1	None

Source: P.M. Paris and R.D. Stewart (eds.). *Pain Management in Emergency Medicine.* East Norwalk, CT: Appleton & Lange, 1988.

ripheral fibers and descending supraspinal tracts. The final experience is subject to a complex series of facilitatory and inhibitory events that precede pain awareness. In Sugeura, et al., we see that the basic premise has been expanded with the identification of postsynaptic, segmental, and suprasegmental influences and the demonstration of specific nociceptors that respond only to, for instance, tissue damage. With this fundamental groundwork laid, our knowledge of pain physiology continues to be greatly expanded by the identification of the neurotransmitters at these sites and other sites in the CNS and their relationship to pain modulation (i.e., opiate receptors). It is now within this context that great hope is held out for new therapeutic interventions.

PERIPHERAL STRUCTURES

Pert, et al., Willis, Mense, and others have described that there are two basic fiber types (Table 44-2) involved in the majority of transmissions of painful stimuli from the periphery: the small myelinated A-group and slower conducting unmyelinated C-fibers. Painful stimuli include thermal and pressure stimuli as well as tissue damage perceived by nociceptors. These types of receptors were identified as mechanosensitive, thermosensitive, and polymodal (mixed) nociceptors. The polymodal unmyelinated fibers formed the largest group and respond to mechanical, thermal, and cutaneously injected substance stimulation. C-fibers form the majority of polymodal nociceptors responding to high-threshold mechanical and thermal stimulation. A-fibers also form mixed groups sensitive to mechanical stimulation, chemical irritation, and thermal perception as well as light touch and are frequently more selective.

VISCERAL STRUCTURES

The exact mechanisms involved in visceral pain are not fully known. There is evidence, as presented by Fields, Mense, and Willis, of particular receptors relating to visceral pain—for example, bladder A-δ and C-fiber afferents—increasing their rate of firing with its distention as well as similar results in other hollow viscera such as the gastrointestinal tract, ureters, and gall bladder. This issue is clouded, however, by the close proximity of these organs to blood vessels also innervated by small-caliber afferent axons. Many of these blood vessels are pain-sensitive, and their input may be a contributing factor to pain within the abdominal cavity.

The viscera receives innervation by way of nerves via the body wall to somatic structures or nerves with primarily autonomic function, or both. Visceral sensory input goes through the splanchnic nerves, which also receive input from the cutaneous field, suggesting a mechanism for the clinical phenomenon of referred pain due to intrathoracic and abdominal structures.

The afferents from the splanchnic nerves enter the spinal cord in the thoracic and upper lumbar regions and end primarily in the dorsal horn laminae I and V. This is in contrast to cutaneous (somatic) nerves in the same areas, which terminate primarily in layers II, III, and IV. However, all neurons in these laminae receiving visceral afferents also receive input from the somatic nerves. This may explain the poor localization properties of visceral pain on clinical examination.

While it remains unclear how or even if these afferents can signal pain, current information strongly suggests that they do. This is supported by the fact that the ascending pathways associated with pain, the spinothalamic and spinal reticular, have been shown to be stimulated by the visceral afference.

DORSAL HORN AND ITS PERIPHERAL PAIN RELATIONS

Nociceptive afferents enter the CNS by way of the dorsal horn of the spinal cord or, in the case of cranial nerves, the brain stem. This is a layered gray matter structure made up of six laminae (Fig. 44-2). The superficial layers (I, the marginal zone; II, the SG) and the deep layers (laminae III–V, the nucleus proprius; VI, the dorsal horn base) were first well defined and named by B. Rexed in 1952 and further elucidated by the work of many, including Cervero and Connell, Craig and Mense, Kuo, et al., and Melzack and Wall.

Skin A-δ fibers synapse with second-order neurons in the first and fifth laminae while C-fibers terminate in laminae I and II. Muscle, viscera, and deep tissues terminate in laminae I, V, and, to a lesser extent, X.

Second-order postsynaptic neurons (Fig. 44-3) ascend one or two levels before crossing to the contralateral lateral spinothalamic tract. This is a white matter tract in the ventral lateral aspect of the spinal cord and is composed of mixed ascending projections in a somatotopic presentation. Each rostral layer pushes the more caudal segments toward the peripheral so that leg spinal thalamic fibers form the most lateral aspects, with the trunk and arms more medially. This has clinical significance in both treatment of intractable

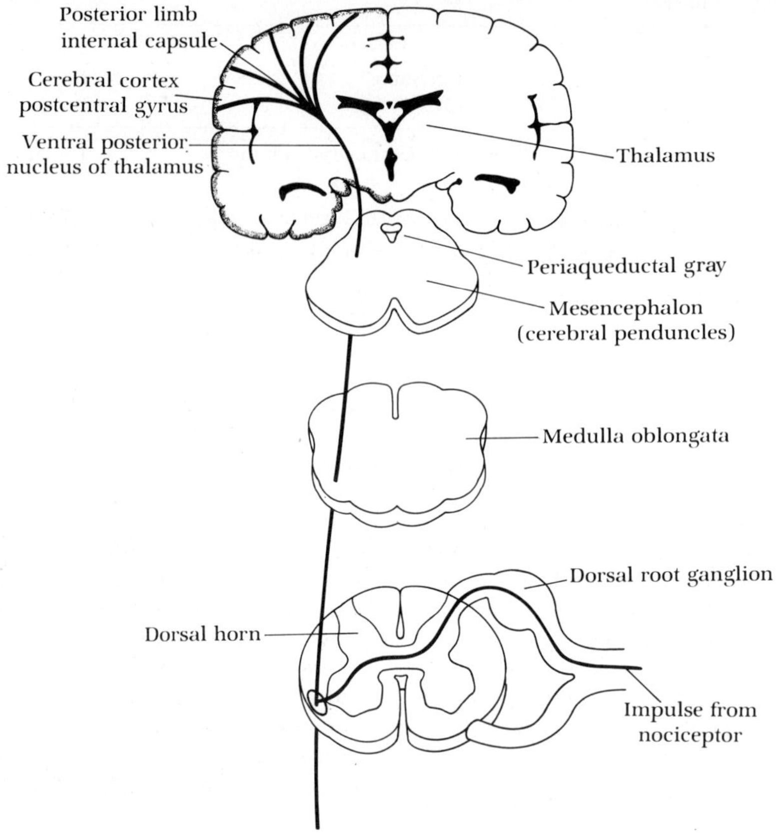

Fig. 44-2. A cross hemisection of the spinal cord. The six laminae composing the dorsal horn are highlighted. (From P.M. Paris and R.D. Stewart [eds.]. *Pain Management in Emergency Medicine.* East Norwalk, CT: Appleton & Lange, 1988.)

pain (e.g., partial cordotomy) and recognition of certain pathologic processes (e.g., syrinomyelia).

PAIN-ASSOCIATED ASCENDING AND DESCENDING TRACTS AND THEIR CENTRAL PROJECTIONS

Maciewicz, Sandrew, and Kelly report that the spinothalamic afferents (Fig. 44-4) are divided into the neospinothalamic tract and phylogenetically more primitive paleospinothalamic tract. The paleospinothalamic portion is a nontopographically distributed and widely branched ending primarily in the caudal brain stem reticular formation with a smaller portion going to the medial and posterior thalamic nuclei. The neospinothalamic segment remains topographic and unbranched and ends in the ventroposteriolateral nucleus of the thalamus. The paleospinothalamic system is believed to be more involved in the emotional and autonomic responses to pain with synapses in a wide variety of cortical and subcortical areas. The neospinothalamic system, on the other hand, synapses with the ventroposteriolateral nuclei of the thalamus, which in turn projects to the primary somatosensory cortex involved in detailing the location, type, and intensity of the painful stimuli.

Sugeura, et al., Maciewicz, Kelly, and others describe how pain sensations are modified by descending systems that modulate the sensory information transmitted from the periphery. This pain modulation, in regions separated from ascending transmissions, implies an independent descend-

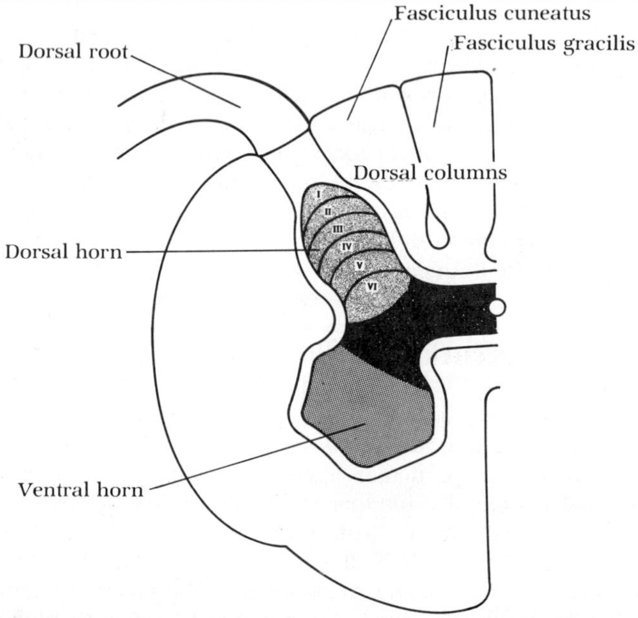

Fig. 44-3. A cross section of the entire spinal cord with all major tracts labeled. (From P.M. Paris and R.D. Stewart [eds.]. *Pain Management in Emergency Medicine.* East Norwalk, CT: Appleton & Lange, 1988.)

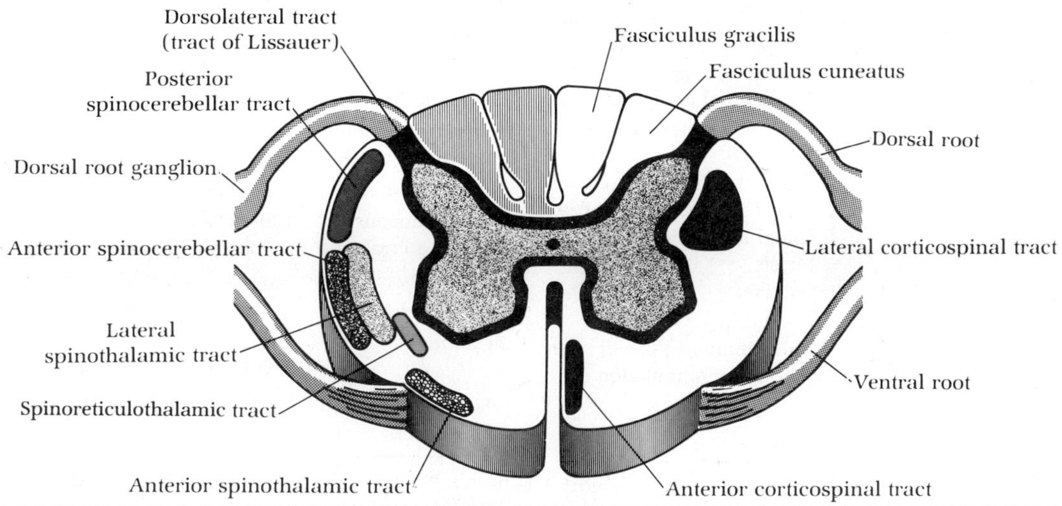

Fig. 44-4. A diagram tracing the path of the major tract that carries pain stimuli to the brain, the lateral spinothalamic tract. (From P.M. Paris and R.D. Stewart [eds.]. *Pain Management in Emergency Medicine.* East Norwalk, CT: Appleton & Lange, 1988.)

ing tract of pain inhibition. Electrical stimulation of the ventral lateral portion of the central gray substance of the mesencephalon and the periventricular gray produces profound analgesia comparable to that produced by opiates. This analgesia may last for 1 hour after stimulation. Also, this analgesia is not associated with depression and cortical functions or vital signs. The analgesia produced may be due to the activation of an inhibitory neurosystem in the spinal cord or other parts of the CNS as outlined by the work of Kosterlitz, et al. One proposed mechanism of pain inhibition involves encephalon release in the dorsal horn. Future efforts to modify pain perception may be directed toward these descending tracts and manipulation of their neurotransmitters.

NEUROCHEMISTRY

Peripheral Afferents and Dorsal Horn

Levin, Stimmel, and Mense have detailed how many chemical mediators may produce the sensation of pain. The traditional mediators of inflammation play a role in the persistent pain of injury and disease. Histamine—the slow-releasing substance of anaphylaxis—kinins, prostaglandins, and leukotrienes, when applied to nerve endings elicit pain. The E and F series of prostaglandins may mediate mild pain independently. Although prostaglandins alone cause only mild to moderate pain, they can significantly potentiate the discomfort of other pain-induced substances such as kinins.

Many other substances have been identified, and there is intensified research in this direction as described by Willis, Mense, and others. Of more recent interest, the role of certain peptides—vasoactive intestinal peptide, calcitonin gene-related peptide, neurotensin, and cholecystokinin—are under investigation. The exact role of these peptides in the transmission or in the inhibition of pain, or both, is unclear. Another undecapeptide, substance P, is released by C-fibers in the superficial laminae of the dorsal horn when stimulated. This neurotransmitter is responsible for pain transmission associated with injury or disease. Drugs that deplete substance P are associated with analgesia. With increasing information, novel pharmacologic approaches may become available to clinicians as the exact role of these neurotransmitters is more clearly identified.

ENDOGENOUS OPIATE PEPTIDES

The most exciting advance in the past 2 decades of pain research has been the discovery and study of endogenous opioid peptides and opiate receptors. These endogenous analgesic systems have stimulated a tremendous amount of basic research as reported by Kosterlitz, Terenius, Pert, Pasternak, Hughes, and many others. The structural specificity and stereospecificity of opiates led many to hypothesize the existence of opiate receptors, but it was not until 1973 that three investigators independently confirmed the existence of opiate receptors. The confirmation of receptor sites capable of binding opiates hastened the search for endogenous substances that would also bind to and function at these receptor sites. The first endogenous opioid peptides to be identified by Hughes and Kosterlitz in 1975 were metencephalon and leu-enkephalin. There are many endogenous opioid peptide substances. Three substances of opioid peptides have been classified: the endorphins, the enkephalins, and the dynorphins. Each of these substances has a protein precursor (Table 44-3). As with other humeral transmitting

Table 44-3. Endogenous opioid peptides and their precursors

Precursors	Opioid peptides
Proenkephalin	Met-enkephalin Leu-enkephalin
Proopiomelanocortin	Alpha-endorphin Beta-endorphin ?Gamma-endorphin
Prodynorphin	Dynorphin A Dynorphin B

Source: P.M. Paris and R.D. Stewart (eds.). *Pain Management in Emergency Medicine.* East Norwalk, CT: Appleton & Lange, 1988.

Table 44-4. Opiate receptors

Receptor	Action
Mu	Supraspinal analgesia Respiratory depression Euphoria Physical dependence Suppression of withdrawal
Kappa	Spinal analgesia Miosis Sedation
Sigma	Dysphoria Hallucinations Vasomotor stimulation
Delta	?
Epsilon	?

Source: P.M. Paris and R.D. Stewart (eds.). *Pain Management in Emergency Medicine.* East Norwalk, CT: Appleton & Lange, 1988.

Table 44-5. Therapies for pain

Modality	Mechanism of action
Opiate analgesics	Binding to opiate receptors in the CNS
Nonsteroidal anti-inflammatories	Block production of prostaglandins
Nerve blocks	Block transmission of nerve impulse
Transcutaneous nerve stimulation	Closes "gate" in dorsal horn of spinal cord; may also be some endorphin component
Acupuncture	Same as transcutaneous nerve stimulation
Nitrous oxide	Calms emotional reaction to pain
Ketamine	Dissociation of thalamoneocortical and limbic systems
Hypnosis	Cognitive reinterpretation of pain stimulus
Biofeedback	Decreases muscle tension

Source: P.M. Paris and R.D. Stewart (eds.). *Pain Management in Emergency Medicine.* East Norwalk, CT: Appleton & Lange, 1988.

substances, the active peptide is cleaved from a larger peptide or protein.

In a situation analogous to adrenergic and histamine reception, subpopulations of opioid receptors are found in varying concentrations throughout the nervous system. These subpopulations of receptors are relatively specific for the opioid ligand that will activate them, as well as being relatively specific for the physiologic alterations that they mediate. All natural and synthetic opiates have been found to bind to opiate receptors. Opiate receptors have been demonstrated throughout the CNS, with the highest concentration at those areas known to be involved with pain pathways. The unique actions of a given opiate are due to the binding interactions with specific subpopulations of opiate receptors. The currently identified subclasses of these receptors are the mu, kappa, sigma, delta, and epsilon receptors. Activation of these receptors is responsible for the different physiologic actions that we identify as being a result of opiates. Table 44-4 lists the current actions attributed to each of these receptors. With further research it is hoped that future opiate agonists will have such receptor activity that analgesia will be accomplished without such side effects as respiratory depression or physical dependence.

PAIN PERCEPTION AND REACTION

The threshold for the perception of a painful stimulus is similar in everyone. This threshold may be lowered by certain chemicals, such as the mediators of inflammation. However, the pathways and actual cognitive processes involved in the interpretation of painful stimuli remain a mystery. The cognitive and emotional reactions to a given painful stimulus are quite variable among individuals and may be affected by culture, personality, past experiences, and underlying emotional state. This reaction can be greatly influenced by many pharmacologic interventions. Drugs such as narcotics have the greatest effect on the reaction to pain and not on the perception of the stimulus itself. Techniques such as distraction and relaxation as well as hypnosis are also effective in diminishing suffering by controlling the cognitive and emotional reaction to noxious stimuli. In chronic pain problems such as chronic low back pain or migraines, these techniques have become valuable adjunctive therapies leading to greater life control and less need for prescriptive analgesics.

PAIN MANAGEMENT

Hypothetical strategies for improved pain management can be proposed for each of the anatomic sites or pathways discussed. Many such strategies are now available, but others will require further research and development. Table 44-5 lists several currently available therapies and their basic mechanisms of action.

The potential site for future pain control intervention may be the superficial laminae of the dorsal horn. In these laminae, both peripheral and central influences are thought to provide a physiologic "denial gate" that prevents nociceptive access to the CNS. Future pharmacologic interventions that may add to current therapies include leukotriene synthesis blockers and polypeptides with unique opiate receptor specificities as proposed by Pert, Willis, and others.

Effective counterirritative therapies have existed for centuries. When low threshold A-alpha and A-beta neurons are excited by counterirritative stimuli, these neurons close the gait to C-neuron transmissions. Yet the counterirritative stimuli does not achieve C-neuron threshold, which could produce pain. Acupuncture is the best known of these therapies, and a modern version is transcutaneous electrical nerve stimulation (TENS).

Less cumbersome techniques that close the gate are needed. The heterogeneity of opiate receptors with respect to location and physiologic function may provide more practical means of "closing the gate." Opiate ligands are being sought that selectively bind and activate subpopulations of opiate receptors that, in turn, "close the gate." Ideally, these ligands should have no possibility of activating those subpopulations of opitate receptors that mediate euphoria or vital function depression as suggested by Crue, Kosterlitz, and Pasternak.

SUMMARY

The physiology of pain transmission and perception has been studied for hundreds of years; however, work in the last 2 decades has uncovered much new information. This has enhanced our understanding and therefore therapies for pain and greatly increased research efforts. However, our improved understanding of pain physiology has not yet been translated into dramatically improved approaches to acute and chronic pain treatment. The practice of emergency medicine can be greatly aided with practical applications of currently available analgesic techniques such as counterirritative therapy and more sophisticated use of narcotic and non-narcotic analgesics. In the 1990s, new therapies should arise from our improved understanding of one of the most complex systems of the human body.

SELECTED READING

Adams, RA, and Victor, M. *Pain in Principles of Neurology.* New York: McGraw-Hill, 1985. Pp. 99–113.

Cervero, F, and Connell, LA. Distribution of somatic and visceral primary afferent fibres within the thoracic spinal cord of the cat. *J Comp Neurol* 230:88, 1984.

Craig, AD, and Mense, S. The distribution of afferent fibers from the gastrocnemius-soleus muscle in the dorsal horn of the cat, as revealed by the transport of horseradish peroxidase. *Neurosci Lett* 41:233, 1983.

Crue, BL (ed), *Pain Research and Treatment.* New York: Academic, 1975. Pp. 7–14.

Fields, HL. *Pain.* New York: McGraw-Hill, 1987.

Hughes, J, et al. Identification of two related pentapeptides from the brain with potent opiate agonist activity. *Nature* 258:577, 1975.

Kelly, DD. Somatic sensory system IV: Central representations of pain and analgesia. In ER Kandel and JH Schwartz (eds), *Principles of Neural Science* (2nd ed). New York: Elsevier, 1985.

Kosterlitz, HW, and Hughes, J. Peptides with morphine-like action in the brain. *Br J Psychiatry* 130:298, 1977.

Kuo, DC, and DeGroat, WC. Primary afferent projections of the major splanchnic nerve to the spinal cord and gracile nucleus of the cat. *J Comp Neurol* 231:421, 1985.

Levin, J. Pain and analgesia: The outlook for more rational treatment. *Ann Intern Med* 100:269, 1984.

Light, AR, and Perl, ER. Spinal termination of functionally identified primary afferent neurons with slowly conducting myelinated fibers. *J Comp Neurol* 186:133, 1979.

Maciewicz, R, and Sandrew, BB. Physiology of Pain. In G. Aronoff (ed), *Evaluation and Treatment of Chronic Pain.* Baltimore: Urban & Schwartzenberg, 1985. Pp. 17–38.

Mayer, DJ, Wolfe, TL, Akil, H, Carder, B, and Liebeskind, JC. Analgesia from electrical stimulation in the brainstem of the cat. *Science* 174:1351, 1971.

Melzack, R, and Wall, PD. Pain mechanisms: A new theory. *Science* 150:971, 1965.

Mense, S, and Prabhakar, NR. Spinal termination of nociceptive afferent fibres from deep tissues in the cat. *Neurosci Lett* 66:169, 1986.

Morley, GK, Erickson, PL, and Morley, JE. The Neurology of Pain. In AB Baker (ed), *Clinical Neurology, Vol. 2.* New York: Harper & Row, 1986. Pp. 1–80.

Muller, J. *Handbuch der Physiologic des Menchen.* Coblenz, 1838.

Paris, PM, Uram, M, and Ginsburg, MJ. Physiological Aspects of Pain. In PM Paris, and RD Stewart (eds), *Pain Management in Emergency Medicine.* East Norwalk, CT: Appleton & Lange, 1988.

Pasternak, GW. Opiate, enkephalin, and endorphin analgesia: Relation to a single subpopulation of opiate receptors. *Neurology* 31:1311, 1981.

Pert, CB, Pasternak, G, and Snyder, SH. Opiate agonists and antagonists discriminated by receptor binding in the brain. *Science* 182:1359, 1973.

Raja, SN, Meyers, RA, and Campbell, JN. Peripheral mechanisms of somatic pain. *Anesthesiology* 68:571, 1988.

Rexed, B. The cytoarchitectonic organization of the spinal cord in the cat. *J Comp Neurol* 96:415, 1952.

Reynolds, DV. Surgery in the cat during electrical analgesia induced by focal brain stimulation. *Science* 164:444, 1968.

Spimmel, B. Neuroregulators and Pain. In Barry (ed), *Pain, Analgesia, and Addiction.* New York: Raven, 1983. Pp. 18–35.

Sugeura, Y, Lee, CL, and Perl, ER. Central projections of identified, unmyelinated (C) afferent fibers innervating mammalian skin. *Science* 234:358, 1986.

Terenius, L. Characteristics of the receptor for narcotic analgesics in synaptic plasma membrane fractions from cat brains. *Acta Pharmacol Toxicol* 33:377, 1974.

Wall, PD. The gate theory of pain mechanisms: A reexamination and restatement. *Brain* 101:1, 1978.

Willis, WD. Pain and dorsal horn neurophysiology of pain. *Ann NY Acad Sci* 531:76, 1988.

45. General Approach to Pain Control

William H. Cordell

Pain is the number one reason that patients seek emergency care. Pain itself is an emergency. Pain, especially acute, severe pain, is a crisis that totally dominates the patient's life. The patient in pain expects the emergency practitioner not only to diagnose the cause of the pain but also to provide immediate relief. These are very compelling reasons that pain control should be one of the most important skills mastered by emergency physicians and nurses and prehospital care providers.

There are many unique aspects of pain control in the emergency setting. Emergency medicine is a time-dependent specialty in which contact with the patient is typically brief and pressured, data are incomplete, and patient follow-up is poor. Patients present to the emergency department with a variety of painful conditions. The management of many of these conditions, including prehospital patients in pain and the excruciating pains of migraine, renal colic, and sickle cell crisis, falls mainly under the purview of emergency specialists. Although other specialties treat patients in pain, what may be true concerning pain management in the operating room, hospice, or pain clinic may not be directly applicable to the patient with migraine headache in the emergency department or the conscious, injured patient trapped under a collapsed parking garage.

Emergency practitioners have little scientific fact to guide them in treating patients in pain. The techniques and skills of pain management are more founded in belief and habit, are shrouded in mystery, and are ritually passed from generation to generation. Fortunately, acute pain management, despite the inherent difficulties of studying such a subjective complaint, is becoming a field of research and education interest, particularly among emergency physicians.

PHYSIOLOGY OF PAIN

An understanding of pain mechanisms, pathways, and biochemistry of pain is slowly evolving and is discussed in greater detail in Chap. 44. Pain involves a physical stimulus, transmission of the impulse to the central nervous system (CNS), and a cognitive response. One theory proposes that a painful stimulus causes the release of local chemical mediators of pain such as prostaglandins, substance P, and bradykinins. These mediators evoke an inflammatory response and incite an electrochemical transmission of the "pain message." This message travels up the spinal cord to the brain, eliciting a conscious response ("ouch!"). Pain itself may also produce deleterious physiologic consequences, including skeletal muscle spasm, vasospasm, and impairment or inhibition of gastrointestinal, genitourinary, and other visceral functions. Thus, the treatment of pain may have more benefit than just humane concerns.

Table 45-1. Pain control menu

Pharmacologic analgesics	Nonpharmacologic pain control
Narcotics	Placebo "effect"
Nonsteroidal anti-inflammatory drugs	Transcutaneous electrical nerve stimulator
Acetaminophen	Acupuncture
Dihydroergotamine (for migraine)	Massage and manipulation
Local anesthesias; nerve blocks	Splinting, rest
Low-dose "general anesthetics" (e.g., nitrous oxide, ketamine)	Heat/cold therapy
	Hypnosis
Placebo medications	Biofeedback

The discrete cognitive processes and pathways involved in the interpretation of a painful stimuli remain a mystery. The cognitive interpretation of pain involves emotions, previous experiences with pain, and cultural background. Recognizing and managing the emotional, cognitive component is vital to effective pain control.

PRINCIPLES OF PAIN CONTROL

The goals of pain control in emergency medicine are threefold: (1) relieve the pain and suffering, (2) rule out life-threatening causes of severe pain, and (3) attempt to diagnose the origins of the pain. All three tasks may be undertaken simultaneously. Often, however, treatment begins prior to a definitive diagnosis, an approach that contradicts traditional medical teaching.

Several avenues of pain control emerge from this simplified schema of the etiology of pain just presented.

1. *Removal of the painful stimulus.* Trephining a subungual hematoma or treating coronary artery spasm or blockage with vasodilators, thrombolytic agents, or angioplasty are examples of removing the pain-provoking stimulus to relieve pain.

2. *Blocking the transmission of the pain message.* Nonsteroidal anti-inflammatory agents block the production of prostaglandins, which are pain mediators. For example, prostaglandin synthesis inhibitors have been used to treat ureteral colic and are commonly used in emergency practice for a wide variety of inflammatory and noninflammatory conditions. Local anesthetics and nerve blocks interrupt the transmission of the nerve impulse and, in addition to their use in wound repair, may provide relief in such conditions as dental pain or rib fractures. Transcutaneous electrical nerve stimulation, counterirritation, and acupuncture block the transmission of pain by "closing the pain gate" in the dorsal horn of the spinal cord.

3. *Centrally acting agents.* Narcotics bind to opiate receptors in the CNS to effect analgesia. Other centrally acting agents such as dihydroergotamine (DHE) and sumatriptan are administered to treat migraine. Ketamine is thought to produce "dissociative anesthesia," analgesia, and amnesia by acting on the thalamoneocorticol and limbic systems in the brain.

Table 45-2. "The Shaman's Touch": Psychological aspects of pain control

"High-touch" vs. "high-tech" approach
Caring, empathic, relaxed demeanor
Nonjudgmental attitude
Listening to the patient
Providing explanations
Soothing, quiet environment
Positive suggestion ("This will make you better")

4. *Modulating the patient's perception.* Headphones and music, suggestion, and guided imagery have been used to "take the patient's mind somewhere else," refocusing his or her attention away from the pain. Modification of the patient's cognitive response to pain might be as simple as putting the patient in pain in a quiet, soothing environment (and not next to the screaming child undergoing laceration repair). How the emergency practitioner approaches the patient, whether it's a pat on the hand or adjusting a pillow, not only demonstrates a caring attitude but can also do wonders to alleviate fear and pain.

Although analgesia is often effected by pharmacologic agents, pain control is not synonymous with administration of medicines (Table 45-1). Our bias as practitioners of a profession named *Medicine* is toward pharmacologic intervention.

In practice, pain control in emergency medicine often involves a combination of drugs, skills, and techniques. Consider the patient who sustains lower rib fractures in a motor vehicle accident and suffers pain severe enough to limit respiratory excursions. Both a peripherally acting nonsteroidal anti-inflammatory agent and a centrally acting narcotic may be prescribed. The patient may be fitted with a transcutaneous electrical nerve stimulator (TENS) unit to diminish the amount of drugs required. Ideally the patient is compassionately treated and continually reassured by the emergency medical technician (EMT), paramedic, emergency physician, emergency nurse, and trauma surgeon involved in his or her care.

PSYCHOLOGICAL ASPECTS OF PAIN CONTROL

It cannot be overemphasized that pain always involves a physical stimulus–neuroanatomic process *and* an emotional reaction evoked by the stimulus. In every clinical encounter, a person who comes to a healer has expectations. The patient seeks medical attention for "a bit of magic and a bit of caring."

Pain relief begins with how the emergency specialist presents him- or herself to the patient and how he or she makes use of the potent influence of the psyche on the patient's perceptions of pain. The shaman achieved cures throughout the ages without advanced technology by instilling a positive, healing attitude in his patients. In Table 45-2, some of the important "art of medicine" aspects of pain management are given.

Placebos are powerful, albeit misunderstood tools for pain control in selected patients regardless of the origin of the pain. One cannot help but be amazed by the analgesic efficacy of placebos in placebo-controlled trials. As many as 30 to 40 percent of patients will have their pain and other subjective symptoms satisfactorily relieved by placebo.

Misconceptions concerning placebo therapy abound. Some physicians incorrectly use placebos to fool the patient or treat disliked patients. Studies indicate that demanding, complaining patients are less likely to respond to placebos than are well-liked patients. Another misconception is equating an analgesic response to placebos with malingering or hysteria.

The concept of a placebo need not be limited to a "sugar pill" or "shot of normal saline." Instead, *placebo effect* implies anything that positively modulates the patient's mental attitude, whether it is a mother's kiss, a warm hand on the shoulder, or a positive reassuring manner on the part of the physician, nurse, or paramedic. Some aspect of placebo effect exists in every clinical encounter. Even in this modern, high-tech age, the "high-touch" art of medicine still plays a pivotal role in pain control.

ANALGESIA: TOO LITTLE, TOO LATE, NOT AT ALL

In every major study done to evaluate the management of pain in the hospital setting, our methods of pain relief have been weighed in the balance and been found wanting. Despite the fact that pain is the most frequent complaint that motivates patients to seek medical care, it is evident from many studies that patients in pain are inadequately treated. Even in the emergency department, where physicians and nurses daily treat large numbers and wide varieties of patients with acute pain or exacerbating pain, analgesia is often inadequate.

In a retrospective review of 198 emergency department patients with painful conditions, more than half received no analgesia while in the emergency department. Of those who did, most waited more than an hour before narcotic analgesia was administered. Furthermore, many received suboptimal equianalgesic doses of narcotics when compared to morphine.

Numerous explanations for why analgesia is inadequate or totally neglected follow:

1. *Inability to objectively measure pain.* Many of the prejudices and misconceptions of pain stem from one simple fact: There is no way to objectively measure pain. Because there are no "painometers" or "serum pain levels" to quantify pain severity, the patient's pain may be underestimated and undertreated. Furthermore, physical examination is unreliable in predicting the presence or absence of severe pain. Although some clinical signs such as tachycardia, diaphoresis, or agitation are consistent with pain, their absence does not mean that pain is not present.

An individual's experience and interpretation of pain is extremely variable. Some patients appear "stoic" in the presence of severe pain, whereas others scream with apparently less pain. Moreover, communicating a painful experience is very difficult for the patient, especially when in severe pain. Similar pains may be described in dissimilar ways. Angina may be described as a "pressure" rather than a "pain." Pain may be expressed as a "hurt," "throb," "sickness," or "sticking," rather than more technical, medical descriptions. The last thing patients in severe pain want to do is repeat the story two or three times. They want relief.

Communication may be further hampered by serious illness or injury, speech or hearing impairment, language barrier, cognitive disorders, or age. Many inconsolable children are expressing their pain by their sole means of communication: incessant crying and irritability.

The severity of pain can be estimated only by various scaling methods, including asking the patient to rate the pain on a 0 to 10 scale. ("If 10 is the worst pain you've ever had and 0 is no pain, how bad is your pain?")

2. *Lack of understanding of pharmacology.* Numerous studies have shown that narcotics are sometimes given in the wrong dose, by the wrong route, and with the wrong frequency of administration. For example, the usual answer to what narcotic dose is required to produce analgesia in adults is "Demerol 75 mg and Phenergan 25 mg IM." The problems with this rote response is that 75 mg of meperidine (Demerol) may not provide adequate analgesia for many patients; promethazine (Phenergan) may be antisynergistic; and serum levels achieved from an intramuscular injection are variable and unpredictable.

Because there are few "average, 70-kg patients," no single, standard analgesic dose or dose schedule can adequately treat everyone's pain. Each patient is unique in his or her response to analgesics. Although usual dosages are quoted in reference books, this does not guarantee efficacy or safety. Some patients, such as those with frequent sickle cell pain crises, have developed a tolerance to narcotics and require seemingly extraordinarily large doses of narcotics for relief. The pharmacology and clinical uses of narcotics is further discussed in Chap. 46.

3. *Fear of side effects.* Narcotic side effects, particularly respiratory depression and hypotension, are rare and may be minimized by intravenous titration and careful patient monitoring. Titration means that incremental doses of the drug are administered by IV push until pain relief is achieved or side effects appear. Patient-controlled analgesia (PCA) electronic pumps with mechanisms that limit dose and frequency allow the patient to titrate his or her own narcotic analgesia.

There are some situations, particularly in the hemodynamically compromised but conscious patient, in which the use of narcotics seems imprudent. Pain control of the hypotensive trauma victim or the woman with a ruptured ectopic pregnancy present major clinical challenges.

4. *Search for etiology supercedes treatment.* Preoccupation with diagnosing the cause of the pain while ignoring or delaying pain treatment is another common error. Patients in severe pain not only want to know the cause of the pain but also want immediate relief. The search for the etiology of the pain can proceed while the patient is receiving analgesia.

5. *Fear of obscuring the physical examination.* "Patients with undiagnosed abdominal pain should never receive analgesia until the surgeon lays on hands" is a frequently quoted dictum of obscure origin and a recurring source of friction between surgeons and emergency physicians. The question as to whether narcotics in particular obscure the abdominal examination is controversial and unsettled but has been challenged in one prospective study.

A cavalier approach to pain control such as "blasting all patients in pain with narcotics" is never recommended. In fact, the approach of juggling pain relief while searching for a diagnosis is more demanding of the skills of the emergency staff. The use of IV titration of narcotic analgesics to make the patient at least comfortable, avoidance of sedation with agents such as promethazine, and open communication with surgical colleagues may prove to be a middle-of-the-road course.

6. *Painful myths.* Analgesia is notoriously inadequate in children and during emergency department surgical procedures. Under the mistaken belief that children do not feel or at least do not remember pain, "we do things to them that by law we can't do to research animals." "Brutane analgesia" is an oxymoron that means no analgesic or anesthetic was used used ("I used Brutane to set that child's broken arm").

The emergency department incision and drainage of abscesses, particularly in the body's exquisitely pain-sensitive areas, including the perineum, perirectum, and axillae, can border on the barbaric. A "this will only hurt a little" attitude is symptomatic of an unempathic attitude toward pain control. For example, ethyl chloride, a topical anesthetic, may be the sole anesthetic used for the incision and drainage, with predictably painful results. Drainage of these abscesses may instead require, in addition to local anesthesia, IV analgesics/amnestics such as fentanyl and midazolam (Versed) or 50:50 nitrous oxide:oxygen inhalation. In the hands of experienced emergency staff and with careful patient monitoring, these techniques can be safely used in an outpatient setting such as the emergency department. Local anesthesia, nitrous oxide, conscious sedation, and pain control in children are discussed further in Chaps. 46–50.

7. *Fear of producing addiction.* The social taboo against addiction is often given higher priority than relieving pain. The overwhelming evidence is that the vast majority of patients with acute pain do not become addicted. Again, the point is not to promote a cavalier approach to narcotic therapy but to promote a realization that even the most potent narcotics in limited numbers for short courses have little potential for addiction.

8. *Concern that the patient is a drug abuser.* Emergency physicians and nurses and prehospital care providers not only treat a broad spectrum of painful conditions but also encounter drug-seeking, hostile, demanding, uncooperative, and other "difficult" patients in a setting of episodic care. Emergency practitioners are not law enforcement agents. Doctors and nurses are patient advocates whose mission is to relieve pain and suffering. Unfortunately, they often find themselves in an adversarial relationship with many patients suspected of "abusing the system" or "trying to trick the staff into prescribing narcotics."

Just as there is no "painometer" or reliable physical examination indicator of pain, there is no accurate stereotype for drug-seeking behavior. Disheveled, smelly, demanding, tattooed patients with needle tracks experience severe pain, and successful, well-coifed suburban business executives feign pain and illness to gain drugs for felonious use. Until a painometer is invented, the emergency specialist must, in these situations, rely on experience and judgment and err on the side of giving the patient the benefit of the doubt.

This should not be misconstrued as advocating indiscriminate prescription of habituating drugs. Commonly abused narcotics such as oxycodone should be judiciously dispensed in limited numbers. Patients claiming to be allergic to "everything but Tylox, Percodan, and Dilaudid" should be scrutinized. Files may be maintained on patients known to be drug seekers. But these are, in the end, compromised, problem-riddled approaches to typical emergency medical pain control problems that lack black-or-white answers.

SUMMARY

Pain control has for too long been shrouded in mystery and perpetuated by habit. Analgesia is often administered too little, too late, or not at all. But the assumptions and beliefs about pain control are being challenged, and more effective, safer methods of analgesia are being sought.

Unique solutions to unique problems of pain control in the emergency setting where questions often lack clear answers must be pursued. At the same time, the basic humanistic principles of compassionate care should be reinforced and the mission never forgotten: Patients call ambulances and go to emergency departments seeking comfort and relief.

Emergency medicine specialists are emerging as leaders and advocates of the treatment, research, and education of proper management of acute pain. The advancement of methods and a system of care that lessen or ablate pain can be one of the specialty of emergency medicine's greatest legacies.

SELECTED READING

Amadio, P. Peripherally acting analgesics. *Am J Med* 77(3A):17, 1984.

Beaver, WT. Combination analgesics. *Am J Med* 77(3A):38, 1984.

Beecher, HK. The powerful placebo. *JAMA* 159:1602, 1955.

Callaham, M, and Raskin, N. A controlled study of dihydroergotamine in the treatment of acute migraine headache. *Headache* 26:168, 1986.

Chudnofsky, CR, et al. The safety of fentanyl use in the emergency department. *Ann Emerg Med* 18:635, 1989.

Doenicke, A, Brand, J, and Perrin, VL. Possible benefit of GR43175, a novel 5-HT1-like receptor agonist, for the acute treatment of severe migraine. *Lancet* 2:1309, 1986.

Graves, DA, et al. Patient-controlled analgesia. *Ann Intern Med* 99:360, 1983.

Holmlund, D, and Sjoden J-G. Treatment of ureteral colic with intravenous indomethacin. *J Urol* 120:676, 1978.

Khalifa, MS, and Sharkawi, MA. Treatment of pain owing to acute ureteral obstruction with prostaglandin-synthetase inhibitor: A prospective randomized study. *J Urol* 136:393, 1986.

Marks, RM, and Sachar, EJ. Undertreatment of medical inpatients with narcotic analgesics. *Ann Intern Med* 78:173, 1973.

Oosterlinck, W, et al. A double-blind single dose comparison of intramuscular ketorolac tromethamine and pethidine in the treatment of renal colic. *J Clin Pharmacol* 30:336, 1990.

Paris, PM. No pain, no pain. *Am J Emerg Med* 7:660, 1989.

Paris, PM, Stewart, RD. Pain Management in Emergency Medicine. Critical Decisions in Emergency Medicine series published by the American College of Emergency Physicians, 1988.

Paris, PM, and Stewart, RD. *Pain Management in Emergency Medicine.* Norwalk, CT: Appleton & Lange, 1988.

Perry, S, and Heidrich, G. Management of pain during debridement: A survey of U.S. burn units. *Pain* 13:267, 1982.

Peterson, LJ. Clinical assessment of new I.V. sedation agents and techniques. *J Dent Res* 63:838, 1984.

Selbst SM, and Clark, M. Analgesic use in the emergency department. *Ann Emerg Med* 9:1010, 1990.

Sloan, JP, et al. Multiple rib fractures: Transcutaneous nerve stimulation versus conventional analgesia. *J Trauma* 26:1120, 1986

Stene, JK, et al. Nalbuphine analgesia in the prehospital setting. *Am J Emerg Med* 6:634, 1988.

Torgerson, WS. What objective measures are there for evaluating pain? *J Trauma* 24:S187, 1984.

Wilson, JE, and Pendleton, JM. Oligoanalgesia in the emergency department. *Am J Emerg Med* 7:620, 1989.

Zoltie, N, and Cust MP. Analgesia in the acute abdomen. *Ann R Coll Surg Engl* 68:209, 1986.

46. Narcotic Analgesics

Larry D. Weiss
Susan M. Dunmire

The relief of pain is a relatively neglected topic in emergency medicine, but in many cases it is our most important intervention. This chapter reviews the systemic administration of narcotic analgesics. A review of basic pharmacology is included, as well as a detailed discussion of the clinical uses of these agents in the emergency department setting.

NARCOTIC AGONISTS

Opiates have been used since ancient times for their sedative and analgesic effects. Opium, the dried extract from opium poppies, contains greater than 20 alkaloids. Of these, four have medicinal value—morphine, codeine, papaverine, and noscapine. Morphine was first isolated in 1803 by Sertuner. Many of the other alkaloids were isolated within the next 50 years.

The term *opiate* refers to the naturally occurring alkaloids of the opium poppy and some semisynthetic derivatives. *Opioid* refers to the synthetic drugs that have morphine-like effects. In the following section, we describe the pharmacologic actions and clinical uses of morphine in detail, since this is a standard by which all other narcotics are compared. Other narcotics are then discussed, with emphasis placed on their clinical application to emergency medicine in comparing their effects with morphine (Table 46-1).

Morphine

Morphine was available for medicinal use by the middle of the nineteenth century. The use of narcotics was generally unrestricted until the early twentieth century. By that time, problems with drug abuse became apparent. In the early 1950s, the first narcotic antagonists were discovered, supporting the hypothesis of specific opiate receptors being responsible for the various actions of narcotics. In 1973, opiate receptors were confirmed by direct measurement using radioimmunoassays.

Opiate receptors are present in many areas of the central nervous system (CNS), with the highest concentration being found in the limbic system, spinothalamic tracts, medial thalamic nuclei, and other regions of pain perception. Each receptor type is coded by a different gene and has distinct biologic functions. The receptors that currently have been identified and their respective functions are listed in Table 46-2.

Oral morphine has only one-sixth the potency of parenteral morphine because of the first-pass effect. However, it is quite efficacious when sufficient oral doses are administered. Oral morphine has found widespread use in cancer patients. When injected intravenously, morphine is rapidly taken up in the tissues. This accounts for morphine's high volume of distribution, which is 3 to 4 times body weight. The drug

Table 46-1. Narcotic agonists

Generic name	Proprietary name	Oral dose (average)	Parenteral dose (average)	Duration	Comments	Precaution
Morphine sulfate	—	30–60 mg	10 mg	3–5 hr	Standard narcotic for all comparisons	Respiratory depression, hypotension, histamine release, sedation
Meperidine	Demerol	250–300 mg	75–125 mg	2–3 hr	See Table 46-3 for comparison with morphine	CNS toxicity; caution if renal or hepatic failure. Avoid with MAO inhibitors
Hydromorphone	Dilaudid	2–6 mg	1–2 mg	2–4 hr	Very soluble, allowing small volumes to be used for injection; available as suppository	Much euphoria
Fentanyl	Sublimaze	Not available	0.1–0.2 mg	1–2 hr	No histamine release; good for short periods	May produce truncal rigidity
Codeine	—	30–100 mg	30–100 mg	4 hr	Excellent cough suppressant; not good for severe pain; abuse relatively uncommon	Much constipation, nausea, and vomiting; decreased with supine position
Oxycodone	Percodan Percocet Tylox	5 mg	15 mg	3 hr	Parenteral form not available in U.S.; very effective	Euphoria predisposes to abuse
Propoxyphene	Darvon-N	100 mg	Not available	3 hr	Very weak analgesic	Overdoses are complicated and serious
Napsylate	Darvocet-N	—	—	—	—	
Alphaprodine	Nisentil	—	25–35 mg	1–2 hr	—	
Methadone	Dolophine	10–20 mg	10 mg	4–6 hr	Analgesic half-life not the same as plasma half-life; not much euphoria	Long plasma half-life may produce cumulative totality
Alfentanyl	Alfenta	Not available	1 mg [v]	1 hr	Minimal cardiovascular side effects; not yet released; shortest half-life of all narcotics	Muscular rigidity in high dose or if administered too quickly
Hydrocodone	Hycodan Vicodan	5–10 mg	Not available	3–4 hr	Excellent cough suppressant; similar potency to codeine; perhaps fewer side effects	Similar to codeine

Source: P.M. Paris and R.D. Stewart. *Pain Management in Emergency Medicine.* East Norwalk, CT: Appleton & Lange, 1988.

Table 46-2. Opiate receptors and their actions

Receptor	Action
Mu	Supraspinal analgesia Respiratory depression Euphoria Physical dependence
Kappa	Spinal analgesia Miosis Sedation
Sigma	Dysphoria Hallucinations Vasomotor stimulation
Delta	?
Epsilon	?

Source: P.M. Paris and R.D. Stewart. *Pain Management in Emergency Medicine.* East Norwalk, CT: Appleton & Lange, 1988.

that is present in plasma is approximately 35 percent protein bound.

The major metabolic pathway is conjugation in the liver with a glucuronic acid. The conjugated drug is excreted by the kidney, with only 10 to 15 percent of the total drug excreted unchanged in the urine or as the conjugated form in the feces. In patients with cirrhosis, morphine may be safer to use than other narcotics, such as meperidine, which are oxidized in the liver. Oxidation appears to be more impaired than conjugation in patients with cirrhosis.

Morphine may be administered by intramuscular (IM), intravenous (IV), subcutaneous (SC), buccal, sublingual, intraspinal, or oral (PO) routes. A sustained-release rectal suppository is under investigation. The IV route has many advantages in the emergency department setting, including rapid onset, accurate titration of dosage, and less pain from administration of the drug. IV access also allows rapid administration of narcotic antagonists if this becomes necessary.

Dosage should be individualized. A common mistake is to administer narcotics in standardized doses at regular intervals. A more practical and efficacious approach is to use small, frequent doses until the desired effect is reached, while closely monitoring patients for side effects. Most adults can be given 2 to 3 mg of morphine IV every 5 to 10 minutes until adequate analgesia is achieved. Most adults require a total of 5 to 30 mg for the initial relief of severe pain. An alternative that may not be practical in the emergency department is patient-controlled analgesia, which allows the patient to self-activate the delivery of a small dose of IV narcotic. This often results in better analgesia with less total medication administered.

Morphine and other narcotics have been used in combination with phenothiazines, hydroxyzine, amphetamines, and nonsteroidal anti-inflammatory drugs (NSAIDs). Considering the efficacy and side effects of using these drugs with narcotics, only the concurrent use of hydroxyzine can be recommended at the current time. Hydroxyzine enhances the analgesic potency of narcotics. It also decreases the nausea caused by narcotics. A disadvantage is that it cannot be administered IV. It must be given orally or by IM injection.

In most patients, the most prominent effects of morphine are on the CNS. Morphine is most often prescribed for its analgesic effects. Continuous dull pain is better relieved by morphine than sharp colicky pain. Other CNS effects include sedation, nausea, euphoria, miosis, and occasional hallucinations and dysphoria. The most serious CNS side effect is a dose-dependent respiratory depression. Morphine causes a reduction of the sensitivity of brainstem chemoreceptors to increases in carbon dioxide tensions. This results in a decrease in respiratory rate and tidal volume. It is the increase in carbon dioxide (and the resultant vasodilation) that is responsible for the increase in intracranial pressure seen after the use of morphine. Many patients who develop respiratory depression after therapeutic doses of morphine have a previous history of impaired pulmonary function from obstructive lung disease or pneumonia.

Morphine causes bronchoconstriction, largely due to histamine release. Pruritis and urticaria at the injection site and generalized flushing may occur. These symptoms are not due to a true allergic response but are direct pharmacologic effects of histamine release by morphine. Aggravation of asthma may occur. Respiratory status should be monitored in these patients, but asthma is not an absolute contraindication to the use of morphine. Fentanyl is an opioid that does not release histamine and may therefore offer an advantage in patients with asthma. Morphine directly depresses the cough center located in the medulla. It is rarely used as a cough suppressant, since more effective and safer antitussives are available (e.g., dextromethorphan, codeine).

Opiate receptors have been found throughout the gastrointestinal tract. Morphine causes a decrease in stomach motility and an increase in antral tone. Both effects delay gastric emptying. In general, tone is increased throughout the small and large bowel. This results in a decrease in peristalsis and an increase in the reabsorption of water. Anal sphincter tone is also increased. The result is a constipating effect. There is also a decrease in pancreatic and biliary secretions.

Morphine causes dramatic increases in biliary pressure due to spasm of the sphincter of Oddi. This is probably due to morphine's ability to cause smooth muscle contraction and may have significant clinical implications. Patients being treated for biliary colic may note an increase in pain following the administration of opiates, and in other patients, biliary colic may be precipitated. It is commonly believed that meperidine causes less spasm than morphine, but this has not been consistently demonstrated in experimental and clinical studies. The opiates that seem to cause the smallest increase in biliary spasm are those in the agonist-antagonist group. Glucagon can be used to reverse biliary spasm. Unlike naloxone, it will not reverse the analgesic effects of opiates. Atropine and nitrates have been studied in this setting with variable results.

The cardiovascular effects of morphine in therapeutic doses are relatively minor. Much of the literature is difficult to interpret, but an increase in venous capacitance has been well established. The resulting decrease in preload can be beneficial in patients with congestive heart failure. In some patients, mean arterial pressure and peripheral vascular resistance may decrease slightly. Morphine causes little change in myocardial contractility or heart rate. At higher doses, patients may become bradycardic. This may be due to central stimulation of the vagus nerve. Morphine probably has no effect on coronary artery flow.

Morphine causes contraction of the smooth muscles of the lower ureters and bladder. This may result in urinary urgency or, conversely, may cause retention in some patients if the tone of the vesicle sphincter increases. Morphine decreases urine production by increasing antidiuretic hormone. Even though morphine causes ureteral spasm, it is still efficacious in patients with ureteral colic because of the potent analgesia it can provide. Studies of ureteral peristalsis show no advantage to using meperidine.

Other Narcotic Agonists

Meperidine

Although morphine is often used in emergency medicine, there are situations when other narcotics may be preferred. Meperidine is the most widely used narcotic analgesic for acute pain in the United States. It was originally promoted as a safer alternative to morphine, but it has the same abuse potential and depresses respiration to the same degree as morphine in equianalgesic doses. Meperidine has one-eighth the potency of morphine when used parenterally. The differences between morphine and meperidine are summarized in Table 46-3.

Meperidine is one of the only narcotics with atropine-like effects; most narcotics have a cholinergic effect. Meperidine may cause an increase in heart rate and may therefore be useful in patients having a myocardial infarction in which a bradycardia has developed. However, this potential advantage of meperidine must be weighed against its mild negative inotropic effect. Meperidine may have less of a spasmogenic effect on smooth muscle than morphine. Even though this has not been consistently demonstrated, meperidine is widely used to treat pain during episodes of biliary and ureteral colic. Studies measuring biliary pressure and ureteral contractions have shown little difference between morphine and meperidine. Meperidine does cause less constipation and urinary retention than morphine. It is a weak cough suppressant but should not be used for this purpose.

Meperidine has long been used in obstetrics because of its relatively short duration of action. However, the agonist-antagonists are probably safer alternatives. Because of its

Table 46-3. Morphine versus meperidine

	Meperidine	Morphine
$t_{1/2}$	$2\frac{1}{2}$–3 hr	3–$3\frac{1}{2}$ hr
Parenteral potency	$\frac{1}{8}$ morphine	—
Oral/parenteral potency	50%	15%
Respiratory depression	Moderate	Moderate
Abuse potential	High	High
Metabolism	Hepatic	Hepatic
Liver disease	$t_{1/2}$ prolonged	$t_{1/2}$ unaffected
Renal disease	Increased CNS toxicity	Unaffected
Histamine release	Yes	Yes
Biliary tract spasm	Significant	Significant
Urinary tract spasm	Yes	Yes
Side effects	Similar to morphine's but higher CNS toxicity; less constipation	See text
Cardiovascular system	Increased pulse, decreased contractility, decreased peripheral vascular resistance	No change or increased pulse, no change in contractility, decreased peripheral vascular resistance
Allergic reactions	Extremely rare	Extremely rare
Constipation	Minimal	Moderate
Cough suppression	Minimal	Marked
Routes of administration	PO, IM, IV, SQ	PO, IM, IV, SQ
Dose–response curve	Very steep	Steep

Source: P.M. Paris and R.D. Stewart. *Pain Management in Emergency Medicine.* East Norwalk, CT: Appleton & Lange, 1988.

lack of cholinergic effects, meperidine may be safer than morphine in asthmatics, but this has not been clearly demonstrated. Like morphine, meperidine does cause histamine release.

The major difference in toxicity between morphine and meperidine relates to the occasional incidence of CNS excitation with meperidine. The adverse CNS effects include nervousness, hyperreflexia, tremors, disorientation, hallucinations, psychosis, multifocal myoclonus, and seizures. Most of these effects are thought to be due to the metabolite normeperidine. Meperidine is contraindicated in patients taking monoamine oxidase (MAO) inhibitors because these drugs interfere with meperidine metabolism.

Parenteral doses of meperidine can be safely administered every 2 to 3 hours. The usual initial dose is 1.0 to 1.5 mg/kg (see Table 46-1). When administered orally, approximately 50 percent of the drug avoids the first-pass effect. The shorter half-life makes meperidine less ideal in treating chronic pain. Metabolism may be slowed in patients with liver disease; therefore, morphine may be preferable in these patients. Patients with renal dysfunction may have CNS toxicity due to elevated normeperidine levels. Hydroxyzine may be administered concurrently to decrease nausea and increase analgesia, but it cannot be administered IV.

Fentanyl

Fentanyl does not release histamine and may be preferable in patients with asthma and reactive airways disease. In other cases, fentanyl may be preferred because it does not depress myocardial contractility. Fentanyl does have a vagal effect similar to that of morphine, resulting in a mild slowing of heart rate, but cardiac index is actually increased.

The short duration of action of this drug makes it ideal for brief procedures in the emergency department. Fentanyl has been shown to be safe and efficacious for sedating children prior to closing facial lacerations. The dose used was 2 to 3 μg/kg IV over 3 to 5 minutes. Fentanyl sometimes causes skeletal muscle rigidity when used in high doses. This should not be of concern with doses used in the emergency department, but intraoperatively it may decrease chest wall compliance and make ventilation difficult.

FENTANYL DERIVATIVES. Alfentanil is very similar to fentanyl but has the advantage of a more rapid onset and shorter duration of action. Sufentanil has a duration of action between that of fentanyl and alfentanil. It has an increased lipid solubility and affinity for the mu opiate receptors that gives it a potency 5 to 10 times that of fentanyl. Currently there is not enough clinical experience to suggest a use for alfentanil or sufentanil in the emergency department.

Hydromorphone

Hydromorphone (Dilaudid) retains much of its potency when administered orally. It is 7 to 8 times more potent than morphine when given parenterally and has a more rapid onset of action and shorter duration. It is one of the few opiates (along with oxymorphone and pentazocine) available as a rectal suppository.

Perhaps its most salient feature is its high solubility. This allows high doses of the drug to be given in small quantities of fluid for SC or IM injection. It is possible to dissolve 330 mg of hydromorphone in 1 ml of water; however, the highest concentration commercially available is 10 mg/ml (Dilaudid HP). In the United States, much of the debate favoring the use of heroin (diacetylmorphine) in cancer patients is based on heroin's high solubility, but since this property is shared

Table 46-4. Narcotic agonist-antagonist analgesics

Generic name	Proprietary name	Oral dose (average)	Parenteral dose (average)	Duration	Comments	Precaution
Pentazocine	Talwin	50–100 mg	30–60 mg	2–3 hr	Suppositories available	Increase stroke work; high incidence of psychotomimetic effects
Nalbuphine	Nubain	40 mg	10–15 mg	3–4 hr	Minimal if any hemodynamic effects; ceiling on respiratory depression; low abuse potential	Can precipitate withdrawal if dependence on narcotic agonist
Butorphanol	Stadol	Not available	1–4 mg	2½–3½ hr	—	Cardiovascular effects similar to pentazocine; can precipitate withdrawal
Buprenorphine	Buprenex	—	0.3–0.6 mg	5–6 hr	A partial agonist can be given sublingually; long analgesic action	Not completely antagonized by naloxone

Source: P.M. Paris and R.D. Stewart. *Pain Management in Emergency Medicine.* East Norwalk, CT: Appleton & Lange, 1988.

by hydromorphone, a suitable alternative exists. This is one of hydromorphone's few unique features, and it would therefore be a drug of choice in cancer patients requiring large IM doses of narcotics.

Oral Narcotics

Oral narcotics are often useful in the emergency department setting for patients who are experiencing considerable pain but who are able to be discharged. The most commonly used oral narcotics are codeine, hydrocodone, oxycodone, and propoxyphene. These drugs are often combined with aspirin or acetaminophen to enhance their analgesic effects.

Codeine retains two-thirds of its activity when given orally. It can be used parenterally, but since it has no advantage over parenteral morphine, it is rarely used by this route. Compared with other narcotics, it has a low abuse potential. It causes little euphoria and is slow to produce dependence. However, it does not appear to be very efficacious in relieving severe pain. Also, it is quite constipating and frequently causes nausea. The usual dosage is 30 to 60 mg with 325 to 650 mg of acetaminophen or aspirin. When prescribing codeine, it is best to provide prophylactic treatment with anticonstipation measures, particularly when using it in the elderly.

Oxycodone (Percocet, Tylox) is a semisynthetic derivative of codeine. It is considerably more potent than codeine on a weight basis and is usually administered with acetaminophen or aspirin. It is a more efficacious analgesic than codeine but has a high abuse potential. It may be preferable to codeine in patients with severe pain.

Hydrocodone (Vicodin, Hycodan) is also a potent semisynthetic derivative of codeine and is usually administered with acetaminophen. It is an excellent antitussive and is less constipating than codeine. Its relative potency and precise indications have not been well delineated due to a relative lack of clinical studies.

Methadone is often used to suppress narcotic withdrawal. It retains much of its potency when administered orally. Because of its delayed onset of action and prolonged activity, it is not well suited for the short-term treatment of acute pain. Propoxyphene is widely prescribed, but many studies have shown that it is no better or only marginally better than placebo. Other studies have shown that it is not better than NSAIDs. Overdoses can be extremely toxic and refractory to treatment, especially when the drug is taken in combination with alcohol. There would seem to be rare indications at best for the use of this drug in the emergency department setting.

NARCOTIC AGONIST-ANTAGONISTS

The development of the agonist-antagonist class of narcotics represents continued attempts to develop safer narcotics, potent analgesics that do not cause respiratory depression or have significant abuse potential. These drugs do cause some respiratory depression, but they seem to have a ceiling effect whereby a plateau of respiratory depression is reached; further increases in dosage do not cause an increase in respiratory depression.

In general, these drugs appear to have a slower onset of physical dependence, a mild withdrawal syndrome, less euphoria (with the possible exception of pentazocine), and a limited abuse potential. Early studies show that these agents cause less of an increase in biliary pressure than a pure agonist drug. These attributes make the agonist-antagonist drugs better suited to the emergency department than are many of the pure agonist drugs. The safe and efficacious use of these drugs for ureteral colic, sickle cell pain crises, and migraine headaches has been described. Table 46-4 compares the agonist-antagonists.

Pentazocine

Pentazocine (Talwin) was the first widely available narcotic agonist-antagonist. The usefulness of this drug is limited by the appearance of psychotomimetic reactions in up to 10 percent of patients. These reactions are seen with other agonist-antagonists but are most common with pentazocine. Significant respiratory depression can occur with high doses. This effect can be reversed with naloxone, but high doses may be necessary. Pentazocine may be useful in the emergency department setting when a suppository is needed or when attempting to avoid smooth muscle spasm (e.g., biliary or renal colic, pancreatitis). The recommended parenteral dose is 30 to 60 mg every 2 to 3 hours.

In some localities, Talwin is widely abused in combination with antihistamines. The combination is commonly referred to as "T's and blues." The pills are ground up and dissolved (often in alcohol) prior to injection. Pentazocine is now available in combination with naloxone (Talwin Nx) to combat parenteral abuse of the tablets. Since naloxone is not orally absorbed, it does not affect oral use of the drug.

Nalbuphine

Nalbuphine (Nubain) is approximately equianalgesic with morphine. It is currently available only for parenteral use in the United States. When administered orally, it is approximately 20 percent as potent as the parenteral form. Nalbuphine has a respiratory depression effect equal to that of morphine at therapeutic doses. However, unlike morphine, it exhibits a ceiling effect. Unlike pentazocine, which increases peripheral vascular resistance and myocardial work, nalbuphine has minimal cardiovascular effects. It is therefore an analgesic of choice in cases of myocardial infarction and in other patients with hemodynamic instability. The recommended parenteral dose is 10 to 15 mg every 3 to 4 hours. The prehospital use of nalbuphine for a variety of indications has been shown to be safe and efficacious.

Nalbuphine is about 3 times more potent than pentazocine as a narcotic antagonist. It may precipitate withdrawal in patients dependent on pure agonists. Psychotomimetic reactions have been reported but occur much less frequently than with pentazocine, probably with an incidence rate of less than 1 percent. Nalbuphine causes less euphoria than most other narcotics and has a low abuse potential. The recommended dosage is 10 mg every 3 to 4 hours.

Butorphanol

Butorphanol is a potent narcotic agonist with moderate antagonist activity. Most of its properties are similar to those described for nalbuphine except the cardiovascular effects, which are similar to those of pentazocine. It is approximately 3.5 to 7 times more potent than morphine on a weight basis. Sedation is a common problem, but psychotomimetic reactions are rare. It has little euphoric effects and, like nalbuphine, is at present not a controlled substance. The recommended parenteral dosage is 0.5 to 4 mg every 3 to 4 hours.

Buprenorphine

Unlike the previously mentioned agonist-antagonists, which are active at the kappa receptors, buprenorphine (Buprenex) is active at the mu receptor. Therefore, buprenorphine is classified as "morphine-like," whereas pentazocine, nalbuphine, and butorphanol are "nalorphine-like." The most significant advantages of this drug are its long duration of action and its proven efficacy when administered by the sublingual route. It is 25 to 30 times more potent than morphine on a weight basis. Its duration of action ranges from 5 to 10 hours. It is not yet clear whether the respiratory depression induced by buprenorphine has a ceiling effect.

Opiate antagonists do not completely reverse the actions of buprenorphine, and high doses of naloxone must be used to partially antagonize respiratory depression. The cardiovascular effects of buprenorphine are similar to those of morphine. Sedation, nausea and vomiting, and diaphoresis are common side effects. It causes little sedation and may precipitate withdrawal in narcotic addicts. The recommended parenteral dose is 0.3 to 0.6 mg every 6 to 8 hours.

SUMMARY

Relief of pain is a high priority in the clinical practice of emergency medicine. Narcotic analgesics are the most efficacious means of relieving severe pain in most patients. Significant side effects are rare when short courses of therapy are used in a judicious manner.

Morphine is the standard by which all other narcotics have been compared, but there are many circumstances when we can take advantage of the unique qualities of some other narcotic agonists. Most of the agonist-antagonists appear to have a limited abuse potential (except pentazocine) and less of a respiratory depressant effect than the narcotic agonists. These characteristics make them well suited for emergency department use.

SELECTED READING

Arguelles, JE, et al. Intrabiliary pressure changes produced by narcotic drugs and inhalation anesthetics in guinea pigs. *Anesth Analg* 58:120, 1979.

Baker FJ, and Sullivan, SN. Effect of morphine and butorphanol on gallbladder emptying. *Can J Surg* 26:70, 1983.

Brash, PG, and Kopriva, CJ. Narcotics and the Circulation. In LM Kitahata, and JG Collins (eds), *Narcotic Analgesics in Anesthesiology*. Baltimore: Williams & Wilkins, 1982. Pp. 91–132.

Berry, FN, Miller, JM, and Levin, HM. Relief of severe pain with acetaminophen in a new drug formulation versus propoxyphene HCl 65 mg and placebo: A comparative double blind study. *Curr Ther Res* 17:361, 1975.

Billmire, DA, Neale, HW, and Gregory, RO. Use of IV fentanyl in the outpatient treatment of pediatric facial trauma. *J Trauma* 25:1079, 1985.

Bovill, JG, Sevel, PS, and Stanley, TH. Opioid analgesics in anesthesia: With special reference to their use in cardiovascular anesthesia. *Anesthesiology* 61:731, 1984.

Economou, G, and Ward-McQuaid, JN. A cross-over study of the effect of morphine, pethidine, pentazocine, and phenazocine on biliary pressure. *Gut* 1:218, 1971.

Gonzalez, ER, et al. Comparison of intramuscular analgesic activity of butorphanol and morphine in patients with sickle cell disease. *Ann Emerg Med* 17:788, 1988.

Goth, A. Narcotic Analgesic Drugs. In A Goth (ed), *Medical Pharmacology: Principles and Practice.* St. Louis: Mosby, 1984. Pp. 319–335.

Graves, DA, et al. Patient-controlled analgesia. *Ann Intern Med* 99:360, 1983.

Hanning, CD, et al. The morphine hydrogel suppository: A new sustained release rectal preparation. *Br J Anaesth* 61:221, 1988.

Heel, RC, et al. Buprenorphine: A review of its pharmacological properties and therapeutic efficacy. *Drugs* 17:81, 1979.

Hopkinson, JH, and Bartlett, FH. Acetaminophen versus propoxyphene HCl for relief of pain in episiotomy studies. *J Clin Pharmacol* 13:251, 1976.

Hsu, HO, Hickey, AR, and Forbes, AF. Morphine decreases peripheral vascular resistance and increases capacitance in man. *Anesthesiology* 50:98, 1979.

Hurst, JW. *The Heart* (5th ed). New York: McGraw-Hill, 1982. Pp. 1079–1080.

Jaffe, JM, and Martin, WR. Opioid Analgesics and Antagonists. In AG Gilman, et al (eds), *The Pharmacologic Basis of Therapeutics* (7th ed). New York: Macmillan, 1985. Pp. 491–531.

Jones, FM, Fiddian-Green, R, and Knight, PR. Narcotic-induced choledochoduodenal sphincter spasm reversed by glucagon. *Anesth Analg* 59:946, 1980.

Kaido, RF, et al. Central nervous system, excitatory effects on meperidine in cancer patients. *Ann Neurol* 13:180, 1983.

Kitahata, LM, Collins, JG, and Robinson, CJ. Narcotic Effects of the Nervous System. In LM Kitahata, and JG Collins (eds), *Narcotic Analgesics in Anesthesiology*. Baltimore: Williams & Wilkins, 1982. Pp. 57–89.

Miller, RR. Clincial effects of parenteral narcotics in hospitalized medical patients. *J Clin Pharmacol* 20:165, 1980.

Miller, RR, et al. Propoxyphene hydrochloride—a critical review. *JAMA* 223:996, 1970.

Pert, CB, Pasternak, GW, and Snyder, SH. Opiate agonists and antagonists discriminated by receptor binding in brain. *Science* 182:1359, 1973.

Radney, PA, et al. The effect of equi-analgesic doses of fentanyl, morphine, meperidine, and pentazocine on common bile duct pressure. *Anaesthetist* 29:26, 1980.

Roebel, LE, Cavanaugh, RL, and Buyniski, JP. Comparative gastrointestinal and biliary tract effects of morphine and butorphanol. *J Med* 10:225, 1979.

Roscow, CE, et al. Histamine release during morphine and fentanyl anesthesia. *Anesthesiology* 56:93, 1982.

Schowalter, CV. Ts and blues. Abuse of pentazocine and tripelennamine. *JAMA* 244:1224, 1980.

Simon, EJ, Hillier, JM, and Edelman, I. Stereospecific binding of the potent narcotic analgesic etorphine to rat brain homogenate. *Proc Natl Acad Sci* 70:1947, 1973.

Staritz, M, et al. Effect of modern analgesic drugs on the bile duct sphincter in man. *Gut* 27:567, 1986.

Stene, JK, et al. Nalbuphine analgesia in the prehospital setting. *Am J Emerg Med* 6:634, 1988.

Stower, MJ, Wright, JW, and Hardcastle, JD. The action of glucagon and the commonly used antispasmodics and analgesics on the canine ureter. *Br J Surg* 70:89, 1983.

Tegerstedt, I, et al. The effect of buprenorphine and oxycodone on the intracholedochal passage pressure. *Acta Anaesth Scand* 25:99, 1981.

Urthaler, F, Isobe, JH, and James, TN. Direct and vagally mediated chronotropic effects of morphine studied by selective perfusion of the sinus node of awake dogs. *Chest* 68:222, 1975.

Zola, EM, and McLeod, DC. Comparative effects and analgesic efficacy of the agonist-antagonist opioids. *Drug Intell Clin Pharm* 17:411, 1983.

47. Nonnarcotic Analgesics

Susan M. Dunmire
Larry D. Weiss
Paul M. Paris

Nonnarcotic analgesics (NNAs) are the most widely used prescription and over-the-counter drugs in the field of medicine today. Aspirin sales alone exceed one billion dollars per year. This class of drugs has a variety of beneficial properties, including analgesic, antipyretic, and antiinflammatory actions. They are useful in treating a wide spectrum of conditions, including musculoskeletal injuries, arthritis, gout, headaches, myalgias, pharyngitis, pleuritis, ureteral colic, dysmenorrhea, and many other painful disease processes.

Traditionally, NNAs are perceived as the "weaker analgesics" for mild to moderate pain while narcotics are the "stronger analgesics." Although this is true to some extent, in several situations the NNA may provide analgesia that is superior to a narcotic agent. NNAs possess antiinflammatory properties that narcotic agents lack and therefore are the drugs of choice in conditions such as gout, pseudogout, pleuritis, and acute flares of rheumatoid arthritis and osteoarthritis. While all NNAs offer antiinflammatory properties, some (indomethacin, aspirin, propionic acid derivatives) are much more potent than others (acetaminophen, diflunisal).

Several studies indicate that indomethacin may be a more effective drug than narcotics in the treatment of renal colic. It is postulated that inhibition of prostaglandin relaxes the ureteral spasm, thus providing pain relief and possibly accelerating passage of the stone. Initial studies were performed with parenteral indomethacin, but similar success has been observed with indomethacin rectal suppositories.

Nonnarcotics have become popular analgesics because of a perceived safety secondary to the absence of central nervous system (CNS) and respiratory depression and lack of abuse potential. This should not lull the physician into a false sense of security. The NNAs have a variety of serious side effects, the most common of which are gastric erosion and gastrointestinal (GI) bleeding. Other potential adverse effects include renal and hepatic dysfunction, hypersensitivity, and drug interactions. In certain situations it may be safer for the patient to use a narcotic agent.

With the constant influx of new NNAs on the market, it is becoming increasingly difficult for the physician to be aware of their properties and side effects. The following guidelines by Kaplan are designed to assist the clinician in selecting the appropriate drug for a particular clinical situation.

1. Most NNAs have significant antiinflammatory actions. Those with the least antiinflammatory action include acetaminophen and diflunisal.
2. Most NNAs possess antipyretic properties. Acetaminophen is the antipyretic of choice for all age groups. Ibuprofen and fenoprofen can be used as alternatives. Aspirin is contraindicated as an antipyretic in children secondary to its possible association with Reye's syndrome.

3. A variety of dosage regimens are available. Piroxicam offers once-a-day therapy, while diflunisal, sulindac, and naproxen are administered twice daily. These agents may offer advantages in the noncompliant patient or in individuals who are receiving chronic therapy.
4. All NNAs can produce GI upset; however, the least irritability is seen with acetaminophen, ibuprofen, naproxen, and sulindac. Indomethacin and aspirin are associated with significant gastric irritation while meclofenamate is frequently discontinued because of diarrhea.
5. Although all NNAs can acutely impair renal function, acetaminophen, aspirin, and sulindac appear to produce the least renal toxicity.
6. Hypersensitivity has been reported with all the NNAs. In aspirin-sensitive individuals, acetaminophen is the safest alternative.
7. Most NNAs are highly protein bound and can displace oral anticoagulants, oral hypoglycemics, and other drugs. Acetaminophen, ibuprofen, naproxen, flurbiprofen, and tolmetin do not appear to interact with either oral anticoagulants or hypoglycemics.
8. The elderly are particularly susceptible to side effects of NNAs and dosage may need to be adjusted.
9. Acetaminophen, aspirin, and tolmetin are approved for use in children.
10. If a given NNA is ineffective for pain after a one- to two-week trial period, it may be helpful to choose another NNA.

The majority of NNAs are classified as nonsteroidal antiinflammatory drugs (NSAIDs)—prostaglandin synthesis inhibitors that possess analgesic, antiinflammatory, and antipyretic properties. The NSAIDs discussed in this chapter include aspirin and salicylate derivatives, ibuprofen, ketoprofen, fenoprofen, flurbiprofen, naproxen, indomethacin, sulindac, tolmetin, meclofenamate, and phenylbutazone. Acetaminophen lacks significant antiinflammatory actions and is not categorized as an NSAID, but will be discussed separately.

In this chapter, an in-depth discussion of mechanism of action, pharmacokinetics, drug interactions, and side effects of NNAs in general will be followed by a brief section on each drug and its particular properties, indications, and dosing regimens. The discussion is designed to aid the clinician in the selection of the best agent for a particular disease state, thus providing optimal pain management.

MECHANISMS OF ACTION

Nonnarcotic analgesics inhibit the enzyme cyclooxygenase, which is involved in the synthesis of prostaglandins. Prostaglandins are compounds found throughout the body that play a role in the production of pain, inflammation, and fever. Studies suggest that prostaglandins as well as other mediators sensitize pain receptors. A variety of prostaglandins have been identified, each with different actions on the body. The specific properties and therapeutic advantages of a particular NNA depend on which prostaglandins are inhibited. The analgesic and antiinflammatory effects of NNAs are thought to be due to the decreased synthesis of the peripherally acting prostaglandin E_2 (PGE_2), whereas the antipyretic properties are thought to be a result of a decrease in centrally acting PGE_1.

PHARMACOKINETICS

There are several chemical classes of NNAs, which differ in potency, duration of action, drug interactions, and side effects (Table 47-1). All agents are rapidly absorbed and peak serum levels are obtained within two hours. All NNAs undergo hepatic metabolism to varying degrees, and the half-life can be significantly prolonged with hepatic dysfunction. Elimination is via renal and fecal routes depending on the drug.

DRUG INTERACTIONS

Most NNAs are highly protein bound and thus may compete with other medications for binding sites. Table 47-2 lists the significant drug interactions. Of note, the NNAs will displace oral anticoagulants, hypoglycemics, lithium, and phenytoin (Dilantin) from their respective binding sites, and therefore prothrombin time, blood glucose, and drug levels should be monitored closely in these patients. In patients who take antihypertensive medications, the blood pressure should be monitored regularly, as NNAs can antagonize the actions of beta-blockers, captopril, and diuretics.

SIDE EFFECTS

Although NNAs offer many beneficial properties, the incidence of side effects is significant and should be weighed against the potential benefits before these medications are prescribed. Gastrointestinal complaints account for the majority of side effects with NNAs; however, a potential also exists for renal, hepatic, and hematopoietic complications.

Gastrointestinal

Nonnarcotic analgesics, through inhibition of gastric prostaglandins, produce a wide spectrum of GI complaints, including nausea, vomiting, abdominal pain, diarrhea, and constipation. All NNAs can produce gastric mucosal irritation, resulting in erosive gastritis, gastric ulceration, and GI bleeding. Certain drugs produce a higher incidence of GI irritation (aspirin, indomethacin, meclofenamate) than others. In one study, chronic administration of aspirin (2,400 mg a day) produced gastric erosions in 40 percent of patients and gastric ulcers in 20 percent. When combined with NNA-induced platelet dysfunction, these gastric erosions can significantly increase the risk of GI bleeding. Highly buffered solutions, enteric-coated tablets, and sustained-release preparations offer improved GI tolerance. Diflunisal, acetaminophen, sulindac, and the propionic acid derivatives are associated with a much lower incidence of gastric irritation than aspirin. Gastric erosions and GI symptoms can be minimized by administering all NNAs with meals, antacids, and/or sucralfate.

Table 47-1. General properties of NSAIDs

Chemical class	Drug	Trade name	Time to peak (hr)	Half-life
Acetylated salicylates	Aspirin		0.75	2–30[a]
Acetaminophen	Acetaminophen	Tylenol	0.5–1.0	2–4
Nonacetylated salicylates	Diflunisal	Dolobid	2–3	12
	Magnesium salicylate	Magan	1.5	2
	Choline Magnesium trisalicylate	Trilisate	1–2	9–17
	Salsalate	Disalcid	4	3.5, 16[a]
Acetic acids	Indomethacin	Indocin	2	4.5
	Sulindac	Clinoril	2	8, 16[b]
	Tolmetin	Tolectin	0.5–1.0	1–6
Propionic acids	Ibuprofen	Motrin Rufen Advil Nuprin Medipren Haltran	1–2	2
	Fenoprofen	Nalfon	1–2	3
	Ketoprofen	Orudis	0.5–2.0	3–5
	Flurbiprofen	Ansaid	1–2	3–4
	Naproxen	Naprosyn	3–4	13
		Na Naprosyn	1–2	
	Suprofen	Suprol	0.5–2.0	2–4
Oxicams	Piroxicam	Feldene	3–5	50
Fenamates	Meclofenamate	Meclomen	0.5–2.0	2–4
	Mefanamic acid	Ponstel	2–4	2–4
Pyrazoion	Phenylbutazone	Azolid Butazolidin	2	50–65

[a]Half-life is dose-dependent.
[b]Active metabolite (sulfide).
Source: P.M. Paris and R.D. Stewart. *Pain Management in Emergency Medicine.* East Norwalk, CT: Appleton & Lange, 1988.

Renal

Nonnarcotic analgesics have the potential to impair renal function, produce acute renal failure, and worsen chronic renal failure secondary to inhibition of renal prostaglandins. Renal prostaglandins have a vasodilatory effect on renal vasculature, counterbalancing the vasoconstricting catecholamines and ultimately contributing to the regulation of renal blood flow and glomerular filtration rate. Inhibition of prostaglandins produces unopposed vasoconstriction, resulting in decreased renal blood flow and fluid retention. Dosage adjustment, careful selection of the appropriate NNA, and close monitoring of renal function are necessary in patients with renal dysfunction. Indomethacin and fenoprofen are associated with the highest incidence of renal impairment, while aspirin, acetaminophen, and sulindac reportedly have a lower incidence.

Hypersensitivity

Hypersensitivity reactions have been reported with all of the NNAs. These reactions range from rhinitis and urticaria to angioedema, acute bronchospasm, and anaphylaxis. Aspirin has been the NNA most widely studied for hypersensitivity. Predisposing factors to aspirin sensitivity include vasomotor rhinitis, chronic urticaria, and nasal polyps. Acute allergic reaction to aspirin is usually manifested by rhinorrhea, conjunctivitis, and a flushing of the face, trunk, and neck. Death has been reported with as little as 300 mg of aspirin.

Indomethacin has a 100 percent cross-sensitivity to aspirin-allergic individuals, whereas acetaminophen has only a 5 percent cross-reactivity. Zomepirac (Zomax) was removed from the market because of a high incidence of anaphylactic reactions and associated deaths.

Acute therapy of an NNA-induced allergic reaction includes antihistamines with or without epinephrine, depending on the age of the patient and severity of reaction. Once a history of NNA hypersensitivity has been elicited from a patient, further use of these agents is contraindicated.

Other Side Effects

Infrequent side effects with NNAs include hepatic dysfunction, pancreatitis, cutaneous reactions, thrombocytopenia, and aplastic anemia. These reactions are usually seen with chronic administration of higher doses of NNAs or in the elderly. Several of the newer NNAs have been removed from distribution by the Food and Drug Administration (FDA) secondary to side effects. Benoxaprofen (Oraflex) was discontinued secondary to hepatotoxicity, and suprofen (Suprol) was removed because of a high incidence of associated renolithiasis.

Table 47-2. Possible drug interactions with nonnarcotic analgesics (NNAs)

Drug	Interaction
Alcohol	May protect against acute acetaminophen poisoning, but chronic alcohol administration may potentiate acetaminophen-induced hepatotoxicity
Antacids	Depending on the antacid and NNA, may delay or not affect absorption
Antihypertensives (e.g., beta blockers, captopril, furosemide, thiazides)	NNA may antagonize the hypotensive action
Cimetidine	May decrease absorption or metabolism of a NNA
Corticosteroids	May increase the clearance of a NNA
Lithium	May elevate lithium levels of a NNA
Methotrexate	NNA may decrease clearance of methotrexate
Oral hypoglycemics	NNA may displace an oral hypoglycemic from its binding sites
Other NNAs	Aspirin may decrease the clearance of a number of NNAs; fatal gastrointestinal hemorrhage has resulted from concomitant treatment with diflunisal and indomethacin
Phenytoin	May be displaced from protein-binding sites
Probenecid	May decrease the excretion of NNAs; NNAs may antagonize uricosuric action of probenecid
Triamterene	Reversible acute renal failure has been reported when administered with indomethacin
Warfarin	May be displaced from its binding sites; increased likelihood of bleeding

Source: P.M. Paris and R.D. Stewart. *Pain Management in Emergency Medicine.* East Norwalk, CT: Appleton & Lange, 1988.

New NNAs continue to be developed and there is a constant influx of new agents into this competitive market. It is the clinician's responsibility to use these new agents cautiously, with close monitoring of potential side effects until their safety has been proved.

ASPIRIN

The use of salicylates as analgesics can be traced back 2,000 years to Hippocrates' use of the bark of the willow tree (*salix*) to relieve fever and pain. The active ingredient of the bark is salicin, from which salicylic acid was produced. In 1853, acetylsalicylic acid, a more soluble and less corrosive form, was synthesized at the Bayer Laboratories in Germany. Today, aspirin is used as an analgesic for mild to moderate pain, and as an antiinflammatory, antipyretic, and antiplatelet agent. It is widely available as an over-the-counter preparation, both alone and in combination with other medications.

Pharmacokinetics

Aspirin is rapidly dissolved in the stomach and absorbed primarily in the small intestine. Some preparations are buffered with magnesium, calcium, or aluminum, which increases solubility, absorption, and gastric pH, leading to less GI distress. Once absorbed the aspirin is rapidly hydrolyzed to salicylate in the gastric mucosa and liver. Peak plasma levels are reached within 2 hours. At low doses of aspirin (250 mg) the half-life is approximately 3 hours, while at higher antiinflammatory doses (2.5–5.0 gm per day) the half-life approaches 12 hours.

Enteric coated aspirin dissolves over a period of at least four hours and demonstrates variable absorption. With these characteristics it should not be used in the treatment of acute pain.

Actions

Analgesic
Aspirin inhibits the enzyme cyclooxygenase, thus blocking synthesis of prostaglandins. It is effective to some extent on any type of pain that is not visceral in origin. Aspirin alone may not be effective in the treatment of moderate to severe pain. In such cases, narcotic analgesia may be indicated, and some studies suggest that aspirin may potentiate the analgesia obtained with narcotics. Analgesic doses of aspirin range from 300 to 2,500 mg.

Antiinflammatory
Aspirin is an excellent antiinflammatory agent because it inhibits peripherally acting prostaglandin PGE_2. Larger doses of aspirin are required to achieve antiinflammatory effects (3–5 gm per day) and therefore the incidence of GI intolerance is increased. Frequently, administration with antacids is necessary to combat this common side effect.

Antipyretic
Aspirin and acetaminophen are excellent antipyretics and are the drugs of choice to combat fever in adults. Studies suggest that combined use of aspirin and acetaminophen produces a greater and longer temperature reduction than each agent used alone. Aspirin has been replaced by acetaminophen as the antipyretic of choice for children, since aspirin has been implicated in the development of Reye's syndrome in children with viral illnesses.

Antiplatelet
Low-dose aspirin therapy (40–100 mg per day) selectively inhibits thromboxane, resulting in decreased platelet aggregation. Aspirin is now FDA approved for use in patients with myocardial infarction (MI) or unstable angina. Studies have shown a decrease in cardiovascular mortality and rate of MI in aspirin-treated patients. Future studies may also prove aspirin to be a valuable therapy in the treatment of transient ischemic attacks and prevention of cerebral infarction.

Side Effects

Aspirin produces many of the side effects discussed in the introductory section on NNAs. A dose-dependent GI intolerance is the most common adverse effect. Chronic administration of aspirin is associated with an increased incidence of gastric ulcers and GI bleeding.

Aspirin is associated with a relatively high incidence of hypersensitivity as compared with other NNAs. The nonacetylated salicylate preparations have a much lower incidence of hypersensitivity. As stated previously, there is a high incidence of aspirin sensitivity in individuals with a history of vasomotor rhinitis, nasal polyps, and chronic urticaria. Future use of NNAs in hypersensitive patients is not recommended.

As little as 40 mg a day of aspirin is needed to irreversibly inhibit platelet thromboxane and elevate bleeding time. Larger doses will inhibit platelet prostacyclin and very large doses of aspirin (6 gm per day) will inhibit prothrombin synthesis and prolong prothrombin time.

Rarely, aspirin will cause a transient elevation of hepatic transaminases and bilirubin. These side effects are dose and duration dependent and usually are reversible on discontinuation of the drug.

DIFLUNISAL (DOLOBID)

Diflunisal is a nonacetylated salicylate derivative that offers the properties of a longer half-life and twice-a-day dose intervals. It has been shown to be at least as potent an analgesic as aspirin, ibuprofen, and acetaminophen with codeine in comparable doses.

Diflunisal offers the advantage of less GI intolerance than aspirin. Disadvantages include a relatively high incidence of dermatologic reactions (10%) and no significant antipyretic properties.

Diflunisal is indicated in the treatment of pain associated with rheumatoid arthritis and osteoarthritis. A loading dose decreases the time necessary to reach peak serum levels.

Dosage

Loading dose is 1,000 mg by mouth. Maintenance dose is 250 to 500 mg every 12 hours.

ACETAMINOPHEN

Acetaminophen, first synthesized in 1878, has become a standard over-the-counter drug, both alone and in combination with other medications, for the treatment of pain and fever. Its actions are achieved through inhibition of the enzyme cyclooxygenase. It has strong effects on this enzyme in the CNS, accounting for its analgesic and antipyretic properties, and weaker actions in the periphery, allowing for its lack of antiinflammatory actions.

Acetaminophen is an excellent analgesic in the treatment of mild to moderate pain. It has been shown to potentiate the effects of certain narcotics (codeine, oxycodone, hydrocodone) and can be used in combination with these drugs in the treatment of more severe pain.

Acetaminophen is also a very effective antipyretic agent, with onset of action within 30 minutes and duration of activity for six hours. It is the antipyretic of choice for infants and children.

Pharmacokinetics

Acetaminophen is rapidly absorbed after oral administration and peak levels are obtained within 60 minutes. Hepatic metabolism results in sulfuric, glucuronic, and cysteine metabolites. Elimination half-life is two to four hours but may be prolonged in neonates and patients with hepatic dysfunction. The half-life is unaffected by renal dysfunction.

Side Effects

Side effects with therapeutic doses of acetaminophen are rare. Allergic reactions, consisting of skin rashes and fever, are reported infrequently.

Drug Interactions

Acetaminophen does not interfere with oral anticoagulants or hypoglycemics.

Dosage

Dosage for children is 10 to 15 mg/kg every four hours. Adults should be given 325 to 650 mg every four to six hours.

PROPIONIC ACID DERIVATIVES

Ibuprofen

In recent years ibuprofen, a prostaglandin inhibitor, has become an extremely popular drug in the treatment of acute and chronic pain, inflammation, fever, and primary dysmenorrhea. It is available in a wide variety of prescription and over-the-counter preparations, including Motrin, Rufen, Advil, Nuprin, Medipren, Haltran, and Midol.

Studies of postoperative and dental pain have shown ibuprofen (400 mg) to be a superior analgesic to aspirin (650 mg) or aspirin or acetaminophen combined with codeine (60 mg). Ibuprofen is also an excellent antiinflammatory agent in the therapy of acute orthopedic injuries, rheumatoid arthritis, osteoarthritis, and acute inflammation.

Side Effects

Although GI intolerance is the most frequently reported side effect, it occurs much less often with ibuprofen than with aspirin. Other side effects include dizziness, vertigo, tinnitus, and, rarely, aseptic meningitis and hepatic and renal dysfunction.

Dosage

For mild to moderate pain, the dosage is 1,200 to 1,600 mg per day in divided doses. For inflammation, 1,600 to 2,400 mg per day should be given in divided doses. The dosage for primary dysmenorrhea is 1,200 to 1,600 mg per day in divided doses.

Naproxen (Naprosyn)

Naproxen and naproxen sodium (Anaprox) are propionic acid derivatives with a longer half-life (13 hours) than ibuprofen and twice-a-day dose intervals. Dental studies have shown naproxen to be at least as potent an analgesic as pentazocine (50 mg), morphine (10 mg), or an aspirin-codeine combination. It is indicated in the treatment of acute pain, primary dysmenorrhea, acute gout, rheumatoid arthritis, and osteoarthritis. Naproxen has a significant incidence of GI side effects, including constipation, abdominal pain, nausea, vomiting, and GI bleeding.

Dosage
For mild to moderate pain, the initial dose is 500 mg, followed by 250 mg every 8 to 12 hours. For rheumatoid arthritis or osteoarthritis, the dosage is 250 mg every 12 hours. For acute gout, initial dosage is 750 mg, followed by 250 mg every 6 to 8 hours until pain has subsided. The dosage should be decreased by one half in cirrhotic patients. Naproxen can be given as a suppository when the patient is unable to tolerate oral intake.

Fenoprofen (Nalfon)

Fenoprofen is a relatively short-acting propionic acid derivative that is equipotent to codeine, Naprosyn, and ketoprofen as an analgesic. It offers the advantage of less GI intolerance than aspirin; however, it is associated with a significant incidence of mild headache, dizziness, confusion, and depression. Fenoprofen has also been associated with dysuria, cystitis, hematuria, and nephrotic syndrome, which is frequently preceded by fever, rash, arthralgias, and proteinuria.

Dosage
Initial dose is 200 mg every four to six hours (up to 3,200 mg per day).

Ketoprofen (Orudis)

Ketoprofen is another of the propionic acid derivatives with a shorter duration of action (half-life, two to four hours). It inhibits both the cyclooxygenase and lipooxygenase pathways. Ketoprofen has similar side effects to all NNAs; however, it is associated with a lower incidence of GI intolerance than aspirin.

Dosage
Initial dose is 75 mg every eight hours or 50 mg every six hours up to 300 mg per day.

Suprofen (Suprol)

Suprol has been taken off the market because of an unacceptably high incidence of associated renolithiasis, thought to be secondary to its uricosuric properties.

Flurbiprofen (Ansaid)

Flurbiprofen is relatively new on the market. It offers the advantage of a rapid onset of action (peak serum levels in 1.5 hours) and a longer duration of action (5.5 hours). Initial studies indicate that flurbiprofen is associated with a higher incidence of GI intolerance than other propionic acid derivatives.

Dosage
Initial dosage is 50 to 100 mg by mouth four times a day.

ACETIC ACIDS

Indomethacin (Indocin)

Indomethacin is a nonsteroidal antiinflammatory indole derivative. It possesses analgesic, antiinflammatory, and antipyretic properties; however, its use is limited because of a high incidence of GI and CNS side effects. Indomethacin is indicated in the treatment of acute gouty arthritis, acute bursitis-tendonitis, moderate to severe rheumatoid arthritis, osteoarthritis, and ankylosing spondylitis.

Pharmacokinetics
Indocin is available in the traditional and slow-release form (Indocin SR). The latter form is designed to release 25 mg initially, followed by sustained release of the remaining 50 mg over 12 hours. Rectal suppositories have more rapid absorption and onset of action than the oral route. Indocin is hepatically metabolized with significant enterohepatic circulation. It is eliminated via renal and biliary excretion.

Side Effects
GASTROINTESTINAL. Gastrointestinal side effects from indomethacin occur in as many as 10 percent of patients within the first few weeks of therapy. Gastritis, GI bleeding, and gastric ulceration have been reported with alarming frequency. Gastric erosion is a dose-dependent phenomenon and a decreased incidence of GI upset has been reported with the sustained-release preparation and indomethacin suppositories. Indocin must be discontinued in more than 30 percent of patients secondary to GI side effects.

CENTRAL NERVOUS SYSTEM. Many patients complain of headaches and dizziness in association with indomethacin therapy. Other CNS disturbances include exacerbation of depression, somnolence, and vertigo.

OCULAR. Corneal deposits and retinal disturbances have been reported with indomethacin. Blurred vision is often the initial symptom and the physician should discontinue therapy and initiate an ophthalmology consult if this occurs.

Dosage
For rheumatoid arthritis and osteoarthritis the initial dosage is 25 mg three times a day. This should be increased 25 mg per day over weekly intervals (maximum, 200 mg per day). The dosage for bursitis-tendonitis is 25 to 50 mg three times a day. For acute gouty arthritis, the dosage is 50 mg three times a day until the pain is tolerable; then it should be rapidly tapered.

Sulindac (Clinoril)

Sulindac is chemically related to indomethacin but offers the advantage of fewer GI side effects. Sulindac is metabolized into an active sulfide form that is a cyclooxygenase inhibitor. Some studies suggest that sulindac may have less effect on renal function than other NNAs because of sparing of renal prostaglandin synthesis. This is still unproven, however.

Dosage
Initial dosage is 100 to 200 mg twice a day (maximum, 400 mg per day). (Sulindac is also available in 200-mg suppositories.)

Tolmetin (Tolectin)

Tolmetin lacks the indole ring of the other acetic acids, which leads to a lower incidence of CNS side effects. It also offers the advantage of being one of the few NSAIDs to be approved for use in children. Tolmetin does produce a significant amount of gastrointestinal side effects, resulting in discontinuation of therapy in five to eight percent of patients.

Dosage
Dosage for adult arthritis is 400 mg three times a day (maximum, 2,000 mg per day). Dosage for juvenile rheumatoid arthritis is 20 mg/kg per day in divided doses (three or four times a day).

PIROXICAM (FELDENE)

Piroxicam, a member of the oxicam family, is a nonsteroidal agent with a prolonged half-life (45 hours), which offers the advantage of once-a-day dosing and steady-state plasma levels. It provides a rapid onset of analgesia; however, antiinflammatory effects may not be seen for 72 hours. Piroxicam offers analgesia equivalent to aspirin, ibuprofen, sulindac, and naproxen.

Dosage
The initial and maintenance dosage is 20 mg per day.

MECLOFENAMATE (MECLOMEN)

Meclofenamate is a nonsteroidal, antiinflammatory agent used for the treatment of rheumatoid arthritis and osteoarthritis. It has very effective analgesic and antiinflammatory actions, but its use is limited because of a high incidence of side effects. The most common adverse effect with meclofenamate is diarrhea, which occurs in 10 to 33 percent of patients.

Dosage
Maintenance dosage is 200 to 400 mg per day in three to four divided doses.

KETOROLAC (TORADOL)

Ketorolac is the first parenteral NSAID made available in the United States. Several clinical trials have shown 30 mg IM of ketorolac to be equivalent with 12 mg IM of morphine or 100 mg IM of meperidine in postoperative patients. The advantages of ketorolac over other nonnarcotics include a rapid onset of action (peak plasma levels at 50 minutes), potent analgesia, and a relatively long duration of action (6 hours). Obvious advantages over narcotic analgesics include a lack of central nervous system and respiratory depression and absence of euphoria and dependence.

Ketorolac has similar side effects to other NSAIDs including gastrointestinal upset and possible gastric erosion with prolonged use. Hypersensitivity has not been a problem. Since the parenteral form of this drug lends itself to sporadic use, side effects are infrequently seen. The oral form of ketorolac is not yet available in the United States. The drug is not currently approved for intravenous use.

Dosage
The loading dose is 30 to 60 mg IM. The maintenance dose is 30 mg every 6 hours.

SUMMARY

Nonnarcotic analgesics are extremely valuable in the treatment of acute and chronic pain, inflammation, and fever. While each agent has distinct characteristics, there is not tremendous variability between agents. Certain NNAs may work better for some individuals than others. The clinician's choice of an agent should be based on his or her clinical experience and comfort with that drug and the patient's response to the medication. If the patient does not experience significant relief within a week, a change to another NNA may be beneficial.

In summary, the physician should be very familiar with a select few NNAs and have a general knowledge of the benefits and side effects of the others. When prescribing an NNA the physician should choose one with which he or she is comfortable and should be aware of potential side effects. Appropriate dose and route of administration are important for adequate analgesia. With proper use, these medications are invaluable tools in the treatment of fever, pain, and inflammation.

SELECTED READING

Ameer, G, and Greenblatt, DJ. Acetaminophen. *Ann Intern Med* 87:202, 1977.

Boardman, PL, and Hart, FD. Side effects of indomethacin. *Ann Rheum Dis* 26:127, 1967.

Brown, CR, Sevelius, H, and Wild, V. A comparison of single doses of naproxen sodium, morphine sulfate and placebo in patients with post-operative pain. *Curr Ther Res* (4):511, 1984.

Carmichael, J, and Shankel, SW. Effects of nonsteroidal antiinflammatory drugs on prostaglandins and renal function. *Am J Med* 80:74, 1986.

Cooper, SA. Five studies on ibuprofen for post surgical dental pain. *Am J Med* 77:70, 1984.

Cooper, SA, Needle, SE, and Kruger, GO. Comparative analgesic potency of aspirin and ibuprofen. *J Oral Maxillofac Surg* 35:898, 1977.

Dunn, MJ. Nonsteroidal anti-inflammatory drugs and renal function. *Annu Rev Med* 35:411, 1984.

Feldberg, W, and Saxena, PN. Fever produced by prostaglandin E_1. *J Physiol* 217:547, 1971.

Filtzer, HS. A double-blind randomized comparison of naproxen sodium, acetaminophen and pentazocine in post-operative pain. *Curr Ther Res* 27:293, 1980.

Flower, RJ, Moncada, S, and Vane, JR. Analgesic-antipyretics and Anti-inflammatory Agents: Drugs Employed in the Treatment of Gout. In AG Gilman, et al (eds), *The Pharmacologic Basis of Therapeutics*. New York: Macmillan, 1985.

Forbes, JE, et al. A twelve hour evaluation of the analgesic efficacy of diflunisal, propoxyphene, a propoxyphene-acetaminophen combination and placebo in post-operative oral surgery pain. *Pharmacotherapy* 2:43, 1982.

Harwig-Otto, H. Pharmacokinetic considerations of common analgesics and antipyretics. *Am J Med* 75:30, 1983.

Holt, LPJ, and Hawkins, CF. Indomethacin: Studies of absorption and the use of indomethacin suppositories. *Br Med J* 1:1354, 1965.

Kaplan, RM, and Levine, RL. Nonnarcotic Analgesics. In PM Paris and RD Stewart (eds), *Pain Management in Emergency Medicine.* East Norwalk, CT: Appleton & Lange, 1988.

Keet, JGM. A comparative clinical trial of diflunisal and ibuprofen in the control of pain in osteoarthritis. *J Int Med Res* 7:272, 1979.

Lanza, FL, Royer, GL, and Nelson, RS. Endoscopic evaluation of the effects of aspirin, buffered aspirin and enteric coated aspirin on gastric and duodenal mucosa. *N Engl J Med* 303:136, 1980.

Lanza, FL, et al. Effects of flurbiprofen and aspirin on the gastric mucosa. *Am J Med* 80:31, 1986.

Lehtonen, T, et al. Intravenous indomethacin in the treatment of ureteral colic: A multicenter pilot study. *Scand J Urol Nephrol* (Suppl):37, 1983.

Masotti, G, et al. Differential inhibition of prostacyclin production and platelet aggregation by aspirin in humans. *Adv Prostaglandin Thromboxane Leukotriene Res* 6:317, 1980.

Moncada, S, and Higgs, EA. Introduction of the mode of action of aspirin. *Aspirin Symposium* Pp 1–9, 1983.

Moncada, S, Flower, RJ, and Vane, JR. Prostaglandins, Prostacyclin, Thromboxane A_2 and Leukotrienes. In AG Gilman, et al (eds), *The Pharmacologic Basis of Therapeutics.* New York: Macmillan, 1985.

Plotz, PH, and Kimberly, RP. Acute effects of aspirin and acetaminophen on renal function. *Arch Intern Med* 141:343, 1981.

Ruedy, J. A comparison of the analgesic efficacy of naproxen and propoxyphene in patients with pain after orthopedic surgery. *Scand J Rheumatol* 2 (Suppl):60, 1973.

Sedor, JR, et al. Effects of sulindac and indomethacin on renal prostaglandin synthesis. *Clin Pharmacol Ther* 36:85, 1984.

Silvoso, GR, et al. Incidence of gastric lesions in patients with rheumatic disease on chronic aspirin therapy. *Ann Intern Med* 91:517, 1975.

Steel, RW et al. Oral antipyretic therapy: Evaluation of aspirin-acetaminophen combination. *J Dis Child* 123:204, 1973.

Szczeklik, A, and Gryglewski, RJ. Asthma and anti-inflammatory drugs. Mechanisms and clinical patterns. *Drugs* 25:533, 1983.

Yee, J, et al. Comparison of intramuscular ketorolac tromethamine and morphine sulfate for analgesia of pain after minor surgery. *Pharmacotherapy* 6:253, 1986.

Yee, J, et al. A comparison of analgesic efficacy of intramuscular ketorolac tromethamine and meperidine in postoperative pain. *Clin Pharmacol Ther* 39:237, 1986.

Zipser, RD, and Henrich, WL. Implications of nonsteroidal anti-inflammatory drug therapy. *Am J Med* 80:74, 1986.

48. Conscious Sedation

Ronald N. Roth

Pharmacologic conscious sedation provides a method of pain management for patients who are seen in the emergency department with pain or for those who suffer pain as a result of a procedure performed in the emergency department. Although the term *conscious sedation* seems paradoxical, "conscious but sedated" is precisely the state that we are trying to achieve. Ideally, the patient who requires a painful procedure or is in pain would be conscious, able to respond appropriately to commands, and able to maintain all protective reflexes, including the maintenance of a patent airway. In addition, the patient would be sedated which would blunt the patient's fear, anxiety, and response to pain. The concept of conscious sedation is outlined in Table 48-1.

Occasionally, painful procedures are performed in the emergency department as lifesaving maneuvers—for example, chest thoracotomy for a tension pneumothorax—and pain control is often neglected or dismissed by the physician because of the acuteness of the situation. However, in the majority of situations, the painful procedures, such as incision and drainage of a skin abscess, are done electively. Unfortunately, even for most elective procedures, pain control is neglected or dismissed. Situations that lend themselves to verbal and chemical preparation are listed in Table 48-2.

The "cure" should be no worse than the "disorder." After suffering the ordeal of a painful procedure at the hands of a well-meaning physician, few patients will be consoled by "you'll thank me later." Conscious sedation serves as an alternative to physical restraint, as an adjunct verbal support, and as local anesthesia.

Although some of the agents used in conscious sedation can be used as analgesics (e.g., narcotics), complete elimination of pain is not the goal in conscious sedation. In fact, attempts at total pain control with most agents used for conscious sedation will result in unconscious sedation (general anesthesia), with loss of patient responsiveness and protective reflexes.

The ideal agent for providing conscious sedation would have the following properties: (1) safety, with minimal side effects and a high therapeutic : toxic dose ratio; (2) effectiveness; (3) convenient administration and storage; (4) rapid onset, with a predictable duration and rapid reversibility; and (5) in common use in the emergency department. Unfortunately, this ideal agent does not exist. As a result, a variety of agents are used for the initiation of conscious sedation, each with their own benefits and drawbacks.

Three major groups of agents are used for emergency department conscious sedation. These include inhalation agents with nitrous oxide : oxygen mix, currently the only clinical agent commonly in use in this group, narcotics, and benzodiazepines. An alternate agent, ketamine, is used to provide a state of "dissociative sedation," which will be discussed later. Agents for conscious sedation can be used individually or in combination. Combining two agents allows

Table 48-1. The concept of conscious sedation

Conscious	Sedated
Able to respond to verbal commands	Reduced anxiety and fear
Intact protective reflexes, including ability to maintain an airway	Blunted response to painful stimuli
	Increased acceptance and cooperation

Table 48-2. Suggested indications for conscious sedation in the emergency department

Cardioversion
Chest tube placement
Incision and drainage of abscesses
Repair of extensive lacerations
Orthopedic procedures, including dislocation reduction and fracture realignment
Procedures requiring significant patient cooperation
Procedures involving children
Central line placement
Burn debridement and dressing changes
Arterial line placement
Debridement of extensive abrasions (road rash)
Anoscopy
Painful conditions such as ureteral colic

the physician to take advantage of the beneficial effects of each agent. However, combinations also potentiate the risk of excessive sedation and loss of protective reflexes. As a precautionary measure, before agents for conscious sedation are administered, resuscitation equipment, including intubation, suction devices, and resuscitation drugs and naloxone, should be immediately available.

NITROUS OXIDE

In a 50 : 50 mixture with oxygen, self-administered nitrous oxide is a "potent" anxiolytic agent with sedative and mild analgesic properties. When self-administered, delivered by way of a demand valve, the potential dangers of loss of consciousness and protective reflexes are minimized. The nitrous oxide : oxygen mixture blunts patients' reactions to pain rather than blocking the pain stimulus itself. This sedative-analgesic mixture has been used for inhospital and prehospital care pain and anxiety management. The nitrous oxide : oxygen mixture appears to be well tolerated by most patients with a variety of painful conditions, including musculoskeletal trauma, burns, and urethral colic, and by patients undergoing incision and drainage procedures.

The keystone to the safety of nitrous oxide as an adjunct to pain control is a self-administered demand-valve system, providing a nitrous oxide concentration of no greater than 50%. At high altitudes or during helicopter transport, nitrous oxide concentrations of up to 70% may be required to achieve an equipotent effect. Clinically important changes in vital signs have not been observed with the use of this gas

Table 48-3. Contraindications to nitrous oxide use

Altered level of consciousness
Pneumothorax
Suspected bowel obstruction
Decompression sickness
Severe chronic obstructive pulmonary disease
Preterm pregnancy?

mixture in clinical practice. However, concomitant administration of narcotics with nitrous oxide can depress cardiovascular function.

The administration of the gas mixture containing 50% oxygen should be used with caution in patients with chronic lung disease, since it carries the potential of depressing their ventilatory drive. Other relative contraindications to the use of the nitrous oxide : oxygen mixture are listed in Table 48-3. The use of nitrous oxide in pregnancy, other than during labor, remains controversial. The unsettled issue of teratogenicity limits the use of nitrous oxide in preterm pregnancy.

When nitrous oxide is administered, trace levels can leak into the surrounding environment. These low levels have been studied and can be minimized with a scavenging device when used in the emergency department.

Nitrous oxide also has the disadvantage of the potential for abuse. Nitrous oxide mixtures must be regulated in a manner similar to that of other potent analgesics used in the emergency department. The demand valve required for use of the nitrous oxide can be kept separate from the cylinder in a locked drug box. A locking mechanism on the delivery unit, with a log containing patient names and amount remaining in the tank after use, is another alternative for security.

The nitrous oxide : oxygen gas mixture can be used for conscious sedation before painful procedures such as splinting, burn dressings, and wound incision and drainage. Patients should be permitted to breathe the gas mixture for several minutes before the procedure is performed. The mixture can be administered via hand-held mask or a mouthpiece held by the patient. Should the patient become drowsy during the procedure, the mask or mouthpiece will fall away, discontinuing the flow of nitrous oxide.

The ease of administration, rapid onset, and quick recovery time of self-administered nitrous oxide : oxygen makes this gas mixture a useful agent for conscious sedation. Because of its potent anxiolytic effect, nitrous oxide is a useful adjunct to local anesthetics. Nitrous oxide conscious sedation may blunt the anxiety and discomfort associated with the injection of local anesthetics.

Clinical trials using a self-administered nitrous oxide : oxygen mixture for relief of acute pain have shown partial to significant pain relief in 80 to 90 percent of patients. In these trials no major side effects were reported. In the Pittsburgh emergency medical services system, more than 3,000 patients have received the mixture since its introduction in 1979 without any untoward reactions.

As was mentioned earlier, nitrous oxide appears to act by blunting the patient's reaction to pain rather than blocking the painful stimulus itself. The sedative and anxiolytic effects of the nitrous oxide mixture are the most evident clinically. Verbal guidance and suggestion during the administration of nitrous oxide can increase its effectiveness. Guiding the patient to think pleasant thoughts or supplying pleasant music by headphones may distract the patient from the emergency department environment and enhance the effectiveness of the nitrous oxide.

NARCOTICS

The ability of narcotics to produce both analgesia and euphoria makes them popular agents for conscious sedation. Narcotics are routinely used and stocked in the emergency department for pain control and advanced life support, and therefore are readily available for use in conscious sedation. The use of narcotics, as opposed to nitrous oxide or ketamine, for conscious sedation in the emergency department is also less likely to provoke unfavorable discussions with colleagues in anesthesia.

Although potentially any injectable narcotic can be used for conscious sedation, meperidine (Demerol) and morphine tend to be the most popular agents because of physician familiarity with these drugs. Both meperidine and morphine can be used via the intramuscular (IM), subcutaneous, or intravenous (IV) route. Drug absorption via the IM route is similar to absorption via the subcutaneous route, although the IM injection is considerably more painful and should be avoided if possible. When the drug is given via the IM route as a single dose, the physician lacks control of drug absorption and the ability to titrate the drug's effect. In addition, supplementation of inadequate initial dose is difficult. If the subcutaneous route is chosen, meperidine, 1 to 2 mg/kg, has been used in children for conscious sedation. In adults, meperidine, 100 mg/70 kg, or morphine, 10 mg/70 kg, can be used for sedation. However, the effective dose of a narcotic analgesic must be tailored to the needs of the individual patient.

Using the IV route, meperidine or morphine can be given in small, incremental IV doses and titrated. When IV narcotics are administered, the end point should not be total pain relief, since this point may be preceded by hypotension, hypercarbia, loss of consciousness, and loss of protective reflexes. A more reasonable end point is reached when the patient notes that pain is present on the initiation of a procedure (i.e., local infiltration of a wound or palpation of a skin abscess), but the pain is tolerable.

Difficulties in using narcotics for conscious sedation are related to the side effects of the narcotic agents. The use of morphine has occasionally been associated with nausea, vomiting, and, rarely, transient bradycardia and hypotension. Bronchospasm can also occur secondary to histamine release. Because of the long half-life of both meperidine (2.5–3.0 hours) and morphine (3.0–3.5 hours), a patient undergoing a brief emergency department procedure who is sedated with these narcotics is committed to a prolonged period of drowsiness and possible need for observation unless the narcotics are reversed.

Fentanyl (Sublimaze) is a synthetic narcotic analgesic with a potency that is approximately 150 times greater than morphine and has a distribution half-life of about 20 minutes. In addition, it has a rapid onset, with a duration of approximately 30 to 40 minutes. These characteristics make fentanyl an ideal agent for conscious sedation in the emergency department, where rapid recovery is desired. Fentanyl reportedly produces a lower incidence of nausea and vomiting than either morphine or meperidine and also produces fewer reactions as a result because of the lack of histamine release. Potential complications of fentanyl use are the problems associated with narcotic use in general. Muscle rigidity can occur after rapid IV administration of fentanyl, causing chest-wall spasm. Fentanyl-induced rigidity is centrally mediated and can impair the ability to assist ventilation if respiratory depression is induced with the drug. The fentanyl-induced rigidity is exacerbated by nitrous oxide but can be prevented by slow IV administration and reduction of the dose of the narcotic.

In their study of the use of IV fentanyl in the outpatient treatment of pediatric facial trauma, Billmire and associates used the agent in 2,000 patients between 1981 and 1984. A dose of 2 to 3 μg/kg body weight was administered slowly to provide conscious sedation for both minor and major facial wounds. Three episodes of apnea occurred in the series, all of which were successfully reversed with naloxone. This dose usually gives 30 to 40 minutes of sedation. Older children tended to require the full 2 to 3 μg/kg, with younger children often requiring less than the calculated dose.

As with other narcotics used for conscious sedation, the dose of fentanyl should be titrated, with adequate time allowed for the drug to take action between doses. It is essential to monitor the patient's respiratory rate during the procedure, as the peak respiratory depression of fentanyl may not occur for 5 to 10 minutes after the injection.

Due to its potency and as a safety precaution, fentanyl, which is available in a concentration of 50 μg/cc (1 cc = 50 μg = 0.05 mg), should be diluted and only the maximum calculated dose placed in a syringe at the patient's bedside. This may prevent inadvertent overdosing of the patient. As with all drugs given for conscious sedation, equipment for respiratory support should be immediately available. In addition, a syringe containing naloxone should be at the patient's bedside. As with the other narcotics, the end point for fentanyl is not complete analgesia but acceptable patient tolerance of the pain during the procedure.

BENZODIAZEPINES

Benzodiazepines have been used for preoperative medication and conscious sedation since the 1960s. Although these agents do not provide analgesia for painful procedures, they possess potent amnestic and anxiolytic effects. Patients about to undergo a painful or anxiety-provoking procedure in the emergency department may benefit from the administration of a benzodiazepine.

Benzodiazepines have the potential of making the patient more comfortable and cooperative for the procedure. In addition, they allow some degree of muscle relaxation and may provide anterograde amnesia, especially when given IV. Benzodiazepines are often used in conjunction with local anesthetics or IV narcotics, or both, before the initiation of a painful procedure. In general, benzodiazepines can be administered orally, IV, or IM. However, IM injection is painful and absorption via the IM route is often variable.

In the past, diazepam (Valium) has been the primary benzodiazepine used for conscious sedation. However, it has

Table 48-4. Conscious sedation versus dissociative sedation

	Conscious sedation	Dissociative sedation
Agents	Nitrous oxide, narcotics, benzodiazepines	Ketamine
Analgesia	Minimal to moderate	Profound
State of consciousness	Relaxed, cooperative	Cataleptic state
Muscle tone	Unchanged or decreased	Unchanged or increased
Amnesia	None to significant	Significant

active metabolites and a long half-life of greater than 24 hours, making it less desirable for brief emergency department procedures. Patients often complain of drowsiness that lasts longer than 24 hours. In addition, diazepam causes pain and venous irritation with IV injection.

Midazolam (Versed), introduced in 1986, is unique among the benzodiazepines in that it is water soluble, resulting in fewer local adverse reactions and less pain after injection. With an elimination half-life of 1½ to 2 hours, midazolam has the potential to produce less drowsiness after a brief emergency department procedure. Midazolam is approximately two to four times as potent as diazepam although there is significant patient variability. The rapidity of action, degree of anxiolysis, sedation, and amnesia of midazolam have been reported as similar or superior to those of diazepam.

The effective dose for midazolam as an agent for conscious sedation before short emergency department procedures range between 0.05 and 0.1 mg/kg. Because of its rapidity of onset, midazolam should be given immediately before the procedure, after the patient and the necessary equipment for the procedure are prepared. The midazolam should be administered in small incremental doses, approximately ½ to 1 mg, over several minutes until the desired effect is obtained (i.e., slurred speech). There is considerable interpatient variability in the dose required to produce conscious sedation. No more than 2.5 mg should be administered over two minutes and an additional two-minute waiting period should be used to fully evaluate the sedative effect of the initial dose. Additional titration of the midazolam dose should be done in small increments, with time allowed in between doses to assess sedation. A total dose of greater than 5 mg is usually not necessary. Doses of more than 0.15 mg/kg can result in an increase of respiratory depression and drowsiness, especially in elderly or debilitated patients.

Midazolam has been associated with respiratory depression and arrest when used for conscious sedation. Therefore, as with all other drugs used for conscious sedation, resuscitative equipment and drugs must be immediately accessible. Midazolam produces minimal decreases in mean arterial pressure and cardiac output comparable to those of other benzodiazepines.

In summary, benzodiazepines are useful agents for conscious sedation because they produce rapid and reliable sedation, amnesia, and anxiolysis. The ability to produce a short period of anterograde amnesia is a useful feature of the benzodiazepines. Patients will have little or no memory of the painful event, but a rapid recovery time allows the patient to be fully awake and able to receive follow-up instructions on discharge. Midazolam's rapid metabolic clearance and lack of tissue irritation on injection provide useful advantages over diazepam.

KETAMINE

Ketamine, a derivative of phencyclidine, has been used in clinical practice since 1970. It has the unique ability to provide more profound analgesia than can be safely and reliably obtained with nitrous oxide, narcotics, or benzodiazepines. Ketamine induces a state in which the patient is disconnected or dissociated from the environment and able to tolerate very painful procedures while maintaining protective reflexes. A comparison of conscious sedation versus dissociative sedation is given in Table 48-4. In addition to providing profound analgesia, ketamine induces a cataleptic state with significant amnesia. While in the dissociative state induced by ketamine, the patient's eyes are often open, and vertical or horizontal nystagmus is seen.

Reluctance to use ketamine stems in part from a reported emergence phenomenon, which can include hallucinations, delusions, excitement, and unusual dreams. The reported rate of incidence of the emergence phenomenon ranges from 3 to more than 30 percent, depending on the premedication technique of administration and total dose of ketamine, as well as the nature of the procedure being performed and the patient's age, sex, and personality. Emergence phenomena tend to resolve within 30 minutes. Large doses (greater than 2.2 mg/kg IV), rapid infusion, lack of premedication, and female sex are usually associated with a higher incidence of the emergence phenomenon. Children rarely experience the emergence phenomenon and benzodiazepines reportedly minimize the incidence of these reactions in adults. Long-term side effects have not been elicited on follow-up studies searching for long-term psychic effects.

The role of ketamine in the emergency department is similar to that of previously described agents used for conscious sedation. Ketamine produces a dissociative state in which the patient is conscious but free of pain and anxiety. In addition, ketamine is able to provide a significantly higher level of analgesia and pain tolerance, allowing many painful procedures to be carried out in the emergency department. For example, a patient with a large perirectal abscess could be made comfortable and cooperative for an incision and drainage procedure that is typically very painful. Dailey and associates reported the successful use of ketamine in the emergency department in children who require laceration repair, foreign body removal, and incision and drainage procedures.

Ketamine can be administered intramuscularly or intravenously; the IM route is the less predictable of the two since the dose cannot be accurately titrated. A dose of 0.5 to 1.0 mg/kg will induce a dissociative state within 5 minutes. The duration of satisfactory sedation will last approximately 20 minutes. Higher doses may be required in patients with high anxiety levels or an inability to cooperate. The most predictable method of providing ketamine sedation is by the IV route, which allows small amounts of ketamine titrated against the patient's response to produce the desired level of sedation. After an IV loading dose of approximately 0.5 to 1.0 mg/kg ketamine, the patient will become calm and cooperative within 10 to 15 seconds. To sustain the dissociative state, 5- to 10-mg doses of ketamine can be administered as needed. A dose of ketamine should be given over 15 to 30 minutes to avoid excessive pressor effect and to minimize respiratory depression.

Ketamine is supplied in the 1%, 5%, and 10% forms. The 1% concentration is preferred for IV administration. At a dose of 1 mg/kg, unconsciousness lasts approximately 3 to 10 minutes. The duration can be extended with additional doses of ketamine. Diazepam (Valium), given at a dose of 0.15 to 0.30 mg/kg IV administered before ketamine sedation, minimizes the occurrence of the emergence phenomenon. Satisfactory results have also been shown when diazepam, 5 mg IV, is given at the completion of a procedure performed under ketamine sedation. The short-acting benzodiazepine midazolam may provide a more useful alternative to diazepam in the prevention of emergence reactions.

Clinically, ketamine appears to be a stimulant to the cardiovascular system, increasing both heart rate and blood pressure. This action may be achieved primarily by sympathetically mediated stimulation of central nervous system (CNS) structures. Ketamine can produce an increase in intracerebral pressure as a result of the rising systemic blood pressure and secondary to cerebral vasodilatation. Therefore, it should be avoided in the emergency department setting in patients with uncontrolled hypertension, significant atherosclerotic heart disease, intracranial disease, or elevated intracerebral pressure. Except when administered in high doses or by rapid infusion, ketamine does not produce respiratory depression in low doses. However, upper respiratory secretions can be increased by ketamine, and adequate airway suctioning and monitoring must not be forgotten. For procedures that last longer than 15 minutes or those that involve the mouth, an antisialagogue can be given before the administration of ketamine. For children atropine, 0.1 mg, has been found to be adequate, while in adults atropine, 0.4 mg, can be administered. Glycopyrrolate, a quaternary ammonium compound, has been recommended over atropine because of its lack of cardiovascular and CNS effects.

Many of the individual drugs used for conscious sedation are often used in combination. Benzodiazepines, used in conjunction with ketamine, can reduce or eliminate ketamine's emergence phenomenon. The anxiolytic, amnestic, and muscle relaxant properties of benzodiazepines can be combined with the analgesic qualities and reversibility of the narcotics. Combining agents often requires reducing the dosages of each individual agent. The physician must be aware that, in addition to potentiating the beneficial effects of the individual drugs, combining agents used for conscious sedation runs the risk of potentiating the unwanted effects of each drug (e.g., the sedation of the benzodiazepines along with the respiratory depression of the narcotics).

SUMMARY

Conscious sedation allows the physician to remove the anxiety, fear, and pain associated with many painful emergency-department procedures and conditions. Patients undergoing procedures with the aid of conscious sedation often describe their experience as pleasant. This may make the patient less reluctant to return for follow-up visits and improve patient compliance and satisfaction.

SELECTED READING

Al-Khudairi, D, Whitwam, JG, and McCloy, RF. Midazolam and diazepam for gastroscopy. *Anesthesia* 37:1002, 1982.

Barclay, JK, Hunter, KM, and MacMillan, W. Midazolam and diazepam compared as sedatives for outpatient surgery under local anesthesia. *Oral Surg* 59:349, 1985.

Bennett, CR, and Stewart, RD. Ketamine. In PM Paris and RD Stewart (eds), *Pain Management in Emergency Medicine.* Norwalk: Appleton & Lange, 1988.

Billmire, DA, Neale, HW, and Gregory, RO. Use of IV fentanyl in outpatient treatment of pediatric facial trauma. *J Trauma* 25: 1079, 1985.

Ceravolo, FJ, et al. Full dentition periodontal surgery using intravenous conscious sedation. *J Periodontol* 57:383, 1986.

Christian, CM, Waller, JL, and Moldenhauer, CC. Postoperative rigidity following fentanyl anesthesia. *Anesthesiology* 58:275, 1983.

Compstock, MK, et al. Rigidity and hypercarbia on fentanyl-oxygen induction. *Anesthesiology* 51:328, 1979.

Corby, JM. Nitrous oxide for outpatient surgery. *Am Intra-Ocular Implant Soc J* 10:232, 1984.

Corssen, G, Reeves, JG, and Stanley, TH. *Intravenous Anesthesia.* Philadelphia: Lea & Febiger, 1988.

Dailey, RH, Stone R, and Repert, W. Ketamine: Dissociative anesthesia—emergency department use in children. *JACEP* 8:57, 1979.

Dundee, JW, et al. Midazolam: A review of its pharmacological properties and therapeutic use. *Drugs* 28:519, 1984.

Flomenbaum, N, et al. Self-administered nitrous oxide: An adjunct analgesic. *JACEP* 8:95, 1979.

Geiderman, J. Benzodiazepines. In PM Paris and RD Stewart (eds), *Pain Management in Emergency Medicine.* Norwalk: Appleton & Lange, 1988.

Herregods, L, et al. A comparison of midazolam and diazepine for sedation during locoregional anesthesia. *Acta Anaesth Belg* 38:97, 1987.

Khanderia, U, and Pandit, SK. Use of midazolam hydrochloride in anesthesia. *Clin Pharmacol Ther* 6:533, 1987.

Michelson, LN, et al. Diazepam and fentanyl as adjuncts to local anesthesia. *Anesth Plast Surg* 11:207, 1987.

Moore, PA, et al. Sedation in pediatric dentistry: A practical assessment procedure. *JADA* 109:564, 1984.

Ochs, MW, Tucker, MR, and White RP, Jr. A comparison of amnesia in outpatients sedated with midazolam or diazepine alone or in combination with fentanyl during oral surgery. *JADA* 113:89, 1986.

Paris, PM, and Weiss, LD. Narcotic Analgesics: Pure Agonists. In PM Paris and RD Stewart (eds), *Pain Management in Emergency Medicine.* Norwalk: Appleton & Lange, 1988.

Paris, PM, et al. A perspective prehospital trial of nitrous oxide use in urban and suburban/rural systems: A study of efficacy and side effects (abstract). *Ann Emerg Med* 17:425, 1988.

Reifkohl, R, Cole, MM, and Cox, EB. The effectiveness of benzodiazepines and narcotics in outpatient surgery. *Anesth Plast Surg* 8:227, 1984.

Scamman, FL, Klein SL, and Choi, WW. Conscious sedation for procedures under local or topical anesthesia. *Ann Otol Rhinol Laryngol* 94:21, 1985.

Stewart, RD. Nitrous oxide. In PM Paris and RD Stewart (eds), *Pain Management in Emergency Medicine.* Norwalk: Appleton & Lange, 1988.

Stewart, RD, et al. Patient controlled inhalation analgesia in prehospital care: Study of side effects and feasibility. *Crit Care Med* 11:51, 1983.

Vinnik, CA. An intravenous disassociation technique to outpatient plastic surgery. Tranquility in the office surgical facility. *Plast Reconstr Surg* 67:799, 1981.

White, PF, Way, WL, and Trevor, AJ. Ketamine—its pharmacology and therapeutic uses. *Anesthesiology* 56:119, 1982.

49. Local Anesthesia

Donald M. Yealy
Ronald D. Stewart

The clinical use of local anesthetics began in the late nineteenth century after the isolation of the alkaloid cocaine from the erythroxlon coca bush. Koller described the topical anesthetic properties of this compound in 1884, and Halsted and Hall reported the first use of cocaine-induced injection anesthesia for minor surgery less than one year later. Although an effective drug for local anesthesia, cocaine was quickly recognized as carrying some risk because of the high incidence of toxicity associated with its use. Procaine was synthesized in 1905 and became the local anesthetic of choice because of its efficacy and safety. Tetracaine and chlorprocaine soon followed and were structurally similar due to their ester linkage.

In 1943, Lofgren synthesized lidocaine, an amide-linked local anesthetic, as an alternative to the procaine-related agents. Lidocaine offered similar or improved safety and efficacy, with a lower risk of allergic phenomenon than the ester class of local anesthetics. Since that time, other amide agents have been developed, including mepivacaine, bupivacaine, prilocaine, and etidocaine. These agents offer varying degrees of potency and clinical duration of action.

TYPES

Local anesthetic techniques can be classified according to the anatomic site of drug placement and subsequent neural blockade. Topical anesthesia is obtained by direct application of an agent to the structures to be anesthetized. It is often employed on mucous membranes or moist surfaces, such as the cornea, although skin structures can also be anesthetized. Infiltration anesthesia, the most common technique employed in the emergency department, refers to injection of an agent into or around painful tissues. Nerve-block anesthesia refers to the injection of a local anesthetic in proximity to a peripheral nerve (or group of nerves) to allow neural blockade of a particular anatomic site. These blocks are useful for dental procedures, large wound repairs, and abscess drainage. Regional nerve blocks involve similar principles, with larger or more central nerve groups targeted for pharmacologic pain impulse interruption. Intravenous regional anesthesia, often employed in the upper extremity for orthopedic manipulation, can render an entire limb anesthetized. Spinal and epidural anesthesia cause blockade of large dermatomal segments after local anesthetic instillation at or near the spinal nerve roots. Although minor peripheral nerve blocks can and should be included in the emergency physician's pain management arsenal, major peripheral nerve trunk, spinal, and epidural anesthesia are best performed by staff specifically trained in such techniques.

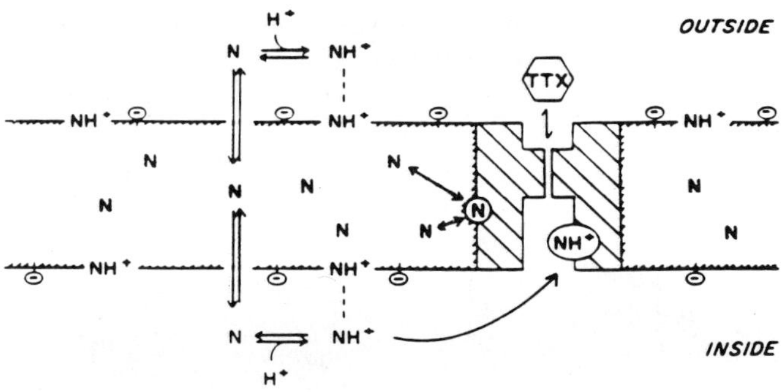

Fig. 49-1. Tertiary amine local anesthetics exist as neutral base (N) and protonated (NH^+) species in physiologic solution. These forms interact in various modes with phospholipids and proteins in nerve membranes: N preferentially partitions into the hydrophobic membrane interior, whereas NH^+ absorbs at the negatively charged membrane surface, through hydrophobic and electrostatic interactions. Two primary reactions with Na^+ channel proteins are shown: rapid binding of the neutral form at the lipid : protein interface and slower binding of the charged form by means of the inner mouth of the channel; the latter depends on the conversion of the channel to open or activated conformations (see text). The natural "local anesthetics" tetrodotoxin (TTX) and saxitoxin bind at the external surface of the channel and have no obvious interactions with local anesthetics. (From M.J. Cousins and P.O. Bridenbaugh. *Neural Blockade in Clinical Anesthesia and Management of Pain* [2nd ed.]. Philadelphia: Lippincott, 1988.)

MECHANISM

Local anesthetics interfere with the excitation-conduction process of peripheral nerve fibers, specifically through interactions with the sodium-potassium cell membrane channels. At rest, an electrical potential of −70 to −90 mV exists between the cytoplasm and the extracellular fluid. This is a result of the ionic asymmetry between the two areas. The intracellular : extracellular concentration gradient for potassium is about 10 : 1, and a similar inverse relationship exists for sodium concentration. These gradients occur as a result of differential ion permeability; at rest, the axonal membrane is highly permeable to potassium ions, but only slightly permeable to sodium ions. Excitation of a nerve causes a membrane change that allows an influx of sodium ions into the intracellular fluid, changing the potential to −50 mV. Once this level is reached, an explosive increase in membrane permeability occurs, allowing massive influx of sodium ions. The membrane potential rises to +40 mV and represents the peak of depolarization. After this peak, the sodium channel begins to assume permeability characteristics similar to those seen in the resting state, restoring the resting potential (repolarizing) to −70 to −90 mV. At the end of repolarization, a slight sodium excess exists within the cell, and an adenosine triphosphate–driven "sodium pump" actively transports sodium across the membrane in exchange for potassium.

Local anesthetics act to decrease the maximal rate of depolarization and thereby impede the propagation of an impulse. Resting membrane potential and repolarization are unaffected by local anesthetics. Lidocaine has been shown to completely inhibit sodium conductance through the membrane, while potassium flux is diminished by approximately five percent.

The actual site of local anesthetic action is still contested, yet most evidence suggests that the commonly used agents bind to receptors on the inner surface of the cell membrane (Fig. 49-1). The binding of the local anesthetic, in the ionic form within the cytoplasm, causes a change within the sodium-potassium channel that interferes with ion flux. Other compounds that act as local anesthetics interact with the sodium-potassium channel differently. Benzocaine and benzyl alcohol penetrate the nerve membrane directly and cause expansion, thus limiting sodium channel size.

In summary, local anesthetics act by: (1) crossing axonal membranes; (2) binding to intracellular membrane receptors in the ionized form; (3) reducing sodium permeability; (4) decreasing the rate of depolarization, which leads to failure to reach threshold; (5) causing a lack of propagation of impulses; and (6) producing neural conduction blockade.

PHARMACOLOGIC PRINCIPLES

The agents used for local and regional anesthesia can be divided into two groups, based on their chemical structures. Common to both groups is the presence of an aromatic lipophilic moiety and a hydrophilic group. The linkage between these two ends provides the chemical basis for classification. Ester-type local anesthetics have an amino-ester link, while amide-type agents have an amino-amide link (Fig. 49-2). The two groups vary in elimination characteristics and allergic potential. Ester-type local anesthetics are hydrolyzed by plasma cholinesterase, forming paraaminobenzoic acid as one metabolite. This is the substance responsible for the vast majority of local anesthetic allergic reactions in the general population. Patients with low plasma cholinesterase levels may have a more prolonged duration of blockade from ester-type local anesthetics. Amide local anesthetics do not undergo hydrolysis and are rarely associated with allergic reactions. The liver enzymatically degrades the amide agents, and the elimination half-lives are generally prolonged when compared to the esters. Table 49-1 lists the

Fig. 49-2. Basic structure of local anesthetics, based on the linkage between the lipophilic and hydrophilic groups. Modification of either the linkage group or the amine and aromatic ends can influence the activity and potency of the agent.

Ester Structure

Aromatic lipophilic group—$COOCH_2CH_2$—amine hydrophilic group

Amide Structure

Aromatic lipophilic group—NHCO—amine hydrophilic group

Table 49-1. Pharmacology of local anesthetics

Agent	pKa	Percent protein bound	Relative lipid solubility[a]	Site of metabolism
Esters				
Procaine	9.0	6	1	Plasma
Tetracaine	8.5	75–85	7	Plasma
Chlorprocaine	9.0	?	0.5–1.0	Plasma
Amides[b]				
Lidocaine	7.7	65	3	Liver
Mepivacaine	7.8	78	1	Liver
Bupivacaine	8.1	95	30	Liver
Etidocaine	7.7	94	130	Liver

[a] Based on relative heptane/buffer partition coefficient derived in vivo.
[b] Note that all amide local anesthetics contain the letter "i" in their prefix.
Source: Modified from M.J. Cousins and P.O. Bridenbaugh. *Neural Blockade in Clinical Anesthesia and Management of Pain* (2nd ed.). Philadelphia: Lippincott, 1988.

Table 49-2. Factors influencing local anesthetic clinical profile

Factor	General effect
pKa	Being closer to physiologic pH (7.4) increases potency
Lipid solubility	Increases potency and block duration
Protein binding	Increasing binding increases the duration of blockade
Intrinsic vasodilator activity	An increase shortens the duration of clinical block
Non-neuronal diffusibility	An increase shortens onset of clinical block

$$N: + H \rightleftharpoons NH$$

Fig. 49-3. Local anesthetics exist as solutions in equilibrium. At a pH that equals pKa, the concentrations of the nonionized base (N:) and the ionized conjugate acid (NH) are equal.

most common local anesthetics and their chemical classification.

The anesthetic profile of a given compound depends on many factors, including pKa, lipid solubility, protein-binding, intrinsic vasodilator activity, and nonnervous tissue diffusibility (Table 49-2). All local anesthetics are weak bases. The pKa of a compound is defined as the pH at which the ionized and nonionized forms are equal in concentration (Fig. 49-3). In solutions, local anesthetics exist as both nonionized bases and ionized cationic forms. In commercial preparations, usually the hydrochloride salt, the solution is made acidic (pH, 4–7) to promote water solubility. All local anesthetics have a pKa greater than the physiologic pH of 7.4, and in general, the amide types have a lower pKa (7.7–8.1) than the esters (8.5–9.0). After injection, the nonionic form of the agent is more lipid soluble and is responsible for diffusion across cell membranes. Hence, agents with a pKa closer to 7.4 will have a higher percentage of the drug in diffusible form in the extracellular space. For example, lidocaine has a pKa of 7.9, and tetracaine has a pKa of 8.9. At the physiologic extracellular pH of 7.4, 35 percent of lidocaine is in the diffusible nonionic form, compared to only 5 percent of tetracaine. The clinical onset of action is shortened in agents with a pKa closer to physiologic extracellular pH. In acidic tissues, such as those in areas of ischemia and infection, a lower percentage of the drug exists in the nonionic form as compared to a similar injection into nonacidic tissue. This may render the block less effective, a situation commonly noted clinically when a local anesthetic is injected into or around an abscess. Once the agent has crossed the cell membrane, the cationic form assumes an important role in impeding pain impulse propagation. The lower intracellular pH shifts the equilibration toward a higher percentage of the drug in the cationic form when compared to extracellular fluid. Carbonation of a local anesthetic (the addition of CO_2, not HCO_3) can increase the effective concentration of the cationic form intracellularly.

Lipid solubility varies greatly among local anesthetics (see Table 49-1) and can be modified by structural changes within the compound. The addition of a butyl group to the aromatic end of procaine creates tetracaine, and a similar butyl addition to the amine end of the mepivacaine creates bupivacaine. Both resulting compounds are more lipid soluble than the parent local anesthetic. In general, higher lipid solubility is associated with greater potency and longer duration of clinical blockade. Tetracaine, bupivacaine, and etidocaine are the most lipid-soluble local anesthetics. Procaine is poorly lipid soluble and requires higher concentrations at the level of the nerve sheath to produce neural blockade similar to that obtained with the other agents.

Similarly, protein-binding can also affect the duration of clinical blockade noted with local anesthetics. Procaine is poorly protein bound and possesses a relatively short duration of action. Conversely, bupivacaine, etidocaine, and tetracaine are highly protein bound and possess a longer duration of anesthesia. The effects of lipid solubility and protein-binding on the clinical characteristics of neural blockade are consistent with the structure of the axon membrane. Analysis of axons reveals that the membrane is composed of approximately 90 percent lipid and 10 percent protein; it follows that agents bound more strongly to the membrane components will exert a longer duration of action than those that are less well bound. Although highly lipid-

Table 49-3. Clinical effect of vasoconstrictors on infiltration block

Agent	Duration without epinephrine (minutes)	Duration with epinephrine (minutes)
Procaine	30–45	60–90
Lidocaine	60–100	120–220
Mepivacaine	70–120	90–150
Bupivacaine	150–240	240–360

soluble and protein-bound compounds possess a longer duration of action and higher intrinsic potency, the onset of action may be delayed when compared to less lipid-soluble and protein-bound compounds. For infiltration anesthesia, the difference is minimal, with onset of anesthesia within one to two minutes for all agents. When nerve or nerve-trunk blockade is performed, the onset of action may be clinically longer, because of the need to overcome the diffusion of the anesthetic into nonneural fatty tissue and binding by nonneural proteins.

All local anesthetics except cocaine are vasodilators. After injection of a local anesthetic, some of the drug will be taken up by the nerve and the rest will be absorbed by the vascular system. The addition of a vasoconstrictor can help decrease local blood flow and reverse the intrinsic vasodilating properties of the local anesthetic, resulting in a more prolonged clinical blockade and lowered systemic toxicity (Table 49-3). Epinephrine is the most commonly employed vasoconstrictor; previous work has shown that a 1 : 200,000 (0.05%) concentration is optimal, with higher doses adding little, aside from increased risk of catecholamine toxicity when used for infiltration or nerve block. Phenylephrine and noradrenaline have also been used to decrease blood flow after local or regional injection; phenylephrine is less effective than epinephrine, and norepinephrine offers little advantage and increased risk of catecholamine toxicity.

Finally, nonneural diffusibility can also influence local anesthetic activity. This diffusibility can vary among agents, with more diffusible compounds demonstrating a more rapid onset of action in vivo. For instance, procaine and chlorprocaine each have a pKa of 8.9 to 9.0 and have a similar onset of action in vitro, although in vivo chlorprocaine has a more rapid onset. A similar relationship exists between lidocaine and prilocaine, with the in vivo onset of action shorter for lidocaine. The reasons behind nonneural tissue diffusibility are not well understood.

In summary, local anesthetic activity is the result of a variety of physiochemical properties of the agents (see Table 49-2). These agents can also be grouped according to duration of action. Short-acting agents last for up to 45 minutes and include procaine and chlorprocaine. Intermediate agents last for up to 120 minutes and include lidocaine and mepivacaine. Bupivacaine and etidocaine are long-acting local anesthetics, with a duration of anesthesia of up to four to six hours. The addition of a vasoconstrictor can prolong the duration in vivo of all local anesthetics, although the effect is more pronounced in the shorter-acting groups (see Table 49-3). Duration of action is also influenced by the type of nerve block, with major peripheral nerve anesthesia lasting longer than local infiltration (Table 49-4).

Table 49-4. Duration of clinical neural blockade as a function of location

Agent	Clinical use	Duration (minutes)
Lidocaine	Infiltration	60–100
	Peripheral Nerve	100–120
	Epidural	100–200
Bupivacaine	Infiltration	120–240
	Peripheral Nerve	240–480
	Epidural	240–360
Mepivacaine	Infiltration	70–120
	Peripheral Nerve	120–180
	Epidural	100–180
Procaine	Infiltration	30–45
	Peripheral Nerve	40–65
	Epidural	40–60

CLINICAL ASPECTS OF NEURAL BLOCKADE

A variety of factors unrelated to the physiochemical properties of the local anesthetic can influence the onset and degree of neural blockade. These factors include fiber size and type, topographic location of fibers, and surrounding tissue structure.

Fiber Size and Type

The diameter and myelinization of a nerve fiber is related to its function and, to a lesser degree, to its sensitivity to local anesthetics (Table 49-5). Pain and temperature are controlled by both the A delta and C (nonmyelinated) fibers. Although the C fibers are smaller, they conduct more slowly because they lack a myelin sheath.

Table 49-5. Characteristics of nerve fibers

Class	Function	Myelin	Diameter (μ)	Conduction speed (m/sec)
A-alpha	Motor	+ + +	12–20	70–120
A-beta	Touch/pressure	+ +	5–12	30–70
A-gamma	Proprioception	+ +	5–12	30–70
A-delta	Pain/temperature	+ +	1–4	12–30
B	Preganglionic autonomic	+	1–3	14
C	Pain/temperature	−	0.5–1.0	1.2

Key: + + + = heavily myelinated; + = mildly myelinated; − = nonmyelinated.

In general, the smaller fibers are blocked at a lower concentration of local anesthetic, and more quickly. Clinically, this is often noted as a loss of pain and temperature sensation before motor and touch sensation during peripheral nerve blockade. There are exceptions to this simplification, for reasons that are not clearly understood.

Topographic Nerve Location

Local anesthetics are deposited near a nerve trunk and depend on diffusion to gain access to the fibers. Axons in large nerve trunks, such as the ulnar nerve at the level of the elbow and the axillary nerve, contain fibers that supply the more proximal areas in the periphery. Clinically, this results in a proximal to distal progression of anesthesia during peripheral nerve block. Increasing the dose of local anesthetic to the surrounding tissue can hasten the onset, yet does not do so in a linear fashion and adds the risk of toxicity. Intravenous regional techniques, such as Bier's block, demonstrate a distal to proximal progression, since the anesthetic diffuses from the vascular channels (located in the center of the sheath) outward.

Surrounding Tissue Structure

Since local anesthetics depend on diffusion to reach nearby nerves, increasing tissue resistance to diffusion can impede neural blockade. Edema, scar tissue, and other physical barriers can markedly reduce the efficacy of a local anesthetic.

Tachyphylaxis

The development of clinical resistance to repeated attempts at neural blockade usually is a result of nonpharmacologic tolerance. Edema and tissue trauma from the injections can impede the diffusion of the local anesthetic. A lower extracellular pH from the tissue trauma and local ischemia as well as the acidic nature of commercially prepared solutions can diminish the amount of local anesthetic in the nonionic form, limiting diffusion across cell membranes.

LOCAL ANESTHETIC TOXICITY

Toxic reactions can occur from local tissue trauma, a true allergic phenomenon, and systemic absorption. Ester-type local anesthetics are associated with the majority of true allergic reactions, with only rare case reports of similar events in the amide group. The paraaminobenzoic acid metabolite of the ester group is believed to be responsible for the reaction. Signs and symptoms can range from local and generalized pruritus, urticaria, and edema to headache, dyspnea, and wheezing. Cardiovascular collapse secondary to hypotension is the most serious manifestation of this reaction. Histamine is the mediator of the reaction, along with slow-reacting substance of anaphylaxis (SRS-A). Treatment is similar to that for other allergic crises, with airway and circulatory support as needed, along with the use of beta-agonists and antihistamines based on symptoms. Patients with a true allergy to esters can safely receive amide agents. Alternatively, a 0.25% solution (25 mg/10 ml) of diphenhydramine can be used for local infiltration.

Table 49-6. Maximum doses, pH, and usual concentration of common local anesthetics for injection[a]

Agent	pH	Maximum single dose (mg)[b]	Usual concentration
Esters			
Procaine	5.0–6.5	1000	1.0–2.0
Chlorprocaine	3–4	800	1.0–2.0
Amides			
Lidocaine	6.5	300–400	0.5–1.0
Mepivacaine	4.5	400–500	0.5–1.5
Bupivacaine	4.5–6.0	175–225	0.25–0.50

[a] The use of epinephrine may increase the maximum single recommended dose by 25% for each agent by decreasing systemic absorption. Also, the proximity of the injection to a major vascular structure will influence the possibility of toxicity from systemic absorption. Infiltrative blocks away from major vascular structures are associated with a lower risk of toxicity.
[b] Based on average 70-kg adult without underlying disease (see text).

Allergic phenomena are also possible from the preservatives used in commercially prepared local anesthetic solutions, such as methylparaben and sodium metabisulfite. The latter is employed as an antioxidant in solutions containing epinephrine. The use of an agent such as lidocaine without these additives is suggested if the history raises suspicions that this reaction might occur. This form can be easily obtained in the emergency department in the resuscitation drug box, where many lidocaine preparations do not contain these additives. The anesthetic should be diluted to the proper concentration to avoid inadvertent excessive doses.

Systemic reactions are more common than allergic reactions and result from serum levels in excess of safe ranges, usually from doses greater than the maximum recommended (Table 49-6). The occurrence of these reactions depends on the specific local anesthetic, the route of administration, the presence of vasoconstrictors, and the underlying medical condition of the patient. Acidosis, hypercarbia, underlying systemic illnesses, and extremes of age are associated with a greater risk of systemic toxicity. Additionally, patients who are being treated with antiarrhythmic lidocaine congeners, such as tocainide and mexiletine, can develop systemic toxicity after a lower total dose of lidocaine as a result of an additive effect from these structurally similar agents. Decreases in elimination ability can also increase the risk in some patients. Those with atypical or diminished plasma cholinesterase levels are at risk for ester systemic toxicity. Impairment of liver function, particularly in acute hepatitis, increases the risk of amide toxicity. Renal failure has minimal effects on the elimination of active local anesthetics.

Route of administration can influence the risk of systemic reactions, with rapid high peaks representing the greatest risk. Intravascular injections, intended or inadvertent, raise levels quickly to a peak, resulting in a high risk of toxicity. Of the techniques used in the emergency department, intercostal nerve blocks result in the highest serum levels of local anesthetics. Conversely, local infiltration and minor peripheral nerve blocks do not usually result in high serum levels and are less commonly associated with systemic toxicity. One exception is in the area of the head and neck, where local vascular injection during attempted nerve block can quickly deliver high concentrations of the agent to the central

Table 49-7. Common topical anesthetics

Agent	Concentration (%)	Duration (minutes)	Primary use	Maximal dose (mg)[a]
Cocaine	2–10[b]	30–60	ENT	150
Tetracaine	0.5	20–40	Cornea	20
Proparacaine	0.5	20–40	Cornea	?
Lidocaine	2–10	10–45	Mucous membranes ? Abraded dermis	300
Benzocaine	14–20	10–20	Mucous membranes	400[c]
TAC	Tetracaine 0.5 Adrenaline 0.05 Cocaine 5.0–11.8	30–45	Skin[d]	200 (cocaine)

[a] Based on healthy 70-kg adult.
[b] Concentrations over 4% not recommended for ENT use because of risk of toxicity.
[c] Two seconds of 14% spray.
[d] Contraindicated for use on end-artery or marginally perfused tissues (fingers, toes, tip of nose, auricular cartilage, penis, skin grafts) and on mucous membranes.

nervous system (CNS). Addition of a vasoconstrictor will increase the duration of anesthesia and lower peak plasma levels and lessen the risk of systemic toxicity.

The two major manifestations of systemic toxicity are seen in the CNS and cardiovascular system. Although most local anesthetics exhibit antiseizure properties in low doses, high serum levels are associated with CNS excitation and tonic-clonic seizures. Aside from the risks already mentioned, toxicity is greater in patients with underlying seizure disorders and with rapid rises in blood levels. Less severe symptoms include numbness, tinnitus and hearing loss, somnolence, muscle-twitching, and difficulty with speech. After the initial CNS excitant effects of local anesthetic toxicity, further increases in blood levels can cause severe depression of cortical function. The CNS toxicity is directly related to the potency of the agents (see Table 49-2). Treatment is routine, consisting of airway stabilization and anticonvulsants as needed. Prophylaxis with oral diazepam (0.25 mg/kg, at least 30 minutes before injection) can raise the seizure threshold in patients at risk. Chlorprocaine has been reported to cause paraplegia in several patients after dural instillation but is considered safe for peripheral nerve blocks.

The cardiovascular toxicity of local anesthetics as used in the emergency department occurs as a result of direct depressant actions on cardiac and smooth muscle, as well as arrhythmogenic properties in high doses. Lidocaine possesses the greatest antidysrhythmic action of all the local anesthetics at low doses, with other agents less well studied. Atrioventricular conduction defects, prolongation of the QRS duration, and atrial or ventricular dysrhythmias are the major electrocardiographic manifestations. Toxicity is increased with all the aforementioned factors but appears to be greater with bupivacaine. This has been seen primarily in patients who received concentrated (0.75%) solutions for epidural anesthesia. Bupivacaine in the concentrations recommended for peripheral nerve and infiltration anesthesia (0.25–0.50%) has an excellent record of safety when maximal doses are not exceeded. Treatment of cardiac toxicity is supportive. Some authors suggest the use of bretylium for treatment of ventricular dysrhythmias, although scientific validation of its efficacy is lacking.

Toxicity can result from other causes, including catecholamine excess and methemoglobinemia. Catecholamine excess, from absorbed epinephrine or cocaine, can result in tachycardia, CNS excitation, seizures, and cardiac ischemia or arrest. Methemoglobin formation is best documented after prilocaine use, as a result of the metabolite toluidine blue O. Additionally, numerous cases have been reported after typical benzocaine use. In therapeutic doses, methemoglobinemia is not noted with the commonly used local anesthetics. Treatment of methemoglobinemia consists of discontinuation of the offending agent, oxygen administration, and intravenous methylene blue (as discussed in Chap. 156).

METHODS AND AGENTS OF ANESTHESIA

The emergency physician is often confronted with the challenge of deciding which local anesthetic, by which technique, is most useful for a given procedure. Based on the previously discussed principles, rational choices can be made. In the following paragraphs the agents suggested for topical, infiltration and nerve block, and intravenous regional anesthesia are discussed.

Topical Anesthesia

The mucous membranes, cornea, and skin are the most common topically anesthetized areas. Although abraded or denuded skin absorbs topical anesthetics more readily than intact skin, new formulations and vehicles have improved the ability of normal skin to be anesthetized. Table 49-7 lists the agents most commonly used in the emergency department for topical anesthesia (see Procedure 37).

For corneal anesthesia, tetracaine and proparacaine are the most popular agents and are associated with minimal risks. These agents can improve the physician's ability to examine the painful eye, add diagnostic information, and relieve discomfort. The onset of action for all ocular agents is within one minute. These agents should not be used for outpatient analgesia because of the risks of retarded healing, masking of important symptoms, and loss of protective reflexes. Proparacaine is believed to be less irritating than the other corneal anesthetics.

For ear, nose, and throat topical anesthesia, 2 to 10% cocaine has a proven record as an excellent anesthetic and vasoconstrictor. However, the risk of toxicity and the logistic difficulties with its availability have limited the usefulness of this agent. Lidocaine is available in concentrations from 2 to 10%, and in a variety of forms (jelly, liquid spray, and viscous solutions), and is the anesthetic of choice in these anatomic areas. Benzocaine also provides good topical anesthesia of the oropharynx and is available in commercially prepared sprays at a concentration of 20%. Caution in avoiding maximal doses must be taken when anesthetizing mucous membranes, since rapid systemic absorption can occur.

Topical anesthesia of the skin can be achieved through the use of 2 to 4% lidocaine jelly, particularly if the stratum corneum has been disrupted. This technique is less effective in intact epithelium, but recent advances have helped improve topical anesthesia in normal skin. A solution of tetracaine, 0.5%; adrenaline, 0.05%; and cocaine, 10.0 to 11.8% (TAC) is useful for topical anesthesia, particularly in children. A gauze pad with the appropriate amount of solution should be held with gentle pressure over the area to be anesthetized. The onset of action is generally within 15 to 20 minutes and lasts for up to one hour. Care must be taken to avoid toxicity, usually due to cocaine, which has been fatal in some cases. Most authors recommend limiting the total amount applied to 2 to 3 ml in adults (200–300 mg cocaine) and less for small children. There have been concerns about suboptimal wound healing after the use of TAC as a result of the vasoconstrictive effects, but this has not been clinically validated. The use of solutions containing similar concentrations of tetracaine and adrenaline without cocaine can provide topical dermal anesthesia, but less reliably. TAC should be avoided on mucous membranes because of the risk of rapid absorption and toxicity. Also, precautions similar to those suggested for epinephrine-containing solutions should be observed when TAC solutions are applied.

Two new formulations of common agents have shown promise for skin topical anesthesia. Liposome-encapsulated tetracaine creams have been evaluated in one small study and offer the promise of safe, rapid (within 30 minutes) anesthesia for up to four hours. Similarly, eutectic 5% prilocaine-lidocaine creams have been efficacious in clinical trials, yet require up to one hour of application before adequate anesthesia is obtained. These agents deserve further research before routine use is recommended. If proved effective, they may render vascular puncture and cannulation a painless experience for most patients.

Infiltration and Nerve-Block Anesthesia

Infiltration and peripheral nerve-block anesthesia are the most common techniques of analgesia before wound repair or incision in the emergency department (see Procedure 38). Additionally, the use of nerve blocks can provide pain relief for nonsurgical conditions, particularly in the dental area, when performed with proper technique and agents. The mechanics of different types of injection anesthesia techniques are discussed in Procedures 38 and 39.

The choice of local anesthetic depends on the area to be injected, the procedure to be performed, and the desired length of anesthesia. In general, more concentrated solutions offer a more reliable block when used for injection, but not in a linear fashion. Additionally, the use of more concentrated solutions adds increased risk of systemic toxicity. Table 49-6 lists the usual concentrations of agents suggested for injection. If a large volume of injectate is needed for infiltration, the lowest effective concentration should be used. If an isolated peripheral nerve is to be blocked, more concentrated solutions are appropriate. Also, the addition of a vasoconstrictor can decrease localized bleeding (especially in the scalp), peak plasma levels, and systemic toxicity, as well as prolonging the duration of blockade. The total dose of epinephrine should not exceed 200 μg (a 1 : 200,000 solution contains 5 μg/ml). Vasoconstrictors are to be avoided in areas with limited arterial supply, such as the penis, external nose, pinna, digits, and skin grafts. Also, gravid patients at term, those with poorly controlled hypertension or diabetes, and patients at risk for ischemic heart disease should probably not receive epinephrine. Commercial solutions with epinephrine are usually 1.0 to 1.5 pH units lower than similar nonepinephrine-containing solutions.

The emergency physician should become familiar with one agent from each class of local anesthetic, based on chemical structure and duration of action. Procaine and chlorprocaine are the most commonly employed short-acting agents and the most popular esters. Lidocaine is an effective and safe intermediate-duration agent and is the most commonly injected local anesthetic. Bupivacaine is gaining popularity in the emergency department as a long-acting local anesthetic and can provide pain relief for hours after discharge. When used for infiltration, the onset of action of each of these agents is within 2 minutes. However, peripheral nerve block with bupivacaine may require a longer time for onset, usually within 10 to 20 minutes. The key for all injection techniques is to place the solution near the nerve and to wait at least 20 minutes before deciding the injection has failed.

Continuous pain on injection and pain that radiates to distal distribution sites of a peripheral nerve are the hallmarks of an intraneural injection. This is to be avoided, not only because of the discomfort but also to lessen the risk of neural damage. Although the elicitation of a paresthesia during nerve block is helpful, the injection should occur near (not within) the nerve.

Local anesthetic solutions are acidic, ranging in pH from 4.5 to 6.0. The addition of sodium bicarbonate to lidocaine has been shown to decrease the pain associated with infiltration. One milliliter from a standard bicarbonate ampule (50 mEq/50 ml) per 10 ml lidocaine is the proper method for alkalinization in the emergency department. This may hasten the onset of anesthesia by raising the pH of the injected solution and increasing the nonionized portion of the drug in the extracellular space. These solutions should not be prepared in advance since the increased pH can diminish the solubility of the drug. Other local anesthetics have not been studied as well as lidocaine and should therefore not be routinely alkalinized. Use of carbonated solutions, not to be confused with alkalinized solutions, can hasten the onset of anesthesia without affecting the perceived pain on injection.

Aside from differences in duration and elimination, each of these agents is well suited for emergency department use.

One author has suggested that bupivacaine may decrease the need for additional oral analgesics after discharge. Although a promising concept, further evidence to support this contention is lacking.

The choice of infiltration versus nerve-block anesthesia depends on the site and size of the wound (or painful tissue) and the presence of infection. Nerve blocks are advantageous when a large area is involved in order to lessen the total volume to be injected and decrease the risk of toxicity. Also, areas of infection are poorly anesthetized by infiltration techniques and are better suited to peripheral nerve block if possible. Certain anatomic areas, such as digits and distal extremities, are particularly easy to anesthetize by peripheral nerve block. Infiltration techniques are useful when multiple peripheral nerves supply the area to be anesthetized and if the area is relatively small. Distention of the edges of a wound can make a more difficult closure after infiltration and can be eliminated by time or the use of a peripheral nerve block.

Intravenous Regional Anesthesia

The use of intravenous lidocaine for regional anesthesia of a limb is common in the operating room and occasionally useful in the emergency department for orthopedic manipulations (see Procedure 40). "Bier's block" refers to the use of this technique in the upper extremity. Although it is not used routinely by emergency physicians, its safety and efficacy in the emergency department has been documented. This technique requires meticulous attention to total dose of local anesthetic, method of vascular depletion of the arm before injection, and maintenance of tourniquet pressure to avoid rapid release of local anesthetic into the systemic vasculature. Lidocaine, in doses of 0.25 to 0.75 mg/kg, is the agent of choice in the emergency department. Prilocaine has a proven record of safety and efficacy in the United Kingdom and is another option in the emergency department.

SUMMARY

Local anesthetics can rapidly diminish the pain of most procedures in the emergency department and add to the emergency physician's arsenal for analgesia in acutely painful conditions. A thorough knowledge of the pharmacologic and clinical characteristics of these agents can allow for safe administration and patient satisfaction.

SELECTED READING

Bernards, CM, et al. Effect of midazolam and diazepam premedication on central nervous system and cardiovascular toxicity of bupivacaine in pigs. *Anesthesiology* 70:318, 1989.

Braid, DP, and Scott, DB. The systemic absorption of local analgesic drugs. *Br J Anaesth* 37:394, 1965.

Brown, DT, Beamish, D, and Wildsmith, JAW. Allergic reactions to an amide local anesthetic. *Br J Anaesth* 53:435, 1981.

Buffington, CW. The magnitude and duration of direct myocardial depression following intracoronary local anesthetics: A comparison of lidocaine and bupivacaine. *Anesthesiology* 70:280, 1989.

Catchlove, RFH. The influence of pCO_2 and pH on local anesthetic action. *J Pharmacol Ther* 181:291, 1972.

Cooper, CM, et al. EMLA cream reduces the pain of venipuncture in children. *Eur J Anaesthesiol* 4:441, 1987.

Covino, BG. Clinical Pharmacology of Local Anesthetics. In MJ Cousins and PO Bridenbaugh (eds), *Neural Blockade in Clinical Anesthesia and Management of Pain* (2nd ed). Philadelphia: Lippincott, 1988. Pp 111–142.

Covino, BG, and Vassallo, HG. *Local Anesthetics. Mechanism of Action and Clinical Use.* New York: Grune & Stratton, 1976.

Daya, MR, et al. Recurrent seizures following mucosal application of TAC. *Ann Emerg Med* 17:646, 1988.

de Jong, RH. Toxic effects of local anesthetics. *JAMA* 239:1166, 1978.

de Jong, RH, and Heavner, JE. Diazepam prevents local anesthetic seizures. *Anesthesiology* 34:523, 1971.

de Jong, RH, Wagman, IH, and Prince, DA. Effect of carbon dioxide on the cortical seizure threshold to lidocaine. *Exp Neurol* 17:221, 1967.

Geszetes, A, and Mezei, M. Topical anesthesia of the skin by liposome-encapsulated tetracaine. *Anesth Analg* 67:1079, 1988.

Hilgier, M. Alkalinization of bupivacaine for brachial plexus block. *Reg Anaesth* 10:59, 1985.

Hopkins, CS, Buckley, CJ, and Bush, GH. Pain-free injection in infants. *Anaesthesia* 43:198, 1988.

Koller, C. On the use of cocaine for producing anesthesia of the eye. *Lancet* 2:990, 1884.

Kotelko, MD, et al. Bupivacaine induced cardiac arrhythmias in sheep. *Anesthesiology* 60:10, 1984.

Lieberman, NA, et al. The effects of lidocaine on the electrical and mechanical activity of the heart. *Am J Cardiol* 22:375, 1968.

McKay, W, Morris, R, and Mushlin, R. Sodium bicarbonate attenuates pain on infiltration with lidocaine, with or without epinephrine. *Anesth Analg* 66:572, 1987.

Moore, DC, et al. Arterial and venous plasma levels of bupivacaine following peripheral nerve blocks. *Anesth Analg* 55:763, 1976.

Moore, DC, et al. Chlorprocaine neurotoxicity: Four additional cases. *Anesth Analg* 61:155, 1982.

Pearson, AC, Labovitz, AJ, and Kern, MJ. Accelerated hypertension complicated by myocardial infarction after use of a local anesthetic/vasoconstrictor preparation. *Am Heart J* 114:662, 1987.

Reynolds, F. Allergy reaction to an amide local anesthetic. *Br J Anaesth* 53:901, 1981.

Schaffer, DJ. Clinical comparison of TAC anesthetic solutions with and without cocaine. *Ann Emerg Med* 14:1077, 1985.

Shuster, MR, et al. Effect on the seizure threshold in dogs of tocainide/lidocaine administration. *Ann Emerg Med* 16:749, 1987.

Smith, AR, Hur, D, and Resano, F. Grand mal seizures after 2-chlorprocaine epidural anesthesia in a patient with plasma cholinesterase deficiency. *Anesth Analg* 66:677, 1987.

Soilman, IE, et al. Comparison of the analgesic effects of EMLA (eutectic mixture of local anesthetics) to intradermal lidocaine infiltration prior to venous cannulation in unpremedicated children. *Anesthesiology* 68:804, 1988.

Spivey, WH, et al. A clinical comparison of lidocaine and bupivacaine. *Ann Emerg Med* 16:752, 1987.

Stevenson, TR, et al. Damage to tissue defenses by vasoconstrictors. *JACEP* 4:532, 1975.

Strichartz, G. Molecular mechanisms of nerve block by local anesthetics. *Anesthesiology* 45:421, 1976.

Tucker, GT, and Mather, LE. Properties, Absorption, and Disposition of local Anesthetic Agents. In MJ Cousins and PO Bridenbaugh (eds), *Neural Blockade in Clinical Anesthesia and Management of Pain* (2nd ed). Philadelphia: Lippincott, 1988. Pp 47–110.

Tucker, GT, et al. Systemic absorption of mepivacaine in commonly used regional block procedures. *Anesthesiology* 37:277, 1972.

White, WB, Iserson KV, and Criss, E. Topical anesthesia for laceration repair: Tetracaine versus TAC (tetracaine, adrenaline, and cocaine). *Am J Emerg Med* 4:319, 1986.

50. Pain Management in the Pediatric Emergency Department

Michael L. McManus
Charles B. Berde

The emergency department can be both a painful and terrifying place for children. In many circumstances the condition that brought the child to medical attention produces pain (e.g., fractures, otitis media). In other circumstances medical, diagnostic, and therapeutic procedures (e.g., venipuncture, suture of lacerations) produce pain, as well as anxiety. Although not all aspects of the emergency department experience can be made pleasant, in many cases provision of analgesia and a calm, supportive approach to the patient can make the encounter more tolerable for patients, parents, and medical staff. In this chapter we review the following topics as they pertain to children: (1) developmental aspects of pain experience; (2) problems associated with pain assessment; (3) pharmacology of analgesics, sedatives, and local anesthetics; (4) behavioral pain management techniques; and (5) specific application in the emergency department setting.

PAIN EXPERIENCE IN CHILDREN

Recent investigations support some generalizations regarding pain perception in infants and children. First, the neural pathways for pain perception are sufficiently developed in early infancy to permit nociception even in preterm infants. Second, there is no evidence to support the view that infants fail to perceive pain; in fact, pain threshold is lower in young infants than in older subjects. Third, although the emotional meaning of pain develops through childhood, there is reason to imagine that pain is experienced as subjective distress at a very early age. Memory of untreated pain can be associated with adverse psychological effects, although there is ongoing dispute about the significance of these effects in early infancy. Finally, children's concepts of pain and its relation to illness vary with age and developmental level.

PEDIATRIC PAIN ASSESSMENT

Assessment and interpretation of pain complaints are essential for management of patients of all ages, both in the establishment of diagnoses and in evaluating effects of treatment. Pain assessment is performed using three types of information: self-report (ask the patient), behavior (observe the patient), and physiologic measures (vital signs, sweating).

Most three-year-olds and some two-year-olds will report the source of their pain with some fluency to their parents although they may be unwilling to do so for medical personnel. Standard visual analogue scales are reliable in children aged seven and above. Other self-report scales are based on either a graded series of pictures (showing children experiencing pain of different intensities, happy-sad faces), a series of icons (e.g., poker chips), or color intensity. These scales appear to assess pain intensity well in the four- to seven-year-old age group. In most circumstances children of these ages, if asked properly, can discriminate pain from fear. Nevertheless, in a clinical setting difficulties in use of verbal pain assessment in infants and toddlers have major ramifications both in terms of using pain as a sign of disease (e.g., diagnosis of appendicitis is commonly delayed in the first year of life), as well as in evaluating responses to analgesic management. In the majority of cases, children aged three to four and above will correctly localize pain to the site of pathology. Particularly in younger children, pain may be referred to contiguous structures. Thus, a three-year-old with a septic hip may complain of knee pain.

Behavioral assessment is useful in all ages and is a major source of information for the pediatrician evaluating infants and toddlers. For example, unwillingness to move an arm or walking with a limp is a clue to pathology. Behavioral scales, such as the Children's Hospital of Eastern Ontario Pain Scale (CHEOPS) or the Objective Pain Scale (OPS), have been used most often to assess pain after operation or painful diagnostic procedures. Behavioral scales may underestimate pain of moderate intensity relative to self-report measures, and they may not discriminate pain from fear or anxiety. As an example, a toddler who is being held down for an ear examination may scream and cry (and thereby score highly on both the CHEOPS and the OPS) despite the fact that the reactions are due to fear or anticipation of pain, rather than pain per se. With many forms of chronic pain, the patient withdraws and pain-related behaviors are inhibited.

Physiologic measures include autonomic signs, such as sweating, tearing, tachycardia, and hypertension, as well as biochemical measures, such as plasma or cerebrospinal fluid levels of endorphins and other neurohumors. The biochemical measures are useful only in a research setting, and, as with the autonomic signs, they can be modified by a number of other factors in addition to pain, including sepsis, asphyxia, and so forth. Autonomic signs are particularly useful in patients receiving general anesthesia and neuromuscular blockade. Autonomic signs may show habituating with chronic pain. In clinical practice corroboration among self-report, behavior, and physiologic signs is needed.

PEDIATRIC PHARMACOLOGY

Clinical investigations regarding the pharmacology of opioid (narcotic) analgesics, sedatives, and general and local anesthetic agents has accelerated in recent years. Thus, the previous argument that there is insufficient information to administer these agents to young children is no longer tenable.

Various physiologic differences between adults and infants affect drug distribution, clearance, and effect. Clinical implications are often significant. First, a proportionally higher total body water volume in infants results in a proportionally higher volume of distribution for some drugs. Thus, water-soluble agents often require *larger* initial doses and longer dosing intervals. Opposing this, in the first week of life, immaturity of the blood-brain barrier permits greater and more rapid penetration of some drugs (such as morphine), necessitating *smaller* doses. Additionally, in the first month there seems to be greater *sensitivity* to opioids (perhaps due to immaturity of respiratory centers) and exaggerated respiratory depression can occur. This is particularly true of premature infants, lasting up to 60 weeks postconception. Finally, in the first three weeks of life, immaturity of hepatic enzyme systems can delay metabolism and lead to accumulation of opioids and other drugs.

In general, there is sufficient physiologic maturation, in most respects by age six months, that responses to analgesics, sedatives, and anesthetics are reasonably well predicted based on experience with adults and extrapolations based on the patient's weight. In most respects this approach will result in appropriate dosing or slight underdosage, not overdosage, for toddlers and younger children.

In infants under age six months, the pharmacodynamics of most medications are poorly understood, and some preliminary studies demonstrate exaggerated responses to even small doses. Thus, it is our practice to employ continuous cardiorespiratory monitoring while slowly titrating potent analgesics in this age group and to avoid their use whenever possible.

LOCAL ANESTHETICS

Local anesthetics are becoming increasingly recognized as important agents in pediatric pain management. Obvious advantages include effectiveness and avoidance of central nervous system (CNS) or systemic effects. Disadvantages include potential toxicity and, in the case of regional blocks, the requirement of experience and technical skills.

Ester anesthetics (tetracaine, procaine, and chloroprocaine) are rapidly metabolized by plasma cholinesterase in patients over six months of age. Newborns and young infants metabolize the drug more slowly because of reductions in enzyme activity. Amide local anesthetics (lidocaine and bupivacaine) undergo primarily hepatic metabolism.

Potential toxicity is determined by total dose, rate of absorption, extent of protein-binding, and developmental sensitivity. Recommended maximal doses for commonly used local anesthetics are listed in Table 50-1. Rate of absorption varies with admininstration site according to vascularity. Tracheally administered anesthetics (such as lidocaine for topical anesthesia during awake intubation) are most rapidly absorbed, while those administered topically to nonmucous membranes or subcutaneously are least rapidly absorbed. Absorption can also be diminished by the addition of a vasoconstrictor such as epinephrine.

Toxicity is the direct result of circulating free drug concentrations and, as such, is influenced by protein binding. Thus, infants less than two or three months of age with lower

Table 50-1. Maximum allowable local anesthetic doses (mg/kg)

Drug	Without epinephrine	With epinephrine
Lidocaine	5	7
Bupivacaine	2	2.5

albumin and alpha-1 lipoprotein levels are at added risk of toxicity from typical doses of highly protein-bound agents such as bupivacaine.

Finally, developmental differences such as seizure threshold, integrity of the blood-brain barrier, and incomplete nerve myelination can theoretically influence dose effect and toxicity. Signs and symptoms of local anesthetic toxicity include tinitus, metallic tastes, dizziness, disorientation, delirium, nystagmus, tachycardia, tachypnea, seizures, and cardiovascular collapse. Aspiration before injection and test dosing are common methods of avoiding significant intravascular injection. It is important to recognize, however, that many of the early signs of toxicity can be easily missed in the preverbal child.

LOCAL ANESTHETIC TECHNIQUES

With an understanding of the pharmacology and toxicities of local anesthetics, the clinician can begin to approach the pain management of selected minor procedures and localized injuries in pediatric patients. Local anesthesia is considered by the emergency physician most commonly when he or she is called to repair a minor laceration. However, the veteran practitioner is aware that local anesthetics are extremely helpful for such common procedures as intravenous (IV) placement and lumbar puncture. In caring for any child, the step of initial importance is reassurance and establishment of a rapport that ensures confidence and cooperation. Perhaps the most difficult and certainly the most time-consuming task, establishment of trust, will generally make the difference between success and failure. Involvement of parents, a pleasant tone of voice, avoidance of terms with frightening connotations (such as "bee sting" or "shot"), as well as keeping equipment out of sight until needed, will aid in this. A younger child or one with whom communications is difficult will likely require some form of restraint or sedation, or both, in addition to local anesthesia.

Classically, local infiltration (accomplished with the smallest needle practical) is performed with concentrations of lidocaine ranging from 0.25% (2.5 mg/ml) to 1% (10 mg/ml). In smaller children with large lacerations, close attention must be paid to the total per-kilogram dose lest toxic quantities be administered. For example, in the 25-kg eight-year-old a safe total lidocaine dose would not exceed 175 mg (7 mg/kg). This dosage would permit only 8 ml of a 2% solution, a volume sometimes reached earlier than one might expect. In an even younger child—the 10-kg one-year-old, for example—an even smaller volume (less than 4 ml) is permitted. Adequate anesthesia is produced equally well by a more dilute solution (usually 0.5%), allowing a greater total volume.

Similarly, when a local anesthetic is administered, attention must be paid to the presence or absence of added epinephrine (often identified by a red package label). Epinephrine is often desirable for its vasoconstrictive properties, producing both a clearer field and prolonged duration of anesthesia (through diminished absorption). Decreased absorption can also limit toxicity. A prudent dose of subcutaneous epinephrine would approximate that routinely employed and well tolerated in the initial treatment of asthma: 10 μg/kg. Epinephrine is commonly added in concentrations of 1 : 200,000 (5 μg/ml) or 1 : 400,000 (2.5 μg/kg). Because epinephrine-induced vasoconstriction is often profound, it is contraindicated in areas without collateral blood supply such as the pinna, penis, and digits.

In any case where total doses of local anesthetics or epinephrine are high, close attention must be paid to the patient's mental and cardiovascular status. In the uncooperative or marginally cooperative child, this may be difficult. Thus, continuous electrocardiographic monitoring and placement of an IV line remote from the site of operation is often advisable.

In addition to simple infiltration with local anesthetics, several more imaginative techniques have been introduced. An oil-in-water emulsion cream of the eutectic mixture of prilocaine and lidocaine (or EMLA, for eutectic mixture of local anesthetics) has been developed and studied for topical use. It has been found to somewhat diminish pain associated with venipuncture in adults and children, yet carries the disadvantages of slow onset time (usually greater than 40 minutes) and somewhat poor penetration (often requiring an occlusive dressing). In a human model of laser-induced pain, the analgesic effect of EMLA was found comparable to that of lidocaine infiltration and was thought to be acceptable for minor skin operations. Similarly, other investigators have achieved adequate anesthesia with EMLA in 96 percent of men and 40 percent of women undergoing thermocautery of genital warts. The possible role of a reliable topical anesthetic in the emergency care of children is obvious.

A composition of tetracaine (0.5%), adrenaline (1 : 200,000), and cocaine (11.8%) (TAC) has been described as a topical anesthetic for the outpatient repair of minor lacerations in children. Applied generously with cotton pledgets, TAC is rapid and effective but has proved hazardous in mucosal application and is subject to the same dosage limitations and toxicities described earlier. Additionally, the possibility of increased infection rates in wounds treated with potent vasoconstrictors has been raised but not clinically verified. The necessity of care in application, attention to dosage, and avoidance of mucous membranes has been sadly emphasized by the death of a $7\frac{1}{2}$-month-old infant from cocaine toxicity after use of TAC in closure of a lip laceration. Obviously, the ideal local anesthetic agent or combination of agents for pediatric application remains to be discovered.

REGIONAL ANESTHETIC TECHNIQUES

A variety of peripheral nerve blocking techniques are useful for emergency physicians and for orthopedic, plastic, and general surgeons. For example, digital blockade and wrist blockade can be useful for a variety of minor hand procedures. The maximum dosing guidelines are given in Table 50-1. Techniques for peripheral blockade are similar to those described for adults. (See Cousins and Bridenbaugh [editors], *Neural Blockade.*)

The use of regional anesthetic techniques is currently gaining considerable popularity in both the intraoperative care of pediatric patients and in postoperative pain management. Additionally, experience is being rapidly gained in some centers in the application of these techniques to the care of children experiencing chronic pain of various causes.

It is likely that in the future many nerve-block techniques will join IV regional anesthesia (Bier's block) as useful in the emergency department for procedures such as fracture reduction and laceration repair. Although peripheral nerve blocks in children may commonly be applied by pediatricians, emergency physicians, and surgical specialists, in most cases, major regional blocks (e.g., brachial plexus blocks) in children should be performed by pediatric anesthesiologists skilled in regional techniques.

SYSTEMIC AGENTS FOR PAIN CONTROL

While much can be accomplished in many patients with local and regional anesthetic techniques, the majority of pain experienced in the emergency department requires systemic medication for adequate control. In the younger child local and regional techniques are often grossly inadequate and impossible for even relatively simple procedures. A crying and struggling child is not only difficult to care for but can on occasion be a danger to himself. Furthermore, agitation can only serve to heighten the already ill or injured patient. Thus, systemic medications are frequently used in the management of pain in the pediatric emergency department patient. As noted previously, the potency and associated properties of the systemic agent employed should be matched to the intensity of the painful stimulus and titrated to effect. In the younger patient, particularly those below one year, multiple physiologic differences must be borne in mind, some of which can significantly affect the uptake, distribution, metabolism, elimination, and, thus, pharmacodynamic effect of the agent.

Nonnarcotic Analgesics

Nonnarcotic analgesics are commonly used in outpatient pediatric patients and are the mainstays of many prescription and nonprescription preparations. The nonnarcotics carry the advantages of wide margins of safety, easy availability, familiarity, and absence of associated tolerance or dependence syndromes. Codeine, though a narcotic, is relatively mild in its effects and carries less of the stigma commonly attached to other opioid analgesics. In many areas, codeine, particularly in combination with acetaminophen, can be prescribed without special Drug Enforcement Administration schedule II prescription forms.

Acetaminophen is useful in the emergency department for management of mild to moderate pain in patients of all ages. As an antipyretic, it is particularly helpful when fever contributes to overall discomfort. It can be administered in oral (PO) or rectal (PR) doses of 10 to 15 mg/kg and 15 to 20 mg/kg, respectively. The rectal route is useful in the uncooperative patient or those unable to take oral medication, although even at the larger 20-mg/kg dose, plasma levels are frequently subtherapeutic.

Acetylsalicylic acid (aspirin) is similar to acetaminophen in analgesic potency and antipyretic actions. It has more specific antiinflammatory action and is frequently employed (in higher doses) in patients with arthritis and related disorders. Disadvantages of aspirin include gastric irritation and irreversible inhibition of platelet function. Also, an epidemiologic association has been made between aspirin use during viral illness and the development of Reye's syndrome (a form of hepatic injury associated with metabolic encephalopathy, coma, and brain swelling). Consequently, use of aspirin in the pediatric population has declined substantially. In our view acetaminophen, not aspirin, should be regarded as the routine pediatric analgesic for mild pain.

Nonsteroidal antiinflammatory agents inhibit prostaglandin synthetase; unlike that in aspirin, this inhibition is reversible. Naproxen (Naprosyn, 5–7 mg/kg per dose PO two or three times a day) and tolmetin (Tolectin, 6–8 mg/kg per dose PO three to four times a day) are approved for pediatric use. Oral elixirs are available. Ibuprofen (4–8 mg/kg per dose PO four times a day) is commonly used in over-the-counter tablets for adolescents and has recently been made available as a pediatric elixir. Like aspirin, these agents are especially useful for pain with an inflammatory component or for musculoskeletal pain. In adolescent girls they are useful for pain associated with menstrual cramping. The risk of gastric irritation is considerable with chronic use. Administration with food is recommended. In long-term use hepatic, renal, and hematopoietic function, as well as signs of occult enteral blood loss, should be monitored regularly. Aspirin should be discontinued at least seven days before invasive procedures are performed; nonsteroidal agents should be discontinued one to two days before procedures, depending on the elimination half-life of the particular agent.

Opioid Analgesics

Opioid analgesics are indicated for the relief of moderate to severe pain in many contexts. All share similar side effects: nausea, histamine release (pruritus, vasodilation), constipation, urinary and biliary retention, sedation, and euphoria. With excessive doses, unconsciousness, respiratory depression, and apnea occur. The primary virtues of narcotics include potency, reliability, predictable dose-response in titration, ease of administration through a variety of routes, and, most important, the existence of specific antagonists for reversal if overdose occurs. Most narcotics are available for IV, intramuscular (IM), subcutaneous (SQ), or PO administration although duration of action, potencies, and bioavailability differ widely. The general use of opioid analgesics in pediatrics has been reviewed by Yaster and Deshpande.

Codeine is commonly used, either alone or in combination with acetaminophen, in the treatment of mild to moderate pain. It has approximately one-tenth to one-twelfth the analgesic potency of morphine; in equianalgesic doses codeine has good equivalent side effects (i.e., respiratory depression) to morphine. Codeine has good bioavailability (roughly 60%) after oral dosing. Typical pediatric dosing is 0.5 to 1.0 mg/kg per dose every four hours.

Morphine has long been the standard to which all narcotics (and indeed all analgesics) are compared. As an analgesic it can be administered IM, PO, SQ, or IV, although the latter route is best for titration and rapid (5- to 10-minute) onset. Peak effects, including respiratory depression, occur in 20 to 30 minutes. In pediatric patients, the standard initial IV-IM analgesic dose of 0.1 mg/kg can be titrated to end points of comfort, sedation, miosis, and respiratory rate. Requirements will vary directly with the intensity of the painful stimulus, and symptoms of overdose can therefore arise if the stimulus is suddenly removed (as by performance of a block). As was noted previously, neonates are particularly sensitive to the respiratory depressant effects of morphine, and alteration of the carbon dioxide response has been demonstrated with doses of 0.05 mg/kg. Additionally, seizures have been reported as complicating morphine administration in neonates. Thus, it is prudent to avoid morphine use in these patients unless it is accompanied by close cardiorespiratory monitoring in a setting where resuscitation equipment and personnel are immediately available.

Meperidine (Demerol) is a synthetic narcotic with roughly one-tenth the potency of morphine. In equipotent doses effects are essentially identical to those of morphine, with the possible exception of those related to respiratory responses in the newborn. Like codeine, oral bioavailability is high, and it is frequently administered in elixir form. Intramuscular dosing is common in combination sedatives or for postoperative pain control with an adjunct such as hydroxyzine. Meperidine differs from morphine in its production of tachycardia and in its association with numerous CNS excitatory side effects mediated through its primary hepatic metabolite, normeperidine. Because of these latter effects, the drug is contraindicated in patients who are receiving monamine oxidase inhibitors. Typical pediatric dosage is 1 mg/kg per dose IV or IM and 2 to 4 mg/kg per dose orally.

Methadone (Dolophine) is equipotent with morphine and clinically differs only in its more prolonged duration of action (6–12 hours). It is useful as a long-acting, potent analgesic in postoperative patients or those with chronic pain syndromes. It has also gained recognition in the management of narcotic dependence. As a long-acting agent, it is ill suited to emergency department use, and prolonged naloxone infusion would be required should overdosage occur.

Hydromorphone hydrochloride (Dilaudid) is a hydrogenated ketone of morphine with approximately seven times the potency of the parent drug. Actions are similar to those of morphine, with onset of analgesia occurring roughly 15 minutes after IV and 30 minutes after PO doses are given. Duration of action is four to six hours and oral bioavailability is approximately 30 percent. Parenteral doses of 0.015 mg/kg are equipotent with 0.1 mg/kg morphine, and oral doses are roughly three times parenteral doses. Orally, the drug is available in 1-, 2-, 3-, and 4-mg tablets; 3-mg suppositories are also available. In our hospital Dilaudid is occasionally employed in the care of patients with severe sickle cell disease and frequent painful crises.

ADJUNCTIVE AGENTS FOR PAIN MANAGEMENT

A variety of nonanalgesic medications have enjoyed widespread use in adults and children for the management of pain. As noted previously, fear, anxiety, and agitation can frequently accompany or be mistaken for pain in the pediatric patient. Occasionally, an anxiolytic agent such as diazepam or a mild sedative such as diphenhydramine can be helpful and appropriate. Rarely, a psychotic component of agitation accompanying pain is best addressed with a phenothiazine. However, more often than not, what is needed most is patience, compassion, and the understanding of the needs of children. In the pediatric patient, as in the adult, it is just as inappropriate to treat pain with a nonanalgesic as it is to treat anxiety with sedative doses of narcotics.

Antihistamines are components of many over-the-counter preparations and are widely used in pediatric patients. For young children, diphenhydramine has significant sedative effects and is occasionally used for this purpose. In doses of 1.0 to 1.5 mg/kg, light sleep is often produced without risk of respiratory depression or loss of protective airway reflexes.

Hydroxyzine is an antihistamine with slightly less sedative effects, yet it is known to mildly potentiate the analgesia of narcotics. Although unavailable for IV use, it is commonly employed IM in combination with a narcotic such as meperidine. A typical dosing schedule is 0.5 mg/kg IM or PO every four to six hours.

Phenothiazines possess little or no analgesic effects, have prolonged elimination half-lives, and can sometimes cause unwanted dysphoric or dystonic side effects. In the emergency department they are useful in the acute management of psychotic patients and for rapid sedation. Drugs such as chlorpromazine (Thorazine) and promethazine (Phenergan) are frequently employed in combination sedatives (see the following section).

In treatment of chronic pain syndromes and migraines, tricyclic antidepressants are gaining popularity in pediatrics. Amitriptyline (0.3–1.5 mg/kg) two hours before bedtime is frequently helpful in this setting. Effects on pain are typically not noted before completion of the first week of treatment, and its use in acute pain management is therefore unwarranted.

SEDATION AND ANALGESIA FOR PROCEDURES

When administering potent analgesics and anesthetics to any patient, the clinician must bear in mind the attendant risks of overdosage, particularly obtundation, respiratory depression, and the loss of protective airway reflexes. Many of these risks are particularly important to consider in the emergency department patient. For example, even if a patient has not recently eaten, gastric emptying is slowed or even stopped in trauma and many illnesses, leading to increased gastric volume, decreased gastric pH, and greatly increased risk of aspiration pneumonitis if obtundation with loss of airway reflexes occurs. Also, in addition to obscuring the neurologic examination, administration of depressant agents to the head-injured patient can potentially raise intracranial pressure through hypoventilation, hypercarbia, and resultant cerebral vasodilation. Even agents frequently valued for their relative preservation of airway reflexes and ventilatory response, such as ketamine, can cause unwanted increases in sympathetic tone and raise intracranial pressure directly.

Ideally, potent agents are avoided in patients with significant head injury, full stomach, or difficult airway (such as craniofacial injuries, neck trauma, injuries of the mouth or mandible, and so forth). However, after weighing the risks and benefits, this is not always possible or desirable. A certain measure of safety is then gained through careful monitoring and slow, careful titration to end points such as comfort, drowsiness, and slurred speech.

Table 50-2. Suggested dosing for conscious sedation*

Nonpainful procedures (e.g., CT scan)
Chloral hydrate 50–75 mg/kg PO or PR
Pentobarbital 1–2 mg/kg IV over 10 minutes; repeat one time to a maximum of 150 mg
Moderately painful procedures (e.g., bone marrow aspiration)
Intravenous line present
Midazolam 0.05 mg/kg IV (may repeat once in 10 minutes)
with
Fentanyl 1 μg/kg IV (may repeat twice every 10 minutes)
Intravenous line absent
Midazolam 0.3 mg/kg PO
with
Meperidine 3 mg/kg PO 35–40 minutes before the procedure

* Dosing guidelines are approximate and should be modified according to individual circumstances.

Unfortunately, in the preverbal child or infant, most titratable end points (other than cessation of crying and sleep) are lost. Additionally, the airway of an infant or young child differs significantly from that of an adult and can, almost by definition, be classified as "difficult" unless managed by one with experience and skill. Certain other disorders in the pediatric population, such as Down's syndrome, the Pierre Robin malformation sequence, and Treacher Collins or Goldenhar's syndromes, can make securing the airway a challenge if overdose occurs. Even the presence of loose deciduous teeth can prove to be a serious hazard if emergency intubation is required.

For all of these reasons, general anesthesia with complete control of the airway is frequently the preferred route for many painful procedures in infants and young children, while conscious sedation may be routine for the same procedure in an adult or older child. If conscious sedation is employed in children, it should be conducted only with careful monitoring, including a nurse or physician whose only responsibility is to administer medications and watch the patient. In the older child verbal contact should be maintained throughout the procedure, while in the younger child level of consciousness and respiratory rate must be followed more meticulously. Continuous pulse oximetry should be employed. "Preoperative" history should include questions regarding medication allergies, family history of anesthetic problems, most recent oral intake, and the presence of loose teeth. A "postoperative" period of observation commensurate with the extent of the procedure, level of sedation, and age of the patient should also not be forgotten. Whenever potent agents are administered, resuscitative equipment, including medications, working suction, appropriately sized oral airways, endotracheal tubes, and laryngoscope blades, as well as a narcotic antagonist (if appropriate), should be immediately available. Some general guidelines for conscious sedation are provided in Table 50-2.

Hypnotics

Barbiturates and chloral hydrate, as hypnotic agents, can be useful for sedation, amnesia, and unconsciousness yet are not true analgesics and therefore have a limited role in emergency department pain management. Anesthetic doses of barbiturates are most commonly used for very brief procedures such as endotracheal intubation (usually in combination with a music relaxant) and cardioversion. Rarely, carefully titrated subanesthetic doses can be used for rapid emergency department diagnosis of certain psychiatric disorders. Chloral hydrate and pentobarbital are commonly used in sedation of small children for relatively nonstimulating procedures (such as detailed physical examination, noninvasive radiologic procedures, and echocardiography).

Rapid intravenous induction of anesthesia in healthy adults is produced by a 3- to 5-mg/kg intravenous bolus of thiopental. A somewhat higher dose, 5 to 6 mg/kg, is necessary for a similar response in children. Clinical duration is brief and limited primarily by redistribution. Methohexital is approximately 2.75 times more potent and undergoes hepatic metabolism more rapidly. It is therefore often selected over thiopental when rapid recovery after large or repeated doses is required. Both agents can be administered rectally and are well absorbed. For its increased potency, methohexital is most frequently selected, thus limiting the total necessary volume. A rectal dose of 20 to 25 mg/kg PR will reliably produce sleep in 5 to 10 minutes, and the typical patient will awaken in 45 to 60 minutes (often sufficient time for a radiographic study). Although asleep while unstimulated, the patient will continue to respond to noxious stimuli such as venipuncture and intravenous line placement. Finally, although spontaneous ventilation is usually maintained, apnea and soft-tissue obstruction of the airway can occur. Thus, these medications are best administered with monitoring similar to that used in the operating room and under the supervision of an anesthesiologist or other physician skilled in their use and capable of securing the airway if necessary.

Barbiturates, particularly when intravenously administered in anesthetic doses, are to be avoided in the hypovolemic or debilitated patient because of their significant cardiodepressant effects. In cases of the hypotensive patient in need of rapid intubation, ketamine is preferred (in the absence of significant head injury).

Chloral hydrate is perhaps the most common hypnotic in pediatric use. Like the barbiturates, it produces sleep and amnesia rather than analgesia and anesthesia. It is conveniently administered either orally or rectally, usually in doses of 50 to 75 mg/kg. Chloral hydrate has been used safely as a sedative in patients of all ages from preterm infants to the elderly. In term infants, 50-mg/kg doses have been demonstrated to cause no significant change in ventilatory drive. Although doses as high as 250 mg/kg have been tolerated in animal studies, toxicity has been reported in preterm infants who received 165 mg/kg over a 16-hour period and in a 2½-year-old who received a single oral dose of 115 mg/kg.

Anxiolytics

Like the hypnotics, benzodiazepines provide little in the way of analgesia yet are useful during painful procedures for anxiolysis, sedation, and amnesia. The agents most commonly employed in the emergency department include diazepam (Valium) and midazolam (Versed), with the latter offering the advantages of water solubility and short duration of action.

Diazepam has been employed in a variety of settings since its introduction in the 1960s. Intravenously, it is useful as an anticonvulsant during status epilepticus and as a potent sedative-amnestic agent. The anticonvulsant dose of 0.1 to 0.3 mg/kg IV can often produce unconsciousness and apnea, particularly when given in combination with other CNS depressants such as barbiturates. Injectable preparations require propylene glycol as a solvent, frequently resulting in burning pain on infusion and occasionally producing thrombophlebitis. Finally, diazepam has a relatively prolonged elimination half-life ($t^{1/2}$; 20–40 hours) and is degraded to active metabolites. Thus, the drug is less than ideal in the management of brief emergency department procedures.

More recently, a short-acting and water-soluble benzodiazepine, midazolam (Versed), has been introduced. Its chemistry is unique in that below pH 4 it exists as a polar, water-soluble molecule, yet at physiologic pH its ring structure closes to produce a lipid-soluble molecule that more closely resembles other benzodiazepines. Injection is therefore painless, yet onset of action is rapid. Metabolism is also rapid via hepatic hydroxylation, and elimination half-life is one-tenth that of diazepam (2.0 to 2.5 hours). Intravenously, the drug may be rapidly titrated to end points of sedation or slurred speech and for unpleasant procedures it is a particularly effective amnestic. It can be administered IV, IM, orally, nasally, or per rectum, although proper doses for the latter routes are under investigation.

In our hospital midazolam is frequently used as a sedative-amnestic agent in the intensive care unit, operating rooms, and critical-care sites. It has been found to be a useful adjunct to painful procedures such as dressing changes, bone-marrow biopsies, thoracentesis, and chest-tube placement, as well as for comfort and amnesia in patients who require prolonged mechanical ventilation.

In pediatric emergency departments, although midazolam offers many significant advantages over diazepam, its potency has limited common intravenous use. In early (adult) experience, occasional respiratory depression and apnea have been described during conscious sedation of debilitated patients. It is likely that as more experience is gained (particularly with PO and PR administration), it will be used much more commonly.

Guidelines for dosing outside of the operating room are somewhat preliminary. Suggested midazolam dosing in our experience would be the following: orally—0.3–0.5 mg/kg (maximum 15 mg) 25 to 35 minutes before the procedure; nasally or rectally—0.2–0.3 mg/kg (maximum 10 mg) 10 minutes before the procedure.

For conscious sedation in our institution, midazolam is administered intravenously with an initial dose of 0.05 mg/kg by a physician capable of securing the airway if overdosage occurs. As with general anesthesia, care is taken that the patient has been NPO before the procedure. Pulse oximetry is maintained throughout, and resuscitative equipment, including an appropriate-sized mask, oral airway, Mapleson circuit, and suction, are at hand. The initial dose is repeated in 5 to 10 minutes if necessary, and additional supplementation with fentanyl, 0.6 μg/kg min is employed thereafter. Just as in the operating room, vital signs are recorded every 5 minutes during the procedure and every 15 minutes thereafter for one hour. Patients are typically alert within the hour and are amnestic for the experience. Use of midazolam in neonates has not yet been adequately studied and is therefore not recommended.

Combination Sedatives

Over the years a variety of sedative medication "mixes" have been concocted and employed in the management of painful procedures in children. Among these are those containing hypnotics (such as pentobarbital), analgesics (such as morphine, meperidine, and fentanyl), anxiolytics (such as diazepam and midazolam), dissociative agents (such as ketamine, droperidol, and phenothiazines), and anticholinergics (such as atropine and glycopyrrolate) in various combinations to be administered IV, IM, or PO.

The most frequent combination analgesic-sedative used in the care of pediatric patients is meperidine, promethazine, and chlorpromazine. The trio is frequently referred to as "pedimix," "lytic cocktail," "DPT" (Demerol/Phenergan/Thorazine), or "Demerol compound" and was developed in the 1950s after reports of synergism between narcotics and phenothiazines. Advantages of the combination include ease of delivery (IM injection), wide experience, fair reliability, and applicability to most age groups in weight-scaled doses.

In our institution "Demerol compound" is frequently employed for sedation and analgesia in the management of painful procedures such as cardiac catheterization, fracture reduction, and laceration repair where sedation and immobility are required. The formulation is available in 1- and 2-ml syringes and includes meperidine, 25.0 mg/ml; chlorpromazine, 6.25 mg/ml; and promethazine, 6.25 mg/ml. Use is limited to patients older than one year and dosage is carefully tailored to the clinical status of the patient. For cardiac catheterization doses of 0.11 ml/kg to a maximum of 2 ml are employed in asymptomatic patients. This dose is halved for cyanotic or debilitated patients. In the emergency department doses of 0.1 ml/kg have been found excessive, resulting frequently in prolonged sedation and occasionally in respiratory depression that requires reversal with a narcotic antagonist. Current practice has therefore involved doses of 0.067 ml/kg (1 ml/15 kg) for healthy children undergoing routine procedures. The majority of procedures are conducted with simple vital sign monitoring and without placement of an intravenous line.

Disadvantages of all sedative combinations include the fixed nature of drug ratios and the inability to titrate to effect. In particular, the DPT combination entails disadvantages of slow onset, variable sedation levels (frequently inadequate or excessive), and occasional side effects such as dyskinesia and hypotension. This has prompted evaluation of newer drug combinations and of single-drug regimens that involve intravenous administration.

Fentanyl

Fentanyl, a relatively new synthetic narcotic with a potency 80 to 150 times that of morphine, has been extensively used by anesthesiologists and is theoretically well suited to the emergency department because of its rapid onset and short duration of action. It is a phenylpiperidine derivative that is approximately 80 percent protein bound in plasma and undergoes primarily hepatic metabolism. Distribution is biphasic, with rapid ($t^{1/2}$ = 1–3 minutes) and slower ($t^{1/2}$ = 5–20 minutes) components, while elimination half-life ($t^{1/2}$)

is two to four hours. The increased lipid solubility over morphine results in more rapid CNS penetration and onset of effects. Potential side effects include those of all narcotics, as well as profound respiratory depression or apnea; muscular, in particular chest-wall, rigidity (especially associated with rapid administration); and bradycardia. Bradycardia is thought to be secondary to a vagotonic effect and can be profound in younger patients or those receiving beta-blockers such as propranolol.

Although several vehicles for fentanyl's administration are in various stages of development (including oral and transdermal forms), the common and most tightly controllable route is intravenous. Billmire and associates have reported their experience with IV fentanyl in 2,000 outpatients with facial trauma. For sedation and analgesia during laceration repair, fentanyl was administered by slow (over three to five minutes) IV push in doses of 2 to 3 μg/kg to patients aged 12 months to 12 years. The area to be repaired was infiltrated with local anesthetic after adequate sedation was achieved. The usual duration of action was approximately 30 to 40 minutes, and supplements were provided on a *pro re nata* (PRN) basis. With this regimen the authors observed three cases of apnea that required a narcotic antagonist and brief bag-and-mask support of ventilation. No patients required subsequent hospitalization. The authors concluded that IV fentanyl was effective and safe for sedation and analgesia in the repair of minor lacerations, noting further that the possible disadvantages presented by the necessary placement of an IV line were, in their view, outweighed by the quality of relaxation provided.

Although the precise monitoring employed in the aforementioned series is not described, the authors note that during injection of fentanyl the patient's speech and respiration are closely watched. They further emphasize that resuscitation equipment and a narcotic antagonist should be readily available when this potent narcotic is administered. It is notable that patients under one year of age were excluded from the study, perhaps because of concerns regarding unpredictable respiratory depression. This question of variable pharmacodynamics and ventilatory response is now being addressed through work such as that of Hertzka and associates, who reported their attempts to correlate ventilatory response, age, and plasma fentanyl concentrations. Their results suggest that ventilatory response in infants older than three months is similar to that of older children and adults. Observed differences in effect and duration are therefore attributable to pharmacokinetic factors. Unfortunately, only one patient less than three months old was studied and exhibited significant respiratory changes despite low plasma fentanyl concentrations. We hope that further work will elucidate this matter. As noted previously, we prefer pulse oximetry or electrical cardiorespiratory monitoring in addition to careful clinical observation in all patients less than six months of age who are receiving potent narcotics.

Ketamine

Ketamine is an anesthetic agent structurally related to phencyclidine (PCP, "angel dust"). First described as producing "dissociative anesthesia" (referring to dissociation of the thalamus, limbic system, and higher centers), it is frequently employed by anesthesiologists for procedures such as endotracheal intubation, cardiac catheterization, minor surgery, endoscopy, and radiologic or radiotherapeutic procedures. Like fentanyl, onset is rapid and duration is short because of high lipid solubility and rapid redistribution. Effects include unconsciousness, amnesia, and profound analgesia even in low doses. Classically, it has been administered intravenously and intramuscularly although PO and PR routes have also been used.

Initial experience with ketamine was most favorable as it was believed to be devoid of respiratory-depressant effects and, at least in low doses, appeared to spare protective airway reflexes. The true picture of ketamine pharmacodynamics has since slowly evolved from clinical reports of apnea and hypoxemia to contemporary quantitative studies. In the pediatric population, it has been demonstrated that ketamine doses decrease the slope of the CO_2 response curve after IV bolus administration and shift the curve rightward (without a slope change) during steady-state continuous infusion. Respiratory depression is principally related to diminished rate, with tidal volume and functional residual capacity retained. Unpredictability of dose-response in children is likely related both to dosage and technique of administration.

Ketamine is desirable as a rapid, short-lived, sedative-anesthetic technique that tends to stimulate the sympathetic nervous system. In hypovolemic shock, blood pressure and heart rate are supported through increased sympathetic tone, although direct cardiodepressant effects may be observed in patients who lack sympathetic reserve. In the asthmatic patient, bronchodilatory effects can be helpful. Disadvantages include increases in intracranial and intraocular pressures (contraindicating its use in severe head trauma and penetrating eye injuries). Significant increases in salivation (necessitating concomitant use of an antisialagogue) and postoperative dysphoria or nightmares are also problems. The latter difficulties lead many anesthesiologists to avoid ketamine in patients with a history of psychiatric illness, although symptoms can be reduced significantly by the concurrent administration of a benzodiazepine.

Dosage requirements of ketamine vary greatly with the intensity and duration of the painful stimulus. Typically, 1 to 2 mg/kg IV or 4 to 5 mg/kg IM is sufficient to produce unconsciousness lasting 15 to 30 minutes. Profound analgesia, amnesia, and sedation, usually with sparing of respirations, can be produced with half of these doses. For painful procedures, consciousness is difficult to assess as the patient will often maintain the eyes open and sometimes move without stimulation even though deeply anesthetized. Verbal contact is usually lost with doses exceeding 0.5 mg/kg IV. Additionally, heart rate and blood pressure elevations can be related either to painful stimuli or the drug itself. Consequently, ketamine in general is an agent best reserved for use by an experienced anesthesiologist with full monitoring and resuscitative equipment available. In small doses (0.25 and 0.50 mg/kg), Hirlinger and Pfenninger have described IV use of ketamine for analgesia in adult emergency department patients suffering from fractures and soft-tissue injuries. They observed effective analgesia within 5 minutes, lasting 10 to 15 minutes, and impairment of consciousness in the higher, but not lower, doses.

Inhalational Analgesia

Nitrous oxide (N_2O) has been widely used in dentistry and surgery for its weak anesthetic, anxiolytic, and amnestic properties since soon after its discovery by Priestly in 1772. It is perhaps the most commonly used anesthetic agent in operating rooms today. In inspired concentrations of 30 to 70%, it is useful in a variety of settings and is particularly suited for emergency department use by its wide margin of safety, rapid onset, and quick elimination.

Nitrous oxide is a clear, colorless, nonflammable gas without detectable odor. Its uptake and elimination are entirely through the lungs, and, dissolved in plasma without protein-binding, distribution is rapid. In anesthetic terms, with a minimum alveolar concentration of 105%, nitrous oxide alone will not reliably produce surgical anesthesia. Although it is capable of depressing protective airway reflexes at high concentrations, little risk of aspiration has been demonstrated when it is used in concentrations of 50% with oxygen (O_2). Nitrous oxide liquefies when pressurized to 750 psi, yet can be further compressed to 1,980 psi without liquefication when mixed 50% with oxygen. This latter property allows commercial production of a 50 : 50 analgesic mixture for delivery via compact, portable devices.

Early research using human (adult) experimental pain models indicated equipotency of a 20% N_2O : 80% O_2 mixture and 15 mg subcutaneously administered morphine sulfate. Subjective reports of patients receiving inhalational analgesia include, in addition to mild analgesia, descriptions of euphoria, lightheadedness, amnesia, and detachment that may supersede true analgesia. Side effects include nausea and vomiting in as many as 15 percent of patients (which may be dose related). Its greater solubility and more rapid diffusion than nitrogen contraindicates its use when the possibility of closed collections of gas exist (such as in patients with bowel obstruction, pneumothorax, or middle ear disease). In our practice, altered mental status or the concurrent presence of CNS depressants (such as ethanol, narcotics, or "street drugs") contraindicate its use. Finally, significant respiratory disease with suspected hypoxemia bars its use.

In our emergency department, nitrous oxide inhalational analgesia is considered for a variety of brief procedures, including laceration repair, orthopedic manipulations, incision and drainage of abscesses, burn debridement, and dressing changes. Administration is limited to cooperative children four years of age or older. To maximize safety, a 50 : 50 mixture of N_2O : O_2 is employed and is self-administered via a hand-held demand-valve mask. In addition to the physician performing the procedure, our protocol requires the presence of an emergency department attending physician to constantly observe the patient. Verbal contact is maintained throughout and equipment necessary for securing the airway (including suction) is within easy reach. Pulse oximetry monitoring and measurement of inspired oxygen concentration (FIO_2) can increase safety.

Once an analgesic state is achieved, infiltration with local anesthetic is performed if possible. At the conclusion of the procedure, 100% O_2 is administered for three to five minutes to minimize the risk of transient hypoxemia due to "diffusion hypoxia" (displacement of alveolar oxygen by rapidly diffusing N_2O). Although investigators have observed no such hypoxemia in a study of 20 adult volunteers after replacement of an inspired mixture of 50% N_2O : 50% O_2 with room air, the case of the pediatric patient with a more than proportionately decreased functional residual capacity and increased oxygen consumption has yet to be studied.

Gamis and associates reported a prospective evaluation of inhalational analgesia (30% N_2O : 70% O_2) versus placebo in 34 children for outpatient procedures. They concluded that nitrous oxide by inhalation is an effective and simple analgesic technique in children aged seven years and above for repair of simple, uncomplicated lacerations. Documentation of analgesia was via an observer-based pain behavior scale, and complications were both rare and minimal. Specifically, the authors noted no episodes of hypoxemia, nausea, vomiting, or oversedation.

MANAGEMENT OF ENDOTRACHEAL INTUBATION

As a stressful and painful procedure, endotracheal intubation warrants a place in any discussion of pediatric emergency department pain management. While an adult patient will undoubtedly receive some form of sedation or topical anesthesia for intubation, the "awake" intubation is often routine in small pediatric patients. In part this is due to concerns regarding the possibly difficult intubation of pediatric patients, with the physician electing to pursue the "safe" course of maintaining alertness, airway reflexes, and spontaneous ventilation throughout.

Unfortunately, awake intubation has some disadvantages: significant sympathetic stimulation, with tachycardia, hypertension, and increased oxygen demand; often significant parasympathetic stimulation with profound bradycardia; transient airway obstruction and hypoxemia; and the ever-present possibility of direct trauma to the oral, pharyngeal, and laryngeal structures of the struggling child. Thus, in our practice, sedation is provided for all conscious patients (regardless of age) who require endotracheal intubation. Appropriate agents and dosages are tailored to the age and physical status of the patient with, as described previously, a barbiturate, ketamine, or narcotic-benzodiazepine combination employed most frequently.

SELECTED READING

Berde, CB, Anand, KJS, and Sethna, NF. Pediatric Pain Management. In G Gregory (ed), *Pediatric Anesthesia.* New York: Churchill Livingstone, 1989.

Berry, FR. Analgesia in patients with fractured shaft of femur. *Anesthesia* 32:576, 1977.

Billmire, DA, Neale, HW, and Gregory, RO. Use of IV fentanyl in the outpatient treatment of pediatric facial trauma. *J Trauma* 25:1079, 1985.

Brewer, EJ, and Arrovo, I. Use of non-steroidal anti-inflammatory drugs in children. *Pediatr Ann* 15:575, 1986.

Cousins, MJ, and Bridenbaugh, PO. *Neural Blockade in Clinical Anesthesia and Management of Pain.* Philadelphia: Lippincott, 1988.

Dailey, RH. Fatality secondary to misuse of TAC solution. *Ann Emerg Med* 17:159, 1988.

Dalens, B. Regional anesthesia in children. *Anesth Analg* 68:654, 1989.

Eyers, RL, et al. Local anesthetic plasma levels in children. *Anesth Intens Care* 6:243, 1978.

Fitzgerald, B. Intravenous regional anesthesia in children. *Br J Anaesth* 48:485, 1976.

Gamis, AS, Knapp, JA, and Glenski, JA. Nitrous oxide analgesia in a pediatric emergency department. *Ann Emerg Med* 18:177, 1989.

Griffin, GC, Campbell, VD, and Jones, R. Nitrous oxide-oxygen sedation for minor surgery. Experience in a pediatric setting. *JAMA* 245:2411, 1981.

Grossbard, GD, and Love, BRT. Femoral nerve block: A simple and safe method of instant analgesia for femoral shaft fractures in children. *Aust N Z J Surg* 49:592, 1979.

Hallen, B, and Upjpffeldt, A. Does lidocaine-prilocaine cream permit painfree insertion of IV catheters in children? *Anesthesiology* 57:340, 1982.

Hamza, J, Ecoffey, C, and Gross, JB. Ventilatory response to CO_2 following intravenous ketamine in children. *Anesthesiology* 70:422, 1989.

Hertzka, RE, et al. Fentanyl-induced ventilatory depression: Effects of age. *Anesthesiology* 70:213, 1989.

Hirlinger, WK, and Pfenninger, E. Intravenous analgesia with ketamine for emergency patients. *Anaesthesist* 36:140, 1987.

Koren, G, et al. Postoperative morphine infusion in newborn infants: Assessment of disposition characteristics and safety. *J Pediatr* 107:963, 1985.

Lynn, AM, and Slattery, JT. Morphine pharmacokinetics in early infancy. *Anesthesiology* 66:136, 1987.

Maunuksela, EL, and Korpela, R. Double-blind evaluation of a lidocaine-prilocaine cream (EMLA) in children. Effect on the pain associated with venous cannulation. *Br J Anaesth* 58:1242, 1986.

Mazoit, JX, Denson, DD, and Samii, K. Pharmacokinetics of bupivacaine following caudal anesthesia in infants. *Anesthesiology* 68:387, 1988.

McGrath, PJ, and Unruh, AM. *Pain in Children and Adolescents.* Amsterdam: Elsevier, 1987.

McNicol, LR. Lower limb blocks for children. *Anaesthesia* 41:27, 1986.

Miser, AW, Miser, JS, and Clark, BS. Continuous intravenous infusion of morphine sulfate for control of severe pain in children with terminal malignancy. *J Pediatr* 96:930, 1980.

Mitchell, AA, et al. Risks to children from computed tomographic scan premedication. *JAMA* 247:2385, 1982.

Morselli, PL, Franco-Morselli, R, and Bossi, L. Clinical pharmacokinetics in newborns and infants: Age-related differences and therapeutic implications. *Pharmacokinet* 5:485, 1980.

Olney, BW, et al. Outpatient treatment of upper extremity injuries in childhood using intravenous regional anaesthesia. *J Pediatr Orthop* 8:576, 1988.

Payne, R. Principles of analgesic use in the treatment of acute pain and chronic cancer pain. Report of a committee to the American Pain Society. Washington: American Pain Society, 1987.

Rich, EC, Marshall, RE, and Volpe, JJ. The normal neonatal response to pin-prick. *Dev Med Child Neurol* 16:432, 1974.

Ronchi, L, et al. Femoral nerve blockade in children using bupivacaine. *Anesthesiology* 70:622, 1989.

Sethna, NF, and Berde, CB. Pediatric Regional Anesthesia. In G Gregory (ed), *Pediatric Anesthesia.* New York: Churchill Livingstone, 1989. Pp. 647–678.

Shanding, B, and Steward, DJ. Regional analgesia for postoperative pain in pediatric outpatient surgery. *J Pediatr Surg* 15:477, 1980.

Shannon, M, and Berde, CB. *Pediatr Clin North Amer* 36:855, 1989.

Small, GA. Brachial plexus block anesthesia in children. *JAMA* 147:1648, 1951.

Soliman, IE, et al. Comparison of the analgesic effects of EMLA. Eutectic mixture of local anesthetics to intradermal lidocaine infiltration prior to venous cannulation in unpremedicated children. *Anesthesiology* 68:804, 1988.

Stang, HJ, et al. Local anesthesia for neonatal circumcision. Effects on distress and cortisol response. *JAMA* 259:1507, 1988.

Way, WL, Costley, EC, and Way, EL. Respiratory sensitivity of the newborn infant to meperidine and morphine. *Clin Pharmacol Ther* 6:454, 1964.

Weil, JV, et al. Diminished ventilatory response to hypoxia and hypercarbia after morphine in normal man. *N Engl J Med* 292:1103, 1975.

Yaster, M, et al. The pharmacokinetics of lidocaine during caudal anesthesia in children. *Anesthesiology* 63:465, 1985.

Yaster, M, and Deshpande, JK, Management of pediatric pain with opioid analgesics. *J Pediatr* 113:421, 1988.

Zeltzer, L, Jay, S, and Fisher, D. The management of pain associated with pediatric procedures. *Pediatr Clin North Amer* 36:941, 1989.

Zeltzer, L, and LeBaron, S. Hypnotic and nonhypnotic techniques for reduction of pain and anxiety during painful procedures in children and adolescents with cancer. *J Pediatr* 101:1032, 1982.

51. The Prehospital Management of Pain

Vincent P. Verdile
Ronald D. Stewart

During the formative years of emergency medical services, the focus was on the delivery of advanced life support (ALS) to patients who were acutely ill or injured in the field. Emergency medical services (EMS) systems have improved the care of medical and surgical emergencies with the implementation of ALS maneuvers such as transcutaneous pacing, decompression of tension pneumothorax, and the availability of extensive pharmacotherapy. Despite sophisticated accomplishments in prehospital medicine, attention has seldom been paid to the management of pain.

Beginning with the work of Pantridge and Geddes on the impact of mobile intensive care units in the prehospital management of patients with myocardial infarction (MI), through the development of advanced aeromedical teams for trauma care as described by Baxt and others, we have demonstrated that EMS systems can deliver effective and at times lifesaving care to the sick and injured in the field. The time has come for emergency physicians to address perhaps the less life-threatening yet important aspects of prehospital patient care, such as the alleviation of pain and suffering. We must turn our attention to providing total care for patients while they are en route to the hospital. Obviously, providing analgesia should never take precedence over the fundamentals of airway, breathing, and support of circulation (ABCs). However, after the ABCs have been taken care of, the management of the prehospital patient's pain must be a consideration. Pain must be recognized as a true emergency.

Studies have shown that acute pain is often inadequately treated in the inpatient population, with patients continuing to suffer needlessly. It is safe to assume that the mismanagement of pain by physicians reflects the lack of sufficient training in and the lack of attention paid to the significance of pain control. How then can physicians involved with EMS train prehospital providers in the assessment and treatment of pain in the prehospital patient? In addition, the most recent text dedicated to emergency medical technician (EMT) training is devoid of a single chapter or even section dedicated to the prehospital management of pain. Granted, EMTs cannot administer ALS interventions such as narcotics; however, basic, as well as advanced, prehospital providers can perform many interventions to reduce pain and suffering.

The perception by the acutely ill or injured patient of a concerned and caring prehospital provider in itself can serve to alleviate anxiety and help reduce pain. Providing the patient with ample information about what is about to occur, how long it will take, and how long it will be until he or she is transported to the hospital will all help the patient cope with the unfamiliarities of prehospital medicine. Just as preoperative information from surgeons, nurses, and anesthesiologists can allay some of the anxiety and fear patients have before operation, communication with the prehospital patient during treatment and transport can be expected to have the same beneficial effect.

The prehospital provider can also use routine splinting and immobilization of an injured extremity, along with the gentle, controlled handling of a patient during transport to the hospital, to help reduce or prevent pain. Neither the caring approach to the prehospital patient nor gentle handling of the patient constitutes an ALS intervention; however, they are two of the nonpharmacologic maneuvers that can add to reduction or elimination of pain.

Very little clinical research has been done to elucidate the ideal analgesic for the prehospital management of pain. The ideal agent would have a rapid onset, minimal side effects, proven efficacy in acute pain, and a short duration of action, and it would not mask the underlying pathology to avoid confounding the inhospital evaluation of the patient. Further challenging the implementation of a field analgesic is the reliance on physician surrogates in the field to assess patients with pain and the severity of that pain. Any emergency physician who has given medical command can attest to the occasional misleading or inaccurate medical report from prehospital personnel. Therefore, the safety of a given agent takes on greater importance when it is to be administered by prehospital providers without direct physician supervision. It is clear that there is a need for EMS medical directors to develop protocols for the management of the patient in pain, analogous to the protocols developed for the management of other prehospital emergencies such as shock or respiratory distress. The patient in pain must also be considered a prehospital emergency.

It is the intent of this chapter to present a current perspective on field analgesia. The paucity of controlled, prospective, blinded studies prevents the declaration of a single ideal agent for prehospital pain control. Nevertheless, the discussion of the prehospital management of pain is both timely and necessary.

ANALGESIC AGENTS

Narcotics

In 1680, Syndenham wrote, "Among the remedies it has pleased Almighty God to give to man to relieve his sufferings, none is so universal and so efficacious as opium." Narcotics remain the most effective agents for producing analgesia in or out of the hospital. Despite their potency for pain relief, however, the negative aspects of narcotic agents are the well-known side effects of hypotension, respiratory depression, nausea, and vomiting. These side effects somewhat limit the prehospital utility of narcotics, particularly in the hands of nonphysician providers. Naloxone has improved safety, although narcotic-induced hypotension in the setting of trauma can unnecessarily confound patient management. Judicious use of narcotics, however, can still be an important aspect of prehospital analgesia.

The intravenous (IV) route of administration of narcotics is preferable because it ensures a rapid and reliable delivery and allows for smaller incremental dosage, thus minimizing untoward side effects. It has been suggested that even when properly administered, narcotics rarely provide complete analgesia. This suggestion underscores the importance of titrating the dose of the narcotic to the patient's response. Individualization of the narcotic dose must be the rule in any prehospital pain protocol.

Morphine sulfate is perhaps the most widely used prehospital narcotic. With minimal effect on cardiac contractility, it is the drug of choice for the management of pain associated with myocardial infarction. For the patient with an isolated injury, no head or central nervous system involvement, and little risk of hypovolemia, morphine sulfate can be used in small 3- to 5-mg IV doses titrated to effect. Again, the total dose of morphine required to produce analgesia will depend on the cause of the acute pain and the individual's response to the pain and the therapy. Morphine is less likely to precipitate narcotic-induced hypotension if it is administered when the patient is supine.

Unfortunately, the lack of prehospital clinical research involving the use and safety of parenteral narcotic analgesia has limited the implementation of new agents into the field. Fentanyl (Sublimaze) offers several advantages over morphine sulfate and warrants investigation. Fentanyl has a relatively short half-life, with a duration of action of 30 to 60 minutes. This short half-life would make it an ideal agent for prehospital use in patients who require painful extrication of a body part that has been trapped in machinery or under a heavy object. Furthermore, fentanyl does not cause histamine release, allowing it to be safely used in the patient with reactive airway disease and limiting the incidence of narcotic-induced hypotension. At higher doses, fentanyl has been known to produce chest wall rigidity; however, this has usually been in anesthetized patients and when it is given rapidly. It is unlikely that this would occur in the dosage range that produces analgesia in adults (150–200 μg, slow IV push), and if it did occur it would be reversible with naloxone. Because of fentanyl's potency, safe and effective dosage regimens must be established for prehospital use.

Agonist-Antagonist

Agonists-antagonists comprise a class of analgesics that are potentially the most well suited for prehospital use. They can provide analgesia without euphoria and, if administered within the recommended dosage range, have a ceiling on respiratory depression and limited hemodynamic alterations. Care must be exercised in using this class of analgesics in opiate-dependent patients to prevent precipitating narcotic withdrawal. Surprisingly, only recently has the use of an agonist-antagonist been investigated in the prehospital setting.

Stene and colleagues studied 46 prehospital patients with moderate to severe pain secondary to trauma, burns, or intraabdominal processes and used intravenous nalbuphine (Nubain) for analgesia. The patients received 15 mg nalbuphine over 15 seconds if they were judged to be 60 kg or less, and 20 mg nalbuphine if they were over 60 kg. Forty-one patients (89%) received partial to complete pain relief and no significant change was noted in vital signs. This study demonstrates the safety and efficacy of conservative doses of nalbuphine in the prehospital setting for patients in moderate to severe pain.

The agonist-antagonist agents as a group offer a promising alternative for prehospital analgesia and warrant more extensive investigation. The fact that some are not considered controlled substances makes the risk of theft and personnel abuse less likely and the general handling and storage of these agents in the prehospital environment easier.

Inhalation Agents

The use of an inhalation agent, such as nitrous oxide, for pain control has several advantages that make it attractive for prehospital use. Rapid onset, patient self-administration, safety, effectiveness, and a relatively inexpensive cost are a few of the properties that make inhalation agents easily adaptable to the field.

Most of the EMS literature dealing with inhalation analgesia focuses on the use of nitrous oxide : oxygen mixtures ($N_2O : O_2$); in a 50 : 50 mixture, they provide mild analgesia, with significant anxiolysis. Repeatedly, studies have shown that between 80 and 90 percent of patients with mild to severe pain have received safe, effective analgesia with this mixture. Because it is self-administered through a demand-valve system, the risk of excessive sedation and loss of normal airway reflexes is greatly reduced. In over 3,000 cases in the City of Pittsburgh EMS system, no major untoward side effects have occurred.

The relative contraindications for $N_2O : O_2$ administration include: (1) an altered level of consciousness, (2) pneumothorax, (3) suspected bowel obstruction, (4) decompression sickness, (5) severe chronic obstructive pulmonary disease, and (6) simultaneous use with narcotics in patients with compromised cardiac output. Although $N_2O : O_2$ is used in labor and delivery, the litigious society in which we practice prevents recommending its routine use in pregnancy, especially in the first-trimester patient with pain. Studies using a 50 : 50 $N_2O : O_2$ mixture in the pregnant patient are lacking and, thus, the fetal risk is unclear.

Once again, it has been our experience that the 50 : 50 mixture of $N_2O : O_2$ is effective in the vast majority of patients who obtain some, if not complete, relief of their pain. The other important property of $N_2O : O_2$ is its anxiolytic effect, which can help patients better tolerate the often stressful prehospital circumstances. Unfortunately, the $N_2O : O_2$ tends to be underutilized by field personnel, and it is often the medical command physician's responsibility to initiate this modality. Making it particularly helpful for prehospital management of pain is its broad and varied potential application. Musculoskeletal trauma is the most commonly treated condition with $N_2O : O_2$; however, it is also routinely used in patients with burns, chest pain, amputations and lacerations, renal colic, and headache. There are several commercially available $N_2O : O_2$ delivery systems, and the patient can choose from either a mouthpiece or face-mask administration setup. For the most complete and up-to-date information concerning the use of $N_2O : O_2$ in emergency medicine, the reader is referred to Stewart's chapter in *Pain Management in Emergency Medicine* and Chap. 48 in this text.

Although other gaseous agents such as enflurane and methoxyflurane have promise for application in the prehospital management of pain, insufficient prehospital clinical research prevents our recommending these agents at this time.

Ketamine

Ketamine is a dissociative anesthetic agent that is structurally related to phencyclidine. A renewed interest has been shown in the use of ketamine hydrochloride in emergency medicine. Low-dose ketamine, 0.3 to 0.5 mg/kg IV, has been demonstrated to be effective in selected patients as an analgesic and anesthetic in the emergency department. Ketamine in low doses is a safe, rapidly active parenteral agent that provides a unique functional and electrophysiologic dissociative state. Dissociative sedation is particularly attractive in the prehospital setting because the patient remains conscious, with intact airway reflexes, cooperative, and with significant pain relief. Besides producing central nervous system effects, ketamine can act as a direct cardiovascular stimulant, increasing heart rate and blood pressure, although some critically ill or injured patients may have unexpected bradycardia and hypotension. In anesthetic doses, there is also an associated increase in intracranial pressure with ketamine administration, which is believed to be secondary to an increase in cerebral blood flow from increased systemic blood pressure and cerebral vasodilation.

Unless administered in high doses or by rapid infusion, ketamine does not produce respiratory depression. Another interesting effect of ketamine is the potent bronchodilation it produces, which can reduce bronchospasm and facilitate intubation in status asthmaticus.

Ketamine has also been noted to produce increased muscle tone, particularly in the masseter muscles, at dissociative anesthetic dose levels. The enhanced muscle tone can produce a state of catalepsy in which the patient can have a self-maintaining position.

A potential unwanted side effect of ketamine is the occasional emergence reaction that occurs in some patients (10–23%). Benzodiazepines, used concurrently, both enhance the sedative properties of ketamine and decrease the incidence of the emergence reaction. The benzodiazepines can also reduce the likelihood of other unwanted side effects as well. In addition, research involving the "d" isomer of ketamine suggests that this form may be more potent and faster acting and have less incidence of the emergence phenomenon and other unwanted side effects. Only a few studies have examined the utility of ketamine in emergency medicine. In 1979, Dailey and associates first reported the use of ketamine in children less than 10 years old as an analgesic for wound repair, foreign body removal, or incision and drainage procedures. For 30 patients, ketamine proved to be a safe and effective agent, and only 3 children had an emergence reaction.

In another report by Dick, et al., 20 traumatized patients were given either 0.5 mg/kg or 1.0 mg/kg ketamine by deltoid injection. These patients, with moderate to severe pain from extremity fractures or burns, received significant analgesia from the intramuscular (IM) injection. It was believed that the higher dose, although producing more analgesia, impaired the level of consciousness to an undesirable degree. No hemodynamic or respiratory complications occurred, and the authors recommended ketamine as an effective, rapidly acting analgesic agent for traumatized patients. The rapid onset after IM injection makes this agent easily adaptable to paramedic field usage.

Based on the pharmacology of ketamine already discussed, the contraindications become obvious: cardiovascular disease (i.e., uncontrolled hypertension, aortic aneurysms, unstable angina, or recent MI) and central nervous system disease (i.e., cerebral trauma, intracerebral mass, or hemorrhage). Because laryngospasm has been known to occur, the drug should not be administered by personnel who are not skilled in advanced airway techniques. A more comprehensive review of the use of ketamine in emergency medicine has been published by Bennett and Stewart.

Transcutaneous Electrical Nerve Stimulators

Transcutaneous electrical nerve stimulators (TENS), although not widely used in emergency medicine, have been shown to be effective in the management of a variety of acute pain conditions, such as acute musculoskeletal pain, rib fractures, low back pain, and angina pectoris. Although never studied in EMS, this modality could prove to be an easily implemented, readily available, nonnarcotic analgesic for use in the prehospital management of some forms of acute pain. TENS will not produce central nervous system or respiratory depression, and analgesia is obtained noninvasively. The patient or paramedic can operate the TENS unit and side effects are minimal. The only absolute contraindication to the use of TENS is in patients with demand cardiac pacers or other implanted electrical devices. Many features of TENS make it potentially suitable for prehospital use, and the opportunity for research in the use of TENS in EMS is plentiful.

PAIN EVALUATION

Pain is so subjective that it does not lend itself to easy evaluation and measurement. Nonetheless, it is necessary, particularly for research purposes, to somehow quantitate pain and pain relief. For our EMS system we have developed a clinical scale in an attempt to "grade" the relief of pain after analgesic use. The patient is the sole determinant of whether sufficient pain relief has occurred, and the patient's behavior is an indication of the analgesic effect of the agent used. All patients with pain are graded as follows:

Grade 0	No pain
Grade 1	Mild pain: patient calm, complains only when asked, no other signs
Grade 2	Moderate pain: patient spontaneously complains of pain, no other signs
Grade 3	Severe pain: patient groans, complains bitterly; nausea, vomiting, diaphoresis, or pallor can occur
Grade 4	Very severe pain: patient groans, writhes, weeps, or screams from pain; nausea, vomiting, diaphoresis, or pallor is usually present

SUMMARY

Unfortunately, neither experience nor research can support the recommendation of a single analgesic for the prehospital management of pain. Furthermore, the subjective nature of pain and the sometimes adverse milieu of the field confound the evaluation of any modality in the prehospital care of patients. The prehospital management of patients in pain must start with gentle handling, proper communication, and professionalism on behalf of the prehospital provider. Several analgesic agents that are currently being used or studied show promise. Whether it be for the patient with trauma, burns, or acute MI, pain relief in the field is a challenge that must be met. A great deal of research must be done to determine the best way to provide pain relief to our patients before their arrival in the emergency department.

SELECTED READING

Amey, BD, Ballinger, JA, and Harrison, EE. Prehospital administration of nitrous oxide for control of pain. *Ann Emerg Med* 10:247, 1981.

Arthurs, GJ, and Rosen, M. Self-administered intermittent nitrous oxide for analgesia for labour. *Anaesthesia* 34:301, 1979.

Baskett, PJF, and Withnell, A. Use of entonox in the ambulance service. *Br Med J* 2:41, 1970.

Baxt, WG, and Moody, P. The impact of a rotocraft aeromedical emergency care service on trauma mortality. *JAMA* 249:3047, 1983.

Bennett, RC, and Stewart, RD. Ketamine. In PM Paris and RD Stewart (eds), *Pain Management in Emergency Medicine.* Norwalk: Appleton & Lange, 1988. Pp 295–310.

Bonica, JJ. Biology, Pathophysiology, and Treatment of Acute Pain. In S Lipton and J Miles (eds), *Persistent Pain: Modern Methods of Treatment.* Orlando: Grune & Stratton, 1985. Pp. 1–30.

Caro, DB. Trial of ketamine in an accident and emergency department. *Anaesthesia* 29:227, 1972.

Cartwright, PD, and Pingel, SM. Midazolam and diazepam in ketamine anaesthesia. *Anaesthesia* 39:439, 1984.

Dailey, RH, Stone, R, and Repert, W. Ketamine dissociative anesthesia: Emergency department use in children. *JACEP* 8:57, 1979.

Dick, W, Hirlinger, WK, and Mehrkens, HH. Intramuscular ketamine: An alternative pain treatment for use in disasters? In C Manni and SI Magalini (eds), *Emergency and Disaster Medicine: Proceedings of the Third World Congress in Rome, 1983.* Berlin: Springer-Verlag, 1985. Pp 167–172.

Domino, EF, Chodoff, P, and Corssen, G. Pharmacologic effects of C 1–581, a new dissociative anesthetic in man. *Clin Pharmacol Ther* 6:279, 1965.

Donen, N, et al. Prehospital analgesia with Entonox. *Can Anaesth Soc J* 29:275, 1982.

Ersek, RA. Relief of acute musculoskeletal pain using transcutaneous electrical neurostimulators. *JACEP* 6:300, 1977.

Fischer, RP, et al. Urban helicopter response to the scene of injury. *J Trauma* 24:946, 1984.

Gal, TJ, Difazio, CA, and Moscicki, J. Analgesic and respiratory depressant activity of nalbuphine: A comparison with morphine. *Anesthesiology* 57:367, 1982.

Heckman, JD, et al. (eds): *Emergency Care and Transportation of the Sick and Injured* (4th ed). Park Ridge, IL: American Academy of Orthopaedic Surgeons, 1987.

Hustead, RF. Nitrous oxide in obstetrics. *Clin Anesthesia* 1:97, 1964.

Jaffe, JH, and Martin, WR. Opioid analgesic and antagonists. In AG Gilman et al. (eds), *The Pharmacological Basics of Therapeutics* (7th ed). New York: Macmillan, 1985. Pp 491–531.

Marks, RM, and Sachar, EJ. Undertreatment of medical inpatients with narcotic analgesics. *Ann Intern Med* 73:173, 1973.

McKinnon, KDL. Prehospital analgesia with nitrous oxide/oxygen. *Can Med Assoc J* 125:836, 1981.

Myers, RAM, Woolf, CJ, and Mitchell, D. Management of acute traumatic pain by peripheral transcutaneous electrical stimulation. *S Afr Med J* 52:309, 1977.

Nordemar, T, and Thorner, C. Treatment of acute cervical pain—a comparative study group. *Pain* 10:93, 1981.

Pantridge, JF, and Geddes, JS. A mobile intensive care unit in the management of myocardial infarction. *Lancet* 2:271, 1967.

Paris, PM, and Blenko, JW. Narcotic Agonist-Antagonist Analgesics. In PM Paris and RD Stewart (eds), *Pain Management in Emergency Medicine.* Norwalk: Appleton & Lange, 1988. Pp 157–168.

Paris, PM, et al. Transcutaneous pacing for bradyasystolic cardiac arrests in prehospital care. *Ann Emerg Med* 14:320, 1985.

Paris, PM, and Weiss, LD. Narcotic Analgesia: The Pure Agonists. In PM Paris and RD Stewart (eds), *Pain Management in Emergency Medicine.* Norwalk: Appleton & Lange, 1988. Pp 125–156.

Paris, PM, et al. A prospective prehospital trial of nitrous oxide use in urban and suburban/rural systems: A study of efficacy and side effects (abstract). *Ann Emerg Med* 17:425, 1988.

Romagnoli, A, and Keats, AS. Ceiling effect for respiratory depression by nalbuphine. *Clin Pharmacol Ther* 27:478, 1980.

Sloan, JPP, et al. Multiple rib fractures: Transcutaneous nerve stimulation versus conventional analgesia. *J Trauma* 26:1120, 1986.

Soliman, MG, Brinale, GF, and Kuster, G. Response to hypercapnia under ketamine anaesthesia. *Can Anaesth Soc J* 22:486, 1975.

Stene, JK, et al. Nalbuphine analgesia in the prehospital setting. *Am J Em Med* 6:634, 1988.

Stewart, RD. Nitrous oxide sedation/analgesia in emergency medicine. *Ann Emerg Med* 14:139, 1985.

Stewart, RD, and Heleniak, SJ. Nitrous oxide in prehospital care (letter). *JAMA* 245:1909, 1981.

Stewart, RD. Nitrous Oxide. In PM Paris and RD Stewart (eds), *Pain Management in Emergency Medicine.* Norwalk, CT: Appleton & Lange, 1987. P. 221–239.

Stewart, RD, et al. Patient controlled inhalation analgesia in prehospital care: A study of side effects and feasibility. *Crit Care Med* 11:851, 1983.

Sundin, RH, et al. Anxiolytic effects of low dosage nitrous oxide–oxygen mixtures administered continuously in apprehensive subjects. *South Med J* 74:1489, 1981.

Thal, ER, et al. Self-administered analgesia with nitrous oxide: Adjunctive aid for emergency medical care systems. *JAMA* 242:2418, 1979.

Twee, WA, Minuck, MS, and Mymin, D. Circulatory responses to ketamine anesthesia. *Anesthesiology* 37:613, 1972.

Verdile, VP, and Paris, PM. Transcutaneous Electrical Nerve Stimulation. In PM Paris and RD Stewart (eds), *Pain Management in Emergency Medicine.* Norwalk: Appleton & Lange, 1988. Pp 471–489.

Waxman, K, Shoemaker, WC, and Lippman, M. Cardiovascular effects of anesthetic induction with ketamine. *Anesth Analg* 59:355, 1980.

White, PF, Way, WL, and Trevor, AJ. Ketamine—its pharmacology and therapeutic uses. *Anesthesiology* 56:119, 1982.

White, PF, et al. Pharmacology of ketamine isomers in surgical patients. *Anesthesiology* 52:231, 1980.

Zorab, JSM, and Baskett, PJF. *Immediate Care.* London: Saunders, 1977. Pp 39–51.

C. Wounds

52. Management of Superficial Wounds

John B. Mulliken

WOUND HEALING

All fresh wounds—regardless of depth, whether open or closed—heal with the same biologic mechanism, classically divided into three phases: inflammation, fibroplasia, and maturation. The process starts with a transient reflex constriction of the local injured vessels and the first signs of *inflammatory response.* Leukocytes adhere to the injured vascular endothelium, particularly in the small venules. Retraction of severed vessels and platelet plugging initiate the hemostatic process. With the injured vessels sealed, the 5- to 10-minute period of vasoconstriction is followed by vasodilation, with increased flow and a concomitant increase in the permeability of the local venules. The endothelial cells appear to swell and pull away from the neighbors, opening gaps through which the serum enters the injured tissues. The inflammatory response is mediated by local substances within the wound. Histamine is responsible for the initial vasodilation and the early permeability changes. Hemostatic factors, released from activated platelets, kinins, complement components, and the prostaglandin system, all participate in sending control signals to initiate cellular activation. Fibronectin seems to promote the adhesion and migration of neutrophils, monocytes, fibroblasts, and endothelial cells into the wound. Although the initial wound exudate contains mainly polymorphonuclear leukocytes, these have a shorter life span than mononuclear leukocytes. In time, monocytes predominate the interstitium, and studies have shown that these cells must be present to trigger fibroblast invasion of the wound. The degree of tension set during suture placement and dressing application should be adjusted with these phenomena in mind.

The *fibroblastic phase* of wound healing actually begins during the inflammatory period. Local histocytes begin to loosen from their perivascular habitat and migrate into the wound along the strands of the recently constructed fibrin network. These activated fibroblasts extrude ground substance (glycosaminoglycans) and tiny collagen fibrils into the wound within 48 hours after injury. At the same time, there is angiogenesis, budding of nearby capillaries, and growth of new vessels into the healing matrix. This primitive capillary bed is only a microscopic finding in closed wounds, which heal *per primum.* Wounds whose edges remain open become filled with "granulation tissue," a granular-appearing bed of capillaries, ground substance, and collagen. By 7 to 10 days after injury, an open wound (providing it is not heavily contaminated with bacteria) begins to close by contraction. The end result may be contracture, a distortion or loss, or both, of function of nearby tissues.

Epithelial cells also participate in the healing process. Within 24 hours, there is mitosis and migration of epithelial cells from the wound margins and from the surviving dermal appendages. The cells migrate as epithelial sheets, flowing in the direction of cytoplasmic extensions of the cells' free edges. Epithelial migration is guided by the orientation of extracellular ground substance and fibrillar scaffolding; this migration stops as the epithelial free margins touch ("contact inhibition"). Epithelium also grows downward along the dermal puncture wounds caused by sutures. In superficial abrasions, epithelialization, both from the wound edges and adnexal structures, can cover a denuded dermal surface within 72 hours. Topical wound care and dressings should be selected to expedite this process.

Fibroplasia increases apace, yet newly formed collagen fibers contribute very little to the strength of a closed wound during the 7 to 10 days after injury. Only the fibrin network, ground substance, and epidermal continuity bind the wound together, but sutures are the mainstays of the wound's tensile strength during this early period.

By 10 days, the healing wound is increasing in tensile strength parallel to increasing collagen production. The gain in tensile strength is most rapid while the collagen-building curve is climbing. By two weeks, however, net collagen production begins to diminish and yet wound tensile strength continues to increase. This phenomenon is the result of formation of intra- and intermolecular cross-linking between collagen fibrils. A skin wound reaches 20 to 30 percent of strength by two to three weeks and 60 percent of strength by four months. Percutaneous sutures should be removed by 7 days after injury to minimize the chance of suture track scars, leaving buried sutures and maturing collagen to secure the wound.

By three weeks, the wound enters its *phase of maturation and remodeling*. Collagen synthesis and degradation are accelerated, with no net increase in collagen content. The collagen fibers, initially deposited in a haphazard fashion, gradually become more organized and arranged into a pattern determined by local mechanical forces. The intrinsic characteristics of the healing tissue and external forces, particularly motion, are well-recognized factors that modulate the collagen weave in a scar. The large numbers of new capillaries that grew into the wound begin to regress. During this phase, the scar becomes indurated, raised, and pruritic and then gradually it softens, over many months, to become pale mature scar. Although careful wound management will affect the eventual quality of a scar, the final appearance is primarily determined by the axis, extent, and location of the wound.

ASSESSMENT

The cutaneous wound usually attracts attention, as a patient is brought into the accident room; however, a detailed assessment of this wound should be deferred until the patient has been evaluated for other, more serious injuries. Lifesaving maneuvers assume first priority. To minimize further contamination, all wounds, however small, should be covered with a dressing shortly after the patient arrives in the emergency unit. If the wound is actively bleeding, a pressure dressing should be applied, held in place by elastic gauze or, if necessary, by an assistant's hand.

History

Once the patient's condition is stable, a careful history should be obtained as to the time, circumstances, and mechanisms of injury (as described in Chap. 42). This information provides clues as to possible associated injuries beyond the obvious wounds and gives indications about the extent and degree of contamination of the wound. The patient's history should also be taken, with attention to any medications or underlying medical conditions.

Examination

The protective dressing, applied to the wound shortly after admission to the accident room, should now be removed for detailed evaluation of the extent of soft-tissue injury. Sterile gloves and mask should always be worn when one examines and treats a wound. The number of observations of the wound should be restricted to minimize the chances for further contamination.

The depth of a laceration should be assessed (Fig. 52-1A), keeping in mind the possibility of injury to underlying structures, such as nerves, tendons, muscles, or bone. Different anatomic areas contain unique structures, which must always be evaluated for possible injury—for example, parotid duct, lacrimal duct, canthal tendon, and seventh cranial nerve in the face (see Chap. 56). Lacerations overlying bones should be probed with a gloved finger to determine whether a compound fracture is present. Small puncture wounds in the head-neck region and thoracoabdominal areas are managed on the premise that penetration and damage have occurred in vital deep structures. Lacerations in the extremities should be viewed as involving the underlying neurovascular structures, tendons, and muscles, until proved otherwise.

A contusion, usually caused by blunt force, is a disruption of dermal continuity, with intact overlying dermis and epidermis. Signs include swelling and ecchymosis, resulting from interstitial edema and hemorrhage, or hematoma formation can occur, with gross extravasation of blood into the subcutaneous space (see Fig. 52-1B). A contusion, like a laceration, can be associated with injury to important underlying structures.

An abrasion is caused by shearing force, with loss of epidermis and a variable thickness of dermis. The depth of an abrasion wound can be assessed by the pattern of bleeding. A deep abrasion exhibits a brisk bleeding pattern from damaged capillaries in the lower dermis (see Fig. 52-1C). Superficial abrasions, at the level of tiny capillaries in the papillary dermis, usually bleed very little.

EMERGENCY DEPARTMENT MANAGEMENT OF SUPERFICIAL WOUNDS

Before treatment of the wound is initiated, one must decide who should be responsible and whether care should be accomplished in the emergency department or in the operating room. Important considerations include the condition of the patient, type of wound, degree of contamination, possibility of damage to deep structures, and presence of associated injuries.

In general, simple and superficial wounds can usually be

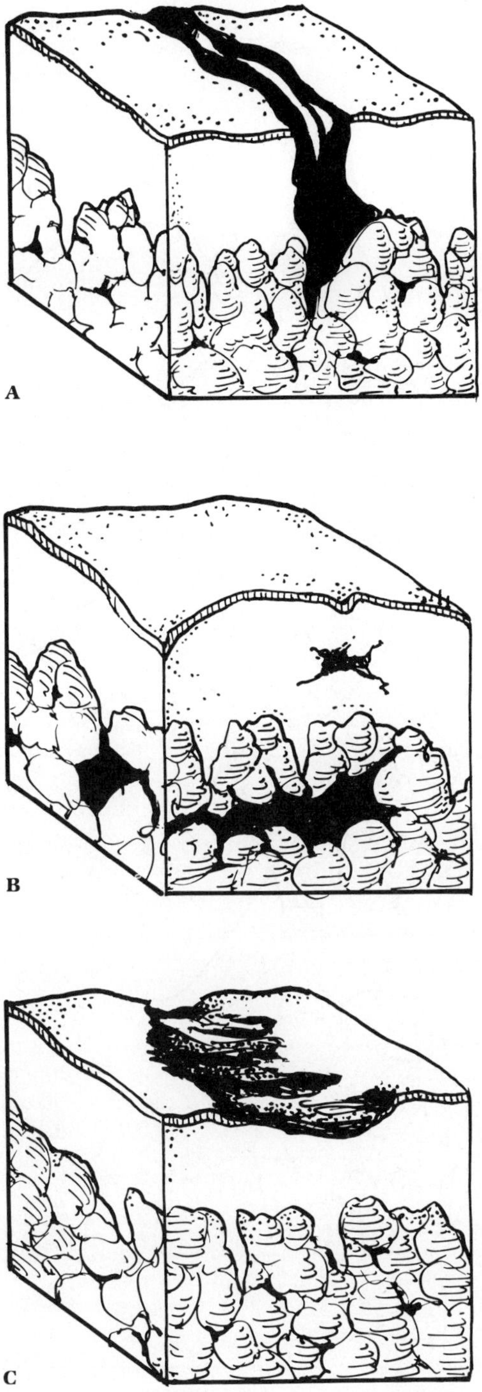

Fig. 52-1. Types of soft-tissue injury. A. Laceration. B. Contusion. C. Abrasion.

managed in the accident room. This statement also holds true for injured children, providing they can be satisfactorily premedicated. Complex wounds, such as bite or bullet injuries, or wounds in which underlying nerves, vascular structures, tendons, or bone are damaged, require admission and surgical consultation. Some avulsion wounds (in which an actual loss of tissue occurs) can be closed in a linear fashion or with a small, split-thickness skin graft by the surgeon in the emergency department; most avulsion wounds are best handled in the main operating theater.

SKIN PREPARATION

Most lacerations of the scalp or beard area are easier to manage if the hair is first clipped or shaved. The small cut hairs should not be allowed to fall into the wound, where they can act as a nidus for infection. Eyebrows should never be shaved.

Antiseptic cleansing of the skin around the wound can be done before or after the wound is anesthetized; usually, it is kinder to the patient if the anesthetic is injected before vigorous skin preparation. An antiseptic, such as 1% povidone-iodine solution or chlorhexidine, should be applied to the skin surface, taking care not to place it into the wound.

LOCAL ANESTHESIA

Local anesthesia permits proper irrigation, debridement, and closure of a wound. Xylocaine (Lidocaine), 0.5% or 1.0%, is the most useful agent. The combination solution of xylocaine and epinephrine, 1:200,000, minimizes troublesome dermal bleeding, decreases the risk of rapid absorption and xylocaine toxicity, and prolongs the anesthetic effect. The local anesthetic should not contain epinephrine when used in the digits or when used to infiltrate thin skin flaps that have a compromised blood supply.

With gloved hands, the physician should inject the local anesthetic solution through a 25- or 30-gauge needle placed through the wound surface; this is less painful than penetrating intact skin. The pain of injections is also less if one slowly infiltrates the subcutaneous layer, waits, and then injects the dermis.

DEBRIDEMENT AND IRRIGATION

Clean wounds—those with minimal tissue destruction and foreign body–bacterial contamination—do not require debridement or irrigation. Untidy wounds—those that contain dirt and other foreign material or that appear six hours or more after injury—are contaminated with bacteria. The number of bacteria, rather than the bacterial type, is the critical determinant of whether or not a wound subsequently becomes infected. The critical level of bacteria is 10^5 organisms per gram of tissue. Below this level, wounds heal, while at levels greater than 10^5 bacteria per gram of tissue, wounds are at high risk of becoming infected after closure.

Debridement, irrigation, and antibiotics all help to reduce the bacterial level of the contaminated wound. All devitalized tissue must be thoroughly excised and, for this purpose, a sharp knife is best. Irrigation reduces contamination by dislodging bacteria and foreign material. The oft-used "physiologic saline" solution is acidic and hyperchloric. Buffered Ringer's solution or commercially available balanced salt solutions—for example, Tis-U-Sol or Physiosol—are more physiologic. A 30-ml syringe fitted with a 19-gauge needle gives 7 lbs per square inch irrigation pressure. At this pressure, bacteria or particles are dislodged and not forced into the tissue.

The volume of the irrigation must be enough to dislodge the dirt and lower the concentration of bacteria. Clean wounds require little or no irrigation, whereas bite injuries and other heavily contaminated wounds can require up to a liter or more. Irrigation with topical antibacterial agents should only be considered in the management of wounds that are heavily contaminated with bacteria.

SUTURE SELECTION

Suture selection is determined by the type of wound, its location, vascularity, viability, and degree of contamination, as well as the physical and biochemical characteristics of available suture material. Absorbable sutures may be indicated for closure of the deep layers of a wound. Gut sutures, which dissolve by phagocytosis, elicit more inflammatory reaction than the synthetic, absorbable sutures, which undergo enzymatic degradation (e.g., polyglycolic acid and polyglactin 910 polymer). These synthetic braided sutures remain longer than gut sutures, although 60 to 80 percent of tensile strength is lost by two weeks. Polydioxanone is a monofilament, synthetic absorbable suture that lasts longer than the braided polymers. This material is useful in situations that require extended wound support or in a potentially infected wound, in which the monofilament suture has less tendency to harbor pathogenic bacteria.

Nonabsorbable sutures can be used in a buried position in clean wounds, particularly in the fascial layer, where it takes considerably more time for tensile strength to approach a normal level. In an effort to minimize widening of a scar, no convincing evidence has been found that dermal closure with nonabsorbable sutures offers any advantage over closure with synthetic absorbable sutures. Nonabsorbable braided sutures, particularly those made of silk, should never be used to close a wound, whether clean or contaminated. Percutaneous silk sutures left in place for over a week incite a perisuture inflammatory reaction and miniabscess formation, which are in part responsible for suture track marks. Monofilament nylon elicits a minimal inflammatory reaction, even with the ingrowth of epithelium along its suture tracks. Braided, coated nylon suture approaches the superior handling quality of silk, while possessing many of the desirable qualities of monofilament suture.

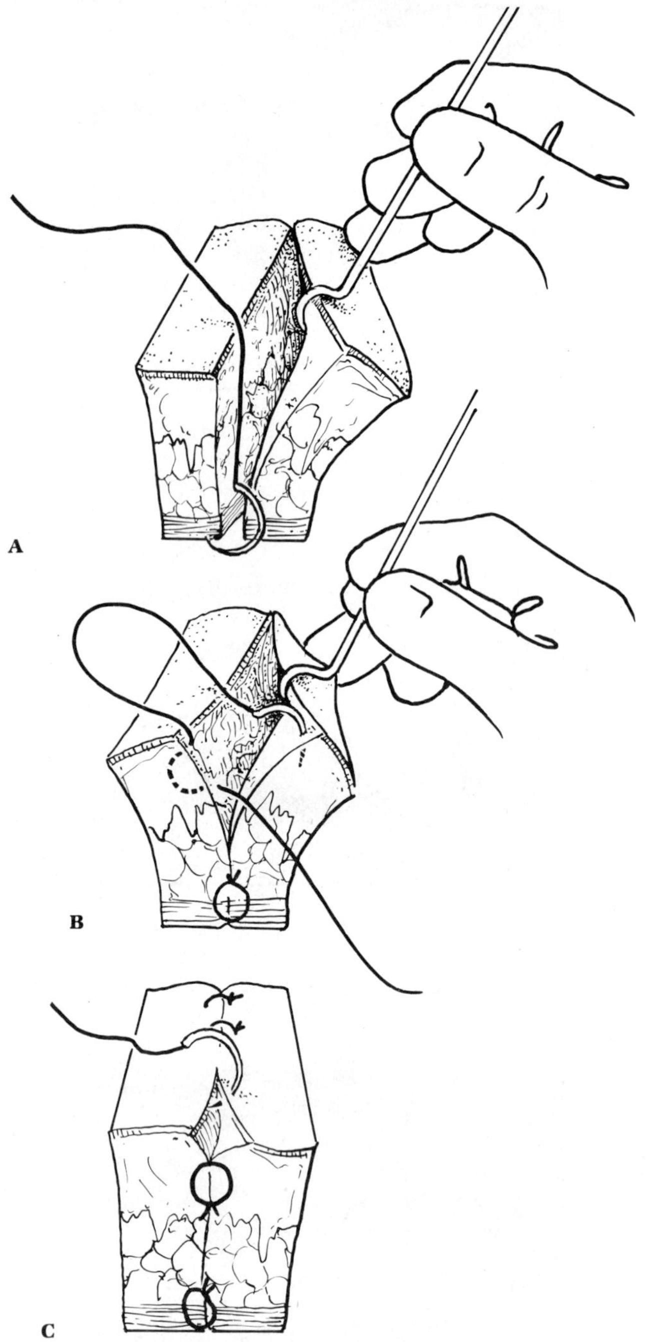

Fig. 52-2. Layered wound closure: placement of fascial (A), dermal (B), and percutaneous (C) sutures. A delicate skin hook helps to evert the wound edge and is less traumatic than forceps.

SUTURE CLOSURE OF SIMPLE WOUNDS

Before undertaking a layered closure, one must have a firm understanding of the various integumentary components and of the proper planes for inserting sutures: the fascial layers, dermis, and dermoepidermal junction. Gentleness in technique of placement is more important than suture selection. The minimum number of absorbable sutures should be used for the deep closure. The fascial layer should be approximated, with the knots tied above (Fig. 52-2A). Torn dermis retracts because of its elastic fibers and it should be definitively sutured. Dermis is the foremost layer for wound strength and its closure apposes the epidermal edges. A cutting rather than a round (taper) needle is preferred, and the knots in the dermal layer should be everted (Fig. 52-2B). Every effort should be made not to include subcutaneous tissue when placing the dermal ("subcuticular") sutures. The buried dermal suture technique is useful for reducing tension, approximating accurately, and providing immediate tensile strength to the healing wound. If the dermis is very thin (e.g., in an infant or in eyelid tissue), a vertical, buried dermal suture may be difficult to place and a horizontal insertion is acceptable. A fine skin hook facilitates placement of an everting suture of either type. In very thin tissues, particularly in recalcitrant infants, percutaneous sutures alone may have to suffice.

Dermal apposition may be so exact that tapes can then be used for epidermal approximation. However, for fine coaptation of the epidermal wound margins, some form of percutaneous suture, usually a fine monofilament nylon, is preferred (see Fig. 52-2C). If the edges are well apposed by intradermal sutures, a running suture technique saves time and simplifies removal (Fig. 52-3). A running percutaneous suture is also useful in controlling the brisk bleeding from the edges of a scalp laceration, but this technique can compromise the circulation of a more poorly vascularized wound margin in other locations. When interrupted stitches are used, each knot should be placed to one side or the other for "fine adjustment" and to aid in eversion of the wound margins. Also, with the knots to one side, less disruption of epidermis will occur when the sutures are removed. When the wound is in lax tissues that are easily approximated, one can choose a running intradermal suture closure, with either absorbable suture or monofilament "pullout" nylon (Fig. 52-3C).

Technical details of suture insertion are important at each layer (Fig. 52-4). Sutures should be placed near the cut edge to prevent strangulation of the enclosed tissue. The layers should be approximated without tension. Eversion of the skin margins is crucial to minimize the formation of a trough-like scar. Eversion is especially critical in closing wounds through anatomic margins, such as the eyelids, ears, nasal columella, and alae, to minimize the tendency for late notching. To achieve eversion of the wound edge, the needle-holder should be held in pronation so that the needle will enter at 90 degrees to the skin surface. At the other wound edge, the needle should enter the cut surface at the corresponding level and emerge equidistant from the edge at an angle of 90 degrees (see Fig. 52-2C). To be certain of the angle of entrance and exit, it is best to take separate "bites" in each wound edge rather than to penetrate both edges with a single thrust. The slight ridgelike "pouting" of the properly everted wound will smooth out with time. The goal is uniform skin eversion along the length of the wound, with minimal tension at the margins.

ADHESIVE TAPE CLOSURE

Adhesive tape closure has been used since the time of the Egyptian Middle Kingdom. Modern Steri-Strips of micropore tape can be used to approximate superficial wounds that have not extended into the subcutaneous layer and for wounds parallel to the "relaxed skin tension lines." Tape closure is particularly applicable to wounds on a flat surface and wounds with thin flaps of tissue for which suturing is difficult, particularly in children. It is sometimes difficult to obtain a fine adjustment of epidermal margins and wound-edge eversion using tape closure. Tape closure alone is unreliable for wounds in areas where there is motion. The application of tincture of benzoin to the skin improves tape adhesiveness.

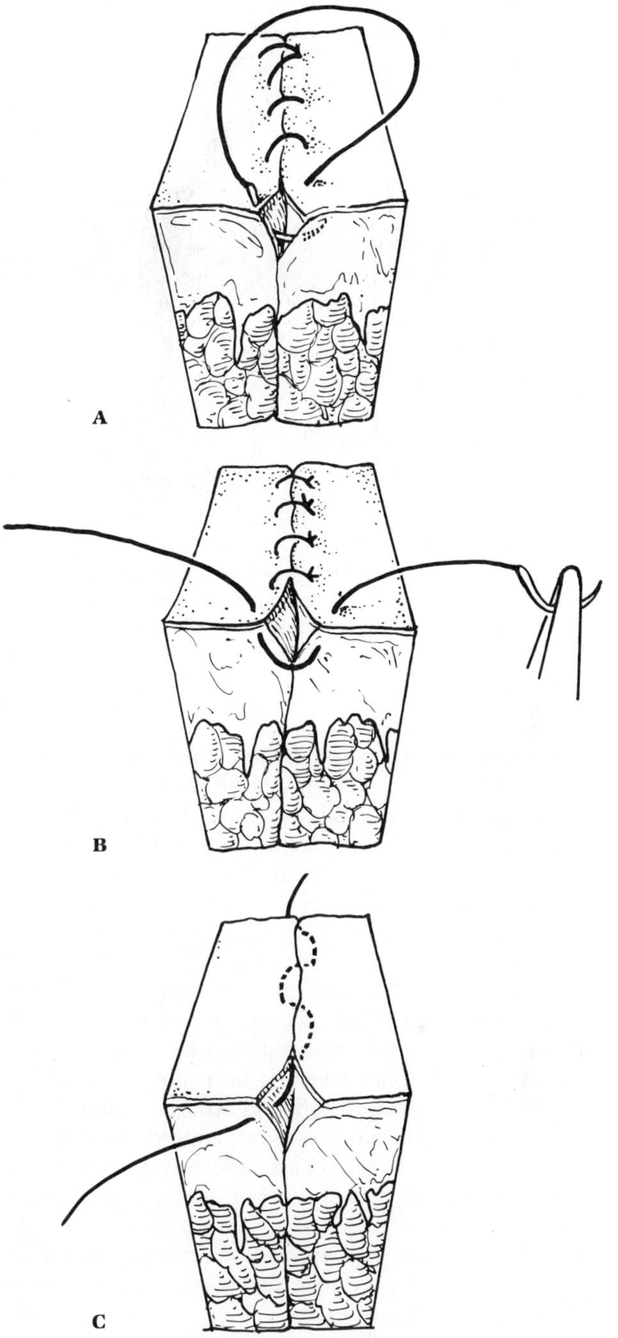

Fig. 52-3. Basic skin-closure techniques. A. Interrupted percutaneous. B. Running percutaneous (continuous). C. Running intradermal ("subcuticular").

DRESSING THE WOUND

Wound management is not complete with placement of the final suture. The dressing should be constructed in a thoughtful manner to aid the healing process. Dressings serve a number of purposes: protection, absorption, immobilization, and compression. A well-conceived and well-fashioned dressing is a reflection of the quality of wound

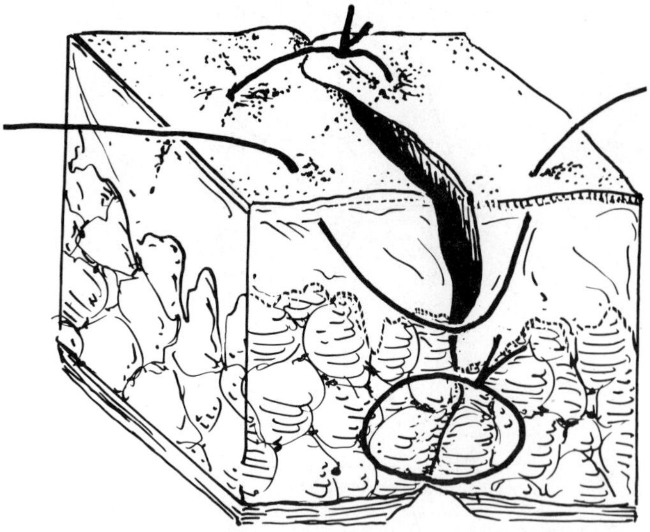

Fig. 52-4. Five common errors of suture placement: (1) failure to close fascia, (2) tight suture in subcutaneous layer, (3) improper angle of entry and exit of skin suture causing inversion of wound edges, (4) tightly tied skin suture, and (5) sutures too far from wound edge.

care and character of the physician. If the sutured wound is relatively dry, protection with a layer of transverse or longitudinal Steri-Strips may suffice. Any blood or serum that collects underneath micropore tape should be expressed to prevent pooling and maceration. A layer of tincture of benzoin helps hold the tape in place until suture removal. Tape fixation is aided by epithelial ingrowth into the micropore interstices.

Tape should not be applied over sutured wounds that ooze serosanguinous fluid. Instead, a nonadhering layer of petroleum-impregnated gauze should be chosen, followed by a layer of absorbent gauze to keep the wound dry and protected. If it is difficult to affix an absorbent dressing—for example, within the hairline—the sutured wound can be left open. Daily application of an antibacterial ointment minimizes crusting and bacterial proliferation around exposed sutures.

So-called pressure or compression dressings are difficult to achieve in practice. Gauze or cotton tends to compact, and experimental studies haye shown that pressure over a wound is quickly dissipated. A pad of polyurethane foam can provide gentle pressure to a wound for a period of time. Elastic tape or elastic cloth wraps can also provide several hours of compression; however, these techniques should be used with care in a circumferential dressing of an extremity.

CLOSURE OF COMPLEX WOUNDS

Stellate and Avulsion Wounds

Wounds in which there is actual loss of tissue (avulsions) and wounds with ragged and traumatized edges present special problems for closure in the emergency department. Wound margins that are thin, ragged, and traumatized should be conservatively trimmed. If a tattered edge is first "scored" with a sharp No. 15 blade, the compromised margin can be easily cut with fine scissors. This two-step trimming technique is more accurate than sawing the wound edge without prior scoring (Fig. 52-5). The beveled-type wound edge also deserves special consideration before suturing. With a sharply angled bevel cut, the edges should be "squared off" before closure, using the scoring technique (Fig. 52-5).

Every effort should be made to carefully align edges of a complicated skin laceration, much like fitting together pieces of a puzzle. The half-buried, horizontal, mattress suture technique is useful when approximating wound edges of which one is ischemic—for example, the distal end of a triangular flap of tissue (Fig. 52-6). The buried loop of the half-buried mattress should be placed through the dermis of the ischemic wound edge, with the knot tied loosely to minimize strangulation of the dermal plexus. It is remarkable how often the edges of a complicated stellate laceration can be neatly apposed when, initially, there appeared to be actual loss of tissue. More complicated is the avulsion wound, in which the retracted wound margins cannot be apposed without undue tension. Undermining the wound edges in the subdermal plane can be useful. However, undermining is always done with a "double-edged sword." This technique can allow a more relaxed closure; however, it also creates more potential "dead space" and can further compromise the vascularity of the elevated skin edges. Rather than resort to undermining, it is usually preferable to try to take the tension off the approximated, or near-approximated, skin margins by the proper placement of deep sutures. Most incised wounds, and some avulsion wounds, can usually be closed by appropriate suturing technique. The accident room physician should not try to get "too fancy" in attempting "plastic" surgical techniques. There is no indication for a Z-plasty flap transposition in the closure of acute wounds.

Major soft-tissue avulsion injuries will necessitate expert consultation to effect primary closure with a skin graft or flap tissue. In special instances, particularly where consultation is not available, it may be best to place an occlusive dressing over a large wound, anticipating delayed primary closure in three to five days.

Contaminated Wounds

Wounds that are seen several hours after injury or those that are heavily contaminated at the time of injury require special attention in an operating theater. The first step is sharp debridement—excision of the contaminated wound surface as well as nonviable or marginally viable tissue. The second step is irrigation of the wound. If the wound is judged to be clean, it can be closed primarily, particularly in areas where there is excellent blood supply, such as the face and scalp. The number of sutures should be kept to a minimum. Even a single extra suture can spell the difference between the development of wound sepsis and primary healing. The sutures should be absorbable, with the fewest possible knots, so as to minimize the interstices for bacterial growth and total amount of foreign material. The common practice of closing off dead space with sutures in the subcutaneous layer has been shown to potentiate sepsis in experimentally con-

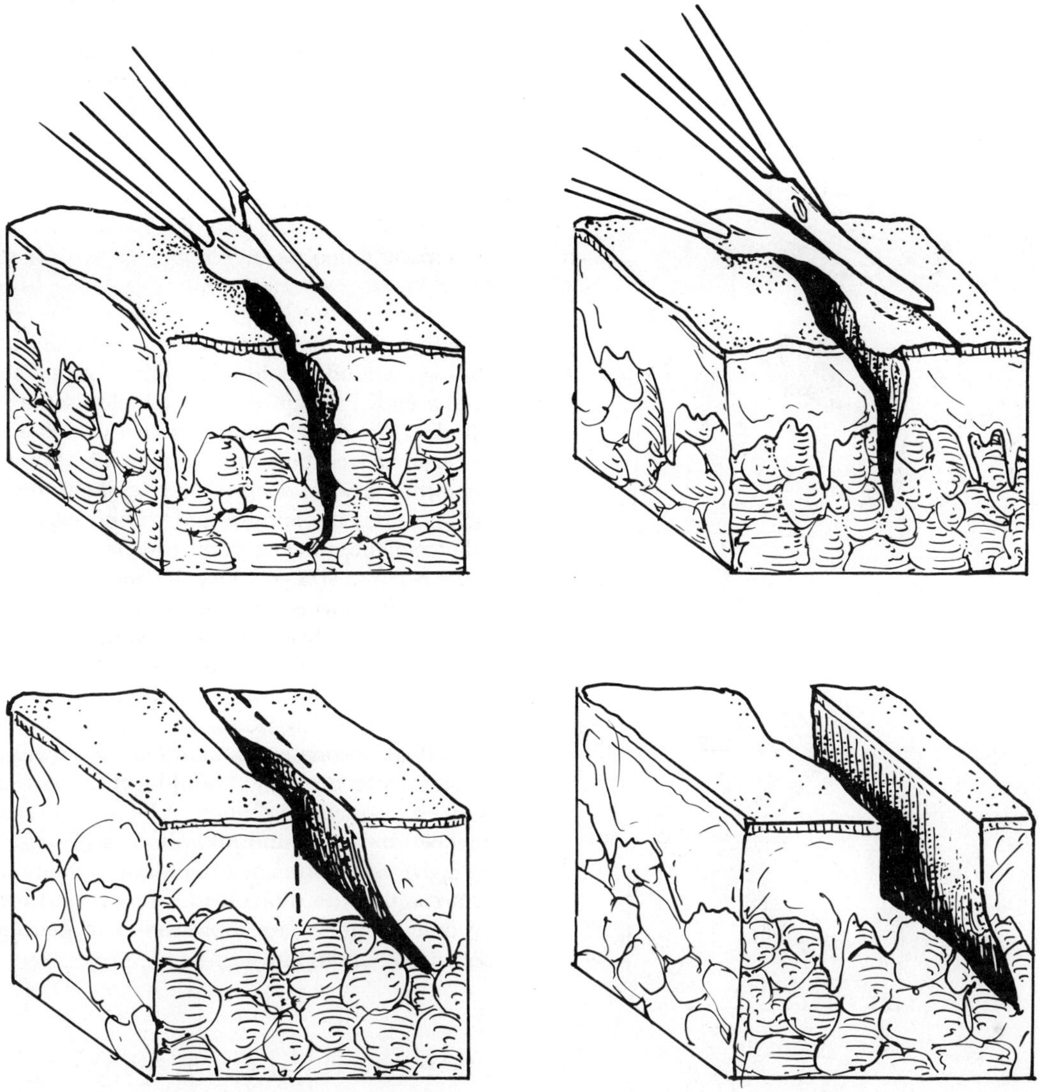

Fig. 52-5. Technique for trimming a ragged wound edge (*above*) and for squaring the edges of a beveled laceration (*below*).

taminated wounds. Preventive antibiotics are usually indicated to supplement host resistance during the crucial posttraumatic period.

If a sterile viable wound cannot be accomplished by debridement and irrigation, delayed primary closure is indicated. After initial treatment, the wound is dressed, often with a drain if equivocally viable tissue or extensive bacterial contamination is present. If the wound appears to be clean, on the second to fifth day it can be closed using an aseptic technique.

Secondary closure is reserved for wounds that manifest obvious infection at the time they are first encountered or for wounds in which sepsis develops during the program, leading to delayed primary closure. Closure is delayed until granulation tissue is well formed within the wound; this usually takes 10 days or longer. Secondary closure can be accomplished by apposition of the wound margins, with or without excision of the granulations, or by application of a thin, split-thickness skin graft to the wound bed.

CONTUSIONS

Once a possible underlying fracture or serious soft-tissue injury has been ruled out, little can be done for a contusion except to splint the area (if appropriate) and apply cold packs to minimize edema formation. If a large hematoma is present, consideration should be given to drainage. One must clearly differentiate between interstitial hemorrhage or ecchymosis (which cannot be evacuated) and true hematoma, which can de drained. Because of the excellent vascularity of scalp tissue, a cephalic hematoma is innocuous, notwithstanding its extent and the degree of tension in the overlying skin. However, even a small hematoma between skin with a poor blood supply—for example, the pretibial region or a compromised flap of tissue—should be promptly evacuated. Evidence has been found that hemoglobin is re-

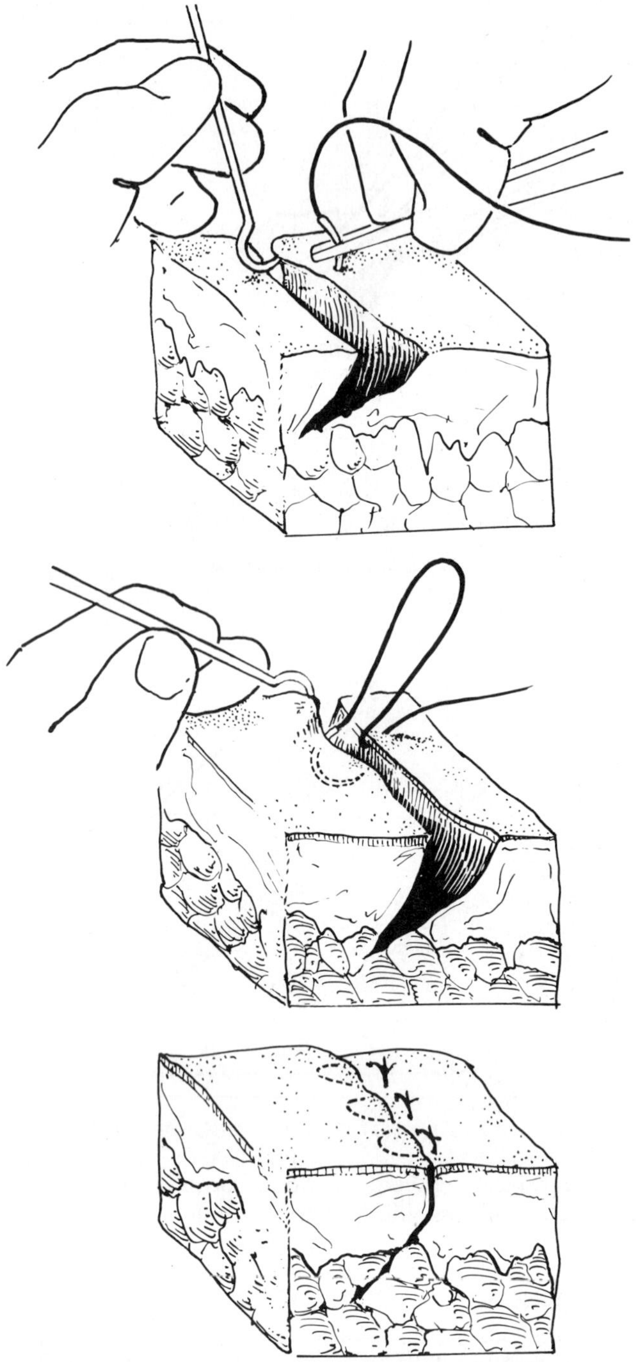

Fig. 52-6. Half-buried mattress suture, useful if there is vascular compromise of one wound edge; the knot is tied on the more healthy margin.

sponsible for generating free radicals that, in turn, cause vasoconstriction and tissue destruction. In addition, a hematoma is known to be an adjuvant in the presence of bacteria and will thus potentiate wound infection. A contused area without any skin loss may need nothing more than simple immobilization. If incision and drainage are necessary, an appropriate absorbent dressing is indicated.

ABRASIONS

Gross particulate matter in a deep abrasion must be removed. The area should be anesthetized first, and then scrubbed vigorously with a brush or the foreign material extracted with fine forceps. If necessary, loupe magnification should be utilized. If the foreign matter is not removed within a short time after the injury, the particles will become encased in the healing wound, resulting in a tattoo. Such a "traumatic tattoo" is exceedingly difficult to remove secondarily.

The proper dressing for an abrasion requires an understanding of the biology of the healing epidermal wounds. An abraded wound should heal rapidly by epidermal migration from adnexal structures (hair follicles, sebaceous and sweat glands). The dressing must protect the exposed wound surface from desiccation. If the abrasion is allowed to dry, forming a thin layer of dead dermis (eschar), the migrating epithelium from the adnexa and wound edges has to produce collagenolytic enzymes to burrow beneath this eschar to find living dermis. This prolongs the time of epithelialization and can cause a thicker scar and more prominent skin-pigment changes. If an abrasion wound is not heavily contaminated with bacteria, a petroleum dressing (e.g., Xeroform gauze) offers protection to the exposed dermis and allows maximum epithelial migration over its surface. Another gauze is needed to absorb serosanguinous drainage and minimize crusting. This dressing should be checked every two to three days for possible infection. The dressing should remain attached to the wound and allowed to separate on its own with the establishment of epidermal continuity. Abrasions in areas that are difficult to keep dressed can be managed by daily cleaning and application of petrolatum ointment containing antibiotic.

PROPHYLAXIS AGAINST TETANUS

Although clinical tetanus is rare today, it is still seen sporadically so that prevention should be considered in all major soft-tissue injuries. Prophylaxis against tetanus requires three intramuscular doses of 0.5 ml adsorbed tetanus toxoid (or as instructed on the label of the package because of product variation in antigen concentration). The second dose is given 6 to 12 months after the initial injection. A booster dose of 0.5 ml adsorbed toxoid is indicated 10 years thereafter. An anamnestic response to a booster dose can occur for as long as 25 years after active immunization, and in many patients it can last a lifetime.

A booster dose is not required for a patient with a clean minor wound, treated early, and when there is a clear history of tetanus immunization within the last 10 years. If the patient has never been immunized or if the history of immunization is unclear, a subcutaneous booster of 0.5 ml toxoid as well as 250 units of human tetanus immunoglobulin should be given. Passive immunity should also be given to patients with old major wounds that are likely to harbor clostridia. In severe neglected wounds, 500 units of tetanus immunoglobulin (human) is recommended. Penicillin prophylaxis is usually indicated for problematic wounds. In addition, removal of devitalized tissue and foreign material is a critical step in prophylaxis against tetanus.

POSTOPERATIVE CARE AND SUTURE REMOVAL

A sutured wound is effectively closed by the healing process within a few hours, while dressings provide protection, comfort, and support. Dressings applied over wounds that ooze and continue to drain after the closure should be changed frequently. If the wound was contaminated before debridement and closure, the dressing should be removed so that the wound can be examined for possible infection at 48 hours. Most dressings usually serve little purpose after 24 to 48 hours; thereafter, the uncovered sutured wound can be cleaned with soap and water. No evidence has been found that getting the sutures wet potentiates wound infection. An occlusion dressing over an abrasion wound should be periodically examined but allowed to separate naturally with epithelialization.

To minimize the formation of suture track scars, percutaneous sutures should be removed by the seventh postoperative day. The timing of suture removal depends on the integrity of the dermal closure and the degree of motion and healing characteristics of the particular body region. For example, sutures in an extremity should remain for 10 days or more unless dermal closure is secure and prolonged splinting is necessary. In the face, with its excellent vascularity and healing, sutures can be removed earlier, usually in 3 to 5 days.

The cut suture should be extracted toward the wound. When withdrawing a percutaneous running suture, one should not pull the exposed portion of a "stitch" into the suture sinus track. When removing interrupted sutures, one should check to be certain that one end of the loop is longer than the other, indicating that the entire suture is out (Fig. 52-7). A one-week-old wound is at less than 10 percent of tensile strength; therefore, Steri-Strips should be applied for another one to two weeks, or even longer, for support and protection and also to minimize scar hypertrophy and widening.

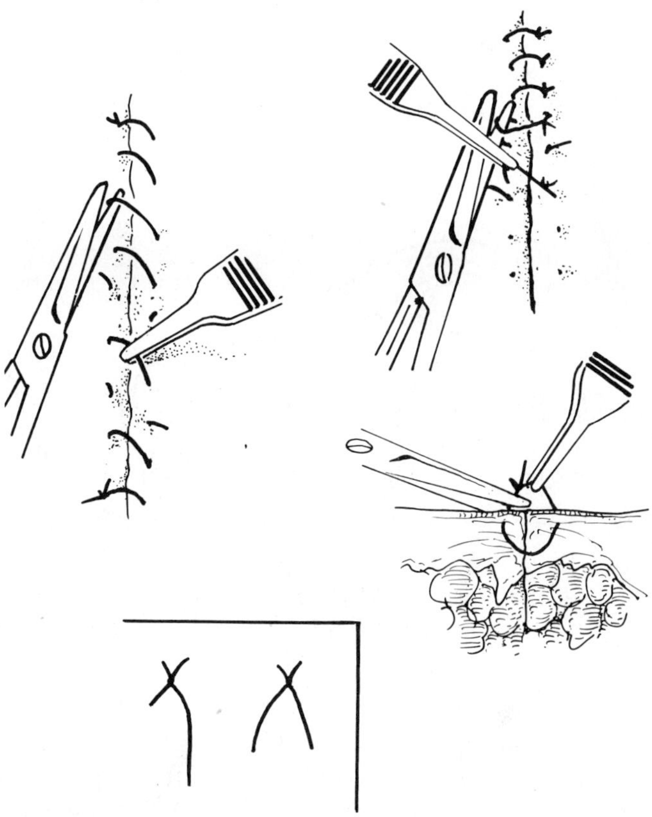

Fig. 52-7. To remove a continuous suture, every other loop is cut. With an interrupted closure, each cut suture should be pulled toward the young wound. The cut suture should be checked for unequal tails, signifying complete removal of the buried portion (*inset*).

SCAR PROGNOSIS

After the wound is repaired, the patient or relatives usually ask, "Will there be a scar?" It is important to emphasize that there will, indeed, be a scar whenever the dermal layer has been breached. The emergency physician should prepare the patient for the expected degree of scarring.

The factors that determine prognosis for the scar are: (1) age of the patient, (2) race, (3) type of injury, (4) location of injury, (5) course of wound healing, and (6) psychological reaction. Lacerations in children less than 1 year of age and in patients over age 60 tend to leave fine scars. Patients with dark skin have a tendency to scar pigmentation, hypertrophic scarring, and possible keloid formation. A true keloid is defined as a heavy scar that extends beyond the confines of the original wound and rarely regresses. A hypertrophic scar is also heavy but does not go beyond the confines of the original wound and improves with time. However, the most important factors in scar prognosis are the type of injury (i.e., the extent of tissue damage and propensity for sepsis) and the location of injury. Wounds with tissue loss and wounds that become infected usually result in prominent scarring. There are regional predispositions to heavy scarring and keloid formation—for example, the anterior chest, shoulders, and ear lobules. Lacerations that parallel the "relaxed skin tension lines" of the face and body tend to close under minimal tension and generally heal with fine scars (Fig. 52-8). Wounds that cross the relaxed skin tension lines or those that cross areas of joint motion—for example, flexion creases—tend to heal with hypertrophic scars and scar contracture.

The technical aspects of wound management, emphasized in this chapter, are also important in scar prognosis. Proper wound management is critical to minimizing the possibility of wound sepsis. Another important determinant in scar prognosis is the patient's perception of the injury. Thus, in addition to wound care, the emergency physician should provide counsel to the patient and family in an effort to minimize anxiety and prevent false expectations.

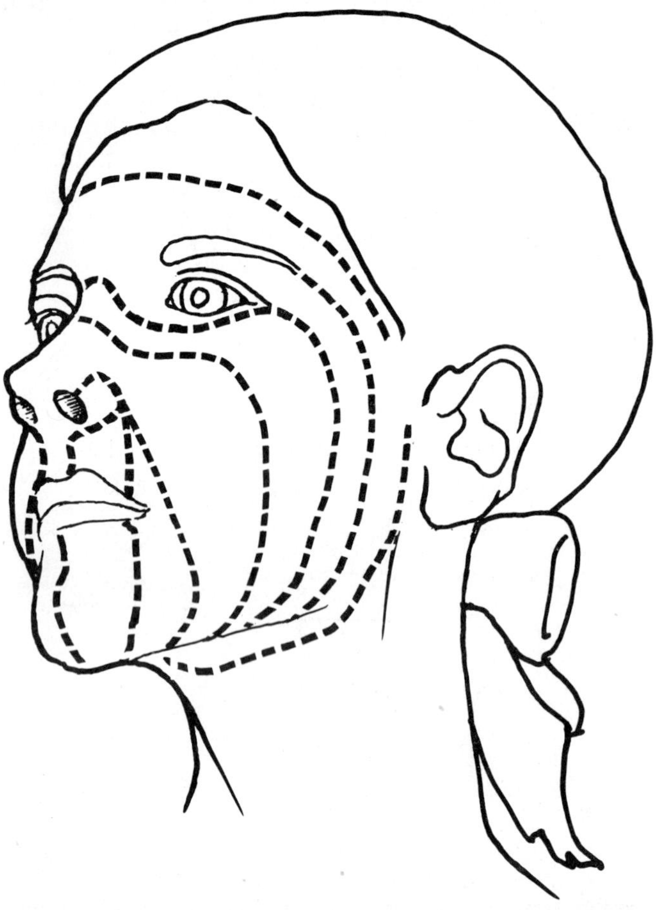

Fig. 52-8. Relaxed skin tension lines (RSTL) of the face; in most instances, they follow wrinkle lines at a right angle to the muscles of facial expression. Lacerations parallel to these lines tend to heal with finer scars than those at right angles to the RSTL.

BITE WOUNDS

Human Bites

Human bite wounds often have an interesting sociologic background. The embarrassed recipient may be reluctant to come to the emergency department. As a result, human bite wounds are frequently seen days after the injury, after home remedies have failed and the wound is infected.

The treatment of human bite injuries depends on the type of wound, location, and time that has elapsed since the occurrence. Human bites can be of a penetrating or avulsive type or a combination. The hallmarks of successful therapy are copious cleaning of the wound and aggressive debridement of damaged tissue and removal of foreign material. With such an approach, some human bite wounds of the face can be closed and will heal *per primum.* A few carefully placed skin sutures are used to anatomically approximate wounds of the nose, eyelids, ears, or lips. On the other hand, wound sepsis is a frequent occurrence after human bites, particularly in the extremities, where the blood supply is not as abundant as in the facial region. Therefore, as a general rule, most human bite wounds should be cleaned, debrided, and covered with a dressing, but not sutured.

Human bite wounds of the upper extremities are particularly worrisome. The patient frequently will prevaricate regarding the circumstances of the injury. Typical locations are the skin over the metacarpophalangeal joints and fingers. These are usually puncture-type wounds, with penetration of the underlying joint space or bone; deep sepsis, tenosynovitis, and even osteomyelitis can result. This injury requires exploration and debridement in the operating room.

Human saliva is filled with a variety of organisms in the concentration of 10^7 bacteria per milliliter, mostly streptococci, *Veillonella,* and fusobacteria. Transient flora, present only intermittently, include staphylococci, *Escherichia coli, Pseudomonas aeruginosa, Eikenella corrodens,* and other coliforms. Notwithstanding the wide variety of microorganisms in contaminating saliva, the most common human bite wound infections occur with streptococcus and penicillin-resistant *Staphylococcus aureus.* Therefore, prophylactic antibiotics should be selected with these specific bacteria in mind (see Chap. 94).

Time is an important factor in the management of human bite wounds, since many patients come to the physician several days after injury. At this stage one must consider incision and drainage of loculated pus, dressings, strict immobilization, and elevation of the extremity, along with systemic antibiotics.

Animal Bites

Only individuals with serious animal bite wounds and litigious recipients come to an emergency unit for treatment. All animal bites are reportable by law. They should be considered in the same category as human bites, with an added potential serious problem—rabies.

Dog Bites

There is indeed some truth in the old maxim, "clean as a hound's tooth." Nevertheless, dog bite wounds must be well irrigated and thoroughly debrided if primary healing is to be expected. The cheek region is a typical location for a dog bite. Although there may appear to be a number of small puncture wounds, on close inspection a large subcutaneous "dead space" is found below the facial skin. This is the result of a shearing pull of the skin away from the underlying aponeurotic fascia. If such a cavity is present, a drain should be placed and brought out through one of the wounds. Occasionally, leakage from a bite wound of the parotid area or its duct will occur (see Chap. 56).

The traumatized edges of a dog bite wound can be trimmed for 1 to 2 mm by a skilled operator. This will remove damaged tissue along with contaminating bacteria. Puncture-type wounds and most dog bite wounds of the extremities should not be sutured. However, with proper wound cleaning, most bites of the facial area can be closed using a minimum number of sutures and micropore tapes. Antibiotics are given routinely; the bacteria in dogs' saliva are sensitive to penicillin. Tetanus prophylaxis should be given to all patients who have been bitten by dogs or other animals.

RABIES. The rare but potentially most dangerous complication of any dog bite is rabies. Knowledge of the biting animal's health is extremely important. If this is unknown, the treating physician is faced with the decision of whether to begin rabies vaccination. Moreover, a rabid dog can be infectious several days before symptoms appear. Therefore, the best policy is to be certain that the animal is confined for observation before antirabies treatment is initiated.

If the confined animal appears healthy, treatment need not be initiated unless signs of rabies develop in the patient, usually within five days of the exposure. If the animal is rabid, or the animal has escaped and the signs in the patient suggest rabies, treatment should be started immediately. There are two methods of treatment: vaccination with duck embryo vaccine and antirabies immune globulin. Duck embryo rabies vaccine produces antibodies by the tenth day; therefore, it is useful in cases in which the incubation period is longer than three weeks. For immediate therapy, when the incubation period is short, passive immunity is confirmed using human antirabies immune globulin. It is given in a single dose, 20 IU/kg. Half of the injection should be infiltrated around the site of injury when feasible, and the remainder is given intramuscularly in the buttocks. The duck embryo vaccine is given in twenty-three 1-ml doses, starting the day that the antirabies serum is given. First, 21 daily doses are given, followed by a 1-ml booster dose at 10 and 21 days after completion of the series. The vaccine should be injected subcutaneously, rotating sites about the trunk and lateral thighs. Therapy can be discontinued if the laboratory examination of the animal shows negative results. Fortunately, only 100 cases of confirmed rabies are reported each year in the United States.

Cat Bites

Cat bites and scratches often become infected. Because of their cleanliness, cats harbor large numbers of bacteria in their mouths. Cat wounds should be cleaned and topical antibacterial ointment applied. *Pasteurella multocida* is a small gram-negative staining rod, a common pathogen in cat as well as dog bites; it is sensitive to penicillin or tetracycline. Preventive antibiotics should be given to a patient with a deep cat scratch or bite wound.

SELECTED READING

Alexander, JW, Kaplan, JA, and Altemeir, WA. Role of suture materials in the development of wound infection. *Ann Surg* 165:192, 1965.

Angel, MF, et al. The etiologic role of free radicals in hematoma-induced flap necrosis. *Plast Reconstr Surg* 77:795, 1986.

Bilos, ZJ, Kucharchuk, A, and Metzger, W. *Eikenella corrodens* in human bites. *Clin Orthop* 134:320, 1978.

Bodvall, B, and Rais, O. Effects of infiltration anaesthesia on the healing of incisions in traumatized and non-traumatized tissues. *Acta Chir Scand* 123:83, 1962.

Borges, AF. Scar prognosis of wounds. *Br J Plast Surg* 13:47, 1960.

Brown, LL, et al. Evaluation of wound irrigation by pulsatile jet and conventional methods. *Ann Surg* 187:170, 1978.

Callahan, M. Prophylactic antibiotics in common dog bite wounds: A controlled study. *Ann Emerg Med* 9:410, 1980.

Conolly, WB, et al. Clinical comparison of surgical wounds closed by suture and adhesive tapes. *Am J Surg* 117:318, 1969.

Craig, PH, et al. A biologic comparison of polyglactin 910 and polyglycolic acid synthetic absorbable sutures. *Surg Gynecol Obstet* 141:1, 1975.

Criklair, G. Skin suture marks. *Am J Surg* 96:631, 1958.

Edlich, RF, et al. Physical and chemical configuration of sutures in the development of surgical infection. *Ann Surg* 177:679, 1973.

Forrester, JC, et al. Wolff's law in relation to the healing skin wound. *J Trauma* 10:770, 1970.

Francis, DP, Holmes, MA, and Brandon, G. *Pasteurella multocida* infections after domestic animal bites and scratches. *JAMA* 233: 42, 1975.

Gillman, T, and Penn, J. Studies on the repair of cutaneous wounds. *Med Proc* 2 (Suppl):121, 1956.

Gross, A, Cutright, DE, and Bhaskar, SN. Effectiveness of pulsating water jet lavage in treatment of contaminated crush wounds. *Am J Surg* 124:373, 1972.

Guba, AM, Jr, Mulliken, JB, and Hoopes, JE. The selection of antibiotics for human bites of the hand. *Plast Reconstr Surg* 56:538, 1975.

Haury, B, et al. Debridement: An essential component of traumatic wound care. *Am J Surg* 135:238, 1978.

Holmlund, DEW. Physical properties of surgical suture materials: Stress-strain relationship, stress-relaxation and irreversible elongation. *Ann Surg* 184:189, 1976.

Krizek, TJ, and Davis, JH. The role of the red cell in subcutaneous infection. *J Trauma* 5:85, 1965.

Krizek, TJ, and Robson, MC. Evolution of quantitative bacteriology in wound management. *Am J Surg* 130:579, 1975.

Levenson, SM, et al. The healing of rat skin wounds. *Ann Surg* 161:293, 1965.

Magee, C, et al. A rapid technique for quantitating wound bacterial count. *Am J Surg* 133:760, 1977.

Malinowski, RW, et al. The management of human bite injuries of the hand. *J Trauma* 19:655, 1979.

McGregor, IA. *Fundamental Techniques of Plastic Surgery* (8th ed). Baltimore: Williams & Wilkins, 1989.

Mulliken, JB, and Healy, NA. Pathogenesis of skin flap necrosis from underlying hematoma. *Plast Reconstr Surg* 63:540, 1979.

Mulliken, JB, Healy, NA, and Glowacki, J. Povidone-iodine and tensile strength in wounds in rats. *J Trauma* 20:323, 1980.

Peacock, EE, Jr. *Wound Repair* (3rd ed). Philadelphia: Saunders, 1984.

Peeples, E, Bostwick, JA, Jr, and Scott, FA. Wounds of the hand contaminated by human or animal saliva. *J Trauma* 20:383, 1980.

Postelthwait, RW, Willigan, DA, and Ulin, AW. Human tissue reactions to sutures. *Ann Surg* 181:144, 1975.

Robinson, DA. Dog bites and rabies: An assessment of risk. *Br Med J* 1:1066, 1976.

Rodeheaver, G, et al. Identification of wound infection potentiating factors in soil. *Am J Surg* 128:8, 1974.

Rodeheaver, G, et al. Wound cleaning by high pressure irrigation. *SG & O* 141:357, 1975.

Rovee, DT, and Miller, CA. Epidermal role in the breaking strength of wounds. *Arch Surg* 96:43, 1968.

Schauerhamer, RA, et al. Studies in the management of the contaminated wound. VII. Susceptibility of surgical wounds to postoperative surface contamination. *Am J Surg* 122:74, 1971.

Schultz, RC, and McMaster, WC. The treatment of dog bite injuries, especially those of the face. *Plast Reconstr Surg* 49:494, 1972.

Tindall, J, and Harrison, C. *Pasteurella multocida* infections following animal injuries, especially cat bites. *Arch Dermatol* 105:412, 1972.

Van Winkle, W, Jr, and Hastings, JC. Consideration in the choice of suture materials for various tissues. *Surg Gynecol Obstet* 135:113, 1972.

Van Winkle, W, Jr, et al. Effect of suture materials on healing skin wounds. *Surg Gynecol Obstet* 140:7, 1975.

Wheeler, CB, et al. Side effects of high pressure irrigation. *SG & O* 143:775, 1976.

Zook, EG, et al. Successful treatment protocol for canine fang injuries. *J Trauma* 20:243, 1980.

53. Deep Wounds: Vascular Injuries

Michael Sobel
John J. Skillman

ARTERIAL RESPONSES TO INJURY

Mechanisms of Injury

Penetrating wounds in a civilian setting are chiefly caused by a low-velocity bullet or shotgun, knife, or a miscellany of other penetrating objects. The tissue injury caused by a bullet depends on the energy forces imparted by the bullet, which are a function of mass and velocity. Because of the relatively low velocity of handguns, tissue injuries they cause are usually limited to a narrow tract surrounding the path of the bullet. High-velocity rifle wounds transfer much greater force to the tissues, producing an expanding swath of tissue destruction that may not be apparent from the entry wound. Blast and shotgun wounds at closer range can produce large soft-tissue defects at the surface of impact. Nerves, arteries, and veins can be injured by direct impact or by the concussive shock wave of the passing bullet. When a bullet impacts bone, secondary missiles of bony fragments can cause additional tissue and vascular injury.

Blunt injuries can also cause significant deeper tissue injury. The thoracic aorta and renal arteries can be disrupted by the forces of severe deceleration. Crush forces are less selective, injuring nerves, muscles, and blood vessels. Fractures and dislocations can frequently injure arteries and veins, both by torsion and by direct injury from fracture fragments.

Vasospasm

The smooth muscle of the normal arterial wall responds to external or luminal injury by vasoconstriction. Arterial injuries that produce complete disruption of the arterial wall may manifest little hemorrhage because of this effective but temporary adaptation by the artery. In contrast, vasoconstriction alone rarely if ever causes the loss of pulses or critical ischemia in the trauma patient. When ischemia is present, a direct vascular injury should always be sought.

Thrombus Formation at Sites of Intimal Injury

Either penetrating or blunt trauma can disrupt the arterial intima, exposing subendothelial tissues on which platelets and fibrin clot accumulate. The growth of the luminal thrombus is determined by the degree of intimal injury and the velocity of local blood flow. The injury can lead to immediate or delayed arterial occlusion, depending on the diameter of the vessel and associated vasospasm. The presence of normal distal perfusion at the time of trauma does not rule out a nonocclusive arterial injury, which can ultimately result in thrombosis, bleeding, or embolism.

Manifestations of Arterial Injury

Bleeding and thrombosis are the most common consequences of major arterial injury. A persistent hole in the artery can produce the symptom of pulsatile hematoma or false aneurysm, contained by the surrounded subcutaneous tissues and fascia. Venous and arterial injuries in close proximity can result in an arteriovenous fistula, usually in association with a false aneurysm. Ischemia from thrombosis can be subtle or profound, depending on the anatomic location of the injury and the extent of the collateral circulation. After brachial artery thrombosis, the hand may appear warm and well perfused, while acute popliteal artery thrombosis almost uniformly produces limb-threatening ischemia. Differences in the extent of ischemia depend on the extent of preformed collateral arterial vessels.

GENERAL PRINCIPLES OF CLINICAL EVALUATION

Although serious vascular injuries frequently rank high in priority for treatment, all trauma patients should be given a comprehensive assessment aimed at stabilization and identification of the most urgent problems. When possible, one should avoid placing intravenous cannulae in injured extremities or at sites where surgical incisions may be necessary. The history and physical examination should assess both the wound itself and the vascular tree.

History

A careful history as to the circumstances and force of injury is important. The greater the force of impact and the faster the velocity and momentum of the missile, the more likely is there to be major destruction of soft tissues, nerves, and vessels. Major trauma to the sternum or cervical spine and dislocations and fractures about the elbow and knee should alert the emergency physician to the presence of potential blunt vascular injuries. Deep wounds frequently involve simultaneous injuries to major arteries and nerves. Precise timing of the age of the injury will be important in assessing the urgency of vascular repair of an ischemic extremity. Irreversible neuromuscular damage begins after four to six hours of ischemia to the extremities. The patient's age and previous vascular history provide important clues as to the presence of preexisting atherosclerotic occlusive disease.

Physical Examination

A complete but expeditious vascular examination should involve palpation of all accessible pulses (including the abdominal aorta), assessment of capillary refilling of fingers and toes, and measurement of the blood pressure in both arms. The degree of clinical ischemia can be determined by the presence or absence of pallor and by the impairment of neuromuscular function. Focusing on the suspected areas of injury, one should inspect for puncture wounds, hematomas (pulsatile?) and bleeding, and auscultate for bruits or the machinery murmur of an arteriovenous fistula. In blunt trauma the intact skin can hide evidence of a more severe underlying soft-tissue or nerve injury. It is important to perform a complete assessment of motor and sensory function to detect peripheral nerve injuries. A diligent search should be made for all entry and exit wounds.

Diagnostic Testing

Plain X-Rays

Plain X-rays are indicated to document fractures and dislocations and to identify bullets and other foreign bodies. All bullets should be accounted for by X-rays and by a tally of entry and exit wounds. Bullet trajectories under the skin are unpredictable. Bullets themselves can embolize once they are inside the vascular tree.

Doppler Ultrasound

Using a hand-held Doppler ultrasound device and a sphygmomanometer, the systolic blood pressure can be objectively measured in most injured extremities. The ratio of systolic pressure in the index extremity to a normal arm should be between 0.9 and 1.0. Ratios less than 0.5 or absolute systolic pressures lower than 55 to 60 mm Hg suggest critical ischemia. The presence of normal arterial signals and normal pressures, however, do not rule out the possibility of a significant but nonocclusive vascular injury.

Angiography

Controversy still surrounds the indications for and timing of angiography in vascular trauma. The standard, accepted indications remain bleeding, ischemia or loss of distal pulses, arteriovenous fistula, and proximity of the injury to major vessels. However, the nature and age of the injury, the patient's condition, and an institution's facilities are such important variables that it is difficult to generalize policies for angiography. The purposes of angiography are to identify injuries that may be occult and to delineate the vascular injury and adjacent anatomy. The first purpose is best served in patients with suspected but unproven vascular injuries for whom a normal arteriogram would obviate unnecessary surgery. The second purpose is best served when the techniques of surgical exposure are complex and dependent on the exact site of injury (e.g., subclavian artery, aortic arch), or when injury is complicated by preexisting vascular disease. These variables emphasize the importance of close consultation between vascular surgeons and radiologists early in the care of patients with suspected vascular injuries.

DIAGNOSIS AND TREATMENT OF SPECIFIC VASCULAR INJURIES

Torso Injuries

Penetrating or blunt injuries of the chest, abdomen, and neck frequently produce multiple internal injuries, including those to major blood vessels. Preoperatively, it is difficult to distinguish isolated vascular injuries from those of visceral organs. Therefore, the evaluation of vascular injuries in these areas should be considered as part of the overall assessment of these complex anatomic sites (see later sections of this chapter).

Extremity Injuries

In contrast to abdominal injuries, vascular wounds of the extremities lend themselves to a more focused evaluation. Not only are there unique physical findings and diagnostic tools, but also the injuries are less often immediately life threatening, allowing time for a more complete vascular assessment.

Penetrating Wounds
Care of major wounds should be managed by a qualified surgeon. All penetrating wounds should be considered contaminated or dirty, according to the missile and method of injury. Therefore, prompt antibiotic prophylaxis, wound cleaning, and debridement are indicated. This wound care is often best accomplished in the operating room. The entrance site of bullet wounds should be debrided back to clean healthy skin, leaving a larger wound that is wide open for drainage. Stab wounds should not be sutured closed if their depth exceeds their width, although exceptions can be made for facial injuries. The role of drains is controversial, as they do not provide hemostasis and are a two-way street for later bacterial contamination. When major bacterial contamination has occurred, delayed primary closure may be preferable.

Major bleeding from wounds should be controlled by direct compression. Tourniquets may have a limited role in cases of near-amputation where direct pressure is not feasible. If the penetrating object (knife, spear, and so forth) is still in place, it should be removed in the operating room when a full surgical team is assembled.

A major vascular injury may be obvious: an expanding pulsatile hematoma, brisk arterial bleeding, an arteriovenous fistula, or loss of distal pulses (Fig. 53-1). For obvious vascular injuries, expeditious preparations for operation should be made. In such cases, many vascular surgeons will proceed directly to surgical exploration for repair of arterial and venous injuries. Preoperative diagnostic arteriography may not be needed, although intraoperative and completion angiography is commonly employed. Stab wounds can frequently be repaired by direct suture of the injured vessel, while gunshot injuries may require interposition bypass grafts because of the extent of vessel destruction. Autogenous saphenous vein is the graft of choice, preferably taken from an uninjured limb.

Angiography is very helpful when a vascular injury is suspected but not proved. Many trauma centers advocate routine biplane angiography when the penetrating wound is in proximity to major vessels. Bullet or knife wounds can produce intimal injury, hematoma of the vessel wall, or even complete transection of the vessel, and yet distal pulses may be present. Missed injuries can result in late thrombosis, embolism, or chronic false aneurysm formation that require more extensive corrective surgery. Normal results on arteriography will effectively rule out major vascular injury. In spite of the risks of occult vascular injuries, more recent experience suggests that careful observation and followup can safely supplant arteriography in selected cases.

Patients with preexisting atherosclerotic occlusive disease present a special problem: Their distal pulses may be chronically absent, and their occlusive disease may require more complex surgical procedures to restore normal circulation.

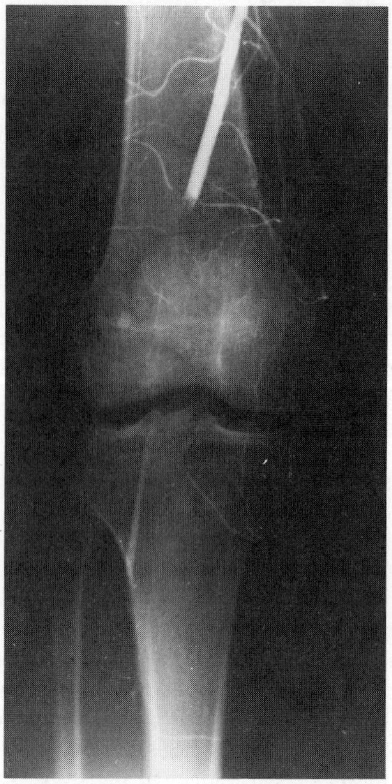

Fig. 53-1. Popliteal artery occlusion from gunshot wound. An arteriogram shows that the popliteal artery is occluded. At surgical exploration both the popliteal artery and vein were found to be completely transected.

Arteriography is especially helpful in delineating the abnormal anatomy and planning vascular reconstruction.

Blunt Injuries
When major nonpenetrating forces are applied to an extremity, complex injuries involving muscles, nerves, bones, and blood vessels can result. The classic physical signs and symptoms of ischemia can be obscured by the associated injuries. Pain can be severe or diminished, depending on the relative damage to sensory nerves. There may be swelling and hematoma formation from bleeding muscles and bones. Fractures can impair active range of motion and diminish the examiner's ability to assess neuromuscular function.

There are three keys to the early identification of major vascular injuries in blunt trauma of the extremity: absence of pulses, diminished Doppler pressures, and a high index of suspicion in fracture-dislocations about the knee and elbow (Figs. 53-2 and 53-3). Reversible compromise of the distal arterial circulation can occur in compartment syndromes (see Chap. 73), or when the arteries are compressed or twisted by fracture-dislocations. These causes for ischemia should be considered diagnoses of exclusion, however. If normal pulses and perfusion do not return after fasciotomy or reduction of the fracture or dislocation, arteriography should be performed. The anatomic course of the popliteal artery makes it especially prone to injury during posterior dislocation of the knee (30% of cases). Distal pulses may

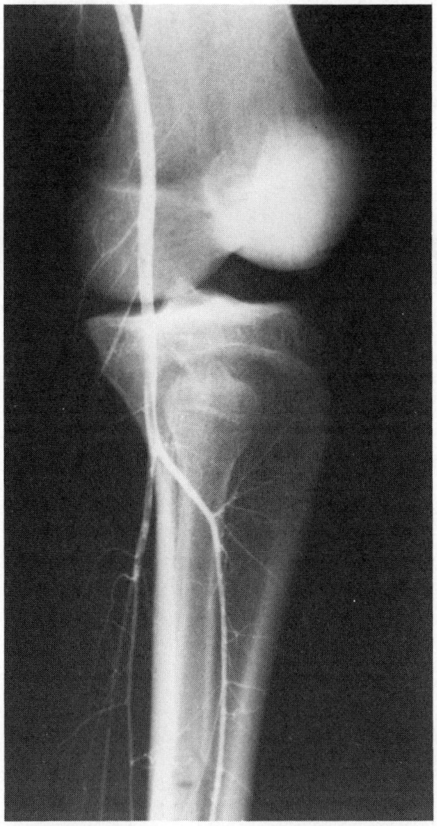

Fig. 53-2. Popliteal artery injury from knee dislocation. This angiogram shows an intraluminal thrombus extending down the tibioperoneal trunk from the site of intimal injury just above the joint. This patient had palpable pulses after reduction of the dislocation.

be present initially, because the vascular injury begins as a nonocclusive tear in the intima. Because of the high rate of limb loss with missed injuries, arteriography is indicated in all patients with knee dislocation, regardless of the status of their pulses (see Fig. 53-2). Diagnostic angiography should also be used liberally in patients with unstable knee joints when the force and mode of injury suggest that the joint may have dislocated and spontaneously reduced.

Pelvic Fractures

Pelvic fractures can cause bleeding from bone, pelvic and sacral veins, and the hypogastric, sacral, and gluteal arteries. Patients with less severe pelvic fractures can lose 2 to 4 units of blood, while those with major injuries are hemodynamically unstable at presentation and can lose 10 to 20 units of blood. Prompt resuscitation with fluid and blood is essential to restore hemodynamic stability. A pneumatic antishock suit (MAST) can be immediately beneficial. While pelvic venous hemorrhage will frequently tamponade, significant arterial injuries may not. When there is persistent pelvic hemorrhage, external pelvic fixation or angiographic embolization of bleeding arteries, or both, can be lifesaving.

Venous Injuries

In penetrating trauma, venous injuries frequently accompany major arterial injuries, and concomitant surgical venous repair is generally advocated. However, if arterial injury or bleeding does not call for surgical exploration, diagnostic venous studies (constant venography or noninvasive testing) are usually not pursued acutely. Isolated surgical venous repair is rarely indicated, because of a lack of proven efficacy in preventing venous thrombosis. All patients with lower-extremity trauma, penetrating or blunt, are very prone to the development of deep venous thrombosis. Even when no direct venous injury is present, silent venous thrombosis can occur in up to 60 percent of patients with major leg injuries. Therefore, prophylaxis against venous thromboembolism is an important part of the comprehensive care of all patients with lower-extremity injuries. When anticoagulants are contraindicated, the use of intermittent pneumatic compression boots is an effective alternative. Postinjury surveillance using noninvasive methods to detect deep venous thrombosis can help to identify patients with silent thrombosis and to prevent pulmonary embolism.

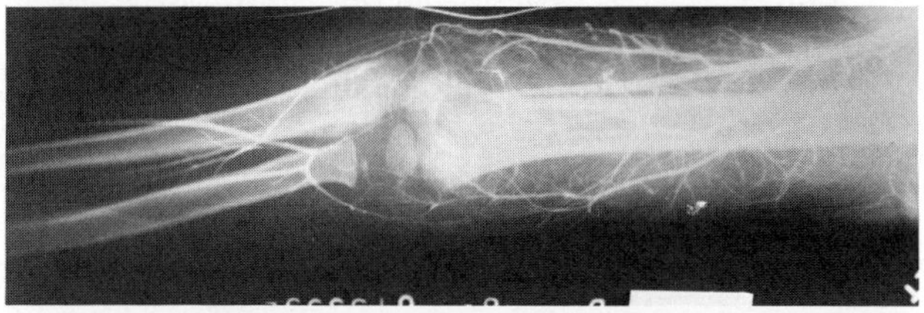

Fig. 53-3. Brachial artery thrombosis from supracondylar fracture dislocation of the elbow. This 6-year-old patient had a warm, asymptomatic hand but wrist pulses were absent. Angiogram shows reconstitution of the radial and ulnar arteries via collaterals.

SELECTED READING

Anderson, RJ, et al. Reduced dependency on arteriography for penetrating extremity trauma: Influence of wound location and noninvasive studies. *J Trauma* 30:1059, 1990.

Ashworth, EM, et al. Lower extremity vascular trauma: A comprehensive, aggressive approach. *J Trauma* 28:329, 1988.

Bergqvist, D, et al. Trends in civilian vascular trauma during 30 years. A Swedish perspective. *Acta Chir Scand* 153:417, 1987.

Collins, PS, et al. Intra-abdominal vascular injury secondary to penetrating trauma. *J Trauma* 28:S165, 1988.

Feliciano, DV, et al. Delayed diagnosis of arterial injuries. *Am J Surg* 154:579, 1987.

Feliciano, DV, et al. Management of vascular injuries in the lower extremities. *J Trauma* 28:319, 1988.

Mattox, KL, et al. Prospective randomized evaluation of the "MAST" garment in hemorrhagic shock. *J Trauma* 26:779, 1986.

McCorkell, SJ, et al. Indications for angiography in extremity trauma. *AJR* 145:1245, 1985.

Meagher, DP, Jr, et al. Vascular trauma in infants and children. *J Trauma* 19:532, 1979.

Meek, AC, and Robbs, JV. Vascular injury with associated bone and joint trauma. *Br J Surg* 71:341, 1984.

Moreno, C, et al. Hemorrhage associated with major pelvic fracture: A multispecialty challenge. *J Trauma* 26:987, 1986.

Nichols, JS, and Lillehei, KO. Nerve injury associated with acute vascular trauma. *Surg Clin North Am* 68:837, 1988.

Rich, NM. Management of venous trauma. *Surg Clin North Am* 68:809, 1988.

Rich, NM, and Hughes, CW. Vietnam vascular registry: A preliminary report. *Surgery* 65:218, 1969.

Rodgers, CM, and Ketch, LL. Management of associated soft-tissue injury. *Surg Clin North Am* 68:823, 1988.

Rosental, JJ, et al. Vascular injuries associated with fractures of the femur. *Arch Surg* 110:494, 1975.

Shannon, JJ, Jr, et al. Peripheral arterial missile embolization: A case report and 22-year literature review. *J Vasc Surg* 5:773, 1987.

Wagner, WH, et al. Blunt popliteal artery trauma: One hundred consecutive injuries. *J Vasc Surg* 7:736, 1988.

White, RA, et al. Peripheral vascular injuries associated with falls from heights. *J Trauma* 27:411, 1987.

D. Injuries of the Head, Neck, and Spinal Cord

54. Head Injuries

Edwin G. Fischer

Head and neck injuries are a major cause of disability and death in Western society, especially among young adults and children. Head injuries occur at an estimated rate of 200 per 100,000 neck injuries at 5 per 100,000 population. Although a majority of the deaths and vegetative outcomes can be attributed to injury to the brain parenchyma at the time of trauma, a significant number are caused by secondary events and may be prevented when detected early and treated promptly. Intracranial hematomas occur in approximately 10 percent of patients hospitalized for head injury and cause delayed deterioration as they expand. Their recognition is a major goal of trauma management. Cervical spine fractures, although not common in patients with severe head injuries, may go unrecognized when a patient is in coma or is agitated and confused, and serious additional neurologic injury may occur if the neck is not properly protected before appropriate x-ray studies are made. Depressed skull fractures or basilar fractures with cerebrospinal fluid (CSF) leak may be overlooked, as may other accompanying injuries that require multispecialty treatment.

PATHOPHYSIOLOGIC CONSIDERATIONS

Injury to Brain Parenchyma

Brain parenchyma and its vasculature may be injured by a number of mechanisms. The most obvious are direct lacerations caused by penetrating objects and in-driven bone. Shock waves from high-velocity missiles may also cause injury to brain tissue. Severe brain injuries may occur when the freely movable head is acutely rotated on its axis at the time of impact. Rotational acceleration creates shearing within the brain that disrupts and deforms brain substance and its vasculature. The cortex alone may be affected, especially the undersurface of the frontal and temporal lobes. Deeper structures may be involved, resulting in diffuse white matter injury and injury to the corpus callosum and superior cerebellar peduncle. The result may be coma, decerebration, and autonomic instability in a clinical picture erroneously interpreted as a pure brainstem injury and from which recovery is usually unsatisfactory. Intracerebral hematomas may develop in areas of torn tissue, either as small scattered lesions or as a single, large mass often in a contracoup location. The temporal and frontal lobes are common locations. Traumatic vasospasm may cause neurologic deficits due to ischemia, and traumatic aneurysms may be responsible for delayed intracerebral hematomas days or weeks after the injury. In children, transient focal neurologic deficits such as blindness have been attributed to local disturbances in cerebral blood flow.

Epidural and Subdural Hematomas

Acute epidural hematomas form between the dura and the inner table of the skull, usually within minutes or hours of the injury. A torn middle meningeal artery in association with a fracture is the most common source of bleeding, and the hematomas are therefore usually located just lateral to the temporal lobe. A fracture is not always present. In children, epidural hematomas may be located in the posterior fossa where the dura is exceptionally vascular. If the hematoma is evacuated before herniation occurs, recovery is excellent because direct injury to the brain parenchyma is usually absent. *Acute subdural hematomas* result from rotational injuries to the skull, which injure superficial cortical arteries or tear veins as they cross from the brain to the dura or sagittal sinus, forming within the potential space between the dura and arachnoid membrane and extending over the entire convexity surface of the hemisphere. They may occur after trivial injuries in patients taking anticoagulants. Accompanying injury to the brain is largely responsible for the high mortality rate (50–80%) and a high incidence of neurologic sequella. *Chronic subdural hematomas* occur more often in the elderly, are often contracoup in location, are frequently bilateral (10–20%) and, because of their slower evolution and the lesser incidence of associated brain injury, have a much better prognosis. They typically develop over days, weeks, or even months and have a clinical course that is similar to that of a brain tumor, with progressive headache, lethargy, confusion, and neurologic deficit.

Brain Edema and Altered Cerebral Blood Volume

Brain swelling caused by brain edema or an expanded cerebral blood volume may increase intracranial pressure and be as life threatening as intracranial hematomas. Brain edema can be caused by direct injury to the vasculature with disruption of the blood–brain barrier and leaking of fluid into the extracellular space. The cytotoxic products of cell injury or death in areas of ischemia or tissue disruption also cause brain edema. Increased cerebral blood volume causes brain swelling following trauma when cerebral autoregulation is lost or when the cerebral arterioles dilate because of retention CO_2 caused by airway or ventilatory problems.

Brain Herniation

Herniation of the medial temporal lobe can often be detected clinically and is immediately life threatening. The uncus of the temporal lobe is pushed or becomes herniated over the medial "free" edge of the tentorium by a laterally placed mass, such as an epidural or temporal lobe hematoma. The displaced uncus first compresses the oculomotor nerve as it runs along the edge of the tentorium toward the cavernous sinus (Fig. 54-1). With further displacement, there is compression of the cerebral peduncle of the midbrain, which contains the uncrossed portion of the pyramidal tract (Fig. 54-2). Sometimes the opposite cerebral peduncle may be pressed against the opposite tentorial edge creating a "Kernohan's notch" (Fig. 54-3).

Clinically, temporal lobe herniation is recognized in its early stages by decreased mental status as intracranial pressure increases and the brainstem is displaced and by a dilated pupil on the ipsilateral side accompanied by pathologic reflexes that are contralateral (unless a Kernohan's notch is created). In approximately 10 percent of cases, both pupils are dilated or the opposite pupil is dilated. As the thalamus and brainstem shift, compression of the third ventricle or the aqueduct will result in CSF obstruction and hydrocephalus, thereby greatly aggravating intracranial hypertension. As midbrain compression continues, spinal cord motor systems are cut off from cortical inhibition, causing decerebrate posturing (opisthotonus, extension and internal rotation of the upper extremities, and extension and plantar flexion in the lower extremities with extension of the big toe). Finally, compression causes ischemia and hemorrhage in the brainstem (Duret's hemorrhages)—an irreversible situation with loss of brainstem reflexes and cardiorespiratory arrest.

When hematomas occur in the posterior fossa, the cerebellar tonsils may herniate through the foramen magnum compressing the medulla and causing cardiorespiratory arrest. Although depression of consciousness is usually present beforehand, there are no warning neurologic signs as there are in temporal lobe herniation.

As masses develop within the skull, displacement of the brain may cause localized vascular obstruction. Herniation of the frontal lobe under the falx can occlude the anterior cerebral artery and cause an infarct in the leg area of the interhemispheric precentral gyrus. Herniation of the inferior temporal lobe over the posterior edge of the tentorium may occlude the posterior cerebral artery as it crosses the posterior edge of the tentorium on its way to the occipital lobe, causing an infarction in the calcarine cortex.

Increased Intracranial Pressure

Any rapidly developing intracranial mass can increase intracranial pressure because the skull is essentially a closed compartment and the two principal mechanisms for buffering pressure—reduction of cerebral intravascular volume and displacement of CSF into the spinal canal—have limited capacity. As intracranial pressure increases, waves of pressure develop, first lasting only a few seconds or minutes and then becoming prolonged (15–20 minutes)—the so-called plateau waves. Cerebral perfusion pressure is the difference between mean arterial pressure and mean intracranial pressure and is normal or adequate when it is 50 mm Hg or more. When intracranial pressure approaches arterial pressure, blood flow to the brain becomes inadequate and eventually ceases, causing cerebral death from ischemia.

SKULL FRACTURES

Linear fractures in themselves do not pose a danger, but they are indicative of the force of impact of a head injury. They may be harbingers of an intracranial hematoma, especially if they cross a major vascular structure such as the groove of the middle meningeal artery, the sagittal sinus, or, in children, the vascular dura of the posterior fossa and foramen magnum. If the margins of the fracture are separated significantly, the dura may be torn, especially in infants in whose skulls the dura is attached to the sutures.

Depressed fractures are often accompanied by injury to the underlying dura or brain. Fractures depressed more than 1 cm or depressed more than the thickness of the skull itself are generally explored and elevated in the hopes of reducing the risk of posttraumatic epilepsy, especially in the region of the central sulcus. Depressed fractures and penetrating objects may tamponade major arteries or veins and should

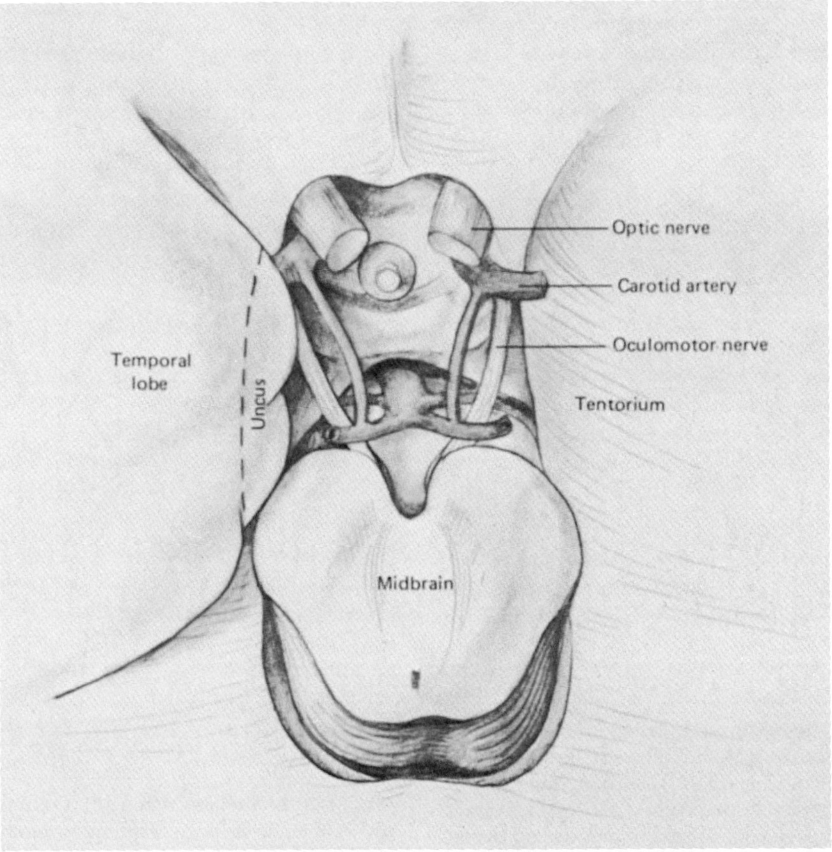

Fig. 54-1. Compression of the ipsilateral oculomotor nerve by the uncus of the temporal lobe as it herniates over the edge of the tentorium.

be manipulated or removed in the operating room, where uncontrolled bleeding can be dealt with with minimal injury to the brain. Depressed compound fractures—that is, fractures associated with scalp lacerations or that traverse the frontal, paranasal, or mastoid sinus air cells—are a potential source of meningitis or brain abscess and must receive neurosurgical management accordingly. Basilar skull fractures may be associated with CSF rhinorrhea and otorrhea; the proper antibiotic management for these is controversial. Broad-spectrum antibiotics may lead to fungal or difficult-to-treat, antibiotic-resistant bacterial infections. Fractures of the temporal bone, often associated with a Battle's sign (ecchymosis over the mastoid region), may cause a surgically correctable dislocation of the ossicles of the middle ear or injury to the facial nerve. Sphenoid bone fractures may be associated with traumatic carotid-cavernous fistula, pituitary or hypothalamic insufficiency, or damage to orbital structures, including the oculomotor or optic nerves.

NEUROLOGIC PRESENTATIONS

Altered Consciousness

Concussion is a transient loss of consciousness following trauma, and its pathophysiology is uncertain. It lasts several minutes or longer and is often associated with retrograde or anterograde amnesia. Since altered consciousness is the most sensitive indicator of increasing intracranial pressure, if consciousness is not regained promptly, the "lucid interval" associated with subsequently evolving intracranial hematomas becomes eclipsed.

A patient may be alert and intact following head injury (the "lucid interval") only to become lethargic or obtunded hours or even days later. The clinical hallmarks of temporal lobe herniation may appear: depressed consciousness, coma, ipsilateral dilated pupil, contralateral hemiparesis, hyperreflexia, or posturing. The clinical presentation is the same for acute epidural hematomas, acute subdural hematomas, intracerebral hematomas, and acutely evolving cerebral edema. In these patients there must be no delay in performing diagnostic studies and instituting appropriate therapy.

Persistent coma is common following head injury and may be accompanied by focal neurologic deficits if there has been localized brain injury such as laceration, contusion, or hematoma. Unless the patient is clearly regaining consciousness, an expanding intracranial hematoma is assumed and the patient is worked up expediently.

In patients who are awake and stable, focal neurologic symptoms form a more prominent part of the clinical problem and there is time for more detailed evaluation. The characteristic pain and paresthesias accompanying spine injuries will not be obscured. When headache and vomiting are prominent, they suggest increased intracranial pressure, but they are frequently present without it, especially in children.

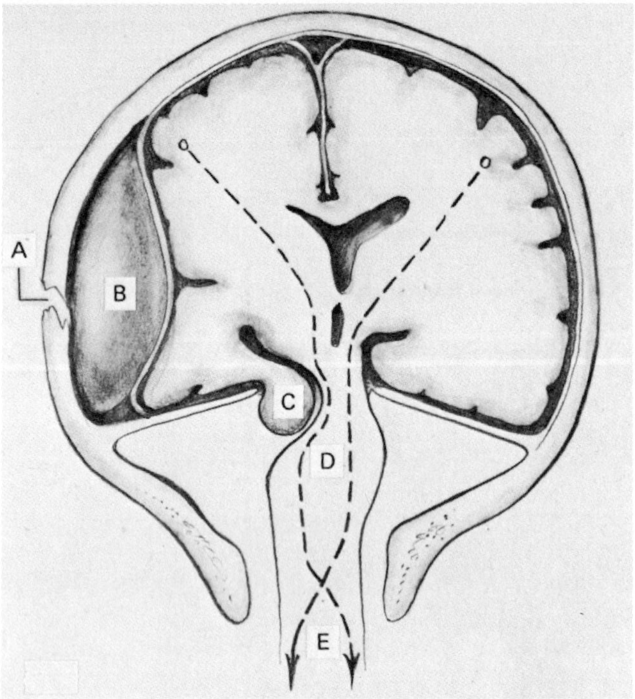

Fig. 54-2. Compression of the midbrain by temporal lobe herniation. A. Temporal bone fracture across middle meningeal artery. B. Epidural hematoma. C. Uncus of temporal lobe herniating over edge of tentorium and compressing descending corticospinal tract (D) at level of midbrain, causing contralateral motor defect. Decussation of the corticospinal tract occurs at spinomedullary junction (E).

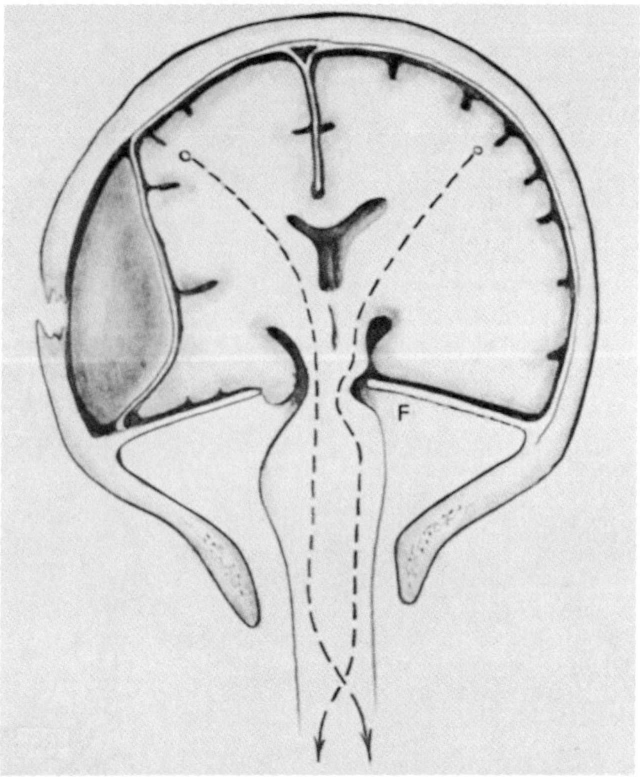

Fig. 54-3. Kernohan's notch (F). Compression of midbrain against opposite tentorial edge resulting in motor deficit on same side as hematoma.

Likewise, seizures may herald an intracranical hematoma but not necessarily. Transient focal neurologic deficits are often found in children without demonstrable pathology and have been attributed to local disturbances in blood flow. Finally, the detection of other injuries is facilitated by the ability to obtain a more complete history and to perform a more thorough examination in an alert patient.

Head Injuries in Infants

Intracranial hematomas in infants may enlarge enough to result in systemic hypotension without intracranial hypertension and coma, because in infancy the cranial sutures can easily separate, allowing the skull to expand. Intracranial pressure can be assessed directly by palpation of the anterior fontanelle if it is open. In infants, the dura is adherent to the skull at the cranial sutures. A diastatic or separated linear fracture may tear the dura, which in the months and years that follow could result in an expanding cystic deformity of skull, meninges, and brain and causing not only deformity of the skull but also seizures and neurologic deficit as the child grows. The most frequent head injuries *during birth* are cephalhematomas, which almost always resolve spontaneously, and "ping-pong" fractures, which are easily elevated. More rarely, the birth process may distort and mold the skull so severely that the tentorium is torn and the tentorial artery injured, causing bleeding into the tentorium, the posterior fossa, and even the upper brainstem. Computed tomography (CT) has made possible early diagnosis of the entity, allowing successful decompression or clot removal. Injuries to the facial nerve, the brachial plexus, and spinal cord may also occur during birth.

Child abuse must be suspected when the cause of head injury is unknown or implausible or when other injuries of varying age are noted by physical examination or by x-rays of the ribs or extremities. These children must be reported by law because there is significant reinjury and mortality when they are returned to their environment unprotected.

Chronic subdural hematomas in infants often occur without a history of trauma. Signs and symptoms are nonspecific and include irritability, fever, poor feeding, seizures, enlarging head, bulging anterior fontanelle, and anemia. The diagnosis is made by CT, and treatment consists of subdural taps, removing, at first, not more than 15 to 20 ml from each side. If fluid persists for more than 1 to 2 weeks despite daily tapping, surgery may be indicated, including irrigation of the subdural spaces through burr holes, drainage by insertion of a subdural-peritoneal shunt, or removal of subdural membranes by craniotomy, when other measures fail.

Cervical spine injuries (see Chap. 55) cannot be detected by clinical criteria in patients who are in coma or who have a compromised mental status. Since there is high likelihood of producing additional cervical cord injury while caring for a head-injured patient who has an undetected cervical spine fracture, the neck should always be protected with a Philadelphia collar or sandbags to keep the neck from moving and in neutral position until a lateral x-ray is taken and all seven cervical vertebra are visualized and shown to be free of injury.

Table 54-1. Emergency department management of head injuries

Initial resuscitation—airway/ventilation/blood pressure
Simultaneously obtain history of accident and of major medical problems and illnesses
Protect neck (Philadelphia collar, sandbags)
General examination—for major injuries
Neurologic examination—looking for temporal lobe herniation
Glasgow Coma Scale (alertness)
Pupils
Motor asymmetry
Cover scalp wounds with sterile dressing, stop scalp bleeding
Blood tests: CBC, electrolytes, BUN, PT, PTT, type and crossmatch
Intravenous lines—give fluids sparingly if blood pressure is stable
Foley catheter
X-rays: Neck, CT scan, cervical spine films, skull x-rays (patient must be monitored closely while having x-rays)
Management of increased intracranial pressure (if comatose or deteriorating)
Intubation and hyperventilation
Mannitol: Loading dose 1–2 gm/kg
Prompt neurosurgical and CT assessment

MANAGEMENT (TABLE 54-1)

History

The details of the injury and of the patient's general health are obtained during the process of resuscitation. Persons accompanying the patient (e.g., family, police, ambulance attendants) are the major source of information about children and unconscious adults. They should not be allowed to leave before these details are obtained.

Neurologic deterioration or loss of consciousness after a posttraumatic "lucid interval," as indicated previously, suggests an evolving intracranial hematoma. Other common factors may also affect consciousness: drug or alcohol ingestion, prior neurologic illness, metabolic disease or its treatment, and hypothermia. History of bleeding disorders, either natural or iatrogenic, of other major illnesses, and of required medications or of drug allergies will be of major importance in management.

Initial Resuscitation

Clear airway, adequate ventilation, and sufficient blood pressure are necessary at the onset. Poor oxygenation and low cerebral perfusion will result in severe, irreversible brain damage within 3 to 5 minutes. Hypoventilation will cause hypercarbia, dilating the cerebral vasculature and thereby increasing intracranial pressure. The mouth and oral pharynx are suctioned and cleared of debris. Ventilation can be assisted by a mask and bag. If the patient requires intubation, a cervical fracture is assumed and the neck is stabilized in a neutral position by an assistant by applying continuous traction on the head along the axis of the spine; otherwise, the neck is stabilized with a Philadelphia collar or sandbags. Once a patient is intubated and paralyzed chemically, the advantage of being able to assess intracranial pressure by level of consciousness or to assess neurologic function is lost and no longer are there clinical guidelines for the urgency of further radiologic evaluation or emergency surgery. Therefore, if a patient is awake or combative and intubation would require administering paralyzing agents, it is usually best to avoid intubation.

Intravenous catheters are inserted for volume expansion or to administer medications or maintenance fluid, remembering that intracranial bleeding, except in infants, does not cause hypotension and that fluid overload can aggravate brain edema and herniation. In the absence of hypotension, fluids are given sparingly. Lactated Ringer's solution or glucose and saline are preferred to glucose and water, and they are given at a rate of 40 to 60 ml/hour in adults and 1 to 2 ml/kg/hour in children. Infants who are in shock from blood loss can be given a transfusion that is one-half their blood volume or 3.5 percent of their body weight.

Blood is drawn for type and crossmatch, hematocrit, platelet count, prothrombin time, partial thromboplastin time, blood urea nitrogen, creatinine, glucose, and electrolytes and for alcohol level and toxic screen when appropriate. The results are obtained as promptly as possible, but it may be necessary at times to begin surgical treatment without them.

A Foley catheter is inserted to monitor urine output and to prevent overdistention of the bladder when hyperosmolar agents are given.

Nasal intubation is to be avoided until there is reasonable certainty that fractures do not exist in the ethmoid and sphenoid areas that might allow inadvertent introduction of nasogastric or endotracheal tubes into the intracranial cavity.

Examination

A general examination of sites of other possible life-threatening injury, including airway, neck, chest, abdomen, pelvis, and extremities is rapidly performed as resuscitative measures are begun (see Initial Resuscitation).

The scalp and face are examined for lacerations, puncture wounds, and underlying bony deformity. The entire scalp must be examined. Lacerations are thoroughly explored for fractures, CSF, and brain tissue. Ears, nose, and throat are also examined for blood, CSF, and brain tissue. Scalp wounds should be covered with a sterile, noncompressive dressing. Bothersome bleeding from scalp vessels can be controlled with hemostats or very gentle pressure, but pressure must not be applied directly over an unstable skull fracture or in an area of potentially unprotected brain. Penetrating objects and fragments of depressed bone should be left alone.

Neurologic examination may of necessity be limited, but a systematic examination is performed focusing on level of consciousness, equality and reactivity of pupils, and motor function of the extremities. The examination is aimed at recognizing increased intracranial pressure, temporal lobe herniation, spinal cord injury, and gross neurologic deficit and should be accurately recorded so that future deterioration or improvement may be easily recognized. The Glasgow Coma Scale (see Table 41-1) has been adopted by most trauma centers to grade the level of neurologic injury. A score of 7 or less defines the presence of coma, and scores of 3 or 4 are associated with a 97 percent chance of death or vegetative outcome. Level of consciousness is the best clinical guide to intracranial pressure and cerebral perfusion. Depressed consciousness with an enlarged pupil on one side usually means a life-threatening temporal lobe herniation caused by an intracranial hematoma. They are generally accompanied by contralateral corticospinal tract dysfunction: depressed motor response, hyperreflexia, Babinski's reflex, or decerebrate posturing. The side of pathology is on the side of the enlarged pupil and contralateral to the motor abnormality but is falsely localized approximately 10 percent of the time. An enlarged pupil in a fully awake patient means peripheral injury to the oculomotor nerve rather than herniation. Spinal cord injury is suggested by bilateral weakness of extremities, intercostal muscle paralysis with abdominal breathing, a sensory level, and bladder distention. The more alert and cooperative the patient, the more detailed the examination can be.

Radiologic Examination

A lateral cervical spine film is done first to rule out a fracture or dislocation. All seven cervical vertebra must be visualized including the odontoid and C7. A swimmer's view or traction on the arms may be required for the latter. Only after this has been done are the neck supports (collar or sandbags) removed.

CT provides the definitive radiologic examination in head trauma. A high-quality scan can identify all the pathology seen on skull films, as long as a limited study is not performed. It can readily demonstrate intracranial hematomas, edema, hydrocephalus, obliteration of CSF cisterns due to increased intracranial pressure, and temporal lobe herniation.

Skull examination consists of a brow-up lateral, anteroposterior, and Towne's views. A fracture crossing the vascular channels of the dura, the groove of the middle meningeal artery, the sagittal sinus, or the posterior fossa increases the possibility of an intracranial hematoma. Depressed fractures are noted by a "double density" of bone and can be further defined by tangential views. Occult penetrating objects may be noted. An air–fluid level in the sphenoid sinus or air intracranially indicates a basal fracture.

Magnetic resonance imaging (MRI) may provide better imaging of the anatomic details of traumatic injuries to the brain, although limited availability and problems of management of complexly monitored patients within the magnetic system have thus far restricted its use in head injuries.

Treatment

Comatose or deteriorating patients are rapidly assessed, resuscitated as indicated previously, and evaluated by CT. Surgical lesions, such as epidural, subdural, or intracerebral hematomas are evacuated promptly, using mannitol or hyperventilation, or both, to reduce intracranial pressure while the operation is in preparation. If hydrocephalus is present, emergency ventriculostomy may be required. If surgery is not indicated, the patient is transferred to an intensive care unit (ICU) where intracranial pressure may be monitored to guide the treatment of cerebral edema when it exists. In the unfortunate circumstance in which CT is not readily available and acute increased intracranial pressure or temporal lobe herniation is suspected clinically, the patient is evaluated by exploratory burr holes and ventriculostomy. Any patient at risk for such intervention should be transferred to the care of a neurosurgeon without delay.

Treatment of increased intracranial pressure may briefly avert brainstem compression from herniation while the comatose patient is being scanned and readied for surgery. These measures are not necessary if the patient is awake or waking up. Hyperventilation by intubation and artificial ventilation reduces intracranial pressure within minutes—the lowered arterial PCO_2 (to 20–25 mm Hg) decreasing cerebral blood volume by causing cerebral arterial constriction. Hyperosmolar agents, such as mannitol, reduce intracranial pressure within 15 to 30 minutes by remaining within the intact intravascular space and selectively dehydrating normal brain. Mannitol is the most effective agent and has the least rebound effect. The loading dose is 1 to 2 gm/kg. Smaller doses can subsequently be given every 4 to 6 hours. Furosemide may enhance its effect. A Foley catheter must be in place to avoid overdistention of the bladder. Steroids, especially dexamethasone, were used in the past to treat head injuries but have been shown to be ineffective. However, the immediate use of high doses of steroids may lessen neurologic deficit in patients with spinal cord injury. Barbiturate coma can reduce intracranial pressure, but its use requires continuous monitoring of intracranial and arterial pressure. Intubation and artificial ventilation must be in place, and the patient's neurologic examination can therefore no longer be used as a clinical guide. Its use is restricted to an ICU setting, and its overall effectiveness for achieving useful recovery is debated.

Compound skull fractures—that is, fractures associated with lacerations of the scalp or depressed fractures that involve paranasal sinuses, especially the frontal sinus—are elevated, debrided, and closed within 12 to 24 hours to prevent continued bacterial contamination of the brain and development of meningitis or a brain abscess. Such fractures are easy to overlook. Loose bony fragments and penetrating objects discovered in the emergency department are covered with a sterile dressing and are manipulated only in the operating room.

Depressed fractures are elevated when they exceed the thickness of the skull or penetrate more than a centimeter, these being the fractures most likely to have torn the dura and to have injured underlying brain. The practice of elevating depressed fractures solely for the purpose of reducing seizures is tradition-bound but not scientifically substantiated.

Seizures at the time of injury are common and may indicate a developing hematoma. During a seizure, the patient should be placed on his or her side to avoid aspiration, keeping the head and neck supported in a neutral position. Phenytoin (Dilantin) may be given intravenously. In adults, the loading dose is 400 to 600 mg IV over 15 to 20 minutes. Cardiovascular collapse may occur at rates greater than 50 mg/minute. In children, the loading dose is 15 mg/kg IV. When seizures are prolonged or repetitive, diazepam or phenobarbitol may be more effective. Both drugs suppress respiration, so that ventilatory assistance should be available during and after their intravenous administration. The dosage of diazepam for adults is 2.5 to 10.0 mg; for children, it is 0.25 mg/kg IV over 1 to 2 minutes and repeated if necessary after 15 to 20 minutes. The dose of sodium phenobarbitol

Table 54-2. Indications for hospitalization

Depressed or declining level of consciousness
Prolonged unconsciousness
Neurologic deficit
Inceasing headache and vomiting
Seizures
Cerebrospinal fluid otorrhea, rhinorrhea
Linear skull fracture crossing the groove of the middle meningeal artery, a venous sinus of the dura, or the foramen magnum
Compound skull fracture or fracture into the frontal sinus
Depressed skull fracture
Bleeding disorder (or anticoagulant therapy)
Non-neurosurgical indications
Intoxication or illness that may obscure neurologic state
Inadequate observation at home
Suspected child abuse

for adults is 400 to 800 mg (dissolved in distilled water); for children, it is 5 to 6 mg/kg. Delayed posttraumatic epilepsy occurs in approximately 5 percent of patients with penetrating injuries and is more common with injuries in the region of the central sulcus. The onset is generally within the first few months or year of the accident but may be much later. There is controversy whether prophylactic anticonvulsants reduce the risk of posttraumatic seizures. When there is clear structural brain injury, they are commonly given for 1 year and then discontinued if the electroencephalogram (EEG) fails to show epileptogenic activity.

Scalp lacerations and penetrating wounds are the source of potential contamination and infection of the brain. They must be thoroughly explored and are often studied by x-ray or CT. A retained foreign body, such as a pencil or stick, may be easily missed, especially if the site of entry is hidden in the orbit, nose, or throat. Significant blood loss may occur from scalp lacerations, and in infants and children, large amounts of blood may collect under the galea. Hair around the laceration is shaved, and the surrounding scalp is cleaned with surgical antiseptic solution. Bleeding from scalp arteries and veins can be controlled with hemostats, self-retaining retractors, or, if there is no skull fracture, direct compression. The entire wound ought to be inspected visually and with a gloved finger. If the skull is intact, the wound can be irrigated, all foreign and necrotic material removed, and the skin edges trimmed and sutured. If the laceration is large, the galea and skin can be closed separately—the galea with 2.0 or 3.0 absorbable suture, the skin with nylon or silk.

Basilar skull fractures associated with CSF otorrhea or rhinorrhea are treated expectantly, often with elevation of the head of the bed and repeated lumbar punctures or even lumbar drainage to reduce intracranial pressure and encourage sealing of the leak. Broad-spectrum antibiotics are not usually given because of the risk of inducing infection by an antibiotic-resistant organism or a fungus. Low doses of penicillin may be used to suppress pneumococcus or streptococcus.

Awake and stable patients, even after seemingly mild injuries, require careful examination. Most will not require hospitalization. It is often desirable to prolong a patient's evaluation in the emergency department so that the early clinical course may be observed and a disposition not be made prematurely. A major portion of preventable deaths occur in low-risk patients, who are likely to receive relatively less immediate attention. In uncertain situations, neurosurgical referral or hospitalization is recommended (Table 54-2). If the patient is hospitalized because of the possibility of developing an intracranial hematoma, it should be to a neurosurgical unit or to a suitably equipped trauma service. It is inadvisable to admit such a patient to a hospital that cannot provide definitive neurosurgical care. If the patient is discharged home, it must be in the care of a responsible person who is adequately warned about the symptoms and signs of a developing hematoma, which include persisent headache, vomiting, lethargy or altered mental state when woken up, unequal pupils, seizures, or neurologic symptoms. Printed instruction sheets are useful for this purpose.

SELECTED READING

Becker, DP, et al. Diagnosis and Treatment of Head Injury in Adults. In E Youmans (ed), *Neurological Surgery*, Vol. 4. Philadelphia: Saunders, 1982. Pp. 1938–2083.

Cooper, PR (ed). *Head Injury* (2nd ed). Baltimore: Williams & Wilkins, 1987.

Ewing, CL (ed). *Impact Injury of the Head and Spine*. Springfield, IL: Thomas, 1983.

Grossman, RS, and Gildenberg, PL (eds). *Head Injury: Basic and Clinical Aspects*. New York: Raven, 1982.

Jennett, B, and Teasdale, G. *Management of Head Injuries*. Continuing Neurology Series, Philadelphia: Davis, 1981.

Klauber, MR, et al. Determinants of head injury mortality: Importance of the low risk patient. *Neurosurgery* 24:31, 1989.

McLaurin, RL. *Extracerebral Collections*. Advances in Neurotraumatology, Vol. 1. New York: Springer, 1986.

Shapiro, K (ed). *Pediatric Head Trauma*. Mt. Kisco: Futura, 1983.

Teasdale, G, and Jennett, B. Assessment of coma and impaired consciousness: A practical scale. *Lancet* 2:81, 1974.

Wilberger, JE, Jr, Deeb, Z, and Rothfus, W. Magnetic resonance imaging in cases of severe head injury. *Neurosurgery* 20:571, 1987.

Wilkens, RH, and Rengachary, SS (eds). *Neurosurgery*, Vol. 2, Part VIII, Trauma. New York: McGraw-Hill, 1985. Pp. 1531–1763.

55. Spinal Cord Injuries

Robert W. Hussey

The primary protection to the spinal cord is the spinal column; therefore, any injury to the spine has the potential for causing injury to the spinal cord. If the cord is damaged, the effects are frequently permanent and extremely disabling. Only 10 to 20 percent of spine fractures result in spinal cord injury, but improper handling can result in damage to the cord, as evidenced by a study of 85 patients with cervical spinal cord injuries at the Massachusetts General Hospital in which eight patients were neurologically worse on admission to the emergency department than they had been at the scene of the accident. Statistics from the National SCI Data Bank indicate that the proportion of patients with neurologically incomplete spinal cord injuries has increased significantly, from 38.1 percent in 1973–1974 to 53.8 percent in 1983–1984. This is believed to be due in large part to management at the accident scene.

The incidence of spinal cord injury is 3.0 to 3.2 per 100,000 population per year. The most frequent causes are motor vehicle accidents (47.7%), falls (20.8%), violence (mostly gunshot wounds) (14.6%), and sports (mostly water sports) (14.2%). Although preliminary reports from some local prevention programs directed mainly at school students have shown decreased incidents, there are not as yet any large incidence studies that reflect the impact of lower speed limits, seat belt usage, and other safety campaigns on the incidence of spinal cord injuries. The initial mortality rate may be as high as 50 percent, occurring mainly before or shortly after arrival at the initial hospital primarily as a result of associated injuries of very high cervical cord injuries at the C1 and C2 levels. Once the patient is admitted and stabilized, the mortality rate is 10 to 20 percent. After completion of the initial hospitalization and rehabilitation, the life expectancy is nearly normal for the person's age.

The primary goals of emergency management of patients with spine and spinal cord injuries are to prevent or minimize spinal cord damage, to stabilize the injured spine, and to treat the associated life-threatening injuries. At the scene of an accident, the main objectives are to recognize a potential spinal cord injury and to manage the patient in such a way as to minimize or prevent injury to the spinal cord. In the emergency department, the objectives are to determine the nature of the spine, spinal cord, and associated injuries and to initiate treatment that will meet the primary goals. This immediate stabilization should be carried out as expeditiously as possible so that the patient with a spinal cord injury can be transferred to a spinal cord injury center within hours of injury. These centers, staffed by professionals experienced in treating patients with such injuries, are equipped to offer the comprehensive care and rehabilitation that facilitates recovery and rehabilitation to the fullest extent possible in a reasonable time period and without preventable complications.

MECHANISM OF INJURY AND PATHOPHYSIOLOGY

Mechanism of Injury

Spinal cord injuries are usually caused by forces exerted on the spine indirectly through other parts of the body. The force may result in flexion, extension, rotation, axial loading, or any combination of these motions. Each type of motion tends to produce a characteristic injury pattern at a particular level of the spinal column. This pattern is related to the anatomy of the vertebrae—in particular, the shape and orientation of facet joints and the size and shape of the vertebral body (Figs. 55-1 and 55-2). Injuries are more common in an area in which a highly mobile segment joins a less mobile segment, such as the lower cervical spine and the thoracolumbar junction (T10 to L1).

The first two cervical vertebrae are unique in their structure, function, and pattern of injury. The first cervical vertebra, or atlas, articulates with the occipital condyles superiorly and the second cervical vertebra, the axis, inferiorly. The atlas is ring-shaped and has no body. Its articular facets are ovoid and are part of the lateral masses. Dislocations between the skull and C1 are rare and even more rarely survivable. The most common injury to the atlas is the "Jefferson fracture," caused by a primarily compressive force in which the ring is broken in several places. This rarely produces spinal cord injury and does not usually result in spinal malalignment or instability.

Fig. 55-1. Normal cervical spine.

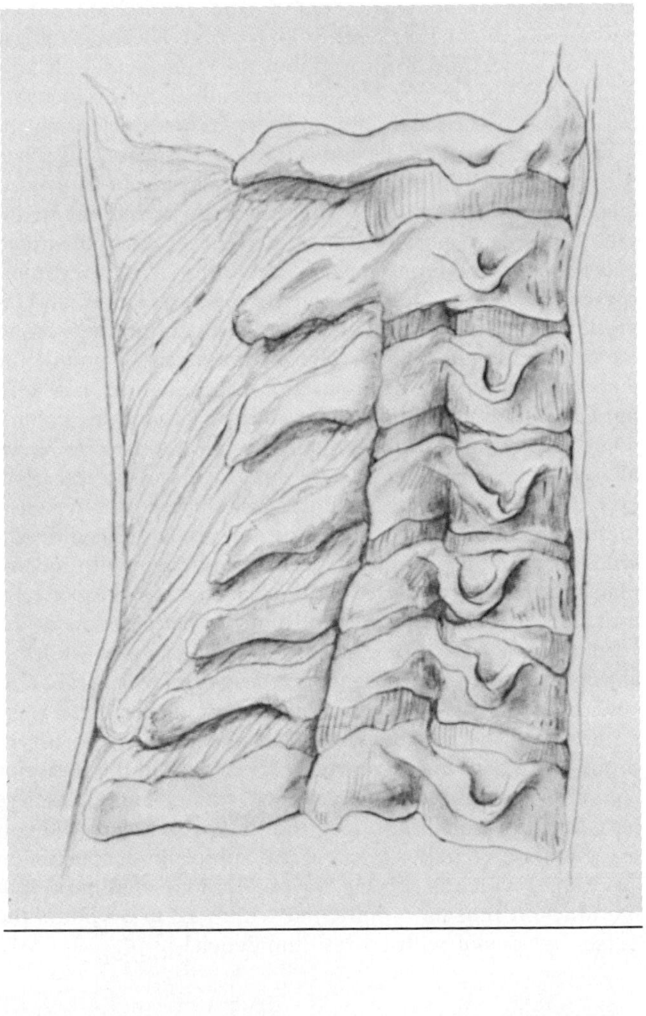

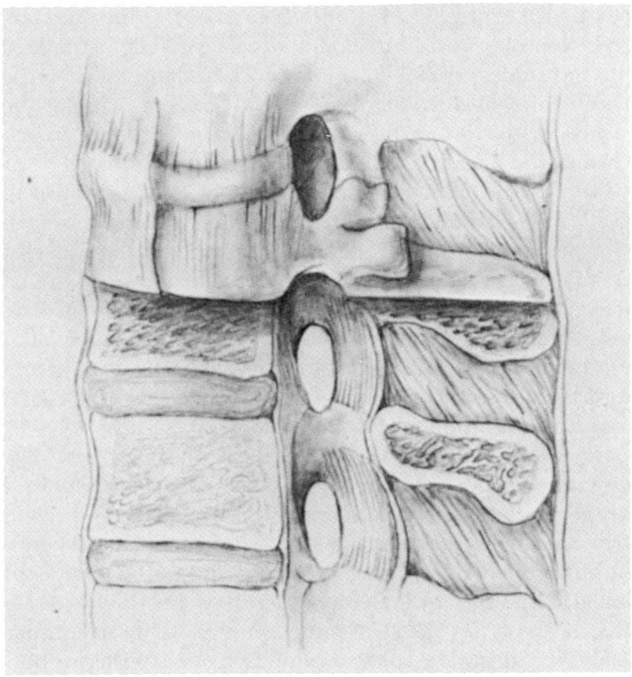

Fig. 55-2. Major spinal ligaments.

The second cervical vertebra, or axis, is distinguished by the peg-shaped odontoid process protruding superiorly, which represents, embryologically, the body of C1. The most common fracture of this vertebra is the "hangman's fracture," which, despite its ominous name, rarely produces spinal cord injury. It is produced by extension force. This fracture got its name from studies of victims of judicial hanging. The difference between what we see clinically and the hangman's victim is the application of traction. This should serve as a warning that one must be extremely careful in applying traction to immobilize injuries to the first two cervical vertebrae so as not to complete the hangman's job.

The C1-C2 articulation is the most unique in the spine. The odontoid process of the axis articulates with the posterior aspect of the anterior ring of the atlas. Excessive flexion force results either in the rupture of the transverse ligament holding the odontoid to the atlas or fracturing of the odontoid process. Either of these injuries is potentially fatal since injury to the spinal cord at this level can result in respiratory paralysis.

The cervical vertebrae are shaped to allow maximum mobility in all planes, but particularly flexion. The facets are oriented obliquely in the coronal plane. The bodies are wider in their transverse diameter than anteroposterior diameter and are sloped inferiorly from posterior to anterior. This makes these vertebra more liable to dislocation without fracture than the other spinal regions. The small size of the vertebral bodies also makes them liable to comminuted body fracture. Flexion and rotation or flexion and mild compression result in the dislocation of one or both facets. If the vertical loading force is greater, the body will fracture. Either of these injury patterns has a high association with major spinal cord injury. Extension forces, except in the extreme, produce posterior subluxation and are generally associated with incomplete spinal cord injury. This is particularly true in middle-aged or older persons with osteoarthritis of the spine in whom the cord is pinched between the spurs anteriorly and the buckled ligamentum flavum posteriorly.

The thoracic spine is relatively rigid due to the stabilizing effect of the ribs and sternum. Except for the first rib, each rib articulates with two adjacent vertebra, and the true ribs are attached to the sternum anteriorly. Much more extreme force is required to cause major spine fracture and is usually associated with major chest injury. An exception is the compression fractures that occur in the osteoporotic spine; these require little force but are rarely associated with spinal malalignment, instability, or risk of spinal cord injury.

The lumbar vertebrae are the largest and strongest. The bodies are cylindrical with nearly equal anteroposterior and transverse diameters. The facets are oriented in the sagittal plane so as to allow relatively free flexion and lateral bending but limited rotation. Based primarily on the computed tomography (CT) examination, Denis proposed the three-column theory for the determination of stability in lumbar fractures. The middle column composed of the posterior portion of the vertebral body and the posterior column composed of the facet joints, and laminae were most important for maintaining spinal stability. Injuries that disrupted these two columns rendered the spine unstable and carried a high risk for spinal cord injury and required either prolonged bed rest or surgical stabilization. These include the burst fracture and flexion-rotation or slice fracture.

Pathophysiology

The spinal cord is composed of a central core of gray matter that contains the neuronal cell bodies and a peripheral layer of white matter in which the major ascending and descending tracts are located. The major tracts, whose functioning can be determined by routine neurologic examination, are illustrated in Fig. 55-3. Blood normally reaches the anterior two-thirds of the spinal cord through the anterior spinal artery and the posterior one-third through the paired posterior spinal arteries. Interconnecting vessels that encircle the spinal cord supply the blood to the periphery of the white matter. Fibers are arranged in a segmental manner, or laminae, within the tracts. The lateral spinothalamic tract and the corticospinal tract are anatomically close to each other and have a common blood supply. If functioning of one tract is impaired, functioning of the other is usually similarly impaired, and the potential of recovery is the same for both. Impairment and recovery of functioning of these two tracts are, however, unrelated to the impairment and recovery of function of the dorsal column. If there is sparing of pain pathways and preservation of motor function in the lateral tract, the patient has a more favorable prognosis than if only the posterior column is not damaged.

A force strong enough to injure the patient's spinal cord initiates a complex series of biochemical and physical events that may completely destroy the functional tissue of the involved segment within a period of 4 to 8 hours. When a 400 gm/cm force is delivered to the exposed spinal cord of a laboratory animal, pericapsular hemorrhages appear in the gray matter within 15 minutes, coalesce, and expand until they involve all of the gray matter and extend into the white matter. These events are accompanied by a decrease in oxygen saturation and intracellular and extracellular edema. Although the histologic changes evolve over several hours, the effect is an immediate and permanent loss of spinal cord function. On the other hand, if less force is applied, the injury is frequently reversible, even though similar biochemical and physical responses occur (Fig. 55-4). The prognosis is better because only a part of the cross section of the cord is affected. The destruction, nevertheless, leaves residual damage in its wake as it recedes.

Spinal cord injuries are classified as follows. If there is no evidence of function distal to the site of injury (i.e., if the patient has no sensation and is totally paralyzed below the level of injury), the injury is *complete.* If no sensation or movement is apparent 12 to 24 hours after the cord is injured, recovery is extremely unlikely. An *incomplete injury* spares some sensory and motor function below the level of the lesion. Because sparing, which is observed most often in sacral segments, is often slight and can be easily overlooked, the patient should be examined closely in this region. This is important for prognosis and treatment planning since significant recovery is possible in incomplete injuries that are managed properly.

The incomplete injuries can be divided into one of five patterns or syndromes, each of which has a different prognosis that can determine the emergency treatment priorities. The most common is the central cord syndrome, and its hallmark is motor and sensory loss, which is greatest at the level of injury and improved function the further distally from the level of injury. It is seen typically in hyperextension injuries of the cervical spine in persons with osteoarthritis of the spine. Its prognosis is variable and has classically been considered an injury best treated nonoperatively. However, there have been reports of increased improvement in instances in which herniated disk material was demonstrated and removed. The anterior cord syndrome is the next most common and shows preservation of touch, position, and vibration sense but loss of pain and temperature sense and motor function. It has the poorest prognosis of any of the incomplete injuries. In this group, the spinal canal is compromised by bone or disk material anteriorly; many recommend emergent or urgent surgery to restore the canal alignment and diameter. There have been no studies, however, that support this concept. Most studies that are cited in support of this concept fail to differentiate the different syndromes but report better results in patients with incomplete syndromes compared with other series or historic controls. The Brown-Sequard syndrome or hemisection of the cord presents with motor loss on the side of injury and loss of pain and temperature sense on the contralateral side. This syndrome has the best prognosis of any of the incomplete syndromes. The fourth syndrome is the posterior cord syndrome, in which motor power is preserved but the posterior column functions of touch, vibration, and position sense are lost. This syndrome is so rare that the prognosis is difficult to determine. Finally, there is the spinal cord concussion syndrome, which is similar to a cerebral concussion in that the function returns rapidly and within 12 to 24 hours the person is normal with no residual deficit.

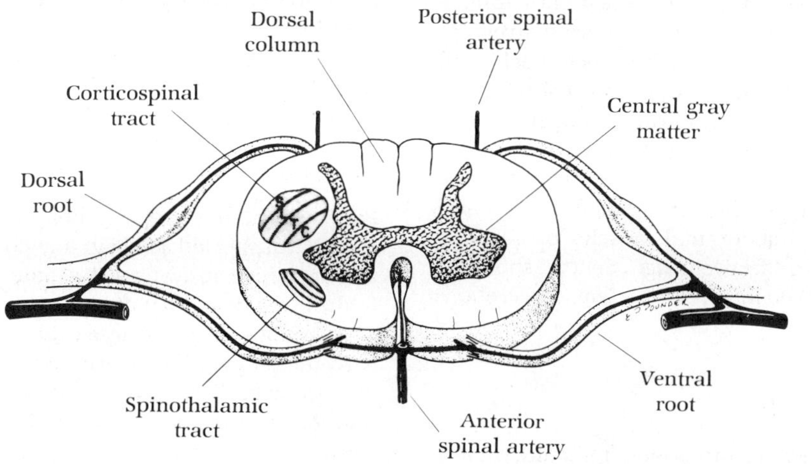

Fig. 55-3. Anatomy of the normal spinal cord. The fibers of the sacral distribution are most lateral in position in both the corticospinal and spinothalamic tracts.

MANAGEMENT AT THE ACCIDENT SITE

Evaluation of the Patient

An evaluation of injuries to the patient's whole body, not just the spine, should begin as soon as the emergency personnel arrive at the site of the accident. The position of the patient and of the parts of the body should be noted, and any external evidence such as bruises, contusions, or lacerations indicating that the spine may have been injured should be sought. Pain in the neck or spine, tenderness of the spine, or paralysis or loss of sensation suggests a spinal injury. In addition, any patient who sustained a head injury, is unconscious, has fallen from a height, has had a driving accident, or is a victim of a high-velocity accident should be assumed to have a spinal injury. These patients should be handled as though the spine is so damaged that the cord is threatened. Although the spine should be inspected specifically for deformity, especially abnormal angulation, no attempt should be made to correct the deformity except to position the body in the neutral anatomic position. This can usually be carried out safely, but forceful manipulation should be avoided. Because the forces that produce injuries are often transmitted through the head, shoulders, or pelvic regions, these areas should be examined closely for additional local injury.

Fig. 55-4. Central damage in an incomplete injury.

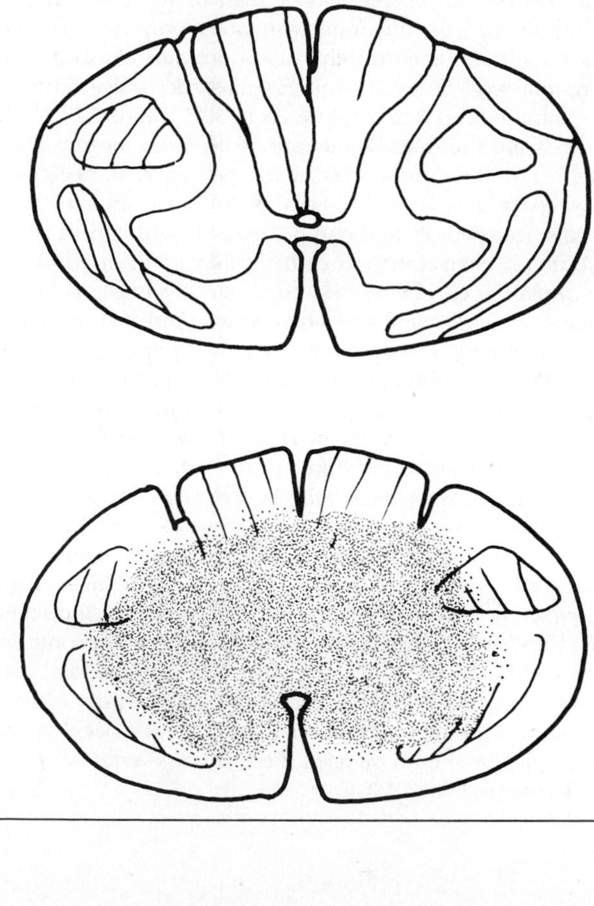

The evaluation should include a search for signs of other injuries, such as labored respiration, which may indicate that the airway is obstructed or the chest is injured; external bleeding; limb deformity, which may suggest a fracture; bleeding from the ears, nose, or mouth; and unequal dilation of pupils, which may be a result of head injury. Because injuries below the level of spinal cord injury may be totally asymptomatic and the patient may be completely unaware of them, a thorough search is essential. Life-threatening conditions should be treated immediately but, whenever possible, without moving the patient or the spine excessively. Other conditions that are uncovered may require special handling. If the patient cannot be fully examined before being immobilized and extricated, the examination should be repeated after extrication but before departure for the hospital, if no life-threatening conditions are present.

Immediate Life Support

All injuries to the spinal cord above the tenth thoracic segment (T10) compromise respiration, which normally requires the coordination of the diaphragm, the intercostals, and the abdominal muscles. The diaphragm is innervated primarily by C3 and C4, the intercostal muscles by T2 through T8, and the abdominal muscles by T8 through T11.

Any complete injury above C3 therefore necessitates application of total respiratory support, and an injury between C4 and C5 may also require respiratory assistance. Lack of innervation of the intercostals causes a paradoxical motion of the chest wall when the lower cervical or upper thoracic spine is injured, decreasing the tidal volume and ventilatory capacity. Oxygen should therefore be administered to patients with cervical and upper thoracic spine injuries. Paralysis of the intercostal and abdominal muscles prevents the patient from producing an effective cough. Suction should be available at all times to keep the pharynx clear of secretions, blood, and vomitus.

History

The personnel at the scene of the accident should elicit as much background information about the accident as possible from witnesses and the patient. Information about how the accident happened, the events that occurred between the time of the accident and the time the emergency personnel first saw the patient, any change in the patient's sensation or ability to move (e.g., was paralysis followed by return of feeling and ability to move, or vice versa?), and the patient's current symptoms (pain and its location or any other abnormal sensation) often provide clues about the type and mechanism of injury. Knowing the mechanism may be useful in deciding how to handle the patient in order to prevent further injury. A good rule of thumb is that the patient should be handled in such a way that he or she is not subjected to the type of motion that seems to have caused the injury. For example, if the injury resulted from flexion, particular attention should be paid in the immobilization to prevent further flexion.

Treatment

Immobilization

The entire spine should be immobilized, preferably with a spine board, before the patient is extricated. A short board is appropriate if the patient is sitting in a confined space such as an automobile. One person should maintain firm but gentle longitudinal traction with the patient's head in the neutral position, and another person should place a cervical collar or other immobilizing device (e.g., rolled up towel or newspaper) around the patient's neck. The patient should then be secured to the appropriate board. If a short board was used during extrication, the patient should then be completely immobilized onto the long board before transportation. If the patient is initially found in a nonconfined location, he or she should be immobilized initially on the long spine board. The standard log rolling technique carried out by three or four people is the preferred method. The essential feature of this method is to move the patient as a single unit without bending or twisting the spine.

Neurologic Examination

A brief check of motor and sensory functions of any patient who is suspected of having spine injury should be carried out by emergency personnel before transporting the patient. This would involve at least observing the patient's ability to move the hands and feet and checking the patient's ability to feel touch and pain sensation in both feet and both hands. These findings should be documented by the emergency personnel.

Transportation

Patients who are properly immobilized with a spine board can be transported safely in any position. The standard position in which to transport a patient is the supine position. In the event of sudden emesis or excessive collection of fluids or secretions in the pharynx that interferes with a clear airway, the patient, if properly secured to the spine board, can be rapidly turned to the side position or even to a semiprone position in order to allow gravity to help maintain a clear airway.

Transportation from the site of the accident to the nearest treatment facility should be as expeditious as possible, but unless the patient is in critical condition because of nonspine injuries or respiratory involvement, high-speed transfer is unnecessary. Indeed, the inevitable bouncing and jolting may further injure the patient's spine and spinal cord.

MANAGEMENT AT THE INITIAL MEDICAL FACILITY

Resuscitation

Priority is given to stabilizing the vital functions when the patient arrives in the emergency department. An intravenous line with a large-bore needle should be inserted, and treatment for shock and blood loss should be initiated as appropriate. Lesions to the cervical or high thoracic spinal cord result in immediate functional sympathectomy. The patient's signs are altered accordingly: blood pressure 70 to 90 mm Hg systolic and 50 to 70 mm Hg diastolic; pulse 50 to 60 beats/minute; and temperature 35 to 36°C (95–97°F). If the patient is alert and conscious and if the urine output is acceptable, treating these vital signs per se is unnecessary. Bradycardia that is severe enough to cause an arrythmia presents occasionally and can be reversed with atropine, 0.4 to 0.6 mg. A central venous catheter may be inserted so that the circulation can be monitored. A blood sample is drawn for routine hemogram and chemistries, and arterial blood gases are obtained to determine whether respiration is adequate. Prompt initiation of intermittent positive pressure breathing helps prevent pulmonary complications, which are the most common cause of early morbidity and mortality. If ventilation requires mechanical support, inserting a nasotracheal or an orotracheal tube is preferable to performing a tracheotomy. Extreme caution must be exercised to avoid extending or flexing the neck of a patient who is suspected of having cervical spine injury. Ideally, an anesthesiologist or another physician experienced in inserting endotracheal tubes should perform this procedure. Using a fiberoptic laryngoscope or a bronchoscope with the endotracheal tube passed down over it is a technique that permits difficult intubation without manipulating the patient's neck. A volume respirator should be used if continuous ventilatory support is required.

Evaluation of the Patient

Physical Examination

After life-threatening conditions have been stabilized, a thorough examination aimed at finding associated injuries should be begun, but it may have to be conducted in stages as treatment progresses. Above the level of neurologic deficit, the examination should be conducted exactly as it would be if the patient's spine were not injured. Below the level of the spinal cord injury, normal symptoms and signs may be modified or absent: Abdominal pain, tenderness, or reflex guarding, for example, may be absent even if injuries are present with intraperitoneal bleeding. Additional diagnostic procedures such as peritoneal lavage or minilaparotomy to check for abdominal bleeding may therefore be necessary. All body surfaces should be inspected, but unless definite evidence of a life-threatening injury is noted, the patient should not be turned to complete the examination until the skeletal lesion has been defined radiographically and the patient has been immobilized appropriately. This examination should be conducted as rapidly as possible, and ideally the patient should remain immobilized on the spine board until the spine has been cleared radiographically. Concomitant injuries should be managed in the usual manner and generally have priority for treatment over the spine and spinal cord injuries. Care must be exercised once again throughout this treatment to protect the spine and spinal cord. A fracture below the level of injury should be immobilized using a well-molded splint or bivalve cast, never a solid circular cast. Because the muscles below the level of injury are usually flaccid initially, skeletal traction is not necessary; in fact, it often makes treatment of the spine injury more difficult and may result in complications.

Neurologic Examination

The presence of paralysis and the level of completeness of injury can be determined by testing the patient's motor and sensory functioning. Precise recording of the findings on a diagram and marking the level of injury directly on the patient facilitates frequent assessment. In addition to checking for paralysis by having the patient make purposeful movements with the hands and feet, the physician should observe the patient's sensory response to pinprick, light touch, vibration, and proprioception.

With the patient fully supine with arms extended in the palm-up position, the physician should begin the examination distally and move proximally. The physician should begin in the perianal region, move down the posterior thighs and then proximally along the anterior leg and thigh and up the trunk in the midaxillary line, down the arms, across the palm, and up the preaxial border of the arm (Fig. 55-5). It is preferable to begin this sensory examination distally and move proximally because the level of injury can be identified more easily by going from an area in which sensation is absent. Because the sensory segments from C5 through T1 are not represented on the anterior torso, it is preferable to move proximally in the midaxillary to anterior axillary line rather than in the midclavicular line. A precise motor level cannot be defined as rapidly as a sensory level, but certain muscles provide a convenient index to level of injury (Table 55-1). Each muscle is innervated by several spinal cord seg-

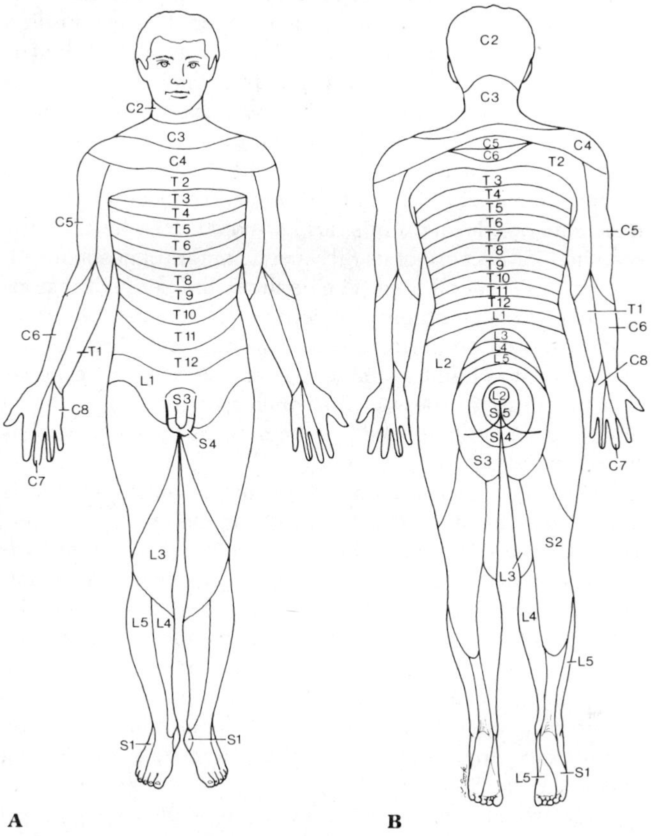

Fig. 55-5. Frontal (A) and dorsal (B) distribution of dermatomes.

Table 55-1. Major index muscles for determining level of motor function

Muscle	Spinal cord segment
Diaphragm	C3
Sternocleidomastoid	C4
Deltoid	C4, C5
Biceps	C5
Extensor carpi radialis	C6
Triceps	C7
Flexor carpi radialis	C8
Extensor digitorum communis	C8
Interossei and lumbricals	T1
Upper rectus abdominis	T8
Lower rectus abdominis	T9, T10
Quadratus lumborum	T11
Iliopsoas	T12, L1
Adductors of the hip	L2
Quadriceps femoris	L3, L4
Tibialis anterior	L5
Gastrocnemius	S1
Gluteus medius and maximus	S2
Sphincter ani	S3, S4

ments. The segments listed in Table 55-1 are the ones that appear to provide the major innervation to the muscles. Thus, if a muscle has a strength of fair (3 out of 5) or better, the major portion of the segment is probably intact. The representation of segments in the lower extremities is much broader and less precise than in the upper extremities.

Any residual sensation or motor function below the level of the lesions signifies that the injury is incomplete. The most common location of sparing, which must be carefully searched for because of its therapeutic and prognostic implications, is the sacral area. The perianal and perineal regions should be tested with pin and light touch, and a rectal examination should be performed to determine whether the patient has any voluntary sphincter response. Sensory response to a pin prick in the sacral segments or motor sparing at any level below the injury has the most favorable prognosis for recovery.

Neurologic deterioration that occurs in an injury that is known to be incomplete is frequently an indication for emergency surgery. The major deep tendon reflexes, the plantar reflexes, and the conus reflexes should be tested. Most patients demonstrate no major deep tendon reflexes below the level of injury, the condition known as spinal shock. The anal wink (contraction of the external sphincter when the skin near the anus is stimulated with a pin) and the bulbocavernosus reflex (contraction of the anal sphincter upon compressing the glans of the penis or clitoris or tugging gently on the Foley catheter) are conus reflexes and frequently are not lost or return a short time after spinal cord injury. The plantar reflex following acute spinal cord injury is extremely variable without regard to the nature or completeness of the injury. This variation is seen in patients with similar lesions and in the same patient at different times after the injury. Reflex testing is important because it occasionally provides evidence that the injury may be incomplete even if no sensory or motor sparing is demonstrated. If hyperactive deep tendon reflex appears soon after injury or if an injury is above the lower thoracic spine and no bulbocavernosus reflex can be elicited, the injury may be incomplete. Such findings do not, however, constitute proof of incompleteness.

Radiologic Examination

After any high-velocity trauma, the spine should be examined radiographically. Many trauma centers have a routine trauma series of x-rays that are obtained in all major trauma victims. In our center, this includes anteroposterior, lateral, and open mouth views of the cervical spine and anteroposterior and lateral views of the lumbar spine. If there is any indication of thoracic trauma or suspicion of vertebral injury on the chest film, a lateral view of the thoracic spine is obtained.

X-ray films of the skull are indicated, particularly if there is any history of unconsciousness, if there is suspicion of head injury, or if skull tongs traction is to be applied. In patients with head and cervical spine injuries, in addition, an open mouth view of the atlas and axis should be performed. Figures 55-6 through 55-9 illustrate the most common types of injury to the cervical and thoracolumbar spines. If x-ray examination reveals that the superior vertebrae is displaced more than one-half the width of the vertebral body below, the patient has sustained a bilateral facet dislocation or a fracture dislocation. A displacement of one-half the width or less of the superior over the inferior vertebral body, on the other hand, suggests that the injury is only a partial dislocation or unilateral facet dislocation. An oblique view of the spine demonstrating the side of the dislocation should be made. This can be accomplished without moving the patient by placing the film flat beneath the patient and angling the x-ray to 50 degrees. This view is also of value in identifying injuries to the pedicles or injuries of the lower cervical spine when the lowest vertebrae are obscured on lateral film by the shoulders. Occasionally, x-ray films do not confirm an injury of the cervical spine that is suggested by neurologic signs. This may result if the entire cervical spine was not visualized, if the injury was caused by extension injury, or if the dislocation spontaneously reduced; occasionally spinal cord injury occurs without demonstrable spine injury. Despite negative initial films, an injury to the spine cannot be ruled out as a possibility, and the patient should be treated as though such an injury had occurred. Neurologic evidence indicating that the spinal cord is injured between C6 and T2 should be confirmed by films of the lower cervical and upper thoracic spine. These areas may be demonstrated radiographically if traction is applied to the patient's arm and shoulders while performing the lateral x-ray. If this method fails, the swimmer's view, taken with one arm over the head and the other at the side, may demonstrate the lesion. Oblique films also can be valuable in this situation, as noted previously. If these methods fail to demonstrate the lower cervical and upper thoracic spine adequately, tomography may be necessary.

Demonstrating a dislocation that has spontaneously been reduced is also possible. Lateral views should be made while the patient's neck is gently flexed and extended. Although flexion up to 20 degrees and extension to 20 degrees seem to impose no significant risk, force should not be applied and the motion should be stopped if it causes any additional pain or neurologic symptoms. These views should be obtained only under the supervision of a physician who is experienced in dealing with patients who have had cervical spine injuries. If this expertise is not available, the patient should be immobilized and transferred to a facility where such physicians are available.

Computed tomography (CT) scan of the injured area of the spine is used to determine more precisely the nature of the bony injury and the degree of canal compromise. In the cervical spine, metrizamide enhancement will help identify disk material that may be impinging on the spinal cord. It will often demonstrate vertebral injuries not apparent on plain radiographs, particularly in the vertebrae adjacent to the injured vertebral. CT scan is the major study used to determine stability applying the three-column theory. Except in evaluating injuries to the odontoid, it has replaced tomography in evaluation of the spine. CT scan should be obtained whenever the plain x-rays do not demonstrate a vertebral injury in a person with neurologic deficit. If possible, a CT scan should be obtained prior to any operative procedure on the spine in the person with spinal cord injury.

Magnetic resonance imaging (MRI) enables one to image the spinal cord directly. The T2-weighted image will show the spinal cord directly and can demonstrate what is thought to be either hemorrhage or edema within the spinal cord and may aid in determining the prognosis. The MRI does not demonstrate bony detail but will show the status of the

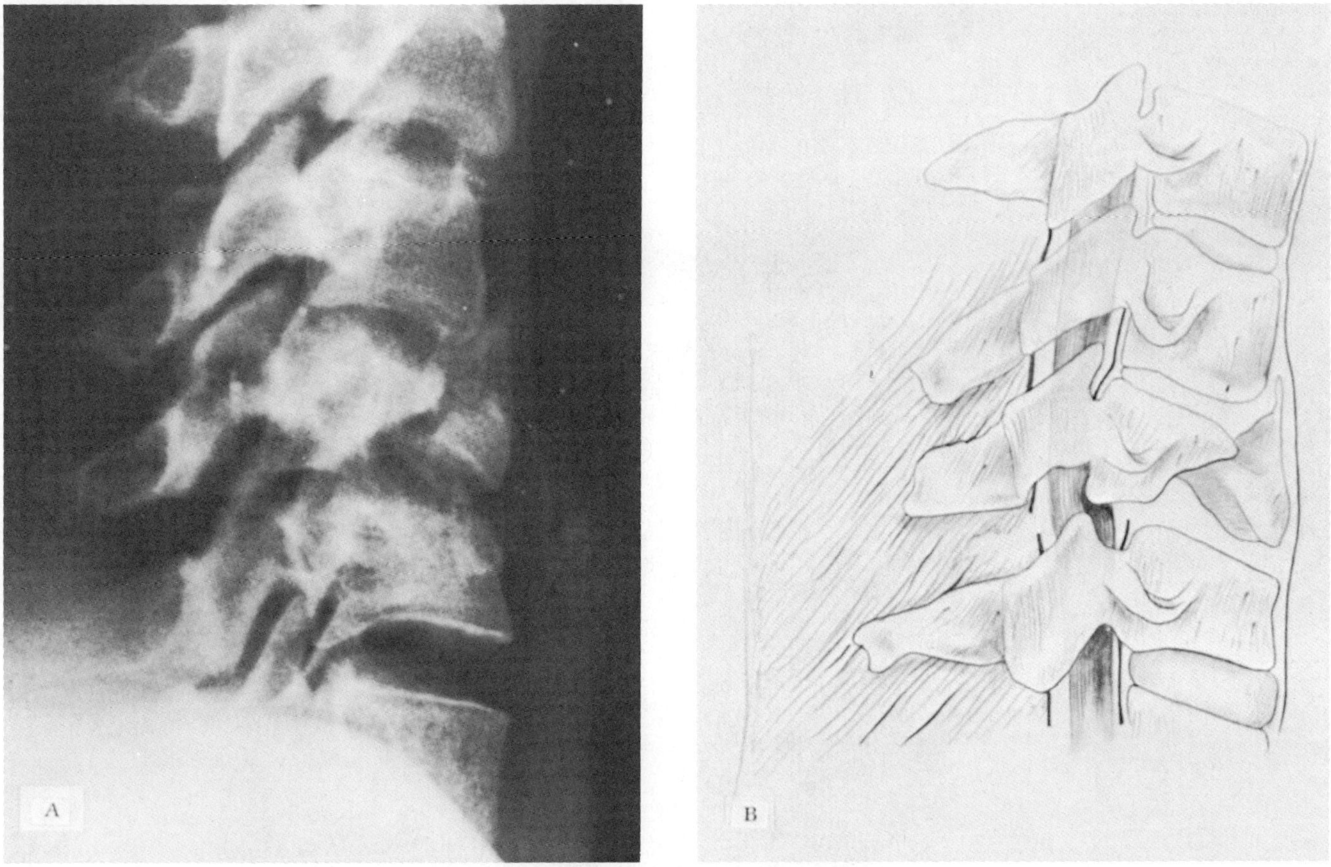

Fig. 55-6. Radiograph (A) and drawing (B) of fracture dislocation of the cervical spine.

ligaments, disk, and other soft tissue in and adjacent to the spine and spinal cord. Since MRI will demonstrate bone disk or hematoma and its relationship to the spinal cord, it can be invaluable in determining the need for surgery. Currently, the major problem with MRI examination of the acutely injured person is the confining nature of the machine, the length of time required to carry out the examination, and the difficulty monitoring the patient during the examination. If our experience with CT scanning is any indicator, we can expect that these logistic problems will be overcome and MRI will become part of the standard examination of acute spinal cord injury. Because MRI does not show bony detail, it cannot replace the CT scan in the examination of the injured spine.

Treatment

Immobilization

A patient with an injured spine should always be immobilized whether or not the spinal cord is injured. Patients with thoracic and lumbar spine injuries are most effectively immobilized in a firm bed with a bed board or in a Striker frame. Patients with cervical spine injuries require traction in addition to postural immobilization. Although head halter traction with a 4.5-kg weight and a cervical collar are acceptable for a short period, skeletal skull traction should be used if traction must be applied for a longer period of time. Several types of cranial tongs (Crutchfield, Cone-Barton, Vinky, Gardner-Wells) are currently available. The choice of device should depend on the physician's experience and on what is available in the hospital. The Gardner-Wells tongs have gained wide acceptance. In addition to being simple to use, they can be rapidly applied. They require no special instruments or skin incisions, and a spring-loaded device built into them indicates when the proper amount of compressive force has been applied. The Gardner-Wells tongs are inserted 2 to 4 cm above the helix of the ear below the point of maximum circumference of the skull in neutral axis of the neck. The neutral axis is estimated to be on a line drawn from the tip of the mastoid process through the external auditory meatus (Fig. 55-10). Unless the patient's hair is long, thick, or dirty, the area need not be shaved. The area selected on each side of the head is prepared with an antiseptic solution such as povidone-iodine. Local anesthesia is given to the patient by infiltration by 1 or 2 percent lidocaine, being certain to infiltrate down to and including the galea and periosteum. The tongs are then placed in the selected position, and the pins are turned by hand on each side simultaneously until they penetrate the skin and soft tissues and are seated firmly in the outer table of the skull. The pins are tightened until the indicator pin on the spring-loaded side protrudes 1 to 2 mm. After the axis of the pins and the lock nuts are tightened, the tongs are moved up and down. The following day, the pins should be retightened to

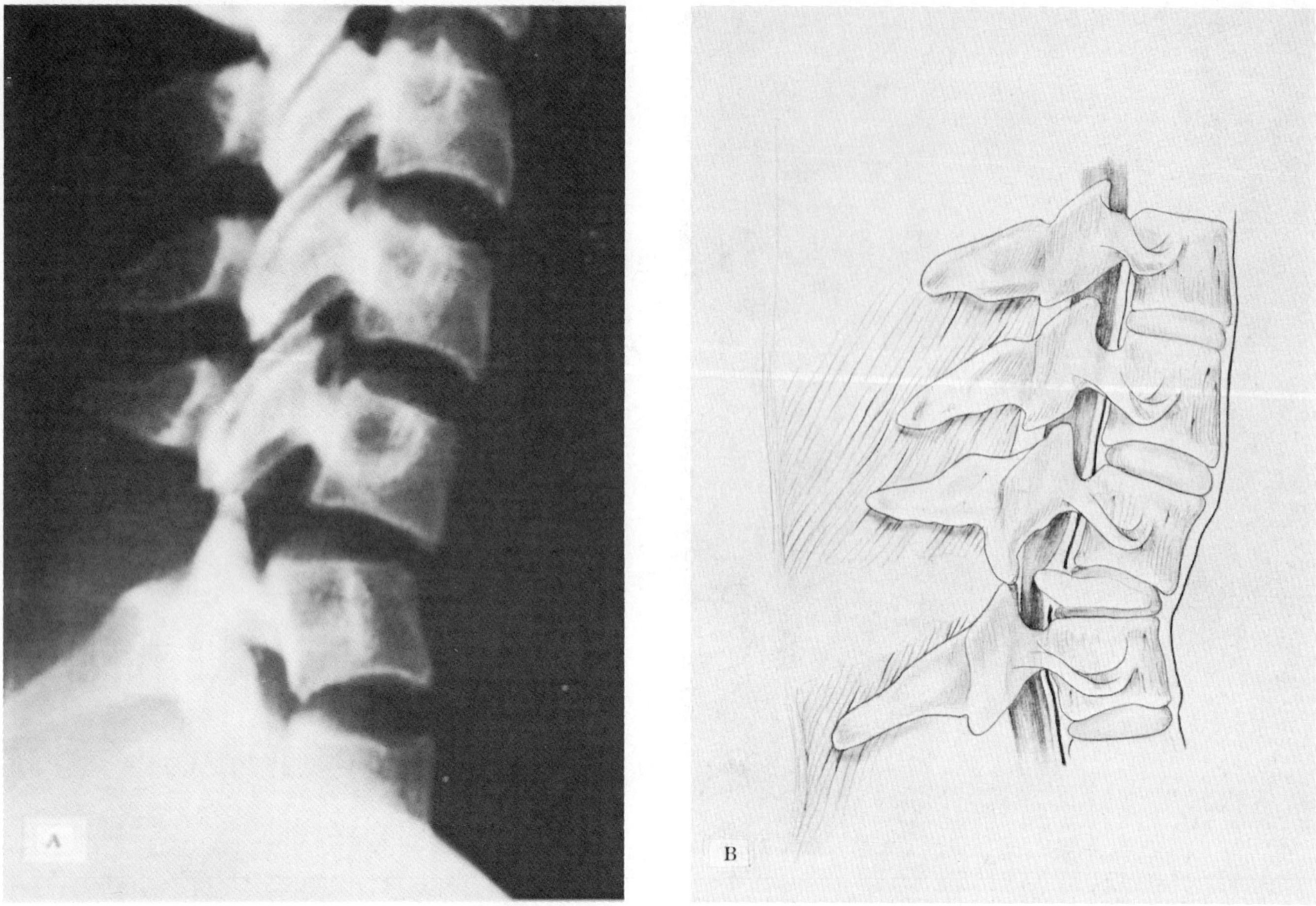

Fig. 55-7. Radiograph (A) and drawing (B) of dislocation of the cervical spine with ligament damage.

be sure that the indicator protrudes 1 to 2 mm. They should not be tightened subsequently.

The patient who presents with symptoms or signs of an injury to the cervical spinal cord should be immobilized with cranial tongs traction whether or not radiographs have demonstrated injury to the cervical spine. This type of immobilization is especially important if a lower cervical or upper thoracic segment has been injured, because these parts of the spine are extremely difficult to visualize radiographically, and a special technique such as laminography may be required to confirm the diagnosis. Cranial tongs traction is also efficacious if the spinal cord is injured only slightly. Experience indicates that a speedier recovery is effected by such immobilization even if the skeletal injury appears not to be severe enough to cause spine instability.

Bladder Management

An indwelling Foley catheter should be aseptically placed in the patient's urinary bladder. This enables close monitoring of urine output and prevents bladder distention during this immediate period when it may be necessary to carry out fluid replacement therapy and to give medications intravenously. Intermittent catheterization is the preferred method of long-term bladder drainage to prevent urinary tract infection and retrain the bladder, but it requires careful control of fluid intake and precise technique. An indwelling catheter can be left in place for up to 48 hours without the bladder becoming infected.

Medication

Based on the recently published study by Bracken, et al., it has now become the standard of care to give all acute injuries treatment with high-dose steroids as soon as possible after injury. This is the first study that, in a controlled trial, has shown the efficacy of any drug treatment program. In this study both complete and incomplete injury showed beneficial effects of treatment. To be effective, treatment must be instituted within 8 hours of injury. If treatment was not started within 8 hours of injury, the results were no different from those in the placebo control group. The dosage schedule is as follows: 30 mg/kg methylprednisolone IV over 15 minutes followed by a 45-minute pause, then 5.4 mg/kg/hour methylprednisolone over the next 23 hours. No statistically significant increase in complications was noted in the treatment group.

Decompression of the Gastrointestinal Tract

A patient should be given nothing by mouth, because ileus usually accompanies any significant spine or spinal cord injury. Nausea, vomiting, or abdominal distention indicates the need for a nasogastric tube, placed either on gravity drainage or low suction. Additionally, a nasogastric tube

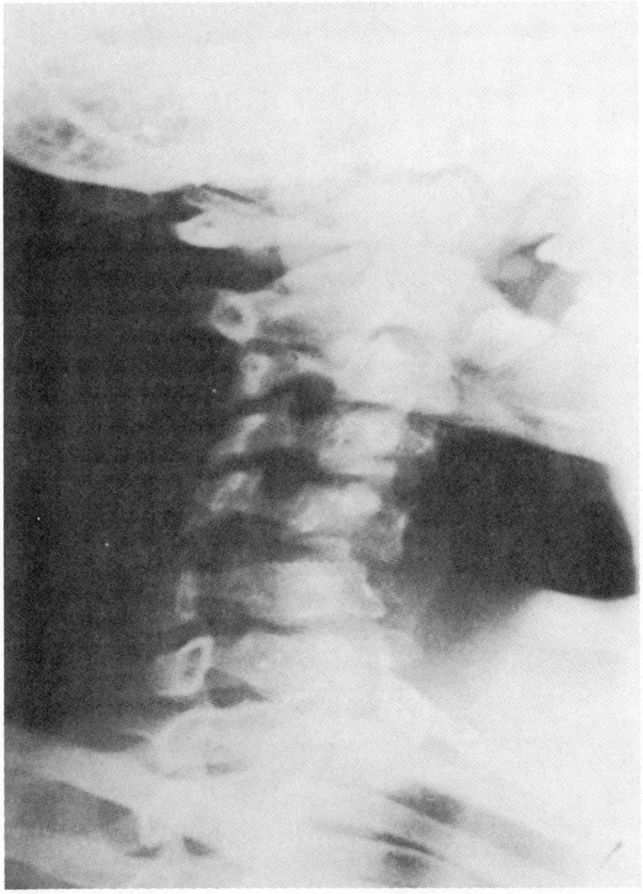

Fig. 55-8. Oblique view of a unilateral facet dislocation of the cervical spine.

should be inserted before the patient is transported to a secondary or tertiary care facility to reduce the risk of vomiting and aspiration during transportation.

Fluids

A crystalloid solution should be administered intravenously; 5 percent dextrose and water or 5 percent dextrose and 0.5 percent normal saline or Ringer's lactate solution are the recommended solutions. These solutions should be given at a rate of not more than 100 ml/hour unless a higher rate is specifically indicated—for example, if there is a large volume of gastric drainage. Blood plasma or colloid solution should be given only if volume replacement is required. The physician must remember that a low blood pressure is normal for a patient with a high spinal cord injury and that patients with spinal cord injuries are extremely sensitive to fluid overload, which is a frequent cause of pulmonary problems as a result of increased secretion and interstitial fluid.

Transfer

Once the patient's condition has been stabilized in the emergency department, plans should be made for transfer to a facility that has the capability for definitive management of spine and spinal cord injuries if such capability is not available at the initial treating facility. Every emergency department should have arrangements and protocols for transferring patients with spinal cord injuries to the nearest spinal cord injury unit or center.

WHIPLASH INJURIES

Soft tissue injuries to the neck present a problem to emergency medical personnel. If patients with a soft tissue or whiplash injury are properly handled at the site of the accident, they should arrive at the emergency department completely immobilized with a collar. Although this procedure may seem to be overtreatment for a benign condition, personnel at an accident site are not equipped to differentiate between a soft tissue injury of the neck and a more serious cervical spine injury. It is the responsibility of the emergency physician to evaluate the patient and rule out the possibility that a more serious injury has not been sustained and to begin appropriate treatment.

A sudden acceleration that causes the head to move backward rapidly and the neck to hyperextend is the most common way in which whiplash injuries occur. This is frequently experienced in rear-end automobile collisions. This type of injury may produce transient cerebral injury and stretch the anterior cervical structures, the esophagus, the neck muscles, and ligaments in the intervertebral disk. These injuries rarely result in a structural instability of the cervical spine or in a spinal cord injury.

Evaluation of the Patient

History

Two-thirds of patients presenting with soft tissue injuries to the neck have cerebral symptoms (confusion, mental dullness, or mild amnesia), and one-tenth are unconscious for a brief period. Neck ache often followed several hours later by soreness and stiffness in the neck and upper shoulders are the most common symptoms. Patients frequently complain of pain radiating to the occiput and forward to the eyes, the upper scapular regions, or into the arms, but the pains do not follow a nerve root or a peripheral nerve distribution and are not accompanied by objective signs of nerve injury.

Physical Examination

The physical examination should include a complete neurologic examination, including state of consciousness, cerebral functioning, cranial nerves, spinal cord function, and peripheral nerve. Except for minor temporary cerebral signs, the findings should be normal if the patient has a soft tissue injury. The neck and upper thoracic spine should be examined for swelling, tenderness, spasm, and restricted mobility. Few if any signs appear in the first hour or two after injury. Spasm and restriction of motion usually do not develop for several hours or even until the day after injury. These symptoms usually subside in 5 to 7 days. In general, the physical findings are rarely proportional to the symptoms.

X-Ray Examination

A suspected diagnosis of soft tissue injury should be confirmed by x-ray film to ensure that no bone or major ligament injury has occurred. The examination should include anteroposterior and lateral views of the entire cervical spine

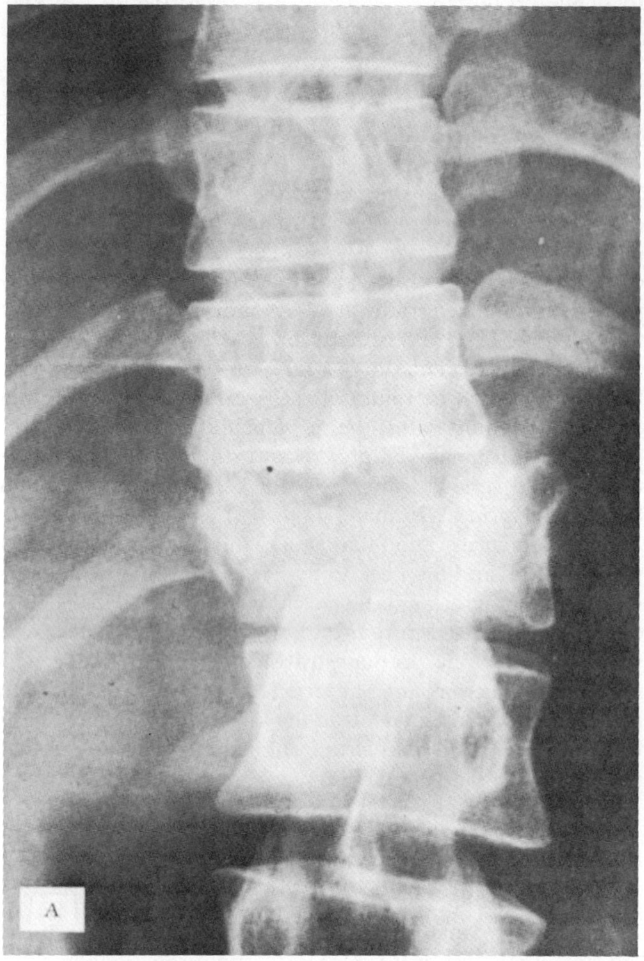

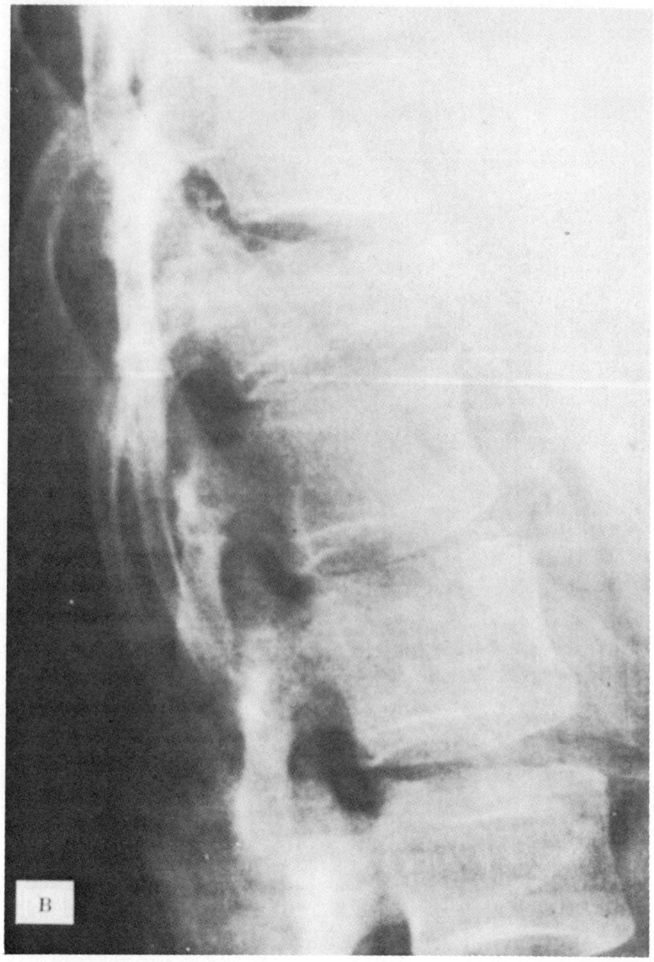

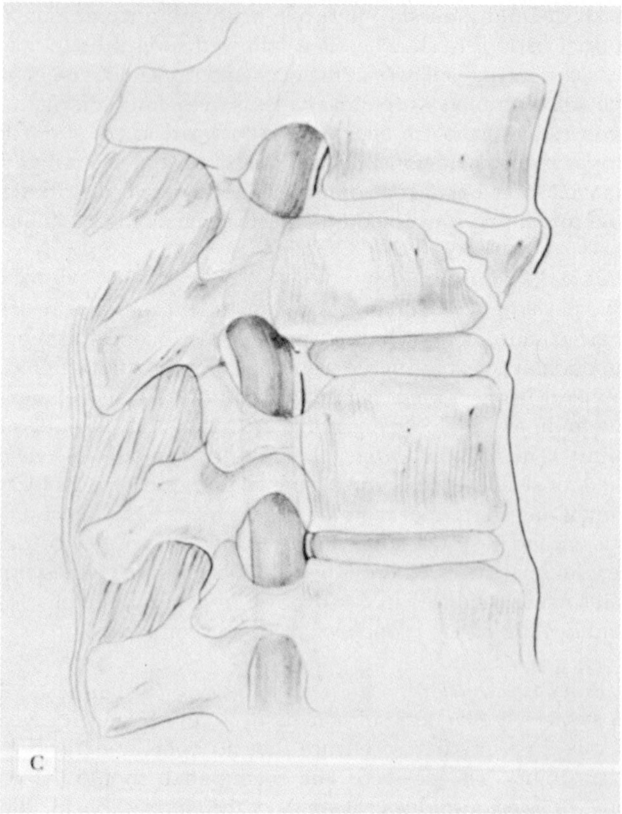

Fig. 55-9. Anteroposterior radiograph (A), lateral radiograph (B), and drawing (C) of B. Fracture dislocation of the thoracolumbar spine.

as well as odontoid views and oblique or pillar views. If the neurologic and film examinations are negative, lateral views of the flexed and extended neck should be made to rule out significant ligament damage. The patient should flex and extend his or her neck rather than have a technician place the neck at the extremes of the range. An abnormal distance between the spinous processes indicates that the posterior ligaments are torn. Signs of soft tissue injury (i.e., abnormal soft tissue shadows such as widening of the perivertebral space), not just of bone injuries, should be looked for on the film. Evidence of preexisting problems such as degenerative disk disease may also be found.

Management
The most important treatment is thorough examination to confirm that the patient has no serious injury. A soft cervical collar, bed rest if spasm is severe, and mild analgesics are usually sufficient to relieve the symptoms. As soon as possible, however, the patient should be weaned from the collar and should begin simple motion exercises in order to resume normal activity. If symptoms and disability persist any longer than 5 to 7 days, the patient should be referred to a specialist

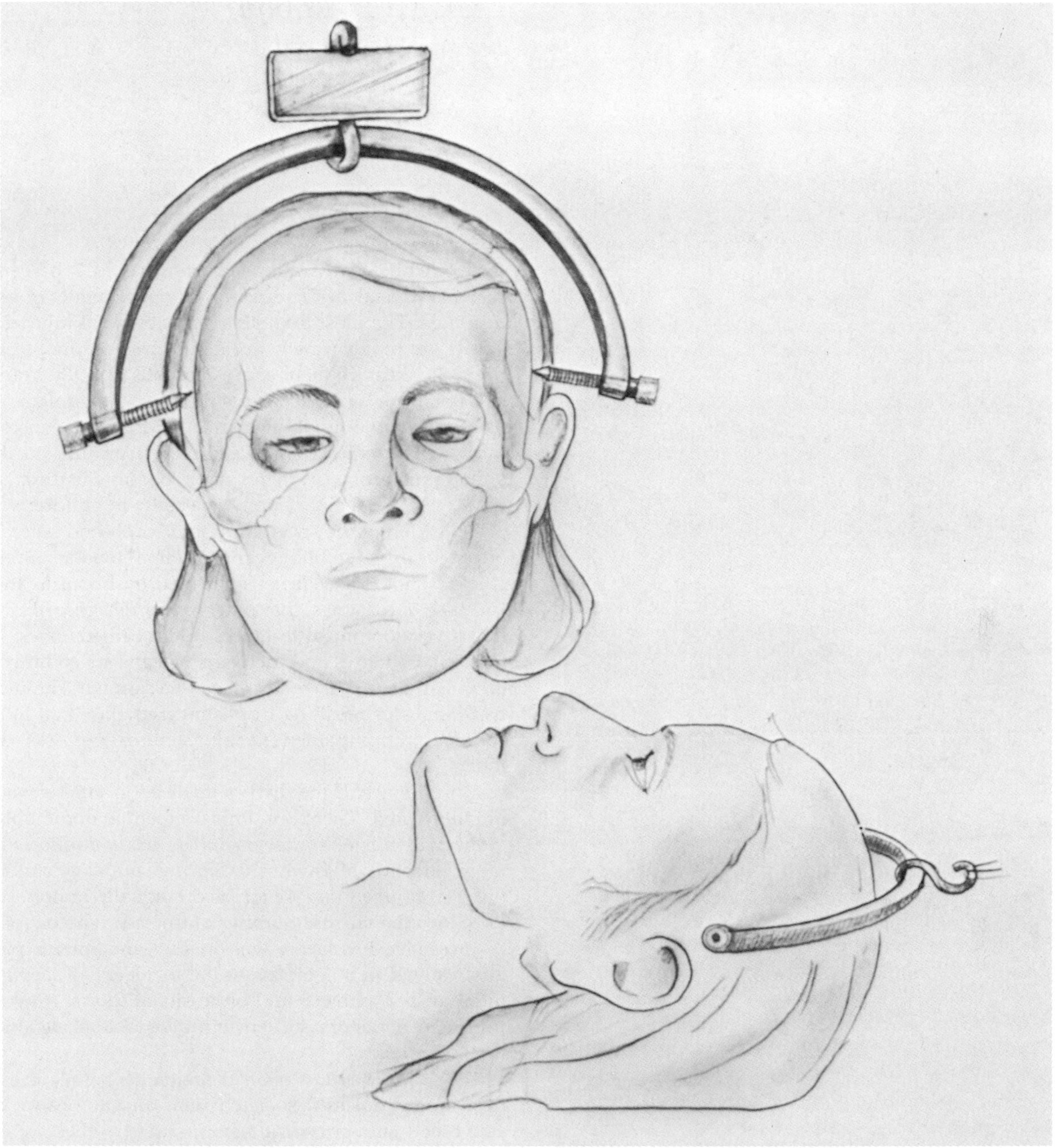

Fig. 55-10. Insertion of Gardner-Wells tongs.

such as a neurosurgeon, orthopedic surgeon, or neurologist for a more specific program.

SELECTED READING

Bedbrook, GM. Spinal injuries with teraplegia and paraplegia. *J Bone Joint Surg* 61B:267, 1979.

Bosch, A, Stauffer, ES, and Nickel, VL. Incomplete traumatic quadriplegia: A ten-year review. *JAMA* 216:473, 1971.

Bracken, MB, et al. A randomized, controlled trial of methylprednisolone or naloxone in the treatment of acute spinal cord injury. *N Engl J Med* 322:1405, 1990.

Guttman, L. *Spinal Cord Injuries: Comprehensive Management and Research.* Oxford: Blackwell Scientific Publications, 1973.

Harris, JH. *The Radiology of Acute Cervical Spine Trauma.* Baltimore: Williams & Wilkins, 1978.

Holdsworth, FW. Fractures, dislocations and fracture-dislocations. *J Bone Joint Surg* 52A:1534, 1970.

Roaf, R. A study of the mechanics of spinal injury. *J Bone Joint Surg* 42B:810, 1960.

Stauffer, ES, and Kauffer, H. Fractures and dislocations of the spine. In CA Rockwood and DP Green (eds), *Fractures.* Philadelphia: Lippincott, 1975. P. 817.

56. Facial Injuries

Leonard B. Kaban
David H. Perrott

People with facial trauma constitute 2 to 7 percent of all patients treated in the emergency departments of large city hospitals. The most frequent causes of facial injuries among adults are motor vehicle accidents; among infants and children, the most frequent causes are falls, usually from a bicycle, porch, or step. Accidents in the home, athletic injuries, fist fights, and animal bites are other frequent causes. Often, intraoral structures alone are injured; trauma to the teeth and dentoalveolar segments are probably the most common injuries in the facial region, especially in children.

Reduction of the speed limit to 55 mph and several recent advances in automobile construction (shatterproof windshields, shoulder seat belts, padded dashboards and roofs, stronger car frames) have helped to decrease the number and severity of facial fractures in the United States. Mandatory seat belt laws and increases of some speed limit's effects on facial trauma have yet to be determined. The major soft tissue injuries resulting from shattered glass that in the past so often accompanied facial fractures are less common today.

More than half the drivers involved in fatal car accidents are inebriated. Therefore, improvement in automobile safety alone will not eliminate facial injuries. Public education, more effective highway monitoring, and law enforcement directed at offending motorists are equally important efforts to reduce the current number of injuries. The increased use of protective headgear, face masks, and mouth protectors has resulted in a decrease in the incidence of facial trauma in organized amateur and professional sports. However, unprotected amateurs still sustain avoidable skeletal and soft tissue damage.

Facial injuries are often dramatic, but they are not life threatening unless associated with airway obstruction, severe blood loss, or central nervous system, chest, or abdominal trauma. These problems must be promptly recognized and treated as the first step in management of the injured patient.

INITIAL ASSESSMENT AND MANAGEMENT

Airway Management

Establishment of a patent airway is the first priority in the treatment of maxillofacial injuries. Airway obstruction may result from intraoral or nasal bleeding; loose teeth, fillings, or dentures; posterior displacement of the tongue and soft tissues associated with fractures of the mandible or midface; swelling of the intraoral soft tissues; or damage to the larynx and trachea.

Foreign bodies, blood, or clots in the mouth or pharynx must be promptly removed by suctioning, by the fingers, or by an instrument. If the patient is able to sit up, he or she should be encouraged to clear the airway by coughing. If unable to sit up, a semiprone position allows for drainage of the oropharynx and proper positioning of the tongue.

Massive swelling of the floor of the mouth or tongue may interfere with respiration. Even if the airway is not obstructed immediately after the accident, it may become blocked as swelling increases or as a hematoma develops in the floor of the mouth, the submandibular region, or pharynx. Oroendotracheal or nasoendotracheal intubation is occasionally necessary if soft tissue swelling continues to interfere with respiration or if the patient is unable to tolerate an oral or nasopharyngeal airway. Only in an emergent situation where intubation is unattainable is cricothyroidotomy or tracheostomy necessary. The physician must remember that a blow forceful enough to fracture the mandible or midface may also result in an injury to the cervical spine. When there is evidence of cervical spine trauma, or when airway management precludes C-spine radiographs, the endotracheal tube should be introduced by threading it over a fiberoptic bronchoscope or laryngoscope, which is guided carefully into the trachea without hyperextending the neck.

In patients with fractures of the mandible, the tongue may be displaced posteriorly, causing airway obstruction. Allowing the patient to bend forward or pulling the tongue forward with a suture or even a towel clip may be lifesaving. If a suspected fracture of the mandibular symphysis is the likely cause of labored respiration, the bone may be stabilized with a wire placed around the teeth adjacent to the fracture site, allowing the mandible and tongue to be supported in a forward position.

Control of Bleeding

Patients rarely become hypotensive when they have isolated facial injuries because bleeding is easy to control with external pressure. Clamping or tying of vessels should be avoided except under very controlled circumstances—that is, in the operating room or in a room with good light and suction. Proper light, exposure, and anesthesia are necessary to avoid inadvertent injury to the facial nerve and parotid or submandibular ducts. Intraoral hemorrhage contributing to airway obstruction can usually be controlled by placing a few sutures or a roll of sterile gauze over the wound and asking the patient to apply pressure by biting. If these measures fail, suction will have to be applied until the bleeding can be controlled. If the nasal hemorrhage is brisk, it is most likely associated with injury to branches of the internal maxillary artery. If this is persistent, it will require placement of posterior and anterior nasal packs (see Procedure 18).

Treatment of Shock

Because the face and scalp can bleed massively and yet rarely cause shock, the physician should not assume that persistent hypotension in the patient is caused by a facial injury. The presence of shock mandates a search for serious injury elsewhere; bleeding into the thorax, abdomen, or retroperitoneum is the most likely source for shock-producing hemorrhage. The necessary intravenous lines must be inserted and proper fluid therapy initiated (see Procedure 9).

Identification of Associated Injuries

As soon as conditions that pose an immediate threat to life have been identified and corrective measures have been initiated, a rapid but complete history and physical examination should be performed to identify associated injuries and to establish priorities of care. Although damage to the face may be the most apparent and anxiety-provoking injury, it may be the least important with regard to immediate survival. It is important that the physician understand the mechanism of injury. How did the trauma occur? What was the impact velocity? Is it likely that there was contamination? How many minutes or hours since the injury? As much information as possible should be obtained from the patient or from witnesses to provide clues to the severity and magnitude of the resulting injury.

Examination of the Face and Oral Cavity

A thorough examination of the face and head, conducted in an orderly manner, must be carried out to evaluate the severity and extent of soft tissue injuries and to diagnose facial fractures. Radiography, although a valuable adjunct, is not an acceptable substitute. Since patients with facial injuries sometimes become involved in personal injury litigation, it is essential that accurate description of the injury and the method of treatment be recorded carefully. Photographs are most helpful. If a photograph cannot be taken, a diagram is useful, including a careful measurement of lacerations and documentation of neurologic deficits.

Since the face is being examined by inspection, palpation, and x-ray, it is essential that the examiner have a basic understanding of facial anatomy, especially as it relates to the underlying skeleton, the course of the seventh (motor nerve to the facial muscles) and fifth (sensory) cranial nerves, the parotid glands, and ducts (Fig. 56-1).

Inspection

Soft tissue injuries are usually apparent. The nature, location, and depth of lacerations should be carefully noted. Debris on the face and in wounds and the status of skin edges of any wound must be carefully observed. If the eyelids are closed, they should be separated and the globes should be observed for blunt or sharp injury (see Chap. 58). The mouth should be opened and examined for lacerations and for areas of swelling or discoloration. Missing teeth should be accounted for to rule out aspiration. If the patient is edentulous, dentures should be located, since they may be helpful in the treatment of maxillary or mandibular fractures. Inspection can reveal many evidences of facial fractures. Facial asymmetry, ecchymoses, areas of swelling or depression, diplopia, epistaxis, malocclusion, sensory deficits, hematomas in the floor of the mouth or the buccal sulcus, and limitation of mandibular movement are among the indications that a fracture is probably present.

Palpation

The processes of inspection and palpation are not separate. While observing the patient, the examiner must also carefully palpate all bony prominences before soft tissue swelling

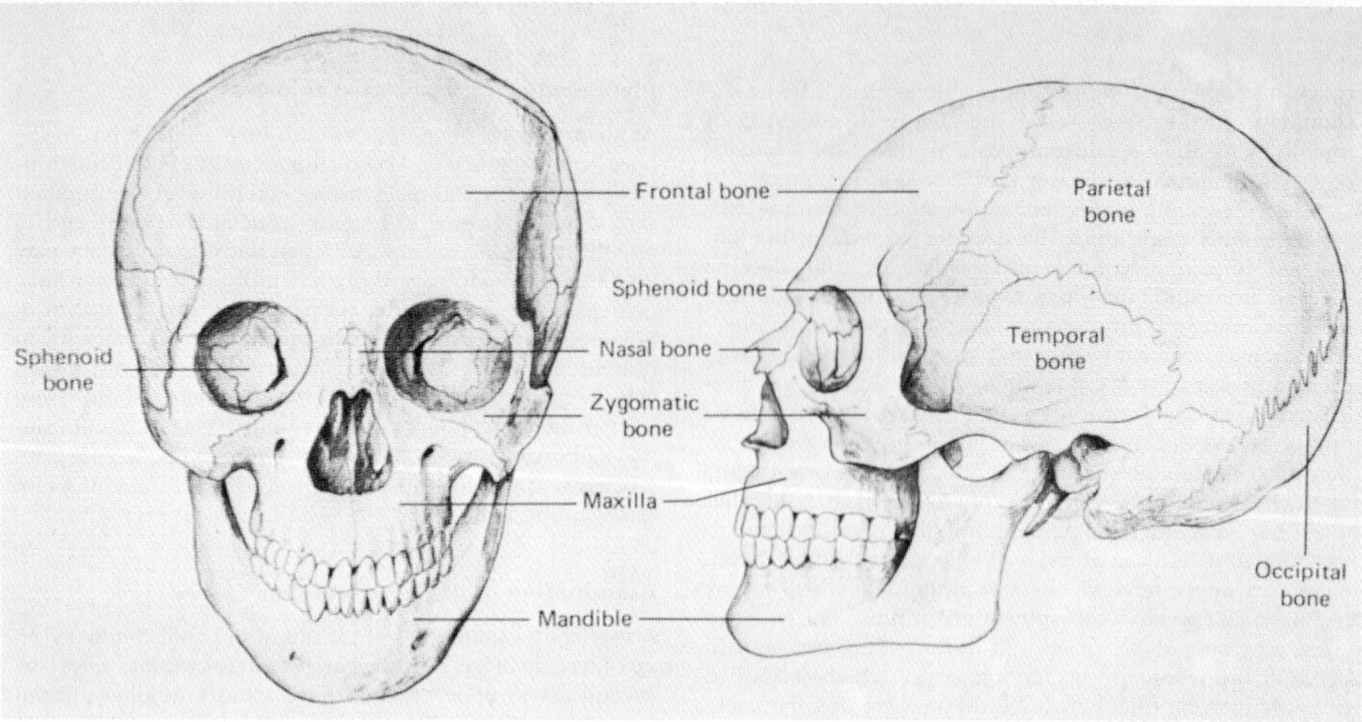

A

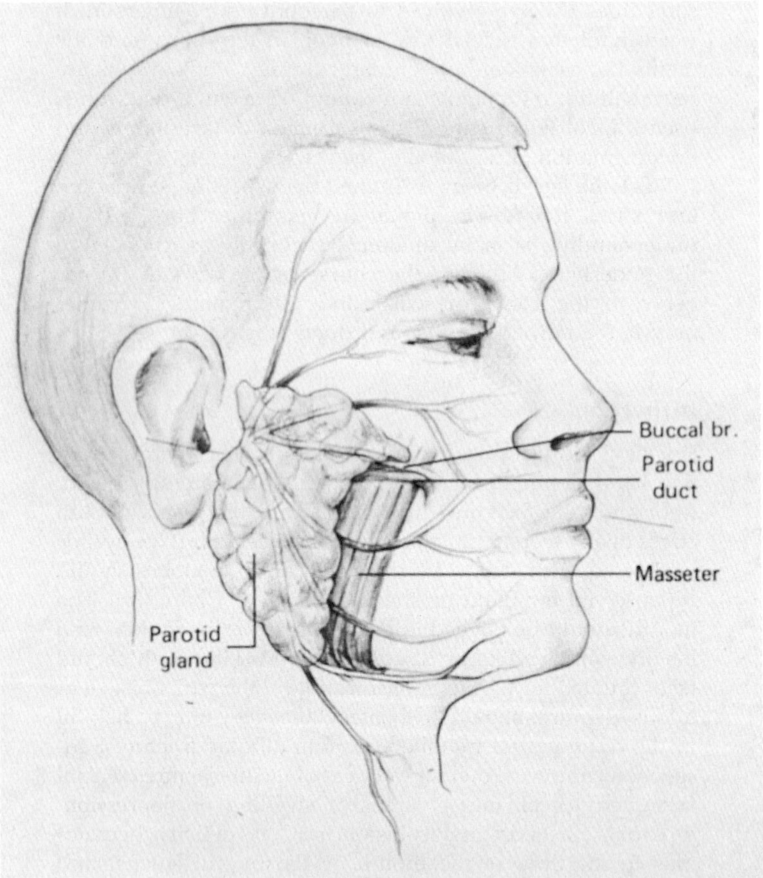

B

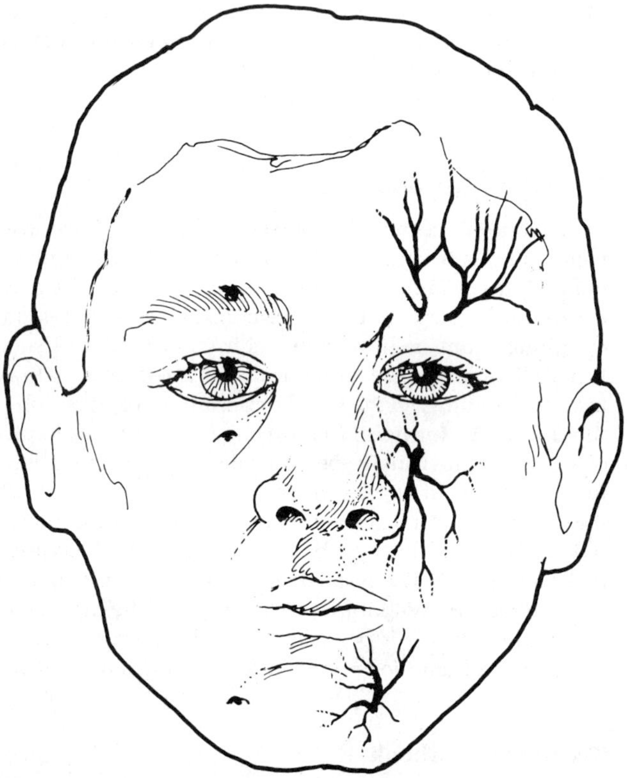

C

Fig. 56-1. A. Frontal and lateral views of a normal skull. B. This lateral view of the face with the superficial lobe of the parotid gland removed shows the facial nerve, deep lobe of the parotid gland, masseter muscle, and the entrance of the parotid duct into the mouth just anterior to the masseter muscle. Note that the course of the parotid duct follows a line from the tragus of the ear to a point about 1 cm above the commissure of the lip. C. Frontal view of the face demonstrating the course of the terminal portions of the first, second, and third divisions of the trigeminal nerve.

of the face obliterates these landmarks. (Details of the examination are described in the section on specific facial fractures.) When there has been trauma to the nasofrontal, nasoethmoidal region and the orbit, the medial canthi should be carefully evaluated, because one or both may be disrupted (Fig. 56-2). One index finger is placed on the medial canthus and the other index finger on the lateral portion of the upper eyelid, which should be stretched laterally. Thus tightened, the intact medial canthus can be palpated. If the medial canthus does not become obviously palpable with this maneuver, disruption of the medial canthus tendon has occurred.

X-Ray Examination

Radiographic examination is only adjunctive and does not take the place of a well-organized and accurate physical examination. In the seriously injured patient, x-rays of the face may be deferred until the patient is stable, since treatment of facial fractures and even of facial lacerations may need to be delayed. In all cases in which facial fractures may have occurred, however, x-rays are required to confirm the presence of suspected fractures and to delineate possible unsuspected fractures. Patients with a suspected cervical spine injury should have a lateral x-ray of the neck before any other x-rays.

Radiographs of the facial bones that are most useful for diagnosis of fractures include the following:

1. Water's view—for fractures of the middle third of the face involving the maxilla, zygomatic bone, and nasal and orbital regions (Fig. 56-3).
2. Posteroanterior view of facial bones—for frontal and zygomaticofrontal fractures.
3. Posteroanterior view of the mandible—for the body of the mandible from angle to angle (Fig. 56-4).
4. Towne's view—for fractures of the mandibular condyles (Fig. 56-5).
5. Lateral oblique view of the mandible—for fractures of the body, angles, and rami of the mandible (Fig. 56-6).
6. Submental vertex (jug-handle) view—for fractures of the zygomatic arches (Fig. 56-7).
7. Lateral nasal and Water's view—for delineation of nasal bones.
8. Computed tomography (CT) facial scans are useful but can require lengthy scanning procedures. Basic radiographs are routinely used for diagnostic procedures, whereas CT scans are used for reconstructive purposes.

Summary

The emergency physician should be concerned with the diagnosis of facial injuries and with the early management of potentially life-threatening complications. The diagnosis of facial fractures can usually be made on the basis of history and physical examination, with radiographs as an adjunct. If the history is that of a blow of limited force, directed to a specific area of the face, attention can be primarily focused there. However, in a situation in which there is a potential for multiple facial injuries, the examination should be thorough and systematic. Treatment of specific facial fractures can be delayed and the patient can be referred to a specialist for definitive care.

EMERGENCY DEPARTMENT MANAGEMENT OF SOFT TISSUE INJURIES OF THE FACE

General Considerations

Many soft tissue injuries of the face can be repaired in the emergency department by the emergency physician. However, if there is extensive soft tissue damage or if there are serious associated injuries, repair should be carried out in the operating room by a specialist. Other injuries that require specialty care include lacerations of the facial nerve, parotid gland or duct, eyelid, canthal tendons, and the lacrimal ducts. A plastic surgeon should be called if there is full-thickness loss of a portion of the ear, or, if soft tissue injury results in exposure of the cartilaginous framework of the ear or nose, a surgeon who is experienced in the care of such problems should be notified.

The general principles of emergency wound care are described in Chap. 52. When repairing facial lacerations, keep in mind the presence of delicate structures in a small area. Tissues should be treated gently, ideally with fine-toothed forceps, sharp small scissors, skin hooks, and small needle holders. Debris and tissue that is obviously dead should be removed; if there is any possibility that tissue is viable, it should be allowed to remain. Since the face of a young patient has little tissue to spare and that which it has has exceptionally good vascularity, debridement should be reserved for only the tissue that is dead or severely contused. The wound must be searched carefully for foreign bodies, and any such material should be removed. If the laceration is deep and could conceivably be associated with a fracture, it is important to make the diagnosis before the wound is closed. The laceration may be used to gain access to the fracture site, and closure may not be necessary in the emergency department.

Fixed facial landmarks, such as the eyebrow line or the Cupid's bow of the vermilion, should be approximated first. Deep lacerations should be closed in layers in order to eliminate dead space and to prevent a widened, depressed scar. Muscle should be approximated with interrupted sutures of absorbable material, either polyglycolic acid (Dexon) or 4-0 chromic catgut. Subcutaneous or dermal sutures should be used so that the skin edges approximate easily without tension; these sutures should be used sparingly. Surgeons differ in their preference, but 4-0 white nylon is acceptable for subcutaneous or subcuticular closure of a clean wound; for skin, 6-0 nylon swedged on small cutting needles should be used.

Complicated Lacerations and Other Soft Tissue Injuries

Complicated Lacerations

Some facial lacerations are irregular in shape, stellate, or form a flap of tissue. When repairing an irregular laceration, do not anticipate a bad scar by performing a Z- or W-plasty to realign the wound in a more favorable direction with respect to skin tension lines. The scar can be revised months

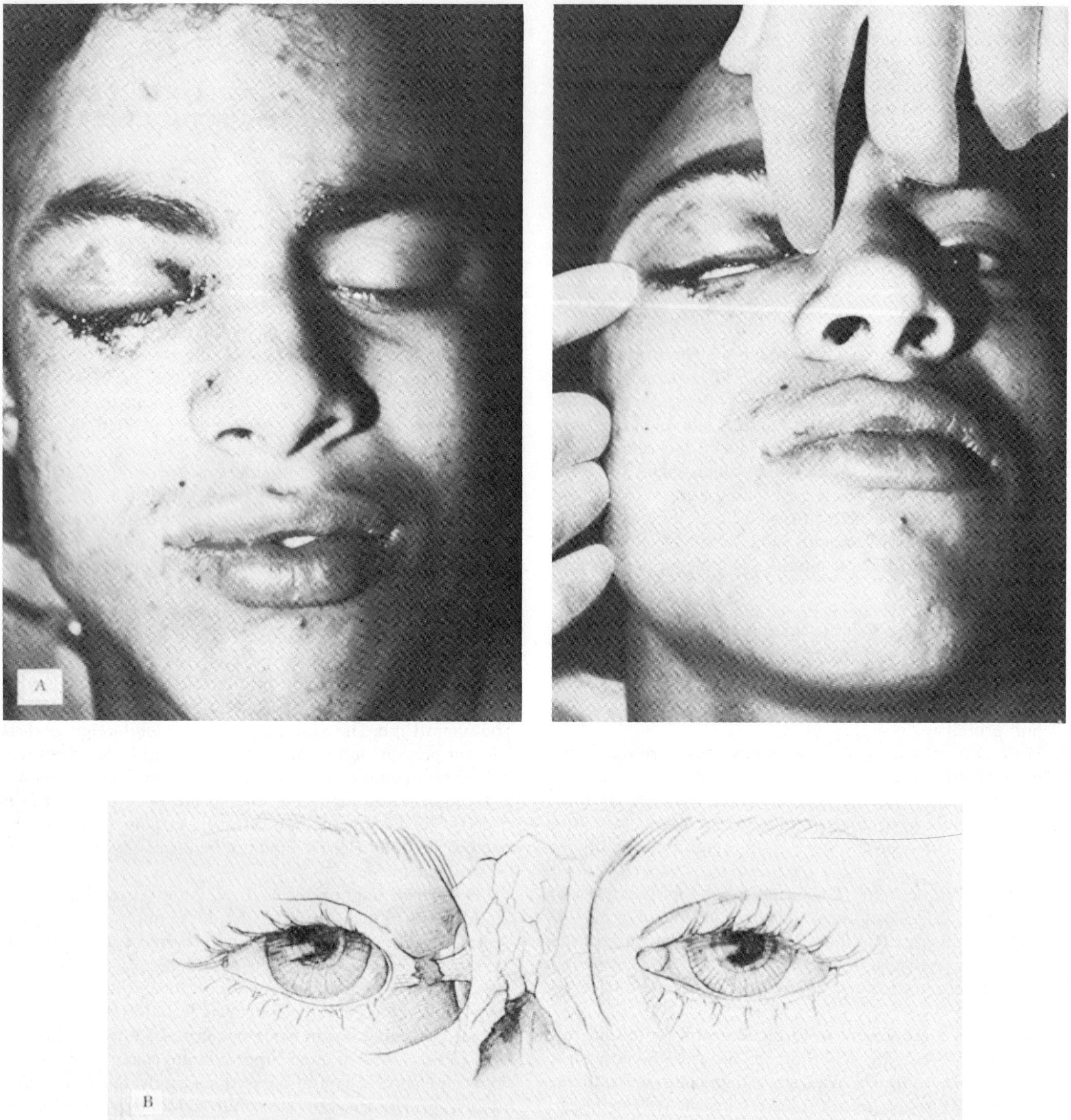

Fig. 56-2. A. The patient shown on the left has sustained a laceration of the medial aspect of the upper eyelid. On the right, examination of the medial canthus is demonstrated. B. This frontal view shows disruption of the medial canthal tendon in association with a nasoethmoidal fracture.

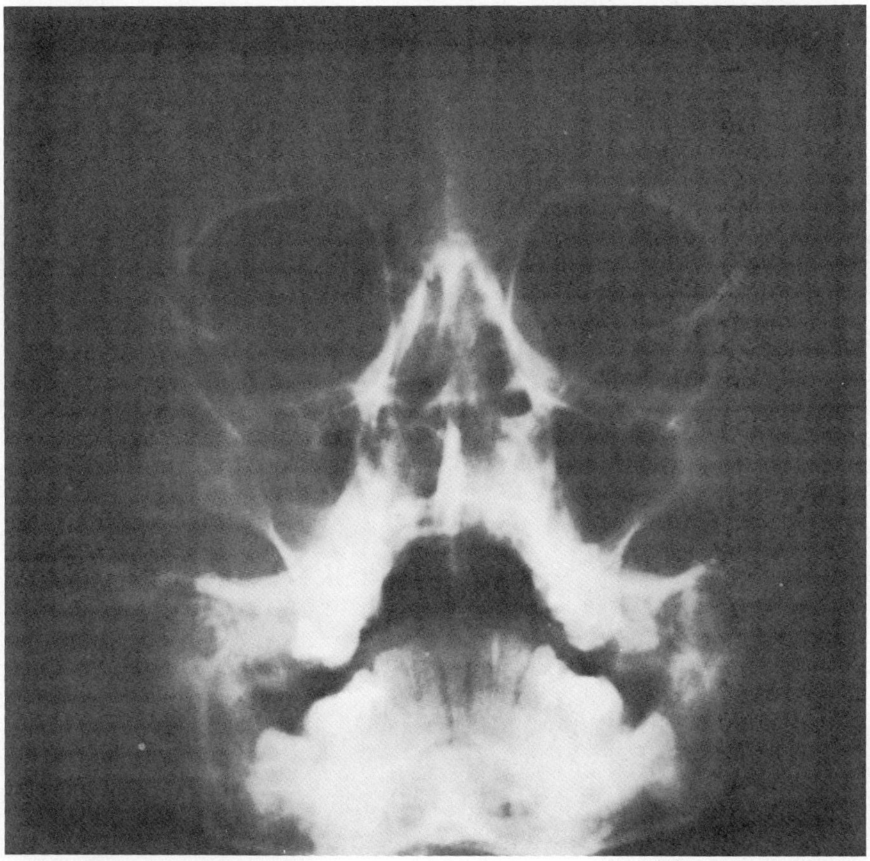

Fig. 56-3. Water's view roentgenogram. The Water's view is a standard radiograph to investigate the zygomatic complex, orbits, maxilla, and midface. It shows the orbits and frontal, ethmoid, and maxillary sinuses, as well as the zygomatic complex. This x-ray demonstrates an opaque maxillary sinus on the right side, indicating fluid in the sinus. The zygomatic bone and orbital rim are intact. The patient has a blow-out fracture of the orbital floor.

later if necessary. As described in Chap. 52, debridement of ragged edges of lacerations should be as conservative as possible, and every effort should be made to fit fragments together. On the other hand, beveled edges must be carefully trimmed. If a flap has been raised by the laceration, it should not be stitched tightly on all sides; otherwise, the blood supply to the tip will be compromised. Sometimes, Steri-Strips provide better closure than sutures for this type of laceration. If the wound is so small that it can be excised and closed primarily without tension, this method of treatment is very satisfactory. The excision should be in the form of an ellipse, with its long axis in the direction of the skin tension line.

Avulsion Wound

Small losses of tissue can sometimes be corrected by primary excision and closure. However, the defect may be so large that it will require skin graft or local flap. Such a procedure should be performed in an operating room by a specialist.

Old or Contaminated Wounds

If a soft tissue wound has been open for more than 6 hours, a decision must be made whether or not to close it. With antibiotic therapy, thorough irrigation, and judicious debridement, a tidy, clean wound can be closed even after 12 to 24 hours. However, the patient and the doctor must be aware that infection is a definite possibility. If in doubt, it is better to leave the wound open and treat it with dressings. In some cases, approximating the wound with Steri-Strips hastens the healing process.

A dog bite produces the most common "dirty wound" in the face. A puncture wound caused by a dog or any other animal should not be sutured, but bites that produce a laceration heal best if repaired primarily. Copious irrigation (at least 1,000 ml of normal saline or Ringer's lactate) is a prerequisite to success. The wound should be carefully debrided and penicillin should be given. If the wound is not recent or if the debridement would require sacrifice of a large amount of tissue, the wound should not be sutured but a surgeon who is experienced in the management of such wounds should be consulted. Careful attention to tetanus prophylaxis is required and any necessary rabies precautions must be observed (see Chap. 52).

Multiple Small Cuts

Multiple small cuts were more common before the shatterproof windshield became widely used, but they still occur. They should be treated by minimal debridement, thorough irrigation, pressure dressing, and only a few sutures. Too many sutures will cause necrosis of the small flaps. Using magnifying lenses, wounds should be inspected carefully for

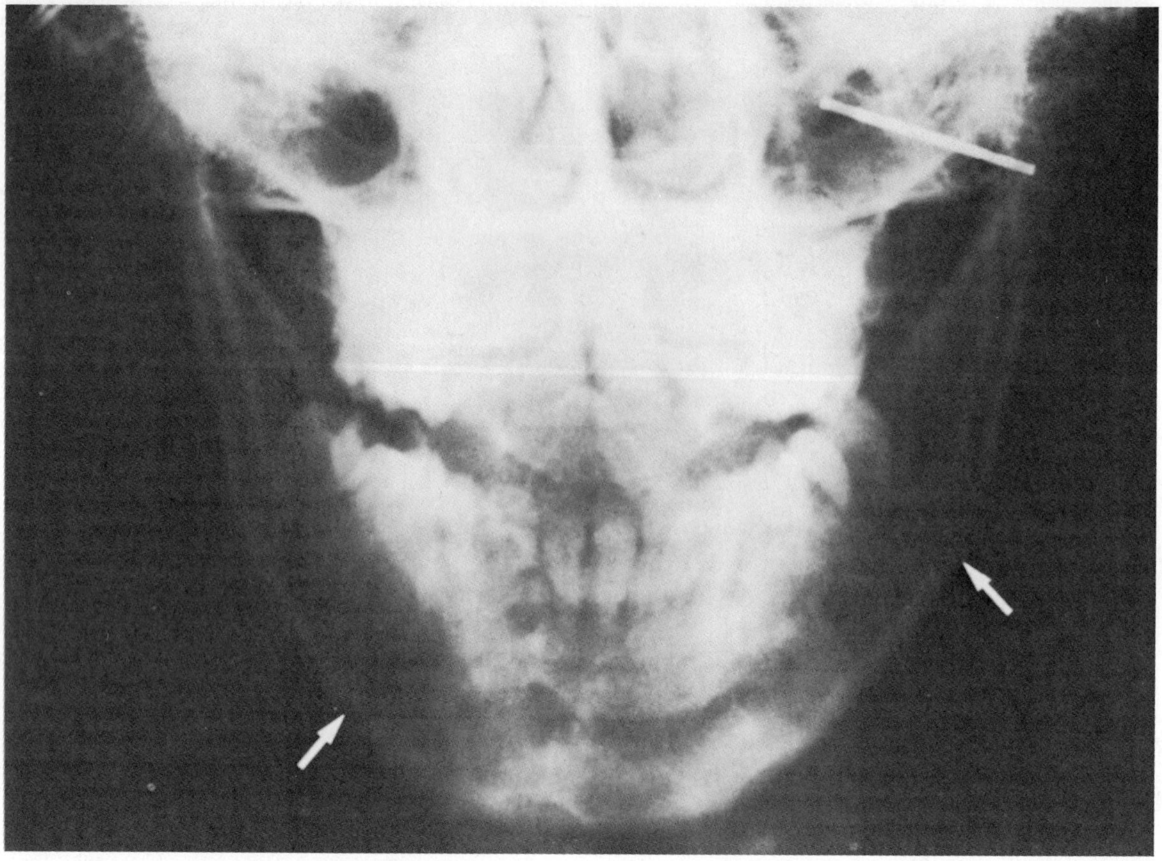

Fig. 56-4. Posteroanterior view of the mandible. This radiograph demonstrates the mandible from angle to angle and shows undisplaced fractures at the left angle and right premolar region (*arrows*). The radiopaque structures are hair pins.

small pieces of glass or other foreign bodies. An attempt should be made to remove all the small fragments, but this is sometimes impossible. The patients should be told that glass may "work its way out," or, if necessary, additional removal may be necessary in the future. Many patients worry that some of the fragments will work their way into the blood stream. They should be reassured that this will not happen.

Tattooing

Asphalt, dirt, grease, and gunpowder may enter the dermal and subcutaneous tissues and should be removed within 12 hours by scrubbing with a stiff, sterile hand brush. If foreign material is not removed carefully, it will remain in the tissue as a permanent tattoo. Local anesthesia can be used if the area is small, but general anesthesia is necessary for more extensive injuries. If the material cannot be completely removed by brush, a No. 11 blade should be used to take the pieces out meticulously under lens magnification. Small amounts of ether or acetone are useful for dissolving grease and paint; the eyes must be carefully protected. If it is not always possible to remove all the debris, the patient should be so informed, because another operation may be necessary. The treated areas should be covered with an antibiotic ointment dressing.

Postoperative Care

If the patient is well enough to be discharged after soft tissue repair, he or she should be instructed in proper wound care. In general, dressings should be light; abrasion wounds can be left open and covered with antibiotic ointment. Initially, diet should consist of only fluids; soft foods may be added later. Chewing and jaw motion may pull skin against stitches and result in a poor scar. Warm saline intraoral rinses every few hours will help keep intraoral wounds clean.

Any patient with a facial injury should be instructed to return to the emergency department or to call if any of the following symptoms develop: increased pain, fever, nausea, vomiting, headache, diplopia, fainting, weakness, paralysis, or slow pulse or any symptoms suggesting intracranial damage or wound infection. A patient at risk for infection—for example, a dog bite victim—should be advised to return in 24 to 48 hours.

Sutures on the face should be removed after 4 or 5 days; permanent "suture tracks" may result if they are left longer than 7 days. If a patient cannot return but is to be followed elsewhere, he or she should be supplied with specific instructions and a summary of the diagnosis and treatment.

Soft Tissue Injuries in Specific Regions

Intraoral Soft Tissue Injuries

For generations, it had been taught that intraoral lacerations should never be sutured. However, with the use of prophy-

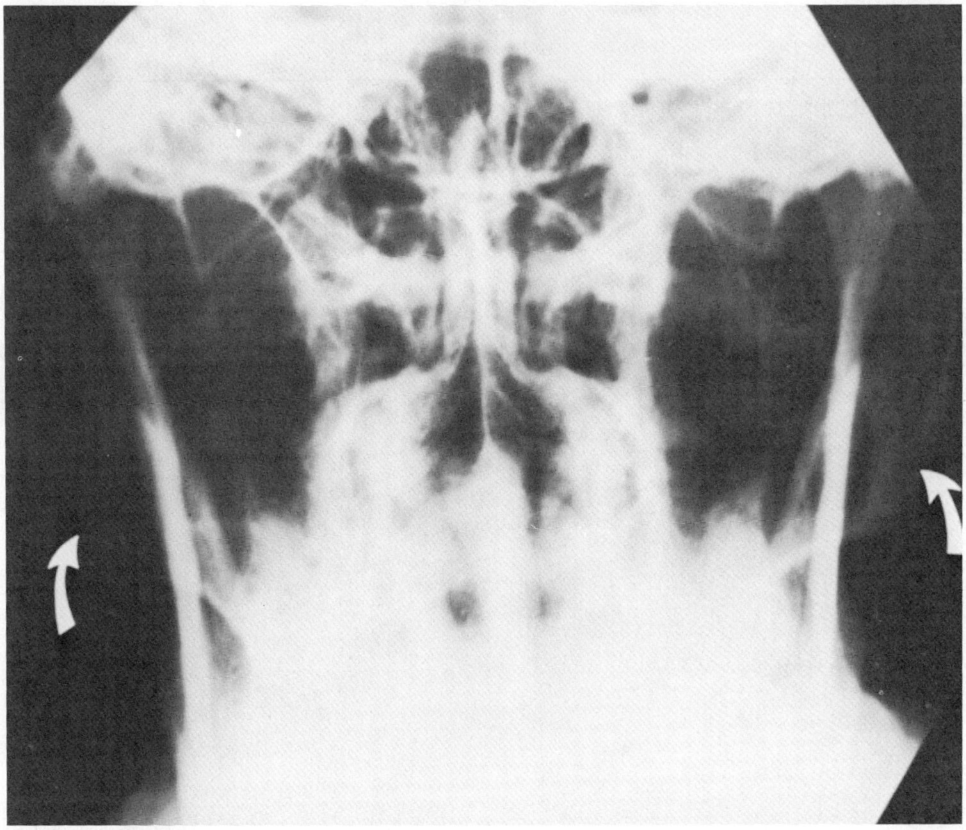

Fig. 56-5. The Towne's view radiograph shows the ramus and condyles of the mandible in the mediolateral plane. In this case, there are no fractures. We can also see the zygomatic arches (*arrows*).

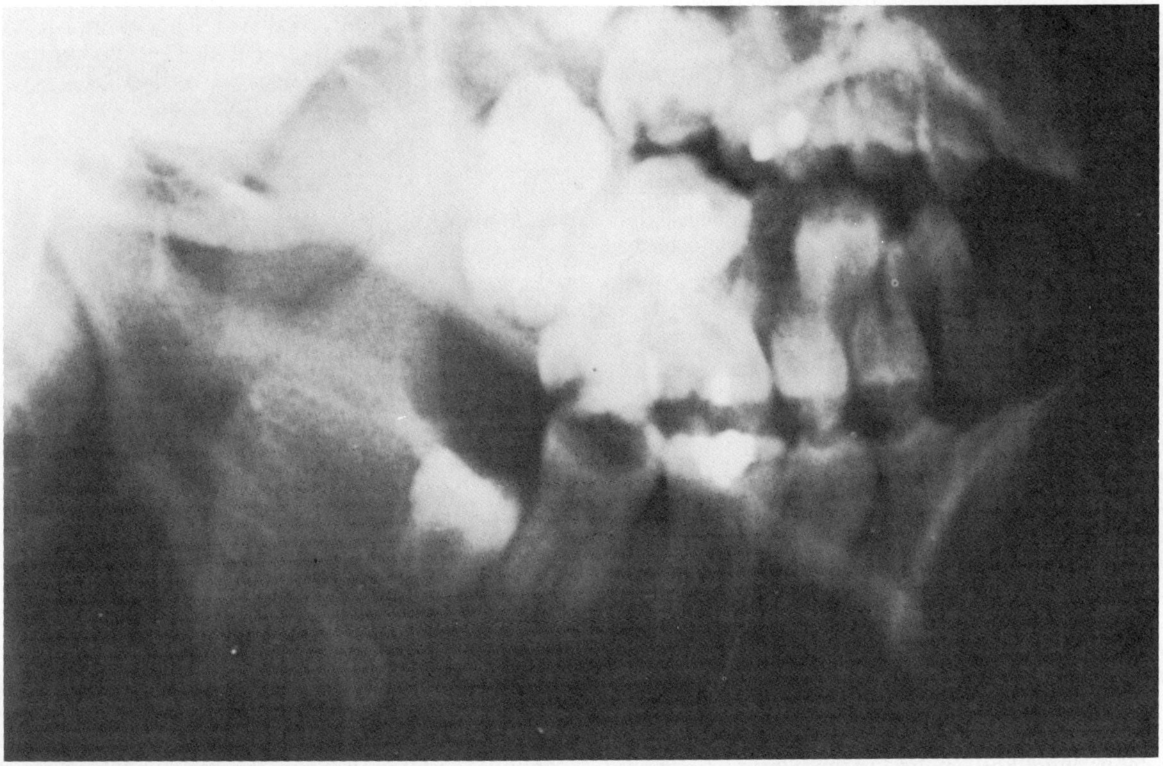

Fig. 56-6. The lateral oblique x-ray of the mandible shows the condyle, sigmoid notch, coronoid process, and the body of the mandible in the molar region.

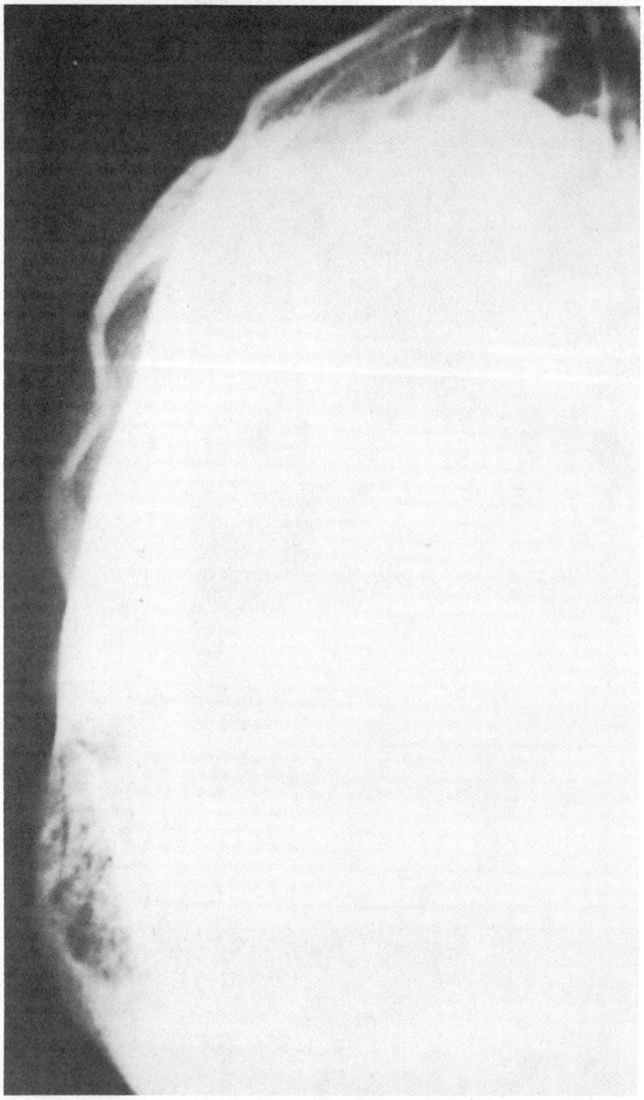

Fig. 56-7. The submental vertex or "jug-handle" view illustrates the zygomatic arch and, in this case, shows a classic V-shaped depression of the zygomatic arch.

lactic antibiotics, these lacerations can be closed. An intraoral wound that is sutured will bleed less and result in improved soft tissue contour and greater comfort for the patient. For most mucosal and tongue lacerations, 4-0 chromic catgut is a satisfactory material. For through-and-through lacerations, the intraoral portion should be sutured loosely first; then the external portion of the wound may be draped and sutured in layers. The patient should be placed on penicillin or erythromycin prophylaxis (250 mg every 6 hours for 5 days), and the mouth should be rinsed with warm saline frequently to maintain optimal oral hygiene.

Lip

Lip lacerations should be repaired in three layers, beginning with mucosa, then muscle and skin (Fig. 56-8). The first skin suture should be in the vermilion border. The mucous membrane, orbicularis, and subcutaneous tissue should be approximated with 4-0 chromic catgut and the skin with 6-0 nylon.

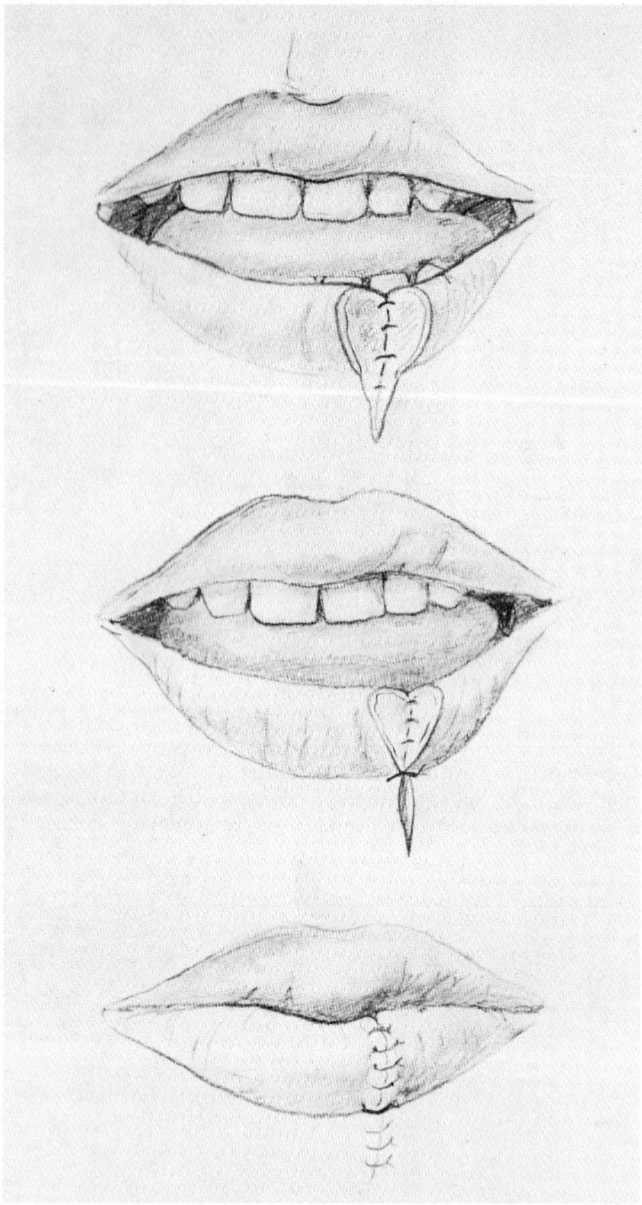

Fig. 56-8. The technique of closure of a through-and-through lip laceration crossing the vermilion border is illustrated. The vermilion border should be tattooed by needle with methyl blue before anesthesia. Once the mucosal and muscle layers are approximated, skin closure can be started. The first skin sutures should approximate the vermilion border.

Electrical Burns of the Mouth

Electrical burns of the mouth occur usually between the ages of 6 months and 3 years. A typical situation involves a mother who is interrupted in her ironing, disconnects the appliance plug, but leaves the connection to the wall outlet. The child places the dangling end in his or her mouth. Although the contacts are not exposed, electrolytes in the saliva allow completion of the electrical circuit and transmit the

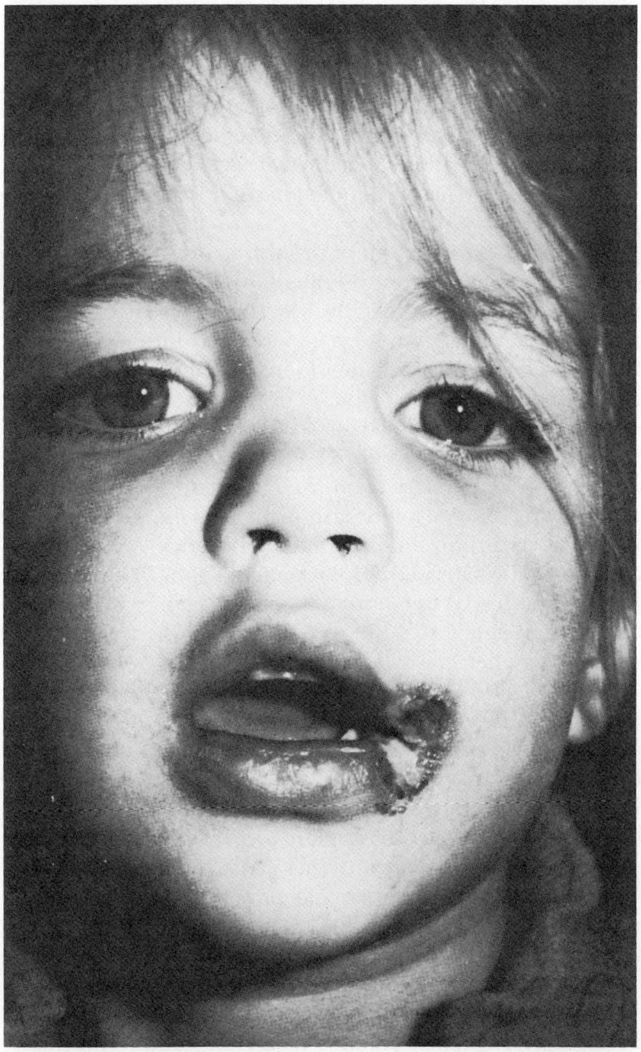

Fig. 56-9. Electrical burn of the lip. This photograph illustrates a young girl with an electrical burn in the left labial commissure. This is a typical location of these injuries in children.

current through the local tissues with considerable destruction.

The oral mucosal burn may appear superficial; however, thrombosis propagates and causes necrosis (Fig. 56-9). Within a few hours, pronounced edema appears and the injury may extend 2 cm or more beneath the visible edge of trauma. As vacuoles form in the vascular endothelium and intima, the likelihood of late rupture of vessels and hemorrhage increases. Significant bleeding may occur any time within 3 weeks in 25 percent of patients; therefore, hospitalization for 6 to 21 days of observation is warranted. Although initial treatment is still controversial, most electrical burns are treated conservatively to allow delineation of necrosis and separation of the eschar. Neosporin or bacitracin ointment may be applied to the injured area 2 or 3 times a day; the patient should be restrained at night to prevent rubbing the burn on the bed coverings and should be fed with a cleft lip feeder. Whenever possible, a plastic surgeon should be called in immediately because what appears to be a superficial burn may result in a severe late deformity.

Nose

Full-thickness lacerations of the nose must be closed meticulously in layers. To approximate the nasal mucosa, 5-0 absorbable interrupted sutures are used; the knots are placed in the nasal cavity. A continuous subcuticular (intradermal) suture with 4-0 nylon can be used to approximate the skin. Alternatively, 6-0 nylon sutures can be placed in the skin.

Ear Laceration

The ear has an excellent blood supply, which frequently protects it even after severe jagged lacerations and partial avulsions. Flaps survive in spite of what appears to be a very narrow pedicle. For this reason, no part of the ear should be excised during debridement unless it is definitely necrotic. It is essential that hemostasis be precise to avoid postrepair hematomas and resultant damage to the underlying cartilage.

Lacerations that involve only the skin can be sutured in the emergency department with 6-0 nylon using a field block around the base of the ear for anesthesia (1% lidocaine with epinephrine, 1:200,000). For a simple laceration involving the cartilage, repair should include reapproximation of the cartilage with 5-0 absorbable sutures. If there has been significant full-thickness loss of the ear, if a large area of cartilage is exposed, or if an avulsed segment of the ear has been brought in for reattachment, a surgeon who is experienced in such care should be called. By means of local flaps or storage of the cartilage, the valuable framework of the ear can be preserved to be used for later reconstruction.

Hematoma of the External Ear

Hematoma of the external ear usually occurs after blunt trauma or a shearing type of injury. The hematoma is subperichondral and is typically fluctuant and purplish in color. Ice packs for 24 hours and oral penicillin, 250 mg 4 times daily for 5 days, are indicated. The patient should be referred to an otolaryngologist or plastic surgeon within 24 hours so that definitive surgical drainage and stenting can be performed.

Careful application of a pressure dressing to an injured ear after it has been repaired is an important factor in the prevention of a seroma or hematoma. A drain between the skin and cartilage may also be used. To create a pressure dressing, moistened pieces of cotton are placed behind the ear and into the convolutions of the auricle. The ear is then covered with fluffed gauze and the head is wrapped with a dressing of "Kling" and Ace bandage. After 48 to 72 hours, the ear is inspected.

Eyelid

Any wound of the eyelid mandates a careful examination of the eye to rule out ocular injury (see Chap. 58). If a laceration involves the tarsal plate of the eyelid at its free edge, or the medial aspect of the eyelid, it should be repaired by an ophthalmologist or a plastic surgeon. Medial injuries of the eyelid are often associated with injuries of the medial canthal ligament or the lacrimal duct, or both. These injuries must be recognized and repaired by a specialist. Simple lacerations of the eyelid skin heal well if carefully cleaned but should never be shaved. The eyelid skin must be carefully aligned to prevent an obvious step deformity. Minimal debridement should be carried out in the region of the eyebrow, even in the presence of complicated lacerations with small flaps. Careful aligning of the fragments will often lead to a good result. Repair is described in Chap. 58.

Facial Nerve Injury

Every patient with facial injuries should receive careful evaluation of facial nerve function, although the facial nerve is damaged rather infrequently because of its position, between the lobes of the parotid gland. Occasionally, paresis of the facial nerve or its branches results simply from hematoma formation or from contusion. When in doubt, the physician should refer the patient to a surgeon experienced in the treatment of facial nerve injuries for diagnosis and repair. Branches of the facial nerve that are severed between the stylomastoid foramen and a vertical line dropped from the lateral canthus of the eyelids should be repaired primarily. The terminal nerve branches anterior to that line will usually regenerate satisfactorily if the soft tissues are approximated. A facial nerve repair should be carried out in the operating room within 72 hours.

Parotid Duct Laceration

The parotid duct lies beneath the middle one-third of a line drawn from the tragus of the ear to the midportion of the upper lip (see Fig. 56-1B). If damage to this duct is suspected because of the location of the laceration, a small polyethylene tube or lacrimal duct probe can be passed into the parotid duct orifice on the buccal mucosa opposite the upper first and second molar teeth. Laceration of the duct is diagnosed by the appearance of the probe or tube in the wound. When possible, the parotid duct should be repaired early; this requires the facilities of the main operating room as well as the skills of a trained specialist. Failure to recognize a parotid duct laceration may result in a sialocutaneous fistula or a sialocele.

Nasal Fractures

DIAGNOSIS. Nasal fractures, the most common facial fractures in adults and children, may occur as isolated injuries or in combination with fractures of other facial bones. The patient who presents with a history of trauma to the nose should be questioned about the direction and nature of the force that caused the injury and about any possible preexisting nasal deformity or nasal obstruction. Nasal fracture may be indicated by deviation or depression of the bone, ecchymosis, swelling, or nosebleed. A deviated septum, constricted airway, or septal hematoma may be seen on intranasal examination, and subconjunctival hemorrhage or periorbital ecchymosis with edema is common several hours after the injury. One must be careful not to miss a nasal fracture in which the cartilage is telescoped up and under the nasal bone. In this type of injury, the nasolabial angle may be increased, and there may be a step deformity at the junction of the septum and nasal bone. The injury site is tender, and crepitus is noted on palpation.

Although the standard x-ray films (lateral nasal and Water's view) are necessary for documenting the injury and are possibly desirable for medicolegal reasons, they are not particularly helpful as a diagnostic tool. Delineating the area radiographically is difficult, and because fracture lines do not calcify as they heal, new fractures cannot be distinguished from old ones.

MANAGEMENT. By nasal speculum examination, the emergency physician must determine whether there is a septal hematoma. A specialist should drain a widened and fluctuant septum within several hours. The patient should be started on antibiotics against the normal gram-positive nasal flora. If a hematoma becomes infected, an abscess forms and the septal cartilage becomes necrotic within 24 to 48 hours, resulting in loss of support of the nasal tip and a saddle-nose deformity.

The results of treatment of nasal fractures are often poor. Since the problem may be a difficult one, even for the experienced physician, it is usually best for these fractures to be treated by surgeons who are experienced in nasal surgery. The emergency physician should instruct the patient to place iced saline sponges or ice packs over the nose and eyes and to keep the head elevated on several pillows when asleep or resting. This will minimize posttraumatic swelling. The patient should be started on dicloxacillin, 500 mg every 6 hours or, for patient's who are penicillin-allergic, the same dosage of erythromycin or cephalexin (Keflex). A decongestant should be started, and the patient should be instructed not to blow his or her nose and not to smoke. The patient should be referred to a surgeon to reduce the fracture in 5 to 10 days, when the swelling has decreased.

If the nasal fracture is to be reduced in the emergency department, the patient should be supine on the operating table. After he or she has been adequately sedated with an agent such as intravenous diazepam or a combination of diazepam and meperidine hydrochloride (Demerol), the face should be washed with plain soap and water. After the exact nature of the deformity has been determined, topical cocaine (5% or 10%) is used to provide anesthesia and to induce vasoconstriction in the mucous membranes. This is applied by 3-inch rolled cotton pledgets soaked with the agent and thoroughly squeezed out to remove excess solution. Under direct visualization, one pack is placed along the floor of the nose, another along the middle turbinate, and a third along the roof. The external nose is anesthetized by bilateral infraorbital nerve blocks with lidocaine, 1 percent, with 1:100,000 epinephrine, and by infiltrating the same agent across the base of the columella and across the glabellar region. It is important to wait 15 to 20 minutes to achieve complete anesthesia before the reduction is carried out.

One hand should hold a closed Kelly clamp, covered with a thin piece of rubber tubing, to mobilize and reduce the nasal fracture while the other hand simultaneously molds the nose under direct palpation. Walsham forceps can also be used for this maneuver. If the septum is deviated, an Asch forceps is the best instrument to use to manipulate the nasal bones and septum into position while the fingers of the left hand palpate the bridge of the nose and function as a guide. After careful observation and palpation confirm the fact that the nasal pyramid and the septum are in the midline, nasal packs of petroleum-impregnated gauze or plastic stent should be inserted into the nasal airway to support the fractured bones (without displacing the nasal bones laterally) and to prevent hematomas. A nasal splint made of plaster of Paris or a commercially available metal or plastic splint should be placed on the external surface of the nose to protect it. The nasal pack should be removed after 48 hours, and the splint after 5 to 7 days. If the septum is injured, the

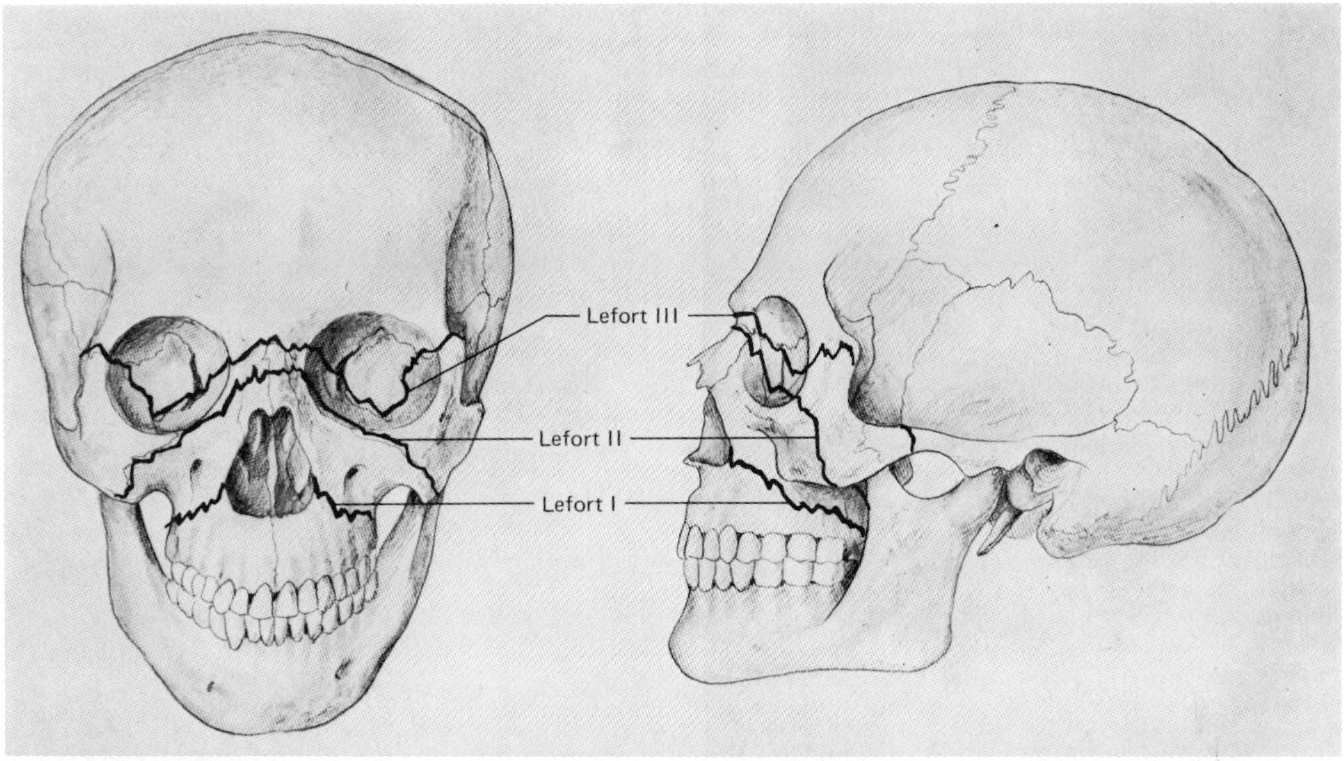

Fig. 56-10. Le Fort fracture line. Frontal and lateral views of the skull illustrating the fracture lines of the Le Fort I, II, and III injuries.

patient should be warned that a nasal deformity may develop gradually over a period of months, and further reconstructive surgery may be necessary.

PROGNOSIS. The prognosis for nasal fractures depends on the severity of injury. In noncomminuted fractures, the prognosis is excellent. After adequate reduction, no further treatment should be necessary. In comminuted fractures and those in which there is septal hematoma, a varying degree of nasal deformity may occur postreduction and may require further reconstructive surgery.

Maxillary and Midface Fractures

Fractures of the maxilla are less common than those of the mandible. They are often the result of high-speed motor vehicle trauma and, as a consequence, are often associated with skull, central nervous system, chest, or abdominal injury. The most common associated problem involves a dural tear manifested by cerebrospinal fluid rhinorrhea or otorrhea.

Because of its relationship to the base of the skull, the maxilla is able to absorb and withstand great compressive forces without being fractured. Therefore, maxillary injuries rarely occur from a blow to the chin driving the mandible upward into the maxilla. Maxillary and midface injuries most commonly occur from a shearing-type blow delivered from an anterior direction. The patterns of midface fractures were investigated and classified at the turn of the century by René Le Fort (Fig. 56-10). The Le Fort I fracture is a transverse fracture of the maxilla above the palate and roots of the teeth. The Le Fort II fracture is one in which the fractured segment, shaped like a pyramid, contains the nasal bones and the frontal process of the maxilla, as well as the palate, teeth, and lateral walls of the maxillary sinus. The fracture lines usually run through the lacrimal bones and inferior rim of the orbit and extend obliquely and inferiorly along the edge of the maxilla toward the pterygomaxillary fissure. The Le Fort III fracture is craniofacial disjunction. The maxilla, nasal bones, and zygomatic bones will move as a unit from the base of the skull.

DIAGNOSIS. The patient with a midface fracture usually has marked swelling of the upper face with periorbital ecchymosis and edema (Fig. 56-11). In fractures at the Le Fort II level, there may be a significant widening of the inner canthus of the eyes. The patient should be observed in profile for elongation of the middle third of the face and for possible telescoping inward of the nose and midface. A midface fracture may cause the nose to look "cute" or "infantile" when actually the nose has been foreshortened by the retrodisplacement of the midportion of the face.

Palpation will reveal a mobile segment containing the upper teeth, the palate, and part of the wall of the maxillary sinus. Intraoral palpation with one hand while placing the other hand at the frontonasal suture will reveal mobility of the lower maxilla and infraorbital rims and the nasomaxillary complex as one unit with movement across the frontonasal suture at the Le Fort II level (Fig. 56-12). Intraoral palpation with one hand while moving the other hand from the frontonasal suture to the frontozygomatic sutures on both sides will reveal movement of the entire midface complex

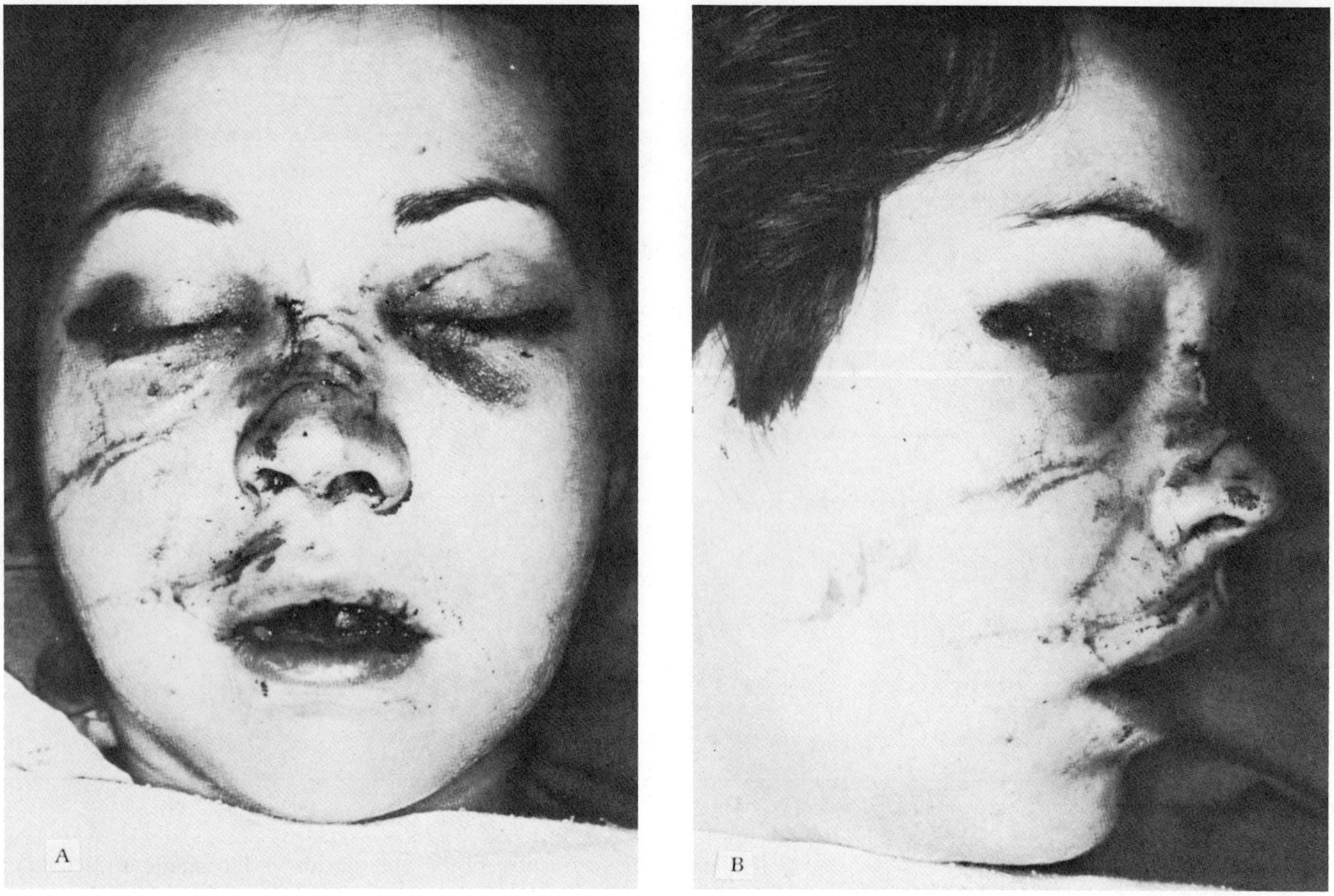

Fig. 56-11. Midface fractures. Examination of this patient with a Le Fort III fracture shows bilateral periorbital ecchymosis and edema (the "panda bear" facies) and elongation of the middle one-third of the face.

in relation to the cranium in the Le Fort III fracture (Fig. 56-13).

Sensation should be tested along the distribution of the infraorbital nerve, which, in the Le Fort II fracture, may be injured at the infraorbital foramen. The patient's occlusion and the occlusal plane should be observed as described for mandibular fractures, and the patient's subjective evaluation of his or her occlusion should also be determined.

Cerebrospinal fluid rhinorrhea, resulting from damage to the cribriform plate, may accompany a midface fracture and should be suspected if watery fluid drains from the nose or if the patient reports a salty taste in his or her mouth. Cerebrospinal fluid may be suspected if the discharge stiffens a fresh piece of linen or tissue paper on drying. Compared with blood, cerebrospinal fluid contains less protein, uric acid, and sugar but more chloride; the high chloride content is responsible for the salty taste.

The initial x-rays should consist of a Water's view to evaluate the status of the orbits, orbital rims, and maxillary sinuses (Fig. 56-14). A posteroanterior view of the skull is helpful in visualizing the frontal sinuses, the supraorbital rims, and the frontozygomatic sutures. In addition, a lateral skull film will illustrate elongation of the midface and tilting of the maxillary occlusal plane.

Although the three patterns of midface fractures described by Le Fort are convenient for classification, variations commonly occur and the fracture should be precisely described. For example, the patient may have a maxillary fracture at the Le Fort III level on one side, but at the Le Fort I or II level on the other side. In addition, there may be fractures in the midline separating the two sides, and there may be severe comminution on one or both sides.

MANAGEMENT. The early treatment of midface and maxillary fractures is similar to that described later in this chapter for mandibular fractures. Oral intake is restricted to clear liquids or is totally stopped. Intravenous penicillin (1,000,000 units) is given every 6 hours, and the patient is placed in a head-upright position with ice packs applied to the upper face bilaterally. Usage of antibiotics with cerebrospinal fluid leakage remains controversial; therefore, consultation with a neurosurgeon is recommended. Close observation is essential for the first 24 to 48 hours because of the possibility of associated central nervous system or other injuries. The definitive treatment of maxillary fractures requires the same concern for occlusion as described in the treatment of mandibular fractures. In reducing these fractures, one must consider the complex interrelationships between the occlusion, the nasomaxillary complex, orbits, the medial and lateral canthi, and facial aesthetics, as well as function. For this reason, definitive treatment should be de-

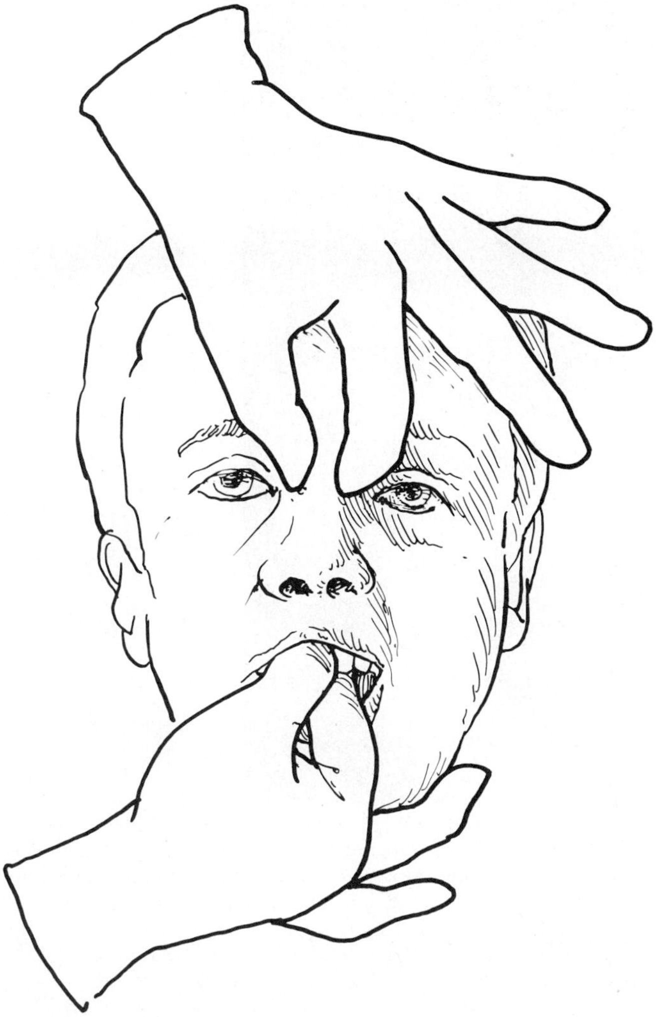

Fig. 56-12. Bimanual palpation of the maxilla for a Le Fort I or II fracture.

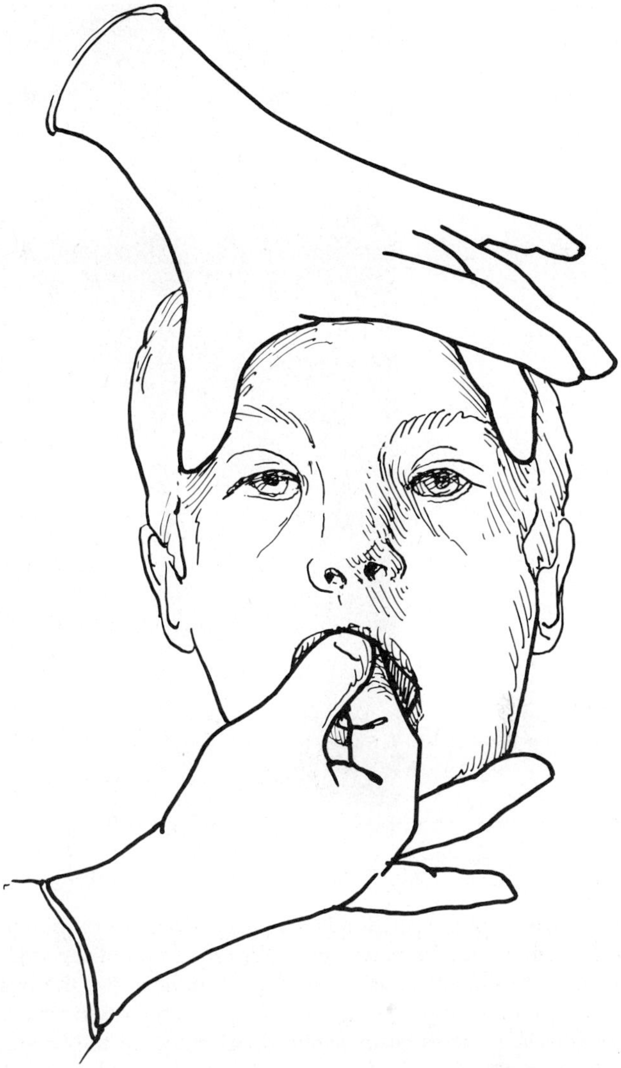

Fig. 56-13. Bimanual palpation of the midface for a Le Fort III fracture.

layed until it can be carried out by an appropriately trained specialist.

PROGNOSIS. The prognosis for midface fractures depends on the severity of the initial injury—that is, the degree of soft tissue damage and the degree of comminution of the bony fragments. There is no question that the best chance for a successful outcome is the first one. It is therefore imperative that a patient with a midface fracture be treated within 5 to 10 days after injury by a surgeon experienced in the treatment of these fractures. If treatment is directed toward reestablishing the correct facial proportions, occlusion, projection of zygomatic bones, and integrity of the orbital floor, the ultimate outcome will be favorable, even if secondary reconstructive procedures are required. Today's newer techniques utilizing rigid fixation allow for immediate restoration of form and function and may negate the need for secondary reconstruction.

Inadequate or poor early treatment, resulting in elongation of the middle third of the face, malocclusion, or enophthalmos, is difficult to correct at a later stage.

Zygomatic Complex and Zygomatic Arch Fractures

The zygoma has a thick, long, central portion known as the buttress and four projections that articulate with the maxilla, temporal bone, greater wing of the sphenoid, and frontal bone (Fig. 56-15). Discontinuity usually occurs at the junction of the zygoma with the other bones. Twenty percent of zygomatic fractures do not result in significant displacement, and 10 percent affect only the zygomatic arch; the other 70 percent result in depression with or without rotation.

DIAGNOSIS. If the zygomatic complex is fractured, swelling and ecchymosis are seen in the periorbital area, and the malar region appears flat, particularly when observed from above (Fig. 56-16). The lateral canthus has an antimongoloid slant resulting from depression of the lateral portion of the orbital floor, and subjunctival hemorrhage and enophthalmos are present (Fig. 56-17). The zygomaticofrontal, maxillary, and temporal sutures are tender, and a separation or step deformity may be appreciated in these areas. The

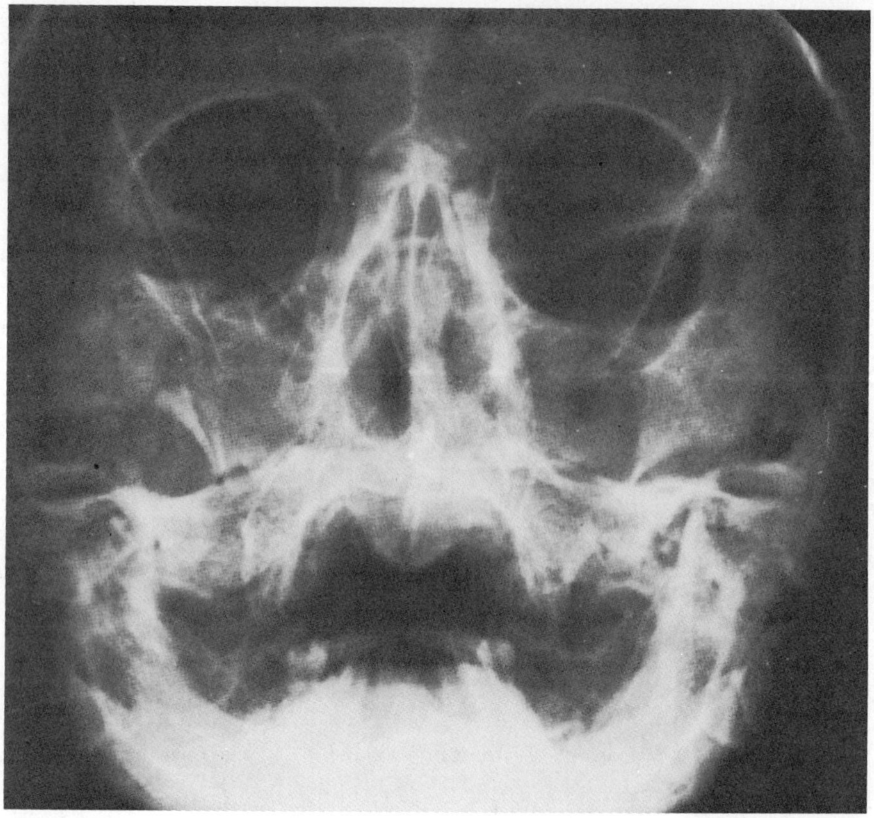

Fig. 56-14. Water's view roentgenogram of a patient with a Le Fort III injury demonstrates fractures at the frontozygomatic suture, the infraorbital rims, the nasofrontal suture, and opacification of both maxillary sinuses.

anterior wall of the maxilla is tender on intraoral palpation, and crepitus may be noted; the inferior portion of the zygomatic buttress may be separated or irregular above the posterior maxillary teeth. Neurologic examination often reveals paresthesia or anesthesia in the distribution of the second division of the trigeminal nerve. A test of extraocular muscle function may indicate entrapment of the inferior oblique and inferior rectus muscles in the fracture of the floor of the orbit.

A fracture confined to the *zygomatic arch* may occur as an isolated injury and is most often secondary to a blow directly over the arch. These fractures present with none of the orbital signs and symptoms associated with a fracture of the zygomatic complex. Rather, the patient may report pain when opening the jaw and limited motion. The arch fracture causes pain when the mouth is opened because of the relationship of the arch to the coronoid process and temporalis muscle. The zygomatic arch may be ignored because of these symptoms, and x-rays of the mandible and temporomandibular joint are incorrectly ordered.

When a zygomatic complex fracture is suspected, it can be confirmed radiologically with a Water's or a submental vertex x-ray (see Figs. 56-3 and 56-7). A submental vertex (jug-handle) view may be helpful in demonstrating the relationship of the zygomatic arch to the coronoid process.

MANAGEMENT. Fractures of the zygomatic bone with significant displacement are usually reduced under general anesthesia. The procedure is usually performed on a semielective basis after the swelling subsides and the facial aesthetics are evaluated. During the waiting period, the patient is placed on decongestants and antibiotics because of the violated maxillary sinus. The antibiotic of choice is usually penicillin, 250 mg by mouth every 6 hours. Zygomatic arch fractures are treated if the fracture prevents jaw opening or if it produces an aesthetic deformity. These fractures can be treated early, prior to the onset of maximum swelling, or after 5 days. They are usually reduced by a specialist.

Blow-Out Fractures

The term *blow-out fractures,* coined by Converse and Smith in 1957, refers to a fracture of the orbital floor without a fracture of the orbital rim or zygoma. The term is now used to include isolated fractures of the medial wall of the orbit. The injury is usually caused by a direct blow from a nonpenetrating object larger than the orbital opening (e.g., a fist or tennis ball). The orbital contents are compressed and driven posteriorly into the smaller portion of the orbital cone. The resultant increased intraorbital pressure causes the weak floor or medial wall to "blow out." It has been shown that blow-out fractures may also result from an oblique or shearing blow to the zygomatic bone.

DIAGNOSIS. Periorbital ecchymosis, edema, and subconjunctival hemorrhage are seen on examination; chemosis is common. Orbital fat may herniate into the maxillary antrum, resulting in enophthalmos. When the inferior rectus

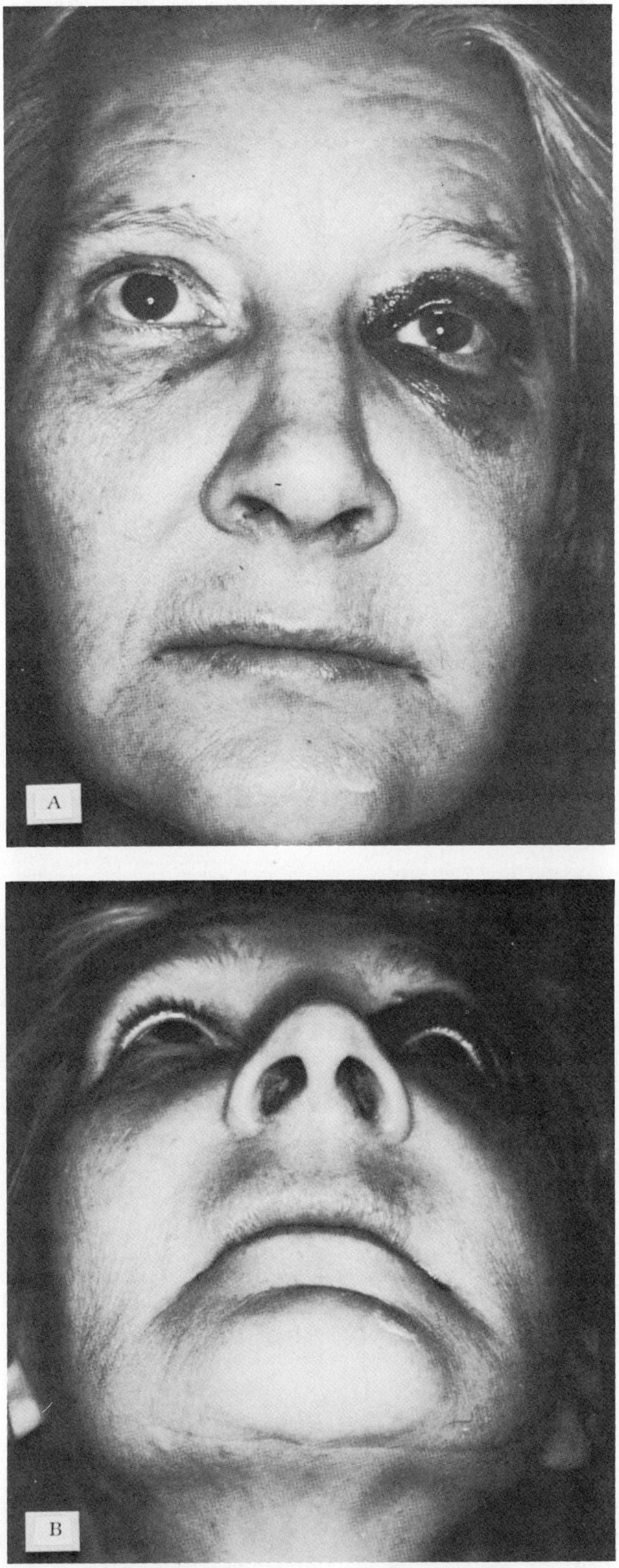

Fig. 56-15. A. Examination of a patient with zygomatic complex fracture reveals periorbital ecchymosis and swelling and antimongoloid slant of the lateral canthus. B. Examination from below reveals the flatness of the left cheek bone.

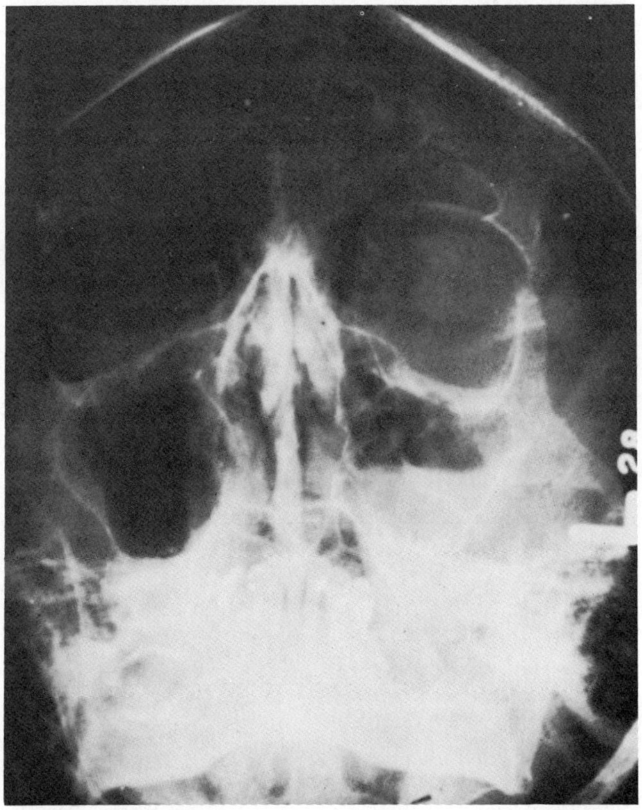

Fig. 56-16. This Water's view roentgenogram demonstrates a left zygomatic complex fracture. Note the inward displacement of the frontozygomatic suture, downward displacement of the infraorbital rim, and the air–fluid level in the left maxillary sinus.

and inferior oblique muscles become entrapped, limitation of ocular movement occurs, particularly in upward gaze (Fig. 56-18). Occasionally, downward gaze is also limited. The presence of diplopia is not necessary for the diagnosis nor is the finding an absolute confirmation of the diagnosis, since transient double vision may occur without fracture.

The eye should be examined very carefully for the presence of hyphema, laceration of the globe, retinal tears, or other injuries (see Chap. 58). In addition, sensation in the distribution of the infraorbital nerve should be tested carefully since paresthesia or anesthesia of this nerve usually occurs (the infraorbital nerve courses along the floor of the orbit before it exits from the infraorbital foramen). Visual acuity should be assessed, and the orbital rim should be carefully palpated to detect a separation or fracture.

A Water's x-ray is helpful in the diagnosis of blow-out fractures (see Fig. 56-3). Typically, the x-ray reveals cloudiness and a "hanging drop" of orbital contents in the maxillary sinus. Orbital tomograms in the posteroanterior and lateral planes or CT scans are often helpful in delineating the size and location of the orbital floor defect.

MANAGEMENT. Whenever a patient sustains trauma to the orbit or globe, or both, an ophthalmologist should be called to evaluate these structures and the patient's vision. Once the diagnosis of blow-out fracture is made, the patient is usually observed for several days while the swelling resolves.

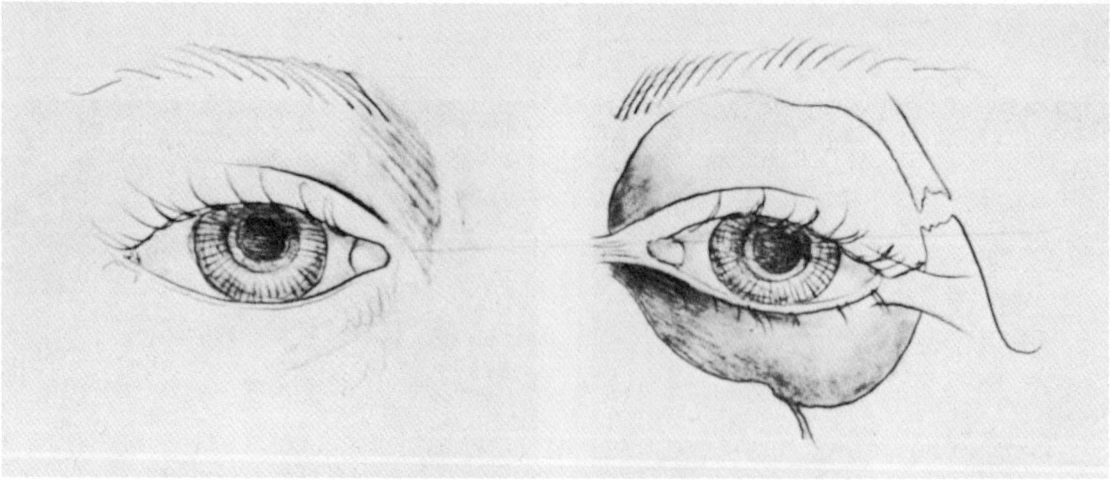

Fig. 56-17. Schematic representation of the underlying injury in the patient in Fig. 56-15.

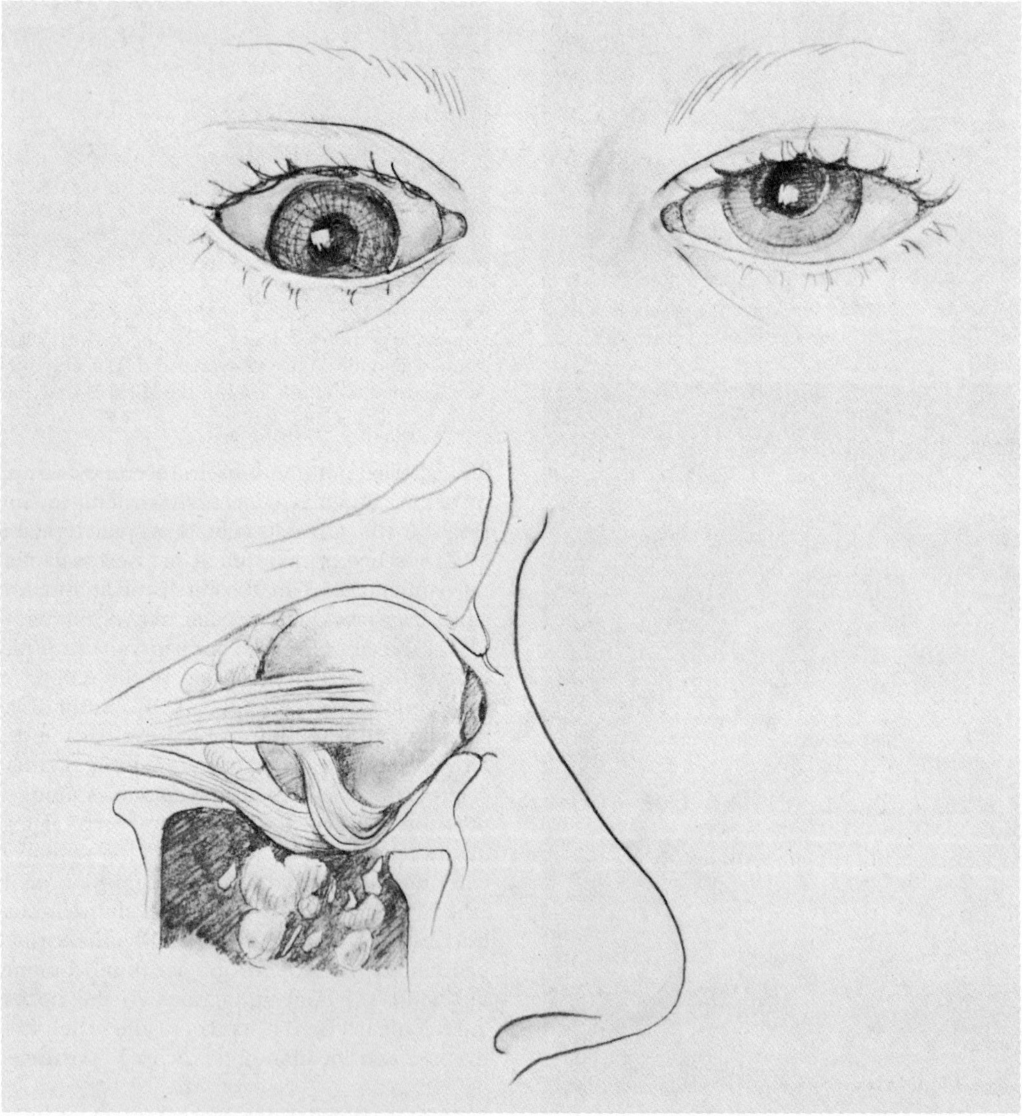

Fig. 56-18. Frontal view (*top*) shows the restriction in upward gaze of the right globe secondary to entrapment of the inferior oblique-inferior rectus muscles. Lateral view (*bottom*) shows the muscles and periorbital fat herniated down into the maxillary sinus.

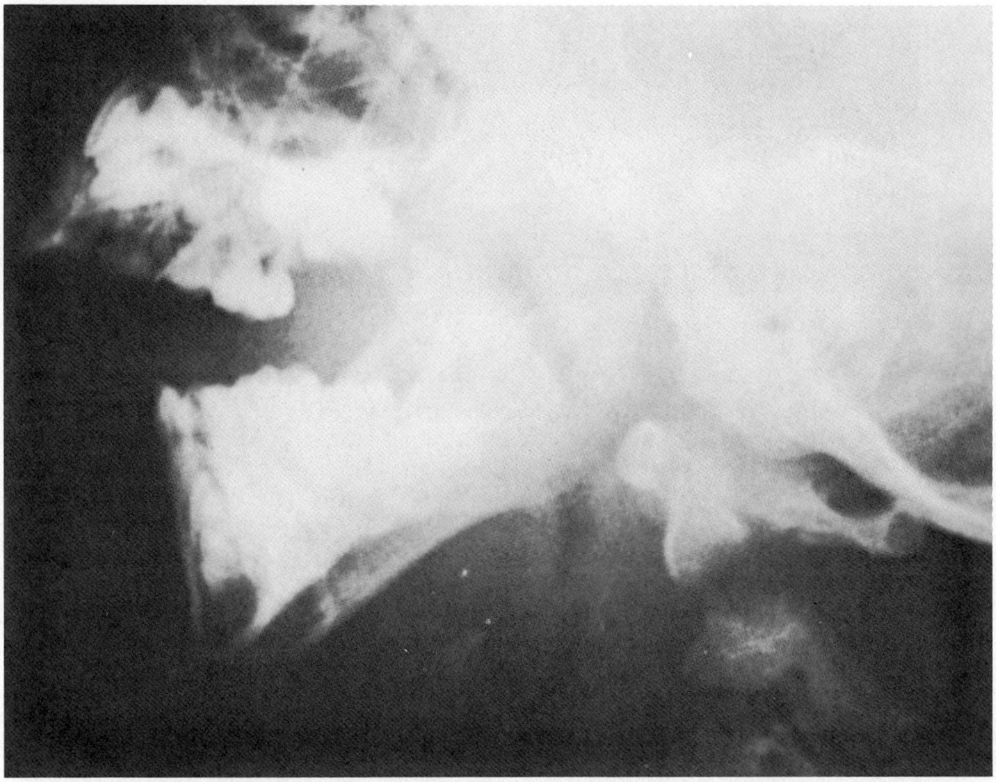

Fig. 56-19. This lateral skull and cervical spine radiograph shows an anteriorly displaced odontoid process (C2) fracture. Note that the mandible is retrognathic and there is an open bite. This is evidence of bilateral subcondylar and mandibular symphysis fractures, although they do not show on this radiograph.

Ice packs or iced compresses should be applied to the orbit, and the patient should be placed on decongestants and antibiotics because of the potential for infection in the violated maxillary sinus. Patients should sleep in a head-elevated position and should not blow their nose; if they do, subcutaneous emphysema may increase and further contaminate the traumatized tissue planes. A decision about surgery is made after several days, when enophthalmos, extraocular muscle function, diplopia, and infraorbital nerve paresthesia have been evaluated. Indications for surgical repair are quite controversial; in brief, however, the decision to operate is usually made on the basis of severe enophthalmos, persistent severe limitation of extraocular muscle movement and persistent anesthesia or paresthesia (see Chap. 58).

Mandibular Fractures

Mandibular fractures are the most common facial fractures that require patients to be admitted to the hospital. Because of the great force required to fracture the mandible, associated injuries are frequently found in these patients. Cervical spine injury should be particularly ruled out when the mandibular symphysis and condyles are involved (Fig. 56-19).

DIAGNOSIS. In the patient with a history of trauma to the mandible resulting in pain, swelling, and difficulty opening the jaw, the most significant finding is the complaint that the bite has changed. Swelling and ecchymosis, contusion, or laceration may mark the site of impact. Gross malocclusion may be visible when the mouth is closed (Fig. 56-20); abnormal interdigitation of the cusps of the teeth or nonalignment or nonocclusion of "wear" facets is evidence of a change in bite and thus a fracture. Ecchymosis and hematoma are seen in the floor of the mouth and in the buccal vestibule near the fracture site; the floor of the mouth may be elevated secondary to hematoma or edema and the gingiva overlying the fracture may be lacerated. Trismus, preventing the patient from opening his or her mouth, may make detection of a fracture difficult. Limited opening or deviation on opening may be due to a fracture in the condylar region, but it may also result from a hematoma in the joint space. On palpation, the site of the blow and, if the condyles are involved, the temporomandibular joint region are tender. The teeth in the line of fracture are mobile and tender, and bimanual palpation demonstrates mobility of the mandible across the fracture site (Fig. 56-21). Neurologic examination reveals paresthesia or frank anesthesia in the distribution of the inferior alveolar nerve (the third division of the trigeminal) on the side of the fracture.

The ramus and subcondylar region, where the bone is thinnest, are the most common sites of mandibular fracture. In fact, two-thirds of all fractures occur within an area bounded by the third molar, the angle, and the condyles. The symphysis, on the other hand, is fractured infrequently because of its thickness. A blow that produces a symphyseal injury drives the mandible posteriorly and superiorly, wedging the condyles against the base of the skull; unilateral or bilateral subcondylar fractures often result. When the symphysis is fractured, the potential for airway obstruction is great and the patient should be positioned with head ele-

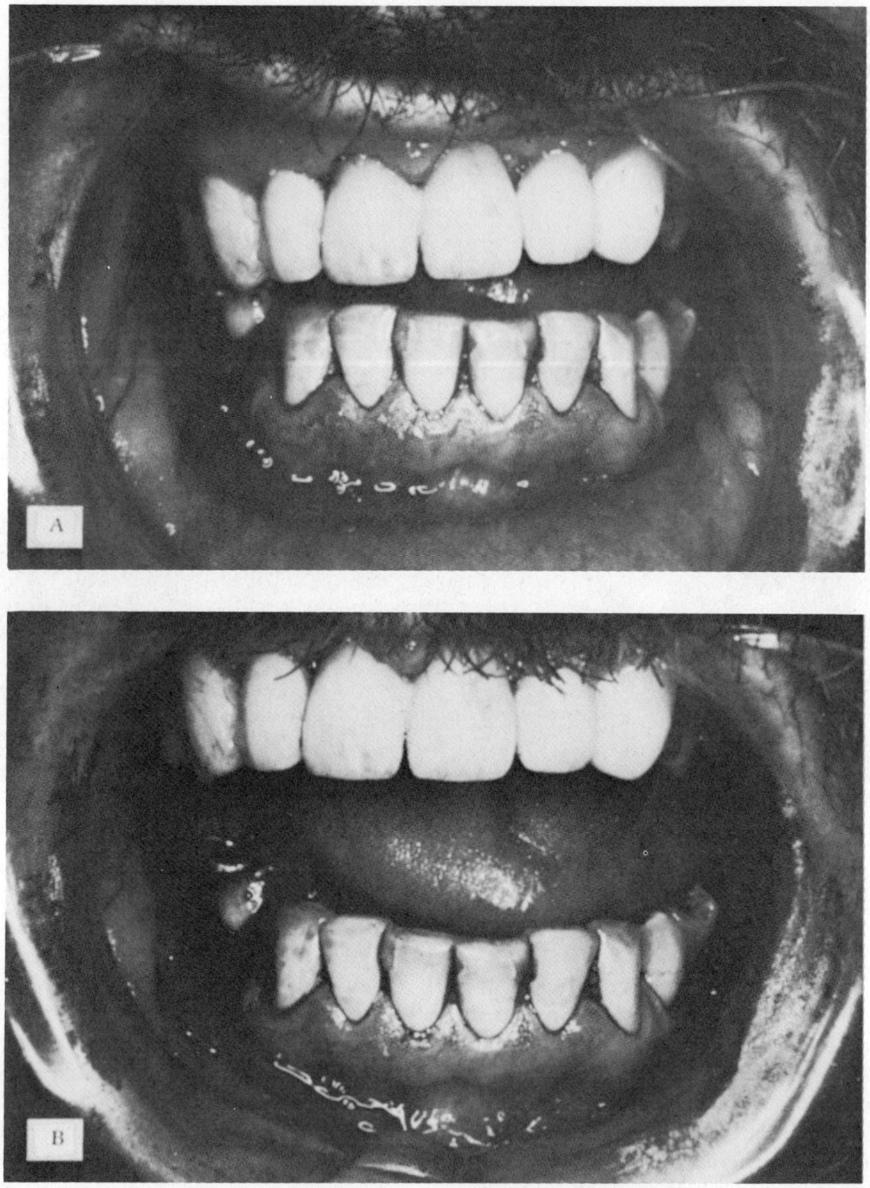

Fig. 56-20. This photograph illustrates the intraoral examination in a patient with bilateral mandibular fractures. A. There is a gross malocclusion with abnormal interdigitation of the teeth and an open bite on one side. B. The limitation of opening of the jaw (trismus) is shown.

vated and should be closely observed for respiratory distress. Temporarily stabilizing symphyseal fragments with a wire wrapped around the teeth on either side of the mandible is often helpful.

Fractures in the subcondylar region may be difficult to detect, particularly when trismus prevents movement of the jaw. A swollen, discolored, or lacerated auditory canal may serve as a clue to this injury. When there is a unilateral subcondylar fracture, the jaw will deviate toward the side of fracture on opening, because of asymmetric lateral pterygoid muscle action. When the fracture is bilateral, an anterior open bite results from the downward rotation of the body of the mandible by the suprahyoid muscles. Retrusion of the mandible is also common in the presence of bilateral subcondylar fractures.

X-rays are a helpful adjunct in the diagnosis of mandibular fractures. The standard mandibular views are the posteroanterior, right and left lateral oblique, and the Towne's view (see Figs. 56-4, 56-5, and 56-6). The posteroanterior radiograph shows the body, from angle to angle. The right and left lateral oblique x-rays show the ramus of the mandible, condyle, sigmoid notch, coronoid process, and the molar regions. The Towne's view is an anteroposterior x-ray with the head tilted to project the petrous ridges and the mastoid processes away from the condyles. In this x-ray, the posterior portion of the ramus of the mandible, the condylar neck, and the head of the condyle can be seen. A panoramic x-ray is very helpful, but many hospitals do not have the machine and the patient must be ambulatory. This view,

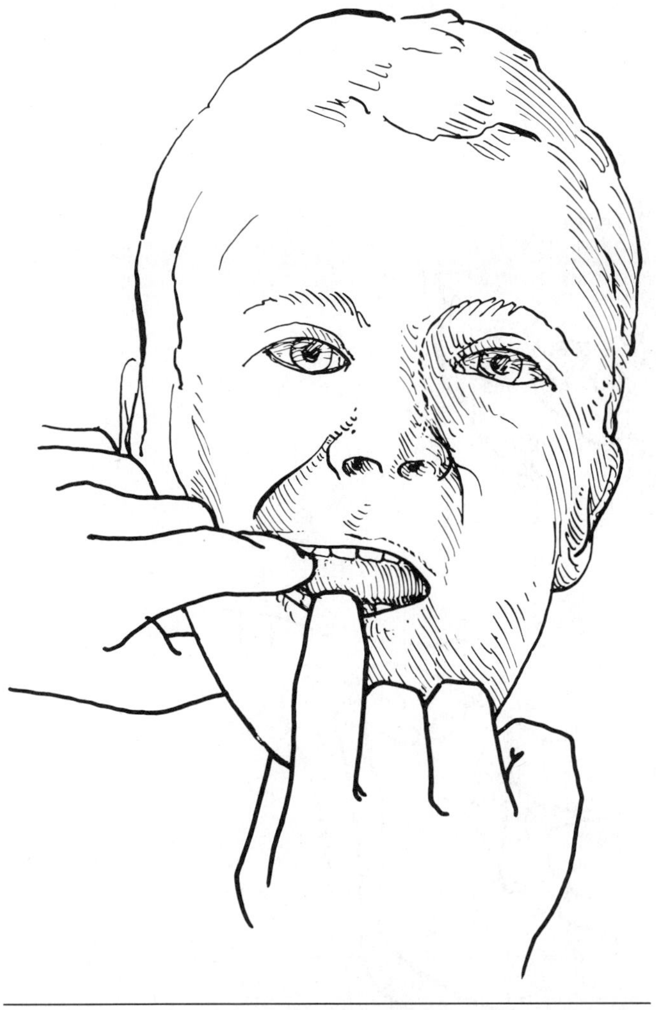

Fig. 56-21. Illustration of the bimanual palpation of the mandible.

however, does give the clearest picture of the mandible and is most helpful diagnostically.

MANAGEMENT. Oral intake is reduced to clear liquids or is stopped. Moving the jaw in an attempt to chew or swallow food tends to pump bacteria into the fracture sites and into any open intraoral wounds. Since almost all mandibular fractures are compound into the mouth and contaminated by oral flora, antibiotic therapy consisting of 1,000,000 units of penicillin G intravenously every 6 hours is begun. Erythromycin, clindamycin, or a first-generation cephalosporin is used in penicillin-allergic patients. Temporary stabilization with a single wire around the teeth adjacent to the fracture site or with an arch should be attempted if a gross malocclusion is present or if there is a fracture of the symphysis of the mandible with collapse of support and respiratory difficulty. This is usually done by a maxillofacial specialist. If the fracture is undisplaced and minimally mobile and the patient is having no respiratory difficulty, temporary stabilization is not necessary and no further treatment need be carried out during the immediate postinjury period. Once the preliminary measures are carried out, the patient is usually referred to a specialist trained in the management of maxillofacial injuries.

The goal of treatment of subcondylar fractures of the mandible is to achieve a mobile, functioning joint and to maintain the height of the mandibular ramus. Immobilization for 4 to 6 weeks in the presence of a high subcondylar or intra-articular fracture may result in a stiff joint with a fibrous or bony ankylosis. To avoid this complication, subcondylar fractures are treated with minimal immobilization. Patients with unilateral subcondylar fractures may be treated with a liquid diet and analgesics alone. They are closely observed and are not immobilized unless a malocclusion develops. Patients with bilateral subcondylar fractures usually require a short period of intermaxillary fixation (2 weeks) and then exercises to maintain function. For patients with isolated subcondylar fractures, the emergency physician need only start the patient on a liquid diet, analgesics, and ice to the area for 24 to 36 hours, followed by heat. The patient should be referred to an oral and maxillofacial surgeon for follow-up within 24 hours.

Mandibular fractures in children are often nondisplaced and are treated conservatively with 3 weeks of intermaxillary fixation using arch bars or interdental wiring. Open reduction is avoided because it may damage tooth buds in the body of the mandible. It is especially important for children to be treated and followed by an experienced specialist because of potential problems with growth.

Dislocation of the Jaw

The mandible articulates with the base of the skull at the temporomandibular joint. This is an unusual joint in that the right and left sides work simultaneously and must be perfectly coordinated. Its anterior aspect is bounded by the articular tubercle of the temporal bone. Initial opening of the jaw occurs on a hinge axis, without anterior translation. Once hinge opening reaches its maximum, however, the mandible translates anteriorly.

Dislocation of the mandible occurs when the condylar head of the mandible moves out of the glenoid fossa and anterior to the articular tubercle. It may be caused by a sudden uncontrolled movement such as yawning, laughing with the mouth wide open, coughing, or vomiting. Other etiologic factors commonly seen are trauma, prolonged wide opening of the mouth during induction of general anesthesia, or involuntary movements in patients taking prochlorperazine (Compazine) or other phenothiazines.

DIAGNOSIS. Dislocation of the jaw has occurred when the jaw is locked in the open position. X-rays of the mandible are helpful only to rule out fractures when the etiology is trauma. A panoramic x-ray is most revealing; if this is not available, however, temporomandibular joint views will suffice.

MANAGEMENT. Therapy for a dislocated mandible is directly related to the anatomy and muscle function. With the patient sitting upright in a chair, the physician should stand above and manipulate the mandible into its normal position. Having another person hold the patient's head is often helpful. Grasped between the thumb and index finger, the mandible is pushed downward until it clears the articular tuber-

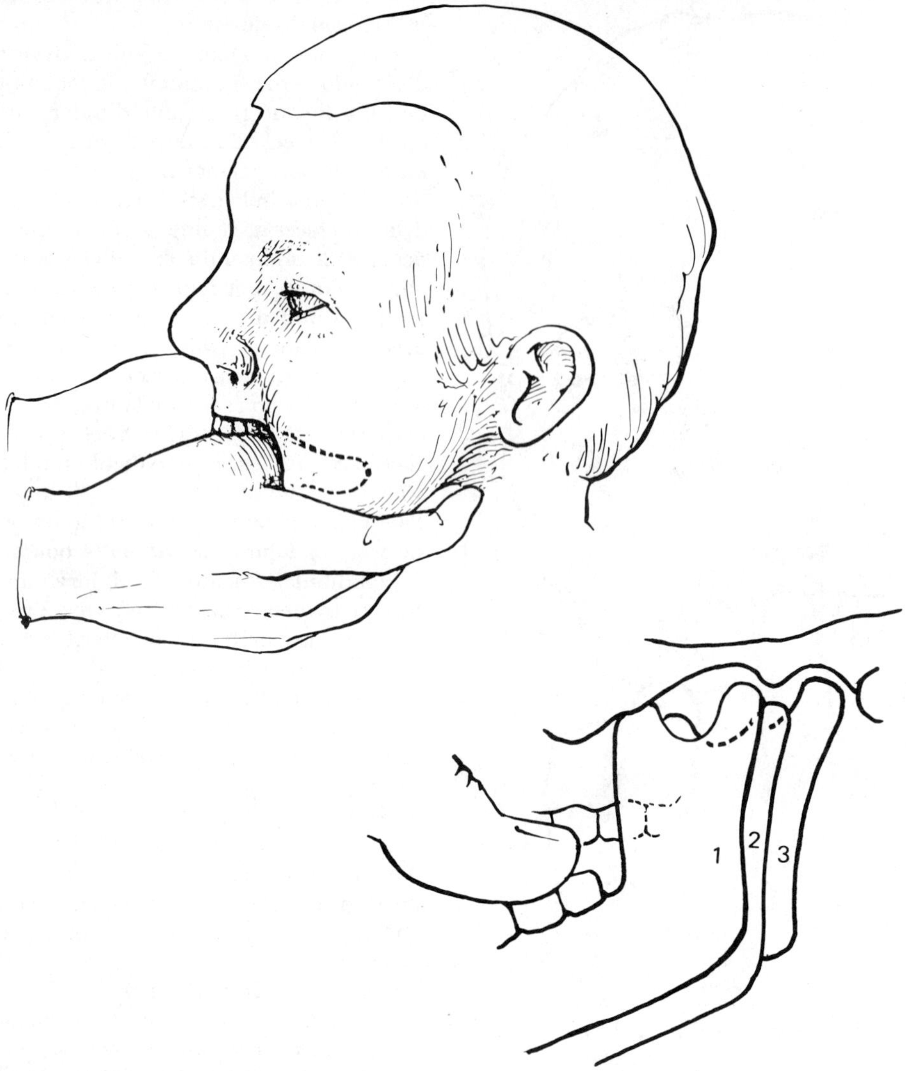

Fig. 56-22. Reduction of a dislocated mandible. The upper drawing demonstrates the method of grasping the jaw in order to relocate it. The lower drawing demonstrates the path taken by the mandible as the bone is pushed inferiorly to clear the articular tubercle. It is then manipulated posteriorly and superiorly back into the glenoid fossa.

cle and is then rotated upward and posteriorly into the glenoid fossa (Fig. 56-22). If bilateral dislocation is present, reduction may be best accomplished one joint at a time. Care should be taken by the person reducing the temporomandibular joint to avoid injuries to his or her fingers by the teeth. The jaw should be held in the patient's proper occlusion. If the lateral pterygoid muscles are in spasm, repositioning the jaw may be difficult or impossible without general anesthesia. Once the mandible has been relocated, movement of the jaw should be limited to minimize the chance of recurrent dislocation. A soft diet and muscle relaxant such as diazepam, 5 to 10 mg twice a day, are appropriate, and heat therapy is helpful. The patient should be instructed to place a fist under his or her chin to prevent the jaw from opening too wide, when he or she yawns, for example. A dislocation that recurs requires immobilization by intermaxillary fixation for 7 days, after which the jaw should be released and returned to function.

The emergency physician should attempt to relocate a dislocated jaw as just described, without premedication. If this attempt is unsuccessful or if the jaw dislocates again, an oral and maxillofacial surgeon should be consulted to treat the patient.

SELECTED READING

Dingman, RO, and Natvig, P. *Surgery of Facial Fractures.* Philadelphia: Saunders, 1964.

Kazanjian, V, and Converse, JM. *Surgical Treatment of Facial Injuries.* Baltimore: Williams & Wilkins, 1974.

Mulliken, JB, Kaban, LB, and Murray, JE. Management of facial fractures in children. *Clin Plast Surg* 4:491, 1977.

Rowe, NL, and Killey, NC. *Fractures of the Facial Skeleton* (2nd ed.). Baltimore: Williams & Wilkins, 1968.

57. Dentoalveolar Injuries

Leonard B. Kaban
David H. Perrott

Trauma to the teeth and dentoalveolar segments are probably the most common injuries in the facial region. They occur most frequently in children and are the result of a direct blow to the dentoalveolar segments. The most common location is the maxillary anterior region, followed by the mandibular anterior region. The posterior dentoalveolar segments are less commonly involved. These injuries may be associated with fractures of the teeth or jaws and with lacerations of the buccal mucosa, gums, or lips.

Dental injuries consisting of fracture or avulsion of teeth are commonly seen in the dental office but may also be seen in the emergency department. They are usually the result of a fall from a bicycle, steps, or jungle gym type of apparatus. Other common etiologic factors include athletic injuries or fisticuffs.

DIAGNOSIS

Dentoalveolar segment injuries are usually quite obvious. The patient complains of a malocclusion, and, on physical examination, the teeth and underlying bony segments are out of position and mobile. The overlying gingiva is usually lacerated (Fig. 57-1). A panoramic x-ray is helpful to document the position of the fractured alveolar segment and to evaluate the status of the teeth within it. A thorough examination is necessary as facial fractures are often associated with dentoalveolar fractures.

A fracture in a tooth may be superficial, affecting only the enamel (the outer covering of the crown), or it may involve the dentin, pulp, or root (Fig. 57-2). The extent of the fracture is important because it affects the initial symptoms and treatment and also the prognosis for the tooth. If only the enamel is involved, the patient is asymptomatic because the enamel is not supplied by nerves. A fracture into the dentin commonly causes sensitivity to changes or extremes of temperature or air or to sweets; the pain is much like that associated with dental caries. The yellowish color of dentin is visible on examination.

Sensitivity when the tooth is percussed or tapped by an instrument is typical when a fracture extends into the pulp, and the pink color of the pulp tissue may be visible. Sensitivity to a thermal, chemical, or physical stimulus and continuous pain are common, and the pulp may bleed.

A fracture of the root can usually be diagnosed by the extreme mobility of the tooth and pain on palpation or percussion. A dental x-ray is necessary to locate the fracture.

Teeth that are extruded or partially avulsed are visibly malpositioned and mobile. Children following a fall often present with intruded primary deciduous teeth. Occlusion may be affected and the patient is aware of the abnormality of his or her bite. Because the root of such a tooth may be

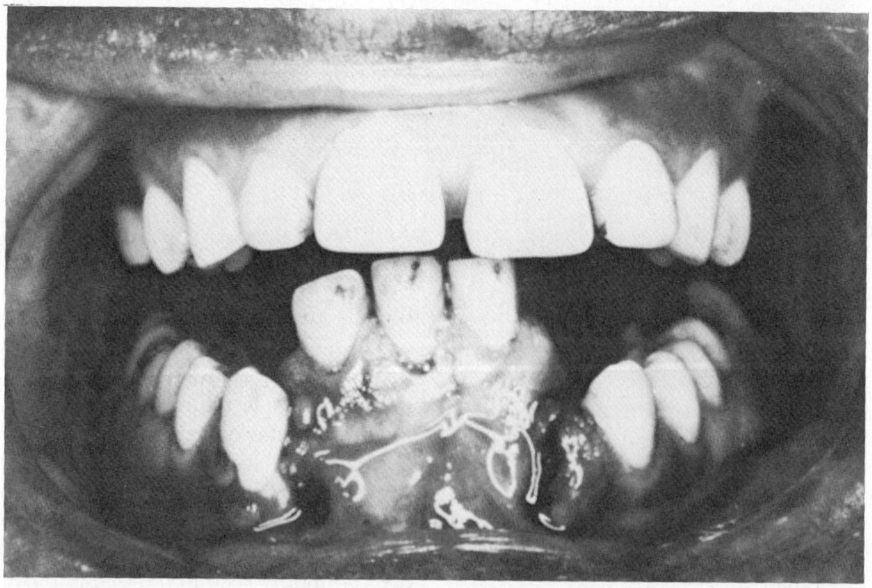

Fig. 57-1. Dentoalveolar segment trauma. Intraoral examination reveals a gross malocclusion secondary to fracture and displacement of the mandibular anterior segment with three incisor teeth. The segment was reduced, then stabilized with an arch bar wired to the mandibular teeth.

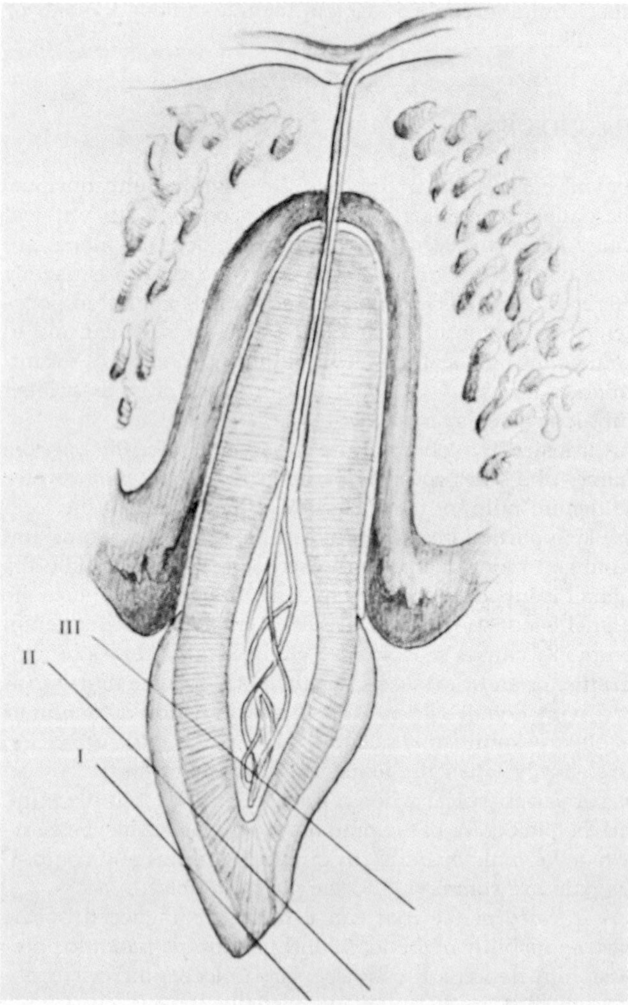

Fig. 57-2. A cross-section of a maxillary incisor tooth showing levels of fracture that may occur. A class I fracture is into the enamel. A class II fracture is into the dentin. A class III fracture is into the pulp.

fractured, x-rays are necessary. Teeth may also be totally avulsed from their sockets.

MANAGEMENT

Dentoalveolar injuries are treated by reducing the fractured segment and stabilizing it with an arch bar or dental restorative material (Figs. 57-3 and 57-4). This procedure should be performed by a dentist or oral and maxillofacial surgeon as soon as possible after the injury in order to salvage the teeth and bone. Occasionally, an acrylic splint is fabricated after dental impressions have been taken. The patient is placed on prophylactic penicillin or erythromycin (250 mg 4 times a day) for 5 to 7 days and should remain on a liquid diet for 3 weeks. The diet may then be advanced and the arch bars removed after 4 weeks. The emergency physician should manually reduce the segment to make the patient more comfortable and reduce bleeding.

Fractures of the teeth should also be treated by a dentist as soon as possible after the injury. Those involving only the enamel will usually be smoothed off with a dental drill, and x-rays should be taken to rule out root fractures. If the dentin is involved, the dentist usually places a sedative dressing, such as zinc oxide and eugenol (oil of cloves) over the tooth. When a small amount of pulp is exposed, a covering with calcium hydroxide and a sedative dressing are sufficient in most cases; the calcium hydroxide causes the pulp to regress and stimulates calcification over the opening. If a large pulpal exposure occurs, the nerve is removed by a dentist and root canal therapy is carried out later.

When a dental root is fractured in the apical third, nothing is done initially, but root canal therapy may be required

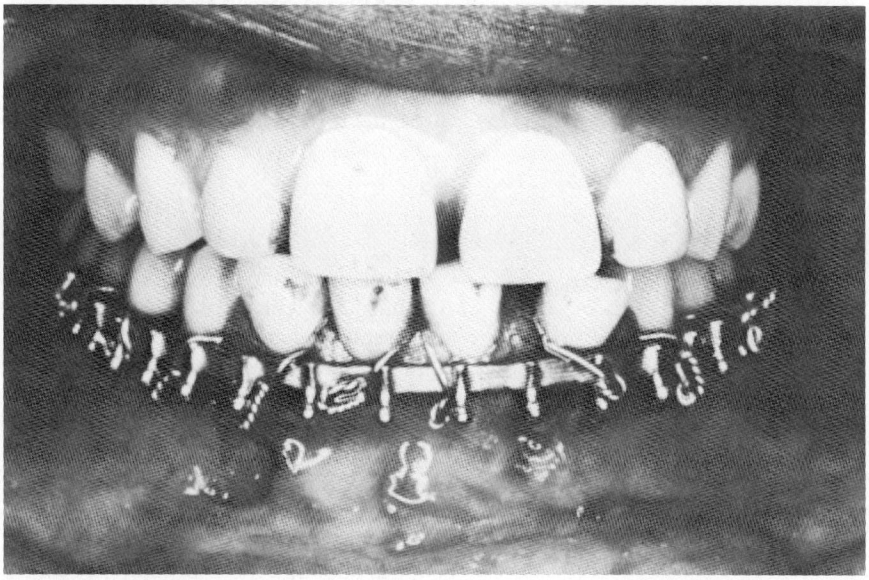

Fig. 57-3. Photograph showing the fracture illustrated in Fig. 57-1, which has been wired and stabilized into its correct position.

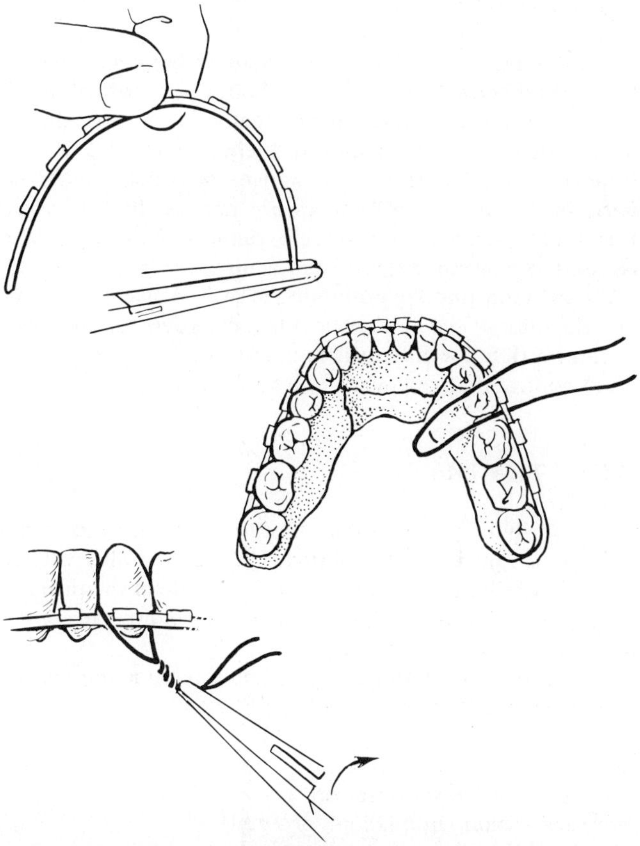

Fig. 57-4. Series of drawings showing the technique of bending an arch bar and wiring it into position around the teeth.

later. When the root is fractured in the middle or cervical third, however, the tooth is usually removed.

Teeth that are displaced or avulsed may be saved. X-rays are taken to rule out root fractures and then the teeth can be manually repositioned into their proper location. The tooth is then fixed and immobilized with an arch bar, interdental wiring, or a composite resin splint to adjacent stable teeth. If a tooth has been totally avulsed from its socket, reimplantation is frequently possible. Therefore, an avulsed tooth should always be brought to the emergency department or to the dentist's office for evaluation. While waiting for the dentist, the tooth should be placed in saline solution. If a dentist is not available, the emergency physician should clean off the tooth, irrigate and debride the socket, then reimplant the tooth.

Because of contamination of the open socket and hematoma at its apex, and because infection almost certainly causes the reimplanted tooth to be lost, the patient should be placed on an antibiotic, penicillin or erythromycin, 1 gm a day for 5 days.

Intruded primary teeth (deciduous) often require no treatment, but the child should be referred to a dentist for definitive treatment.

SELECTED READING

Andreasen, JO. *Traumatic Injuries of the Teeth* (2nd ed). Philadelphia: Saunders, 1981.

Peterson, LS, et al. *Contemporary Oral and Maxillofacial Surgery*. St. Louis: Mosby, 1988.

58. Injuries to the Eye and Adnexa

Roger V. Ohanesian

Most traumatic eye injuries may be categorized as blunt, sharp, or chemical. They can range from mild to sight threatening, and the immediate action of the emergency physician may determine the ultimate vision of the patient.

Examination of the traumatized eye may be brief or lengthy depending on the extent of injury and the ability of the patient to cooperate. Great care must be taken in this examination, for if the eye is lacerated or even punctured, manipulation can result in the prolapse of the inner contents of the globe.

If possible, the examination outlined here should be conducted in the following order:

Visual acuity of each eye
Penlight or slit lamp examination
External ocular motions
Ophthalmoscopy

Of these tests, *visual acuity is the most important test to determine disorders of the eye.* It should be recorded on all patients with ocular emergencies. Acuity of each eye should be recorded using the standard Snellen chart at a 20-foot distance (6 m). Glasses for distance correction should be worn since "raw vision" scores are useless. If glasses are broken or otherwise not available, pinhole vision should be assessed to determine best visual acuity.

Visual acuity and the remaining tests are basically to compare the injured eye to its mate. Most disorders are monocular, and a difficult diagnosis is made easier by comparison to the nontraumatized eye.

BLUNT TRAUMA

The majority of complaints of blunt trauma are associated with sports injuries, automobile accidents, and altercations; the order of frequency depends on the locale of the primary care center. Trauma of this nature can affect any part of the eye, from the lids to the optic nerve.

The history after blunt trauma should include the following pertinent information:

Size of object causing injury
Place of contact (eye, nose, brow)
Decreased vision (immediate, gradual)

Patients with obvious blunt trauma injuries should be questioned as to the size of the object producing the trauma. A softball may cause facial fractures but rarely injures the globe, which is protected within the orbital recess. In contrast, a golf ball or elbow may cause a blow-out fracture of the orbital floor as well as global injuries.

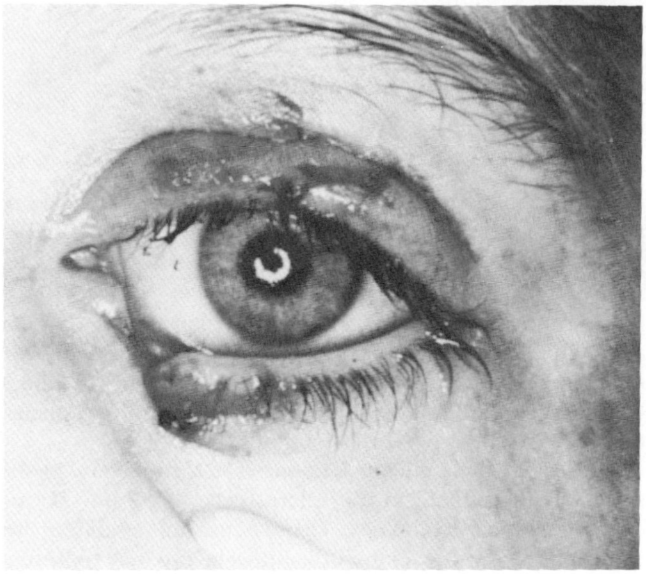

Fig. 58-1. Tear duct laceration exposed with lid retraction.

Patients often consider injuries to the bridge of the nose or the brow as trauma to the eye. It is important to ascertain the point of contact, since an indirect blow to the orbit does not cause as severe a visual injury. Immediate decrease of vision indicates vascular compromise or retinal involvement and carries a worse prognosis than gradual decrease in vision, most commonly resulting from corneal edema or hyphema.

Laceration of the Lid and Tear Duct

Laceration of the eyelid commonly accompanies blunt injury to the eye. If the wound is medial, a tear duct laceration should be suspected and is far more ominous than a superficial lid laceration.

Diagnosis

Injuries of the lid should be closely examined with the aid of a penlight or slit lamp. Lid lacerations frequently appear to be little more than abrasions, but on careful retraction of wound margins, the true extent of the laceration may be seen to involve the tear duct or lid margin (Fig. 58-1). All lid lacerations must be considered to be associated with global injuries until proven otherwise.

Management

Lacerations of the lid margin or tear duct deserve the attention of a specialist; they must be closed layer by layer to prevent disfiguring lid notching or chronic tear problems. Surgery should be performed within 24 hours. A deep wound of the upper lid may sever its levator muscles, causing a resultant ptosis if not adequately repaired.

Blow-Out Fractures

Following blunt injury from a small diameter ball, club, or fist, the eye may be forced posteriorly into the socket, causing a bursting to its surrounding walls, known as a blow-out fracture.

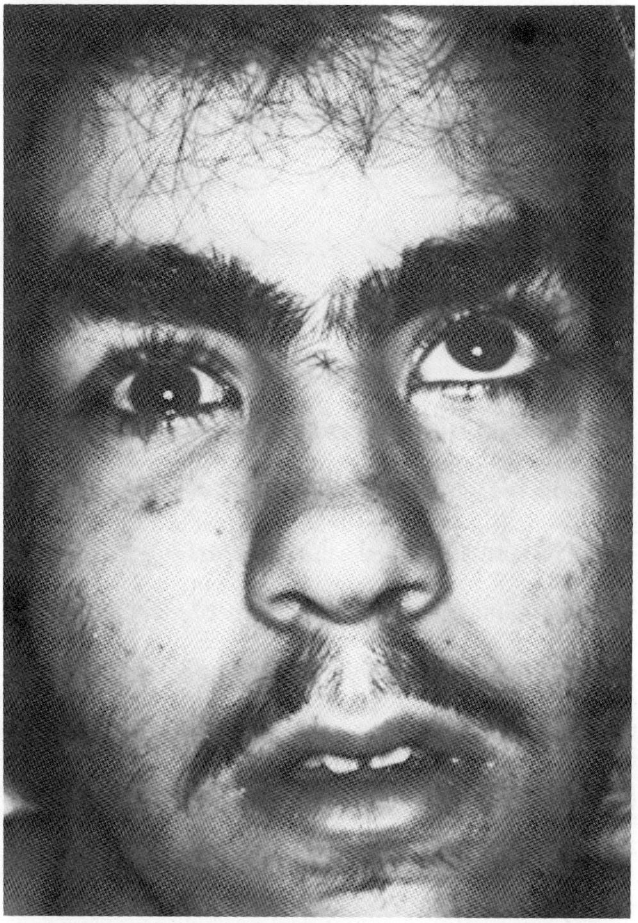

Fig. 58-2. Upward gaze limitation in blow-out fracture with inferior rectus muscle entrapment.

Diagnosis

After blunt injury to the globe, the orbital contents are compressed and may result in fracture of one of the orbital walls. The most common sites to fracture are the medial or inferior walls. Inferior wall fractures are associated with much more pathology than the relatively benign medial wall fractures. If the inferior rectus muscle becomes entrapped in the fracture site, vertical eye movement will be limited (Fig. 58-2) and is often associated with pain. Horizontal gaze is usually unaffected after inferior wall blow outs. Reduced tactile sensation of the lower lid, cheek, and alveolar ridge are diagnostic signs of a fracture involving the inferior orbital nerve. X-ray film evidence, especially in Water's view, frequently demonstrates opacification or soft tissue density within the maxillary sinus of the affected side (see Fig. 56-3). This finding should make the emergency physician suspicious of the possibility of a fracture of the floor of the orbit.

Management

An ophthalmologist, otolaryngologist, or plastic surgeon should be consulted for patients with blow-out fractures. Coughing, sneezing, or nose blowing should be discouraged to avoid contamination of the posterior orbit with the nasal contents. Usual treatment is topical with systemic antibiotics and surgical repair within 2 weeks. Delay of diagnosis or treatment, or both, beyond this time increases surgical risks because of the increased vascularity of fibrosing tissue. Not all cases of blow-out fracture require surgical repair.

Scleral Rupture

A blow that is strong enough to retroplace the eye may cause the globe instead of the orbital walls to burst. A stronger blow may cause a blow-out fracture as well as a ruptured globe.

Diagnosis
A scleral rupture may be the underlying result of an apparent simple lid injury. The conjunctiva may have evidence of hemorrhage that indicates the site of injury to the globe. This subconjunctival bleeding frequently masks the underlying scleral rupture. Blood beneath the conjunctiva in this condition causes a much greater reaction and is often so pronounced that it prevents lid closure. A ruptured sclera may also show abnormal pigmentation beyond the circumference of the cornea, representing herniated uveal pigment. This rupture may occur at the site of trauma, at the limbus, or at a weak area of the globe. In cases in which this diagnosis is suspected, no further examination of the globe should be performed by the emergency physician. Further attempts at examination may cause extrusion of orbital contents through the wound.

Management
An ophthalmologist should be consulted to complete the examination and to repair the wound under general anesthesia in the operating room. Until the ophthalmologist arrives, the patient should be sedated and given appropriate systemic analgesics and a metal shield to prevent rubbing of the eye.

The emergency physician may cause great harm and eventual loss of the eye by inappropriately applying antibiotics to a ruptured globe, since topical ointments are oil based and are intensely reactive to the inner eye.

Corneal Edema

Trauma of a lesser magnitude may cause only corneal injury yet may be intensely painful tó the patient.

Diagnosis
Corneal edema may occur after a contusion of the globe by blunt trauma. Alone it may reduce visual acuity to the 20/400 level, but it is often associated with injuries to other ocular structures. Penlight or preferably slit lamp examination reveals a loss of the crisp architecture of the iris when seen through the cloudy cornea.

Management
An ophthalmologist should be called to assist in the management of this disorder, since subtle signs of other injuries may escape detection by the primary care practitioner.

Corneal edema, frequently associated with corneal abrasion, may require eye patching for several days in order for the patient's eyesight to return to clarity. Pain medication, dilators, and sleeping pills may become necessary. Often a bandage soft contact lens is necessary to reduce pain and allow corneal epithelial regrowth.

Hyphema

If the blow caused the iris diaphragm to be retroplaced or avulsed, bleeding into the anterior chamber may occur.

Diagnosis
Blunt trauma often causes a hyphema, blood in the anterior chamber (Fig. 58-3), which is classified as gross or microscopic. The former is readily diagnosed, but, in the latter, the blood has not settled and the anterior chamber appears normal to all but slit lamp biomicroscopy.

Both types of hyphema demonstrate a reduction in the visual acuity, which, in the microscopic type, may be the only indication of pathology. Visual acuity in the injured eye that is one line worse than in the opposite eye may represent a microscopic hyphema and call for further investigation by an ophthalmologist.

Management
A patient with a hyphema is usually sedated, with the eye patched, and placed on strict bed rest. This disease has a potential for rebleeding from the injured iris vessel 4 to 5 days after the initial trauma. Rebleeding frequently causes the anterior chamber to fill with blood, producing a severe glaucoma that may result in irreversible loss of vision. The prognosis of this potentially grave disease rests entirely on the primary care physician who must suspect a hyphema in all cases of reduced visual acuity after eye trauma.

Retinal Edema or Choroidal Rupture

Diagnosis
Retinal edema may develop after blunt trauma and is a result of a contrecoup injury to the fundus. Pupillary dilation is often necessary to examine the fundus and may be performed by the topical application of 1 drop of tropicamide, 1 percent. Pallor is clinically obvious by direct ophthalmoscopy in the involved retinal tissue. If the macula is involved, vision is reduced to 20/200 or less. A choroidal rupture may also occur in worse cases of blunt trauma. A semicircular white line with adjacent subretinal hemorrhage marks the rupture site, which is often near or through the macula.

Management
Consultation with an ophthalmologist is necessary to determine medical treatment. If the edema or rupture does not involve the macula, prognosis for the return of vision is good. If the macula is involved, prognosis is guarded.

Retinal Detachment

Tears in the peripheral retina followed later by retinal detachment commonly occur after blunt trauma to the eye. Frequently, patients have previously existing retinal holes that develop into detachments after a sudden blow to the eye. The sudden onset of flashes of light or floating spots

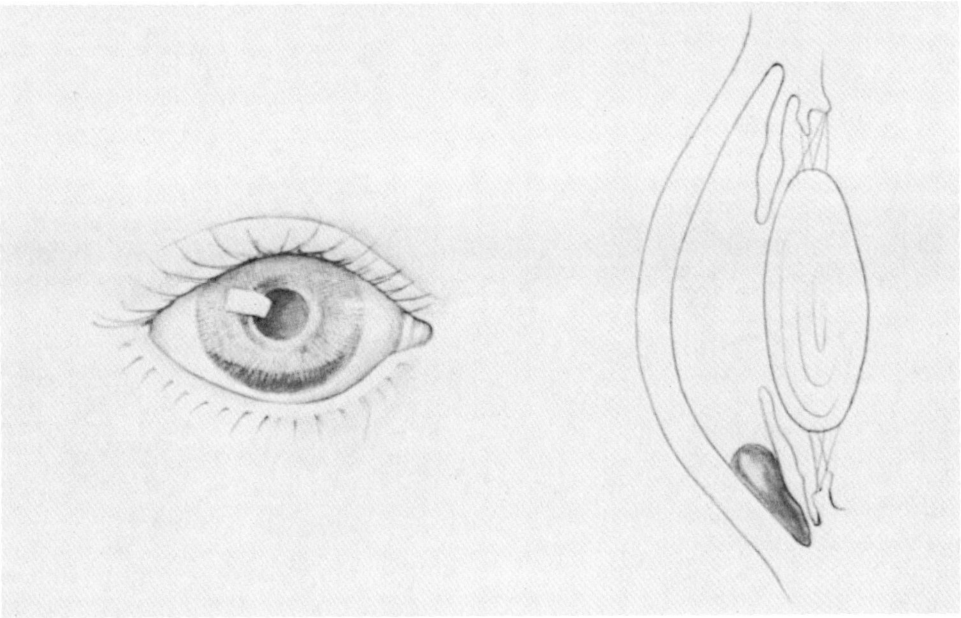

Fig. 58-3. Gross hyphema—layered blood in anterior chamber.

after trauma is a frequent symptom of a break in the retina. A veil or curtain in front of the vision is the usual complaint of detachment of the retina. The peripheral retina should be examined carefully, especially at the site of contact.

If the central retina is uninvolved, vision will be normal but is in jeopardy since a detachment may continue to progress to the macular region. Once the macula is detached, prognosis for return of normal vision is markedly reduced.

Diagnosis

The emergency physician should be aware that even with a dilated pupil and a direct ophthalmoscope, it may be possible to see only to the equator of the eye and that most retinal tears are beyond the physician's view. Retinal detachments, however, can often be seen with the direct ophthalmoscope.

On examination, the vessels overlying the detached retina will be tortuous and out of focus compared to the attached portion. Occasionally, blood will accompany the tear or detachment and make the diagnosis easier. If the retina is greatly detached, it will be pale and appear bullous and billowing with eye movements. There will be no vision in the detached portion.

Management

Patients with suspected detachments should be calmed and placed on a flat bed in a supine position and told to avoid excessive eye or head movements until an ophthalmologist can confirm the diagnosis and schedule operative repair. Prognosis is improved if there is early treatment and an uninvolved macula. Avoid the use of ointments as they will obscure future examination of retina.

SHARP TRAUMA

The vast majority of cases of sharp trauma are associated with industrial accidents. The most important determination in this category is whether the eye has been perforated. Although the globe is extremely resistant to foreign body penetration, sharp trauma is more likely to occur under certain conditions.

The history taken after sharp trauma should include the following pertinent questions:

What was the immediate preinjury activity?
  (welding, grinding, hammering)
Were glasses or other eye protectors worn?
  Are they present? Intact?
What was the nature of the object?
  (metallic, steel, brass, thorn)

Foreign bodies that penetrate the eye are often the result of high-speed missiles and are frequently metallic. Slivers from a hammered wedge or grinder wheel frequently create hot steel particles that may penetrate the eye, as will shards of glass from shattered spectacles or a thorn from a snapped twig.

In most cases of perforation, patients are unaware of the severity of the injury and consider it of minor consequence. The emergency physician must suspect penetration in all patients who present a history of a propelled foreign body striking the eye.

Corneal or Scleral Perforation

Despite the severity of the injury, many patients with corneal or scleral perforation present with only a mild foreign body sensation.

Diagnosis

On examination, visual acuity is occasionally normal but is usually reduced by at least a line or two of the Snellen chart. By penlight examination, the site of entry of a scleral wound is often masked by overlying conjunctival hemorrhage. If the cornea is perforated, a surface irregularity may be visible at

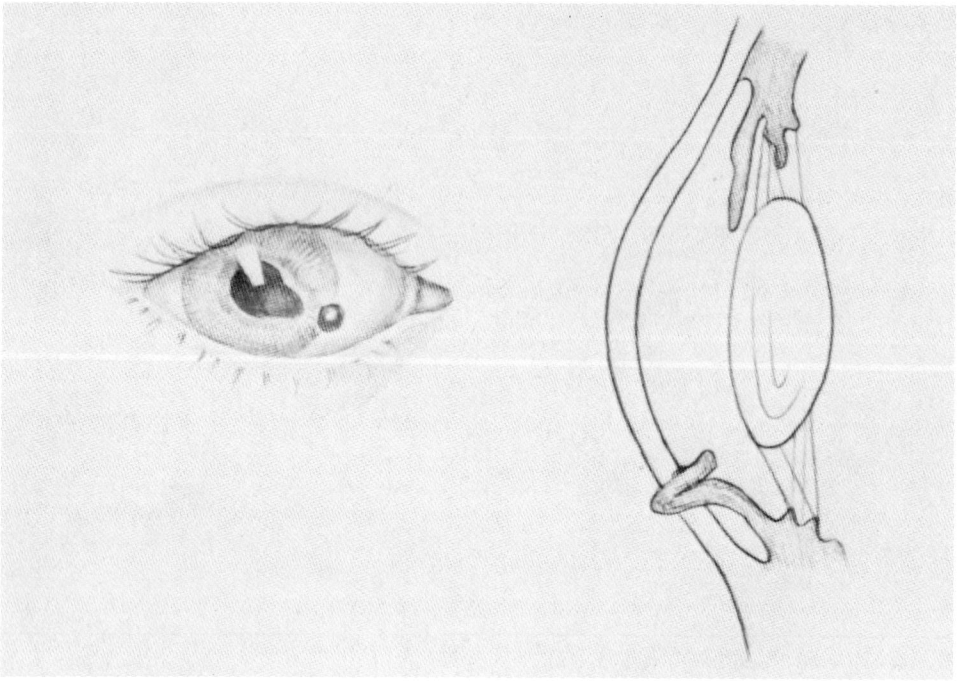

Fig. 58-4. Penetrating injury with iris prolapse into the wound resulting in peaked pupil.

the entry site. Often a brown elevation having a foreign body appearance obscures the wound margins. (Fig. 58-4). This is actually a prolapsed iris that has herniated, thereby plugging the wound.

This iris prolapse is a diagnostic sign of corneal perforation, producing an irregular pupil that "points" to the site of the wound. In many cases, the prolapse is small and indistinguishable without the aid of a slit lamp.

Management

Once the diagnosis of corneal or scleral perforation is made, the primary care physician should discontinue the examination. Children and anxious adults are especially prone to squeezing their lids, thus elevating ocular pressure, and this may eviscerate the entire global contents through a small wound. Surgical repair by an ophthalmologist may be necessary, depending on the size of the perforation and its location. Prognosis should always be guarded because of the grave dangers of infection and latent ocular disease.

Lens Penetration

Diagnosis

When the lens is penetrated by a foreign body, it may rapidly turn opaque. This traumatic cataract may form within 1 hour, become quite dense, and prevent further view of the fundus. Usually the opacity begins at the site of the lens penetration and provides a clue to the position of the foreign body within the eye.

Management and Prognosis

The lens capsule, once penetrated, usually causes a dense cataract to form. Extraction of this traumatic cataract may be performed at the time of the initial operative repair or may be delayed for months or years.

Prognosis for vision depends on other ocular injuries. After cataract extraction, a contact lens or lens implant is usually necessary for the return of adequate visual acuity.

Posterior Pole Foreign Body

A severe injury from a foreign body is usually quite obvious and results in a profound loss of vision; there is little difficulty in making the diagnosis.

Diagnosis

A foreign body that has come to rest in the posterior pole may be seen as a grey opacity out of focus to the remaining fundus. Intraretinal and choroidal hemorrhage may be seen in the adjacent tissue.

The position of the foreign body and any bleeding should be noted on the patient's chart (e.g., in the periphery of the 3 o'clock position) since a cataract may form so quickly after lens penetration that the first fundus examination may be the only one.

X-ray films of the orbit, especially Water's view, will identify an intraorbital metallic foreign body in suspicious cases. In unquestionable cases of foreign body penetration, x-ray films should be requested with caution since the added manipulation of transportation and positioning to take an x-ray film may cause increased orbital pressure and result in the further prolapse of intraocular contents.

Management

Until the ophthalmologist arrives, the patient should be calmed and given appropriate systemic analgesics, and the eye should be lightly patched with a metal shield. *No topical ointments* should be applied since they are oil based and reactive to intraocular structures and may cause the eventual loss of an eye if applied to a penetrated globe. Prognosis is generally guarded because of the high risk of endophthalmitis, hemorrhage, and detached retina, although with the use of modern microscopic instrumentation for intraocular surgery, many patients who were previously considered to have little hope of retaining vision have had adequate visual acuity returned.

CHEMICAL TRAUMA

Because of the ubiquitous appearance of toxins in our environment, chemical burns to the eye may occur in the household or in an industrial setting and in people of any age, sex, or race. *The emergency care administered during the first few minutes is worth more than the treatment during the first few years.*

Chemical burns represent the most dangerous cases in ophthalmology, and their entire course may be determined by the emergency physician. Treatment should be immediate and is the same for all types of chemical trauma—in a word, *irrigation.*

At the time that treatment is being initiated, the history can be obtained and should include pertinent questions such as the following:

What was the nature of the substance?
(acid, alkali, dry, liquid form)
Was there prior treatment?
How soon after the injury?
For how long?

Alkaline Burns

Alkaline burns represent the most serious eye emergencies. The degree of damage is determined by the strength of the alkalinity and the time between injury and irrigation. The most common alkaline burns are from lye (NaOH or KOH), lime (CaO), and ammonia (NH_4OH). A pH hydron paper can be used to determine initial alkalinity and can later confirm neutrality. Of importance is whether the chemical was splashed into the eye or propelled from guns, cartridges, or grenades at close range.

Diagnosis
Examination of an eye recently burned by a chemical may reveal surprisingly few positive signs, but this should not deter initiation of complete treatment.

In severe cases, blanching of the conjunctiva and corneal opacities are present before irrigation.

Management and Prognosis
The hydroxyl radical rapidly infiltrates all layers of the cornea and may appear in the aqueous fluid within 1 minute after injury. It is therefore essential to dilute the alkali with large volumes of *available fluid.* Water *from any source* that can be directed onto the exposed eye should be immediately and copiously used for at least 1 hour. Although the patient's eyelids may be opened manually for instillation of anesthetic drops and initial lavage, a speculum or lid retractor is necessary for long-term irrigation.

Lids and conjunctiva should be examined quickly and carefully for alkaline particles that adhere to the lash margins and mucosal surfaces. A wet cotton-tip swab is used to sweep fornices and dislodge these particles with surrounding blebs. The pH within these blebs will cause further corneal damage if the bleb is not ruptured and the particle removed.

Treatment should be 2,000 ml of normal saline or irrigating fluid for at least 1 hour. This may be performed or started by the physician and may be continued by an experienced nurse.

The order of treatment should be as follows:

1. Instillation of anesthetic drops into each eye (avoid repeated use).
2. Sweep of the undersurface of each lid with a wet cotton-tipped applicator with removal of all easily dislodged particles.
3. Retraction of lids with a speculum.
4. Irrigation for 1 hour with the tip of the tubing directly over the cornea.
5. Evert upper and lower lids, rupture blebs, and remove remaining particles—test fluid within bleb with pH paper to confirm neutrality.
6. Continue irrigation until resumption of neutrality.

The disastrous effect of alkaline burns usually makes the prognosis very poor. The speed and length of treatment become critical determinants of the patient's final vision.

Prognosis is improved if irrigation is performed at the accident site and continued for at least one-half hour. When advising treatment over the phone, care should be taken to require that the patient open his or her eyes during irrigation.

Late corneal transplantation, necessary for badly scarred corneas, is hazardous because of highly vascular host tissue.

Acid Burns

Acid burns, although considered as devastating by the patient, are usually less severe than alkaline burns. A coagulum of precipitated protein prevents the acid radical from infiltrating beyond the first few corneal layers. Exceptions to this relatively benign course are strong acids such as hydrofluoric acid, which inflict far more serious corneal damage.

Diagnosis
As with alkaline burns, the patient is often well aware of the particular substance that caused the injury. An exploding automotive battery is a frequent occurrence and may result in an ocular penetrating wound as well as an acid burn.

On examination, the lids and conjunctiva are edematous and erythematous, often with copious tearing. In more severe cases, the cornea will lose its transparency due to surface necrosis. Removing the opaque epithelium with a cotton-tipped swab reveals an underlying clear cornea.

Management
Hydron paper again is helpful—first, in establishing the acidity and, later, following treatment, in confirming neutrality. Irrigation should be performed as in the treatment of

alkaline burns, but the consequences of an acid burn are far less damaging. The order and process of treatment should be similar to that listed previously. Corneal epithelium may become edematous and slough, causing delayed corneal healing. In most cases, after irrigation the eye may be given antibiotic drops, dilated with homatropine, 2 percent, and may be firmly patched with two eye pads. Analgesics and sleeping pills will be necessary to assist patients through the night if they are to be sent home and seen by an ophthalmologist on another day.

Other Toxic Substances

Other toxins of unknown substance can cause irritation to the surface of the eye and, even if not alkaline, can cause severe damage if propelled into the eye.

Diagnosis

Tear gas discharge from an exploding device at close range causes an infiltration of toxin into deeper corneal layers, producing damage as severe as that of an alkaline material. Since particulate matter often accompanies propelled substances, consideration should be given to the possibility of ocular perforation. Examination of the globe should be performed as described under sharp trauma.

"Crazy" glue will often adhere to lids and lashes that are dry but very rarely causes damage to the "wet" corneal surface.

Aerosol sprayed toxins such as mace, deodorants, and hair sprays are usually nonalkaline and cause only localized corneal and conjunctival epithelial damage.

Ultraviolet burns from a welder's torch or sunlamp are familiar to most primary care practitioners. The appearance of these unfortunate patients tearing profusely while being led to the examining room by a friend is all too familiar. After 1 drop of anesthetic, however, they are usually relieved to a point where visual acuity and a complete eye examination can be performed without discomfort.

In all of these cases, visual acuity of the affected eye is often slightly reduced. Periorbital and conjunctival edema varies, as do corneal surface changes. Fluorescein staining is often the only way to appreciate minute erosions of the cornea. The remaining examination is usually normal.

Management and Prognosis

Eyes that have been contacted by a toxin should be managed by irrigation similarly to the treatment mentioned earlier for alkaline burns. Eyelid eversion and sweep with a cotton-tipped applicator is necessary to remove concealed particles. Touching the affected tissue with pH paper is helpful to confirm the acid–base balance and postlavage neutrality. These results should be noted on the patient's chart.

Lids or lashes that are glued together should be treated conservatively with warm soaks. Unnecessary damage can be done by attempting to remove crusted glue, which will dislodge spontaneously within 3 to 5 days.

In cases in which a toxin was propelled into the eye, an ophthalmologist should be consulted and asked to take over the care of the patient after emergency treatment. Those patients with severely injured eyes often require admission to the hospital for medical or surgical care.

Ultraviolet burns to the cornea are managed differently since irrigation and lid eversion are unnecessary and counterproductive. In these cases and others with extreme photophobia, dilation should be performed with homatropine, 2 percent, to prevent intraocular inflammation. Patients should be warned that blurred vision and dilated pupils will persist for a few days.

In milder cases of chemical or ultraviolet burns, ophthalmic antibiotic ointment and eye patching provide sufficient treatment. Two eye patches should be applied to the affected eye; the first patch should be folded to conform to the ocular recess. By this method, a pressure dressing will be created that will allow a greater degree of comfort.

As with other corneal surface injuries, patients may require analgesics and sleeping capsules to assist them through the acute stages of their illness.

Prognosis in all but propelled toxins is good. The pain produced is often disproportionate to the long-term effect. People so affected should be reassured that within a few days their vision and pain should be vastly improved. If progressive improvement is not achieved within a few days, patients should be advised to seek follow-up care from an ophthalmologist.

SELECTED READING

Baylis, H et al. Repair of the lacerated canaliculus. *Ophthalmology* 85:1271, 1978.

Bettman, J. Medical Problems Associated with Litigation. In *Ophthalmology the Art, the Law and a Bit of Science.* New York: Aesculapius, 1977.

Bettman, J. Medicolegal aspects of ophthalmology. *Int Clin Ophthalmol* 20:137, 1980.

Brown, S, Tragakis, M, and Pearce, D. Treatment of the alkali-burned cornea. *Am J Ophthalmol* 74:316, 1972.

Duke-Elder, RNO. *System of Ophthalmology.* St. Louis: Mosby, 1972.

Gambos, G. *Handbook of Ophthalmologic Emergencies.* Garden City, NY: Medical Examination Publishing, 1973.

Grove, A. Orbital trauma and computed tomography. *Ophthalmology* 87:403, 1980.

Irvine, RA. Old and new techniques combined in the management of intraocular foreign bodies. *Ann Ophthalmol* 13:27, 1981.

Laigson, P, Oconor, J (trans). Explosive tear gas injuries to the eye. *Am Acad Ophthalmol Otolaryngology* 74:811, 1970.

Minatoya, H. Eye injuries from exploding car batteries. *Arch Ophthalmol* 96:477, 1978.

Paton, D, and Emery J. Injuries of the Eyelids and the Orbit. In W Ballinger, R Rutherford, and G Zuidema (eds), *The Management of Trauma* (2nd ed). Philadelphia: Saunders, 1973.

Paton, D, and Goldberg, M. *Management of Ocular Injuries.* Philadelphia: Saunders, 1976.

Pico, G, and Boyd, B. Lacrimal Pathway Trauma. In *Highlights of Ophthalmology* (25th ed). Panama City: Arcata, 1981.

Putterman, A, et al. Nonsurgical management of blowout fractures of the orbital floor. *Am J Ophthalmol* 77:232, 1974.

Runyan, TE. *Concussive and Penetrating Injuries of the Globe and Optic Nerve.* St. Louis: Mosby, 1975.

Ryan, S, and Boyd, B. Management of Trauma. In *Highlights of Ophthalmology* (25th ed). Panama City: Arcata, 1981.

Stasior, OG, and Sorsby, A (eds). Blowout Fractures. In *Modern Ophthalmology.* London: Butterworth, 1974.

Vinger, P. Ocular sports injuries. *Int Ophthalmol Clin* 21:21, 1981.

Wergeland, L, and Brenner, E. Solar retinopathy and foveomacular retinitis. *Ann Ophthalmol* 12:5, 1973.

Wilson, F. Traumatic hyphema pathogenesis and management. *Ophthalmology* 87:910, 1980.

59. Neck Injuries

Charles J. McCabe
J. Dugan Mahoney
Alasdair K. T. Conn

The list of vital contents in the neck is impressive and consistent with the significant morbidity and mortality that can result from trauma in this anatomic region. The emergency department physician is well aware and cautious of cervical spine trauma, but injury to the other structures are more common and require equal attention. Both blunt and penetrating forces may result in trauma to all the structures listed in Table 59-1. The mechanism of injury is environmentally and ethnically dependent.

The injuries that most emergency department physicians are familiar with are those that result from penetrating forces (SW—stab wound, GSW—gunshot wound, and SGW—shotgun wound). However, more and more trauma is being seen that results from blunt forces—for example, strangulation, hanging, motor vehicle accidents, and altercations. Both varieties can present subtly and then rapidly result in death because of the vital structures involved. In this chapter, the discussion will be divided into penetrating injuries to each of the three "zones of the neck" (Fig. 59-1) and to blunt trauma. Prehospital care, evaluation and management in the emergency department, and the final disposition of the patient will be discussed.

PREHOSPITAL CARE

The care of the patient with neck trauma *must* begin in the field with protection of the airway, control of external hemorrhage, and immobilization of the cervical spine to prevent flexion and extension. The latter is particularly true in patients with blunt trauma or gunshot wounds; the incidence of cervical spine fractures in patients with stab wounds is considered to be low, but immobilization should still be provided to unconscious or obtunded patients or those with a neurologic deficit. The emergency medical technician (EMT) or paramedic must perform proper examination for sensation and motion and document the initial neurologic status. All patients are assumed to have a cervical spine injury until it has been proved otherwise if the mechanism of injury is appropriate. Neck immobilization is probably best provided by taping the head across the forehead to a shortboard with sandbags or some restraining device on each side of the neck. A rigid collar will add some additional immobilization. (Commercial products are available that provide similar neck stabilization.)

One of the major dilemmas in prehospital care is the provision of a patent airway in a patient with suspected or documented spinal trauma. In this situation, hyperextension, flexion, and rotation of the neck must be avoided. The patient should be positioned so as to prevent airway obstruction from secretions or blood. Suctioning may be frequently

Table 59-1. Structures in the neck

Musculoskeletal	
Cervical spine	Platysma muscle
Hyoid bone	Sternohyoid muscle
Sternocleidomastoid muscle	Sternothyroid muscle
Scalene muscles	Omohyoid muscle
Digestive	
Pharynx	
Esophagus	
Respiratory	
Trachea	
Larynx	
Nervous	
Brachial plexus	
Spinal cord	
Phrenic nerve	
Vagus nerve/sympathetic ganglia	
Recurrent laryngeal nerves	
Hypoglossal nerve	
Vascular	
Carotid, Vertebral, Innominate	Arteries and branches
Internal, External	Jugular veins and branches
Glandular	
Thyroid	
Parathyroid	

necessary, and oxygen should be administered by face mask or bag valve mask. Patients with airway compromise require more aggressive airway management. Endotracheal intubation without neck movement is possible with a nasotracheal approach in the breathing patient. Oral intubation is possible as long as in-line manual immobilization is maintained to prevent flexion and extension. Special attention must be given to patients with blunt neck trauma since laryngeal fracture, elevation of a mucosal flap, or partial or complete transection of the airway may have occurred. Nasal and oral intubation can be impossible or may complete a partial transection leading to total airway obstruction.

External hemorrhage is controlled by digital pressure, which is usually sufficient. Obviously, universal precautions with gloves, masks, and goggles are recommended whenever body fluids or blood is potentially handled. The goal in the prehospital environment is to provide the absolutely necessary care and to be in transport within "the golden 10 minutes." Any delays that might be precipitated by potentially unnecessary and unhelpful procedures should be avoided. The emergency physician providing on-line or off-line medical control must impress upon the ambulance team that rapid transport is essential!

Fig. 59-1. Zones of the neck.

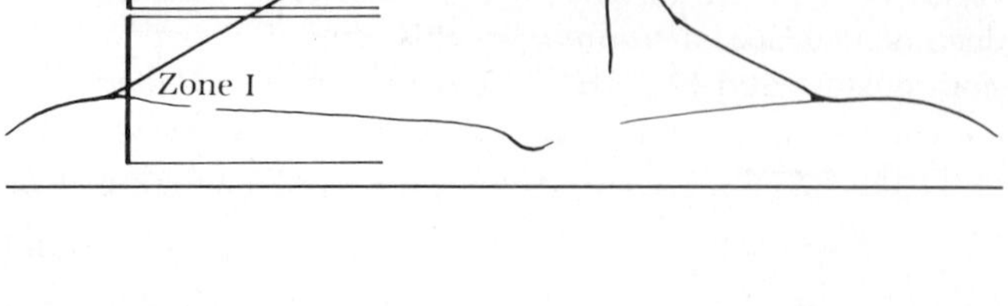

EMERGENCY DEPARTMENT CARE AND EVALUATION

The principles of emergency department management have been very well standardized and include the primary survey, resuscitation, secondary survey, and definitive care. It is important that the emergency department physician not overlook associated injuries while concentrating specifically on those of the neck. Blunt and penetrating trauma to the neck can result in injuries that may be life-threatening, causing laryngeal fractures, tracheal disruptions, or neck hematomas with acute airway occlusion and respiratory compromise. Carotid artery lacerations may result in a large pulsatile cervical hematoma causing airway compression or external exsanguination if the injury is open. Hemic drowning from hemorrhage into the oropharynx or trachea can occur secondary to lacerated vessels, strap muscles, or the thyroid gland.

Rule: Maintain the airway

Proper airway management is essential. If necessary and technically possible, nasal or oral endotracheal intubation should be performed. Cervical spine injury should be suspected, and immobilization of the neck is essential in gunshot wounds and blunt trauma. The larynx and trachea may have been damaged, and blind or laryngoscopically guided intubation may disrupt the already tenuous airway; alternative techniques of airway management should be considered, including intubation using the fiberoptic laryngoscope, needle or surgical cricothyrotomy, or formal tracheostomy below the injury. The emergency physician must recognize that with an expanding or pulsatile hematoma, placing an incision in the neck runs the risk of exsanguinating hemorrhage. The needle cricothyrotomy has demonstrated effectiveness but unfortunately is not frequently used. It should probably be the first alternative to endotracheal intubation. The technique is easily performed by inserting a 12- to 14-gauge catheter over a needle, through the cricothyroid membrane or into the trachea below the injury. The catheter is then directed caudally. During insertion, air should be freely aspirated once the tracheal lumen has been entered. The needle is then removed, and the catheter is connected to oxygen extension tubing and oxygen at flush and under 50 PSI of pressure. Oxygen is then insufflated for 1 second, and 4 seconds is allowed for exhalation. The fully inflated lung will provide its own force of exhalation by the normal elastic recoil of the lung, and the partially occluded trachea will provide the lumen. This technique is satisfactory for approximately 45 minutes. CO_2 retention with respiratory acidosis will occur if used for longer time periods. The catheter *does not* provide a large enough lumen for exhalation.

As a result, if the trachea is totally occluded, the lungs will be overinflated, resulting in parenchymal rupture and tension pneumothorax.

In penetrating trauma, there is a low incidence of spinal cord injuries with stab wounds, and an oral endotracheal intubation is usually quite safe. Gunshot wounds to the neck, on the other hand, cause spinal cord trauma in 10 to 15 percent of cases. Spinal precautions should be used.

Intravenous lines are inserted into the antecubital veins. If there is any suspicion of an interruption of the superior vena cava or subclavian veins, lower extremity sites should be chosen. Antibiotics covering gram-positive organisms and a tetanus toxoid should be administered. A chest x-ray and cervical spine films are obtained with special attention for air in the neck or mediastinum.

It is rare for isolated neck injuries to cause hypotension unless major external hemorrhage has resulted or if injuries to the spinal cord have occurred. External hemorrhage from the carotid artery may be significant and quickly lethal and is best controlled with digital pressure; clamping of the bleeding site is ill-advised. Major venous injuries must be occluded to prevent air emboli. Hypotension and tachycardia are consistent with hemorrhage, whereas spinal cord injuries will result in hypotension with a normal heart rate with motor paralysis and sensory deficit.

TYPES OF INJURIES

Rule: Look for a reason to explore the neck

Once the emergency evaluation and stabilization have been completed, attention should be focused on defining the injury. Injuries to the neck should be divided into two categories: penetrating and blunt. Penetrating injuries should be subdivided into stab wounds and gunshot wounds. The goal of the emergency department physician after controlling or ruling out life-threatening injuries is to determine whether significant injury to the esophagus, trachea, spinal cord, and cervical blood vessels has occurred (aerodigestive or neurovascular systems). In penetrating trauma, carotid artery and jugular venous injuries account for 4 to 6 percent of the reported cases, larynx/tracheal for 4 percent, and the pharynx/esophagus for 5 to 7 percent. Spinal cord trauma has been reported to occur in 12 to 15 percent of gunshot wounds to the neck and rarely secondary to stab wounds. The exact incidence of similar injuries secondary to blunt trauma is unknown.

Penetrating Injuries

Rule: Do not probe penetrating injuries of the neck

For diagnostic and therapeutic reasons, the neck is divided into three zones (see Fig. 59-1). The approach to the patient with penetrating injuries to these three zones is controversial and will vary depending on not only the anatomy of the injury and the weapon but also the protocol established by the emergency department physician and the consulting surgeon. The long-held dictum that any wound that penetrates the platysma should undergo formal neck exploration has recently been challenged.

It is essential to abide by *one* rule in handling penetrating wounds to the neck: They should *not* be probed in the emergency department. This maneuver can dislodge fresh clot and result in significant hemorrhage. Gentle and superficial examination of the wound can usually determine whether the platysma has been penetrated. Some clinicians argue that there is no benefit to wound examination since it will be the clinical evaluation of the patient, not the depth of the wound, that determines whether formal neck exploration is necessary.

The emergency department physician and consulting surgeon must develop a protocol as to the management of knife injuries. In some situations, the patient will need immediate surgery or evaluation in the operating room. Most clinicians would agree that a pulsatile or expanding hematoma, external hemorrhage, subcutaneous air, hematemesis, or hemoptysis require surgical exploration of the neck.

If the patient is hemodynamically stable without obvious signs of injury, the emergency department physician and surgeon have three options (Fig. 59-2). The first is to admit the patient to the surgical floor for clinical observation. Close observation for the development of neck pain, subcutaneous emphysema, pain on swallowing, or other clinical evidence of significant injury would indicate the need for surgical exploration. The second option is the "nonsurgical exploration" of the patient. This would include Gastrografin swallow, arteriography, and endoscopy of the trachea and esophagus (Table 59-2). The last option, and one that was originally held, is to explore all wounds of the neck that penetrate the platysma. The surgeon and the emergency department physician must decide which of the three options is to be selected in the stable patient without clear-cut indications for exploration. Different situations probably require different modes of management.

The fear in the nonoperative management of stab wounds of the neck is that a delay in diagnosing significant injury will occur. This is particularly important with injuries to the esophagus. The esophagus and mediastinum are in the same fascial plane, and an unrecognized perforation of the cervical esophagus will allow contamination of the mediastinum and mediastinitis. Routine exploration of all neck penetrating injuries permits the surgeon to examine the esophagus, trachea, and carotid sheath and its contents. Repair of any injured structure and drainage of the neck is possible early. The proponents of expectant management point out that most of the mandatory neck explorations are not therapeutic (50–60%) and result in longer hospital stays and higher medical costs and subject the patient to the potential risks of general anesthesia and surgery. At surgery, the injury may still remain occult (4%) (Obeid et al). These proponents believe that patients requiring exploration will identify themselves early, and no increase in morbidity will result from the delay.

The middle course of evaluation (see Table 59-2) carries with it the risks of endoscopy, general anesthesia, and angiography; also to be considered is the chance of false-negative results, particularly with esophageal studies.

Rule: Patients with unstable zone I injuries should be managed in a level I trauma center

The diagnostic and therapeutic options are considerably influenced by the location and mechanism of the injury (see

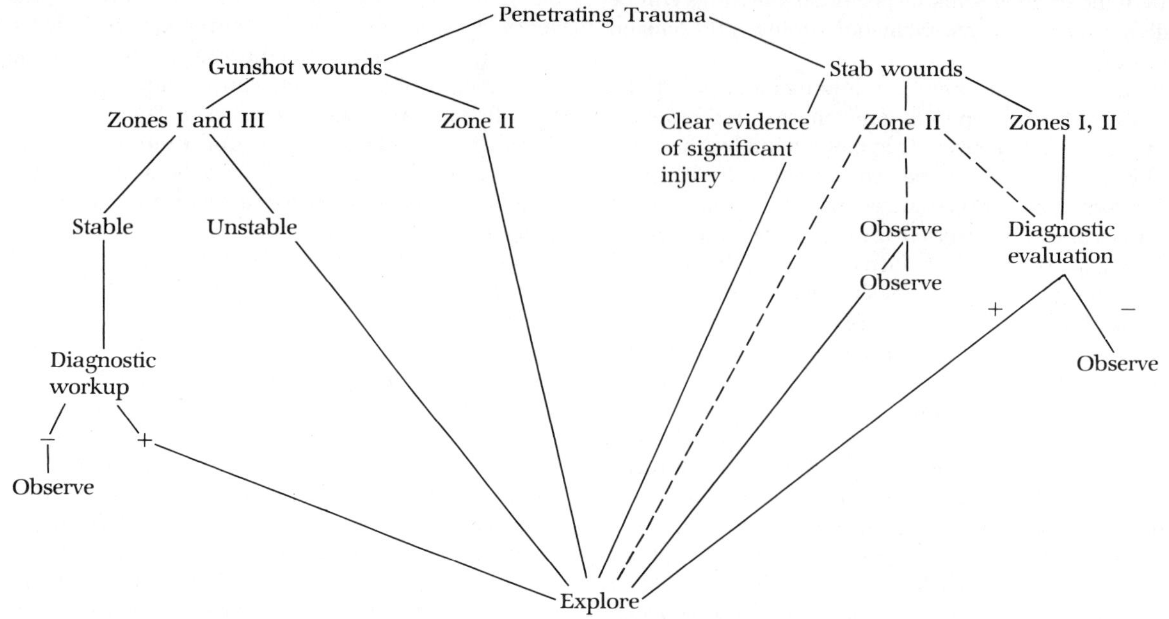

Fig. 59-2. Suggested management of penetrating injuries.

Table 59-2. Nonsurgical exploration

Gastrografin barium swallow
Esophagoscopy
Laryngosopy
Bronchoscopy
Angiography
Computed tomography

Fig. 59-2). Zone I and III injuries are very difficult to explore surgically and thus are best evaluated by the diagnostic methods mentioned. Angiography is essential in the *stable* patient. An unstable patient with a penetrating wound of zone I has likely suffered an injury to a blood vessel in the thoracic outlet (innominate or carotid) and may have significant intrathoracic hemorrhage. Resuscitation, chest x-ray, chest tube insertion, and autotransfusion may be necessary with a rapid transfer to the operating room. These patients are often unstable before arrival in the emergency department, and, when facilities do not permit immediate chest exploration, the injuries are usually lethal. Stable patients with zone I injuries may have tamponaded the hemorrhage by formation of a false aneurysm or an arteriovenous fistula. Probing of these wounds may disrupt this tamponade and lead to exsanguinating hemorrhage. An arteriogram will demonstrate these injuries and permit planned emergency surgical repair.

In a similar fashion, zone III injuries are very difficult to expose surgically. As a result, nonsurgical exploration as described is ideally used to evaluate these injuries. Clinical observation may also be satisfactory. If an arterial injury of this area is identified, it may be controlled and managed by proximal ligation or balloon occlusion. Some unique surgical procedures may allow exposure of these injuries and repair.

The appropriate management of zone II penetrating injuries probably remains the most controversial. Many studies have demonstrated that exploration and appropriate intervention can be easily and safely performed. The alternative "selective management" with the use of diagnostic studies and operation when positive has also proved successful. Both options are probably appropriate depending on the situation and clinical setting.

Gastrografin studies and endoscopy are used to identify or rule out esophageal injuries (Fig. 59-3). It is again important to recognize that false-negative results do occur predominantly with injuries to the proximal esophagus (approximately 10–20% with Gastrografin, and can be as high as 50% with endoscopy). If an injury is identified, neck exploration and attempted repair of the esophagus is required. Ideally, esophageal repair should be performed in 6 to 8 hours from the injury. Injuries to the trachea are usually obvious with the presence of subcutaneous air and blood bubbling from the open neck injury. Bronchoscopy will confirm the injury.

Rule: Explore all zone II gunshot wounds

Gunshot wounds can be evaluated nonsurgically in the same way as knife wounds but are probably best managed by neck exploration. The zone of injury around the bullet track will depend on the velocity of the bullet and type of gun but can cause much more damage than is initially apparent. Stable zone I and III injuries should be managed similarly to knife wounds, but high-velocity zone II injuries should all probably be routinely explored after noninvasive studies. A neck x-ray will be of benefit to define the path of the bullet (Fig. 59-4).

Nonpenetrating Trauma

Nonpenetrating trauma may result from altercations, impalement against the dashboard or steering wheel in a motor

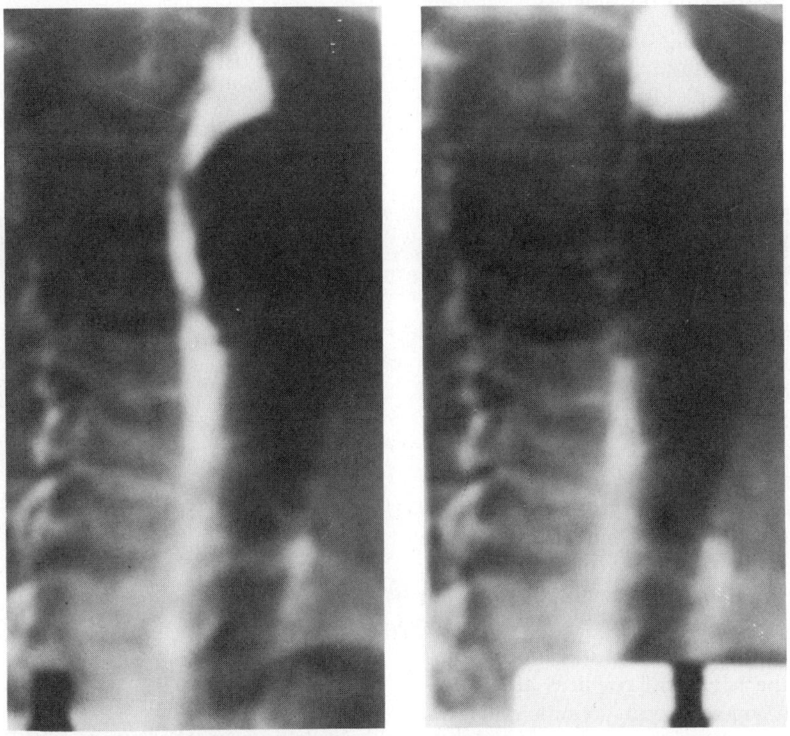

Fig. 59-3. Gastrografin swallow reveals extravasation from the proximal esophagus; the patient suffered a gunshot wound to zone I.

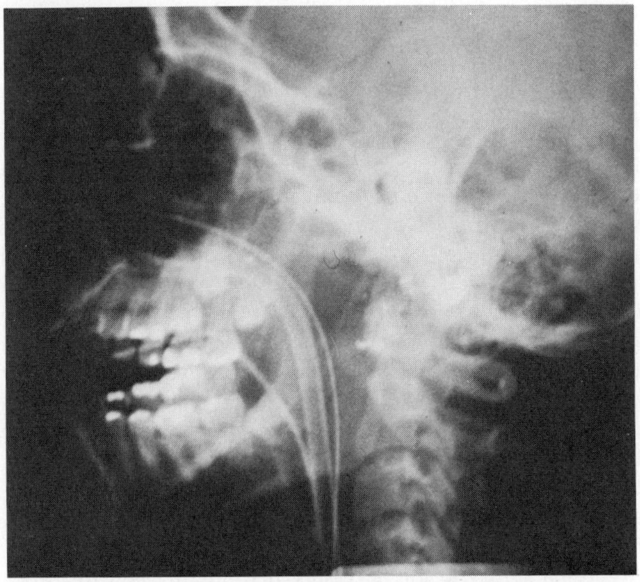

Fig. 59-4. Lateral cervical spine film reveals destruction of C1 and multiple bullet fragments after a gunshot wound to the neck.

vehicle accident, by hyperextension injuries of the neck, or from hanging or strangulation. Blunt laryngotracheal injuries are infrequent owing to the mobility and compressibility of the trachea. Motor vehicle accidents are probably responsible for the majority of those seen. The forehead of the unrestrained motorist strikes the windshield causing neck hyperextension. The injury results when the neck directly impacts the steering wheel or dashboard. Rupture of the trachea may also occur from forced exhalation against a closed glottis. A unique pathophysiology is the bicycle or snowmobile operator who drives into a clothesline or cable, which strikes him or her across the trachea. These injuries may present subtly, and the patient may be quite stable complaining of only neck pain and perhaps aphonia and hoarseness. This benign presentation clouds the underlying tracheal, esophageal, and recurrent laryngeal nerve transections. A thorough physical examination and evaluation is essential. Cervical contusions, ecchymosis, subcutaneous emphysema, and respiratory distress should signal tracheolaryngeal trauma. Initial evaluation should not relegate these patients to the stable area of the emergency department or to x-ray as the airway, although not apparent, may be in acute jeopardy.

Blunt injuries can include laryngeal fracture (physical examination will reveal absence of the Adam's apple), separation of the trachea and the larynx at the cricothyroid membrane, esophageal laceration, and tearing of the recurrent laryngeal nerve. All these injuries result in a very tenuous airway and one that can be compromised at any time. If time permits, separation of the larynx and trachea may be implied by elevation of the hyoid bone on lateral cervical spine film. Stable patients might be best evaluated by an ear, nose, and throat specialist. A laryngeal computed tomography (CT) will be helpful. The airway is often maintained solely by the soft tissue surrounding the trachea, and attempts at intubation are unsuccessful if the trachea is completely separated. In this situation, intubation using the fiberoptic endoscope is possible, or an acute surgical tracheostomy might be necessary. Attempts at cricothyrotomy will identify the transection.

Rule: Auscultate the carotid arteries

In patients without life-threatening injuries, nonsurgical evaluation is reasonable. This would include Gastrografin swallow, tracheal and esophageal endoscopy, and angiography. Auscultation over the carotid arteries is important since hyperextension injuries of the neck can result in stretching of the carotid body or the carotid artery across the transverse process of the vertebral body, resulting in the development of an intimal flap and a bruit (Fig. 59-5). If not diagnosed and repaired early, internal carotid artery and bifurcation injuries may thrombose and result in devastating long-term morbidity. Horner's syndrome is often associated with this type of injury owing to the anatomic proximity of the superior cervical ganglion and the internal carotid artery. If trauma to the carotid artery is suspected, an arteriogram is absolutely indicated. Therapy will depend on the arteriographic findings and neurologic status. The emergency physician must be aware of this potential injury in any patient with Le Fort fractures or head trauma. Neurologic sequelae usually occur at a delayed time from the accident, implying that the emergency physician has the opportunity to prevent them.

The cervical spine should be evaluated in blunt trauma and gunshot wounds to the neck and requires anteroposterior (AP), lateral, and open mouth odontoid views. (Oblique and stress views may also be necessary.) A single lateral spine film is not sufficient. ("One film is no film.") Soft tissue swelling can be identified, implying visceral injury (Figs. 59-6 and 59-7). Immobilization should be maintained until cervical spine injury has been ruled out.

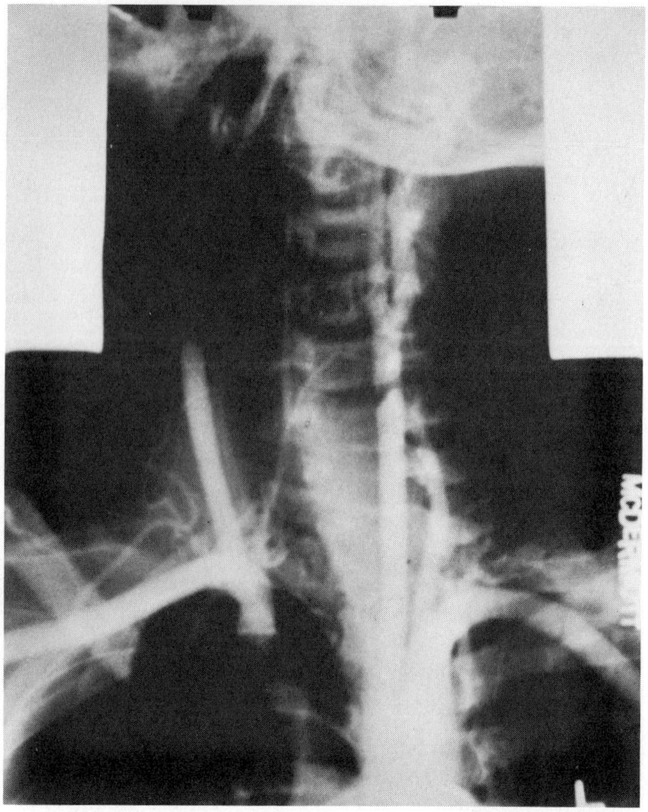

Fig. 59-5. Blunt head trauma (Le Fort III) resulting in hyperextension of the neck and a carotid artery injury. The intimal flap proximal to the bifurcation of the common carotid artery is demonstrated. The patient presented with a carotid bruit.

Nerve Injuries

Nerve injuries secondary to penetrating trauma are much more common than after blunt injuries. They often require very careful physical examination once life-threatening injuries are managed. Major injuries to the spinal cord will usually be obvious and present with motor and sensory deficits. Injury to the vagus nerve in the neck will affect the recurrent laryngeal nerve and cause vocal cord paralysis on the affected side. In the stable patient, indirect laryngoscopy will prove the deficit by demonstrating a paralyzed midposition cord on the affected side. Phrenic nerve injuries are more common following penetrating trauma than after blunt trauma and will result in a paralyzed diaphragm on the affected side. This can be recognized on chest x-ray. The hypoglossal nerve can be injured and evidenced by tongue deviation. Injury to the accessory nerve will result in trapezius muscle weakness. In blunt trauma, particularly with carotid artery injuries, the superior sympathetic ganglion may be avulsed, resulting in Horner's syndrome (ptosis, meiosis, and anhydrosis). Brachial plexus injuries can occur secondary to both blunt or penetrating trauma. Avulsion of the brachial plexus nerve roots from the spinal cord can result from traction forces applied at the shoulder and sternoclavicular joint. Separation of this joint on an AP chest x-ray is suspicious (Fig. 59-8). The physical examination of the extremity will reveal an insensate and paralyzed or paretic arm. Subclavian artery injuries are often associated with this type of trauma.

DEFINITIVE CARE

The emergency department physician will be responsible for the control of the immediate life-threatening conditions that have been described. The need for surgical intervention may be obvious, or the diagnostic studies are positive. In penetrating injuries to zone I, the emergency department physician should recognize the need to perform a left or right anterior thoracotomy in an attempt to control exsanguinating hemorrhage. These injuries obviously require operating room surgical intervention.

Injuries to the esophagus require surgical repair and drainage of the paraesophageal area. The injuries are evident by chest x-ray (air in the mediastinum), extravasation of contrast, or a positive endoscopy. Antibiotics and surgical therapy with drainage are standard. The approach is usually by an incision anterior to the sternocleidomastoid with exposure and two-layer repair. Early repair is essential. Mortality rates for injuries repaired beyond 12 hours may increase by fourfold. Injuries to the larynx require involvement of an otolaryngologist and surgical repair. The otolaryngologist, thoracic surgeon, and trauma surgeon are usually comfortable with tracheal repairs. Simple suture approximation is often all that is necessary. Injuries to the cervical vessels are managed in variable ways depending on the location of the

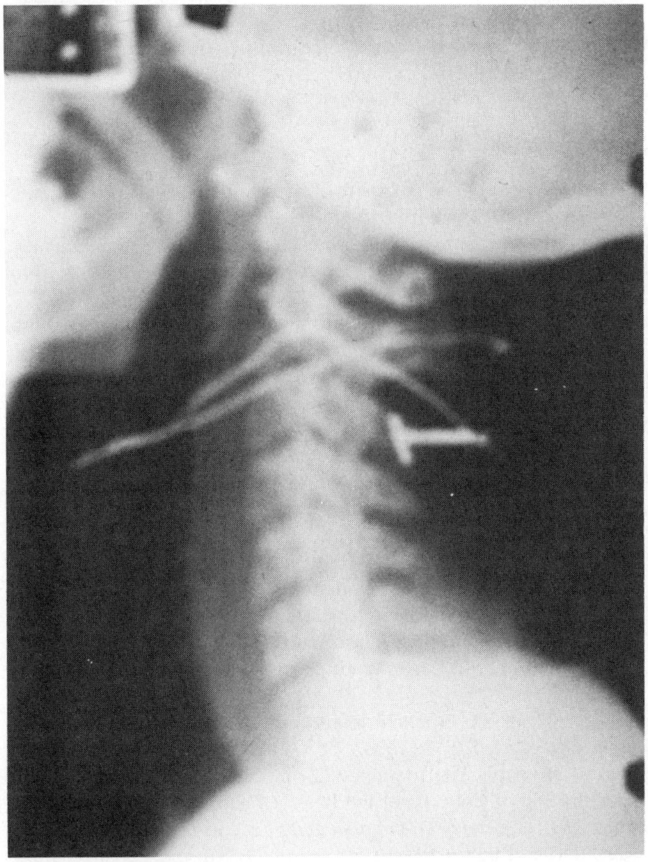

Fig. 59-6. This lateral cervical spine film reveals an increase in the prevertebral space.

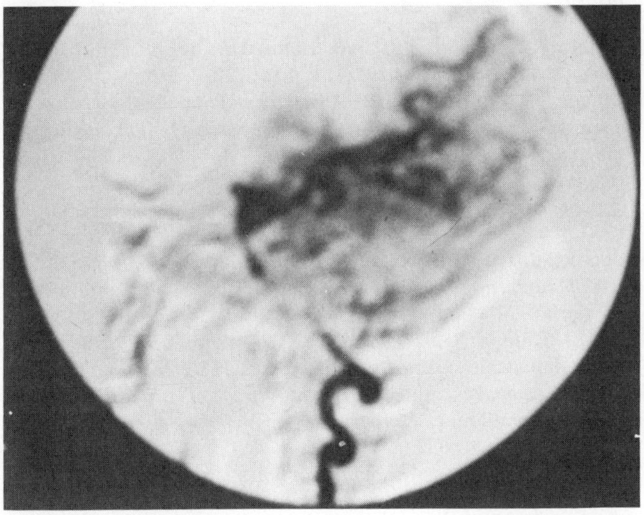

Fig. 59-7. An arteriogram demonstrating vertebral artery disruption in the same patient as in Fig. 59-6.

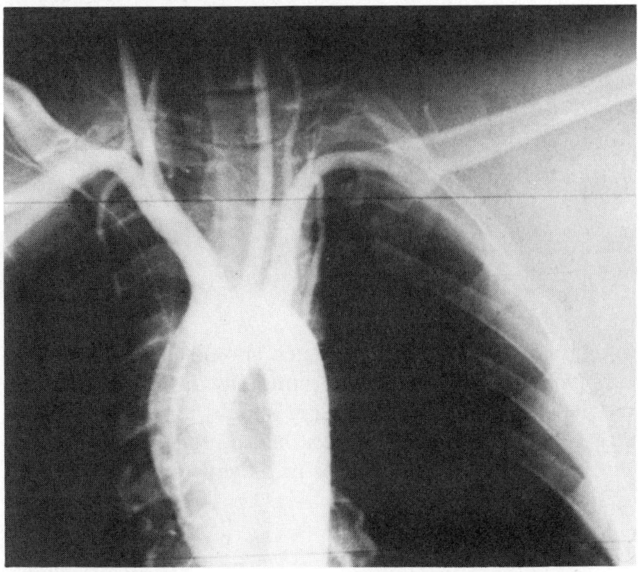

Fig. 59-8. Separation of the sternoclavicular joint in a patient with severe upper extremity traction injury. The left arm was insensate and paralyzed. The arteriogram reveals a left subclavian artery occlusion.

injury, the patency of the vessel, and the neurologic status of the patient. Surgical repair of any identified injury is ideal. Carotid artery repairs are best managed by surgeons familiar with arterial surgery. Arterial injuries have been the subject of much controversy as to whether surgical repair should be performed. If a patient presents with a carotid injury without neurologic deficit, vascular repair should be undertaken, but, if the artery requires ligation, it is anticipated that no deficit should result. In a patient with a neurologic deficit and carotid transection or occlusion, the fear has been expressed that reestablishing inflow would result in hemorrhage and potentiation of the deficit. This fear, however, is probably unfounded, and most would agree that vessel repair, if possible, should be undertaken. Vertebral artery injuries are very difficult, and the lack of exposure often makes repair impossible. As a result, proximal ligation may be necessary. Angiographic balloon occlusion has been successful. The venous injuries can usually be directly repaired by a lateral venography. Unilateral ligation of the jugular vein is well tolerated.

SKIN AND SOFT TISSUE REPAIR

The neck is in an obvious location so that cosmetic repairs of lacerations should be performed when possible. Gunshot wounds, in general, are not amenable to primary closure and normally require debridement and drainage. Since they often require exploration in the operating room, vigorous irrigation and debridement can be performed there. Knife injuries, on the other hand, will sometimes not require surgical exploration in the operating room; proper management in the emergency department is essential. Necrotic tissue should be debrided and hemostasis obtained before closing. Vigorous irrigation is important. Closure is often possible with a subcuticular layer of absorbable suture material (5-0 or 6-0). If this is neither possible nor appropriate, closure should be performed using 5-0 or 6-0 nylon. Drains, if placed, should be brought out at the inferior margin of the wound. Skin suture should be removed within 3 to 5 days, and the wound may be reinforced with Steri-Strips.

SUMMARY

An aggressive diagnostic approach should be taken toward both penetrating and blunt trauma to the neck, and the emergency department physician should approach the patients with the utmost of respect. Life-threatening difficulties may quickly expose themselves in patients who initially appear "stable."

SELECTED READING

Cervical Spine

Bachulis, BL, et al. Clinical indications for cervical spine radiographs in the traumatized patient. *Cervical Spine Radiographs and Trauma* 153:473, 1987.

Cline, JR, Scheidel, E, and Bigsby EF. A comparison of methods of cervical immobilization used in patient extrication and transport. *J Trauma* 25:649, 1985.

Dick, T, and Land, R. Spinal immobilization devices. Part 1: Cervical extrication collars. *JEMS* 1:26, 1982.

McGuire, RA, et al. Spinal instability and the log-rolling maneuver. *J Trauma* 27:525, 1987.

Podolsky, S, et al. Efficacy of cervical spine immobilization methods. *J Trauma* 23:461, 1983.

Reid, DC, Henderson, R, and Saboe, L. Etiology and clinical course of missed spine fractures. *J Trauma* 27:980, 1987.

Ross, SE, Schwab, W, and David, ET. Clearing the cervical spine: Initial radiologic evaluation. *J Trauma* 27:1055, 1987.

Carotid Artery Injuries

Brown, MF, et al. Carotid artery injuries. *Am J Surg* 144:748, 1982.

Burrows, PE, and Tubman, DE. Multiple extracranial arterial lesions following closed craniocervical trauma. *J Trauma* 21:497, 1981.

Golueke, P, et al. Vertebral artery injury: Diagnosis and management. *J Trauma* 27:856, 1987.

Karlin, RM, and Marks, C. Extracranial carotid artery injury. *Am J Surg* 146:225, 1983.

Krajewski, LP, and Hertzer, NR. Blunt carotid artery trauma. Report of two cases and review of the literature. *Ann Surg* 191:341, 1980.

LeBlanc, KA, and Benzel, EC. Trauma to the high cervical carotid artery. *J Trauma* 24:992, 1984.

Welling, RE, Kakkasseril, JS, and Peschiera, J. Pseudoaneurysm of the cervical internal carotid artery secondary to blunt trauma. *J Trauma* 25:1108, 1985.

Welling, RE, Saul, TG, and Tew, JM, Jr. Management of blunt injury to the internal carotid artery. *J Trauma* 27:1221, 1987.

Neck Injuries

Bishara, RA, et al. The necessity of mandatory exploration of penetrating Zone II neck injuries. *Surgery* 100:655, 1986.

Golueke, PJ, et al. Routine versus selective exploration of penetrating neck injuries: A randomized prospective study. *J Trauma* 24:1010, 1984.

Hermon, A, et al. Complete cricotracheal separation following blunt trauma to the neck. *J Trauma* 27:1365, 1987.

Jurkovich, GJ, et al. Penetrating neck trauma: Diagnostic studies in the asymptomatic patient. *J Trauma* 25:819, 1985.

Meyer, JP, et al. Mandatory vs selective exploration for penetrating neck trauma. *Arch Surg* 122:592, 1987.

Noyes, LD, McSwain, NE, and Markowitz, IP. Panendoscopy with arteriography versus mandatory exploration of penetrating wounds of the neck. *Ann Surg* 204:21, 1986.

Obeid, FN, Haddad, GS, and Horst, HM. A critical reappraisal of a mandatory exploration policy for penetrating wounds of the neck. *Surg Gynecol Obstet* 160:517, 1985.

Ordog, GJ. Penetrating neck trauma. *J Trauma* 27:543, 1987.

Ordog, GJ, et al. 110 bullet wounds to the neck. *J Trauma* 25:238, 1985.

Roberge, RJ, et al. Tracheal transsection following blunt trauma. *Ann Emerg Med* 1:47, 1988.

Sclafani, SJ, et al. The management of arterial injuries caused by penetration of Zone III of the neck. *J Trauma* 25:871, 1985.

Stanley, RB, Crockett, DM, and Persky, M. Knife wounds into the air spaces of the laryngeal trapezium. *J Trauma* 218:101, 1988.

Stroud, WH, and Yarbrough, DR. Penetrating neck wounds. *Am J Surg* 140:323, 1980.

Weigelt, JA, et al. Diagnosis of penetrating cervical esophageal injuries. *Am J Surg* 154:619, 1987.

Airway

Behrendt, RE, Kidwell, KG, and Rund, DA. Surgical and needle airways. *Am J Emerg Med* 2:474, 1984.

Brantigan, CO, and Grow, JB. Cricothyroidotomy: Elective use in respiratory problems requiring tracheotomy. *J Thorac Cardiovasc Surg* 71:72, 1976.

Christopher, KL, Spofford, BT, Brannin, PK, and Petty, TL. Transtracheal oxygen therapy for refractory hypoxemia. *JAMA* 256:494, 1986.

Jorden, RC, Moore, EE, Marx, JA, and Honigman, B. A comparison of PTV and endotracheal ventilation in an acute trauma model. *J Trauma* 25:978, 1985.

McGill, J, Clinton, JE, and Ruiz, E. Cricothyrotomy in the emergency department. *Ann Emerg Med* 11:33, 1982.

Neff, CC, Pfister, RC, and Van Sonnenberg, E. Percutaneous transtracheal ventilation: Experimental and practical aspects. *J Trauma* 23:84, 1983.

Sise, MJ, et al. Cricothyroidotomy for long-term tracheal access. A prospective analysis of morbidity and mortality in 76 patients. *Ann Surg* 200:13, 1984.

E. Torso Injuries

60. Thoracic Injuries

J. Kenneth Koster, Jr.
John H. Sanders, Jr.
Richard M. Stromberg

GENERAL CONSIDERATIONS

Thoracic injuries are common in a busy emergency department, and many prove to be relatively minor. All thoracic injuries, however, demand a constant awareness that any injury with the potential to significantly impair cardiorespiratory function may rapidly become life threatening. Key considerations are *anticipation* and *recognition*. Anticipation requires a clear knowledge of the spectrum of possible intrathoracic injuries that might be present in a given situation. Recognition requires the ability to appreciate the clinical manifestations of serious intrathoracic pathology following trauma. Once the situation has been properly defined, relatively simple means such as endotracheal intubation, placement of a chest tube, or pericardiocentesis will often suffice to meet the immediate demands of the emergency.

INITIAL ASSESSMENT AND MANAGEMENT

In cases of major thoracic trauma, there frequently will be multiple injuries that are not necessarily isolated to the chest. First, attention should always be directed toward those conditions producing immediate compromise of cardiorespiratory function, and the initial patient evaluation must frequently be conducted in conjunction with resuscitative measures. Often, the available history is limited since the patient may be agitated or even unconscious. Learning (at the least) the nature of the injuring agent and the circumstances of the injury is useful in allowing some estimate to be made of the possible extent of the patient's injuries.

To avoid distraction by the many simultaneous activities required in instituting care of a seriously injured patient, it is exceedingly important that the physical examination be conducted in an orderly manner. *The examiner should have a mental checklist of potential injuries that may complicate a given situation and look for signs of them.* Such a discipline makes it less likely that serious injuries that may not be immediately obvious, such as an aortic transection, will not be overlooked. Great reliance must be placed on intelligent interpretation of physical signs and the chest x-ray.

ENSURING A PATENT AIRWAY

The initial step in the care of any trauma patient is to ensure a patent airway. Prolonged asphyxia from airway obstruction will rapidly produce permanent central nervous system injury, rendering other resuscitative measures useless. A rapid assessment of the adequacy of ventilation should be made by observing the patient's level of consciousness and the rate and quality of respiratory efforts, and noting stridor or other sign of difficulty. In the obtunded patient, the hypopharynx must be checked and cleared of vomitus, blood, or dislodged dentures. If the degree of obtundation is such that protective reflexes are lost, or if there is any question as to the adequacy of ventilation, *endotracheal intubation* using a cuffed tube should be performed immediately. In circumstances in which proper equipment for tracheal intubation is not immediately available, the patient's jaw should be pulled forward, and in the absence of a possible cervical spine injury, the neck should be extended to prevent the base of the tongue from obstructing the pharynx. An oropharyngeal or nasopharyngeal tube will provide a patent pharyngeal airway for bag-mask ventilation but will *not* protect against aspiration. In the unusual circumstance in which passage of an endotracheal tube is impossible because of extensive maxillofacial trauma or laryngeal disruption, a *cricothyroidotomy* will provide the most rapid and effective airway. The cricothyroid membrane, palpable as a subcutaneous indentation immediately inferior to the thyroid cartilage, can be incised with a sharp instrument, allowing placement of the tube directly into the trachea. Later, if there is concern over the potential for cricoid erosion, a standard tracheostomy may be performed electively.

With major blunt trauma, cervical spine injury must always be considered until radiographically ruled out, and the head and neck should be immobilized. In the circumstance of severe hypoxemia, the need for adequate ventilation justifies the risk of rapidly providing it, but this risk should be minimized. If an artificial airway must be established prior to x-ray clearance, stabilization of the cervical spine is best provided by an assistant's holding the head and neck in the midline. The manipulation required for orotracheal intubation poses some hazard, even with attempts at stabilization, and consideration should be given to the feasibility of blind nasotracheal intubation.

Lower airway obstruction from aspirated material, intrapulmonary bleeding, or mucoid secretions must also be considered once control of the upper airway is ensured. In severe blunt chest injuries, intrabronchial accumulations of excessive bronchial secretions and a bloody alveolar transudate rapidly compound the initial respiratory functional impairment of the edematous, contused lung parenchyma (traumatic wet lung). Vigorous catheter suction of the excessive secretions through the endotracheal tube or bronchoscopic lavage with removal of gross clot and other aspirated material is indicated. Bronchoscopy should be performed in those instances in which there is any question of major bronchial obstruction or disruption.

INTRAVENOUS ACCESS AND FLUID REPLACEMENT

When a patent airway has been ensured and any immediately obvious life-threatening condition such as a sucking chest wound (see below) or severe external bleeding has been treated, venous access should be established using large-bore catheters. This should include a central venous line for critically injured patients. In those cases with an obvious, serious intravascular volume deficit, the sheaths normally used for Swan-Ganz catheter placement may be bilaterally introduced into the subclavian veins to provide large-bore infusion sites. An alternative route for rapid volume replacement may be provided by saphenous vein cutdowns in the proximal thigh to allow passage of sterile intravenous tubing directly into the femoral veins. Lower extremity cutdowns at the ankle or groin can also be used when the extent of thoracic trauma makes the subclavian route impractical. Although Ringer's lactate and plasma fractions will suffice for initial volume resuscitation, massive volume infusions obviously also include restoration of the red cell mass. In critical situations, this may be done with O-negative blood. Uncrossmatched *type-specific blood* should be obtainable within 10 to 15 minutes after the blood bank receives a clot and can be administered to bridge the time until fully crossmatched blood is available.

PHYSICAL EXAMINATION

Once a patent airway is ensured and adequate venous access established, an orderly physical examination is performed, and an early chest film with the patient as upright as possible is obtained. This film should be made at the earliest opportunity *while the patient remains in the emergency department.* Vital signs and, particularly, any upward or downward trends should be closely observed. The examination should begin at the neck and thorax with the patient fully unclothed. The neck should be examined for tracheal deviation and fullness of the external jugular veins. A quick check of each hemithorax for breath sounds should be followed by a careful inspection of the chest wall for contusions, abrasions, symmetry, and any paradoxical motion. When penetrating trauma is involved, entrance and exit wounds should be noted. Such wounds provide a *rough* estimate of the track of the missile through the body suggesting central regions of injury. Special organ injury within these areas must be ruled out by systematic investigation, remembering that the extent of penetrating thoracic injuries can be highly unpredictable. The chest wall should be palpated for fractures, areas of instability, or subcutaneous emphysema. Hyperresonance or dullness with percussion may suggest either a large pneumothorax or collection of pleural fluid. Auscultation of the heart may demonstrate a number of important signs, including diminution of the heart sounds because of intrapericardial blood, cardiac murmurs, or the characteristic crunch of mediastinal air.

SPECIAL STUDIES

If there is suspicion of a major intrathoracic injury, early thoracic surgical consultation should be obtained. Special studies such as aortography should be undertaken only after such consultation. In any event, patients with potential major chest injuries should never be sent from the emergency department for specialized studies without being *constantly* attended by a person qualified to reliably assess any change in status.

BLUNT THORACIC TRAUMA

Most blunt chest injuries are seen in victims of automobile accidents, although some result from falls, contact sports, physical assaults, and other types of accidents.

Awareness of the potential intrathoracic injuries possible in a given situation is a large factor in the recognition of such injuries. With blunt chest injuries, both the direct force of impact and decelerative stress dictate the pattern and extent of injury. Significant pulmonary contusion, myocardial contusion, and disruptions of the great vessels, tracheobronchial tree, or diaphragm are more likely to be seen in victims of vehicular accidents that involve motorcycles, pedestrians, or high-speed automobiles. So-called simple rib fractures are not infrequently complicated by pneumothorax, hemothorax, or pulmonary contusion. The likelihood of these complications is greatly increased if the fractures of the ribs are multiple. When fractures involve the lower rib cage, blunt intra-abdominal injuries, such as lacerations of the spleen and liver, must be considered. Shock in multiple-trauma patients with blunt chest injury often originates from associated abdominal injuries. Because of the relatively protected position of the upper ribs, a fracture, particularly of the first two ribs, indicates that the chest has received very severe trauma. The possibility of serious intrathoracic injury must be seriously entertained when there are such fractures, and thoracic surgical consultation is advisable.

Chest Wall Injury

Contusions

Contusions of the chest wall, although painful, are usually not serious in themselves. When uncomplicated, chest wall contusions require only analgesics and an ice bag. However, they should alert one to the possibility of intrathoracic injury even in the absence of rib fracture. This is especially true in young people whose relatively flexible rib cages can often sustain a heavy blow without fracture.

Subcutaneous Emphysema

Subcutaneous emphysema, a condition usually not intrinsically significant, is an indication that air has dissected from some disruption of the upper or lower airway along deep fascial planes into the subcutaneous tissue. In patients with major blunt trauma, it may be a marker of bronchial injury, but, much more commonly, air enters these fascial planes from a pneumothorax associated with some disruption of the mediastinal or parietal pleura. Less frequently, air reaches the subcutaneous tissue through the mediastinum by way of retrograde dissection along the bronchial tree from a bronchopulmonary air leak without a pneumothorax. Subcutaneous air may also be a sign of an accidental tear of the hypopharynx or proximal esophagus following attempts at endoscopy or intubation. Treatment of subcutaneous emphysema is directed at identifying and controlling the source of the air leak. In most instances, this involves reexpansion of a pneumothorax with a chest tube. In the absence of identifiable pneumothorax, or a bronchial or pharyngeal injury, the condition is usually self-limiting.

RIB FRACTURES

Rib fractures are usually related to external trauma, although they are occasionally seen in osteoporotic persons following the stress of coughing. Because a considerable force is usually required to produce a rib fracture, one must be alert to the occurrence of associated injuries such as pneumothorax, hemothorax, and pulmonary contusion. The injured rib is usually quite painful, leading to splinting of the affected side and shallow respiration. Pain is intensified by breathing, coughing, or moving. There is marked point tenderness over the fracture site, and, occasionally, crepitus or grating of the fractured bone can be palpated. Rib detail x-rays may be obtained specifically to demonstrate the fracture, although certain fractures, especially those located anterolaterally, may be difficult to identify on film. In such cases, a clinical diagnosis will suffice. A standard chest film should always be taken in instances of suspected rib fracture to ensure that there is no associated intrapleural air or fluid, or pulmonary injury.

Management

In the absence of underlying injuries, the primary treatment goal of an isolated rib fracture is the relief of pain. Immobilization of the rib is not required for healing. Strapping the chest with tape or an elastic rib belt is only variably effective in pain relief and can potentially produce atelectasis by limiting chest wall excursion. Pain relief is most effective with an *intercostal nerve block* (Fig. 60-1). This is best performed by infiltrating several milliliters of a long-acting anesthetic (0.25% bupivacaine with epinephrine 1:200,000) at the inferior margin of the ribs posteriorly slightly medial to the frac-

Fig. 60-1. Intercostal nerve block. A 22-gauge needle is used to infiltrate the tissues at the inferior margin of the rib with a long-acting local anesthetic such as bupivacaine.

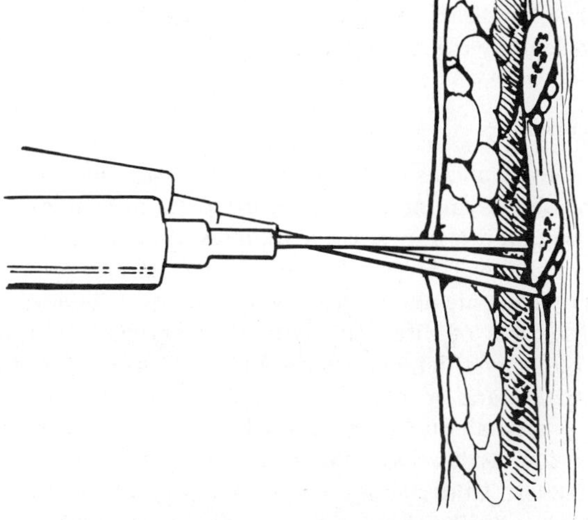

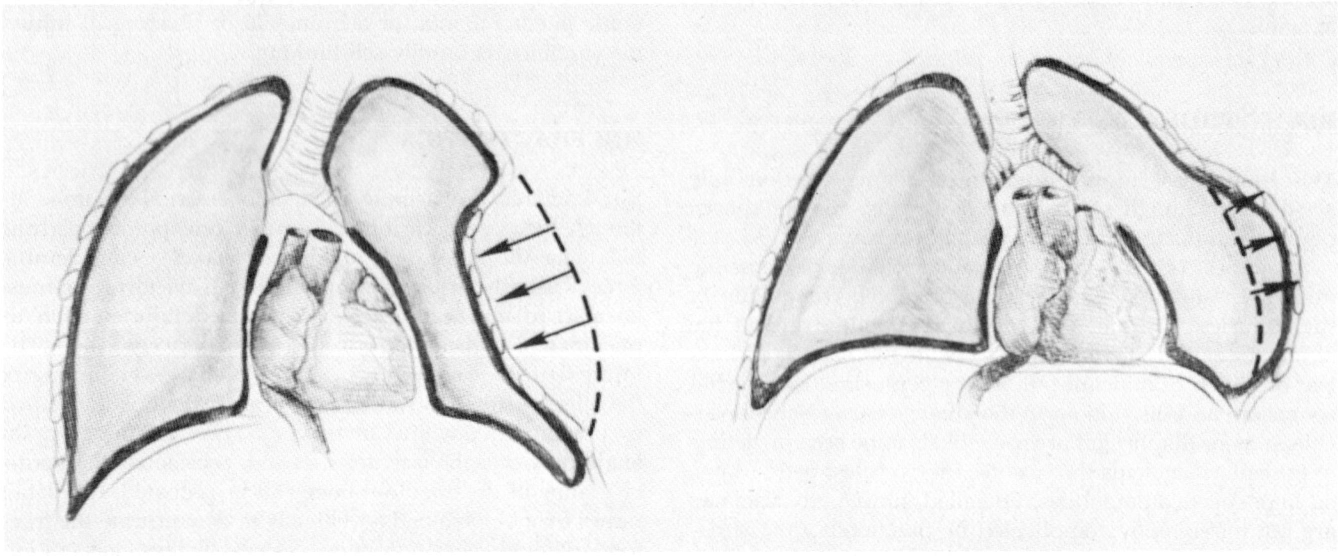

Fig. 60-2. Flail chest. Instability of a chest wall section during respiratory effort destroys the effectiveness of the thoracic bellows, thereby limiting the generation of negative intrathoracic pressure with inspiration.

ture site for two interspaces above and below. This approach has the disadvantage of lasting only hours, but it may be repeated if the pain from the fracture continues to be intolerable despite the use of oral analgesics. In the elderly, or in patients with obstructive airway disease, the pain and muscular splinting associated with rib fractures may further diminish already compromised functional lung volumes and lead to atelectasis and retention of secretions. Hospital admission for these patients may be warranted to ensure that adequate pain relief and proper pulmonary toilet are maintained.

FLAIL CHEST

Multiple rib fractures secondary to major blunt chest injury may render a significant portion of the chest wall unstable and allow it to move parodoxically inward with inspiration and outward with expiration (Fig. 60-2). Such instability, called a *flail chest,* may greatly compromise respiratory mechanics by impairing the ability of the thoracic bellows to generate negative inspiratory pressures and, thus, greatly increase the work of breathing.

Diagnosis

The chest wall instability that results from such fractures is not always immediately apparent because of muscular splinting, and it may become manifest only on repeated examinations over several hours or even days as progressive muscular fatigue allows chest wall mobility. Whenever there are fractures of three or more ribs, especially if anterior and posterior fractures are combined, instability should be anticipated and specifically sought with repeated examination. A sternal fracture of costochondral cartilaginous disruption in association with rib fractures may also produce a flail chest. Underlying pulmonary injury, particularly pulmonary contusion, frequently complicates the flail chest. Ineffective ventilation, secondary to the unstable chest wall, may, in combination with the alveolar edema of the underlying contused lung, rapidly precipitate severe respiratory insufficiency.

Management

Initial therapy is directed toward stabilization of the flail segment of the chest wall. Several approaches have been used: (1) immobilization of the unstable segment with either compression or external traction, (2) endotracheal intubation with positive pressure ventilation, or (3) surgical fixation. Endotracheal intubation and positive pressure ventilation are considered to be definitive therapy. The decision to institute mechanical ventilation should be based on objective findings of respiratory insufficiency—not on the presence of multiple rib fractures alone. When a patient with multiple rib fractures is placed on the ventilator, a chest tube should be inserted on the injured side, even in the absence of an obvious pneumothorax. In this setting, the lung can be injured by bony spicules, and a pulmonary air leak produced with positive pressure ventilation can rapidly generate a tension pneumothorax. Any decision regarding surgical fixation of the flail segment is deferred until the patient has been well stabilized and other possible significant intrathoracic injuries, such as myocardial contusion, have been considered.

STERNAL FRACTURE

Fractures of the sternum occur much less frequently than rib fractures, but they are not rare and are often diagnosed belatedly. In certain cases, they may be caused by hyperflexion, but the majority result from a direct blow to the anterior chest. Most often, they are transverse and nondisplaced. Sternal fractures represent a significant injury, because with the great force required to fracture the sternum, there is a high likelihood of associated major intrathoracic injury. The possibility of myocardial contusion, thoracic aortic tear, pulmonary contusion, and other serious injuries requires that the patient with the sternal fracture be admitted to the hospital and investigated.

Diagnosis

A nondisplaced sternal fracture is usually marked by local tenderness and possibly crepitus. Overlying ecchymosis may be absent. Pain is variable but often significant and exacerbated with efforts to breathe or move. The best radiographic demonstration of a sternal fracture is usually with a lateral chest film, although tomograms may be required.

Management

In most cases, the pain from sternal fractures can be controlled with analgesics or injections of local anesthetic agents into the fracture site. Operative reduction and fixation are necessary only if the fracture is severely displaced or unstable and is undertaken only after the treatment of other more pressing injuries.

PULMONARY CONTUSION

Pulmonary contusion frequently complicates blunt chest trauma. This often serious injury is occasionally initially overlooked in the rush of caring for a victim of multiple trauma. Although the mechanism of pulmonary contusion has not been completely elucidated, it appears that transmission of an abrupt compressive-decompressive wave across the lung parenchyma from a strong force that has distorted the chest wall will produce alveolar and interstitial edema and hemorrhage. Transudation of fluid from an ongoing pulmonary capillary leak, in combination with the reflex increase in bronchial mucous secretion, impedes local gas exchange and produces bronchiolar obstruction and atelectasis. Adverse alterations in pulmonary blood flow worsen hypoxemia. The clinical presentation depends in great part on the extent of pulmonary parenchymal injury. When the area of contusion is relatively localized, it may be manifest only by a small, patchy infiltrate on x-ray with the patient exhibiting little or no sign of respiratory functional impairment. An important point is that pulmonary contusions that initially seem to be of only moderate severity may significantly worsen in their clinical manifestations over the first few hours after injury.

Diagnosis

Patients who have lesser degrees of contusion may be asymptomatic or only slightly dyspneic and tachypneic when first examined. Scattered rales may be heard over the area of injury, and there may be coughing or mucoid or even blood-tinged material. The chest film will usually show an infiltrate that tends to be patchy, irregular, and streaky. With milder injuries, the PaO_2 is normal or only slightly depressed, whereas the $PaCO_2$ may be low because of tachypnea. With severe contusions, the degree of obvious respiratory difficulty is greater. In the worst injuries, the patient may be severely dyspneic or cyanotic and coughing frothy, bloody fluid on arrival in the emergency department. Such patients show significant arterial desaturation and, usually, metabolic acidosis. The most severe injuries are marked by an ominous elevation of the $PaCO_2$. Respiratory function frequently deteriorates during the initial period of injury. Patients who at first have signs of only mild respiratory difficulty may become desperately ill over several hours. Careful monitoring and repeated observation are necessary. Radiographic changes do not necessarily correlate well with changes in the patient's clinical status and often lag behind them. Serial blood gas determinations augmented with continuous oximetry are the only accurate measures of the severity of a pulmonary contusion and its response to treatment.

Management

It cannot be overemphasized that therapy for pulmonary contusion is most effective when begun as soon as possible after injury. Early consultation with a pulmonary specialist is advisable in suspected cases of pulmonary contusion. Good bronchial toilet should be maintained through vigorous chest physical therapy, including, if required, nasotracheal suctioning and therapeutic bronchoscopy. Intercostal nerve blocks will help alleviate chest wall pain to aid coughing and lessen the requirement of narcotic analgesia. For patients with a milder degree of contusion, supplemental oxygen should be given by mask or nasal catheter to maintain the PaO_2 at normal levels. For patients with more serious injuries, manifest by significant arterial desaturation at the time of admission (PaO_2 <70 mm Hg on nasal oxygen), there should be early institution of respiratory support through mechanical ventilation. Positive expiratory pressure should be added if the PaO_2 cannot be maintained at greater than 60 mm Hg with an FIO_2 of 0.5.

Avoiding *intravenous fluid overload* while replenishing intravascular volume deficits is of particular importance in the management of pulmonary contusion. Careful hemodynamic monitoring, including measurement of the pulmonary capillary wedge pressure, should be instituted to determine when adequate but not excessive cardiac filling pressures have been restored. The withholding of crystalloid solutions, "drying-out" the patient with diuretics, and raising the plasma oncotic pressure with blood and plasma fractions does not alter the capillary leak in the damaged lung. Although much of the care of pulmonary contusion occurs in the intensive care unit, the final outcome is heavily influenced by the events in the emergency ward—early diagnosis of the condition, early institution of measures to ensure adequate pulmonary toilet, and the principle of adequate but not excessive intravascular volume restoration.

DIAPHRAGMATIC RUPTURE

Because of the great force required to produce diaphragmatic rupture, coexistent injuries are frequent and may dominate the initial clinical picture. Most tears are in the central portion of the hemidiaphragm, with the overwhelming majority involving the left side. The right hemidiaphragm seems to be protected somewhat by the bulk of the liver. The manifestations of the diaphragmatic laceration itself depend on the size of the disruption and the degree of visceral herniation into the chest. A small tear may initially be largely unapparent only to yield in time to late herniation. Massive prolapse of abdominal viscera through a large tear may fill the chest to such an extent as to produce collapse of the lung, shift of the mediastinum, and respiratory distress.

Diagnosis

The x-ray findings with diaphragmatic rupture are usually nonspecific, and many diaphragmatic tears are first diagnosed through abdominal exploration for associated injuries. The possibility of diaphragmatic rupture is suggested by radiographic findings of an elevated or otherwise obscured contour of the hemidiaphragm, pleural fluid, and, possibly, visceral gas shadows in the lower chest. Attempted passage of a nasogastric tube may indicate upward angulation of the stomach. Contrast studies of the stomach and colon may aid the diagnosis through demonstrating superior displacement. Surgical repair is indicated.

TRACHEOBRONCHIAL INJURY

Blunt tracheobronchial injuries are not frequent, but they may present difficult management problems. The usual bronchial injury consists of an incomplete circumferential disruption of the cartilaginous portion of a mainstem bronchus, whereas the less frequent intrathoracic tracheal injuries are usually longitudinal posterior tears near the carina. Tracheobronchial injuries result from severe trauma, usually in high-speed vehicular accidents, and frequently there are other serious injuries.

Diagnosis

Several clinical presentations are possible. Hemoptysis may be caused by bronchial arterial injury, and occasionally it is severe. A complete transection of the bronchus may produce total obstruction at the point of injury with distal atelectasis. The much more commonly observed *partial* bronchial separations are usually marked by large air leaks, either into the mediastinum or into the pleural cavity. If the mediastinal pleura remains intact, air tends to dissect into the soft tissues of the chest and neck, producing subcutaneous emphysema that may reach remarkable proportions. If the airway tear freely communicates with the pleural space, the resultant pneumothorax is complicated by a continuing large air leak. This leak may be so great that closed tube thoracostomy is inadequate to fully reexpand the lung. In extreme cases, the great loss of gas volume through the disruption may make it impossible to adequately ventilate the patient. A tension pneumothorax may result if the pleura overlying the bronchial tear acts as a one-way valve permitting only an outward air leak into the pleural cavity. On occasion, the peribronchial tissue will maintain continuity of the airway despite even a complete tear of the bronchial wall, and the injury may pass undetected until healing results in late bronchial stenosis.

Management

Following closed thoracic trauma, the possibility of a tracheobronchial injury should be considered in patients who have hemoptysis, develop mediastinal and subcutaneous emphysema, or have a large or persistent air leak following evacuation of a pneumothorax with a chest tube, especially if the lung remains incompletely expanded. In such patients, bronchoscopy is indicated at some point to allow identification of any bronchial injury. The timing of this procedure, in part, depends on the extent of the patient's associated injuries and general condition. Operative repair of tears of the central bronchus is necessary and, in circumstances in which the large air leak after chest tube placement compromises ventilation, must be done as an emergency procedure.

PNEUMOTHORAX

Normally, the lung is held fully expanded against the chest wall with negative pressure within the potential space between the opposed smooth visceral and parietal pleural surfaces. Disruption of the seal between these surfaces by the entry of air into the space either from a leak from the lung (closed pneumothorax) or through a chest wall defect (open pneumothorax) will allow collapse of the lung to a variable degree.

Closed Pneumothorax

Spontaneous closed pneumothoraces are relatively common. Most occur in otherwise healthy young adults and are the result of a rupture of a small subpleural pulmonary bleb. Rupture of such blebs often appears to be unrelated to any particular exertion since many people have the onset of symptoms in the course of normal activity or when at rest.

Diagnosis

Variable sudden sharp chest pain and some degree of dyspnea usually mark the onset of a spontaneous pneumothorax. Dyspnea is related to both the extent of lung collapse and any preexisting pulmonary disease. Healthy people may experience little sense of breathlessness with total collapse of one lung, whereas others with extensive pulmonary parenchymal disease may be quite dyspneic with even a relatively small pneumothorax. Physical signs vary with the size of the pneumothorax and may be limited to only a slight diminution of breath sounds on the affected side. With larger pneumothoraces, there may be ipsilateral hyperresonance. The chest radiograph confirms the diagnosis and allows an estimate of the degree of lung collapse.

Management

In the absence of complicating factors, treatment of a patient with a closed pneumothorax can be generally individualized. An asymptomatic small pneumothorax of less than 20 to 25 percent in an otherwise healthy patient can be safely observed in most instances. A somewhat larger pneumothorax can often be managed with simple aspiration (see Procedure 19) using an Intracath with an attached three-way stopcock, placed through the second intercostal space anteriorly. The inclination to use aspiration rather than a chest tube is strengthened if the time span from the onset of symptoms along with the finding of an incompletely collapsed lung suggest that the initial air leak has sealed. If an x-ray film taken after aspiration of air from the pleural space demonstrates virtual full expansion of the lung, it is reasonable to assume that there is no further pulmonary air leak, and a reliable patient may be released and instructed to return in 24 hours for a follow-up chest film (or earlier if symptoms supervene). In those cases in which the degree of pulmonary collapse is significantly greater than 50 percent, in which aspiration has been ineffective, or in which an ongoing air leak is otherwise suspected, closed tube thoracostomy is necessary (see Procedure 20). A chest tube is also advisable when the pneumothorax results from a small pulmonary laceration incurred from thoracentesis or placement of a central venous line. In the absence of significant pleural fluid, a No. 22 French chest tube in the second intercostal space at the midclavicular line is generally satisfactory. For women, a better cosmetic result may be obtained through placement immediately posterior to the lateral margin of the pectoralis muscle and up through the third intercostal space. The chest tube is connected to an underwater seal system, and approximately 20 cm of suction is applied to facilitate lung reexpansion.

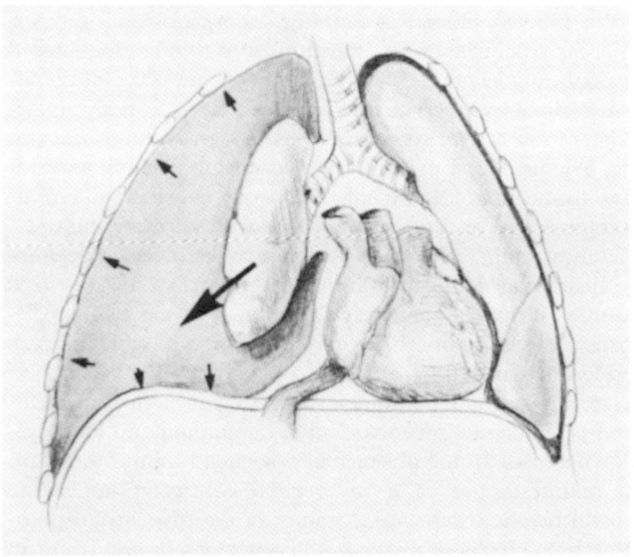

Fig. 60-3. Tension pneumothorax. Progressive one-way air leak of air into the pleural space increases the intrathoracic pressures, angulating and compressing the great veins in the mediastinum, thus hindering venous return to the heart.

Tension Pneumothorax

In certain circumstances, the tissue around an air leak from the lung will, by acting as a one-way valve, allow air to enter the pleural space during inspiration but not to escape during expiration. Such progressive accumulation of intrapleural air under pressure will produce marked collapse of the ipsilateral lung and a contralateral shift of the mediastinum, causing some compression of the contralateral lung (Fig. 60-3). As the accumulation of intrapleural air under pressure increases, systemic venous return to the heart is impeded by increasing positive intrapleural pressure and, possibly, mediastinal angulation. If this process continues unchecked, progressive hypoxemia and a falling cardiac output will lead to marked dyspnea, tachycardia, cyanosis, and vascular collapse. A tension pneumothorax may arise from rupture of a pulmonary bleb, a missile wound, or a lung laceration of virtually any size. A tension pneumothorax may complicate any condition in which there is a pulmonary air leak into the pleural space and will invariably do so when the patient is on positive pressure ventilation. Respirator patients, especially those requiring high inspiratory pressures or positive end-expiratory pressure (PEEP), are particularly at risk of developing a spontaneous tension penumothorax through rupture of a bleb, and this possibility should always be considered if there is sudden unexplained deterioration of a patient on a ventilator.

Diagnosis

Physical signs in patients with tension pneumothorax are usually more striking than those observed in patients with a simple closed pneumothorax—diminished or absent breath sounds, hyperresonance over the involved hemithorax, tracheal shift away from the affected side, and, in alert patients, some degree of dyspnea. Although an x-ray film will confirm the diagnosis, if the patient is symptomatic and a tension pneumothorax is suspected, one should proceed with decompression of the pleural space on the basis of the physical findings alone.

Management

Immediate placement of a chest tube in the second anterior interspace is indicated. In cases in which the patient is severely symptomatic, simply placing an 18-gauge needle through a high anterior interspace will convert the tension pneumothorax to a simple pneumothorax and will allow more leisurely placement of the chest tube.

BLUNT CARDIAC INJURY

Major blunt chest trauma may produce a variety of severe cardiovascular injuries either through decelerative stresses or by direct compressive forces. The spectrum of potential injury is broad, including myocardial contusion and rupture, cardiac valvular disruption, pericardial tamponade, and tears of the intrathoracic great vessels. Of these, myocardial contusion and aortic disruption are by far the most frequent. Initial physical findings may be surprisingly subtle and few, especially in view of the severity of the intrathoracic pathology. In addition, the signs may be relatively nonspecific, such as hypotension and tachycardia. An awareness of potential cardiovascular injuries in a given setting together with a careful and orderly evaluation of the patient is necessary to avoid overlooking significant lesions.

MYOCARDIAL CONTUSION

In any patient with severe blunt chest trauma, the potential for cardiac injury and, particularly, myocardial contusion, should be considered. The signs associated with myocardial contusion may be few and transient and easily overlooked in the process of caring for other more obvious injuries. Whereas fractures of the sternum or multiple ribs should particularly alert one to the possibility of myocardial contusion, serious intrapericardial injuries may exist with no evidence of chest wall bony fractures or cartilaginous disruption. The heart is most subject to contusion from an anterior blow that causes it to be either abruptly decelerated against or compressed by a posteriorly displaced sternum and anterior chest wall (steering wheel injury). However, because the heart's suspension within the pericardial sac allows it mobility, it may be forcefully driven against the spine posteriorly or sternum anteriorly in any situation in which abrupt decelerative forces are applied to the chest.

The myocardial pathologic lesion can range from scattered petechiae to intramyocardial hematoma and local cellular necrosis. In the absence of associated injury, the clinical manifestations of a myocardial contusion appear to depend on the extent and location of the myocardial damage. The majority of myocardial contusions do not result in gross functional cardiac impairment, and the outcome is good. In a few instances, necrosis is so severe as to result in delayed cardiac rupture or late aneurysm formation.

Diagnosis

Although it is possible that patients may have no cardiac symptoms, many will complain of precordial pain similar to that experienced in pericarditis or myocardial infarction. Chest wall pain from the injuring blow may obscure this discomfort. Failure of the pain to be exacerbated with palpation or movement of the anterior chest wall may be differential diagnostic clues. Most myocardial contusions seem to be of minor or no clinical significance. Clinical evidence of congestive heart failure is uncommon, although experimental studies have demonstrated that contusion can produce loss of cardiac functional reserve. The physical signs of uncomplicated contusion may be few, the most common one being sinus tachycardia. The diagnosis may be supported by electrocardiographic changes consistent with focal pericarditis or myocardial infarction. Focal changes may not be immediately present and may be delayed for up to 48 hours. In most instances, they never develop. If present, these focal changes do not tend to persist as long as those observed in typical myocardial infarction. Measurement of creatine phosphokinase–myocardial fraction (CPK-MB) seems to be an insensitive measure of myocardial contusion. Radionuclide ventriculography appears to be the most sensitive test for myocardial contusion but is not readily applicable to the typical trauma setting. Two-dimensional echocardiography seems to be the most sensitive test readily adaptable to the trauma setting, but it should be generally reserved for situations in which there is concern about cardiac functional deterioration. Prognosis for myocardial contusion is usually that of complete recovery.

Management

Because cardiac arrhythmias represent the most commonly observed complication of myocardial contusion, patients with this diagnosis should have continuous electrocardiographic monitoring during the initial period of hospitalization. Although ectopic atrial and ventricular beats are most common, virtually all arrhythmias, including heart block, ventricular tachycardia, and ventricular fibrillation, have been observed. Standard antiarrhythmic therapy is indicated. If cardiac functional compromise is apparent, pericardial tamponade should be ruled out with echocardiography and measurement of intracardial pressures with a Swan-Ganz catheter.

Nonurgent surgical procedures requiring general anesthesia should be delayed in patients with myocardial contusion during the initial weeks of myocardial healing.

OTHER BLUNT CARDIAC INJURIES

Nonpenetrating cardiac injuries other than myocardial contusion are much less common. Hemopericardium from epicardial bleeding following blunt trauma is not rare but is usually limited and only infrequently produces pericardial tamponade. Two-dimensional echocardiography is particularly useful in demonstrating intrapericardial fluid. Valvular injuries from blunt trauma are rare. Tears or detachments of the aortic valve leaflets may produce aortic insufficiency. Disruption of the papillary-chordal attachments of the atrioventricular valve may render them incompetent. Interventricular septal rupture, either acutely or following softening of a severe contusion, may produce a ventricular septal defect. Coronary arterial thrombosis is also possible with nonpenetrating trauma, although, again, it is rare.

NONPENETRATING VASCULAR INJURIES

Blunt trauma, usually resulting from vehicular accidents, may injure any of the intrathoracic great vessels. The aorta is the most frequently involved by far. Of the less commonly injured vessels, the innominate and subclavian arteries are vulnerable to avulsion or tears, particularly in their more proximal segments. Autopsy studies of victims of automobile accidents have shown that blunt aortic injuries may involve any segment, but, in the group of patients who survive to reach emergency care, the majority of aortic tears are in the proximal descending aorta immediately distal to the origin of the left subclavian artery. The typical aortic injury is a relatively sharp tear that is generally transverse or spiral. Occasionally, the injury may consist of several closely grouped tears. The frequent localization of aortic disruptions at the isthmus suggests that the mechanism of injury is related to decelerative stresses at this junction of the more mobile transverse arch and the relatively fixed descending aorta (Fig. 60-4A). Initial survival with aortic tears is permitted only when the tear is not completely transmural and the adventitia and periaortic tissue contain the hematoma for an unpredictable period. If the aortic injury is unrecognized, it is virtually certain that the resulting false aneurysm will progress to rupture, producing exsanguination during the first few days or weeks after the accident.

Diagnosis

The clinical presentation of blunt aortic injuries is varied. Frequently, there are coexisting severe injuries in other areas

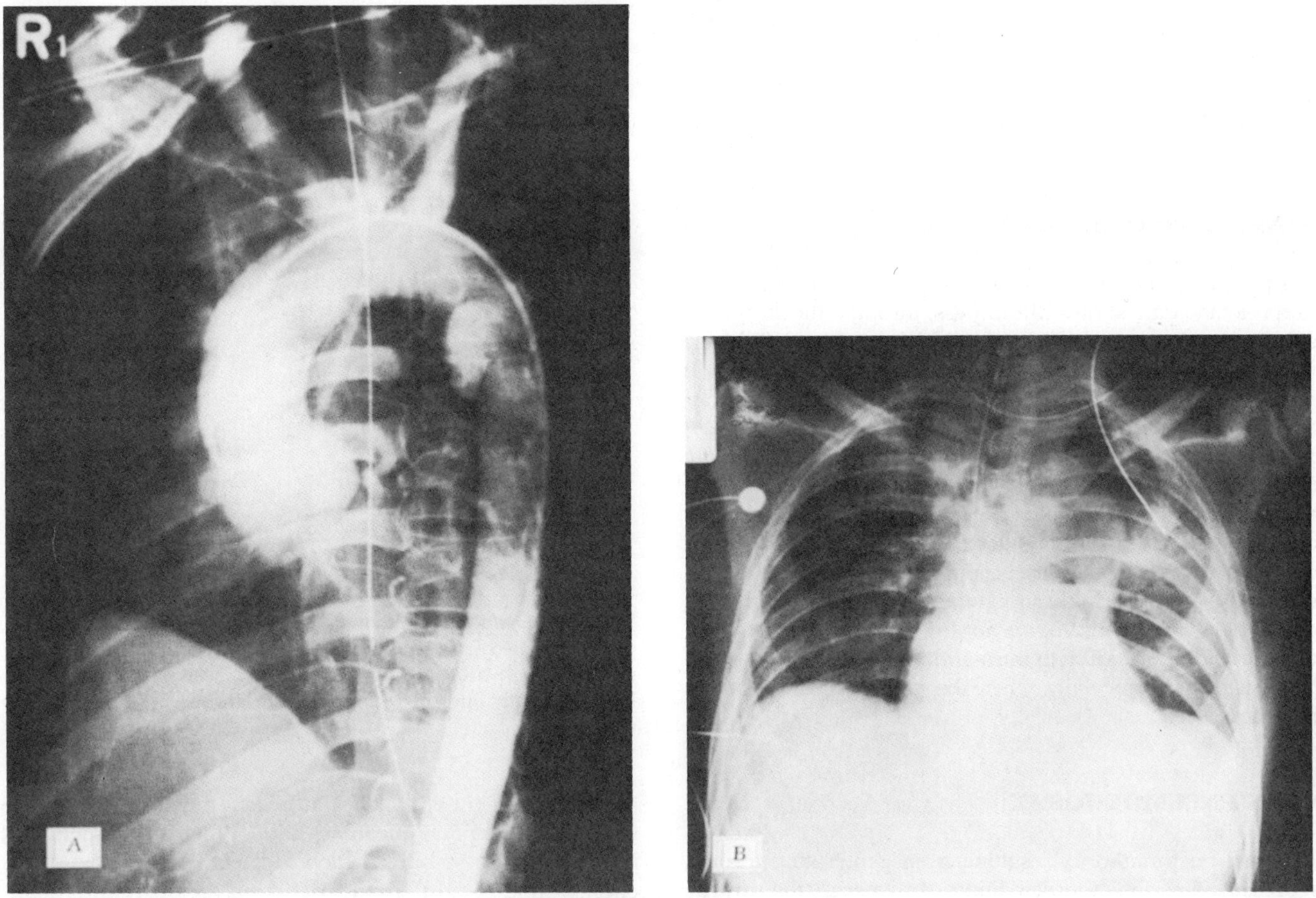

Fig. 60-4. A. Traumatic disruption of the thoracic aorta. Note hematoma surrounding aortic knob, inferior displacement of left mainstem bronchus, and left apical hemothorax. B. Thoracic aortogram showing disruption of the thoracic aorta distal to the left subclavian artery with false aneurysm formation.

that also require assessment and treatment. It is surprising, especially considering the magnitude of the internal derangement, that specific physical findings with aortic rupture may be quite subtle or even nonexistent. For this reason, the potential for an aortic tear should be considered for *any* patient who has sustained high-speed decelerative trauma. The suspicion of aortic injury may be heightened if there is evidence of severe trauma to the thorax, such as fractures of the sternum or upper ribs, but it should be remembered that a significant percentage of aortic disruptions occur with no striking external evidence of chest injury. Similarly, the physical findings that have been associated with aortic disruption—upper extremity hypertension, posterior thoracic systolic bruit, and diminution of distal pulses, all resulting from partial aortic obstruction by the periaortic hematoma at the site of injury—are more frequently absent than present.

The chest radiograph often provides the first evidence suggestive of traumatic aortic disruption. Several radiographic signs have been correlated with aortic injury, although none is diagnostic or even specific for aortic rupture. The periaortic hematoma may produce superior mediastinal widening, tracheal deviation to the right, inferior displacement of the left main stem bronchus, obliteration of the sharp outline of the descending aorta or aortic knob, and opacification of the clear region between the aorta and pulmonary artery. Extrapleural dissection of blood over the left pulmonary apex may produce a "cap," and weeping or leak of blood through the mediastinal pleural may produce a left pleural effusion (Fig. 60-4B). In a small percentage of cases, the initial chest radiograph may be virtually normal.

Management

Angiography is the best means of providing a definitive preoperative diagnosis of traumatic disruption of the aorta or of any other great vessel. For this reason, angiography should be used in any case in which there is a reasonable suspicion of this possibility. Most aortic disruptions are demonstrable on the aortogram as contained pseudoaneurysms immediately distal to the origin of the left subclavian artery. If the diagnosis of aortic rupture or other major vascular injury is confirmed, an operation should follow immediately.

When a patient presenting with signs suggesting blunt aortic injury cannot be satisfactorily stabilized in the emergency department, steps should be taken to facilitate direct transfer to the operating room without aortography. If there is an indication of abdominal injury, the possibility of intra-abdominal bleeding as the source of the shock must be considered and appropriate consultation obtained. The return of gross blood from diagnostic peritoneal lavage combined with the absence of exsanguinating hemorrhage from the chest tubes could reasonably dictate laparotomy for control of bleeding prior to any further thoracic study or procedure, even when there is a strong suspicion of a *contained* aortic transection.

PENETRATING CHEST TRAUMA

Most penetrating chest injuries are produced by knives or low-velocity gun shots. Many pass through the lung, resulting in a hemopneumothorax, which is often definitively treated simply with closed-tube thoracostomy. Wounds of the heart, aorta, and great vessels may be partially tamponaded by the pericardium, surrounding tissue, or accumulation of clot, allowing an initial period of survival. Bleeding from the lung and chest wall is often self-limited. Plotting the course of the bullet from the entrance wound and point of lodgement or exit wound allows some estimate to be made of what structures may have been injured, although the missile path is not invariably straight and one is frequently surprised at what is and what is not injured. Possible penetration of the diaphragm with intra-abdominal injury must also be considered, especially when the wound is at or below midchest level.

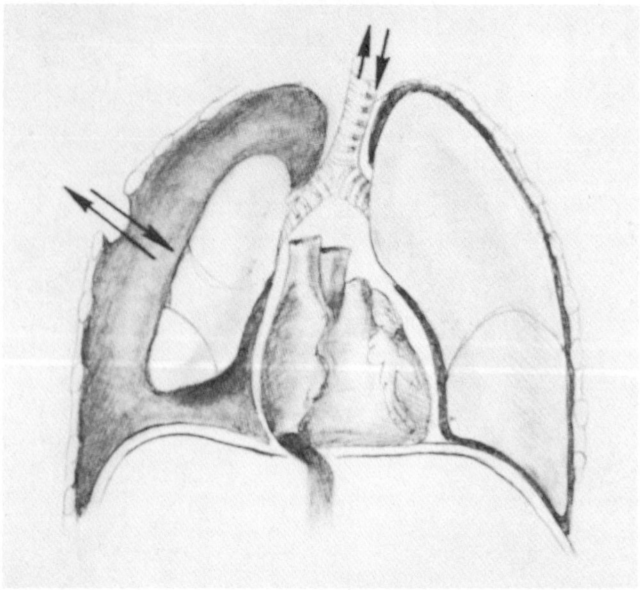

Fig. 60-5. Open pneumothorax. Airflow through the chest wall defect into the pleural space with inspiration minimizes development of intrathoracic negative pressure. Tracheal airflow into the lungs is greatly limited by the lack of an inspiratory negative pressure gradient.

OPEN PNEUMOTHORAX

An open pneumothorax resulting from penetrating trauma represents a serious thoracic injury. In general, the severity of the clinical problem is a function of the size of the chest wall defect. This is not absolute since even a small stab wound that causes no other intrathoracic injury may produce a tension pneumothorax in the course of lacerating the lung. An open pneumothorax becomes especially critical in cases in which the chest wall defect is large enough to allow free communication of the pleural space with the outside atmosphere (sucking chest wound). Severe respiratory insufficiency may rapidly result. Intrapleural pressure on the side of the injury becomes atmospheric, and respiratory excursions of the chest move air in and out through the defect, diminishing the tidal volume passing through the glottis into the lungs (Fig. 60-5). Moreover, as air is drawn into the pleural space with inspiration, the mediastinum shifts toward the uninjured hemithorax, in which there is still negative intrapleural pressure, and returns with expiration (mediastinal flutter). The combined effect is to move increasingly stagnant air in a to-and-fro manner from the aerated to partially collapsed lung, further diminishing the effective tidal volume.

Management

Therapy is directed at immediate occlusion of the chest wall defect. This is usually done with a pack of sterile plain or petrolatum gauze. However, if no sterile materials are readily available, a clean wadded cloth held in place is adequate. It is best to occlude the defect at end expiration to evacuate as much air as possible from the pleural cavity. Closure of the sucking wound stabilizes the situation and allows placement of the chest tube at a point away from the wound to reexpand the lung fully. When the patient has been otherwise stabilized, debridement and closure of the chest wound should be undertaken in the operating room.

HEMOTHORAX

Hemothorax frequently complicates both blunt and penetrating thoracic trauma. Excluding blunt rupture of the aorta, larger collections of pleural blood generally follow penetrating trauma. Because the source of bleeding may be the chest wall, the lung, or the heart and great vessels, it is difficult to categorize treatment of hemothorax rigidly as an isolated entity. Bleeding from the lung and chest wall veins is often self-limited, whereas that from the heart and arteries requires operative control.

Diagnosis

On physical examination, intrapleural blood is characterized by dullness to percussion and diminished or absent breath sounds. In cases of larger hemothoraces, there may be mediastinal shift and tracheal deviation away from the involved hemothorax. A chest film provides the best estimate of the amount of intrapleural blood. The chest film should be rapidly obtained with the patient as upright as possible, because several hundred milliliters of blood layered posteriorly may produce only a faint haziness on a supine film.

Management

Generally, once detected, any significant collection of pleural blood should be evacuated in coordination with other resuscitative measures, including intravascular volume replacement. In the usual trauma setting, closed tube thoracostomy with at least a No. 28 French tube is advisable. Satisfactory drainage can usually be obtained with chest tube placement through the fifth intercostal space in the midaxillary line. This insertion point minimizes the risk of diaphragmatic injury in the emergency situation. The initial volume of blood obtained from the chest or the rate of continued bleeding indicates either conservative therapy or the necessity of exploratory thoracotomy. If chest tube placement is followed by the immediate drainage of 1,000 ml or more of blood, immediate thoracotomy should be undertaken because of the great likelihood of a major intrathoracic injury that will not stop bleeding spontaneously. Similarly, after tube placement, an operation for surgical control of bleeding should be performed if, after the first hour, the drainage for any hour exceeds 400 ml or if the bleeding does not appear to be diminishing after the first 4 hours. The patient with a hemothorax and penetrating trauma to the chest who remains in shock after vigorous resuscitative measures should be transferred to the operating room for immediate thoracotomy. For the patient who arrives in the emergency department in extremis, endotracheal intubation should immediately be followed by left anterolateral thoracotomy through the fifth interspace. Although such an approach is aggressive, it offers the only small hope of saving a patient who would otherwise die from the injury. Pericardial tamponade may be relieved by the direct evacuation of blood and clot, and effective open-chest cardiac massage may be instituted. Massive bleeding from tears or gunshot wounds in the heart and great vessels may possibly be temporarily controlled with application of direct pressure, application of vascular clamps, or suture while intravascular volume is being replaced.

PERICARDIAL TAMPONADE

The limited space between the heart and the surrounding relatively inelastic pericardium is normally occupied by only a few milliliters of serous fluid. A chronic slow increase in the volume of fluid within the pericardial space up to several hundred milliliters can be accommodated by a gradual stretching of the pericardium with minimal hemodynamic consequence. In contrast, the capacity of the pericardium to adapt to rapid accumulations of intrapericardial fluid by stretching is limited. When fluid accumulates at a rate or to a volume that exceeds the capacity of the pericardium to enlarge, intrapericardial pressure will increase and impede diastolic filling of the heart. When inflow is limited, cardiac output progressively falls, and the atrial and central venous pressure will rise. The severity of the derangement depends on the degree of intrapericardial pressure elevation. Pericardial tamponade may be severe and life threatening, or it may be mild and, although hemodynamically demonstrable, not necessarily clinically significant in terms of requiring pericardial drainage.

Pericardial tamponade may complicate virtually any pathologic process that produces an intrapericardial fluid accumulation. This includes effusions associated with the full spectrum of infectious pericarditis, malignancy, autoimmune disease, uremia, and other metabolic disorders. In certain cases, tamponade is the first manifestation of previously unrecognized pericardial disease. Intrapericardial hemorrhage from blunt and, especially, penetrating chest trauma may produce tamponade. In cases of penetrating wounds of the heart, tamponade occasionally may, in a sense, be initially lifesaving by preventing immediate exsanguination into the chest, thereby allowing a short period of survival during which the patient may reach medical care.

Diagnosis

The clinical signs of pericardial tamponade may be subtle or dramatic. Sustained tachycardia indicates compensation for a diminished stroke volume. The signs of arterial hypotension and an elevated central venous pressure indicate a falling cardiac output and increased cardiac filling pressure. The rapidity of the progression of these signs depends on the rate of intrapericardial pressure rise. If the onset of tamponade is gradual, signs of compensatory adrenergic activity such as peripheral vasoconstriction and cool, clammy skin may precede a significant fall in blood pressure. Neck vein distention from the elevated central venous pressure (CVP) may or may not be observable depending on neck anatomy and the degree of intravascular volume depletion. Direct measure of the CVP should be obtained for any patient suspected of having pericardial tamponade unless the urgency of the situation does not allow it. In normal circumstances, the systolic blood pressure diminishes slightly with inspiration. When this inspiratory fall in pressure exceeds 10 mm Hg, it is termed *pulsus paradoxus* and is highly suggestive of pericardial tamponade. However, pulsus paradoxus is not invariably present with pericardial tamponade, and its absence should not argue against the diagnosis if there is other evidence to the contrary. Although the heart sounds may be muffled or distant with pericardial fluid collections, such a finding should be considered as being quite relative and equally dependent on other factors such as chest wall thickness and the amount of overlying lung tissue.

The chest film may demonstrate an enlarged globular pericardium with chronic effusion. In acute tamponade following trauma, however, the pericardial silhouette is often relatively normal. When the situation allows, echocardiography is the most reliable means of confirming the presence of pericardial fluid.

Management

In situations in which pericardial tamponade with hemopericardium is suspected following thoracic trauma, immediate pericardiocentesis (see Procedure 21) is indicated. With penetrating thoracic trauma in which the missile has possibly passed through the pericardium, the combination of elevated venous pressure and arterial hypotension virtually ensures the diagnosis of cardiac tamponade. Aspiration of even a small quantity of blood may be marked by significant hemodynamic improvement. Although controversy exists as to the subsequent management of patients after initial successful pericardiocentesis, many thoracic surgeons believe that early thoracotomy in the operating room before the reaccumulation of blood should be undertaken for definitive control of the bleeding point and certain evacuation of the intrapericardial blood clot rather than relying on repeated pericardial aspiration. If there is continued severe hemodynamic deterioration despite pericardiocentesis, time may be insufficient to get the patient to the operating room. Consideration should be given to opening the chest in the emergency department, either via anterior thoracotomy or through a subxiphoid approach.

In contrast, when pericardial tamponade complicates the various forms of effusive pericarditis, repeated pericardiocentesis may be more useful, and surgery may be reserved for those cases in which there is refractory reaccumulation or considerable risk of late constriction.

AIR EMBOLISM

Venous Air Embolism

The accidental introduction of small volumes of air into the venous system is tolerated without apparent effect in the absence of a right-to-left shunt. This probably occurs in the course of central venous cannulation with a greater frequency than is generally recognized. Larger volumes (>300 ml) passing through the right heart may obstruct the right ventricular outflow tract or pulmonary artery producing sudden cardiovascular collapse. Such volumes may enter with surprising rapidity through the large-bore introducer sheaths used to insert Swan-Ganz catheters, temporary dialysis catheters, and transvenous pacemaker leads. The risk of venous air embolism is especially great when the patient is breathing spontaneously and the central venous pressure is low. To minimize this hazard during central venous cannulation, the patient should be placed in slight Trendelenburg position to raise intrathoracic venous pressure. The end of the sheath or catheter being introduced must be carefully controlled, and the patient should be instructed not to breathe during manipulation. Sudden complaints of dyspnea and chest pain associated with tachycardia, tachypnea, wheezing, or chest pain in the course of central venous cannulation should alert one to the possibility of air embolism. A churning cardiac murmur has been reported with venous air embolism, but the realization that air has entered the catheter and the patient has suddenly deteriorated may be the best diagnostic clues. If the portable fluoroscope is being used to position a pacemaker lead or Swan-Ganz catheter, air may possibly be seen as lucency in the right ventricular outflow tract or the pulmonary artery.

Treatment

Symptomatic air embolism should be treated by placing the patient in steep Trendelenburg position with the right side of the body turned well up to allow the air to move away from its obstructing position in the right ventricular outflow tract. If this is successful, the patient should be kept in this position until the air is resorbed. Such resorbtion can be hastened by placing the patient on 100 percent oxygen. Some air may possibly be aspirated through the catheter being inserted. In truly *desperate* circumstances where there is relative certainty that the air embolism has occurred and the patient remains unimproved by respositioning, the only remaining measure is immediate thoracotomy for open cardiac massage and direct needle aspiration of air from the right ventricle and pulmonary artery. With severe cardiovascular collapse, the difficult decision to open the chest would have to be rapidly reached and expertly carried out to prevent anoxic brain injury.

Arterial Air Embolism

Very small volumes of air entering the arterial circulation can have a disastrous effect with passage into the coronary or cerebral arteries. In the emergency department, the potential to see arterial air embolism is probably greatest when positive pressure ventilation is required for patients with injuries that have produced pulmonary parenchymal disruption. Air under pressure may pass from disrupted small bronchioles into torn pulmonary venous branches to the left heart and into the arterial circulation.

Recognition

In a patient with penetrating pulmonary injury, there may be several causes for sudden occurrence of bradycardia, ventricular ectopy, and hypotension. Arterial air embolism requires consideration, particularly if there are neurologic symptoms suggesting stroke or seizure. Treatment consists of minimizing positive airway pressures while the chest is opened on the injured side. The pulmonary hilum is clamped to stop further embolism of air, and air is aspirated from the ascending aorta. The wounded segment of lung is then resected.

ESOPHAGEAL INJURIES

Esophageal perforations, particularly those that occur within the intrathoracic segment, represent extremely serious injuries. The entry of saliva containing anaerobic mouth organisms into the visceral spaces of the neck and mediastinum or into the pleural cavity produces a rapidly progressing infection in areas in which there are few barriers to extensive spread. Any delay in the recognition and treatment of such injuries seriously jeopardizes the potential for favorable outcome.

Blunt injury to the esophagus has been reported, but it is rare. Penetrating injury is also infrequent because of the deep and central position of the esophagus. A contrast study of the esophagus should be routinely performed if it appears that a penetrating missile may have traversed the mediastinum. Spontaneous esophageal rupture from retching, although not common, occurs more frequently than is generally recognized, and the diagnosis is often made only after a significant delay. Severe substernal or epigastric pain associated with an episode of vomiting requires radiographic study of the esophagus unless there is unequivocal evidence of other intrathoracic pathology to explain the symptoms, such as an acute myocardial infarction.

Most esophageal perforations result from penetration of the esophageal wall from within, infrequently by swallowed foreign bodies such as a pin or a small bone, but much more commonly from an endoscopic accident. Instrumental perforation usually occurs proximal to a stricture, a tumor, or a point of natural esophageal narrowing such as is encountered at the diaphragmatic hiatus.

The clinical manifestations of esophageal perforation depend on the site of injury and the degree of periesophageal contamination with digestive juices. Cervical perforations are characterized by early pain with swallowing followed by progressive cervical tenderness and crepitation to palpation. Intrathoracic perforations are usually accompanied by variable substernal pain and, especially with pleural contamination, some degree of dyspnea. Early physical signs are limited when there are intrathoracic perforations. Cervical crepitation may be a late development as gas dissects superiorly through the mediastinum. Auscultation may demonstrate a "mediastinal crunch" within the soft tissues. Fever and tachycardia usually develop within a few hours. Radiographic studies are necessary to confirm esophageal disruption. When cervical perforation is suspected, early anterior, posterior, and lateral films will usually demonstrate air within the soft tissues of the neck. X-ray film taken later in the process might show a periesophageal fluid collection, edema of the prevertebral tissues, and even superior mediastinal widening. When the esophageal perforation is within the intrathoracic segment, mediastinal widening, pleural effusion, and mediastinal air may be visible on the plain film; however, all are inconstant early findings, and contrast studies with a water-soluble medium should be obtained any time there is suspicion of an esophageal injury.

When the diagnosis of an esophageal perforation is suspected, early surgical consultation should be obtained to expedite any necessary surgical drainage and repair.

SELECTED READING

Glinz, W. *Chest Trauma: Diagnosis and Management.* Berlin: Springer-Verlag, 1981.

Hood, RM, Boyd, AD, and Culliford, AT. *Thoracic Trauma.* Philadelphia: Saunders, 1989.

61. Abdominal Injuries

Dennis P. Orgill
Robert T. Osteen
Frederick W. Ackroyd

Before the twentieth century, an abdominal injury was a mortal wound. Not until exploratory laparotomy and repair of damaged organs became possible and safe did a person with an injury of the abdominal viscera survive—except by good fortune.

Physicians and surgeons in civilian practice see fewer major penetrating injuries than do military surgeons in wartime. What physicians in civilian emergency departments witness is a sad byproduct of our high-speed society: the blunt trauma of automobile accidents. Urban violence contributes to the casualty list, but the family automobile is the major culprit. In a review of civilian experience, 67 percent of patients with abdominal injuries had sustained blunt trauma from automobiles, farm equipment, or athletic injuries; 17 percent had been stabbed; and 14 percent had been shot.

As in other fields of medicine, prevention is more desirable than treatment. The Roman legionnaires in Gaul, the crusaders at Tyre, and, most recently, the United States servicemen in Vietnam all wore body armor. Unfortunately, the knife fighter in the street and the victim of the ubiquitous "unknown assailant" are not so well protected. Even though automobile manufacturers are gradually devoting attention to safety features, many of these devices have their own innate problems. For example, the use of seat belts often trades neurologic trauma for abdominal injuries. Finally, patients in the hospital are not always safe from abdominal injury. The increasingly effective and aggressive diagnostic use of endoscopes, needle biopsies, and vascular catheters is accompanied by a small but disturbing number of injuries.

INITIAL ASSESSMENT AND MANAGEMENT

The arrival of a patient with abdominal injuries in the emergency department is usually accompanied by clamor and confusion proportional to the severity of the injuries. The physician on duty must transform this disorderly scene into an efficient task force in order to provide the appropriate sequence of diagnostic and therapeutic maneuvers. A quiet room without unnecessary chatter is essential.

First and foremost one must remember to treat the immediate life-threatening injuries. A useful way to organize this effort is to remember the ABCs of trauma: specifically, to obtain an *a*irway with cervical spine immobilization, to assure adequate ventilation (*b*reathing), and to restore *c*irculating blood volume. At that point, a detailed physical examination and appropriate x-ray studies and consultations can be obtained. A time-proven principle in caring for the trauma patient is the "golden hour." During this first hour, all resuscitative measures and x-ray studies in the emergency department should be completed. Anyone who has worked in an emergency department for any period of time has witnessed apparently stable trauma patients whose condition quickly becomes hemodynamically unstable.

As early as possible, an assessment should be made of the staff and specialists available to provide the care required for an injured patient. Any time there is a patient with severe abdominal trauma, a surgeon should be called. A patient with pelvic trauma invariably requires that the emergency physician consult with an orthopedist, a urologist, and a general surgeon. Many hospitals have a disaster plan that can be activated when emergency facilities become overloaded. A train wreck or other large-scale accident is not the only circumstance in which the plan should be implemented. Indeed, the facilities of the hospital can become saturated by the victims of a two-car collision.

It is impossible to separate completely the multiple features of resuscitation and diagnosis. Initial management of the patient with abdominal trauma may combine resuscitative and diagnostic measures. For example, the response to fluid therapy is an important indicator of intraabdominal bleeding. It may not be possible to make the diagnosis of an injury to a specific organ. Diagnoses tend to be more generic, such as "ruptured viscus" or "continuing intraabdominal hemorrhage." Central to the process of diagnosis and treatment is the decision of whether there is a need for laparotomy.

Immediate Measures

The patient must be completely undressed. Unless the patient is awake and cooperative, the clothing should be cut away to minimize the chance of displacing an unsuspected fracture or vertebral injury. An unconscious patient should be viewed with a high index of suspicion for abdominal and spinal cord injuries.

Combative, intoxicated patients present a problem. Although they may have serious abdominal injuries, definitive evaluation may have to be delayed until they are calmed; minimal light and noise and the sedative effects of the alcohol may help to achieve this. During this period, however, their vital signs should be monitored if they will cooperate. The urge to use drugs to tranquilize such patients must be avoided.

The lighting in the examining room should be adequate to assess the patient's true color. The patient's level of consciousness and breathing characteristics can be determined at a glance. If breathing is impaired, patency of the airway must be ensured and, if necessary, ventilatory support provided. The stability of the patient's chest can be tested by gentle compression of the sternum and the lateral thoracic walls.

All patients suspected of having intraabdominal injuries should have two large-bore intravenous lines and tubes to decompress the stomach and bladder. Nasogastric (NG) tubes can generally be placed but are contraindicated in patients with facial fractures or with suspected injuries of the cribriform plate. There have been several reports of NG tubes that have been placed intracranially in such patients. Foley catheters should be placed unless there is blood at the meatus, a high-riding prostate on rectal examination, or pelvic fractures. The urine should be checked for the presence of blood. Blood samples should be drawn when the intravenous lines are placed. A blood count, a chemistry profile, a toxic screen when indicated, clotting parameters, and a clot to the blood bank are sent.

Patients should be given oxygen, placed on an ECG monitor, and have frequent vital signs monitored. Automatic blood pressure cuffs and portable pulse oximetry devices are available in many emergency departments. These can be very useful, especially when procedures or diagnostic tests are being performed. Lateral cervical spine, chest, and AP pelvis films are frequently performed early after admission to the emergency department to help prioritize additional therapy.

Details of the accident or assault should be obtained from the patient and any available witnesses. The patient's position when shot may give some indication of the course of the bullet. A small penknife is less likely to penetrate the peritoneal cavity than is a long butcher knife or a stiletto. With an eye toward the patient's subsequent course, a few routine questions should be asked. A history of allergies, immunizations, and medications should be obtained. The time of the patient's last meal should be established since this may influence the anesthesiologist's technique of intubation if the patient needs an operation. If cranial trauma can be ruled out by history, a clouded sensorium may be an early indication of cerebral hypoperfusion secondary to internal blood loss.

A complete physical examination must be performed. All information, including pertinent negative findings, should be recorded in detail. Because the process of diagnosis may take many days and involve many people who will not have seen the patient immediately after the accident, the initial examiner's observations are crucial to evaluate changes in the patient's condition. The physician must bear in mind that surgical exploration may be necessary at any time from the moment that the patient is first seen. Evidence of peritoneal irritation or bleeding signals the need for surgery. Such physical findings, which often appear within several hours, include gradually disappearing bowel sounds, systemic evidence of infection, or abdominal tenderness. Particularly in the setting of blunt trauma, the signs of intraabdominal injury may evolve slowly, and examination of the abdomen should be repeated frequently by the same examiner.

Laboratory Tests and Diagnostic Studies

In most civilian emergency wards, the patient is seen soon after the injury and before fluid shifts have diluted the hematocrit, before peritonitis has raised the white blood cell count, before amylase has been absorbed from the peritoneal surface, and before massive fluid replacement has diluted the serum sodium. Although the initial tests have little diagnostic value, they do provide baseline levels against which later results can be compared to evaluate changes in the patient's condition. Normal values should never be used to support an attitude of complacency toward the patient who demonstrates clinical evidence of abdominal injury. After an episode of major blood loss, dilution of the remaining red-cell mass begins immediately, but the hematocrit may not be significantly lowered for several hours. The process of hemodilution continues for approximately three days after a single episode of bleeding. A rising serum amylase may suggest injury to the pancreas or duodenum. An early leukocytosis should not be interpreted as anything more specific than evidence of major trauma.

Blood in the urine is a major indicator of urinary tract trauma. Gross or microscopic hematuria should be pursued with appropriate radiologic studies, including cystography and intravenous urography.

An electrocardiogram (ECG) should be performed to establish the baseline condition of the patient's heart. There is no electrocardiographic finding, including myocardial infarction, that would contraindicate a laparotomy in a patient who has evidence of significant intraabdominal trauma.

Roentgenography

In general, plain roentgenograms of the abdomen are of little diagnostic value for assessing abdominal trauma. Some subtle signs of organ damage or intraperitoneal bleeding may be seen, but they must be interpreted in light of the evidence from the physical examination. Chest films should always be ordered to check for a pneumothorax and to look for free air under the diaphragm. Radiographic views of the urinary tract can be extremely helpful and should be used to investigate any degree of hematuria.

Roentgenographic studies should not be attempted until the patient is resuscitated. At that time, and in consultation with the involved specialist and the radiologist, the appropriate studies can be ordered. Some particularly well-equipped emergency departments have x-ray facilities in their resuscitation rooms. In too many hospitals, the patient must be moved from the brilliantly lighted, well-staffed, and well-equipped emergency room to a small, dim x-ray cubicle where only the x-ray technician is in attendance. If intraabdominal bleeding continues, the recently resuscitated patient can slide back into shock. In the radiology department, vital signs and the ECG of the patient should be monitored and a person skilled in the diagnosis of hypovolemia should be present. A physician qualified to make decisions regarding transfusion and the need for immediate laparotomy should be available. Adequate support and observation must be provided while adequate x-ray studies are performed. The use of portable x-ray equipment in the emergency department is a compromise in the evaluation of abdominal trauma. The quality of a portable x-ray film is never as good as that of one taken by regular x-ray equipment.

Computed Tomography

Computed tomography (CT) provides an excellent noninvasive technique for accurately assessing, simultaneously, injuries of the head, neck, thorax, abdomen, pelvis, and extremities. The patient need not be moved from one position, and the study can be serially repeated as necessary. The body scanner provides images of the liver, spleen, kidneys, bladder, bowel, and bony skeleton. These views demonstrate findings characteristic of organ disruption, subcapsular hematoma, and bleeding, permitting rapid assessment of patients with multisystem trauma. Pancreatic injuries are well demonstrated, and the addition of intravenous contrast media outlines the abdominal vasculature. This technique is valuable in evaluating patients with blunt trauma, and a negative scan may permit a more cautious, nonoperative approach, rather than emergency operation. The CT scans can be interpreted with confidence, and decisions in management can often be made without multiple additional tests, since CT is, in many cases, the most sensitive and specific for the various conditions.

The use of CT in the assessment of intraabdominal trauma depends on having a competent radiologist present to interpret the films. CT scans should not be performed in a patient whose condition is hemodynamically unstable or in patients in whom the decision to explore the abdomen has already been made. Body CT is particularly convenient in patients who require CT scans for concomitant head injuries.

Urography and Cystography

Intravenous urography and cystography are important techniques to be considered in abdominal trauma and are discussed in detail in Chap. 62.

Peritoneal Lavage

Peritoneal lavage is a sensitive and specific technique for diagnosing intraabdominal hemorrhage and can also be diagnostic of a perforated viscous, pancreatic, or biliary injury. It is particularly useful in blunt trauma and has been used selectively in managing stab wounds to the abdomen. It has the advantage over CT scans in that it can be used with simple equipment available in all emergency wards. It also tends to be more expeditious than CT scan, particularly in unstable patients.

BLUNT INJURIES

The definitive evaluation and management of abdominal injuries differs depending on the wounding agent. There are two major divisions of injuries—blunt trauma and penetrating wounds. *Blunt trauma* presents a difficult diagnostic problem in that a blow to the abdominal wall may not produce significant visceral injury. Furthermore, bleeding into or irritation of the peritoneum may be insufficient to produce symptoms until many hours after the accident. Patients who have sustained blunt abdominal trauma may be asymptomatic at first even though they have significant injuries. Indeed, many patients initially deny that they are injured, though a short time later they gradually begin to perceive the severity of their injuries. Injury to solid organs such as the liver or spleen is more likely to cause rapid blood loss and early appearance of the signs of hypovolemia. Injury to the hollow gastrointestinal (GI) tract may cause symptoms of peritonitis initially, and hypovolemic symptoms may develop later.

Assessment of Blunt Trauma

History

An estimation of the potential for significant visceral injury can be made from the history of the accident. The faster the automobile was traveling or the greater the distance of the fall, the more likely a severe injury has occurred. The history of a sharp blow to the left flank will focus the examiner's attention on the spleen and kidney. Cross-lap seat belts have been associated with mesenteric tears, small-bowel lacerations, and rupture of the gravid uterus. The accident victim who is unconscious for any period of time should be a suspect for abdominal as well as intercranial injuries simply because of the force involved. Even an asymptomatic patient who has sustained a major impact should be admitted to the hospital for 24 hours of observation.

Physical Examination For Blunt Trauma

The best single approach for the evaluation of blunt abdominal trauma is a series of careful physical examinations. Close observation and monitoring of vital signs are essential. The initial physical examination is performed in the emergency department by the emergency physician.

After immediate measures are taken to provide an adequate airway and to stabilize the patient, a complete physical examination is performed. The abdomen, flanks, and back should be inspected for abrasions and discoloration. Bluish discoloration of the flanks can indicate bleeding into the retroperitoneum. Similar discoloration arising from the pelvic area or perineum can result from a pelvic fracture. Abrasions or contusions of the lower abdominal wall can be caused by a seat belt. The lower part of the rib cage is inspected for ecchymoses and is palpated for crepitance. Fractured ribs are not diagnostic of abdominal trauma, but they do indicate that major trauma has occurred. A blow that is forceful enough to fracture the lower left ribs could also rupture the spleen or kidney by direct puncture, crushing against the vertebral column, or shearing (see Fig. 40-11).

The examination of the abdomen for tenderness must be done so gently that pain from a fractured rib or vertebra does not interfere with the evaluation of peritoneal irritation. Light percussion is a better test for rebound tenderness than is the sudden release of pressure after deep, bimanual palpation. Concurrent spinal cord injury will eliminate abdominal muscle tone and blunt the perception of pain, making the evaluation of peritoneal irritation difficult. Patients with spinal cord injuries will feel abdominal discomfort relayed through the autonomic nervous system, but sensations from the peritoneum that has somatic innervation may be obliterated. X-ray film studies, selected on the basis of clinical evidence, are helpful when the patient's condition permits. Peritoneal lavage or a CT scan plays a valuable role in the evaluation of comatose patients or stable patients with suggestive but not conclusive evidence of intraperitoneal injury.

Injury to the abdominal wall with bleeding from epigastric vessels can produce a tender abdomen associated with a visible and palpable mass in the abdominal wall. Guarding and tenderness should not be ascribed to a rectus hematoma unless a mass is present. If the abdominal wall is the source of the patient's discomfort, tensing the abdominal muscles will increase pain, but if the pain is from an intraabdominal injury, tensing the abdominal muscles will lessen it.

The physician should listen for bowel sounds. Because bowel sounds may persist for a while after the intestine has ruptured and because ileus is common after chest trauma, even when the abdominal contents have not been injured, the presence or absence of bowel sounds initially is not diagnostic. However, the gradual disappearance of sounds is suggestive of intraabdominal injury.

A rectal examination should be performed in men, and rectal and pelvic examinations should be performed in women. Blood in the rectum indicates damage to the colon or rectum.

Pelvic fractures should be suspected when gentle pressure on the iliac crests or symphysis pubis causes pain. One leg may occasionally be noticeably shorter than the other. Pelvic fractures can be associated with injuries to the rectum, bladder, or male urethra. The short female urethra is rarely injured. Trauma to the bladder causes hematuria that is not usually associated with frank bleeding from the urethral meatus. Blood at the tip of the urethral meatus is a sign of urethral injury and a contraindication to catheterization until the continuity of the urethra has been confirmed. The urethra can rupture on either side of the urogenital diaphragm. Anterior rupture of the urethra typically causes extravasation of blood and urine through Buck's fascia into the superficial tissues of the perineum, scrotum, penis, and anterior abdominal wall with swelling and discoloration of those structures. Rupture of the posterior urethra (on the bladder side of the urogenital diaphragm) is associated with less obvious physical findings because the extravasation of blood and urine is into the retroperitoneum and tissues surrounding the bladder. The hematoma from a posterior urethral rupture may be palpated on rectal examination as a fullness that obliterates the normal feel of the prostate (Fig. 61-1). If the posterior part of the urethra is completely transected and there is rupture of the puboprostatic ligaments, the prostate is no longer fixed in its normal position and cannot be palpated. In young men who normally have a small, barely palpable prostate, the absence of a palpable prostate is not a reliable sign.

Although the initial physical examination is performed in the emergency department by the emergency physician, consultation with a general surgeon should be sought when the signs and symptoms indicate intraabdominal injury or when the magnitude of the force or the nature of the accident was such that the patient should be admitted for observation even though he or she lacks significant evidence of visceral injury. In the unstable patient, exploratory laparotomy is carried out when there is evidence of continued blood loss with persistent or recurrent signs of hypovolemia despite vigorous fluid administration. In the stable patient, exploratory laparotomy is performed if there are signs of peritoneal irritation, intraperitoneal bleeding diagnosed by peritoneal lavage or CT, and roentgenographic evidence of rupture of a hollow viscus.

Specific Injuries

Although the need for laparotomy rests on evidence of continued occult blood loss or signs of peritoneal irritation, or both, there are some differences in the presentation of various injuries. It is not always possible to make a diagnosis of specific organ injury preoperatively, but an understanding of the special considerations relating to specific organs is helpful.

Spleen

The spleen is the organ most susceptible to injury by blunt trauma, which is seen frequently after motor vehicle accidents and falls. There is a high association of splenic injury with left-sided rib fractures. The spleen can be crushed by a force that deforms the left side of the lower part of the rib cage, or the spleen's ligamentous attachments can be torn by rapid deceleration.

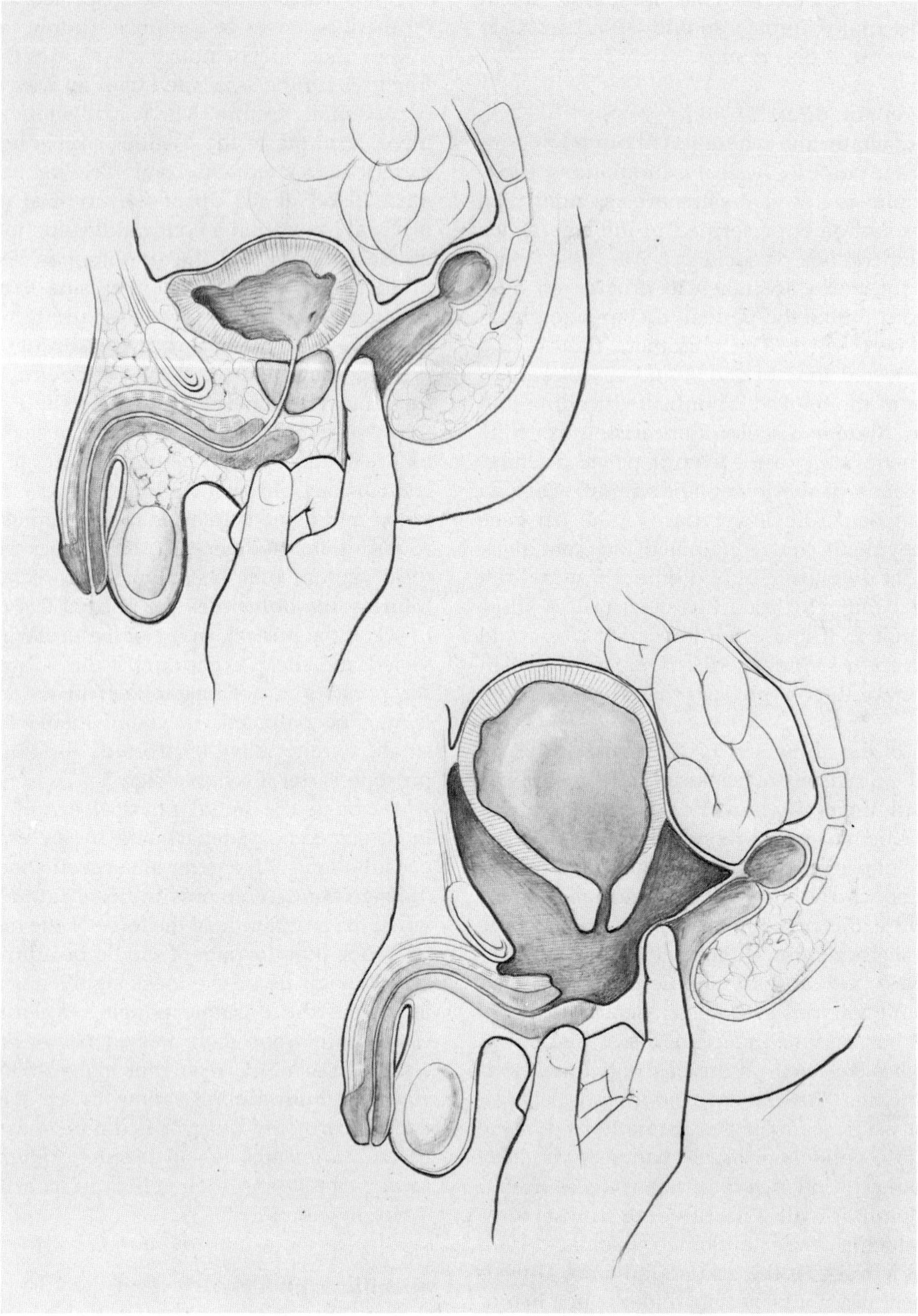

Fig. 61-1. Normal rectal examination (*top*) when the palpable prostate is in normal position. When there is urethral disruption, the prostate is not palpable and spongy consistency is present because of retroperitoneal hematoma (*bottom*).

DIAGNOSIS. Deep, left-sided abdominal pain with coughing and pain in an epaulet pattern distributed over the left shoulder are characteristic of spleen injuries. Subcapsular hematomas can cause pain without significant blood loss. Most ruptured spleens are found in patients who have multiple trauma, with obvious hemoperitoneum seen on laparotomy. For more stable patients, the abdominal CT scan has generally replaced liver-spleen scanning as the diagnostic modality of choice.

MANAGEMENT. Because the spleen plays a major role in the immune response of children, many pediatric surgeons try to avoid removing demonstrably ruptured spleens in children who are hemodynamically stable. Children and young adults are often carefully monitored in an intensive care unit with serial hematocrits. If a nonoperative approach is taken, bed rest in the hospital for 10 days is advised, with a repeat CT scan before discharge.

In adults the immune function seems to be less important, and a ruptured spleen is generally considered to be an indication for splenectomy although many authors advise splenorrhaphy in patients in whom bleeding can be controlled. It is not clear what action should be taken when a subcapsular hematoma can be demonstrated by CT scan, but there is no compelling reason for an immediate operation. A subcapsular hematoma may progress to a delayed rupture days or months after the original injury, but no data are available to estimate that risk. At the present time, conservative, expectant treatment seems to be advisable for the asymptomatic patient.

PROGNOSIS. Patients who have isolated ruptures of the spleen have an excellent prognosis. If an operation is performed before the secondary problems of hypervolemia complicate the situation, the patient should survive.

Education of patients after splenectomy is very important to avoid death from postsplenectomy sepsis.

Liver

Trauma to the liver can be as inconsequential as a minor self-limiting laceration or as severe as exsanguinating hemorrhage from major vessels.

DIAGNOSIS. Injuries to the liver frequently result from a direct crushing force to the right upper quadrant of the chest with fractures of the ninth to the twelfth ribs on the right (see Figs. 40-8 and 40-13) or laceration of the diaphragm. Right-upper-quadrant pain and evidence of intraabdominal bleeding are the signs of liver injury. Like the spleen, the liver can contain a subcapsular hematoma. In stable patients, an abdominal CT scan is the diagnostic method of choice.

MANAGEMENT. When the liver has ruptured, laparotomy is necessary to control bleeding and to debride devitalized parenchyma. Small cracks in the liver capsule can be treated by simple drainage. Controlling bleeding from tears in the liver parenchyma, the porta hepatis, and the hepatic veins where they join the inferior vena cava may be difficult.

PROGNOSIS. Patients who have small injuries with all nonviable tissue removed have an excellent prognosis. Patients who have more complex injuries that require debridement of large portions of the liver and are associated with trauma to other organs have a high mortality.

Duodenum and Pancreas

The duodenum and pancreas are usually damaged when forces crush them against the rigid vertebral column. Death is common unless the injury is treated promptly.

DIAGNOSIS. Establishing the diagnosis of duodenal or pancreatic injury may be difficult. Because the organs are retroperitoneal, the usual signs of intraperitoneal bleeding may be absent.

In a stable patient, an abdominal CT scan with GI contrast is the initial study of choice. If duodenal rupture (i.e., retroperitoneal air on a plain film or increased serum amylase) is suspected, water-soluble contrast material should be used. An upper-GI series with water-soluble contrast may follow.

Elevation of the serum amylase can indicate pancreatic trauma, but the amylase may be normal if only the duodenum is ruptured. Signs and symptoms, when they do appear, may be delayed for 12 to 24 hours, and peritoneal lavage may be negative.

Pancreatography can often be performed at the time of operation by injection of contrast into the gallbladder. If this is unsuccessful, the ampulla can be cannulated directly through a duodenotomy.

MANAGEMENT. A distal pancreatectomy or a pancreaticoduodenectomy is sometimes necessary for the treatment of major injuries to the pancreas or duodenum, or both. The hematoma that occasionally develops in the duodenum from an injury that is less than transmural may show up as a gastric outlet obstruction several days after the accident as bowel sounds return and oral alimentation resumes. Only nasogastric suction and supportive care are required to treat a patient with a hematoma.

PROGNOSIS. The high mortality associated with pancreaticoduodenal injuries is in part a result of massive trauma involving other systems, especially the brain, and of delays in diagnosis.

Small and Large Intestines

Trauma can perforate the bowel or shear it from the mesenteric vessels. Perforation usually results from a direct crushing force that pinches the bowel against the vertebral column or from high pressures that develop suddenly within an air-filled loop and cause a blowout. The colon can be punctured by a spicule of bone from a pelvic fracture. Shearing injuries are produced by decelerating forces and are frequently associated with wearing seat belts.

DIAGNOSIS. Perforation of the bowel is usually detectable early. Signs of peritoneal irritation are manifested soon after the accident, and free intraperitoneal air is seen on x-ray films. Perforation from the ischemic bowel that has been sheared from the mesenteric vessels may not occur for several days.

MANAGEMENT. Surgery is always necessary for intestinal rupture. If the pelvis is fractured and laceration of the rectum is even suspected, a colostomy is necessary to divert the fecal stream because the contamination of a pelvic hematoma is frequently fatal.

PROGNOSIS. Patients who have isolated injuries of the small intestine or colon have a good prognosis. The prognosis is more guarded when intestinal injury is associated with trauma to other systems.

PENETRATING INJURIES

Gunshot Wounds

The prevalent use of handguns is distressing but persistent. The severity of a gunshot wound depends on the energy expended by the bullet as it passes through the tissue. The expended energy is related to the velocity, weight of the missile, and the tendency of the missile to deform. Soft-nose bullets become deformed and expend all of their energy before exiting, whereas steel-jacketed bullets can pass easily through the tissues, giving up less energy and causing less injury. The velocity of the bullet is inversely related to the distance from the gun. The bullet's weight generally increases with increasing caliber. Shotguns present a different problem in that the pellet pattern is tightly grouped at short range but rapidly widens, and the energy rapidly decreases as the distance from the gun increases. Whereas shotgun wounds inflicted at close range are devastating, shotgun wounds from 55 m away may be trivial at the edge of the pattern. In addition to the pellets, shotgun wounds may contain the paper or plastic wadding. At close range, shotgun wounds can cause a major tissue loss from the abdominal wall, resulting in external blood loss as well as evisceration of abdominal contents. Bullets are sterilized by the heat generated in passage through the weapon and the air, and they need not be retrieved from a patient simply because they are foreign bodies.

Assessment

Initially, it is safest to assume that a bullet wound of the trunk may have injured anything in the abdominal or thoracic cavities. The physician's priorities are for airway maintenance, ventilatory stability, and blood volume support. From knowledge of the caliber of the weapon, the position of the patient, and the distance from the weapon, inferences can be made regarding the extent of injury.

Bullet wounds of the lower part of the chest are difficult to evaluate. During expiration, the dome of the diaphragm can rise as high as the fourth interspace and bullets that enter the chest can penetrate the peritoneal cavity through the diaphragm. When the patient is stable, the entrance and exit wounds can be marked with radiopaque markers for comparison with the level of the diaphragm on inspiratory and expiratory chest films. Peritoneal lavage may be helpful to establish the diagnosis of peritoneal penetration in the patient who has been shot in the lower part of the chest. The consulting surgeon can perform a peritoneal lavage either in the operating room if the patient is undergoing thoracotomy or in the emergency department if the chest injury is not severe enough to require a thoracotomy.

The other major preoperative diagnostic problem is whether the kidneys and ureter have been damaged in the retroperitoneum. Injuries to the bladder are usually apparent when the abdomen is explored. It is preferable not to explore the retroperitoneum; consequently, preoperative knowledge that the urinary tract is uninjured may obviate the need to explore that area. In the stable patient with adequate renal perfusion, an intravenous urogram can be ordered by the consultant in order to simplify the operation.

Since injuries to the colon are likely, patients should be advised of the possibility of a temporary colostomy.

Management and Prognosis

All patients who are shot in the abdomen should have an exploratory laparotomy. Intraoperative management consists of inspection and repair of all damaged organs.

Patients who survive long enough to reach the operating room will usually survive the injury. The mortality for intraabdominal injuries from gunshot wounds is about 12 percent. Death is usually caused by blood loss in patients who never reach the operating room or are in refractory shock from major-vessel injury when they do reach the operating room.

Stab Wounds of the Abdomen

Many stab wounds do not penetrate the peritoneal cavity, and many wounds that do penetrate the peritoneum do not injure the abdominal contents. Except for gaping wounds with protruding intestines or omentum, the size and characteristics of the entrance wound give no information regarding possible visceral injury. The length of the weapon and the force with which it was wielded determine the potential for injury.

Assessment and Management

The physical examination of patients with stab wounds is confusing because there is always some tenderness and rigidity around the entrance site whether or not peritoneal irritation is present. Tenderness at a distance from a stab wound can increase. Most surgeons now have a selective policy on exploring stab wounds to the abdomen. Many wounds in asymptomatic patients can be explored in the emergency department with the patient under local anesthesia. Wounds that penetrate the fascia can be taken to the operating room for exploration. In stable patients with wounds lateral to the anterior axillary line, a contrast-enhanced CT scan can help select injuries that require exploration. Until better guidelines are available for selecting patients to be managed without surgery, laparotomy and closure of perforated bowel appear to be the safest course of action.

Gastroscopy

Fiberoptic gastroscopy also carries a small risk of perforation. Some patients with free air in the peritoneal cavity after fiberoptic gastroscopy fail to demonstrate extravasation when radiologic studies are made with a water-soluble contrast medium, and no perforation is found in some patients who undergo laparotomy. Because the stomach is empty during endoscopy and because gastric juice is sterile, small perforations of the stomach can frequently be managed with nasogastric suction and antibiotics. However, if an endoscope is passed through a tear in the stomach, laparotomy to close such a large perforation is advisable.

Needle Biopsies or Cholangiography

Needle biopsies of the liver or kidneys can cause intraperitoneal bleeding that should be treated with transfusion and observation. If the transfusion requirement exceeds three units, laparotomy is indicated. Percutaneous cholangiography carries the added risk of bile leakage from penetration of distended biliary radicles.

SELECTED READING

Blaisdell, F N, and Trunkey, D D. *Trauma Management*, vol 1. New York: Thieme-Stratton, 1982.

Cook, D E, et al. Upper abdominal trauma: Pitfalls in CT diagnosis. *Radiology* 159:65, 1986.

Dauterive, A H, Flanebaum, L, and Cox, E F. Blunt intestinal trauma. A modern-day review. *Ann Surg* 201:198, 1985.

Davis, J J, Cohn, I, and Nance, F C. Diagnosis and management of blunt abdominal trauma. *Ann Surg* 183:672, 1976.

Ecker, M D, et al. Benign pneumoperitoneum after fiberoptic colonoscopy. *Gastroenterology* 73:226, 1977.

Fabian, T C, et al. A prospective study of 91 patients undergoing both computed tomography and peritoneal lavage. *J Trauma* 26:602, 1986.

Federle, M P, et al. Evaluation of abdominal trauma by computed tomography. *Radiology* 138:637–644, 1981.

Lucas, C E. The role of peritoneal lavage for penetrating abdominal wounds. *J Trauma* 17:649, 1977.

Luna, G, and Dellinger, E P. Nonoperative observation therapy for splenic injuries. *Am J Surg* 153:462, 1987.

Mattos, R L, Moore, E D, and Feliciano, D V. *Trauma.* Norwalk, CT: Appleton & Lange, 1988.

Maynard, A de L, and Oropeza, G. Mandatory operation for penetrating wounds of the abdomen. *Am J Surg* 115:307, 1968.

McLelland, B A, et al. Analysis of peritoneal lavage parameters in blunt abdominal trauma. *J Trauma* 25:393, 1985.

Parvin, S, et al. Effectiveness of peritoneal lavage in blunt trauma. *Ann Surg* 181:255, 1975.

Root, H D, et al. Diagnostic peritoneal lavage. *Surgery* 57:633, 1965.

Shafton, G W. Indications for operation in abdominal trauma. *Am J Surg* 99:657, 1960.

Shires, G T, et al. Trauma. In S I Schwartz (ed), *Principles of Surgery* (5th ed). New York: McGraw-Hill, 1989.

Tom, W W, et al. A nonoperative approach to the adult ruptured spleen sustained from blunt trauma. *Am Surg* 51:367, 1985.

Trunkey, D D, and Lewis, F R. *Current Therapy of Trauma 1984–85. Abdominal Trauma.* Philadelphia: B. C. Decker, 1984.

62. Genitourinary Injuries

Gary P. Kearney
Charles E. Horton, Jr.
David Allegra

The management of genitourinary injuries has undergone significant change since the publication of the first edition. Board-certified emergency physicians and dedicated trauma surgeons have greatly improved the quality of emergency care, and more lives are being saved. Abdominal computed tomographic (CT) scanning has replaced conventional intravenous urography to define renal injury with increased sensitivity while at the same time ruling out other intraabdominal injury. This chapter will review genitourinary trauma and the recent urologic literature, with emphasis on the treatment of injuries to the upper urinary tract, bladder, urethra, and genitalia.

KIDNEY INJURY

The individuals who are most likely to sustain genitourinary injuries are generally male and young. There has been a substantial decrease in mortality due to renal injuries over the past three decades. In large part, this is a result of the overall management of abdominal trauma rather than specific problems associated with injury to the kidney itself. Renal trauma alone rarely causes death. An individual who demonstrates abnormal physical findings in the back, flank, abdomen, pelvis, genitalia, or perineum should be suspected of having sustained injury to the urinary tract. Any individual who demonstrates hematuria, abnormal urinary output, an abdominal mass, or a penetrating wound, or who is struck by an automobile, requires a urologic evaluation.

Approximately 90 percent of all kidney injuries are the result of blunt injury and only 10 percent are from penetrating trauma. Nunn classified renal injuries into five categories based on the clinical radiographic findings. While these classifications are of interest, only class IV, a complete fracture of the kidney, and class V, a vascular pedicle injury, are of importance in terms of management since the lesser classifications can all be treated expectantly.

Blunt Renal Injury

It has been well established that blunt renal trauma can be managed in a conservative fashion. Recent trends are away from diagnostic studies for minor degrees of microscopic hematuria. Klein and associates performed a retrospective analysis of 134 patients and correlated the findings of intravenous pyelography (IVP) and nephrotomography with the magnitude of hematuria on urinalysis, associated injuries, management, and outcome. They concluded that IVP and nephrotomography should be reserved for patients with greater than 30 red cells per high-powered field on admission urinalysis.

Hardeman and associates prospectively evaluated 506 consecutive patients with blunt trauma and hematuria. All patients underwent excretory urography (EU); of the 506 patients, 25 had detectable urinary tract injuries that were confirmed either by initial studies or by CT, angiography, or direct intraoperative inspection. Diagnoses included seven renal contusions; seven renal lacerations (one major and six minor); one renal artery, three intraperitoneal bladder, and five extraperitoneal bladder ruptures; and two urethral injuries. Of the 25 patients, 21, including all of those with lower urinary tract injuries, had gross hematuria. One of 4 patients with microscopic hematuria was hospitalized in shock; of the remaining 3 patients, with no shock, 1 had a minor renal laceration and 2 had renal contusions. All 3 patients were managed conservatively and all 3 were hospitalized, chiefly for nonurologic injuries. If the patients with microscopic hematuria and no shock were excluded from the initial radiographic evaluation, one minor renal laceration and two renal contusions would have been missed. The message taken from these studies is that if radiographic imaging is deferred for patients with minor degrees of microscopic hematuria who are clinically well, operative injury will not be missed.

Urologic Imaging

If urologic imaging of the upper urinary tract is indicated, obtaining an IVP with nephrotomography or abdominal CT scan has been recommended. Halsell and associates performed prospective studies designed to evaluate the reliability of excretory urography (EU) in excluding renal damage in patients with blunt abdominal trauma, using contrast-enhanced CT (CECT) as the "gold standard" of diagnostic studies. Sixty patients with indications for genitourinary evaluation and with a normal EU underwent CECT. Five renal injuries were demonstrated by CECT in patients with a normal EU: one contusion, one subcapsular hematoma, two perirenal hematomas, and one renal laceration. All of these lesions resolved with conservative management. The conclusion was that CECT did not alter treatment for these five patients, but, CECT was more sensitive than EU.

The advantage of abdominal CT scanning is that it provides significant information regarding other intraabdominal organs, such as the liver and spleen, that conventional EU would not. Meredith and Trunkey have concluded that CT scanning has become an important adjunct in the evaluation of patients with blunt abdominal trauma. It provides quantitative information about hemoperitoneum as well as qualitative information about its source (Fig. 62-1). Computed tomographic scanning also evaluates retroperitoneal organs and retroperitoneal hematoma more accurately than other available imaging techniques. Like any other diagnostic tool, the CT scan must not be overutilized or abused. This technique should be applied only to stable patients in institutions with up-to-date equipment in the CT scan suite and a committed radiologic-surgical staff. If proper techique is used, high-quality scans can be obtained that, if interpreted by experienced personnel in the light of clinical findings, can improve the management of selected trauma patients.

The CT scan has also been used to distinguish between urinary extravasation due to ureteropelvic disruption secondary to blunt trauma and renal parenchymal injury (Fig. 62-2). In three cases of isolated ureteropelvic disruption, the renal parenchyma was intact, contrast medium excretion was normal, and no perinephric hematoma was present. Contrast medium extravasation was confined predominantly to the medial perirenal space. The ipsilateral ureter was not opacified in three of the four cases of ureteropelvic disruption. The authors believed that, when these findings are present on CT scan performed for trauma, the diagnosis of ureteral disruption can be made (Fig. 62-3). Hematuria from trauma in the pediatric patient differs from that in the adult population only in its higher incidence of anomalies (i.e., congenital ureteropelvic junction obstruction).

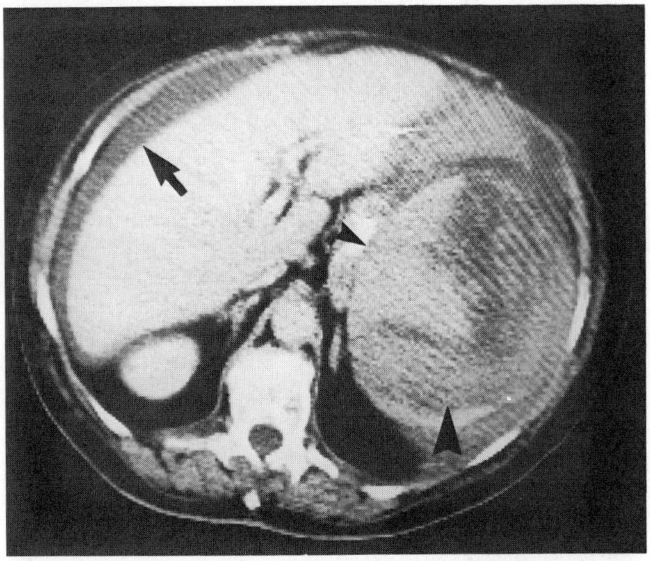

Fig. 62-1. Unsuspected splenic laceration is identified on upper abdominal slices. Enhancing splenic parenchyma (*small arrowhead*), subcapsular hematoma (*large arrowhead*), and a moderate amount of hemoperitoneum (*arrow*) are seen.

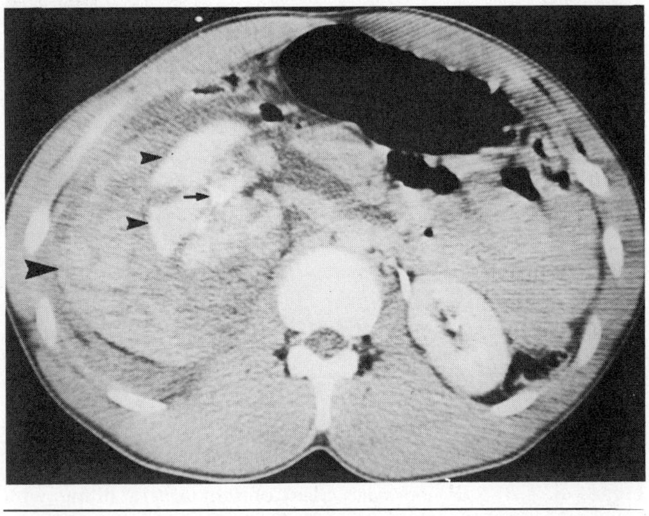

Fig. 62-2. Contrast-enhanced CT demonstrates upper pole parenchymal "fracture" (*small arrowheads*), with contrast excretion seen in the collecting system (*arrow*), and perinephric hematoma (*large arrowhead*).

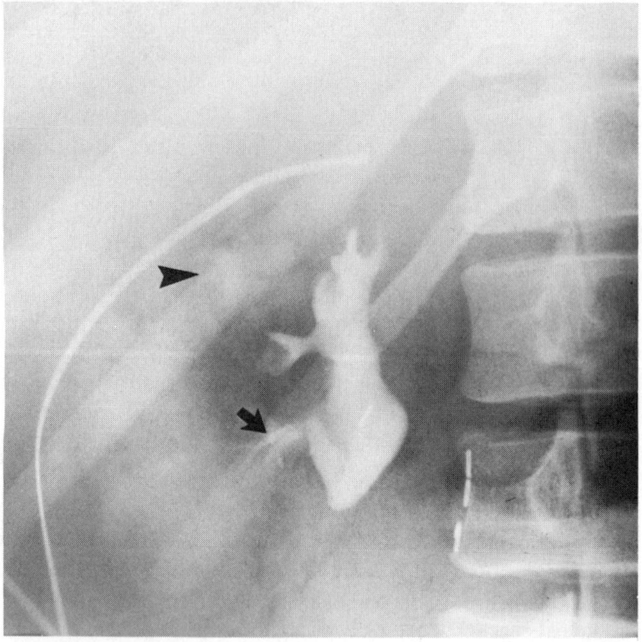

A

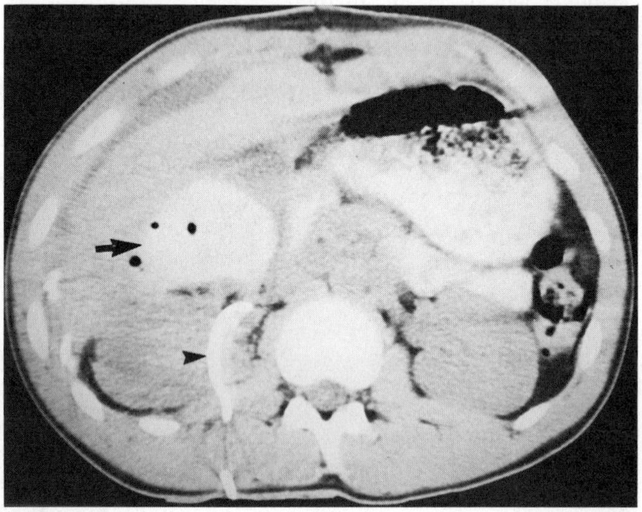

B

Fig. 62-3. A. IVP demonstrates a lack of right ureteral filling, with contrast extravasation (*arrowhead*) and reabsorption of contrast into renal veins (*arrow*). B. Delayed CT scan reveals large collection of extravasated contrast anterior to the right kidney (*arrow*). A nephrostomy tube has been placed (*arrowhead*).

Management

Renal artery thrombosis remains a rare complication of blunt abdominal trauma; however, controversy exists as to whether early surgical intervention will improve renal salvage. In patients with a solitary kidney or with a bilateral injury, intervention may be appropriate, whereas in patients with two functioning kidneys, conservative therapy is indicated. In an effort to resolve the controversy, Spirnak and Resnick reviewed the literature on injuries due to blunt trauma that resulted in complete occlusion of the renal artery documented by roentgenographic means. Avulsion injuries

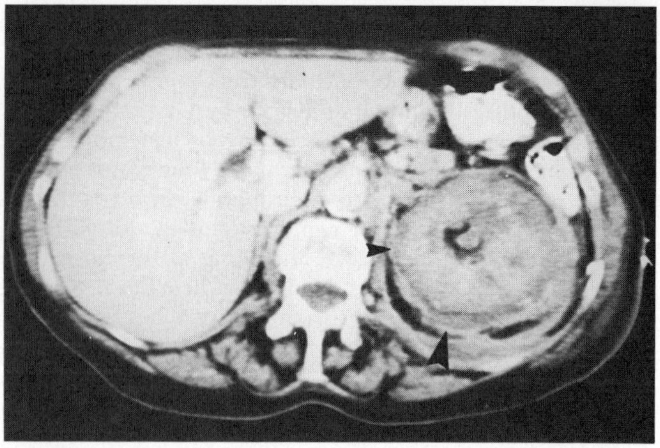

Fig. 62-4. Contrast CT scan demonstrates a swollen, nonenhancing left kidney (*small arrowhead*) compatible with renal infarction. A small amount of perinephric fluid is present (*large arrowhead*).

and incomplete occlusion or branch artery injuries were excluded. To be classified as a surgical success, postoperative documentation of renal function and a patent renal artery were required. Nine successfully performed vascularization procedures were identified. There were four instances of bilateral obstruction with a postoperative serum creatinine level ranging between 1.7 mg/dl and 7.1 mg/dl. All required postoperative dialysis, ranging from three days to three months. Thirty-five patients with unilaterally obstructed renal arteries underwent attempted revascularization. Five patients, all with presumed ischemic time of less than 12 hours, had successful outcomes. Postoperatively, four patients demonstrated either a decrease in size or function of the injured kidney. Thirteen patients eventually required nephrectomy. Revascularization in unilateral obstructed renal arteries has approximately a 14 percent success rate, although of these successes, the majority will have some evidence of decreased function.

Meyrier and associates reported severe hypertension in four patients who sustained blunt renal trauma 2 to 32 years previously. A protracted period of normal blood pressure separated the renal injury from the onset of hypertension. Angiography disclosed lesions that had been previously underestimated by IVP. These lesions consisted of traumatic dissection of branches of the renal artery, leading to renal infarct (Fig. 62-4). In three cases, unilateral high renin secretion was demonstrated. In one case this was confirmed by immunofluorescence with an antirenin antiserum, which demonstrated abundant renin granules within the infarcted zone. In all patients, total or polar nephrectomy was followed by return of blood pressure to normal or near normal levels. This report emphasizes the importance of evaluating patients with significant renal trauma over prolonged periods of time. Hypertension can be caused by arteriovenous fistulas (Fig. 62-5), ureteropelvic junction obstruction with hydronephrosis, infundibular stricture with partial hydronephrosis, or perinephric scarring, in addition to narrowing of the renal vasculature.

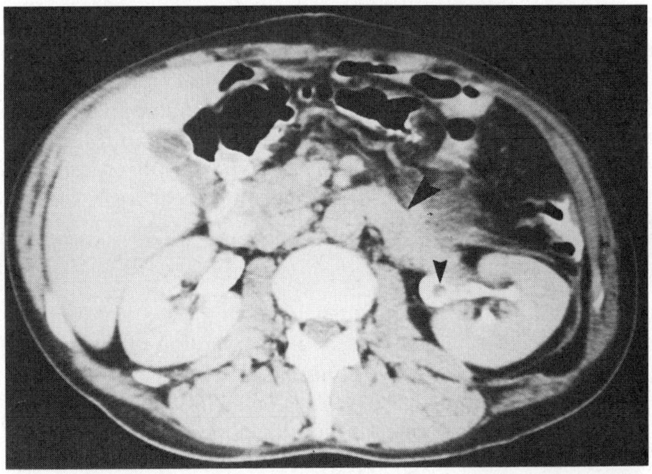

A

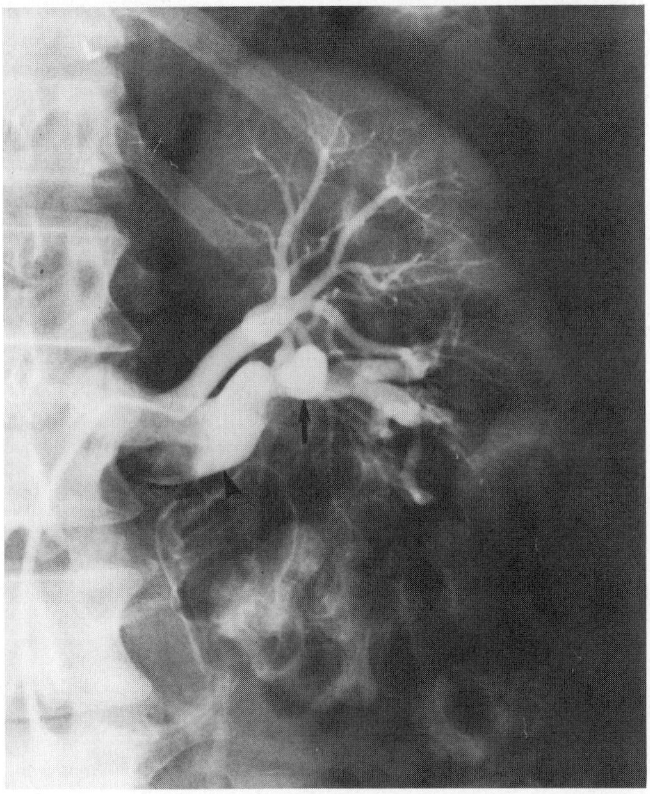

B

Fig. 62-5. A. Contrast CT demonstrates normal parenchymal enhancement, with clot in collecting system (*small arrowhead*) and enlarged left renal vein (*large arrowhead*), a clue to the presence of an arteriovenous fistula. B. Selective arteriogram demonstrates site of fistula (*arrow*) with early draining vein that is enlarged (*arrowhead*).

Penetrating Renal Injuries

In assessing patients in the emergency department, it is important to note that of those patients with renal trauma, 80 percent had an associated injury; 65 percent were of the musculoskeletal system, whereas one-third were injuries involving the liver, spleen, colon, stomach, chest, pancreas, small intestine, duodenum, and great vessels. Injuries occurring above the hepatoduodenal ligament carry the highest mortality.

Deaths from genitourinary trauma occur generally in patients with multiple injuries. In four reported cases, one death occurred early in the postinjury period from continued severe hemorrhage resulting from a ruptured kidney that was managed conservatively; the remaining three died six to eight weeks after injury from sepsis with a pelvic abscess secondary to a ruptured urethra or bladder.

Delayed hypertension occurring in renal trauma can be seen with Goldblatt or Page kidneys. The Goldblatt kidney is one with a narrowed major renal vessel and a Page kidney (Fig. 62-6) is one with a subcapsular lesion that causes hypertension from parenchymal compression.

Computed Tomography

Federle and associates reviewed 27 consecutive patients with stab wounds to the back and flank who were thought to be at risk for renal injury. Twenty-two patients were studied by CT, 11 by excretory urography, and 3 by angiography. No correlation was found between the presence and amount of hematuria and the extent of renal injury. Computed tomography gave an accurate assessment of the extent of parenchymal injuries, perirenal hemorrhage, extravasation of urine, and extrarenal injuries. Excretory urography was of little use because the extent of renal parenchymal injury was underestimated, overestimated, or indeterminate in many cases. Angiography was rarely required to better define renal vascular injuries. Only 7 of the 27 patients required surgical repair. The 20 patients managed nonoperatively included 7 patients with renal lacerations, considered minor by CT scan. The authors concluded that most patients with penetrating renal trauma did not require surgical exploration and that a combination of clinical evaluation and CT scan criteria allowed confident management in all cases.

If indications for contrast imaging of the urinary tract are present, the patient must be stable, not in shock, without severe volume depletion, and without significant preexisting renal disease that would render the patient more susceptible to renal failure with the infusion of contrast material. Noniodinated contrast media are currently not indicated unless the patient has a history of severe anaphylaxis.

Patients who are at increased risk for developing contrast material nephropathy include those with preexisting renal disease, multiple myeloma, diabetes mellitus, shock, and dehydration. Possible mechanisms that can lead to renal failure include tubular toxicity, renal ischemia, intertubular obstruction, and unknown immunologic factors.

Noncontrast CT scan in the unstable patient can provide valuable information while stabilization is awaited. In this setting, the need for surgical exploration after initial resuscitation may be necessary, with intraoperative imaging carried out.

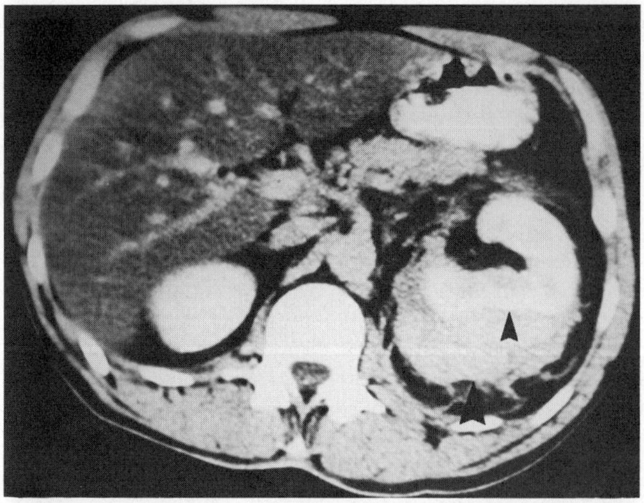

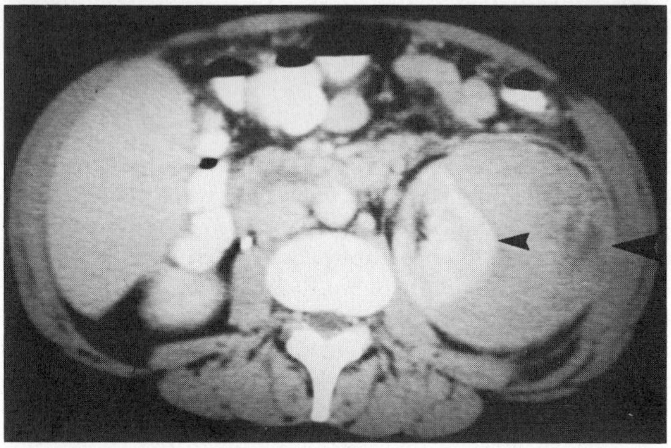

Fig. 62-6. Two patients with contrast CT scans demonstrating perinephric hematoma (*large arrowheads*), with compression of the enhancing renal parenchyma (*small arrowheads*).

With urography the infusion of 1 ml/kg body weight of 30% iodinated contrast is frequently utilized. For adults, 100 ml 60% solution of meglutamine diatrizoate (Renografin) can be used; for children, 2 ml/kg body weight of 50% sodium diatrizoate (Hypaque) is recommended. Films should be taken at 1-minute intervals for nephrographic visualization of the renal cortex and at 5-, 15-, and 20-minute intervals for excretion of contrast from the collecting system and to rule out extravasation from the upper urinary tracts.

Selective renal arteriography for the upper urinary tract may be required to define the anatomy, especially in the patient with a solitary kidney and as a road map for delayed exploration for severe renal laceration. Cystoscopy and retrograde pyelography are rarely indicated for the evaluation and management of renal injury.

Magnetic Resonance Imaging

The role of magnetic resonance imaging in the management of trauma with genitourinary patients is undergoing study. There does not appear to be any significant advantage of this technology over CT at the present time in the management of patients with renal trauma.

Renal Scan

Renal scan and ultrasonography are generally not used for the emergency evaluation of patients with renal trauma but can be excellent tools for evaluating and following the presence of perinephric hematomas or urinomas in patients who are observed with nonsurgical management in mind. Renal scan is also useful for mapping out blood supply to the various parts of the kidney and for detecting recovery or loss of function of renal parenchyma.

Management

Until recently, the management of penetrating trauma has been exploration. If early surgical intervention of the kidney is carried out, the nephrectomy rate is higher than when operation is delayed.

Advocates of early intervention for patients with deep parenchymal or collecting system lacerations believe that a significant decrease in complications can be achieved. They believe that by excising and debriding devitalized tissue and draining extravasated urine and blood, complications are decreased, healing is more rapid, and hospitalization is shortened.

In a combined series of three authors, 81 percent of 120 patients with penetrating injury underwent operation; 35 percent required nephrectomy in the aggressively managed group, whereas only 6 percent needed nephrectomy in the conservatively treated group. It should be pointed out that the aggressively managed series of patients were treated in the 1950s and the conservatively treated group in the mid-1970s.

In summary, most patients with renal trauma have minor injuries and can be treated conservatively. Of those patients with severe hematuria, complete renal fracture, or vascular pedicle injury, 5 to 10 percent will require immediate operation, and the remainder can be observed or undergo delayed exploration, depending on surgical judgment. The management goal of operative intervention for renal trauma is to maximize renal preservation of tissue and function without adding to the morbidity in patients who have associated abdominal injuries.

URETERAL INJURY

Most ureteral injuries, either from blunt trauma or penetrating wounds, are seen infrequently, are iatrogenic, and occur during operative surgery. Most often, these injuries are of gynecologic origin. The close proximity of the urinary tract to organs of the female reproductive system often results in injury to urinary tract structures during extirpative surgery for gynecologic cancers. Hysterectomy carries the risk of both ureteral and bladder trauma. During radical (Wertheim's) hysterectomy, the ureters are injured in a small percentage of cases. Ureterovaginal fistulas also can occur; they can have a delayed presentation and may be seen in the emergency department weeks after initial operation. When external ureteral injury occurs, frequent multiple body injuries are associated with it, involving the small bowel, colon, and fracture of the bony pelvis with or without vascular involvement. It is of interest that the gastrointestinal tract is involved over 50 percent of the time when the ureter is injured.

A penetrating ureteral injury is more common than a

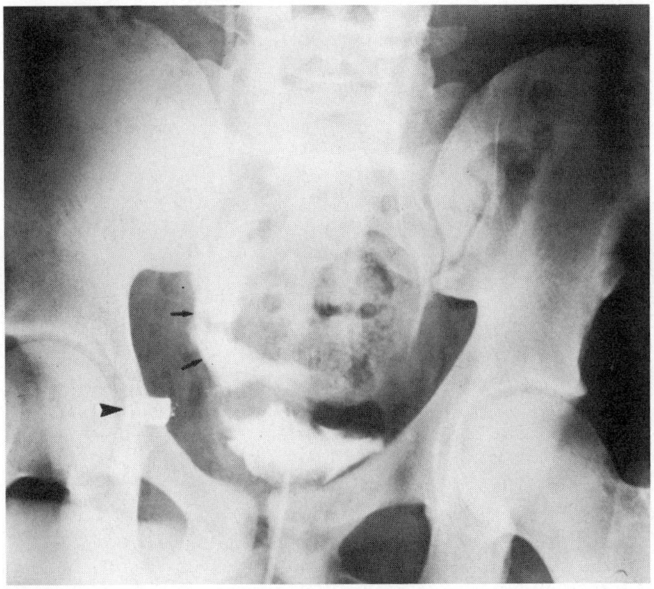

Fig. 62-7. Intravenous pyelography demonstrates extravasation of contrast at the distal right ureter (*arrows*). Ureteral laceration was due to gunshot wound (*arrowhead* points to bullet).

blunt injury. As might be anticipated, most ureteral injuries occur with military operations. The difficulty with ureteral injury is that frequently few symptoms are present. Injury to the ureter in the upper abdomen occurs from penetrating trauma, such as a gunshot or a knife wound (Fig. 62-7). Closed blunt trauma resulting in ureteral injury is less common and is caused by compression of the ureter against the spinal column, as in an automobile injury or lateral flexion of the trunk. Experimental studies have shown that an automobile rolling over the abdomen causes injury at the level of L2 through L4. In pelvic fractures, the ureter is injured at the pelvic brim, where its intimate relationship with the bone can cause contusion or puncture by fragments or avulsion. In a large series, only one-third of the patients showed no hematuria, 28 percent had microscopic hematuria, and the remainder had gross hematuria.

Since most ureteral injuries are associated with abdominal injury, early recognition is rare unless it is diligently searched for. It is not uncommon for recognition to result from complications that arise after failure to diagnose the primary ureteral injury, such as expanding retroperitoneal urinoma, fever, or urocutaneous fistula occurring at an exit point of a gunshot or knife wound. A mass in the abdomen associated with fever, chills, urgency of urination, and abnormalities of urinary sediment should raise the suspicion of a ureteral injury.

When there is clinical suspicion of a ureteral injury, an IVP should be obtained. Because of fluid resuscitation of the injured patient, concentration and opacification of the collecting system may be poor, especially when the injury is at the ureteropelvic junction. Extravasation of contrast can occur within Gerota's fascia around the kidney, which would suggest laceration of the kidney, renal parenchyma, or pelvis. In this setting, in a stable patient in whom suspicion cannot be confirmed by intravenous urography, cystoscopic examination with a retrograde pyelogram may be necessary to define the anatomy. Nephrotomography with high-dose contrast can avoid this intervention.

Whenever ureteral disruption is present, surgical intervention is required. Franco and associates reported 21 cases of penetrating trauma, 17 gunshot wounds and 4 stab wounds seen in a New York hospital over a nine-year period. Early urologic complications included urocutaneous fistula. Reoperative surgery was required in 50 percent of patients with a proximal ureteral injury but was less common when nephrostomy and stent were utilized at the time of repair. This review also confirmed that stenting with nephrostomy reduced a 91 percent complication rate to 15 percent in the upper ureter. The difference between stenting and nephrostomy was less obvious in midureteral injuries, in which the rate of urologic complications was lower. Repair of proximal, penetrating ureteral injuries should include stenting and nephrostomy as well as a generous debridement, watertight closure, and retroperitoneal drainage of any ureteral injury. Surgical options for "bridging the ureteral gap" are many and are often dictated by the level and extent of ureteral injury. Options for primary repair include ureteroureterostomy, ureteroneocystostomy with or without bladder flap, and transureteroureterostomy. If the injury is extensive, proximal diversion via nephrostomy tube for four to six weeks and subsequent ureteral replacement with ileum or renal autotransplantation may be required. Associated injuries of the gastrointestinal, pancreatic, and major vascular structures, regardless of location, also argue for proximal diversion and ureteral stenting.

A 15-year personal experience by Peterson and Schulze evaluating 157 penetrating and 225 blunt urologic injuries included 2 instances of simultaneous upper and lower tract involvement, for a 0.5 percent incidence rate. Review of 750 cases in the urologic literature yielded 17 patients with simultaneous upper and lower urinary tract injuries, for an incidence rate of 0.6 percent. In all but one of these 17 patients, injury was caused by blunt trauma. This suggests that comprehensive radiologic evaluation of hematuria in patients with blunt injury may be unnecessarily expensive and that one should routinely limit evaluation in the areas of maximum injury rather than evaluating areas not obviously involved by the trauma. There is abundant literature indicating that delay in diagnosis results in nephroureterectomy in a majority of cases.

A separate review by Peters in 1976 revealed that a significant percentage of ureteral injuries were unrecognized, with the patient discharged from the hospital without a diagnosis being made. This fact emphasizes to emergency department personnel that patients with abdominal trauma, fever, and flank mass should be evaluated for ureteral injury.

BLADDER INJURY

Most bladder injuries occur in patients with a distended bladder and result from blunt trauma following pelvic compression from automobile accidents, such as pedestrians being hit. When the bladder is not distended, it is well protected by the rectus abdominis anteriorly, the rectum, the coccyx, and the lateral pelvic sidewalls. When the bladder is full, it rises out of the pelvis. Compression of the anterior abdominal wall transmits pressure on the bladder, which

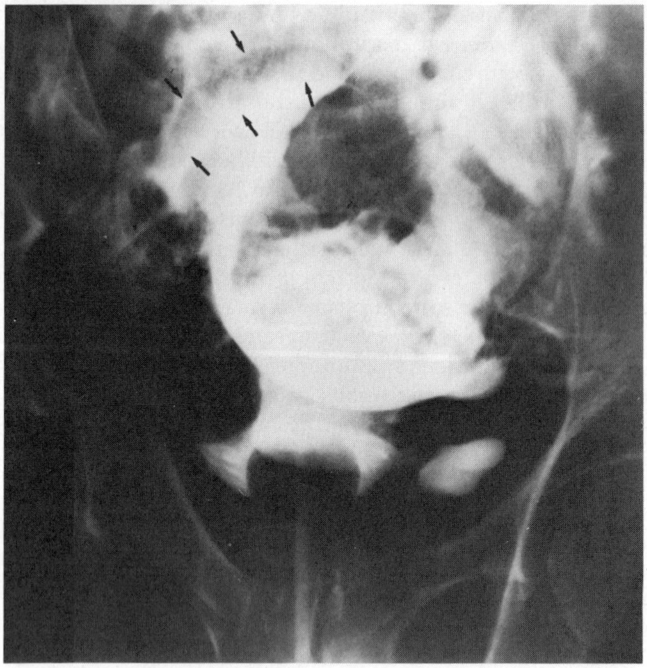

Fig. 62-8. Postdrainage cystogram film reveals both intra- and extraperitoneal rupture of the bladder. Bowel loop impression is seen on the extravasated contrast (*arrows*).

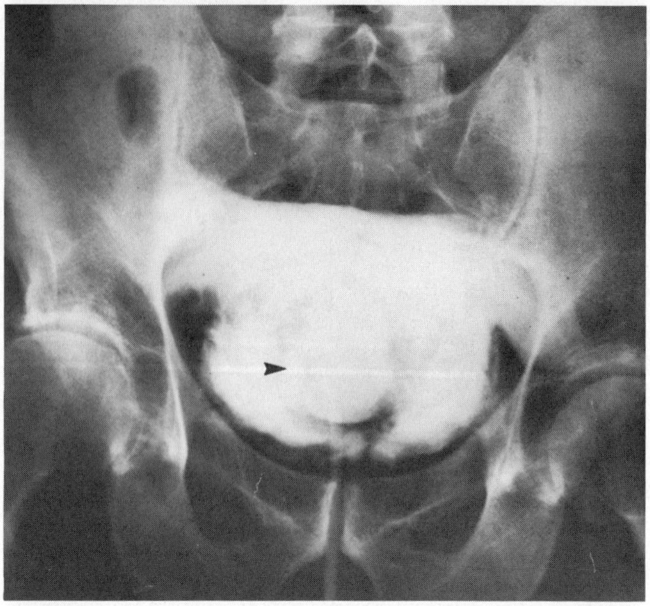

Fig. 62-9. Postdrainage cystogram film reveals an extraperitoneal rupture (*arrowhead*, bladder). Impression of bowel loops on the extravasated contrast is not seen. (Courtesy of Robert C. Sarno, MD, Department of Radiology, Tufts–New England Medical Center Hospital, Boston, MA.)

can result in a contusion or tear, causing intraperitoneal or extraperitoneal rupture or a combination of both injuries.

Intraperitoneal rupture of the bladder can be catastrophic and can result in pelvic peritonitis, and later abscess formation and death if it goes unrecognized (Fig. 62-8). Most intraperitoneal ruptures occur on the posterosuperior bladder wall where the peritoneum is attached.

Extraperitoneal bladder rupture occurs where the bladder is not covered by peritoneum, and extravasation can occur in any direction, including as high as the umbilicus and space of Retzius anteriorly and below to the anterior thigh (Fig. 62-9). Urine can dissect into the retroperitoneum, up and around the kidney, or pass to the sciatic notch, to the buttocks, to the obturator foramen, into the thighs, the inguinal region, or the scrotum. Undrained urine can result in absorption, suppuration, or even death.

Symptoms associated with intraperitoneal bladder rupture include suprapubic pain, peritoneal signs, ileus, or a strong desire to void. The pain is constant and hematuria is usually present. If these symptoms are unrecognized after 24 to 48 hours, the patient will become toxic and will show constitutional symptoms. In penetrating bladder injuries, associated visceral injuries involving the rectum, small bowel, and pelvic vessels should be considered. Extraperitoneal bladder rupture can present similar symptoms without peritoneal signs. Bimanual examination may reveal a mass containing extravasated blood in the urine. Combined intraperitoneal and extraperitoneal bladder rupture is relatively uncommon.

In a review of 100 cases of bladder rupture, the majority were due to blunt trauma. Of these ruptures, 62 were extraperitoneal, including 59 (95%) with associated pelvic fractures. Twelve patients had an associated urethral injury and five had a concomitant intraperitoneal bladder rupture. It is noteworthy that complex injuries with extravasation outside the perivesical space were noted in 42 percent of the patients. Forty-one of these patients were treated with catheter drainage alone and did well.

In another series of 164 cases of bladder rupture from external trauma, 145 (88%) patients suffered blunt trauma, 59 (36%) suffered intraperitoneal rupture, 93 (57%) had extraperitoneal rupture, and 12 (7%) experienced both types of rupture. Bladder perforation due to blunt trauma was caused by a compression-type injury in all patients with intraperitoneal rupture and in 24 percent of those with extraperitoneal rupture. In the remaining instances of extraperitoneal rupture, pelvic bone fragments corresponded to the site of injury. Nonoperative catheter management of extraperitoneal rupture was successful in most cases.

Assessment

Early diagnosis by the physician of the possibility of intraperitoneal bladder rupture is important. While uncommon, spontaneous or idiopathic rupture of the bladder has been reported 84 times without known trauma. The common cause in most of these cases was intraperitoneal rupture, with diagnosis being made at autopsy after surgical exploration. Indwelling Foley catheters, alcohol, medications such as bethanechol or methamphetamine, a neuropathic bladder, pseudodiverticulum, chronic infection, or a combination of these factors have been implicated as predisposing factors. The symptoms of pain, difficulty or inability to void, rigidity of the abdominal wall, and elevation of the blood urea should produce a high degree of clinical suspicion of intraperitoneal rupture.

Clinicians should suspect intraperitoneal rupture of the bladder in patients with pelvic or abdominal trauma in the presence of elevated blood urea nitrogen (BUN), potassium, abnormal serum creatinine, and decreased mean serum sodium levels. In reviewing 20 patients with intraperitoneal bladder rupture, Heyns and Rimington noted that patients seen more than 24 hours after intraperitoneal bladder rupture had increased serum urea, creatinine, and potassium levels and a decreased mean serum sodium and carbon dioxide content. After laparotomy and repair of the bladder rupture, the serum urea, creatinine, and BUN level abnormalities reversed themselves.

The diagnosis of intraperitoneal rupture can be difficult because of the presence of distended small-bowel loops. An opaque linear band outlining the peritoneal reflection, colon, spleen, diaphragm, or liver with dye between loops of small bowel indicates intraperitoneal rupture.

In cases of extraperitoneal rupture, the diagnostic study is the postdrain film after gravity cystography. In these cases, dye can be seen in streaks or lines with various patterns.

A "stress cystogram" in addition to the gravity cystogram is produced by adding 50 ml water-soluble contrast agent to the filled bladder, followed by a drain film. This may demonstrate a perforation that was not apparent on gravity cystogram alone because omentum or clot had sealed off the perforation.

Cystography

Once a urethral injury has been ruled out, a gravity cystogram is performed by filling the bladder with water-soluble contrast agent through a urethral catheter. Most important is obtaining anteroposterior, oblique, and lateral films when possible with the contrast-filled bladder. The most important film is the postdrain film to rule out extravesical extravasation. Cystography may demonstrate a normal bladder outline or teardrop-shaped bladder from compression of the lateral bladder wall by hematoma or urinoma, or both (Fig. 62-10).

Computed tomography in bladder rupture has diagnostic limitations, as illustrated by case reports by Mee and associates, in which a Foley catheter was inserted and clamped during CT to ensure bladder filling. In two patients, no opacified urinary extravasation was demonstrated in one and only subtle evidence was seen in the other. Cystography in these two patients subsequently revealed gross intraperitoneal extravasation of opacified urine in both. The authors concluded that retrograde cystography, including a drainage film of the distended bladder, remains the most reliable test in suspected bladder rupture.

Cystoscopy

Cystoscopy is rarely indicated in this setting. Minor injuries to the bladder without perforation that result in hematuria are treated with observation or catheter drainage after irrigation for clots until the urine becomes clear.

Since 10 percent of pelvic fractures have associated bladder injury, radiologic studies should be carried out to determine the presence or absence of bladder injury, especially in patients with hematuria. A plain film of the abdomen (KUB: kidneys, ureters, bladder) may show a diffuse ground-glass appearance of the pelvis, displacement of obturator flat line by pelvic hematoma, or one or more of the following: urinoma, ileus, fractured pelvis, or air within the bladder.

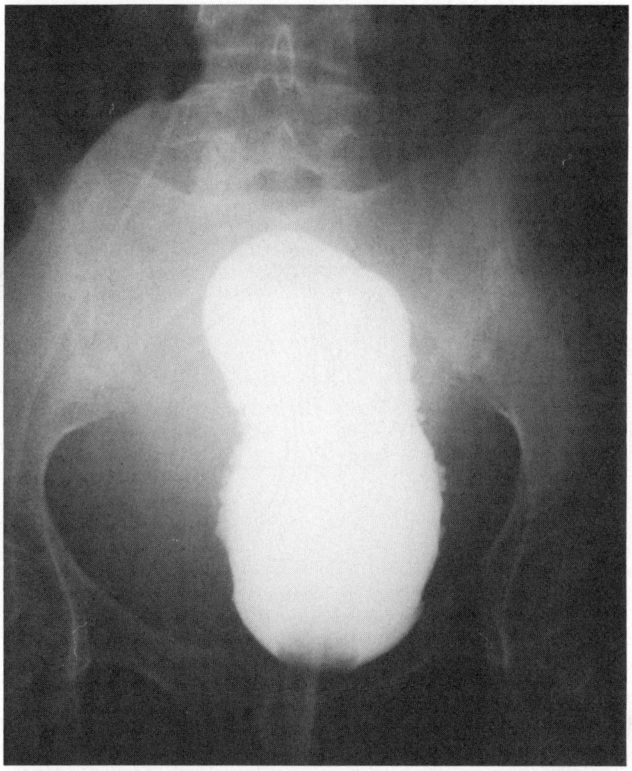

Fig. 62-10. Cystogram showing teardrop-shaped bladder from surrounding massive pelvic hematoma with intact urethra. (Courtesy of Robert C. Sarno, MD, Department of Radiology, Tufts–New England Medical Center Hospital, Boston, MA.)

In all patients with blood at the meatus in a setting of pelvic injury, one must consider that the urethra might be injured as well as the bladder. A sterile retrograde urethrogram with water-soluble contrast agent should be obtained to rule out urethral injury before a catheter is passed.

Management

Intraperitoneal rupture from an especially complex injury with intraabdominal trauma, such as rectal injury, and especially in the presence of major urethral injury should generally be treated with surgical repair and catheter drainage. When patients require operative management for blunt trauma, mortality related to associated injuries is high. Most blunt traumas result from motor vehicle accidents. Flancbaum and associates described 29 patients with multiple injuries who required operative treatment for blunt trauma. Motor vehicle accidents accounted for 86 percent of the injuries. Hypotension and gross hematuria were the most prevalent features, 68 and 97 percent, respectively. Pelvic fractures occurred in 93 percent of these patients and intraabdominal injuries in 48 percent. The majority (72%) of the bladder ruptures were intraperitoneal and mortality was high (34%), attesting to the magnitude of injury sustained by the patient.

There has been a significant trend away from operative intervention of extraperitoneal bladder rupture using cathe-

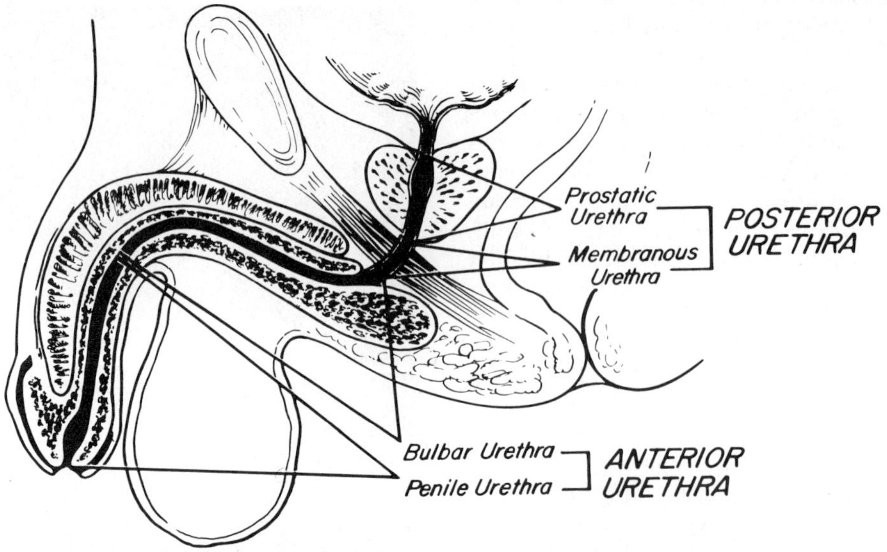

Fig. 62-11. Cross-sectional anatomy of normal male urethrae. Total rupture of urethrae generally occurs at junction of membranous and prostate urethra.

ter drainage, with excellent results. In patients with bladder perforation who have infected urine without associated rectal injury, percutaneous drainage of the prevesical space should be carried out. If any concomitant urethral or rectal injury is present, a suprapubic cystotomy should be considered. Patients with large extraperitoneal ruptures must be observed carefully for signs of sepsis. Prevesical drainage and antibiotics with or without suprapubic drainage should be considered until such time as the extraperitoneal rupture has closed, as proved by gravity cystography.

Patients who require prolonged catheter drainage for bladder injury are at risk of developing urethral stricture secondary to the Foley catheter. If prolonged bed rest in the male patient is anticipated, suprapubic drainage should be considered in significant pelvic trauma. Any prolonged period of catheter or suprapubic drainage can result in bladder calculi, with encrustations around the catheter or fractured bony spicules, or both, from pelvic fracture left within the bladder. Urethral stricture should be sought in the presence of abnormalities of urinary sediment six to eight weeks after removal of the suprapubic tube or Foley catheter.

The mortality associated with bladder ruptures has decreased significantly as a result of modern management techniques. Emergency physicians are cautioned that highest mortality occurs in patients in whom diagnosis is delayed because of an absent history of trauma.

URETHRAL INJURY

Injuries in the Male Patient

The male urethra is divided by an anatomic boundary of the urogenital diaphragm into the anterior and posterior urethrae. This fascial layer attaches anteriorly to the pubic symphysis and posterior to the perineal body and ischial tuberosities laterally to the inferior ischium. The posterior urethra lies within and above the urogenital diaphragm and includes the membranous and prostatic urethrae. The anterior urethra, located below the urogenital diaphragm, includes the bulbous and penile urethrae. The prostatic urethra attaches to the urogenital diaphragm and posterior pubic symphysis by the puboprostatic ligaments, which may be disrupted when laceration avulsion of the prostatic urethra is present (Fig. 62-11).

The mechanisms of injury involving the anterior and posterior urethrae are different, resulting in different clinical presentations, and are treated independently. Injuries that disrupt the urogenital diaphragm occur with the most severe pelvic trauma. Anterior bulbar urethral straddle injuries occur when the urethra is crushed between the inferior border of the pubis. This results in considerable pain and can cause bleeding at the meatus and perineal discomfort with swelling. Voiding may be impossible. Later, perineal edema, ecchymoses, and sepsis can occur as a result of extravasated urine within the penile shaft.

Assessment

The clinical presentation depends on whether Buck's fascia is intact. With disruption of this fascial covering, extravasated urine can extend superiorly on the abdominal wall under Scarpa's fascia up to the clavicles, or into the scrotum when Scarpa's is contiguous with Colles' fascia; however, the urine is limited from traveling inferiorly by attachment of Scarpa's fascia to the fascia lata. When Buck's fascia is not violated, the extravasated urine remains locally confined to the penile shaft.

Posterior urethral injuries are usually a result of the patient being struck by an automobile or suffering an injury from a motorcycle. These injuries are associated with pelvic fracture and can result in transection of the urethra at the prostatic apex. Blood is present in the urethral meatus and the patient is unable to void. A boggy, high-floating prostate from hematoma or extravasated urine has been described but is rarely clinically useful in confirming the diagnosis.

When posterior urethral injury is suggested by the presence of blood at the urethral meatus and the patient is unable to void, a retrograde urethrogram should be obtained before instrumentation unless intravenous urography demonstrates a high-riding bladder that confirms the diagnosis. Standard radiosoluble contrast agent, 10 to 20 ml, is drawn up in a syringe and injected into the urethral meatus under scrupulous sterile conditions for anterior, posterior, and oblique x-rays.

Urethral injuries are infrequent in genitourinary trauma, but when they involve massive pelvic trauma, the potential exists for significant morbidity as a result of urinary extravasation, unrecognized colon injury below the pelvic peritoneum, and massive pelvic bleeding, which can be difficult to control. The pelvic girdle is a stout ring of pelvic bones in the adult. The vascular supply to these bones themselves and to the extremities and pelvic viscera can result in massive retroperitoneal blood loss. Despite the fact that this is a major blood loss, it can be controlled arteriographically, and surgical intervention is rarely indicated. When the peritoneum is allowed to remain intact, minor degrees of pelvic bleeding will usually be tamponaded.

On examination pelvic fracture should be suspected when compression of the iliac wings, pressure on the symphysis pubis, or rotation of the hip causes pain. Fractures can sometimes be palpated on rectal or pelvic examination and the diagnosis confirmed by plain x-rays.

Management of Urethral Injuries

Posterior Urethral Injury

Injuries involving the posterior urethra often require surgical intervention. In abdominal injury, the majority of patients will be explored by the general surgeon and a suprapubic tube will be placed at that time. Percutaneous placement is possible but may be difficult when the bladder contour is abnormal because of associated pelvic hematoma, and great care must be taken to ensure proper placement.

Complications from posterior urethral injury include stricture, incontinence, and impotence. If the bladder neck is intact, urinary incontinence is generally not a problem. Stricture formation depends on the extent of urethral injury, the presence of infection, and the distance between the obstructed urethra and the normal urethra. Sexual function is influenced by factors that still remain unknown but damage to vessels and nerves, especially the pudendal arteries and the branches to the bulbocavernosus, cavernosal bodies, and deep penile artery, can affect erectile function. The pudendal nerve supplies sensation to the glans penis and motor function to the bulbocavernosus and ischiocavernosus muscles, while the autonomic sacral plexus, S2–S4, supplies the cavernous nerves responsible for erection. Fortunately, recent techniques using artificial erection with pharmacologically active drugs and state-of-the-art prosthetics provide options for individuals with sexual dysfunction after pelvic injury, which occurs most frequently in young men.

In patients with posterior urethral injury, anywhere from 30 to 50 percent of patients are either partially or totally impotent. There appears to be a higher incidence of sexual dysfunction with bilateral pelvic ramus fracture as opposed to impotence occurring after single pelvic fracture or symphyseal separation.

Urethral injuries from knives or guns are uncommon, but foreign body injury does occur in emotionally disturbed individuals. For example, safety pins, razor blades, and paper clips, which are removed cystoscopically or by urethrotomy, can result in urethral stricture formation.

Anterior Urethral Injury

When anterior urethral injury is present, the choices for urinary diversion are a small catheter (No. 14–16 French) placed transurethrally or suprapubic cystotomy, either by the percutaneous route or by placement in the operating room. Diversion should be maintained until it is determined that the urethral injury is completely healed. Pericatheter urethrography using an angiocath or a small feeding tube alongside the Foley catheter will determine whether or not urethral healing is complete before removal. Generally, two to three weeks are required to allow sufficient healing to take place.

Catheterization itself can be a cause of anterior or posterior urethral tear. In patients with pelvic trauma and hematuria, placement of a urethral catheter should be carried out by a urologist because of the possibility of converting a partial to a complete urethral tear. Alternatively, in patients who will require prolonged bed rest or immediate surgical intervention, percutaneous or operative placement of a cystotomy tube will avoid urethral injury or the potential infection of a pelvic hematoma. In a diagnosis of complete posterior urethral disruption, instrumentation should be avoided. The patient may require prolonged hospital care for massive complex injury. A suprapubic catheter is preferable to urethral drainage to avoid catheter-induced urethral stricture. Use of specialized techniques such as filiforms and followers should be carried out only by individuals who are trained in the indications and limitations of their use. Broad-spectrum antibiotic prophylaxis should be used to ensure coverage against diphtheroids, staphylococcus, and streptococcus, in addition to gram-negative organisms.

Management of Pelvic Hematoma

Pelvic hematoma complicates the diagnosis of intraperitoneal injury since blood from the hematoma seeps through small rents in the peritoneum and will lie free in varying quantities within the peritoneal cavity. Peritoneal lavage in this setting is of limited use. Pain from the pelvic injury and reflux ileus also obscures physical findings. Arteriography is indicated to control pelvic bleeding when bleeding continues or the patient's condition is unstable, or both. The celiac axis and mesenteric vessels can be studied at the same time when required. Contrast agent given at the time of arteriography can be used to provide detail of the renal parenchyma and collecting system if follow-up films are timed appropriately.

A direct surgical approach on the hematoma releases the tamponading effect of the peritoneum. Exploration is rarely successful in locating a single bleeding source. Ligation of the hypogastric arteries has been used in the past but with modern arteriographic techniques, the bleeding vessels can be more precisely identified and selectively embolized by techniques such as a balloon or coils, or both, for effective control of bleeding.

Patients are usually hospitalized for a number of months after massive pelvic trauma involving injury to the urethra. Late potential complications are infection of the pelvic hematoma, which can result in sepsis and multiple organ system failure. Contamination of this hematoma by a urethral or rectal source should be scrupulously avoided. Attempted catheterization in the presence of an unrecognized urethral injury is a source of this contamination.

Another source for pelvic hematoma is unrecognized rectal injury below the pelvic peritoneum. A diverting colostomy and irrigation of the colon contents should be considered in a patient with massive pelvic trauma or pelvic hematoma with or without urethral injury.

Injuries in the Female Patient

Massive pelvic trauma and urethral injury in the female patient is very uncommon but should be considered when perineal injury or pelvic fracture is present. Pelvic examination should be carried out with palpation for bone fragments. Urethral injury can occur in association with vaginal injury and laceration. Cystography may delineate the injury.

GENITAL INJURY

Genital trauma can be characterized as penile, scrotal, and testicular injury. These injuries result from multiple causes and often involve both the urologist and plastic surgeon in their repair.

Penile Injury

Injuries to the penis range from minor lacerations and contusions to degloving and complete amputation. Incarceration of the glans penis is seen in neonates due to scalp hair encircling the penis and can cause minor penile edema to near complete amputation. Constricting devices must be removed and the injury followed conservatively until delineation of the injury has been established. Adolescents and young adults have placed various objects, including metal rings, around the penis in efforts to induce prolonged erections. Accidental injuries to the penis in small children may be a manifestation of child abuse, and a high index of suspicion should be maintained with this clinical finding.

Incarcerated penile problems can generally be solved under local anesthesia. Ring cutters may be necessary to remove foreign objects and should be available. Reconstruction of the penis should be delayed until an eschar forms or gangrene defines itself to make sure that viable tissue is not excised by error. In severe penile burns, swelling can result in a compartment syndrome (similar to that of other extremities) and may require a longitudinal escharotomy to preserve circulation. The corporal blood supply is separate from the penile shaft and may be preserved even though penile skin sloughs and requires grafting. Therefore, a delicate balance must be maintained between aggressive primary management and maximal preservation of potentially viable tissue.

Degloving injuries may require skin grafting after proper cleaning and debridement. In cases of partial degloving, any remaining distal penile shaft skin should be removed before grafting, as its lymphatic drainage has been interrupted and misguided attempts to preserve this skin will result in a lymphedematous "horse-collar" deformity. Usually, split-thickness grafts are used. Meshed split-thickness grafts work well on the scrotum and head, with the appearance of normal scrotal rugation.

Amputation of the penis can now be handled with reimplantation, plastic reconstruction, or reshaping of the amputated penis. Reimplantation requires a sophisticated knowledge of penile blood supply. The arterial blood supply is generally not a problem. However, venous engorgement from a thrombosis can occur, requiring the facilities and expertise of both urologist and microsurgeon. The amputated phallus should be placed in sterile saline and the patient referred to a center that has the capability of performing this reconstructive procedure. If the organ cannot be salvaged, then total phallic reconstruction using microsurgical free-flap techniques is a realistic option.

"Flail penis" or traumatic rupture of the corpora cavernosum occurs when the tunica albuginea is fractured during vigorous sexual activity when the penis is in the erect state. Frequently, a cracking sound is heard, followed by localized pain and hematoma. Voiding is usually possible since the urethra is not injured. The best treatment is open exploration, debridement, and surgical repair. The incidence of permanent deformity, suboptimal coitus, or impaired erection in conservatively managed patients is estimated at approximately 10 percent.

Pneumatic lymphangitis of the penis is a self-limiting disease caused by frequent intercourse and masturbation. Sexual abstinence usually results in spontaneous remission of this condition.

Thrombosis and thrombophlebitis of the dorsal vein of the penis are associated with a history of direct trauma. The condition results in pain and swelling but is self-limited, and patients can be reassured that there are no long-term sequelae.

Testicular Injury

Testicular injuries can include contusion with localized orchitis, hematocele with blood within the tunica vaginalis, and laceration and fracture of the tunica albuginea with rupture of the testis (Fig. 62-12). An emergency physician must define whether or not the tunica albuginea is intact. Ultrasound examination in the presence of a large hematocele is the only way to confirm the continuity. When disruption of the testicle cannot be established or discontinuity has been defined by ultrasonography, or both, surgical exploration should be carried out, with repair of the tunica albuginea and evacuation of the hematoma. Symptoms of testicular rupture include severe pain, nausea, vomiting, and even urinary retention. At times, with complete disruption, there will be no scrotal skin changes to indicate this since the blood has not had a chance to dissect into the soft tissues overlying the testicle.

Scrotal Injury

When gangrene is present over the scrotal skin as a fulminant process involving the scrotal tissues, the testicle is spared because of its separate blood supply. This condition is commonly found in diabetic or immunocompromised patients. Gangrene may begin with instrumentation, catheterization, mild degrees of scrotal trauma, or lymphedema and rapidly progresses to a subcutaneous emphysema involving

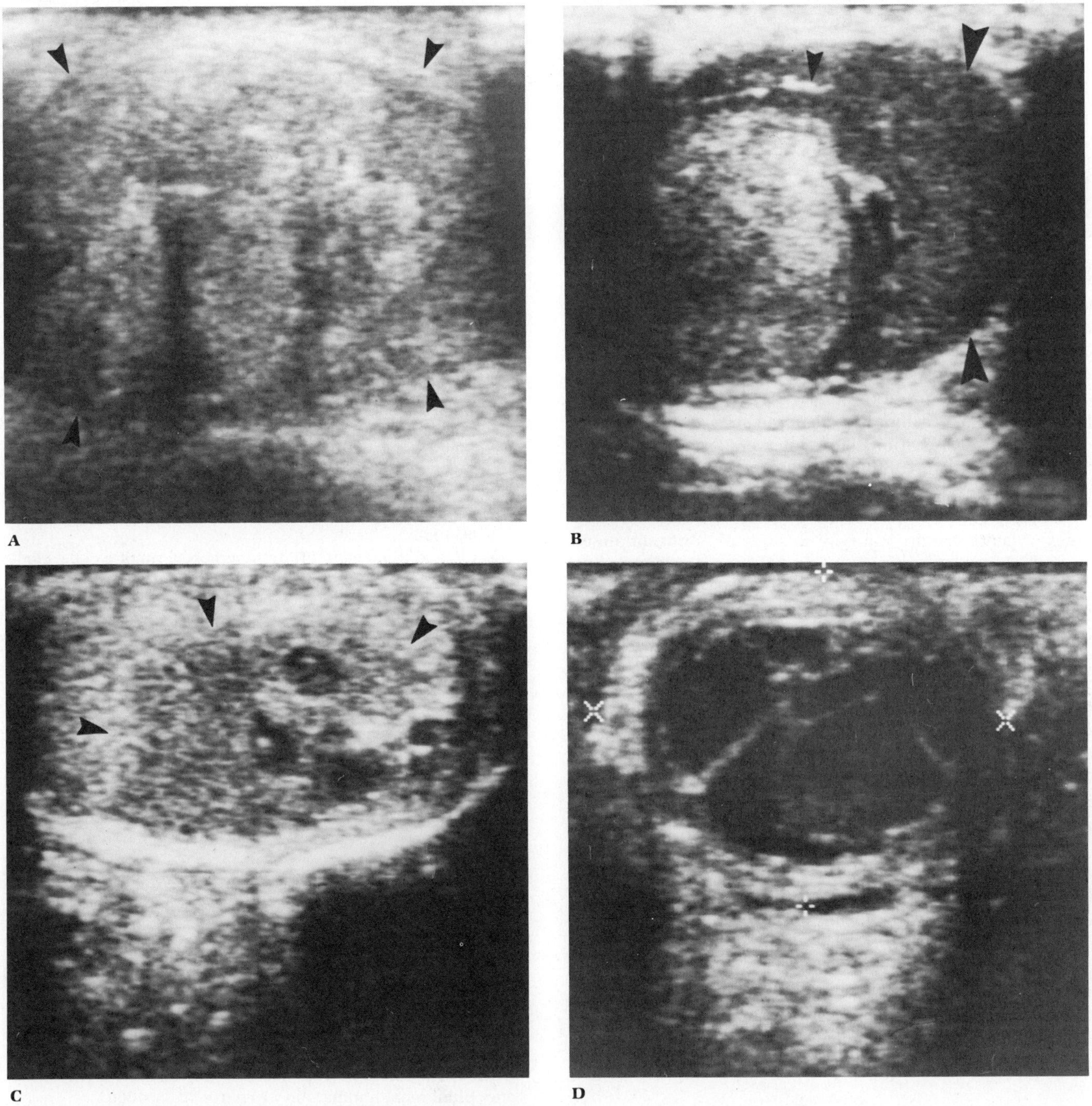

Fig. 62-12. A. Diffuse contusion of testis (*arrowheads*). No normal echogenic pattern is recognizable. B. Disruption of the echogenic tunica of the testis (*small arrowhead*) is seen with hematocele (*large arrowhead*). C. Early intratesticular hematoma (*arrowheads*). D. Organizing intratesticular hematoma. (Courtesy of Frederick J. Doherty, MD, Department of Radiology, Tufts–New England Medical Center Hospital, Boston, MA.)

the scrotal skin, inguinal regions, and lower abdominal wall. Early diagnosis, debridement with incision and drainage using Penrose skin bridges, cultures of the tissues with infectious disease consultation, intravenous antibiotics, and frequent debridement will reduce the high mortality associated with this condition. Microaerophilic streptococci or other anaerobic organisms are responsible for this rare but fulminant condition.

Other conditions of the scrotal tissue can involve scrotal skin loss, but because of the redundant amount of scrotal tissue, frequently the lost tissue can be bridged by surrounding scrotal skin. It is rarely necessary to remove testicles to cover the skin defect although split-thickness skin graft or a vascularized pedicle to bridge any significant loss can be used.

In a 10-year review by Bertini and Corriere, 70 patients with trauma to the genitalia were treated; treatment involved 42 penile, 38 scrotal, and 16 testicular injuries. Patients with severe multisystem or extensive genital wounds were successfully managed by early conservative debridement and delayed definitive repair.

SUMMARY

It is important to realize that when significant injuries to the urinary tract occur, in most patients, associated intraabdominal injuries will be present that will involve trauma and emergency physicians. Attention to the cardiovascular and respiratory systems and neurologic status will take precedence over genitourinary injury. When the patient's condition is stabilized, a thorough genitourinary evaluation can generally be carried out before intervention. On occasion, the urologist will be notified that the patient is en route to the operating room.

Radiologic studies should be performed based on likely areas of genitourinary injury. The study of nontraumatized areas of the urinary tract is rarely productive. When injury occurs to the upper abdomen, CT scan should be performed instead of intravenous urography, which will provide further information regarding the liver and spleen.

If a pelvic fracture is present, the lower urinary tract should be assessed by cystography after urethral injury has been ruled out. When there is blood at the urethral meatus, retrograde urethrography or other imaging should be carried out to determine whether the urethra has been injured. Great care should be taken that the retrograde urethrogram is carried out in a sterile fashion to obviate against contaminating a pelvic hematoma in urethral injury.

In the setting of trauma, evaluation and treatment of the genitourinary tract involves a multidisciplinary team of trauma surgeons, emergency physicians, neurosurgeons, orthopedic surgeons, the blood bank, and anesthesiologists. Coordination of the efforts of these various disciplines is important in the management of the patient. Aggressive diagnostic evaluation of the patient should lead to early recognition of injuries, with renal preservation and avoidance of the complications of delayed bleeding, urinary extravasation, abscess formation, and multiorgan failure.

SELECTED READING

Allison, RC. Urethrography in pelvic trauma. *J Urol* 111:778, 1974.

Baker, RJ. Newer techniques in evaluation of injured patients. *Surg Clin North Am* 55:31, 1975.

Banowsky, LH, et al. Considerations in diagnosis and management of renal trauma. *J Trauma* 10:587, 1970.

Bertini, JE, Jr, and Corriere JN, Jr. The etiology and management of genital injuries. *J Trauma* 28:1278, 1988.

Brunschwig, AF. Urinary tract fistulas following radical surgical treatment of carcinoma of the cervix. *Am J Gynecol Obstet* 72:479, 1975.

Campbell, MF, and Harrison, JH. *Urology,* vol 2 (3rd ed). Philadelphia: Saunders, 1970.

Cass, AS, and Godec, CJ. Urethral injury due to external trauma. *Urology* 11:607, 1978.

Cass, AS, and Luxenberg, M. Features of 164 bladder ruptures. *J Urol* 138:743, 1987.

Cass, AS, et al. Deaths from urologic injury due to external trauma. *J Trauma* 27:319, 1987.

Corriere, JN, and Sandler, CM. Mechanisms of injury, patterns of extravasation and management of extraperitoneal bladder rupture due to blunt trauma. *J Urol* 139:43, 1988.

Evans, RA, and Smith, MJ. Violent injuries to the upper ureter. *J Trauma* 16:558, 1976.

Federle, MP, Brown, TR, and McAninch, JW. Penetrating renal trauma: CT evaluation. *J Comput Assist Tomogr* 11:1026, 1987.

Flancbaum, L, et al. Blunt bladder trauma: Manifestations of severe injury. *Urology* 31:220, 1988.

Franco, I, et al. Value of proximal diversion and ureteral stenting in management of penetrating ureteral trauma. *Urology* 32:99, 1988.

Haddad, FS, and Wachtel, TL. Spontaneous intraperitoneal rupture of the bladder. *Urol Int* 42:467, 1987.

Halsell, RD, et al. The realiability of excretory urography as a screening examination for blunt renal trauma. *Ann Emerg Med* 16:1236, 1987.

Hardeman, SW, et al. Blunt urinary tract trauma: Identifying those patients who require radiological diagnostical studies. *J Urol* 131:99, 1987.

Heyns, CF, and Rimington, PD. Intraperitoneal rupture of the bladder causing the biochemical features of renal failure. *Br J Urol* 60:217, 1987.

Hodges, CV, et al. Renal trauma: A study of 71 cases. *J Urol* 66:627, 1951.

Kenney, PJ, Panicek, DM, and Witanowski, LS. Computed tomography of ureteral disruption. *J Comp Assist Tomogr* 11:480, 1987.

Kiracofe, HL, et al. Management of nonpenetrating distal urethral trauma. *J Urol* 114:57, 1975.

Klein, S, Johs, B, and Fujitani, R. Hematuria following blunt abdominal trauma. The utility of intravenous pyelography. *Arch Surg* 123:1173, 1988.

Lieu, TA, et al. Hematuria and clinical findings as indications for intravenous pyelography in pediatric blunt renal trauma. *Pediatrics* 82:16, 1988.

Marberger, H. Trauma to the urinary tract. *Br J Urol* 48:145, 1976.

McKay, HW, et al. Management of the injured kidney. *JAMA* 141:575, 1949.

Mee, SL, McAninch, JW, and Federle, MP. Computerized tomography in bladder rupture: Diagnostic limitations. *J Urol* 137:207, 1987.

Mendez, R. Renal trauma. *J Urol* 118:698, 1977.

Meredith, JW, and Trunkey, DD. CT scanning in acute abdominal injuries. *Surg Clin North Am* 68:255, 1988.

Meyrier, A, Rainfray, M, and Lacombe, M. Delayed hypertension after blunt renal trauma. *Am J Nephrol* 8:108, 1988.

Mitchel, JP. Trauma to the urinary tract. *Br Med J* 2:567, 1971.

Monstrey, SJ, et al. Urinary tract injuries in children: Are they different from adults? *Z Kinderchir* 43:31, 1988.

Morehouse, DD, et al. Rupture of the posterior urethra. *J Urol* 107:225, 1972.

Nunn, IN. Management of closed renal injury. *Aust NZ J Surg* 31:263, 1962.

Orkin, LA. Evaluation of the merits of cystoscopy management of the injured kidney. *JAMA* 141:575, 1945.

Persky, L, and Hoch, WH. Genitourinary tract trauma. *Curr Probl Surg* 1–64, 1972.

Peters, PC. Management of trauma to the urinary tract. *Adv Surg* 10:197, 1976.

Peterson, NE, and Schulze, KA. Selective diagnostic uroradiography for trauma. *J Urol* 137:449, 1987.

Pumphrey, JD, et al. Missile wounds of the ureter. *J Trauma* 2:89, 1962.

Reznichek, RC, et al. Ureteral avulsion from blunt trauma. *J Urol* 109:812, 1973.

Richter, MW, et al. Radiology of genitourinary trauma. *Radiol Clin North Am* 11:593, 1973.

Salvatierra, O, et al. Penetrating ureteral injuries. *Surg Gynecol Obstet* 128:591, 1969.

Simpson-Smith, A. Traumatic rupture of the urethra: Eight personal cases with a review of 381 recorded ruptures. *Br J Surg* 24:309, 1936.

Sonda, LP, and Wang, S. Evaluation of male external genital diseases in the emergency room setting. *Emerg Med Clin North Am* 6:473, 1988.

Spirnak, JP, and Resnick, MI. Revascularization of traumatic thrombosis of the renal artery. *Surg Gynecol Obstet* 164:22, 1987.

Todd, IA. The genitourinary complication of blunt pelvic trauma. *Can J Surg* 7:43, 1964.

Tomlanovich, M. Blunt pelvic trauma with urethral injury in the female. *J Emerg Med* 2:2, 1984.

Turner-Warwick, R. A personal view of the management of traumatic posterior urethral strictures. *Urol Clin North Am* 4:111, 1977.

Wallis, NE, et al. Blunt ureteral trauma with perineal urine fistulization: Review of the literature. *J Urol* 114:942, 1975.

Waterhouse, K, and Gross, M. Trauma to the genitourinary tract: A five-year experience with 251 cases. *Trans Am Assoc Genitourin Surg* 60:162, 1968.

Wesolowski, S. Bilateral ureteral injuries in gynaecology. *Br J Urol* 41:666, 1969.

F. Skeletal and Soft-Tissue Injuries

63. Musculoskeletal Injuries: General Principles of Assessment and Management

David W. Lhowe

The emergency physician will be called on to evaluate a wide spectrum of musculoskeletal injuries, occurring in young athletes on the school playing field, among the elderly in nursing homes, or in individuals with multiple injuries from motor vehicle or industrial accidents. Whereas the ultimate treatment for these injuries can be complex, requiring specialized skills and knowledge, the initial management follows basic principles and can significantly affect the patient's ultimate outcome.

Most extremity injuries are obvious, but many, including the most severe, can be overlooked. Frequently deformity, swelling, pain, and local skin changes will be clues to the presence of injury. This is especially true of injuries in the arm and leg. However, injuries to the spine, pelvis, hip, and shoulder are often unaccompanied by these signs because of the thicker soft tissue layer covering these bony structures. Accordingly, injuries to these areas are frequently missed. In addition, if the patient is unable to cooperate and provide information, the evaluating emergency physician must suspect injuries based on the circumstances of the trauma. Each bone should be palpated and all joints put through a range of motion. All unconscious patients with trauma should have an x-ray of the chest, pelvis, and entire spine taken.

There is a tendency for the busy emergency physician to rely too heavily on radiographic evaluation. Although x-ray films are an important aid to diagnosis, the absence of x-ray abnormality should not suggest the absence of injury. Ligamentous injuries and neurovascular compromise will not be apparent on radiographs, but will be evident on a quick but thorough physical examination. Furthermore, the presence of a fracture on x-ray examination should not prevent the emergency physician from making a complete evaluation of the associated soft tissue injuries.

Soft tissue evaluation is extremely important because these tissues comprise the ligaments, muscles, nerves, and blood vessels, which are critical to ultimate function of the extremity. The state of the soft tissues at the time of injury should be noted and documented. Frequently, the associated soft tissue injuries will evolve during the first few hours after an injury. For example, a compartment syndrome that results from a crush injury may not be seen at the time of initial evaluation. The documentation of extremity swelling, induration, and motor/sensory status will be of great importance in determining the next stage of management.

INITIAL ASSESSMENT

The evaluation of patients with musculoskeletal injuries must be methodical and organized to prevent oversights and to be efficient. The patient's airway, circulatory status, and vital signs will always take precedence over injuries of the extremities. This does not mean, however, that the extremities should be completely ignored during the care of higher-priority injuries. Unstable fractures or severe ligamentous disruptions need to be protected during resuscitative efforts in order to prevent further injury. Adhesive tape, pillows, and sandbags can easily provide this modicum of stability and allow the emergency physician to attend to the higher-priority injuries in the multiply injured patient.

Present emphasis in care of polytrauma victims is on management of extremity and skeletal injuries concurrently with head, chest, and abdominal injuries. Multiple clinical studies have demonstrated the systemic benefit derived from aggressive treatment of extremity trauma in patients with multiple system injury.

History

A clear and chronologic history is unquestionably important. The physician should assume that the patient might lapse into unconsciousness at any moment, and therefore should first establish the presence of allergies, medication use, and preexistent medical problems. Thereafter, the details of injury can be obtained. It is of particular importance to document prior treatment in patients who are seen several days after initial injury.

The magnitude of the trauma should be established. If the patient cannot provide this information, the examining physician should discuss the details of the accident with emergency personnel who attended the patient at the scene of the injury, or, if possible, individuals who observed the injury itself. With higher-energy injuries, such as high-speed motor vehicle accidents or falls from heights, the index of suspicion for associated injuries must be raised. (Conversely, low-energy injury that results in a major fracture should alert the emergency physician to a preexisting pathologic condition of the bone, such as osteoporosis or, less commonly, a metastatic tumor.) Witnesses may be able to provide details of the injury that suggest the presence of a head injury, seizure disorder, or even a cardiac arrest. Whenever possible, the patient's preinjury status should be established; this is particularly helpful in the case of elderly patients as regards their ambulatory status. This knowledge will help determine treatment and predict functional outcome.

Physical Examination

Examination of the musculoskeletal system can be performed quickly and with a minimum of discomfort for the patient. Clothing must be removed, along with any constricting jewelry (rings, bracelets) present on the involved extremity.

The examination should follow the format outlined in Table 63-1. The initial examination should be an observation of the extremity or spine, looking for asymmetry, deformity, and changes in the appearance of the skin. After this, each bone of the affected area and each joint should be palpated and each joint gently put through a range of motion and checked for ligamentous stability. Motor testing with emphasis on the ability to initiate active motion should follow. Vascular status should then be established, followed by an assessment of sensation to light touch. Further neurologic testing depends on the clinical situation.

Table 63-1. Outline of musculoskeletal examination

1. Observation: deformity, asymmetry, skin changes
2. Palpation of bones and joints: tenderness, crepitus, defects, instability
3. Range of motion of joints
4. Motor function: ability to initiate joint motion
5. Vascular assessment: pulses, temperature, color
6. Sensory assessment: light touch stimulus

The examiner can note asymmetry by comparing one side to the other. Areas of abrasion or ecchymosis suggest underlying pathology. For example, when there are abrasions on the forehead, a cervical spine injury should be suspected, while significant abrasions of the knee should suggest the possibility of knee or hip dislocation or patella fracture. Each bone of the affected area should be palpated, looking for discontinuity, tenderness, false motion, or crepitus. The examiner should start at the top of the cervical spine, feeling each spinous process. The clavicles should then be palpated from their sternal attachments to the acromioclavicular joints. The thoracic and lumbar spine should be palpated, followed by bimanual compression of the iliac crests and palpation of the pubic rami. The long bones are palpated, starting proximally and extending to the digits. Next, each joint should be put through a range of motion, actively by the patient if possible, but gently assisted by the examiner if necessary. The presence of significant injury as suggested by obvious deformity, instability, or crepitus will limit this phase of the examination until after radiographs have been obtained. Any suspicion of cervical spine injury by history or gentle palpation requires at least an emergency lateral radiograph of the cervical spine (and preferably an anteroposterior and open-mouth view as well) before any motion of the neck is permitted.

Many methods of measuring joint motion exist, and most are satisfactory, provided the examiner is consistent throughout the recording. The American Academy of Orthopaedic Surgeons has established a standardized range-of-motion format based on the "zero-extended position." By this method, the extended anatomic position is recorded as "zero degrees" of motion. For example, Fig. 63-1 shows this method applied to the elbow, which is measured at zero degrees when fully extended. For more detail, the reader is referred to the selected reading list at the end of this chapter.

The motor examination should test for active motor function. Whenever possible, the physician should have the patient perform the functions actively, which thereby establishes normal motor pathways from cerebral cortex through the spinal cord and peripheral nerve to muscle. The presence of active motion is more important than the actual degree of motor strength since the strength of contracture depends on many variables, including pain and the presence of preexistent disease. Therefore, there is little value in grading muscle strength in the acutely injured extremity. The exception to this is spinal cord injury; in these injuries the estab-

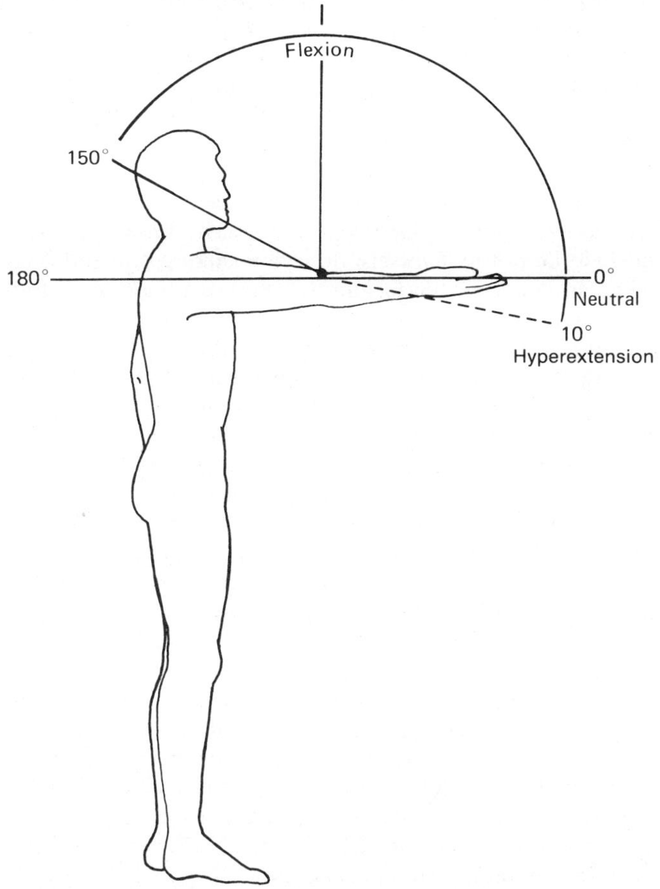

Fig. 63-1. The zero-extended position of measuring joint range of motion as adopted by the American Academy of Orthopaedic Surgeons. Note that hyperextension refers to extension beyond the usual range of motion for the joint. A wrist joint would have both flexion and extension from zero whereas the elbow and knee normally do not extend beyond the neutral position; therefore, further extension is referred to as "hyperextension."

lishment of specific initial motor status is important since the patient's neurologic condition may evolve in the first several hours after injury.

The circulatory status of the extremity should be examined next. The presence or absence of peripheral pulses, color, temperature, and the state of capillary filling should be recorded on the patient's chart. This is especially important before any manipulation of an injured extremity in order to ascertain whether the manipulation produced a change in the neurovascular status. Frequently, a Doppler unit is required to detect pulses in swollen extremities. *The presence of normal pulses does not rule out a compartment syndrome,* as is detailed in Chap. 73. Pulse volume recording, where available, is another method of objectively assessing the circulatory status.

Testing for sensation can vary from the crude to the elegant, but in the acute traumatic situation light touch is usually a sufficient screening examination of the sensory system. If abnormality is disclosed on light touch testing, a more detailed sensory examination is indicated. The use of a pin for sensory testing is a poor choice since it can often be felt, even in the presence of major neurologic compromise.

Table 63-2. Symptoms or signs that suggest injury

Symptom or sign	Associated injury
Unconscious patient who sustains high-energy trauma	Spine-pelvic fracture Hip dislocation
Shoulder pain with limited external rotation	Posterior dislocation of shoulder
Elbow pain after fall on outstretched hand	Radial head fracture
Wrist pain localizing to radial aspect	Scaphoid fracture
Back pain in the elderly	Compression fracture of thoracic-lumbar vertebral body, possibly pathologic
Lateral knee or calf contusion	Peroneal nerve palsy
Calf pain	Rupture of medial gastrocnemius muscle or plantaris tendon
Posterior lower calf–ankle pain	Achilles tendon rupture
Heel pain after fall	Calcaneus fracture
Midfoot pain and/or deformity	Tarsometatarsal dislocation Rupture of posterior tibial tendon
Disproportionate extremity pain, sensory loss, soft tissue induration	Compartment syndrome

Associated Injuries

A number of musculoskeletal symptoms and signs suggest specific orthopedic injuries. In addition, certain specific injuries are well associated with other injuries, to the extent that the presence of one should initiate a directed search for the other (Tables 63-2 and 63-3).

When the patient is unconscious, the presence of a spine fracture, pelvic fracture, or hip dislocation must be suspected. Clavicle fractures can injure the brachial plexus or subclavian vessels and, when located in the distal half, can be associated with acromioclavicular disruption. Shoulder pain accompanied by an inability to externally rotate and an apparently normal anteroposterior x-ray may well represent a posterior dislocation, particularly in patients with a history of seizure or electrical shock. Scapular fractures that result from high-energy trauma are often associated with first rib or clavicle fractures or a pneumothorax. The close approximation of the radial nerve to the middle and distal humerus puts it at risk in the setting of displaced or angulated fractures of this bone. Supracondylar fractures in children are well known to be associated with brachial artery disruption and can even produce a forearm compartment syndrome, particularly if the elbow is held in a flexed position as postinjury swelling increases. In the forearm, the fracture of one bone can produce a dislocation of the other at either its proximal or distal end. In proximal ulna shaft fractures, one should look particularly for a dislocation of the radial head, while a fracture of the distal radial shaft requires a careful inspection of the distal radioulnar joint. Patients with wrist trauma and radial-sided wrist pain, despite normal x-ray views, should be suspected of having a nondisplaced scaphoid fracture.

Table 63-3. Commonly associated injuries

Diagnosed injury	Associated injury
Clavicle fracture	Brachial plexus or subclavian vessel injury Acromioclavicular joint disruption
Scapular fracture	First-rib fracture Pneumothorax
Anterior shoulder dislocation	Axillary nerve palsy
Middle or distal third humerus fracture	Radial nerve palsy
Supracondylar humerus fracture	Brachial artery laceration Forearm compartment syndrome
Ulnar shaft fracture (proximal)	Radial head dislocation
Radial shaft fracture (distal)	Distal radioulnar joint dislocation
Displaced Colles' fracture	Median nerve palsy
Posterior hip dislocation	Sciatic nerve injury Acetabular fracture
High-energy patella fracture	Posterior hip dislocation Acetabular fracture
Knee joint dislocation	Popliteal artery injury
Calcaneus fracture	Lumbar compression fracture

In the lower extremity, a posterior hip dislocation can injure the posterior acetabular wall or the sciatic nerve. Patients who sustain a high-energy patellar fracture, particularly when they are seated in an automobile, must have a posterior hip dislocation ruled out by examination and possibly x-rays. Any knee dislocation, even if it has spontaneously reduced before presentation, requires arteriography to rule out popliteal artery injury. Calf pain, if proximal, should suggest gastrocnemius muscle injury and, if distal, rupture of the Achilles tendon. Calcaneus fractures often result from forces sufficient to also cause a compression fracture of the lumbar spine. Midfoot pain and swelling can represent a Lisfranc (midfoot) dislocation, and x-rays may be difficult to interpret, particularly if they are oblique in their projection. Comparison views of the opposite foot may be helpful. Finally, any patient with extremity trauma who shows induration, sensory loss, or disproportionate pain must have a compartment syndrome ruled out by compartmental pressure measurement.

Radiographic Evaluation

The details of radiographic examination are addressed in the specific chapters that follow. Several principles that are applicable to the interpretation of any film of the musculoskeletal system are described here.

One should always inspect the soft tissue densities first. Soft tissue swelling causes abnormal contours and helps confirm or localize the injury. One should remember that blood and muscle appear identical on plain x-rays, but fat is more radiolucent than either. Fat pads are frequently found in and about joints, and an effusion within that joint can change the position of the fat pad, producing a lucent line such as the posterior "fat pad sign" in the case of elbow effusion.

Next, the bones should be examined. Each bone should be inspected individually, following the cortical margin completely around the bone until the starting point is reached again. Any lucent break in the contour must be explained as either a nutrient vessel, an overlying shadow from another bone (especially in the hand and foot), or, in the case of children, a physeal (growth) plate. Lucent lines that represent acute fractures tend to be sharp edged and angulate abruptly. Gently curving lucent lines are more likely to be nutrient vessels, overlying shadows, or old fractures. In children, the location of physeal plates is predictable, although fractures frequently involve these physes, making radiographic interpretation difficult. Comparison views of the uninjured side are helpful in these situations.

Correlation of the suspected fracture with the site of tenderness is helpful in evaluating the film. A lucent line involving the tibial shaft is not likely to represent an acute fracture if it is absolutely without tenderness on examination. Avulsion fractures, common about the foot and ankle, are probably old if they are not tender on examination.

If there is still question of fracture despite normal routine x-rays, then oblique films or tomograms can be obtained. Technetium bone scans will reliably show locally increased uptake within 48 hours of fracture, and usually sooner. Under certain circumstances, such as a suspected hip fracture, it is more important to completely establish the diagnosis since immediate treatment decisions depend on it. In other cases, such as suspected fractures of the radial head, no change in therapeutic plan results whether the nondisplaced fracture of the radial head is suspected or confirmed, and therefore no bone scan is necessary.

Description of Extremity Injury

Since communication by phone is frequent, the description of an extremity injury needs to be accurate and concise. As documentation is becoming increasingly important, recording of injuries should be as complete as possible.

Soft Tissue Injury

A skin injury is described as contusion, abrasion, or laceration, with the first term implying that the dermis is intact. The location and extent of injury and swelling are important to record, particularly if the injury is located near a fracture or bony prominence (Fig. 63-2). Any underlying muscle defect should also be described, localizing the muscle involved as specifically as possible.

Sprains are defined as tearing of the ligamentous fibers that stabilize the joint. The generally accepted grading scheme is: I, minor tearing of fibers with resultant tenderness and swelling but no instability on examination; II, more fibers disrupted with detectable instability on examination that is limited by a definite end point; III, complete tearing of the ligament with gross instability and no detectable end point on examination (Fig. 63-3). Often, the completely disrupted ligament will be less painful when examined than a partial disruption, due to the absence of tension forces on the injured but still intact ligament fibers.

Strains are defined as injuries to the musculotendinous unit that result from contraction of that muscle ("pulled muscle") or the forceful stretching of the musculotendinous unit by an exogenous force. The spectrum of injury for

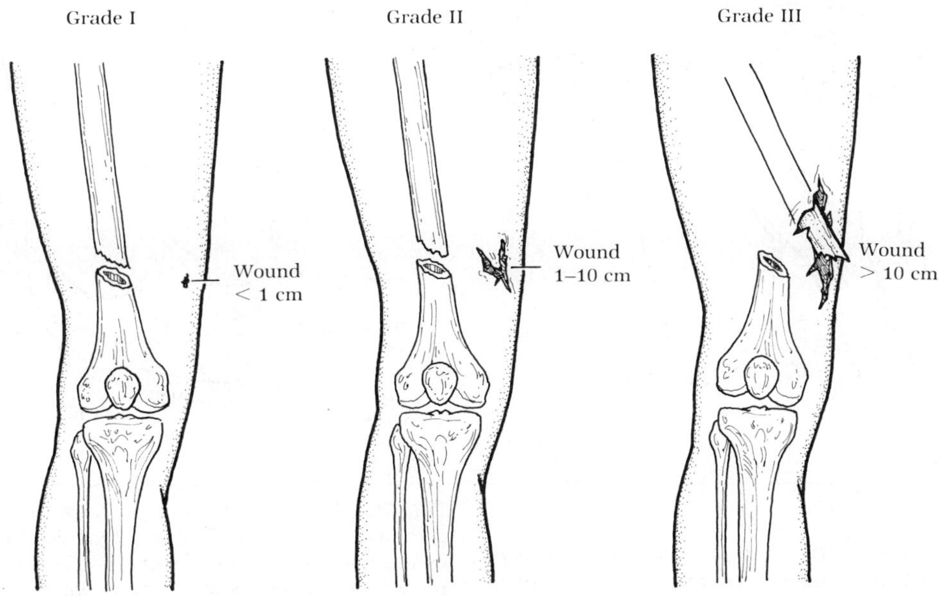

Fig. 63-2. Grading of soft tissue injuries associated with open fractures. Grade I refers to a wound less than 1 cm in length. Grade II describes a wound that is 1 to 10 cm in length. Grade III refers to a wound greater than 10 cm in length. It is equally important to note the condition of the surrounding soft tissues, which, while not lacerated, may have sustained crush, contusion, or abrasion. The degree and type of contamination by foreign material are also important to describe.

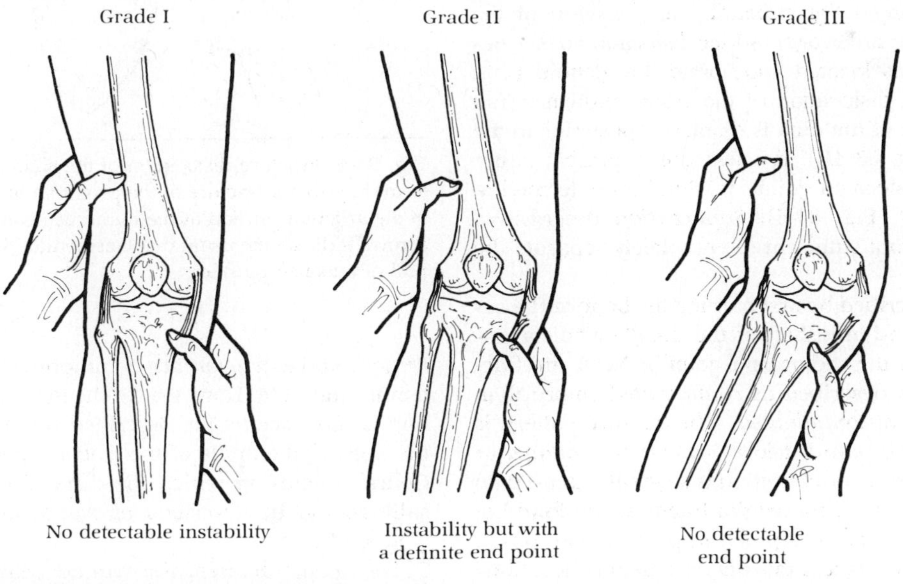

Fig. 63-3. Grading scheme for ligamentous injuries as illustrated for the knee. Grade I indicates a mild sprain with definite tenderness along the course of the ligament and pain with stretch of that ligament but no instability detectable by the examiner. Grade II implies a detectable amount of instability with a definite end point to motion. Grade III refers to a complete disruption of the specific ligament with no detectable end point. Such complete disruptions may be less painful with stretching.

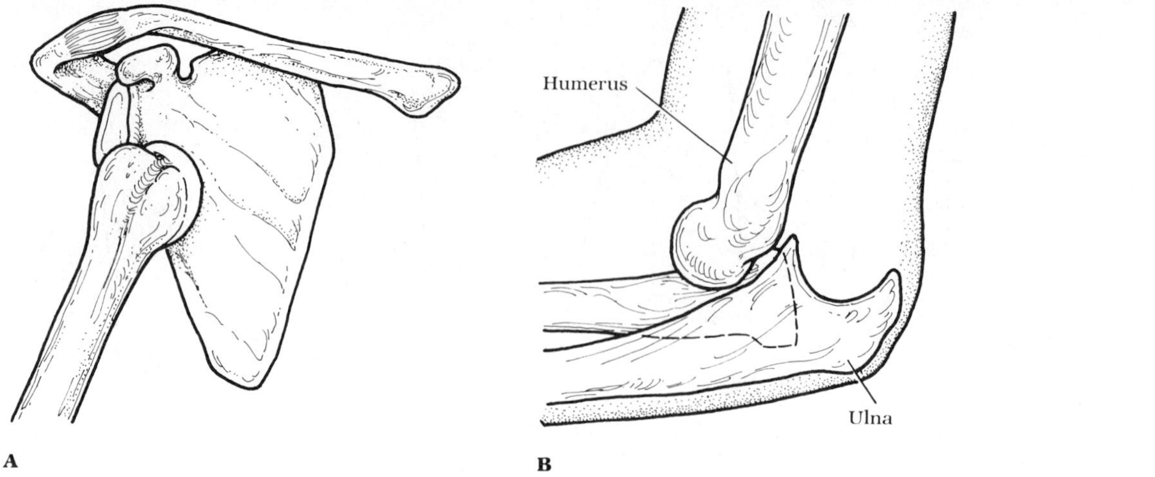

Fig. 63-4. A. The bony anatomy of an anterior shoulder dislocation is shown. Note that the humeral head lies anterior to the glenoid by this description. B. The posterior elbow dislocation describes a posterior displacement of the ulna relative to the humerus, as shown.

strains is continuous, from minor to severe, but numerical grading is rarely applied. At the most severe end of the spectrum are muscle strains, which represent a complete disruption of the musculotendinous unit, such as a distal quadriceps or Achilles tendon rupture.

Neurovascular status needs to be documented in nearly all cases of musculoskeletal trauma. Anesthetic-hypesthetic areas should be noted and correlated with the appropriate spinal cord level, nerve root, or peripheral nerve involved. Abnormal motor function, particularly where paralysis exists, should be similarly correlated. Distal color, temperature, and pulses should be recorded.

Bone and Joint Injuries

Dislocations should be described by naming the joint involved and modifying it by indicating the position of the distal bone. Thus, an anterior shoulder dislocation describes the humeral head as located anterior to the glenoid (Fig. 63-4A). A posterior dislocation of the elbow indicates that the semiulnar notch of the ulna is displaced posterior to the distal humerus (Fig. 63-4B). If a fracture is present either near or into a dislocated joint, it should be termed a *fracture-dislocation* (Fig. 63-5). *Subluxation* describes a partial dislocation, not sufficient to completely separate the joint surfaces.

Fractures are described by first naming the bone and location within the bone ("midshaft of the tibia" or "distal radius, extending into the radiocarpal joint"). Next, the fracture pattern itself is described as *comminuted* (more than two fragments) or *noncomminuted*. The fracture pattern is also described by the path it takes: *transverse, oblique,* or *spiral*. In certain cases, comminution is so great that no path is discernible. In other cases, several fractures are found at intervals from each other—a *segmental* pattern (Fig. 63-6).

If the fracture is displaced, this displacement is described by the position of the distal fragment relative to the proximal fragment (medial/lateral, anterior/posterior). In the forearm and hand, the terms *ulnar, radial, volar,* and *dorsal* are used preferentially. In the foot, *plantar* and *dorsal* are used, also by convention. If there is shortening of the bone, due to overriding of the fragments, this should be noted and measured from the x-ray.

If the fracture is angulated, the terms *varus, valgus,*

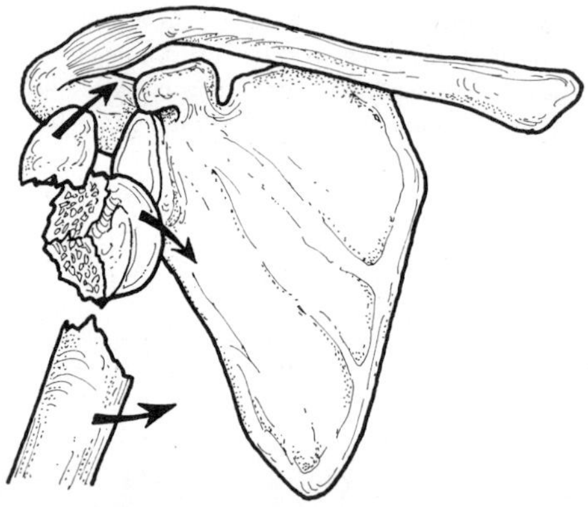

Fig. 63-5. Fracture-dislocation of the shoulder. Specifically, this term describes a fracture of the proximal humerus with dislocation of the articular portion of the humerus away from the glenoid. The arrows indicate the usual displacement of the fragments due to the pull of attached muscles.

flexion, and *extension* are commonly used for the humerus, femur, and tibia. However, in the forearm and wrist, angulation is most accurately described by the direction in which the apex of the angle of the fracture points. For example, a Colles' fracture in which the distal fragment is facing dorsally should be described as "angulated with apex volar" (Fig. 63-7).

For open fractures, the wound description is especially critical. By convention, open fractures are graded by the size of the visible soft tissue wound: grade I (<1 cm), grade II (1–10 cm), and grade III (>10 cm); see Fig. 63-2. One should be suspicious of even small wounds that are somewhat removed from the fracture site, since they are often produced by a spike of bone piercing the overlying tissue while in the deformed position. With the fracture relatively reduced, the soft tissue injury becomes removed from the

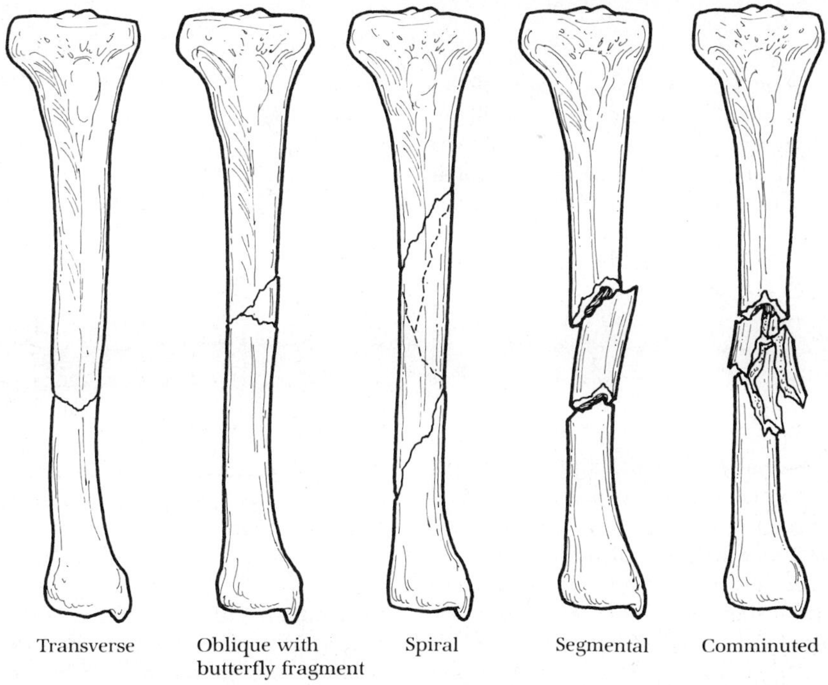

Fig. 63-6. Fracture patterns as seen in the tibia. These patterns may be more or less displaced than is shown in specific instances. In these drawings the transverse, oblique, and spiral fractures would be considered nondisplaced, while the segmental fracture would be described as having minimal displacement with slight angulation of the middle fragment. Note that the degree of displacement, angulation, and comminution correlates with the amount of energy absorbed by the bone at the time of fracture.

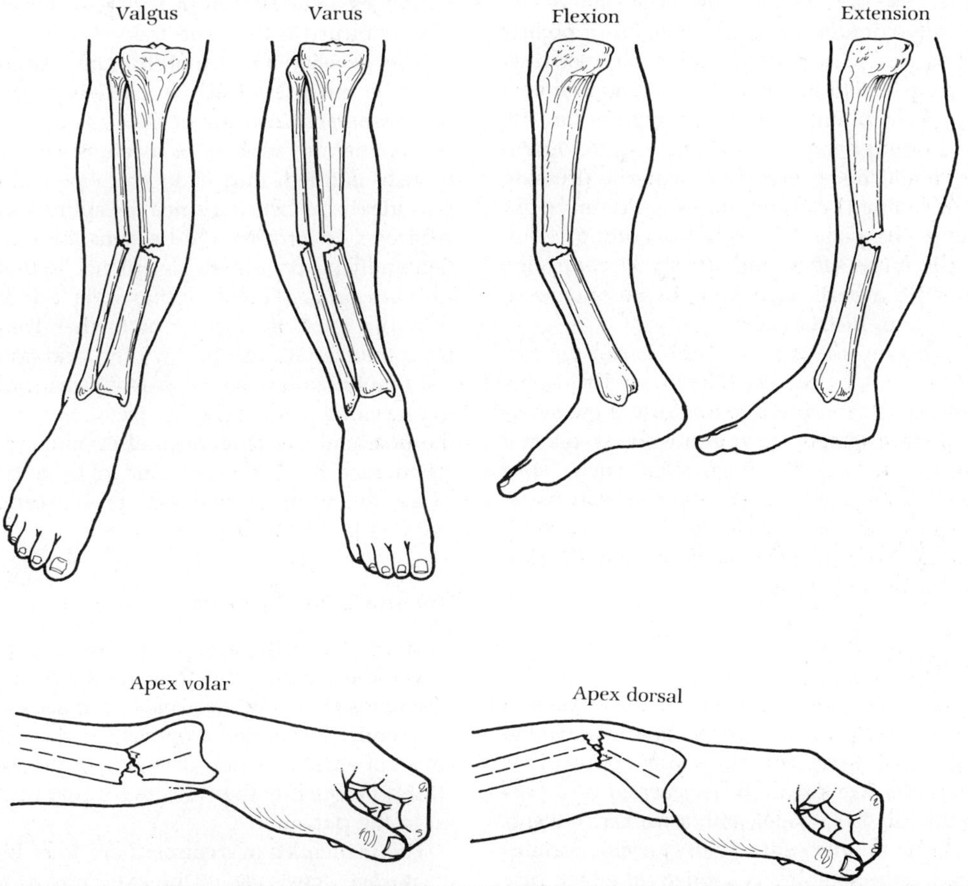

Fig. 63-7. Angulation as seen in the tibia and distal radius. The terms *valgus* and *varus* are well understood and used nearly universally. When in doubt, particularly in a region not commonly described by these terms, a more consistent method is to describe the angulation by the direction in which the apex of the fracture points. This method is particularly helpful in the description of forearm and wrist fractures.

fracture site. More important than the exact length of the wound is the general condition of the soft tissue itself. Is there evidence of a crushing injury with a great deal of skin loss and contamination? It is not hard to imagine that a long, clean skin laceration over a fracture could be a lesser injury than a crushing injury with minimal break in the skin, even though the former injury would rate a grade III classification and the latter a grade I.

INITIAL MANAGEMENT

Initial Handling

The injured extremity, especially when the injury is the result of a fracture or crush, must be handled carefully. The patient will not have normal muscular control of the arm or leg because of reflex inhibition of the controlling musculature or direct injury to the nerves or muscles themselves. The extremity is at risk of further injury due to uncontrolled movements in the presence of sharp, bony fracture fragments. Increased bleeding, pain, and contamination of the wounded area can result from inadequate protection.

The examiner must handle the injured extremity with good control to prevent further deformity. This will often require an assistant to lift and hold the patient while the examiner removes clothing and dressings to assess the limb. If large open wounds are present, especially over a fracture, the examiner should use sterile gloves and a face mask and should not probe the wounds. Such introduction of objects into a wound will only increase contamination and bleeding, and there is very little benefit in terms of additional clinical information. Wound swabbing for bacterial culture has not been found to yield useful data. Wounds that require operative debridement should be covered with a sterile dressing soaked in povidone-iodine (Betadine) and should not be inspected further until the patient is in the operating room. Pulsatile bleeding is more safely and effectively controlled by direct pressure with a sterile pack than by an attempt to clamp the vessel with an instrument.

As long as the vascular status of the limb is satisfactory, gross deformity should not be corrected before radiographic evaluation is obtained. An exception to this rule is the situation in which a bony fragment or prominence is placing substantial pressure on the overlying skin, such as a fracture-dislocation of the ankle where the thin soft tissue over the malleolus can easily become ischemic. If the prominence is not promptly reduced, ischemic damage to the skin and a resultant skin slough can occur.

Uncomplicated Sprains

For grade I and II sprains, typically involving the ankle and knee, the principles of rest, ice, compression, and elevation (RICE) apply (Fig. 63-8). Crutches are usually appropriate, although children under age six are better carried by a parent, and elderly individuals are safer with a walker. Patients should be instructed to ambulate with partial weight-bearing as tolerated, unless a splint is applied, in which case non–weight-bearing is indicated. Elevation should be nearly continuous for the first 48 hours, since swelling will tend to increase during this period. Application of ice should be

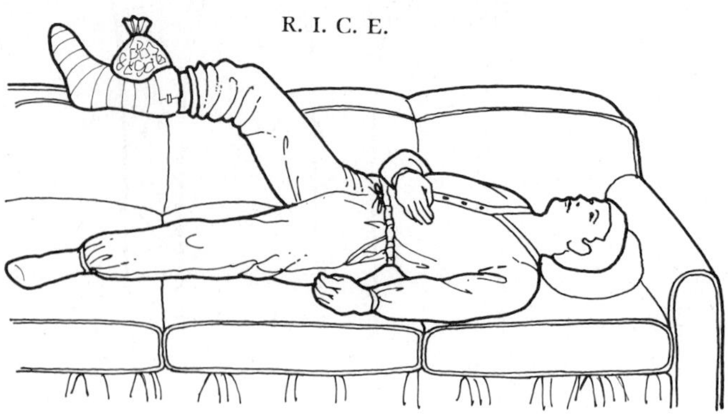

Fig. 63-8. The principles of rest, ice, compression, and elevation (RICE) are illustrated.

intermittent (30–60 minutes at a time), using crushed ice placed in a plastic bag. If the extremity is not wrapped or splinted, this ice bag should be covered with a cloth so that the bag does not contact that skin directly. Ace bandage wrapping can be used to provide gentle compression, but patients should not be encouraged to keep the bandage tightly wrapped. If an Ace wrap is to be used by the patient, it is recommended that it be removed at least twice a day to check the underlying skin during the first 48 hours. Ace bandages alone do not provide any support or immobilization, contrary to the expectations of many patients.

The decision to immobilize an extremity with a splint must be individualized for each patient. There are several disadvantages: The site of injury is obscured, the splint can be too tightly applied or become constrictive if not adequately padded, and it does not permit the resumption of partial weight-bearing since the splint itself will break when subjected to any weight-bearing forces. Furthermore, patients suffer a certain inconvenience in mobility and bathing. The advantages of immobilization are stabilization of the unstable joint, avoidance of further trauma and swelling from inadvertent use of the joint, and pain relief.

Immobilization is most safely provided by splinting. Casting has almost no use in the treatment of acute sprains since the potential disadvantages of circumferential plaster (constriction of the extremity) outweigh its benefits. An appropriate follow-up period for sprains serious enough to be splinted is 7 to 10 days as a rule.

Uncomplicated Muscle Strains

Uncomplicated muscle strains are common injuries of the musculotendinous unit that fall short of complete rupture. The hamstrings and gastrosoleus muscles are involved most frequently. Pain often worsens the day following injury because of spasm, which develops in the 24 to 48 hours after strain. Frequently the causative injury or overuse seems trivial to the patient.

The principles of treatment are to reduce discomfort and encourage active use of the extremity as tolerated. Application of ice is helpful for the first 48 hours, but less consistently than for persons with acute sprains. After 2 days, local heat delivered for 30 to 60 minutes at a time by means of a heating pad, hot-water bottle, or bath can reduce the surrounding spasm, which is the source of much of the patient's discomfort. "Antispasmodic" medication is of little proven benefit, and some such medications have substantial sedative effects, about which patients should be warned. Rest is important, with crutches the mainstay for lower extremity strains. Immobilization is usually not possible or desirable. Patients should be encouraged to put the joints powered by the affected muscle through a gentle range of motion daily, beginning as soon as tolerable. Follow-up examination should be recommended if symptoms fail to improve over 7 to 10 days.

Fractures

All acute fractures need immobilization in the emergency department. This applies to patients who will be admitted as well as those who are being discharged. Splinting is usually the method of choice, although fractures are sometimes acutely reduced and placed in circumferential plaster by orthopedic surgeons, particularly when hospital admission for elevation and observation is anticipated. In most instances, the recommendation is for splinting acutely, with subsequent casting at a later date.

The other principles of treatment are similar to those for sprains. Elevation is the most important and ice should be applied over the fracture site intermittently. If surgical treatment is being considered at a subsequent date, the patient being discharged needs to understand that operation will be feasible only if the swelling has sufficiently resolved. Failure to elevate or the premature resumption of weight-bearing activity is certain to prolong the swelling and could easily delay a planned surgical procedure.

IMMOBILIZATION

While many useful prefabricated splints and immobilizers are available, it is important to understand how to fashion splints from plaster of Paris and cast padding since these materials are available in any emergency department and can be fashioned to accommodate an extremity of any size. Casting plaster solidifies when wet by an exothermic reaction. The speed of setting is a characteristic of the specific plaster itself and varies between manufacturers. Any given plaster will set more rapidly in warm than in cold water.

Splints consist of a sandwich of plaster covered by several layers of cast padding on either side. As a rule, at least 10 thicknesses of plaster are necessary. This splint is then overwrapped with an Ace bandage, which holds it closely to the patient's extremity.

Splints are made by measuring the length required and adding a little extra (5%) to allow for shrinkage as the plaster is wetted. After the plaster is folded, but before it is wetted, cast padding is torn to identical lengths at least two thicknesses on each side, and preferably three to four thicknesses on the side to contact the skin. Only the plaster is dipped into warm water, just long enough to wet it, and next squeezed until damp. It is then laid out on one set of cast padding lengths, with the second set placed on top (Fig. 63-9).

The assembled splint is then placed on the extremity and held in position as an Ace bandage is overwrapped, using just enough tension to hold the splint in position. The extremity must be kept motionless as the plaster hardens or else the splint will be weak and fail prematurely. The length of the splint should be checked as it may extend too far in one direction and need trimming to allow adjacent joints to move fully.

Upper-Extremity Splints

Volar or Dorsal Wrist Splint
Materials for a volar or dorsal wrist splint include a four-inch plaster roll, four-inch cast padding, and 2 three-inch Ace bandages. The wrist is positioned at 30 degrees of dorsiflexion (Fig. 63-10). It should be noted that the splint ends just at the midpalmar crease. The metacarpophalangeal (MCP) joints must be free to move. Alternatively, this splint can be applied dorsally, producing less interference with finger motion.

Radial Gutter Splint ("Thumb Spica" Splint)
Materials for a radial gutter splint include a four- or five-inch plaster roll, four- or five-inch cast padding, and 2 three-inch Ace bandages. This splint immobilizes the wrist and thumb. It can be used for suspected or confirmed scaphoid fractures or de Quervain's tenosynovitis (Fig. 63-11). It should be noted that the MCP joints other than the thumb are not immobilized. The wrist is positioned at 30 degrees dorsiflexion and the thumb is positioned as if the patient were holding a can of soup.

Ulnar Gutter Splint
Materials for an ulnar gutter splint include a four- or five-inch plaster roll, four- or five-inch cast padding, and 2 three-inch Ace bandages. This splint is most typically used for ring- and little-finger metacarpal fractures (Fig. 63-12). It is extended out to the distal interphalangeal (DIP) joints of the ring and little fingers. The wrist is positioned at approximately 30 degrees of dorsiflexion and the metacarpophalangeal (MCP) joints should be held in at least 70 degrees of flexion.

Sugar Tong Splint
Materials for a sugar tong splint include four-inch plaster rolls, four-inch cast padding, and 2 three-inch Ace bandages. This splint can be used alone or to augment one of the other splints (Fig. 63-13). It provides elbow immobilization and should be placed with the elbow flexed 90 degrees and the forearm in neutral pronation-supination.

Coaptation Splints with Collar-and-Cuff
Materials for a coaptation splint include two to three rolls of four-inch plaster, four-inch cast padding, 2 four-inch Ace bandages, and three feet of cast liner (stockinette). These splints are used for fractures of the middle and distal humerus to provide alignment. They are most effective when used in conjunction with a collar-and-cuff, which allows the weight of the arm to provide a gentle distal traction force. Alternatively, a sling can be used in place of the collar-and-cuff (Fig. 63-14).

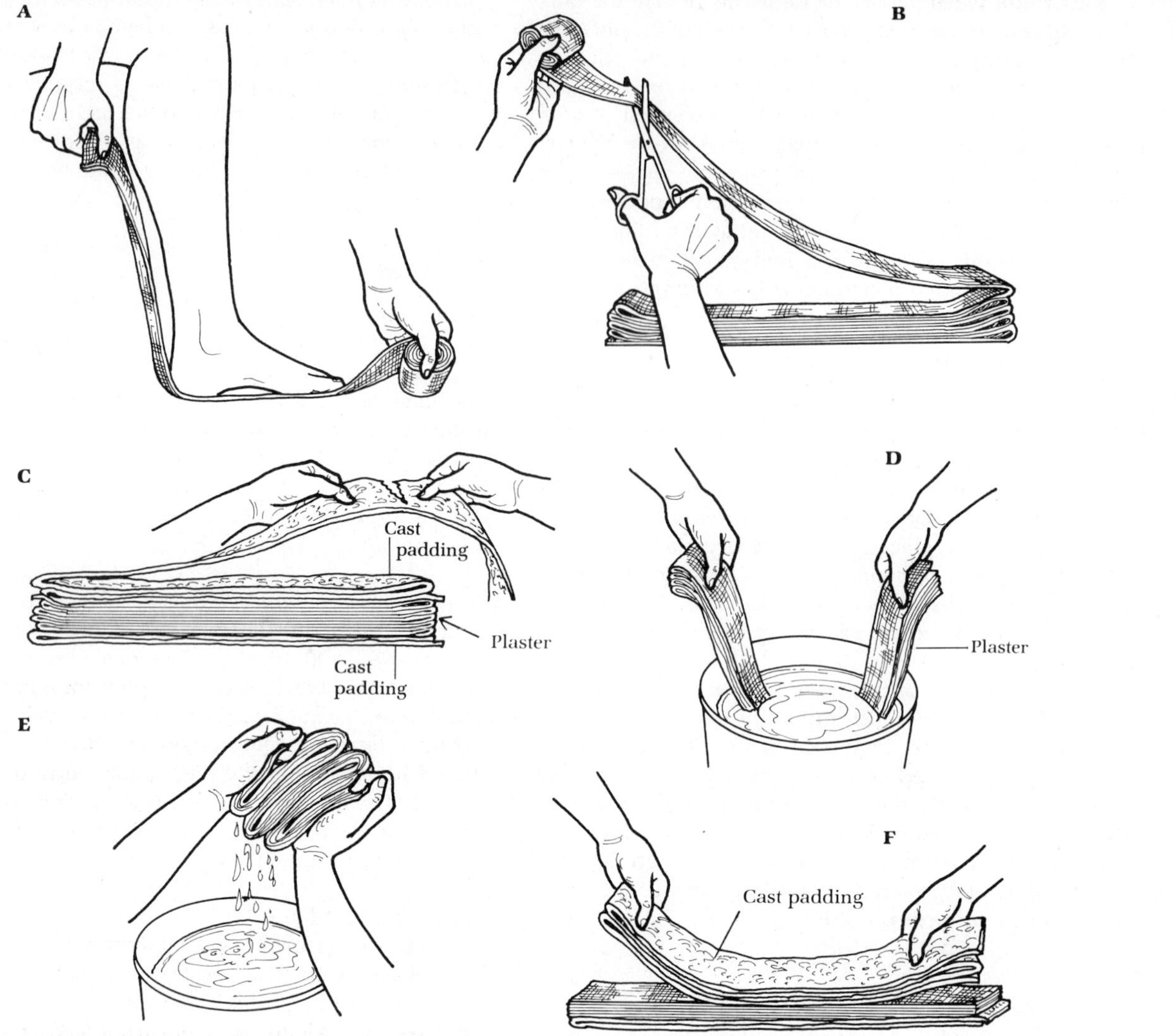

Fig. 63-9. Fabrication of splints from plaster and cast padding. A. The plaster is measured directly against the area to be immobilized, allowing an extra five percent for shrinkage caused by wetting of the material. B. Using this length, the plaster is folded multiple times on itself until at least 10 thicknesses are achieved. C. Cast padding of equivalent length and width is then torn to match the folded plaster. At least 2 thicknesses are needed for the side away from the extremity, while 3 to 4 thicknesses against the extremity will provide adequate protection from the rigid plaster. These lengths of cast padding are then set aside. D. Only the plaster is then firmly grasped at each end and dipped into warm (100°) water sufficient to wet it through all thicknesses. E. The plaster is then carefully folded into an accordion configuration and gently pressed to expel excess water, leaving the plaster damp. The damp plaster is next extended and laid on the cast padding and gently smoothed. F. The second set of cast padding lengths is then placed on top of the wet plaster, creating a padding-plaster-padding composite. The splint is now ready for application to the extremity. The speed at which it will harden depends on the particular plaster used and the temperature of the water.

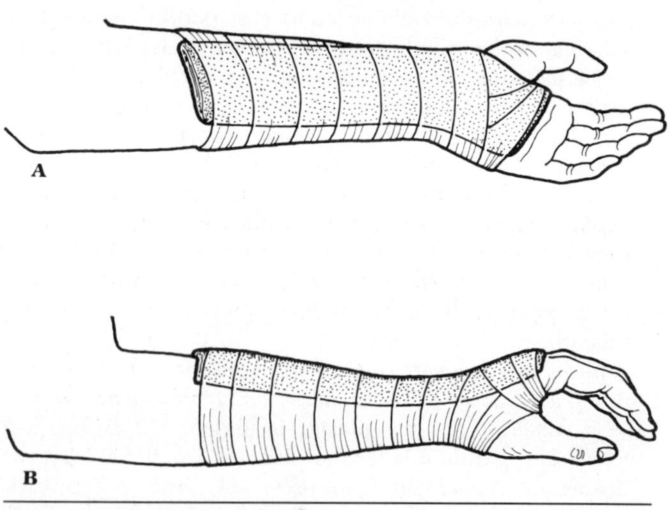

Fig. 63-10. A. Volar wrist splint. B. Dorsal wrist splint. The most common practice is to apply the splint to the volar aspect, but a dorsal application will produce less interference with finger motion. Note particularly that the splint ends proximal to the MCP joints. The wrist should be positioned at approximately 30 degrees of dorsiflexion and not radially or ulnarly deviated.

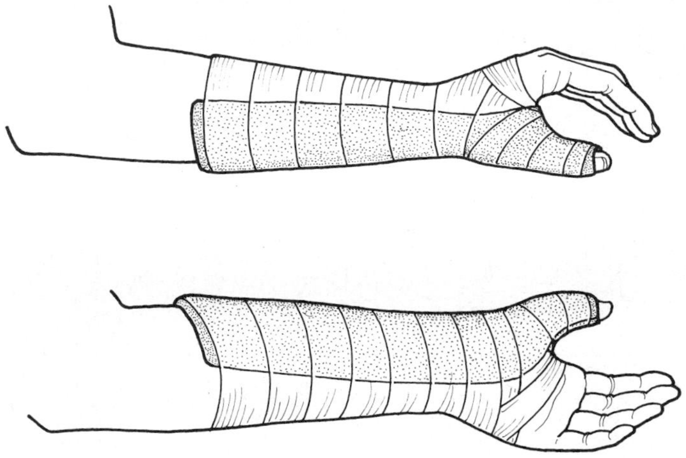

Fig. 63-11. Radial gutter or "thumb spica" splint. This splint is placed along the radial aspect of the forearm and can be brought around the thumb in order to immobilize it in cases of suspected scaphoid fracture or de Quervain's tenosynovitis. Note that the tip of the thumb is left exposed and the thumb is positioned as though the hand were grasping a can of soup.

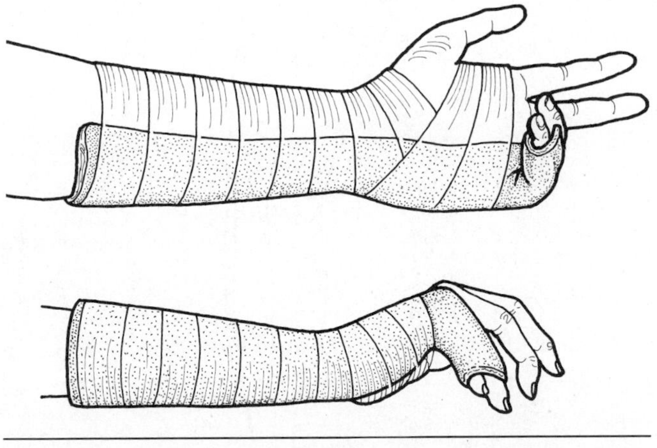

Fig. 63-12. Ulnar gutter splint. This is the splint most commonly used for metacarpal fractures. The wrist is held at approximately 30 degrees of dorsiflexion while the metacarpophalangeal joints are flexed at least 70 degrees. It is important to obtain an x-ray after splinting since the actual position of the MCP joints will be less flexed than is appreciated visually. The thumb, index, and middle fingers are left completely free.

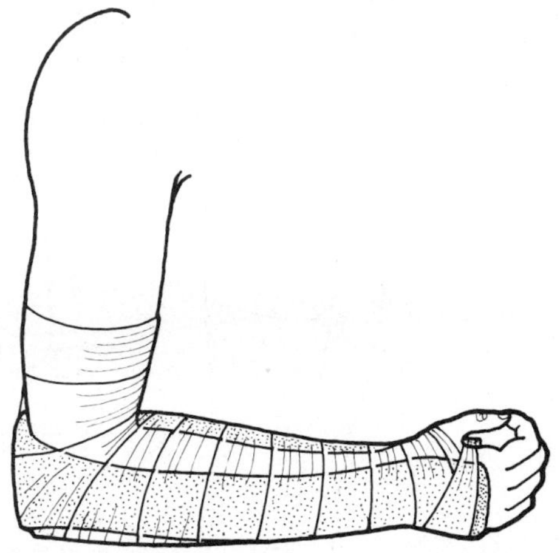

Fig. 63-13. Sugar tong splint. This splint can provide simultaneous immobilization of both the wrist and elbow and can be used alone or in conjunction with other short arm splints such as a radial gutter splint. When used with the volar wrist splint, the sugar tong splint should end proximal to the MCP joints and allow them to flex and extend fully. The usual position of the forearm is in neutral pronation-supination, as shown.

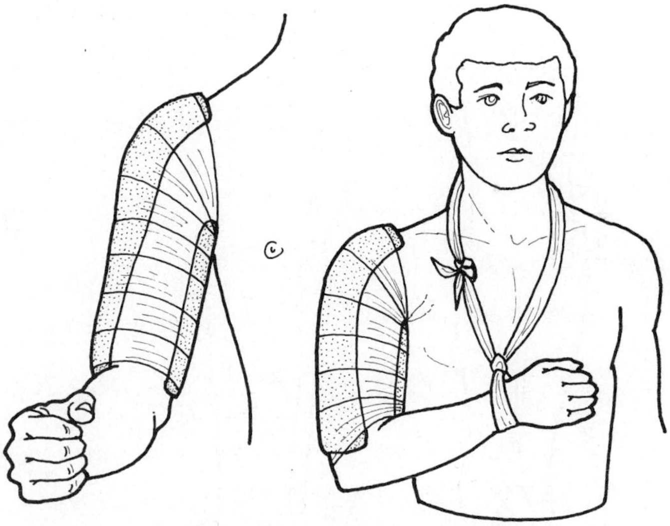

Fig. 63-14. Coaptation splints with collar-and-cuff. The medial splint should be placed as proximal as possible although not so proximal as to cause skin irritation or neurovascular compression in the axilla. X-rays obtained after splinting will often demonstrate a less proximal position of the medial splint than is appreciated at the time of application. The collar-and-cuff should be positioned so that the knot is not pressing at the back of the patient's neck and the wrist is not too tightly constricted.

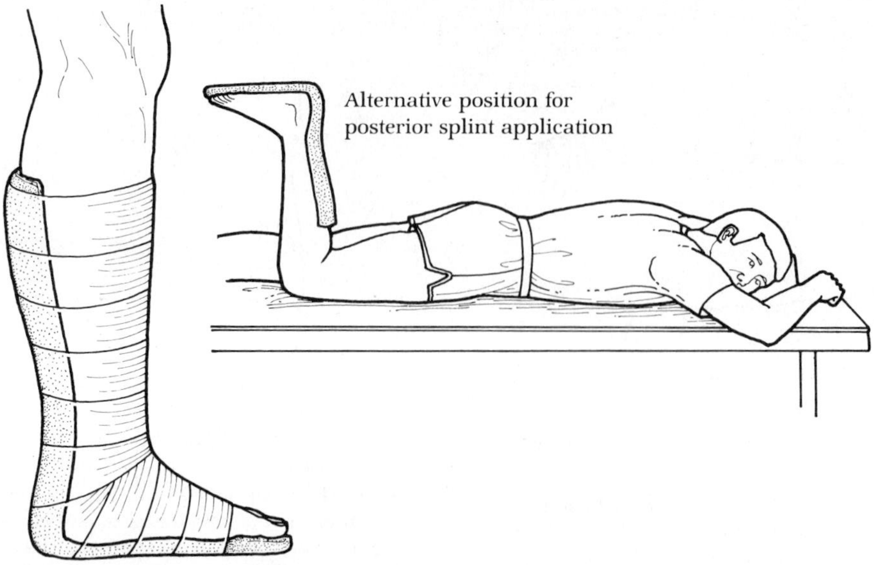

Fig. 63-15. Posterior splint of the lower leg. Note that the splint does not extend so proximally as to interfere with knee motion. The ankle is held as close to neutral as possible. Application of the splint and positioning of the ankle in the neutral position are both facilitated by placing the patient prone with simultaneous knee flexion. This relaxes the gastrosoleus muscles and allows easier positioning of the ankle into neutral.

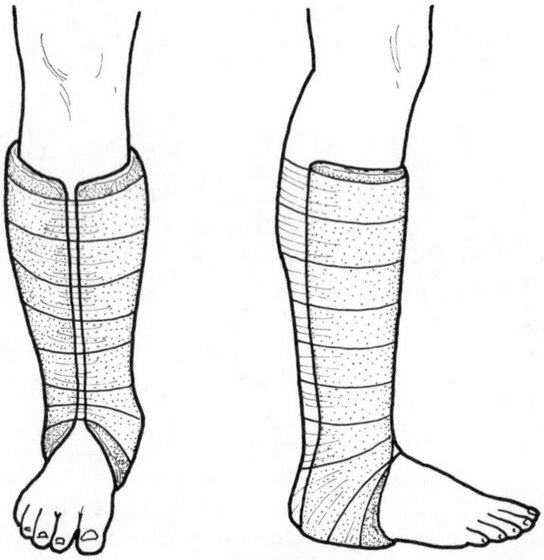

Fig. 63-16. Stirrup splint. This splint can be used alone or in conjunction with the posterior ankle splint to provide greater stability for ankle injuries. Care must be taken not to mold it too firmly over the malleoli in order to prevent skin ulceration. Care must also be taken not to place pressure over the common peroneal nerve near its course around the fibular head.

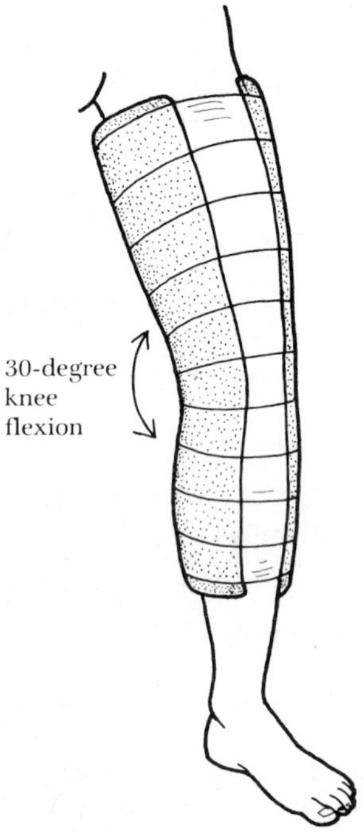

Fig. 63-17. Medial/lateral knee splints. These splints will effectively immobilize a knee, and the typical position is 30 degrees of flexion. These splints should be molded in the supracondylar region of the femur and along the middle and distal calf. Pressure should not be placed in the region of the fibular head, in order to avoid traumatizing the peroneal nerve. This splint can be combined with a posterior splint for the ankle in cases in which both knee and ankle immobilization is desired.

Lower-Extremity Splints

Posterior Splint

Materials for a posterior splint for the ankle include 2 four-inch plaster rolls, four-inch cast padding, and 2 four-inch Ace bandages. For the ankle and knee, 4 four- to five-inch plaster rolls, four-inch cast padding, and 3 to 4 four-inch Ace bandages are needed. For immobilizing the ankle, this is the simplest splint available. It can be carried above the knee when appropriate to provide rotational stability for an unstable ankle fracture or a tibiofibula fracture. The ankle should always be positioned as close to neutral as possible and the knee flexed approximately 30 degrees (Fig. 63-15). One particularly helpful maneuver is to have the patient lie prone with the knee flexed when the splint is applied. If the knee is not to be immobilized, one must be certain that the splint does not press into the popliteal fossa as the knee is flexed. If immobilization of the knee is desired, the splint can be carried up to the posterior thigh, but this does not offer the same rigidity across the knee as medial/lateral splints (described later).

Stirrup Splint

Materials for a stirrup splint include 2 to 3 four-inch plaster rolls, four-inch cast padding, and 2 four-inch Ace bandages. This splint can be used to augment the simple posterior splint just described and will provide much greater stability although it is more complicated to apply (Fig. 63-16). Care must be taken not to mold the stirrup too closely to either medial or lateral malleolus or over the common peroneal nerve, just below the fibular head. As for the simpler posterior splint, placing the patient in the prone position will facilitate application (see Fig. 63-15).

Medial/Lateral Knee Splints

Materials for medial/lateral knee splints include 4 four- or five-inch plaster rolls, four-inch cast padding, and 2 to 3 four-inch Ace bandages. This splint can effectively immobilize a knee in any position, but 30 degrees of flexion is the choice for most injuries as it allows the greatest intraarticular volume to accommodate a traumatic effusion (Fig. 63-17). When applying these splints one should be careful not to press over the fibular head and common peroneal nerve. Instead the splint should be molded more firmly in the supracondylar region and mid-to-distal calf. Extra cast padding should be placed over the fibular head and peroneal nerve.

SELECTED READING

American Academy of Orthopaedic Surgeons: Joint Motion—Method of Measuring and Reading. Chicago, 1965.

Charnley, J. *The Closed Treatment of Common Fractures* (3rd ed). Edinburgh: Churchill Livingstone, 1974.

Crenshaw, AH (ed). *Campbell's Operative Orthopaedics* (7th ed). St. Louis: Mosby, 1987.

Hoppenfeld, S. *Physical Examination of the Spine and Extremities.* New York: Appleton-Century-Crofts, 1976.

Iverson, LD, and Clawson DK. *Manual of Acute Orthopedic Therapeutics.* Boston: Little, Brown, 1977.

64. Shoulder Injuries

Brian J. Awbrey

Injuries of the shoulder are seen frequently in the emergency department or office setting. Sudden and forceful trauma can produce a dramatic injury such as the anteriorly dislocated shoulder. On the other hand, one can see a much more subtle presentation of shoulder dysfunction, without an obvious antecedent event, such as subacromial bursitis. This latter condition also represents an injury to the shoulder—one that occurs incrementally over a prolonged interval. Thus, the spectrum of shoulder injury is very broad.

Accurate diagnosis and the initiation of appropriate early treatment are the goals of the emergency physician. Errors in diagnosis and delayed or inappropriate treatment have particularly severe consequences in the shoulder, which is the most mobile of all the body's joints.

FUNCTIONAL ANATOMY

The shoulder obtains its great mobility from an absence of bony constraints. Unlike the hip's ball-and-socket joint, the shoulder joint is composed of a "ball-and-saucer" that obtains stability and a remarkably large range of motion from a massive cuff of muscles that arises primarily from the upper back region. Further stability is provided by the joint capsule itself. During motion, the shoulder is critically dependent on the free gliding of these supportive, closely approximated soft-tissue layers (Fig. 64-1A). These muscles include the latissimus dorsi, teres major, subscapularis, infraspinatus, supraspinatus, deltoid, pectoralis major, and the long and short heads of the biceps and triceps. In addition, these soft tissues are reinforced by a very strong shoulder capsule and associated ligaments (Fig. 64-1B).

This freedom of movement comes at a cost, however. Because the shoulder depends on the surrounding soft tissues for its stability, tearing or stretching of these structures can result in dislocation (or more subtle subluxation) of the glenohumeral joint. Furthermore, these soft-tissue layers must move past one another over a large distance, and this motion can be easily compromised by inflammation or adhesions. The result is restricted and painful shoulder motion.

Bony Structures

The most dramatic and painful injuries of the shoulder are fractures. These can involve any of the three bones that make up the shoulder girdle: the clavicle, the scapula, or the proximal humerus (see Fig. 64-1B).

The *clavicle* is an S-shaped bone that serves as a protector of the brachial plexus and also acts as a strut to maintain the shoulder girdle at the desired distance from midline. Because of its subcutaneous location, the clavicle is frequently fractured, usually in its middle third, with characteristic upward displacement of the medial fragment produced

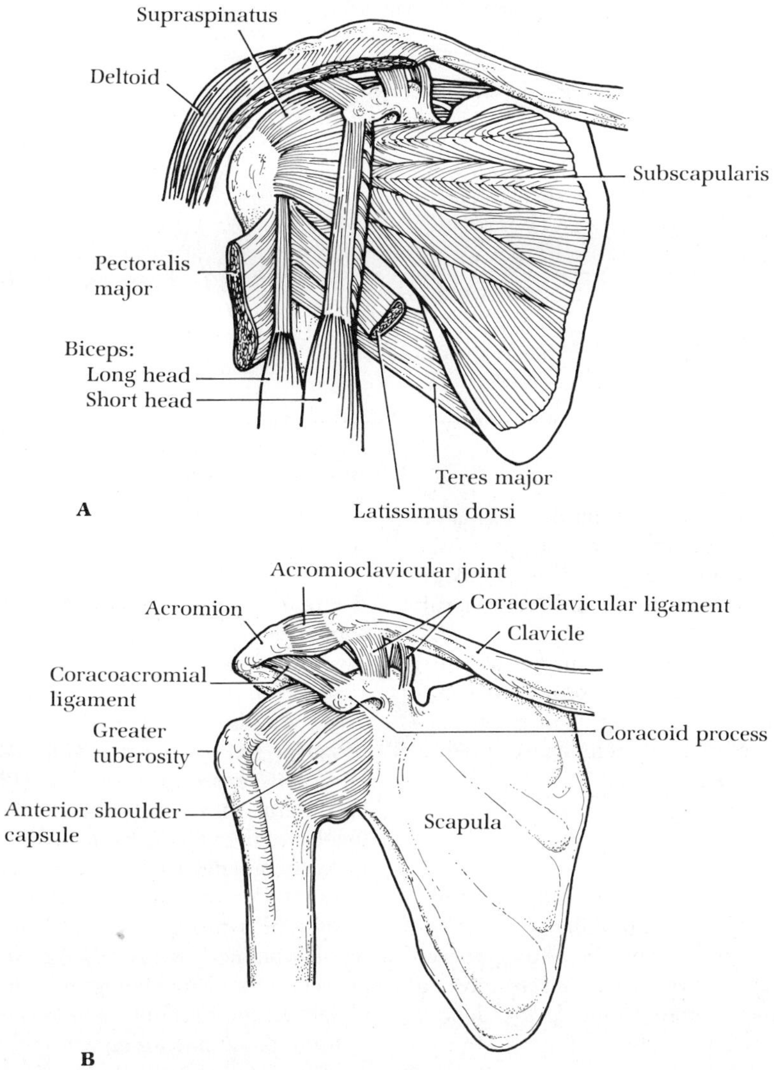

Fig. 64-1. The shoulder is critically dependent on the supportive soft-tissue layers of ligaments, capsule, and numerous muscle groups. An anterior view of the muscles (*A*) and capsule and ligaments (*B*).

by the sternocleidomastoid muscle. The lateral fragment is pulled downward by the weight of the arm, through the coracoclavicular ligaments. At the medial and lateral ends of the clavicle are found the sternoclavicular and acromioclavicular joints respectively. Of the two, the acromioclavicular joint is most frequently involved in injury to the shoulder region.

The *scapula* serves primarily for muscular attachment and has no bony connection to the thorax. It is a large and flat bone with two important bony landmarks, the acromion and the coracoid process (see Fig. 64-1B). It is from the scapula that the muscles of the rotator cuff take their origin. The scapula also provides an articulation with the proximal humerus at the glenoid and with the clavicle at the acromioclavicular joint (Fig. 64-2). In addition, the function of the scapula is facilitated by the significant motion at the sternoclavicular and acromioclavicular joints (Fig. 64-2).

The *proximal humerus* is formed from epiphyseal centers that unite by adolescence to form the humeral head, its greater tuberosity, and its lesser tuberosity. Fractures of the proximal humerus usually occur between these former epiphyseal centers. In the anterior portion of the humeral head, there is a depression between the tuberosities, the bicipital groove, through which runs the tendon of the long head of the biceps.

The *rotator cuff*, or musculotendinous cuff, of the shoulder is the name given to the common tendon that surrounds the nonarticular portion of the humeral head. In this cuff, four muscles are fused into a broad insertion. They are the subscapularis, supraspinatus, infraspinatus, and teres minor. The function of these muscles is to hold the humeral head in position in the glenoid during shoulder abduction and arm elevation, thus permitting raising of the arm without dislocation. This permits clearance of the greater tuberosity beneath the acromial arch as the shoulder is both abducted and elevated. Inflammation or small tears in the rotator cuff can produce painful and restricted motion of the glenohumeral joint while large tears of the cuff can result in the loss of active abduction and forward flexion.

The *superficial muscle layer* consists of the deltoid mus-

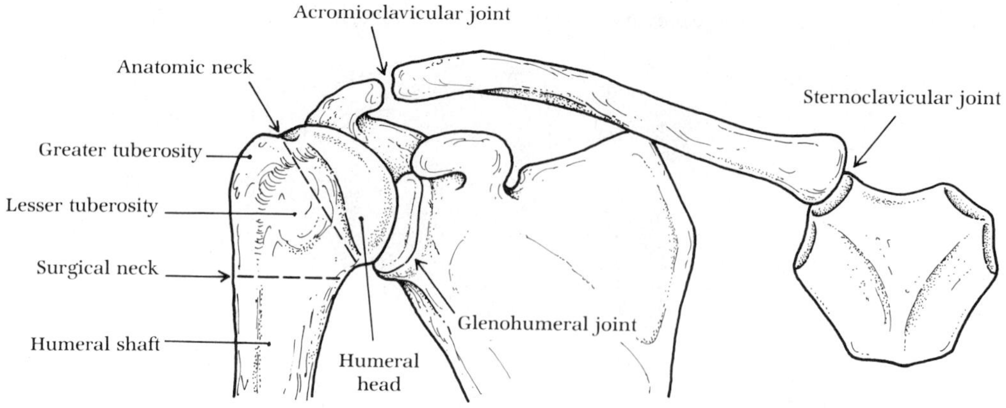

Fig. 64-2. The bones and joints that are a part of the shoulder girdle, and anatomic landmarks of the proximal humerus, as shown from an anterior perspective.

cle, which originates on the clavicle and scapula and inserts at the junction of the proximal and middle thirds of the humerus. Strains and contusions of this muscle are commonly seen in the emergency department and rarely result in long-term dysfunction.

The *subacromial bursa* is located in the interval between the rotator cuff and the overlying bony acromion. It facilitates the gliding motion of the rotator cuff as it passes beneath the bony arch and is of clinical significance when it becomes inflamed (subacrominal bursitis).

Associated Structures

Other important soft-tissue structures adjacent to the shoulder joint include the brachial plexus and axillary artery (inferior), the cephalic vein (anterior), and the axillary nerve (posterolateral). The axillary nerve provides sensation to the lateral shoulder and motor information to the deltoid muscle.

FRACTURES

Clavicle Fractures

The clavicle is a frequently fractured bone and possibly the most common pediatric fracture seen in the emergency department. Fractures of the clavicle are classified according to their location in either the medial, middle, or lateral third. The vast majority are middle third clavicle fractures, with the medial and lateral third fractures accounting for 5 and 15 percent of the total, respectively. Furthermore, fractures of the lateral third of the clavicle are functionally divided into three types according to the mechanism of fracture and treatment requirements (Fig. 64-3). Type I is nondisplaced or minimally displaced, with ligaments intact; type II is displaced with obvious deformity of the proximal fragment; and type III is a fracture across both sides of the acromioclavicular joint.

Evaluation

The patient with a clavicle fracture will complain of tenderness directly over the clavicle and will hold the arm against the body to protect against any motion of the shoulder. Initial inspection may reveal a deformity along the anterior shoulder region with evidence of swelling over the clavicle and shoulder. There may be palpable motion of the fracture fragments and localized crepitus.

When a clavicle fracture is suspected, two radiographic views should be obtained. The first is a standard anteroposterior (AP) projection (Fig. 64-4A) and the second is a 30- to 45-degree lordotic view (Fig. 64-4B). If a fracture of the lateral third of the clavicle is identified or suspected, involvement of the acromioclavicular (AC) joint and damage to AC ligaments are best evaluated by taking an AP x-ray of the shoulder with the patient in the standing position. This x-ray will better demonstrate associated soft-tissue damage if it is obtained by decreasing the x-ray voltage intensity by 20 percent and by having the patient hold a 5- to 10-pound weight in the hand of the affected shoulder.

Immediate assessment for possible neurovascular injury is of the utmost importance. Fortunately, these injuries are extremely rare despite the proximity of the brachial plexus and subclavian artery to the clavicle. Pneumothorax is also rare but should be suspected and appropriately evaluated in high-energy injuries.

Treatment

For fractures of the middle third, treatment can be started within the emergency department. A figure-of-eight strap is most commonly used (Fig. 64-5). Perfect reduction of clavicle fractures is impossible to maintain by any nonoperative therapy and is not necessary. Attempting to manipulate the ends of a fractured clavicle into anatomic alignment is extremely painful and can result in skin necrosis if excess pressure is placed by the strap. For best results, the figure-of-eight splint should be applied with the patient sitting in an upright military recruit (shoulders back, chest out) position. The strap should be slowly tightened and the buckle attached so that it is snug, placing about as much pressure onto the shoulder as would the straps of a moderately heavy backpack (Fig. 64-5). A reliable family member should be instructed to tighten the strap, as needed, twice daily during the subsequent few days to maintain the fit initially achieved in the emergency department. Patients should be instructed to take several days of rest, in which the patient lies in a

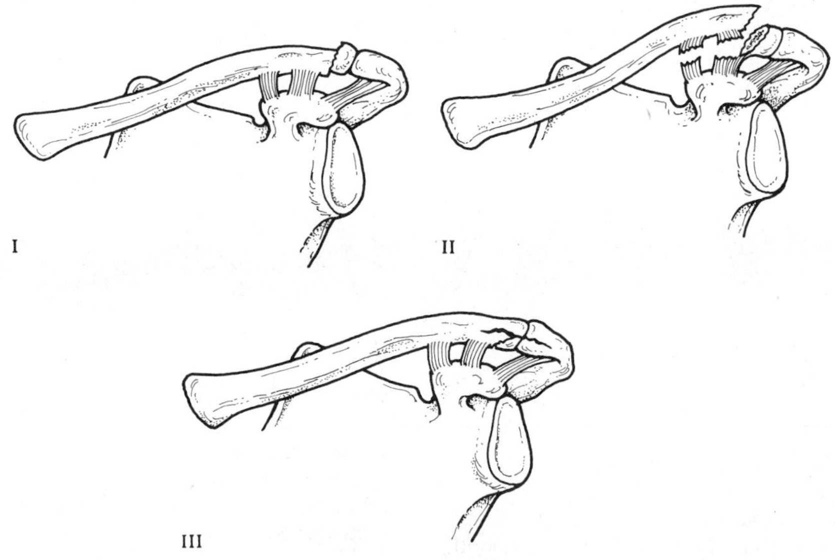

Fig. 64-3. Classification of fractures of the lateral third of the clavicle, as originally described by Neer (see text). (Redrawn from C.S. Neer, II. Fractures of the distal third of the clavicle. *Clin. Orthop.* 58: 43, 1968.)

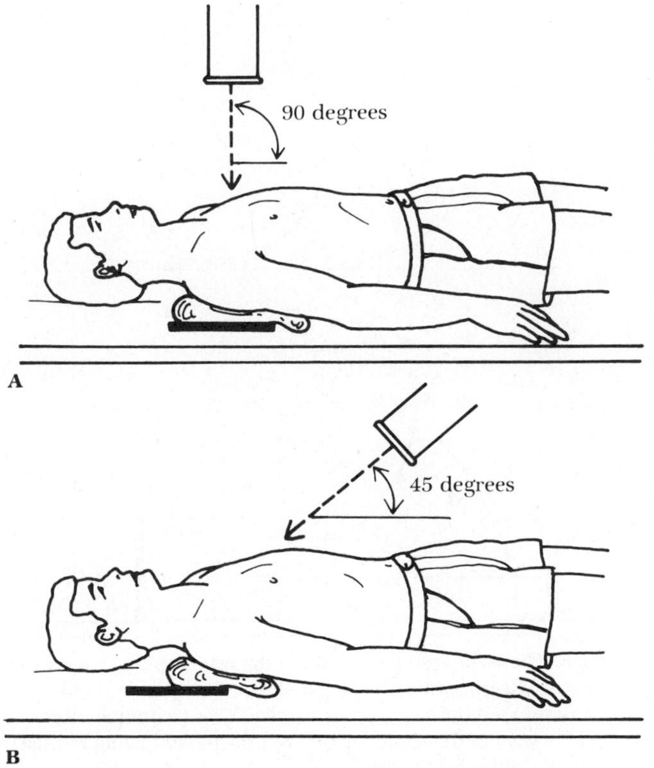

Fig. 64-4. The technique for obtaining two radiographic views of the clavicle. The anteroposterior view (A), shooting directly through the clavicle, and the 45-degree lordotic view (B), angling the x-ray beam toward the head with the film plate placed superior to the first view.

semireclining position in a chair or bed, with the arm supported by a pillow. Analgesics should be prescribed and the patient referred for orthopedic follow-up examination in three to five days. Fractures of the medial third of the clavicle should be treated with a supportive sling placed and analgesics given, with orthopedic follow-up in three to five days.

For fractures of the lateral third of the clavicle, treatment depends on the occurrence of displacement of the fracture or involvement of the acromioclavicular joint (see Fig. 64-3). For nondisplaced fractures, type I, a sling (not a figure-of-eight strap) and analgesics are provided, with follow-up evaluation as for other clavicle fractures. If the fracture is displaced, type II, or if it enters the acromioclavicular joint, type III, the orthopedist should be contacted at the time of presentation. Further treatment recommendations in type III fractures may be for either operative or nonoperative treatment.

For neurovascular compromise, even if transient, orthopedic and vascular consultations should be sought, since further study in the form of angiography may be necessary, and admission for observation should be considered. For open injuries or for skin over the clavicle, compromise orthopedic evaluation is necessary in the emergency department.

Although nonunion and complications of clavicle fractures are uncommon, prominence of the bone at fracture site, particularly in thin individuals, is common and usually permanent. The majority of clavicle fractures achieve union within six to eight weeks of injury in adults and three to four weeks in children. Formal physical therapy is rarely needed in the majority of clavicle fractures, but close follow-up study as to union and restoration of shoulder function is essential.

Scapula Fractures

Scapula fractures are relatively uncommon and usually occur as the result of high-energy trauma to the shoulder. There are two types: fractures of the body of the scapula, due to direct high-energy impact, and fractures about the glenoid, occurring as a result of avulsion injury or disloca-

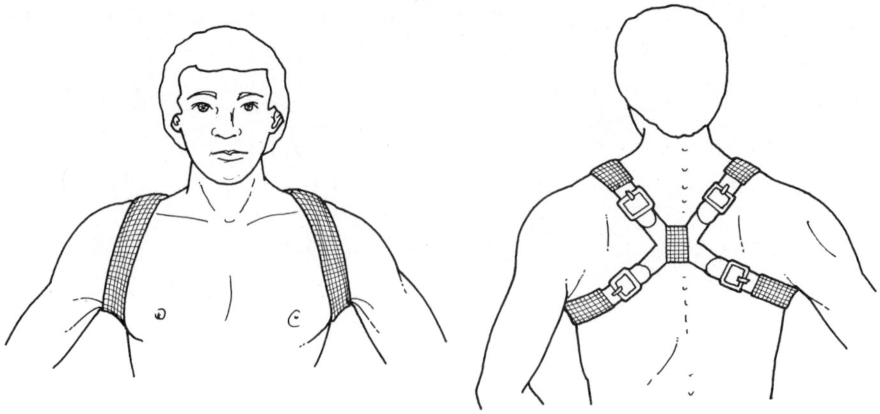

Fig. 64-5. The figure-of-eight clavicle strap. The strap is positioned like a backpack strap, with the patient in a sitting position, and each portion is tightened posteriorly until it applies firm pressure on the distal clavicle.

tion of the humeral head. Scapula fractures can be difficult to visualize radiographically but should be suspected with associated fracture of the first rib, pneumothorax, and even head and visceral injuries. It is common to discover these fractures incidentally, subsequent to admission, in the polytraumatized patient.

Evaluation

The patient will complain of pain of a diffuse nature about the shoulder and scapula region that may increase with attempts to lift the affected arm. Radiographic evaluation of the scapula should be by full chest x-ray, comparing the two scapulae. In addition, anteroposterior and transscapular lateral (Neer) x-ray views (Fig. 64-6) are helpful in diagnosing both scapula fractures and associated thoracic injuries. The incidence of other injuries associated with scapula fractures is very high, and the examiner should look for evidence of rib fracture, clavicle fracture, pneumothorax, and flail chest. In cases in which the fracture involves the glenoid, tomograms and computed tomographic scanning may be necessary to adequately image the fracture, but such studies are rarely necessary in the emergency department.

Treatment

For fractures of the scapular body, treatment is a simple sling or shoulder immobilizer, also known as "sling-and-swathe" (Fig. 64-7), for several weeks. This is followed by range-of-motion exercises, which can be initiated as tolerated. Prolonged immobilization is not required, and these fractures rarely displace because of the surrounding soft tissues (see Fig. 64-1A), which tend to stabilize, rather than displace, the fracture fragments. As was noted previously, these fractures occur in severely injured patients, and hospital admission is common.

For fractures of the glenoid, orthopedic consultation should be obtained at the time of presentation. Small avulsion fractures are rarely treated surgically, but open reduction and internal fixation of the glenoid may be indicated for significant angulation or displacement of the fracture or disruption of the articular surface as noted by x-ray examination. If the patient with a glenoid fracture is to be released from the emergency department, a sling or shoulder immobilizer should be placed and referral made to an orthopedic surgeon in two to three days.

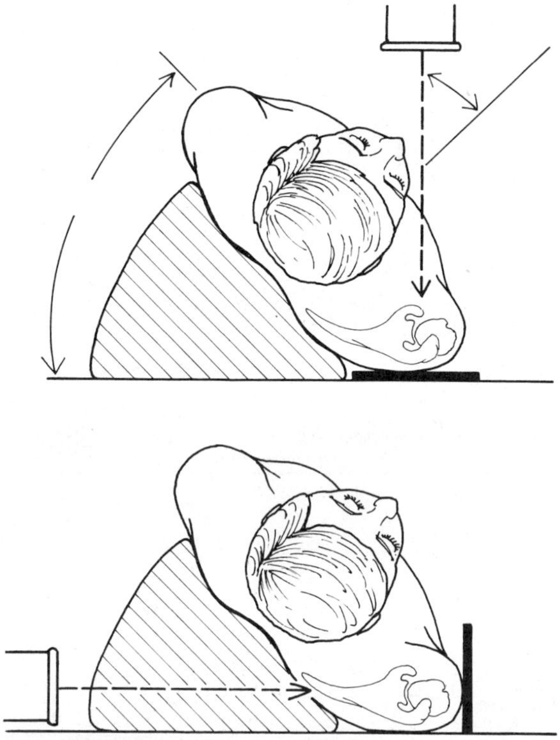

Fig. 64-6. The technique for obtaining the AP (*top*) and transscapular lateral (Neer; *bottom*) radiographs of the shoulder, with the patient positioned on a 45-degree bolster. This technique allows 90-degree views of the shoulder without the patient being required to move the injured shoulder.

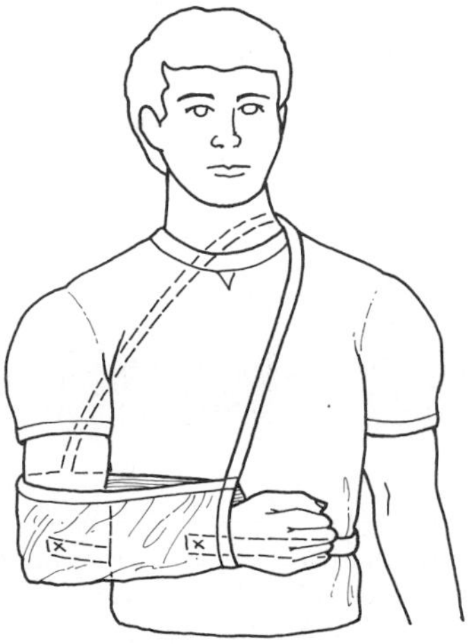

Fig. 64-7. The proper application of a universal shoulder immobilizer. The arm sling should first be positioned, then the body strap should be placed.

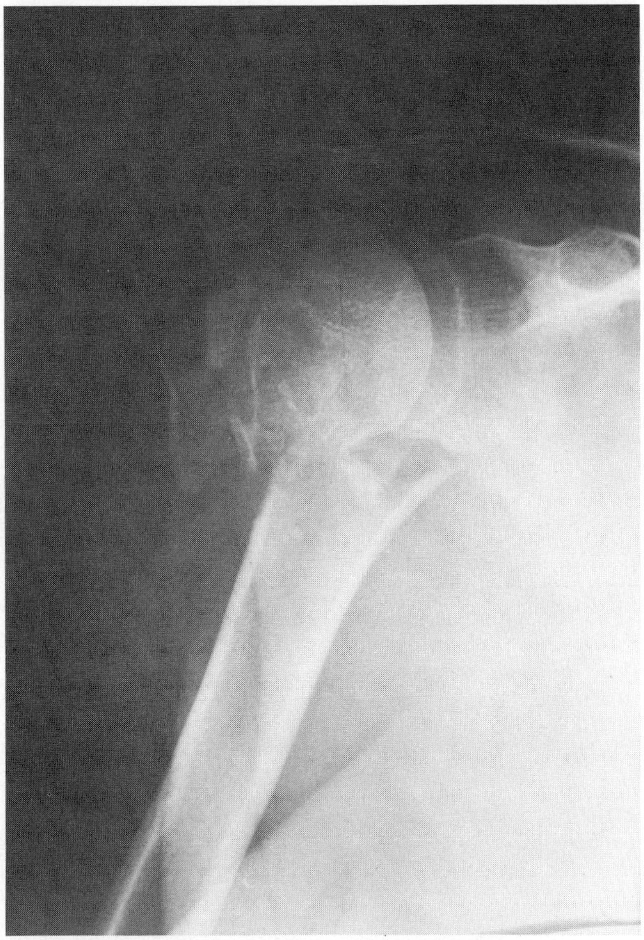

Fig. 64-8. A minimally displaced, two-part, proximal humerus fracture. There are two fragments: the humeral head and the humeral shaft. Early treatment consists of immobilization with a sling combined with a swathe if needed for comfort. This is followed by early range of motion, before complete fracture healing.

Supervised physical therapy is almost always required for scapular body and glenoid fractures, whether treated operatively or not. Some loss of motion is to be expected, particularly in older patients, but a functional range of motion is usually achieved.

Proximal Humerus Fractures

Fractures of the proximal humerus are most commonly seen in elderly patients after a fall onto the outstretched arm or directly on the shoulder. Most of these fractures are stable injuries in which the shaft of the humerus has been driven into the humeral head, with minimal displacement of the fracture fragments (Fig. 64-8). The majority of these fractures occur at the level of the surgical neck (see Fig. 64-2). These fractures are best described using the Neer classification system, which divides the humerus into four anatomic parts: the head, lesser tuberosity, greater tuberosity, and shaft (see Fig. 64-2).

Displaced fractures are described according to the number of displaced fracture fragments. A separate fracture of each part (articular surface, greater tuberosity, lesser tuberosity) is thus called a two-part, three-part, or four-part fracture depending on anatomic involvement. A two-part fracture is one in which either the head, greater tuberosity, or lesser tuberosity is displaced in relationship to the shaft. A three-part fracture is one in which two of these fragments are displaced relative to the shaft. A four-part fracture is one in which all three fragments are significantly separated from each other and the shaft of the humerus. Such severe displacement can occur as the result of large injury forces, osteopenic bone, or both.

Evaluation

The patient with a proximal humeral fracture will complain of severe pain and tenderness about the shoulder. There may be inability to move the shoulder, although the elderly patient with a stable fracture may have little pain or restricted motion on initial examination.

Radiographic evaluation should consist of two views of the shoulder: a true AP view (see Fig. 64-9A) and either a lateral scapula (Neer) view (see Fig. 64-6) or an axillary view (see Fig. 64-9B). The AP and lateral views can be obtained with the patient sitting with the arm in a sling, and no motion of the shoulder joint is required. These two views will show not only the presence of fracture, but also an associated glenohumeral dislocation, if present.

Treatment

For nondisplaced-impacted fractures of the humeral neck or minimally displaced (<1 cm) fractures of a single major segment, the initial treatment is a sling or sling-and-swathe for comfort (Fig. 64-10). An absorbent pad should be placed in the axilla and changed daily to prevent skin maceration due to moisture. Analgesics are prescribed as appropriate, but with care in the case of elderly patients. Orthopedic follow-up study should be arranged within 7 to 10 days.

For all displaced fractures, or fractures consisting of multiple fragments, orthopedic consultation at presentation is advised (Fig. 64-11). In some cases, treatment will be identical to that for nondisplaced fractures. However, a large num-

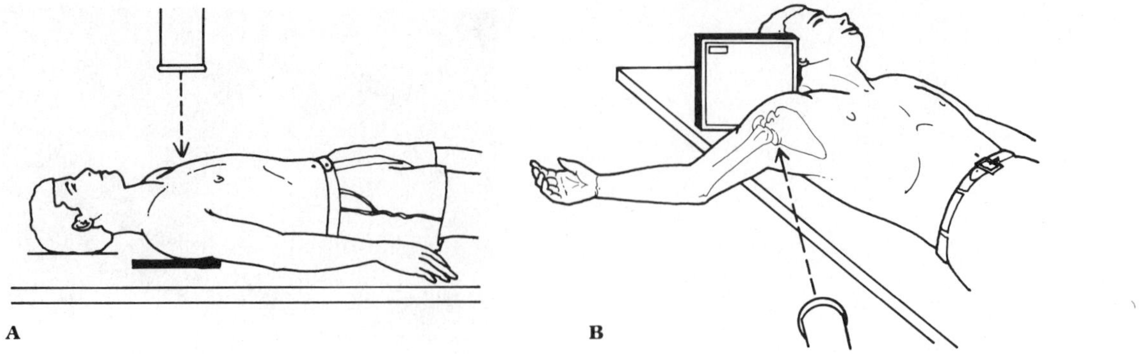

Fig. 64-9. The technique for obtaining AP (A) and axillary lateral (B) views of the shoulder joint. The axillary lateral view requires the patient to be able to abduct the shoulder, with the x-ray beam aimed at the axilla and the film placed superior to the shoulder.

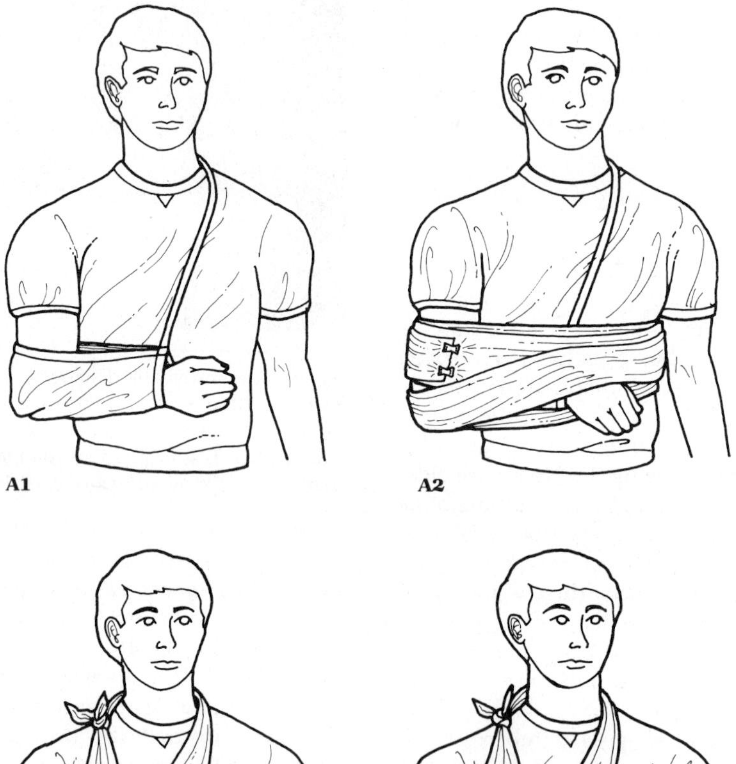

Fig. 64-10. The proper technique of application of a sling-and-swathe bandage for shoulder injuries using a standard sling (A) or a triangular bandage sling (B). The swathe should be applied so as to allow free use of the involved hand.

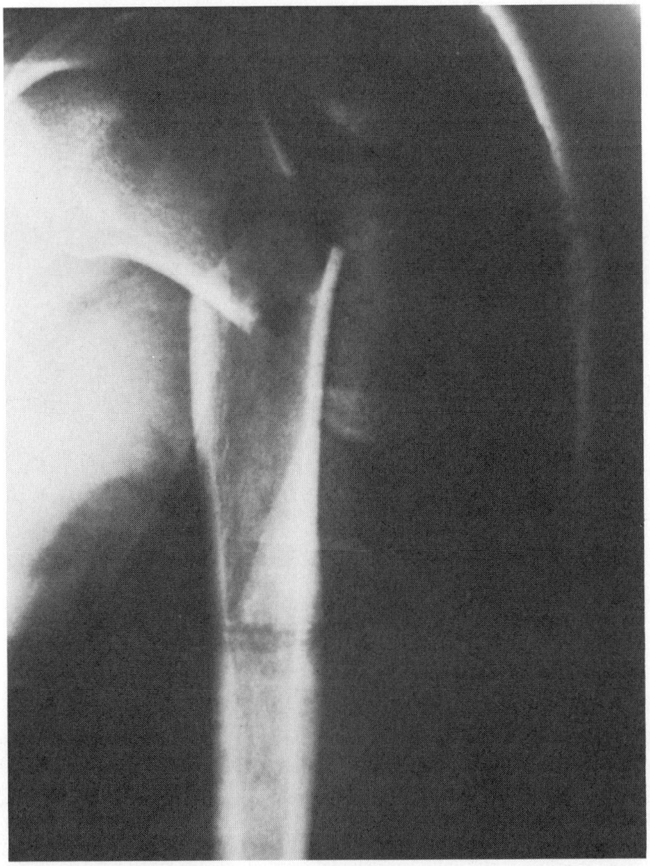

Fig. 64-11. Anteroposterior radiograph of a low humeral neck fracture with unacceptable angulation. This fracture requires a reduction maneuver and immobilization. Orthopedic consultation at the time of presentation is advised.

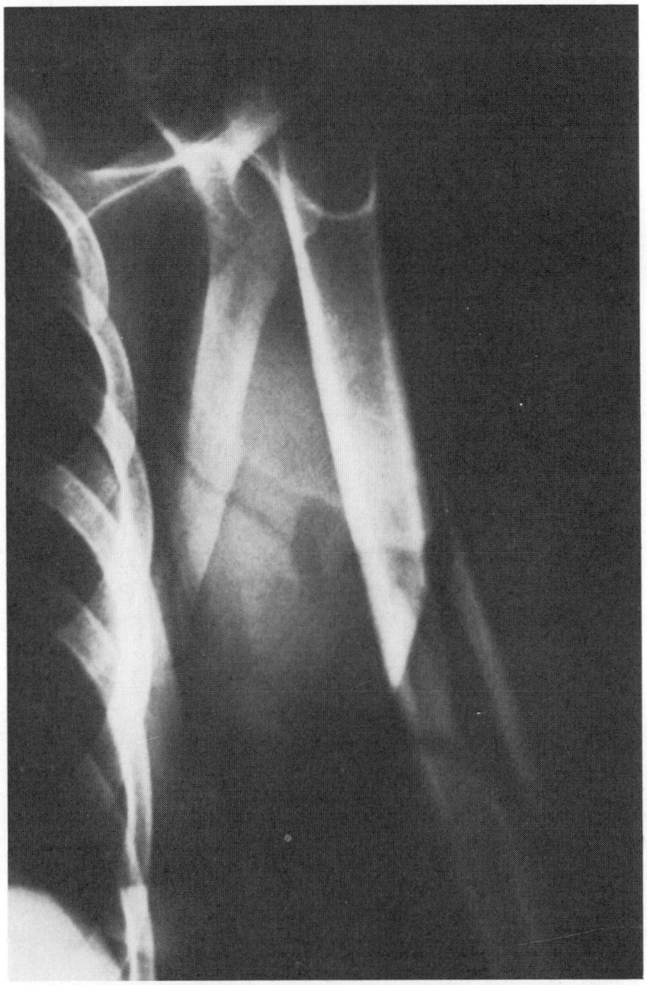

Fig. 64-12. Anteroposterior radiograph of the humerus showing an oblique midshaft fracture with a single, large comminuted fragment. The status of the radial nerve should be checked in all such fractures.

ber of these fractures are treated more aggressively, either by manipulation, internal fixation of the fracture fragments, or, when severe displacement has occurred, prosthetic replacement of the proximal humerus. The decision to proceed with surgical management is best made early, so in these cases the orthopedic consultation should not be delayed. Prolonged immobilization of the shoulder in the elderly is to be avoided at all costs since it could result in later adhesive capsulitis and loss of shoulder motion.

Some degree of permanent loss of shoulder motion is the rule after proximal humerus fractures. Close supervision of physical therapy is essential and success is critically dependent on the patient's effort and persistence in therapy during the first three months. Associated tears of the rotator cuff can often accompany displaced fractures and can impair the long-term function of the shoulder. These are diagnosed and assessed after shoulder motion has been started. The tears can be treated surgically in younger individuals but are rarely so treated in the elderly. Union of fractures of the proximal humerus occurs reliably.

Humeral Shaft Fractures

Humeral shaft fractures occur as the result of a fall onto the outstretched arm, or as the result of direct trauma to the arm itself. They are usually located below the level of the deltoid insertion (Fig. 64-12).

The posterior humeral shaft gives origin to the medial and lateral heads of the triceps. The radial nerve runs in close proximity to the posterior humeral shaft, particularly at the midshaft (Fig. 64-13). Anteriorly, the humerus is covered by the origin of the brachialis muscle and, superficial to this, the biceps muscle. With fractures of the diaphysis of the humerus, the fracture fragments usually displace as a direct result of muscular forces. Thus, angulation and shortening can occur.

Evaluation

Diagnosis is rarely difficult, except in cases where a nutrient artery is mistaken for a nondisplaced fracture line. X-rays in two planes, with palpation of the shaft to localize the tenderness, will usually resolve this question.

Fractures of the middle and lower thirds of the humeral shaft require careful examination of the upper extremity for possible radial nerve injury, because of the proximity of bone and nerve at these levels. The radial nerve can be damaged

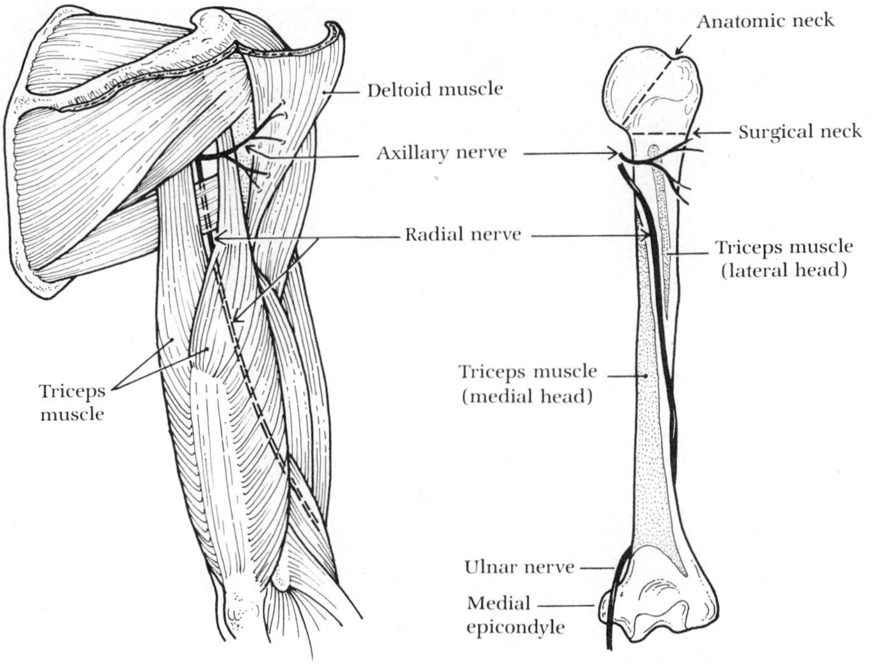

Fig. 64-13. The posterior aspect of the humeral shaft gives origin to the medial and lateral heads of the triceps. The radial nerve courses in close proximity to the humeral shaft throughout the entire central third and can be damaged or entrapped by fractures in this region of the humerus.

at the time of fracture, or at any time in the subsequent transport or treatment of the patient, by becoming entrapped within the fracture site (see Fig. 64-13). Active extension of the fingers, dorsiflexion of the wrist, and extension of the thumb must be documented. In addition, sensation over the dorsum of the thumb and first web space of the hand should also be tested.

Patients with humeral shaft fractures should have the injured arm splinted with a sling-and-swathe against the chest wall before x-rays are obtained (see Fig. 64-10). Although this immobilization can hamper the effort to obtain certain views, it is safer and less painful to the patient. If specific views are needed, the sling can be released and the arm carefully positioned on the x-ray table by the physician.

Treatment

Orthopedic consultation is indicated for all humeral shaft fractures at the time of presentation. Immobilization can be obtained by coaptation splints or possibly a hanging cast that utilizes the weight of the arm plus a cast to provide continuous gravity traction on the fracture fragments. The majority of humeral shaft fractures can be managed in such a closed fashion. If angulation cannot be adequately controlled, open reduction and internal fixation of the fracture may be recommended.

As a rule, a radial nerve injury that occurred at the time of the fracture should be observed, with recovery of function expected within 6 to 12 weeks of injury. On the other hand, if radial nerve function was initially present and is later lost, either during transport of the patient or during reduction of the fracture, then exploration of the nerve may be recommended if prompt return of function does not occur. This is because nerve function that is lost after the time of the initial injury is more likely due to mechanical compression or laceration than it is to neuropraxic "stretch" and will more likely require the surgical release or repair of the radial nerve.

Union of humeral shaft fractures can be expected at six to eight weeks and is seldom delayed. Angulation and shortening are rarely a problem, and excellent return of shoulder and elbow function should be anticipated if a supervised physical therapy program is followed.

DISLOCATIONS

Glenohumeral Joint Dislocation

Dislocations of the glenohumeral joint (Fig. 64-14) are extremely common injuries, most frequently seen as a result of athletic activity. Dislocation occurring in patients under age 20 is associated with a higher incidence of recurrence, and the eventual need for surgical repair is frequent. Patients who have a first dislocation after age 20 will have a much lower incidence of recurrence, but mild restriction of shoulder motion is more likely to develop.

As described earlier in this chapter, the remarkable range of motion and versatility of the shoulder joint are owed to its ball-and-saucer configuration. The large articular surface of the humeral head is only congruent with the glenoid over a third of its surface at any given time. Because of the need for massive soft-tissue support of the joint, any breach in the supporting structure about the joint can lead to instability and possible dislocation.

Acute shoulder dislocations are primarily (95%) anterior dislocations. Of these, the subcoracoid anterior dislocation is the most common, with the humeral head lying just infe-

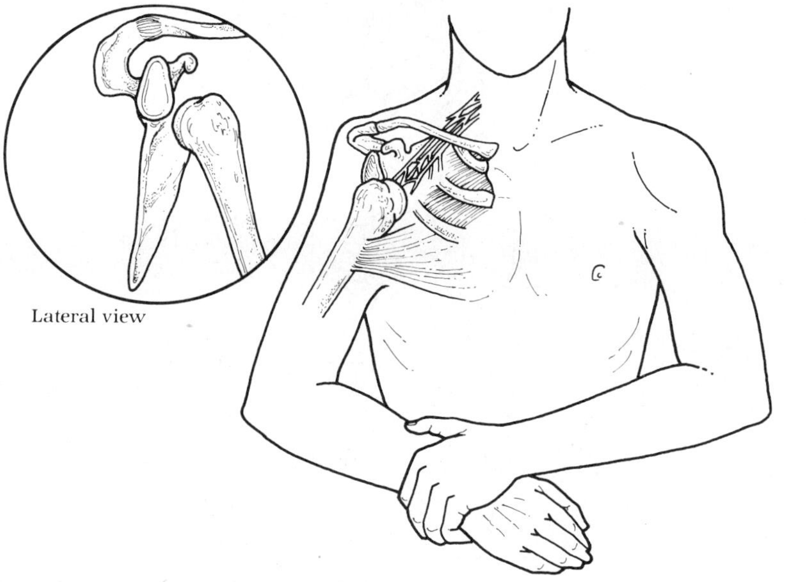

Fig. 64-14. Acute shoulder dislocations are primarily anteroinferior dislocations in which the patient will be seen in great pain, holding the injured arm. Anterior shoulder dislocations can lead to neurovascular injury as a result of pressure of the humeral head in the region of the brachial plexus and subclavian artery and stretching of the axillary nerve.

rior to the coracoid process. On rare occasions, a subclavicular or intrathoracic anterior dislocation is seen. Posterior shoulder dislocations occur almost exclusively as the result of seizures, electrical shock, or forced internal rotation of the arm, such as when it is placed in a "hammer lock."

Evaluation

Patients with acute shoulder dislocations arrive at the emergency department in extreme distress, most often holding the injured arm by the chest in an attempt to splint the shoulder and prevent any motion. In a case where previous dislocation has occurred, careful attention should be paid to the neurovascular examination since past injury to the axillary nerve or brachial plexus, or both, may have occurred.

Observation of the affected shoulder will reveal a fullness anteriorly due to the anterior dislocation or, in the case of the posterior dislocation, a fullness posteriorly. A noticeable step-off or squaring at the lateral acromion may be seen. In the case of anterior dislocation, there is a palpable "hollow" lateral to the acromion. The heavily muscled or obese individual may have no reliable visible sign of shoulder dislocation.

Initial examination should consist of attention to the distal neurovascular function, particularly that of the axillary nerve (Fig. 64-15). The axillary nerve supplies the deltoid muscle as well as a patch of cutaneous sensation over the lateral deltoid (Fig. 64-16).

Although the temptation to reduce the apparent dislocation immediately is strong, it is not a wise procedure and should be deferred until AP and transscapular lateral (Neer) radiographs are obtained (see Fig. 64-6). The transscapular (Neer) view will confirm whether the dislocation is anterior

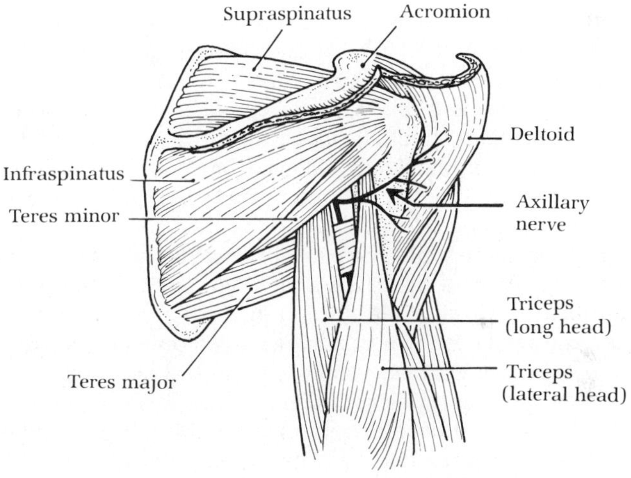

Fig. 64-15. The posterior musculature of the shoulder. Note the location of the axillary nerve coursing close to the posterior shoulder capsule, exiting the quadrilateral space over the lateral head of the triceps and innervating the deltoid and the skin overlying the deltoid insertion.

or posterior, and is an essential part of the evaluation. If an associated fracture or nerve injury is present, reduction should be deferred to the orthopedic surgeon, who should be summoned immediately.

One should be particularly aware of the potential for posterior dislocation. The most consistent clinical finding is an inability to externally rotate. The anterior and posterior dislocations are best determined on the transscapular (Neer) x-ray view. Posterior dislocations are often chronic and the patient may have little pain. If a chronic dislocation is suspected by history, it may be best to obtain orthopedic consultation before a reduction is attempted. In the case of chronic dislocation, reduction may not be possible or desirable.

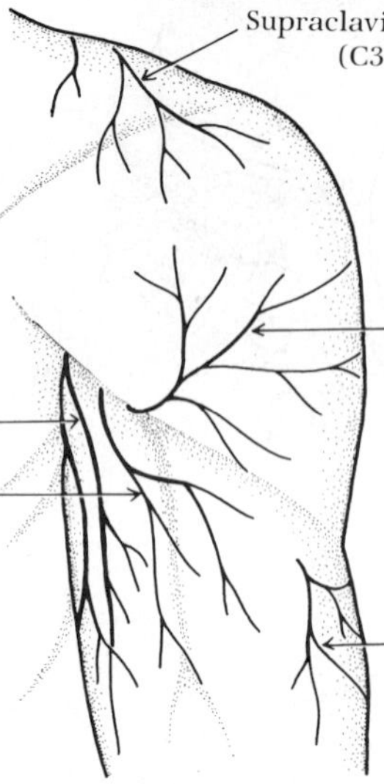

Fig. 64-16. The supply of skin sensation overlying the posterior shoulder. Note the area of cutaneous innervation by the axillary nerve, also known as the superolateral cutaneous branch.

Treatment

For uncomplicated acute anterior dislocations, reduction should be performed as soon as possible. Initially, an intravenous line should be placed and analgesics given in the form of meperidine or morphine. It is helpful, but not necessary, to supplement this with diazepam. Administration of these medications should be under the direct guidance of the physician and immediately followed by a gentle reduction maneuver. The simplest and most effective maneuver is one whereby the elbow is extended and the arm is held adducted against the chest wall. The patient's chest is stabilized with a sheet firmly held by an assistant (Fig. 64-17). The physician then provides gentle traction in the line of the arm in one hand while the arm is gently elevated over the patient's head. At 90 degrees of elevation, the humeral head will usually relocate. The physician's opposite hand can be used to push the humeral head into position. By this maneuver, the muscular structures that hold the humeral head in a dislocated position are relaxed.

There are also several other ways to reduce the dislocated shoulder. One is the modified Kocher maneuver whereby instead of applying traction while the arm is elevated, the elbow is flexed and a second sheet is applied around the elbow and the waist of the physician performing the reduction, such that, by a combination of direct traction, internal rotation, and pressure directly over the humeral head, reduction is accomplished. Another appropriate reduction, requiring less force, is one in which the patient is placed prone on the examination table and is asked to hold up to 15 pounds of traction weight in the involved hand while the physician applies a force of downward traction and internal rotation. Successful reduction is heralded by pain relief but not always a marked reduction "clunk." With reduction, the previous lateral acromial hollow should be full. If reduction is unsuccessful after several attempts, an orthopedic surgeon should be contacted, as occasionally a general anesthetic is required, particularly in a heavily muscled individual.

After reduction, the patient will normally experience tremendous pain relief. At this point, neurovascular status should be rechecked. A shoulder immobilizer or simple sling-and-swathe should be applied to hold the arm in internal rotation against the chest wall (see Fig. 64-10). An absorbent pad should be placed in the axilla. Postreduction x-rays are mandatory and should consist of an anteroposterior and transscapular lateral (Neer) view. If the reduction is well maintained and no fracture has appeared, the patient can be discharged, with instructions to change the axillary pad daily and to seek orthopedic follow-up examination within a week of injury.

For the dislocation associated with fracture of the humeral head or glenoid, or the presence of a chronic bony defect in the humeral head (Hill-Sachs lesion), evaluation by an orthopedic surgeon before reduction is indicated. The Hill-Sachs lesion is a frequent complicating fracture of shoulder dislocations and is caused by glenoid pressure compressing into the posterior humeral head (Fig. 64-18). Certain fractures require operative management, and involvement of the surgeon from the outset is best.

All dislocations require repeated orthopedic follow-up evaluation. Patients should be instructed to keep the arm immobilized and to change the axillary pad daily. Redislocations during treatment occur occasionally. First-time dislocations in patients under age 20 are kept immobilized for four weeks, and should be followed by supervised physical therapy. Older patients and those with recurrent dislocations are immobilized for shorter periods. For patients with recurrent instability, surgical reconstruction can offer a stable shoulder with minimal loss of mobility.

Acromioclavicular Joint Injuries

Acromioclavicular joint injuries often occur as the result of a direct blow to the lateral aspect of the shoulder, typically in athletics or falls onto the shoulder itself. These injuries are commonly referred to as "shoulder separations." The AC joint permits motion between the clavicle and acromion

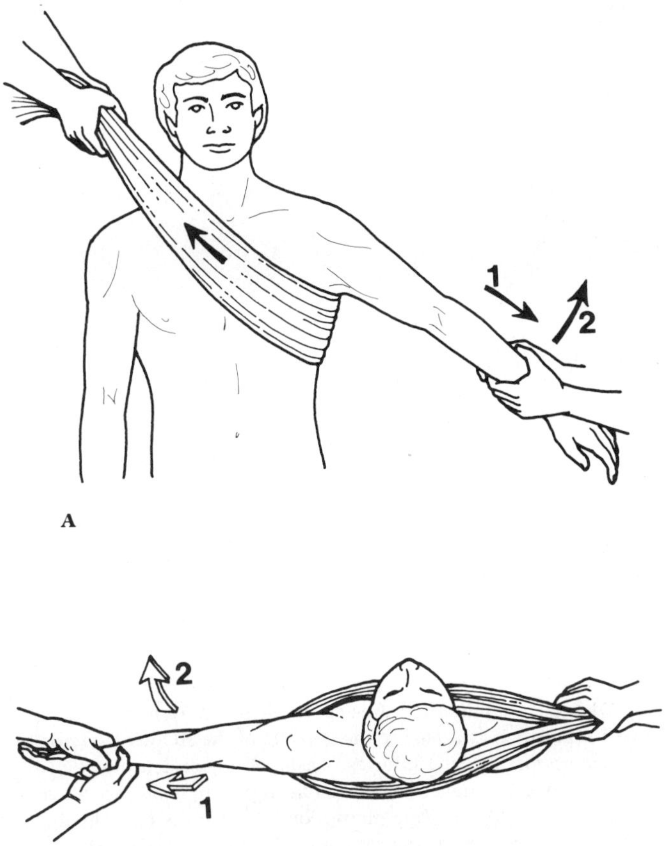

Fig. 64-17. One recommended maneuver for the reduction of shoulder dislocation, shown from an anterior (A) and lateral (B) view. After administration of adequate analgesics and muscle relaxants, the physician applies traction to the arm in the adducted position. An assistant stabilizes the patient's chest with a sheet in the axilla, which is either held or tied around the assistant's waist. The physician applies constant gentle traction for several minutes while the arm is slowly elevated over the patient's head and the physician's opposite hand is used to push the humeral head into position. At 90 degrees of elevation, the humeral head will usually relocate.

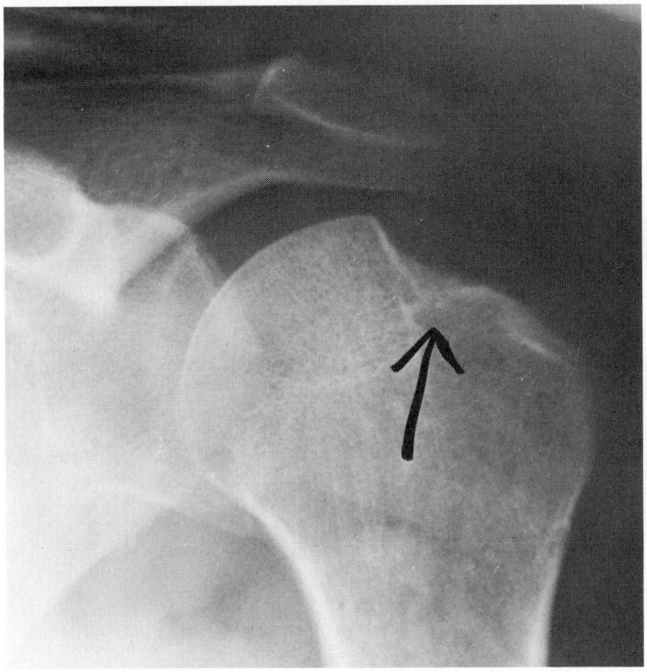

Fig. 64-18. Radiographic demonstration of a compression fracture of the humeral head occurring at the time of shoulder dislocation. This is known as a Hill-Sachs lesion and is associated with long-term shoulder instability. It is advisable to obtain orthopedic consultation at the outset when such a fracture is identified.

during movements of the shoulder, particularly with over-the-shoulder use of the arm.

The joint is reinforced by two sets of ligaments: the horizontally directed AC ligaments and the stronger vertically directed coracoclavicular ligaments (see Fig. 64-1B). Tears of the AC ligaments will allow increased motion in the anteroposterior direction but do not result in gross dislocation of the AC joint. The coracoclavicular ligaments are suspensory ligaments of the upper extremity and, if torn, the result is a dislocation, or separation, of the AC joint (Fig. 64-19).

Evaluation

The patient usually complains of tenderness and pain directly over the AC joint and hesitates to move the shoulder, although some motion can be accomplished if the elbow is supported. Swelling or a noticeable step-off at the distal end of the clavicle may be present.

X-ray evaluation of suspected AC injuries should consist of reduction of the usual radiation voltage by 20 percent, allowing better visualization of the joint. Comparison views of the uninjured shoulder can help in diagnosis. The addition of weights to both hands is usually not required to demonstrate a separation between the distal end of the clavicle and the acromion, although this maneuver is very helpful in accentuating a discrepancy if the diagnosis is in doubt. Conversely, if a patient is mistakenly allowed to support the arm while the film is being taken, an AC joint dislocation or separation can be masked.

The appearance of the x-ray will help distinguish the degree of ligamentous disruption about the joint (see Fig. 64-19). First-degree (type I) shoulder separation consists of a partial or complete tear of the capsule of the AC joint without visible separation of the joint radiographically. Second-degree (type II) AC separation involves a complete AC joint capsular tear and partial coracoclavicular ligament tear, resulting in a step-off both on x-ray and by physical examination. Third-degree (type III) AC separations are the most severe and include not only a capsular tear but also complete disruption of AC and coracoclavicular ligaments. The resulting shoulder deformity can be so marked as to be mistaken for a clavicle fracture.

Treatment

For first- and second-degree AC separations, emergency treatment should consist of a sling to support the elbow, analgesics, and the early application of ice to the shoulder. Follow-up examination by an orthopedic surgeon is appropriate at one week from injury.

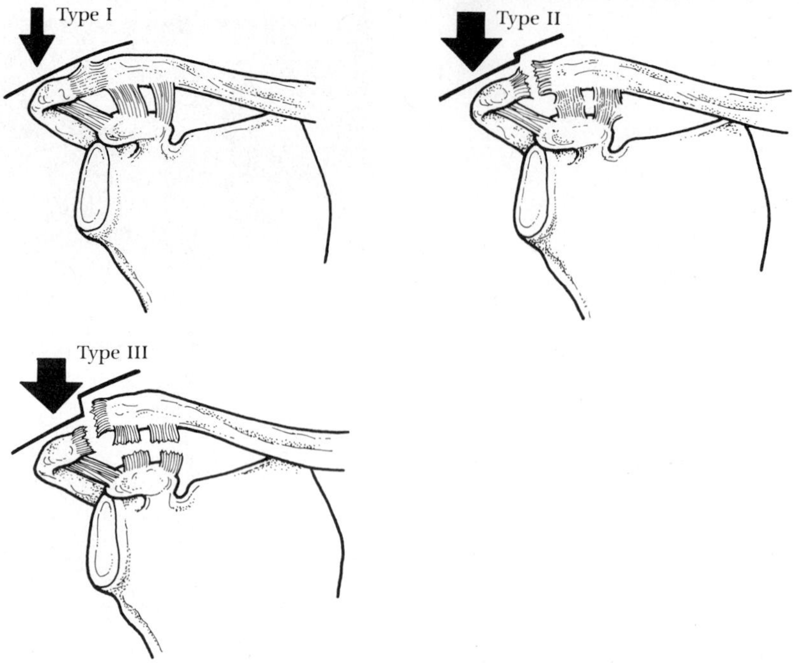

Fig. 64-19. Anatomic diagrams of shoulder AC joint separations. Type I separation is a tear of the capsule of the AC joint without joint separation. Type II injuries consist of a complete AC joint disruption with partial coracoclavicular ligament tear. Type III separations consist of complete disruption between the clavicle and scapula with marked displacement of the distal clavicle.

For third-degree AC separations, closer follow-up study is indicated and the orthopedic surgeon should be contacted by the emergency physician. The reason for this is that controversy exists regarding the management of this injury, with some consultants preferring to treat with surgical repair or to employ a more complex type of brace, designed to hold the AC joint in a reduced position. These patients need to be seen earlier for examination and discussion of treatment options.

Prognosis for this injury is excellent, with only occasional patients reporting chronic shoulder pain. A number of corrective surgical procedures are available for patients with long-standing symptomatic AC dislocation.

Sternoclavicular Joint Dislocations

The sternoclavicular joint dislocation is a rare injury and is usually the result of either massive trauma or a direct blow about the shoulder, delivered through the clavicle. Because the sternoclavicular joint is inherently much more stable than the AC joint (see Fig. 64-2), these injuries are more frequently associated with thoracic pathology, including rib fractures and injuries to the lung or heart. The posterior sternoclavicular dislocation is a clear warning sign of possible further intrathoracic pathology, which warrants extensive evaluation and appropriate consultation.

Evaluation

The patient will complain of chest pain or pain and swelling over the sternoclavicular joint and will be reluctant to fully abduct the shoulder. In many cases, associated thoracic injury can divert attention from the sternoclavicular joint dislocation.

Diagnosis is made by AP chest x-ray and 45-degree lordotic view since the dislocation is often not revealed by a single AP radiograph. Posterior dislocations of the clavicle must be particularly evaluated for the presence of intrathoracic injury.

Treatment

Once associated injuries have been ruled out (especially with posterior dislocations), a gentle reduction maneuver can be attempted. A rolled towel is placed between the scapulae of the supine patient and the shoulders are allowed to fall back. If reduction is obtained, then a sling can be placed and the patient referred for orthopedic follow-up examination within one to two days. If the reduction is unsuccessful, orthopedic consultation should be obtained for possible further attempts at reduction. Once reduced, the posterior dislocations tend to be stable, although anterior dislocations frequently are not. Fortunately, chronic unreduced anterior dislocation produces little long-term functional disability.

MUSCLE AND LIGAMENTOUS INJURIES

Rotator Cuff Tears

Ruptures or tears of the rotator cuff occur as the result of trauma associated with resisted abduction, or direct trauma to the shoulder in younger persons. For individuals over age 50, in whom degenerative changes in the rotator cuff are frequently present, a relatively minor injury can result in a rotator cuff tear. It is commonly believed that rotator cuff pathology, bursitis, and tendonitis of the shoulder have a common origin and involve progressive degrees of inflammation about the shoulder joint, although they are distinct anatomic structures. During the course of rotator cuff disease, severe inflammation of the subacromial bursa ("bursitis") may be the presenting finding, leading to inflammation of the rotator cuff. If this inflammatory process progresses, it can lead to degenerative tears of the rotator cuff and further inflammation of the subacromial bursa.

Evaluation

Patients with rotator cuff tears have pain in the shoulder and generally a history of minor to moderate trauma. They may have a prolonged history of bursitis. The pain is frequently referred to the insertion of the deltoid and is described as being of an "achy" nature and increased with attempts at abduction of the shoulder. In general, the routine AP and lateral radiographs of the shoulder appear normal. Occasionally, with massive tears, the humeral head is elevated relative to the glenoid; this is particularly notable when compared to films of the opposite shoulder. With large rotator cuff tears, there may be profound weakness of the shoulder such that the involved arm can be abducted to 90 degrees passively; however, the patient is unable to maintain this position. Confirmatory testing in the form of arthrogram or ultrasound examination is rarely indicated in the emergency department.

Treatment

Emergency department management should consist of a sling and analgesics, with application of ice to the shoulder during the first several days. The patient should be referred to an orthopedic surgeon for follow-up examination at 7 to 10 days, sooner for young patients with suspected large tears since surgical repair is frequently recommended. For patients with associated fracture or neurovascular injury, or both, immediate orthopedic evaluation is required.

The majority of patients with small rotator cuff tears regain satisfactory strength and motion of the shoulder within 8 to 12 weeks of injury. If strength and function are not improved by 6 weeks, arthrogram or ultrasound examination of the shoulder is usually performed as a diagnostic procedure.

Incomplete tears of the rotator cuff can produce thickening of the subacromial bursa and a chronic condition known as "impingement syndrome." Symptoms are classically a painful crepitus with forward flexion of the shoulder between 70 and 135 degrees but can be more subtle. Internal rotation of the shoulder with forward flexion or abduction will usually accentuate the pain. If these symptoms persist, a partial resection of the anterior acromion (acromioplasty) combined with bursectomy and release of the coracoacromial ligament often proves successful.

Bursitis and Tendonitis of the Shoulder

A large subacromial (subdeltoid) bursa covers the entire rotator cuff (Fig. 64-20). Its primary function is to maintain a gliding surface between the rotator cuff, the acromion, and the coracoacromial ligament. The bursa serves as a smooth and efficient lubricating and cushioning surface for the shoulder joint, as long as the rotator cuff remains intact and unharmed. The major tendon of the shoulder is the long head of the biceps coursing over the anterior glenohumeral joint. In addition, there are numerous smaller bursae about the shoulder region, which aid in the cushioning and gliding of one musculotendinous group on the other.

Evaluation

If the subacromial bursa is injured due to overuse, rotator cuff pathology, or an inflammatory arthropathy, this bursa can become extremely painful and disabling. Subacromial bursitis in the region of the deltoid is to be distinguished from acute tendonitis of the tendon of the long head of the biceps, which courses over the anterior shoulder joint. Both of these situations represent severe inflammatory conditions

Fig. 64-20. The anatomic position of the muscles of the rotator cuff and subacromial bursa. A. Posterior view. B. Lateral view. If treatment requires injection of the subacromial bursa, a reliable approach is injection at the posterolateral edge of the acromion (x).

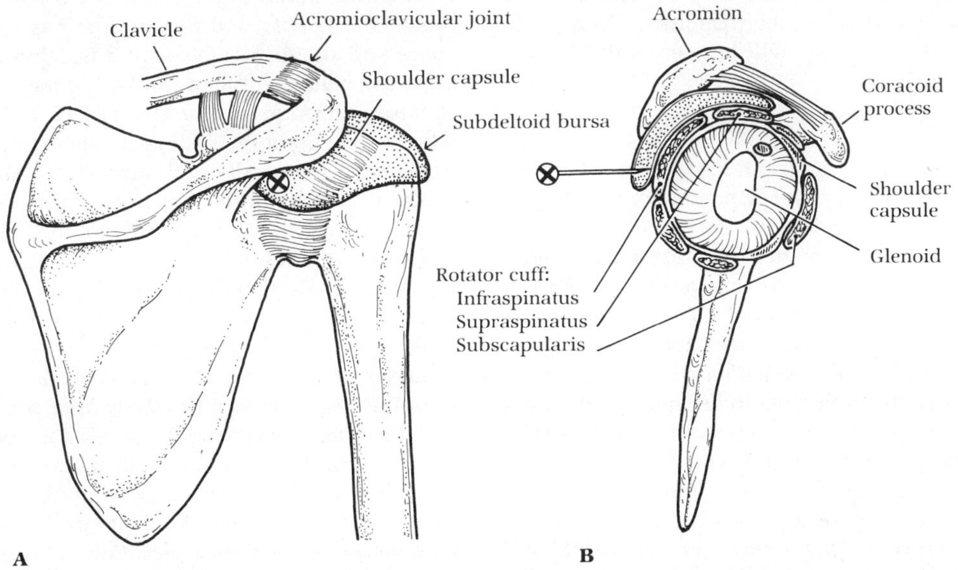

of the soft tissues of the shoulder and are differentiated primarily by anatomic location. One of the most common causes of acute pain in the shoulder is irritation of the subacromial bursa or nearby tendons, causing subacromial or anterior shoulder pain and resultant loss of movement. The onset of these conditions can be both rapid and extremely painful and will be considered by the patient to be an emergency condition. The typical patient is middle aged and gives a history of unusually excessive use of the shoulder in activities such as raking leaves, playing tennis, or repetitive overhead reaching. The history, however, may only vaguely suggest such activity or injury. A past history of similar episodes is helpful in making the diagnosis.

On examination the shoulder will be warm and slightly swollen, and exquisite tenderness may be found just distal or lateral to the acromion in the case of subacromial bursitis. Shoulder motion is markedly limited because of this pain and is usually most affected in abduction and external rotation. The area of tenderness about the shoulder aids in differentiating this condition from bicipital tendonitis. Although lateral and superior tenderness is most typical for bursitis, anterior shoulder pain and tenderness are more characteristic of bicipital tendonitis. The presence of fever and leukocytosis in association with the patient holding the involved shoulder rigidly to the side requires further evaluation, including aspiration of the joint to rule out septic arthritis. It is of utmost importance to differentiate septic arthritis from acute bursitis in the emergency setting, and this can only be done by aspiration.

Diagnostic x-rays of the shoulder should consist of the standard AP projection, but three other views should be obtained. Internal rotation, external rotation, and axillary views (see Fig. 64-9) of the proximal humerus are extremely helpful. The axillary view is performed by abducting the extremity to 45 to 90 degrees, placing the x-ray cassette against the lateral neck and shoulder superiorly and the x-ray tube at the level of the patient's waist, and aiming through the axilla (see Fig. 64-9). The only positive radiographic finding with subacromial bursitis may be small, fluffy calcific deposits, which are most frequently located in the supraspinatus tendon (Fig. 64-21). The presence of such deposits suggests a chronic inflammatory condition but is by no means necessary to make the diagnosis. Usually, no abnormal radiographic findings will be seen with bicipital tendonitis.

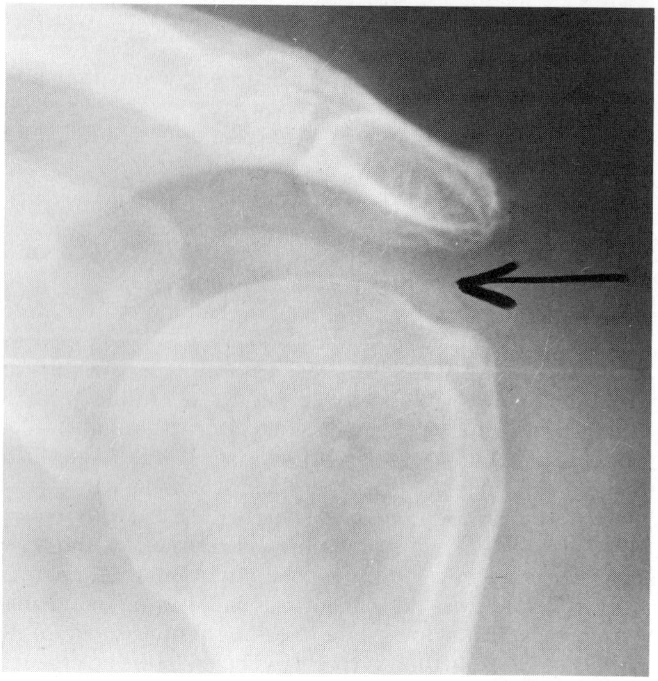

Fig. 64-21. Radiographic demonstration of calcific deposits within the supraspinatus tendon consistent with calcific subacromial bursitis. The presence of a calcific deposit suggests a chronic inflammatory condition but is not necessary to make the diagnosis of bursitis.

Treatment

Emergency management of bursitis and tendonitis should be based on function and symptoms. For patients who exhibit a fair range of motion, a great deal of relief can be provided by use of a sling, ice, and nonsteroidal antiinflammatory medications. On occasion, narcotic analgesics may be appropriate. On rare occasions, injection of the subacromial bursa with a combination of local anesthetic and corticosteroid can be used. Injections are indicated when the diagnosis of acute bursitis has been positively established, when infection has been ruled out, and conservative measures by the patient have provided little relief. There are no indications for injection of the shoulder joint itself. Injections to the subacromial bursa require strict sterile technique and a knowledge of the underlying anatomy (see Fig. 64-20) but can be accomplished by the treating physician in the emergency department. An injection should not be given if infection is suspected.

The simplest and most reliable method for injecting the subacromial bursa is to approach it posteriorly at the posterolateral edge of the acromion (see Fig. 64-20). An alternative site of injection is anteriorly just below the acromion (see Fig. 64-20). The patient should sit with the arm held loosely in the lap. The area to be injected should be prepared in a sterile fashion and the needle introduced so that it passes beneath the acromion into the bursa itself. On entering the bursa, the needle will feel as if it has come into an open space and should not feel as if it is being impeded by either bone or rotator cuff tendon. Asking the patient to move the shoulder through a few degrees of motion will confirm whether the tip of the syringe has penetrated the rotator cuff itself, since the needle will move as the shoulder is ranged.

The bursa should be distended with a relatively large volume of solution. A suggested combination is 5 ml long-acting local anesthetic, such as 0.5% bupivacaine; 5 ml short-acting anesthetic, such as 1% lidocaine; and 1 ml corticosteroid preparation, such as dexamethasone, 8 mg/ml. After the injection, the area should be massaged and the shoulder gently ranged to disperse the solution about the bursa. If the injection has been into the appropriate area and the diagnosis is correct, the relief the patient experiences can be dramatic and shoulder motion improves considerably. The emergency treatment should be followed by use of ice packs to the shoulder but never the use of heat, which may increase the discomfort. Follow-up examination with an orthopedic surgeon in three to five days is recommended, particularly for confirmation of the diagnosis and for further treatment, which will usually be required. Prolonged (greater than 2 weeks) immobilization of the shoulder in elderly patients is to be avoided because of the possible loss of shoulder motion.

The majority of patients who have episodes of acute subacromial bursitis or associated bicipital tendonitis describe isolated events that resolve quickly over five to seven days. For patients with recurrent episodes of shoulder bursitis, evaluation by an orthopedic surgeon for the possible presence of rotator cuff tears, hypertrophy of the anterior edge of the acromion, and "impingement syndrome" is indicated.

A small number of patients may have, after one or several episodes of bursitis, marked restriction of the motion of the shoulder as a result of adhesive capsulitis, commonly referred to as "frozen shoulder." This condition is more common in middle-aged women than men and can result from a relatively minor injury. It is difficult to treat and can lead to severe permanent loss of motion in the shoulder. Adhesive capsulitis requires management by multiple modalities, usually under the direction of an orthopedic surgeon or physiatrist.

Biceps Tendon Rupture

Biceps tendon rupture is an acute condition that occurs in two groups of patients: elderly individuals in whom a degeneration of the tendon has occurred, resulting in rupture with minimal or no trauma, and younger individuals engaged in heavy labor, specifically elbow flexion–forearm supination. In the latter case, a history of obvious trauma is more likely to be obtained.

Evaluation

Patients will often report that a "snapping" sensation occurred at the onset of their symptoms. Pain is usually present over the proximal portion of the biceps muscle. Examination discloses a prominent bulge of muscle, usually distal to the typical location of the contracted biceps muscle. In patients first seen several days after injury, a substantial ecchymosis of the upper arm may be present. Elbow flexion motion will be somewhat impaired by pain, but may be near normal since the long head of the biceps contributes a relatively small proportion of elbow flexion strength. X-rays are of limited diagnostic value but may show an elevation of the humeral head. Distal ruptures of the biceps tendon occur, although less frequently. They are more consistently associated with an acute traumatic event and may show a proximal retraction of the biceps muscle on physical examination.

Treatment

Symptomatic treatment is the appropriate emergency care. Application of ice and use of a sling are helpful. Analgesics should be given as necessary and appropriate. Young patients who may be candidates for surgical repair should be referred within the first 3 to 5 days, while elderly patients, in whom operation is rarely indicated, can be seen in 10 to 14 days.

The long-term function is quite good, but some strength of elbow flexion and supination may be lost. The functional significance of this depends on the daily demands placed on the extremity by the patient.

SELECTED READING

Armstrong, CP, and Van der Spuy, J. The fractured scapula: Importance and management, based on a series of 62 patients. *Injury* 15:324, 1984.

Bjerneld, H, Hovelius, L, and Thorling, J. Acromioclavicular separations treated conservatively. *Acta Orthop Scand* 54:743, 1983.

Cofield, RH. Tears of the rotator cuff. *AAOS Instructional Course Lectures* 30:258, 1981.

Neviaser, RJ. Symposium on disorders of the shoulder. *Orthop Clin North Am* 11:185, 1980.

Pavlov, H, et al. The roentgenographic evaluation of anterior shoulder instability. *Clin Orthop* 194:153, 1985.

65. Elbow Injuries

Jonathan T. Deland

Elbow injuries are seen in all age groups. The most significant injuries occur in pediatric patients and in adults with considerable trauma, but even elderly patients with minor trauma can sustain severe elbow injuries. Common modes of injury include a fall on the outstretched hand as well as a direct blow to the elbow.

The elbow is an intrinsically stable joint with a great deal of bony stability. While purely ligamentous injuries are rare, bony injuries are not. However, radiographic examination of the elbow can be difficult, and fractures are easily missed. This is particularly true for pediatric patients, and the reader should carefully review the chapter on pediatric injuries (see Chap. 160).

The elbow has a propensity to become stiff after injury, particularly if immobilization is prolonged. Permanent loss of elbow motion can be very debilitating, as the elbow provides an essential part of upper-extremity motion, allowing the hand to be properly positioned in space. Normal elbow range of motion is 0 to 150 degrees of flexion, with 75 degrees of pronation and 85 degrees of supination. The functional range of motion needed for activities of daily living is 30 to 130 degrees of flexion, combined with a total of 100 degrees of forearm rotation, the rotation being equally divided between pronation and supination. This functional range will allow patients to reach their face and perineum for essential activities.

FUNCTIONAL ANATOMY

The elbow joint is composed of three articulations (Fig. 65-1). They are the humeroulnar, humeroradial, and radioulnar joints; all three are contained within one synovial cavity. The proximal end of the ulna is composed of the olecranon and the coronoid process; together they form the semilunar notch, which articulates with the trochlea of the humerus. Lateral to the ulna, the radial head articulates with a rounded protuberance of the distal humerus, the capitellum. Proceeding down the radius, the annular (or orbicular) ligament stabilizes the radius and maintains its relationship with the ulna (Fig. 65-2). Just distal to this ligament is the bicipital tuberosity of the radius, the location of the biceps tendon insertion. The eccentric location of this insertion is what makes the biceps muscle a powerful forearm supinator as well as an elbow flexor.

Medial and lateral stability of the elbow are provided by the interlocking joint surfaces and the collateral ligaments. The lateral collateral ligament runs from the lateral epicondyle of the humerus to both the radius and the ulna, blending with the annular ligament (see Fig. 65-2B). The medial collateral ligament arises from the medial epicondyle of the humerus to the medial surface of the olecranon and coronoid process (see Fig. 65-2A). The anterior band, in particular, provides the major stability of the elbow joint.

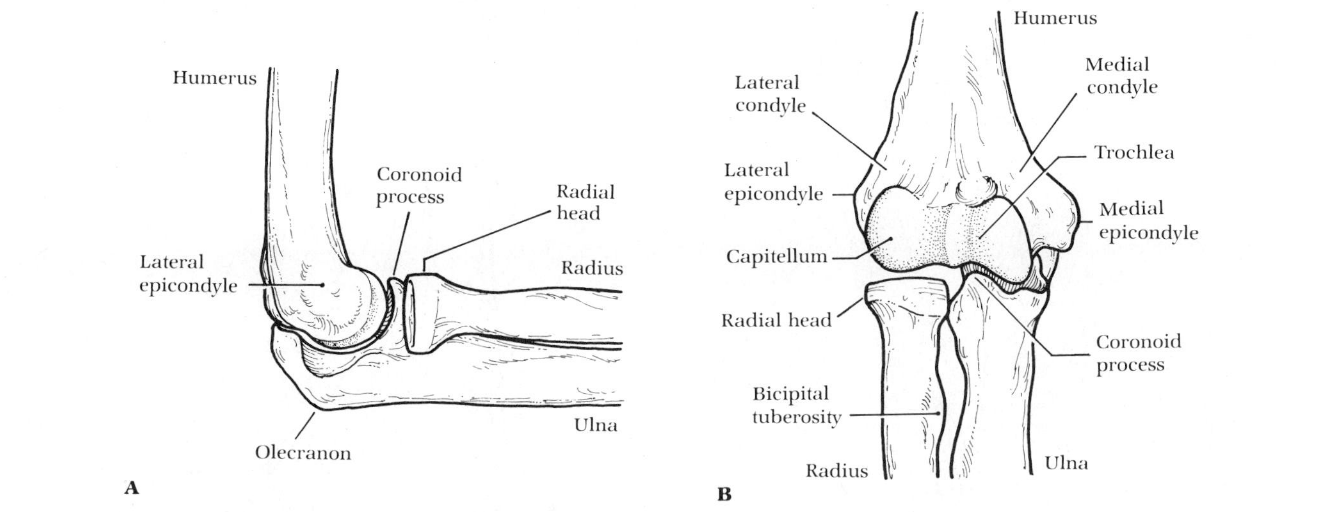

Fig. 65-1. The bony anatomy of the elbow as seen in the lateral (A) and anteroposterior (B) projections.

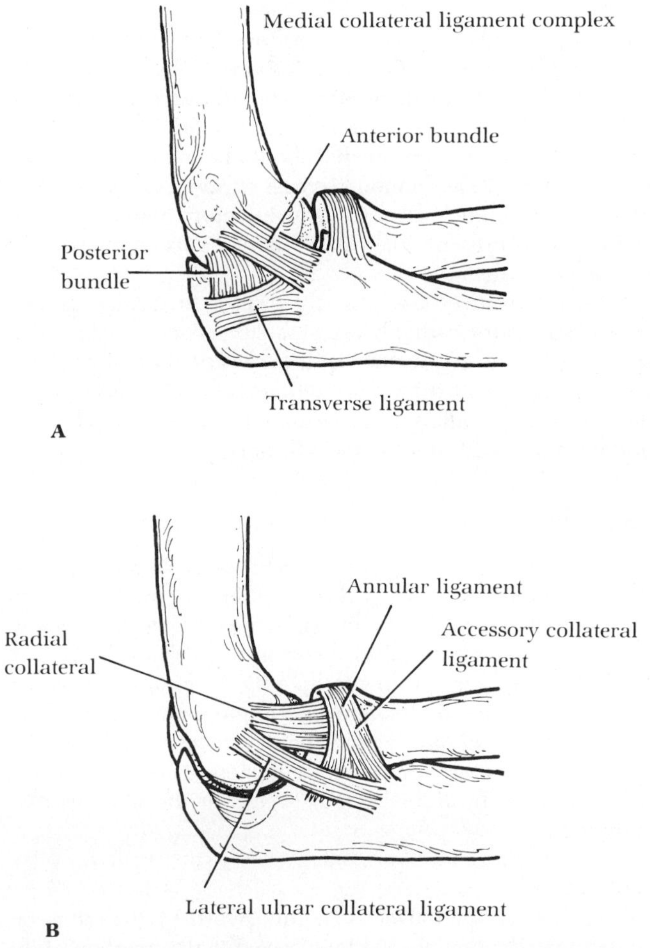

Fig. 65-2. The ligamentous anatomy of the elbow as seen from the medial (A) and lateral (B) sides.

Because there is so little subcutaneous tissue, surface landmarks of the elbow are easily palpated. The olecranon, the medial and lateral epicondyles, and the radial head are all easily located by gentle palpation (see Fig. 65-1). The radial head is most effectively examined by placing a thumb directly over it while pronating and supinating the forearm. Careful palpation of the bony landmarks will often help direct the attention of the examiner to particular parts of the x-ray and thus ensure that a fracture is not missed. Other surface landmarks include the biceps tendon and brachial artery, both of which can be palpated anteriorly (Fig. 65-3). In the groove behind the medial epicondyle, the ulnar nerve can be felt superficially.

FRACTURES AND DISLOCATIONS ABOUT THE ELBOW

Radial Head and Neck Fractures

Although radial head and neck fractures can occur in pediatric as well as elderly patients, they are most commonly seen in middle-aged patients who fall on their outstretched hands. Most of the injuries are due to the force that travels up the pronated forearm, driving the radial head against the capitellum. Long-term disability from the injury is not common.

Evaluation

Radial head and neck fractures should be suspected when tenderness is found on palpation of the radial head. Palpation can be performed as described in the section on functional anatomy, using the normal elbow for comparison. Tenderness over the radial head and pain on pronation-supination out of proportion to that with flexion-extension suggest a radial head fracture.

X-rays occasionally do not have a visible fracture line. With proper positioning and exposure, x-rays will almost always demonstrate a posterior "fat-pad sign," a lucent area caused by fat just posterior to the distal humerus. This area of low density is produced by a joint effusion, which elevates the posterior fat pad away from the olecranon fossa of the

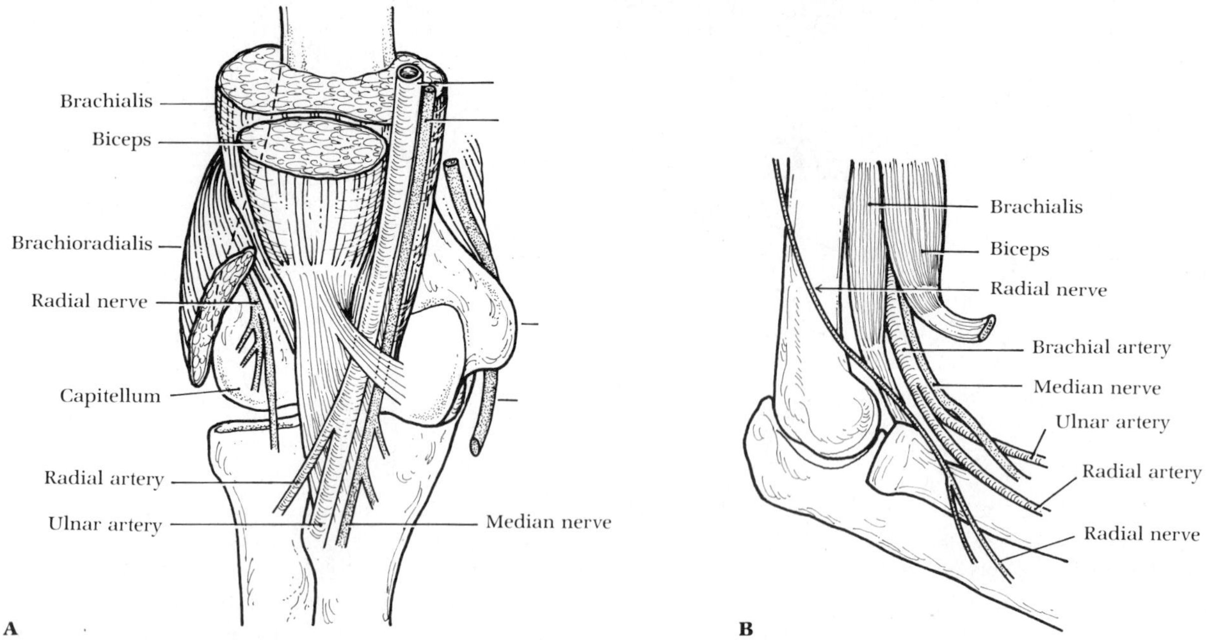

Fig. 65-3. The soft structures adjacent to the elbow as seen on the anteroposterior (A) and lateral (B) views. Note particularly the proximity of the radial and ulnar nerves to the distal humerus.

humerus (Fig. 65-4). It is evidence of intraarticular fracture. Patients can also have an anterior fat-pad sign; however, this sign may also be seen in normal elbows.

Radial head and neck fractures are classified into three types (Fig. 65-5). Type I fractures are nondisplaced. Type II fractures have a displaced articular fragment in the case of a head fracture or less than 30 degrees of angulation in the case of a neck fracture. Type III fractures have comminution, with multiple head fragments or more than 30 degrees of angulation of the neck. Complete displacement of the head, even if it remains intact, is classified as a type III fracture.

It is always important to evaluate the wrist for any signs of tenderness, since the distal radioulnar joint can be subluxed or dislocated with radial head or neck injuries. Additionally, elbow motion should be gently checked for any mechanical block, which may be caused by a loose cartilaginous or bony fragment. Aspiration of the elbow joint by the emergency physician is helpful if the elbow joint is too painful to assess motion. This is described in Procedure 32. After aspiration of the hemarthrosis, 3 to 4 ml 1% lidocaine (Xylocaine) is injected through the same needle. After 10 minutes, the elbow is usually well anesthetized and much easier to examine. Range of motion can then be assessed without guarding by the patient. With adequate anesthesia, at least 50 percent of flexion-extension and pronation-supination should be present. If it is not, a mechanical block should be suspected.

Treatment

Type I fractures are treated with a sling and gentle early motion, beginning as soon as tolerated by the patient. In cases in which a great deal of pain and swelling are present, the sling can be augmented with a posterior splint (see Chap. 63). Follow-up examination of these fractures should be at 7 to 10 days after injury to be certain that motion has been started and is progressing.

Type II fractures are most typically treated like type I fractures but should be referred for orthopedic follow-up examination within three to five days for closer observation. If in the emergency department 50 percent of the normal motion cannot be demonstrated despite adequate anesthesia, immediate referral to the orthopedist should be made. Loose bodies that block elbow motion are best removed early. In addition, if an articular fragment involving more than 30 percent of the head is present, internal fixation or early removal may be recommended.

Type III fractures are generally treated surgically, usually by excision of the radial head. Since the propensity for myositis ossificans is greater when surgery is performed between 2 and 21 days after injury, immediate referral to an orthopedic surgeon will allow the operation to be performed at the optimal time, within 48 hours of injury.

Olecranon Fractures

These proximal ulnar fractures occur most often in middle-aged and older patients. A direct fall on the posterior tip of the elbow is the usual mechanism. On occasion, the fracture can occur as a result of an avulsion force from the pull of the triceps muscle on an osteoporotic olecranon. In either case, the triceps remains attached to the proximal fragment and causes proximal displacement. Because this is an intraarticular fracture, anatomic reduction is critical. Starting elbow motion by three to four weeks at the latest is also important.

Evaluation

The diagnosis is relatively straightforward by lateral x-ray. Particular attention should be directed to the function of the ulnar nerve, which can be injured as a result of its location near the fracture. It is important to be certain that the radial

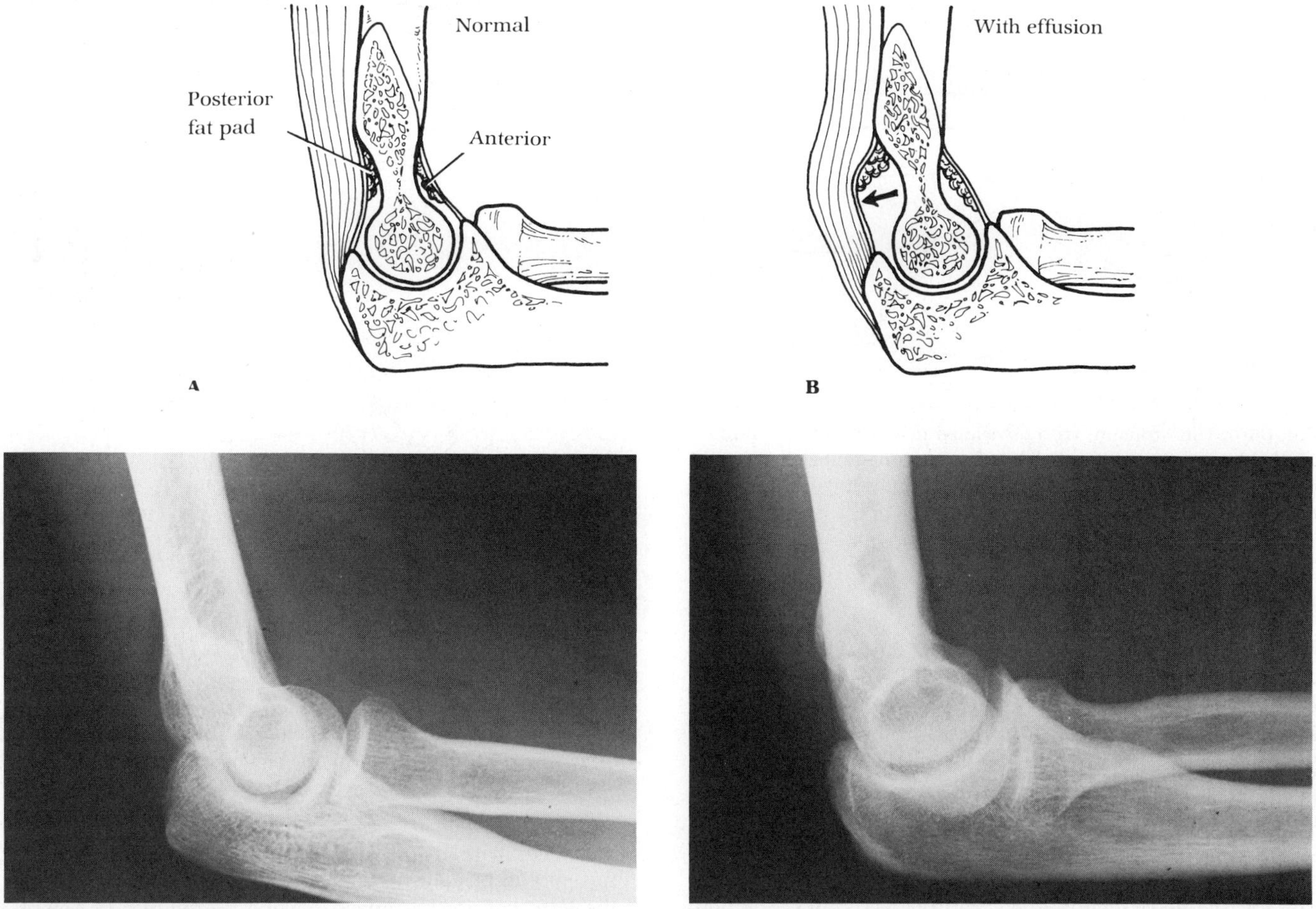

Fig. 65-4. Cause of the fat-pad sign. A. In the normal joint the fat pad is not visible since it lies within the olecranon fossa and cannot be seen on a lateral x-ray. B. With a joint effusion, the fat pad is pushed out of the olecranon fossa, producing a lucent area between bone and overlying muscle. C. X-ray of normal elbow. D. X-ray of elbow with anterior and posterior fat-pad sign.

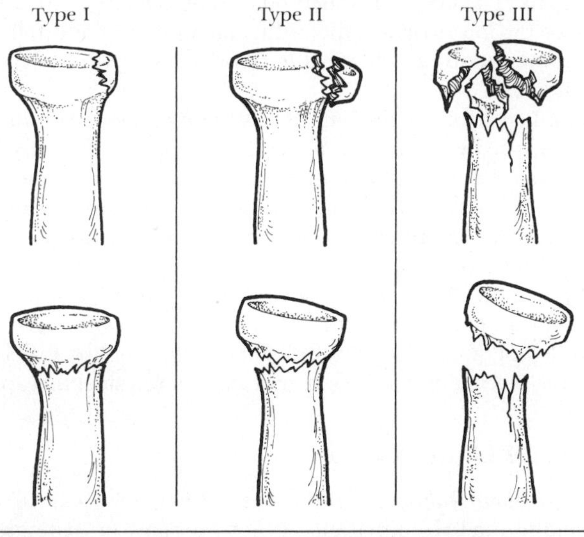

Fig. 65-5. Classification of radial head and neck fractures (see text).

head is not dislocated. The combination of an ulna fracture and radial head dislocation is known as Monteggia's fracture (Fig. 65-6). The diagnosis of radial head dislocation is sometimes missed. One should check that a line drawn down the center of the radial shaft lines up with the capitellum in all views. This will verify that the radial head is not dislocated.

Treatment

Nondisplaced olecranon fractures can be treated in a posterior splint and sling with the elbow positioned at 45 to 90 degrees of flexion. See Chap. 63 for details on splint application.

Displaced fractures (more than 2 mm between fragments) require operative treatment, usually consisting of open reduction and internal fixation of the fracture. In cases in which the olecranon is severely comminuted or osteoporotic, up to 75 percent of the olecranon can be excised and the insertion of the triceps advanced more distally onto the ulna. For patients who are to be treated surgically, placement of a well-padded posterior splint at 30 to 60 degrees of elbow flexion will stabilize the injury, protect the soft tissues from further trauma, and decrease the skin tension. The splinted elbow should then be placed at or above the heart level by means of pillows. This will help keep swelling to a minimum and avoid postoperative wound problems.

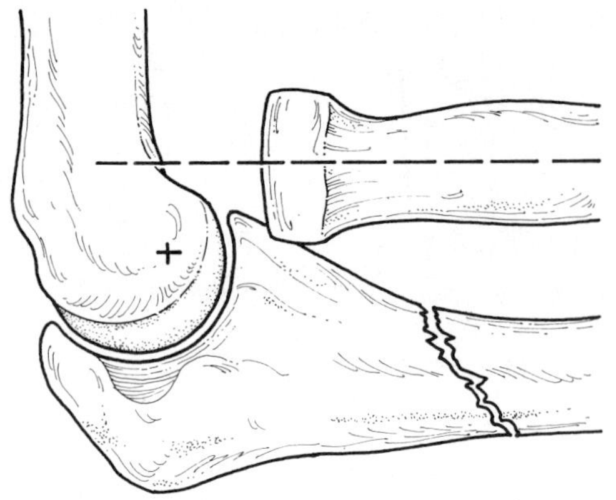

Fig. 65-6. Ulna fracture with associated dislocation of the radial head (Monteggia's fracture). A line drawn through the center of the radial shaft passes above the capitellum, confirming dislocation of the radial head.

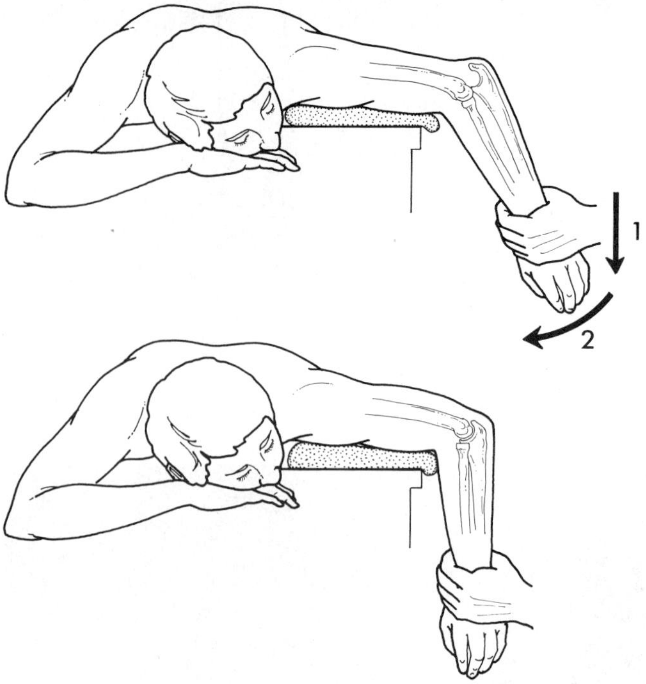

Fig. 65-7. Maneuver used for reduction of posterior elbow dislocation. If an assistant is available to hold the humerus, reduction can be performed with the patient in the sitting position.

Elbow Dislocation

Elbow dislocation is a very common joint injury in adults and in children under the age of 10. The usual mechanism of injury is a fall on the outstretched hand, with the elbow in some degree of flexion. With flexion, the force of the impact is transmitted through the forearm, pushing the ulna posteriorly. The frequency of occurrence of posterior dislocation is therefore much greater than that of anterior dislocation. Small joint surface fractures, neurovascular injury, and compartment syndrome can occur. For these reasons, prompt, gentle reduction and careful assessment of the neurovascular status before and after manipulation are important.

Evaluation

A gross physical deformity is usually seen at the elbow, although this may be somewhat obscured by soft-tissue swelling or obesity. With a posterior dislocation, a very prominent olecranon is noted, whereas with an anterior dislocation, the normal olecranon prominence is absent. Comparison with the normal side is helpful. A careful neurovascular and radiographic examination should be completed before any reduction is performed. Median or ulnar nerve injury may be present and associated fractures of the humerus or forearm should not be missed. Although arterial injury is not common in this setting, it must be ruled out.

Treatment

For posterior dislocations, some form of sedation is usually required for reduction. Intravenous diazepam with morphine under close observation is usually satisfactory. It is best to have control of both the forearm and the humerus. Reduction is started by distal traction on the forearm as the humerus is held by an assistant. Alternatively, when no assistant is available, the patient can lie prone with the affected arm over the side of the stretcher. Humeral countertraction can then be provided by the stretcher itself (Fig. 65-7). With either method, the elbow is held in slight flexion and then distal traction is applied. As traction is maintained, the elbow is progressively flexed until reduction is achieved.

The reduction is usually felt and often seen. After this, the elbow should be gently ranged to check for adequate motion. If the joint cannot be moved beyond 60 degrees of flexion, an incomplete reduction or intraarticular fragment should be suspected. Regardless, postreduction x-rays should be obtained. If motion is adequate, the elbow should be placed in a well-padded posterior splint and flexed to 90 degrees. Repeat neurovascular examination is mandatory.

For mediolateral dislocation, the technique is similar, with the use of traction, elbow flexion, and appropriate medial or lateral pressure. For anterior dislocations, gentle flexion is used to disengage the olecranon from the anterior humerus. The forearm is then pushed posteriorly, with some further flexion to obtain the reduction. Splinting and follow-up examination are identical to those used for posterior dislocations.

In all types of dislocations, if reduction cannot be obtained after one or two attempts, referral to an orthopedic surgeon is indicated. Repeated attempts at reduction increase the risk of myositis ossificans by increasing the soft-tissue trauma.

Follow-up examination with an orthopedic surgeon is indicated within 7 to 10 days of the reduction to check for any redislocation. Patients should be told from the outset that some permanent loss of motion is inevitable, although it is usually not of functional significance. Active motion is begun at three weeks, under the supervision of a physical therapist.

Fractures of the Distal Humerus (Adult)

Several distal humerus fracture patterns can occur in the skeletally mature individual. It is important to distinguish between them (Fig. 65-8). An *intercondylar* fracture (Fig.

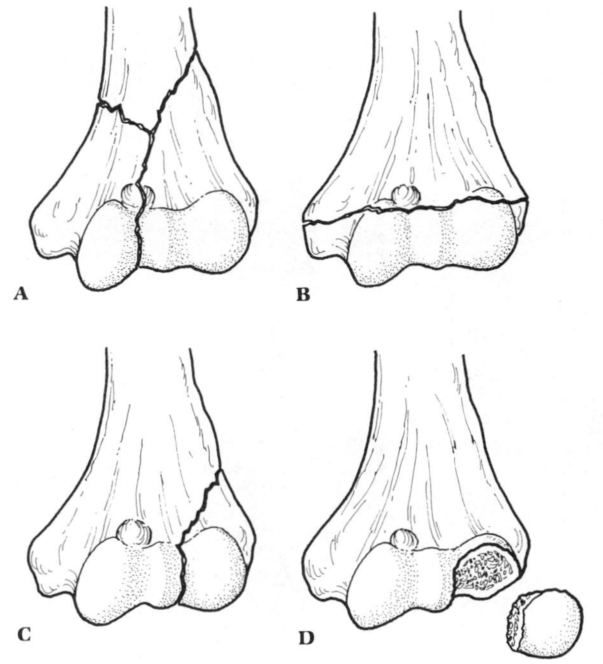

Fig. 65-8. Distal humerus fractures. A. Supracondylar-intercondylar pattern. In adults, this combined fracture may be mistakenly called a "supracondylar fracture." B. Transcondylar fracture. C. Condylar fracture. D. Capitellar fracture.

65-8A) involves the area between the capitellum and the trochlea. The fracture line then extends into the supracondylar region, producing a Y- or T-shaped pattern. In adults, this fracture pattern is often termed "supracondylar," although it is more properly defined as "supracondylar-intercondylar." A *transcondylar* fracture (Fig. 65-8B) extends transversely through a line just above the capitellum and trochlea. This particular fracture is most often seen in osteoporotic bone, typically in elderly women. The *condylar* fracture (Fig. 65-8C) involves only one of the humeral condyles, either medial or lateral. These fractures are more often the result of a direct blow than a fall on the outstretched arm. The *capitellar* fracture (Fig. 65-8D) is in the coronal rather than the sagittal plane and involves only the articular surface.

Evaluation

On physical examination, the neurovascular status of the arm should be carefully assessed. As can be seen in Fig. 65-3, the major neurovascular structures are susceptible to injury in distal humerus fractures. A common error is to have the patient extend the fingers with the wrist palmar flexed and to assume that this represents intact radial function. To adequately test the radial nerve, the wrist must be slightly dorsiflexed before active extension of the fingers is tested. A forearm compartment syndrome can develop in association with distal humerus fractures, especially in fractures associated with substantial trauma or dislocation. Signs of a developing compartment syndrome include pain with passive extension of the fingers, hypesthesia of the hand, and increasing swelling and tension in the forearm. Peripheral pulses are not a reliable indicator of forearm muscle perfusion. Their presence does not rule out a compartment syndrome. Measurement of forearm compartment pressures is the most valuable test available (see Chap. 73).

On radiographic examination, anteroposterior and true lateral x-rays of the elbow are needed without the distortion caused by an overlying plaster splint. Plastic radiolucent splinting materials are satisfactory, although the best x-rays of this critical region are obtained by careful removal of the splint and positioning of the elbow by the physician.

Treatment

Since all of these fracture patterns involve disruption of the joint, early operative treatment is the rule. The severely comminuted fracture in osteoporotic bone is the exception and can be treated with initial splinting followed by early motion, since operative fixation of multiple osteoporotic fragments is often unsuccessful. The emergency physician should stabilize distal humerus fractures in a well-padded posterior splint at 30 to 60 degrees of flexion and contact the orthopedic surgeon.

In cases in which neurovascular compromise is noted in the presence of a displaced fracture, a gentle reduction can be performed. This is best left to the orthopedist, unless the emergency physician is experienced in such manipulations.

Supracondylar Fractures (Children)

Because the metaphysis of the distal humerus in a child is small in relation to the other parts of the bone, a supracondylar fracture without the intercondylar component is seen most frequently in this age group. These fractures are treated with great respect by the orthopedist, given their potential for neurovascular complication and malunion. They are discussed in Chap. 160.

Condylar and Epicondylar Fractures (Children)

Fortunately, neurovascular compromise is unusual in condylar and epicondylar fractures. However, these fractures present a greater diagnostic challenge than the supracondylar fracture, since much of the growing child's distal humerus is cartilaginous and therefore difficult to image by plain x-ray. These fractures are discussed in Chap. 160.

Subluxation of the Radial Head (Nursemaid's Elbow)

Very young children with unexplained elbow pain may have subluxation of the radial head. The history is helpful in making the diagnosis. The child is usually between the ages of one and five years, has tenderness in the radial head area, and refuses to use the upper extremity after sustaining a longitudinal pull on it. The subluxation can usually be reduced by extending and supinating the elbow and then maintaining supination as the elbow is flexed. This condition is discussed in Chap. 160.

SOFT-TISSUE AND OVERUSE INJURIES

Many patients sustain injuries to the elbow from overuse or repetitive trauma, as with the shoulder. Several of the most common conditions are described in this section.

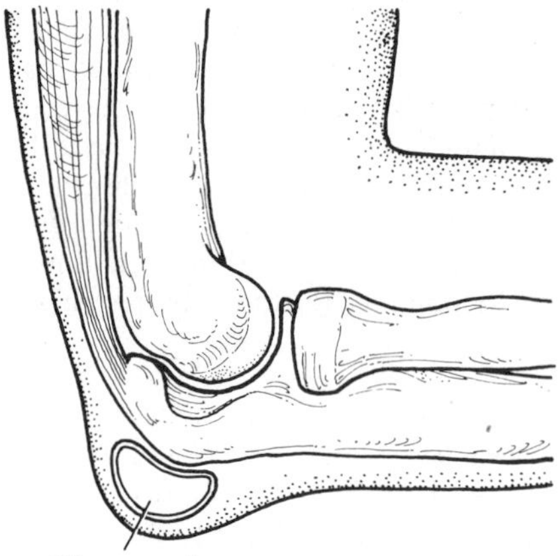

Fig. 65-9. Location of the olecranon bursa over the posterior tip of the olecranon. This figure depicts the bursa in its inflamed condition, since it is virtually without volume in its normal state.

Olecranon Bursitis

The olecranon bursa is illustrated in Fig. 65-9. Because it is located at the tip of the elbow (an area frequently subjected to pressure), inflammation of this bursa is common. It is most often seen in individuals who give direct repetitive contact to the elbows in athletic or industrial settings. Other reasons for olecranon bursitis include sepsis, gout, and rheumatoid arthritis. Rarer causes (and less likely to be encountered in the emergency department) are chondrocalcinosis, pigmented villonodular synovitis, and xanthoma.

Evaluation

Before categorizing the bursitis as traumatic, sepsis and other conditions need to be ruled out. A routine traumatic olecranon bursitis can be warm, with pink skin, and tender to palpation. However, bursitis that is exquisitely tender and has any one of the following signs should be aspirated: parabursal cellulitis (usually red), an elevated peripheral white blood cell count, fever, tender axillary lymph nodes, or visible pus. Aspiration of the bursa should be performed under strict sterile conditions since careless aspiration of a traumatic bursitis can produce infection. While aspiration for gouty crystals may help in the diagnosis of gout, aspiration is not recommended if rheumatoid arthritis is strongly suspected. A patient will usually have other stigmata of rheumatoid arthritis, thereby obviating the need for diagnostic aspiration.

Treatment

For nonseptic bursitis, a bulky dressing and sling are applied for one to two weeks. This will usually result in some shrinkage of the bursa, though perhaps not complete resolution. Nonsteroidal antiinflammatory medication is helpful, especially in patients with significant inflammation and tenderness. Avoidance of any direct pressure on the elbow and the long-term use of elbow padding may be necessary to prevent recurrence. The best recommendation is alteration of the activity that has brought about the bursitis. Cases that do not respond within one to two weeks should be referred for orthopedic follow-up examination. On occasion, formal drainage is performed with excision of the bursa, but this is the exception.

For septic bursitis, orthopedic consultation is indicated. If an adequate diagnostic aspiration has been performed, intravenous antibiotics can be started. Since staphylococcus species are the usual pathogens, an intravenous course of cefazolin is begun, pending the results of aspirate culture.

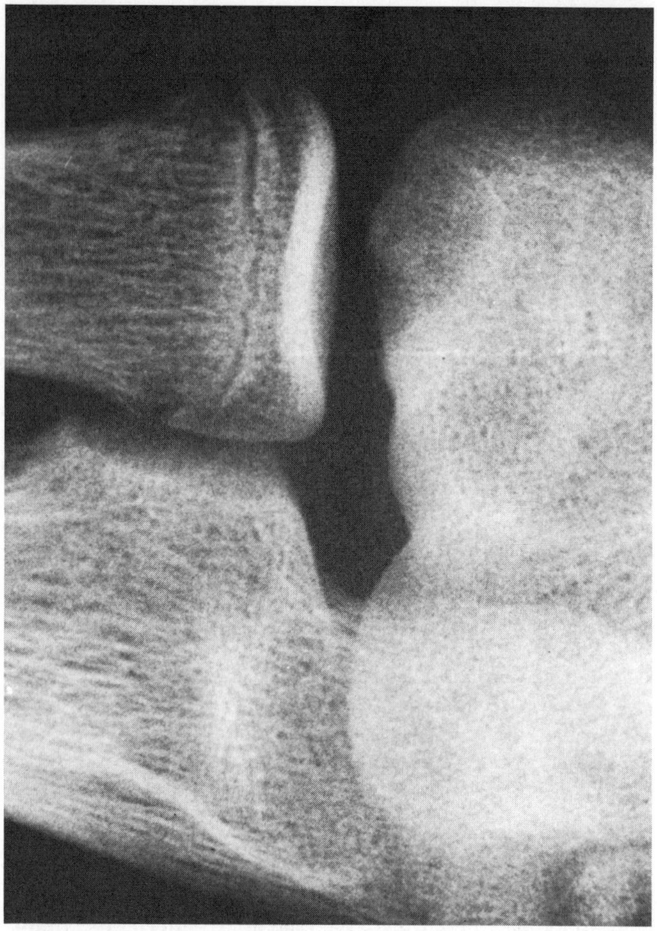

Fig. 65-10. This film shows a lucency in the capitellum consistent with osteochondritis dissecans.

Osteochondritis Dissecans

Osteochondritis dissecans involves necrosis of the subchondral bone and overlying cartilage. It typically occurs in adolescents or young adults and involves the capitellum. The first symptom is elbow pain, often with a flexion contracture of insidious onset. The etiology is unknown, but inadequate osseous blood supply, trauma, or a combination of both are the most likely causes.

Evaluation

Results of initial x-rays may be normal. Tomograms may therefore be required, although this is not necessary in the emergency department setting. The lesion can usually be seen as a defect in the capitellar articular surface (Fig. 65-10). There can be an accompanying bone island, which represents the necrotic bone piece. It may be relatively radiodense or radiolucent in comparison to the surrounding bone. Osteochondritis dissecans should be differentiated from Panner's disease, which is the fragmentation of the entire capitellar ossific nucleus that occurs in young children. Panner's disease is usually acute in onset, treated conservatively, and has a better prognosis than osteochondritis.

Treatment

Osteochondritis should be treated by immobilization in a posterior splint for a three-week period, followed by range of motion exercises. Follow-up examination with an orthopedic surgeon at the time of splint removal is appropriate, and the usual advice will be to avoid physical stress, such as throwing sports, until symptoms have resolved. In cases in which a necrotic fragment of bone has broken free into the joint, operative excision of the fragment is often recommended. In osteochondritis, the healing phase can require several years, either with or without operative treatment.

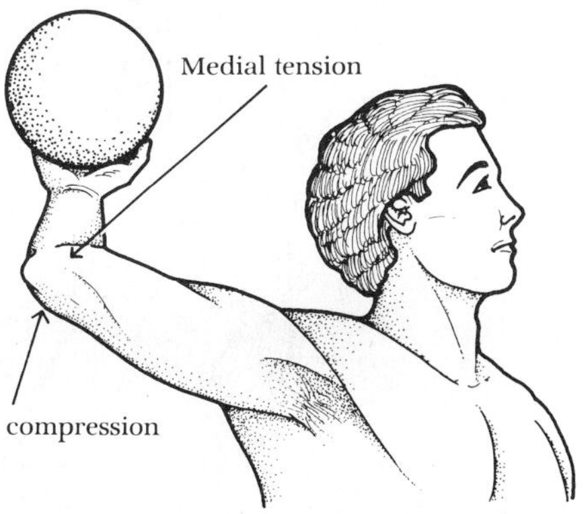

Fig. 65-11. The elbow in the act of overhand throwing. Note the valgus strain in throwing, which produces tension stresses medially and compression stresses laterally.

"Little League Elbow"

The elbow of the throwing arm in overactive athletes is a common source of pain whether the patient is preadolescent or skeletally mature. The terms *baseball elbow* or *Little League elbow* are not diagnoses but do help direct the physician toward the area of probable pathology. Osteochondritis dissecans is not the most frequent diagnosis in these patients. Rather, the condition represents a composite picture of injury that results from chronic valgus stress at the elbow. In the act of throwing, the elbow is positioned and stressed in such a way as to place compression across the radial head and capitellum and tension along the medial collateral ligament (Fig. 65-11). Lateral compression can result in injury to the capitellar articular surface and the production of intraarticular loose bodies (Fig. 65-12). The loose bodies may or may not be visible on plain x-ray. On the medial side, stretching of the medial collateral ligament can occur, resulting in instability and formation of a traction spur (Fig. 65-12).

Evaluation

On physical examination, the examiner should note the precise area of maximal tenderness and determine whether the muscle, ligament, or bone is injured (Fig. 65-13). If the tenderness is in the muscle, as in the flexor pronator group of the medial side, the injury may be a muscle strain resulting from the valgus stress. If tenderness is in the ligament, it is usually a chronic instability with attenuation, rather than an acute ligamentous rupture. Some tenderness may be noted over a traction spur. If bony tenderness is found, an avulsion fracture should be carefully checked for on x-ray.

On the medial side, instability can be from either a ligamentous injury or an avulsion fracture. If an avulsion fracture is suspected, it is best to obtain x-rays before stress testing since valgus stressing can cause further displacement. If no fracture is found, one should check for instability by placing a valgus stress on the elbow when it is flexed approximately 20 degrees. Comparison with the patient's normal elbow should be made. On the lateral side, tenderness may be noted over an injured capitellum or over posterolateral loose bodies.

Fig. 65-12. "Little League elbow" showing medial collateral ligament attenuation and ulnar traction spur. Posterior loose bodies can also be seen. The necrosis of the capitellum is probably traumatic in origin. (Redrawn from D.A. Barnes and H.S. Tullos. An analysis of 100 symptomatic baseball players. *Am. J. Med.* 6:62, 1978.)

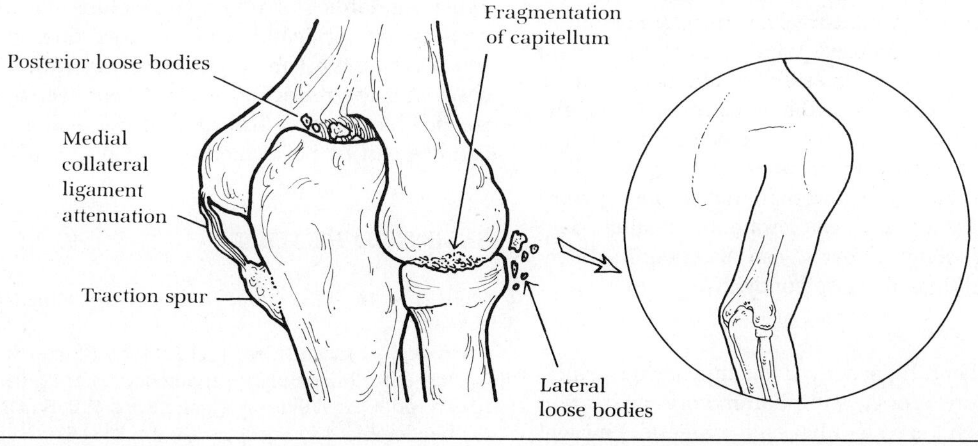

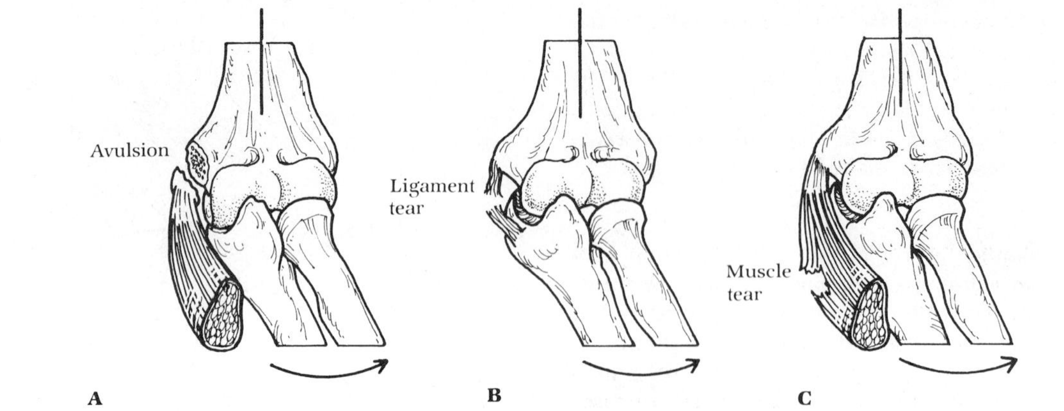

Fig. 65-13. Possible causes of lateral tenderness in "Little League elbow." The tenderness can represent avulsion fracture (A), ligamentous tear (B), or muscle injury (C).

Treatment
In the rare case of a large, displaced avulsion fracture, early referral to an orthopedist for possible operative treatment is indicated. In the majority of patients, application of a sling combined with active range of motion exercises should be the initial treatment. Throwing sports must be discontinued until evaluation by an orthopedic surgeon is arranged. The urgency in seeking orthopedic consultation will often seem greater to the patient who needs to give up a particular activity than it is to the examining physician.

Epicondylitis

Perhaps the most famous overuse syndrome of the elbow is lateral epicondylitis, or tennis elbow. Although not found only in tennis players, the condition classically is seen in active adults who repetitively strain the wrist extensors at the elbow. The history is one of pain that begins insidiously at or near the origin of the extensor carpi radialis brevis (ECRB) on the lateral epicondyle (Fig. 65-14). Epicondylitis can occur on the medial side of the elbow, and tenderness in this case is located at the origin of the flexor pronator group on the medial epicondyle.

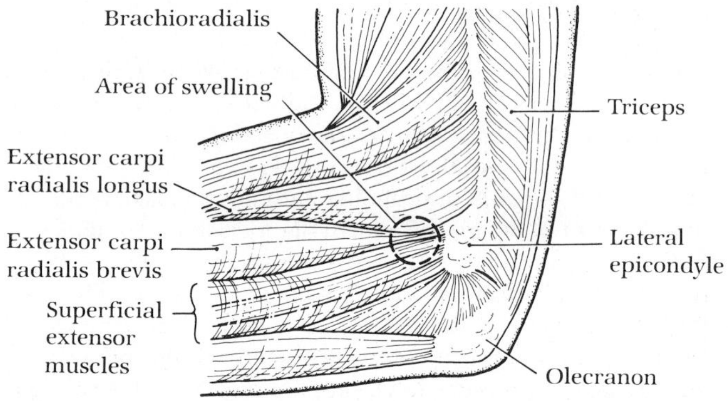

Fig. 65-14. View of elbow joint with overlying muscle insertions. Location of tenderness in lateral epicondylitis is at the origin and most proximal portion of the extensor carpi radialis brevis.

Evaluation
The patient should be able to localize the pain to either side of the elbow. Tenderness should be most severe close to the epicondyle. With lateral epicondylitis, pain will often be produced by wrist dorsiflexion against resistance. With medial epicondylitis, palmar flexion of the wrist against resistance should produce pain. X-rays are usually normal.

Epicondylitis can be confused with neural entrapment syndromes of the radial nerve (laterally) or the median nerve (medially). In these conditions, the tenderness is usually more distal than for lateral or medial epicondylitis, being located over the supinator and pronator teres muscles, respectively. Neurologic changes and pain that are most prominent with resisted supination or pronation (rather than wrist dorsiflexion or palmarflexion) can also help in differentiating these conditions from epicondylitis.

Treatment
Avoidance of the offending activity is the underlying principle of treatment. Nonsteroidal antiinflammatory medication can be of some benefit, even if only as an analgesic. Physical therapy for active and passive stretching of the affected muscle-tendon unit is often utilized and is particularly helpful when loss of motion is present. A "tennis elbow strap" or wrist splint can be used and is believed to function by decreasing the tension at the origin of the affected muscle.

Referral to an orthopedic surgeon should be made for individuals who do not show substantial improvement over three weeks' time. The condition can be difficult to treat. Other modalities of treatment include corticosteroid injections or the application of hydrocortisone cream with ultrasound treatment (phonopheresis). On rare occasions (those cases that are refractory to treatment over a 6- to 12-month period), excision of a portion of the tendon origin and epicondyle can be performed with good results.

SELECTED READING

Morrey, F. *The Elbow and its Disorders.* Philadelphia: Saunders, 1985.

Rockwood, C A, and Green, D P (eds). *Fractures in Adults,* vol 1 (2nd ed). Philadelphia: Lippincott, 1984. Pp 559–652.

Rockwood, C A, Wilkins, K E, and King, R E. *Fractures in Children.* Philadelphia: Lippincott, 1984. Pp 363–576.

66. Wrist and Forearm Injuries

Peter Waters

WRIST INJURIES

Injuries of the wrist are usually secondary to a fall or, less commonly, from direct trauma. The type and severity of injury depend on many factors, including the age and muscular coordination of the patient, energy of the impact, position of the extremity at the time of injury, and the degree of osteoporosis present. The majority of these injuries occur in the position of dorsiflexion, resulting in compression stresses dorsally and tension stresses on the palmar side. These forces can result in either a sprain of the wrist ligaments or a variety of fractures and dislocations, including epiphyseal plate injury in the child, scaphoid fracture or carpal dislocation in the young adult, or Colles' fracture in the older individual.

FUNCTIONAL ANATOMY

The wrist is comprised of the area between the carpometacarpal joints distally and the insertion of the pronator quadratus onto the radius proximally. The carpus itself is divided into a proximal row (lunate, triquetrum) and distal row (capitate, hamate, trapezoid, trapezium), with the scaphoid (formerly the navicular) serving as the stable linkage between proximal and distal rows (Fig. 66-1A). In addition to the bony stability provided by the scaphoid, the carpus is further stabilized by volar and dorsal ligaments, the most important of which are the volar radioscaphocapitate, radiolunate, and radioscapholunate ligaments (Fig. 66-1B).

The major articulations of the wrist are the radiocarpal and radioulnar joints. While wrist dorsiflexion and palmar flexion occur largely at the radiocarpal and intercarpal joints, pronation and supination occur at the radioulnar joints as the radius rotates about the fixed ulna (see Fig. 66-13). The integrity of these articulations is critical, and they must be carefully evaluated in any fracture or dislocation about the wrist.

The normal range of motion for an adult is 70 degrees of dorsiflexion, 75 degrees of palmar flexion, 20 degrees of radial deviation, and 30 to 60 degrees of ulnar deviation. A "tenodesis effect" on the fingers occurs with wrist motion—that is, wrist dorsiflexion results in finger flexion and wrist palmar flexion produces finger extension. This action permits easier grasp and release function. Pronation and supination can normally be performed to 80 degrees each and are most reliably measured with the elbows flexed at 90 degrees and held against the side of the trunk.

Although the wrist and hand are generally well perfused with blood, the scaphoid bone has a tenuous blood supply that can easily be disrupted by a fracture, resulting in os-

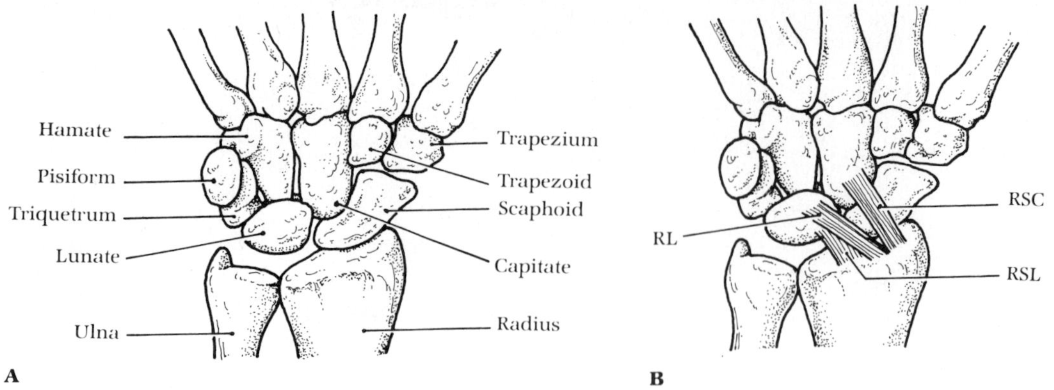

Fig. 66-1. A. Bony anatomy of the carpus. B. Ligamentous anatomy of the carpus showing volar radioscaphocapitate (RSC), radiolunate (RL), and radioscapholunate (RSL) ligaments.

teonecrosis of the devascularized proximal segment. Scaphoid fracture healing can also be delayed or prevented by this process.

FRACTURES AND DISLOCATIONS ABOUT THE WRIST

Distal Radial Fractures

Distal radial fractures are predominantly dorsiflexion injuries with dorsal displacement of the distal radial fragment, commonly termed *Colles' fractures.* This is an extremely common fracture in the elderly, in whom it can occur with a relatively minor injury force, typically a household fall. This injury is less commonly seen in younger patients, in whom a substantial amount of energy is required to produce such a fracture. The tendency to label all distal radial fractures as Colles' fractures is convenient but misleading. The term is correctly applied only to metaphyseal fractures of the distal radius in which the distal fragment is dorsally displaced.

Evaluation

The patient has pain and swelling, a deformity of dorsal displacement and radial deviation of the wrist—the "silver fork" deformity (Fig. 66-2A). Median nerve dysfunction may be present and must be evaluated before any reduction maneuver is performed. Uncommonly, puncture wounds of the skin can be caused by the fracture fragment, usually the proximal portion of the radius as it is pushed toward the volar side of the wrist. After a brief neurovascular examination with special attention to the median nerve, a volar splint should be applied (radiolucent plastic is best) while the patient awaits radiographs in order to lessen the discomfort, swelling, and soft-tissue trauma from fracture motion.

Anteroposterior (AP) and true lateral radiographs (Fig. 66-2B) are necessary to determine the extent of injury and planned treatment. It is important to assess whether the fracture involves the radiocarpal joint, the distal radioulnar joint, or both. An associated ulnar styloid fracture may be present as well. The lateral radiograph should show the radius and ulnar superimposed and should be scrutinized to determine the displacement of the distal radial fragment and the presence of any dorsal displacement of the ulnar head. As with all wrist injuries, the forearm and elbow joint must also be included on the cassette to rule out proximal fractures or dislocations.

It is imperative that the emergency physician distinguish between the commonly seen dorsal displacement of Colles' fracture and the rarer volar displacement of a Smith's fracture (Fig. 66-3). This latter injury is secondary to a fall on a palmar flexed wrist and results in palmar displacement and comminution. Although a much less common pattern, it can be mistaken for a typical dorsal displacement injury. The fracture will be suggested by the position of the hand at the time of injury as well as the appearance of the wrist on initial examination. The hand will be displaced to the palmar side of the wrist and the ulnar head will be prominent on the dorsal surface. In contrast to dorsally displaced fractures, closed reduction is frequently unsuccessful in these distal radial fractures and surgical reduction and fixation are often required.

Analysis of AP and lateral radiographs for the degree of dorsal displacement, dorsal comminution, and intraarticular extension of the fracture guides the treating physician in management decisions. The AP radiographic view (Fig. 66-4B) is assessed for the extent of radial shortening and articular involvement caused by fracture extension into the radiocarpal joint. The lateral radiographic view (Fig. 66-4A) is assessed for dorsal displacement, apex volar angulation, and the integrity of the distal radioulnar joint. Comparison with the opposite, uninjured wrist is often useful. In describing the injury to the orthopedist, it is helpful to report the specifics of articular incongruity, radial shortening, dorsal displacement, and apex volar angulation (Fig. 66-4). (See Chap. 63 for further details regarding fracture description.)

Minimally displaced or angulated fractures can be treated without reduction by application of a volar splint (see Chap. 63). Closed reduction and immobilization are indicated for displaced, angulated fractures. External fixation or open reduction–internal fixation may be indicated for fractures with severe comminution or radiocarpal articular incongruity.

Closed reduction is performed with the patient under local anesthetic block, either by injection of the acute hematoma with 1% lidocaine (Xylocaine) or by means of an intravenous regional block (see Procedure 40). A hematoma block can be safely placed by the following technique: The dorsal skin

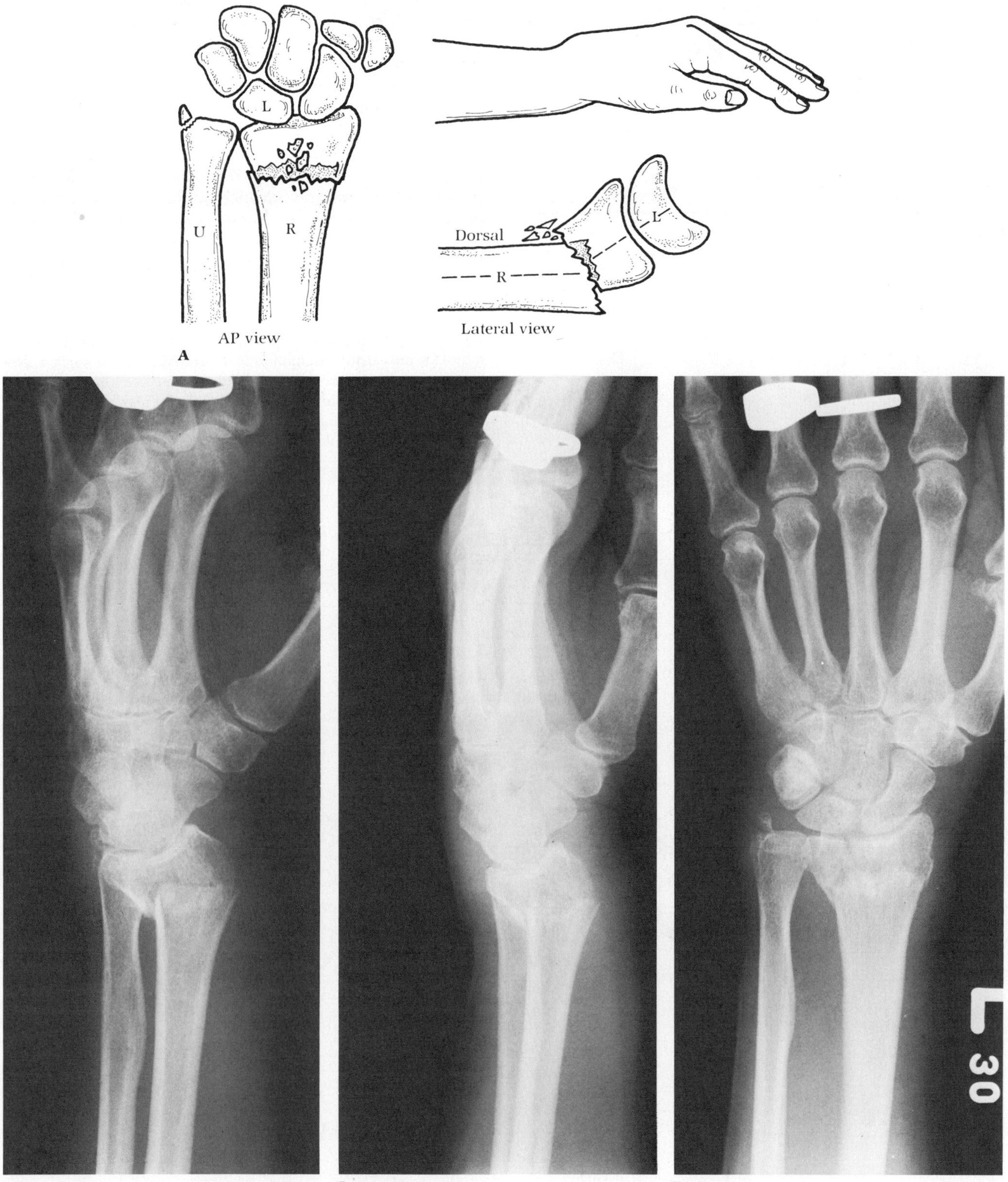

Fig. 66-2. A. Colles' fracture showing metaphyseal location, apex volar angulation, dorsal displacement and comminution, and associated ulnar styloid fracture. A typical silver-fork deformity is depicted. (U = ulna; R = radius; L = lunate.) B–D. Anteroposterior and lateral x-rays of Colles' fracture.

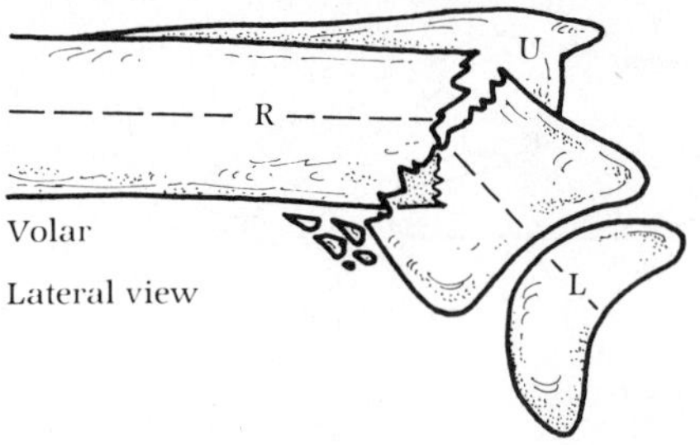

Fig. 66-3. Smith's fracture showing apex dorsal angulation with volar displacement and comminution. (R = radius; U = ulna; L = lunate.)

is scrubbed with alcohol and painted with iodine. A sterile, gloved technique is used thereafter. The fracture is located by gentle palpation, correlated with the lateral radiograph. It will usually be more proximal than expected. The skin is anesthetized dorsally, 1 to 2 cm proximal to the fracture site, and a 20-gauge needle is then introduced at an angle of approximately 45 degrees to the skin surface (Fig. 66-5). The needle is gently advanced to the dorsal surface of the radius, just proximal to the fracture. It is then angled slightly more parallel to the arm and advanced until it reaches an area of no resistance, the fracture hematoma. Gentle aspiration will produce a flush of blood in the syringe, confirming that the hematoma has been found. At this location, 5 ml 1% Xylocaine (without epinephrine) is gently injected. At least 10

Fig. 66-4. A. Schematic lateral view of the radius showing technique for measuring angulation of the radial articular surface. Note that fracture angulation is described by the direction in which the apex of the fracture angle points. This figure shows apex volar angulation. B. Schematic AP view of distal radius illustrating method of measurement of radial length.

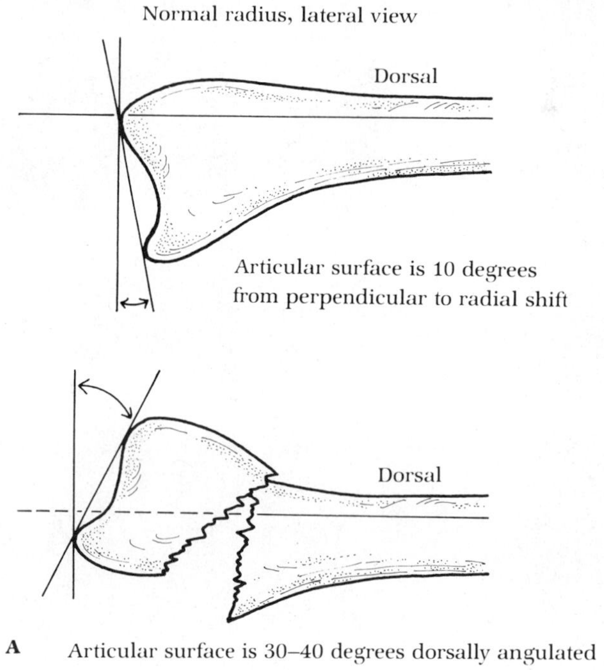

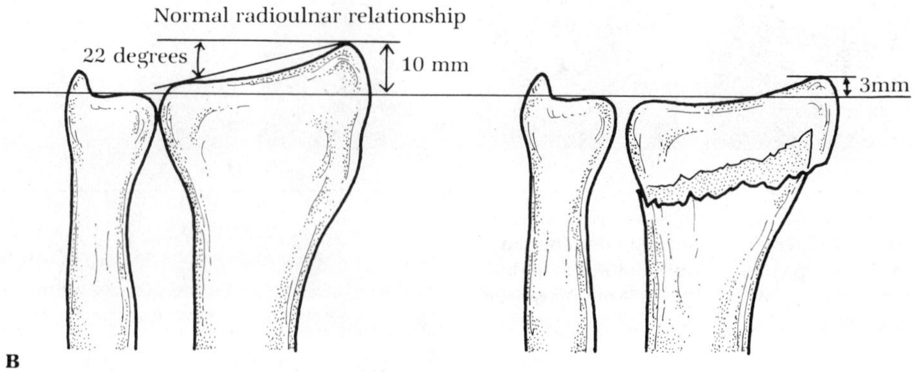

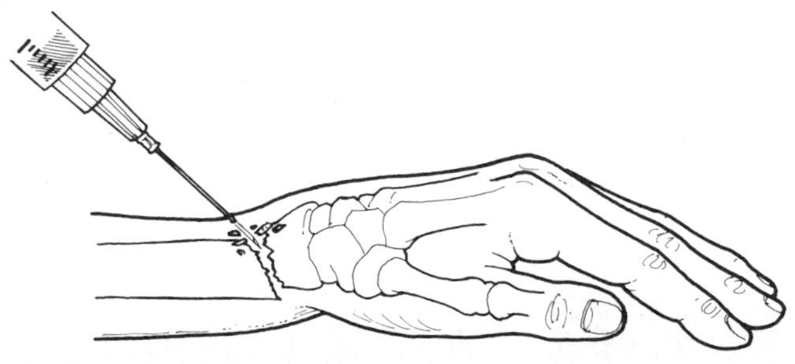

Fig. 66-5. Technique of hematoma block.

minutes are required for the anesthetic to take effect. If an associated ulnar styloid fracture is present, injection of 3 to 5 ml 1% Xylocaine into the fracture in a sterile fashion will further lessen the patient's discomfort during the reduction.

Reduction of the fracture is greatly facilitated by distal traction, which will disimpact the fracture fragments. An acceptable means of achieving this is by finger traction (Fig. 66-6). Ten to fifteen minutes of traction with up to 10 pounds of weight across the upper arm will usually disimpact the fracture and reduce muscle spasm, allowing a reduction to be performed (Fig. 66-6A, B). For the dorsally displaced distal radius fragment, gentle downward pressure with simultaneous wrist flexion and ulnar deviation will usually reduce the fracture (Fig. 66-6C). If no movement is felt and the deformity appears unchanged (Fig. 66-6D), it may be necessary to hyperextend the wrist at the fracture and then apply downward pressure on the distal fragment (Fig. 66-6E, F). After reduction, the wrist is held in slight flexion and ulnar deviation and a noncircumferential plaster splint, such as a Charnley splint, is applied (see Chap. 63). Repeat AP and lateral radiographs are then obtained and the neurovascular status is rechecked. If the reduction is satisfactory, the splint is extended proximally to immobilize the forearm in neutral or slight supination by means of a "sugar tong" extension, as described in Chap. 63. A sling is fitted.

For volarly displaced fractures (Smith's fractures) or fractures with involvement of the radiocarpal or radioulnar joints, or both, orthopedic consultation is advisable, since reduction and immobilization methods will vary considerably. Application of an external fixator or open reduction and internal fixation of the fracture may well be recommended, particularly in active patients.

All patients should be strongly advised to elevate the extremity and apply ice for the first 48 hours. Ice should be applied using a waterproof liner to avoid damage to the plaster and maceration of the underlying skin. It should be applied dorsally for approximately 20 minutes every 1 to 2 hours while the patient is awake. All patients with distal radial fractures must be checked within 24 hours for swelling and neurovascular dysfunction, regardless of whether a reduction maneuver was performed. Referral to an orthopedic surgeon, if not made at the time of the presentation, should be arranged for two to three days from injury for possible readjustment of the splint and repeat x-rays. Loss of reduction can occur, particularly in the comminuted fracture patterns, and repeat reduction is more easily accomplished early than late.

Dislocation of the Distal Radioulnar Joint

A dislocation of the distal radioulnar joint is frequently missed on initial assessment. The typical history is a twisting fall with the forearm in the position of pronation at the time of impact. The distal radioulnar joint dislocates, with the ulnar head typically moving dorsally (Fig. 66-7). An ulnar styloid fracture may be present as well.

Evaluation

Examination reveals a dorsally prominent ulnar head, with tenderness and swelling over the distal radioulnar joint. The deformity is pronounced in pronation and usually absent in supination, as the joint will spontaneously reduce as the forearm is supinated. Confirmation is obtained by a true lateral radiograph in pronation and supination, showing the dorsal dislocation of the distal ulna. Comparison views of the opposite wrist are helpful. At times a CT scan of the radioulnar joint in pronation and supination aids in diagnosis and management.

Treatment

In the acute stage, treatment consists of placement of a long arm cast with the elbow flexed 90 degrees and the forearm in supination. Swelling is not usually severe, but if this is a concern, a posterior splint extending from the upper arm to the dorsum of the metacarpophalangeal joints can maintain the wrist in the identical position.

Referral to an orthopedic surgeon within five days is recommended. The usual course of treatment is six weeks in a long arm cast. Chronic radioulnar dislocation, if symptomatic, can be treated surgically, although for most individuals the dislocation is of more cosmetic than functional significance.

Carpal Fractures and Dislocations

Fractures of the scaphoid are the most common carpal injuries. Less common are fractures of the other carpal bones and subluxation-dislocation of the intercarpal joints. Scaphoid fractures can occur in a variety of situations, including minor falls from a standing position. Carpal dislocations, however, usually require more force and are more typically the result of a high-energy injury such as a motor vehicle accident or a fall from a height.

Evaluation

Careful inspection and palpation will usually localize tenderness in the setting of acute injury. Tenderness dorsally in the anatomic snuffbox (Fig. 66-8) or volarly at the distal scaphoid tubercle can be taken as clinical evidence of a scaphoid fracture. If pain seems localized to another part of the carpus, then this area should be most carefully scrutinized on the x-ray films.

Radiographs are usually diagnostic but may require inclusion of a "scaphoid view" (Fig. 66-9A) or "stress views" of the wrist: AP views in radial and ulnar deviation, AP "clenched fist" view, and lateral views in dorsiflexion and palmar flexion. Films must be examined carefully for fractures, particularly of the scaphoid. The AP view may show shortening of the scaphoid along its long axis due to either rotation of the scaphoid as a whole or angulation of the distal

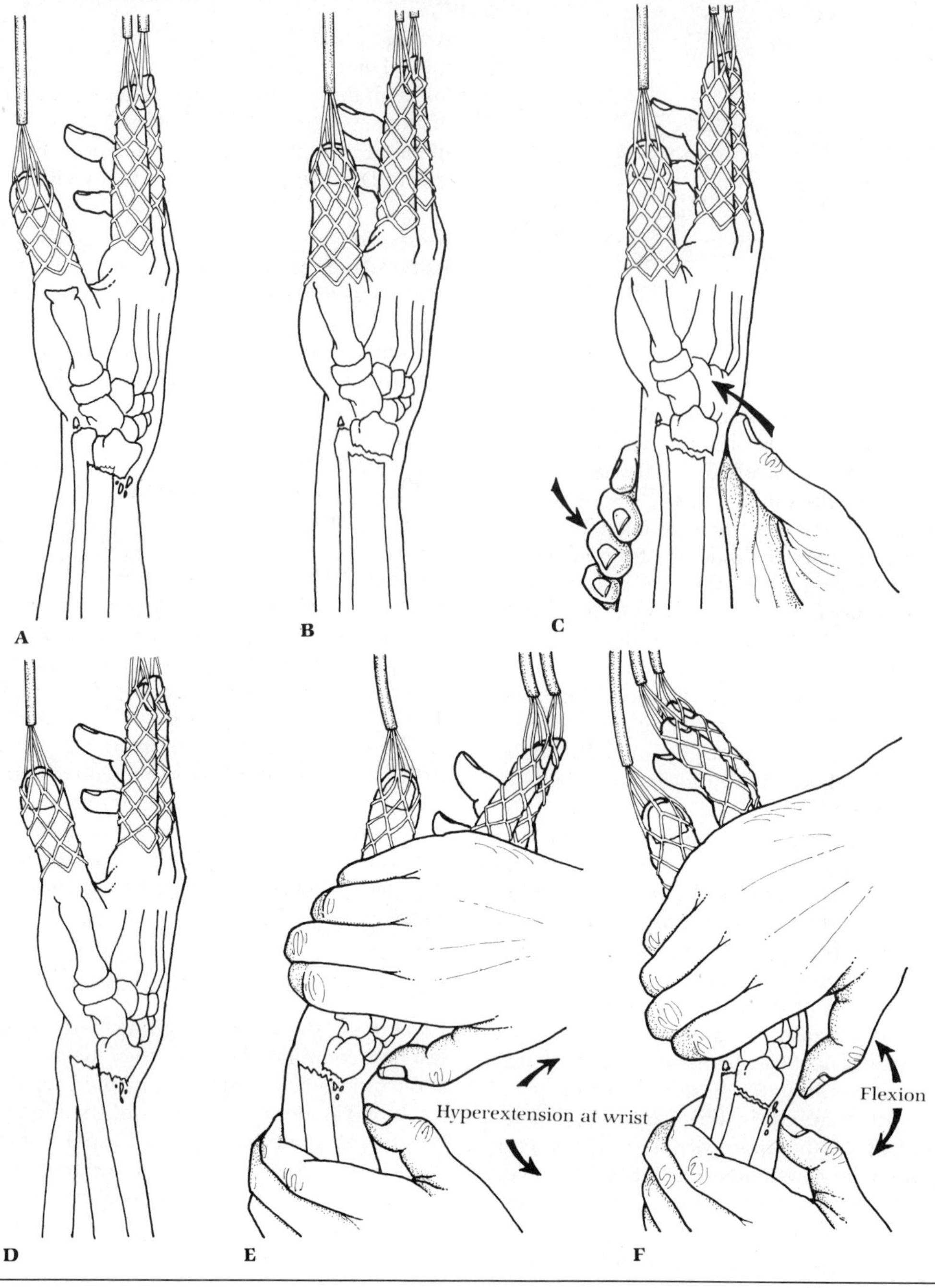

Fig. 66-6. Method of closed reduction of distal radial fracture using finger-trap traction. A. The displaced-impacted fracture is placed in finger-trap traction and distraction force is applied by means of counterweight across the elbow. B. After 10 to 15 minutes, disimpaction of the fracture has occurred. C. Reduction is performed with traction by pushing on the dorsally displaced fragment. D–F. If no reduction is achieved, the fracture is hyperextended and the distal fragment is simultaneously pushed in a volar direction. The fracture site is then flexed, and reduction is maintained by holding the wrist in flexion and ulnar deviation as the finger traps are removed.

fragment of a scaphoid fracture. Another sign of intercarpal dislocation is an increased space (>3 mm) between the lunate and the scaphoid, as seen on the AP view (Fig. 66-9B). This results from rotation of the scaphoid into an abnormally vertical alignment. The lateral view should be checked to see that the radius, lunate, and capitate are all collinear and that the scapholunate angle is between 30 and 60 degrees (Fig. 66-10).

Two patterns of intercarpal instability should be recognized. One is dorsiflexed intercalated segment instability (DISI), which is present when the capitolunate angle is greater than 20 degrees dorsally and the scapholunate angle is greater than 70 degrees. Volar flexed intercalated segment

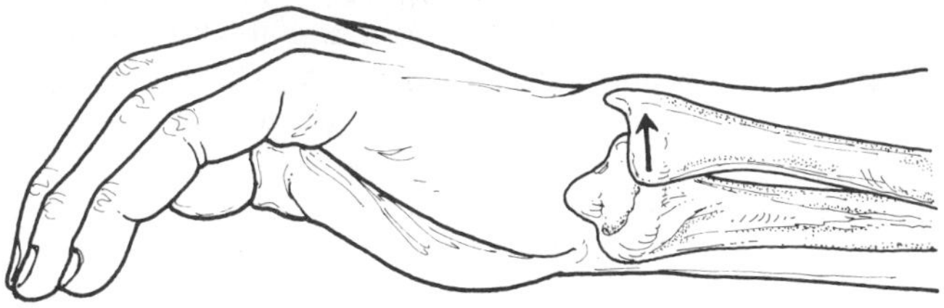

Fig. 66-7. Distal radioulnar joint dislocation.

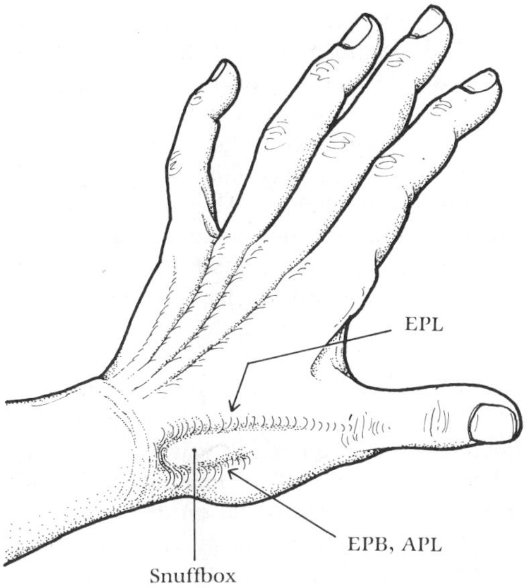

Fig. 66-8. Illustration showing the location of the "snuffbox." (EPL = extensor pollicis longus; EPB = extensor pollicis brevis; APL = abductor pollicis longus.)

instability (VISI) produces the opposite pattern, with a scapholunate angle decreased to less than 30 degrees and a capitolunate angle of greater than 20 degrees volarly. The key to recognition is the direction in which the lunate points; that is, if the crescent is angled with its concavity pointed dorsally, a DISI pattern results. If the concavity points volarly, a VISI pattern is produced (see Fig. 66-10). If all wrist and carpal films are examined in this systematic fashion, carpal fractures and dislocations are not likely to be missed.

Treatment

For nondisplaced scaphoid fractures, immobilization in a long arm splint with radial gutter to immobilize the thumb is recommended (see Chap. 63). Follow-up examination with an orthopedic surgeon is appropriate within 7 to 10 days. Immobilization will usually be required for a minimum of 12 weeks and often longer, depending on radiographic evidence of union over time. If a scaphoid fracture is suspected by clinical examination but not seen on x-ray, immobilization in a radial gutter splint or short arm-thumb spica cast is indicated until repeat films can be obtained in 10 days. Often, a nondisplaced fracture will become visible during this interval as a result of bony resorption at the fracture site. For nondisplaced fractures of the other carpals,

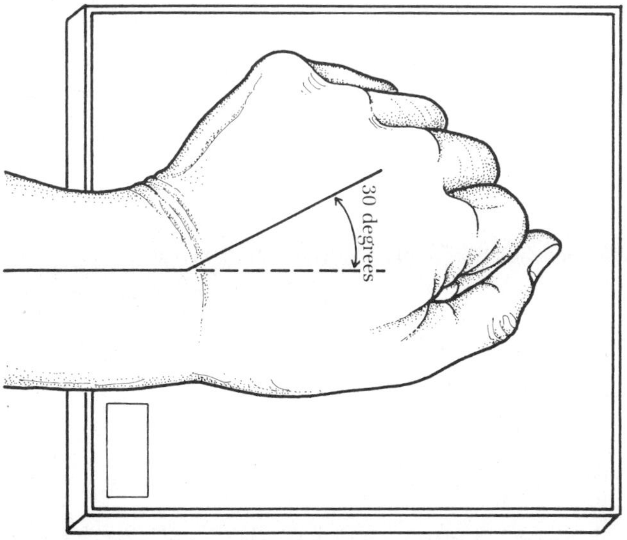

A

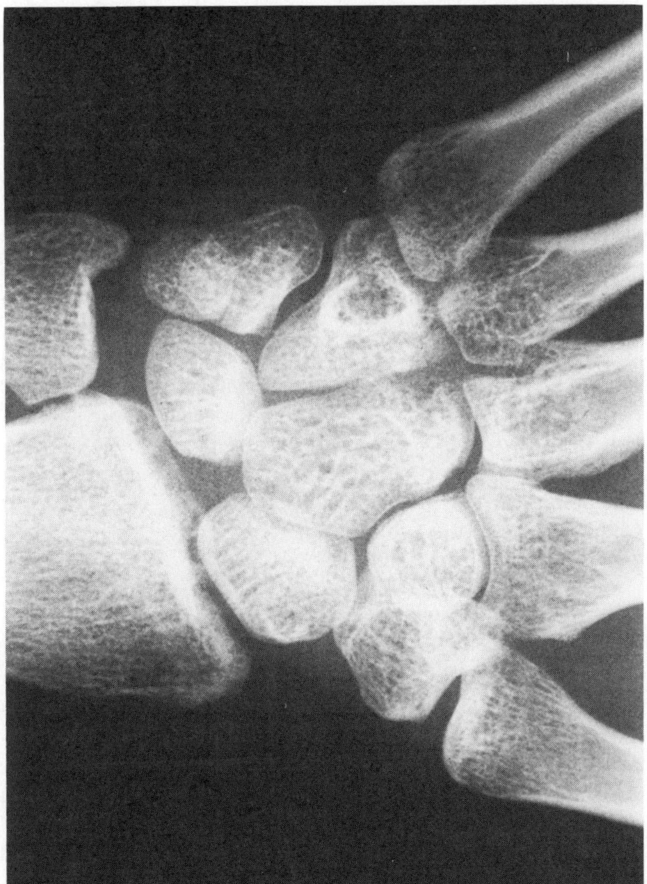

B

Fig. 66-9. A. The wrist is maximally ulnar deviated to obtain scaphoid view. B. Anteroposterior x-ray of scapholunate dislocation with greater than 3-mm gap between scaphoid and lunate.

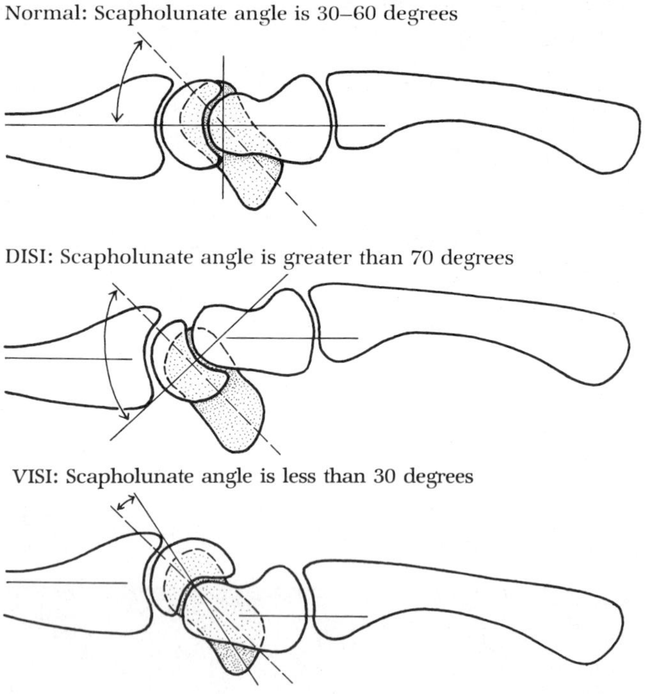

Fig. 66-10. A. Lateral view of the wrist showing measurement of the normal scapholunate angle. B. DISI pattern showing a scapholunate angle of greater than 70 degrees. C. VISI pattern showing scapholunate angle reduced below 30 degrees.

a volar splint and orthopedic follow-up examination in 7 to 10 days are recommended.

For displaced scaphoid fractures or intercarpal dislocations, orthopedic consultation is advised in the emergency department. Reduction and pinning of scaphoid fractures can be undertaken, and carpal dislocations must be adequately reduced and stabilized for optimal long-term wrist function. A further discussion of carpal injuries is found in Chap. 67.

WRIST SPRAINS

If results of x-ray evaluation are normal and neurovascular examination is intact, the injured wrist can be treated as a sprain by placement of a volar splint, either made from plaster or prefabricated. Ace bandages are often used, but while they control swelling to a degree, they do not offer much support. The ideal position for splinting is approximately 30 degrees of dorsiflexion, and the splint should not be carried beyond the metacarpophalangeal joints (see Fig. 63-9). Finger motion should be encouraged to reduce stiffness. As for all sprains, elevation and periodic application of ice are most important for the first 48 hours. Orthopedic consultation within 7 to 10 days is necessary to be certain that ligamentous disruption with carpal instability has not occurred. If untreated, this condition can lead to long-term carpal instability.

The exception to this rule is when a scaphoid fracture is suspected by clinical examination. In this case the volar splint is better modified in such a way as to immobilize the thumb (see Fig. 63-10). The plaster should be carried out to just beyond the distal interphalangeal joint of the thumb, maintaining the thumb in the position it would assume if grasping a small paper cup. Repeat x-rays at 7 to 10 days are mandatory to rule out a scaphoid fracture.

FOREARM FRACTURES

The forearm is injured less commonly than the wrist. The most frequent causes are falls on an outstretched arm or direct blunt trauma, such as when lifting the arm to deflect a blow aimed for the head. Significant contusions are occasionally seen; compartment syndromes of the forearm are well described and can be permanently debilitating (see Chap. 73). The most important acute injuries of the forearm are fractures and fracture-dislocations. The majority of these fractures need immediate orthopedic referral because management often involves open reduction and internal fixation.

The radius and ulna articulate both proximally at the elbow and distally at the wrist. They are parallel throughout their length, connected by the interosseous membrane. While the ulna is relatively straight, the radius has a lateral bow, alignment of which is critical for pronation and supination, a motion that occurs as the radius rotates about the fixed ulna (Fig. 66-11).

Forearm fractures fall into several categories (Fig. 66-12). These include (1) fractures of both the radius and ulna, (2) isolated fracture of the ulna ("night-stick fracture"), (3) proximal ulna fracture with dislocation of the radial head (Monteggia's fracture), (4) distal radial fracture with dislocation of the ulnar head (Galeazzi's fracture), and (5) green-stick fractures of the forearm in children.

Evaluation

Most patients with forearm fractures will have obvious pain and deformity, although in children the pain of a buckle fracture may be minimal and the deformity undetectable by examination. In these more subtle cases, careful palpation along the radius and ulna will usually localize the tenderness and suggest the diagnosis of fracture.

Inspection of the forearm for an occult puncture wound is important. Open fractures carry a different prognosis and require immediate treatment, which might be delayed if they are not diagnosed promptly. If the forearm is tensely swollen, compartment pressures should be measured (see Chap. 73). Neurovascular function should be documented in all cases and serially with any suspicion of elevated compartment pressures.

Radiography should be performed as expeditiously as possible after the forearm is splinted. The wrist and elbow must both be visualized in two projections, since forces are frequently transmitted the length of the forearm, resulting in both proximal and distal injury. Radial head dislocation can be associated with proximal ulnar fractures (Monteggia's fractures) and can be missed if the radiographs are not carefully inspected. The radial head should align with the capitellum in all views; otherwise a radial head dislocation is present. Similarly, distal radioulnar joint disruption can occur with distal radial fractures (Galeazzi's fractures). A true lateral radiograph of the wrist in pronation will best demonstrate a distal radioulnar joint subluxation, if it is present.

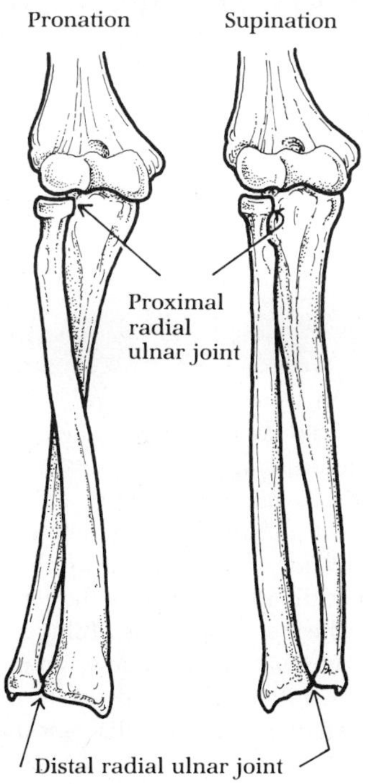

Fig. 66-11. The forearm in pronation and supination showing the interrelationships of the two shafts plus articulations, both proximally and distally.

Treatment

For nondisplaced fractures, such as buckle fractures in children and undisplaced night-stick fractures in adults, no reduction will be performed and initial treatment will consist of application of a long arm plaster splint or cast (see Chap. 63). In most distal buckle fractures in children, a short arm splint or cast is adequate.

In children, displaced forearm fractures are treated with closed reduction. This is detailed further in Chap. 160.

In adults, displaced forearm fractures are treated operatively. This is because the potential for remodeling in the skeletally mature individual is minimal and any malunion will produce substantial loss of pronation and supination. One should be highly suspicious of an isolated ulnar fracture, particularly when angulated or displaced, since an associated radial head dislocation can easily be missed.

Night-stick fractures or the extremely rare, nondisplaced, isolated radial fractures are treated with initial immobilization in a long arm splint for comfort. Current treatment recommendations for ulnar fractures involve early motion with bracing in a reliable patient, whereas radial fractures are generally immobilized for six weeks in a cast, with repeat x-ray examination to check for displacement. Both of these injuries need close orthopedic follow-up and should be seen within five days of injury.

For any question of neurovascular compromise or elevated compartment pressures, emergent consultation is needed. If a compartment syndrome is suspected, any dressing present should be loosened or removed and the extremity placed at the level of the heart, *not elevated*. This is because elevation will immediately reduce arterial pressure more than venous pressure, thus aggravating the underlying problem of inadequate perfusion of muscle. Serial evaluations of sensory and motor status and the tolerance of passive finger extension should be made. Peripheral pulses are not useful in evaluation for compartment syndrome (see Chap. 73).

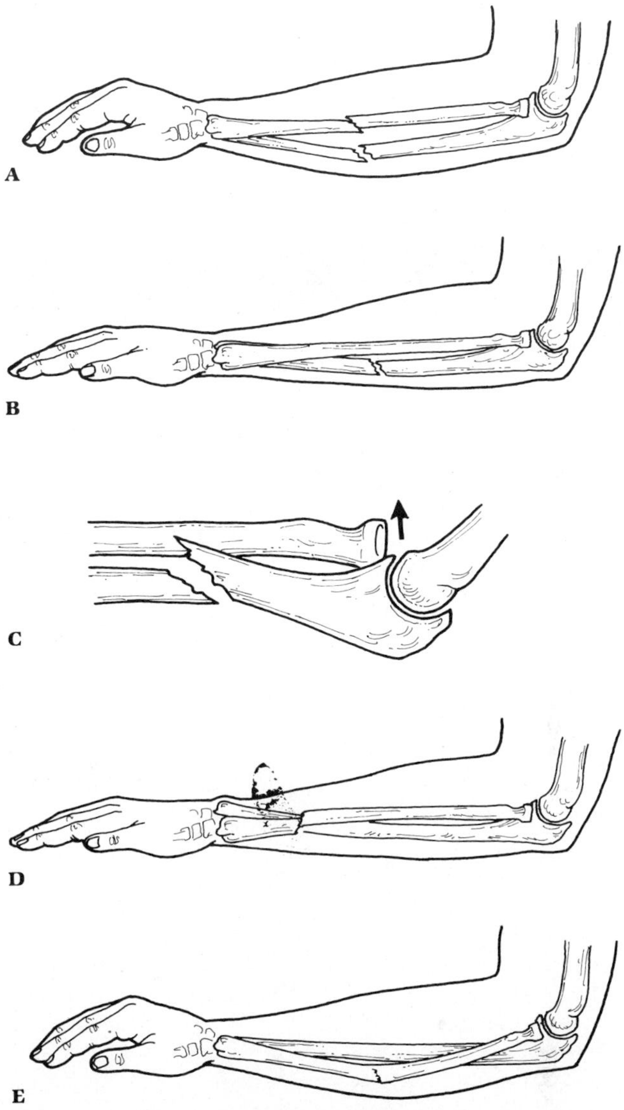

Fig. 66-12. Forearm fractures. A. Fractures of both radius and ulna. B. Isolated fracture of the ulna ("night-stick fracture"). C. Proximal ulnar fracture with dislocation of the radial head (Monteggia's lesion). D. Distal radial fracture with dislocation of the ulnar head (Galeazzi's fracture). E. Green-stick fractures of both forearm bones, as seen in children.

SELECTED READING

American Society of the Hand. *The Hand: Exam and Diagnosis* (3rd ed). New York: Churchill Livingstone, 1990.

American Society of the Hand. *The Hand: Primary Care of Common Problems*, 1985.

Green, DP (ed). *Operative Hand Surgery*. New York: Churchill Livingstone, 1988. Pp. 813–1026.

Rockwood, C, Jr, and Green, D. *Fractures*. Philadelphia: JB Lippincott, 1984. Pp 411–558.

67. Hand Injuries and Other Acute Disorders of the Hand

Paul Feldon
Edward A. Nalebuff

The outcome of an injury to the hand is often determined by the care provided in the emergency department. Hand injuries are common, comprising over 30 percent of all industrial accidents. Seventy-five percent of the injuries that result in permanent partial disability involve the hand. Optimal initial care of hand injuries can minimize the physical and emotional handicaps as well as the loss of productivity that results from these injuries. The ability to make an accurate diagnosis—that is, to determine what can be treated by the primary physician in the emergency department and what should be referred to a specialist—is the key to providing optimal care.

EVALUATION OF THE PATIENT

First aid for patients with injured hands should be provided before a detailed history and physical examination are undertaken. Watches, bracelets, and especially rings should be removed immediately so that thay will not become tourniquets as swelling occurs. Open wounds and massive injuries of the hand should be wrapped in a dry, sterile bandage while the patient is waiting for clinical or x-ray examination. The hand should *not* be immersed in a pan of water to soak.

History

The mechanism, time, place, and other circumstances of the injury must be determined. A snap or pop at the time of injury suggests a ligament disruption or a fracture. Prolonged copious bleeding from a finger wound suggests neurovascular bundle division. Injuries from glass can result in damage to deep structures that is not apparent from the superficial wound or can result in fragments of glass being retained in the soft tissue. Hands that are caught in machines may sustain a combination of lacerations and crush and thermal injuries, depending on the type of machine and nature of the moving parts. The exact nature of the substance that caused chemical burns will affect the choice of treatment. The age, occupation, avocations, hand dominance, and general health of the patient should be recorded. The patient should specifically be asked about the use of daily medications, the status of tetanus immunization, and oral intake before and after the injury. The patient should be asked about old hand injuries or any preexisting disability of the hand. If a patient has unexplained swelling and tenderness consistent with infection but no obvious source of contamination, he or she should be asked about puncture wounds, insect bites, or possible medical conditions, such as gout, that can imitate infection.

Physical Examination

Proper diagnosis of the injured hand requires a knowledge of its functional anatomy—the locations and functions of the muscles that control it, the skeletal framework, and the major and "minor" nerves that supply the hand. It is acceptable, even advisable, to use an anatomic atlas to refresh one's memory. Potentially dangerous exploration or probing of open wounds should not be undertaken in the emergency department to establish a diagnosis; the diagnosis should be made by clinical and x-ray examination. A systematic examination should be carried out with the following questions in mind:

1. What is the extent and nature of the skin wound?
2. Has a neurovascular bundle been injured?
3. Is there tendon damage?
4. Is there bone, joint, or ligament damage?

In general, one should assume that all longitudinal structures crossing the site of an open wound are divided and that swollen joints have unstable ligament disruptions or dislocations until proved otherwise.

The stance of the hand is important for quickly discovering major tendon and joint injuries. The normal posture of the fingers in relation to each other and to the palm is familiar and can be checked by comparing the injured hand against the noninjured hand or the examiner's hand. The fingers normally lie in sequence with each joint in slight flexion (Fig. 67-1). Loss of continuity of one or more tendons, or an alteration in skeletal alignment, changes this stance. Gentle palpation of the hand will reveal areas of local tenderness, skeletal irregularity, or joint instability. An alteration in skin moisture suggests damage to the sensory nerves in the affected area. The skin loss, the amount of tissue crushed, and the presence of cleanly incised wounds, ragged lacerations, or combinations of these will determine where and how the injuries must be handled. The amount of bacterial contamination that has occurred should be estimated and, if indicated, cultures should be obtained. Occasionally, the amount of dirt present obscures the nature of the wound and preliminary cleaning must be done. Soap and water usually are best for cleaning the skin adjacent to the wound, although occasionally degreasing agents such as ether or a solution of hydrogen peroxide to remove coagulated blood is required. The wound itself should be cleaned only by irrigation with a physiologic solution, such as Ringer's solution or normal saline in amounts sufficient to remove superficial contaminants and foreign material from the wound (usually 1–2 liters).

Vascular Examination

Examination of the circulatory status of the hand should not be neglected, particularly if the nature of the injury is such that the vascular structures are at risk—for example, lacerations on the volar aspects of the wrist, hand, or digits or crush injuries, or both. The hand has an excellent vascular supply via the ulnar and radial arteries, which join to form the superficial and deep vascular arches in the palm. Multiple collateral vessels are found at the wrist and hand levels, but few in the distal palm and in the individual digits. It is easy to overlook an ischemic digit, especially in massive injuries when the injured hand is covered with dried blood from open wounds, when the hand or digits have been stained by grease or other material, or when the adjacent digits have intact circulation.

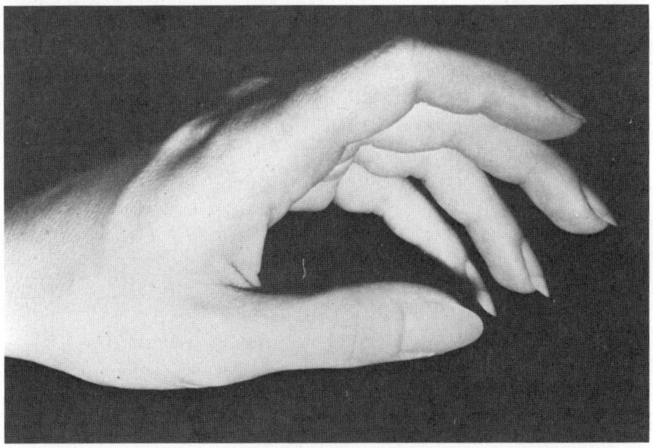

Fig. 67-1. When the hand is at rest, the fingers lie in slight flexion. Note the normal "cascade" of progressive flexion from the index to the small fingers.

The injured hand should be examined for circulation after it has been cleaned and after adequate anesthesia has been obtained, if necessary. Brisk capillary filling at the distal pulp or of the nail bed after light compression of the fingertip usually indicates adequate blood flow. Blanched or cyanotic digits should be examined in more detail, as should those with a decrease in turgor of the pulp compared to noninjured digits. Doppler flowmeters with small vascular probes can be used to check individual digital arteries. Electronic temperature sensors provide accurate measurement of skin temperatures at the fingertips and are a sensitive and accurate reflection of digital blood flow that can be used with ease in the emergency department. This equipment usually is available from the anesthesia department or neonatal pediatric unit. The temperature of the tips (pulps) of the digits in question is compared to that of digits that have brisk capillary refill on either the ipsilateral or contralateral hands. Skin surface temperatures below 30°C suggest compromised vascular function.

Examination of Tendons

A loss of tendon function after upper extremity injury can be secondary to transection of the tendon, rupture of the tendon, or paralysis of the muscle unit. Tendon transection must be suspected in any open wound of the hand. Complete division of the tendon must be differentiated from partial or incomplete transection. A laceration in the appropriate anatomic area, pain from active or passive motion of the finger, and tenderness over the tendon, without loss of the normal finger posture or active motion, suggest a partial tendon laceration. These must be treated to prevent subsequent rupture or adherence. Open wounds should not be probed in an attempt to detect tendon damage. Rather, a careful detailed examination should be performed.

Flexor tendon ruptures can occur and must be suspected when tendon function is suddenly lost in the absence of an open wound. The flexor digitorum profundus tendon of the

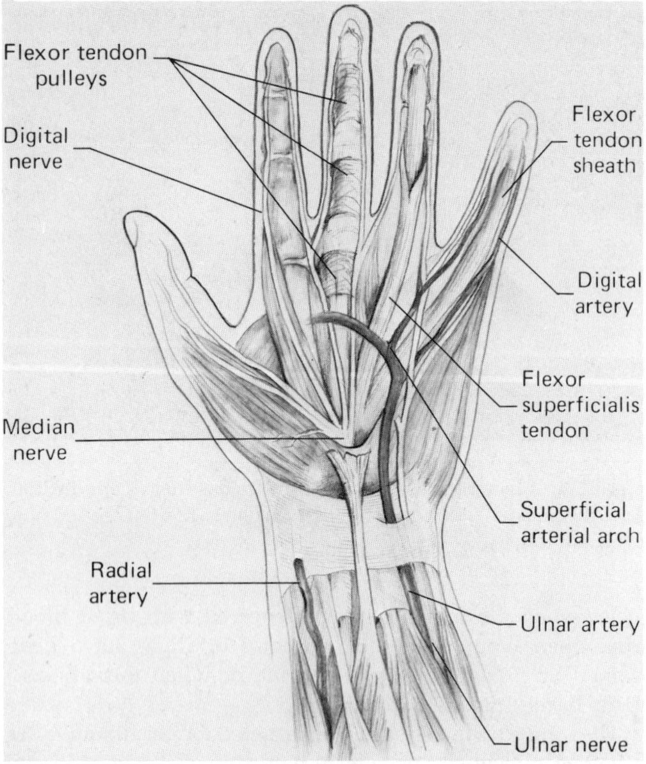

Fig. 67-2. The flexor aspect of the hand. The locations of the digital nerves and arteries are illustrated in the index and small fingers, the flexor tendon and sheath and pulley mechanism are shown in the long finger, and the superficial and deep flexor tendons are illustrated in the ring finger.

ring finger is not uncommonly avulsed from its distal attachment in football players holding on during a tackle. This can occur either with or without an avulsion fracture of the distal phalanx. Any sudden extension force applied to the hand during grip can cause tendon rupture, although significant force is required.

A tendon's function also can be lost if the nerve innervating its muscle belly is damaged. Thus, the integrity both of the tendon and the nerve supplying the musculotendinous unit must be determined.

FLEXOR TENDONS. Each finger has two flexor tendons: the *flexor digitorum superficialis,* which inserts on the middle phalanx and flexes the proximal interphalangeal (PIP) joint, and the *flexor digitorum profundus,* which inserts on the distal phalanx and flexes both the distal and proximal interphalangeal joints (Fig. 67-2). The thumb has one extrinsic flexor tendon, the flexor pollicis longus, which inserts on the distal phalanx and flexes the interphalangeal (and metacarpophalangeal) joint. Division of one or more of these tendons will alter the posture or stance of the finger with respect to the other fingers and will result in the inability to flex the digit fully. The tendons are tested by asking the patient to make a fist. The tips of all of the fingers should touch the distal palm crease. The thumb tendon is tested by asking the patient to touch the head of the fifth metacarpal with the tip of the thumb. The inability to flex a finger actively at the PIP joint suggests division of both the superficial and deep flexor tendons (Fig. 67-3). The diagnosis of damage to a single flexor tendon in the finger is more difficult since the remaining tendon has considerable functional capacity and the posture of the digit can be altered only slightly. Thus, each deep and superficial tendon must be tested individually.

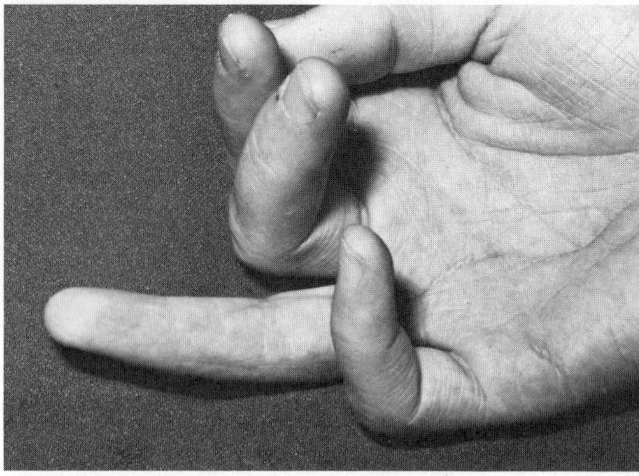

Fig. 67-3. Stance of the ring finger when both superficial and deep flexor tendons are cut.

The profundus tendon is tested by stabilizing the PIP joint in extension and asking the patient to flex the tip of the finger (Fig. 67-4). The profundus is the only tendon that can flex the distal interphalangeal (DIP) joint, and the absence of this function is diagnostic. Each finger and the thumb are tested in sequence. Isolated injuries of the sublimis (superficial) tendon are more difficult to detect since the profundus tendon is capable of flexing the digit fully by itself. Therefore, the posture of the finger may not be changed, and full active motion may be present in spite of damage to this tendon. Testing the sublimis tendon requires that the profundus tendon action be eliminated. This is done by holding all of the fingers not being tested in extension (Fig. 67-5). This limits profundus tendon action in the finger being tested because of the interdigitation of the profundus muscle bellies in the forearm. Any motion of the PIP joint now is the result of sublimis tendon action alone. The exception to this will occur in a patient with an independent profundus tendon in the index finger. Since this usually is present bilaterally, the uninjured side should be tested.

EXTENSOR TENDONS. Extension of the fingers is accomplished by a complex structure composed of interlacing fibers from the extrinsic extensor tendons (extensor digitorum communis, extensor indicis proprius, and extensor digiti quinti) and from the intrinsic muscles (interossei and lumbricals) (Fig. 67-6). The long or extrinsic extensor tendons are responsible for extension of the metacarpophalangeal (MP) joints, whereas the intrinsic tendons combined with the extrinsic tendons act to extend the interphalangeal (IP) joints. The combination of the extrinsic extensor tendons and the intrinsic tendons is called the *extensor mechanism.* The ability to extend the fingers fully at all joint levels suggests that there is no interruption in the continuity of this mechanism. However, a lag in extension of the MP joint suggests an injury of the extrinsic extensor tendons. Finger

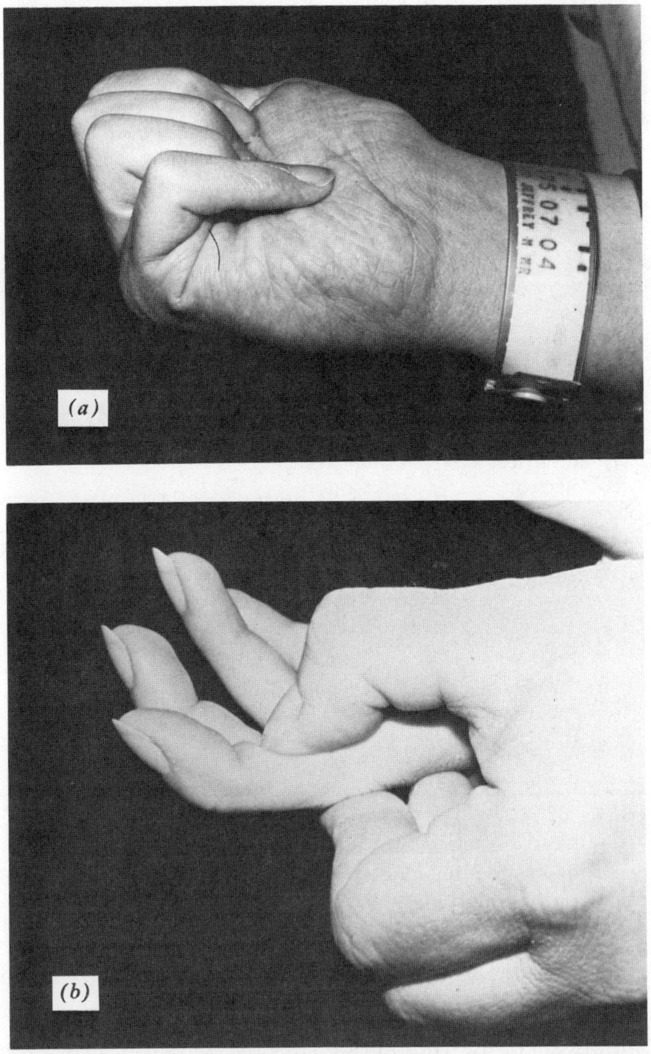

Fig. 67-4. (*a*) The appearance of the hand during maximum active finger flexion with a complete division of the deep flexor tendon to the small finger. Note the absence of flexion of the DIP joint. (*b*) Method for testing for deep flexor tendon function. The PIP joint is held in extension and the patient is asked to flex the DIP joint actively.

extension should be tested against resistance because of the juncturae that interlink the extensor digitorum communis tendons at the midmetacarpal level and that can provide weak extension in the case of a divided tendon. A lag in extension of the PIP or DIP joints suggests an injury of the extensor mechanism distal to the MP joints. Closed as well as open injuries on the dorsal aspect of the digit can damage the extensor mechanism and result in finger deformity (see section on closed tendon injuries). The extensor pollicis longus tendon should be tested by palpating the tendon at the wrist level during active extension, since the IP joint of the thumb can be extended by the intrinsic muscles and complete division of the extensor pollicis longus may be manifested only by incomplete extension of the thumb MP joint.

Nerve Examination

Nerve function should be assessed before any form of local anesthetic is used. Sensory function can be evaluated quickly

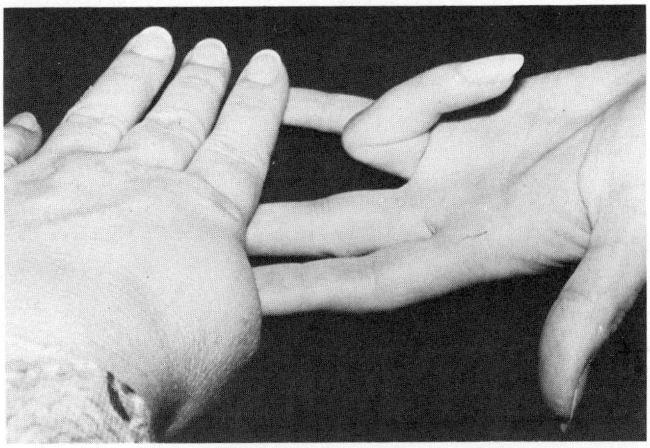

Fig. 67-5. Test for superficial flexor tendon function. All fingers except the one being tested are held in extension to eliminate the effect of the deep flexor tendon. If the superficial flexor tendon is intact, the finger can be flexed actively at the PIP joint.

by testing both sides of each digit using light touch, either by the examiner's finger or with a wisp of cotton, and comparing the patient's report of subjective sensation to that on the adjacent or contralateral (noninjured) fingers. Sharp pins are not necessary to test sensibility and can cause discomfort when nerve function is intact. In children this discomfort will make the frightened child uncooperative. We should not ask, "Do you feel this?" but rather, "Does this feel the same as the other side (or finger)?" Sympathetic denervation at the time of sensory nerve damage results in cessation of sweating. Therefore, areas of dryness on the volar surfaces of the digits are very suggestive of nerve damage. The pattern of dryness can help determine which nerves have been injured when the clinical examination is difficult (such as with a child or an unconscious patient) or when nerve damage proximal to the digit is suspected. Injuries proximal to the digits require that the function of the three major nerves supplying the hand be tested (Fig. 67-7).

Tests of two-point discrimination can be performed using a paper clip unbent to form a U-shaped caliper with the points of the caliper about 15 mm apart. The points of the caliper are pressed longitudinally along the radial and ulnar sides of the pulp of the digit with just enough pressure to momentarily blanch the skin, and then are lifted away. The patient (with eyes closed) is asked to report whether one or two points were perceived on the fingertip. The points are moved closer and closer together with each trial until the patient reports perceiving only one point. The ability to perceive two points 5 mm apart is considered normal, while two-point discrimination greater than 6 mm is considered abnormal. This test requires cooperation of the patient and an experienced examiner in order to be reliable. For these reasons, this test is of less value in the emergency department than those described previously.

MEDIAN NERVE. The median nerve in the hand provides sensibility to the volar surfaces of the thumb, index, long, and one-half of the ring fingers, as well as to the dorsal surfaces of these fingers distal to the MP joints. It innervates

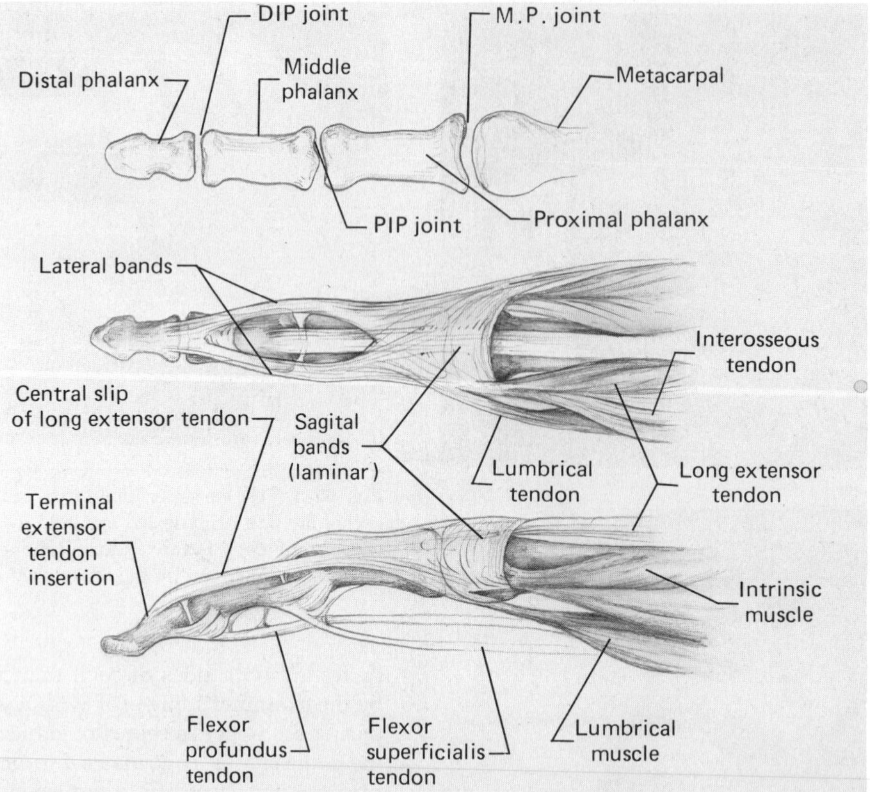

Fig. 67-6. The complex extensor mechanism drapes over the proximal portion of the finger and is composed of interlacing fibers with contributions from the long extensor tendon that terminates in the central slip inserting at the base of the middle phalanx and from the interosseous and lumbrical tendons that terminate in the lateral bands.

the thenar muscles (opponens, abductor pollicis, and one-half of the flexor pollicis brevis) and the lumbricals of the index and long fingers.

To test for thenar muscle function, the patient should place the hand palm up on a flat surface. Then he or she should be asked to point the thumb to the ceiling. The ability to perform this maneuver confirms function of the opponens and abductor pollicis brevis muscles. Contraction of these muscles can be palpated adjacent to the thumb metacarpal during the test. Only an intact opponens and abductor pollicis brevis will abduct the first metacarpal bone away from the plane of the palm and rotate the pulp of the thumb to oppose that of the small finger. However, one must observe carefully during thenar muscle testing. An intact ulnar nerve will allow a patient with a divided median nerve to bring the tip of the thumb toward the small finger. However, in this case, the patient will "oppose" the tip of the thumb and small finger by flexing both digits, rather than by bringing the thumb away from the palm to meet the small finger in space (Fig. 67-8). Rarely, all of the thenar musculature is innervated by the ulnar nerve. If present, this anomaly can confuse the physical examination.

ULNAR NERVE. The ulnar nerve provides sensibility to the volar surfaces of the ulnar half of the palm, the ulnar half of the ring finger, and to the entire volar surface of the small finger. The dorsal branch of the ulnar nerve arises 3 to 5 cm proximal to the wrist flexor crease and innervates the dorsal skin on the ulnar half of the hand and on the ring and small fingers. The motor portion of the ulnar nerve innervates the hypothenar muscles, the dorsal and volar interossei, the lumbricals of the ring and small fingers, half of the flexor pollicis brevis, and the adductor pollicis muscle. In the forearm, it innervates the profundi to the ring and small fingers and the flexor carpi ulnaris muscles.

Damage to the ulnar nerve can result in a claw deformity of the ring and small fingers, which is manifested by hyperextension of the MP joints and incomplete extension of the IP joints (Fig. 67-9). Weakness of abduction and adduction of the fingers (spreading and closing the fingers) and flexion of the IP joint of the thumb during pinch are also indicative of ulnar motor nerve damage (Fig. 67-10).

RADIAL NERVE. The sensory branch of the radial nerve provides sensibility to the radial aspect of the dorsum of the hand. Transection of branches of the sensory portion of this nerve can cause exquisitely sensitive subcutaneous neuromas or painful dysesthesias, or both. The radial nerve provides three major motor functions distal to the elbow: wrist extension, MP joint extension, and thumb extension and abduction.

Tests for radial nerve motor function should include active wrist extension, MP joint extension, and active firing of the extensor pollicis longus (demonstrated by palpation of the tendon rather than IP joint extension for the reason discussed previously). One should not assume that the ability

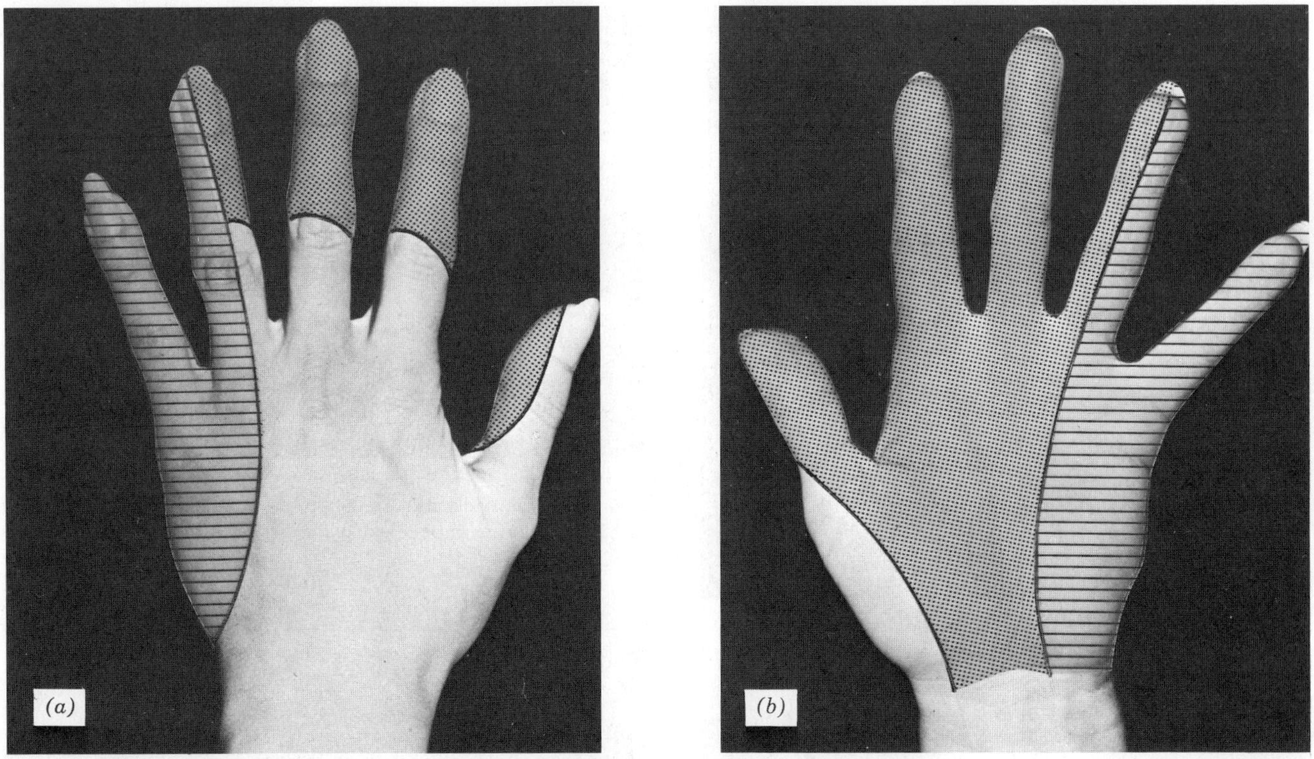

Fig. 67-7. (*a*) The sensory innervation on the dorsum of the hand is a combination of contributions from radial, ulnar, and median nerves. (*b*) The sensory innervation on the volar aspect of the hand is divided between median and ulnar nerves.

to extend the PIP and DIP joints of the fingers implies an intact radial nerve since this function is shared with the median and ulnar nerves and remains present in the absence of radial nerve function.

Examination of the Skeletal System

Deformities, tenderness, and areas of soft-tissue swelling signal skeletal injury. X-ray films confirm the diagnosis and provide information about the nature and location of the fracture or dislocation.

Injured joints will be swollen and tender. Localization of tenderness to the dorsal, volar, or lateral sides can aid diagnosis of the structures injured and can be facilitated by the use of a small blunt object (such as the eraser of a pencil) for palpation. Joints should be stressed gently in the anteroposterior (AP) and lateral planes to detect gross instability. Occasionally, examination under local anesthesia is warranted. The most common joint injuries involve partial damage to the ligamentous supporting structures of the joint—the volar plate and collateral ligaments.

Collateral ligament injury occurs as the result of lateral stress. If the collateral ligament has been damaged, there will be tenderness over the involved structure on the side of the joint. If the ligament has been stretched severely or avulsed, some instability of the joint in the lateral plane can result. This can be detected by gentle stress testing as described previously. The amount of instability should be compared to the same joint in an uninjured finger since people may normally be "loose jointed" or "tight jointed" (Fig. 67-11).

The volar plate supports the volar aspect of the joint. This fibrocartilaginous structure can be injured by hyperextension stress (catching a ball or falling with the fingers extended). Tenderness is most marked on the volar capsule of the joint, and the joint may be held flexed because of pain.

Complete dislocation of a joint is usually evident and most commonly is lateral or dorsal. Complete dislocations are most common at the IP joints of the fingers and at the MP joint of the thumb. Carpometacarpal joint dislocations occur but often are overlooked since they may present with minimal deformity and only slight or moderate swelling over the joints. These dislocations can be missed on routine film views, and oblique views may be required.

X-Ray Examination

X-ray examination of the hand or wrist, or both, is indicated after any penetrating injury of the hand to detect retained foreign material. Retained metal fragments will always be visible, but materials such as glass, wood, and plant thorns are more difficult to detect. In the latter cases, the x-ray technique can be modified to enhance the soft-tissue image if the x-ray technician is made aware of the clinical problem.

X-ray examination of the hand and wrist also is indicated after any musculoskeletal trauma that is severe enough to bring the patient to the emergency department. If there is any question of bone or joint damage, it is better to obtain x-rays of the part than to forego such examination. This is particularly true after wrist injuries in young patients. It is

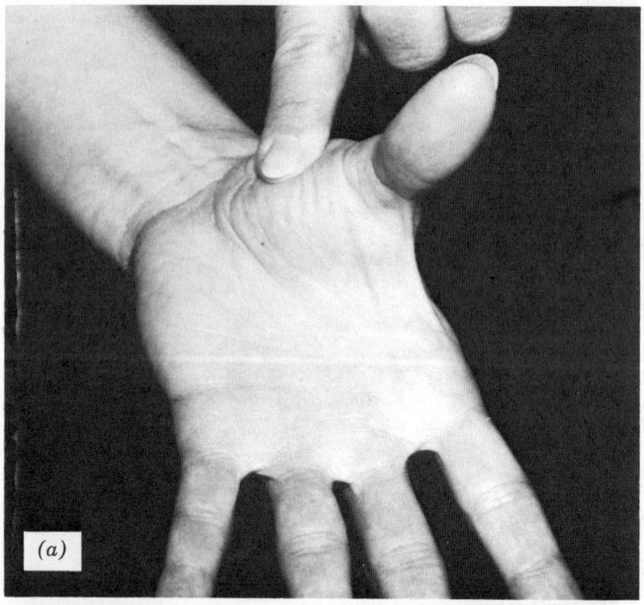

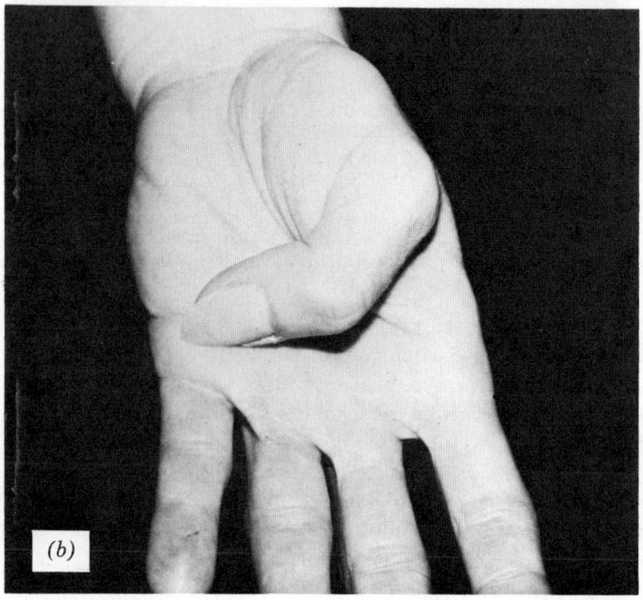

Fig. 67-8. (*a*) The thenar musculature innervated by the median nerve is tested by asking the patient to point the thumb toward the ceiling with the dorsum of the hand resting on a flat surface. Active firing of the median nerve–innervated thenar muscles can be palpated during this maneuver. (*b*) "False" test of the median nerve–controlled thenar musculature. This motion can be accomplished using only the ulnar nerve–innervated thenar muscles to flex the thumb.

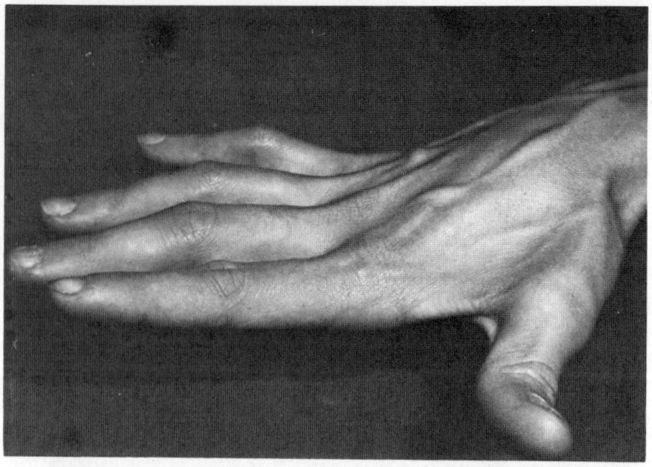

Fig. 67-9. Claw deformity of the fingers with hyperextension of the MP joints and incomplete extension of the PIP joints.

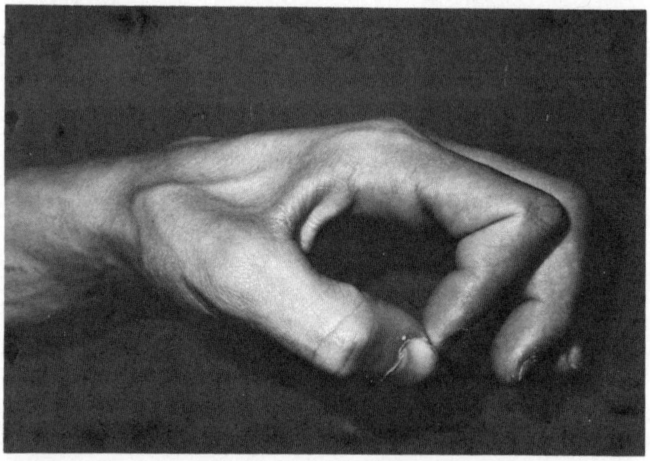

Fig. 67-10. Test of pinch strength demonstrating flexion deformity of the IP joint of the thumb (Froment's sign) as the result of weak ulnar nerve–innervated intrinsic hand muscles after damage to the ulnar nerve. Note atrophy of the first dorsal interosseous muscle.

not uncommon to find carpal scaphoid bone fractures after falls on the outstretched hand, even when the clinical examination reveals minimal swelling, tenderness, or ecchymosis.

X-rays should be obtained before attempts are made to reduce dislocations or displaced fractures, or both, of the hand or wrist. A digit with compromised circulation is the exception to this. Posteroanterior (PA) and lateral views of the fingers and thumb should be obtained. Lateral views are facilitated by using the "fan" position of the hand, with progressive flexion from the index to the small fingers, or by placing cardboard cassettes between the fingers. Oblique views of the metacarpal bones are helpful (Fig. 67-12).

Although x-ray findings usually are straightforward, pit-

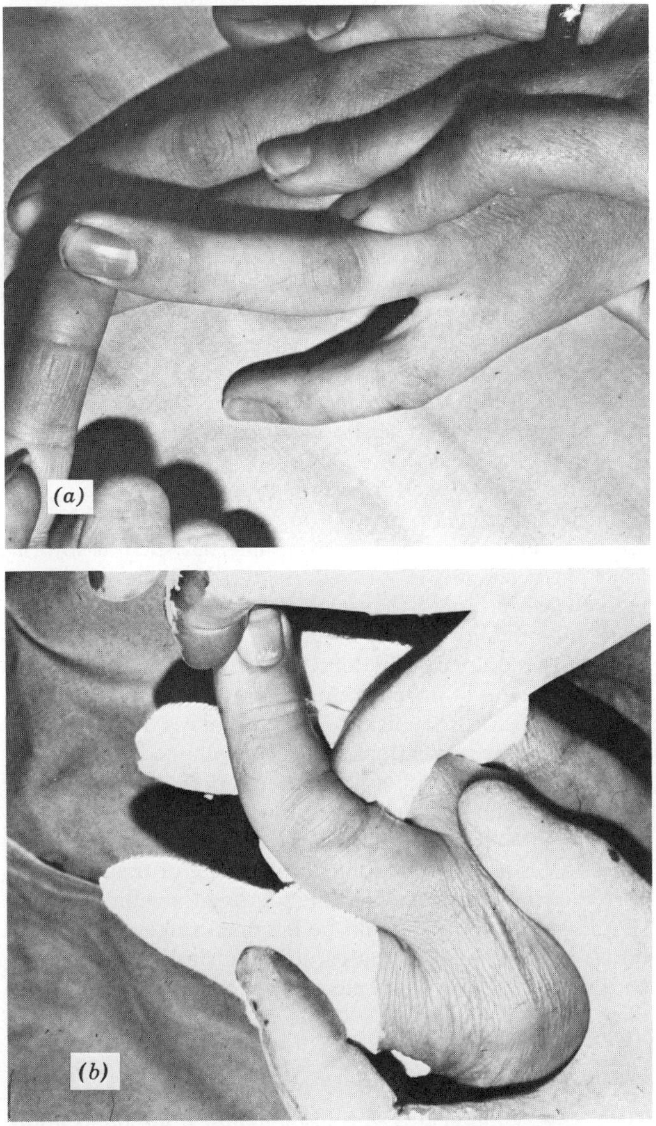

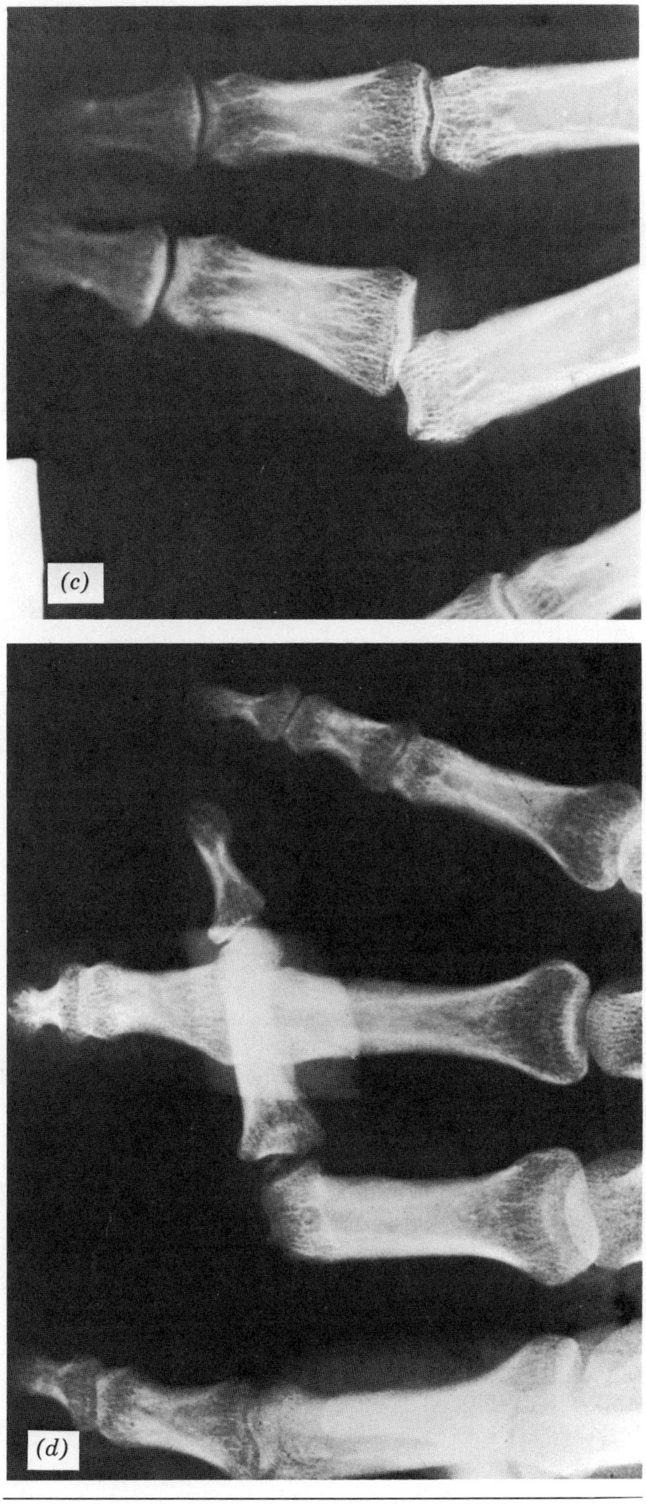

Fig. 67-11. (*a*) Moderate instability of the PIP joint collateral ligament demonstrated by a stress test. (*b*) Gross instability of the PIP joint collateral ligament when stress tested. Stress roentgenograms show partial (*c*) and complete (*d*) collateral ligament instability.

falls are possible. Multiple views may be necessary to detect carpal injuries. Fractures of the carpal scaphoid may not appear on the initial films and may become apparent only after bone resorption at the fracture site has occurred. Epiphyseal lines must be recognized as such. Nutrient vessels penetrating the cortex are occasionally mistaken for hairline fractures. Avulsion or chip fractures are indications of complete ligament avulsion and alert the examiner to the need for careful evaluation of a specific joint. If there is a question regarding the significance of a radiograph, a comparison view of the uninjured part can be obtained. Communication with the technicians and radiologist will enhance the information obtained from the radiographs.

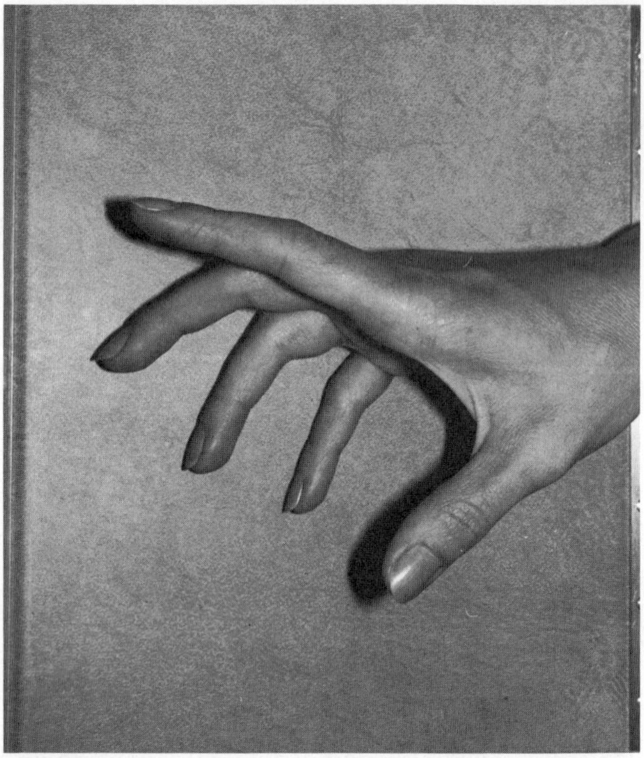

Fig. 67-12. Hand placement on a film cassette for obtaining a "fan" lateral view of the hand.

MANAGEMENT

Massive Hand Injuries

Severe, mutilating injuries of the hand involving multiple fracture, skin or bone loss, and damage to neurovascular structures and tendons will require care by an experienced surgeon. In the emergency department, the wound should be cultured and dressed with a dry sterile dressing and roller bandage and, if necessary, a plaster splint. The hand consultant and the operating room team are notified, and the patient is admitted to the hospital. An intravenous line should be started and a broad-spectrum antibiotic (such as a cephalosporin) begun. Tetanus antitoxin or toxoid, or both, should be given. If bleeding is profuse, blood should be typed and cross-matched. X-ray films should be obtained, through the dressing if necessary. The appropriate laboratory studies required before general anesthesia should be obtained to minimize delay in transporting the patient from the emergency department to the operating room.

Uncomplicated Hand Injuries

Open Wounds

Commonly, the emergency physician is the primary physician in the treatment of minor hand injuries. The care of superficial hand lacerations is similar to that of lacerations elsewhere on the body.

The wound should be cleaned of blood and foreign material as described earlier (see section of physical examination). If an open or puncture wound of the hand has occurred, tetanus toxoid or human immune globulin, or both, should be administered according to the guidelines set forth in Chap. 52 after the status of the patient's tetanus immunization has been determined.

The decision to close an open wound of the hand and the type of closure to be used depend on the extent and nature of the wound and the extent of damage to structures underlying the skin. If the wound is a sharp laceration without division of underlying structures or excessive skin damage or loss, primary closure can be performed in the emergency department. In most hand or finger lacerations, a single-layer closure of the skin with 5-0 nylon is all that is required. Layered closures rarely are indicated. The use of vertical mattress sutures will prevent overlapping of the skin edges in the palm and the inversion of skin edges in loose dorsal skin. In children, the use of 5-0 or 6-0 plain gut suture for skin closure will obviate the need for suture removal after the wound has healed.

Hand wounds generally heal with minimal scarring, particularly if there is no tension on the wound. Wounds with the potential for retained foreign material, such as injuries from glass, should be x-rayed, using soft-tissue technique, before closure. Ragged lacerations have variable degrees of contamination, as well as damage to circulation in the skin. These will require careful debridement and closure, perhaps by combination of primary suture, skin graft, and local flap coverage. Slicing or avulsion wounds that result in flaps (especially distally based flaps) must be evaluated carefully for viability of the flap, rather than sutured primarily as a matter of course. Although the arterial blood supply of these flaps may be sufficient, venous drainage may not be, and flap necrosis can result. If significant crushing of tissue has occurred or if there is considerable soft-tissue swelling without skin loss, the wound should be left open rather than closed under tension. In these cases, a bulky sterile dressing can be applied and secondary closure performed in five to seven days.

Special Wounds

There is very little extra skin in the hand. If the hand injury has resulted in skin loss, it is not advisable to bring the skin edges together under excessive tension. Skin loss can be treated either by allowing the wound to heal secondarily by granulation or by adding skin in the form of a graft or flap. Allowing the wound to granulate is acceptable only for small areas of skin loss (up to 5 mm in diameter) or for small wounds in children. Skin grafts can be either split or full thickness.

SKIN GRAFTS. *Split-thickness grafts* are indicated most commonly and are the simplest method to obtain closure of hand wounds. They can be used to provide a physiologic cover in severe wounds, even through revision or replacement with more suitable skin may be required later. Small grafts often can be applied by the emergency physician. These grafts can be taken freehand with a sterile surgical blade or with a dermatome. Portable, battery-operated dermatomes are now commonly available in emergency departments and allow even a neophyte to harvest a good graft. Larger grafts will require the expertise of a specialist.

The donor site of a split-thickness skin graft leaves a scar that is noticeable and occasionally unsightly, particularly if the graft is thick. For this reason, the donor site must be chosen with care. The forearm, although convenient, should not be used since the scar in this area is often the source of patient discontent. Ideally, the donor site should be from an area covered by a bathing suit. Usually, the upper thigh or buttocks are suitable. The grafts can be sutured in place or held with Steri-Strips. A gentle pressure dressing and immobilization are essential since a hematoma under the graft will elevate the graft from its base and shear stress on the graft will disrupt capillary ingrowth.

Full-thickness grafts are indicated less frequently in emergency situations. If there is any doubt about the ability of the full-thickness graft to survive, it is preferable to apply a split-thickness graft. If the area of skin loss uncovers bone or a joint, an alternative method of skin closure is required. Free grafts, split or full thickness, will not survive over joint surfaces, cortical bone, or bare nerve or tendon. Coverage by a flap will be necessary. This is best done by an experienced surgeon.

TOURNIQUET. The debridement and repair of hand injuries in a bloodless field is essential, whether done in the emergency department or in the operating room. The emergency physician who treats hand injuries should be familiar with the use of a tourniquet and should not hesitate to use an appropriate tourniquet when indicated. If bleeding has stopped or is minimal, a tourniquet is not necessary. If bleeding is profuse, a tourniquet should be used.

A ¼- or ⅜-in. Penrose drain placed about the base of the digit without excessive tension and held in place with a hemostat can be used as a tourniquet if necessary. However, the pressure applied is uncontrolled with this method. If it is used, only the minimal tension necessary to control bleeding should be applied to the drain, and in no case should the digital tourniquet be left in place for longer than one hour. The bulk of the drain and clamp makes the possibility of forgetting that the tourniquet is around the finger unlikely. Other methods used for finger tourniquets, such as rolled glove fingers or rubber bands, are not bulky and can easily be forgotten, with disastrous results. The use of the latter materials for digital tourniquets is not recommended because of the irreversible ischemia that could occur if such a tourniquet were inadvertently left in place for a prolonged period.

The use of a blood pressure cuff applied to the upper part of the arm is also risky. These instruments were not designed to maintain sustained pressures in the range of 250 to 300 mm Hg. Pressure usually is lost slowly, and the tourniquet changes from an arterial to a venous tourniquet. This not only allows arterial bleeding in the field but also increases venous congestion and edema and is worse than no tourniquet at all. Modern pneumatic tourniquets designed for use in the upper extremity should be used. The upper part of the arm is padded with two to three layers of circumferentially wrapped 4-in. cast padding, and the tourniquet is applied snugly around the arm. Tourniquet pressure should be maintained in the range of 250 to 300 mm Hg (depending on arm size) in adults and 200 mm Hg in children. Before application of the tourniquet, blood is expressed from the hand and arm with an elastic rubber bandage. Most patients can tolerate 15 to 20 minutes of tourniquet pressure with minimal discomfort.

Nerve Injuries

Lacerations of digital nerves in the fingers are not uncommon, but they are frequently missed because of inadequate examination at the time the finger wound is closed in the emergency department. Prompt recognition will allow a considered decision regarding primary, delayed primary, or secondary repair of the nerve by the appropriate consultant. In addition, patient discontent will be avoided if the correct diagnosis is made at the time of the initial visit rather than days or weeks later.

Nerve repair should not be attempted in the emergency department. Optimal results from digital nerve repair require fine suture material (8-0 to 10-0), magnification, and an experienced operating room team. As with flexor tendons, it may be advisable to close clean wounds with underlying nerve damage and refer the patient to an experienced surgeon for definitive care.

We prefer to repair divided nerves with five to seven days after injury. After this time, the retracted nerve ends become fixed to adjacent soft tissue and it is harder to restore the normal length of the nerve. In addition, after this period it is necessary to resect more tissue from the ends of the divided nerve to expose normal-appearing fascicles. This increases the amount of nerve gap that must be overcome during the repair.

Damage to major nerves at the wrist level requires the same surgical techniques described for digital nerves. The care of mixed motor and sensory nerves (the median and ulnar nerves) is even more difficult because of the necessity of accurately aligning and matching major fascicular groups (motor to motor and sensory to sensory). This so-called grouped fascicular repair of mixed nerves requires high-power magnification.

Damage to the superficial radial nerve on the dorsoradial aspect of the wrist deserves special mention. This nerve supplies sensibility to the dorsal and radial aspects of the hand. Its integrity is not critical to the function of the hand. However, damage to this nerve or its terminal branches can result in either an exquisitely painful neuroma or a chronic pain syndrome (causalgia or reflex sympathetic dystrophy) that may either be limited or cause dysfunction of the entire upper extremity. For this reason, we recommend that acute laceration of this nerve be repaired primarily in an attempt to minimize both symptomatic neuromata or minor or major causalgia, or both. Injuries on the dorsum of the hand and wrist require a high index of suspicion combined with routine sensory examination of the dorsal and radial aspects of the hand.

Tendon Injuries

Closed Tendon Injuries

Closed injuries of the extensor mechanism are common and result in characteristic deformities that make the diagnosis straightforward. The common levels of injury are at the DIP and PIP joint levels.

MALLET DEFORMITY. A mallet deformity results from avulsion of the terminal portion of the extensor tendon from the distal phalanx, either with or without a flake of bone. The patient is unable to extend the DIP joint actively. If

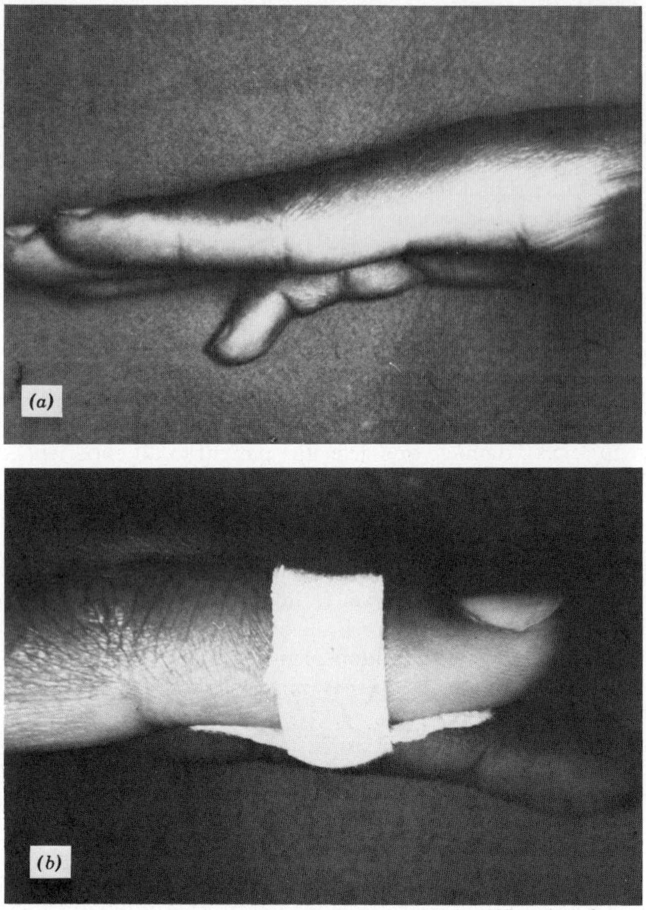

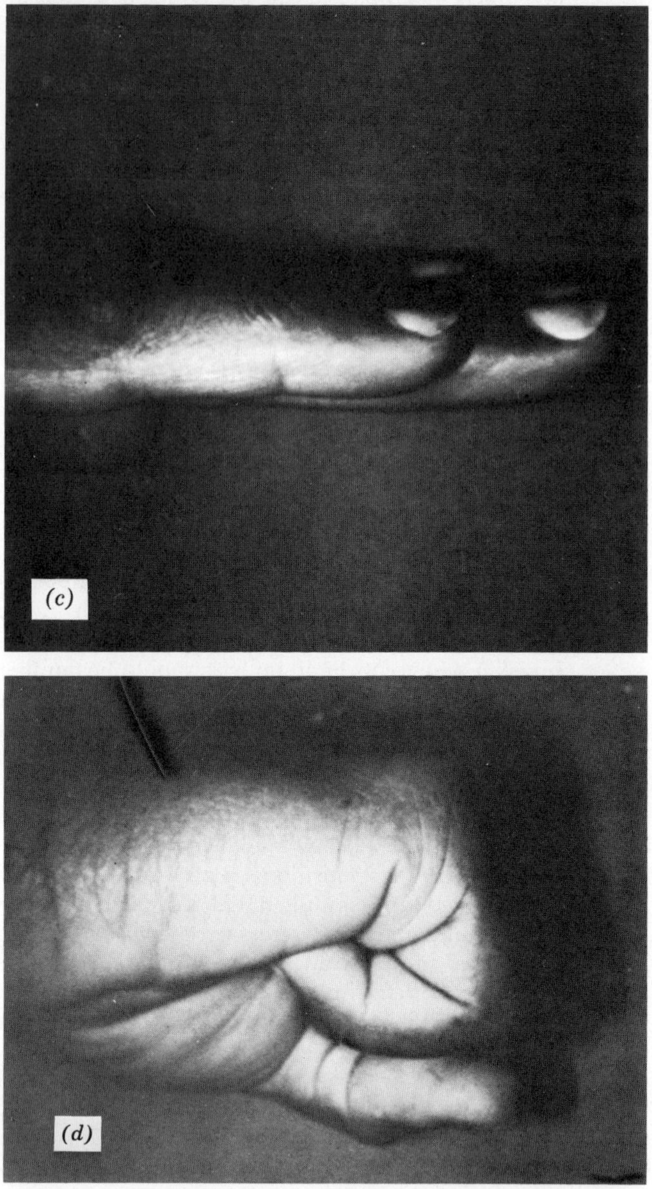

Fig. 67-13. (*a*) Mallet deformity of the small finger with inability to extend the DIP joint. (*b*) Volar splint used to keep the DIP joint in extension. (*c*) Active extension of the DIP joint after eight weeks of splinting. (*d*) Active flexion of the DIP joint after splint has been discontinued.

x-ray reveals a large fragment of displaced bone or volar subluxation of the distal phalanx, or both, the injury should be considered a fracture-dislocation and the patient should be referred for treatment. Most injuries, however, result in only a small avulsion fracture or a pure tendon avulsion. These can be treated by splinting the distal joint in full extension with a volar or dorsal metal splint (Fig. 67-13). It is not necessary to splint the PIP joint. However, these injuries require splinting for prolonged periods—8 to 10 weeks—and premature discontinuation of splinting can result in recurrence of the deformity. Even after the full course of treatment, splinting should not be discontinued abruptly but should be weaned over a two-week period. The patient will need to change the splint daily to prevent maceration of the dorsal skin and should be instructed to keep the DIP joint extended when doing this. Even when the patient is not seen for several weeks after the initial injury, these deformities sometimes can be improved by splinting. Treatment can be started by the emergency physician, and the patient can be referred to the appropriate consultant for follow-up care. Occasionally, a swan-neck deformity of the fingers (hyperextension of the PIP joint combined with extensor lag of the DIP joint) can occur after mallet injuries secondary to extensor mechanism imbalance in individuals with lax volar plates. In open mallet injuries, the tendon can be repaired, as will be described later, but prolonged splinting is still necessary.

BOUTONNIÈRE DEFORMITY. A laceration or a closed injury of the "central slip" of the extensor mechanism overlying the PIP joint (see Fig. 67-6) can result in a deformity of the finger characterized by flexion of the PIP joint and hyperextension of the DIP joint (the boutonnière). Recognition of this injury is important since inadequate initial treatment can lead to progressive deformities that are very difficult to treat secondarily. Again, a high index of suspicion may be necessary with injuries on the dorsal aspect of the PIP joint since the deformity may be very subtle or even absent initially but progresses as the PIP joint is flexed repeatedly. Closed injuries should be splinted with the PIP in full extension and the DIP joint left free (Fig. 67-14). Active flexion of

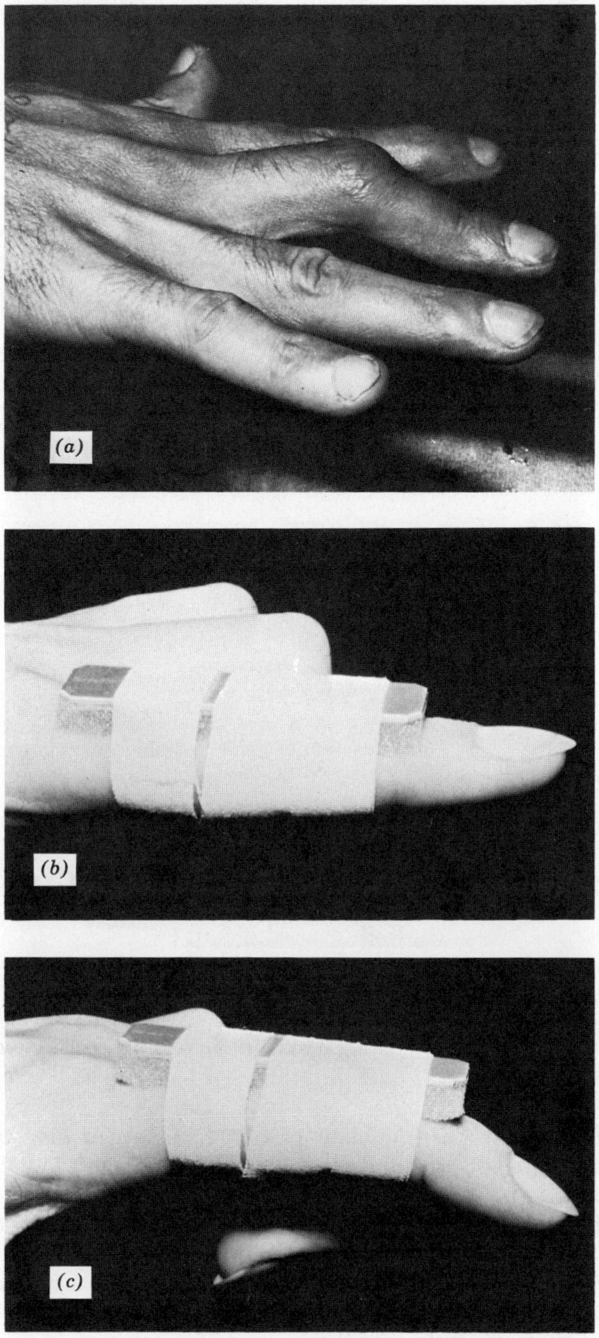

Fig. 67-14. (*a*) Boutonnière deformity (flexion deformity of the PIP joint and hyperextension of the DIP joint) as a result of damage to the extensor mechanism overlying the PIP joint. (*b*) Method of splinting closed injuries of the extensor mechanism that have resulted in a boutonnière deformity. The PIP joint is held in full extension. (*c*) The splint should allow flexion of the DIP joint. This motion is encouraged to prevent adherence of the extensor mechanism.

the distal joint will preserve balance between the central slip and the lateral band portions of the extensor mechanism. Splinting of the PIP joint in full extension is continued for at least four weeks, after which active, but protected, flexion is started. The patient should be referred for follow-up observation and care.

CLOSED FLEXOR TENDON INJURIES. Rupture of the flexor digitorum profundus in young athletes has been described previously (see section on examination of tendons). Early recognition of these injuries allows recovery and repair of the avulsed tendon. Delayed recognition, even for several days, often precludes definitive repair because of retraction and scarring of the tendon. The complaint of inability to flex the distal joint actively and an appropriate clinical history should be heeded.

Open Tendon Injuries

Open tendon injuries can occur with apparently superficial skin wounds as well as with extensive open injuries to the hand. Therefore, careful examination of tendon function of every patient who has an open wound in the hand or fingers, or both, should be undertaken.

EXTENSOR TENDONS. Laceration of the extensor tendons can occur either proximal or distal to the juncturae tendinae, the cross-connections between the extensor digitorum communis tendons at the level of the necks of the metacarpal bones (Fig. 67-15). Lacerations proximal to these interconnections will allow the tendon to retract and preclude repair in the emergency department since extensive exposure may be necessary to retrieve the tendon. However, if a laceration of the extensor tendon has occurred distal to the interconnections, the tendon will not retract and repair can be carried out primarily by the emergency physician. The ends of the tendon should be approximated with either one or more simple interrupted sutures or with a horizontal mattress suture using nonabsorbable material such as 4-0 nylon. The affected joint is splinted in extension. The type of suture material used is not important as long as it is *not silk*. Recently, 4-0 polyglycolic acid (Dexon) or polyglactin (Vicryl) has been used with satisfactory results. Postrepair immobilization *is* important to prevent the repair from pulling apart if the finger flexes.

FLEXOR TENDONS. Since there are two flexor tendons in each finger (see Fig. 67-2), the problems of treating flexor tendon injuries differ completely from those of treating extensor tendon injuries. From the distal palm to the midportion of the middle phalanx, these tendons are surrounded by the so-called fibroosseous tunnel, which is a tight tunnel composed of bone and volar plate tissue on one side and the flexor tendon sheath with its pulley mechanism on the other side. Surgery within this delicate area is difficult, and even skilled surgeons may find that the results of tendon repair are compromised because of adhesions, joint stiffness, and limited active motion. Although flexor tendon lacerations distal and proximal to the fibroosseous tunnel are easier to repair and the prognosis for good postoperative tendon function is better all tendon surgery on the flexor aspect of the hand should be performed in a completely equipped operating room by a surgeon experienced in flexor tendon

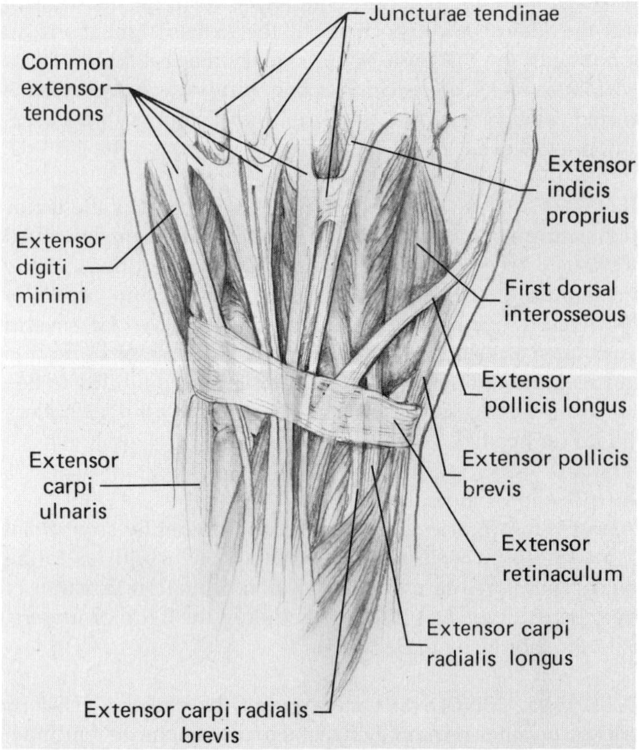

Fig. 67-15. Arrangement of the extrinisic (long) extensor tendons on the dorsum of the hand. Note the juncturae that interconnect the extensor tendons just proximal to the MP joints.

surgery. If in doubt, it is wiser to close the skin of a tidy wound and refer the patient rather than to attempt primary repair under suboptimal conditions.

While it is preferable to repair divided flexor tendons as soon as possible (within several days), satisfactory primary repair can be accomplished up to three weeks after the injury. If both a digital nerve and a flexor tendon have been divided, repair of both structures within seven days is advisable for the reasons outlined in the previous section on nerve injuries.

Fractures

Because bones of the hand are small, the consequences of injury to them often are minimized. However, improper treatment of finger and hand fractures can result in prolonged morbidity, and frequently the resulting malunion and stiffness are amenable only to surgical treatment.

Precise rotatory alignment of phalangeal and metacarpal fractures is necessary to prevent overlap of the fingers during flexion (Fig. 67-16). Even a small residual rotatory displacement can interfere significantly with hand function. Fractures that appear stable and nondisplaced on x-ray and even on cursory clinical examination may have significant rotatory displacement.

Rotary alignment is tested by flexing the finger into the palm and noting proper alignment of each finger with the next. Although fingernail alignment and/or alignment of the fingers with the pulps pointing toward the carpal scaphoid bone are useful guides, the final check can be done only with the fingers in nearly full flexion.

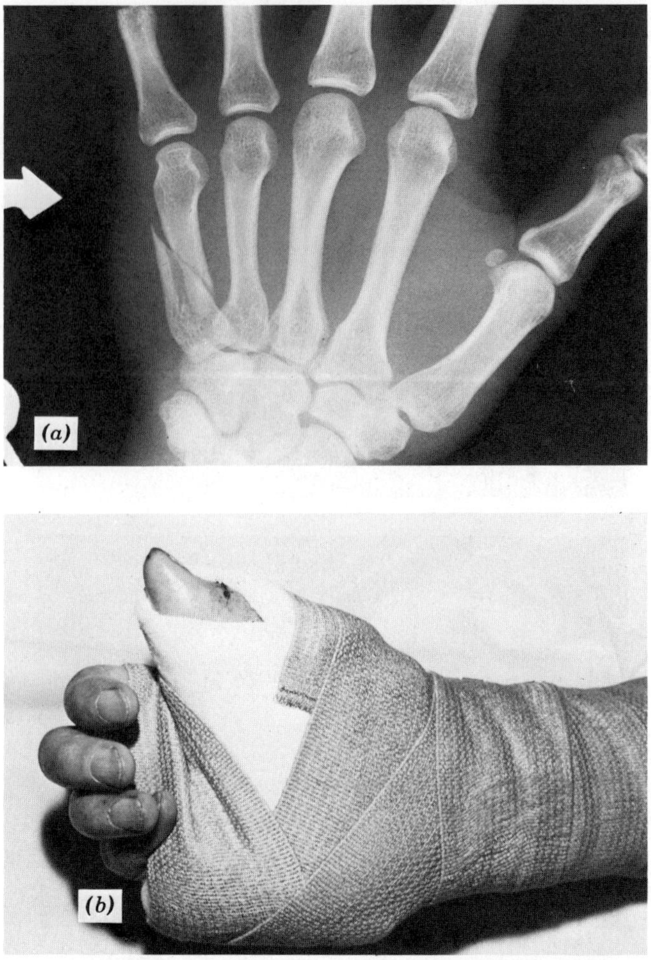

Fig. 67-16. (*a*) Spiral fracture through the midshaft of the fifth metacarpal bone with rotatory malalignment. (*b*) Overlap of the small and ring fingers during flexion as the result of rotatory malalignment.

Satisfactory determination of rotary alignment may require digital or proximal nerve block anesthesia to allow the patient to flex the finger fully without limitation because of pain. Such examination also may require removing part or all of the material used to immobilize the finger. If there is any question of residual rotatory deformity after a tubular bone fracture in the hand, the patient should be referred to an orthopedic or hand surgeon for follow-up examination. Angular deformity is easier to detect, both clinically and radiographically.

Fracture healing can result in adherence of the tendon to the bone because of the proximity of the extensor and flexor tendons of the fingers to the phalanges. This will limit tendon excursion and, thus, finger motion. Prolonged immobilization compounds the problems of tendon adherence and can cause joint stiffness as well. Therefore, early motion is necessary when dealing with patients who have finger and hand fractures. The adage of six weeks of immobilization for a fracture does not apply in the hand; its use will complicate and prolong rehabilitation of the hand. Follow-up care for patients with even simple fractures is necessary to obtain satisfactory functional recovery.

The treatment of fractures of the small bones of the hand

is simplified by classifying them as stable, unstable, and intraarticular.

Stable Fractures

Stable fractures usually involve linear "cracks" of the shaft of a phalanx or metacarpal or fractures of the distal phalanx after a crush injury. They are stable either because there is no tendon pull across the fracture site to displace the fracture or because the periosteum and soft tissue surrounding the fracture are intact and are sufficient to counteract any forces tending to displace the fracture. They do not require reduction. *Any fracture that is displaced enough to require reduction should be considered unstable and treated as described in the following section.*

Stable fractures cause no deformity of the hand other than soft-tissue swelling. Films of these fractures show minimal, if any, displacement. The treatment of these fractures consists of a brief period of immobilization until the acute pain and swelling subside, followed by early active motion of the adjacent joints. These fractures are "clinically" united before the x-ray film demonstrates complete bone healing. Complications of this group of fractures are most often the result of prolonged immobilization. Molded plaster or metal splints are used, and as little of the hand as possible is immobilized. The metacarpophalangeal joints should be splinted in flexion to keep collateral ligaments at their maximum length and thereby prevent extension contractures. The fingers should *not* be immobilized with both the metacarpophalangeal and the interphalangeal joints in full extension. Thus the use of straight splints such as tongue blades is precluded. Cotton or a gauze sponge is placed between adjacent fingers that are splinted together to prevent skin maceration. Follow-up films within the first week are mandatory to ensure that no change in alignment has occurred. Immobilization for 10 to 21 days is necessary before the splint is removed and an exercise program to regain motion is started. Full use of the hand should be restricted for four to six weeks.

Crush fractures of the distal phalanx are common. However, these fractures are stable and are treated as soft-tissue injuries rather than as fractures. Reduction is not required, and a protective splint with immobilization of the DIP joint for two to three weeks is all that is necessary. The frequent subungual hematoma that occurs after this injury should be treated as described later to provide relief of pain.

Unstable Fractures

Unstable fractures require immobilization to prevent displacement or maintain reduction. Closed reduction under adequate anesthesia should be attempted. However, if satisfactory position of the fracture cannot be obtained or if position is lost either immediately or within the first week, open reduction with internal fixation may be indicated. The stability achieved by open reduction and internal fixation will allow earlier motion and reduce the risk of tendon adherence and joint stiffness. If any question remains after initial care of a hand fracture, the patient should be referred for appropriate consultation and follow-up. Traction in the treatment of hand fractures is mentioned only to condemn its use.

Common unstable fractures include displaced and angulated fractures of the shafts of the metacarpals and of the proximal and middle phalanges, supracondylar fractures through the neck of the middle phalanx, fracture-dislocations of the PIP joint, and fracture-dislocations of the thumb carpometacarpal joint (Bennett's fracture) or of the carpometacarpal joint of the small finger ("baby" Bennett's fracture) (Fig. 67-17).

Intraarticular Fractures

Intraarticular fractures are difficult to treat and require experienced judgment for decisions regarding operative versus nonoperative treatment. Several fracture-dislocations usually require percutaneous wire fixation or open reduction and internal fixation. Bennett's fractures (fracture-dislocation of the base of the thumb metacarpal), "baby" Bennett's fractures (fracture-dislocation of the base of the fifth metacarpal), and those mallet fingers that are the result of the avulsion of a significant portion of the dorsal articular surface of the distal phalanx and/or result in volar subluxation of the DIP joint fall into this category, and these patients should be referred.

Open Fractures

Open fractures, which are those fractures that communicate with an external skin wound, require surgical debridement, and patients should be referred to the appropriate consultant whether the fractures are stable, unstable, or intraarticular. Minimally displaced fractures of the neck of the fifth metacarpal associated with either tooth marks or a cut on the dorsal skin overlying the bone should be considered and treated as a human bite (see section on human bites).

Carpal Injuries

The carpus consists of eight small bones arranged in two horizontal rows and linked to one another by their contours and a complex set of dorsal, volar, and interosseous ligaments. Carpal bones bear tremendous stress during both direct and indirect trauma and thus are easily injured. The nature of the injury, the bone involved, and bony versus ligamentous injury depend on many factors, including the age of the patient and the position of the wrist and forearm at the time of the injury. Most carpal injuries occur after a fall on the outstretched hand or a twisting injury—for example, when a tightly gripped steering wheel is suddenly twisted as the vehicle's wheels strike an obstruction or pothole, or when the torque of a power drill motor rotates the hand and wrist when the bit binds. High-energy injuries such as falls from ladders and other heights as well as motorcycle injuries cause more significant fractures, ligamentous injuries, or fracture-dislocations of the wrist.

Carpal injuries may appear trivial initially if they present with minimal swelling and deformity, moderate pain, and subtle changes on routine x-ray examination. Therefore, a high index of suspicion is necessary so that carpal injuries can be detected and treated at the onset, rather than when the sequelae of these injuries (nonunions, collapse deformities, and posttraumatic arthritis) have occurred.

Carpal scaphoid bone fractures are the most common carpal fractures and typically occur in young men (14–40 years of age) after a fall on the outstretched hand. Clinically, these patients have tenderness to palpation in the "anatomic snuffbox" (the triangular hollow area at the base of the thumb

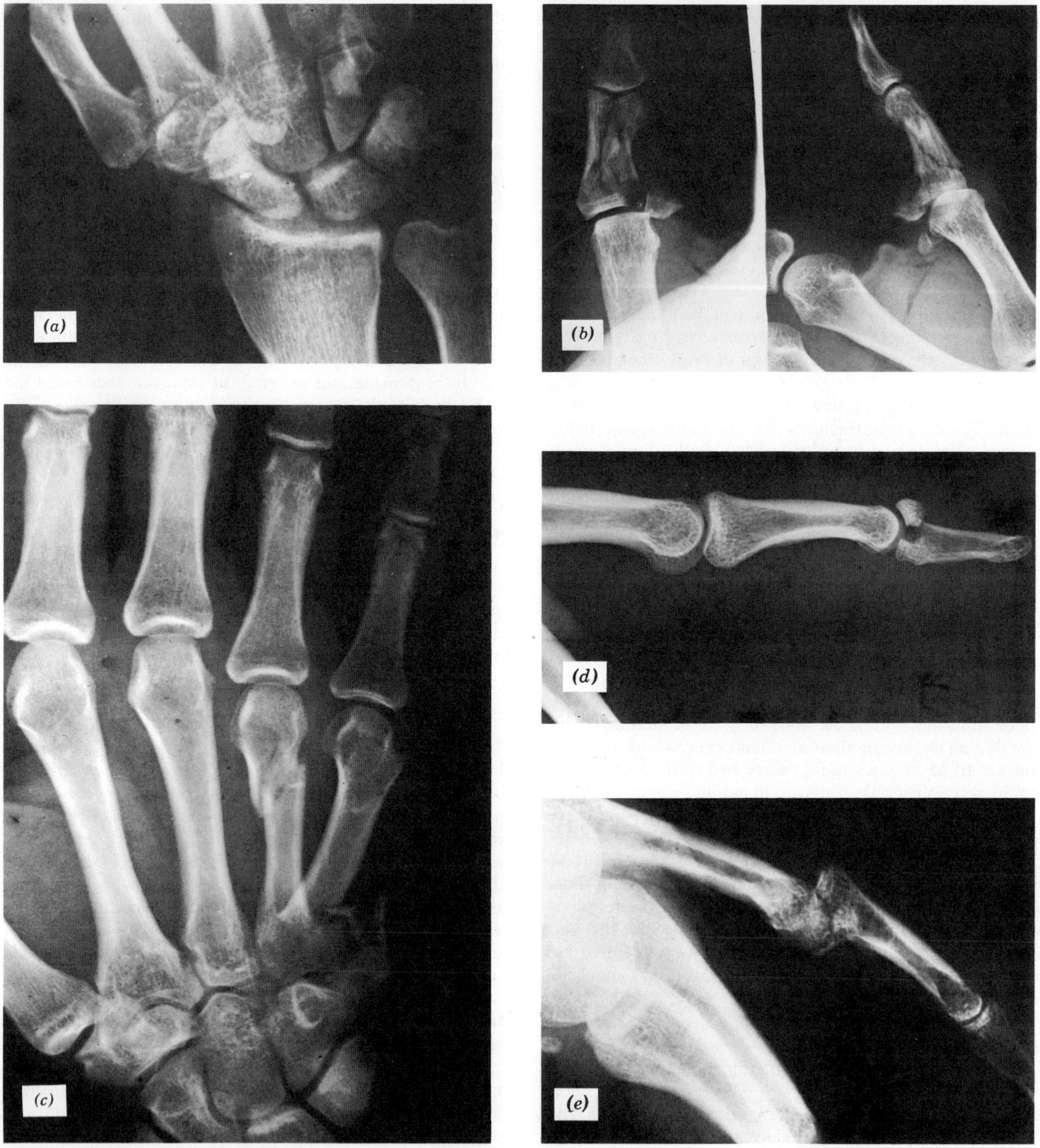

Fig. 67-17. Examples of unstable fractures of the hand. (*a*) Fracture-dislocation of the carpometacarpal joint of the thumb (Bennett's fracture). (*b*) Intraarticular fracture of the metacarpal joint of the thumb. (*c*) Fracture-dislocation of the carpometacarpal joint of the small finger ("baby" Bennett's fracture). (*d*) Mallet fracture avulsion of the insertion of the extensor tendon from the distal phalanx with a displaced intraarticular fracture of the dorsal lip of the distal phalanx. (*e*) Fracture-dislocation of the PIP joint.

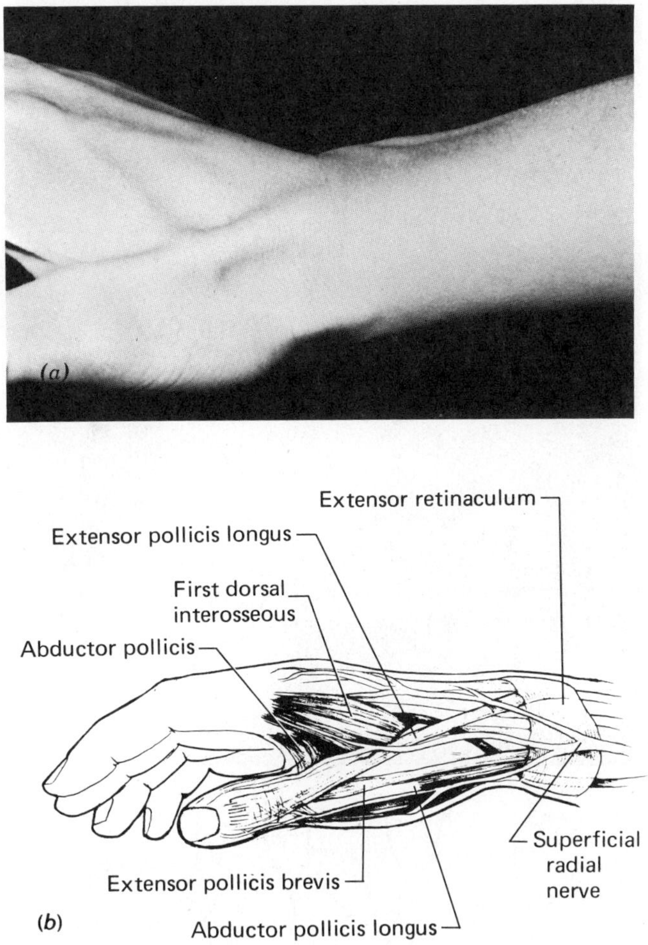

Fig. 67-18. (*a*) The radial aspect of the hand showing the extensor pollicis longus and brevis tendons, the abductor pollicis longus tendons, and the "anatomic snuffbox." (*b*) Drawing of the anatomy of the tendons described, as well as the location of the superficial branch of the radial nerve and its divisions.

outlined by the outcropping tendons of the thumb) (Fig. 67-18). The waist of the scaphoid bone lies directly beneath this area and thus can be palpated through the overlying soft tissue. Films may or may not show a fracture line through the bone. As described previously, if the fracture remains undisplaced, the fracture line may not be detected for two to four weeks, until bony resorption on either side of the fracture has occurred. For this reason, a wrist with a scaphoid fracture suspected by clinical examination but not confirmed by films should be immobilized and the patient referred for follow-up evaluation. Failure to do so may increase the already significant tendency of the scaphoid bone not to heal.

Even if a scaphoid fracture is not present, other serious ligamentous injuries with subtle clinical and x-ray findings may be present. These include rotatory subluxation of the scaphoid bone, which produces a decrease in the normal height of the scaphoid bone and a gap greater than 2 mm between the scaphoid and lunate bones on the PA film; injuries of the ligaments stabilizing the lunate, triquetrum, and hamate bones; and damage to the triangular fibrocartilage, the junction of the distal ulna, and the carpus. Carpal avulsion fractures represent ligamentous injuries that may or may not be significant (Fig. 67-19). Therefore, any wrist injury about which the emergency physician is not entirely sure should be splinted and reevaluated in several days or the patient should be referred to the appropriate specialist for evaluation.

Dislocations and fracture dislocations of the wrist require immediate care. The emergency physician should suspect these injuries on the basis of the history alone—for example, a fall from a height or a motorcycle injury. Films of the wrist with these injuries may be difficult to interpret or may show subtle findings, but in any case they will not look normal when compared to that of an uninjured wrist. A lunate dislocation can be accompanied by paresthesias and numbness in the median nerve distribution since the volarly dislocated bone impinges the median nerve within the carpal tunnel. Lateral roentgenograms will show the dislocation clearly. Lateral films usually are the most important views of the wrist and the emergency department x-ray examination is not complete without them.

Joint Injuries

Collateral Ligaments

Collateral ligament injuries result from forceful lateral stress applied to the extended digit. The radial aspect of the PIP joint is injured more frequently than the ulnar side. In the thumb, the ulnar collateral ligament is at risk and is injured more frequently than the radial side ligament, resulting in the so-called "gamekeeper's thumb." The thumb MP joint should be tested for stability in both flexion and extension (Fig. 67-20). If there is more than 45 degrees of instability in flexion, operative repair of the ligament is indicated. Acute repair of these ligaments is much more satisfactory than secondary reconstruction.

X-ray examination is important and will confirm suspected ligament injuries with small avulsion fractures. Both AP and lateral stress should be applied gently to the injured joint. A complete tear will allow the joint to open easily. Pain during this maneuver is suggestive of a stretched ligament, and digital block anesthesia may be required to determine the degree of joint laxity. Joint laxity varies from person to person, and the degree of laxity found in the injured digit should be compared to that in a noninjured digit. Stress films of both the injured and the noninjured joint may be helpful. If the joint is stable to lateral stress or opens only minimally, the injury is, at most, a partial tear and nonoperative treatment is indicated (see Fig. 67-11).

The finger with an incomplete collateral ligament injury can be immobilized with a padded volar aluminum splint positioned in slight flexion for 10 days. Gentle, gradual joint motion is begun after this period, although the joint can be protected from lateral stress by "buddy" taping the finger to the adjacent digit for an additional 10 days. Full function is not regained for four to six weeks, and some residual enlargement of the joint may persist permanently. If the joint is unstable to lateral stress, a complete tear is present and surgical treatment is required. Nonoperative treatment of complete collateral ligament tears often is followed by permanent joint laxity, instability, and chronic synovitis. The

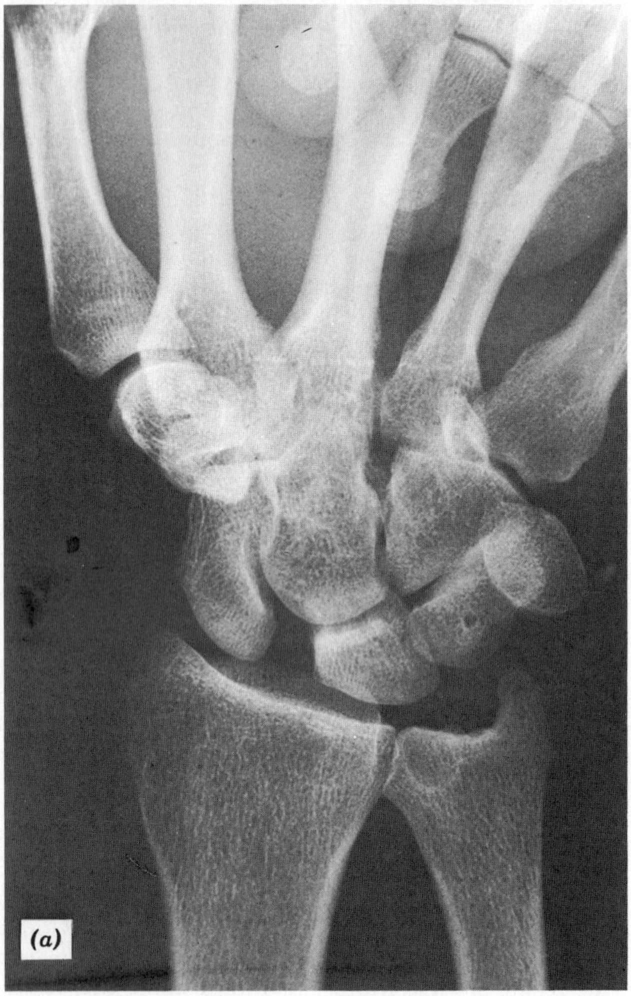

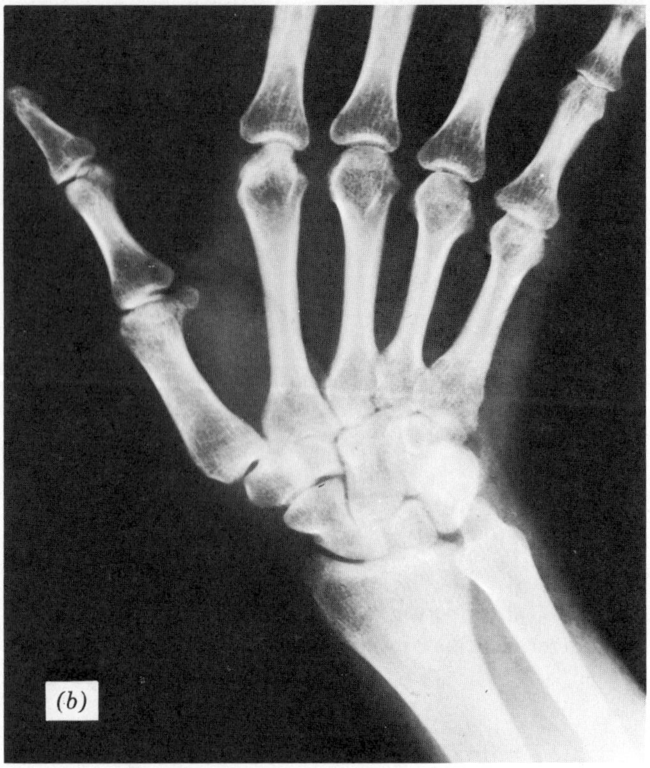

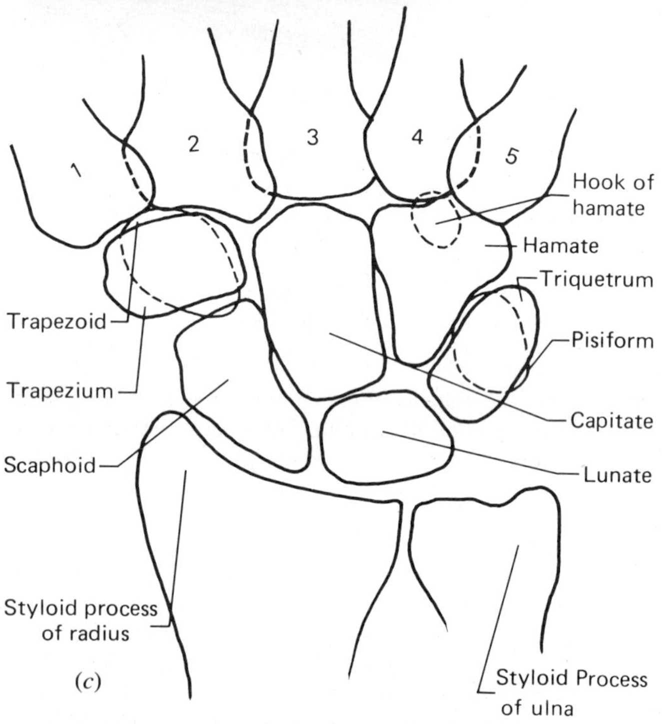

Fig. 67-19. (*a*) Posteroanterior roentgenogram of the wrist showing a wide gap between the scaphoid and lunate bones indicating severe ligamentous damage and scapholunate dissociation. (*b*) Posteroanterior roentgenogram of the normal wrist. (*c*) Nomenclature and positions of carpal bones.

late sequelae of these injuries can be degenerative arthritis and stiffness. If there is any question of significant joint injury, the joint should be splinted and the patient referred.

Dislocations

Dislocations of a joint represent the end stage in soft-tissue injury. They usually are either dorsal or lateral, and damage to the volar plate and collateral ligaments is assumed. Dislocations can be classified as either simple or complex. *Simple dislocations* can be reduced by closed methods, whereas *complex dislocations* have interposed soft-tissue structures that prevent reduction except by open methods. Dislocations in the fingers occur most often at the IP joints. Dislocations of the thumb usually occur at the MP joint. Dislocations of the MP joints of the fingers can occur but are rare. Carpometacarpal joint dislocations can occur but are often overlooked because of the subtle clinical findings. These are most common at the fourth and fifth carpometacarpal joints.

PIP JOINT DISLOCATIONS. Interphalangeal joint dislocation, when seen early (before swelling and muscle spasm occur), can usually be reduced by gentle traction and manipulation. When traction is applied, the deformity is increased slightly to release trapped soft tissues. The joint

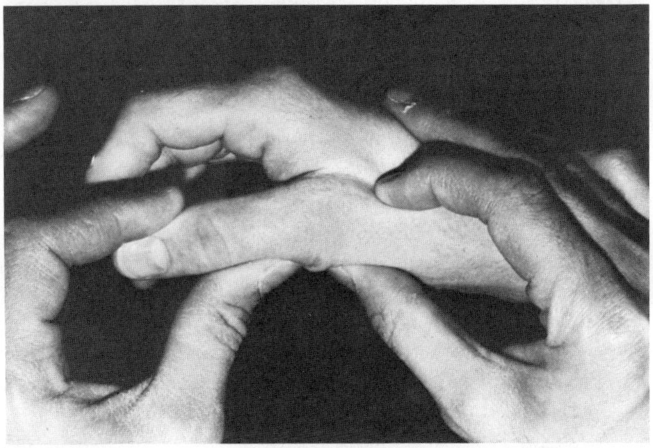

Fig. 67-20. Method of testing the stability of the ulnar side collateral ligament of the thumb metacarpophalangeal joint. Comparison of laxity on the injured and noninjured sides should be made.

is then flexed to accomplish the reduction. Occasionally, these can be reduced without anesthesia, although a digital block is preferable. Multiple attempts to reduce the joint should be avoided, and brute strength should not be used. The emergency physician should attempt a closed reduction once. A dislocation that cannot be reduced closed will require open reduction. If reduction is accomplished in the emergency department, the joint should be stress tested and carried through a complete range of motion. Joint laxity or incomplete motion signals a more serious injury. Stable PIP dislocations are immobilized in slight flexion for 14 days, after which gentle motion is started. As with other ligament injuries, full function will not be regained for four to six weeks.

The *DIP joint dislocations* are frequently unstable after reduction, and the joint may sublux if the reduction is not maintained with a small Kirschner's wire for several weeks. Patients with joints that are unstable after reduction should be referred to the appropriate specialist. Open joint dislocations are less frequent, but when they occur they require immediate surgical care.

Metacarpophalangeal joint dislocations usually reduce easily, but occasionally they are complex and require open reduction. Closed reduction of these joints is performed in a manner similar to that described for the MP joint of the thumb. Persistent volar dislocations of the MP joints of the fingers can cause pressure on the digital nerves resulting in a neuropraxia.

Metacarpophalangeal joint dislocation of the thumb is a relatively common injury resulting from a hyperextension force that tears the volar plate and allows the metacarpal head to herniate through the capsule. These often are complex dislocations and cannot be reduced by closed methods. One attempt to reduce this dislocation closed is justified. If this fails, the patient should be referred for open reduction.

Dislocations of the carpometacarpal (CM) joint of the thumb without fracture can occur—usually with hyperextension stress. If treated early by closed reduction and immobilization in abduction, healing can occur with satisfactory stability. Occasionally there is disruption of the deep ulnar ligament of the carpometacarpal joint. In these cases, chronic laxity with subluxation of the CM joint can result and ligament reconstruction is required.

Dislocations of the carpometacarpal joints of the fingers are usually the result of significant trauma. Recognition of this injury is important since soft-tissue swelling can obscure the deformity. X-ray findings tend to be overlooked, but careful review of the PA films shows a loss of normal joint space, and a lateral or oblique view will show the dorsally displaced metacarpal. Localized tenderness over the CM joints is the clue to injury, and comparison films may be very helpful. These dislocations are deceptive in that they are easily reduced (when treated early) but are very difficult to maintain in the reduced position. Patients with these injuries should be referred for temporary Kirschner's wire fixation.

VOLAR PLATE INJURIES. A hyperextension stress applied to the joint of a digit can damage the volar plate. A complete dorsal dislocation usually results in a tear of the volar plate. However, tears can occur without joint dislocation. These are more difficult to diagnose. A tiny avulsion fracture on the volar aspect of the joint seen in the lateral x-ray view may be present. In most volar plate injuries, the stability of the joint is maintained. The joint should be splinted in slight flexion while the plate heals. Healing with some laxity of the ligament is desirable so that a fixed flexion contracture does not occur. On the other hand, complete instability or marked laxity of the volar plate can result in hyperextension of the joint or a swan-neck deformity.

Nail Injuries

The fingernail provides support for the volar skin and pulp of the finger and is important during pinch and other fine hand functions. Injuries to the nail are often overlooked, either because the damage is considered to be minimal or because of other associated and more serious-appearing injuries of the hand. However, damage to the nail bed can permanently affect nail growth and result in deformity of the nail plate, fingertip, or both.

Nail Plate Avulsion

Partial avulsion of the nail plate without damage to the underlying bed should be treated by trimming and replacing the nail into its normal position. It can be held in place with a dressing. The damaged nail will gradually be replaced by a new nail. In complete nail avulsions, the nail should not be replaced, but the bed should be protected by a nonadherent dressing (petrolatum, Xeroform, etc.). A firm membrane will form over the nail bed in one to two weeks. When this has occurred, the nonadherent dressing can be removed. The skin fold (eponychial fold) surrounding the nail margin must be preserved if the nail is completely avulsed. This is done by packing petrolatum or other nonadherent gauze between the skin fold and the bed. The raw nail bed is quite sensitive, and anesthesia by digital block may be necessary to perform this procedure. Failure to preserve this space can result in a deformed nail. Patients who have lost a nail plate should be told that new nail growth occurs very slowly and that four to five months are required before a completely new nail is present.

The patient should be advised that several nail genera-

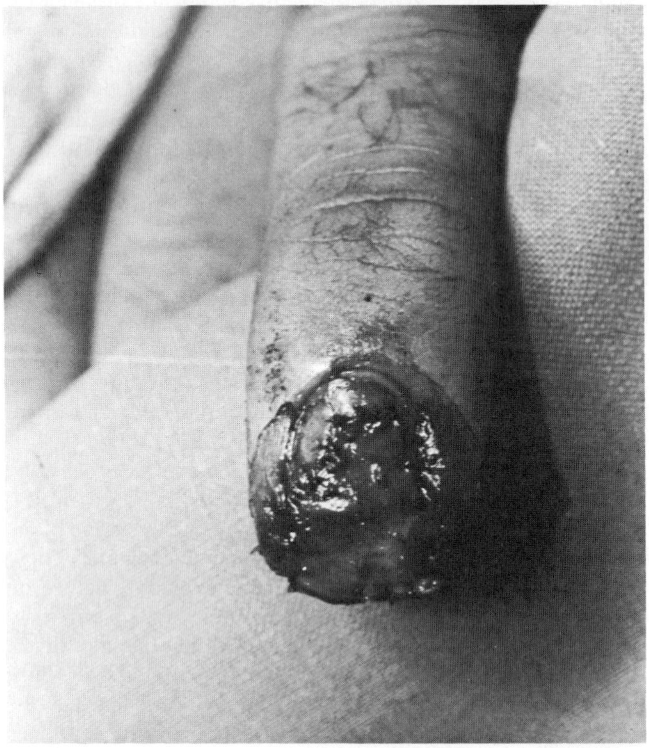

Fig. 67-21. Laceration of the nail bed repaired with fine absorbable sutures (6-0 or 7-0 gut or Vicryl). The eponychial fold is packed open with petrolatum-impregnated gauze and a nonadhering dressing is applied to the nail bed.

tions are necessary after an injury before the nail plate will look as good as possible. Therefore, one year or more may elapse before nail plate appearance is optimal, even through a new nail will have grown out within several months.

Nail Bed Injury

Lacerations of the nail bed should be repaired carefully and accurately, using closely spaced 6-0 or 7-0 absorbable sutures after the damaged nail plate is removed (Fig. 67-21). Occult nail bed lacerations are easy to overlook if the nail plate has not been avulsed by the injury. The physician should have a high index of suspicion for nail bed lacerations underlying an intact or mostly intact nail plate in fingertips injured by crush mechanisms, or in fingers that show displaced fractures of the distal phalanx on x-ray. It is more useful to lift up the nail plate under digital block anesthesia and inspect the underlying nail bed than to allow a nail bed laceration to remain untreated, as scarring of the nail bed can result in nail deformity or in arrest of distal nail growth. Loss of nail bed tissue should be covered by a split-thickness skin graft. These procedures will prevent or minimize subsequent nail plate deformities.

Injury loss of the germinal matrix or nail root will result in complete or partial arrest of nail plate growth. Because the amount of damage to this germinal tissue cannot be determined clinically, the patient should be advised of this possibility. Reconstructive procedures may be required in the future if the amount of nail deformity is unacceptable either functionally or cosmetically.

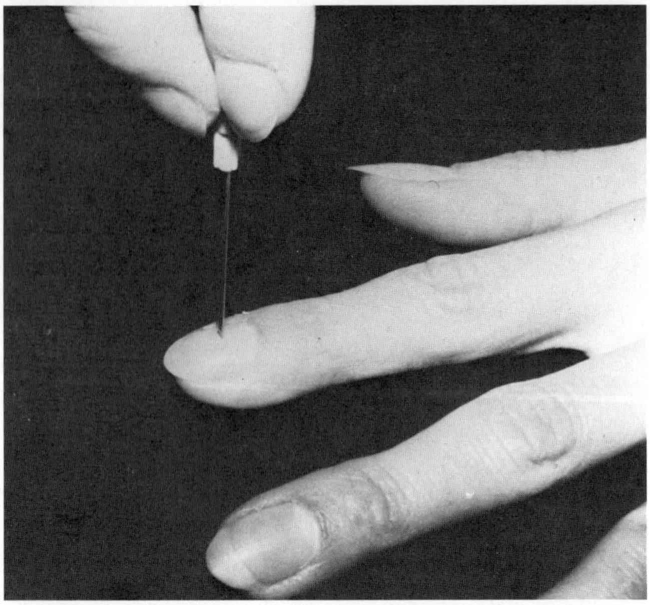

Fig. 67-22. Subungual hematoma decompressed by drilling through the nail plate with a No. 18 needle. The point of a No. 11 scalpel blade also can be used.

Subungual Hematoma

Subungual hematomas occur after blunt trauma and crush injuries, either with or without fractures of the distal phalanx. These are painful and should be drained to provide relief. A hole in the central portion of the nail plate can best be made using a No. 18-gauge needle. This can be drilled through the nail plate without the need for excessive (and painful) pressure on the nail. Some emergency departments have a battery-operated instrument that provides an electrically heated filament that will burn a hole in the nail quickly and painlessly (Fig. 67-22).

Subungual Splinter

Subungual splinters are also painful. The splinter should be removed using a splinter forceps or fine straight hemostat or a No. 20 needle or No. 11 scalpel blade under digital block anesthesia. Attempts to remove the splinter without anesthesia will not be tolerated by the patient. Occasionally a small portion of the nail must be removed so that the splinter can be retrieved.

Fingertip Injuries

Fingertip injuries with pulp damage or loss occur frequently. Small areas of skin or pulp loss (particularly in children) can be cleansed, dressed, and allowed to granulate. Larger areas of pulp loss or partial amputation of the tip will require coverage by skin grafts or local flaps. In these cases, exposed bone should be trimmed with a rongeur. Flap procedures are best done in the operating room by surgeons familiar with these techniques. However, most fingertip amputations can be debrided and covered with a split-thickness skin graft in the emergency department. Reconstruction can be done secondarily, if necessary. Many such injuries covered by split-thickness skin grafts result in functional digits

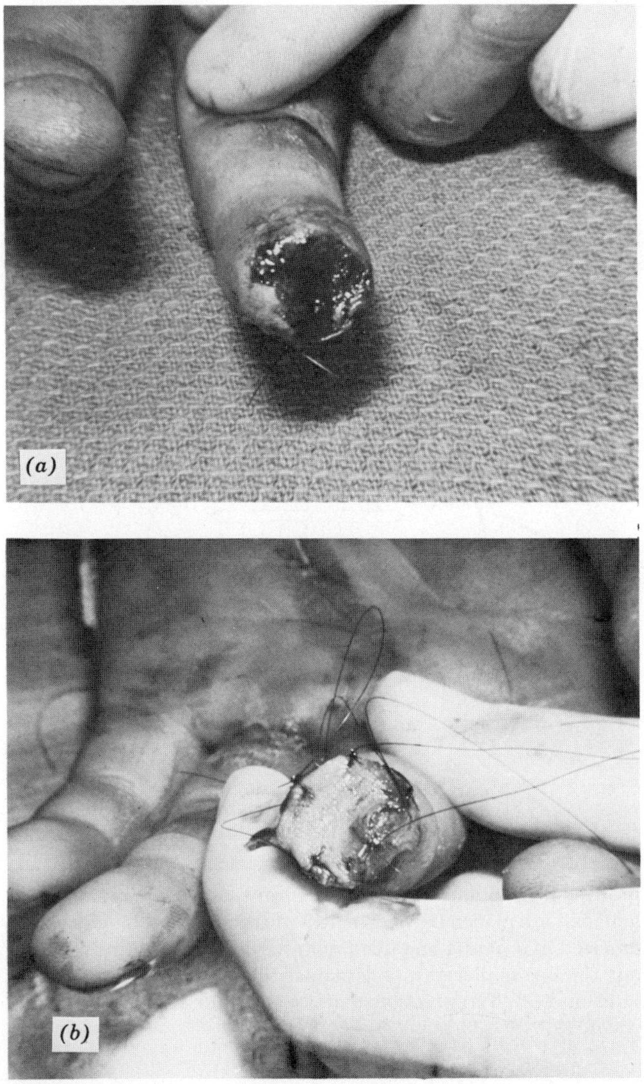

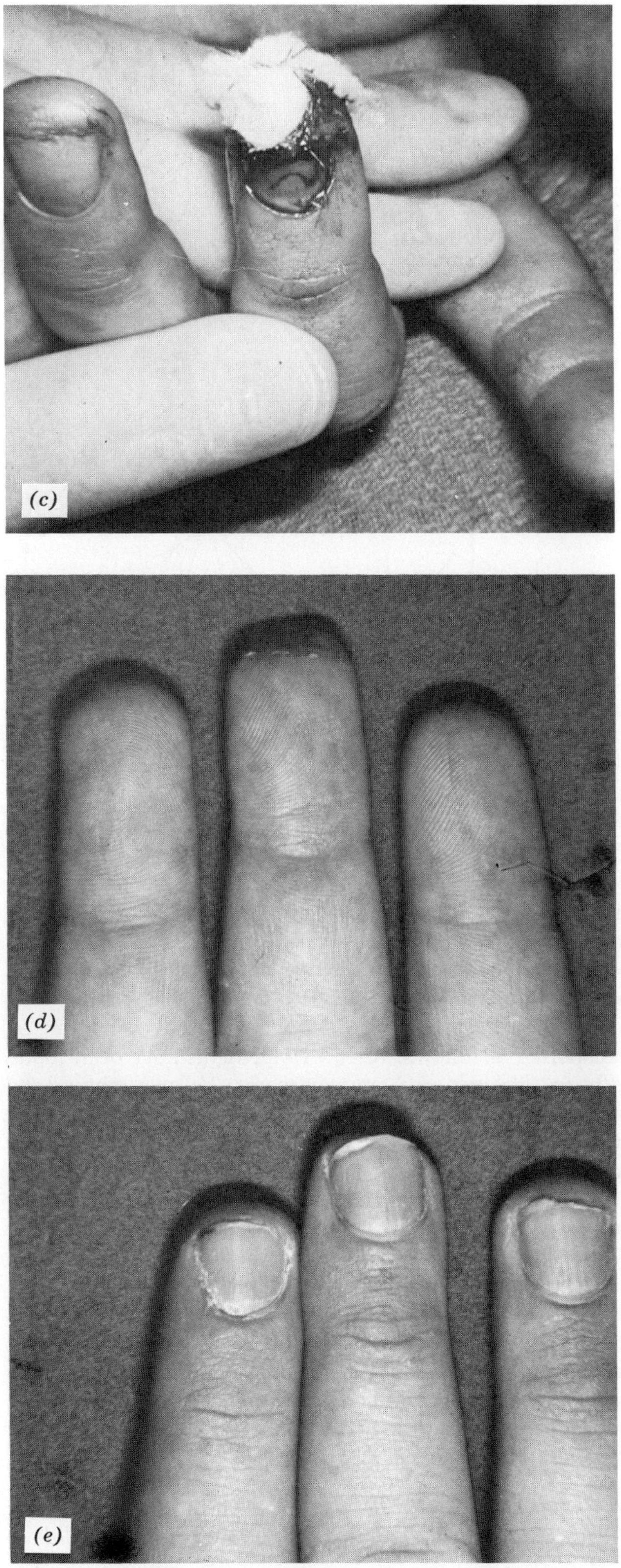

Fig. 67-23. (*a*) Fingertip injury with loss of soft tissue from the distal portion of the pulp. (*b*) Split-thickness skin graft from the lateral thigh applied to the area of tissue loss and sutured in place. (*c*) Stent dressing tied over graft for compression. (*d*) After healing, there has been contraction of the bed to which the graft was applied resulting in satisfactory appearance and function of the distal pulp without the need for revision. (*e*) Normal nail plate growth and appearance after healing.

because of the tendency for the graft bed to shrink and draw normal pulp skin in from the edges of the wound (Fig. 67-23). Bone directly under a split-thickness skin graft or large areas of insensate skin will not be functional and will require revision.

Amputations

Partial or complete amputations of the hand or digits must be evaluated in the light of recent advances in microsurgical techniques and the possibility of revascularization or replantation of the injured parts. Massively traumatized, crushed, or severely contaminated injuries usually are not suitable for these procedures. Cleanly amputated parts or those with

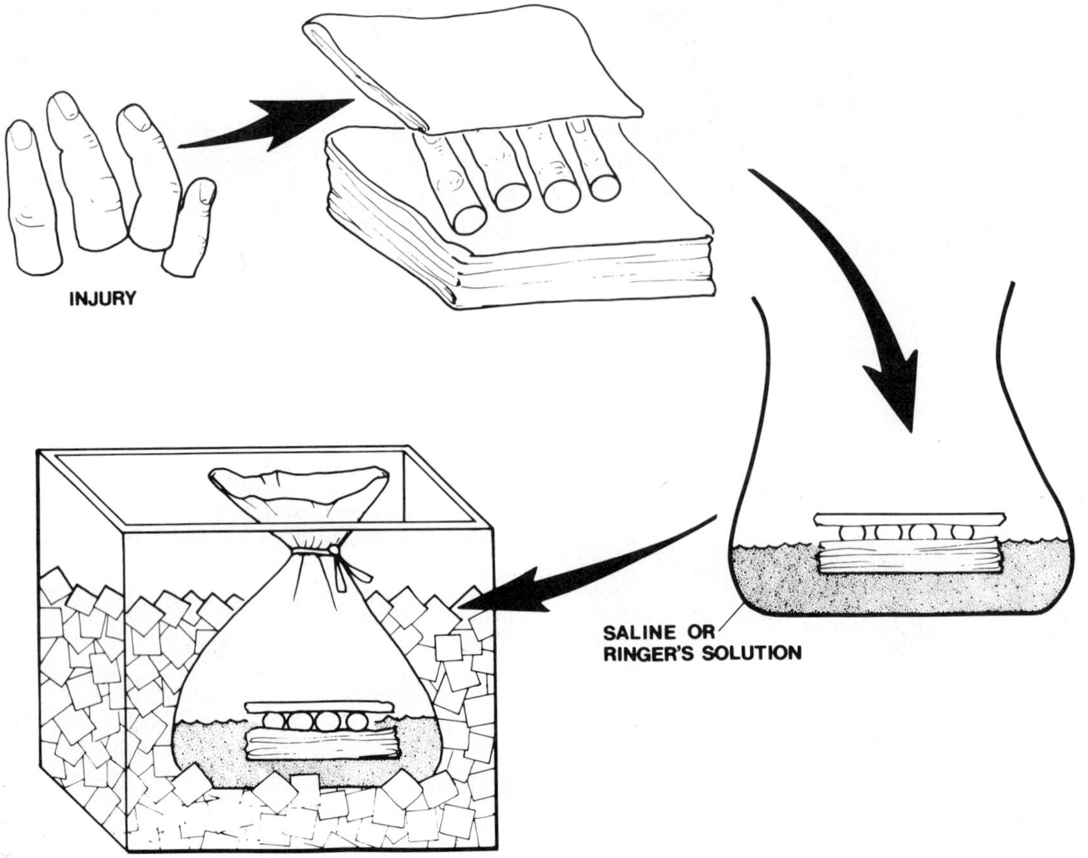

Fig. 67-24. Amputated fingers to be transported for possible replantation are placed between stacks of sterile 4-by-4 in. gauze and immersed in a plastic bag filled with sterile saline or Ringer's solution. The bag is placed in a container filled with ice. (From R.K. Daniel and J.K. Terris. *Reconstructive Microsurgery.* Boston: Little, Brown, 1977. P 130.)

mild crushing can be preserved and transported with the patient for evaluation by a microsurgical team, even though relatively long periods of time may elapse between the initial injury and the definitive surgery.

Parts considered appropriate for replantation should be transported as follows: After arrangements have been made with the nearest replantation team, the part should be washed carefully with normal saline, wrapped in a sterile dressing moistened with normal saline, placed into a plastic bag, and then placed into an ice chest filled with regular ice. Freezing of the tissue must be avoided; thus direct contact of the part with ice or the use of dry ice is precluded (Fig. 67-24).

Amputations that are not suitable for replantation or partial amputations that are not suitable for revascularization should be closed in the operating room under controlled conditions. Occasionally, the cleanly amputated finger can be closed in the emergency department using local skin or split-thickness skin grafts. The patient should be referred for follow-up care or revision, if necessary.

Burns

The depth and extent of a burn wound determines what treatment is necessary. The extent of the burn is determined by the nature of the injury; a flash or flame burn will involve more of the hand than a burn produced by contact with a hot object. The depth of a burn often is difficult to ascertain and can vary within the same wound. Burn wounds can be classified as partial or total thickness. In a *partial-thickness burn* (first or second degree), some dermal elements remain viable and reepithelization is possible if the wound is kept clean and sterile. In these injuries, the skin appears erythematous but blanches with pressure. Sensibility is present and the wound is painful. Blisters or raw weeping surfaces may be present. In a *total-thickness burn* (third degree), there is destruction of all dermal elements, and wound debridement and skin replacement are necessary. Areas of total burn appear blanched, gray, or charred. Sensibility over the wound is absent, and the wound is painless. The skin on the dorsal surface of the hand is thin, and total-thickness burns with damage to the underlying extensor tendons are common. In contrast, the palmar skin is thicker and more often burn injuries in this area are only partial.

Small areas of burn with partial skin loss can be treated in the emergency department with a topical dressing such as silver sulfadiazine (Silvadene) or mafenide acetate (Sulfamylon), a sterile dressing, elevation, and careful follow-up. Debridement and skin grafting may be required during the recovery period.

The treatment of burn blisters has changed in recent years. In the past, it was recommended that the burn blisters be opened and debrided to remove devitalized tissue and to avoid the growth of bacteria in the blister fluid. Now it is recommended that the blisters be left intact unless they appear ready to burst or unless the blister fluid has become cloudy, indicating bacterial contamination. The thin blister membrane is thought to act as a biologic dressing, and antibiotics have been found to diffuse into the blister fluid.

A small contact burn with total skin damage but without damage to underlying structures can often be excised and closed primarily in the emergency department. However, if any questions of the extent of damage remain or if extensive damage is present, the patient should be referred to a specialist. Hospitalization under these circumstances is advisable to minimize hand dysfunction as a result of tissue loss or scar formation.

Chemical Burns

Chemical burns (contact with acid or alkali agents) are treated initially by copious irrigation with water to dilute and remove the agent. Dilute neutralizing agents can be used (with care) for irrigation; dilute acetic acid is used for alkali burns and sodium bicarbonate solution is used for acid burns. Alkali burns require copious and prolonged irrigation since these chemical agents are difficult to remove from the skin. Hydrofluoric acid burns are very serious and must be neutralized by injecting the wound area with 10% calcium gluconate. If there is any question that hydrofluoric acid was the agent involved, the place of work should be contacted and detailed information should be obtained from a knowledgeable source.

Electrical Burns

Although high-voltage electrical burns may cause only a small area of superficial tissue damage, extensive deep-tissue damage may be present. For this reason, the injury may be far worse than it appears initially. Vascular damage may be widespread, resulting in thrombosis, ischemia, and ultimately tissue death. Because the extent of high-voltage electrical burns will only become apparent after several days, patients with these injuries should be hospitalized and observed. Low-voltage burns to small areas are not as serious and can be cared for as thermal burns.

Frostbite

Prolonged cold exposure in temperatures below freezing will cause ice crystal formation in dermal cells. Fingers are particularly prone to this injury. The resultant cell damage or death turns the affected skin white or grayish. The initial treatment for the frostbitten part is rapid rewarming to body temperature by immersion in water heated to 42°C (107.6°F). Debridement should not be done until the affected areas are allowed to demarcate. In contrast to high-voltage electrical injuries, the damage often is more superficial than the initial appearance indicates. Patients with minor areas of frostbite should be referred for follow-up care after rewarming and application of a sterile bulky dressing. Patients with major frostbite injuries should be hospitalized.

The fingers of children are at risk from subclinical damage to the epiphyses from cold exposure. Although no clinical signs or symptoms may be present initially, the subsequent growth impairment of the fingers becomes manifest near the end of the growth spurt at puberty. Parent education about the danger of prolonged unprotected cold exposure will minimize these injuries.

Bites

Animal Bites

Animal bites on the hand are particularly dangerous because of the potential for deep closed space infections, joint infections, and tendon sheath infections. After aerobic and anaerobic cultures are obtained (if possible), these wounds should be washed thoroughly with soap and water or hydrogen peroxide. Ragged skin edges should be debrided. Primary closure usually is not indicated. The wound should be dressed and treated open. Antibiotics should be given prophylactically. Penicillin is the drug of choice because of its efficacy against *Pasteurella multocida*, a common infection-producing bacteria found in the mouths of dogs and cats. Follow-up care is advised so that infections of the bone, joints, or tendon sheaths can be detected early.

Human Bites

Human bites can occur either as the result of altercations or, occasionally, during the emergency care of patients having seizures, dental procedures, cardiac arrest, and so forth. Most commonly, the "bite" is an open wound over the dorsal aspect of the fingers or hand from a tooth as a clenched fist strikes an opponent. Because of the virulent nature of the flora in the human mouth, these wounds must be treated as potentially serious infections. The wounds should be washed, debrided if necessary, and dressed open. Broad-spectrum antibiotics such as penicillin, ampicillin, cephalosporin, or lincomycin should be started after the wound is cultured. The patient should be made aware of the serious nature of the injury and the necessity for frequent follow-up examination. Unreliable patients should be hospitalized for observation. Established infections from human bites are limb threatening and will require hospitalization, intravenous antibiotics, and surgical drainage and debridement.

Injection Injuries

Small puncture wounds on the tips of the fingers caused by high-pressure grease guns, paint spray guns, or broken hydraulic lines may initially appear innocuous to both the patient and the emergency physican. However, the fluids carried by these devices are injected deep into the tissues under very high pressure and are forced along the tissue planes of least resistance, sometimes all the way from the fingertip into the forearm. These fluids cause an extensive chemical inflammatory reaction with subsequent tissue necrosis. Hydraulic fluid is hot and will cause thermal as well as chemical damage. Several hours after the injury, the injured finger and hand will begin to swell and become severely painful.

Patients with these injuries will require emergency surgical exploration, decompression, and debridement of the involved finger and hand far beyond the point of penetration. Failure to do this can result in such extensive tissue necrosis that amputation may be required.

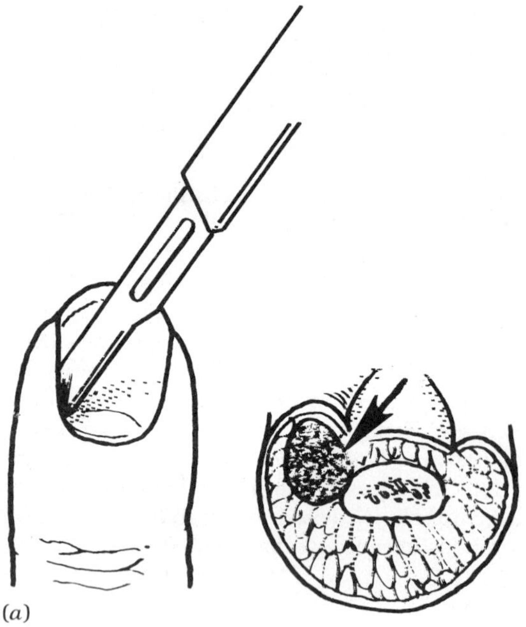

(a)

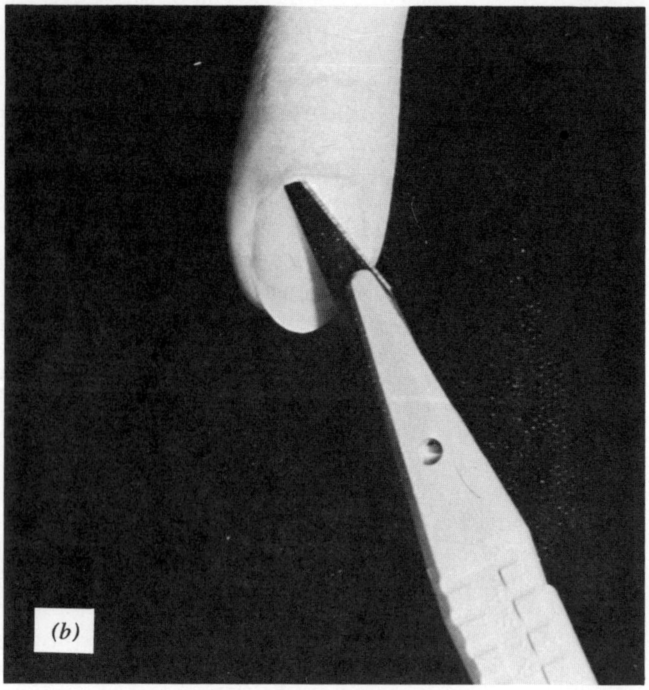

(b)

Fig. 67-25. (*a*) Diagram of the method used to drain a collection of pus beneath the nail fold (paronychia). (*b*) Scalpel blade is inserted beneath the fold parallel to the nail plate.

Infections of the Hand

Acute Paronychia

Acute paronychia is an infection of the skin fold surrounding the nail plate. It is manifest by reddened and swollen tissue adjacent to the nail on the dorsal aspect of the finger. Early cases can be treated by oral antibiotics and soaks. If the infection is established or if the treatment described previously fails, surgical drainage is necessary. This is accomplished by passing a scalpel blade between the skin fold and the nail plate at the point of maximum swelling or erythema (Fig. 67-25). Occasionally a portion of the nail plate must be removed to drain the infection adequately. This is done under digital block anesthesia by passing a straight, sharp, pointed scissor blade longitudinally along the lateral one-fourth of the base of the nail on the affected side between the nail bed and the nail plate. Occasionally both edges of the nail plate must be removed. The patient is then instructed in dressing changes and soaks two to three times daily until all symptoms have resolved. Antibiotics are usually not necessary once the infection has been drained.

Subungual Abscess

Subungual abscess is the collection of pus under the nail plate that results from the volar extension of an acute paronychia. The diagnosis is suspected when the fingertip appears inflamed and the fingernail is opaque, discolored, or lifted away from its bed. The treatment of subungual abscess requires removal of the base of the nail plate under digital block anesthesia. The distal portion of the nail can be left in place. A 7- to 10-day course of oral antibiotics (dicloxacillin or cephalosporins) is given, and the patient is instructed in daily dressing changes as described previously.

Felon

A felon is an infection of the pulp tissue of the finger, usually as the result of a puncture wound. The septae of the pulp form closed spaces, which, when infected, cause the pulp to become swollen, tender, erythematous, and acutely painful. These infections require prompt surgical drainage. This can be done under digital block anesthesia. A straight incision is made 3 mm volar to and parallel with the nail plate on each side of the fingertip. A hemostat is passed from side to side to open the pulp space, and a slip of Penrose drain or Silastic sheeting is passed through the open space and left protruding through each skin incision (Fig. 67-26). The finger is dressed and oral antibiotics are prescribed. The drain can be removed in three to five days, and the patient should be instructed in dressing changes. A "fish mouth" incision should not be used. If the abscess is pointing at one location on the surface of the pulp or has broken through the pulp, drainage can be accomplished by incising directly over the area. Necrotic skin and pulp should be removed and the wound dressed open and allowed to granulate. Untreated or advanced cases of felon can result in osteomyelitis of the distal phalanx. X-rays should be taken if there is any question of bone involvement. Unless the emergency physician is familiar with the surgical drainage of felons, patients with this condition are best referred to a consultant.

Herpes Simplex

Herpes simplex infection of the finger (herpetic whitlow) can be mistaken for a paronychia or felon with erythema and tenderness of the fingertip. However, small vesicles containing clear or turbid fluid usually are present on the sur-

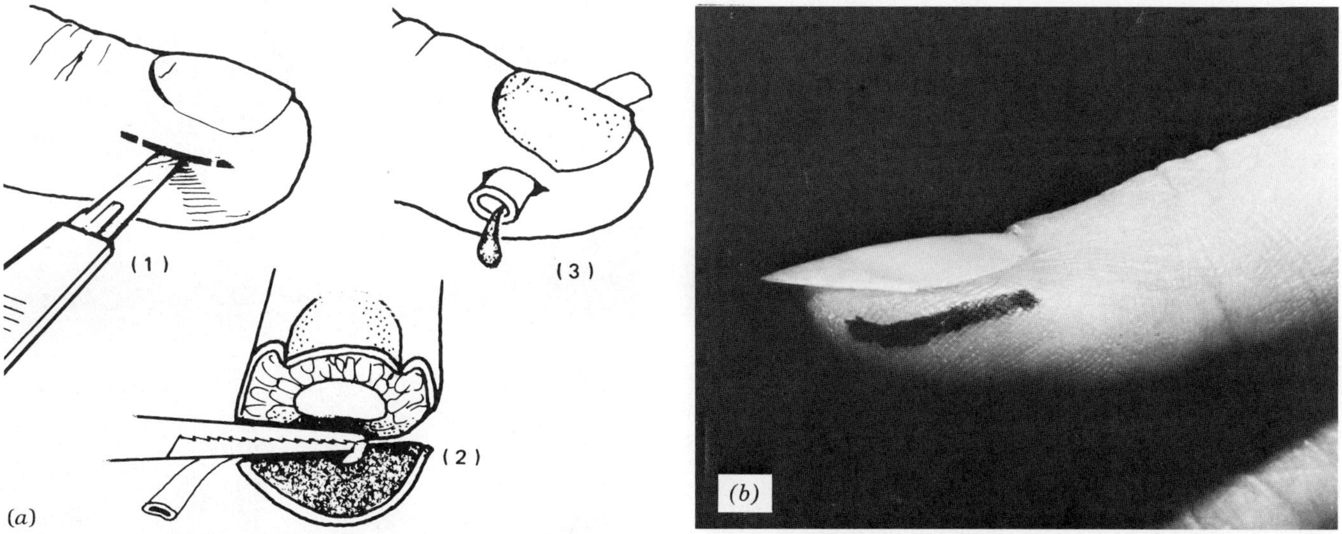

Fig. 67-26. (*a*) Drainage of a felon. (1) Parallel incisions are made on either side of the finger just volar to the nail plate. (2) A hemostat is inserted through the incisions and spread to open the septa of the finger pulp. (3) A through-and-through drain is inserted. (*b*) Incision used to drain a felon. The "fish mouth" incision should not be used.

face of the inflamed areas. The occupation of the patient is the diagnostic clue since these infections occur most often in dentists, dental hygienists, physicians, and nurses, whose fingers are exposed to contamination by saliva or other secretions or excretions containing herpesvirus. The condition is self-limited and will resolve spontaneously in two to three weeks if the affected finger is kept clean and dry. Occasionally, secondary bacterial infection occurs and must be treated with antibiotics. However, attempting to incise and drain fingers affected with herpes is contraindicated. This will delay healing and can increase the risk of bacterial infection.

Deep Infections of the Hand

Bacterial tenosynovitis, web space infections, subepithelial abscesses (collar button abscesses), and palmar space infections are serious infections of the hand. They present with painful swelling and erythema over the affected part. Palmar space infections may present with marked dorsal swelling because the dorsal skin and soft tissues are more distensible. Tenosynovitis presents as a swollen, erythematous finger with tenderness over the tendon sheath and pain with active and passive motion of the finger.

Surgical drainage of established infections in these areas is necessary in order to prevent serious functional impairment of the hand. Drainage of an acute bacterial tenosynovitis is a surgical emergency since the increased pressure in the closed tendon sheath from pus accumulation compromises the vascular supply of the tendon and can result in tendon necrosis. These procedures should be done in the operating room under controlled conditions. Attempts to drain these infections in the emergency department by inexperienced personnel can damage underlying structures. The use of improper incisions can cause excessive scarring or joint contractures. Early or incipient infections can be treated by antibiotics, immobilization and elevation, and frequent follow-up visits.

Hand Dressings

Minor wounds will require a minimal dressing, for example, bandages or tubular gauze. However, more extensive injuries can best be dressed using a bulky compression dressing, usually with a volar or dorsal plaster splint to immobilize the wrist and to protect and position the fingers. This dressing is multifunctional. It will diminish pain by limiting motion of the hand and wrist, it will limit edema by applying gentle compression, and it will protect the injury site. The dressing can be used for temporary immobilization of massive hand injuries or for injuries that require transport of the patient to another facility. It can be used along with multiple fracture or with infections with edema, as well as after surgical repair of injuries.

The "safe" position of the hand places the MP joint at 90 degrees of flexion and the interphalangeal joints in slight flexion. The thumb is abducted to preserve the first web space. This position will diminish the possibility of joint contractures by keeping collateral ligaments in their positions of maximal length. The positioning of the hand, fingers, and wrist can be modified for specific purposes or injuries.

Open wounds should be covered with a nonadhering dressing. The bulky dressing is applied by placing a single layer of 4-by-8 in. gauze between each finger and multiple layers in the first web space. Gauze is placed in the palm to provide bulk. The first layers are held in place with roller gauze. Excessive pressure should not be used in applying the roller dressing. However, gentle compression is advantageous if applied with care. A padded plaster splint made of 10 to 12 thicknesses of 4-in. plaster is applied either volarly or dorsally. This should immobilize the fingers in the desired position and should extend far enough down the forearm to immobilize the wrist, usually in slight dorsiflexion (Fig. 67-27).

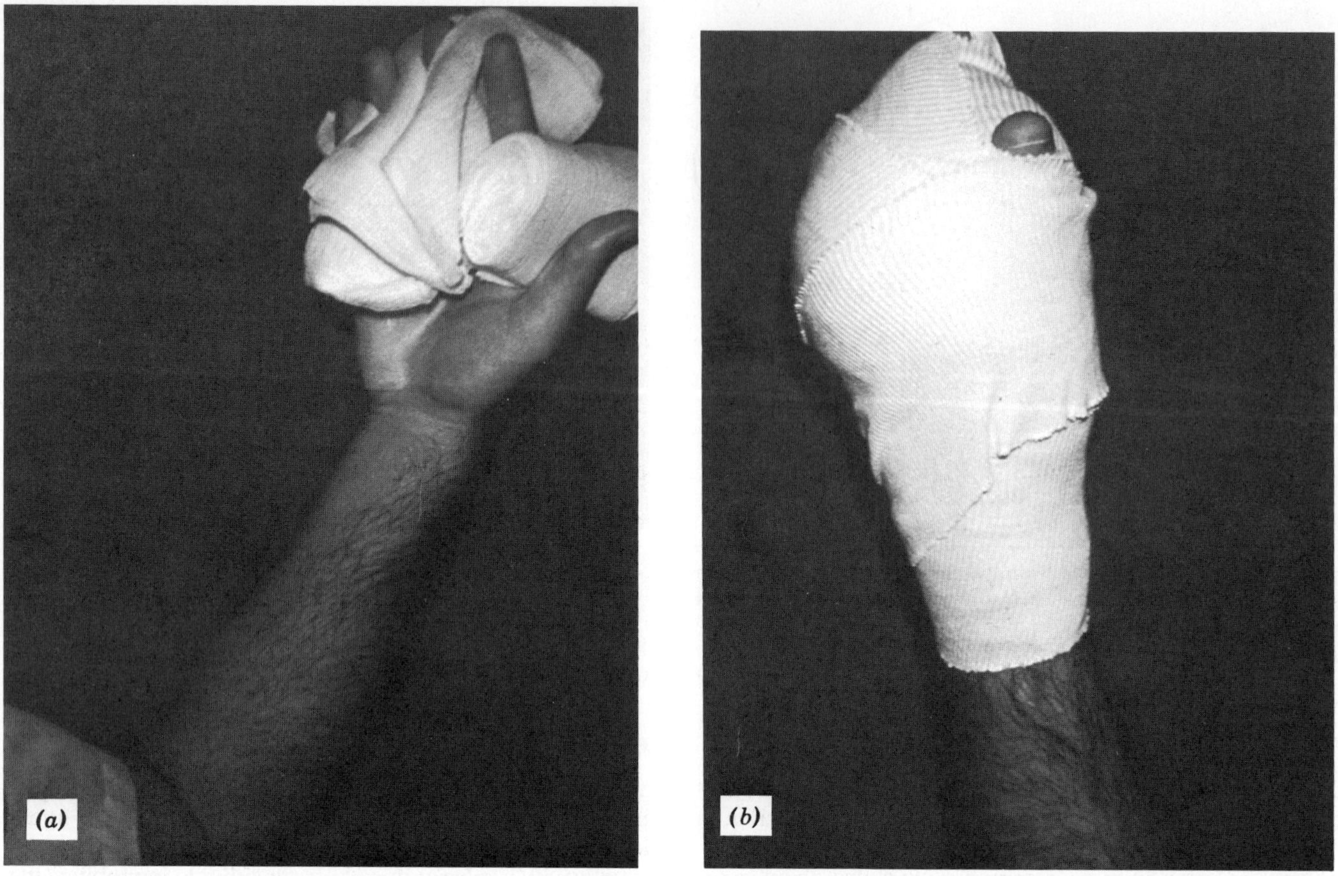

Fig. 67-27. Bulky compression hand dressing with a dorsal plaster splint. (*a*) Sterile gauze dressings are placed between each finger to prevent skin maceration. The first web space is maintained by placing the thumb in abduction and extension (opposition). The MP joints are positioned in 60 degrees of flexion and the PIP and DIP joints in nearly full extension. (*b*) The initial dressing is held in place with bias-cut stockinet or a roller bandage. (*c*) A dorsal plaster splint is applied from the tips of the fingers to the proximal forearm and held in place with bias-cut stockinet or a loosely wrapped elastic bandage. The wrist usually is held in slight dorsiflexion. (*d*) Completed dressing with fingertips exposed for inspection of color and sensibility.

Post–Emergency Department Instructions for Patients with Hand Injuries

Hand elevation is important in minimizing both pain and swelling. In general, a sling will position the hand below the level of the heart and thus will not provide optimum venous drainage. The patient should be instructed to keep the hand at eye level. Usually the patient's arm muscles are sufficient to maintain this position while the patient is ambulatory, although occasionally a modified sling can be applied. When the patient is at home or in bed, pillows can be used to support the forearm and hand. The elbow and shoulder should be moved through their ranges of motion (unless other associated injuries or casts or dressings preclude this) several times a day to prevent stiffness. This is particularly important in older patients.

The patient should be advised to call the physician or return to the hospital if progressive loss of sensation in the fingers occurs, if pain is uncontrolled by minor analgesics, or if a fever, erythema, swelling, or other signs of infection develop. At least one follow-up visit is necessary for most injuries to ensure that healing is proceeding satisfactorily and that hand motion and function have been regained.

THE PAINFUL HAND

Several painful, but not necessarily traumatic, conditions of the hand may be seen by the emergency physician. Recognition of these will allow a diagnosis to be made and reassurance or symptomatic care, or both, provided. The patient can be referred to the appropriate consultant unless urgent care is indicated.

Nerve Compression

Carpal Tunnel Syndrome

Compression of the median nerve as it passes through the carpal canal (a tunnel formed by the carpal bones and the thick transverse carpal ligament—see Fig. 67-2) can occur either acutely as the result of swelling associated with hand, wrist, or forearm trauma or chronically with no apparent underlying cause. It can occur temporarily during pregnancy as the result of swelling secondary to fluid retention or in association with tenosynovitis of the flexor tendons as the result of rheumatoid arthritis or other systemic conditions. It is commonly referred to as *carpal tunnel syndrome.*

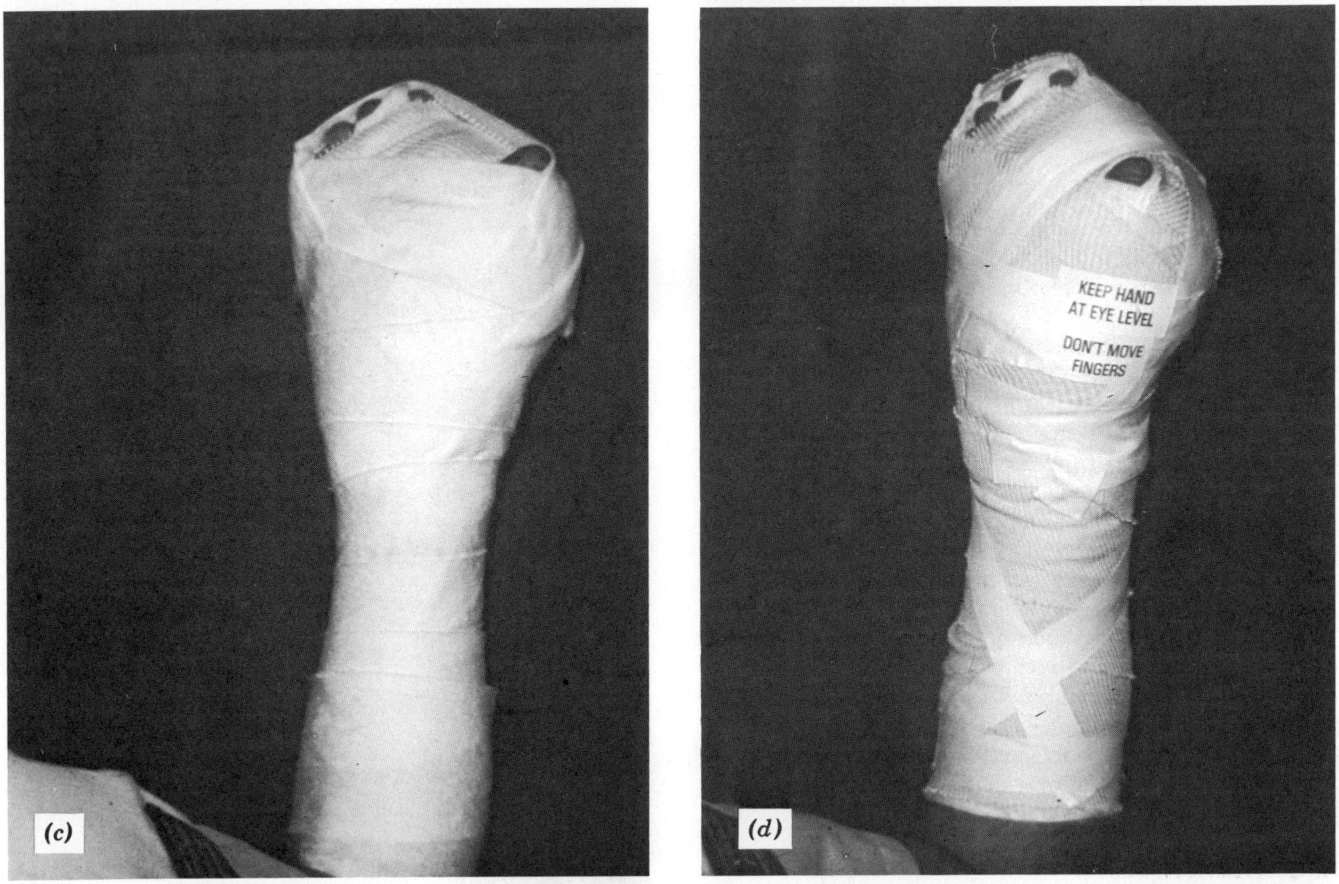

Fig. 67-27. (continued)

The predominant symptoms of carpal tunnel syndrome are paresthesias and numbness in the distribution of the median nerve in the hand associated with pain and discomfort in the hand and forearm at night. These symptoms may be worse after vigorous use of the hand or after driving. The discomfort may be described as aching pain that radiates to the palm, wrist, or forearm. It frequently awakens the patient at night and may be partially relieved by shaking or wringing the hand, immersion in hot or cold water, or changing the position of the wrist. Patients may complain that they frequently drop objects and are "clumsy" or have difficulty in handling or picking up small objects.

Physical examination may reveal either no objective changes in the hand or a combination of signs including impaired sensibility in the median nerve distribution, diminished or absent sweating with resultant dry skin in this distribution, tenderness to percussion over the volar aspect of the wrist, increased numbness or paresthesias when the wrist is held in acute flexion (Phalen's test), and, in advanced cases, atrophy of the thenar musculature.

The treatment of this chronic condition in the emergency department is explanation and reassurance, as well as a plaster or commercial splint to maintain the wrist in a slightly dorsiflexed position. The patient should be referred to a consultant for follow-up and, if necessary, definitive care.

Acute Compression

Acute compression of the median nerve can occur after injuries to the hand, wrist, or forearm that result in swelling or after the application of dressings or rigid casts to the upper extremity following trauma. In these cases, the dressing should be split or removed immediately. Casts should be bivalved with a cast cutter or "univalved" by removing a longitudinal strip 1 cm wide from one surface of the cast. The cast padding is split to the level of the skin, and the edges of the cast are spread apart. The patient's primary treating physician should be notified. Although mild nerve compression may be relieved by the procedures already described combined with elevation of the extremity, occasionally surgical decompression of the nerve on an urgent basis is required.

Compression neuropathy of the median and ulnar nerves can occur after severe closed injuries such as crush injuries by rollers, heavy machinery, or washing machine wringers or by prolonged compression of the upper extremity by the patient's body during periods of unconsciousness (usually resulting from intoxication by drugs or alcohol). These injuries cause soft-tissue damage that results in marked swelling and thereby compression of the neurovascular structures in the closed fascial compartments of the forearm and ischemia of nerves and muscles. Occasionally, compression syndromes of the forearm result from acute hemorrhage in patients with a coagulopathy or in those who are taking anticoagulant medication for other conditions. These closed compartment compression syndromes are surgical emergencies and require urgent decompression by extensive fasciotomy to avoid permanent damage to the nerves and muscles and a deformed functionless extremity (Volkmann's ischemic contracture).

Stenosing Tenosynovitis

Trigger Finger
Patients with painful motion of a finger or thumb associated with tenderness over the proximal portion of the digit or distal portion of the palm and with snapping or locking of the digit during active motion may have stenosing tenosynovitis or "trigger finger." The symptoms may be referred to the proximal interphalangeal joint. The condition is caused by impingement of the flexor tendon on the proximal portion of the tendon sheath (first annular pulley) as the tendon glides in the sheath (see Fig. 67-2). It occurs most commonly in women and results from thickening of the flexor tendon, either from repetitive trauma, infiltration of the tendon by rheumatoid synovium, or occasionally from a partially lacerated or otherwise damaged tendon.

Temporary immobilization and antiinflammatory medication may give relief in very early or mild cases. Steroid injection into the tendon sheath can be used in moderately severe cases, although care must be taken so that no additional damage is done to the flexor tendon by the needle tip. Advanced cases will require surgical release of the proximal portion of the tendon sheath.

De Quervain's Disease
Stenosing tenosynovitis can also occur on the radial aspect of the wrist as the tendons of the first dorsal compartment (the extensor pollicis brevis and the abductor pollicis longus) pass through a tight tendon sheath (see Fig. 67-18). Stenosing tenosynovitis of the first dorsal compartment is known as de Quervain's disease and again occurs most commonly in women. It is the result of chronic inflammation of the tendon sheath and can occur with repetitive use of the thumb or as the result of direct trauma. Patients have pain and tenderness localized to the area of the radial styloid bone or pain radiating along the radial aspect of the thumb, hand, and forearm. These symptoms are worse during use of the thumb and hand, especially during grasp and pinch.

Physical examination reveals maximum tenderness to palpation over the radial styloid of the radius and along the first dorsal compartment of the wrist. There may be mild swelling in this area. Abduction and extension of the thumb against resistance result in pain. Passive forced flexion of the thumb with concomitant ulnar deviation of the wrist results in pain (Finklestein's test).

Mild cases may respond to splinting, antiinflammatory drugs, or the local injection of a steroid solution. The splint should be of the thumb spica type to immobilize both the wrist and the thumb. Advanced or persistent cases require surgical decompression of the first dorsal compartment.

Reflex Sympathetic Dystrophy

Reflex sympathetic dystrophy, also known as *causalgia,* is a pain syndrome that occurs most often in the upper extremity and is thought to be related to a disorder of the autonomic nervous system that results in excessive and prolonged sympathetic response to painful stimulation. The syndrome was originally described following major injuries to peripheral nerves, but it is now known to occur in varying degrees in response to painful trauma of any type in susceptible individuals. Even minor injuries such as superficial cuts, contusions, and bites or fractures or surgical procedures can elicit the syndrome. In addition to the severe pain already described, the patient may complain of severe dysesthesias of the involved area. These may be so severe as to preclude contact of the area by anything, including air currents, clothing, bed sheets, or an examiner's hand. The joints of the involved parts are held motionless, and attempts to move these joints actively or passively result in severe pain. There may be mild erythema, swelling, or stiffness and even deformity in addition to the pain. However, the patient may have few, if any, of the objective signs described previously. Patients affected with reflex sympathetic dystrophy often have a history of multiple return visits to the emergency department

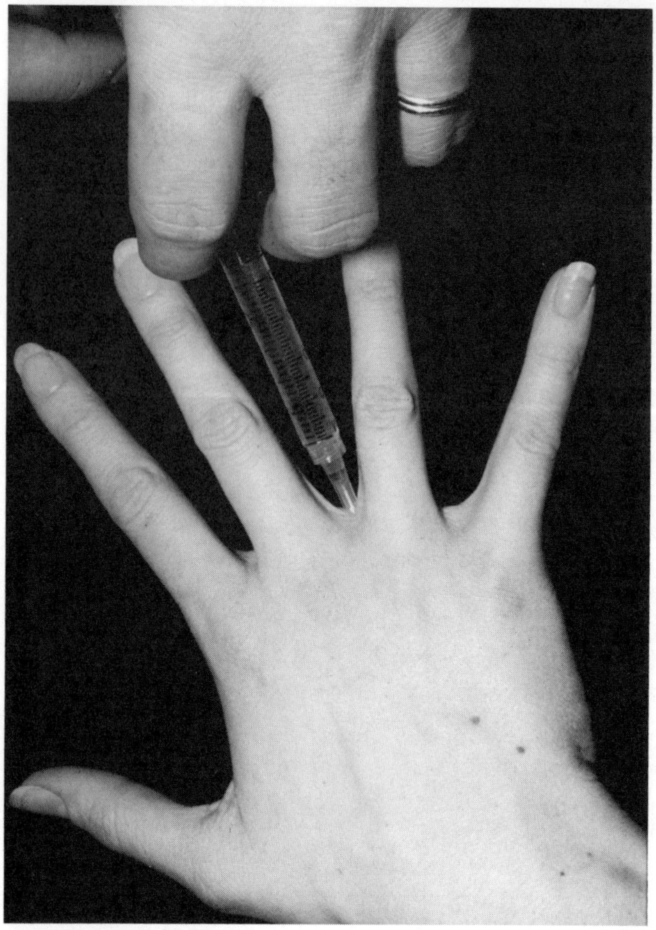

Fig. 67-28. The digital nerves to the thumb are more anterior and closer together than those of the fingers. The thumb can be blocked with a single injection of anesthetic solution by inserting the ⅝-in. needle through the volar skin from radial to ulnar with the needle held parallel to the volar surface of the thumb at the MP joint flexion crease.

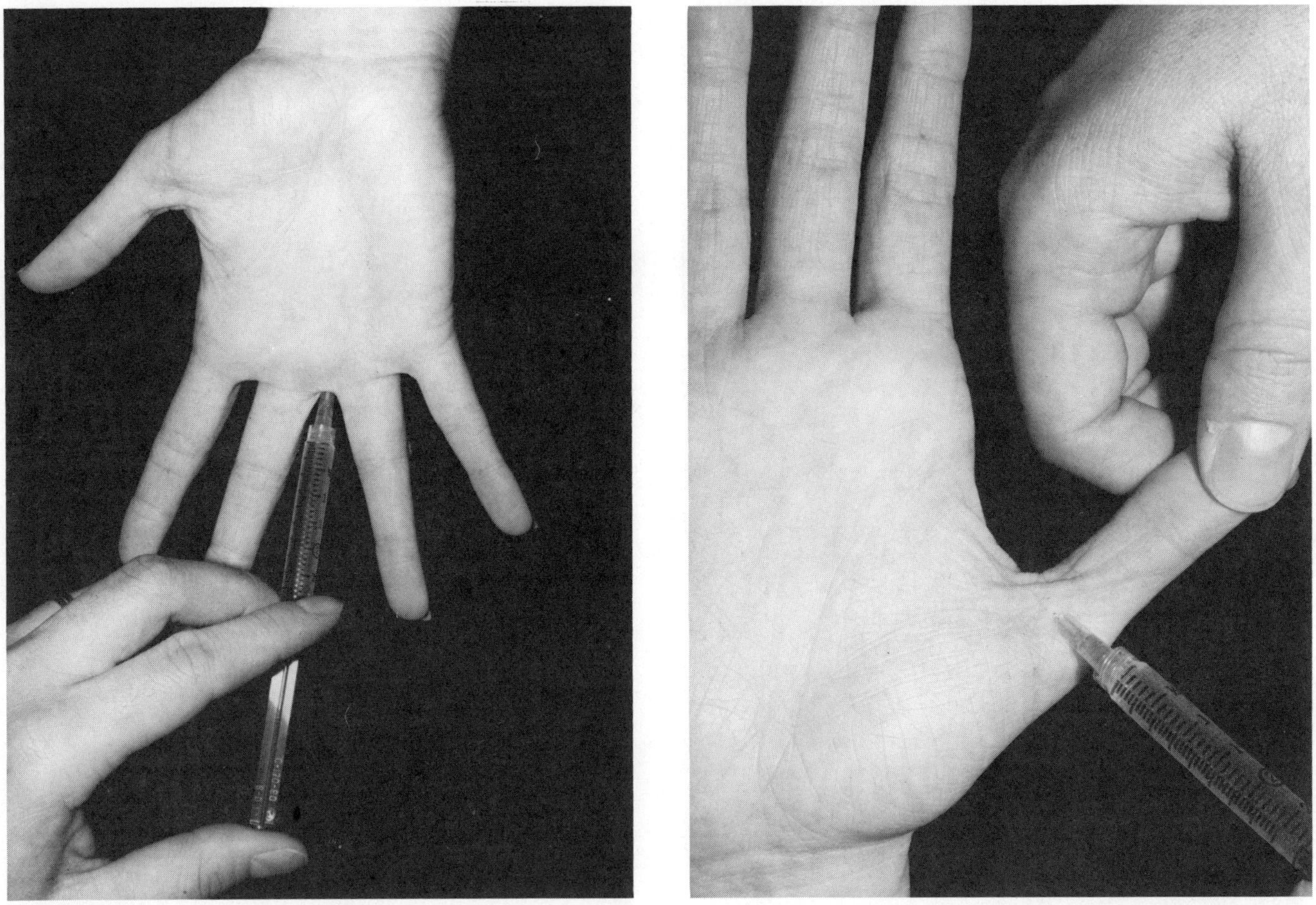

Fig. 67-28. (continued)

because of pain for which no reason can be found. They are often mislabeled as neurotic personalities or drug abusers if the correct reason for their complaints is not recognized.

The care of reflex sympathetic dystrophy is difficult and requires the expertise of an experienced consultant. The basis for proper treatment is early recognition. Sympathetic blockade to relieve pain and carefully supervised active hand exercise are the cornerstones of the treatment program. Failure of diagnosis or treatment results in a chronic pain syndrome accompanied by stiffness and deformity of the extremity that is very refractory to any mode of treatment.

ANESTHESIA

Local infiltration anesthesia and local block anesthesia are used for the control of pain in the emergency department. Occasionally peripheral nerve blocks are necessary and can be administered in the emergency department. However, extensive wound repair or the incision and drainage of infections require more complete and prolonged anesthesia that can be provided only by intravenous regional, axillary block, or general anesthesia. These procedures are best reserved for use in the operating room where experienced help is available for patient monitoring.

Local Infiltration

A solution of 1% lidocaine (without epinephrine) infiltrated into subcutaneous tissue provides satisfactory anesthesia for the suture of lacerations of the palm or the dorsum of the hand. Insertion of a small-gauge needle (25-, 26-, or 30-gauge) through the wound edge rather than through the intact skin minimizes discomfort associated with the procedure. Local lidocaine infiltration is useful in obtaining small skin grafts from donor sites in the arm, groin, or thigh. The injection of large volumes of solution into a digit should be avoided because of the possibility of compression of the neurovascular bundle within the closed space of the digit.

Digital Block (Web Space or Metacarpal Block)

If extensive anesthesia of a digit is required, the digital nerves can be blocked in the distal palm. While this method of anesthesia frequently is referred to as a "digital block," it is better described as a *web space* or *metacarpal block*. The latter terms refer to the site of injection used to achieve blockade of the two sensory nerves that serve each digit. Local anesthetic solution should not be injected into a digit because of the possibility of compression of the digital arteries or nerves, or both, within the closed fascial spaces of the digit. Such compression could lead to a neurapraxia or ischemia, or both, of the digit.

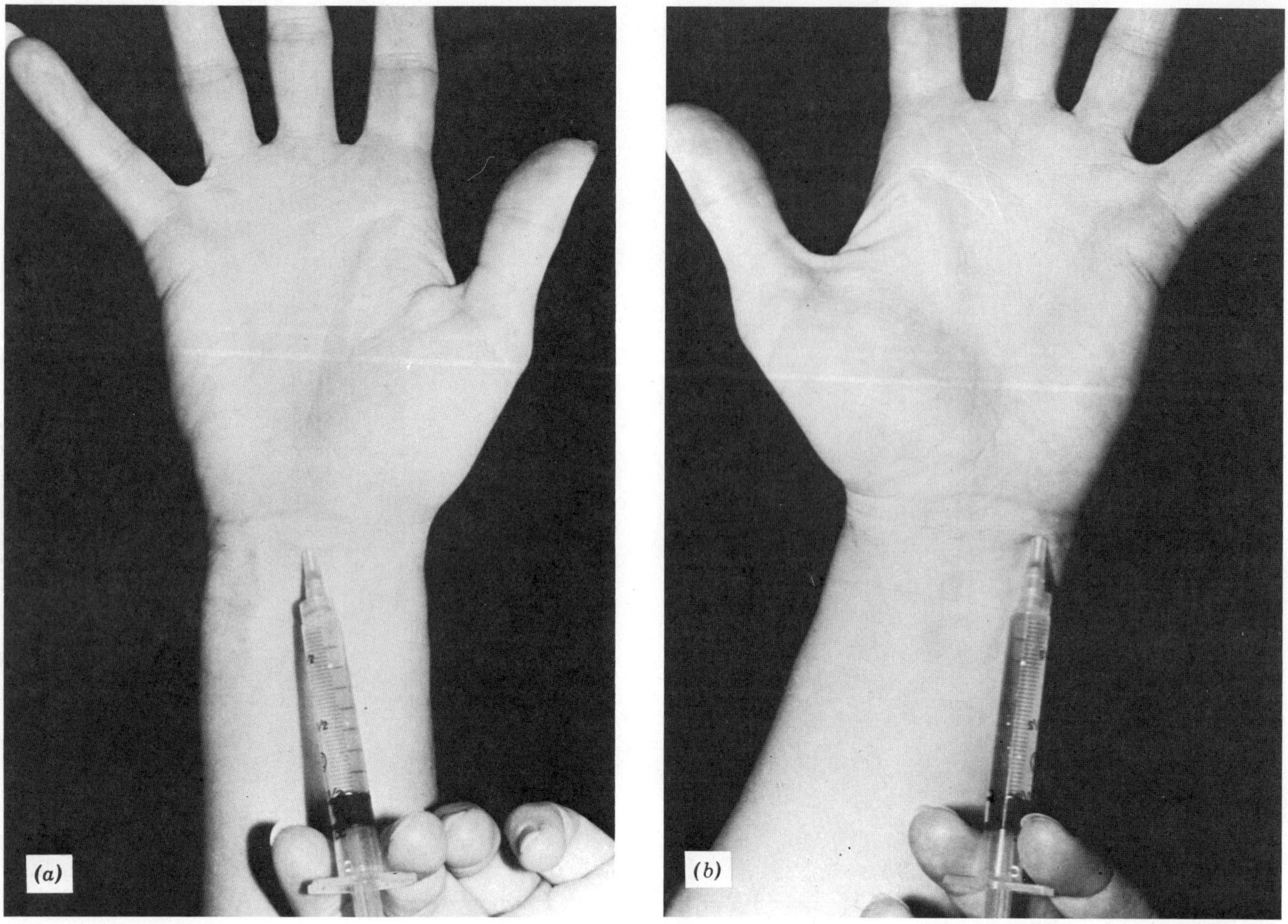

Fig. 67-29. Peripheral nerve block technique. (*a*) Site of needle insertion for median nerve block at the wrist. (*b*) Site of injection for ulnar nerve block at the wrist. (*c*) Site of needle insertion for radial nerve block at the wrist. Note the proximal injection to block the main branch of the superficial nerve as well as its branches (see Fig. 67-18).

For the fingers, the metacarpal or web space block is done by injecting 2 to 3 mm 1% or 2% lidocaine (Xylocaine) without epinephrine or 1.5% or 2% mepivacaine (Carbocaine) into the web space between the fingers through the thin dorsal skin using a 5/8-in. 25-gauge needle (Fig. 67-28). The 5/8-in. needle inserted to its hub and aimed volarward places the anesthetic solution in the proper location to achieve nerve blockade without the risk of neurovascular compression. Two separate injections are required since both the ulnar side and the radial side nerves for each digit must be blocked to obtain complete anesthesia. In the thumb, the digital nerves are more anterior and the block can be administered with a single subcutaneous injection through the volar skin with the needle held parallel to the volar aspect of the thumb at the level of the MP joint flexion crease, as shown in Fig. 67-28. Lidocaine has a rapid onset and provides anesthesia for 30 to 45 minutes. Mepivacaine also has a rapid onset, but its effect lasts for two to three hours. The increased duration of action of mepivacaine may be an advantage in the emergency department setting. Epinephrine-containing anesthetic solutions are not used in the digits because of the risk of ischemia from contraction of the terminal vessels.

Peripheral Nerve Block

If multiple fingers must be anesthetized, peripheral nerve block may be more satisfactory than multiple digital blocks. Two percent lidocaine should be used since lower concentrations often are not effective in blocking large-diameter nerves. The median, ulnar, and radial nerves can be blocked at the wrist (Fig. 67-29).

The *median nerve* lies directly underneath the deep fascia beneath the palmaris longus tendon. A 25-gauge needle is inserted through the skin directly overlying the tendon and advanced through the fascia. If this results in paresthesias, the tip of the needle should be withdrawn slightly before injection of 1 ml plain lidocaine. This technique usually, but not always, provides satisfactory anesthesia in the thumb, index, and long fingers. If anesthesia is incomplete, it can be supplemented using the digital block technique described previously.

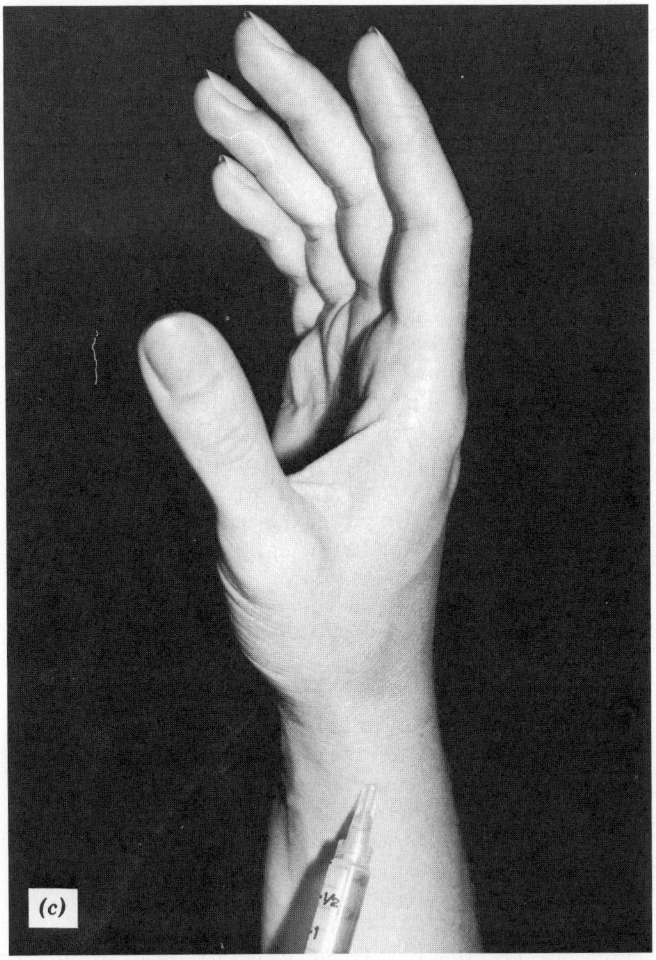

Fig. 67-29. (continued)

The *ulnar nerve* can be blocked at either the wrist or the elbow to provide anesthesia of the ring and small fingers. The ulnar nerve lies just beneath and parallel to the flexor carpi ulnaris tendon. The tissue adjacent to the nerve is infiltrated as described previously, using the palpable flexor carpi ulnaris as the landmark. The nerve also can be blocked at the elbow, where it is palpable in its groove in the medial epicondyle.

The *sensory branch of the radial nerve* divides into several small branches at the wrist. These can be blocked by the subcutaneous infiltration of 1% lidocaine in the region of the radial styloid. However, a median nerve block must be done to provide complete anesthesia of the digits supplied by this nerve.

SPECIAL PROCEDURES

Removal of Fishhooks

The skin surrounding the fishhook should be cleaned. Anesthesia is obtained either with local infiltration or digital block. The hook is then grasped with a plier or needle holder and advanced until the barb end protrudes through the skin at a point separate from that of the entrance wound. The barb is cut off with a wire cutter and the remainder of the hook backed out of the wound. If the hook is too deeply embedded or is embedded in an area adjacent to vital structures, such as the neurovascular bundle, surgical excision of the hook may be required. Prophylactic antibiotics are used because of the contaminated nature of the wound.

Removal of Rings

If finger swelling is minimal and there is no damage to the digit, a ring often can be removed by lubricating the finger with a solution of detergent and water and sliding the ring distally with a twisting motion. If finger swelling is moderate and the method just described does not work, the finger can be wrapped tightly with ¼-in.-wide umbilical tape to compress the soft tissues from distal to proximal. The tape is pulled beneath the ring with a small curved hemostat. The tape then is unwound from proximal to distal, sliding the ring with it. If there is vascular compromise or an open wound, if time is of the essence, or if excessive swelling precludes the use of other methods, the ring should be cut with a commercially available ring cutter and removed.

SELECTED READING

American Society for Surgery of the Hand. *The Hand—Examination and Diagnosis* (2nd ed). New York: Churchill Livingstone, 1983.

American Society for Surgery of the Hand. *The Hand—Primary Care of Common Problems.* Aurora, CO: American Society for Surgery of the Hand, 1985.

Buck-Gramcko, D, Hoffmann, R, and Neumann, R. *Hand Trauma—A Practical Guide.* New York: Thieme, 1986.

Flatt, A E. *The Care of Minor Hand Injuries* (4th ed). St. Louis: Mosby, 1979.

Lister, G. *The Hand: Diagnosis and Indications.* Edinburgh: Churchill Livingstone, 1984.

Milford, L. *The Hand* (2nd ed). St. Louis: Mosby, 1988.

Mittelbach, H R. *The Injured Hand.* New York: Springer-Verlag, 1979.

Romanes, G J. *Cunningham's Manual of Practical Anatomy* (14th ed). London: Oxford University Press, 1976.

Weeks, P M, and Wray, R C. *Management of Acute Hand Injuries—A Biological Approach* (2nd ed). St. Louis: Mosby, 1978.

68. Fractures of the Pelvis

Roger H. Emerson
David W. Lhowe

Pelvic fractures occur in three very distinct patient populations. The first (and largest) group is the elderly, who sustain pelvic fractures in the course of falls, usually minor in nature. Fortunately, this type of fracture has a good prognosis and a return to baseline function can be expected. However, pelvic fractures (or, more accurately, the unexplained falls that often cause them) may have prognostic significance in a frail patient. The occurrence of a pelvic fracture can mark the onset of a progressive physical deterioration, resulting in death within weeks to months, usually for reasons unrelated to the fracture itself.

The second group, relatively small in comparison to the elderly, is the young athletic population. Individuals in this group often have pain about the ischial tuberosity or anterior inferior spine of the pelvis. The history may disclose either a single abrupt injury or a pattern of chronic overuse. The fracture pattern is one of avulsion of bone from the pelvis, produced by muscle tension forces.

The third group is the smallest in size but by far the most challenging for the emergency physician. This group consists of individuals who sustain high-energy trauma, most commonly from motor vehicle accidents, with falls from heights the next most common cause. Crush injury in the industrial setting also occasionally occurs. Pelvic fractures in this setting are major in nature and occur most commonly as one part of a constellation of severe bone and soft-tissue injuries.

FUNCTIONAL ANATOMY

From a clinical standpoint, the pelvis should be thought of as two hemipelvis components connected posteriorly through the sacrum and anteriorly by the pubic symphysis. Posteriorly, there are two articulations, the sacroiliac joints. Anteriorly, there is a single pubic symphysis (Fig. 68-1).

The rigid bony pelvis provides a solid foundation for sitting as well as standing and walking. The symmetry of the ischial tuberosities and sacrum is responsible for comfort in the sitting position. Pelvic deformities affect leg length and hip alignment, especially rotation, and can have a marked effect on gait.

Weight-bearing forces are transmitted down the spine and pass through the sacrum across the pelvis to the hip joints and into the lower extremities. In other words, the major forces are posteriorly oriented across the pelvis and the posterior structures (both bony and ligamentous) are accordingly stouter than the anterior structures in the pelvic ring. Forces that are capable of disrupting posterior pelvic anatomy will necessarily be greater than forces capable of only anterior disruption. It follows, therefore, that the posterior pelvic disruptions are the ones most likely to be associated with other major injuries.

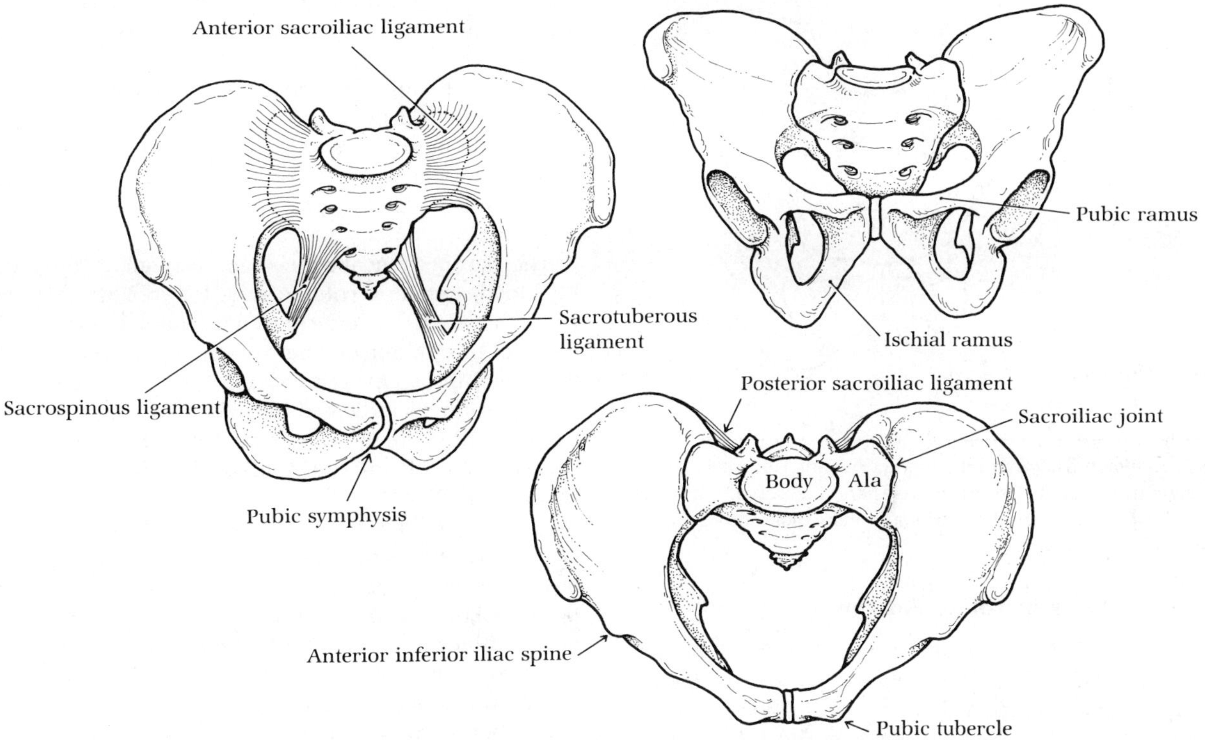

Fig. 68-1. Bony and ligamentous anatomy of the pelvis. The pelvis is seen in three projections. Note particularly the ligamentous structures that stabilize the posterior portion of the pelvis: the anterior and posterior sacroiliac, sacrospinous, and sacrotuberous ligaments.

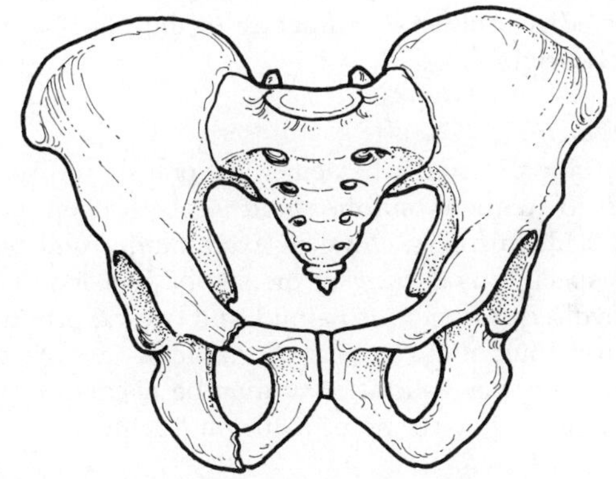

Fig. 68-2. Nondisplaced pelvic ramus fractures.

It may come as a surprise to learn that the stability of the pelvis is largely due to ligamentous supports rather than a complete bony ring (see Fig. 68-1). In the presence of a major ligamentous disruption, even without fracture, the stability of the pelvis is lost. Analysis of pelvic injury is based on the realization that any ring structure must be interrupted in two places, usually anteriorly and posteriorly. In minor pelvic fractures, the visible injuries are anterior and the posterior disruption is typically ligamentous and of such a minor degree as to be invisible on plain radiographs. The nature of the posterior disruption varies but in postmortem studies, a vertical fracture of the sacrum or disruption of the sacroiliac ligaments was the injury pattern most frequently encountered.

MINOR PELVIC INJURIES

Osteopenic Fractures in Elderly Patients

Osteopenic fractures are commonly seen, usually shortly after a minor fall. If the fall is unexplained, a syncopal episode must be ruled out and further evaluation may be indicated, either immediately or on an outpatient basis.

Evaluation

The physical examination will usually disclose tenderness but no instability of the pelvis—that is, the two iliac wings will appear symmetric and cannot be moved relative to each other. Most fractures occur anteriorly and involve either the pubic or ischial ramus, and sometimes both (Fig. 68-2). Posterior tenderness, unless from a soft-tissue contusion, is rare. X-rays are usually diagnostic, and bone scans or tomograms are rarely required.

Treatment

Symptomatic treatment is indicated, with weight-bearing as tolerated. Hospitalization is often needed for the frail, dehydrated, or socially isolated individual, usually to ensure that self-care needs are being addressed. Analgesia may be required but should be used with extreme caution in these patients. Although severe hemorrhage does not occur, the fractured bone surfaces can ooze sufficiently to cause hypotension, particularly if patients are not adequately hydrated. Ambulation is best started early to avoid the complications of prolonged bed rest.

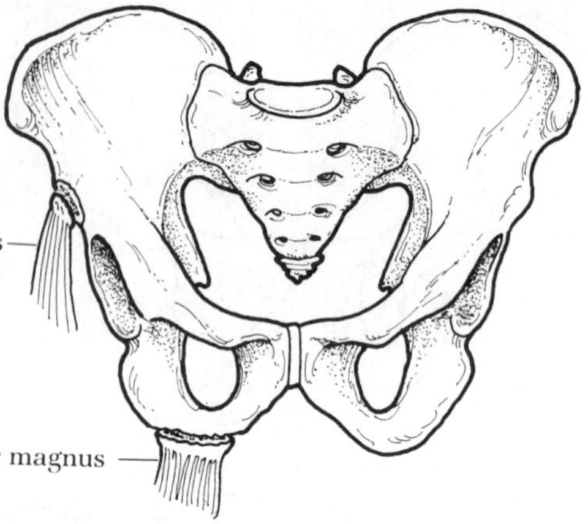

Fig. 68-3. Avulsion fracture of the pelvis. The anterior inferior iliac spine (origin of the rectus femoris muscle) and the ischial tuberosity (origin of the adductors and hamstrings) are the most common sites for these avulsion fractures.

Avulsion Fractures in Young Patients

Athletic individuals with pain and tenderness about the pelvis, usually following forceful or repetitive flexion-extension of the hip, should be suspected of having avulsion fractures. The most common locations are the anterior inferior iliac spine (origin of the rectus femoris muscle) and the ischial tuberosities (origin of the hamstrings) (Fig. 68-3). The mechanism is one of an avulsion force, occurring either once or repeatedly, producing a fracture of the pelvis at the site of muscle origin.

Evaluation

The history will usually be acute, but one should pay close attention to frequent, subthreshold stresses, such as might be seen with hurdlers. Physical examination will typically disclose specific tenderness at the site of avulsion. Traction on the avulsed fragment is painful and can be produced by gentle stretching of the suspected muscle. X-rays are usually diagnostic, but an oblique view may be needed, especially for the anterior inferior spine avulsion fractures.

Treatment

Symptomatic treatment is recommended. Specifically, crutches should be used if ambulation is painful, until weight-bearing can be tolerated. Avoidance of the offending or similar activity is advised for six weeks. Follow-up examination is recommended within 7 to 10 days, and symptoms are usually much improved by that time.

MAJOR PELVIC INJURIES

Severe pelvic fractures are high-energy injuries, commonly from motor vehicle accidents or falls from a height. The significance of severe pelvic fractures comes from the high mortality of injuries associated with them, estimated at 10 percent when the fractures are closed and as high as 40 percent when they are open. The discrepancy in mortality between closed and open pelvic fractures is due to the increased number of associated injuries present in open fractures, since the energy required to produce an open pelvic fracture is greater than that required for a closed fracture, and the number of associated injuries is correspondingly higher.

The major causes of mortality for patients with pelvic fractures are central nervous system (CNS) injury and hemorrhage. CNS injury is usually recognized early and neurosurgical consultation is appropriately obtained. Management of hemorrhage is usually the responsibility of the emergency physician.

The retroperitoneal space can accommodate up to 4,000 ml blood, and this volume may be even greater once the pelvis is widened by a displaced fracture. The most common cause of bleeding is oozing from open cancellous bone surfaces, and torn veins but major arterial bleeding can occur. Arteriography is indicated in cases in which blood loss cannot be controlled. Arteries commonly involved include the superior gluteal, internal pudendal, obturator, and lateral sacral (Fig. 68-4).

Apart from CNS injury and hemorrhage, injuries to the musculoskeletal system, thorax, and abdomen are commonly present. The urinary tract is of particular concern in pelvic fractures and disruption of the urethra, bladder, ureter, or kidney can occur. Loss of lumbosacral nerve function needs to be looked for, particularly where posterior pelvic disruption is substantial and compromises the adjacent nerve roots or plexuses.

Evaluation

In the emergency department, the presence of life-threatening head injury, thoracoabdominal trauma, or exsanguination will direct the investigation appropriately. Pelvic fractures are frequently passed by on the initial patient survey, since the associated deformity may be well disguised by the overlying soft tissues. Further, more obvious injuries will demand the immediate attention of the emergency physician.

Patients will usually complain of pelvic pain, which can be referred to the groin or buttock regions. Localized tenderness is usually present. The emergency physician must keep in mind the possibility of hip dislocation and femoral neck fracture in addition to pelvic disruption.

Abdominal examination is mandatory in major pelvic fractures, and evidence of intraabdominal hemorrhage should be carefully sought. The accuracy of peritoneal lavage is limited in the presence of pelvic fracture, since the fracture itself can produce an elevated red cell count in the lavage fluid. Gross blood, however, is *not* typically the result of pelvic fracture alone.

On examination of the pelvis, areas of swelling, asymmetry, and ecchymosis should be sought. The iliac wing, pubis, and sacroiliac (SI) joints should be gently palpated for instability or crepitus. The perineum must be inspected since this is the location where most of the open fractures will penetrate the skin. With severe pelvic fractures, especially when involving displaced rami or a vertical shear pattern, a pelvic examination should be performed, and blood in the vagina should lead to a careful examination for mucosal tear by fracture fragments. The urethral meatus should be inspected for signs of blood and the bladder palpated for evidence of gross distention, with either finding strongly suggestive of urethral injury. All patients should undergo rectal examination, looking for an elevated, "floating" prostate in men.

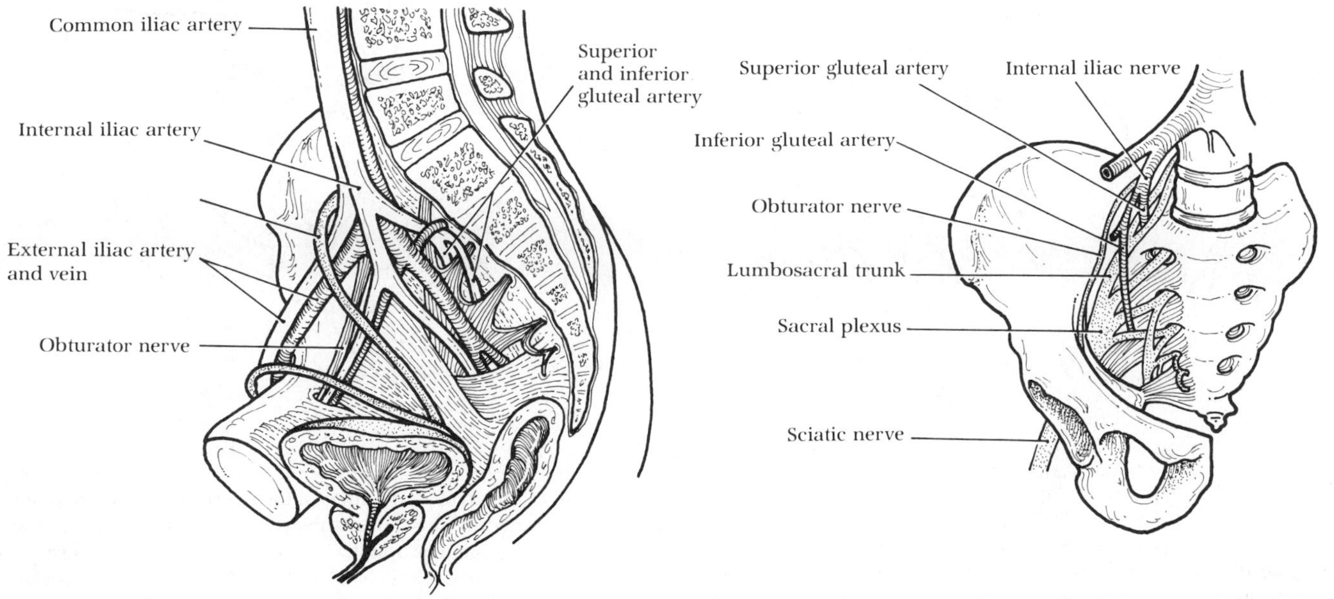

Fig. 68-4. Major pelvic neurovascular structures. The sacral nerve roots and plexus are located just anterior to the lateral sacrum and sacroiliac joint region. With posterior pelvic disruption or fracture, these nerves can sustain either traction injury or outright avulsion.

Neurologic evaluation of the lower extremities is important if posterior disruption occurs, since the lumbosacral plexus can be injured. It is very helpful to know if the neurologic deficit was present at the time of arrival in the emergency department or whether it developed afterward. The most common deficit is that of the L5 nerve root, which is indicated by weakened dorsiflexion of the ankle and great toe, or decreased sensation along the lateral calf and dorsum of the foot.

Urinary bladder catheterization should *not* be performed if there is any sign of urethral injury: blood at the meatus, gross hematuria, distended blader with inability to void, or a floating prostate in male patients. If any of these signs is present, a retrograde urethrogram needs to be performed *before* catheterization is attempted. A common technique is to place a urinary catheter in the meatus and to inject a contrast agent, followed immediately by an anteroposterior (AP) x-ray. If contrast agent is seen flowing into the bladder without extravasation, the catheter can then be advanced.

Radiographic Evaluation

An AP view of the pelvis must be included with the lateral cervical spine and AP chest x-ray for all multiply traumatized patients. In cases in which urethral injury is suspected, the AP pelvic view can be taken immediately after the urethra is injected with contrast medium. A more complete radiographic examination of the pelvis includes the AP view combined with 45-degree inlet and outlet views (Fig. 68-5). The patient does not have to be moved for this series of films as they can be obtained by simply angling the x-ray tube. The inlet view provides more information about the integrity of the SI joints and any rotational deformity of the pelvic ring. The outlet view displays the sacrum and particularly highlights any vertical fracture displacement (shear) that has

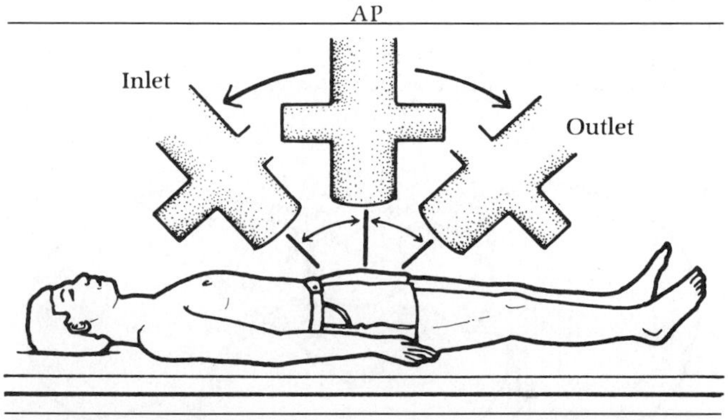

Fig. 68-5. Orientation of x-ray beam for inlet, AP, and outlet views of the pelvis.

occurred posteriorly. Computed tomographic (CT) scanning of the pelvis is not necessary at the time of initial management but can be obtained subsequently. It is particularly helpful in determining the extent of posterior injury when physical examination and plain radiographs are not conclusive.

Three fracture patterns are typically seen in major pelvic injuries. The AP compression fracture is the result of compression that is usually delivered anteriorly, with a typical pattern of a widened symphysis pubis, an "open book" fracture (Fig. 68-6). The second pattern is due to lateral compression and, as suggested, results from a blow delivered from the side, as might be expected when an automobile passenger is struck from the side as his or her vehicle door is caved in by an oncoming car. The radiographic pattern is that of an inward rotation of either hemipelvis, usually associated with several ramus fractures (Fig. 68-7). The third (and most unstable) type is that of the vertical shear pattern (Fig. 68-8). This pattern is recognized by superior displacement of either hemipelvis and requires both posterior and anterior disruption, caused by a vertical shear force.

After considering the physical examination findings and evaluation of radiographs, taking into consideration the type

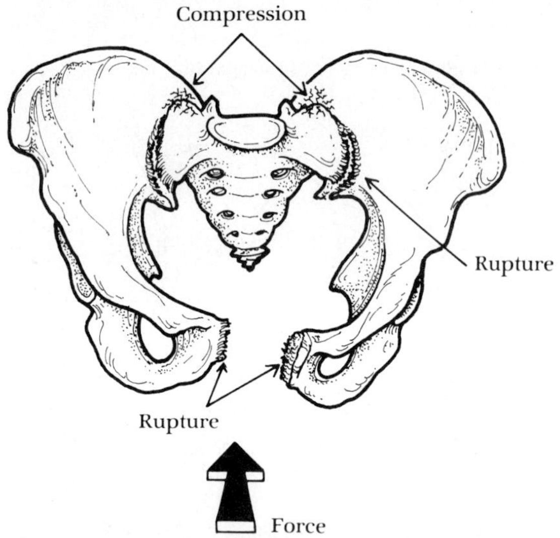

Fig. 68-6. "Open book" fracture pattern. These pelvic fractures are usually the result of anterior-posterior compression force, delivered as indicated by the arrow. The typical pattern results in either a diastasis of the symphysis pubis, as shown, or displaced fractures of the pubic rami. Posteriorly, there is usually rupture of the anterior sacroiliac ligaments with compression posteriorly, typically sparing injury of the posterior sacroiliac ligaments.

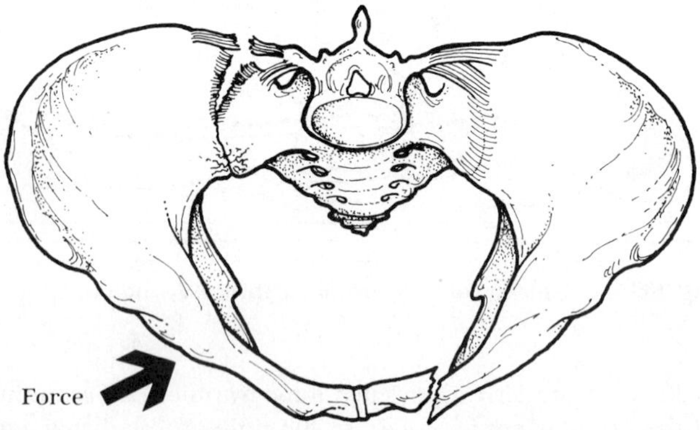

Fig. 68-7. Lateral compression fracture of the pelvis. In this fracture pattern the force is delivered from the lateral aspect, as might be expected when an automobile passenger sustains the force of an oncoming car striking his or her vehicle door. There is relative inward rotation of the affected hemipelvis, resulting in ramus fractures and ligamentous disruption of the sacroiliac joint, usually involving the posterior sacroiliac ligaments. This fracture pattern may be stable or unstable, depending on the amount of posterior pelvic disruption that has occurred.

of injury sustained, the emergency physician must decide whether the fracture pattern is stable. As a general rule, displaced fracture patterns are more unstable than undisplaced patterns. Although gross bony disruption can be seen in the form of displaced fracture fragments, ligamentous disruption may not be so obvious. A subtle sign of severe ligamentous disruption, in the absence of gross deformity, is an avulsion fracture of the ischial spine or the transverse processes of L5. Such avulsion fractures do not occur without substantial forces, usually directed in a vertical shear pattern.

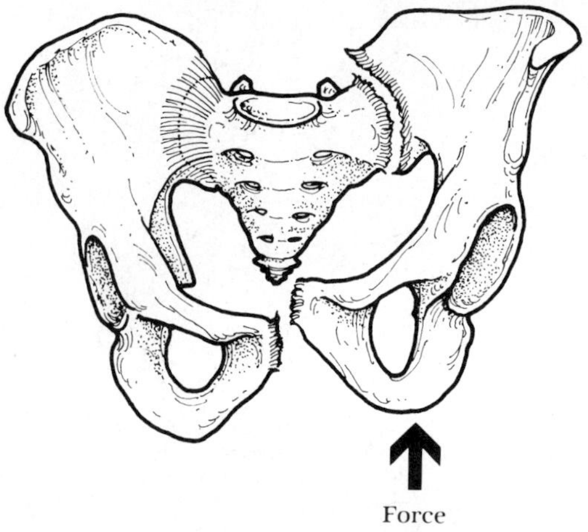

Fig. 68-8. Vertical shear fracture of the pelvis. This fracture pattern is characterized by superior displacement of either hemipelvis and requires substantial disruptions both anteriorly and posteriorly. The direction of the injury force is usually vertical, resulting in a shearing of one hemipelvis against the other. This fracture represents the most unstable pattern, and operative fixation is frequently indicated.

By pattern, AP compression and lateral compression injuries may or may not be unstable. The accepted threshold for AP compression instability is more than 2.5 cm of widening at the pubic symphysis. Widening of the symphysis beyond this threshold implies a significant posterior disruption. In lateral compression pattern injuries, the guidelines are less clear, but the amount of internal rotation of the affected hemipelvis will correlate with the amount of posterior ligamentous disruption of the corresponding SI joint. Vertical shear fracture patterns are all unstable and consist of a posterior disruption (either SI joint dislocation, posterior ilium fracture, or sacral fracture) combined with a vertical or posterior displacement.

Treatment

Due to the magnitude of force necessary to produce a major pelvic frature, it should be assumed that these patients have multiple injuries and will need a systematic evaluation of each organ system before one embarks on treatment of the pelvic fracture alone. A large transfusion requirement should be anticipated. These patients should be moved only with extreme care to minimize both discomfort and further bleeding, since motion of the fracture surfaces tends to dislodge clot and produce another large episode of bleeding from bone surfaces or vascular lumina. A transfusion requirement beyond five to six units is ominous and usually represents severe ongoing bleeding. Immediate management of this rapid hemorrhage can be produced with full MAST trousers, which tend to both stabilize the fracture and produce decreased intrapelvic volume, thereby having a tamponade effect on the bleeding sites.

In the presence of significant bleeding from pelvic fracture, three options for control exist. One is formal open exposure and control of the bleeding vessel, presumably after radiographic localization. Another is arterial embolization under radiographic control. The third method is reduction of the pelvic disruption and stabilization by means of an

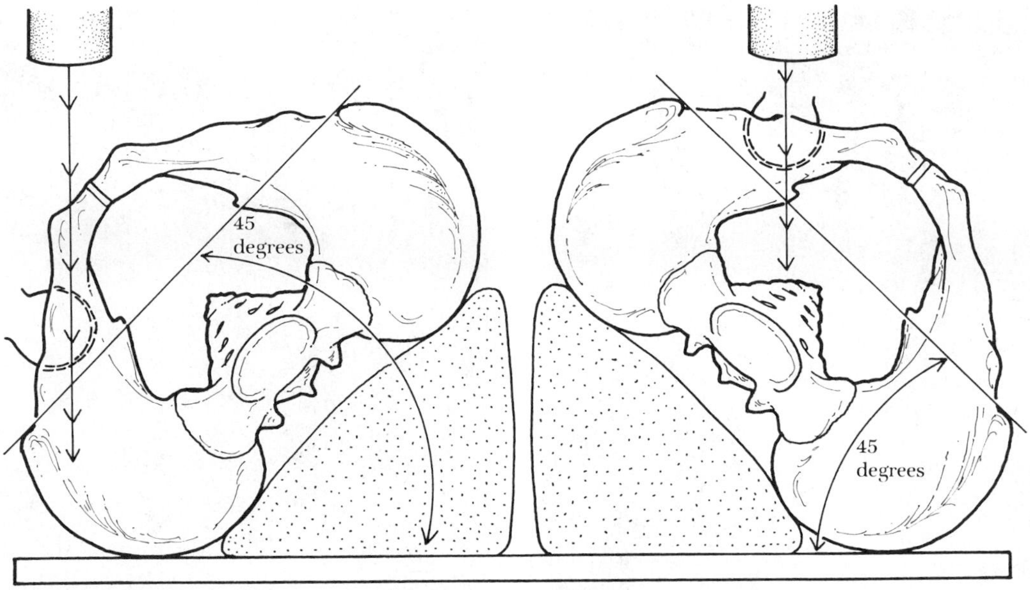

Fig. 68-9. Position of the pelvis for Judet views of the acetabulum. By obtaining oblique views of the acetabulum, it is possible to isolate more accurately the region of bony disruption. The iliac oblique view will show the posterior column of the acetabulum in relief by moving it away from the anterior column and femoral head. Similarly, the obturator oblique view allows the anterior column to be more clearly visualized (see Fig. 68-10).

external frame. Certain fracture patterns, such as the stable AP compression injury and many lateral compression injuries, can be adequately reduced and stabilized with an anterior frame. However, with significant posterior displacement, a simple anterior frame may be insufficient for full control of the disrupted pelvic ring. There is value in applying an anterior frame, even in this setting, since the fracture can be grossly controlled, the pelvic volume reduced, and ongoing bleeding from vessel and bone surfaces decreased. The time required to place such a frame is usually less than one hour, and the ability of the orthopedist to place it is usually dictated by the overall status of the patient. If significant posterior instability remains, it is usually addressed in the subacute period, after major bleeding has been controlled and the patient's overall clinical status has stabilized.

FRACTURES OF THE ACETABULUM

Fractures of the acetabulum may be seen in combination with major pelvic disruptions, although they are more typically found as isolated fractures or in combination with another lower-extremity fracture. The mechanism is usually a motor vehicle accident, although falls from heights are also responsible. A typical motor vehicle setting is a fracture of the posterior wall of the acetabulum in combination with a patellar or tibial plateau fracture. The sequence of events is that of the unrestrained front seat passenger being thrown forward, striking the dashboard with the knee. The force is then transmitted up the femoral shaft with sufficient magnitude to drive the femoral head against the back wall of the acetabulum. Depending on the direction of the force transmitted by the femur, the femoral head can either dislocate without fracture, fracture the posterior acetabular wall, or be driven through the medial wall of the acetabulum, coming to rest inside the pelvis.

Evaluation

Patients with acetabular fractures will complain of pain in the groin or buttock and be reluctant to move the hip. One should look closely for signs of injury about the knee, which indicate that force was delivered there while the patient was in the seated position. The hip will be held internally or externally rotated if the head has been displaced out of the acetabulum. Sciatic nerve function must be assessed, since injuries of this structure are common, particularly with posterior acetabular fractures.

A single AP view of the pelvis will usually disclose that the acetabulum has been disrupted. One should look for loss of congruence of the hip socket or any displacement of the femoral head relative to the acetabulum. The most complete information is obtained from Judet views (45-degree oblique views) (Figs. 68-9 and 68-10). The AP and Judet views can give a complete picture of the acetabular fracture and will define it as basically an anterior or posterior pattern. Injuries to both the anterior and posterior columns can occur but are less common. CT scanning may show loose fragments of bone within the joint and disclose otherwise unrecognized injuries such as nondisplaced femoral head fractures. The use of CT scans is now standard practice for evaluation of acetabular fractures (Fig. 68-11).

Treatment

When the acetabular fracture presents as an isolated injury, accurate diagnosis is essential, particularly recognition of persisting femoral head dislocation. If present, this will require emergent reduction to prevent an increased incidence

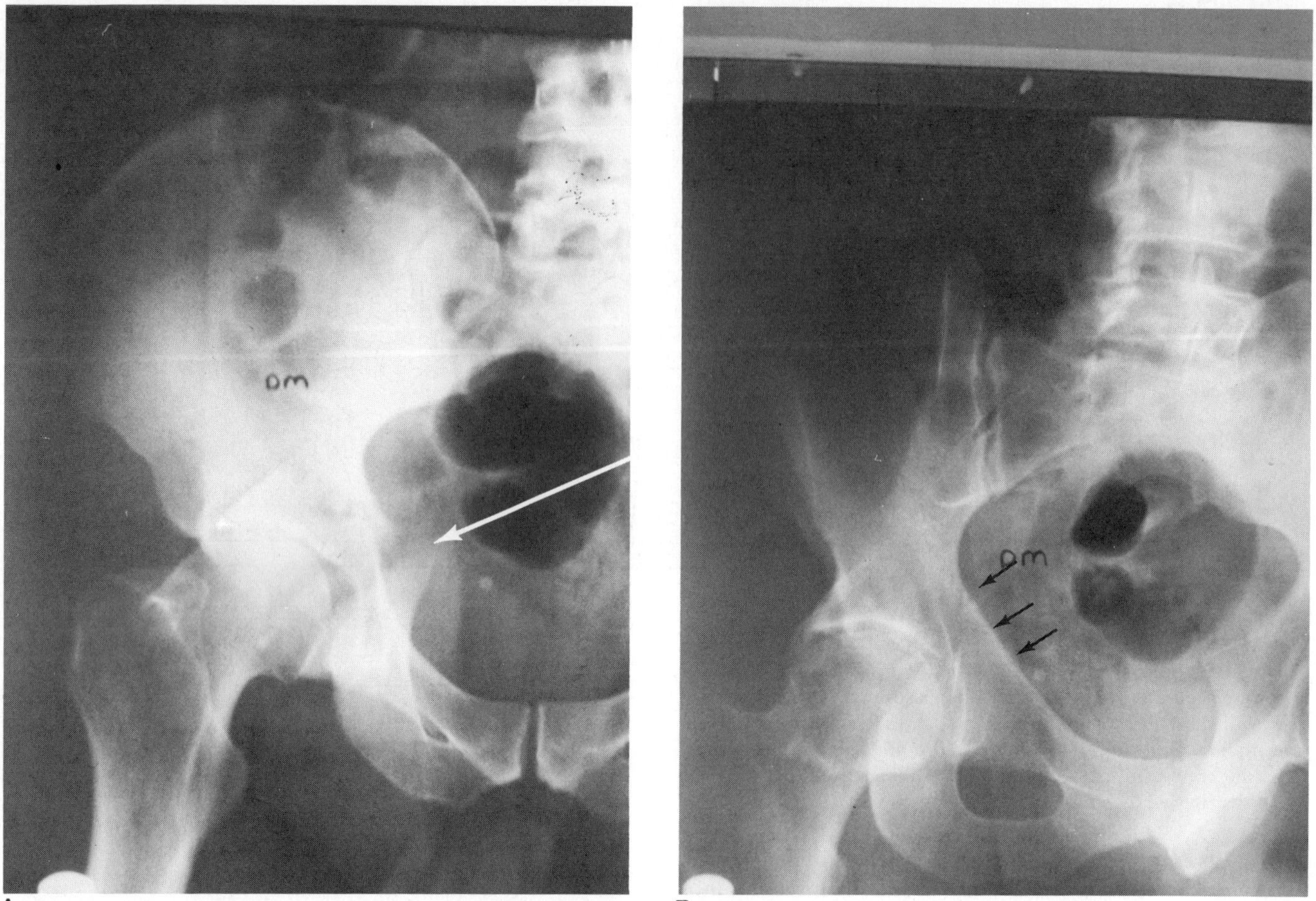

A B

Fig. 68-10. A. Iliac oblique view of a 39-year-old man with a right acetabular fracture involving the posterior column. Note the disruption seen in this iliac oblique view, which allows the posterior column to be visualized medial to the acetabulum itself (*arrow*). B. Obturator oblique view of the same patient. Note how the anterior column is well visualized and without fracture (*arrows*).

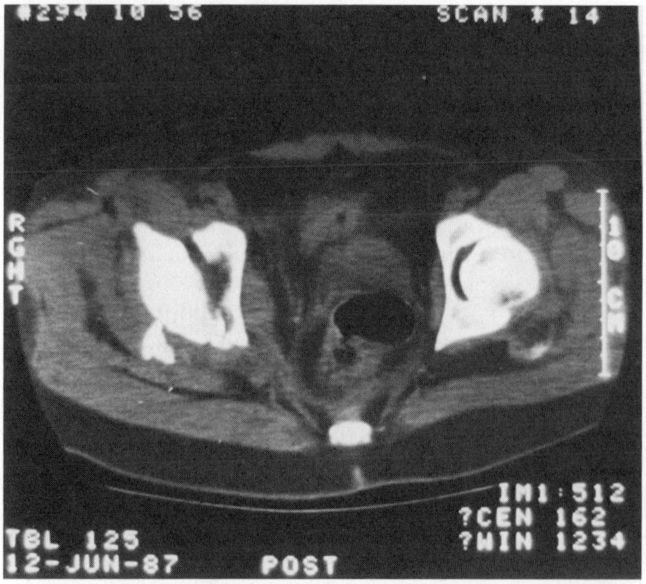

Fig. 68-11. Computed tomographic scan of right acetabular fracture. This scan is made through the acetabular dome on the right, slightly lower on the left. Note the fracture extending through the right acetabulum from anterior to posterior, showing approximately 1 cm of displacement through the weight-bearing dome of the acetabulum.

of osteonecrosis of the femoral head. Acetabular fractures all require hospital admission for either bed rest or operative treatment. The fracture pattern and patient's age will usually dictate the type of treatment rendered.

In a multiply injured patient, the acetabular fracture naturally receives less attention. This is generally unavoidable, but two situations merit more emergent treatment. The most critical is the dislocated femoral head, as noted previously. This should be reduced as soon as possible. The other circumstance is an intrapelvic position of the femoral head, such as occurs when the femoral head is driven through the medial wall of the acetabulum into the pelvis. This situation is rare but should be treated early with skeletal traction, since reduction is more easily obtained early than late.

SELECTED READING

Kane, WJ. Fractures of the Pelvis. In CA Rockwood and DP Green (eds), *Fractures in Adults* (2nd ed). Philadelphia: Lippincott, 1984. Pp 1093–1210.

Tile, M. Fractures of the pelvis. *J. Bone Joint Surg.* 70B:1–15, 1988.

69. Hip and Thigh Injuries

Stephen B. Trippel

Hip and thigh disorders that require emergency management can be broadly classified as traumatic or nontraumatic. The traumatic conditions are the more common and include fractures, dislocations, and soft-tissue injuries. However, a number of nontraumatic conditions may present acutely in the emergency setting. These include certain developmental, metabolic, and idiopathic abnormalities with which the emergency physician must be familiar. Although not injuries by the strictest definition, their clinical presentations can simulate those of traumatic conditions and are therefore appropriately discussed in this chapter.

FUNCTIONAL ANATOMY

The femur is the bone primarily involved in most hip and thigh injuries. Due to the exceptional variation in anatomy over its length from the hip to the knee, the femur is subject to a variety of injury patterns, each with its own mode of treatment. To permit hip motion, the femoral neck must be narrow and oriented at a specific angle to the femoral shaft (Fig. 69-1). The femur is prone to significant mineral loss during aging, and its neck is in the unfortunate position of bearing high levels of stress in a poorly coordinated fall. As a result, it is among the most commonly fractured bones of the body. By contrast, the femoral shaft, with its thick cortex and expansions proximally and distally, is normally resistant to all but high-energy trauma.

The muscles of the hip and thigh region are the most massive in the body and provide an element of protection against open injuries (Fig. 69-2). Compare this with the soft-tissue cuffs surrounding the tibia and it is easy to understand why the prevalence of open fractures of the femur is relatively low. Because of the substantial muscles that run the length of the femur, stabilization of femoral shaft fractures requires substantial traction force compared to that needed for tibial fractures.

The blood supply of the femur is extensive with the exception of the femoral head. The retinacular vessels that supply the femoral head are easily torn by a displaced fracture of the femoral neck. After infancy, these retinacular vessels provide the femoral head with most and, in some cases all, of its blood supply. If disrupted in the course of a fracture, the femoral head can undergo osteonecrosis and the fracture may fail to heal, with poor vascular supply contributing to both conditions.

The major vessels of the thigh, the femoral artery and vein, are relatively well protected within the anteromedial musculature. Perforating branches of the profunda femoris artery supply most of the quadriceps musculature and are responsible for the substantial blood loss often associated with femoral shaft and intertrochanteric hip fractures.

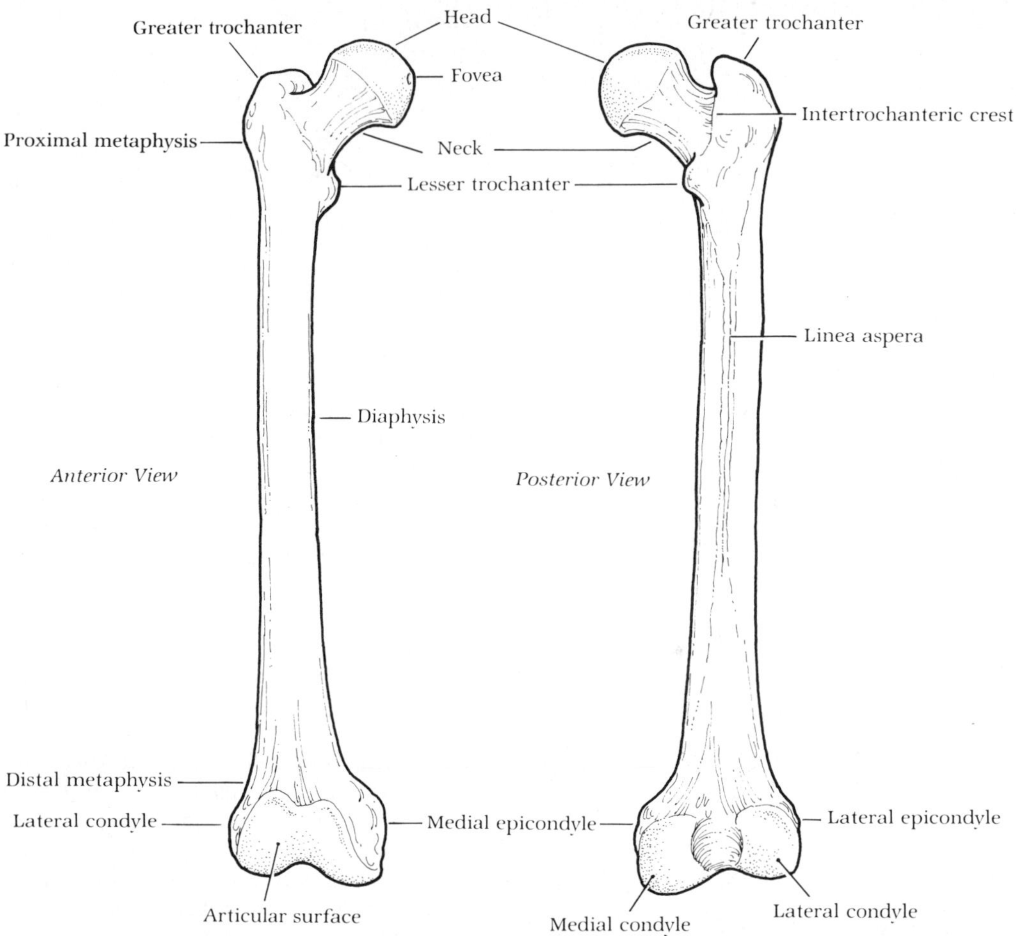

Fig. 69-1. Femur as viewed from anterior and posterior. Important bony landmarks are indicated. Note particularly the neck shaft angle, which ranges between 130 and 140 degrees in most individuals.

The sciatic nerve traverses the sciatic notch of the ilium and passes directly posterior to the hip joint, a vulnerable position in posterior hip dislocations and posteriorly displaced fractures (Fig. 69-3). For this reason, an assessment of the peroneal and tibial distributions of this nerve in any suspected injury of the hip is an important part of the emergency department evaluation. The other major nerve crossing the hip is the femoral nerve, which lies anteriorly and is occasionally injured with a femoral shaft fracture or anterior hip trauma.

FRACTURES

Fractures About the Hip

The term *hip fracture* is a misnomer since the hip joint itself is generally not involved. However, this term has become so widely accepted as denoting fractures of the femoral neck or intertrochanteric region that we continue this usage in the present chapter. Fractures of the acetabulum are discussed in Chap. 68.

Fractures of the hip can be classified as either subcapital (femoral neck) or intertrochanteric (Figs. 69-4 and 69-5). Although these two fracture patterns lie in close proximity to each other, their pathophysiology, treatment, and prognosis are very different. One reason for this is that femoral neck fractures are intracapsular and intertrochanteric fractures are extracapsular. While both fracture types interrupt the intraosseous blood supply to the proximal femur, intracapsular fractures may also disrupt the extraosseous blood supply to the femoral head and neck (Figs. 69-4 and 69-5). This loss of both the intraosseous and extraosseous blood supply is most likely to occur in displaced femoral neck fractures and effectively devascularizes the head-neck fragment. In this setting, the incidence of nonunion of the fracture or osteonecrosis of the femoral head with later collapse of the weight-bearing surface is increased (Fig. 69-6). In marked contrast, intertrochanteric fractures that occur through the thick cancellous bone, distal to the retinacular vessels, heal reliably and are rarely associated with osteonecrosis of the femoral head.

Both fracture patterns occur typically in elderly patients, with the mean age of intertrochanteric fractures being slightly higher than that of femoral neck fractures. Women are more commonly affected than men, probably reflecting a greater degree of osteoporosis and the prolonged life expectancy for women versus men. Both fracture types are

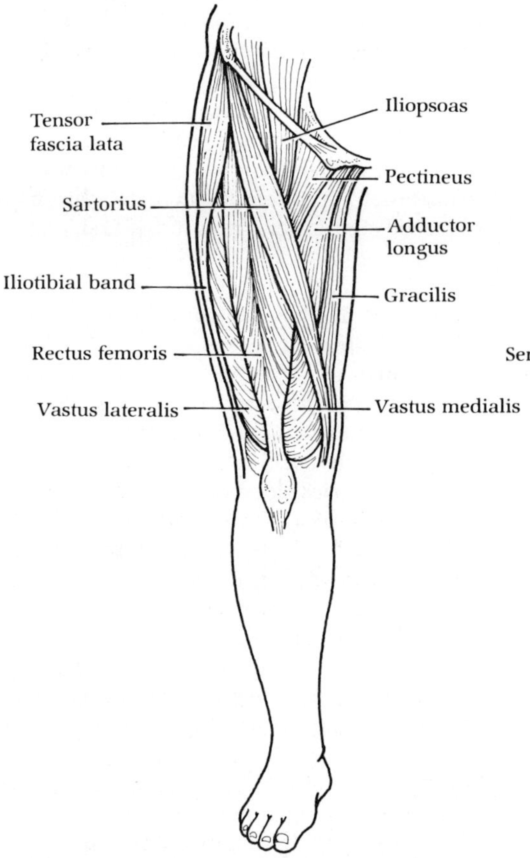

Fig. 69-2. Muscles of the hip-thigh as seen from anterior and posterior views. Not seen is the sciatic nerve, which lies deep to the biceps femoris.

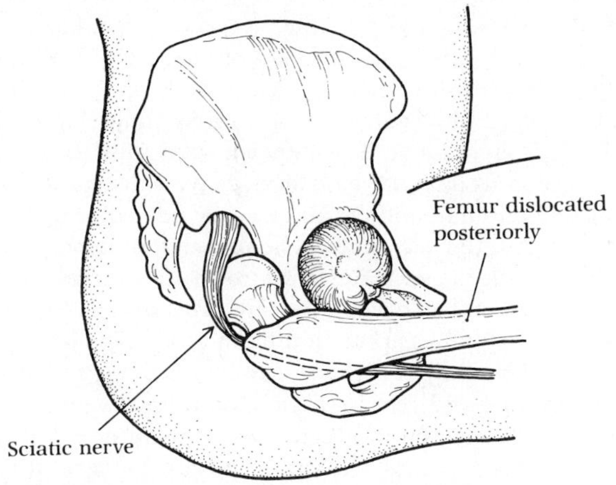

Fig. 69-3. Location of sciatic nerve. The sciatic nerve exits the pelvis through the sciatic notch and passes directly posterior to the hip joint. A posterior dislocation of the hip can place tension on the sciatic nerve, resulting in a partial or complete palsy.

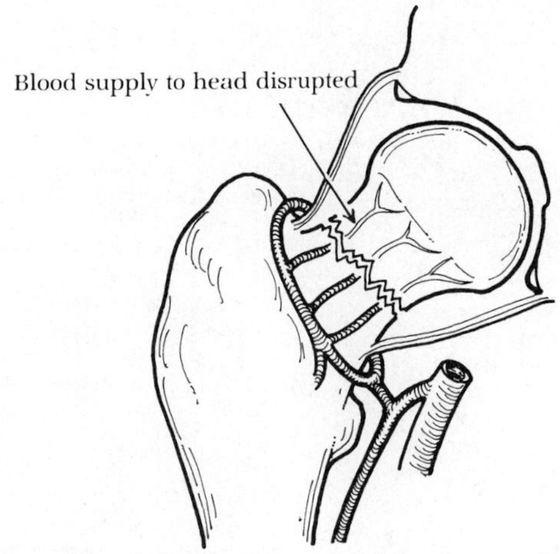

Fig. 69-4. Intracapsular hip fracture. Fractures that occur within the hip capsule (femoral neck fractures) have the potential to disrupt the blood supply to the femoral head through injury to the retinacular vessels, which course along the femoral neck. In general, the degree of injury to these vessels is proportional to the amount of displacement of the femoral neck fracture.

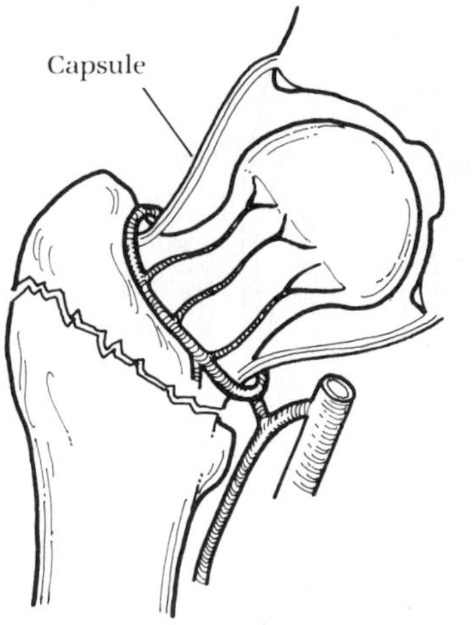

Fig. 69-5. Extracapsular hip fracture. In contrast to a femoral neck fracture, an intertrochanteric fracture does not disrupt the retinacular blood vessels. Osteonecrosis of the femoral head does not occur.

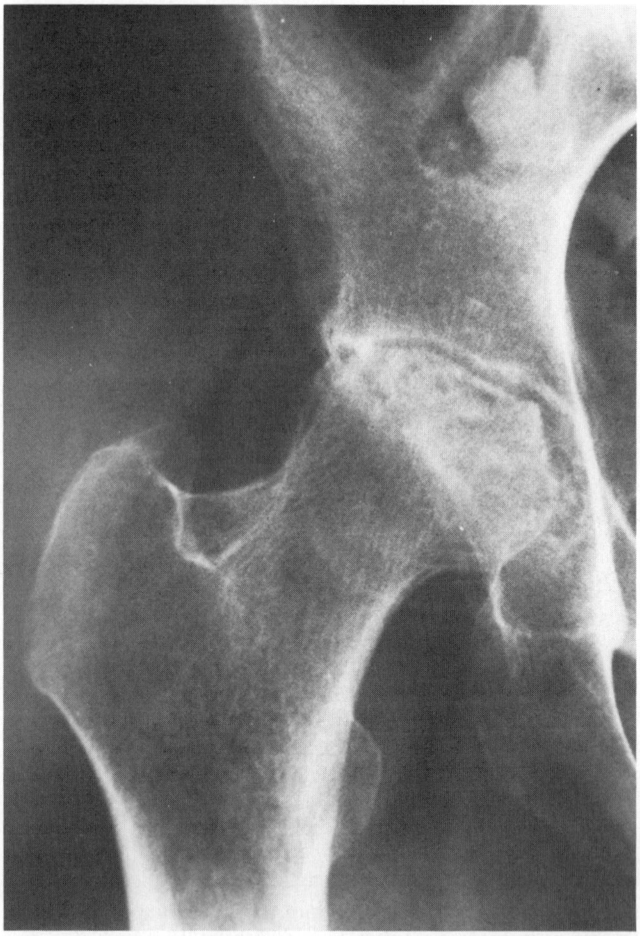

Fig. 69-6. Osteonecrosis of the femoral head. Radiograph demonstrating a typical pattern of osteonecrosis with collapse of the underlying bone, resulting in deformity of the articular surface, and secondary arthritic change.

usually sustained in falls, although it is possible that the proximal femur can simply fail under load during weight-bearing, with the fall being a secondary phenomenon rather than the causative injury.

Several studies have shown that hip fractures in the elderly are associated with a one-year mortality in the range of 25 percent, most often for reasons not directly related to the hip fracture itself. It is safe to say that a hip fracture is a poor prognostic sign in an aging individual.

Evaluation

Establishing the mechanism of injury is important in the initial evaluation of these patients. The elderly individual who stumbles on a rug and falls must be differentiated from the patient who sustains a transient loss of consciousness and falls. Similarly, a young adult with a hip fracture after a motor vehicle accident should be carefully evaluated for associated injuries since substantial force is required to generate this type of fracture in younger individuals. Fractures that occur in the presence of minimal trauma should raise the possibility of metastasic or metabolic bone disease. Stress fractures of the femoral neck, while unusual, do occur in younger individuals, particularly runners.

On examination, the patient is usually unable to walk or bear weight. Straight leg raising is generally painfully difficult if not impossible, and hip range of motion, even passive, is painful. Although intertrochanteric fractures and displaced femoral neck fractures may show shortening and external rotation of the limb, impacted and stress fractures will show little visible shortening on examination. Neurovascular status is usually intact but should be carefully checked for all patients with hip fractures. Patients with undisplaced, impacted, or stress fractures of the femoral neck may be remarkable for their absence of signs on examination and may require tomographic or nuclear medical imaging to be confirmed.

Radiographs include a standard anteroposterior (AP) view of the pelvis, including both hips and a true ("shoot-through") lateral view of the affected hip (Fig. 69-7). While displaced fractures of either type are easy to spot, nondisplaced fractures can be subtle in their radiographic appearance. The AP view alone is insufficient and must be augmented with a good quality lateral view, since posterior displacement and angulation can be easily missed or underestimated by the AP view alone. A helpful sign is incongruity in the head-neck curve (Fig. 69-8), seen in femoral neck fractures. Relative lucency in the intertrochanteric region may be the only radiographic finding in a nondisplaced intertrochanteric fracture. Early stress fractures may yield negative radiographs and require a bone scan for diagnosis.

A useful classification of femoral neck fracture is that of Garden (Fig. 69-9). Classification of intertrochanteric fractures is usually based on the number of "parts" (fracture segments) present—that is, two-part, three-part, or four-part (Fig. 69-10). Intertrochanteric fractures are also classified on the basis of intrinsic stability. Fractures that are minimally displaced, consist of a single fracture line, and show no change in the angulation between neck and shaft are considered stable fractures. Intertrochanteric fractures that consist of multiple displaced fragments or show varus angulation, or both, are unstable (Fig. 69-10).

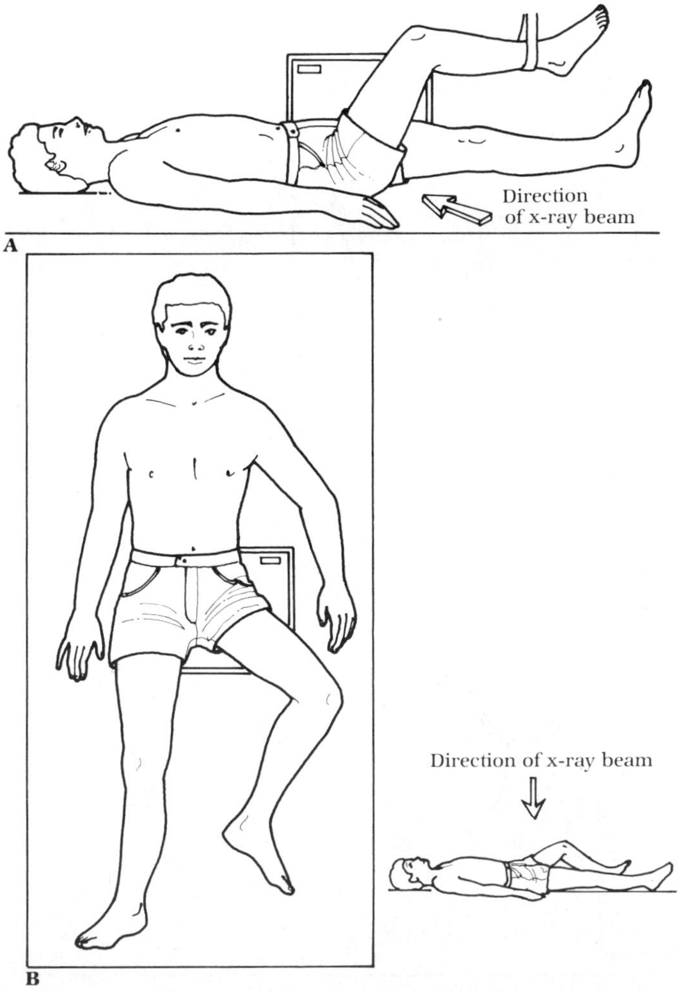

Fig. 69-7. Positioning of patient to obtain "true" lateral (A) and "frog" lateral (B) views of the left hip. Whenever possible, a "true" lateral view should be obtained. The "frog" lateral may be of further value, particularly in cases in which the diagnosis is in doubt.

In cases in which a hip fracture is suspected by the history and physical examination but is not seen on x-ray, further investigation is required. A technetium bone scan will usually become positive within 24 to 48 hours after fracture and should be ordered in cases in which plain radiographs do not support the clinical impression. In elderly patients the scan may remain negative until a week after trauma. It is important not to miss the diagnosis of a nondisplaced femoral neck or intertrochanteric fracture since the later displacement that often occurs usually creates a less favorable position and prognosis. If a technetium bone scan is not available, AP tomograms of the affected hip may help disclose a fracture line.

Treatment

In all cases, initial management consists of resting the limb and preventing further displacement of the fracture. This may be accomplished by applying a foam boot with 5 lbs. of traction through the foot and supporting the leg in pillow suspension (Fig. 69-11).

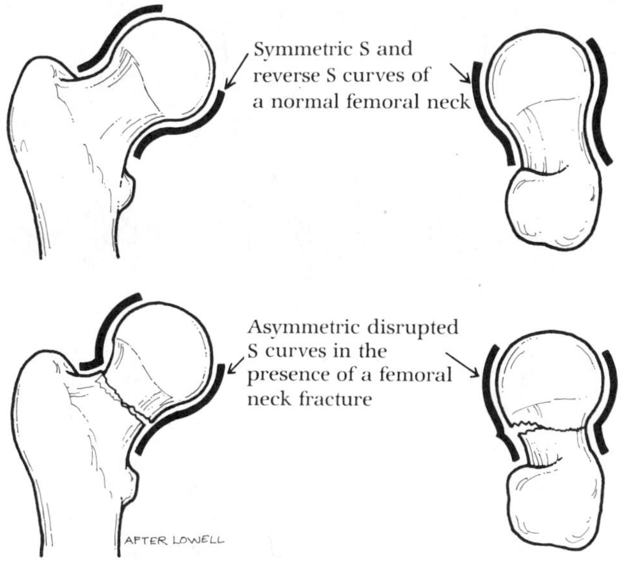

Fig. 69-8. Incongruity of head-neck curve in presence of hip fracture. For femoral neck fractures in particular, the diagnosis may be missed if the fracture is minimally angulated-displaced. Careful review of the AP and lateral x-rays will usually disclose a discontinuity in the curve of the head-neck region. (After J. D. Lowell. Results and complications of femoral neck fractures. *Clin. Orthop.* 152:162–172, 1980.)

For femoral neck fractures, definitive treatment will usually be surgical. For nondisplaced or minimally displaced femoral neck fractures (Garden I, II), internal fixation is typically recommended. For displaced femoral neck fractures (Garden III, IV), the fractured head-neck fragment is more often resected and replaced with a hemiarthoplasty such as an Austin Moore or bipolar endoprosthesis. The advantages of hemiarthoplasty are the avoidance of osteonecrosis and nonunion coupled with immediate mobility at near-full weight-bearing.

Younger individuals with displaced femoral neck fractures constitute the most controversial treatment group. Every effort should be made to retain the head-neck fragment whenever possible. It appears that, particularly in young patients, the risk of osteonecrosis and nonunion is decreased by early reduction and internal fixation. Such patients should be treated as true surgical emergencies and every effort should be made to hasten their preparation for surgery. For patients with incomplete femoral neck fractures whose weight-bearing status can be reliably controlled, such as the runner with a stress fracture, avoidance of weight-bearing for six weeks, with interval radiographs taken to check for displacement, is the usual recommended treatment.

For intertrochanteric fractures, surgical treatment is also the generally recommended modality. Blood loss from the fracture site and at subsequent operation is generally greater than for patients with femoral neck fractures, so appropriate provision for transfusion, possibly even preoperatively, should be made. Although the urgency in surgically treating intertrochanteric hip fracture is not as great as for a displaced femoral neck fracture, where the head is at risk for

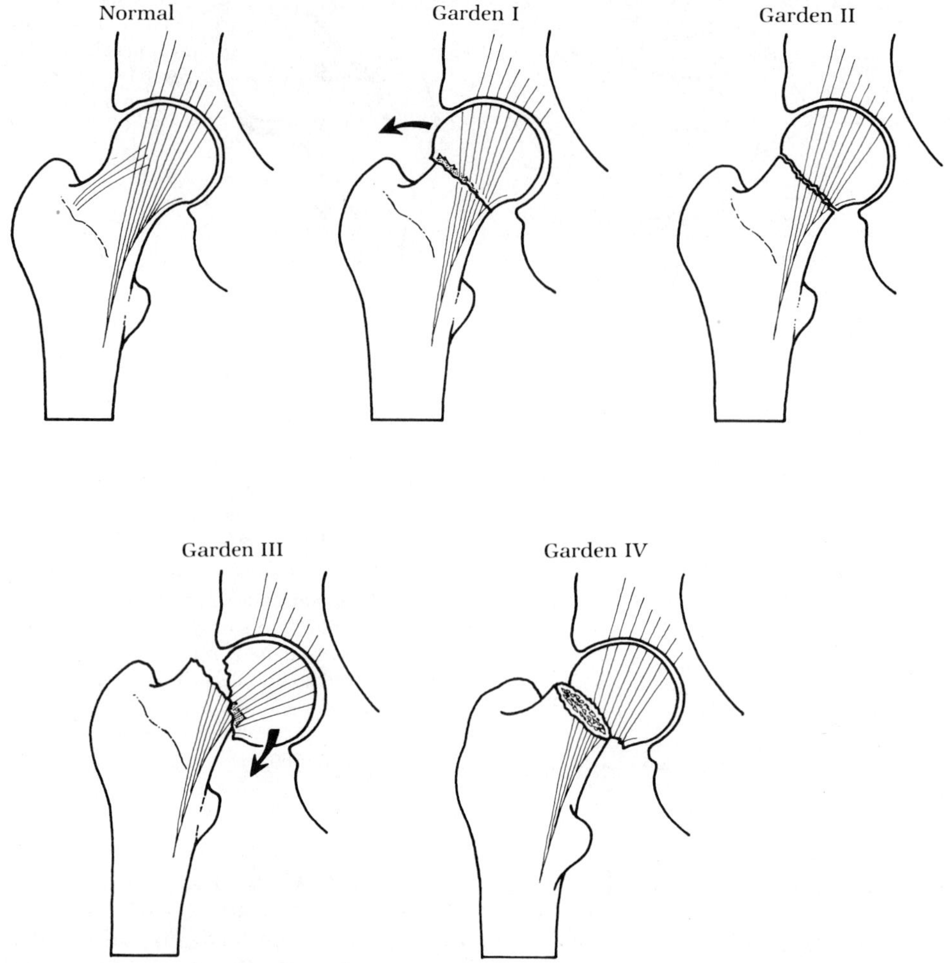

Fig. 69-9. Garden classification of femoral neck fractures. Garden I represents an impacted fracture, angulated slightly into valgus with preservation of medial cortical alignment. Although the Garden classification describes the class I fracture as incomplete medially, it is often more accurately described as nondisplaced medially. Note how the trabecular pattern (fine lines) shows incongruity between the head and neck fragments and between the head and acetabulum. Garden II fractures are nondisplaced. Trabecular alignment is congruous. Garden III fractures are angulated and somewhat displaced; trabecular lines are incongruous in a direction opposite that of the impacted class I fracture. Garden IV fractures are completely displaced and the head fragment is free to rotate back to its normal position, thereby allowing the trabecular pattern of the head to line up with that of the acetabulum. Careful interpretation of the AP and true lateral radiographs is particularly helpful in assessing these fractures.

osteonecrosis, it is generally best to prepare patients for operation as soon as possible. This is largely due to the fact that elderly patients placed at bed rest will often be poorer candidates for surgery after several days than they are on admission. Beyond the initial diagnostic evaluation, including a search for concomitant injuries, a central role of the emergency physician is to identify correctable fluid and electrolyte imbalances and to make a general assessment of the patient's cardiopulmonary status to determine if and when the patient can be taken to the operating room for definitive treatment. These patients may require more extensive evaluation than might be suggested by the hip fracture. If a pathologic fracture is suspected, an evaluation to identify a potential primary neoplasm should be initiated. Adult respiratory distress syndrome or its variants can occur, and a low threshold for obtaining arterial blood gases should be maintained.

In certain isolated instances, these fractures are treated conservatively by bed rest followed by a period of bed-chair immobilization. Such treatment is usually reserved for patients who were nonambulatory at the time of injury.

Avulsion Fractures

The greater and lesser trochanters of the femur represent sites of major tendon insertion for the hip abductors and

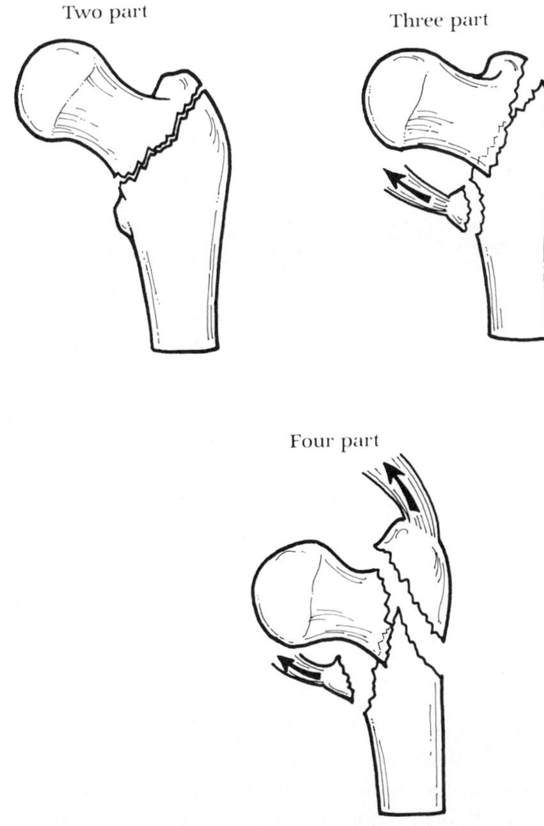

Fig. 69-10. Intertrochanteric hip fractures. Classification is frequently based on the number of individual fracture fragments present. Three- and four-part fractures tend to be more unstable and are more apt to displace into a varus angulation between neck and shaft due to fracture of the medial cortex.

flexors, respectively. In the skeletally immature individual, the greater trochanter is separated from the remainder of the femur by a cartilage bridge, which is relatively weaker than the surrounding bone. With skeletal maturity this cartilage bridge disappears and avulsion fractures are less likely to occur. With advancing age and increasing osteoporosis, the incidence of fracture again rises (Figs. 69-12 and 69-13).

Two major mechanisms of avulsion fracture are relevant. One is the true avulsion caused by pull of either the abductors or flexors on the greater or lesser trochanters, respectively. The other is direct trauma, a mechanism that acts only on the greater trochanter because of its more exposed position.

Evaluation

The history is generally one of a fall or sudden passive force directed against the hip abductors or flexors. On examination, the patient may complain of medial (lesser trochanter) or lateral (greater trochanter) hip pain, and there may be local trochanteric tenderness to palpation when the greater trochanter is involved. Passive stretching of respective muscle-tendon groups can produce pain at the corresponding sites. With complete avulsion the patient may be unable to flex or abduct the hip against gravity.

Treatment

Whether the mechanism is true avulsion or direct trauma, conservative treatment is usually recommended. Bed rest followed by protected weight-bearing as tolerated gives consistently good results in most patients. The need for hospital admission is usually determined by the patient's ability to function at reduced weight-bearing status in the home. Rarely, internal fixation of these fractures is appropriate, but this treatment is usually limited to athletic individuals with more than 2 cm of displacement.

Fig. 69-11. Pillow suspension for acute hip fractures. Such a position allows maximal patient comfort. Small amounts of distal traction help relieve spasm in the muscles about the hip joint.

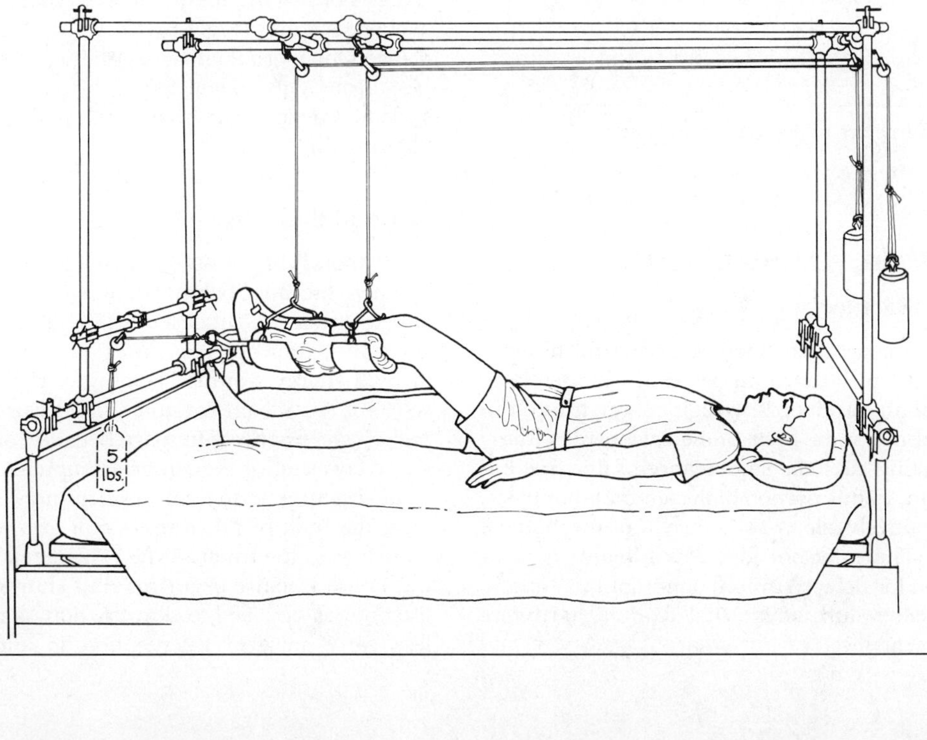

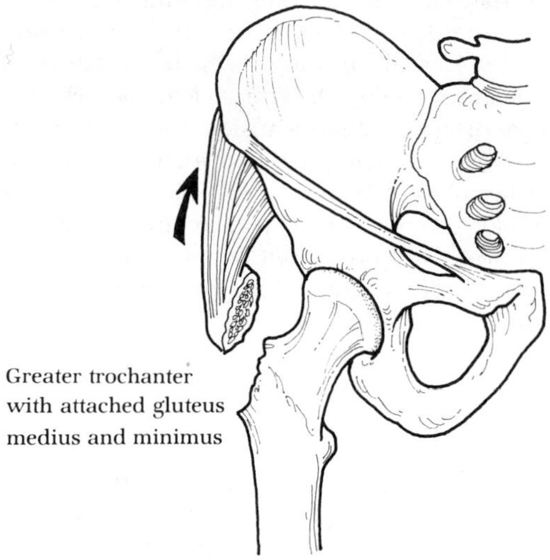

Fig. 69-12. Avulsion fracture of the greater trochanter.

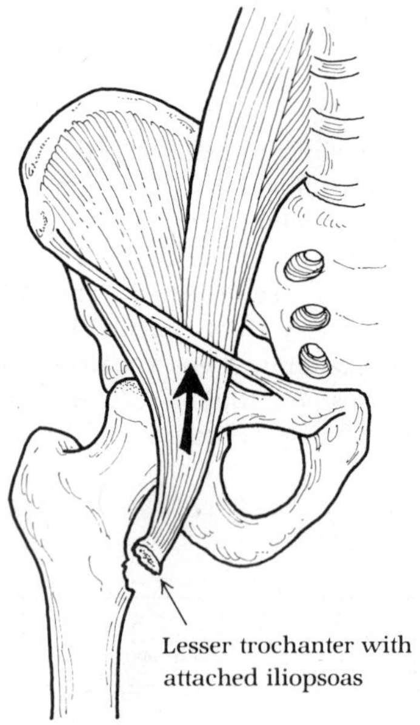

Fig. 69-13. Avulsion fracture of the lesser trochanter.

FRACTURES OF THE FEMORAL SHAFT

Subtrochanteric Fractures

A subtrochanteric fracture is defined as a femoral fracture that occurs in the 5 cm distal to the lesser trochanter (Fig. 69-14). It is commonly produced by high-energy trauma in young individuals but can be seen in the osteopenic elderly patient after a twisting fall. The significance of this fracture relates to its location. In this portion of the femoral diaphysis, bony union is relatively slow to occur and mechanical stresses are high. These factors give this fracture a well-deserved reputation for delayed union, nonunion, malunion, and late mechanical failure of internal fixation hardware after operation.

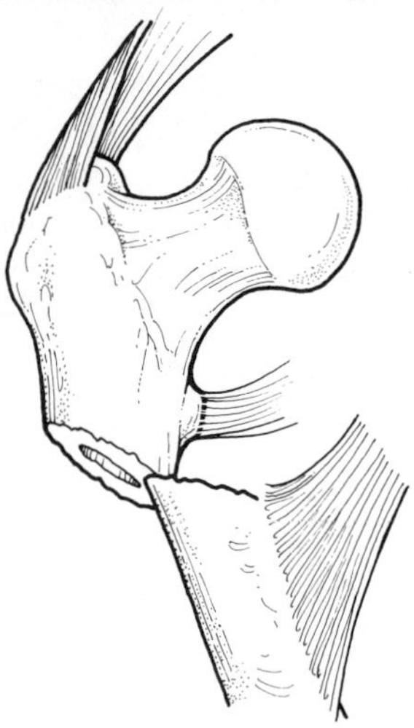

Fig. 69-14. Subtrochanteric fracture of the femur. Such fractures are either two part or more comminuted. In general, they represent a higher-energy injury than intertrochanteric or femoral neck fractures. Healing of this fracture is much less predictable, largely because of the displacing mechanical forces that act across the fracture site.

Evaluation

In younger patients who sustain high-energy injuries, a careful evaluation for associated trauma is required. In the elderly individual in whom the fracture represents an isolated injury, hemodynamic stability of the patient remains a concern because the one to two units of blood that are commonly lost into the thigh may represent a substantial blood loss for a frail, dehydrated individual. Radiographic diagnosis is made by standard AP and lateral radiographs.

Treatment

The vast majority of these patients will be treated with internal fixation, either by plate and screws or an intramedullary device. Before definitive treatment, emergency management consists of placing the patient in balanced suspension using a Thomas splint (Fig. 69-15). If the operation is going to be delayed for more than several hours, placement of a traction pin through the distal femur or proximal tibia to provide skeletal traction can help maintain comfort, stability, and alignment.

Femoral Shaft Fractures

The femoral diaphysis is composed of thick cortical bone in a nearly tubular configuration, rendering it relatively resistant to fracture. Thus, femoral shaft fractures, particularly comminuted or open fractures, are almost always the result of high-energy trauma. Femoral shaft fractures in the absence of significant trauma should raise the possibility of a pathologic fracture. In part because of the extensive soft-tissue covering of the femoral diaphysis, healing of femoral shaft fractures is the rule rather than the exception. However, the bulk of this muscle cuff also applies a substantial force across the fracture site. This tends to produce overriding of the fracture segments and shortening. Thus, skeletal traction, as opposed to skin traction, is usually required unless early surgical intervention is anticipated. Transport

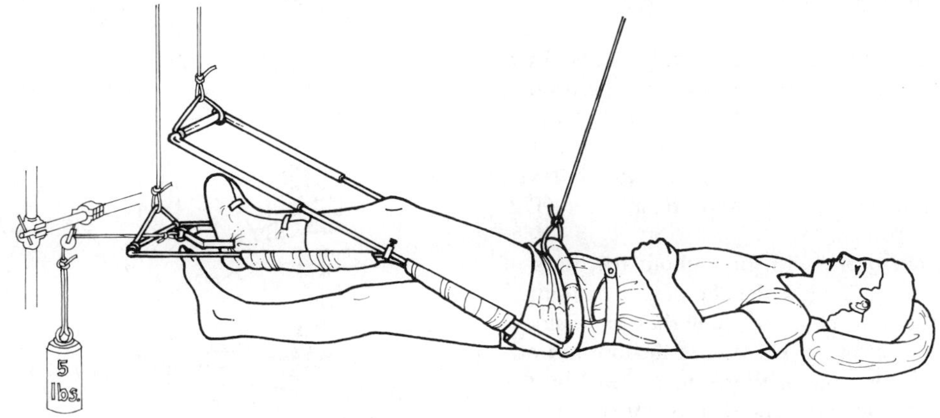

Fig. 69-15. Balanced suspension. In this illustration, the Thomas splint with Pierson attachment below the knee is illustrated. Traction is provided by means of a boot attached to a moderate amount of weight (5 lbs.). Where more traction force is required, it is more safely applied by means of a traction pin placed through the distal femur. (See text for description of traction pin placement.)

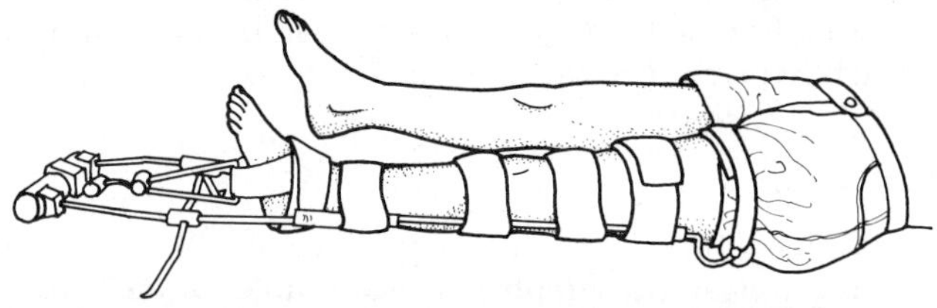

Fig. 69-16. Hare splint. Such splints are suitable for infield immobilization of femur fractures. They achieve traction by using counterpressure against the ischium of the pelvis, and, therefore, their application is limited to relatively brief periods of time to avoid injury to the skin overlying the ischium or foot, or both.

splints, such as the Hare splint, widely used by ambulance personnel (Fig. 69-16), are satisfactory for infield immobilization and transportation but are limited by the fact that they place a great deal of pressure on the foot and ischial tuberosity and can cause a skin slough if left in place too long.

Evaluation

The injured limb is usually shortened, rotated, and, unless seen early, swollen. In the absence of splints or traction, the fracture is usually angulated with its apex anterior and lateral, producing a prominent bulge in the thigh. The ends of the fracture may be palpable beneath the skin, a sign that the quadriceps musculature has been penetrated.

Radiographs should include AP and lateral views of the hip and knee because femoral shaft fractures may be accompanied by hip dislocation or femoral neck or knee fractures. As for other femur fractures, evaluation of hemodynamic status is important. A substantial amount of blood can be sequestered within the compartments of the thigh, resulting in a significant depletion of intravascular volume.

Treatment

Early stabilization of the fracture is required to minimize further soft-tissue trauma and bleeding and provide patient comfort. External splinting with pillows is usually ineffective, and provisional stabilization of these fractures generally requires traction. The Hare splint (Fig. 69-16) is adequate for infield use but must not be left on indefinitely, for the reasons noted previously. If a delay in operation is anticipated, management with balanced suspension and skeletal traction is preferred (see Fig. 69-15).

Traction pins are appropriately placed while the patient is in the emergency department. The pin can be placed either in the distal femur or proximal tibia. The distal femur will tolerate greater traction loads because traction forces are not transmitted across the ligaments at the knee and can be used in the presence of known or suspected knee or proximal tibial injury. While this is the more versatile position, the proximal tibia should be considered if, for example, a distal surgical approach to the fracture is anticipated.

Pin placement is performed using strict aseptic technique and local anesthesia. The medial and lateral femoral epicondyles are palpated and the pin inserted immediately proximal to them through metaphyseal bone using a hand drill. A large-diameter, threaded Steinmann pin reduces the risk of the pin cutting out of bone and of loosening, but for short-term use a thinner smooth pin with a tensioner will reduce soft-tissue trauma. Care is taken to avoid straying posterolateral (peroneal nerve), posteriorly (femoral-popliteal artery), or distally (knee joint). After pin placement, the entry and exit sites are dressed and the sharp pin ends are protected with corks or tape.

In children, definitive management is usually by traction, although children under five years old are increasingly being considered candidates for early application of spica casts. Adolescents and adults are almost universally treated with internal fixation, usually in the form of an intramedullary rod. In the polytraumatized patient, stabilization of such long-bone fractures is critical. Early fracture fixation has been shown to decrease morbidity through a beneficial effect on pulmonary status.

Femoral shaft fracture can occur just below the stem of total hip replacements or just above the femoral component of total knee replacements. Because these fractures often require specialized management involving both the joint replacement and the fracture, early participation of the treating orthopedist is required for these injuries.

DISLOCATIONS OF THE HIP

The hip is a deep ball-and-socket joint, firmly bound by a substantial capsule and thick ligaments. As such, it is among the most stable joints in the body and considerable force is required to dislocate it. When dislocations do occur, they are usually posterior, reflecting a force applied to the flexed hip and knee, as in striking the dashboard of a car (Fig. 69-17).

Hip dislocations can occur with or without fractures of the acetabulum or femur. The greater the degree of adduction and flexion of the hip, the more likely that the dislocation will occur without fracture. Increasing flexion and adduction produces less coverage of the femoral head by the acetabulum so that the head may be driven out posteriorly without causing acetabular fracture.

Anterior dislocations of the hip tend to occur when the hip is abducted and externally rotated and when force is delivered from behind. One such mechanism is a fall from a height wherein the patient lands on the buttocks.

Evaluation

Knowledge of the direction of applied force will help make the diagnosis and differentiate between anterior and posterior dislocation. The position of the hip at the time of injury and the direction from which force was applied can usually be determined by questioning the patient and examining the extremity for the location of impact. Impact at the anterior aspect of the knee that occurs while an unrestrained patient is seated in a car suggests a posterior dislocation. A patient who has fallen, with resulting soft-tissue injury to the buttock, is likely to have an anterior hip dislocation. As a rule, in posterior dislocations the limb is internally rotated, and in anterior dislocations the limb is externally rotated.

A careful neurovascular examination is essential, looking particularly for sciatic or femoral nerve dysfunction. Associated injuries may well be present, including patellar fracture, knee dislocation, or associated femoral fracture.

Initial radiographs should include an AP view of the pelvis and a true lateral view of the hip. The lateral view is not dispensable since, on occasion, a dislocation is difficult to discern on a single AP view. If a force has been transmitted through the knee, knee radiographs (AP and lateral) are necessary.

Treatment

Early reduction of the dislocated hip is critical since the incidence of osteonecrosis is proportional to the period of time that the femoral head remains displaced, compromising its retinacular blood supply. Furthermore, the sciatic nerve may be stretched with a posterior dislocation and will fare poorly with prolonged mechanical stretch. Reductions are optimally performed with the patient under general or spinal anesthesia but, if necessary, can be performed under adequate sedation in the emergency department. Multiple reduction attempts are to be avoided, and if a good attempt under sedation is unsuccessful, the next should be performed under anesthesia, with muscle relaxation. If a dislocation cannot be reduced by closed means, surgical reduction should be performed without further delay.

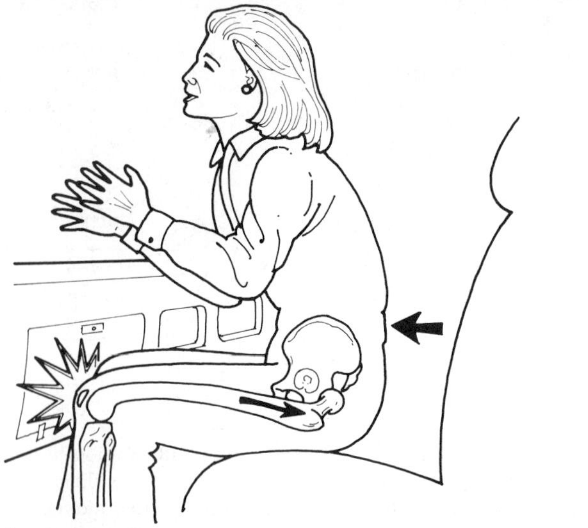

A

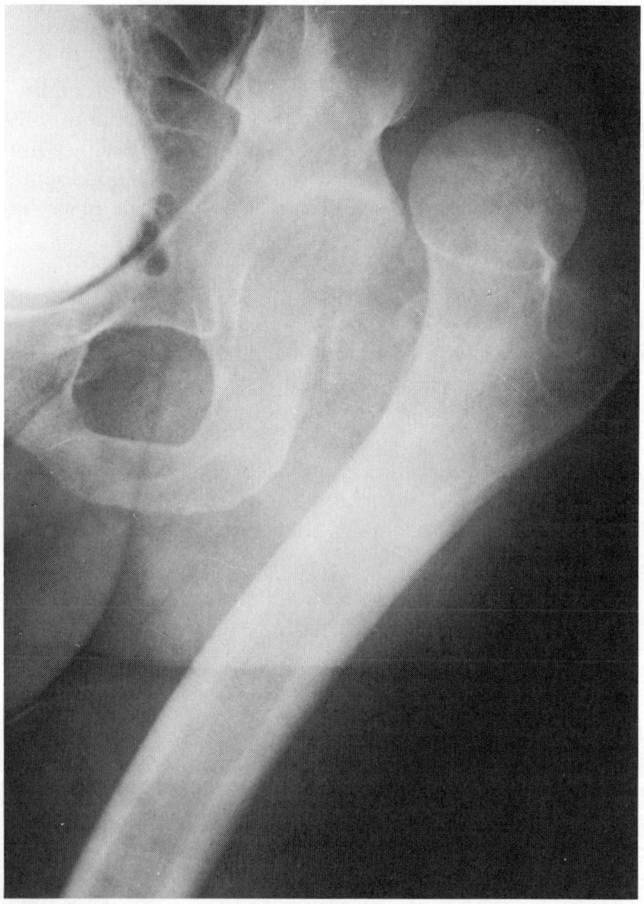

B

Fig. 69-17. Posterior hip dislocation. A. A typical mechanism that occurs in motor vehicle accidents is illustrated, wherein the knee strikes the dashboard, with the hip flexed and perhaps in slight adduction. One should be alert to the possible presence of posterior hip dislocation in patients with anterior knee injuries that result from contact with the dashboard. B. Radiograph of posterior hip dislocation.

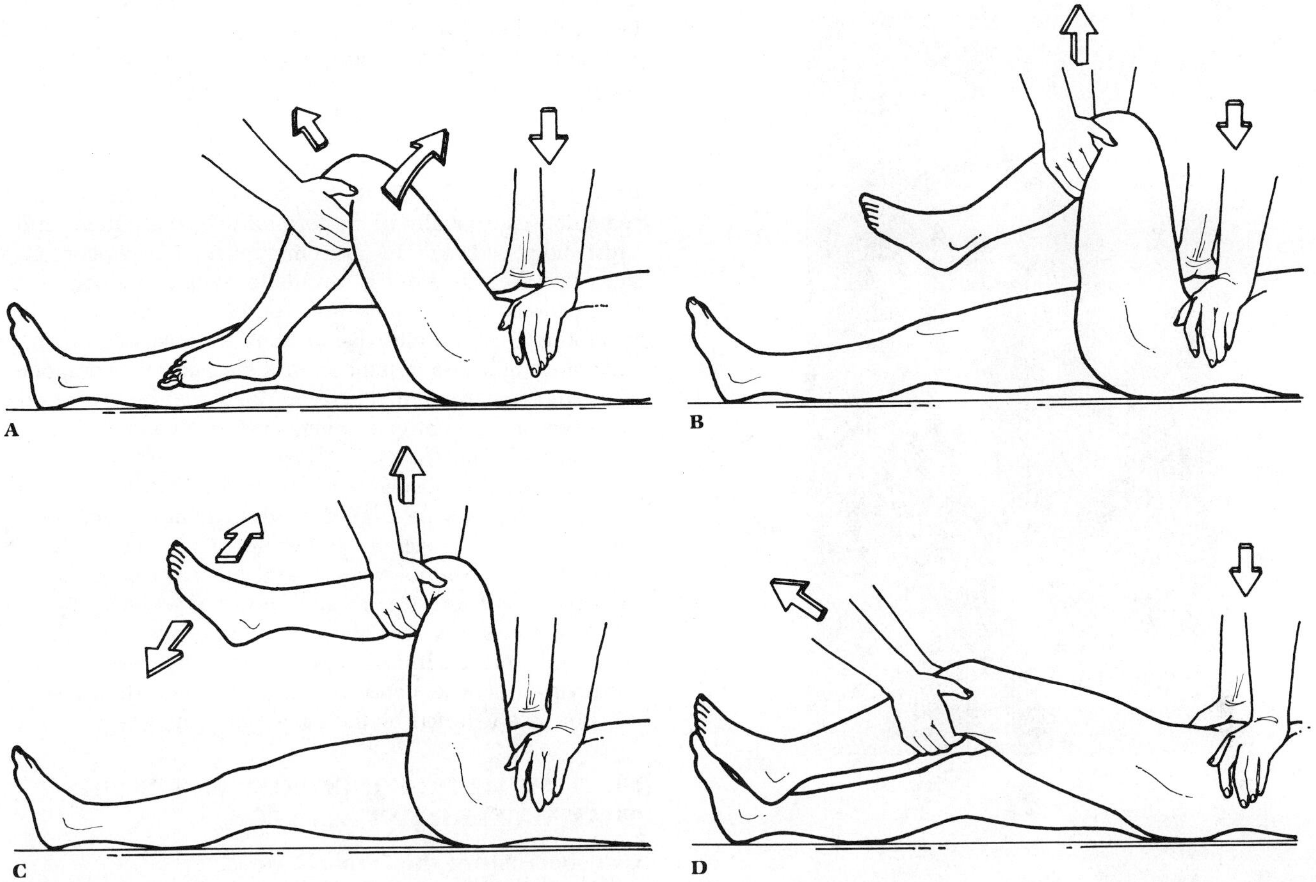

Fig. 69-18. Allis maneuver for reduction of posterior hip dislocation. Two persons are required for this maneuver, with the assistant stabilizing the pelvis by downward pressure on both iliac crests. A. The initial maneuver is to place gentle distal traction on the extremity and slowly bring the hip into flexion. B. Next, the hip is further flexed up to 90 degrees, maintaining distal traction at the same time. C. If reduction has still not occurred, gentle internal-external rocking of the hip joint will often allow the head to slip back into the socket. D. After reduction has been achieved, the hip should be brought back into extension and positioned in slight abduction–external rotation. (From J. C. Delee. Fractures and Dislocations of the Hip. In C. A. Rockwood, Jr., and D. P. Green (eds.), *Fractures in Adults* (2nd ed.). Philadelphia: Lippincott, 1984. Pp 1211–1356.)

Posterior dislocations can be reduced by any of several methods; perhaps the simplest is the Allis maneuver (Fig. 69-18). This maneuver is performed on the supine patient by two persons. After satisfactory intravenous sedation or anesthesia, the assistant stabilizes the pelvis by pushing downward firmly on both iliac crests. The physician, placing longitudinal traction on the flexed knee, gradually flexes the hip. The reduction is achieved with gentle rotation internally and externally and can be facilitated by gentle adduction. Reduction of the hip is usually apparent as a sudden movement of the femoral head and is usually obvious to both the physician and awake patient. After reduction, the limb is extended in slight external rotation and abduction and then placed in balanced suspension with approximately 5 to 10 lbs. of traction through the foot.

Anterior dislocations, much less frequent in occurrence, are reduced in much the same manner. The key to a successful reduction is longitudinal traction combined with gentle internal and external rotation.

Postreduction films are essential and should be carefully scrutinized for fractures not initially seen, intraarticular fragments, or a nonconcentric reduction. CT scanning has been shown to be particularly valuable in detecting intraarticular fragments and in helping to define fracture patterns in associated acetabular fractures (see Chap. 68).

Dislocation of Total Hip Replacements

With the ever-increasing incidence of total hip replacements, there has come an increasing incidence of dislocated total hip replacements. These are commonly seen in the emergency setting and can occur with minimal or no trauma. Such dislocations are usually seen within the first six weeks after arthroplasty, although chronically unstable hips can dislocate at any time. The vast majority of such dislocations are posterior. Occasionally, particularly when the surgical approach has been anterior or anterolateral, the dislocation may be anterior.

Evaluation

Radiographic evaluation is essential before any manipulation of the limb, even if the dislocation has occurred previously. The first determination to be made is the type of implant, specifically whether it is a total hip arthroplasty, a standard unipolar hemiarthroplasty (e.g., Austin Moore), or a bipolar hemiarthroplasty (Fig. 69-19). Fracture or dislodg-

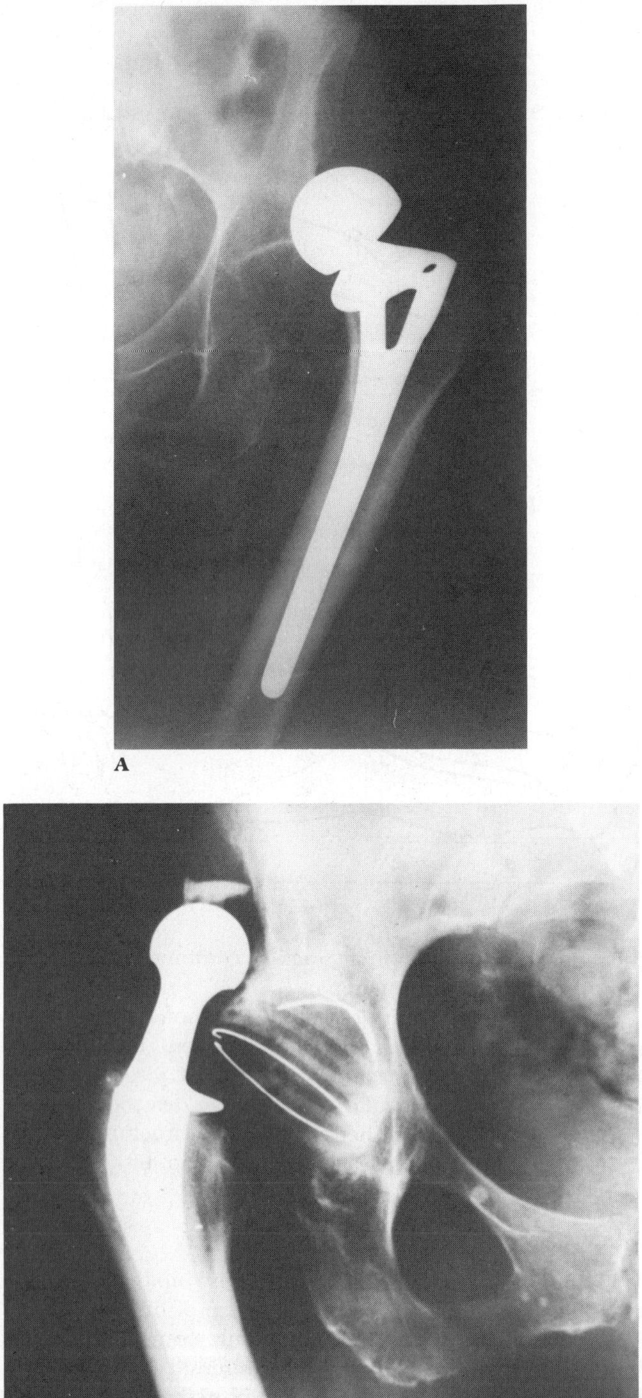

Fig. 69-19. A. Radiograph of dislocated hip hemiarthroplasty. B. Radiograph of dislocated total hip arthroplasty. Note displaced fragment of cement superior to femoral head.

ment of either the femoral or acetabular component should be sought and, if found, reduction should not be attempted. Just as for traumatic dislocations, careful neurovascular examination is required.

Treatment

For dislocated total hip replacements in which both components (femoral and acetabular) remain well fixed to bone, reduction can usually be performed with the patient under satisfactory sedation in the emergency department. Care must be taken to avoid a traumatic reduction since misdirected forces can damage the components or cause their loosening. Occasionally, dislocations are associated with, or occur through, loss of fixation of the acetabular component of the hip replacement. These are identified by loss of position of the acetabular component and are treated by surgical revision of the implant.

For hemiarthroplasties, such as an Austin Moore or bipolar, reduction may be more difficult to achieve since the hip capsule, which is usually preserved at operation, may be trapped within the joint space and prevent replacement of the component into the acetabulum. A disengaged bipolar endoprosthesis in which the two components have become separated from each other and from the hip socket usually requires surgical reduction and manipulation should generally not be attempted by the emergency physician.

NONTRAUMATIC CONDITIONS OF THE HIP THAT MAY PRESENT ACUTELY

Osteonecrosis of the Femoral Head

Osteonecrosis, also termed *avascular or aseptic necrosis,* is a disorder of uncertain cause, characterized by death of varying amounts of the femoral head. Its clinical significance in the adult lies not in the loss of bone viability per se but in the subsequent collapse of the articular surface, with resulting incongruity of the hip joint, cartilage degeneration, and pain. In children, this process is known as *Legg-Perthes disease,* and its natural history differs somewhat from that in adults (see Chap. 160).

A major cause of osteonecrosis in adults is the displaced femoral neck fracture, which presumably interrupts both the intraosseous and extraosseous blood supplies of the femoral head. Other conditions associated with osteonecrosis include alcoholism, corticosteroid use, gout, hemoglobinopathies, caisson disease (exposure to elevated pressure such as in underwater divers and caisson workers), and Gaucher's disease. Some patients have no known associated risk factors.

Evaluation

The typical patient has pain or stiffness, usually of gradual onset, in the absence of recent trauma. Pain is generally localized to the groin and is increased with motion and weight-bearing. Examination reveals pain and limitation of hip motion, particularly internal rotation. In early phases of the disease, x-rays are normal. Later, x-rays demonstrate a subchondral lucency in the femoral head known as the "crescent sign" and mottling of the trabecular bone within the head (see Fig. 69-6). With further progression of the disease, the femoral head begins to collapse and the articular surface becomes irregular, facilitating the radiographic diagnosis.

Treatment
If osteonecrosis is clinically suspected or radiographically confirmed, emergency management consists of instituting non–weight-bearing activity and referral for orthopedic follow-up evaluation. Although definitive management of the early stages of osteonecrosis is controversial, patients may be treated by decompression of the proximal femur, accomplished by drilling through the lateral cortex of the femoral neck and into the femoral head. Once collapse of the femoral head and secondary changes at the joint have occurred, osteotomy, prosthetic replacement, or fusion is usually required for control of symptoms.

Septic Arthritis of the Hip

Septic arthritis is primarily a pediatric disease, most commonly involving the hip joint. The infection begins as a hematogenous osteomyelitis of the proximal femoral metaphysis. Since this portion of the femoral neck is within the hip capsule, the infection easily spreads into the joint space, where rapid destruction of articular cartilage can occur. This condition is a true surgical emergency and is described in more detail in Chap. 160.

Slipped Capital Femoral Epiphysis

Slipped capital femoral epiphysis is a disorder that exclusively affects the growing child and adolescent. The femoral head becomes displaced posteriorly and inferiorly on the femoral neck through the cartilaginous proximal femoral growth plate. The cause of this condition is not known, but in some cases trauma precipitates the slip. See Chap. 160 for a complete discussion.

SOFT-TISSUE DISORDERS ABOUT THE HIP

Quadriceps Contusion

Contusions of the quadriceps are usually caused by direct impact. As might be expected, the severity of these injuries depends on the magnitude of the trauma. In the most severe cases, these injuries can be regarded as partial ruptures through the substance of the quadriceps muscle, and their significance should not be underestimated. Outright rupture of the quadriceps tendon usually occurs near its insertion into the patella and is discussed in more detail in Chap. 70.

Evaluation
The patient is seen with thigh pain and tenderness over the quadriceps. In a mild contusion, there is localized quadriceps tenderness but no alteration in gait and preservation of at least 90 degrees of knee motion. The patient is able to perform a deep knee bend. A moderate contusion is characterized by a tender quadriceps with localized swelling, antalgic gait, less than 90 degrees of knee motion, and considerable pain with attempted deep knee bends. A severe contusion is manifested by a markedly swollen and tender thigh with ill-defined muscle contours. A severe limp and inability to bear weight are present with less than 45 degrees of knee motion.

Active straight leg raising must always be tested and, if the patient is unable to lift the limb, rupture of the quadriceps should be suspected. Radiographs should be obtained to rule out the presence of fracture.

Treatment
Emergency treatment consists of rest, elevation, and application of ice for 24 to 48 hours, followed by partial weight-bearing on crutches and gradual range of motion exercises. Orthopedic evaluation should be obtained early in this program to initiate and supervise rehabilitation. Patients with severe contusions may face up to six months of disability as a result of their injury. Myositis ossificans (a disorder of uncertain cause in which traumatized muscle becomes infiltrated by ectopic bone) is a frequent complication of quadriceps contusion. Its incidence increases with severity of injury and, though not well documented, may be further increased by forced range of motion exercises during healing. Thus, the usual recommendations for rehabilitation include avoidance of passive stretching, with concentration on active hip and knee flexion instead. For patients with a severe quadriceps injury, in which the continuity of the quadriceps mechanism is in doubt, orthopedic consultation in the emergency department is needed.

Hamstring Injury

The principal function of the posterior thigh muscles, termed "hamstrings," is flexion of the knee. As for quadriceps injuries, hamstring trauma is manifested as local pain, swelling, and tenderness. Injuries are generally the result of forced muscle contraction against resistance and take the form of local avulsion of the muscle attachments at the pelvis or knee or, more commonly, a partial tear in muscle substance in the thigh.

Evaluation
On examination, the patient has pain with resisted knee flexion that may be increased by resisted hip extension. The site of injury is tender and palpation may help define the anatomy of the injury, with posterolateral localization suggesting biceps femoris involvement and posteromedial tenderness indicating semitendinosus or semimembranosus injury. Thigh circumference should be measured to assess swelling. Radiographs will rule out fracture or other bony pathology and are particularly useful in diagnosing avulsion fractures of the muscle origins and insertions at the pelvis and knee.

Treatment
Rest, elevation, and ice are the mainstays of emergency care of these injuries. The patient should use crutches, avoiding hamstring stress until symptoms have subsided. Orthopedic follow-up evaluation should be performed at approximately one week to assess progress and initiate rehabilitation, if indicated.

Trochanteric Bursitis

Positioned between the bony prominence of the greater trochanter and the overlying tensor fascia lata, the trochanteric bursa is susceptible both to contusions and chronic inflammation. Inflammation of the bursa can also be caused by previously inserted hardware, including trochanteric wires

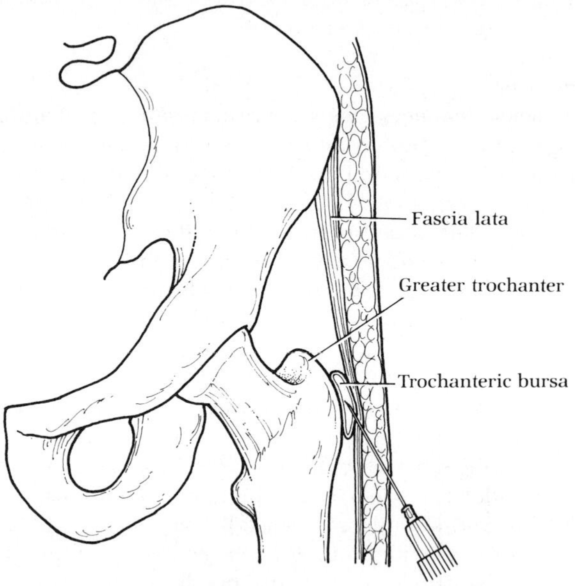

Fig. 69-20. Injection of trochanteric bursa. In normal hips, the trochanteric bursa is merely a potential space, but with inflammation, the bursa can become distended with fluid. In such cases, it can be injected with corticosteroid as shown.

used in total hip arthroplasty or plates inserted for retreatment of hip fractures.

Evaluation

A history of direct trauma is only occasionally present. The patient's complaint is pain over the lateral aspect of the hip in the region of the greater trochanter. The pain is exacerbated by lying on the affected hip and often by climbing or weight-bearing, since these actions increase the pressure of the tensor fascia lata on the bursa. Pain can extend down the lateral thigh, mimicking sciatica, but without associated neural symptoms or signs.

The diagnosis is suggested by localized tenderness over the greater trochanter and pain with resisted hip abduction. Radiographs of the hip are usually normal but may reveal calcification in the peritrochanteric soft tissues. Relief of pain with local infiltration of 1% lidocaine (Xylocaine) substantiates the diagnosis.

Treatment

Treatment consists of relieving stresses on the trochanteric bursa and tendinous attachments to the greater trochanter. Depending on the severity of the symptoms, this may require only the use of a cane or possibly touchdown weight-bearing using two crutches. A nonsteroidal antiinflammatory medication or injection of the trochanteric bursa with corticosteroid (Fig. 69-20) may be helpful. Even when trochanteric bursitis is treated by corticosteroid injection, symptoms often subside slowly and follow-up examination with an orthopedic surgeon is not urgent.

"Snapping" Hip

A close relative of trochanteric bursitis, the "snapping hip" is produced by the fascial band overlying the greater trochanter and trochanteric bursa. This taut structure can snap as it rides over the trochanter during hip flexion-extension range of motion. With local inflammation, such motion becomes painful. Primary treatment consists of rest, including crutches if needed to achieve comfort, and reduced activities involving the hip.

SELECTED READING

American Academy of Orthopaedic Surgeons. *Orthopaedic Knowledge Update 2.* Park Ridge, IL: AAOS, 1987. Pp 331–382.

Barnes, R, et al. Subcapital fractures of the femur. A prospective review. *J Bone Joint Surg* 58B:2, 1976.

Delee, JC. Fractures and Dislocations of the Hip. In CA Rockwood, Jr, and DP Green (eds), *Fractures in Adults* (2nd ed). Philadelphia: Lippincott, 1984. Pp 1211–1356.

Jackson, DW, and Feagin, JA. Quadriceps contusions in young athletes. Relation of severity of injury to treatment and prognosis. *J Bone Joint Surg* 55A:95, 1973.

Mooney, V, and Claudi, BF. Fractures of the Shaft of the Femur. In CA Rockwood, Jr, and DP Green (eds), *Fractures in Adults* (2nd ed). Philadelphia: Lippincott, 1984. Pp 1357–1428.

Rankin, A, and Baker, GI. Complications of Treatment of Fractures of the Femoral Shaft. In CH Epps, Jr (ed), *Complications in Orthopaedic Surgery* (2nd ed). Philadelphia: Lippincott, 1986. Pp 513–536.

William, RM, and Winter, WG. Complications of Treatment of Fractures and Dislocations of the Hip. In CH Epps, Jr (ed), *Complications in Orthopaedic Surgery* (2nd ed). Philadelphia: Lippincott, 1986. Pp 469–512.

70. Knee Injuries

John M. Siliski

Knee injuries are among the most common orthopedic problems that present in the emergency department. They can range from minor sprains to limb-threatening fractures and dislocations. Basic knowledge of the functional anatomy of the knee is essential for the emergency physician to be able to perform the knee examination and make the correct diagnosis. The physical examination is extremely helpful with injuries around the knee, since the soft-tissue coverage is relatively thin. Once a diagnosis has been made, initial treatment is usually straightforward.

FUNCTIONAL ANATOMY

The distal femur, proximal tibia, and patella are the three bones that make up the knee joint proper (Fig. 70-1).

The patella is a sesamoid bone and is contained within the tendon structure of the extensor mechanism over the front of the knee. The articular surface of the patella glides in a groove on the anterior aspect of the distal femur, called the trochlear groove. The patellofemoral joint makes up one of the three articular portions of the knee and functions like any load-bearing joint surface.

The other two articular portions of the knee are the medial and lateral compartments, which are the major weight-bearing parts of the joint. The area between the medial and lateral compartments is a non–weight-bearing region and contains the anterior and posterior cruciate ligaments.

The proximal portion of the fibula does not form part of the synovial compartment of the knee joint but is a functional component of the knee, serving as the site of attachment of the lateral collateral ligament and the biceps femoris tendon. There exists a separate small joint between the proximal ends of the fibula and tibia, which occasionally may become dislocated.

There is no inherent stability to the knee joint, and the joint totally depends on ligamentous structures for stability (Fig. 70-2). Ligament structure and function has certain complexities in that there are additional accessory ligaments and each ligament performs more than a single role in knee stability. For the acutely injured knee, however, it is necessary to know the anatomy and function of the four main ligaments. The anterior cruciate ligament (ACL) is located in the anterior portion of the intercondylar notch and prevents anterior subluxation of the tibia relative to the femur. The posterior cruciate ligament (PCL) has the opposite position and function, preventing posterior subluxation of the tibia; the PCL is the strongest of all ligament structures about the knee. The lateral collateral ligament (LCL) runs from the lateral epicondyle of the distal femur to the proximal end of the fibula. It can be palpated as a cord on the posterolateral side of the knee. The LCL prevents opening of the lateral side of the joint on varus stress to the knee. The medial

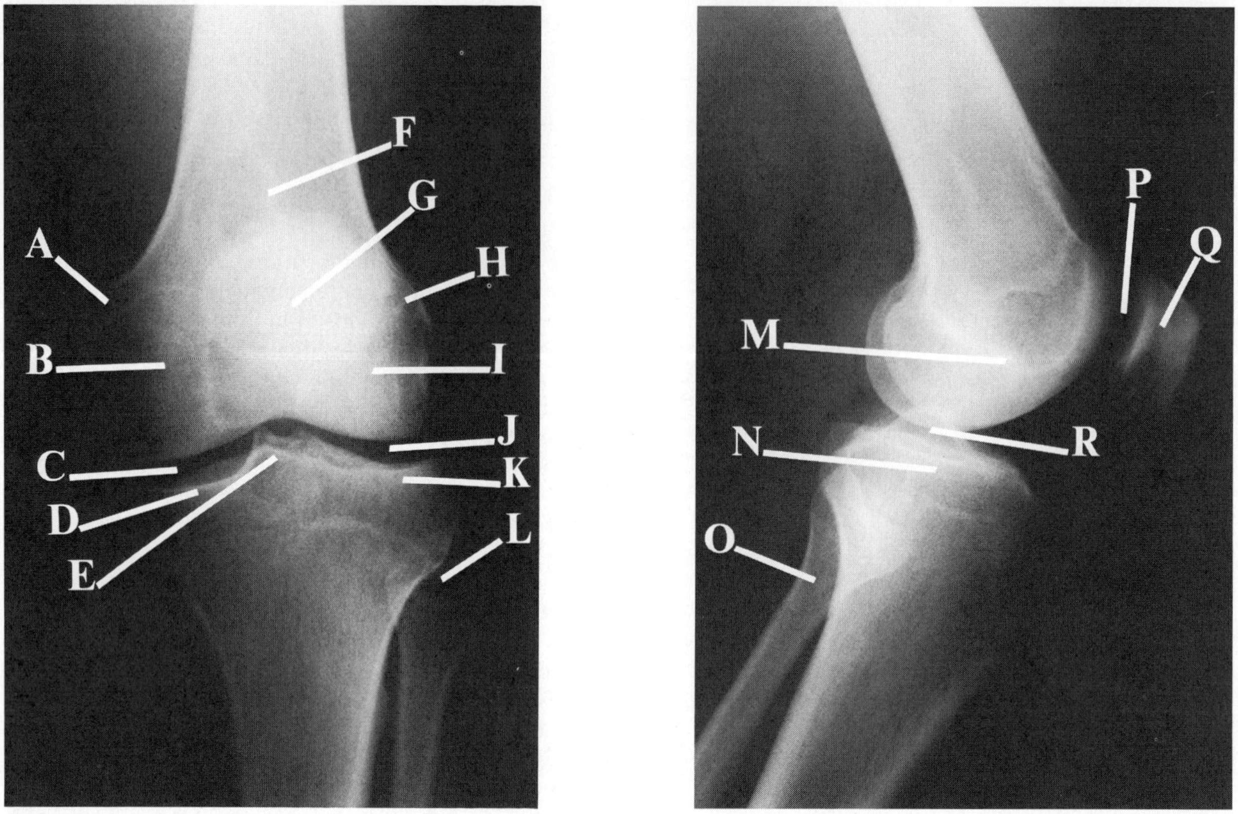

Fig. 70-1. Anteroposterior and lateral x-ray views of the knee demonstrating bony anatomy. A. Medial epicondyle. B. Medial femoral condyle. C. Medial joint space. D. Medial tibial plateau. E. Tibial eminence. F. Femoral metaphysis. G. Patella. H. Lateral epicondyle. I. Lateral femoral condyle. J. Lateral joint space. K. Lateral tibial plateau. L. Fibular head. M. Overlapping femoral condyles. N. Overlapping medial and lateral tibial plateaus. O. Fibular neck. P. Patello-femoral joint space. Q. Patella. R. Joint space with overlapping tibial eminence.

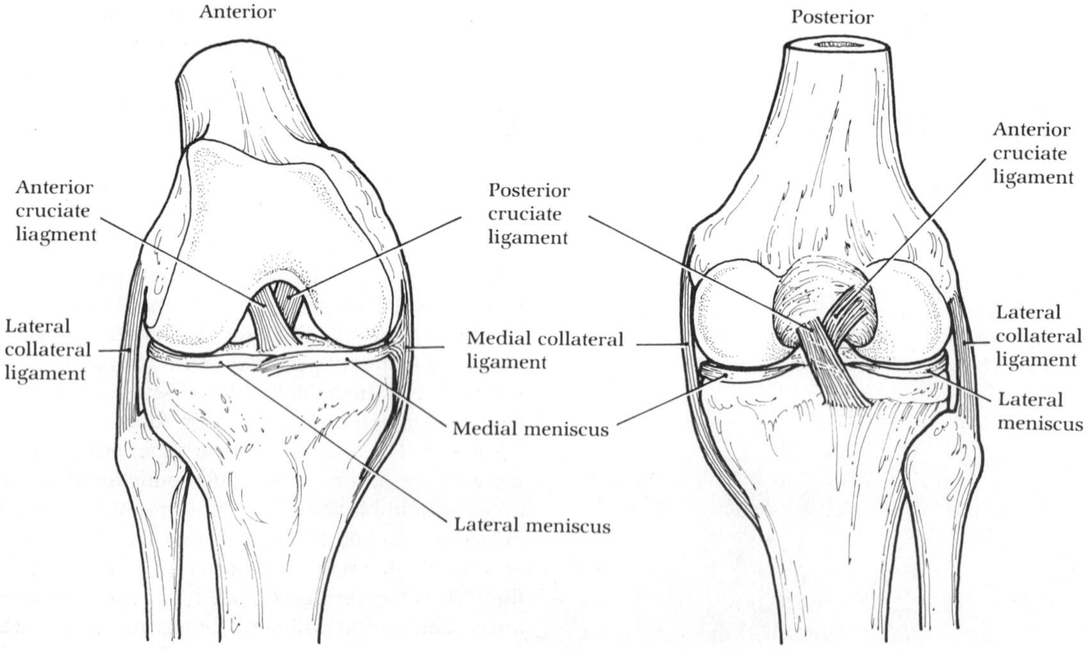

Fig. 70-2. Anteroposterior and lateral views of the knee demonstrating the collateral and cruciate ligaments and the peripheral edges of the menisci with the joint capsule removed.

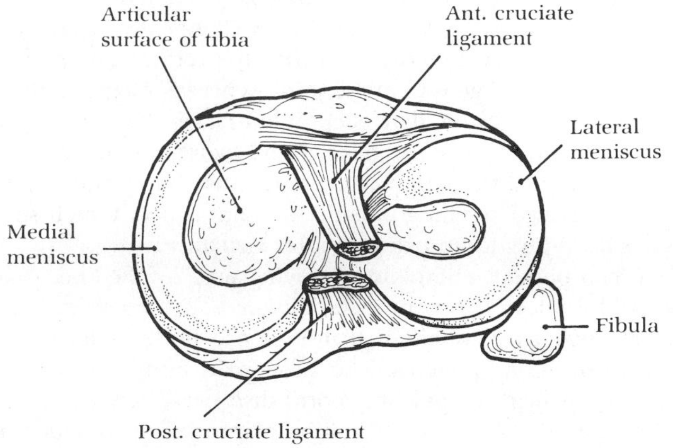

Fig. 70-3. Superior view of the proximal tibia showing the coverage of the peripheral weight-bearing compartments by the menisci and the insertion of the cruciate ligaments in the non–weight-bearing, central portion of the knee.

collateral ligament (MCL) has a deep and a superficial layer, running from the medial epicondyle of the distal femur to the proximal portion of the medial tibia. It is a much flatter structure than the LCL but can be examined directly over its entire length. The MCL prevents opening of the medial side of the joint on valgus stress to the knee.

The medial and lateral menisci (Fig. 70-3) are fibrocartilaginous structures contained within the joint. They have a "C" shape, with the periphery attached to the capsule, and the central edge forming a free border within the joint. The menisci provide additional stability to the joint and also serve to take up some of the forces that would otherwise be borne by the articular cartilage. Because of their location sandwiched between the femoral and tibial condyles, the menisci are commonly torn due to rotational and shear forces. This is the "torn cartilage" injury commonly reported in the popular press.

Muscles and tendons (Fig. 70-4) are the structures that provide motion and dynamic stability to the joint. The quadriceps muscle, which covers the anterior half of the thigh, provides the motor function for the extensor mechanism of the knee, which is described in the following paragraph. The hamstring muscles (Fig. 70-5) cover the posterior thigh and are the primary knee flexors. The tendon of the biceps femoris attaches to the proximal fibula. The medial hamstrings have a broad insertion over the medial capsule and tibia. The medial hamstrings consist of the semimembranosus, semitendinosus, and gracilis. The popliteus muscle and tendon (Fig. 70-5) cross the posterolateral side of the knee and are too deep to palpate. The popliteus internally rotates the tibia on initiation of flexion to "unlock" the knee for motion. The iliotibial band crosses the lateral side of the joint. It rarely sustains acute injury but may become inflamed from overuse. The proximal tendons of the medial and lateral heads of the gastrocnemius muscle cross the posterior surface of the knee and, along with the hamstring tendons, outline the diamond shape of the popliteal fossa.

The extensor mechanism (see Fig. 70-4) of the knee is that group of structures involved with dynamic extension of the joint. The four portions of the quadriceps muscle cover the

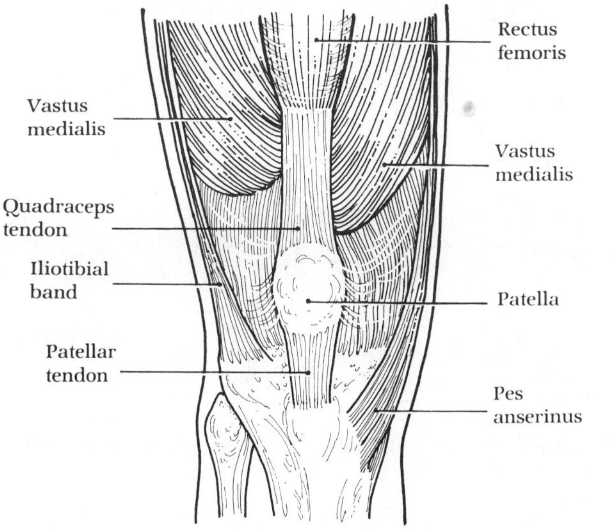

Fig. 70-4. Anterior view of the knee showing the extensor mechanism, anterior capsule, and tendinous structures across the anterior half of the joint.

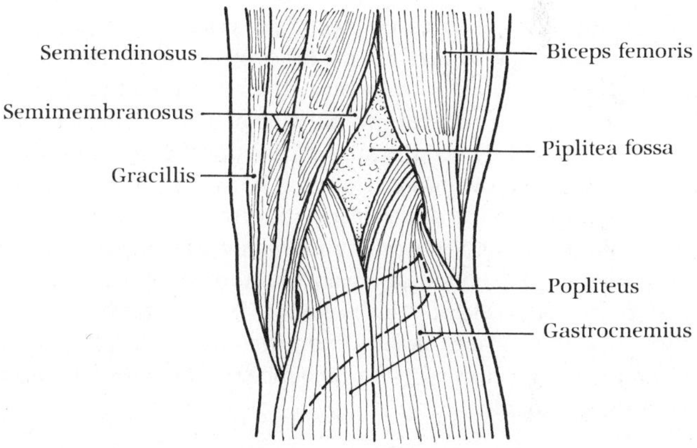

Fig. 70-5. Posterior view of the knee.

anterior thigh. These muscles insert into the quadriceps tendon, which in turn attaches to the upper end of the patella and the adjacent medial and lateral retinaculum of the joint capsule. The patellar tendon, or ligament, attaches the inferior pole of the patella to the tibial tubercle, the prominence easily felt on the upper anterior end of the tibia. Because of the very high tension forces that pass through the extensor mechanism, it is possible to disrupt the mechanism as a quadriceps tendon tear, transverse patellar fracture, or patellar tendon disruption. Because the patella tracks in a relatively shallow groove on the femur, it may sublux or dislocate laterally. More commonly, shear forces in the patella femoral joint can cause articular cartilage injury, such as chondromalacia ("soft cartilage"), which often presents as acute anterior knee pain.

The neurovascular structures about the knee are usually injured only with severe trauma. The popliteal artery courses posterior to the knee joint and, just distal to the joint, trifurcates into the three major arteries of the calf (Fig. 70-6). The popliteal artery is susceptible to injury ranging from

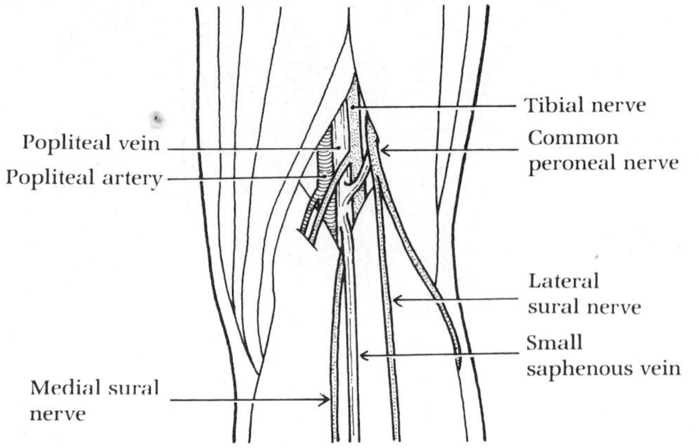

Fig. 70-6. Neurovascular structures on the posterior side of the knee.

an intimal tear to complete transection in association with displaced fractures and knee dislocations. The sciatic nerve separates into the tibial and peroneal divisions just proximal to the knee joint (Fig. 70-6). The tibial nerve tracks along with the popliteal artery through the popliteal fossa. The tibial nerve may be injured by the same major fractures and dislocations that cause popliteal vessel damage. The peroneal nerve tracks from posteriorly around the lateral side of the knee where it may be palpated at the fibular neck before it enters the muscle compartments on the anterior and lateral sides of the calf. Because of its superficial location, it may be injured by either a direct blow or by laceration more readily than the other deeper neurovascular structures. Major ligamentous disruptions involving the lateral side of the joint can place enough tension on the nerve that a peroneal palsy may result. Any patient who has had a major injury about the knee must be examined in the distal portion of the lower extremity for the presence of normal nerve and circulatory function.

EVALUATION

Although particular key points of the history, examination, and x-ray findings are given for the specific disorders discussed later in this chapter, this section will be devoted to performing a systematic knee evaluation.

The history can be exceedingly helpful in limiting the differential diagnosis. Occasionally, patients present because of an aggravation of a previously diagnosed and treated injury, which, of course, must be confirmed by examination. High-energy injuries, such as those incurred from motor vehicle accidents and falls from heights, produce the more severe injuries, such as fractures, dislocations, and multiple ligament injuries. Low-energy injuries, such as those encountered in sports, are more commonly associated with meniscal tears, patellar dislocations, and less severe ligament injuries. A "popping" or "tearing" sensation is often reported by patients in association with meniscal tears and complete ligament tears. Immediate deformity and instability are often reported by patients with major ligament injuries but are not typically a feature of isolated meniscal tears.

The rate of development of an effusion may also provide a clue as to whether the patient has sustained a cruciate ligament tear versus a meniscal tear. Classically, a cruciate ligament tear will almost immediately produce an effusion due to hemorrhage within the joint, whereas meniscal tears produce an effusion that accumulates over the first 12 to 24 hours after injury. By history and examination, effusion representing fluid within the joint must be distinguished from localized swelling outside the joint space, which suggests an injury to an extraarticular structure.

When patients complain of "giving way" of the knee, one should think of ligament instability or an internal derangement such as a meniscal tear or loose body in the joint. However, many patients who have pain from any source, such as arthritis or patellofemoral disorders, may complain of giving way due to an inhibition of quadriceps function at the moment that they experience their episodic pain. Sometimes asking whether pain precedes the giving way may help distinguish these conditions.

Locking of the knee joint is a symptom in which there is intermittent inability to fully extend the joint. It typically is due to either a meniscal tear or a loose body catching in the joint and mechanically preventing full extension. To relieve locking, the patient often manipulates the joint him- or herself until the structure caught between the femur and tibia slips to a more peripheral location in the joint. Many patients will claim to have locking of the knee when they have no true mechanical block to extension, but rather episodic pain or rubbing of an arthritic articular surface that results in temporary and voluntary inhibition of full motion.

Pain is such a common complaint with all types of knee injuries and disorders that its presence alone is not helpful. However, localization of the site of pain can be very helpful. If one knows what structure is causing the pain, the differential diagnosis becomes much smaller. Asking the patient to point with a single finger to the site of maximal pain may greatly simplify history taking.

The knee examination should start with a visual inspection of the lower extremity. Old scars from previous surgery should be noted. Localized swelling and ecchymosis should be distinguished from the presence of a joint effusion, which obliterates the usual indentations seen around the medial, lateral, and superior edges of the patella. If a large effusion is present, the patella is elevated from the femur by the fluid; ballotment of the patella against the femur is possible by direct pressure to the outer surface of the patella. If a small effusion is present, it may be difficult to detect. The following maneuver can be helpful. The effusion can be "milked" from the recesses about the medial and superior edges of the patella to the lateral side of the patella. By then pushing the fluid suddenly from the lateral recess, a fluid wave can be seen appearing to the medial side of the patella. Lacerations should be carefully noted, as they can communicate with the knee joint or with a fracture. Methylene blue (1 ml in 50 ml sterile saline) may be injected under sterile technique (Procedure 32) into the knee joint; if the methylene blue drains from the laceration, the joint is open and potentially contaminated. Gross deformity about the knee suggests fracture, major ligament disruption, tibiofemoral dislocation, or patellar dislocation.

Palpation is most helpful in localizing the site of tenderness. Most of the structures about the knee can be directly examined. The bones of the knee can all be tested for tender-

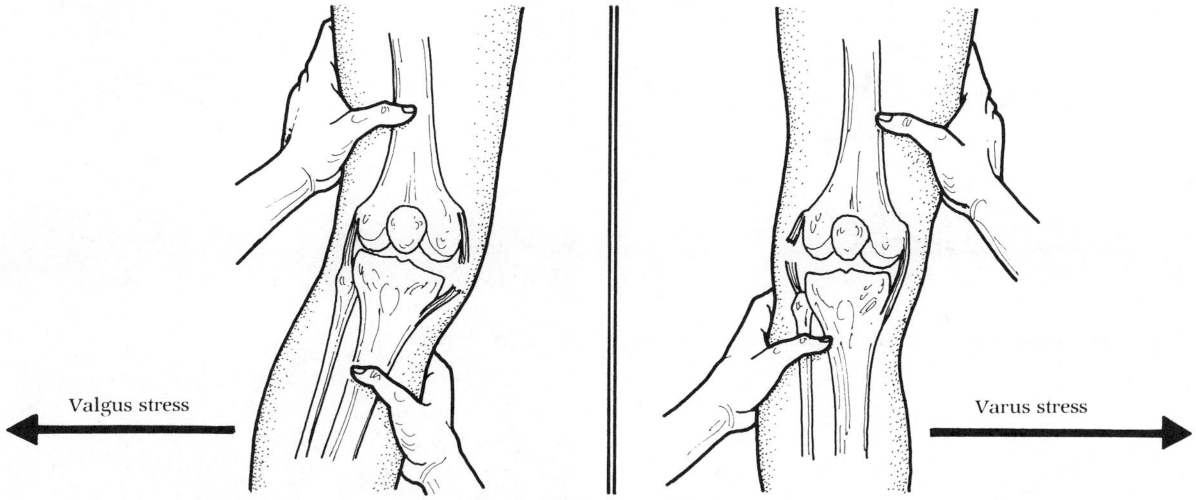

Fig. 70-7. Testing the stability of the collateral ligaments by flexing the knee to 20 degrees and applying a valgus stress to test the MCL (A) and a varus stress to test the LCL (B).

ness by direct pressure. Tenderness along the joint lines raises the suspicion of a meniscal tear. The collateral ligaments can be felt along their entire courses from the femur to the tibia and fibula. The cruciate ligaments, however, are not palpable as they are within the intercondylar notch and can be assessed only by stress testing.

Range of motion should be assessed, providing no obvious fracture or deformity is present. The normal knee will move from 0 to 150 degrees of flexion. The patient's uninjured knee will provide a norm for the individual patient, as some knees may normally hyperextend or have less than 140 degrees of flexion. Full extension and flexion may be limited by the presence of pain or effusion. A torn meniscus or loose body that is caught between the femur and tibia may limit full extension by approximately 20 degrees and may also prevent full flexion.

Provocative tests may be performed, looking for specific disorders. If disruption of the extensor mechanism is suspected, the patient should be asked to actively extend the knee. If complete disruption has occurred, the patient will be unable to extend the knee against gravity. Meniscal tears may be elucidated by tests that load the affected compartment during motion. McMurray's test is done by having the patient lie supine with the knee fully flexed. The knee is internally rotated to check the medial meniscus and externally rotated to check the lateral meniscus. The flexed and rotated knee is then gradually extended to 90 degrees. Pain or clicking within the joint suggests a meniscal lesion. Another way to look for signs of a meniscal lesion is Appley's test. With the patient in the prone position, the knee is flexed to 90 degrees, and the tibia is used to load force across the knee. The joint is then simultaneously rotated, and flexed and extended. Clicking or pain produced by this maneuver increases the likelihood of there being a meniscal lesion. Absence of positive findings on these tests does not rule out a meniscal tear, however.

Ligament stability should be assessed in the emergency department by identifying the presence or absence of major ligament disruption and instability. Fine gradations of the degree of instability are much less important than determining the presence or absence of instability. Familiarity with a few key ligament stress tests is essential to avoid a missed diagnosis. One should first examine the uninjured knee to determine the patient's normal degree of joint laxity, as there is a wide variation from one patient to another. The injured knee is then examined systematically. The knee is brought into full extension. Hyperextension of the joint suggests posterior cruciate injury, with possible anterior cruciate injury as well. In maximal extension, varus and valgus stress applied to the knee should reveal no opening of the medial or lateral sides of the joint, as all ligaments become taut in full extension. If there is medial or lateral instability in full extension, a major injury involving the cruciate and collateral ligaments is to be suspected. The knee should then be examined at 20 degrees of flexion. In this position, the cruciate ligaments are normally relaxed enough to allow evaluation of the collateral ligaments. A varus stress is applied to evaluate instability of the lateral collateral ligament, and a valgus stress is applied to evaluate the medial collateral ligament (Fig. 70-7). Also at 20 degrees of flexion, a Lachman test is performed by grasping the distal femur with one hand and the proximal tibia with the other. An anterior force is applied to the tibia to see whether it will sublux anteriorly, signifying laxity or disruption of the ACL (Fig. 70-8). At 90 degrees of flexion, a posterior drawer test is performed by grasping the tibia and pushing it posteriorly on the femur (Fig. 70-8). If the tibia subluxes back more than the opposite normal knee, the test is positive and indicates laxity of the PCL.

Other tests may be performed to look for cruciate ligament insufficiency and rotatory instabilities of the knee. These tests, such as the pivot shift test, are more difficult to perform and interpret in an emergency department shortly after injury because of the patient's pain and guarding, and are also more difficult to perform and interpret than the simpler provocative tests for ligament insufficiency described previously. It is best that the emergency physician be familiar

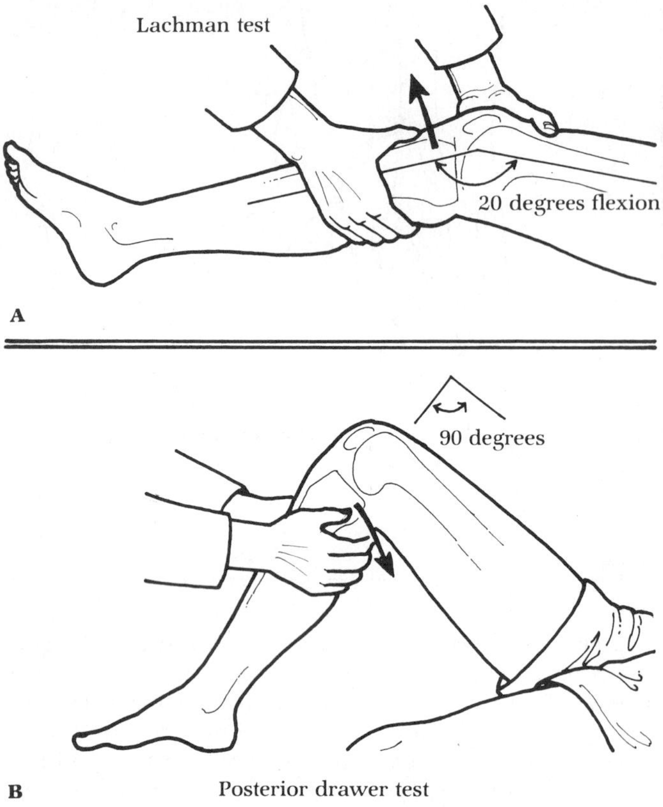

Fig. 70-8. Examination of the knee at 20 degrees using the Lachman test for ACL laxity (A) and at 90 degrees using the drawer test for PCL laxity (B).

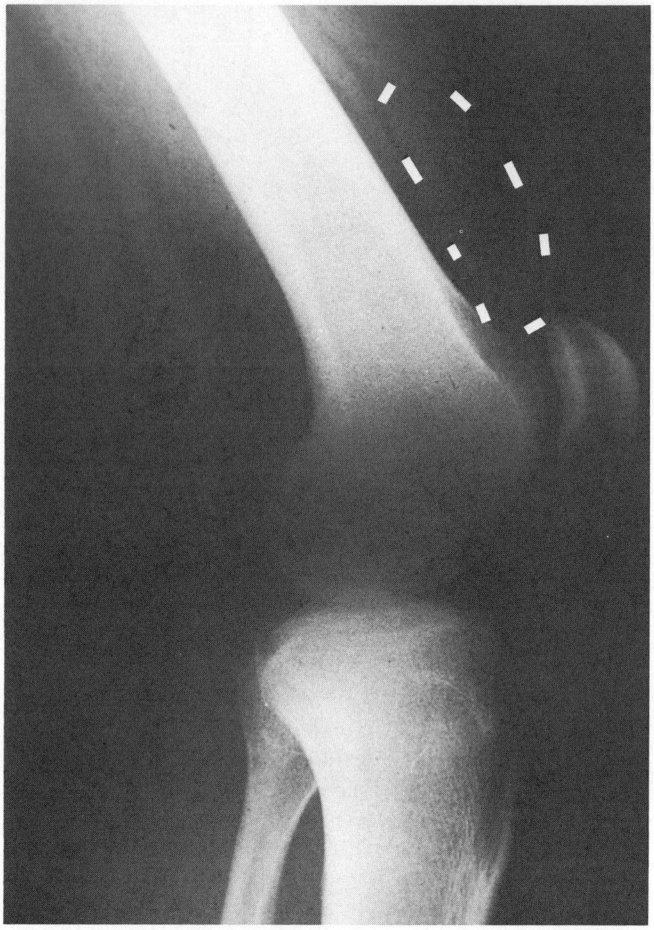

Fig. 70-9. Effusion in the knee seen on the lateral x-ray, with dots marking the extent of the effusion.

with the simpler instability tests, as they will allow identification of major ligament tears in the acute setting.

X-rays are indicated in most cases of knee injury. Anteroposterior (AP) and lateral views (see Fig. 70-1) are the basic screening films. A "skyline" view may be added in cases with patellofemoral symptoms. "Tunnel" views, which image the intercondylar notch, can be helpful in picking up small loose bodies within the notch, or osteochondritis dissecans involving the distal femoral condyles. Forty-five-degree oblique views of the knee may be useful in assessing tibial plateau fractures.

Small avulsion flecks from the rim of the tibial plateau or the tibial spines are a sign of ligament avulsion. Calcified areas within the joint may represent chondrocalcinosis or loose bodies. These should be distinguished from the fabella, a normally occurring sesamoid bone in the tendon of the gastrocnemius muscle, posterior to the knee. A small fleck of bone from the lateral edge of the trochlear groove of the femur suggests that the patient has experienced patellar subluxation or dislocation. A bipartite patella is the result of a second, unfused ossification center. Typically, the superolateral pole of the patella is separated from the main portion of the patella by a fine line, which can be difficult to distinguish from a fracture line. When bilateral, the diagnosis is usually easy. If the x-ray finding is only in the injured knee and there is tenderness over the patella, tomograms may be necessary to distinguish a bipartite patella from a fracture. Radiographic signs of osteoarthritis may explain the new onset of pain in a patient who had been asymptomatic but had a minor injury precipitate onset of symptoms. Often, the only abnormality on an x-ray of the knee is an effusion. This is best seen on the lateral view as an extra soft-tissue density proximal to the patella and anterior to the femur (Fig. 70-9).

Fractures involving the distal femur, patella, and proximal tibia will usually be obvious by x-ray, but films should be studied carefully. Nondisplaced fractures may be relatively subtle on x-ray, and tomograms may occasionally be performed early in the evaluation, particularly in the case of tibial plateau fractures. Tomograms are not, however, a screening test and are most often ordered by the orthopedic surgeon who will be managing a fracture case.

Joint aspiration is occasionally indicated in the evaluation of knee injuries, especially when the patient's history is vague or when the history and examination do not result in a clear diagnosis. Joint aspiration must be performed as a sterile technique (Procedure 32). If bloody fluid is obtained, this indicates fracture or torn soft tissues, such as the anterior cruciate ligament. A nonbloody effusion suggests a torn meniscus.

A full joint fluid analysis is indicated to rule out septic arthritis or crystalline arthritides in situations where patients present with effusion, pain, and minimal (if any) history of trauma.

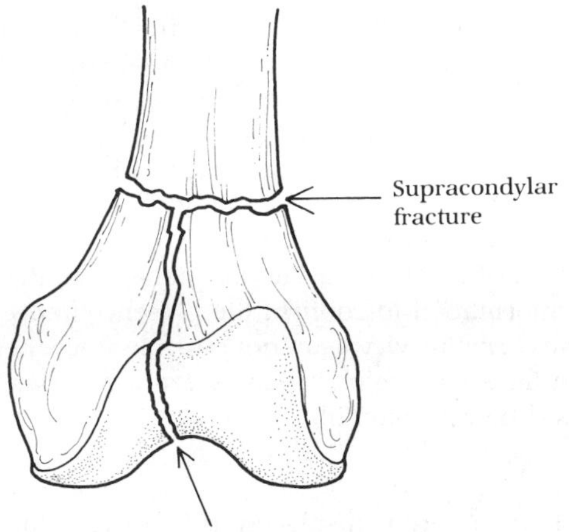

Fig. 70-10. Patterns of distal femoral fractures. These may be supracondylar and therefore extraarticular, or may pass into the articular surface of the distal femur.

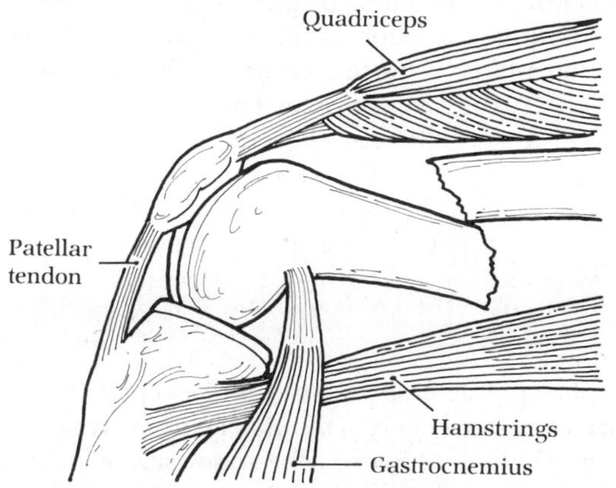

Fig. 70-11. Distal femoral fractures are pulled into angulation with the apex posterior due to the pull of the gastrocnemius muscle on the distal fragments.

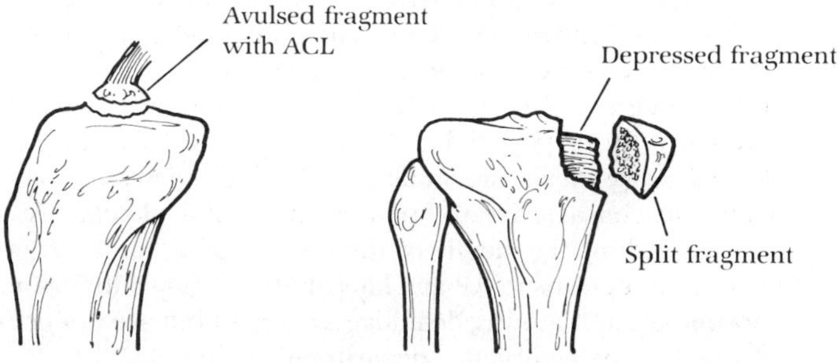

Fig. 70-12. Fractures of the proximal tibia. Lateral view shows avulsion fragment of the tibial eminence, with the ACL attached. Anterior view shows depression and split components of weight-bearing region of tibial plateau.

All fractures and dislocations about the knee should at least be discussed with an orthopedic surgeon by telephone. In some instances, the patient may be treated in the emergency department and released. More commonly, the patient will require urgent treatment in conjunction with an orthopedic surgeon, with admission to the hospital.

Fractures of the Distal Femur

These injuries are usually due to major trauma, such as motor vehicle accidents in young patients or to falling episodes in older, osteoporotic patients. Distal femur fractures should be described as involving the supracondylar region, the articular surface, or both (Fig. 70-10). The pull of the gastrocnemius muscle on the distal fragment(s) tends to displace the fracture as shown in Fig. 70-11.

Evaluation

Pain and swelling are localized to the distal femur. These fractures are usually displaced; therefore, a clinical deformity, including angulation, rotation, and shortening, may be noted. Open wounds communicating with the fracture are common, especially after motor vehicle accidents. The open wounds are usually anterior, where the sharp end of the proximal fragment pierces the extensor mechanism and skin. Neurovascular injuries are uncommon in distal femoral fractures, in contrast to their occurrence in knee dislocations and tibial plateau fractures. However, an initial check of the neurologic and vascular status of the calf and foot is mandatory. X-rays should be taken in the AP and lateral views. Other orthopedic injuries in the same lower extremity often accompany distal femoral fractures, and a thorough examination and appropriate x-rays should be obtained to diagnose these associated injuries.

Treatment

If an open wound is present, its size, location, degree of contamination, and tissue destruction and exposure of deep structures should be noted; the wound should then be sterilely dressed as further evaluation and treatment proceed. If there is a gross angular or rotational deformity, it should be corrected with gentle manipulation by placing longitudinal traction on the lower portion of the limb. A knee immobilizer or medial and lateral plaster splints should be applied, even before x-rays are obtained so that the patient is more comfortable and so that gross displacement of the fracture does not occur during transport and evaluation. An orthopedic surgeon should be contacted soon after the diagnosis has been made. Definitive treatment may consist of traction with skeletal pins, or open reduction and internal fixation.

Fractures of the Proximal Tibia and Fibula

Fractures in this region can be divided into two basic groups (Fig. 70-12). Fractures of the tibial eminence (tibial spine) are avulsion fractures at the insertion of the ACL and occur by mechanisms that also cause ACL tears. Most tibial eminence fractures occur in children, since their ligaments are stronger than their bone. Eminence fractures may be minimally displaced; careful study of the x-ray is required to rule out this injury in children with trauma and a swollen knee (see Chap. 160).

Fractures of the tibial plateau (articular surface of the proximal tibia) are relatively common fractures. They occur in adults of all ages and result from a variety of mechanisms.

One or both condyles may be involved. These fractures may simply split off a portion of the plateau, have a depressed area in the middle of the tibial condyle, or have both patterns of injury. Tibial plateau fractures often have associated meniscal tears and ligament injuries, which must be considered at the time of definitive treatment. Proximal fibular fractures may occur with proximal tibial fractures but rarely require any specific treatment beyond that for the tibial fracture.

Evaluation

Tibial plateau fractures present with local pain and swelling after trauma. If only part of the plateau is involved, deformity may be minimal. However, the more severe fractures are unstable and may be grossly deformed. Neurovascular injuries are more common with tibial plateau fractures than with distal femoral fractures; examination of the lower portion of the extremity is essential. Lateral plateau fractures are often associated with tears of the MCL. Tenderness and ecchymosis over the course of the MCL should be sought.

The standard AP and lateral views of the knee are usually sufficient to confirm the presence of a tibial plateau fracture. Occasionally, a nondisplaced fracture line may run in an oblique plane and be missed on the two standard views. If a fracture is suspected based on the clinical evaluation, oblique x-ray views are indicated. Oblique views are also helpful to characterize the pattern of a tibial plateau fracture, including the depth of depression of articular fragments. Tomograms in AP and lateral planes may add further information in planning definitive treatment but are not usually part of the emergency department evaluation.

Treatment

As with distal femoral fractures, gross angular or rotational malalignment should be corrected with gentle manipulation while longitudinal traction is applied through the calf. Temporary stability is best provided by a knee immobilizer while further evaluation is completed. An orthopedic surgeon should be contacted after the initial evaluation and stabilization have been completed. Definitive treatment will depend on the patient's age and activity level, the fracture pattern, and risk factors for anesthesia and surgery. Nonoperative methods include casting and functional bracing. Open reduction and internal fixation techniques can reconstruct the articular surface and decrease the risk of posttraumatic arthritis.

Fractures of the Patella

Vertical fracture lines through the patella are caused by direct blows to the bone. This pattern is usually nondisplaced and stable. Transverse and comminuted fractures most commonly are caused by a combination of tension forces with a direct impact as the patient falls onto the anterior surface of the flexed knee. This group of patellar fractures is one type of extensor mechanism disruption, which is further discussed in the section on soft-tissue injuries (see Fig. 70-16). Transverse and comminuted fractures usually have displacement of the fragments and associated disruption of the medial and lateral joint capsule.

Evaluation

Hemorrhage from the fracture results in a hemarthrosis and ecchymosis. There is commonly an abrasion over the patella, and any laceration through the skin should be presumed to communicate with the fracture as the patella is so superficial in location. An injection of methylene blue into the joint (Procedure 32) may be performed if it is unclear whether or not the fracture is of the open type.

X-rays in the AP and lateral planes usually provide enough information to confirm the presence and pattern of the fracture. Skyline views are not possible since they require flexion of the knee, which in the presence of a patellar fracture would be very painful.

Treatment

If a patellar fracture is displaced, it is because the extensor mechanism is disrupted and the quadriceps muscle has pulled the proximal fragment upward. No manipulation can reduce such a fracture, and initial treatment is simply to apply a knee immobilizer, which will make the patient comfortable. Given crutches and a secure immobilizer, the patient with a patellar fracture may be partial weight bearing if there is a strong reason for the patient to be released from the emergency department. In most cases, however, the patient with a displaced patellar fracture will be admitted to the hospital for surgical treatment. Open reduction and internal fixation can be achieved with wiring techniques or screws, or both. If comminution is severe, a primary patellectomy may be performed.

Nondisplaced vertical and transverse fractures may be treated in the emergency department with the application of a knee immobilizer or long leg cast. The patient should be given crutches and allowed to be partial weight bearing as tolerated. Since the patella is a part of the extensor mechanism, weight bearing through the femur and tibia produces minimal forces on the patella when the knee is in extension.

DISLOCATIONS ABOUT THE KNEE

There are three types of dislocations that occur about the knee, and since they all have different findings, treatments, and results, each will be discussed individually.

Dislocation of the Knee (Tibiofemoral Joint)

Dislocation of the knee is usually the result of motor vehicle accidents and falls from heights, although it can happen during sports. Disruption of both cruciate ligaments and at least one collateral ligament must occur for the knee to become dislocated. Approximately 25 percent of knee dislocations have associated damage to the popliteal artery, making this a limb-threatening injury. Forty percent of knee dislocations have peroneal nerve palsies due to traction at the time of displacement. Although this is a severe injury, it is, fortunately, an uncommon one.

Evaluation

If the knee remains dislocated until evaluation in the emergency department, gross deformity and swelling will be noted. Since the knee may be dislocated in any of four directions, the appearance of the deformity may be variable. If the knee has been reduced prior to arrival in the emergency department, no deformity will be noted, but the knee will be very unstable on stress testing (see section on evaluation). Any knee that has major instability of the cruciate ligaments and a collateral ligament may have been dislocated and should be evaluated with a high degree of suspicion. The distal portion of the extremity should be examined for neurovascular function and for the presence of a compartment syndrome. If there is any evidence for ischemia or compartment syndrome, the time that has passed since the injury occurred should be noted, as each hour that passes lessens the chance of saving a functional limb.

X-rays should be obtained quickly after initial clinical assessment. If the knee is reduced, small avulsion fragments from the sites of ligament insertion may be noted. If the knee is dislocated at the time of the x-ray, the displacement will be obvious.

Treatment

Knee dislocations are limb-threatening injuries because of the associated vascular injuries and compartment syndromes. Immediately after the diagnosis is made, an orthopedic surgeon should be contacted; a general or vascular surgeon should also be made aware of the case. If the knee is dislocated at the time of arrival to the emergency department, a closed reduction should be attempted to relieve any kinking of vessels and tension on nerves that may be present. Longitudinal traction applied to the calf is usually sufficient to reduce the joint. A knee immobilizer should then be applied to prevent redislocation.

Popliteal artery injuries are common enough that many orthopedic and vascular surgeons consider an arteriogram to be mandatory in the evaluation of knee dislocations. The decision to perform an emergency arteriogram should be made by the orthopedic and general surgeons who assume care of the patient.

The associated neurologic injuries are palsies caused by traction. The only treatment for these is to reduce the knee as early as possible to minimize the degree of injury.

Treatment of the orthopedic aspect of the dislocation may be either surgical or nonoperative and will depend on the patient and the surgeon's preference and experience. If treatment is nonoperative, the knee is ultimately placed into a long leg cast after closed reduction. If treatment is surgical, reattachment and repair of the damaged knee ligaments, capsule, and menisci are performed.

Dislocation of the Patella (Patellofemoral Joint)

Most dislocations about the knee are dislocations of the patella out of the trochlear groove of the femur. The patella dislocates laterally, coming to lie over the lateral femoral condyle. Most of these injuries occur during sports and include, as part of the pathology, a tearing of the medial retinaculum. Some patients are predisposed to patellar subluxation and dislocation. Factors such as the following increase the likelihood of patellar dislocation: (1) a small, proximally positioned patella, (2) a shallow trochlear groove, (3) a valgus knee with a laterally placed tibial tubercle, and (4) poor quadriceps strength.

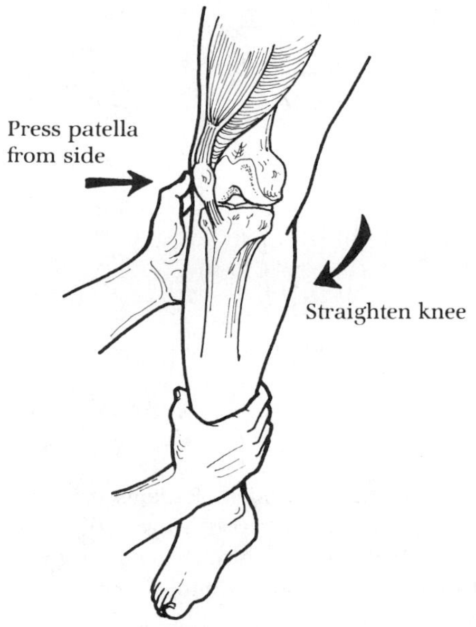

Fig. 70-13. Lateral dislocation of the patella may be reduced in the emergency department by simultaneous extension of the knee while the patella is pushed medially back into the trochlear groove of the femur.

Evaluation

Most patients will give a history of a sports injury, although occasionally the dislocation may occur with a minor event such as arising from a sitting or squatting position. The patient will have been unable to walk on the leg because of pain and the distortion in the extensor mechanism.

If the dislocation persists until the time of presentation in the emergency department, a gross deformity of the anterior knee will be obvious. The patella will be noted over the lateral femoral condyle, and there will be a void over the distal anterior femur so that the trochlear groove may be palpated through the soft tissues. The knee typically is held partially flexed, and the patient will resist both full extension and further flexion.

If the dislocation has reduced spontaneously, the physical findings will consist of swelling about the patella and tenderness of the medial retinaculum, which has been torn or stretched.

X-rays will show an obvious lateral dislocation of the patella if it has not been reduced. Postreduction films are recommended to check for osteochondral fracture fragments that may be loose in the joint.

Treatment

Closed reduction of the dislocated patella should be performed in the emergency department. To decrease pain and muscle spasm, appropriate premedication is recommended. Simultaneous extension of the knee and medial displacement of the patella should be performed as a quick maneuver to slip the patella up the side of the femoral condyle into the trochlear groove (Fig. 70-13). The patient and physician are immediately aware of a successful reduction. The knee should be placed into a knee immobilizer or medial and

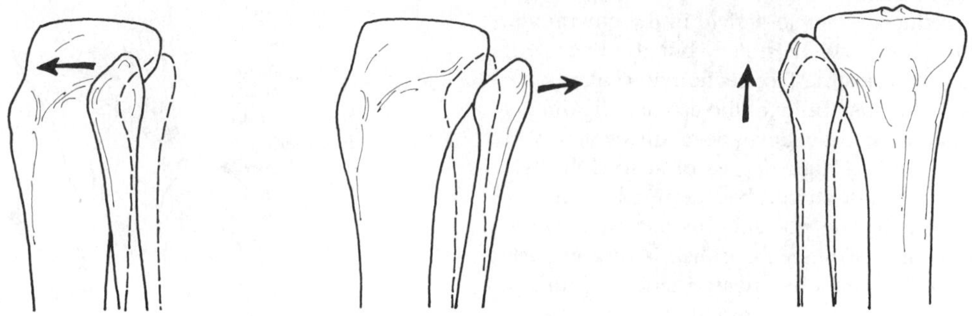

Fig. 70-14. Dislocation of the proximal fibula may be anterior, posterior, or superior.

lateral splints in full extension. Patients can safely be full weight bearing in extension, but most will be made more comfortable and confident if discharged on crutches for partial weight bearing. Follow-up with an orthopedic surgeon at 1 to 2 weeks is recommended. Physical therapy for muscle strengthening and patellar braces for sports are the usual treatment to avoid recurrences. Surgical procedures to stabilize the patella may be indicated if frequent recurrent dislocations occur.

Dislocation of the Proximal Tibiofibular Joint

The small joint between the proximal ends of the tibia and fibula may be dislocated in an anterior, posterior, or superior direction (Fig. 70-14). Shearing blows to the proximal fibula are the usual cause of anterior and posterior dislocations, whereas superior dislocations imply a more severe injury with disruption of all soft-tissue connections between the tibia and fibula, including the ligaments at the distal end of the bones.

Evaluation

There will be pain and swelling localized to the proximal fibula. Careful palpation of the region with comparison to the uninjured side should lead to the diagnosis. Peroneal nerve function should be checked in the lower portion of the extremity. X-ray evaluation should include AP and lateral views of both knees, avoiding differences in rotation of the lower extremities. Comparison of the films of the two knees should confirm the displacement of the fibula relative to the tibia. If the films of the two knees are not taken with identical positioning, an error in interpretation may occur.

Treatment

As a general rule, an orthopedic surgeon should be consulted from the emergency department, since reduction is not always possible in the emergency department. Anterior dislocations can usually be reduced by direct pressure on the fibular head and usually remain stable. Posterior dislocations are more difficult to reduce and are less stable; they may require open surgical procedures. Superior dislocations have disruption of both the proximal and distal tibiofemoral joints and require reduction at both levels.

SOFT-TISSUE INJURIES ABOUT THE KNEE

This section covers sprains of the collateral and cruciate ligaments, tears of the menisci, and disruptions of the extensor mechanism.

Collateral Ligament Sprains

Isolated sprains of the MCL are common. They result from valgus stress to the knee. Conversely, isolated sprains of the LCL are uncommon. Whenever a collateral ligament injury is diagnosed, one should also consider the possibility of an ACL or meniscal tear.

Evaluation

Medial cruciate ligament sprains have tenderness in the ligament at the level of the sprain, and there may be local swelling and ecchymosis. Valgus stress to the knee at 20 degrees of flexion (see Fig. 70-7) will produce pain, but no medial instability will be present unless there has been moderate to complete disruption of the MCL. An effusion suggests an associated intra-articular injury, such as an ACL tear or meniscal tear.

Lateral cruciate ligament sprains have tenderness on the posterolateral side of the knee along the course of the ligament; local swelling and ecchymosis may be present. Varus stress to the knee at 20 degrees of flexion will produce LCL pain, and, if the ligament is disrupted, abnormal opening of the lateral side of the joint will be noted, as shown in Fig. 70-7. A joint effusion implies an associated intraarticular injury.

Treatment

Isolated MCL and LCL sprains of all degrees may be initially stabilized in a knee immobilizer. Evaluation by an orthopedic surgeon is recommended during the first week after injury, so that the diagnosis is confirmed and definitive treatment is planned. Most of these injuries will be treated by splint, brace, or cast immobilization. If there is a question about meniscal or cruciate ligament tears, an early arthroscopy may be recommended by the orthopedic surgeon.

Cruciate Ligament Sprains

Anterior cruciate ligament tears are common injuries and are commonly associated with MCL sprains and meniscal tears. PCL tears are uncommon injuries, but when they do occur, they are commonly associated with LCL sprains.

Evaluation

Anterior cruciate ligament tears usually occur from a rotatory force to the knee, and the patient often recalls a "pop" or "tear" within the joint. The patient is unable to continue sports and frequently reports an immediate sense of instability in the knee as he or she tries to walk. The knee usually swells during the first hour as a bloody effusion develops. By the time the patient arrives in the emergency department, there is usually a large effusion present, and pain and guarding are sufficient to limit the examination. The knee can often be checked only for instability at 20 degrees of flexion (see Fig. 70-8). X-rays are negative unless an avulsion fleck has occurred.

Posterior cruciate ligament tears usually occur from a force that drives the tibia posteriorly on the femur, such as a dashboard injury. There is usually a history of an immediate sense of instability, and pain and swelling develop quickly. In the emergency department, pain, swelling, and guarding may limit stress testing to the examination at 20 degrees. A posterior drawer sign at 20 and 90 degrees is diagnostic of a PCL tear.

Treatment

The most important role of the emergency physician in the case of cruciate ligament injuries is the identification of the patient who has or may have ligament instability. Patients with suspected cruciate ligament tears should be seen within the first few days of injury by an orthopedic surgeon so that the option of arthroscopy and early surgical repair is possible. A knee immobilizer and crutches are appropriate temporary immobilization.

Meniscal Tears

Meniscal tears typically present after a twisting injury to the knee, although many minor events, such as arising from a squatting position, can cause these tears. Many different patterns of meniscal tears have been described, but, for the emergency physician, only two basic types need to be considered (Fig. 70-15). "Bucket handle" tears produce a large fragment that is attached anteriorly and posteriorly but is free centrally. If the fragment shifts toward the intercondylar notch, it may become lodged there, causing "locking" of the knee. The other basic type of meniscal tears are those that produce some irregularity of the free edge of the meniscus, such as "parrot beak" tears. This type of tear can cause pain and effusion but not true locking.

Evaluation

Acute meniscal tears usually produce a nonbloody effusion that develops slowly over the first 12 to 24 hours. The joint line is usually tender in the region of the tear. If the knee extends fully, a displaced bucket handle tear does not exist. If the knee does not extend fully, the limitation may be due

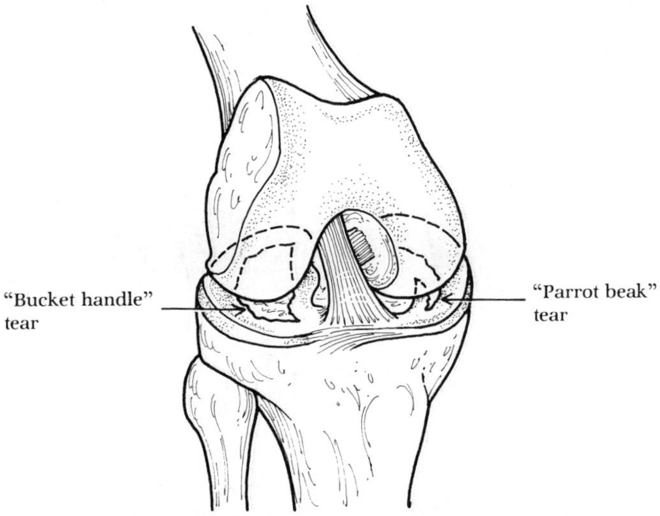

Fig. 70-15. Two types of meniscal tears are demonstrated. A "bucket handle" tear produces classical locking if the semidetached portion becomes lodged in the intercondylar region. A "parrot beak" tear typically produces recurrent pain and effusion without locking.

to either a displaced bucket handle tear (true locking) or the pain and effusion of any type of meniscal tear. It may be difficult in the acute setting to distinguish between true and apparent locking. McMurray's and Appley's tests (see section on evaluation) are most helpful in diagnosing meniscal tears that are producing recurrent symptoms, including joint line pain, clicking, giving way, and swelling. X-rays do not show any abnormalities related to meniscal tears except for an effusion.

Treatment

If a meniscal tear is suspected, the patient should be referred to an orthopedic surgeon within 7 to 10 days. The patient with a locked knee should be seen within a few days, because this patient will usually require early arthroscopic surgery to remove the bucket handle tear and relieve symptoms. A displaced bucket handle tear can sometimes be manipulated out of the intercondylar notch, but this is a temporizing maneuver, as recurrent symptoms are likely. The patient with an acute meniscal tear is usually made more comfortable by being placed on crutches; a knee immobilizer may be added if the patient complains of severe pain with motion.

Patellar and Quadriceps Tendon Tear

Disruption of the extensor mechanism (Fig. 70-16) will be obvious on x-ray if there is a fracture through the patella or tibial tubercle. When the disruption is through the tendons of the extensor mechanism, clinical evaluation becomes more important.

Evaluation

A tear through the quadriceps tendon produces local pain and swelling, with a palpable defect in the tendon. The patient is unable to actively extend the knee against gravity.

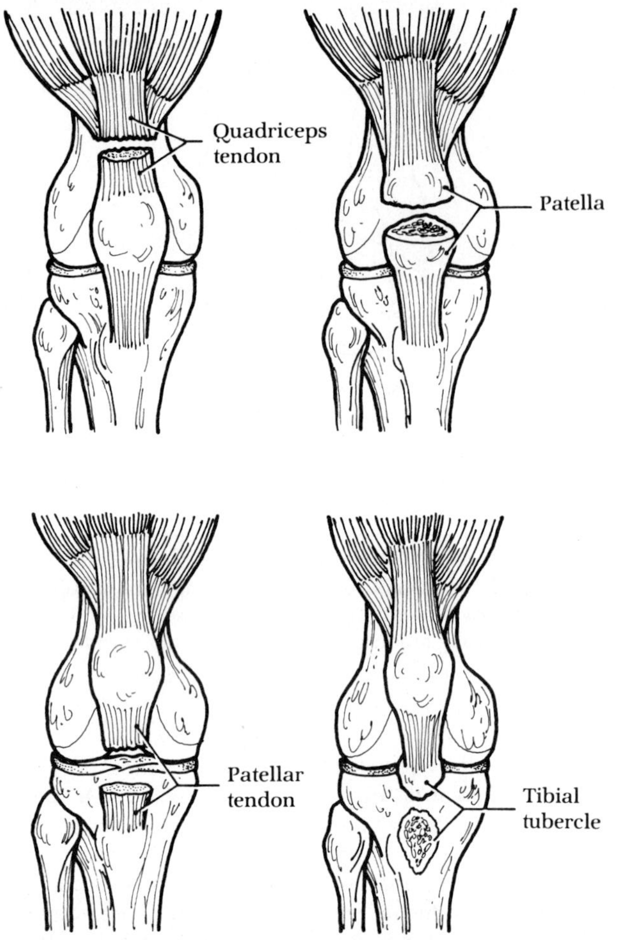

Fig. 70-16. Disruption of the extensor mechanism may occur through the quadriceps tendon, the patella, the patellar tendon, and tibial tuberosity. In all cases, the patient has limited active extension of the knee. Because the disruption may be through soft tissue, a normal x-ray does not rule out a significant injury.

A tear through the patellar tendon also produces local pain and swelling, with a defect in the tendon. In this case, the patella will be displaced proximally by the pull of the quadriceps muscle. X-rays of both knees will confirm the displacement. The patient is unable to actively extend the knee.

Treatment

Surgical repair is necessary for all disruptions of the extensor mechanism. The knee should be stabilized with an immobilizer or plaster splints, and the patient should be admitted to the hospital under the care of an orthopedic surgeon.

NONTRAUMATIC KNEE PAIN

Patients with knee disorders often enter the emergency department for evaluation without a history of injury. Most of them will have pain as their main complaint, and most will be found to have conditions that are not true emergencies. However, since nontraumatic knee pain is commonplace, and since occasionally patients have a disorder that requires urgent diagnosis and treatment, it is essential that the emergency physician be able to evaluate such disorders.

Anterior Knee Pain

Four disorders account for almost all anterior knee pain. A brief discussion of each is included in this section.

Chondromalacia Patellae

The term *chondromalacia patellae,* translated into English, is "soft cartilage of the patella." Clinically, it may range from minimal softening of the articular cartilage of the patella to full-thickness cartilage loss in the patellofemoral joint. Pain is retropatellar, although at times the patient and physician may have difficulty in precisely localizing symptoms. Activities that place high stress across the patellofemoral joint, such as sports, stair climbing, squatting, and even driving, aggravate the pain. Although pain is usually of a mild degree, it can be severe and acute. If there is substantial roughing of the articular surface with debris in the joint, synovitis and effusion can develop. On examination, the patient may exhibit an apprehension sign, with withdrawal and guarding on attempted manipulation of the patella. Compression of the patellofemoral joint during active and passive motion may produce pain and crepitation. The diagnosis is a clinical one, and there are no x-ray findings on which to rely. Treatment in the acute setting should include discontinuation of the precipitating activity and the use of nonsteroidal antiinflammatory drugs (NSAIDs). The patient may be referred to an orthopedic surgeon on a nonemergent basis. Chronic symptoms are treated by activity modification, quadriceps strengthening, NSAIDs, patellar bracing, and surgery.

Quadriceps Tendonitis

Quadriceps tendonitis is an uncommon condition, but it can produce severe, acute knee pain at the insertion of the quadriceps tendon to the patella. Localized swelling and tenderness are present, and pain is produced by active extension and passive flexion. Treatment consists of NSAIDs and rest, which may be achieved by either a knee immobilizer or crutches.

Patellar Tendonitis and Bursitis

The patellar tendon may become inflamed from overuse in sports or from frequent kneeling, which applies direct pressure. Localized tenderness in the tendon makes the diagnosis. Prepatellar bursitis presents as pain, tenderness, and circumscribed swelling over the front of the patella. These conditions should be treated with rest and NSAIDs.

Plica Syndrome

A plica is a fold, or "shelf," in the synovial lining of the knee. It is a normally occurring structure, and one or more of these synovial "shelves" are present in most knees. The medial parapatellar plica, located just medial to the patella, rubs over the medial femoral condyle during knee motion and may become inflamed. The patient complains of anteromedial knee pain and has well-localized tenderness as the examiner compresses the plica against the underlying condyle. The plica runs in a horizontal direction and is best located by flexing the knee to 20 degrees and rubbing a fingertip vertical over the medial femoral condyle adjacent to the patella. The plica, if present, feels similar to an elastic band in the soft tissue. An inflamed plica should be treated with rest and NSAIDs. If pain is recurrent, an orthopedic surgeon is able to resect the plica with arthroscopy.

Medial Knee Pain

Pain on this side of the knee may be caused by chronic pain from a medial meniscal tear or MCL sprain. Medial compartment osteoarthritis is discussed in a later section. Pes bursitis must be distinguished from these other conditions.

Pes Bursitis

There is a bursa located between the proximal medial tibia and the tendon group (pes anserinus) that crosses the medial side of the knee to insert into the tibia. Inflammation in the pes bursa is usually an overuse syndrome. The patient has tenderness and, at times, swelling, localized to the pes bursa about 4 to 5 cm distal to the medial joint line. Treatment includes rest and NSAIDs.

Lateral Knee Pain

Pain on this side of the knee with a history of frequent use of the joint may be due to iliotibial band tendonitis.

Iliotibial Band Tendonitis

The iliotibial band is the extension of the tensor fascia lata of the thigh. The band crosses the lateral side of the knee to insert into Gerdy's tubercle, a bony prominence lateral to the patellar tendon. As the band crosses the joint, it rubs over the underlying rigid bony structures during motion. Athletes are prone to develop tendonitis in the band. Treatment starts with rest and NSAIDs; if pain is persistent, physical therapy may be beneficial.

Posterior Knee Pain

Pain on the posterior side of the knee is rarely a primary complaint. Chondromalacia patellae and conditions that have produced effusions may cause a sense of posterior pain and tightness, but there are other symptoms and findings that should lead to the correct diagnosis. Deep vein thrombosis may present with pain and tenderness in the popliteal space.

Hamstring Tendonitis

The lateral or medial hamstring tendons may become inflamed with overuse. Localized tenderness confirms the diagnosis. The patient will usually have tightness of the hamstring muscle group, tested by flexing the hip with the knee in full extension. Treatment consists of rest, NSAIDs, and hamstring stretching.

Baker's Cyst

Baker's cysts form in the popliteal fossa and occasionally may be large enough to be palpated as a round mass. These cysts are thought to form because of a one-way valve that allows joint fluid to be "pumped" into the cysts, but not back into the joint. The cysts are more likely to occur if a condition, such as a torn meniscus or osteoarthritis, exists in the joint that produces a chronic increase in joint fluid. Two clinical presentations occur with a Baker's cyst. An unruptured cyst produces posterior knee pain and a circumscribed rubbery mass. The patient may be referred to an orthopedic surgeon for further evaluation and advice, but usually the cyst does not require surgical treatment. A ruptured cyst releases synovial fluid into the posterior knee and calf, producing swelling and tenderness that may be difficult to distinguish clinically from deep vein thrombosis (DVT). Appropriate vascular studies may be necessary to rule in or out the more serious condition of DVT. A ruptured Baker's cyst is treated with rest and NSAIDs. Initial pain is often severe enough to require crutches. Nonemergent follow-up with an orthopedic surgeon is appropriate, as the recovery is often slow and requires an exercise program to rehabilitate the knee and calf.

Diffuse Knee Pain

Certain conditions may produce symptoms and findings that are not localized. Since symptoms may be severe, and since a quick diagnosis may be required so that treatment is not delayed, a knowledge of these arthritides is essential to the emergency physician.

Osteochondritis Dissecans

This condition occurs primarily in young, active men. A fragment of subchondral bone and its overlying articular cartilage separates from the underlying bone of the femur. If the fragment remains in position held by fibrous tissue, symptoms consist of recurrent pain and effusion. No localizing findings may be noted on examination. X-rays reveal an abnormality, which is usually on the medial portion of the lateral femoral condyle. If the diagnosis is suspected, a tunnel view is recommended, as it is most likely to reveal the area of osteochondritis.

If the fragment has completely separated from the femur, it becomes a loose body. Patients are then more likely to complain of intermittent "catching" and "giving way" of the knee. They may report that they sometimes palpate the loose body as it circulates within the joint. On examination, findings may include an effusion, a locked knee, or a loose body palpable in the joint recesses around the patella. X-rays reveal a defect in the medial femoral condyle and a loose body. Occasionally, the bony portion of the fragment may be small and the loose body difficult to find by x-ray.

Patients with this condition should be referred on a nonemergent basis to an orthopedic surgeon, as recurrent symptoms are likely and there is a substantial role for surgical intervention.

Osteoarthritis

This common condition usually has an insidious onset and is treated in the office. Moderate-to-severe osteoarthritis is easily diagnosed by the findings of crepitation, limited motion, deformity, and characteristic x-ray changes. In the emergency department the most common type of patient with osteoarthritis is the previously asymptomatic person who twists or otherwise injures his or her knee and develops knee pain. X-ray changes may be minimal or absent. Such patients are often given diagnoses of sprains or meniscal tears. If the diagnosis of osteoarthritis is made, nonemergent follow-up with a primary care physician, rheumatologist, or orthopedic surgeon is appropriate, as the condition is chronic and progressive.

Inflammatory Arthritis

Aseptic inflammatory arthritis may produce acute pain and swelling bringing the patient to the emergency department for diagnosis and treatment. Examination reveals synovitis, warmth, an effusion, and limited motion. The x-ray is normal. Most patients are women and will ultimately be given the diagnosis of rheumatoid arthritis. The development of symptoms over several days and the absence of fever help in distinguishing this from crystalline arthritis and septic arthritis. If the latter conditions are suspected, the knee should be aspirated for fluid analysis, Gram stain, and culture. Patients with inflammatory arthritis should be referred to an internist or rheumatologist for long-term treatment.

Crystalline Arthritis

Gout and pseudogout produce acute and usually severe knee pain, with an effusion and limited motion. Most patients are men, and, in the case of gout, the blood uric acid level is almost always elevated. X-rays have no diagnostic findings. The diagnosis is made in both cases by finding the characteristic crystals for each condition in joint fluid aspirated from the joint. Treatment consists of rest and NSAIDs, although colchicine may be prescribed for gout.

Septic Arthritis

Septic arthritis is the one cause of nontraumatic knee pain that is a true emergency. Delay in diagnosis and appropriate treatment permits the toxic effects of bacterial infection to destroy articular cartilage, resulting in permanent loss of normal joint function. The diagnosis should be considered in all patients who have acute onset of knee pain and swelling. A history of antecedent infection elsewhere in the body adds to the suspicion of infection in the joint. The examination reveals fever, a warm or hot joint with diffuse tenderness and effusion, and marked limitation of motion. The x-ray is unremarkable. The erythrocyte sedimentation rate and white blood cell count are usually elevated. If the diagnosis is suspected, a joint aspiration is mandatory. A Gram stain should be done and examined in the emergency department searching for bacteria, including gram-negative diplococci. A white cell count of greater than 100,000 strongly suggests infection; most of the white cells are polymorphonuclear leukocytes. Fluid should be sent for culture, including gonococci, although results will take one or more days. If the diagnosis of septic arthritis is still suspected after the initial emergency department work-up, an orthopedic surgeon and infectious disease physician should be consulted to treat the case. Joint irrigation, now commonly done in the operating room via the arthroscope, should be strongly considered to lower the bacterial level and wash toxins from the joint. Intravenous antibiotic therapy should be started as soon as fluid for culture has been taken from the knee.

SELECTED READING

Hohl, M, Larson, RL, and Jones, DC. Fractures and Dislocations of the Knee. In CA Rockwood, Jr, and DP Green (eds), *Fractures*. Philadelphia: Lippincott, 1984.

Insall, JN (ed). *Surgery of the Knee*. New York: Churchill Livingstone, 1984.

Sisk TD. Knee Injuries. In AH Crenshaw (ed), *Campbell's Operative Orthopaedics*. St. Louis: Mosby, 1987.

71. Injuries of the Lower Leg

Daniel J. Berry

Bony and soft tissue injuries of the lower leg are common. The tibia is the most frequently fractured long bone in the body. The prevalence of such injuries in the emergency department makes a thorough understanding of these conditions essential for the emergency physician. The lower leg's vulnerable position to injury in combination with specific anatomic features of the leg results in a variety of conditions, some of which present acutely; others may present an interval of time after the injury itself.

FUNCTIONAL ANATOMY

The bony anatomy of the lower leg is relatively simple, consisting of the tibia and fibula. The tibia functions as the main weight-bearing bone, carrying 80 to 90 percent of body weight. As is well known to anyone who has struck his or her anterior leg, the tibia is poorly covered with soft tissue over its anteromedial aspect. This lack of muscle covering makes the tibia more prone to open fracture than any other bone in the body. Additionally, the lack of surrounding muscle results in a tenuous blood supply, which increases the rates of both osteomyelitis and nonunion following tibial fracture. By contrast, the fibula is well covered throughout most of its length except at the ankle where it becomes subcutaneous and is easily palpable. Proximally, the fibular head can be palpated laterally, just distal to the lateral joint line of the knee.

Uniting the tibia and fibula is a fibrous band, the interosseous membrane. This structure has particular importance at the distal portion of the lower leg where it is responsible for keeping the tibia and fibula closely approximated to provide a stable ankle joint. Disruption of this membrane occurs with certain ankle fractures and with displaced fractures of the midshaft of both tibia and fibula. Disruption of the interosseous membrane is of clinical significance when it results in associated disruption of the ankle joint, causing a widening of the distance between tibia and fibula.

The muscles of the lower leg exist in four separate compartments: anterior, peroneal, superficial posterior, and deep posterior (Fig. 71-1). The muscles of the anterior compartment are the dorsiflexors of the foot and toes, which receive motor innervation from the deep branch of the peroneal nerve. The peroneal compartment consists of the peroneus longus and brevis muscles, which evert the foot and receive their motor innervation from the superficial branch of the peroneal nerve. The superficial posterior compartment contains the gastrocnemius and soleus muscles, the very strong plantar flexors of the ankle, innervated by the tibial nerve. The deep posterior compartment contains the posterior tibial muscle as well as the long plantar flexors of the toes. These muscles are also innervated by the tibial nerve. Each compartment has a sensory nerve that runs through it; this anatomic fact can be used to help diagnose an incipient compartment syndrome (see Chap. 73).

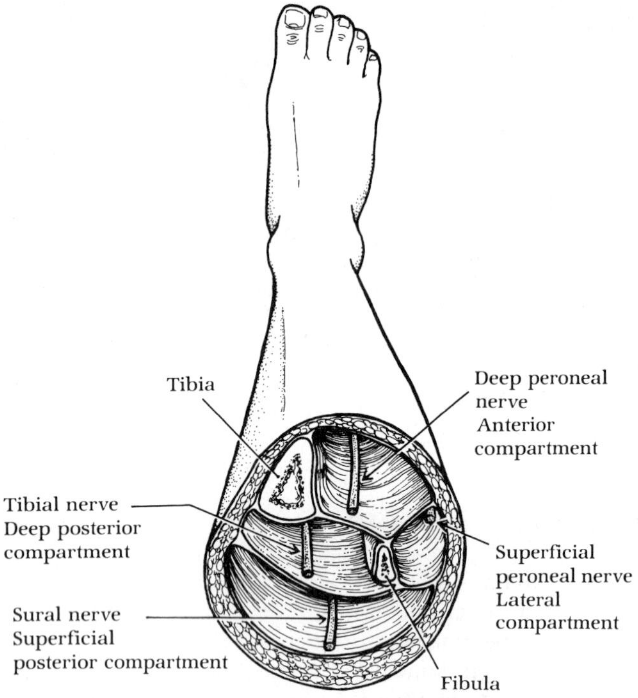

Fig. 71-1. Compartment anatomy of the lower leg. This figure shows each compartment with its associated motor/sensory nerve. The sensory distribution of these associated nerves may be used to help diagnose elevated compartment pressures occurring in any individual compartment. (Redrawn from S.J. Mubarek and C.A. Owen. Double incision fasciotomy of the leg for decompression in compartment syndrome. *J. Bone Joint Surg.* 59A: 184, 1977.)

The vascular supply of the lower leg develops from the popliteal artery, which trifurcates to form three branches: (1) the anterior tibial artery, which passes into the anterior compartment over the top of the interosseous membrane; (2) the posterior tibial artery, and (3) the peroneal artery. The patency of the anterior tibial artery can be assessed by palpating the dorsalis pedis artery pulse over the dorsum of the foot, while the posterior tibial artery pulse can be palpated posterior to the medial malleolus. Doppler instruments may be helpful in documenting the function of these vessels when pulses are weak. In cases of severe ischemia of the foot, angiography may be required to assess arterial supply.

Because the compartmental anatomy of the lower leg is defined by bony and relatively nonyielding fibrous structures (fascia), it is possible to elevate pressures within compartments to levels that exceed the pressure found in the small arterioles that supply the musculature. This condition, known as a *compartment syndrome*, occurs most frequently in the lower leg and is described in more detail in Chap. 73. The emergency physician must remain vigilant for compartment syndrome and should examine the lower leg carefully with this possibility in mind.

FRACTURES OF THE TIBIA, WITH AND WITHOUT ASSOCIATED FIBULA FRACTURE

The tibia is the most frequently fractured long bone in the body, and a greater percentage of tibial fractures are compound (open) than are fractures of any other bone. With sufficient force, the fibula will also be fractured, although often at a level remote from the tibial fracture.

While numerous classification schemes exist for tibial and fibular fractures, perhaps the most important distinctions that the emergency physician can make are (1) whether the fracture is open or closed, (2) whether the fracture represents a high-energy or low-energy injury, and (3) whether the fracture involves the knee or ankle joint. Tibial plateau fractures and proximal fibula fractures are discussed in Chap. 70, and tibial and fibula fractures involving the ankle joint are discussed in Chap. 72.

Evaluation

On presentation to the emergency department, initial evaluation of the injured leg should include a determination of the mechanism of injury, how long prior to presentation the injury occurred, and the nature of any treatment that may have been rendered prior to arrival.

Physical examination should begin with inspection, noting any gross deformity, swelling, or ecchymosis. A meticulous examination should be undertaken to determine whether any breaks in the skin—representing an open fracture—are present. This examination should be directed particularly to the anteromedial portion of the lower leg where the tibia lies subcutaneously. If an open fracture is identified, it may be classified according to the severity of associated soft tissue injury. Type I open fractures have less than a 1-cm skin wound and usually occur when bone transgresses skin from inside to out. Type II open fractures have skin wounds greater than 1 cm in size and have an intermediate degree of soft tissue injury. Type III open fractures are high-energy injuries and have extensive soft tissue trauma involving skin and muscle. They are further subclassified: Type IIIA fractures have extensive soft tissue trauma, but the bone itself is satisfactorily covered by tissue; type IIIB fractures have extensive soft tissue stripping of the bone, sufficient to impair coverage of the exposed fracture, and type IIIC fractures have an associated arterial injury that requires repair.

After visual inspection of the injured leg, a careful neurovascular examination must be documented. The accuracy of this examination is of critical importance in further management of the patient, since it will serve as a baseline against which subsequent examinations must be compared. Pedal pulses, sensory examination to light touch, and active motor function of the foot and ankle must be carefully documented and any deficits noted. Because the peroneal nerve is frequently damaged in lower extremity injuries, its function should be assessed. Motor function of the peroneal nerve is checked by testing active ankle and toe dorsiflexion (deep peroneal nerve function) and active foot eversion (superficial peroneal nerve function). Sensory function of the peroneal nerve is documented by testing sensation in the first dorsal web space of the foot (deep peroneal nerve distribution) and sensation over the dorsal lateral foot (superficial peroneal nerve distribution).

Gentle palpation of the lower leg should be performed, looking for tense swelling. Although such palpation is not an accurate way to measure compartment pressures, it can be a useful clue that compartment pressures are elevated

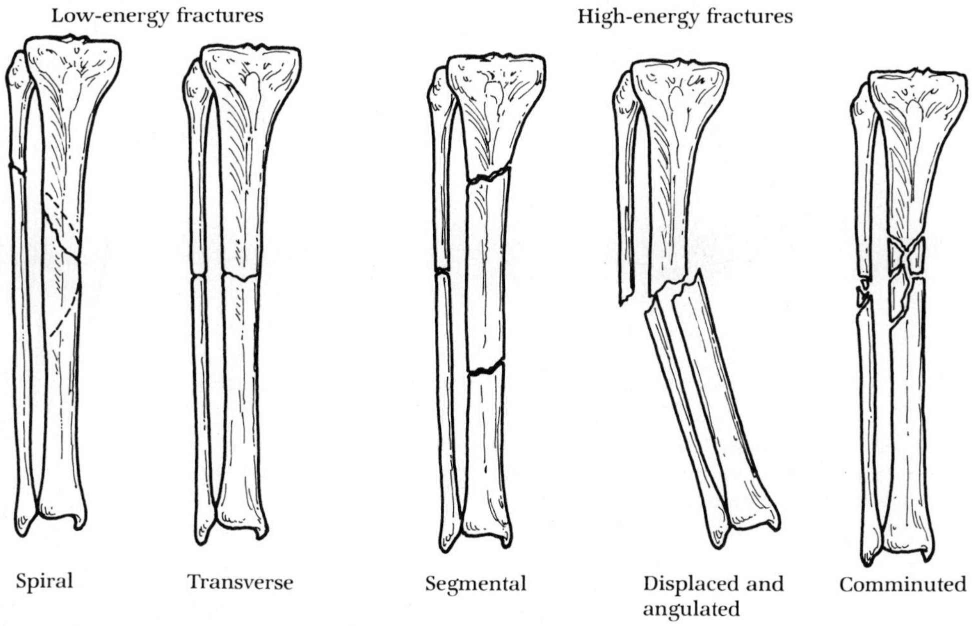

Fig. 71-2. Tibial fracture patterns. In general, the amount of comminution and displacement will be proportional to the energy the bone absorbed at the time of fracture. The distinction between a low-energy and high-energy fracture is important because, in addition to bony disruption, a high-energy fracture involves more injury of the overlying soft tissue.

above normal. The uninjured extremity may be used for comparison. Compartment syndrome is also suggested by severe unrelenting pain in the extremity at rest or extreme pain with passive motion of the toes or ankle (see Chap. 73).

After applying a splint to the lower extremity (from the foot to above the knee), radiographs in two planes should be obtained. The knee and ankle *must* be included in both views. Once films have been obtained, the amount of fracture angulation and displacement, as well as the fracture pattern, will usually be apparent. Fracture patterns that suggest low-energy injury are those fractures that are either spiral or transverse, particularly when the fibula is intact. High-energy injury is reflected in fracture patterns that are segmental, greatly displaced, or severely comminuted (Fig. 71-2). Open fractures more frequently occur with high-energy injuries, but even low-energy fractures may be open due to violation of the thin soft tissue covering the anteromedial tibia.

Treatment

Gross alignment of an angulated or malrotated limb should be obtained; this is most safely done by gentle axial traction through the foot. Open fractures should *not* be debrided or probed in the emergency department; this is more effectively done in the operating room under adequate anesthesia and sterile conditions. Obtaining a culture swab of the open fracture site is appropriate and should be routinely performed. After cultures are obtained, the open fracture should be covered with a sterile dressing and intravenous antibiotics administered, as described below. If tetanus immunization is not current, appropriate tetanus prophylaxis should be given.

For type I open fractures, intravenous antibiotic prophylaxis using a first-generation cephalosporin is recommended (e.g., cefazolin, 2 gm on admission, then 1 gm every 8 hours). For type II and type III open fractures, a loading dose of an aminoglycoside may be given in addition to the first-generation cephalosporin. Any open fracture occurring in an agricultural setting should also be treated with intravenous penicillin (2 million units of penicillin G) for possible clostridial contamination. Patients with open fractures should be made ready for hospital admission and surgical debridement as soon as possible, because the incidence of osteomyelitis is in part related to the delay between contamination and definitive debridement of the open fracture site.

Definitive treatment of open tibia fractures (following initial debridement) remains one of the most controversial topics in orthopedics. At the present time, type III open fractures are most frequently treated with an external fixation frame that stabilizes the bone fragments and allows simultaneous access to the soft tissue injury (Fig. 71-3). Types I and II open fractures may be treated with cast immobilization, internal fixation devices, or external fixation frames depending on the clinical circumstances.

For closed tibia fractures, cast treatment is the mode most frequently used, although internal fixation with an intramedullary nail or a plate is performed in some cases. Most patients with tibial shaft fractures are admitted to the hospital for observation and enforced elevation of the extremity. The orthopedic surgeon should be consulted at the time of presentation. At admission, most patients will initially be treated with a long leg splint, as a circumferential cast in the acute fracture may increase the risk of compartment syndrome in all but the most minimally injured leg.

Tibial fractures are slow to heal, usually requiring a minimum of 12 weeks of cast immobilization. Nonunion occurs with greater frequency than for any other long bone in the body.

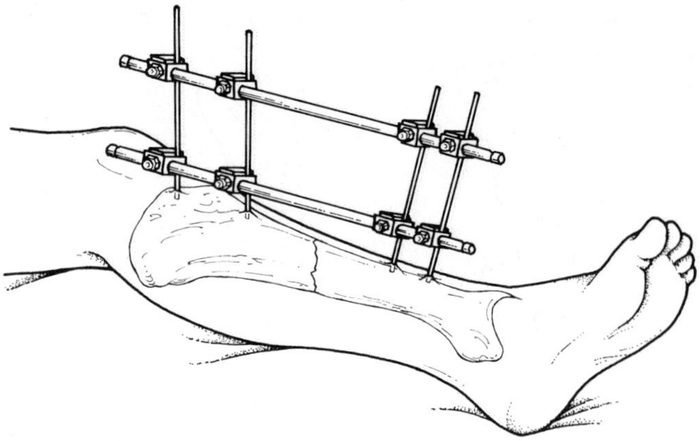

Fig. 71-3. Tibial fracture stabilized by external fixation frame. Such frames are commonly used for open tibia fractures to stabilize the bone and to allow simultaneous access to the soft tissue for observation and treatment.

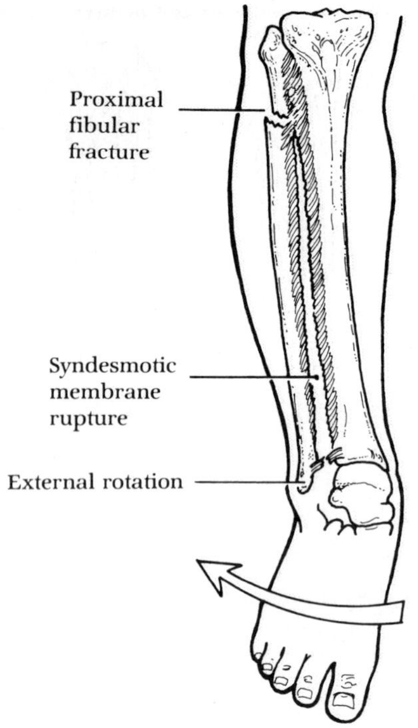

Fig. 71-4. Maisonneuve fracture. This injury results from an external rotation force applied to the ankle, causing tearing of the interosseous membrane and a fracture of the fibula proximally. Palpation of the entire fibula is necessary in all cases of ankle injury, since this fracture can easily be missed if attention is directed only to the ankle itself.

Isolated Fractures of the Shaft of the Fibula

Evaluation

Isolated fractures of the fibular shaft occur as the result of a direct blow to the lateral aspect of the leg. An exception to this is the Maisonneuve fracture, which is a proximal fibular fracture that results from an external rotation stress at the ankle (Fig. 71-4). Therefore, careful evaluation of the ankle is essential for any apparently isolated fibular shaft fracture, just as palpation over the entire fibula should be performed whenever significant ankle injury is present. The common peroneal nerve courses in the subcutaneous tissue around the proximal neck of the fibula where it is vulnerable to injury. Thus, in proximal fibula fractures, particular attention should be paid to peroneal nerve evaluation, as discussed previously.

Treatment

Isolated fractures of the fibular shaft are treated for comfort, since the intact tibia provides satisfactory stability and bears the vast majority of weight through the lower leg. Nondisplaced or minimally displaced fibula fractures do not necessarily require cast immobilization; in many cases, wrapping the foot and leg with an elastic bandage to minimize swelling will be sufficient treatment. The patient should be instructed to elevate the extremity, apply ice periodically, and remain non–weight bearing until a small amount of weight can be tolerated. Weight bearing may then be advanced progressively, as tolerated. Follow-up with an orthopedic surgeon is appropriate at 7 to 10 days. As for any injury of the lower leg, the patient must be instructed to watch for symptoms of elevated compartment pressure. If the patient notes increasing pain, numbness of the foot, or the development of motor deficits, immediate return to the emergency department is necessary.

For severely displaced fibular shaft fractures or those fractures with an associated peroneal nerve deficit ("foot drop"), orthopedic consultation is indicated. The usual treatment will be similar, but follow-up may be scheduled at a shorter interval from injury. Cast immobilization may offer the patient some comfort, but it is often not recommended in cases with concomitant nerve injury.

For Maisonneuve fractures, orthopedic consultation is indicated and an accurate mortise view of the ankle joint is essential. If the ankle mortise is disrupted, surgical treatment may be recommended.

Stress Fractures of the Tibia and Fibula

Stress fractures of both the tibia and fibula occur. The typical population at risk includes athletes or any individual who undertakes a substantial increase in the level of his or her physical activity. Examples include a recreational runner who, after doubling the distance he or she runs, notes leg pain with weight bearing, or a sedentary office worker who begins daily delivery of documents by foot, then develops leg pain that is severe by evening.

Evaluation

Symptoms usually begin with gradual onset of pain associated with activity and may progress to more severe or persistent pain. Findings include pain with weight bearing and localized tenderness. Swelling may or may not be present over the stress fracture, and ecchymosis is rarely seen. Radiographs may be normal at presentation but may eventually show the presence of localized periosteal reaction (Fig. 71-5). If the diagnosis is suspected from history and physical examination but cannot be confirmed by x-ray, a technetium bone scan may confirm the presence of a stress fracture.

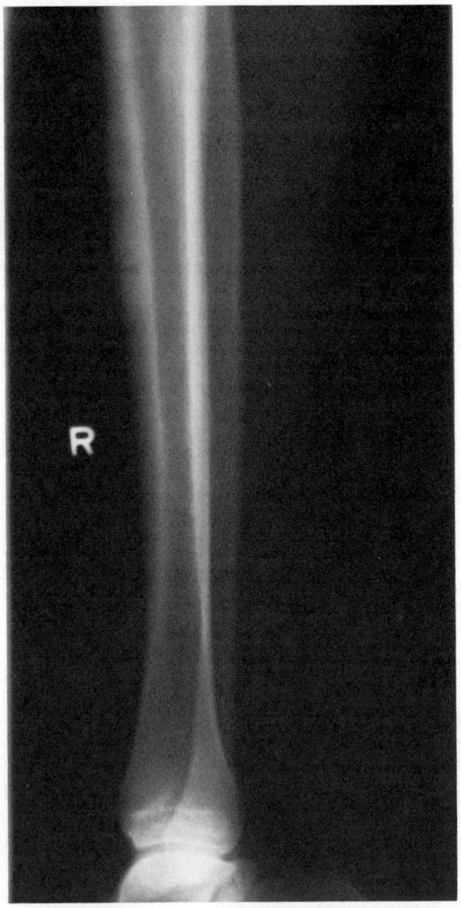

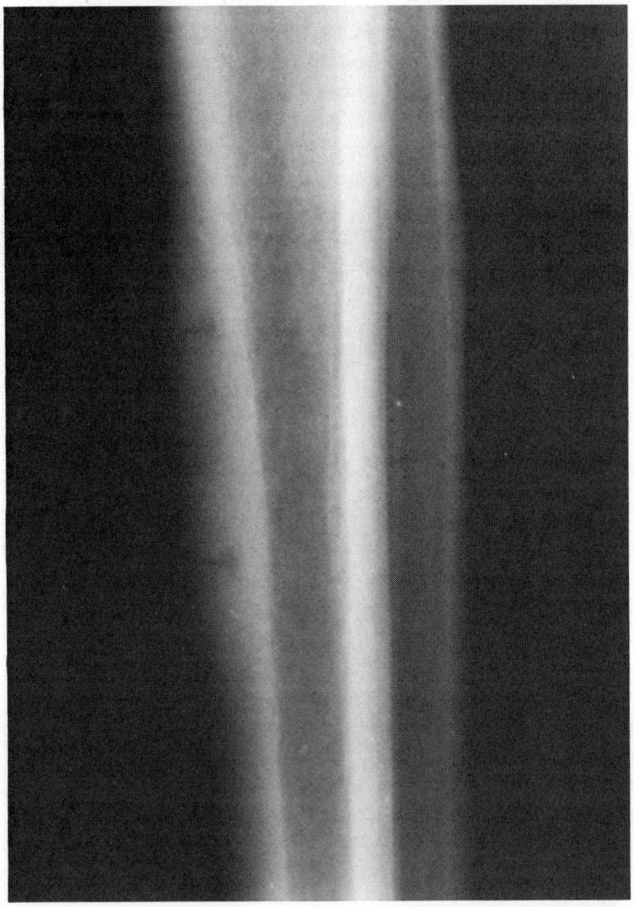

A B

Fig. 71-5. Stress fracture of tibia. Such fractures are quite difficult to see on x-ray and may require multiple oblique views and possibly a technetium bone scan to document.

Treatment
Patients should be told to refrain from vigorous physical activity and to use crutches, bearing approximately 25 percent of their body weight on the injured leg initially. Orthopedic follow-up should be arranged within 2 weeks of presentation. A cast may be used if it permits more comfortable ambulation.

SOFT-TISSUE INJURIES INVOLVING THE LOWER LEG

Contusions

Blunt trauma to the lower leg is quite common, and the blow is usually received anteriorly or anterolaterally. Patients often present late with symptoms of increased pain, swelling, or ecchymosis.

Evaluation
The history is most important. Questions should elicit how the injury was sustained—was it a blow delivered by bumping into a stationary table, or was the leg caught between two car bumpers, even if only briefly? Crushing injuries have a greater propensity to result in elevated compartment pressures than do more focally directed blows. The interval from injury is also important, since most compartment syndromes will develop within 72 hours of injury and are less frequent thereafter.

The physical examination should include palpation of the lower leg, looking for point tenderness or induration involving an entire compartment. Careful motor and sensory examinations are critical. Passive stretching of all muscle groups should also be performed, looking for pain associated with the stretching of ischemic musculature, although this is difficult to differentiate from the pain of muscle contusion itself. X-rays should be obtained if the contusion is significant or if any bony tenderness or deformity is present.

Treatment
With a normal neurovascular examination and no clinical evidence of compartment syndrome, treatment is symptomatic with elevation, periodic application of ice, and protected weight bearing using crutches. Patients should be instructed to watch for signs of developing compartment syndrome and to return to the emergency department immediately if such signs are noted.

Patients who show any evidence of compartment syndrome, as manifested by motor or sensory abnormalities, pain with passive stretch of the musculature, or palpably increased pressures in any compartment, should undergo compartment pressure measurement (see Chap. 73 for this technique). If compartment pressures are normal after accurate measurement, the patient may be discharged from the emergency department with instructions for elevation, application of ice, and protected weight bearing. Follow-up with the patient's primary physician on a symptomatic basis is usually adequate, provided that the patient is aware of the symptoms of developing compartment syndrome. If compartment pressures are elevated in the presence of physical symptoms or signs of compartment syndrome, the patient must be admitted for treatment or observation. Any patient with a major crush injury to the leg should also be admitted to the hospital for observation to ensure that compartment syndrome does not develop, even if compartment pressures are not initially elevated.

Rupture of the Plantaris Tendon or Medial Head of the Gastrocnemius Muscle

The medial head of the gastrocnemius muscle ruptures more frequently than was previously suspected. In the past, it was thought that the plantaris tendon could rupture during forceful ankle plantar flexion. This is now believed to be a rare occurrence; the common site of injury is believed to be within the medial portion of the gastrocnemius muscle. Rupture of the medial head of the gastrocnemius muscle should be distinguished from Achilles tendon rupture. Patients with Achilles tendon rupture typically present with weakness of ankle plantar flexion and have findings of tenderness and swelling over the Achilles tendon itself. Diagnosis and treatment of Achilles tendon rupture is discussed in greater detail in Chap. 72.

Evaluation

Patients present with a history of sudden onset of midcalf pain following forceful dorsiflexion of a plantar flexed foot, such as when stepping down from a height or during a sporting event.

The physical examination usually reveals tenderness and swelling over the midcalf, just medial to midline. Occasionally, a palpable gap in the calf muscle may be present, but this may be obscured by bleeding and edema within 1 to 2 days of injury (Fig. 71-6).

It may be difficult to differentiate a patient with partial gastrocnemius rupture from one with a deep vein thrombophlebitis except by the history of the abrupt onset of symptoms. Venography or noninvasive tests for venous thrombosis may resolve this particular differential and should be obtained in cases where the history and physical examination suggest venous thrombosis.

Treatment

Initial measures include gentle elastic bandage wrapping of the leg and foot or possibly a short posterior splint (to below the knee) for the more uncomfortable patient. Application of ice, elevation, and protected weight bearing using crutches are the recommended measures. Activity may be advanced as tolerated 3 to 5 days after the injury. Follow-up with the patient's primary physician or an orthopedic surgeon at 7 to 10 days is appropriate.

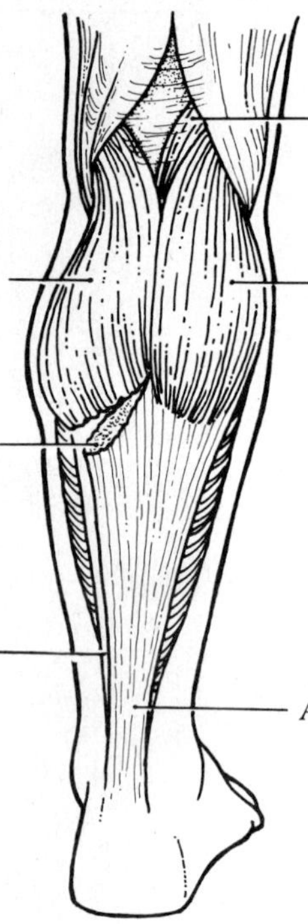

Fig. 71-6. Rupture of the medial head of the gastrocnemius muscle. The typical site of injury is illustrated. Rarely, the tear may be palpable; usually, however, the defect will be obscured by edema and hemorrhage within 24 hours. (Redrawn from J.G. McClure. Gastrocnemius musculotendinous rupture: A condition confused with thrombophlebitis. *South. Med. J.* 77: 1143, 1984.)

Shin Splints

So-called shin splints probably represent a periostitis of the medial tibia. The condition is common in athletes, especially in runners. Shin splints, tendonitis, stress fractures, and chronic compartment syndromes occur in a similar patient population and share presenting complaints of chronic exercise-induced leg pain. Careful physical examination and appropriate testing can be used to distinguish between these diagnoses.

Evaluation

Shin splints typically present with medial tibial pain brought on by exercise or ambulation. Examination usually reveals diffuse medial tibial tenderness, and radiographs are usually normal.

Treatment

Symptomatic treatment emphasizing limitation of the aggravating physical activity and antiinflammatory medication is recommended. Pain that persists requires further workup, including repeat radiographs and possibly a bone scan to rule out stress fracture. Orthopedic follow-up at 3 weeks is appropriate if symptoms persist.

Chronic Compartment Syndromes

In recent years, there has been increasing documentation of exercise-induced transient compartment pressure elevations in certain individuals. The patients afflicted are often runners who experience exercise-related pain in one or another compartment of the lower leg, with the anterior and deep posterior compartments being most frequently involved. Such transient compartment syndromes do not have the same clinical implications as an acute compartment syndrome developing shortly after substantial soft tissue injury.

Evaluation

Patients with chronic compartment syndrome classically describe a history of lower leg pain following exercise and, in some cases, may also relate symptoms of transient numbness involving the foot. The diagnosis is rarely made in the emergency department, since it requires documentation of elevated compartment pressures during exercise. It is important to rule out other potential causes of the symptoms such as shin splints, stress fracture, or a tendonitis about the ankle.

Treatment

Avoiding the offending activity seems the simplest advice, but often these individuals are quite committed to their exercise program and are reluctant to discontinue the activity in question. Referral to an orthopedic surgeon, preferably one with an interest in sports injuries, is appropriate. Rarely, these patients will undergo elective surgical fasciotomy.

SELECTED READING

Chapman, MW. Fractures of the Tibial and Fibular Shafts. In CM Evarts (ed), *Surgery of the Musculoskeletal System* (2nd ed). New York: Churchill Livingstone, 1990.

Gustillo, RB, Merkow, RL, and Templeman, D. The management of open fractures. *J Bone Joint Surg*, 72A: 299, 1990.

Leach, RE. Fractures of the Tibia and Fibula. In CA Rockwood, Jr, and DP Green (eds), *Fractures in Adults*. Philadelphia: Lippincott 1984.

Matsen, FA, III, Mubarak, SJ, and Rorabeck, CH. A Practical Approach to Compartment Syndromes. In CM Evarts (ed), *Instructional Course Lectures*, Vol. 32, American Academy of Orthopaedic Surgeons. St Louis: Mosby, 1983.

Schatzter, J, and Tile, M. *The Rationale of Operative Fracture Care*. Berlin: Springer, 1987.

72. Foot and Ankle Injuries

Brian J. Awbrey

Injuries of the ankle and foot may be the most frequent orthopedic condition seen in the emergency department. The range of injuries extends from minor contusions and sprains to severe crush injuries, which can result in amputation.

The physician having initial contact with this group of patients is in an ideal position to render care appropriate for minor injuries and thus reduce the period of disability. For more severe injuries requiring consultation and possibly operative treatment, early diagnosis and institution of initial, if not definitive, treatment can facilitate the total care of the patient and thereby have a beneficial effect on the outcome.

ANKLE INJURIES

Functional Anatomy

The ankle joint is composed of the talus, surrounded on three sides by the distal tibia and fibula. The joint is a stable one in which the talus is locked into the ankle "mortise" formed by the medial and lateral malleoli. In addition to buttressing the talus, the malleoli serve as pulleys for the major tendons of the foot and as attachment points for the ligaments of the ankle joint (Figs. 72-1 and 72-2).

As is common with other large joints, the capsular ligaments of the ankle joint are weak anteriorly and posteriorly but have strong medial and lateral ligaments providing stability to the joint. The major medial ligamentous structure is the deltoid ligament, which attaches to the medial malleolus and fans out distally to attach to the talus, navicular, and calcaneus (Fig. 72-2). Also on the medial side of the foot is the spring ligament, extending from the medial side of the calcaneus to the navicular. It provides added support to the head of the talus during weight bearing.

The lateral aspect of the joint is stabilized primarily by the anterior and posterior talofibular ligaments and the calcaneofibular ligament, which lies between the two talofibular ligaments (see Fig. 72-1). It is these lateral structures that are most frequently injured, particularly the anterior talofibular ligament (see Figs. 72-1 and 72-9). Between the tibia and fibula, a strong fibrous membrane, the interosseous membrane, maintains the tibia and fibula in close apposition, which is critical for the functioning of the ankle joint (Figs. 72-1 and 72-3).

The muscles that control ankle and foot motion are primarily within the calf and pass through long tendon sheaths held in place about the ankle by thickenings of the crural fascia. Anteriorly, these fascial reinforcements consist of the superior extensor retinaculum and a heavier inferior extensor retinaculum. Medially, the flexor retinaculum covers the tendons and runs from the medial malleolus to the calcaneus (Fig. 72-4). Laterally, it is the superior peroneal retinaculum from calcaneus to fibula that overlies the tendons of the peroneus longus and brevis (Figs. 72-4 and 72-9).

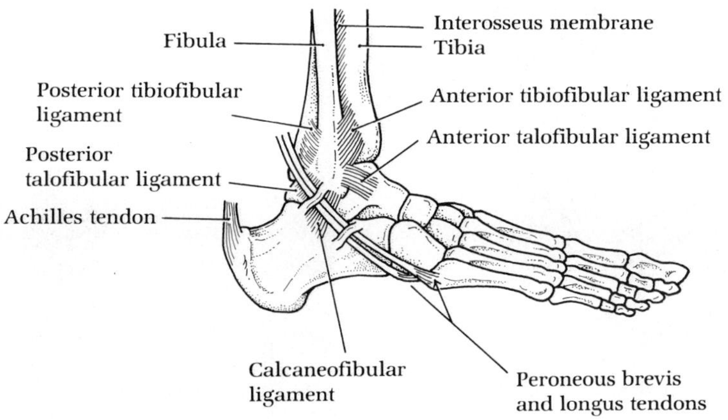

Fig. 72-1. The lateral bone and deep soft tissue anatomy of the ankle, showing the major ligaments and the relationship of the peroneal tendons to the fibula.

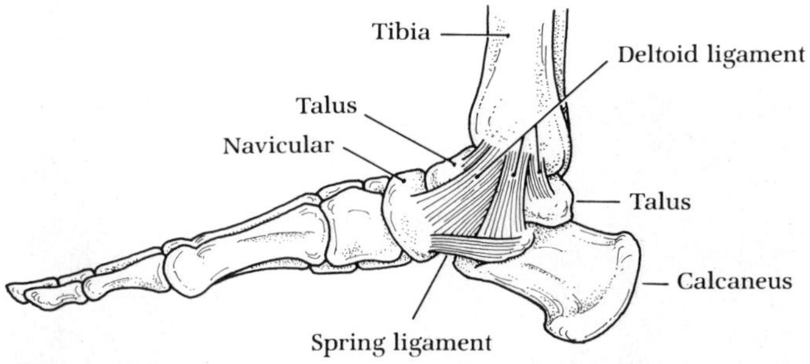

Fig. 72-2. The medial bone and deep soft tissue anatomy of the ankle, showing the deltoid ligament and spring ligament.

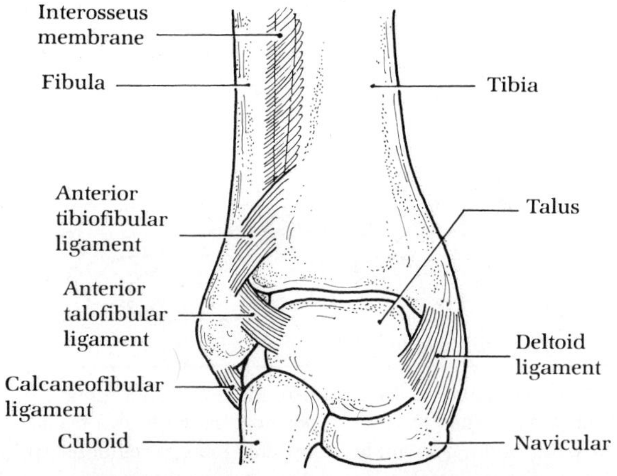

Fig. 72-3. The anterior bone and deep soft tissue anatomy of the ankle, showing the relationship of the medial and lateral supporting ligaments, the ankle mortise, and the interosseous membrane of the tibia and fibula.

There is very little subcutaneous tissue over the entire ankle joint, and because of this, ligamentous injuries to the ankle may present with massive swelling, which can compromise the overlying skin. It is therefore important to evaluate the integrity of the soft tissue when there is significant ankle injury.

Ankle Fractures

Any injury about the ankle must be considered as a possible ankle fracture when bony tenderness, instability, or pain with weight bearing is present. Any disruption of the articulating surfaces of the tibia, fibula, or talus can lead to joint incongruity and resultant degenerative arthritis. Because of this, all ankle fractures except the most minimal avulsion fractures should be referred for orthopedic care to ensure that the fracture alignment is satisfactory and remains so during the healing phase.

Evaluation

Frequently, ankle fractures cannot be differentiated from ankle sprains by gross inspection. Careful palpation of soft tissues and bony landmarks will often reveal crepitus or true bony tenderness rather than ligamentous tenderness, suggesting the presence of a fracture. Obviously, the most important diagnostic tool is the x-ray, which will document the presence of fracture and even certain types of ligamentous instability. To adequately evaluate the ankle, three views are *always* necessary: (1) an anteroposterior (AP) view, (2) a lateral view, and (3) a 20-degree internal rotation view, which is referred to as the *mortise* view. The mortise view reveals the bony arch surrounding the talus, which is critical for the congruity of the ankle joint (Figs. 72-3 and 72-5). The neurovascular status of the foot and the condition of the soft tissues should always be assessed and attended to before the patient is sent for x-rays of the ankle. Any obviously unstable or deformed ankle should be splinted prior to x-rays. Radiolucent splinting with plastic or fiberglass material is preferred when available.

Particular care should be given to rule out the diagnosis of Maisonneuve fracture, in which there is widening of the ankle mortise due to interosseous membrane rupture (see Figs. 72-1 and 72-3) associated with a fracture of the *proximal* fibula. These injuries are frequently missed in the emergency department because palpation and x-ray examination were limited to the ankle joint itself. If a widened ankle mortise due to interosseous membrane rupture is not diagnosed and treated appropriately, the potential for a disrupted ankle joint and posttraumatic arthritis is increased.

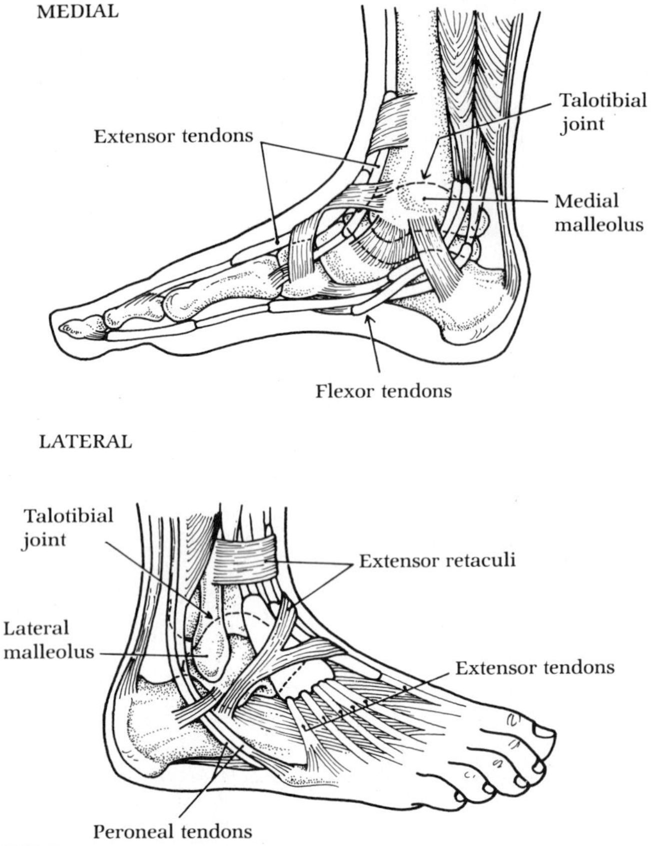

Fig. 72-4. The muscles that control ankle and foot motion pass through tendon sheaths held in position by the crural fascia. Note the position of the true ankle (talotibial) joint in relationship to the medial and lateral malleoli and the extensor retinaculi.

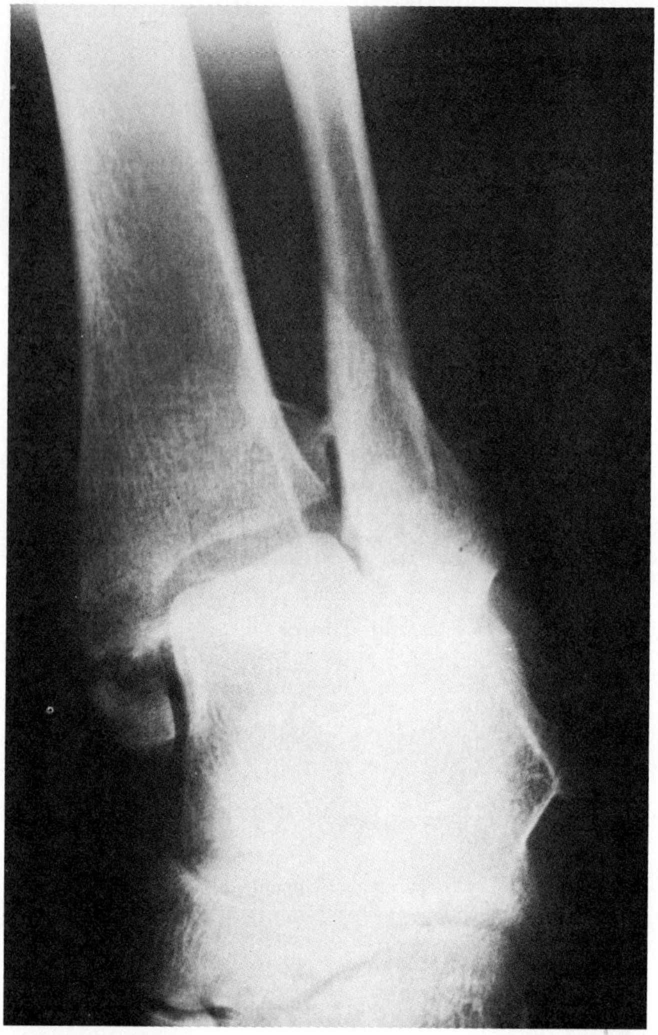

Fig. 72-5. A mortise view of an ankle fracture. There is a transverse fracture of the medial malleolus at the level of the plafond of the tibia, as well as an oblique angulated fracture of the fibula.

Fractures about the ankle are often associated with dislocations of the ankle joint itself and are properly termed *fracture-dislocations* when the talus is displaced from the disrupted mortise. Such injuries are usually quite obvious on initial examination and should be reduced promptly after x-ray confirmation to prevent both vascular compromise and excessive pressure on the overlying skin.

The majority of fractures about the ankle involve displaced or minimally displaced fractures of the distal fibula. These generally occur at three separate levels. The first level of fracture includes fractures below the tibiofibular ligaments (Fig. 72-6A) and is termed a *Weber class A fracture*. The second level consists of fractures at the level of the tibiofibular ligaments, often involving comminution of the fibula at the level of the ligament (Fig. 72-6B). The third level includes fractures above the level of the ligaments and involving disruption of the interosseous membrane as well as rupture of the tibiofibular ligament (Fig. 72-6C).

Chondral (cartilage) fractures should be considered when there are signs of joint pain and effusion and no obvious fracture on x-ray examination. Chondral fractures on the superolateral border of the talar dome are most common and result from dorsiflexion-inversion injuries, particularly in young people. An example would be when a jumper comes down hard onto the inverted foot. Chondral fractures are frequently missed in the initial evaluation and may not be diagnosed until much later in the course of treatment. A radiograph of the ankle in which there is a suspected chondral fracture *may* show a crater or particle of bone that appears opaque about the lateral or medial aspect of the talar dome similar to that shown in Fig. 72-7.

Ankle fractures in children occur primarily at the distal tibia. The physes ("growth plates") are the weakest structure in the bone-ligament complex, leading to a fracture pattern different than that in adults and a different pattern of radiographic findings. In children, fracture, physeal injury, and ligamentous injury can all be present to varying degrees. Because of this, if a fracture is suspected, views should be taken of both ankles. The fracture patterns of the distal tibia in children can be classified into five basic types, as shown in Fig. 72-8. These fracture patterns fit the Salter classification system of radiographic identification, as follows: demonstration of a physeal separation as a type I (Fig. 72-8), a metaphyseal fracture with partial physeal separation as type II, a metaphyseal-epiphyseal fracture as type IV, and a physeal crush injury as type V. Any of these fracture types in children

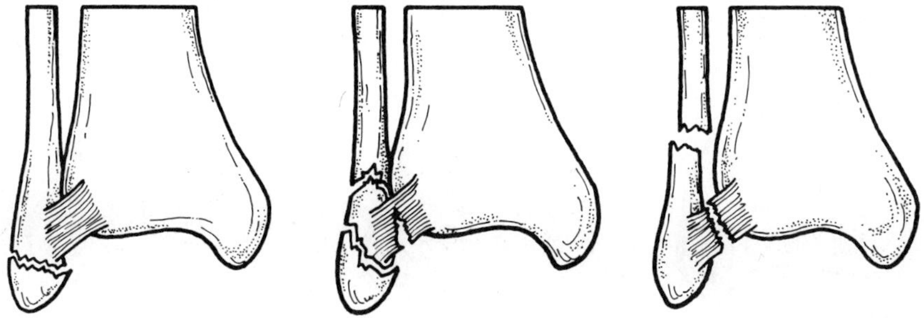

Fig. 72-6. The Weber classification of lateral malleolus fractures of the ankle according to anatomic site. Those fractures below the tibiofibular ligament are transverse (A), those at the level of the ligament are oblique and sometimes comminuted (B), and those above the ligament will involve a tear of the ligament and interosseous membrane as well as fracture (C) and should be treated appropriately.

can be serious and could represent significant injury to the growth plate of the distal tibia.

Treatment

In every case, these patients should be referred for orthopedic consultation since posttraumatic arthritis is more likely to result if proper reduction of an ankle fracture is delayed or inadequate. If the ankle presents with a gross deformity, the emergency physician should realign the foot promptly to prevent ischemic damage to the overlying skin. This can usually be deferred until after x-rays are obtained, but in cases in which the injury is several hours old or when radiographic evaluation is going to be delayed, reduction should be performed immediately.

To perform reduction of a grossly displaced ankle fracture, the safest maneuver is to grasp the heel and forefoot and apply steady traction for 20 to 30 seconds in line with the leg. In most cases, this will realign the talus beneath the tibia. A posterior splint should then be applied. If there is resistance to reduction, further manipulation should not be performed until x-rays are obtained. Interposed soft tissue or bone fragments can prevent reduction from being obtained, and vigorous, blind manipulation can exacerbate the injury.

For nondisplaced fractures of a single malleolus with no widening of the ankle mortise, a posterior splint from foot to below the knee with compressive dressing is sufficient treatment. The patient should be instructed to remain non–weight bearing using crutches with strict elevation of the injured extremity until seen by an orthopedic surgeon 48 to 72 hours from injury.

For displaced fractures about the ankle, a reduction is required. This is most easily performed within the first few hours after injury and should be performed by the orthopedic surgeon.

Despite the best of treatment, posttraumatic arthritis of the ankle will develop to some degree in a sizeable minority of patients. Predisposing factors to posttraumatic arthritis include inaccurate reduction, comminution of the weight-bearing surface of the tibia, and increasing age of the patient. However, the symptoms of posttraumatic arthritis are often minimal and intermittent, and patients may retain an excellent functional range of motion of the ankle joint.

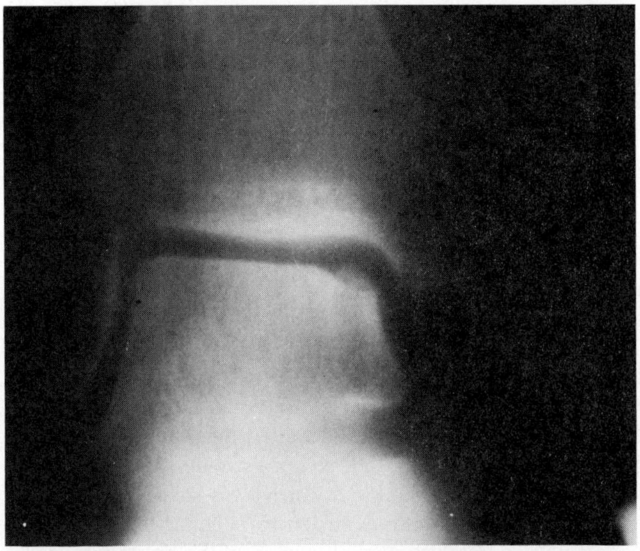

Fig. 72-7. Radiograph of an osteochondral fracture of the talar dome. The mortise view of an ankle suspected of such a fracture may show a crater or particle of bone that appears opaque about the lateral or medial aspect of the talar dome, similar to the one shown here.

Sprains

Sprains of the ankle are caused by either inversion or eversion stresses across the ankle joint, with inversion injuries accounting for almost 85 percent of the total number of ankle injuries. Whenever possible, it is important to note the position of the foot and the direction of the force applied at the time of injury.

The structure most frequently injured with an inversion stress is the anterior talofibular ligament, but with sufficient force, the calcaneofibular ligament will also be torn (Figs. 72-1 and 72-9). Injuries to the posterior talofibular ligament are unusual since it is stronger and stressed only with forced dorsiflexion of the ankle, an unusual stress in most ankle sprains. Sprains about the medial malleolus are much less common, in part due to the strong elastic nature of the deltoid ligament (see Fig. 72-2). Eversion forces are actually

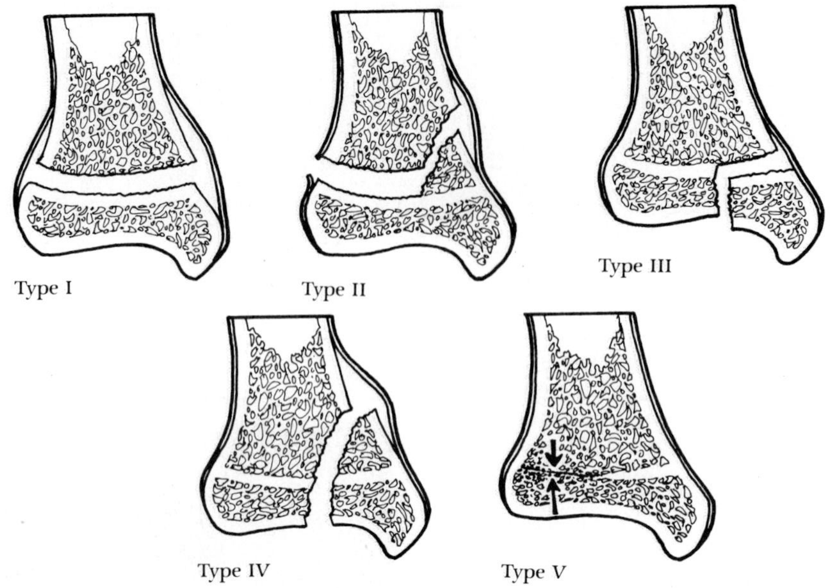

Fig. 72-8. A diagrammatic representation of fracture of the distal tibia involving physeal injuries, according to the Salter classification. Type I is a physeal separation; type II is a metaphyseal fracture with physeal separation; type III is an epiphyseal fracture with physeal separation; type IV is a metaphyseal-epiphyseal fracture; and type V is a physeal crush injury.

more likely to produce an avulsion fracture of the medial malleolus than they are a partial or complete rupture of the deltoid ligament. Rotational forces, however, can produce deltoid ligament tears since these forces tend to shear the ligament.

Injuries of the ligaments of the ankle are classified as first-degree, second-degree, and third-degree sprains, based on their severity. A first-degree sprain results in little or no functional loss in the ankle and involves stretching without tearing of the ligamentous structure (Fig. 72-9). A second-degree sprain involves partial tearing of the ligaments, associated with swelling, local hemorrhage, and pain. A third-degree sprain is defined as a complete tear of the ligament involved; swelling, tenderness, and instability are demonstrable at the time of the examination. With any complete ligamentous rupture, there may be less pain produced with passive motion since there are no intact ligamentous fibers to be painfully stretched.

Evaluation

The initial physical examination should begin at the knee joint, with special attention to the proximal fibula since ankle trauma can produce a proximal fibular fracture by forces transmitted through the interosseous membrane. Avulsion of the lower leg musculature may also be missed if the examination is confined to the ankle itself.

In examining the ankle, the examiner should start by palpating away from the side of the greatest swelling and pain by first gently compressing the contralateral malleolus and palpating the bony prominences for suspected fractures. Next, palpation across the front of the ankle joint to each side of the extensor tendons should be performed. This area represents the anterior capsule of the ankle joint, which can be involved in more severe sprains. Next, the examiner should palpate directly over the ligaments of the uninjured side and, finally, extend palpation to the ligamentous structures on the involved side. There will be point tenderness at the site of ligament sprain.

Next, x-rays should be obtained at the ankle. The decision to obtain x-rays of the knee and proximal fibula should be determined by the presence or absence of bony tenderness. If there is any question of tenderness and pain proximally, these areas must also be x-rayed.

If there is no evidence of fracture, distinction between second-degree (partial tears) and third-degree (complete tears) sprains should be made by stress testing of the ankle joint. This is best done by clinical examination, although stress radiographs can be obtained to document these results. First, the practitioner should examine the opposite ankle to determine the normal ligamentous stability for the patient. The foot should be held in a neutral position and the ankle subjected to inversion stress and anterior drawer stress (Figs. 72-10 and 72-11). Inversion stress is produced by applying a gentle force through the midfoot as shown in Fig. 72-10. The anterior drawer test should be performed with the patient sitting or supine, keeping the knee at 90 degrees of flexion. One hand is placed about the distal tibia anteriorly, and the other hand cups the back of the heel and gently draws it forward, subjecting the ankle to an anterior drawer stress as shown in Fig. 72-11. If the ankle remains appropriately stable (using the opposite side as a rough guide), it is unlikely that complete ligamentous disruption has occurred.

Some second-degree sprains are associated with what appears to be a small flake of bone in the area of the lateral malleolus on x-ray. This finding may represent a small avulsion fracture of the distal tip of the fibula but may just as well represent calcification within the anterior talofibular or calcaneofibular ligament, consistent with previous injury. History and careful palpation distinguish between these two possibilities. In most cases, small avulsion fractures will not be treated any differently than first- and second-degree ankle sprains.

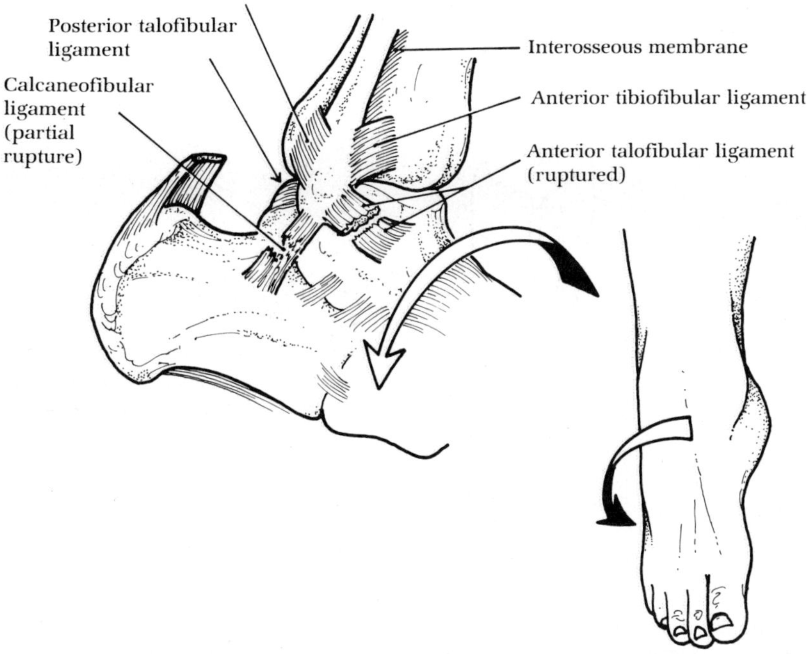

Fig. 72-9. The mechanism of sprain of the lateral ligament complex of the ankle. These structures are most often injured by inversion force, frequently tearing the anterior talofibular ligament, but, with sufficient force, the calcaneofibular ligament will also be torn.

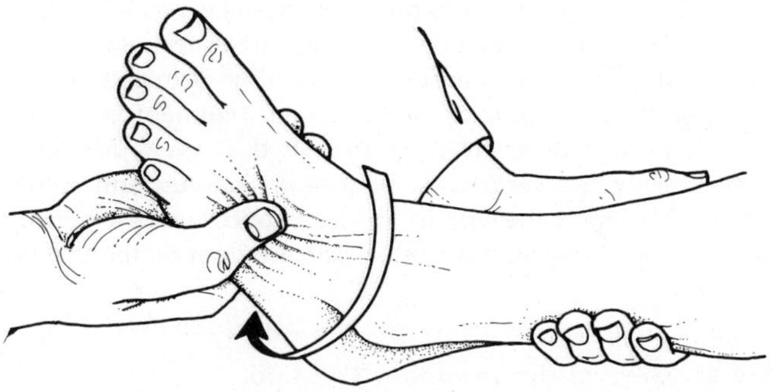

Fig. 72-10. Evaluation of the lateral ligament complex of the ankle for ligament sprain. The foot should be held in a neutral position, and the ankle is subjected to a steady, forceful inversion stress. Comparison should be made with the opposite normal ankle to determine the normal ligamentous stability for the patient.

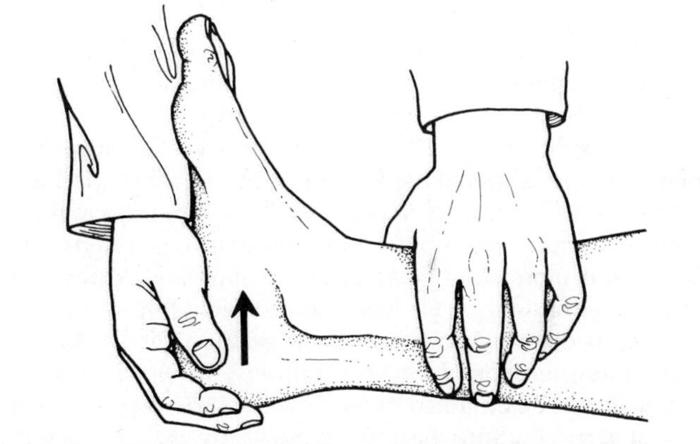

Fig. 72-11. Evaluation of the ligament complex of the ankle for ligament sprain. The anterior drawer test should be performed with the patient sitting or supine, with the knee at a 90-degree angle. One hand is placed over the distal tibia anteriorly, and the other hand is at the back of the heel drawing forward. This subjects the ankle to a firm anterior drawer stress. Comparison should be made with the opposite ankle.

Treatment

For first- and second-degree ankle sprains, initial treatment in the emergency department may be definitive. If the patient can exhibit a nearly full range of motion of the joint and has moderate tenderness limited to one side of the joint, treatment should consist of use of an elastic compressive bandage, crutches (or cane for the elderly patient), ice, and elevation for 72 hours. Thereafter, progressive return to full activities is permitted. After the initial 24 hours, heat and use of aspirin or other nonsteroidal anti-inflammatory agents are helpful for reducing pain and swelling. For best results, the elastic wrap should extend from the tips of the toes to at least midcalf to provide adequate compression and to prevent edema from forming just above the ankle. A slightly more effective compression dressing for more swollen ankles may be achieved by using layers of cast padding alternating with Ace bandages (Jones dressing). Although complete weight bearing can begin after 72 hours, if swelling persists, the patient should be instructed to rewrap the elastic bandage twice per day for 24-hour use. Patients should be instructed to seek orthopedic consultation if not ambulating comfortably by 7 to 10 days.

For more severely sprained ankles—that is, markedly painful second-degree and all third-degree injuries—the pa-

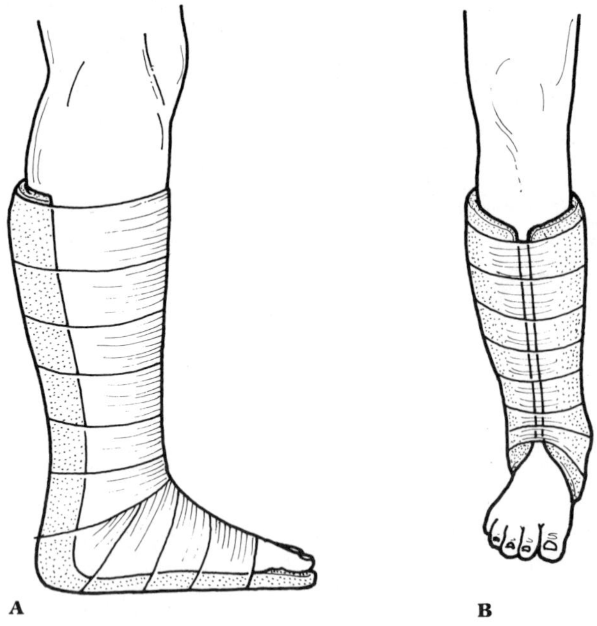

Fig. 72-12. A. The posterior ankle splint fashioned of 10 thicknesses of 4-inch plaster and applied with an elastic bandage will provide rigid immobilization of the ankle in the dorsi-plantarflexion planes. B. For further immobilization, the addition of a stirrup, a U-splint, will prevent motion in the inversion-eversion planes.

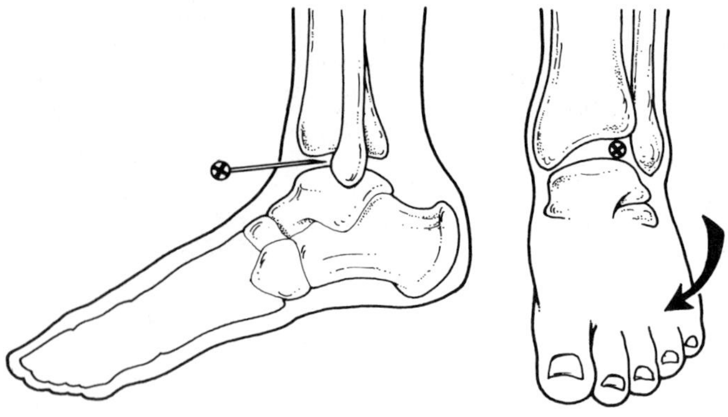

Fig. 72-13. The anterior approach for aspiration of joint effusion of the ankle. The anterior tibiotalor joint region should be prepped and draped with a sterile towel. A wheal of 1 percent lidocaine should be raised in the lateral third of the joint anteriorly with the ankle held in inversion. A 19- or 20-gauge needle can then be used to enter the ankle joint from an anterior approach.

tient will require more rigid immobilization for comfort and adequate treatment. In the emergency department setting, a posterior splint using 10 to 12 thicknesses of 4- to 5-inch plaster or prefabricated splint roll, applied with an elastic bandage, will be adequate (Fig. 72-12A). For additional stability, a second stirrup or U-splint may be added (Fig. 72-12B). A more strict regimen of elevation and application of ice is required than for lesser sprains, and follow-up with an orthopedic surgeon is indicated within 7 to 10 days. If there is any question of a gross instability, orthopedic consultation should be obtained at the time of presentation regardless of x-ray findings because gross laxity associated with rupture may be an indication for acute surgical repair.

Although ankle sprain is a common injury and heals without incident in the majority of cases, the underdiagnosed and undertreated sprained ankle may go on to chronic instability and recurrent ankle sprains. Differentiation between stable and unstable ankle sprains at the time of injury will likely prevent this problem from occurring.

Ankle Tenosynovitis

Synovitis about the ankle is less of a problem than it is at the knee, yet some degree of synovitis may occur with any injury involving the capsule of the ankle joint or tendons (anterior tibial, posterior tibial, peroneus longus-brevis, and extensor digitorum longus). In acute tenosynovitis, which may follow either an injury, an infection, or a metabolic disturbance such as gout, the ankle can be painful, swollen, and hot. In some cases, the tenosynovitis may be localized by palpation to the tendons, but in other cases, the entire ankle joint may appear inflamed.

If a joint effusion is present by palpation, or if the diagnosis of septic arthritis is being considered, aspiration of the ankle joint is required (Fig. 72-13). In aspiration of the ankle joint, the anterior aspect of the joint should be prepped and draped with a sterile towel. A wheal of 1 percent lidocaine should be raised in the lateral third of the joint anteriorly with the ankle held in inversion, as shown in Fig. 72-13. A 19- or 20-gauge needle can then be used to enter the ankle joint from an anterior approach. Following analysis of the aspirated fluid for cell count (hematology laboratory), culture/sensitivity, gram stain, and presence of crystals (bacteriology laboratory), systemic antibiotic treatment should be instituted if infection remains a possibility. If infection does not appear to be present, appropriate treatment based on the underlying cause should be instituted. General principles of rest, ice, compression, use of nonsteroidal anti-inflammatory agents, and elevation are recommended; weight bearing should not be permitted until it can be done without limp or pain.

Subluxation of the Peroneal Tendons

Subluxation and even dislocation of the peroneal tendons is an unusual, but not rare, painful condition of the lateral ankle (Fig. 72-14). When acute, peroneal tendon subluxation is often misdiagnosed as a sprain of the lateral ankle ligaments. The patient with acute subluxation will give a history of having sustained a violent blow to the posterior aspect of the lateral malleolus while the foot was held in dorsiflexion or eversion. This ruptures the crural ligaments at the lateral malleolus, allowing subluxation of the peroneal tendons over the distal fibula (Fig. 72-14).

Evaluation

On examination, there is diffuse tenderness directly over the peroneal tendons, which can often be confused with tenosynovitis if an adequate history is not obtained. Since there is little subcutaneous tissue in this region, tendon subluxation can usually be appreciated by both observation and palpation if present. Dorsiflexion of the ankle will usually demonstrate the pathology, although with chronic subluxa-

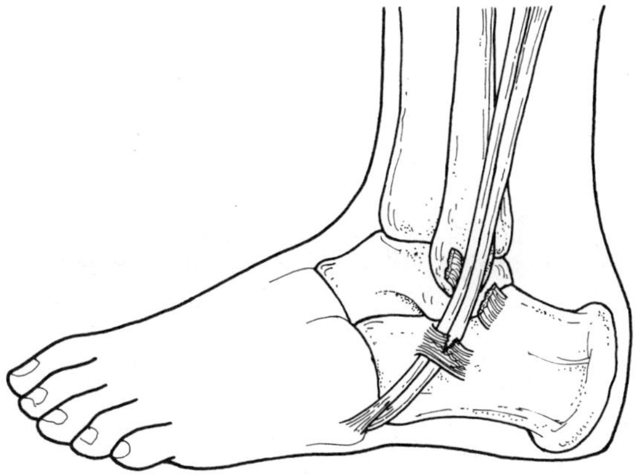

Fig. 72-14. Subluxation of the peroneal tendons is a cause of pain, clicking, and swelling at the lateral ankle. The patient will give a history of violent dorsiflexion or eversion of the ankle. On examination, dorsiflexion of the ankle will usually demonstrate the pathology.

tion the patient can usually describe the position that produces subluxation of the tendons over the fibula.

Treatment

For patients who have demonstrable subluxation and associated symptoms of pain or instability, referral to an orthopedic surgeon for possible reconstruction is indicated. If there is pain without detectable subluxation of the tendons, initial treatment should be anti-inflammatory medication and immobilization in a posterior splint and elastic wrap with orthopedic follow-up in 7 to 10 days.

Achilles and Plantaris Tendon Rupture

Although the Achilles and plantaris tendons are not anatomically located within the ankle, partial or complete rupture or inflammation of these tendons frequently results in complaints and swelling about the ankle. Partial and complete ruptures of these two tendons generally occur at the junction of the tendon with muscle (Fig. 72-15A). The patient will give a history of sudden pain or a sensation of being "kicked" in the back of the calf, followed shortly thereafter by pain and swelling.

Evaluation

Partial tears are more common than complete ruptures, causing calf and ankle pain and swelling. Complete Achilles tendon ruptures generally exhibit marked swelling, inability to plantarflex the foot against resistance, but remarkably little pain. There is generally point tenderness directly at the anatomic site of partial or complete tendon rupture for both of these tendons. Point tenderness is the guide to differentiating which tendon is involved and ruling out involvement of

Fig. 72-15. A. Partial and complete ruptures of the Achilles and plantaris tendons generally occur at the junction of the tendon with muscle. Point tenderness is the guide to differentiating which tendon is involved and ruling out involvement of ankle ligaments (sprains), calf muscle strain, tenosynovitis, or even phlebitis. B. Partial or complete rupture can be differentiated in two ways: palpation of a defect within the tendon, and inability to plantarflex the foot. The examination is best performed with the patient kneeling on the end of an examination table with the toes hanging over the edge. A maneuver of squeezing the calf, the Thompson test, will always cause the foot to plantarflex with an intact or partially disrupted Achilles tendon but will not if there is a complete rupture.

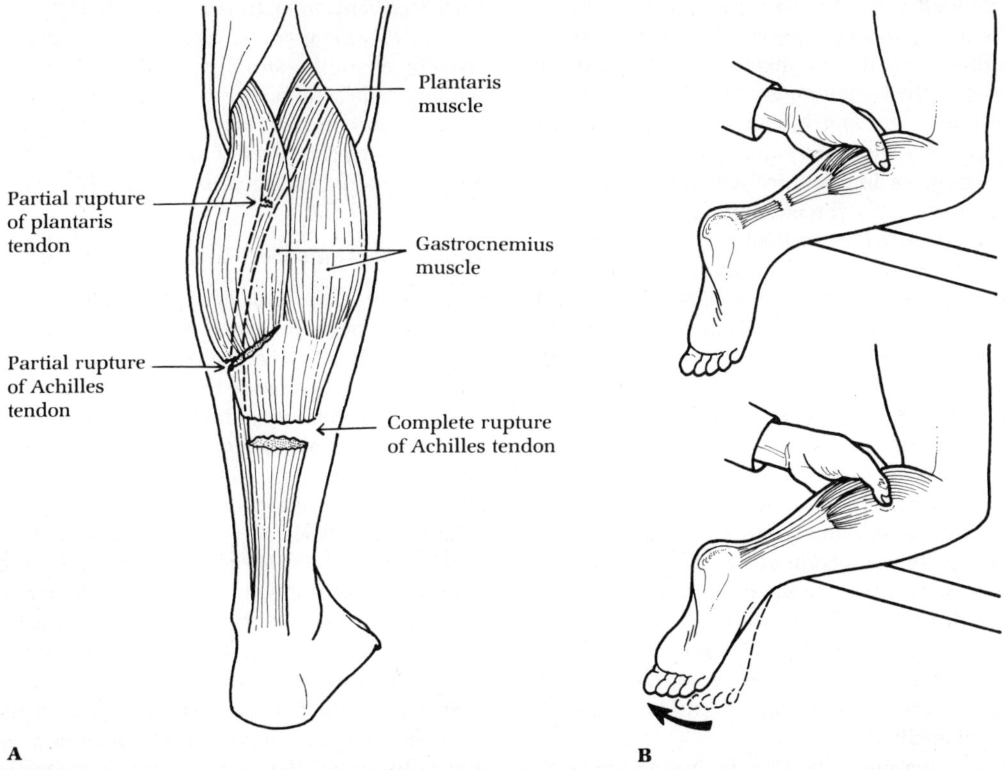

ankle ligaments (sprains), calf muscle strain, tenosynovitis, or even phlebitis.

Treatment of the Achilles tendon rupture is based on the diagnosis of a partial or complete rupture. This can be differentiated in two ways: palpation of a defect within the tendon and inability to plantarflex the foot. The examination is best performed with the patient kneeling on the end of an examination table with the toes hanging over the edge (Fig. 72-15B). In this position, if there is a complete rupture, a defect can usually be palpated in the tendon at 10 to 15 cm proximal to the calcaneus, but, more important, the maneuver of squeezing the calf will not produce the characteristic passive plantarflexion of the ankle (Fig. 72-15B). This maneuver, the Thompson test, will always cause the foot to plantarflex with an intact Achilles tendon but will not if there is a complete rupture.

Treatment

Plantaris and partial Achilles tendon ruptures should be treated by the application of ice, compressive dressings, and elevation, combined with partial weight bearing on crutches. The treatment should be guided by the symptoms. Complete Achilles tendon ruptures should be referred for orthopedic consultation at the time of presentation. There are two acceptable methods of treatment of Achilles tendon rupture: the first requires surgical repair, the second requires casting of the ankle and foot in plantarflexion. Application of either treatment method is at the discretion of the surgeon and based somewhat on the life-style requirements of the patient.

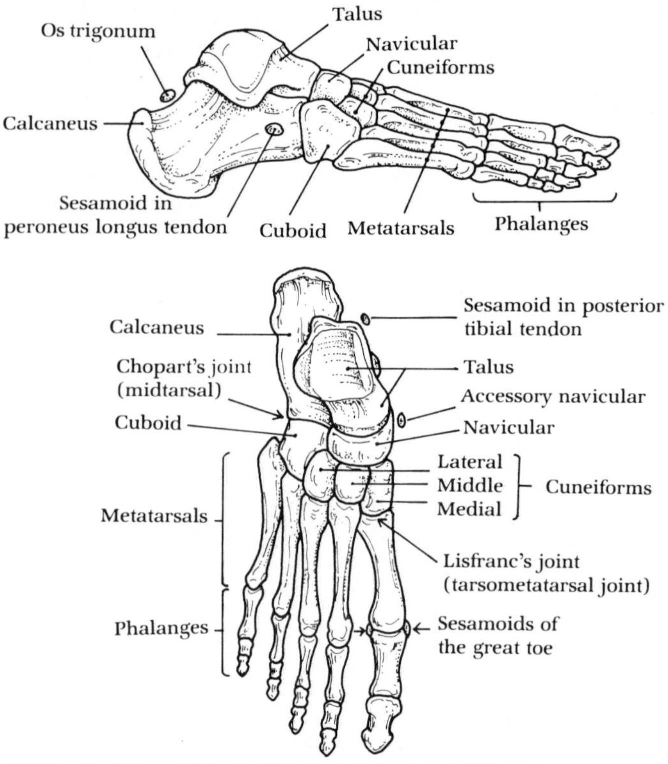

Fig. 72-16. The bones and joints of the foot. The division of the hindfoot and midfoot is the Chopart's joint, while the division of forefoot with midfoot is the Lisfranc's joint. Note the accessory bones of the foot, which sometimes may be mistaken as fracture fragments.

FOOT INJURIES

Functional Anatomy

The foot can be divided into three parts: the *hindfoot,* consisting of the talus and calcaneus; the *midfoot,* consisting of the navicular, cuboid, and three cuneiform bones; and the *forefoot,* consisting of the metatarsals and phalanges (Fig. 72-16). Each portion of the foot has characteristic motion and biomechanical properties that contribute to the type of injury produced. Hindfoot injuries are usually of the compressive type such as when the force of body weight is borne through the leg directly into the hindfoot region. In the midfoot, the injuries are usually of an avulsion type, as the foot is forced through a range of motion beyond its capacity and sustains either ligamentous tears, bone fractures, or both. In the forefoot, the injuries are more varied and may result from crush, torsional, or angular forces.

The entire foot is firmly bound together by ligaments from the talus to the metatarsal heads. Although multiple joints are present and critical to proper functioning of the foot, the individual range of motion in most cases is quite small. Exceptions to this are the subtalar joint and the metatarsophalangeal joints. The general contour of the foot is that of a longitudinal arch resting proximally on the bottom of the calcaneus and distally on the metatarsal heads. The integrity of this longitudinal arch is preserved by the bones, ligaments, and muscles of the foot. Like the ankle, the foot has very little subcutaneous tissue, so deformity and swelling are poorly tolerated and easily detected.

Knowledge of the anatomy of the foot, including the position of tendons, bones, and joints, is important in diagnosis *since localization of tenderness over a particular anatomic structure is the greatest aid in making an accurate diagnosis.* For example, strains of the foot can be pinpointed by palpation directly over the involved musculotendinous unit. Sprains can be diagnosed by localizing tenderness over a joint, rather than a bony structure, and thereby decreasing the likelihood of a fracture diagnosis.

Foot Contusions, Strains, and Sprains

Contusions of the foot are a frequent occurrence and may be caused by any sort of direct trauma. Contusion of the dorsum of the foot may be quite painful due to the extremely thin subcutaneous tissue that overlies the tendons, blood vessels, and nerves, affording little protection to these critical structures. Contusions to the undersurface of the foot, although less frequent, may produce longer term dysfunction due to the pain associated with weight bearing.

Strains are especially common in the foot and are defined as damage to the muscle-tendinous unit, usually at the musculotendinous junction. These are classified as either overuse (chronic strain) or overstress (acute strain) conditions. The severity of strain is related to the violence of the force delivered to the musculotendinous unit.

Sprains of the foot may occur, just as in the ankle. Sprain is defined as a partial or total disruption of the ligaments that hold any of the bones of the foot together. This injury can occur either individually or in combination with fractures or dislocations.

Evaluation
Diagnosis of foot injuries is first made by taking a history. The patient will complain of pain, and, in many cases, a specific localization of the pain will be possible. The examiner should try to pinpoint the area of maximum pain and correlate this with tenderness to palpation. Ecchymosis should be noted, although in injuries that present late, ecchymosis may be misleading as blood can dissect between fascial planes and become visible considerably distal to the point of injury.

Examination of the foot should start with the hindfoot and progress to the toes. The heel should be cradled with both palms and rocked from side to side to estimate the subtalar motion. Next, by supporting the heel and holding it stationary, the rest of the foot may be brought from side to side and may be slightly twisted to determine motion and discomfort in the joints of the midfoot. The first and fifth metatarsals are easily moved about and palpated throughout their length. The middle metatarsals and cuneiform bones can be similarly examined. The "ball of the foot" represents the metatarsal heads, which are palpable on the sole of the foot. The individual toes and metatarsophalangeal joints should be examined last.

Following the physical examination, x-rays should be obtained if there is bony tenderness, crepitus, any sense of instability, or a history of substantial force. Films should include an AP, a lateral, and an oblique view of the foot. Most foot fractures will be apparent on x-ray. The foot has numerous accessory ossicles that can appear to represent chip avulsion fractures. Again, the physical examination will help resolve this uncertainty, since localized pain and tenderness will correlate with any acute avulsion fracture.

Treatment
Strains, sprains, and contusions of the foot should be treated like ankle sprains. Initial treatment should consist of rest, ice, compression, and elevation with or without the use of anti-inflammatory agents. Some degree of splinting is often necessary and may be accomplished with a Jones dressing or, in more severe cases, a posterior plaster splint (see Fig. 72-12). Weight bearing should be advanced as tolerated, but remember that a posterior splint will not withstand weight-bearing forces and must be removed as ambulation is begun.

For those patients who are not ambulating comfortably within 7 to 10 days, further follow-up by an orthopedic surgeon is indicated.

Plantar Fasciitis/Heel Pain

Although this is by nature a chronic inflammatory condition, patients may present with *sudden* onset of heel pain due to plantar fasciitis. There is generally no specific traumatic event, although many patients will report that the pain began when they first arose from bed and began to bear weight on the heel.

Evaluation
The diagnosis is aided by localized tenderness at the anteromedial aspect of the calcaneus, specifically at the attachment of the plantar fascia to the bone itself. With passive dorsiflexion of the toes, the pain may be accentuated. The pain and tenderness may radiate through the longitudinal arch diffusely.

If the symptoms and findings are more posterior and follow the Achilles tendon, Achilles tendonitis is the more likely diagnosis. If the symptoms are lateral, along the course of the peroneal tendons, suspect peroneal tendonitis, particularly when the pain is worsened with subtalar motion and crepitus is present over the tendon sheaths themselves.

Treatment
Heel pain of an inflammatory nature is best treated initially with anti-inflammatory medication and use of arch support. For the majority of patients whose symptoms persist beyond 7 to 10 days, referral to an orthopedic surgeon or podiatrist is indicated. These disorders are often difficult to treat, and modalities of shoe accommodations, orthotic support, and corticosteroid injections are sometimes used. A review of the various approaches is beyond the scope of this text. In the acute setting, there is currently no evidence that invasive treatment by injection or surgery is superior to conservative management. If the problem is chronic, it should be managed by referral for orthopedic or podiatric consultation.

Midfoot Pain

Pain of the midfoot, arch, and dorsum of the foot generally presents with a history of slow and chronic onset. There is usually not a well-recognized antecedent event, except in the case of posterior tibial tendon rupture where a weight-bearing injury to the midfoot followed by pain and a new and prominent flatfoot deformity is noted.

Evaluation
The diagnosis of the cause of midfoot pain is aided first by observation of both feet in stance, the localization of point tenderness, and next by radiographic examination. Acute and violent trauma may lead to fractures of dislocations across the midfoot. Patients with peripheral neuropathies, as may be associated with alcoholism or diabetes, may suffer from swelling and numerous small fractures of the midfoot consistent with Charcot arthropathy without history of trauma. Minor weight-bearing trauma associated with marked pronation and flatfoot deformity of one foot and tenderness along the posterior tibial tendon is consistent with acute rupture of the posterior tibial tendon. Chronic pain in the arch region of the midfoot with flatfoot deformity is consistent with acquired flatfoot and severe plantar fasciitis.

Treatment
Treatment of fractures and dislocations of the midfoot in the acute setting is by use of Jones dressing and posterior plaster splint (see Fig. 72-12) with orthopedic consultation at the time of presentation. These fractures or dislocations will often require reduction or operative repair. The acute treatment of posterior tibial tendon rupture and acquired flatfoot is with the use of posterior splint, minimal weight bearing on crutches, and follow-up by an orthopedic surgeon. Specific cases of these two disorders may require operative correction, but usually not in the acute setting.

Forefoot Pain

As for heel pain, forefoot pain may often present as an acute condition, even though its underlying cause is often chronic.

Evaluation
In the emergency setting, certain acute causes need to be ruled out. Stress fractures (see below) are a common source of pain and often present without a history of trauma. Infection from a remote and now-forgotten puncture wound also needs to be considered. The metatarsophalangeal joints can be the source of acute conditions such as septic arthritis, and, again, localization of the pain by physical examination is critical. Once acute causes are ruled out, the diagnostic possibilities enlarge considerably. Callosities can be painful and may represent either viral infection or biomechanical imbalance in the weight-bearing distribution between the metatarsals. Interdigital neuroma (Morton's neuroma) tends to localize between the metatarsals, classically (although not exclusively) in the third interspace (between the third and fourth metatarsal). Diabetic neuropathy can present with diffuse forefoot pain.

Treatment
As for heel pain, initial treatment of forefoot pain is determined by the acute cause. Acute metatarsalgia and great toe sesamoiditis should be treated with partial weight bearing, analgesics, anti-inflammatory agents and footwear accommodation. Those patients with forefoot pain that is not acutely caused and persists beyond 7 to 10 days will need referral for orthopedic or podiatric evaluation.

Puncture Wounds

Puncture wounds of the foot frequently present late, often after infection has been established. In recent years, it has become more widely accepted that a large number of these infections are due to *Pseudomonas* species, which thrives in footwear.

Treatment
For patients presenting immediately after puncture wound, the wound should be cleansed and irrigated thoroughly. Prophylaxis for tetanus is mandatory. X-rays should be obtained to rule out the presence of a retained radiopaque foreign body. If the puncture is deep or obviously contaminated with foreign material, a more extensive irrigation and debridement should be performed using local anesthetic and enlarging the wound slightly to permit adequate irrigation of deeper tissues. A posterior tibial nerve block placed at the ankle will be helpful in this effort (Procedure 39). Antibiotic prophylaxis by oral route is appropriate and may be augmented by an initial intravenous loading dose in the emergency department. Close follow-up is indicated, and the patient should return for reexamination in 48 hours or sooner if symptoms or signs of infection arise.

For patients who present several days or weeks following puncture wound, increasing pain or swelling are the usual symptoms and deep infection must be ruled out. X-rays are needed, and the examination should attempt to localize the tenderness and define any abscess, if present. Deep foot infection requires evaluation by a general or orthopedic surgeon, since formal surgical drainage may be required. In many cases, the depth of the infection may not be obvious and decision may be made to admit the patient for intravenous antibiotics, elevation, and observation, reserving surgical exploration for those patients who do not respond to nonoperative measures.

Accessory Bones

Patients may present with painful "lumps" of the midfoot region, particularly about the medial side. Such a lump frequently represents an accessory navicular bone that has become tender or swollen as a result of local injury or mild sprain associated with avulsion force through the posterior tibial tendon. In evaluating the foot, it is important to remember that there are many small accessory bones and that these are not pathologic (see Fig. 72-16). Commonly, accessory bones are present at the posterior aspect of the talus (os trigonum), at the navicular, and the inferior surface of the cuboid in the peroneus longus tendon. Additionally, it is possible to have a bipartite condition of the sesamoid bones of the great toe, which may appear as a fracture of the sesamoid.

Evaluation
As emphasized previously, the physical examination is most important in correlating the suspected "fracture" with the physical findings. In this way, differentiation between accessory bones and actual avulsion fractures can usually be made.

Treatment
Whether the bony finding represents a fracture or merely an incidental accessory ossicle, treatment is symptomatic. Rest, ice, compression dressing, and elevation are recommended, with referral for orthopedic or podiatric follow-up in 7 to 10 days if still symptomatic. In rare instances, an accessory navicular may be surgically resected if persistently painful.

FOOT FRACTURES

Any of the 28 bones of the foot are prone to fracture, and these fractures account for approximately 10 percent of all fractures seen in the emergency department setting. The majority of these fractures heal uneventfully, but several are associated with long-term disability.

Hindfoot and Midfoot Fractures

Evaluation
The diagnosis of foot fracture is made by taking a careful history of the injury and performing an examination directed at eliciting the areas of greatest tenderness. Diagnosis is confirmed by radiographic means, correlating the x-ray findings with those of physical examination. These fractures are usually the result of compressive loading of the foot in falls from significant height and are, more often than not, associated with significant soft tissue injury (Fig. 72-17). Hindfoot fractures are usually associated with other injuries, particularly lumbosacral fracture and pelvis injuries, so the patient

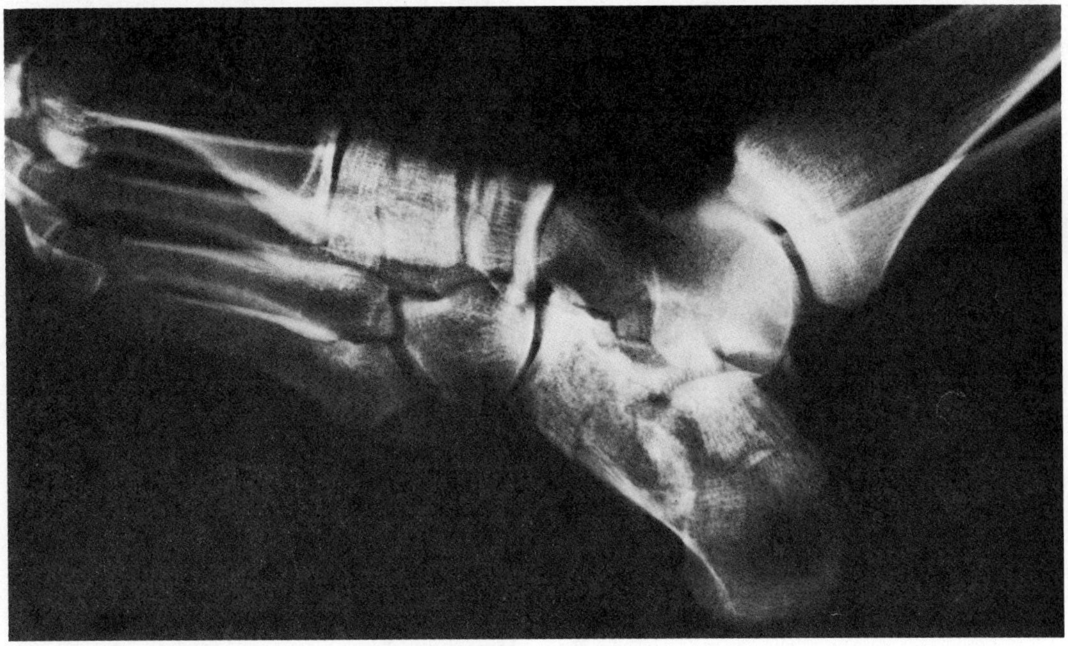

Fig. 72-17. Lateral radiograph of a comminuted intra-articular calcaneous fracture. The normal alignment of the subtalar joint has been completely disrupted.

should be carefully evaluated with these possibilities in mind.

Treatment

For fractures of the hindfoot, involving either the talus or the calcaneus, immediate orthopedic consultation is generally indicated. A displaced fracture of the talus needs urgent reduction and possible internal fixation since disruption of the blood supply to this bone can frequently occur, resulting in osteonecrosis and subsequent collapse of the articular surface of the talus. Fractures of the calcaneus are occasionally treated operatively or possibly manipulated in closed fashion to achieve a better restoration of the longitudinal arch (Fig. 72-17). In both instances, careful evaluation of the soft tissue overlying the site of injury is critical, since a slough of the overlying skin can result in greater disability than the fracture itself. Immobilization in a well-padded splint (see Fig. 72-12), elevation, and application of ice should be instituted while awaiting orthopedic consultation.

For fractures in the midfoot area, the soft tissues must again be carefully evaluated. Since these fractures are often due to a crushing force applied to a very thin layer of skin and subcutaneous tissue, ischemia can occur when the contused skin is further compromised by gross swelling. Nondisplaced fractures will generally be treated with a Jones dressing and elevation, whereas displaced or severely comminuted fractures of the midfoot warrant immediate orthopedic consultation.

In all cases of midfoot trauma, it is important to evaluate the integrity of the Lisfranc joint, dividing the metatarsal bases from the cuneiform bones (Fig. 72-16). If tenderness and swelling are present in the midfoot, careful review of the foot films must be performed to rule out dislocation of the metatarsal bases. These dislocations are frequently missed and can result in long-term disability if not treated early. Of particular importance is the location of the second metatarsal base. It normally occupies a recessed position between the first metatarsal base and the medial cuneiform, and this should be verified on films. Tomograms are usually not necessary but can be obtained if the diagnosis is in doubt. These injuries can occur with minimal trauma, such as stepping down hard from a high curb, and should be suspected whenever significant midfoot pain and swelling presents without an obvious fracture.

Metatarsal Fractures

Evaluation

The metatarsals are long bones spanning the arch of the foot and are prone to injury from both falls and falling objects. Metatarsal fractures can also occur in the absence of an acute traumatic event; these fractures tend to be localized to the distal portions of the middle metatarsal shafts and are called *stress fractures* (Fig. 72-18). The radiographic findings in either acute or stress fractures may be subtle, and careful correlation with the point of tenderness of physical examination is most important.

The most frequent metatarsal fracture is that of the proximal portion of the fifth metatarsal, usually in the setting of an inversion stress that actually pulls the bone apart through the force of the peroneus brevis tendon (Fig. 72-19). This common fracture must be differentiated from the true Jones fracture, which is actually a transverse fracture through the proximal shaft of the metatarsal, requiring more stringent immobilization and avoidance of weight bearing.

Treatment

For isolated, nondisplaced single metatarsal fractures, the treatment is a Jones dressing with instructions for ice and elevation. Follow-up with an orthopedic surgeon should occur in 3 to 5 days, at which time a wooden shoe or short

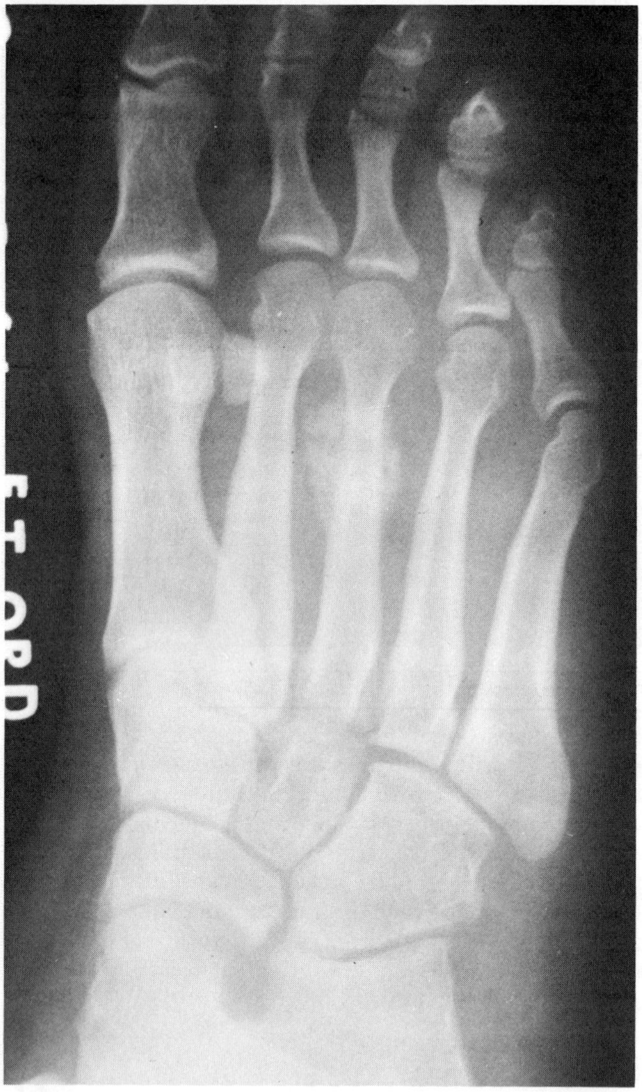

Fig. 72-18. A halo of periosteal new bone formation is seen at the site of a stress fracture of the metatarsal. The fracture line is not evident, although the exuberant repair callus is.

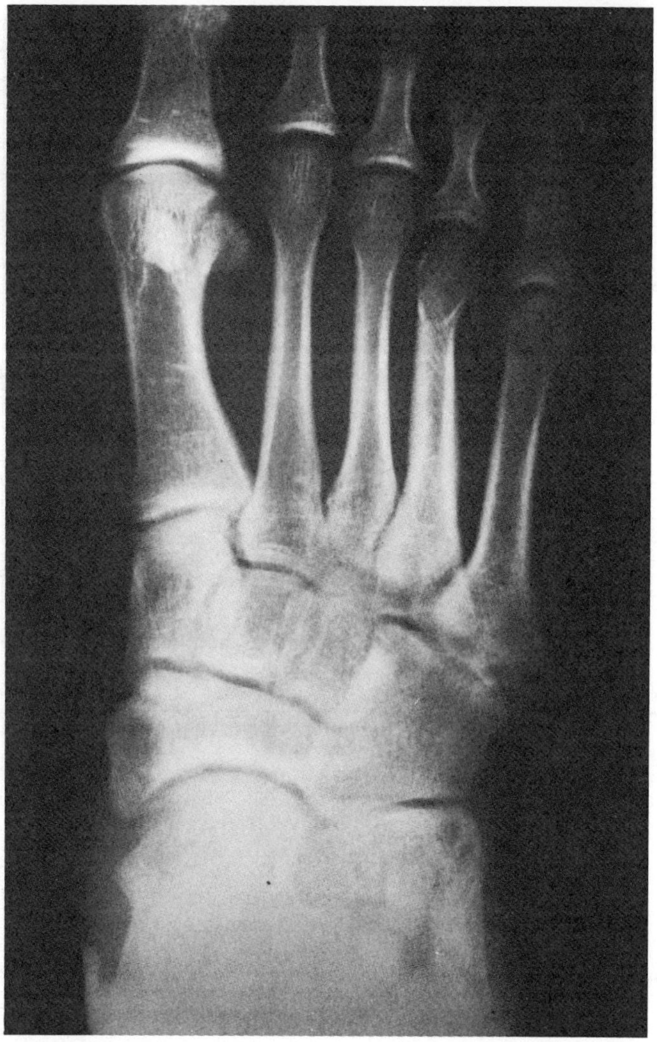

Fig. 72-19. AP radiograph of the foot showing a fracture at the base (proximal aspect) of the fifth metatarsal. The fracture shown here is an avulsion fracture. It should be differentiated from the more unstable proximal diaphyseal fracture of the fifth metatarsal, known as a Jones fracture.

leg walking cast may be prescribed. True Jones fractures must be kept non–weight bearing, although partial weight bearing is permitted for other single metatarsal fractures.

For patients with displaced or multiple fractures of the metatarsals, orthopedic consultation is indicated in the emergency department. Fractures that result in displacement of the metatarsal heads can cause long-term forefoot pain and are frequently treated by closed-open reduction and pinning.

Toe Fractures

Toe fractures are a frequent presenting complaint in the emergency department and are often the result of a blunt blow such as the bare foot striking a table leg or a crush injury (which is usually more serious).

Evaluation

The soft tissues must be evaluated, particularly to rule out the presence of a subungual hematoma. X-rays are then obtained and must be examined looking not only for fracture but also for dislocation of metatarsophalangeal (MTP) or interphalangeal (IP) joints.

Treatment

For phalangeal fractures not involving the MTP joints or the IP joint of the great toe, treatment is by gentle manipulation and taping to the adjacent toe, known as "buddy taping." In these cases, the visual alignment of the toe is more important than the x-ray appearance.

If a subungual hematoma is present and symptomatic, drainage is indicated. This may be performed by using a hot wire, usually with immediate relief of discomfort. The procedure should be performed under sterile conditions and is safe to perform even above a phalangeal fracture without incurring increased risk of osteomyelitis. An undrained subungual hematoma can result in necrosis of soft tissue due to impaired blood supply and should not be ignored.

For severely displaced phalangeal fractures or those involving the MTP joints or IP joint of the great toe, orthopedic consultation is advised. Occasionally, open reduction and pinning of these fractures is indicated, but usually closed reduction is recommended.

For dislocations of the MTP or IP joints, a closed reduction is recommended. The dislocations usually present with the distal portion of the joint dorsal and the proximal portion volar. Reduction can be performed using a local block of 1 percent Xylocaine to anesthetize the interdigital nerves. With the usual pattern, a reduction can be effected by distal traction on the toe combined with hyperextension of the joint and gentle pressure on the dorsum of the joint. If unsuccessful on one or two attempts, or in the setting of fracture-dislocation, orthopedic consultation is advised. Following a successful reduction, the toe should be stabilized by taping to the adjacent toes as described previously.

Follow-up with an orthopedic surgeon or primary care physician within 7 days is indicated for all of the aforementioned injuries.

SELECTED READING

Arrowsmith, SR, Fleming, LL, and Allman, FL. Traumatic dislocations of the peroneal tendons. *Am J Sports Med* 11:142, 1983.

Mann, RA, and Thompson, FM. Rupture of the posterior tibial tendon causing flat foot. *J Bone Joint Surg* 67A:556, 1985.

Niedermann, B, et al. Rupture of the lateral ligaments of the ankle: Operation or plaster cast? *Acta Orthop Scand* 52:579, 1981.

Nistor, L. Surgical and nonsurgical treatment of Achilles tendon rupture: A prospective randomized study. *J Bone Joint Surg* 63A:394, 1981.

Pettrone, FA, et al. Quantitative criteria for prediction of the results after displaced fracture of the ankle. *J Bone Joint Surg* 65A:66, 1983.

73. Compartment Syndrome

David W. Lhowe

Acute compartment syndromes can result from crush injury, fractures, arterial disruption, prolonged limb compression, or burns. Even seemingly minor soft-tissue trauma by history can result in elevated compartment pressures. Chronic compartment syndromes can occur recurrently after exercise in a variety of individuals.

It is in the diagnosis of the *acute* compartment syndrome that the emergency physician can recognize and prevent some of the most permanently disabling (and avoidable) sequelae of extremity injury. The loss of function caused by an unrecognized compartment syndrome is, without exception, greater than that due to the original injury itself. Early diagnosis is facilitated by a high index of suspicion on the part of the emergency physician, who, more than anyone else, is in a position to promptly recognize this potentially disabling complication.

DEFINITION

A compartment syndrome occurs when increased pressure within a muscle compartment produces a significant decrease in the arteriovenous pressure gradient. At this point, the perfusion of muscle is reduced below the minimum needed to maintain viability. The injury to muscle becomes irreversible in proportion to the duration and magnitude of the pressure elevation, as well as other factors, such as anemia and hypoxia, which may also be present.

ETIOLOGY

Skeletal muscles are enclosed in fascial envelopes, which have relatively little "give." Furthermore, these muscle compartments may also be bounded by bone, which is absolutely unyielding in the face of elevated intracompartmental pressures.

Injury to muscle, whether it be due to fracture, burn, crushing trauma, ischemia from arterial disruption, or prolonged compression, results in edema and hemorrhage into the compartment. This causes increased pressure, which reduces perfusion of the muscle. In turn, this results in further muscle injury, further edema, and still further increase in intracompartmental pressure (Fig. 73-1). In the early phase, when a compartment syndrome is impending, it may be possible to break the cycle simply by treating the underlying cause. For example, getting the patient's weight off a limb that has been compressed during coma may be sufficient in itself to restore adequate perfusion to the involved musculature. However, once a compartment syndrome is established, it is necessary to provide immediate decompression of muscle and nerve by performing a fasciotomy, thereby immediately reducing the intracompartmental pressure. If

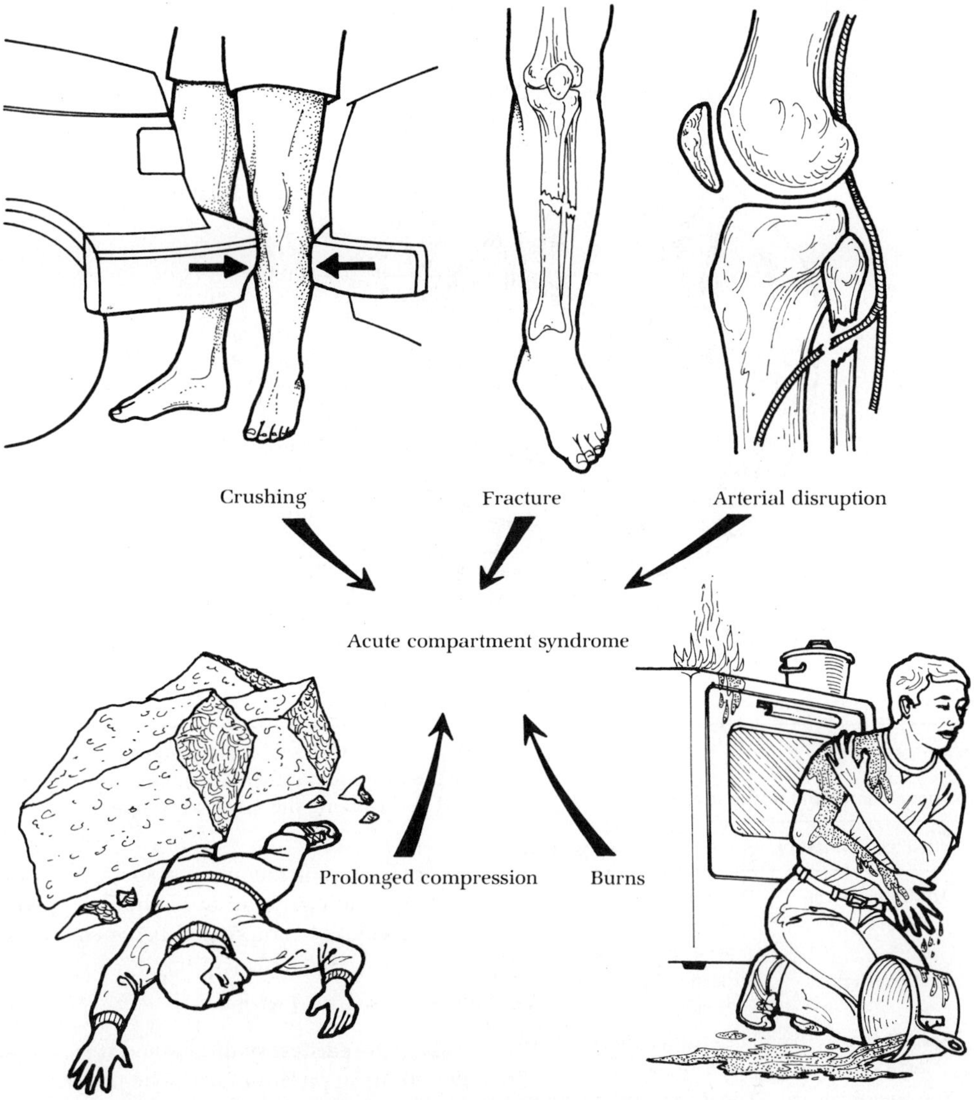

Fig. 73-1. Causes of acute compartment syndrome. The most common causes are fracture and crush injury although the other causes pictured can also produce muscle injury, with resultant edema, hemorrhage, and increased compartmental pressure, which cause reduced perfusion of muscle, ultimately progressing to muscle necrosis.

decompression is performed before necrosis of muscle has occurred, a good functional outcome can be expected. If not, the severity of weakness and contracture will be proportional to the amount of muscle that undergoes necrosis and replacement by nonfunctional scar tissue.

DIAGNOSIS

Location

Although compartment syndromes can occur in any extremity compartment, certain anatomic compartments are more commonly involved as a result of their propensity for injury and the more restrictive boundaries that enclose them. The most common location is the lower leg and the most common setting is a tibial fracture. Contrary to a widely held belief, an open fracture does *not* obviate the possibility of a compartment syndrome through a "traumatic fasciotomy." It is likely that the fascial tearing caused by an open fracture will be unpredictable and probably incomplete, quite possibly leaving sufficient fascia intact to provide a restrictive envelope for the swelling that follows. The emergency physician should also beware of the possibility of elevated compartment pressures after what appears to be a minimally traumatic injury to the lower leg. A classic example is the child who gets his or her leg transiently caught between two car bumpers, sufficient to produce a substantial muscle crush but not enough to result in a fracture or visible soft-tissue laceration. Such a patient can well develop a compartment syndrome, which could be misdiagnosed as a simple contusion if the examining physician is not adequately suspicious.

The anatomy of the lower leg is described in Chap. 71. Pertinent to the present discussion is an understanding of the compartmental anatomy of this region. The most frequently involved compartment within the leg is the anterior compartment, although the peroneal compartment is often involved

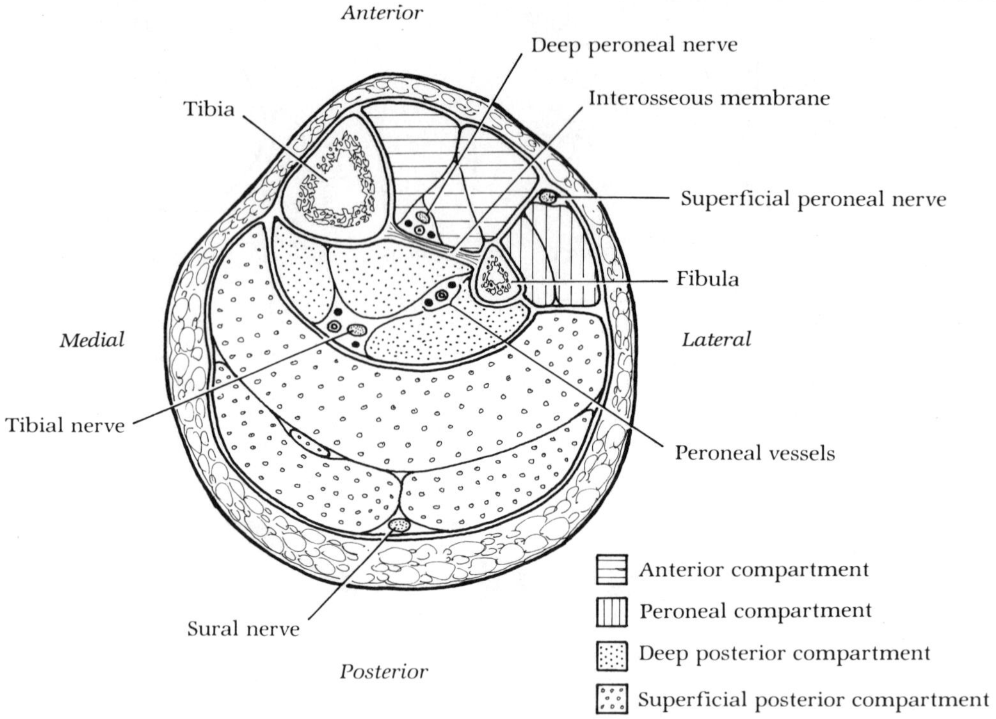

Fig. 73-2. Cross-sectional anatomy of the lower leg. Note that each of the four compartments contains a specific sensory nerve that will aid in localizing the involved compartment.

Table 73-1. Compartmental anatomy of the lower leg

Leg compartment	Muscles involved	Associated sensory nerve
Anterior	Ankle-toe dorsiflexors	Deep peroneal nerve (web space between great and second toes)
Peroneal	Foot everters	Superficial peroneal nerve (dorsum of foot)
Superficial posterior	Ankle plantarflexors	Sural nerve (lateral border of foot)
Deep posterior	Toe flexors Foot inverters	Tibial nerve (plantar surface of foot)

in association with it. The deep posterior compartment is less frequently the site of a compartment syndrome, but it is more difficult to diagnose due to its deeper location. The superficial posterior compartment is infrequently involved. Each of these four compartments is associated with a specific sensory nerve, a fact that helps in making the diagnosis of compartment syndrome (Fig. 73-2, Table 73-1).

After the lower leg, the next most common location for compartment syndrome is the forearm, which contains two compartments. The volar compartment contains the wrist and finger flexors while the dorsal compartment houses the wrist and finger extensors. As in the lower leg, particular nerves are associated with each of these two compartments, which will help in making a diagnosis by clinical examination (Fig. 73-3, Table 73-2).

Compartment syndromes should be looked for in any injured extremity, in addition to the leg and forearm. The buttock is frequently involved in unconscious patients (e.g., drug-overdose patients) who have lain motionless for prolonged periods of time. The thigh can also be a site of increased compartmental pressures if prolonged pressure is applied, such as in an individual trapped in an automobile whose thigh is compressed between seat and dashboard.

Symptoms and Signs

Pain is the earliest symptom and it is typically out of proportion to the apparent injury. The patient with a tibial fracture in whom worsening pain develops 6 to 12 hours after the fracture has been reduced and splinted may well be experiencing pain from ischemic muscle. Although compartment syndromes can develop as late as 72 hours after initial insult, most will be seen within the first 24 hours. The pain is often described as a deep, throbbing sensation.

Pressure is the only truly objective sign of a compartment syndrome. Palpation of the involved compartment will usually disclose the swelling and tension that reflect the underlying increased pressure. Palpation is a notoriously inaccurate method of determining actual compartment pressures and must be supplemented by actual pressure measurements, as described later in this chapter.

Paresthesia is usually present and often progresses to hypesthesia or anesthesia. Since most compartments contain a specific sensory nerve, a careful sensory examination can localize the compartment involved.

Passive stretching that produces pain is a less reliable symptom, since it is found in nearly all patients with significant extremity injury. No specific quality differentiates the pain of ischemia from the pain of contusion or fracture by this maneuver.

Paresis of muscle is also less reliable since it, too, can result from involuntary guarding after contusion or nerve

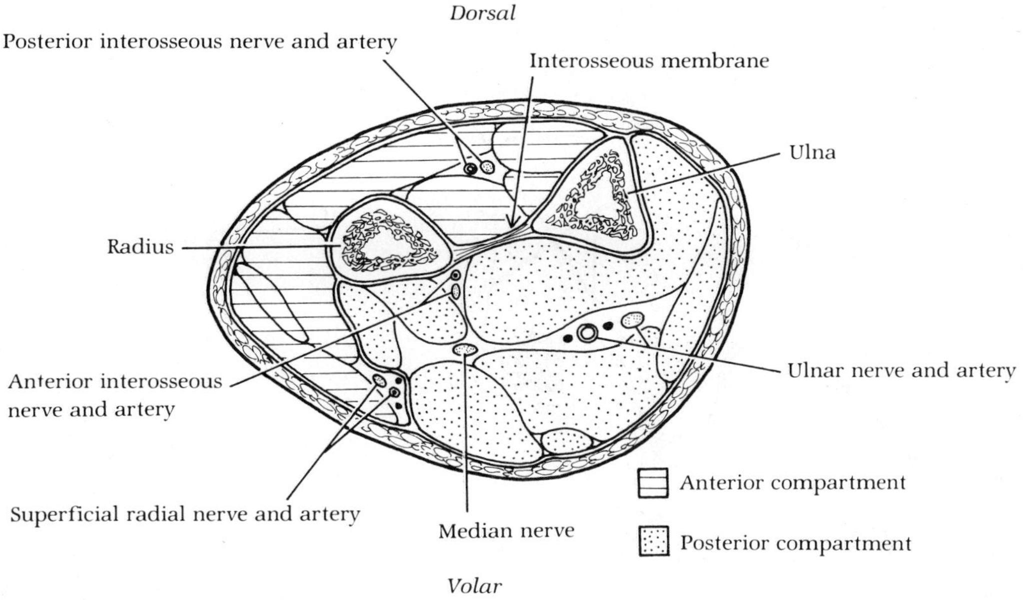

Fig. 73-3. Cross-sectional anatomy of the forearm. The dorsal and volar compartments are shown. Note that the dorsal compartment contains the superficial branch of the radial nerve, innervating the dorsum of the radial side of the hand, while the volar compartment contains the median and ulnar nerves, which supply sensation to the entire palmar surface of the hand and all five fingertips.

injury rather than from muscle ischemia. Therefore, the finding of an inability to voluntarily contract specific muscle groups does not differentiate between contusion and ischemia.

Pulses are absolutely without value in the diagnosis of compartment syndrome. Since the large arteries that traverse the involved compartment usually remain patent (since the small muscle arterioles are first involved), it is quite possible to have a warm and pink foot with bounding pulses below an ischemic leg.

MEASUREMENT OF COMPARTMENT PRESSURES

Compartment pressure measurement is indicated: (1) in a patient in whom symptoms and signs point to a possible compartment syndrome, in order to confirm a clinical impression; (2) in an uncooperative or unreliable patient in whom adequate examination cannot be performed; (3) in an unconscious patient with a history of an appropriate extremity injury who has even the suggestion of increased pressure by palpation; and (4) in a patient who has nerve dysfunction due to other causes, making diagnosis by physical examination more difficult. The technique of compartment pressure measurement can be easily performed by the emergency physician and requires no special equipment. Although a number of proprietary devices for pressure measurement are becoming increasingly available to the emergency physician, it is essential to know how to measure compartment pressures with simple equipment, readily available in any emergency department.

Table 73-2. Compartmental anatomy of the forearm

Forearm compartment	Muscles involved	Associated sensory nerve
Dorsal	Wrist–finger extensors	Superficial radial nerve (dorsum of radial side of hand)
Volar	Wrist–finger flexors	Median and ulnar nerves (palm of hand, all fingertips)

To perform compartment pressure measurements, the physician needs only a basic understanding of regional anatomy to place the needle in the proper location. The needle is introduced just below the fascia, a depth that makes neurovascular injury unlikely. The very remote possibility of neurovascular injury during such an examination must be weighed against the progressive amount of muscle damage that occurs during the delay between onset of compartment syndrome and definitive treatment.

The equipment required includes a sphygmomanometer (preferably with a mercury manometer), a three-way stopcock, a length of intravenous extension tubing, a 10- to 20-ml syringe, a supply of 18-gauge needles, and a bottle of sterile saline (Fig. 73-4). The equipment is assembled as shown in Fig. 73-5. The cuff is removed from the sphygmomanometer and the three-way stopcock is fitted to the open tube. Onto the two remaining ports of the stopcock are fitted the syringe and the intravenous (IV) extension tubing. Only the 18-gauge needle, which goes on the very end of the IV extension tubing, and the saline solution need to remain sterile. The stopcock is first turned so that the manometer, syringe, and needle are all open to each other to equalize the pressure within the system. The stopcock is then turned to close off the manometer and the needle is placed into the sterile

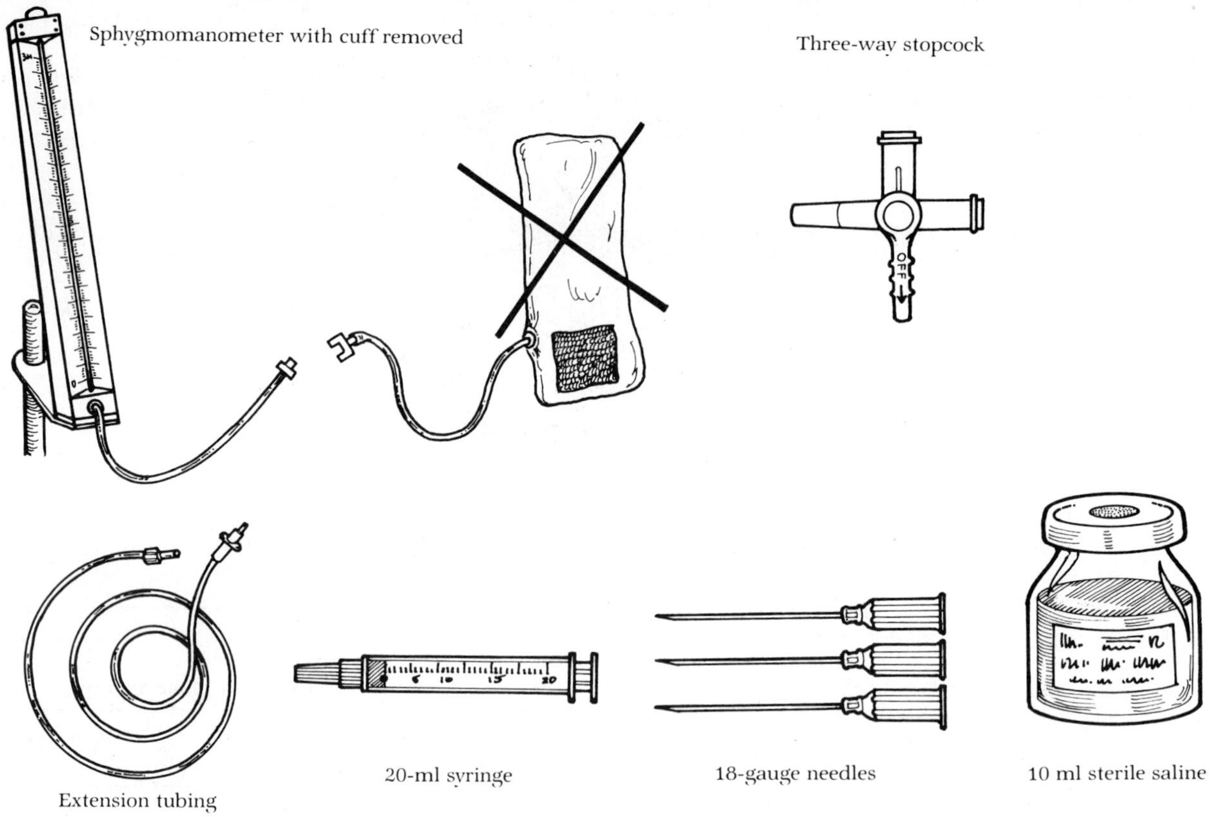

Fig. 73-4. Equipment for compartmental pressure measurement. These items are readily available in any hospital emergency department. The sphygmomanometer should have its cuff removed. Only the 18-gauge needles and saline solution need to remain sterile.

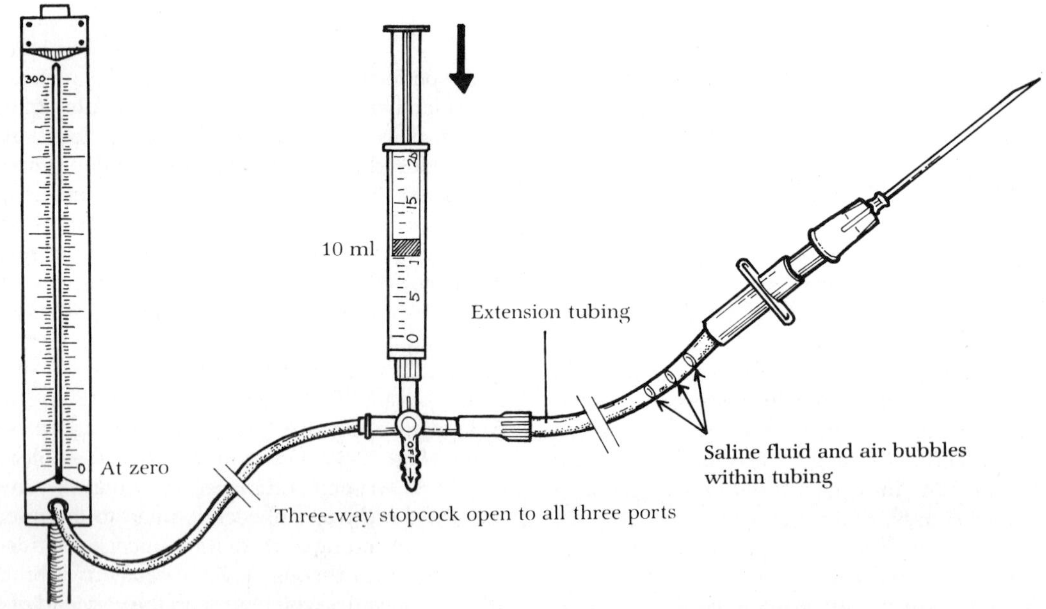

Fig. 73-5. Apparatus assembled for compartmental pressure measurement. Note the several drops of saline fluid within the tubing, which will move toward the end of the needle as the system pressure rises above that of the measured compartment.

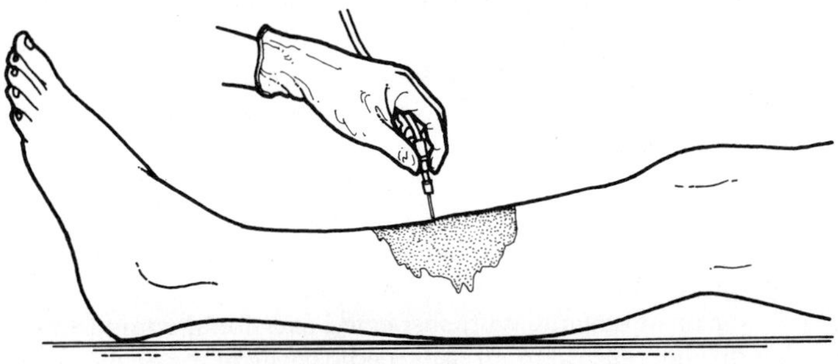

Fig. 73-6. Technique of needle insertion. The leg is sterilely prepped with an iodine solution and sterile gloves are worn. The needle is introduced at right angles to the skin with a single deft motion, penetrating just below the fascia, which can usually be detected as a slight "pop."

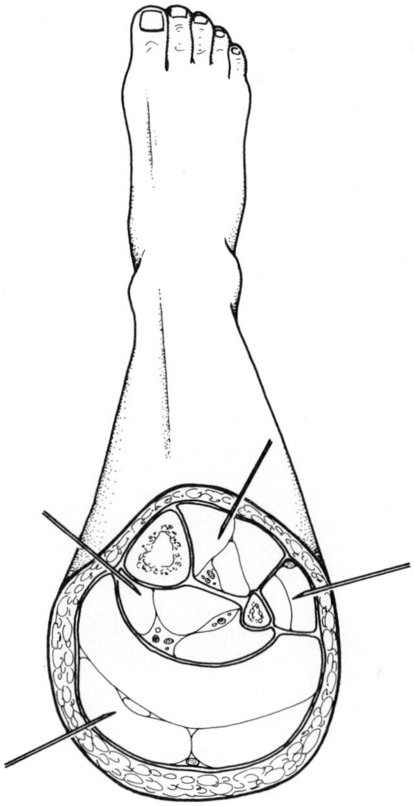

Fig. 73-7. Needle position for leg compartmental pressure measurements. The tibial crest is the most important landmark. Lateral to it lies the anterior compartment, while directly posterior is the deep posterior compartment. The fibula is the landmark used for the peroneal compartment. The superficial posterior compartment is the easiest to localize, although the leg may need to be rotated to expose its posterior surface.

saline as a small amount of fluid is drawn up into the tubing. This fluid serves as a visible marker during the measuring process. Next, the stopcock is again turned so that needle, syringe, and manometer are all again in continuity.

Next, the leg is sterilely prepped with an iodine solution and sterile gloves are worn (Fig. 73-6). A new needle is fitted to the tubing and it is introduced into the compartment in question at right angles to the skin with a single deft motion. The fascia can usually be felt as a slight "pop" when traversed by the needle (Fig. 73-6). Local anesthesia is not necessary and the discomfort is equivalent to that of venipuncture. The landmark most helpful in the lower leg is the anterior tibial crest. Immediately to its lateral side is the anterior compartment. Immediately medial and posterior is the deep posterior compartment. The superficial posterior compartment is large and most easily approached either posteromedially or posterolaterally by advancing the needle just below the fascia of the calf muscle. The peroneal compartment is most reliably entered by aiming at the fibula just proximal to the junction between the middle and distal thirds where the bone first becomes palpable (Fig. 73-7).

With the needle in position, attention is directed to the tubing and manometer. The barrel of the syringe is slowly advanced as the tubing is observed. When pressure in the tubing (as indicated by the manometer reading) exceeds the pressure in the compartment, the fluid in the tubing will begin to move toward the needle. The manometer reading at this point *is* the compartment pressure.

It is recommended that each compartment be measured several times in several different locations. It is also recommended that all four compartments of the leg or both compartments of the forearm be measured whenever the diagnosis is suspected. Frequently, more than one compartment is involved, and such information is critical in guiding treatment.

INTERPRETATION OF PRESSURE MEASUREMENTS

The normal compartment pressure in a resting extremity is less than 5 mm Hg. Exercise can elevate pressure to over 50 mm Hg, but it falls rapidly on cessation of the activity. A generally accepted threshold for compartment syndrome is 40 mm Hg, and when combined with other positive clinical findings, fasciotomy is usually warranted.

TREATMENT

Suspected compartment syndrome should first be treated by removal of any constricting dressings and loosening of any cast. It is important that the cast padding also be cut since it can be a constricting force even after the cast is loosened by cutting and spreading the plaster. If pain and paresthesia do not improve promptly thereafter, compartment pressure measurements should be made and the patient should be admitted for observation.

Impending compartment syndrome (compartment pressures in the range of 15–40 mm Hg) should be treated by placing the extremity at the level of the heart. It has been shown that elevation immediately reduces arterial pressure more than venous pressure, thus further compromising muscle perfusion. Intermittent application of ice (20 minutes on, 10 minutes off) is indicated for acute injuries but should not produce pressure by the weight of the ice pack itself. Repeat pressure measurements should be taken every several hours, or sooner if symptoms or signs warrant it. Hospital admission is indicated.

Established compartment syndrome (pressures > 40 mm Hg) require emergent consultation with an orthopedic or general surgeon. The decision to perform fasciotomy will usually be made by weighing all the information available: the severity of the pain/paresthesia, the duration of time from injury, the trend of the symptoms, and the reliability of the patient, as well as the actual compartmental pressure measurement.

CHRONIC COMPARTMENT SYNDROME

Individuals with chronic reproducible pain in an extremity, usually the lower leg, associated with exercise should be suspected of having a chronic exertional compartment syndrome. The etiology is a supranormal and sustained elevation of compartmental pressure with exercise, resulting in muscle ischemia and pain. Only rarely will neurologic deficit be present.

This syndrome does not result in muscle injury unless the exercise is continued well beyond the onset of pain. In these very rare instances, an acute compartment syndrome can manifest itself.

For most patients with suspected exertional compartment syndrome, referral to an orthopedic surgeon for further evaluation is indicated. It is rarely useful to measure compartment pressures of such patients in the emergency department.

SELECTED READING

Matsen, FA, et al. A practical approach to compartmental syndromes. *Instructional Course Lectures* Vol. 32. St. Louis: Mosby, 1983. Pp 88–113.

Whitesides, TE, et al. Tissue pressure measurements as a determinant of the need for fasciotomy. *Clin Orthop* 113:43, 1975.

74. Partially or Totally Severed Parts

Joseph Upton

Recent technological improvements in instrumentation, in operating microscopes, and especially in the mass production of microsutures have transformed small-vessel (0.5–2 mm) surgery into a clinical reality. Although applications of microsurgery have been developed in virtually all surgical subspecialties, the most dramatic and widespread is the reattachment of severed parts. Initial assessment and management of patients who require this procedure are the first critical steps in a successful replant* effort.

Microsurgery is surgery performed under high-powered magnification that in the clinical setting involves loupe magnification or operating microscopes. A *revascularization* procedure restores arterial and venous flow to a partially severed part, which if left alone would not remain viable. *Replantation* is the reattachment of a totally severed part. Revascularization of partially severed extremities outnumbers replantation efforts 5:1.

THE REPLANTATION TEAM

Teamwork is critical. Each member of the team must make a major personal commitment, and the hospital must make a significant institutional commitment. In the United States, most microsurgery has become regionalized in large cities and major academic centers. There are, however, many smaller community hospitals where these procedures are also performed. Because most amputations involve limbs, the management is usually within the orthopedic or plastic surgical hand service of the hospital. Busy general surgical trauma services may also become involved with extremity and other amputations. The team must be available 24 hours a day and staffed with enough trained people to handle whatever emergency presents. The leaders must be experienced surgeons in the management of major trauma and in all aspects of acute and reconstructive hand surgery. The decision of these individuals to reattach or revascularize salvageable parts to preserve function will require great flexibility, experience, and frequently innovation. To have the necessary expensive and delicate microinstruments and microscopes; the properly equipped operating rooms, recovery rooms, and rehabilitation centers; and the trained nursing personnel, the hospital must make a major commitment to microsurgery. Operating suites and individual surgical services must be ready to delay or reschedule elective cases to accommodate these often lengthy procedures. Enough physicians must be trained and coordinated into units to avoid

*The terms *replant* and *reimplant* are inaccurate because nothing was really planted initially. They are, however, colloquial terms that are commonly used.

frustration and fatigue. Older, more experienced surgeons who may not be enthusiastic about working all night must nevertheless be on the team. Their input will undoubtedly improve the care of the patients.

CARE OF THE PATIENT

Initial Assessment

The patient usually arrives in the emergency department with a towel or handkerchief wrapped around the injured extremity. Profuse bleeding in the palm or digit can always be controlled with direct pressure and elevation. The same is true for the scalp and facial and perineal regions. Blind clamping of vessels will often inflict unneccesary damage to adjacent nerves. Careful ligation of major vessels in the forearm or upper arm may be necessary to avoid severe hemorrhage and hypovolemia. Large-vessel hemorrhage for proximal limb amputations may require several tourniquets. The initial estimation of blood loss is notoriously inadequate.

Multiple trauma patients must be carefully assessed for associated injuries. Sometimes the extremity amputation may be a low-priority injury. More often, preoccupation with the amputation may cause the examining physician to overlook a ruptured spleen, a pneumothorax, or other potentially life-threatening injuries.

Initial resuscitation should include placement of intravenous lines, monitoring of vital signs, and a careful physical examination, regardless of the extent of the injury or level of amputation.

The decision to reattach or revascularize a severed part should be made by the surgical team. Emergency department staff personnel must refrain from promising the patient too much (or too little) before the condition of the patient and amputated part has been thoroughly evaluated.

History

An accurate and complete history will pay tremendous dividends for the surgeon responsible for making the decision regarding the feasibility of a reattachment effort. During recent decades, a great deal of controversy has existed around the indications for replantation, much of which will undoubtedly be refined over the next 10 to 15 years. Currently, experts in the field differ, and absolute guidelines cannot be established. Many factors should be considered in the decision. The ultimate goal is to restore as much function as possible without jeopardizing uninjured parts of the limb. The following items should be included in the history of all patients:

1. Associated injuries
2. Age
3. Level of amputation
4. Digit involved
5. Mechanism of injury
6. Hand dominance
7. Occupation
8. Past medical history
9. Psychological and intellectual status
10. Socioeconomic factors

Associated Injuries
Closed- and open-head trauma and major cardiopulmonary injuries often negate the feasibility of limb reattachment efforts. In addition, other small fractures, contusions, adhesions, dislocations, and other less dramatic injuries are often missed and may become the source of the patient's primary long-term disability.

Age
Younger patients achieve much better long-term results, probably secondary to superior sensory return and motor function. Every effort should be made to reattach major parts that have been amputated in children.

Level of Amputation
Very proximal amputations in the upper arm or midforearm contain a significant amount of muscle tissue that is quite susceptible to warm ischemia. Major parts that have been amputated are considered to be poor candidates for reattachment when muscle ischemia time has exceeded six hours. In addition, avulsion-traction amputations involving the brachial plexus achieve poor secondary motor and sensory recovery. Amputations at the level of the proximal phalanx pose difficult challenges in terms of flexor tendon function. In contrast, distal amputations at or beyond the level of proximal interphalangeal joints may do remarkably well after reattachment. The level of amputation correlates well with the feasibility of reattachment efforts.

Digit Involved
The mobile thumb is essential to all functioning hands and should be reattached if at all possible. Most present controversy surrounds the isolated border digit amputation of the index or fifth finger. Often, reattached border digits are subsequently amputated at the request of the patient because the reattached finger has been "functionally neglected." Stiffness in any of the ulnar three fingers will significantly limit strength because of the common origin of the profondus tendons.

Mechanism of Injury
A detailed description of the circumstances surrounding the injury may be very helpful initially in determining the need for bone shortening or vein grafting. The type of injury probably correlates best with the ultimate prognosis of a successful reattachment effort. Injuries have been classified into the following four categories, each with a different prognosis:

SHARP, GUILLOTINE INJURIES. Sharp injuries are usually civilian amputations from knives, glass, meat cleavers, industrial cutting machines, or band saws. Minimal debridement is required for structures that are minimally traumatized. Prognosis is usually excellent, especially in digital amputations beyond the level of the proximal phalanx.

LOCALIZED CRUSH INJURIES. Accidents involving industrial presses, farm machinery, saws, and slammed doors are often the cause of localized crush injuries. More extensive debridement, shortening of the digit, and intercalated vein grafts are necessary. The prognosis is not very favorable.

AVULSION INJURIES. Avulsion injuries, which are often combined with crush injuries, are the most difficult to manage. Degloving amputations, ski rope amputations, rip saw injuries, and many pediatric amputations fall into this category. Children often instinctively withdraw a hand, finger, or foot that has become caught within a door or elevator. Small vessels and nerves have been stretched over long segments and must be carefully evaluated under magnification and often replaced with autogenous nerves or vein grafts. Although viability can be predictably restored with vein grafts, sensory return is often poor with these injuries. Avulsion of digital arteries may often result in "red streaks" along the midlateral border of the digits, which is a grave prognostic sign. The prognosis for upper-arm and forearm amputations is poor because of prolonged ischemia time and frequent postoperative vascular thrombosis.

DIFFUSE CRUSH AND/OR EXPLOSION INJURIES. Bomb blasts, firecracker accidents, vehicular accidents, and severe industrial crush accidents predominate. The tissue damage often exceeds the initial evaluation. Multiple-level injuries are often found. Initial revascularization attempts may result in thrombosis and tissue demarcation after three to four days as injured tissue becomes more edematous and congested. Although the prognosis is guarded, these patients should always be evaluated, if possible and practical. Portions of the traumatized and/or amputated part may be salvageable and useful as part of a primary reconstruction procedure—for example, to reattach an amputated but nontraumatized fifth finger to the index position to function as an index finger.

Hand Dominance
Indications for reattachment become much more critical in bilateral injuries and in injuries to the dominant hand, especially the thumb. In bilateral injuries, priority should be given to the dominant hand.

Occupation
The functional demands of the patient are important. The thumb is critical to all functioning hands, and in most evaluation scales it accounts for 40 to 50 percent of total hand function. The demands of a left index finger of a concert violinist, who requires precision pinch, may vary tremendously from those of a manual worker, who requires power grip and grasp. Careful individualization of each patient and his or her functional needs becomes quite important.

Past Medical History
Besides obtaining careful tetanus immunization and allergy history, a thorough review of systems regarding cardiac, pulmonary, and peripheral vascular systems is important in adults. In children with sickle cell disease (not sickle cell trait), the use of pneumatic tourniquet is contraindicated. Children with a personal history or family history of malignant hyperthermia should be anesthetized with analeptic techniques. Patients with a history of collagen-vascular disorders as well as many other medical problems may be poor candidates for prolonged surgery, and subsequent immobilization and extensive rehabilitation. History of bleeding problems should always be obtained when the use of anticoagulants is anticipated.

Psychological and Intellectual Status
It may be unwise to reattach an isolated digit (not a thumb) on the hand of a manual laborer, farmer, or other worker who needs to return to work immediately. Psychiatrically unstable patients, specifically schizophrenics, are often poor candidates for cooperation in postoperative rehabilitation. Mental retardation is not a contraindication for these procedures, but considerable ancillary services must be available to help the patient through the difficult postoperative rehabilitation. Although patients with self-inflicted amputations are often poor candidates for reattachment efforts, they must be considered individually since a portion of the amputated part may be useful to provide a well-padded amputation stump.

CARE OF THE AMPUTATED PART

Once the patient has arrived in the emergency department, the amputated part should be located and labeled. If the part has not been obtained, attempts should be made to retrieve it. Asking a scuba diver to search the bottom of a lake or pool or a mechanic to dismantle a machine or car may not be an unreasonable request when the amputated part has a favorable chance for reattachment. Once located, debris should be gently washed away with cold water or isotonic saline. Prolonged irrigation should be avoided. Small remaining skin or soft-tissue bridges should not be incised from partially severed extremities. Often subcutaneous veins and arteries are present that will help sustain flow. An x-ray film of both the injured extremity and the amputated part should be obtained.

The amputated part should then be wrapped in a sponge moistened in a physiologic solution, placed in a plastic bag, and inserted into an ice bath at 2 to 4°C. Direct placement on ice cubes will not afford cooling as homogeneous as that of the ice bath. Dry ice will crystallize and destroy cells. The fluid within any container in the hospital should be checked to avoid inadvertent placement into formalin. The ice bath should then be transported in a cooler along with the patient. Eventual survival of the reattached part depends greatly on the ischemia time and the anoxic tissue damage. Immediate cooling is essential. Muscle tissue is the most sensitive and undergoes irreversible damage after 6 hours of ischemia time at room temperature (20–25°C). Fingers and thumbs contain no muscle tissue and have survived 20 to 30 hours of cold anoxia.

FAVORABILITY FOR REATTACHMENT

Recent publicity given to this dramatic type of reattachment surgery has both educated the public and created often unrealistic expectations. Each individual case must be carefully evaluated with the preceding criteria in mind. Special consideration must be given to the *prognosis for sensory return,* which correlates best with the ultimate functional result.

Favorability for reattachment is difficult to summarize, but general guidelines are listed below.

If possible, all of the following should be reattached:

1. Mid- or distal forearm amputations with low ischemia time
2. Wrist amputations
3. Transmetacarpal or hemihand amputations
4. Major thumb amputations, including those distal to the interphalangeal joint
5. Multiple digit amputations
6. Major amputations in a child
7. Scalp amputations

The following cases should be carefully evaluated on an individual basis:

1. Proximal forearm, elbow, and upper-arm amputations
2. Isolated digital amputations, especially border digits (index and small fingers) excluding the thumb
3. Ring avulsion injuries at all levels
4. Any amputation in elderly patients (over 60 years of age), patients with history of collagen disease, peripheral vascular disease, or any chronic illness
5. Amputations with prolonged ischemia time
6. Amputations with excessive contamination of tissues
7. All avulsion injuries
8. Pediatric lower-limb amputations with good prognosis for sensory recovery

One should not consider reattachment in the following under ordinary circumstances:

1. Gross mangle, explosion, or crush injuries at any level
2. Toe amputations
3. Self-inflicted penis amputations at any level
4. Multiple-level amputations
5. Patients with significant life-threatening associated injuries

TRANSPORTATION OF THE PATIENT

After communicating with the replant team, the following specific instructions regarding transfer should be given:

1. Stop hemorrhage with elevation, pressure dressing, and/or vessel ligature if necessary
2. Place intravenous line to control hypovolemia and to administer antibiotics
3. Monitor vital signs
4. Provide adequate analgesia
5. Make sure patient is accompanied by a qualified ambulance attendant, especially if intravenous fluids are being infused

SUMMARY OF MANAGEMENT

1. Resuscitate the patient, evaluate associated injuries; tetanus prophylaxis
2. Obtain accurate history, including type of injury, level of amputation, ischemia time, condition and location of amputated part
3. Contact replantation team and gain more specific instructions regarding transfer
4. Care for the amputated part: wash debris, put in sterile wrap, insert in plastic bag, and place within ice bath
5. Transfer patient
6. Notify receiving team of exact estimated time of arrival

SELECTED READING

Biemer, E, et al. Early experiences in organizing and running a replantation service. *Br J Plast Surg* 31:9, 1978.

Lister, GD. Replantation. In JW Smith and SJ Aston (eds), *Grabb and Smith's Plastic Surgery* (4th ed). Boston: Little, Brown, 1991.

Manktelow, RT. What are indications for digital replantation? *Ann Plast Surg* 1:366, 1978.

O'Brien, B McC. *Microvascular Reconstructive Surgery*. Edinburgh: Churchill Livingstone, 1977.

G. Environmental Trauma and Other Environmental Injuries

75. Management of the Burn Patient

Robert H. Demling

Burn injury is a very common but extremely complex injury and requires a discussion of cardiovascular, pulmonary, and microcirculatory physiology; metabolism and nutrition; endocrinology; and immunology for any reasonable understanding of appropriate therapy. The pathophysiology also changes with time after the burn, with early physiologic and biochemical changes that are markedly different from those that occur later. The focus of this chapter is on early management—that is, care that is provided in the emergency department. The discussion of pathophysiology focuses on pulmonary changes, mostly from smoke, and the hemodynamic, metabolic, and specific wound-related changes caused by the body burn itself.

PULMONARY CHANGES

Pulmonary dysfunction is a major cause of morbidity and mortality in the burn patient. A decrease in arterial oxygen tension (PaO_2) is frequently seen on admission. Alterations in lung function in the early period are not caused by increased lung water in the absence of smoke inhalation or gross fluid overload. The lack of a significant increase in lung water early after the burn in the absence of smoke inhalation injury has been verified in humans. This assumes that an accurately controlled volume replacement is performed, as even a normal lung can become edematous if massive fluid overload is initiated. Some modest lung circulatory and ventilatory changes in large burn injuries include a transient increase in pulmonary artery pressure and a modest but significant decrease in PaO_2. Ventilatory changes include increases in closing volume and airway resistance, indicating pathology of the small airways. A number of bronchoconstrictor and vasoactive mediators are released from burn tissue. These agents, which have an effect on smooth-muscle constriction in the lung, include histamine, serotonin, and thromboxane $A_2(TxA_2)$. The role of the mediators, particularly TxA_2, in the early lung changes remains to be clearly defined.

Pulmonary insufficiency resulting from heat and smoke inhalation is the major cause of mortality in the fire victim, accounting for over 50 percent of fire-related deaths. The magnitude of the problem has only been well recognized in recent years. The addition of new synthetics in home furnishings has resulted in a more complex form of injury, because of the extremely toxic combustion products of these technologic advances. The various components of this complex injury are discussed in the order in which they normally are seen by the clinician.

Hypoxia, Carbon Monoxide, and Cyanide

The inspired air in a fire has a decreased oxygen content because of oxygen utilization during combustion. Exposure to this hypoxic environment, estimated at a fraction of inspired oxygen as low as 0.1, can cause severe organ dysfunction, in particular to the brain and myocardium. Impaired oxygen delivery to burned tissue will further magnify the heat-induced tissue damage. While oxygen is being used, carbon monoxide (CO) is being released as a basic by-product of combustion. Carbon monoxide is rapidly transported across the alveolar membrane to bind preferentially with the hemoglobin molecule in place of oxygen. The presence of CO on hemoglobin also impairs unloading of oxygen, if present on the same molecule, resulting in a major impairment in oxygen delivery. With prolonged exposure, CO can also saturate the cell, binding to cytochrome oxidase and thereby impairing mitochondrial function and energy products. Hydrogen cyanide released from burning polyurethane (e.g., in upholstery) also binds to mitochondrial cytochrome oxidase, inhibiting cellular respiration.

Symptoms are those of decreased tissue oxygen utilization, with manifestations of impaired cerebral oxygenation the most prominent early sign. Symptoms of CO toxicity are, in general, subtle even with moderately severe intoxication (carboxyhemoglobin levels of 20–40%). These include headache, dizziness, confusion, and nausea. Angina can occur when preexisting heart disease is present. When 40 to 50 percent of the hemoglobin is bound with CO, severe intoxication will produce a semicomatose state as a result of the severe brain hypoxemia. The hypoxemic episode is usually fatal when carboxyhemoglobin (HbCO) levels are greater than 60 percent. Although the oxygen content of blood is reduced, the PaO_2 remains normal, as CO does not alter the amount of oxygen dissolved in plasma. Tachypnea is therefore frequently absent because the carotid body presumably is responsive to oxygen tension rather than oxygen content. The color of HbCO is bright red. Cyanide toxicity presents in a very similar fashion. A persistent metabolic acidosis in the face of adequate blood volume is characteristic of both CO and cyanide. If the cytochrome system is also bound by CO as a result of prolonged exposure, the degree of toxicity may not be totally reflected by the HbCO levels, as CO can be displaced from hemoglobin more rapidly than from the enzymes of the cytochrome system.

Thermal Injury

Direct heat injury caused by the inhalation of air heated to a temperature of 150°C or higher ordinarily results in burns confined to the face, oropharynx, and upper airway (above the vocal cords). Even superheated air is cooled rapidly before reaching the lower respiratory tract because of the tremendous heat-exchanging efficiency of the oropharynx and nasopharynx.

Heat produces an immediate injury to the airway mucosa, resulting in edema, erythema, and ulceration. Flame exposure sufficient to produce a facial burn and singed nasal fibril is often associated with temperatures high enough to produce mucosal damage. A life-threatening upper-airway obstruction can result. Concomitant burns to the face result in massive facial and oropharyngeal swelling, thereby impairing the ability to manage oral secretions. Although these mucosal changes may be anatomically present shortly after the burn, physiologic alterations will not be seen until the edema is sufficient to produce hoarseness or evidence of early airway obstruction. This may not occur for several more hours. It has now been clearly determined that the presence of a body burn magnifies the injury to airways in direct proportion to the size and depth of the skin burn, as evidenced by increased airway edema and collapse in the early stages, followed in later stages by increased lung sepsis. The massive fluid requirements necessary to treat the skin burn are, in part, responsible.

Table 75-1. Toxic elements in house fire smoke

Gas	Source	Effect
Carbon monoxide	Any organic matter	Tissue hypoxia
Carbon dioxide	Any organic matter	Narcosis
Nitrogen dioxide	Wallpaper, wood	Bronchial irritation Dizziness Pulmonary edema
Hydrogen chloride (phosgene)	Plastics (polyvinyl chloride)	Severe mucosal irritation
Hydrogen cyanide	Wool, silk, nylons (polyurethane)	Headache Respiratory failure Coma
Benzene	Petroleum plastics	Mucosal irritation Coma
Aldehydes	Wood, cotton, paper	Severe mucosal damage Extensive lung damage
Ammonia	Nylon	Mucosal irritation

Chemical Injury

Chemical inhalation injury is generally much more serious than that produced by heat alone. Toxic gases contained in smoke as well as carbon particles coated with irritating aldehydes and organic acids can result in injury of both the upper and lower airways. The location of injury will depend on the duration of exposure, the size of the particles, and the solubility of the gases. A partial listing of these agents is presented in Table 75-1.

The unconscious patient, however, loses this airway protection, thereby increasing the smoke exposure. This results in a more severe injury to the lower airways. Water-soluble gases found in smoke from burning plastics or rubber, such as ammonia, sulfur dioxide, and chlorine, react with water in mucous membranes to produce strong acids and alkalis that lead to irritation, bronchospasm and mucous membrane ulceration, and edema. Severe impairment of the ciliary mechanism of the mucosa occurs, leading to impairment of mucus removal. Lipid-soluble compounds, such as nitrous oxide, phosgene, hydrogen chloride, and various toxic aldehydes, are transported frequently to the lower airways on carbon particles, which, in turn, adhere to the mucosa. All these agents produce cell membrane damage. There is a marked early increase in bronchial blood flow, measured to be 10- to 20-fold in experimental animals with chemical inhalation injury. This marked increase in blood flow to an injured microcirculation accentuates the edema formation.

Symptoms consist of early bronchospasm due to smooth-muscle constriction in the injured airways, which is manifested by wheezing. The measured increased airway resistance is due primarily to mucosal edema. Studies on humans using the multiple inert gas technique have demonstrated an early increased dead space as well as increased airway resistance. Vasospasm due to the previously described mediators released from burn tissue is a likely explanation. This is followed in several hours by a decrease in the $\dot{V}/\dot{Q}$ ratio indicative of alveolar derecruitment from bronchospasm and peribronchiolar edema. True intrapulmonary shunting is not severe during this period, indicating that alveolar edema is not a major component of the disease state and therefore not responsible for the impaired gas exchange. An intense bronchorrhea for injured airway mucosa is clearly present, as are markedly increased oral and nasal secretions. Alveolar flooding in these cases may well be due to retrograde flow of bronchiolar mucosal edema. The airways are perfused by the bronchial vessels from the systemic circulation. There is no clear evidence that the integrity of the pulmonary microcirculation is altered with smoke inhalation, except with certain toxins, such as some hydrocarbons, which are absorbed and recirculate to the lung. A body burn also markedly potentiates the inhalation-induced lung dysfunction caused by chemical injury.

EFFECTS OF THE SKIN BURN

Skin Function

The skin is the largest organ of the body, ranging from 0.25 sq m in the newborn to 1.8 sq m in the adult. It consists of two layers, epidermis and dermis (or corium) (Fig. 75-1). The outermost cells of the epidermis are dead cornified cells that act as a tough protective barrier against the environment. The second, thicker layer, the dermis (0.06–0.12 mm), is composed chiefly of fibrous connective tissue. The dermis contains the blood vessels and nerves to the skin and the epithelial appendages of specialized function. Since the nerve endings that mediate pain are found in the superficial portion of the dermis, partial-thickness injuries, which expose the nerves, will be extremely painful, whereas full-thickness burns are usually anesthetic, as the nerves have been heat destroyed. The dermis also acts as a barrier to prevent loss of body fluids by evaporation and loss of excess body heat. Sweat glands help to maintain body temperature by controlling the amount of heat lost by evaporation. Both the continued loss of water through burned skin and loss of heat play a major role in the pathophysiologic changes seen after a burn. The skin is also our primary protective barrier against invasive infection, preventing penetration of microorganisms into the subdermal tissues. Burn wound infection is a major cause of mortality and morbidity in the later postburn period. The skin also adapts to changes in the physical environment initiated by sensory nerve endings in the dermis, which detect the sensations of touch, pressure, pain, cold, and heat. Loss of this function will lead to long-term impairments that must be appreciated. The degree of impairment in these protective characteristics of normal skin depends on the depth of burn injury and the extent of injury—that is, the size of the burn relative to that of total body surface (TBS) area.

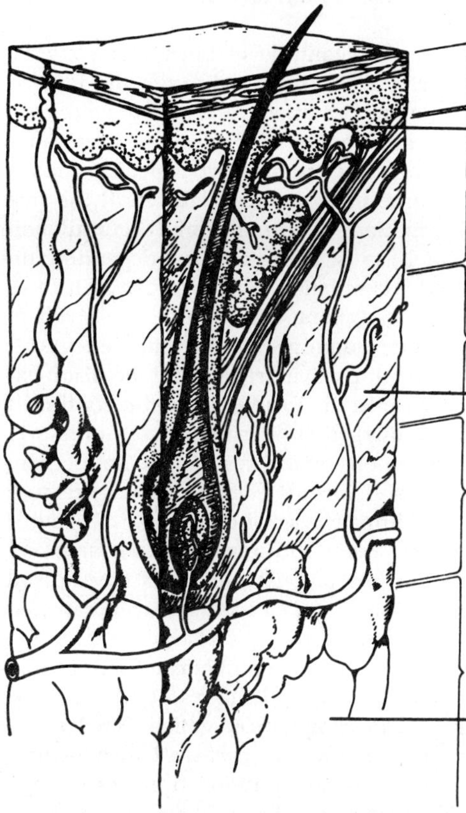

Fig. 75-1. The depths to which skin damage extends with burns of varying degrees. (From R.H. Demling. Burn Care in the Immediate Resuscitation Period. In D. Wilmore [ed.], *Care of the Surgical Patient.* New York: Scientific American, 1987.)

Burn-Induced Microvascular Changes

The burn results in marked changes in the skin vasculature. Although the exact pathophysiology of the postburn vascular changes and volume shifts remains to be determined, it is known that two processes are involved: an increase in microvascular fluid flux into the interstitium, both local to the burn and generalized, and a generalized impairment in cell membrane function, resulting in cell swelling.

It is clear that protein permeability in the burn microcirculation is increased. Some controversy remains as to the role of direct heat injury versus that produced by vasoactive substance released from burn tissue. The concept of a mediator-induced injury is of considerable importance as this would allow for possibly modulating the degree of burn edema by mediator inhibition.

An important factor affecting burn fluid and protein flux is the vascular hydrostatic pressure and microvascular surface area perfused. As with any microvessel with increased protein permeability, very small increases in hydrostatic pressure produce very large changes in fluid transport and, in turn, edema formation. The degree of postburn edema depends on the amount and rate of fluid infused. Since the permeability injury allows macromolecules to cross in excess of 100 A radius, the type of initial resuscitation fluid appears to have little effect on the edema in burn tissue as long as the same pressures and flow are maintained until microvascular integrity is restored. This is not the case in nonburned tissue, in which edema formation is markedly affected by the type of fluid used.

The time course and magnitude of burn tissue edema depends on the degree of blood flow through the injured microcirculation. Edema formation in a small wound is maximum at about 8 to 12 hours after injury, whereas after a larger injury, the degree of systemic hypovolemia, caused by fluid loss into a large burn surface, will retard the rate of further edema formation. Maximum fluid accumulation will usually occur at 18 to 24 hours or later, depending on the adequacy of fluid resuscitation. Since burned skin loses its elasticity, it is less compliant and unable to stretch to accommodate increasing quantities of interstitial edema. If burns are circumferential, particularly around the distal extremities, a tourniquet effect is produced by the continued accumulation of interstitial fluid, elevating tissue pressure. This initially impedes venous return, resulting in an increase in capillary pressure and further edema. Tissue pressure can then increase and impair arterial blood flow. Once this process becomes severe enough to impede arteriolar blood flow, as reflected by a loss of pulsatile blood flow, distal tissue necrosis can result if an incision is not performed through burn tissue—that is, an escharotomy to decrease tissue pressure. The loss of tissue compliance also occurs in the burned chest wall, and severe edema results in a marked impairment in chest-wall compliance, which can lead to severe respiratory compromise. A chest-wall escharotomy may be required, with the patient positioned in a semi-erect fashion, if possible, to decrease the impairment of ventilation.

Generalized soft-tissue edema is a characteristic finding after a major burn. Edema formation in nonburned tissues is evident in patients with burns that exceed 30 percent of the TBS; it can be measured experimentally in less severe injuries.

The edema appears to be due, at least in part, to an alteration in the microvascular interstitium. Protein washout appears to increase the compliance of the interstitial space or the ease of water transport across the microvascular membrane, resulting in edema formation without an alteration in the balance of Starling forces—that is, capillary hydrostatic pressure and the colloid osmotic pressure (COP) gradient. The edema formation can be prevented by maintaining plasma and interstitial protein levels. However, protein content in the first six to eight hours is difficult to maintain due to the early, rapid protein losses after a major burn. After the first 8 hours, protein content in plasma can be more readily maintained with protein infusions. Nonburn edema can also be prevented by using nonprotein colloids if the COP gradient is increased above normal. However, once the colloids are discontinued and cleared, edema will again develop as a result of the persistent hypoproteinemic state.

Fluid requirements are decreased by up to 50 percent if nonburn edema is experimentally prevented in a large burn. This would indicate that a substantial portion of the resuscitation fluid goes to the production of nonburn edema.

Changes in Cell Function

The second process that occurs after a deep partial-thickness or full-thickness burn greater than 30 percent of TBS is a decrease in cell transmembrane potential in tissue distant from the burn, particularly prominent in muscle. This causes a shift of extracellular sodium and, in turn, water into the intracellular space, producing cell swelling while decreasing extracellular volume. The degree of intracellular fluid shift appears to be considerably less than that seen in the interstitium.

Systemic Hemodynamic Changes

Clinically evident cardiovascular instability arises from the microvascular and cell membrane alterations just described. A noticeable early reduction in plasma volume is seen. This plasma loss, measured by Mason and associates, was greater than 30 percent of TBS. There is no functional semipermeable membrane in burn tissue to allow for maintenance of a COP gradient generated by protein. Therefore, functional plasma volume within burn tissue can only be restored with expansion of the extracellular space as well. During this period, some extracellular sodium and water are also being depleted by a shift into the cells. The quantity of sodium lost from the extracellular space during the 24-hour period after the burn has been measured to be 0.4 to 0.5 mEq/kg body weight × the percentage of body burn. The rate of loss of plasma volume is the greatest during the first 4 to 6 hours, decreasing substantially by 18 to 24 hours if adequate perfusion has been restored. Edema in nonburned tissue occurs later in the resuscitation period out of phase with burn edema, indicating a different mechanism of formation.

Cardiac output is initially depressed, primarily because of hypovolemia and the increased systemic and, to a lesser extent, pulmonary vascular resistance due to vasoactive mediators such as catecholamine. Decreased cardiac contractility due to a circulating myocardial depressant factor has also been reported; the factor has yet to be identified and its presence remains controversial. Myocardial depression is most evident in deep burns that cover more than 40 percent of TBS, and is greater for third-degree than for second-degree burns. Positive-pressure ventilation, frequently required in the early postburn period, can further decrease output. Cardiac output is usually restored toward normal before restoration of a normal plasma volume, as a result of an increased heart rate typical of the increased stress response. Central venous pressure and pulmonary artery wedge pressure usually remain low even when cardiac output and perfusion are adequate, indicating less than normal blood volume.

This fact is important to recognize when selecting appropriate resuscitation monitors, as an overzealous attempt at restoring blood volume over and above that necessary for adequate perfusion can markedly accentuate edema-related complications. Fluid and protein losses in burn tissue are markedly aggravated by increases in venous pressure produced by excessive fluid infusion or by the released venoconstrictor mediators. Blood volume in severe burns can remain decreased for days in view of the ongoing losses. Even with massive fluid replacement, blood hematocrit of 50 to 55 percent is not uncommon in the early postburn period. Volume cannot be completely restored until the leak begins to slow at about 18 to 24 hours after the burn.

Temperature Change

With a deep burn, the barrier to water loss by evaporation is markedly impaired. The loss of the evaporation barrier also means loss of the barrier to heat loss, a fact extremely important to recognize in the resuscitation period. The protective mechanism vasoconstriction in the skin is absent. Body heat is lost by the mechanisms of convection, conduction, and radiation, all of which are magnified after burns diminish the skin barrier. Transfer of heat to a moving system such as air or water is known as *convection.* If body surface temperature is higher than air temperature, heat flows from body to air until the gradient is gone. However, warm air rises and is replaced by cooler air. The faster the air moves across the skin, the greater the gradient and the greater the heat loss. Air movement by a fan or by a laminar airflow unit or air-fluidized bed can play a major role in heat loss depending on the size of the gradient. Heat loss can be decreased by closing the wound under dressings, thereby limiting the air movement and decreasing the air-wound temperature gradient.

Heat is also exchanged by direct content with an object—for example, bed or dressing table. This process is known as *conduction,* and heat loss again depends on the temperature gradient. The rate of loss of body heat in water (wet dressings or hydrotherapy) is 25 times greater than that in air due to increased heat conductivity in water. Radiation is emission of energy from the body surface as heat. The amount of loss depends on body heat production, surface blood flow, and surface area. Radiation losses are increased after burn as a result of hypermetabolism and increased blood flow. Both of these processes are not maximized until the inflammation stage. Heat loss by any or all of these mechanisms will lead to hypothermia, an exaggerated stress response, and the increased energy requirements needed to correct the problem.

Metabolic, Immunologic, and Hematologic Changes

The immediate postburn period is known as the *ebb phase,* as nutrient flow and oxygen delivery to cells are decreased, leading to a decrease in metabolic rate. A massive catecholamine release occurs immediately after burn injury, both from the adrenal medulla and the autonomic nervous system. The catechol discharge is, in large part, responsible for the systemic vasoconstriction and increased vascular resistance. Glucagon is released during the same response, as well as corticosteroids, which results in the conversion of liver glycogen to glucose, and thereby a hyperglycemia. The only readily available energy store is liver glycogen, which is rapidly depleted during the resuscitation phase. The effect of the insulin released in response is overwhelmed by these antiinsulin hormones. Burn-induced hypovolemia increases renin production by the kidney and, in turn, increases aldosterone production. The net result is a decrease in free water clearance and a concentration of urine with conservation of sodium. Pain and anxiety will potentiate the stress response. Loss of body heat due to the removal of the skin barrier can add yet another stimulus to the release of these stress hormones, thereby accentuating the physiologic alterations. Hypothermia, which will be accentuated by a cold or wet environment, will stimulate muscle shivering, utilizing any residual glucose to restore body temperature. Anaerobic metabolism will ensue if oxygen demands are further increased, leading to a metabolic acidosis.

Early alterations in both the cellular and humoral components of the immune system appear proportional to the degree of burn injury. Early changes in the function of the polymorphonuclear leukocyte have been identified. Burn-induced monocyte and macrophage defects have been found to alter the lymphocyte response both by a decrease in interleukin-2 production and by an impairment of antigen presentation on the macrophage surface to the lymphocyte. Early alterations in the humoral system also occur. Immunoglobulin of the IgG class and fibronectin, responsible for opsonization of particles and bacteria, are decreased initially, in part due to loss into the burn wound.

As for hematologic disorder, evidence of hemolysis is frequently seen, particularly after deep third-degree burns or any prolonged exposure to a heat source, with free plasma hemoglobin and hemoglobinuria. Increased cell-wall lipid peroxidation is evident and fragmented cells are often seen on smear. Many of these injured red cells will have a markedly shortened life span, leading to an anemia beginning in the first week. Red cell hematopoiesis is markedly impaired and remains so until the burn is closed, resulting in a persistent anemia. Frequently, a hypercoagulable state is seen in the initial period in moderate burn injuries. A hypercoagulable state, reflected in a depletion of clotting factors, can be seen with massive burns.

EVALUATION AND TREATMENT

Neutralization of the Source of the Burn

Clothing

The first objective is to stop the burning process because the deeper the burn, the greater the potential for mortality and morbidity. With chemical burns, chemicals can remain in fabric and on skin for long periods. With a flame or scald burn, clothing can retain heat for a considerable time, and thus rapid removal of clothing is essential. Clothes are often still smoldering when the patient arrives at the emergency department. If clothing is burned or melted into the tissues, the surrounding fabric can be cut off. Adherent clothing can be removed after admission, when further wound cleaning and debridement are performed.

Chemical Burns

Removal of the chemical is urgent. Acid burns should be irrigated for up to 30 minutes with tepid tap water. For burns resulting from alkali contact, lavage for up to one hour may be beneficial. If necessary, particles of corrosive powders should be surgically removed before the wound is irrigated. The skin burn itself is not the only concern, because the absorption of certain chemicals can lead to systemic toxicities such as neurologic dysfunction, red cell hemolysis, and liver and kidney failure. It is important to avoid severe hypothermia during irrigation because hypothermia results in significant morbidity. Therefore, once the burn source is removed, the patient should be covered with clean, dry dressings or sheets.

Table 75-2. Symptoms of carbon monoxide intoxication

Carboxyhemoglobin level (%)	Symptoms
0–15	None
15–20	Headache, confusion
20–40	Disorientation, fatigue, nausea, visual impairment
40–60	Hallucination, combativeness, coma, shock
60+	Death

Establishment of Airway and Adequate Ventilation

Diagnosis and Treatment of Carbon Monoxide Toxicity

Patients who were injured in a closed space or who have inhalation injuries should be suspected of inhaling carbon monoxide (Table 75-2). Carbon monoxide toxicity is determined by a high index of suspicion and by measuring the carboxyhemoglobin (CO-HgB) level. Persistent metabolic acidosis in a patient with adequate volume resuscitation and adequate cardiac output indicates persistent impairment by CO or cyanide of oxygen utilization and delivery. The chemical alteration of hemoglobin or of the cytochrome system by CO will not affect the amount of oxygen dissolved in plasma, and arterial oxygen tension will thus remain relatively normal. However, the measured oxygen saturation of hemoglobin will be markedly decreased relative to the oxygen tension.

Treatment of CO toxicity consists of the early displacement of CO from hemoglobin by administration of 90 to 100 percent oxygen until the CO-HgB level is less severe than 7 percent. If 20 percent oxygen is administered, the half-life of CO-HgB is about 90 minutes; if concentrated high-flow oxygen is administered, the half-life is 20 to 30 minutes. The concentration of CO-HgB is thus reduced by approximately 50 percent every 20 to 30 minutes if an oxygen concentration of 90 to 100 percent is used. Hyperbaric oxygen (2–3 atm) produces an even more rapid displacement, particularly from the cell cytochrome system, but is rarely required to treat CO exposure.

Diagnosis of the Presence and Extent of Inhalation Injury

Inhalation injury should be suspected in (1) individuals who were injured in a closed space; (2) patients with extensive burns or with burns of the face; (3) patients who were unconscious at the time of injury; (4) patients with singed nasal hairs, hoarseness, or wheezing; and (5) patients who are coughing up carbonaceous sputum. Pulmonary changes are best classified according to cause: thermal injury (heat) or chemical injury (incomplete products of combustion).

A number of techniques have been used to assess the degree of injury and to determine the need for endotracheal intubation. Fiberoptic bronchoscopy or laryngoscopy will reveal physical evidence of mucosal injury. Spirometry detects early obstructive patterns in the airways, but reliable data can be obtained only in a cooperative patient without severe facial burns. Because edema is progressive during the first 18 to 24 hours, none of these tests accurately predicts the severity of subsequent airway compromise, and serial studies must be performed.

Diagnosis of chemical injury is complicated by the fact that the facial burns or other signs evident in heat injury may be absent; indeed, the patient may not have been exposed to heat. Fiberoptic bronchoscopy detects the reddened, sometimes ulcerated mucosa that indicates the presence, but not the severity, of chemical injury. Ventilation-perfusion lung scans using xenon-135 reportedly detect early changes in the small airways, as do analyses of flow-volume curves and a simple one-second forced expiratory volume (FEV_1). Preexisting lung disease, however, will alter the interpretation of findings. Measurement of lung water is of minimal benefit because major changes in water content usually occur only in an alveolar injury in which early respiratory failure is prominent. Initial chest x-ray, blood gas levels, and physical examination results are frequently normal.

Intubation

Endotracheal intubation is indicated for deep facial burns—especially of the lips, mouth, neck, or oropharynx—because subsequent edema will impair airway patency; cases of smoke inhalation in which heat or chemical burns to the airway have been demonstrated by laryngoscopy or bronchoscopy; and massive body burns, especially in the presence of circumferential chest burns, because ventilatory support is needed. Deep burns of the face, mouth, or neck can compromise the airway by anatomic distortion and compression from the burn-edema process. Edema-induced distortion peaks at 18 to 24 hours after a burn; airway patency and the ability to clear secretions are impaired. As edema increases, it becomes much more difficult to secure an airway. Endotracheal intubation is thus preferably performed on admission, before the development of severe edema. A patient with inhalation injury can be closely monitored for upper-airway obstruction without a tube, preferably with the head elevated at 30 degrees, only if intubation will be technically possible later. However, if anatomic distortion from face and neck burns is increasing to a point where safe intubation might soon be precluded, the procedure is carried out immediately. Tracheostomy through burned tissue is contraindicated because the risk of infection, both in the wound and in the airway, is substantially increased. Heat injury usually heals in a few days to a week, as the mucosal edema resolves and the relatively superficial mucosal injury heals.

Positive end-expiratory pressure (PEEP) is frequently necessary to keep the edematous airways open and to maintain an adequate functional residual capacity; it is also often used in the early management of severe CO toxicity (CO-HgB $>$ 40). Prophylactic endotracheal intubation and PEEP have been reported to decrease deaths from early pulmonary complications after severe burns and smoke inhalation. A large enough tube (approximately 7.5 mm internal diameter in adults) should be used because very thick secretions develop as the lung injury becomes manifest, and changing tubes in the presence of edema is very dangerous. Therefore, although the nasotracheal route may be more comfortable for the patient, the route of placement must be based on the tube size required.

Initiation of Aggressive Pulmonary Support
Continuous administration of humidified oxygen is indicated to maintain adequate oxygen delivery as well as to assist in the clearance of secretions. If the patient's hemodynamic condition will tolerate it, elevation of the head and chest by 20 to 30 degrees is helpful in reducing neck and chest wall edema. The early addition of bronchodilators, usually by aerosol, is especially advantageous in managing the bronchospasm seen after chemical injury. The β_2-sympathomimetic agent metaproterenol (via nebulizer) is an effective bronchodilator. Intravenous aminophylline, although helpful, is frequently limited in its use because of the tachycardia seen in the early postburn period.

Beginning about 18 to 24 hours after a burn, however, increasing airway resistance (which develops as a consequence of airway edema) responds better to further increases in PEEP. Above a PEEP of 10 cm H_2O, significant problems in cardiac output will occur. Prophylactic antibiotics are not indicated to prevent a lung infection after smoke injury. Steroids have not been found to be helpful in limiting the extent of inhalation injury and, to the contrary, are actually deleterious in the presence of a major burn.

Close monitoring of the adequacy of gas exchange by serial blood gas determination is necessary, particularly during the early evolution of complications from the inhalation injury. An indwelling arterial line is indicated in the presence of severe injuries. If placement of such a line is not possible, a pulse oximeter is very useful if an unburned finger or earlobe is available. The pulse oximeter reads arterial oxygen saturation by means of a photosensor, which detects the color of the blood flowing beneath the probe.

Gastric ileus, commonly seen with a major burn, can persist for several days. The gastric distention increases the risk of aspiration and impairs lung excursion. Placement of a nasogastric tube solves these problems.

Chest Wall Escharotomy
A full-thickness burn of the anterior and lateral chest wall can lead to severe restriction of chest-wall motion as edema develops beneath the nonviable tissue (eschar), even in the absence of a completely circumferential burn. Chest wall escharotomy is required to relieve the restriction; the incision must penetrate completely through the eschar so that the subeschar space can expand and decrease tissue pressure. In a full-thickness burn, nerve endings are destroyed along with the entire epidermis and dermis. Analgesics are thus usually not necessary for escharotomy. The escharotomy incisions are placed along the anterior axillary lines with bilateral incisions connected by a subcostal incision (see Fig. 75-1). Occasionally, another incision from the suprasternal notch to the xiphoid process is needed. Bleeding can usually be managed by pressure and occasional use of the electrocautery unit.

Restoration and Maintenance of Hemodynamic Stability

Estimation of Burn Size
Fluid requirements depend on the size of the burn. A simple determination of the burn surface area can be made using the rule of nines: Each arm is considered to be 9 percent of

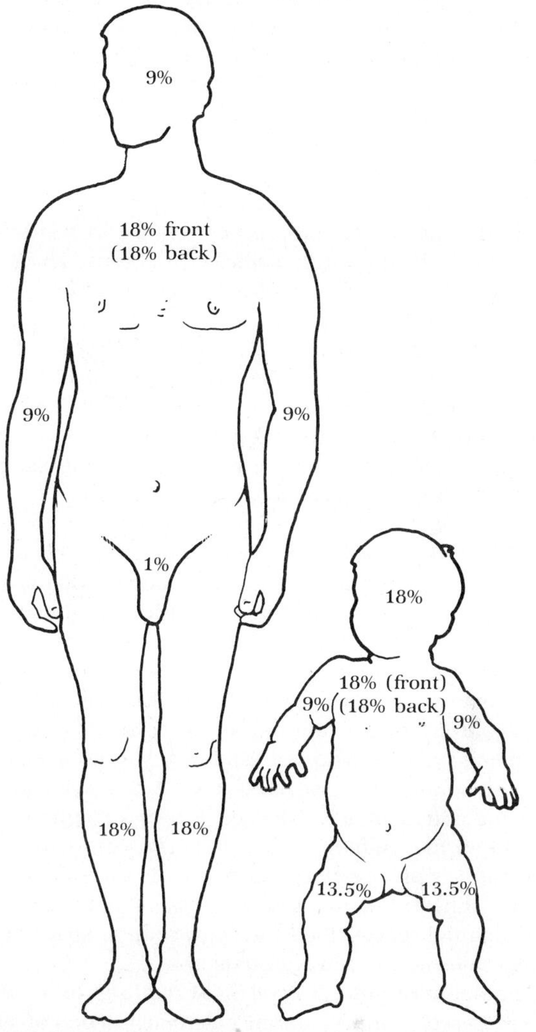

Fig. 75-2. The rule of nines to calculate the percentage of body surface area involved with the burn injury is shown for adults and for children under 12 months of age.

TBS, each leg to be 18 percent, the anterior trunk 18 percent, the posterior trunk 18 percent, and the head 9 percent (Fig. 75-2). In small children, the determination must be modified because the head approaches 18 percent of TBS.

Intravenous Access
A peripheral vein catheter through unburned tissue is the preferred route for fluid administration. A central venous line or pulmonary arterial line is only occasionally needed to monitor the patient during the initial resuscitation period and is removed as soon as it is no longer needed. These lines are usually only required in elderly patients or in patients who have severe heart disease. An extremely high complication rate reportedly accompanies the use of central catheters in burn patients because of infection and embolic episodes related to a hypercoagulable state. Because of the high infection rate, an intravenous catheter should not be placed through burn tissue unless every other possible route has been ruled out. Central line sites not completely dedicated to total parenteral nutrition (TPN) should be rotated every

four to five days to minimize the risk of infection. Arterial lines should also be rotated according to a similar schedule. (A line that is dedicated to TPN should be completely isolated from the burn wound and cared for by covering the entrance site with an occlusive dressing.)

Resuscitation Fluids

In general, fluids containing salt in quantities at least isotonic with plasma are appropriate for use in resuscitation after burn injury if given in sufficient amounts. These fluids should be free of glucose because burn patients exhibit early glucose intolerance as a result of the early release of catecholamines and other stress hormones. The oral route can be used in the case of smaller burns, but intestinal ileus frequently occurs after deep burns in excess of 20 percent of total body surface. A number of intravenous fluids, including colloids, are used to decrease edema in unburned tissues and to maintain a higher blood volume.

CRYSTALLOID. Crystalloid, in particular lactated Ringer's (LR) solution, with a sodium concentration of 130 mEq/liter, is the most popular resuscitation fluid in the United States. The loss of large quantities of sodium and water from the vascular space into the burn wound is well described. Isotonic crystalloid, if given in sufficient amounts, can restore cardiac output toward normal in most patients, the exceptions being patients who are extremely young or extremely old, those whose burns are massive, and those with superimposed inhalation injury. Lactated Ringer's solution is preferred to normal saline because of its physiologic pH of 6.5, versus saline's pH of 5.0. Because isotonic salt solutions generate no differential in osmotic pressure between plasma and interstitial spaces, the entire extracellular space must be expanded to replace intravascular losses.

The amount of isotonic crystalloid required in the first 24 hours is based primarily on the calculated deficit of sodium from the extracellular space. This amount has been estimated by Baxter to be 0.5 to 0.6 mEq sodium/kg/percent burn, which is equal to 4 ml/kg/percent burn of LR solution. The quantity of crystalloid needed is also determined by measuring the parameters used to monitor resuscitation. In most burn centers, a urine output of 0.5 ml/kg/per hour is considered an indication of adequate perfusion. The patient will require about 3 to 5 ml/kg/percent burn in the first 24 hours; about half of this amount is given in the first 8 hours (Table 75-3).

Sodium is apparently the key element in crystalloid infusion; water is primarily the solvent. Solutions with increased sodium concentration therefore have a theoretic advantage because less water is infused. Hypertonic salt solutions used clinically have a milliosmolar content of 400 to 600 (280–300 mOsm is isotonic); such solutions thereby transiently generate potential osmotic pressures of several thousand mm Hg relative to the normal isoosmolar state. Hypertonic salt solutions have been known for many years to be effective in treating shock states, including burns, basically by borrowing intracellular water to fill the extracellular space deficit. Infusion of hypertonic solutions thereby limits edema, compared with treatment by infusion of isotonic solutions.

Hypertonic solutions have also been reported to increase myocardial contractility, produce precapillary dilatation, and decrease vascular resistance by a direct effect on the capillary smooth muscle. Current practice is to use a solution with a sodium concentration of approximately 240 mEq/liter, which is prepared by adding two ampules of sodium lactate to each liter of normal saline. It is recommended that serum sodium levels not be allowed to exceed 160 mEq/liter during infusion of the solution. Complications of hypertonic saline administration relate primarily to hyperosmolarity. A more isotonic solution should be instituted if a hyperosmolar state develops. Free water cannot be given during infusion, because such action will simply lead to a more isotonic solution and, in turn, no decrease in total administered fluid. Increased water retention is likely to occur with the institution of hypotonic solutions beginning on the second postburn day, at least until isotonicity results.

Table 75-3. Fluid resuscitation

Recommendations
3–4 ml Ringer's lactate/kg body weight/% TBS burned
Administer one-half the required volume in the first 8 hours after the burn
Administer one-half the required volume during the next 16 hours
Monitor
Blood pressure (systolic > 90 mm Hg; mean > 80 mm Hg)
Pulse (<120 beats/min)
Urine output (30–50/ml/hr)
Arterial blood gases (PO_2 > 90 mm Hg)
pH (>7.35)
Adjust fluid administration in response to circulatory requirements
Diminish fluid administration if hemodynamic stability is achieved at these infusion rates
or
Add colloid if adequate hemodynamic stability is not achieved at 4 ml/kg/% TBS burned

COLLOIDS. Unburned tissue appears to regain normal permeability very shortly after injury. Because hypoproteinemia can accentuate edema in uninjured tissues, protein restoration should begin 8 to 12 hours after a burn if nonburn edema and total fluid requirements are to be minimized. This method is particularly advantageous in patients who have massive burns and in elderly patients.

Although fresh frozen plasma contains all the protein fractions needed to provide oncotic properties, disease transmission has become a major consideration in limiting its use. It is therefore now strongly recommended that fresh frozen plasma or human plasma fractions be used only to correct documented clotting abnormalities caused by factor depletion and not simply as a volume expander. Volume expansion can usually be accomplished as effectively using an albumin solution.

The amount of protein to be infused remains undefined. Many investigators have arbitrarily used between 0.5 and 1.0 ml/kg/percent burn during the first 24 hours. The amount depends on the magnitude of the injury and on the degree of hemodynamic instability. The protein should be infused at a constant rate (see the section on adjustment of infusion rate); pulsed infusion will transiently increase pressure and the rate of edema formation.

If early adminstration of colloids is required because hemodynamic instability persists despite the infusion of large quantities of crystalloid (about 4 ml/kg/percent burn), nonprotein colloids are more economic. Although the weight of dextran 70 (70,000 MW) is almost identical to that of albumin, dextran's molecular size is considerably larger because of its branched configuration. A standard 6% solution of dextran 70 exerts an oncotic pressure more than twice that generated by a 6% albumin solution. This property makes the compound advantageous as a volume expander. Dextran 40 (40,000 MW) in a 10% solution infused at about 2 ml/kg per hour is an even more potent volume expander because it generates a COP six to eight times that of a protein of comparable weight. To prevent platelet deficits, the total dose of dextran 70 during any 24-hour period should not exceed 33 ml/kg; the total dose of dextran 40 should not exceed 15 ml/kg during any 24-hour period. Therefore, these preparations are usually used in the early resuscitation period and are replaced by protein in the later resuscitation period. The use of the hapten PROMIT, a dextran of 1,000 MW, before the dextran solution essentially precludes allergic reactions to the dextran molecule.

Hetastarch, a 6% starch solution, has colloid properties very similar to those of a 6% protein solution and generates a comparable oncotic pressure. Hetastarch molecules are much larger than those of most dextrans, and vascular clearance is therefore much slower. This solution is being used with increasing frequency as a volume expander.

BLOOD. Because there is no actual early red cell deficit with a burn alone, blood replacement is usually not needed during this period unless severe hemolysis occurs. Occasionally, however, blood can be a very useful volume expander to restore cardiac output if perfusion is not adequately maintained by other resuscitation fluids.

Adjustment of Infusion Rate

Fluids should be infused at a constant rate because rapid fluid challenge transiently increases pressure above the level required for adequate perfusion and contributes to edema formation. Fluid requirements in the first 6 to 8 hours after a burn will clearly exceed those in the subsequent 18 hours because the largest fluid shifts occur early. Approximately half of the total amount of fluid required in the first 24 hours will be given in the first 8 hours. During those first 8 hours, once a fluid infusion rate is reached at which adequate perfusion is maintained, only minor changes should be made so as to avoid large hemodynamic fluctuations. Beginning 8 to 10 hours after a burn, when fluid requirements begin to diminish, an attempt should be made to decrease the infusion rate gradually and to determine the least amount of fluid(s) necessary to maintain adequate perfusion. The rate required in the 12- to 24-hour period must usually deliver approximately 50 to 60 percent of the initial requirements. Fluid requirements during the first 24 hours usually range from 3 to 4 ml/kg/percent burn, depending on the type of fluid, the patient's age, and the presence of other injuries (see Table 75-3).

Parameters to Monitor

PERFUSION. Blood pressure is a poor indicator of perfusion during the early postburn period because a pronounced release of catecholamines results in increased systemic vascular resistance, causing normal blood pressure to be maintained despite the presence of significant hypovolemia. Tachycardia, therefore, is a better indicator of hypovolemia. A heart rate of 110 to 120 beats per minute in the young patient usually reflects an adequate blood volume and an appropriate stress response. A heart rate of 130 beats per minute or greater usually reflects either inadequate volume or an excessive stress response (e.g., to uncontrolled pain or extreme anxiety). Elderly patients with burns frequently do not demonstrate the same degree of tachycardia and require an assessment of multiple clinical parameters (e.g., urine output, central venous pressure, and, perhaps, pulmonary artery pressure) to determine whether perfusion is adequate.

VENOUS PO_2. During the first 24 hours after a burn, the extraction of oxygen from hemoglobin reflects the adequacy of oxygen delivery. Measurements of mixed venous PO_2 are useful if a central or pulmonary artery line is in place. A venous PO_2 below 35 mm Hg indicates marginal perfusion; venous PO_2 below 30 mm Hg indicates inadequate perfusion. Lactic acidosis measured in pH changes in arterial blood samples is definitive evidence that perfusion is inadequate and resuscitation readjustment is necessary. One should monitor body temperature to obtain information about whether the lactic acidosis may be partly the result of rewarming.

CARDIAC OUTPUT. Cardiac output is initially depressed, primarily because of hypovolemia and increased systemic vascular resistance. Decreased cardiac contractility from a circulating myocardial depressant factor has also been reported, but the factor remains unidentified. Decreased cardiac output is greater in third-degree than in second-degree burns and is most evident in deep burns that cover greater than 40 percent TBS. Decreased output is further aggravated by positive-pressure ventilation. Output is usually restored toward normal before restoration of a normal plasma volume as a result of the increased heart rate that is typical of the early postburn period. It is important to recognize that central venous pressure and pulmonary wedge pressure usually remain low even when cardiac output and perfusion are adequate. An overzealous attempt at resuscitating to an arbitrarily determined value for filling pressures, which may be above the value necessary for adequate perfusion, can markedly accentuate the edema process. Elderly patients with a limited ability to increase heart rate will invariably require more fluid for the same burn size.

URINE OUTPUT. Urine output via a Foley catheter is a valuable indicator of adequate renal blood flow, if the urine is nonglycosuric acid and if output has not been increased by administration of solutes (e.g., mannitol or dextran). An output of 0.5 ml/kg per hour in adults or 1.0 ml/kg per hour in children is adequate. Antidiuretic hormone and aldosterone are automatically released in response to the burn stress; therefore, a urine output greater than 0.5 to 1.0 ml/kg/per hour may necessitate a rate of fluid infusion far higher than that necessary to maintain perfusion, and excess edema will result.

Electrical injury can cause extensive damage to underlying tissue that may not be apparent at the time of initial evaluation. Because the area of cutaneous injury may be significantly less than the underlying necrosis, resuscitation needs are based on requirements to maintain urine output. Urine output in patients with electrical injury should be maintained at 75 ml/per hour. Initial fluid resuscitation with a saline solution should begin at 4 ml/kg per hour. An osmotic diuretic (e.g., mannitol, 12.5 gm/liter solution) may be required to maintain urine output after adequate volume replacement. Failure to maintain urine flow can result in the precipitation of hemochromogens in the renal tubules, which in turn can result in acute renal failure.

Inotropic Support

Inotropic support in the first 24 hours is indicated if inadequate perfusion persists despite vigorous fluid resuscitation. This situation is most common in the elderly burn patient. If improved renal blood flow is the major goal, low-dose dopamine (1–4 μg/kg per minute) is preferred. Middle-range dopamine (5–10 μg/kg per minute) or dobutamine will increase contractility and improve cardiac output. Dobutamine results in less tachycardia. Digoxin is not recommended in the immediate postburn period, because the rapid fluid shifts during this period can lead to digitalis toxicity; in addition, digoxin is generally a less potent inotropic agent than dopamine or dobutamine.

Diuretics

Diuretics are rarely indicated in the first 24 hours of resuscitation. The exceptions are when hemoglobinuria or myoglobinuria is present, as can occur after electrical injuries.

Initiation of Wound Management

Cooling the Wound

Cooling will increase heat loss, and neutralizing the heat source is a primary goal of initial management. Immediate cooling of the burn also decreases edema, apparently by stabilizing skin mast cells, thereby preventing histamine release. This effect, however, is short-lived. After the first 30 minutes, the benefit of cooling with water that is approximately 20°C is principally that of pain relief in superficially burned tissues. Prolonged cooling is only indicated for pain relief in second-degree burns of less than 15 percent TBS. Ice should never be used directly on the skin because a freezing injury can result.

After a deep burn, the normal protective mechanism of skin vasoconstriction is absent. The barrier to water loss by evaporation—and hence the barrier to heat loss—is markedly impaired, an extremely important problem to recognize in the resuscitation period. The rate of loss of body heat in water (wet dressings or hydrotherapy) is 25 times greater than in air because of increased heat conductivity in water. Once hypothermia develops, rewarming is extremely slow, and decreased body temperature can affect cardiac output and perfusion of vital organs.

Assessment of Burn Depth

At this point, more precise assessments of burn size and depth are needed to determine the manner of burn care and the need for transfer to a burn facility. Burn depth is classified by degree of injury (Table 75-4). The size of second- and third-degree burns must be determined relative to total body surface (see Fig. 75-2).

Table 75-4. Physical characteristics of burns

Cause	Appearance	Depth	Pain
Hot liquids			
Short exposure	Wet; pink; blisters	Second degree	Severe
Long exposure	Wet; dark red	Second to third degree	Minimal
Flames			
Flash exposure	Wet; pink; blisters	Second degree	Severe
Direct contact	Dry; white; waxy	Third degree	Minimal
Chemicals			
Acid, alkalis	Light brown to light gray	Second degree (converts to third degree)	Severe

FIRST-DEGREE BURNS. A first-degree burn involves only the thinner, outer epidermal layer and is characterized by erythema and mild discomfort. Tissue damage is minimal and protective functions of the skin are intact. Pain, the chief symptom, usually resolves in 48 to 72 hours and healing takes place uneventfully. The pain is probably caused by local vasodilator prostaglandin production. In 5 to 10 days, the damaged epithelium peels off in small scales, leaving no residual scarring. The most common causes of first-degree burns are overexposure to sunlight and brief scalding by hot liquids.

SECOND-DEGREE BURNS. Second-degree burns are those in which the entire epidermis and variable portions of the dermis have been destroyed by heat. A superficial second-degree burn involves heat injury to the upper third of the dermis. The microvessels that perfuse this area are injured, and permeability is increased, thus resulting in the leakage of large amounts of plasma into the interstitium. This fluid in turn lifts the thin, heat-destroyed epidermis, forming blisters. Despite the loss of the entire basal layer of the epidermis, a superficial second-degree burn will heal in 7 to 14 days because of repopulation by the epithelial cells that line the hair follicles, sweat glands, and other skin appendages anchored deep in the dermis. Minimal scarring occurs because the wound closes rapidly; consequently, inflammation, which stimulates excessive collagen deposition, is short lived. A deep, dermal second-degree burn extends well into the dermal layer; fewer viable epidermal cells remain. Epithelialization is extremely slow, sometimes requiring months. Blister formation is not characteristically seen because the layer of dead tissue is sufficiently thick and adherent to underlying dermal collagen that it cannot be readily lifted off the surface. Exceptions occur in very young or very old patients, who have an extremely thin dermis. The surface of the wound is usually red in appearance, with some evidence of plasma leakage from remaining intact blood vessels. Blood supply to the burned tissue is marginal; thus, the probability is high that tissue damage will deepen with time. Pain is present but to a lesser degree than in more superficial burns. Fluid losses and the metabolic effects of deep dermal burns are basically the same as those seen with third-degree burns. Dense scarring usually results if skin grafts are not performed.

THIRD-DEGREE BURNS. In a full or third-degree burn, the entire epidermis and dermis are destroyed; no residual epidermal cells remain to repopulate or epithelialize. Areas of the wound not closed by wound contraction will require skin grafting. A characteristic appearance of avascular burned tissue is a waxy white color typical of any avascular tissue. If the burn extends into the fat or if contact with a flame source has been prolonged, the leathery brown or black appearance of charred tissue is seen. The most common cause of third-degree burns is a short exposure to a very high temperature, such as direct contact with a flame. However, prolonged contact with only moderately hot liquids (e.g., water at 125°F), as seen with intentional scalding, can result in a third-degree burn. This type of prolonged contact with hot liquid will also lead to red-cell hemolysis and release of myoglobin from underlying muscle, resulting in a red pigment deposition in the wound. The red-pigmented wound can be mistaken for viable dermis after a flame burn. Therefore, although a dark-red appearance in a scald burn may represent a full-thickness injury, the same appearance in a flame burn would represent only a deep second-degree injury. The microvessels are not immediately thrombosed in second-degree injury and therefore continue to leak plasma for days. In full-thickness flame burns, however, injured capillaries are usually immediately occluded by thrombosis. The absence of pain sensation in full-thickness burns is the result of heat destruction of nerve endings. This sensory deficit distinguishes a third-degree burn from a partial-thickness injury.

Full-thickness chemical burns are light gray to brown in appearance. Pain is usually extreme because retained chemicals prolong the burning process; these retained chemicals commonly convert partial burns to full-thickness burns.

In the early postburn period (24–72 hours after the burn), a zone of ischemia is usually present below the dead tissue and above the deeper living tissue. The vasculature to this area has been injured. Some vessels are thrombosed; others are patent but have endothelial cell damage. The marginally viable tissue can readily convert to eschar if blood flow is further decreased because of local mediator release or infection. A deep second-degree burn (in which healing is still possible) can therefore progress to a third-degree burn. Wound conversion is prevented or minimized with prompt, adequate resuscitation.

Assessment of Burn Severity

Severity is determined by burn depth, burn size, age, and complicating factors such as the presence of inhalation injury, trauma, or chronic disease (Table 75-5).

Pain Medication

Pain medication is necessary for partial-thickness burns, particularly when the wounds are cleaned. Pain control should be initiated before aggressive wound manipulation because it is important to minimize the subsequent stress response. With minor burns, oral or intramuscular narcotics may be adequate if given about 30 minutes before wound care. For major burns, intravenous narcotics in small doses are appropriate; erratic absorption from the gastrointestinal tract, skin, and muscles makes these routes of administration both ineffective and dangerous.

Table 75-5. Classification of severity of burn injury

Critical burns
Second-degree burns involving >30% TBS
Third-degree burns involving >10% TBS
Any burns complicated by respiratory tract injury, fractures, or involvement of critical areas (i.e., the face, hands, feet, perineum)
High-voltage electrical burns
Lesser burns in patients with significant preexisting disease
Moderate burns
Second-degree burns involving 15–20% TBS (if the face, hands, feet, or perineum are not involved)
Third-degree burns involving 2–10% TBS (if the face, hands, feet, or perineum are not involved)
Minor burns
Second-degree burns involving <15% TBS (if critical areas are not involved)
Third-degree burns involving <2% TBS (if critical areas are not involved)

Removal of Foreign Bodies and Loose Nonviable Tissue

When a patent airway, breathing, and circulation are ensured, the wound can be debrided and cleaned. Soot and dirt are best removed with a mild dilute detergent such as a chlorhexidine product. Gross debris, loose sloughed skin, or skin overlying broken blisters should be gently removed with forceps and scissors. Rough scrubbing should be avoided to prevent further harm to the injured tissues. Ground-in dirt will gradually work its way to the surface with daily dressing changes. The surrounding skin should be shaved to facilitate local wound care. Large intact blisters can be left in place for 48 hours, which will decrease the risk of underlying dermal desiccation.

If a hydrotherapy tank is to be used at this time for wound cleaning, the patient must be hemodynamically stable because good hemodynamic monitoring will be impossible during the procedure. Sequential cleaning of the various burned areas at bedside, which allows continuous monitoring and minimizes hypothermia, is thus a safer approach. A warm environment during burn care, preferably 30 to 35°C (86–95°F), is necessary to avoid heat loss.

Tar burns present unique problems. Tar removal is particularly difficult because the heat of the tar (150–200°C) usually results in a deep burn, and the rapid cooling leads to adherence to the skin. Tar can be gently removed without further tissue damage by means of repeated applications of petroleum-based ointments (such as Neosporin), which also contain surface-active emulsifying agents that dissolve the tar and make it easier to remove.

Tetanus Prophylaxis

As with any large wound, the risk of tetanus must be minimized using standard measures.

Prophylactic Antibiotics
Numerous studies have demonstrated that prophylactic systemic antibiotics do not decrease the rates of wound infection in either minor or major burns. The blood supply to the relatively avascular deep burn is insufficient to provide adequate tissue antibiotic levels. In addition, any open wound will become colonized with bacteria. The only exception to the dictum against prophylactic systemic antibiotics is prophylaxis against beta-hemolytic streptococcus with low-dose penicillin, particularly if the patient is at high risk for infection with this organism (i.e., if the patient is a carrier or has recently been exposed).

Early Infection Control
TOPICAL ANTIBIOTICS. Because topical antibiotics decrease the rate of wound healing (in particular, the rate of epithelialization) as compared with biologic dressings or other forms of temporary skin substitutes, these agents are most useful for deep burns with eschar present and are less helpful in superficial or clean, healing burns. Topical agents are applied to the wound, which is then covered with dressings or left open to the environment. Both techniques are used, but the closed dressing technique is employed more often because pain, heat, and fluid loss are decreased if dressings are applied. In addition, residual dermis is less likely to desiccate under a dressing.

The deep burn must be protected from early bacterial invasion, which can rapidly convert the wound to a still deeper injury. Topical antibiotics that are sufficiently water soluble to penetrate the burn eschar will temporarily control bacterial growth in the wound. The half-life of the currently available topical agents is only a few hours; therefore, the agent must be applied at least twice a day to achieve a reasonable level of antibacterial protection.

Silver sulfadiazine (Silvadene) is the most commonly used topical agent because it has good antibacterial properties and fewer complications are associated with its use. This agent, however, penetrates thick eschar less readily than some other agents and is therefore better used to prevent rather than to treat an established infection. Antibacterial properties are primarily directed against gram-negative organisms, with some antifungal effects. The primary complication of silver sulfadiazine is leukopenia as a result of a transient bone marrow suppression. A white blood cell count of 2,000 to 3,000 can be seen after application is begun. The effect is transient; the white-cell count returns toward normal after several days, even if the agent is continued.

Mafenide (Sulfamylon) is the most effective agent in its ability to penetrate burn eschar. It also has the most potent antibacterial properties and is particularly effective against gram-negative organisms. The agent has some antifungal properties as well. However, mafenide, a carbonic anhydrase inhibitor, can potentiate pulmonary insufficiency and metabolic acidosis; hence, this agent also produces the most significant complications. In addition, application is painful in many cases. This agent is used primarily as a second line of defense or as a primary treatment for small, infected wounds.

Providone-iodine (Betadine) ointment is usually used only on relatively thin eschar because its tissue penetration is not very good. The active agent is iodine, which is quite effective against both bacteria and fungi. Agents such as gentamicin and bacitracin can be used for more selective infections, but systemic toxicity can occur if these agents are used over large open wounds. Bacitracin is reasonably effective against wound colonization with gram-positive organisms. Bacitracin and gentamicin, however, have no antifungal properties, and prolonged use on an open wound can precipitate fungal growth.

TEMPORARY SKIN SUBSTITUTES. Drying of exudate on a superficial or partial-thickness wound with resulting scab or eschar formation has been shown to retard epithelialization. Wounds have been shown to epithelialize more rapidly and with less pain and inflammation when they are occluded and a thin layer of wound fluid is maintained over the surface. The sealed wound is also a more favorable environment for wound defense mechanisms to clear the surface of bacteria. Heat loss and evaporative water loss can also be decreased. A number of temporary skin substitutes have been developed to improve healing of partial-thickness wounds as well as to protect clean, excised wounds when autografts are not performed immediately. Skin substitutes allow excision of burned tissue even if insufficient skin for autograft is available, thus permitting more rapid removal of devitalized tissue.

The properties required of temporary skin substitute have been well defined. Most important, it must adhere to the wound to maximize the epithelialization rate and minimize inflammation and fibrosis. In addition, the dressings must be nonpermeable to bacteria and yet be permeable to water vapor and oxygen to avoid producing a totally anaerobic environment at the wound surface. Elasticity and durability are also major advantages. The biochemical structure must be nonantigenic and nontoxic to prevent local rejection reactions, and the risk of disease transmission via the skin substitute must be low.

There are two types of temporary skin: biologic and synthetic. Biologic dressings are from previously living tissue, including amniotic membranes, xenografts, allografts, and cadaver skin, although the last is only of limited availability and is used primarily to cover excised wounds. A number of synthetic skin substitutes have been developed that have the advantages of ready availability, long shelf life, and minimal risk of disease transmission. After the initial cleaning, these products should be applied to the wound under some modest tension to minimize wrinkling and maximize infection. Synthetic dressings adhere poorly to the grossly contaminated wound.

Subeschar Edema in Extremities
The increased pressure that accompanies the development of subeschar edema is of particular concern in extremities with circumferential burns. In such cases, if the increasing pressure cannot be dissipated, a decrease in venous outflow results; this effect speeds the rate of edema formation and further elevates tissue pressure until there is marked impairment of arterial blood flow to the tissues distal to the obstruction.

Immediate elevation of the burned extremity decreases the magnitude of tissue edema. Perfusion is best monitored by the Doppler flowmeter or by assessment of capillary refill.

Immediate escharotomy is indicated if there is a decrease in pulsatile flow beyond the burn.

Transfer to Specialized Burn Facility

Patients whose burns are critical should be transferred to specialized burn facilities as early as possible after their injury, once the initial assessment and resuscitation have begun (see Table 75-5). Moderate burns require hospitalization but may be manageable outside a burn facility if a local surgeon with an interest or expertise in burns will accept responsibility for the patient's care. Minor burns may be manageable on an outpatient basis.

A major reason for the impressive progress made in the field of burn therapy has been the expansion of the concept of specialized centers for burns. There are now more than 150 burn units in the United States, as compared with a mere dozen 20 years ago. About 21,000 burn patients—approximately one-third of all hospitalized burn patients—are treated each year in these 1,700 specialized burn-care beds. The centralization of patients has made possible not only improved care but also multidisciplinary research.

SELECTED READING

Agarwal, N, Petro, J, and Salisbury, RE. Physiologic profile monitoring in burned patients. *J Trauma* 23:577, 1983.

Alexander, JW. Nutrition and infection: New perspectives for an old problem. *Arch Surg* 121:96, 1986.

Alexander, JW, et al. The importance of lipid type in the diet after burn injury. *Ann Surg* 204:1, 1986.

Atnip, RG, and Burke, JF. Skin coverage. *Curr Probl Surg* 20:623, 1983.

Blank, IH. What are the functions of skin lost in burn injury that affect short- and long-term recovery? *J Trauma* 24:S10, 1984.

Cahalane, M, and Demling, RH. Early respiratory abnormalities from smoke inhalation. *JAMA* 10:771, 1984.

Carlson, RG, et al. Fluid retention during the first 48 hours as an indicator of burn survival. *J Trauma* 26:840, 1986.

Clark, CJ, et al. Mortality probability in victims of fire trauma: Revised equation to include inhalation injury. *Br Med J* 292:1303, 1986.

Cohen, IK. How do the methods and timing of debridement affect the quality of repair? *J Trauma* 24:S25, 1984.

Demling, RH. Burns. (Medical Progress.) *N Engl J Med* 313:1389, 1985.

Demling, RH. Effect of early burn excision and grafting on pulmonary function. *J Trauma* 24:830, 1984.

Demling, RH. Fluid resuscitation after major burns. *JAMA* 250: 1438, 1983.

Demling, RH. Improved survival after massive burns. *J Trauma* 23:179, 1983.

Engrav, LH, et al. Early excision and grafting vs nonoperative treatment of burns of indeterminant depth: A randomized prospective study. *J Trauma* 23:1001, 1983.

Fisher, JC. Skin: The ultimate solution for the burn wound. *N Engl J Med* 311:466, 1984.

Gallico, GG, et al. Permanent coverage of large body burns with autologous cultured human epithelium. *N Engl J Med* 311:448, 1984.

Goodwin, CW, et al. Randomized trial of efficacy of crystalloid and colloid resuscitation on hemodynamic response and lung water following thermal injury. *Ann Surg* 197:520, 1983.

Hatherill, JR, et al. Thermal injury, intravascular hemolysis, and toxic oxygen products. *J Clin Invest* 78:629, 1986.

Heimbach, DM, et al. Burn depth estimation: Man or machine. *J Trauma* 24:373, 1984.

Herndon, DN, et al. The effect of resuscitation on inhalation injury. *Surgery* 100:248, 1986.

Herndon, DN, et al. The quality of life after major thermal injury in children: An analysis of 12 survivors with greater than or equal to 80% total body, 70% third-degree burns. *J Trauma* 26:609, 1986.

Hunt, J, Purdue, G, and Spicer, T. Management of full-thickness burns of the scalp and skull. *Arch Surg* 118:621, 1983.

Libber, SM, and Stayton, DJ. Childhood burns reconsidered: The child, the family, the burn injury. *J Trauma* 24:245, 1984.

Luterman, A, et al. Infections in burn patients. *Am J Med* 28:45, 1986.

Mason, AD, Jr, et al. Association of burn mortality and bacteremia: A 25-year review. *Arch Surg* 121:1027, 1986.

Matsuda, T, et al. The importance of burn wound size in determining the optimal calorie:nitrogen ratio. *Surgery* 94:562, 1983.

Monafo, WW, et al. The role of concentrated sodium solutions in the resuscitation of patients with severe burns. *Surgery* 95:129, 1984.

Pittelkow, MR, and Scott, RE. New techniques for the in vitro culture of human skin keratinocytes and perspectives of their use for grafting of patients with extensive burns. *Mayo Clin Proc* 61:771, 1986.

Pruitt, BS, Jr, and Levine, NS. Characteristics and use of biologic dressings and skin substitutes. *Arch Surg* 119:312, 1983.

Pruitt, BA, Jr, and McManus, JT. Opportunistic infections in severely burned patients. *Am J Med* 76:146, 1984.

Roi, LD, et al. Two new burn severity indices. *J Trauma* 23:1023, 1983.

Tompkins, RG, et al. Prompt eschar excision: A treatment system contributing to reduced burn mortality. *Ann Surg* 204:272, 1986.

76. Cold Injury

Nicholas O'Connor

There are basically two kinds of cold injuries—hypothermia and cold-induced tissue injury. There are three categories of the latter—namely, frostbite, trench foot, and immersion. Hypothermia may be associated with tissue injury and vice versa.

HYPOTHERMIA

Accidental hypothermia, whether from exposure to cold air or cold water, simply reflects an imbalance between the heat produced by the body and the heat lost from it. By adjusting rates of heat production and heat loss, we maintain a stable core body temperature range for optimal enzyme functioning. For example, for each 1°C temperature drop biochemical activity is decreased about 10 percent. The normal core body temperature is in a narrow range of 36.4 to 37.5°C. Heat may be convected, conducted, radiated, or released by evaporation from the body surface. Control of the environment and the use of protective clothing are our major defenses against heat loss. The physiologic adjustments to protect ourselves from loss of body heat include exercise, shivering, basal thermogenesis under the control of the hypothalamus, and peripheral vasoconstriction. For example, shivering can increase the basal metabolic rate four or five times the normal rate.

There are basically three types of accidental hypothermia: acute, subacute, and chronic. A person who is plunged into cold water that causes his or her core body temperature to drop swiftly experiences acute immersion hypothermia. A person who, for example, is lost in a sparsely populated area or is incapacitated for some reason and much of the night lies exposed to snow or rain in cold weather with insufficient clothing or shelter to maintain body core temperature suffers from subacute hypothermia. Chronic hypothermia in which the cooling occurs over several days is more frequent in a person who, as a result of drugs, disease, or failure of the body's temperature-regulating mechanism, perhaps combined with age, experiences a slow but nonetheless potentially lethal cooling over a period of days. This may occur without the person ever leaving his or her living quarters if the room temperatures are lower than the person can safely tolerate. Patients with chronic hypothermia almost always have some other serious disease.

Accidental hypothermia is defined as the pathologic state that occurs after core body temperature is reduced below 35°C as a result of accidental cold stress. If there is continuing stress, the condition may be progressive and fatal unless body temperature is restored and the concomitant metabolic aberrations are corrected. The diagnosis is made by taking a rectal temperature with a low-reading thermometer. Axillary and oral temperatures are misleading. If the body temperature is below 35°C, shivering and vasoconstriction become very intense, and the patient loses manual dexterity but is still relatively well oriented. At this stage, the hypothermia is easily reversible. If the body temperature is below 32°C, the hypothermia becomes severe; shivering is replaced by marked muscular rigidity and stiff movement. The patient is obtunded and is progressing to full stupor. The blood pressure may not be detectable at this time, but a strong carotid or femoral pulse can be palpated. Breathing becomes shallow and irregular and the heart rate begins to slow. If the body temperature is below 27°C, the hypothermia is profound, and the patient experiences deep coma and rigidity. Pulmonary edema can occur, and there is great risk of ventricular arrhythmia.

The most devastating effect of hypothermia occurs when the core temperature drops below 24°C. Below this temperature, ventricular fibrillation generally will occur, and as the core temperature falls below 20°C asystole will occur. If the hypothermia has been acute there may be only relatively mild associated acidosis. If the hypothermia has been chronic a more serious acidosis may accompany cardiac arrest.

Treatment

As soon as hypothermia is recognized, wherever the patient may be, action must be taken to prevent further cooling in the patient. Wet clothing must be removed and the patient placed in a dry blanket. Rewarming should begin as soon as possible but only in hospital facilities where medical resources are available to deal with any resulting complications. This is especially true for patients with severe and profound hypothermia. Patients with mild hypothermia can have heat from external sources, such as from the bodies of warm companions, applied; can be given hot drinks; and can be encouraged to do some isometric exercises.

In rewarming patients with severe or profound hypothermia, it is important, if possible, to warm the core of the body before the shell. If the shell or periphery of the body is warmed first by immersing the patient in warm water, peripheral vasodilation occurs. As the cool blood returns centrally, the core body temperature will drop further, and rewarming shock will occur when the supercooled heart cannot return the amount of blood that the rewarmed skin demands. The most effective way of rewarming the patient's core is to use peritoneal dialysis or lavage. This is carried out by inserting a peritoneal dialysis catheter and using isotonic peritoneal dialysate that is heated by a blood-warming coil to 35 to 37°C. Two liters of the dialysate are exchanged every 20 to 30 minutes in order to raise the rectal temperature above 30°C as soon as possible to obviate the danger of refractory ventricular fibrillation. At the same time, an endotracheal tube should be inserted to protect the airway since vomiting may ensue with central rewarming. Once the rectal temperature exceeds 30°C, a hypothermia pad or warm-water bath can be used to raise the temperature more slowly. The patient will require an infusion of saline to support blood pressure as the periphery becomes rewarmed. Furthermore, any associated acidosis should be corrected carefully; overcorrection with resultant alkalosis should be avoided. Although the prognosis for survival is poor with core temperatures below 25°C, there are many case reports of patients with profound hypothermia and cardiac arrest who have been successfully treated using prolonged cardiopulmonary resuscitation and rewarming.

COLD-INDUCED TISSUE INJURIES

Frostbite

Except in rare instances frostbite is restricted to the extremities of the body or to areas such as the chin, cheeks, nose, and ears. The severity of the injury is influenced by the intensity of the initial exposure and the length of time before adequate circulation can be restored.

The type and duration of contact are the two most important factors in determining the extent of frostbite injury (Table 76-1). For example, touching cold wood is not nearly as dangerous as coming into direct contact with metal, particularly if the hands are wet or even damp, because metal is an excellent thermal conductor. Air itself is a very poor thermal conductor. Cold air alone is not nearly as dangerous as a combination of wind and cold. Hence, the chilling effect of 20°F (−6.7°C) combined with a 45-mph wind is identical to that of −40°F (−40°C) temperature with no wind.

The susceptibility to injury is influenced by training, geographic background, and cold adaptation. During the Korean War, black soldiers had a six times greater incidence of frostbite than white soldiers, and Southern whites had an almost two times greater incidence than Northern whites. Furthermore, general physical condition influences susceptibility; for example, injured soldiers were much more susceptible to frostbite no matter what their initial injury was.

Two types of reaction occur when tissue comes in contact with cold. First, the superficial tissue at the site of contact actually freezes to a depth that depends on the degree of cold and the duration of contact. When this freezing occurs ice crystals grow between cells, and if the source of cold is not removed, these crystals continue to grow, dehydrating and severely damaging the adjacent cells. Intense freezing causes crystals to form within the cells, damaging them immediately.

Second, arteriolar vasoconstriction occurs in the tissue adjacent to the frozen layer, thereby rapidly reducing the blood flow in this zone. When there is arteriolar constriction, shunts occur that allow blood to bypass the affected capillary bed, and if the source of cold is not removed, the whole area begins to freeze.

Diagnosis

The following is a retrospective classification designed by the United States Army during the Korean War. This classification divides frostbite injury into four degrees of seriousness: (1) erythema and swelling with no blister formation, (2) erythema and swelling with blisters, (3) full-thickness injury with gangrene and no loss of part, (4) com-

Table 76-1. Types of cold-induced tissue injuries

Type of contact	Duration of contact	Temperature
Frostbite	Minutes to 16 hours	−60 to +7°C
Trench foot	2 hours to 14 days	− 7 to +10°C
Immersion foot	12 hours to 7 days	− 4 to +16°C

plete necrosis with loss of part. This classification is useful in reporting frostbite injuries, but a more useful classification is to divide frostbite injuries into superficial or deep, determined before the injured part has been thawed. *Superficial frostbite* involves only the skin or the tissues immediately beneath it. The frozen part is white and firm on the exterior but soft and resilient below the surface when depressed gently and firmly. After rewarming, the frostbitten area will first become numb, mottled blue, or purple and will then swell, sting, and burn for some time. In more severe cases, blisters will occur beneath the epidermis after 24 to 36 hours. These blisters slowly dry up and become hard and black after about two weeks. General swelling of the injured area will occur and subside in the same period of time. After the swelling disappears, the skin will peel and remain red, tender, and extremely sensitive to even mild cold, and the area may perspire abnormally for a long time.

In *deep unthawed frostbite,* a much more serious injury, the injured part is hard and solid and cannot be depressed at all. The damage not only involves the skin and subcutaneous tissues but also goes deep into the tissue beneath (even including bone) and is usually accompanied by the formation of huge blisters. These blisters may take from three days to one week to develop. Swelling of the entire hand or foot will take place and last for one month or more. After rewarming, blue, violet, or gray discoloration takes place, and throbbing pains may occur and last for up to eight weeks. The blisters eventually dry up, blacken, and slough off, leaving an exceptionally sensitive red, thin layer of new skin that will take months to return to normal. In extreme cases of deep frostbite, the area, with thawing, turns a lifeless gray and remains cold. If blisters and swelling occur, they will appear along the line of demarcation between the acutely frostbitten area and the remainder of the limb. In one or two weeks after the injury, the tissue becomes black, dry, and shriveled right up to the beginning of the healthy tissue, and eventually the injured tissue will fall off. If this dead tissue becomes infected it will become wet, soft, and inflamed, causing the remainder of the limb to become painful and swollen, and increasing the eventual loss of tissue.

It is noteworthy that tendons and bones are resistant to frostbite, whereas nerves, muscles, and particularly blood vessels are highly susceptible.

Treatment

The first and most important principle in treating frostbite is rapid rewarming of the injured part. This can be done by inserting the injured part into either a large bucket or bathtub filled with water that is carefully kept at a temperature between 37 and 40°C. A thermometer should be used to keep a check on the temperature of the water. Rewarming by immersion in 37 to 40°C water usually takes only 20 minutes; rewarming for a longer period is not thought to be helpful. Using water at higher temperatures than those mentioned can be harmful. Rewarming is painful, and if the patient's condition is otherwise good, he or she can be given pain medication. After the injured part is warmed, it should be carefully covered with sterile bandages to minimize any friction or trauma to the injured part. It is critically important to protect the injured tissue at this stage. A frozen part should never be rubbed before, during, or after rewarming.

Other measures that can be used are much the same as those used for a patient with a burn injury. That is, the patient should be given tetanus toxoid, should be placed on penicillin for several days, and can be given intravenous fluids if necessary. The administration of low molecular weight dextran to help improve circulation to the injured part and heparin to prevent further thrombosis of small vessels in the injured area is sometimes carried out and largely depends on the circumstances of the patient. Once the patient is admitted to the hospital, the use of alpha-blocking drugs and sympathectomy can be considered. Finally, one should never debride or amputate any tissue because it is very difficult at first to determine eventual viability in a cold-injured extremity. The prognosis in most cases of frostbite is excellent.

Trench Foot and Immersion Foot

Trench foot and immersion foot are the subacute and chronic variations of frostbite. The eventual tissue injury can be as severe as with frostbite, and therefore these injuries should be cared for in the same way. Trench foot and immersion foot are rare in civilian life.

SELECTED READING

Renler, JB. Pathophysiology, clinical settings and management. *Ann Intern Med* 89:519, 1978.

Towne, WD, et al. Intractable ventricular fibrillation associated with profound accidental hypothermia. *N Engl J Med* 287:1135, 1972.

Washburn, B. Frostbite. *N Engl J Med* 266:974, 1962.

77. Electrical Injuries

Mary Ann Cooper

Electrical injuries account for four percent of burn unit admissions each year in the United States. Many of these injuries are devastating "composite" injuries that involve deep damage to multiple types of tissues, often necessitating major amputations and drastically changing the victim's way of life. The incidence of fatal injuries is close to 1,000 per year and the incidence of nonfatal injury is nearly five times that amount.

High-voltage injuries, which are classified as those that occur with a voltage of over 1,000 V, are more likely to have severe burns associated with them than are lower-voltage injuries. Unfortunately, however, even low-voltage injuries can cause significant morbidity, long-term sequelae, cardiac arrhythmias, and, under proper conditions, death, and should not be underestimated.

Electrical and construction workers make up the majority of those injured. Those doing careless home repair, farmers, and hobbyists make up a smaller number, and pranksters, vandals, and children who suck on extension cords or play with electrical outlets an even smaller number. The vast majority of those injured are male.

Electrical injuries may involve not only burns, shock, and cardiac damage and arrhythmias but also renal failure, contractures, infection, cataracts, and neurologic damage. Since many of these injuries will involve a protracted hospital course and almost all will have litigation involved, it is essential that the initial evaluation of the patient be well documented, including not only the circumstances of the injury but also a complete description of injuries, neurologic status, neurovascular status of the extremities, and cardiac evaluation.

PATHOPHYSIOLOGY

Exposure to high-voltage electrical currents causes damage in two primary ways: short-circuiting of the body's electrical systems (i.e., cardiac arrhythmias, neurologic damage) and thermal damage to soft tissues in the form of burns. The burns from high-voltage electrical injuries differ from flame burns in that the vast majority of the damage is internal as the current courses through the body after breaking down the skin. Thus, the rule of nines cannot be used to calculate fluid needs and the treatment and evaluation cannot be limited to the surface of the body.

Six factors determine the severity of the damage that will be seen with any electrical injury: type of current, voltage, amperage, resistance, pathway, and duration of exposure. Alternating current is three times more dangerous than direct current of the same magnitude, especially when the hand is the contact point for the current. A direct-current shock tends to force the victim away from the source by causing an opisthotonic contraction of the body, throwing

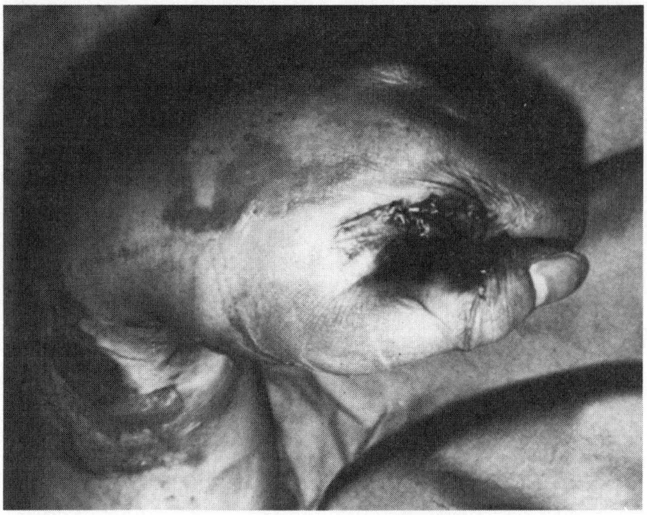

Fig. 77-1. Electrical hand burn.

Table 77-1. Effects of amperage

Amperage	Effect
0.001–0.01	Tingling sensation
0.01–0.02	Freezing to the circuit, chest tetany
0.02–0.05	Respiratory arrest
0.05–0.10	Ventricular fibrillation

Table 77-2. Resistance by tissue

Least resistance
Nerves
Blood vessels
Muscles
Skin
Most resistance
Fat
Tendon
Bone

Table 77-3. Resistance of tissues

Tissue	Resistance (ohms/cm^2)
Mucous membranes	100
Volar arm, inner thigh, other vascular areas	300–10,000
Other skin	10,000–40,000
Sole of foot	100,000–200,000
Heavily calloused palm/sole	1,000,000–2,000,000

the arms away from the source. Alternating current, on the other hand, has a frequency of 60 cps, well within the range of frequencies that will cause continuous or tetanic muscle contraction. Since the flexors of the hand are stronger than the extensors, the hand tends to contract around the current source, freezing the victim to the circuit and causing prolonged exposure and often severe damage to the hand (Fig. 77-1).

Voltage, the second factor, usually causes damage proportionate to its magnitude. The higher the voltage, in general, the more severe the damage seen.

The thermal damage caused by an electrical current is related to amperage and is described by Joule's law:

$$\text{heat} = \text{amperage}^2 \times \text{resistance}$$

Low amperage may cause only a tingling sensation, while higher amperages will cause pain and often severe burns. In addition, amperage can be related to body reactions proportionate to its magnitude (Table 77-1).

Voltage and amperage are related to each other and to resistance by Ohm's law:

$$\text{voltage} = \text{amperage} \times \text{resistance}$$

Each tissue has a different resistance related to its water content and density (Table 77-2). In general, electrical current does not flow well over the outside of the body but does its damage by flowing through the tissues. For a significant amount of electric current to enter the body, the skin must be broken down at the entry site. The resistance of the skin, too, varies with its density and water content, so that the skin of mucous membranes and of the inner arm and thigh offers the least resistance and the calloused sole and palm offer the most (Table 77-3). Electrical current tends to flow through the tissues with the lowest resistance once the skin has been burned through. As a result, often a large amount of muscle, nerve, and blood vessel damage occurs under the surface of the skin that may not be apparent from the surface initially. Conceptually, electrical injuries can be likened to the "tip of the iceberg." Thus, using the rule of nines can result in grossly underestimating the volume of resuscitative fluid that is needed. In addition, because of the large amount of muscle damage that often occurs, myoglobinuria and subsequent renal failure can result unless large amounts of resuscitative fluid are used to perfuse the kidneys. In this sense, electrical injuries resemble crush injuries more than they do thermal burns.

Resistance can be decreased by wetting the skin, so that soapy or sweaty skin may have a resistance of only 1,000 to 1,500 ohms/cm^2. A victim of a bathtub electrocution may have no external burns because of the large surface area over which the electricity could enter as well as the tremendously lowered resistance of the wet skin. In this instance, the death is primarily due to interruption of the cardiac cycle by the electrical current rather than to thermal damage.

Electrical current may have other special effects depending on the pathway that it takes. Passage through the brain or brainstem can have electrical effects as well as thermal damage, causing not only respiratory arrest but also intracranial hemorrhage and coagulation of tissues. The victim who has electrical current pass close to the head will often develop electrical cataracts and must be evaluated for them. The pathway that an electrical current takes can be irregular, acting more like a bouncing bullet than taking a direct path. Thus, damage at distant or unpredictable sites should be expected. The duration of exposure to the electrical current will also determine the extent of injury suffered.

Both entry and exit burns are common with electrical injuries, and the patient should be completely undressed for evaluation. As with other burns, the sites of injury may take a few hours to "mature" so that not all sites may be visible at first. Unlike the case in thermal burns, however, the media and intima of the vessels supplying a burned area are often damaged to such an extent by the internal passage of current that the vessels, which initially appear to be patent, may thrombose over a period of hours to days, leading to what appears to be progressive ischemia. This is particularly devastating in extremities, which must have serial neurovascular checks to ascertain the necessity for fasciotomies if vascular compromise occurs.

INJURIES BY SYSTEM

Four types of burns can occur with electrical injuries. *Contact* burns occur when the victim is in direct contact with the current. These can vary from minimal erythema in low-voltage, short-duration injuries to massive charring and mummification of extremities in high-voltage, prolonged-duration contact. *Flash* burns can occur when the victim is close to an electrical explosion and are usually minor partial-thickness burns. *Arc* burns occur when an electrical current arcs from the source onto the victim, making him or her part of the circuit. Since the temperature of an arc is at least 2,500°C, these burns may be very deep, full-thickness burns. Unfortunately, flash and arc burns are often difficult to tell apart initially so that careful observation and follow-up study of the victim are essential. Regular *thermal* burns from ignition of clothing can occur. Combinations of these four types are not uncommon.

As was previously noted, burns should be evaluated for depth, expecting that deep damage may have occurred. All extremities need frequent neurovascular checks and evaluation for fasciotomy. It is not uncommon for fractures and dislocations to occur as the muscles are thrown into strong contraction by the current.

Cardiovascular effects include arrest, multiple types of arrhythmias, coronary vessel spasm or damage leading to a myocardial infarction–like picture, blocks, and symptoms of cardiac ischemia including constricting chest pain and palpitations. Pulmonary hemorrhage and contusion have been reported.

As was previously mentioned, myoglobinuria can cause renal failure in a victim of electrical injury. In addition, renal failure can result from shock and lack of perfusion during the injury and resuscitative phase.

Gastrointestinal damage can occur from direct burns to the abdominal wall, from blunt injury from a fall or being thrown by the current, and from spasm of vessels with distal ischemia. Gallbladder necrosis has been reported on several occasions. Curling's ulcers are more common with electrical injuries than they are with regular thermal burns. Prolonged ileus should always prompt the physician to suspect intra-abdominal damage rather than to write it off to burn ileus.

Neurologic damage can be sustained from direct injury to the skull, a common point of entry, as well as from blunt injury or cardiovascular collapse and resulting brain ischemia. In addition, spinal artery spasm can cause injuries that mimic transection, transverse myelitis, or amyotrophic lateral sclerosis. Seizures are not uncommon, and peripheral nerve damage often occurs. Decreases in mental ability may be seen as late sequelae.

The eyes may develop cataracts if electrical current passes near the head of the victim. Infection, particularly clostridial myositis, is a common complication of electrical burns, and tetanus prophylaxis should be provided.

EVALUATION AND MANAGEMENT

Historical elements that are useful in evaluating the patient when they are available are listed in Table 77-4. The patient with electrical injuries should have an assessment of vital signs and respiratory status performed first. Injuries usually fall into two categories: life threatening and minor.

In the severe or life-threatening injury, airway protection and cardiopulmonary resuscitation, if indicated, are essential. Cervical spine and spinal precautions are usually indicated, even if a history of a fall or blunt injury is not apparent since spinal fractures from severe muscle contractions alone have been reported. Treatment of cardiac arrhythmias is routine, with the exception of the intravenous fluid, which should be Ringer's lactate or normal saline. Multiple, large-bore intravenous lines should be started as indicated by the degree of shock and the severity of the burn injury.

With extensive burns and muscle damage, it is customary to alkalinize the resuscitative fluid by adding an ampule of bicarbonate to each liter. Some centers also use mannitol or furosemide to ensure adequate kidney perfusion and decrease the chances of myoglobinuric renal failure. Arterial blood gas determinations may be helpful not only in evaluating the respiratory status of the patient but in keeping the pH at 7.35 or above. Urinary output should be at least 1.0 to 1.5 ml/kg per hour if the urine is pigmented and 0.5 to 1.0 ml/kg per hour after the urine has cleared. A urinary catheter is useful in monitoring output. A Swan-Ganz, central venous pressure monitor, or arterial line may be invaluable.

Nasogastric intubation is helpful in decreasing vomiting and distention secondary to burn ileus. Complete neurologic

Table 77-4. Useful history

Circumstances
Voltage, amperage
Duration
Fall, blunt injury
Past medical history
Allergies
Tetanus status
Other medical illness
Medical condition at the scene
Vital signs
Level of consciousness
Cardiac/respiratory arrest
Resuscitation efforts so far
Splinting efforts

and neurovascular evaluations of all extremities should be documented. The physician must not forget that these patients often have suffered blunt injury in addition to the electrical-thermal injury and should evaluate the head, chest, and abdomen accordingly. A decreasing level of consciousness should lead the physician to scan the brain for intracranial injury and hemorrhage.

After the patient's condition is stabilized, evaluation and care of fractures, dislocations, and burns can be instituted. Normally, the patient should be stabilized before he or she is sent to the operating room for debridement or amputation, if possible. On occasion, this may be difficult due to the outpouring of toxic materials from massive extremity burns. Tetanus prophylaxis is indicated.

Treatment of burns should include estimation of the depth and extent of the burns, again recognizing that the rule of nines cannot be used to calculate the fluid volume for resuscitation. Burns will need to be cleaned and debrided. The dressing of choice for deep burns is mafenide acetate (Sulfamylon) due to its superior ability in penetrating eschar. In lesser burns in individuals who will be treated as outpatients, silver sulfadiazine, nitrofurazone (Furacin), or other antibacterial creams can be used.

DISPOSITION

The severely injured victim should be transferred to a burn center staffed by professionals who are familiar with electrical injuries and their care. Because of the composite nature of these injuries, it is important to provide not only appropriate burn management, but physical therapy, occupational therapy, and psychiatric counseling. Due to the high incidence of major amputations, these patients are often unable to continue their former profession and must be retrained. In addition, body image and role within the family are often changed, necessitating counseling for the entire family to achieve the maximal recovery.

Minimal injuries can often be treated at local hospitals and, depending on the extent of the injury, can be taken care of on an outpatient basis with appropriate follow-up care. In the past, patients with minimal injuries were routinely hospitalized for cardiac monitoring. Recent studies indicate that this is probably not necessary and is not cost effective. Unless the patient has complaints referable to the cardiac system, simple monitoring in the department and an electrocardiogram may be enough to determine that the patient does not have signs of ischemia or arrhythmias. The burns should be referred to a surgeon who is familiar with their care and the patient should receive instructions in wound care.

Children with lip burns from sucking on electrical cords are treated as inpatients by some authorities because of the high incidence of labial artery hemorrhage on separation of the eschar. Referral to an oral or plastic surgeon who is familiar with the care of electrical burns is necessary, as these injuries usually require special splinting to prevent contracture of the mouth.

SELECTED READING

Budnick, LD. Bathtub-related electrocutions in the United States, 1979–1982. *JAMA* 252:918, 1984.

Butler, ED, and Gant, TD. Electrical injuries, with special reference to the upper extremities. *Am J Surg* 134:95, 1977.

Christensen, JA, et al. Delayed neurologic injury secondary to high-voltage current, with recovery. *J Trauma* 20:166, 1980.

Hammond, J, and Ward, CG. Myocardial damage and electrical injuries: Significance of early elevation of CPK-MB isoenzymes. *South Med J* 79:414, 1986.

Hirschfeld, JJ, and Assael, LA. Conservative management of electrical burns to the lips of children. *J Oral Maxillofac Surg* 42:1978, 1984.

Housinger, TA, et al. A prospective study of myocardial damage in electrical injuries. *J Trauma* 25:122, 1985.

Josell, SD, et al. Extraoral management for electrical burns of the mouth. *J Dent Child* 51:47, 1984.

Kay, NRM, and Boswick, JA. The management of electrical injuries of the extremities. *Surg Clin North Am* 53:1459, 1973.

Kinney, TJ. Myocardial infarction following electrical injury. *Ann Emerg Med* 11:622, 1982.

LaBorde, TC, and Meier, RH. Amputations resulting from electrical injury: A review of 22 cases. *Arch Phys Med Rehab* 59:134, 1978.

Levine, NS, et al. Spinal cord injury following electrical accidents: Case reports. *J Trauma* 15:459, 1975.

Luce, EA, et al. High tension electrical injury of the upper extremity. *Surg Gynecol Obstet* 147:38, 1978.

Miller, FE, Peterson, D, and Miller, J. Abdominal visceral perforation secondary to electrical injury: Case report and review of the literature. *Burns* 12:505, 1986.

Nichter, LS, et al. Oral cavity electric burns. *Curr Concepts Trauma* Spring, 1984. Pp 11–17.

Oleszewski, SC, and Nyman, JS. Electric cataract: A rare clinical entity. *Am J Optom Physiol Opt* 61:279, 1984.

Parshley, PF, et al. Aggressive approach to the extremity damaged by electric current. *Am J Surg* 150:78, 1985.

Purdue, GF, and Hunt, JL. Electrocardiographic monitoring after electrical injury: Necessity or luxury? *J Trauma* 26:166, 1986.

Rouse, RG, and Dimick, AR. The treatment of electrical injury compared to burn injury: A review of pathophysiology and comparison of patient management protocols. *J Trauma* 18:43, 1978.

Saffle, JR, Crandall, A, and Warden GD. Catatracts: A long-term complication of electrical injury. *J Trauma* 25:17, 1985.

Tarquino, T, Weinstein, ME, and Virgilio, RW. Bilateral scapular fractures from accidental electric shock. *J Trauma* 19:132, 1979.

Williams, D, and Karl, RC. Intestinal injury associated with low-voltage electrocution, *J Trauma* 21:246, 1981.

78. Lightning Injuries

Mary Ann Cooper

Lightning injuries account for a large number of environmental injuries seen in the United States each year, more than those that occur from floods, forest fires, earthquakes, or volcanoes put together. The number of fatalities has been estimated at 100 to 200 per year and morbidity statistics indicate that at least five times that number are injured annually.

The majority of those injured used to be farmers and construction workers, but in the last few years those seeking the outdoors for recreational purposes have been involved more frequently. Lightning injuries occur most commonly during "lightning season," May through October, most commonly during the afternoon when people are outside in an open or rural setting rather than in urban areas. Most victims are still male. Surprisingly, a number of injured individuals have been indoors but have suffered from backflashes through plumbing or telephones during thunderstorms.

Lightning injuries have a large amount of myth and superstition accompanying them that have been difficult to dispel. In addition, lightning injuries are mistakenly often treated like high-voltage electrical injuries from manmade sources, an error that can result in further morbidity for the patient.

PATHOPHYSIOLOGY

Lightning causes injuries primarily from its electrical properties and rarely produces the severe burns that are seen with manmade high-voltage injuries. While high-voltage injuries tend to involve deep burns, shock, cardiac, and subsequent renal damage, lightning is primarily a medical illness involving the cardiac and nervous system.

Because it is a form of electrical energy, lightning follows the same laws of physics that govern high- and low-voltage electricity (see Chap. 77). However, because of substantial differences in the magnitude of some of the factors (Table 78-1) and their complex interaction, injuries from lightning are usually very different from those caused by manmade electricity.

While the voltage and amperage of lightning are very large compared to those of manmade electricity, the duration of current flow is very short, making the total amount of energy delivered to the victim quite small. In addition, because of some technicalities of wave forms and other electrical engineering principles, lightning tends to flash over the outside of a victim rather than going through the internal structures of the body as high-voltage electricity has a tendency to do.

The flashover phenomenon has been reported by Ohashi and associates in small animals and in a collection of case reports in Japan. If flashover occurs, the victim is several times more likely to survive the stroke than is a victim who does not experience flashover. Little has been studied on the physical effects of lightning outside of collected series of case

Table 78-1. Lightning versus high-voltage electrical injuries

Factor	High voltage	Lightning
Voltage	1,000–70,000 V	10,000,000–30,000,000 V
Amperage	1,000–5,000 amps	30,000–300,000 amps
Pathway	Deep, internal	Flashover
Duration	Seconds to minutes	1/10,000–1/1,000 sec
Blunt injury	Common from falls	Rare from "explosion"

Table 78-2. Differential diagnosis of lightning injuries

Intracranial hemorrhage
Myocardial infarction
Seizure
Spinal cord injury
Overdose or toxic exposure

reports by physicians and by cloud physicists and engineers. It is difficult to say whether the effects of lightning on the human body are because of direct lightning strike, microleakages of current internally, internal current changes within the body due to induction by the flashover current, or electromagnetic fluxes within the body induced by the current. Nevertheless, a lightning strike produces some fairly predictable outcomes.

Lightning has an effect on the human body both because of its electrical effect and because of the explosive shock wave generated by the thunder that often occurs with the lightning strike. Lightning can injure a person by several mechanisms:

1. Direct strike
2. Contact voltage, in which the person is touching an object that lightning hits
3. Splash or side-flash, in which the victim is standing near an object or person that is hit by lightning and part of the energy "splashes" onto him or her
4. Step voltage or ground current, in which lightning strikes the ground; it spreads out for quite a distance, sometimes catching people or animals in its energy fields, and causes injury or death
5. Blunt injury from the explosive force of the thunder or lightning energy, causing instantaneous expansion of gases about its path with resultant implosion of the pathway as the air rapidly cools

The injuries seen with lightning incidents include:

1. *Cardiac.* Cardiopulmonary arrest at the time of the incident is the predominant cause of death. Even if the victim is successfully resuscitated, significant brain damage and other sequelae can occur. Arrhythmias and ischemic changes have been reported, although the electrocardiographic changes usually resolve over several months. The patient may have transient hypertension, which usually does not need to be treated and resolves spontaneously.

2. *Neurovascular.* The patient often is unconscious, with mottled, cold, blue, pulseless extremities, more frequently the lower than the upper extremities. This is probably due to sympathetic instability and vascular spasm, and usually clears within a few hours with no intervention necessary. Occasionally, the patient may have permanent paresis and paresthesias. Pulses and blood pressure may be difficult to evaluate. Seizures can occur and should be treated with appropriate oxygenation and ventilation and routine pharmaceutical measures; these seldom persist. Intracranial injuries have been reported and should be suspected if the patient does not begin to become more alert. Patients may be comatose, confused and hysterical, or alert, but are almost universally amnesic for the event and suffer anterograde amnesia similar to that of patients who have had electroshock therapy for depression.

3. *Skeletal and soft tissue.* Blunt injuries, including contusions to lung, liver, and gastrointestinal tract, have all been reported. Fractures and dislocations are less common with lightning injuries than with electrical injuries. Burns are almost always superficial and seldom need care. The clothes may have been exploded off of the victim and serve as a clue to the injury if history is absent. Myoglobinuria and hemoglobinuria are extremely rare since deep muscle damage is seldom encountered, so that renal failure from myoglobinuria is also rare. Fluid loading, use of mannitol or furosemide, and fasciotomies are contraindicated with most lightning victims unless they are one of the rare victims in which the injuries are similar to those seen with high-voltage, manmade electrical currents.

4. *Sensory organs.* The tympanic membranes of lightning victims are ruptured in over 50 percent of the cases. Cataracts from lightning are more common than with high-voltage electrical accidents.

DIFFERENTIAL DIAGNOSIS

Lightning injuries may be confused with several other types of injuries and medical illnesses (Table 78-2). A history of a thunderstorm in the area is helpful but not always possible to obtain.

EVALUATION AND MANAGEMENT

The patient who has suffered a lightning injury may be in cardiac arrest, in which case standard cardiopulmonary resuscitation should be instituted or continued. While the respiratory arrest that occurs with a lightning injury may last longer than the cardiac arrest, there is no reason to believe that the resuscitation of a lightning victim should continue for an inordinate amount of time.

The patient who is comatose, with mottled, cold, blue, pulseless extremities, should be treated expectantly and supportively with airway management, oxygenation, and limited fluid resuscitation. Intracranial lesions may need to be ruled out, but usually the patient will begin to wake up and respond in a few hours. Normally, the patient continues to be confused as to the event for several hours to days and may have anterograde amnesia similar to that of an individual who has undergone electroshock therapy. Sometimes permanent paresis or paresthesias, or both, will develop in extremities affected by the lightning strike.

A search should be made for blunt injuries, fractures, and dislocations, and appropriate therapy should be rendered. Burns are seldom of a degree that require more than superficial cleaning, tetanus prophylaxis, and sometimes a dressing. Only rarely does the lightning victim have burns similar to those seen with high-voltage electrical injuries, and the reader is referred to Chap. 77 for their care. Usually, fluid restriction is the rule, both because the patient seldom needs fluid resuscitation and because of the incidence of cerebral edema, which can be worsened by overly aggressive fluid management. Tympanic membrane rupture should be assessed and the patient referred to an appropriate otolaryngologist for continuing care and reconstruction, if necessary.

DISPOSITION

The care of the lightning victim is usually expectant and supportive. Most lightning victims, with the exception of those with cardiac arrest, live and recover a useful level of function. The physician seldom has to take special measures in their behalf. If the patient continues to be confused, such as is seen in a head-injured patient, observation in the hospital is probably warranted. Otherwise, if there is a responsible party to whom the patient can be released, discharge may be appropriate in many cases in which the patient's condition is otherwise stable. An unfortunate sequela of lightning is the development of paresthesias in affected extremities and, sometimes, fine mental status or personality changes similar to post-traumatic stress disorder. Since these cannot be foretold with certainty at the time of treatment and have little chance of successful treatment, the patient should be warned that they may occur. Referral for psychometric studies and therapy may be necessary.

SELECTED READING

Bergstrom, LV, et al. The lightning-damaged ear. *Arch Otolaryngol* 100:117, 1974.

Burda, CD. Electrocardiographic changes in lightning stroke. *Am Heart J* 72:521, 1966.

Castren, JA, and Kytila, J. Eye symptoms caused by lightning. *Acta Ophthalmol* 41:139, 1963.

Chia, BL. Electrocardiographic abnormalities and congestive cardiac failure due to lightning stroke. *Cardiology* 68:49, 1981.

Cooper, MA. Lightning injuries: Prognostic signs for death. *Ann Emerg Med* 9:134, 1980.

Cooper, MA. Lightning Injuries. In P Auerbach and E Geehr (eds), *Management of Wilderness and Environmental Injuries* (2nd ed). St. Louis: Mosby, 1989.

Kotagal, S, et al. Neurologic, psychiatric, and cardiovascular complications in children struck by lightning. *Pediatrics* 70:190, 1982.

Ohashi, M, Kitigawa, N, and Ishikawa, T. Lightning injury caused by discharges accompanying flashovers—a clinical and experimental study of death and survival. *Burns* 12:496, 1986.

ten Duis, HJ, and Klasen, HJ. Keraunoparalysis, a "specific" lightning injury. *Burns* 12:54, 1985.

Woods, JD. Spinal atrophic paralysis following lightning stroke. *S Afr Med J* 26:92, 1952.

79. Blast Injuries

Joel Geiderman

The term *blast injury* conjures images of the violence born of the late 1960s, 1970s, and 1980s: pubs and courthouses bombed in London and Belfast; buses blown up in Jerusalem; collapsed barracks in Beirut; an embassy destroyed in Kuwait; shoppers maimed in the streets of Paris; and airlines blown out of the sky over the Indian Ocean or Lockerbie, Scotland. And although terrorist bombings have yet to reach American shores, bomb threats are commonplace and military weaponry is just beginning to filter onto the streets of our inner cities.

Indeed, it appears that mankind is becoming more angry and violent, certainly less civilized and more savage, and more ready to use a bomb as the weapon of choice to express hatred or to draw attention to a cause.

Blast injuries may also occur in the military during war per se or during training. The occasional relic of war such as the forgotten mine or bomb may meanwhile produce injury to the civilian population. Finally, blast injuries may result from industrial or mining accidents or may occur in the home, office, or workplace as the result of a gas leak, for instance. Thus, it is not unlikely that a practicing emergency physician will be "called to the radio" (telemetry station) sometime during his or her career only to hear that victims of a blast will be brought to the emergency department. Blast injuries are unique in some aspects but are also usually accompanied by traumatic injuries well known to the emergency physician. The sociology, pathophysiology, injuries, injury patterns, treatment, and disposition of blast trauma are described in this chapter.

TERRORISM

Lenin said that the purpose of terror is to terrorize. That being the case, an explosive device is the perfect instrument of terror. First, because it can be small and can be detonated by timer or remote control, it can go off anywhere or anytime and therefore can be used to create a general threat in a populace that cannot be easily reasoned away.

Second, the detonation itself, with the noise, dust, and debris it produces and the subsequent screams and breaking glass creates a scene of panic, regardless of the actual damage or injuries. Third, the potential injuries, including notorious amputations, lacerations, blindness, and deafness are so dreaded that they produce an increased psychological effect on a population that fears a bomb attack.

Finally, there is something about being "blown up" that makes death itself more horrifying. One suspects that if the space shuttle Challenger had crashed into a mountain as do numerous training missions, there would have been less of a national convulsion in the general population who saw the seven astronauts "blown up."

Physics and Pathophysiology

A blast occurs when an explosive material, solid or liquid, is suddenly converted into a gaseous form, with a massive increase in volume and subsequently in pressure and temperature. This results in a wave of intensely positive pressure spreading outward from the site of explosion at supersonic speed.

In the immediate vicinity of the blast, the shock wave is *brisant,* or capable of blowing to bits all the matter immediately surrounding the detonation itself. Victims of such effects are rare in civilian bombings and are beyond medical care. Beyond the zone of brisance within which everything is disintegrated, the shock wave has great effectiveness but quickly loses its force and then becomes merely a sound wave.

The blast wave is characterized by a steep-fronted positive pressure phase ("overpressure") that rises rapidly, on the order of milliseconds, to reach pressures of hundreds or even thousands of pounds per square inch, and then decays over a longer period to a minimum less than the previous ambient pressure (but which cannot exceed atmospheric pressure of ~15 psi); finally, environmental pressure returns to baseline. An idealized blast wave is depicted in Fig. 79-1.

Transient winds accompany the pressure variation previously described. Because of the low density of air, even small changes in pressure can create winds of high velocity, and small light objects can be accelerated rapidly over short distances. This "displacement wave" will cause large objects to accelerate less, although this may be significant close to an explosion. In a high-energy detonation with a theoretical peak pressure of 15 psi, a 75-kg person could have an instantaneous acceleration of 450 feet/second. On the other hand, small terrorist bombs are usually not of this magnitude, and displacement of the victim is not significant.

Biological Response

The pathophysiology of explosive injury was first studied in the eighteenth century by Pierre Jars, who first correctly described the mechanism of death as "la grande et prompt dilation d'air." The biological response to a shock wave is now known to be dependent on the peak overpressure and the duration of the positive phase of the overpressure. Several factors will affect these variables:

1. *The size of the explosion.* A larger explosive charge produces shock waves of greater velocity and longer duration.
2. *The distance from the explosion.* The magnitude of the explosion is inversely related to the cube of the distance from the source. Therefore, peak overpressure decays rapidly as the shock wave propagates through the air. Consequently, in a small explosion (as with most handheld terrorist bombs, or from an antipersonnel land mine), the victim must be close to the device to suffer traumatic amputation of limbs from the explosion itself.
3. *The medium conducting the blast.* Explosions in water produce shock waves of greater peak pressure and longer duration of action because the wave travels at the corresponding speed of sound, which is 5 times greater in water than in air. Victims exposed to such a wave after abandoning a ship under attack suffered a high incidence of serious injuries. These are termed *immersion blasts,* as opposed to atmospheric blasts.
4. *The orientation to the blast.* One's position relative to a reflecting surface affects susceptibility to a blast. A person situated close to a wall may be subjected to at least twice the incident overpressure. Indoor detonations tend to be associated with especially severe blast injuries because of a geometric increase in the pressure wave as it is reflected off walls, floors, and ceilings. This may reflect the increased incidence of critical injuries and mortality in Bologna, Chu Chi, the Birmingham and Billingham pubs, and Beirut, compared with those events in essentially outdoor locales or with relatively small explosive force such as the Old Bailey, Craigavon, Jerusalem, or Belfast bombings. Reflected shock waves have even caused death in victims around the corner from an explosion. On the other hand, the body of one human may absorb and prevent the transmission of the blast wave so as to protect another individual. Thus, as has been observed, the common cinematic practice of the hero throwing himself on a live hand grenade to protect others, although not particularly self-serving, is probably effective in protecting others.

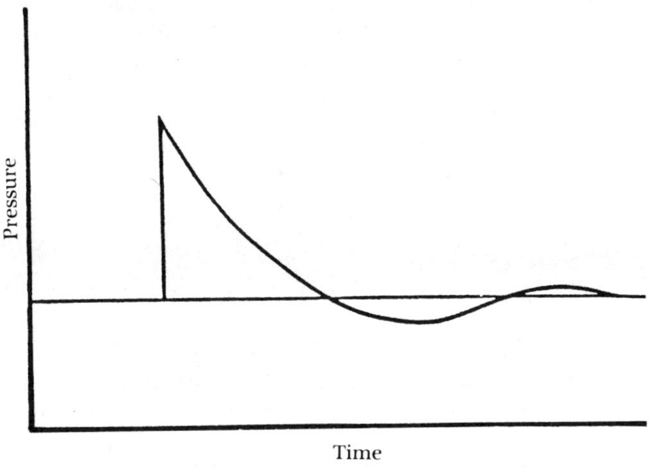

Fig. 79-1. Idealized representation of pressure time history of an explosion in the air.

Blast Wave Transmission

The shock wave passes through the surrounding medium at speeds that vary indirectly with the compressibility of the medium. The particles constituting the medium are not displaced by the wave but merely oscillate about equilibrium points; they may, however, be greatly displaced by the expanding gases resulting from the explosion.

When a shock wave passes from one medium to another, it is changed accordingly and may displace surface particles at the interface; this phenomenon is referred to as *spalling.* One should think of the wave of an underwater explosion that on reaching the surface disrupts surface particles and raises a dome of gas and water. This occurs long before the displaced gases reach the surface and produce a geyser-like plume.

As a blast wave moves through a liquid medium that contains air bubbles or air cavities, the energy is converted into kinetic energy at the liquid-air interface, causing maximal compression of air within the cavity. When the blast wave passes, the air bubble implodes.

In the human body, similar effects occur. Since soft tissues have the physical characteristics of water, spalling and implosion will occur whenever there is an interface with gas. namely in the lungs and the intestines.

TYPES OF INJURIES

Direct exposure to a blast wave results in *primary* blast injuries. As can be inferred from the previous discussion, air-containing organs are most susceptible to injury, and those individuals closest to the blast are most susceptible.

Blast lung is a term often used to describe injuries to that organ. Alveolar parenchymal tissue is torn most frequently by the pressure wave, but there may also be tears to the visceral pleura as well as bullae and alveolar-venous fistulae formation.

Clinical signs will derive from extravasation of edema fluid and blood into the interstitial space and alveoli, with resulting hemoptysis, shortness of breath, and hypoxemia. Radiologic findings are those characteristic of pulmonary contusion and edema. Air embolism and pneumothorax are rare complications. Positive-pressure ventilation may also predispose to these problems but should not be withheld when necessary.

In a large study of survivors of terrorist bomb victims from "the troubles" in Northern Ireland, blast lung was rare. However, this was a common injury in another study of those who died, usually as a part of a pattern of mixed injuries. A cumulative study of 3,357 patients from multiple bombings from Belfast to Beirut corroborated the impression that primary blast injury to the lung was rare among survivors of air blasts (0.6% of 2,934 survivors). It is theorized that those victims close enough to an explosion to be susceptible to blast injury would most likely be killed by secondary and tertiary blast effects.

Bowel injuries (usually colon) are also rare in atmospheric blasts but are common in underwater blasts, which may be experienced by sailors. Twenty-four of 32 patients exposed to an immersion blast in one incident suffered bowel injuries requiring laparotomy, with four subsequent deaths. Fortunately, immersion blasts are of little significance to the emergency physician.

The ear is commonly affected by a blast wave. This is not surprising since the ear is designed to collect and amplify pressure waves, converting acoustic energy to mechanical displacement. Tympanic membrane rupture is frequent and bilateral 50 percent of the time when present. The injury usually heals well with conservative treatment. Sensorineural hearing loss to the point of deafness may occur but usually resolves quickly. Tinnitus is also common and may be severe early on. Tinnitis usually resolves with the recovery of hearing.

Concussion is the most common neurologic manifestation. Epidural and subdural hematomas have also been reported. The most common injury seen in the fatally wounded is brain damage, although multiple injuries (chest and abdomen being next most common) are suffered by virtually all fatalities. These are the same injuries that most commonly cause death in all forms of trauma and may reflect the tolerance of these body systems to severe injury.

Head injuries caused the largest number of late deaths in survivors of terrorist bombings (52%), followed by injury to the chest and abdomen, and traumatic amputations.

Penetrating and Nonpenetrating Impact of Blast-Energized Debris

Secondary blast injuries are caused by the penetrating and nonpenetrating impact of blast-energized debris. Within confined spaces, debris may include shattered glass, splintered wood, plaster, and even large pieces of furniture (e.g., table legs) that can attain velocity sufficient to penetrate the body. Such projectiles are a major source of serious and nonserious injury in civilian bombings. Bruises, lacerations, and small missile entry holes are the most common injuries from these events. The collective profile of injury patterns seen in multiple blast incidents is depicted in Fig. 79-2.

High-velocity dust may embed in the skin and produce dust-tattooing. Clothing is protective, as evidenced by an increased proportion of these injuries occurring to the head and neck and the legs of adult women.

The aforementioned debris are termed *secondary fragments*. Fragments from metal bomb casings or hand grenades are termed *primary fragments,* and these may produce serious injury, depending on their velocity and the end-organ involved.

BLAST-INDUCED WHOLE-BODY DISPLACEMENT. Strong shock waves may displace persons, resulting in impact against a rigid object or decelerative tumbling. These are termed *tertiary* blast injuries. Skull and limb fractures occur frequently as a result of this mechanism.

BURNS FROM THE FLASH AND HOT GASES AND BURNS FROM THE COMBUSTION OF SURROUNDINGS. Serious skin burns may result from the flash produced by the detonation of an explosive. Heat is transferred by radiation, conduction, and convection. Flash burns generally appear in the exposed part of the body, as clothing provides good protection. More extensive burns usually imply that the clothing or occupant space caught fire. While the temperature of a fireball is high, the heat content is low. As a result, burns of the upper respiratory tract are uncommon.

INHALATION OF NOXIOUS GASES PRODUCED BY DETONATION OR COMBUSTION. No generalization can be made about these kinds of injuries. However, this possibility should be considered in special circumstances, such as industrial explosions. Rescue personnel should also be aware of the possibility of leaking gases and should wear appropriate self-contained breathing devices in such circumstances.

COLLAPSE OF THE BUILDING. This sight became all too familiar with the bombings in Lebanon, Kuwait, and elsewhere, where vehicles laden with explosives were detonated. Prior to these events, most terrorists' bombs were small, perhaps 2 to 30 lb, carried in a parcel or suitcase, and were not capable of collapsing buildings.

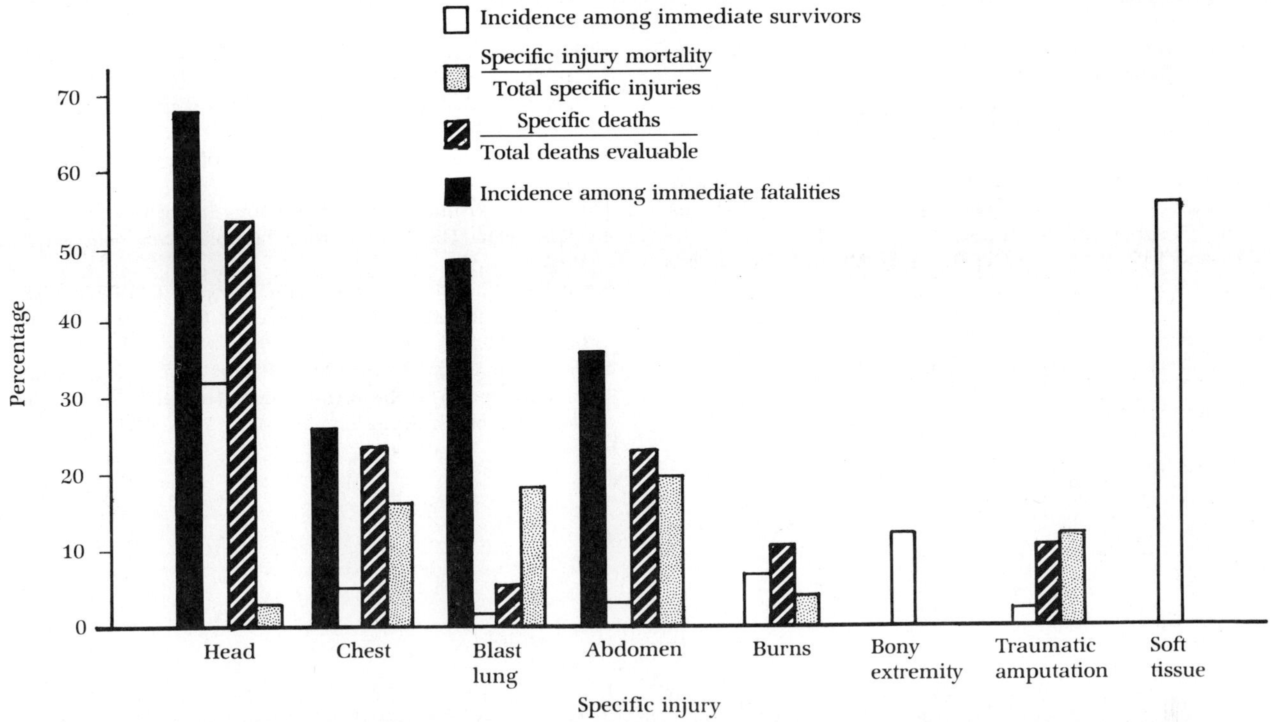

Fig. 79-2. Collective profile of injury patterns among 3,357 terrorist bombing victims. (From E.R. Frykberg and J.J. Tepas. Terrorist bombings. *Ann. Surg.* 208:569, 1988.)

DESTRUCTION OF AN AIRBORNE VEHICLE. Even small, hand-carried, or hidden devices can wreak enormous damage when the explosion occurs on an airplane in flight. Although aircraft have withstood such attacks, depressurization and destabilization of the aircraft can be expected to bring it down in most cases.

EVALUATION AND MANAGEMENT

Prehospital

There are several prehospital care considerations that should be taken into account. First, it is important for someone to maintain order at the scene of the blast, since panic is likely and may be out of proportion to the magnitude of the injuries. Second, patients should be rapidly removed from possible exposure to secondary injury from leaking gas lines, downed power lines, and so on, as soon as possible. Third, paramedics must use caution so that obvious disfiguring injuries of the limbs do not distract them from whole-body evaluation. Finally, paramedics should be reminded of the high incidence of deafness and, if necessary, should communicate on note pads to help distinguish the deaf from those who are head injured.

Emergency Department

In addition to the points listed previously, the emergency physician has a few special considerations. First, an effort should be made to assess the magnitude of force of the explosion and the positioning of the victim relative to the explosion. Considering these factors, the emergency physician should then assess the likelihood of occult or delayed blast lung. If this injury is suspected, positive pressure ventilation should be avoided when possible and used with care when necessary. Other than that, a usual trauma workup should ensue, considering the possibilities of cervical spine injury and occult blunt trauma to the chest or abdomen. Air embolism is another rare event that one must have a high index of suspicion for, lest it be missed with devastating consequences.

Management of the psychological needs of the victims and their families will require a team approach and should not be forgotten, since there is a high incidence of psychological stress in survivors of blasts.

Finally, blast will probably produce at least a minidisaster and will tax the management skills of even the most experienced emergency physician. Maintaining order, privacy, and decorum; communicating articulately with the press; and not neglecting other emergency department patients are all part of the emergency physician's responsibilities.

CONCLUSION

Perhaps humans will someday turn away from violence as a means of expression and of settling differences. For now, the tendency toward the use of violence to express hatred, to draw attention to one's cause, or to retaliate for some real or perceived wrongdoing seems to be increasing. At the same time, for acts of random terror, the bomb seems to be the weapon of choice. Emergency personnel should therefore be familiar with the effects of blast.

SELECTED READING

Adams, DB, and Schwab, CW. Twenty-one-year experience with land mine injuries. *J Trauma* 28:S159, 1988.

Adler, J, et al. Terrorist bombing experience during 1975–79. Casualties admitted to the Shaare Zedek Medical Center. *Isr J Med Sci* 19:189, 1983.

Brismar, B, and Bergenwald, L. The terrorist bomb explosion in Bologna, Italy, 1980: An analysis of the effects and injuries sustained. *J Trauma* 22:216, 1982.

Caro, D, and Irving, M. The Old Bailey bomb explosion. *Lancet* 1:1433, 1973.

Cooper, GJ, et al. Casualties from terrorist bombings. *J Trauma* 23:955, 1983.

Frykberg, ER, and Tepas, JJ. Terrorist bombings. *Ann Surg* 208:569, 1988.

Hadden, WA, Rutherford, WH, and Merrett, JD. The injuries of terrorist bombing: A study of 1532 consecutive patients. *Br J Surg* 65:525, 1978.

Huller, T, and Bazini, Y. Blast injuries of the chest and abdomen. *Arch Surg* 100:24, 1970.

Kennedy, TL, and Johnston, GW. Civilian bomb injuries. *Br Med J* 1:382, 1975.

Kerr, AG, and Byrne, JET. Blast injuries of the ear. *Br Med J* 1:559, 1975.

Phillips, YY. Primary blast injuries. *Ann Emerg Med* 15:1446, 1986.

Scott, BA, et al. The Beirut terrorist bombing. *Neurosurgery* 18:107, 1986.

Stapczynski, JS. Blast injuries. *Ann Emerg Med* 11:687, 1982.

Tucker, K, and Lettin, A. The Tower of London bomb explosion. *Br Med J* 3:287, 1975.

Waterworth, TA, and Carr, MJT. Report on injuries sustained by patients treated at the Birmingham General Hospital following the recent bomb explosions. *Br Med J* 2:25, 1975.

80. Radiation Injury

David E. Drum
Carol B. Jankowski

Accidental injuries involving radiation are rare. Radiation exposure, skin or wound contamination, and inhalation or ingestion may occur alone or in combination as a consequence of a number of mishaps during the following activities: (1) transportation of radioactive materials, (2) use of radioisotopes or radiation sources in medical research or treatment, (3) commercial use of radiation sources for radiography, (4) operation of radiation-producing machines such as accelerators or cyclotrons, (5) noncombat military operations, and (6) operation of research or commercial nuclear reactors. The Joint Commission on Accreditation of Health Care Organizations, which recognizes these potential sources of radiation accidents, requires all hospital emergency departments to have a written procedure for treating patients exposed to radiation or contaminated by radioactivity. Because the initial emergency care of such victims and precautions for the personnel present at the accident site may be critical, it is essential that every health care provider be familiar with the principles of handling such problems.

CLINICOPATHOLOGIC CONSIDERATIONS

Physical Biology

Definitions

Radiation is energy in the form of particles or electromagnetic waves. *Alpha* and *beta particles* are charged emissions from the nuclei of radioactive atoms; *neutrons* are uncharged particles of the same origin. *Gamma rays*, also known as photons and physically identical to x-rays, are a kind of nonparticulate radiation of the electromagnetic spectrum. *Radioisotopes* are unstable forms of elements that emit radiation. Each has a characteristic rate of decay described by its half-life, a unique array of radioactive emissions, and physiologic properties defined by its elemental nature.

The quantity of any radioisotope is measured in *curies* (Ci), a unit representing 3.7×10^{10} radioactive disintegrations per second. Radiation exposure is quantified in terms of the *roentgen* (R), a measure of ionization produced in air. The *rad* is a measure of absorbed dose determined by the nature of the radiation and by the characteristics of the tissue being irradiated. The *rem* (roentgen equivalent-man) is a special unit of absorbed dose used to indicate the biologic consequences of a given absorbed dose. For most beta, gamma, and x-rays of low energy, the rem is used as if it were equivalent to the rad.*

*The following new universal units are now supplanting all of those mentioned above: 1 becquerel (Bq) = $\text{second}^{-1} \simeq 2.7 \times 10^{-11}$ Ci; 1 gray (Gy) = 100 rad; 1 sievert (Sv) = 100 rem.

Because radiation cannot be identified by any of our senses, instruments such as Geiger-Müller counters are necessary for detecting the presence of radiation and are calibrated either in counts per minute (cpm) or milliroentgens per hour (mR/hr). The film badge or thermoluminescent dosimeter (TLD) worn by radiation workers registers cumulative radiation dose in millirem. Other dosimeters often worn by radiation workers or emergency personnel working with radioactivity include pen dosimeters, which allow an immediate readout of cumulative exposure, and ring badges, which reflect finger doses more accurately.

Pathogenesis

The biologic consequences of radiation depend somewhat on the type of radiation involved. Charged particles interact with tissues very rapidly and deposit most of their energy in the skin; generally they are not dangerous unless their parent isotopes gain entrance into the body by inhalation or ingestion. For example, alpha particles emitted by heavy transuranic isotopes such as uranium 238 have a maximum range of less than 1 mm in tissue and will not penetrate even the outer layers of skin. The smaller beta particles are attenuated within several millimeters of tissue. Tritium (hydrogen 3), the best known beta emitter, is the isotope most commonly used in research and is the most abundant component of low-level radioactive waste.

Neutrons are an extremely dangerous form of radiation and are usually generated either in a reactor or by high-energy x-ray machines or linear accelerators. They cause exposure damage only, never contamination, and hence do not require precautions in the emergency department.

Gamma rays and machine-produced x-rays are highly penetrating, reach all parts of the body with increasingly hazardous effects as the exposure increases, and are the most common source of accidental overexposures. Many radioisotopes emit mixed radiation—for example, iodine 131 decay produces both gamma and beta emissions.

The direct cellular effect of radiation is to ionize or dissociate water molecules to form reactive radical species with unpaired electrons. These then destroy parts of protein side chains or DNA molecules, disrupting normal cell function. Thus, tissues most susceptible to radiation injury are those that depend on rapid turnover of nucleic acids and on proper control functions within the cells—that is, the bone marrow, the gastrointestinal epithelium, the embryo/fetus, and the developing gametes.

Types of Radiation Injury

Radiation injury may result from two circumstances: (1) accidental *exposure* to a large radioactive source or radiation field, or (2) *contamination,* either internally or externally, caused by the presence of radioactive gas, liquid, or particulate material within or on the body. The distinctions must be clear because management differs markedly.

Whole-body Exposures

Perennially, the most serious radiation accidents have been the overexposure of industrial workers to unshielded radioactive sources (cobalt 60, cesium 137, iridium 192). These accidents have occurred at industries using sealed radioisotope sources for radiography or sterilization. Within seconds or minutes, depending on the level of radioactivity, the workers may receive a whole-body dose requiring definitive medical treatment. An approximate estimate of absorbed dose can usually be made by the industrial health physicist at the scene and by quick processing of the victim's dosimeter. More rarely, explosions at weapons research or reprocessing facilities have caused fatal exposures along with equally fatal blast and thermal injuries.

Local Exposures

Overexposures to extremities, especially hands, the most common type of accident, are usually not disabling, and are probably frequently unreported. They arise from carelessness during industrial radiography (commonly used in shipbuilding and metal fabrication), x-ray diffraction work, power plant maintenance, and handling of accelerator target materials. Generally no other significant injuries accompany localized radiation overexposures.

Internal Contamination

Radioactive material may gain entrance to the body by way of inhalation (e.g., during a fire or explosion), ingestion (i.e., oral intake of accidental, therapeutic, or suicidal origin), and absorption from an open wound, a burn, or a puncture wound. Internal contamination should elicit prompt therapeutic measures to prevent permanent deposition within a critical organ.

External Contamination

External contamination denotes the presence of radioactive material on the body or clothes of the victim, or in a wound, or complicating a burn. There may be embedded radioactive fragments or particles emitting considerable radiation. The entire outer body may be contaminated, or only a single extremity may be involved. Surface contamination is generally of less medical significance to the patient than acute exposure or ingestion, but it is necessary to conduct appropriate decontamination procedures for the following reasons: (1) to prevent further radiation and internal contamination of the patient, (2) to minimize exposures of attending staff, (3) to prevent spread of radioactive materials elsewhere, and (4) to document, by sampling, the nature and location of radioisotopes contributing to surface contamination.

Accidental contact of the skin with radioactive material in liquid commonly occurs during laboratory and maintenance work in hospitals, universities, and many industries. Serious contamination would be anticipated only in situations of an explosion, valve leakage, apparatus breakage, fall onto a contaminated area, or container rupture. Transportation accidents involving trucks carrying medical isotopes or contaminated ion-exchange resins from nuclear power plants offer a potential contamination hazard.

PLANNING AND PATIENT TREATMENT

General Considerations

In a radiation emergency there are four medical objectives: in order of priority they are as follows: (1) to establish adequate airway, respiratory, and circulatory functions; (2) to minimize any internal contamination that may increase the

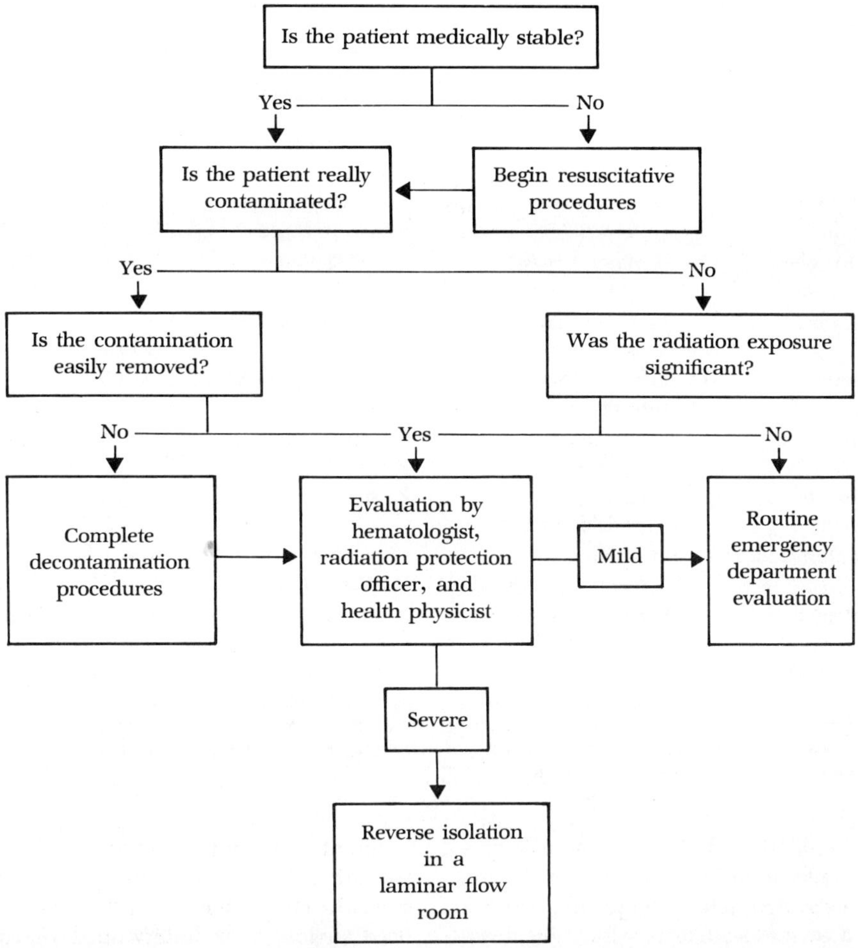

Fig. 80-1. Flowchart for management of radiation injuries.

patient's later risk of leukemia or other cancer; (3) to minimize spread of unsealed radioisotope contamination; and (4) to evaluate and treat any serious exposure.

Immediate care for the seriously injured patient should follow standard medical practice; secondary consideration should be for the patient's surface radiation levels. It would be rare that sufficient surface contamination would be present so as to preclude lifesaving emergency care.

The first action when dealing with any radiation accident is to ensure that the patient is medically stable—that is, circulation is intact, airway is open, and immediately life-threatening conditions are corrected (Fig. 80-1). While major life-support measures are being initiated, a quick report outlining the injuries and nature of radiation exposure and contamination may be elicited from accompanying attendants or police officers. It should be determined whether the level of radioactivity is sufficient to be hazardous to attending staff; it is highly unlikely that surface contamination would emit enough radiation to present an immediate health hazard. Only a metal fragment or foreign body (e.g., cobalt 60) could be so highly radioactive as to require immediate removal. Priority for treating injuries before decontamination depends on the judgment of the emergency physician in consultation with available radiation experts.

Reassurance of the victim, an essential step, is especially important because the victim may not understand the need for extraordinary precautions and may be deeply concerned about the subsequent consequences of an exposure despite the absence of any symptoms.

Treatment of anxiety is always a challenge, whether required for the accident victim, his or her family, or workers. Even persons remote from the accident site may appear in the emergency department "to be checked for radiation."

Whole-Body Exposures

Because patients whose injury is simply overexposure to radiation are not in any way radioactive, initial management can be accomplished within the framework of general emergency department practice.

The acute affects of radiation exposure on the body should rarely contribute to symptoms or treatment needs in the early minutes after an exposure. Treatment of the victim's other injuries, if present, should predominate. Exposures below 100 R rarely cause any physiologic symptoms, but the victim may be extremely upset by the situation. His or her acute anxiety may be mistakenly interpreted as a symptom of more severe overexposure; therefore, it is important to get a calculated estimate of exposure dose. If the exposure is significant (> 50–100 R), evaluation by a hematologist or other health physics professional is warranted to decide whether and when appropriate supportive measures should be instituted.

Table 80-1. Sources and treatment of internal contamination

Radionuclide		Likely accident sources	Recommended treatment	
Class	Example		Alert patient	Unconscious/airway injury
Iodines	Iodine 131	Hospital; transport; reactor; laboratory	SS Kl, 10 drops	$NaClO_4$, 200 mg IV
Tritium	Hydrogen 3	Reactor coolant; laboratories	Water diuresis	Water diuresis
Noble gas	Xenon 133	Hospital; reactor	Air ventilation	Air ventilation
Diagnostic	Technetium 99m	Hospital; transport	Water diuresis	Water diuresis
Fission products	Cesium 137	Reactor coolant or deionizers	Emesis, purgatives: *Gaviscon 30 ml every 2 hr,	Lavage, purgatives: Gaviscon 30 ml every 2 hr,
	Strontium 90	Reactor coolant or deionizers	†Neutraphos 60 ml every 4 hr	Neutraphos 60 ml every 4 hr
Corrosion products	Manganese 54	Reactor coolant or deionizers	Same as above	Same as above
	Cobalt 60	Reactor coolant or deionizers	Same as above	Same as above
Uranium	Uranium 238, 235	Metallurgical laboratories; mines	$NaHCO_3$, 45 mEq IV every 4 hr Water diuresis	Same as for an alert patient
Transuranics	Plutonium 239	Reprocessing plants; weapons accident	Zn-DPTA, 1 gm IV in 500 ml 5% D/W in 30 min	Same as for an alert patient
	Americium 241	Reprocessing plants; industry; laboratory	Zn-DTPA, 1 gm IV in 500 ml 5% D/W in 30 min	Same as for an alert patient

*An aluminum hydroxide-magnesium carbonate antacid containing sorbitol, sodium alginate, and edetate sodium.
†Neutraphos powder (potassium phosphate) reconstituted solution.

Exposures in the range of 100–200 R will generally produce early signs of the acute radiation syndrome, including nausea, vomiting, and fever. A baseline complete blood cell count (CBC) should be drawn as soon as possible. The absolute lymphocyte count is the most practical and effective biologic dosimeter of the radiation exposure and indicator of prognosis. A lymphocyte count less than 1,500 within 48 hours indicates a significant exposure; after severe exposures, the lymphocyte count may dip beneath 500, indicating a poor prognosis. Significant radiation exposures may require subsequent reverse isolation in a special facility, such as a laminar airflow room, designed to minimize infection.

At exposures over 1,200 R to the whole body, prognosis is poor and survival may not be expected even with the best treatment. Such an exposure should be evident very early by central nervous system damage manifest as lethargy, somnolence, ataxia, and seizures, which obviously complicate the differential diagnosis.

Local Exposures

Regional exposures, such as those restricted to a hand, are the most common single form of radiation accidents; they never constitute a therapeutic emergency. Although the appearance may resemble a thermal burn, a careful history may be needed to identify the causal agent as radiation. Redness, swelling, and blistering indicate very serious injury, but these signs may not be apparent for several days following exposure. Slow ischemic necrosis will proceed for months. Local exposures of less severity (< 500 R) may not exhibit any topical changes, but the patient should be followed up for some time.

Initial treatment of patients with local exposures is nonspecific and identical to that of patients with burns of similar severity. The patient should be counseled in regard to the need for long-term follow-up. Progressive friability and necrosis requiring amputation may develop months after hand or foot exposures over 1,000 R.

Internal Contamination

Patients who have ingested or inhaled radioactive material also may be treated in the emergency deparment without special precautions if there is no possibility of external contamination. Someone familiar with radiation survey instruments should be available in case such measurements are necessary. The gamma cameras located in all nuclear medicine departments should be used to identify the internal location of significant contaminants.

A whole-body counter may be useful for detecting very minimal quantities of radioisotopes, but its use could be delayed several days. Moreover, the presence of *any* external or intraluminal gastrointestinal contamination would interfere with interpretation of data from whole-body counting. Table 80-1 summarizes the likely sources for the most common isotopes implicated in internal contamination. It should be emphasized that deliberate therapeutic (e.g., iodine 131 for thyroid cancer) and diagnostic (e.g., technetium 99m for bone scans) internal contamination is commonplace in medical practice.

Radioisotopes that have long half-lives and that emit beta or alpha particles only become real biologic hazards when they have been ingested or inhaled. Pulmonary deposition may be anticipated during a fire if respiratory protective devices are not available or are not properly used. If a victim accidentally inhales or swallows radioactive gas, fluid, or particulate matter (as in a fire), it is essential that procedures be initiated *immediately* to eliminate the radioactive material from the body.

Therapy depends on the particular radioisotope involved (Table 80-1); a careful history is important. Research laboratories primarily use tritium (hydrogen 3), phosphorus 32, carbon 14, and iodine isotopes. A truck delivering medical diagnostic isotopes may contain technetium 99m, molybdenum 99, gallium 67, and thallium 201. Metallurgical industries use depleted uranium, a flammable heavy metal that emits low energy x-rays and beta particles.

Treatment generally involves water diuresis, emesis or lavage, purgation, or administration of a specific blocking or chelating agent. For example, if radioiodine is a suspected contaminant, saturated solution of potassium iodide, 10 drops in liquid, is administered orally as soon as possible. For patients who are unconscious or have head injuries, sodium perchlorate (200 mg intravenously) is effective for blocking any uptake of radioiodine by the thyroid gland.

Most inhaled particulates are coughed up and reach the gastrointestinal tract. For this reason, much of the treatment effort is aimed at emptying the stomach or intestines and preventing absorption (see Chap. 155).

Patients with internal contamination alone do not emit sufficient radiation to require attending medical personnel to use extensive protective measures. All body waste fluids and serial blood samples should be handled with gloves, labeled as radioactive, and saved for later analysis to help determine the quantity of material incorporated.

External Contamination

Managing patients with surface contamination is quite different from managing those with exposures or internal contamination alone. It requires coordination of several health care disciplines and careful preparation of the treatment area. Preparation and logistical responsibilities generally are assigned to the nursing service. In an emergency, the physician may have to fulfill or delegate many roles; these roles ideally may be segregated as follows: (1) medical—to direct the patient's management; (2) radiology—to interpret radiation measurements and to ensure staff protection (a health physicist or nuclear medicine technologist who is familiar with survey meters could serve as monitoring technician. Many fire fighters and police personnel have been trained to use survey meters, although they may be unfamiliar with the interpretation of the measurements); (3) nursing—to give direct patient care and provide overall logistical support; (4) maintenance—to set up and isolate an emergency treatment area and to assist with the final cleanup after completion of the emergency; (5) security—to restrict public access to the accident site or to the emergency department during the initial excitement; (6) public relations—to provide the news media with accurate information concerning the casualty.

Once the patient is medically stable, either local officials or hospital administrators may request assistance, if needed, from their state departments of public health or from the Regional Coordinating Office for Radiological Emergency Assistance of the U.S. Department of Energy. Consultation is also available by phone directly from the Radiation Emergency Assistance Center at Oak Ridge, Tennessee. If the injury occurs offsite (e.g., a highway accident), emergency medical care would take priority, and the area should be immediately secured until radiation surveys establish the presence or absence of area contamination.

Because most medical personnel are unfamiliar with the procedures of dealing with contaminated radiation casualties, it is essential that a written procedure manual delineating detailed job descriptions be available. Periodic drills involving scenarios with contamination should be conducted by health centers or emergency teams who may conceivably attend accident victims.

MANAGING THE CONTAMINATED PATIENT

Notification of the Accident

When possible, it is important to ascertain from the accident site personnel whether contamination is present, what isotopes were involved, and whether there was major whole-body exposure. When the nature of the accident is unknown, preparations must be made to deal with the presence of surface radioactivity. If radioiodine is a suspected contaminant, such as in any nuclear power plant accident or in a thyroid laboratory accident, all attending personnel should take potassium iodide (KI) solution in advance. For unannounced or undefined radiation casualties, it is advisable to keep the victim in the ambulance or at the accident site, depending on his or her medical status, until the area and personnel are adequately protected. If medical attention must be given or if contamination is discovered after admission to the hospital, any area through which the victim has passed must be considered contaminated.

Radiation Emergency Treatment Area

It is preferable to use a treatment area or room separate from other patients as the radiation emergency treatment area (REA), but there should be ready access to emergency equipment and supplies. A marked buffer zone should be designed adjacent to the REA to permit the receipt of needed supplies and discharge of samples and contaminated materials. Ideally, such an area designed as part of an emergency department would have a separate negative pressure air circulation to filter particulates selectively and thereby prevent spread of airborne contaminants. Otherwise, covering the return air vent would suffice. Control of access to the area is necessary to prevent interference by or contamination of nonessential people.

The question always arises as to whether the washings should be contained or should be discharged into the sanitary sewer system. There are no federal statutory limits to sewer disposal of contaminated washings *from a patient* in a general hospital. In addition, radioisotopes disposed of in such a manner may be integrated theoretically over an entire year's volume of sewer water output. Hence, it would be extremely unlikely that institutional disposal limits for even occupational activities would ever be exceeded.

Preparation of the Radiation Emergency Area

The focus of area preparation is the provision of strict containment of all radioactive materials and the assembly of essential emergency supplies. Ideally the floor or topsoil of the area should be covered to prevent contamination, and plastic bags should be available in which to put clothing and rags or towels. Used wash water may be collected from a stretcher top pan in large plastic containers for later radionuclide analysis and disposal. Radiation survey meters, with probes covered by plastic wrap to prevent contamination, should be available and operational in order that frequent radiation surveys can be made.

Details of protective measures to be taken by the medical staff should be modified only by the radiation specialist on site. Personnel in direct contact with the victim will need protective clothing, such as gowns, plastic aprons, head and shoe coverings, masks, and double gloves. Although this clothing does not protect against penetrating radiation, it does prevent skin and airway contamination. All personnel should use film or TLD badges, and those with close contact should wear ring badges and pen dosimeters if anticipated surface radiation is greater than 50 mR/hr.

Radiation Surveying and Sampling

Initially, the entire body is surveyed in detail to determine the extent and location of radioactivity. A probe should be passed *slowly* over the surface, and at the same distance, approximately 3 to 5 cm, from the skin. Readings should be recorded on a body chart analogous to a burn diagram. Most contamination will be removed when the victim's outer clothes and shoes are removed and are placed in plastic bags. Swab samples are then taken from all body orifices, those skin areas exhibiting excess radiation measurements, and any wounds. Clippings of hair, paper tissues into which the nose is blown, and samples of clothing and metal accessories such as a ring or watch are useful sources for identifying the specific contaminating radionuclide and whether neutrons were involved in the exposure. These samples are also important because alpha and low-energy beta particles may not be detected by conventional survey equipment. Samples should be labeled according to their sites of origin, placed in glass or plastic containers, and identified as radioactive for later analysis. The identifying number for each sample should be written on the patient's body chart to identify the origin of the samples. Most general hospitals have laboratory radioisotope counters capable of detecting the presence (not the specific type) of gamma-emitting isotopes.

Decontamination

If surface contamination is present, ambulatory patients may remove it by taking a shower and washing with soap and water after sampling of the skin surface is completed. A large pan with controlled drainage fitted on top of a mobile stretcher should be used for the more seriously injured victim who must be washed down while injuries are being treated. Careful and prolonged washing of body surfaces should eliminate all but a trace of contamination. It is essential that contaminated wash water not be internalized by mouth or other orifices. Irrigation of the eyes should be done, if required, to avoid ingestion.

If there is a serious open wound or burn, the area should be considered contaminated until sampling proves otherwise. Contaminated wounds must be irrigated thoroughly with a surgical detergent, and only repeated sampling and analysis can determine when the wound is completely decontaminated. Puncture wounds that deposit long-lived alpha emitters, such as americium 241, may require excision to remove the radioactive source. The wound should be decontaminated before the rest of the body by irrigation and debridement such as would be appropriate in any case. When the area is clean, it should be temporarily sealed off by plastic wrap to avoid recontamination while washing off other areas. Further removal of radioactivity is accomplished by washing the body surface with any mild detergent in lukewarm water. Soft brushes or 4 × 4's can be used on the skin; care must be taken not to abrade the skin, which would allow the radioactive material to enter the body.

Irrigation of nose and ears with water should follow general procedures, and care should be taken to save all washings for analysis. Hair may require several washings and even trimming. Frequent surveys will rapidly determine the progress in removing contaminants. If residual radioactivity (i.e., more than twice true background cpm or 0.02 mR/hr) remains on the surface after several minutes of washing, the area may be covered with plastic wrap and labeled as slightly radioactive. Final decontamination may be conducted later with reducing, oxidizing, or chelating agents, depending on the nature of the contaminating radioisotope and advice from radiation medicine specialists. Scintiphotos taken in nuclear medicine may be useful to rule out internal contamination as the source of persistent surface radiation. Except for the Chernobyl accident, thermal burn injuries have rarely been contaminated by isotopes other than hydrogen 3 (as water). Radiation burns may be distinguished from thermal burns by the absence of a painful initial event and their more indolent course.

Personnel Monitoring and General Cleanup

Once the patient is finally decontaminated and monitoring shows little more than background radiation levels, the patient may be transferred without precautions to an area for definitive care of any injuries. Strictest conformance to measures for containment of residual radioactivity in the REA must be followed. The attending staff should be carefully surveyed for radioactivity after degowning. All supplies, lines, and equipment that have been in close proximity to the patient should be secured in plastic bags that are surveyed and clearly marked if found to be radioactive. These materials should be removed to the radioactive waste disposal room of the hospital or picked up by government or industry representatives.

Minimizing Radiation Exposure to Attending Personnel

Many procedures for handling a patient contaminated with radioactive material are no different from those for handling

Table 80-2. Working time limits for 125 mR exposure at a distance of 1.5 ft

Survey meter reading*		
cpm	mR/hr	Time personnel may work (hr)
30,000	10	12.5
75,000	25	5
300,000	100	1.25

*The relationship of counts per minute (cpm) and milliroentgens per hour (mR/hr) varies according to the nature of the radiation source and the calibration of the survey meter.

a patient suspected of hepatitis or AIDS. It is the presence of radioactivity that uniquely distinguishes this care. Its hazard, albeit minor in the short run, is continuous and cannot be neutralized. Throughout the care of such a victim, an underlying legitimate concern of staff is that of personal radiation exposure. However, it is most unlikely that any accident victim would ever exhibit surface radiation levels sufficient to cause emergency personnel to receive exposures greater than statutory limits for nonoccupationally exposed workers.

For patients who are extensively contaminated or who have a highly radioactive fragment, *minimizing time* of exposure and *maximizing distance* from the patient are extremely effective protective measures. Because most significant contaminants emit medium-energy gamma rays, lead aprons are *not* effective protective measures.

As shown in Table 80-2, the radiation survey information given by the survey meter is a useful approximate guide to the time that attending personnel may be permitted to work safely near the patient. Needless to say, an offscale survey meter reading on the least sensitive scale should *always* be interpreted as "Danger—High Radiation Field—Move Away" until proven otherwise.

Experience with Radiation Accidents

A balanced appreciation of the spectrum of radiation accidents may be derived from a review of their history. Table 80-3 is a tabulation of all the known major radiation accidents worldwide since 1944. There have been 337 such incidents, with 111 fatalities; these numbers translate to about seven events and two deaths per year. The total number of individuals involved is heavily weighted by the large number who received over 25 rem each from the release of fission products after Russian accidents at Chernobyl and at Kyshtym.

With the exception of mixed injuries (group V), these accident victims suffered from external exposures or internal contamination only. They would not have required any decontamination, nor would emergency personnel have needed special protective procedures in the emergency department.

Perennially, the most common serious accident category is group III, local extremity radiation injuries from exposures to very high-dose rate sealed sources or radiation-producing machines.

In fact, most emergency physicians will see no radiation accident victims during their practicing lifetime. Our experience is that occasionally much less serious accidents arise within our own university teaching hospital or come to community hospitals from nearby industries known to possess and use radioisotopes or radiation-emitting devices.

SUMMARY

Emergency management of accident victims with skin areas contaminated by radioactive material is based on goals of minimizing further injury to the patient, containment of contaminating nuclides, and provision of a safe environment for attending personnel. The procedures are guided by use of radiation survey meters, and prior written plans periodically tested in drills are essential for effective action.

Radiation injuries caused by accidental exposures or internal contamination require medical treatment appropriate to the severity of exposure and specific isotopes involved and do not require special efforts to protect the medical staff. No radiation injury ever preempts immediate airway and circulatory support. The consultative services of radiation medical specialists are available and should be planned for in advance.

Table 80-3. Major radiation accidents worldwide, 1944—March 1991

Injury	Number of accidents	Number of individuals	Fatalities
I. Whole-body ≥ 25 rem	68	660	24
II. Whole-body ≥ 25 rem plus local ≥ 600 rem	44	281	37
III. Local ≥ 600 rem	167	313	24
IV. Internal dose ≥ MPBB	50	98	10
V. Mixed *	8	1,680	16
	337	3,032	111

*This category reflects predominantly the Russian accidents at Chernobyl and at Kyshtym plus the incident at Goiânia, Brazil.
Key: MPBB = maximum permissible body burden
Source: Modified from tabulations of Dr. Shirley Fry, Oak Ridge Associated Universities.

SELECTED READING

Adelstein, SJ, and Dealy, JB. Hematological responses to human body irradiation. *Am J Roentgenol* 93:927, 1965.

American Medical Association. *A Guide to the Hospital Management of Injuries Arising from Exposure to or Involving Ionizing Radiation.* Chicago, IL, 1984.

Conklin, JJ, Walter, RI, and Hirsch, EF. Current concepts in the management of radiation injuries and associated trauma. *Surg Gynecol Obstet* 156:809, 1983.

Hübner, KF, and Fry, SA. *The Medical Basis for Radiation Accident Preparedness.* New York: Elsevier North-Holland Inc, 1980.

International Atomic Energy Agency. *Manual on Early Medical Treatment of Possible Radiation Injury,* Safety Series 47. Vienna, IAEA, 1978.

International Commission on Radiological Protection. *The Principles and General Procedures for Handling Emergency and Accidental Exposures of Workers,* Publication 28. Elmsford, NY: Pergamon, 1978.

Leonard, RB, and Ricks, RC. Emergency department radiation accident protocol. *Ann Emerg Med* 9:462, 1980.

Lushbaugh, CC, Hübner, KF, and Ricks, RC. Medical aspects of nuclear radiation emergencies. *Emergency* 10:32, 1978.

Mettler, FA, Rocco, FG, and Junkins, RL. The role of EMTs in radiation accidents. *Emerg Med Serv* 6:22, 1977.

Mettler, FA, Kelsey, CA, and Ricks, RC (eds). *Medical Management of Radiation Accidents.* Boca Raton, FL: CRC Press, 1990.

Moore, PH, and Mettler, FA. Skin decontamination of commonly used medical radionuclides. *J Nucl Med* 21:475, 1980.

National Council on Radiation Protection and Measurements. *Management of Persons Accidentally Contaminated with Radionuclides.* Report No 65. Washington, DC: NCRP, 1980.

Ricks, RC, and Fry, SA (eds). *The Medical Basis for Radiation Accident Preparedness II. Clinical Experience and Follow-up Since 1979.* New York: Elsevier North-Holland, 1990.

81. Insects, Ticks, and Spiders

Francis P. Renzi

The phylum Arthropoda contains the largest number of organisms in the animal kingdom. This success results from their adaptation to a wide variety of environments and their ability to defend themselves. Although their benefits to humans are numerous, they are one of our greatest competitors and result in significant worldwide morbidity and mortality.

The classes of arthropods of importance with regard to bites or stings are Arachnida and Insecta. The medical consequences following exposure to these arthropods can range from annoying bites or infestations to life-threatening envenomations. In addition, complications such as secondary bacterial infection or disease transmission such as Lyme disease or Rocky Mountain spotted fever may occur. Although toxic reactions to venoms from bites or stings can be serious, it is usually the autopharmacologic response of the individual to the venom that is life threatening.

PATHOPHYSIOLOGY

Allergic reactions can result from many biting or stinging insects; however, major allergic responses in the United States usually result from Hymenoptera (bees, wasps, hornets, yellow jackets, and fire ants) stings. The venom contains amines such as histamine and serotonin, which produce a local sting reaction, while venom polypeptides and proteins induce an IgE-antibody response. On reexposure to the venom, antigen-antibody interaction releases mediators such as histamine, leukotrienes, eosinophilic chemotactic factor, bradykinins, and prostaglandins. Generally, these mediators result in increased capillary permeability and vasodilatation. In hypersensitive individuals, this response can produce a pronounced local reaction or systemic reactions ranging from mild, such as generalized pruritis and urticaria, to severe, such as anaphylaxis with bronchospasm, laryngeal edema, hypotension, coma, and death. It is estimated that about 4 percent of the population experiences a systemic sting reaction with 0.4 percent experiencing anaphylaxis.

HYMENOPTERA

Evaluation

The majority of hymenoptera stings produce only a local reaction and present with itching, redness, wheal formation, and pain at the site. An erythematous papule surrounded by a ring of edema may be seen as well as a stinger with or without the venom sac attached (the honeybee is the only species that leaves its stinger). With systemic reactions, symptoms usually occur within minutes but may be delayed for an hour or more. Generally, the later the onset of reaction, the less severe it is. Cutaneous manifestations may begin with generalized flushing and pruritis and progress to urticaria and angioedema. Upper respiratory complaints such as hoarseness, throat tightness, or dysphagia may progress to complete airway obstruction. Wheezing, cough, shortness of breath, and chest tightness can represent lower airway obstruction. Gastrointestinal symptoms of cramping, nausea, vomiting, or diarrhea are common. Cardiovascular dysfunction may be secondary to hypoxia, myocardial depression, loss of intravascular volume, and peripheral vasodilation. Physical findings may include cyanosis, pulmonary edema, hypotension, tachycardia, or vascular collapse.

Management

In patients with a local reaction, the skin should be inspected for the presence of a stinger and removed by scraping the skin with a scalpel without crushing the apparatus, thus preventing further envenomation.

Generalized allergic response requires immediate management of the cardiorespiratory system with supplemental oxygen, large-bore intravenous catheters, and fluid resuscitation as necessary. Epinephrine subcutaneously in mild to moderate reactions (0.3–0.5 ml 1:1000) or intravenously (2–5 ml 1:10,000) in severe reactions has been the mainstay of therapy. If symptoms persist or progress, repeat doses of epinephrine can be administered as necessary every 20 to 30 minutes or an intravenous infusion can be utilized. A tourniquet should be placed proximal to the sting site to reduce the rate of venom absorption. Bronchospasm can be treated with inhalational bronchodilators, and if wheezing persists, aminophylline, 5 to 6 mg/kg, should be given intravenously. Evidence of upper airway obstruction must be monitored continuously and may require endotracheal intubation. Intubation should also be considered in patients with central nervous system depression or shock. Aggressive volume replacement with crystalloids is necessary in the hypotensive patient. Antihistamines such as diphenhydramine will help limit urticaria and edema, whereas corticosteroids may prevent later recurrence of signs or symptoms of an allergic response. Tetanus prophylaxis should be provided as needed.

Disposition

Patients with local reactions can be discharged with wound care precautions and oral antihistamines. Patients with systemic reactions or a history of anaphylactic reaction who become symptom-free after observation in the emergency department can be discharged home. In addition to antihistamine therapy, it may be beneficial to include a brief course of corticosteroids. Instructions should be provided to return immediately if wheezing, dyspnea, hives, or dizziness occurs. All other patients should be admitted to the hospital for further therapy.

Patients with a systemic reaction should be provided with a prescription and instructions for an insect sting kit and referred to an allergist to be evaluated for desensitization immunotherapy.

All patients should be educated on prevention of future stings by wearing shoes when outdoors and avoiding perfumes and bright-colored clothing, which may attract insects. Hypersensitive individuals should also be advised to wear an identification medical tag or bracelet.

TICKS

Tick bites most often cause only local reactions with the formation of a pruritic papule that subsides in a few days. Occasionally, a secondary bacterial infection occurs or a granuloma may form if there is retention of the tick's mouthparts in the skin. Ticks may also act as a vector for significant systemic illnesses (Table 81-1) and may cause tick paralysis. The more common problems are discussed in the following sections.

Lyme Disease

Lyme disease is caused by a spirochete (*Borrelia burgdorferi*) carried by the deer tick (Ixodid species) and has become the most common tick-transmitted infectious disease reported in this country. Since the first description of the disease in Lyme, Connecticut, in 1975, cases have been reported in most states and in many other countries. Because of the tick's small size, the majority of patients with Lyme disease have no history of tick exposure. The disease has been characterized by three stages that can overlap or occur alone: first, with the appearance of erythema chronicum migrans (days to weeks); second, with the development of neurologic or cardiac manifestations (weeks to months); and third, with the development of arthritis (weeks to years). If left untreated, patients may develop fatal myocarditis, respiratory failure, and permanent neurologic deficits.

The optimal antibiotic regimen for Lyme disease is not known. Treatment of early disease can be accomplished with doxycycline (100 mg twice a day) or tetracycline (250–500 mg four times a day) for 10 days to 3 weeks. In children less than 8 years old and for pregnant or lactating women amoxicillin (250–500 mg three times a day or 20–40 mg/kg/day in three divided doses for children) is preferred. In patients with Lyme arthritis or with mild neurologic or cardiac disease doxycycline, tetracycline, or amoxicillin can be used but should be continued for 3 weeks to a month. For more serious central nervous system or cardiac disease ceftriaxone (2 gm/day IV for 10–21 days) or penicillin G (20–24 million units/day IV for 10–21 days) should be used.

The diagnosis of Lyme disease is based on clinical features and a high index of suspicion. Confirmation can be aided by the use of an indirect immunofluorescence assay.

Rocky Mountain Spotted Fever

Rocky Mountain spotted fever has been reported in nearly all states of the United States and results from the intracellular organism *Rickettsia rickettsii,* which produces widespread small vessel vasculitis in humans. The triad of fever, rash, and a history of tick exposure is present in only 60 percent of patients. After an incubation period of about 7 days, patients may develop a fever, severe headache, myalgia, abdominal pain, nausea, and vomiting. The rash appears on the fourth febrile day and may be the most reliable diagnostic sign. The lesions progress from pink macules located on

Table 81-1. North American tick-borne infectious diseases and their causative microorganisms

Rocky Mountain spotted fever	*Rickettsia rickettsii*
Lyme disease	*Borrelia burgdorferi*
Tularemia	*Francisella tularensis*
Colorado tick fever	*Arbovirus*
Relapsing fever	*Borrelia* species
Babesiosis	*Babesia microti*
Q fever	*Rickettsia burnetii*

the wrists, ankles, palms, and soles and spread centrally becoming confluent and hemorrhagic. If clinically suspected, treatment with tetracycline (25–50 mg/kg/day) or chloramphenicol (50–100 mg/kg/day) either orally or intravenously for a period of 7 to 10 days can prevent progression of the disease to vasomotor collapse and death. Various diagnostic serologic tests are available (Weil-Felix, latex agglutination, indirect fluorescent antibody) but may not be positive in the acute phase of the illness.

Tick Paralysis

In the case of tick paralysis, a neurotoxin is secreted in the saliva of several species of ticks, which acts on spinal and bulbar nuclei, slowing motor nerve conduction. Most cases occur in children during late spring and summer and begin with ataxia and areflexia that progresses to an ascending symmetric flaccid paralysis. The paralysis is progressive as long as the tick is present. Treatment involves removal of the tick and its mouthparts, with complete recovery usually within 48 hours.

Tick Removal

Many anecdotal methods have been described to remove ticks. The major considerations are to avoid crushing the tick, which would result in additional contamination of the wound, and to remove completely the tick and its mouthparts. The use of a curved forceps placed as close as possible to the skin and gently pulled steadily upward may be the most effective method. One should always wear gloves when removing ticks with the fingers and dispose of the tick appropriately.

Prevention of Disease

Prevention is best accomplished by avoidance of areas where tick bites are likely to occur. Otherwise, protective clothing, insect repellent, careful self-examination, and prompt careful removal of ticks will help reduce the incidence of reaction.

BLACK WIDOW SPIDER

Lactrodectus mactans, the black widow spider, has a body length of about 15 mm and is shiny black with red markings on its ventral abdomen. The venom from this spider releases neurotransmitters from both noradrenergic and cholinergic nerve endings. The bite itself may be unnoticed, but within 30 minutes to 3 hours, local symptoms of pain, numbness, and muscle fasciculations progress to generalized muscle rigidity. Examination of the bite site may reveal a halo lesion with two central puncture wounds. The patient will be restless, often with diaphoresis, lacrimation, and increased salivation. Symptoms from envenomation peak 1 to 6 hours after their onset and may last for several days. Muscle relaxants such as methocarbamol or a benzodiazepine can be used to control the muscle spasm, while narcotic analgesics can be used for pain. Treatment in the past included calcium gluconate given intravenously, which may be diagnostic as well as therapeutic. Hospitalization is not usually necessary unless pain or other symptoms persist or if the diagnosis is not certain.

Black widow spider antivenin is derived from horse serum and thus carries the risk of hypersensitivity and should be reserved for severe reactions in high-risk individuals (e.g., infants, elderly).

BROWN RECLUSE SPIDER

Loxosceles reclusa has a body length from 7 to 12 mm long, is brown in color, and has a dark brown to yellow violin-shaped marking on the dorsum of its cephalothorax. The venom from this spider causes direct destruction of cell walls, and its effect is perpetuated by release of vasoactive substances, complement activation, and vascular thrombosis.

The bite wound begins as a central macule or vesicle and progresses into a hemorrhagic blister with central necrosis within 12 to 24 hours. This lesion may enlarge over the following days to weeks. Although many bites have a relatively benign course, systemic symptoms of fever, chills, malaise, headache, and gastrointestinal distress may develop 12 to 24 hours after envenomation. Hemolysis may result in hemoglobinuria, thrombocytopenia, disseminated intravascular coagulation, renal failure, and death.

Treatment of the cutaneous reaction is controversial, with conservative management using pain medications, ice, elevation, and splinting becoming more popular. Dapsone, a polymorphonuclear leukocyte inhibitor, may be helpful in adults with rapidly progressive severe envenomations. Management of systemic arachnidism involves mainly symptomatic and supportive care. Corticosteroids are recommended by many authors and may protect red cells from hemolysis.

MISCELLANEOUS

Many other species of arthropods are responsible for victims seeking emergency department evaluation.

Flea bites, scabies, and lice infestation result in intense pruritis predisposing to secondary infection. Mosquito bites produce an immediate redness and wheal formation with itching and act as vectors for diseases such as encephalitis and malaria.

Although a bite from a tarantula or sting from a scorpion evokes great fear, it usually results in only a local reaction except for the bark scorpion (Centruroides sculpturatus), whose venom can be lethal.

The fire ant, which now exists in the southern United

States, bites its victim and pivots in a circular fashion, inflicting multiple stings. The stings produce a sterile pustule with local burning, redness, and itching. Several species of caterpillars and beetles are capable of producing a dermatitis. In the northeastern United States, the gypsy moth caterpillar has resulted in outbreaks of a pruritic urticarial rash.

SELECTED READING

Barr, SE. Allergy to Hymenoptera sting. *JAMA* 228:718, 1974.

Dattwyler, RJ, et al. Ceftriaxone as effective therapy in refractory Lyme disease. *J Infect Dis* 155:1322, 1987.

Elliot, DL, et al. Pet-associated illness. *N Engl J Med* 313:985, 1985.

Haller, JS, and Fabara, JA. Tick paralysis. *Am J Dis Child* 124:915, 1972.

Hattwick, MA, O'Brien, J, and Hanson, BF. Rocky Mountain spotted fever: Epidemiology of an increasing problem. *Ann Intern Med* 84:732, 1976.

Lichtenstein, LM, and Fauci, AS. *Current Therapy in Allergy and Immunology*. Philadelphia: B.C. Decker, 1983–1984. Pp. 70–83.

Mueller, HL. Further experiences with severe allergic reactions to insect stings. *N Engl J Med* 261:374, 1959.

Needham, GR. Evaluation of five popular methods of tick removal. *Pediatrics* 75:997, 1985.

Patterson, R, and Valentine M. Anaphylaxis and related allergic emergencies including reactions due to insect stings. *JAMA* 248:2632, 1982.

Rees, R, et al. A comparison of surgical excision versus dapsone and delayed surgical excision. *Ann Surg* 202L:659, 1985.

Steere, AC, et al. The early clinical manifestations of Lyme disease. *Ann Intern Med* 99:76, 1983.

Wasserman, GS, and Anderson, PC. Loxoscelism and necrotic arachnidism. *J Toxicol Clin Toxicol* 21:451, 1983–1984.

Wong, RC, Hughes SE, and Voorhees, JJ. Spider bites. *Arch Dermatol* 123:99, 1987.

Wright, SW, and AT. North American tick-borne diseases. *Ann Emerg Med* 17:964, 1988.

82. Snake Bites

Dee Hodge III

The basic human fear of snakes is locked in our primordial consciousness. Although snake bites are not as common as some would believe, there are 7,000 to 8,000 incidents reported per year in the United States. The case fatality rate is less than 1 percent, but the number of permanent deformities and amputations is reportedly much higher. Of the approximately 120 species in the United States, only 20 are venomous. We discuss here only those venomous animals commonly found within the continental United States. These venomous snakes fall into two families: The Crotalidae (pit vipers) include the rattlesnakes, copperheads, water moccasins, and cottonmouths and account for 98 percent of bites in the United States; and the Elapidae, or coral snakes. Most bites occur between April and October in the afternoon and early evening. The highest bite rates are found in North Carolina, Arkansas, Mississippi, and Louisiana. Of all bites, 90 percent are on the extremities. Eighteen-to-28-year-old men are most susceptible, accounting for 50 percent of all bite victims.

ETIOLOGY

The venomous snakes found in the continental United States are listed in Fig. 82-1.

The pit vipers are so-named because of the heat-sensitive pit located between and below the level of the eye and nostril on each side of the head. This heat sensor allows the snake to locate warm-blooded prey. Other characteristics of the pit vipers include the triangular-shaped head, elliptical pupils, single row of subcaudal plates, and the anal plate (Fig. 82-2).

The venom apparatus is composed of three parts: the gland, the duct, and the fangs. The gland is homologous to the human parotid gland. The discharge of venom is controlled by the contraction of muscles, which controls the amount of venom injected. The duct is loosely connected to the fang sheaths. The fangs are two elongated, hollow upper maxillary teeth about 8 to 19 mm long in the adult. The fangs fold against the roof of the mouth and are rotated forward during the strike.

The coral snakes are the only elapids native to North America. The distinctive banding of red next to yellow separates these snakes from nonvenomous mimickers. These snakes have small fixed fangs rather than rectractable fangs.

The venom is structurally complex, containing 5 to 15 enzymes and 3 to 12 nonenzymatic proteins and peptides. All venoms contain a combination of vascular toxins, neurotoxins, cardiotoxins, and hemotoxins. Toxicity varies with the species, individual-to-individual variations, time of the year, age of the snake, and environmental conditions. Twenty-five to 75 percent of the gland's venom is discharged

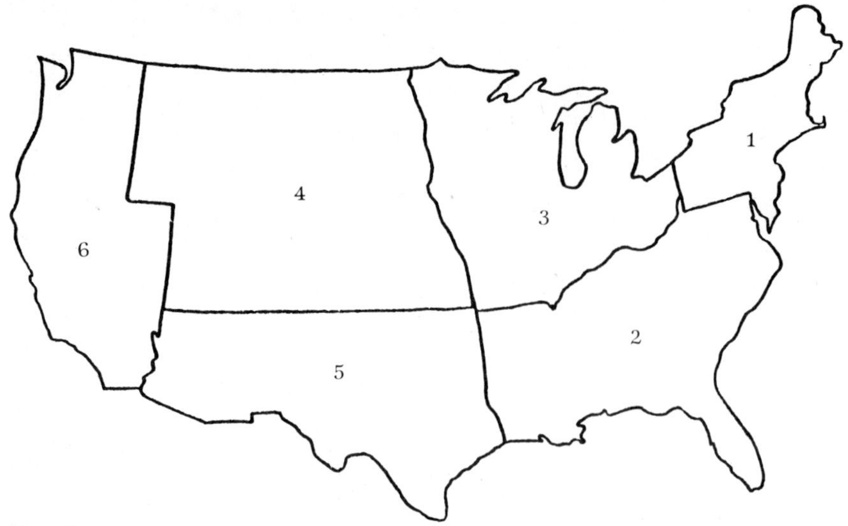

Common name	*Region*	*Common name*	*Region*
Western rattlesnake (*Crotalus viridis*)	4,5,6	Cottonmouth (*Agkistrodon piscivorus*)	2,3,5
Western diamondback (*Crotalus atrox*)	5,6	Copperhead (*Agkistrodon contortrix*)	1,2,3,4,5
Sidewinder (*Crotalus cerastes*)	5,6	Massasauga (*Sistrurus catenatus*)	3,4,5
Mojave rattlesnake (*Crotalus scutulatus*)	5,6	Pigmy rattlesnake (*Sistrurus miliarius*)	2,5
Eastern coral snake (*Micrurus fulvius*)	2	Eastern diamondback (*Crotalus adamonteaus*)	2
coral snake (*Micrurus euryxanthus*)	5	Timber rattlesnake (*Crotalus horridus*)	1,2,3,5

Fig. 82-1. Some venomous snakes of the United States by region. (Modified from F. E. Russell. *Snake Venom Poisoning.* Great Neck, NY: Scholium International Press, 1985.)

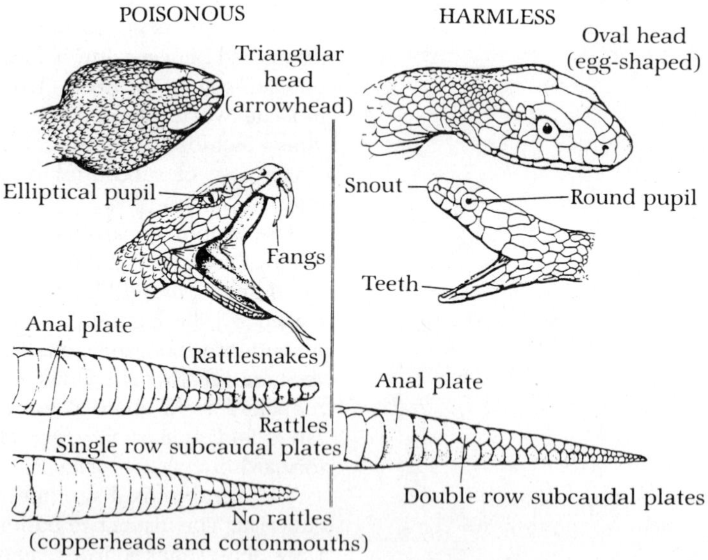

Fig. 82-2. Comparison of poisonous and nonpoisonous snakes. (From G. R. Fleisher, et al. [eds.]. *Pediatric Emergency Medicine.* © 1988, the Williams & Wilkins Co., Baltimore.)

during a strike. The amount injected varies with the weight and size of the animal bitten.

PATHOPHYSIOLOGY

The pathogenesis of the clinical features seen in envenomation is related to the constituents of the venom: local necrosis of tissue, hemolysis of red blood cells, defects in coagulation with disseminated intravascular coagulation (DIC), increase in prothrombin time, and decrease in the platelet count and active bleeding. Hemoconcentration is secondary to the plasma loss caused by the injury to intimal linings of blood vessels, including the lung. There is also pooling of blood in capillary beds. The most toxic constituents are the neurotoxins, which make up a large fraction of the venom of the Mojave rattlesnake. These toxins are related to phospholipase A and bind the nicotinic acetylcholine receptors and thus prevent the depolarizing action of acetylcholine.

CLINICAL FEATURES, SIGNS, AND SYMPTOMS

Rattlesnake and moccasin bites are characterized by one or two fang punctures with immediate pain, swelling, tingling, and numbness. The signs, symptoms, and severity of poisoning depend on the age and size of the patient, the species and size of the snake, depth and location of bites, the length of time the snake holds on, the amount injected, the condition of the fangs, the patient's sensitivity to the venom, and the degree and timing of the first aid. Table 82-1 lists the full range of symptoms.

Not all bites result in envenomation: 10 to 20 percent of bite victims have minimal or no signs of envenomation. The snake may also inject up to 90 percent of the contents of the gland. Multiple variables, including the individual's clinical response, is the only way to judge the severity of envenomation.

The bites of the pit vipers are consistently associated with immediate pain in the affected area. This does not hold true for the coral snakes and some other exotic snakes. The degree of pain is related to the amount of venom injected. The pain is followed by swelling, which gradually spreads proximally to involve the entire extremity. Swelling may continue up to 48 hours. Other local symptoms include erythema, ecchymosis, and bleeding at the bite site. Necrosis of the skin and subcutaneous tissue is a late sign and most often noted when inadequate doses of antivenin are administered. Generalized symptoms are many and varied (see Table 82-1). Hypotension commonly occurs after envenomation and is secondary to the disruption of the coagulation mechanism with DIC and increased capillary membrane permeability. Deaths from pit viper bites are due to DIC, hypotension, and massive pulmonary edema.

The signs and symptoms of coral snake bites and the bites of the Mojave rattlesnake are different because the venom contains neurotoxin, which has a direct effect on cardiac and skeletal muscle. Little or no pain or swelling may occur at the site of the bite. Symptoms and signs include ptosis, paresthesias, fasciculations, dysphagia, dysarthria, increased salivation, and proximal muscle weakness.

Table 82-1. Signs and symptoms of pit viper envenomation

Local
Fang puncture marks
Pain
Swelling
Vesicles
Erythema with progression to ecchymosis
Bleeding at bite site
Necrosis at bite site
Generalized
Perioral tingling
Metallic taste
Weakness
Syncope
Nausea and vomiting
Muscle fasciculation
Hypotension
Coagulopathy with bleeding
Respiratory distress
Renal failure

Other signs of snake bites result from secondary infection. Cellulitis, gas gangrene, tetanus, and osteomyelitis have all occurred in cases of snake bite with and without envenomation.

MANAGEMENT

The aim of treatment in all snake bites is simple:

1. Do no harm.
2. Retard the absorption of venom.
3. Neutralize venom as quickly as possible.
4. Prevent complications, including tetanus and secondary infections.

First aid measures for the bite victim involve immobilization of the bitten part and transport as quickly as possible to a medical facility. First aid measures as outlined in cowboy movies such as "snake bite medicine," surgical incisions of bitten extremities, oral suction, tourniquets, cryotherapy, and so on are based in folklore and are associated with a high morbidity at best.

Hospital management should proceed according to the following protocol:

1. *Establish a physiologic baseline.* Establish whether the patient has been bitten by a poisonous snake. Rapidly evaluate presenting signs and symptoms. Gather information regarding the event, including the approximate time of the bite, first aid measures, previous episodes of bites and treatments used, known allergies, and the date of the last tetanus immunization. Collect blood for a complete blood count, hematocrit, clotting screen, and type and crossmatch and obtain a urinalysis. Vital signs are obtained and recorded at regular intervals. Finally, measure and record the circumference of the injured extremity at the leading point of edema and 10 cm (4 in.) proximal to this level every hour for 12 hours.

2. *Determine the severity of envenomation.* Reactions are graded as follows:

No envenomation: Fang marks are present. There is no local swelling or hemorrhage and no paresthesia.
Minimal envenomation: Fang marks with local swelling are limited to the hand or foot and are not progressing. No systemic reactions occur.
Moderate envenomation: Swelling progresses rapidly beyond the site of the bite. Systemic reactions and laboratory changes are noted. There is a history of bite by a large snake or highly toxic species (eastern or western diamondback, Mojave rattlesnake).
Severe envenomation: There is pronounced and rapidly progressive swelling, ecchymoses, severe generalized symptoms, and laboratory abnormalities. History of multiple bites, large snake, and toxic species are noted.

3. *Start intravenous infusions in two extremities.*
4. *Do a skin test if envenomation has occurred to determine sensitivity to horse serum.* Follow the instructions in the brochure enclosed in the package. The skin test is not infallible, and the results should be used only as a precautionary guide.
5. *Administer an adequate amount of antivenin intravenously.*

No envenomation—no antivenin and no skin test.
Minimal—5 vials.
Moderate—10 vials.
Severe—15 or more vials.

The above amounts should be diluted 1:4 with 0.5N saline solution. The infusion should be started at a very slow rate—15 drops per minute. If no reaction occurs in 15 minutes, the rate may be increased so that the infusion is completed over a 2-hour period. The initial dose of antivenin should be repeated every 2 hours until the progression of the swelling has stopped. Children who weigh less than 45 kg should receive a larger dose by 50 percent. The total dose is the amount required to neutralize the poison as measured by the clinical response. Antivenin should be given within 4 hours of the bite, but it may be efficacious in symptomatic patients for at least 48 hours after a bite.

In serum-sensitive individuals, anaphylactoid reactions may be avoided by premedicating patients with 50 to 100 mg (children 1 mg/kg) of diphenhydramine hydrochloride (Benadryl) given intravenously 15 minutes before giving the antivenin, then administering diluted antivenin at a slow initial rate. If the patient is seriously envenomated, however, antivenin may be successfully administered by diluting to 1:10, decreasing the rate of administration, premedicating the patient with diphenhydramine, and titrating the response by giving epinephrine, 1:10,000 0.01 ml/kg. A consultation through one of the regional poison control centers is recommended if this procedure is required.

6. *Prevent secondary infection with appropriate broad-spectrum antibiotics.*
7. *Prevent tetanus.*
8. *Monitor and support vital functions.* This includes meperidine for pain, plasma expanders for shock, oxygen and ventilatory support, if needed, and dialysis. Local wound care is important but fasciotomy is not recommended.
9. *Prepare to treat serum sickness.* Serum sickness can be seen up to 21 days after administration of antivenin if more than seven vials were given. Corticosteroids are the drug of choice at a dose for prednisone of 10 mg qid or 1 mg/kg/day in children. Steroids are given until all signs and symptoms have subsided for 24 hours.
10. *Report all illegally possessed reptiles to the police or to the appropriate fish and game agency.*

A wall chart for emergency department snake identification and treatment is available from Arizona Poison Information Center, University of Arizona, 1501 North Campbell Avenue, Tucson, AZ 85724. In addition, the Oklahoma Poison Center can provide valuable information as well as a resource for available antitoxins for exotic snakes at 1–405–271–5454.

SELECTED READING

Banner, W. Bites and stings in the pediatric patient. *Curr Probl Pediatr* 18:1, 1988.
Christopher, DG, and Rodning, CB. Crotalidae envenomation. *South Med J* 79:159, 1986.
Ennik, F. Death from bites and stings of venomous animals. *West J Med* 133:463, 1980.
Pennell, TC, Babu, SS, and Meredith, JW. The management of snake and spider bites in the southeastern United States. *Am Surg* 53:198, 1987.
Picchioni, AL, et al. Management of poisonous snakebite. *Vet Hum Toxicol* 26:139, 1984.
Russell, FE. *Snake Venom Poisoning.* Great Neck, NY: Scholium International Press, 1985.
Russell, FE, and Picchioni, AL. Snake venom poisoning. *Clin Tox Con* 5:73, 1983.
Russell, FE, et al. Snake venom poisoning in the United States; experiences with 550 cases. *JAMA* 233:341, 1975.
Simon, TL, and Grace, TG. Envenomation coagulopathy in wounds from pit vipers. *N Engl J Med* 305:443, 1981.
Sprenger, TR, and Bailey, WJ. Snakebite treatment in the United States. *Int J Dermatol* 25:479, 1986.
Stewart, ME, et al. First aid treatment of poisonous snakebite: Are currently recommended procedures justified? *Ann Emerg Med* 10:331, 1981.
Watt, CH. Poisonous snakebite treatment in the United States. *JAMA* 240:654, 1978.
Wingert, WA, and Chan, L. Rattlesnake bites in Southern California and rationale for recommended treatment. *West J Med* 148:37, 1988.
Wingert, WA, and Wainschel, J. Diagnosis and management of envenomation by poisonous snakes. *South Med J* 68:1015, 1975.

83. Dangerous Marine Bites, Stings, and Ingestions

Dee Hodge III

In this chapter, the clinical diagnosis and management of injuries resulting from the bites and stings of commonly encountered marine animals are discussed. There is little information on the incidence of these injuries. The increasing popularity of boating, surfing, wind surfing, snorkeling, and scuba diving provide for increased contact with marine organisms. Emergency department personnel in coastal areas must be prepared to treat these injuries. Because of public and private marine aquaria inland, health care providers in these areas may also be called on to treat marine injuries. Those venomous marine animals encountered within the tidal zone or commonly washed ashore within the continental United States, Canada, and Hawaii are discussed here. Poisoning from ingestion of marine organisms is also discussed.

The type of injuries seen can be used to help identify the offending marine organism. Table 83-1 provides the reader with a quick reference to the injuries and the group of organisms associated with them.

In general, any patient with a suspected bite or sting should undergo an overall assessment, including vital signs, location and size of bite or sting marks, pain, swelling, color of the surrounding skin, and any systemic symptoms. General care, especially meticulous local wound care, is mandatory. The offending species should be identified if possible to determine whether it is a venomous animal and to determine the physiologic effects of the specific venom on humans. Once this is established, definitive care can be rendered.

The marine environment can provide an excellent inoculum for wound infections. Most common marine bacteria are heterotrophic, motile, and facultatively anaerobic gram-negative rods. Common organisms include *Vibrio* species, *Erysipelothrix rhusiopathiae*, and *Mycobacterium marinum.* No antibiotic prophylaxis is recommended in normal individuals, but vigorous irrigation with saline, wound debridement, and leaving the wound open, unless suturing is required for cosmetic reasons, are the basic tenets for management. Infected wounds should be cultured, and surgical incision and drainage should be performed. Antibiotic treatment of minor infections can be done on an outpatient basis. Trimethoprim-sulfamethoxazole or tetracycline are the antibiotics of choice except in wounds with an erysipeloid appearance, in which case erythromycin is indicated. If hospitalization is required, parenteral gentamicin, tobramycin, or amikacin are recommended prior to culture and sensitivity results.

Table 83-1. Injuries associated with marine organisms

Lacerations
- Invertebrates
  - Coral (phylum Cnidera)
- Vertebrates
  - Sharks
  - Barracudas
  - Moray eels
  - Stingrays

Stings
- Invertebrates
  - Portuguese man-of-war
  - Jellyfish
  - Sea anemones
  - Sea corals

Puncture wounds
- Invertebrates
  - Sea urchins
- Vertebrates
  - Stingrays
  - Scorpion fishes

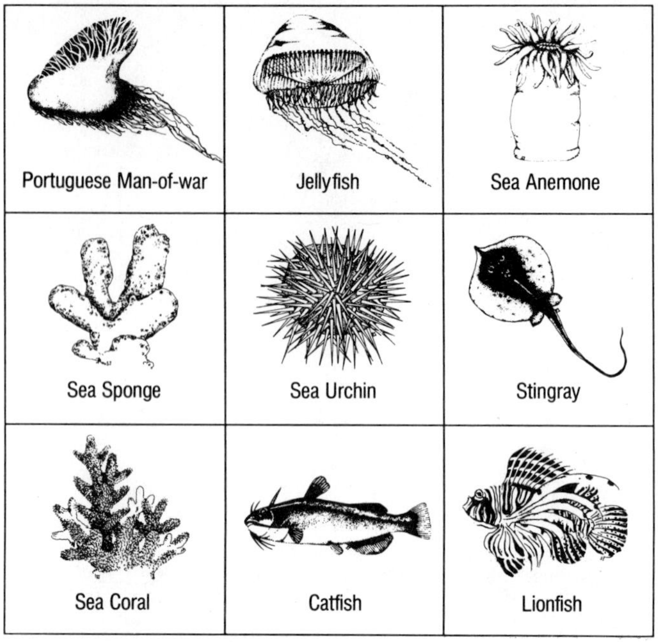

Fig. 83-1. The various marine animals are depicted that can inflict wounds, bites, or stings on unwary swimmers, snorklers, and scuba divers. (From C.L. Rosson and S.W. Tolle. Management of marine stings and scrapes. *West J. Med.* 150:97,1989.)

MARINE INVERTEBRATES

Phylum Cnidera (Coelenterata)

The primitive creatures in the phylum Cnidera are a diverse group encompassing some of the most beautiful as well as deadly marine animals. The phylum is divided into three large classes: the Hydrozoa (hydras, Portuguese man-of-war), Schyphozoa (true jellyfish), and the Anthozoa (soft corals, stone corals, and anemones) (Fig. 83-1).

All members of the phylum have nematocysts—organelles specialized to entangle, penetrate, anchor, and poison prey (Fig. 83-2). Firing of the nematocysts is not fully understood; the process may be protein or cation mediated. Whatever the exact mechanism, weakening of the nematocyst capsule releases a hollow barbed thread containing toxin. The nematocysts of most species cannot penetrate human skin; therefore, although cnidarian stings are the most frequent envenomations encountered in the marine environment, most stings are mild to moderate skin irritations only. Those that do penetrate cause severe pain, serious illness, or even death. Most nematocyst venoms consist of a mixture of peptides or proteins varying in both chemical and physical properties among coelenterate species. Stings from sessile forms are not as severe, in general, as stings from free-floating forms.

Toxic effects include hemolysis, dermatonecrosis, paralysis, and cardiac conduction abnormalities. Burning pain and urticaria are secondary to the presence of serotonin, histamine, or histamine-releasing agents found in the cytoplasm.

Class Hydrozoa and Class Schyphozoa

The more commonly encountered species of the hydrozoa and schyphozoa are:

Class Hydrozoa
- *Physalia physalis*—Portuguese man-o-war

Class Schyphozoa
- *Pelagia noctiluca*—Purple jellyfish
- *Chrysaora guinguecinda*—Sea nettle
- *Cyanea capillata*—Lion's mane

Stings from both classes share many of the same clinical manifestations. These manifestations can be grouped and listed as follows:

- Acute local reactions
  - Eruption and pain due to toxin
  - Exaggerated local angioedema
  - Delayed reactions up to several hours
  - Recurrent eruptions up to four episodes
  - Distant site reactions
  - Papular urticaria
- Chronic reactions
  - Keloids
  - Pigmentation
  - Fat atrophy
  - Contractions
  - Gangrene, vascular spasm
  - Mononeuritis
  - Autonomic nerve paralysis
  - Urticaria
- Generalized reactions
  - Toxin-induced
    - Immediate cardiac arrest
    - Rapid respiratory arrest
    - Renal hypotension
  - Anaphylaxis
  - Respiratory acidosis

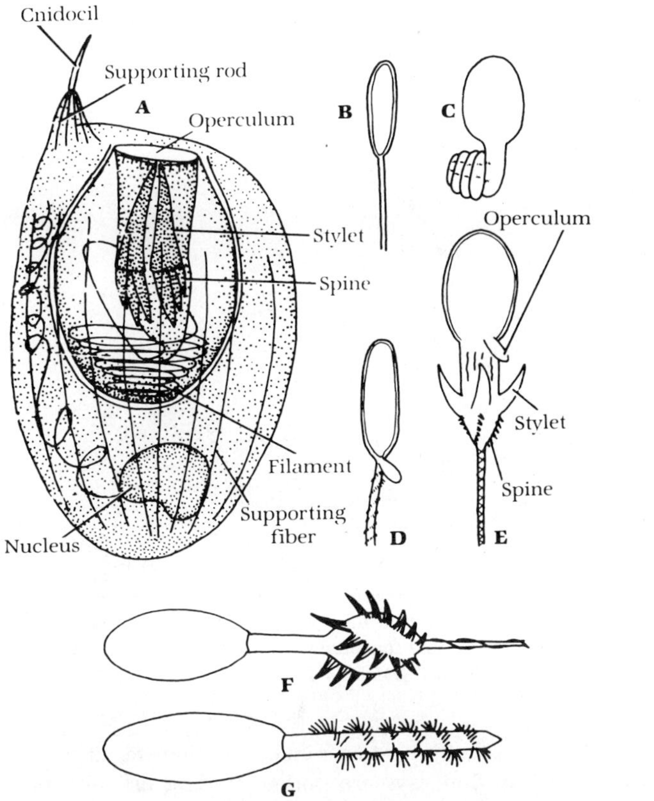

Fig. 83-2. Cnidoblast and nematocysts. A. A schematized cnidoblast containing an undischarged nematocyst. B–G. Discharged nematocysts: B. *Hydra* atrichous isohiza (streptoline glutinant). C. *Hydra* desmoneme (volvent). D. *Hydra* holotrichous isorhiza (steroline glutinant). E. *Hydra* stenotele (penetrant). F. Eurytele. G. Amastigophore. (From P.A. Meglitsch. *Invertebrate Zoology* [2nd ed.]. New York: Oxford, 1972.)

Management of schyphozoan and hydrozoan stings should meet two objectives: (1) to minimize the number of nematocysts being discharged, and (2) to reduce the immediate harmful effects resulting from the discharged nematocysts. Any adhering tentacles should be removed carefully. The unexploded nematocysts should be inactivated by topical application for 30 minutes with vinegar (3% acetic acid) or a slurry of baking soda, or meat tenderizer (papain). The area should be washed with sea water, and corticosteroid cream or lotion should be applied.

In controlling systemic effects, oxygen and intravenous fluids may be required. Severe pain should be controlled with intramuscular codeine or meperidine. The cardiac status should be monitored. Ten percent calcium gluconate intravenously may relieve painful muscle spasms.

Class Anthozoa

The anemones found within the tidal zone of the United States are only mildly toxic. Coral cuts and stings are a problem for swimmers off the Florida and Hawaiian coasts. The severity of coral cuts is due to a combination of laceration of tissue, nematocyst venom, foreign debris in the wound, and secondary bacterial infection. Cellulitis, lymphangitis, fever, and malaise commonly occur.

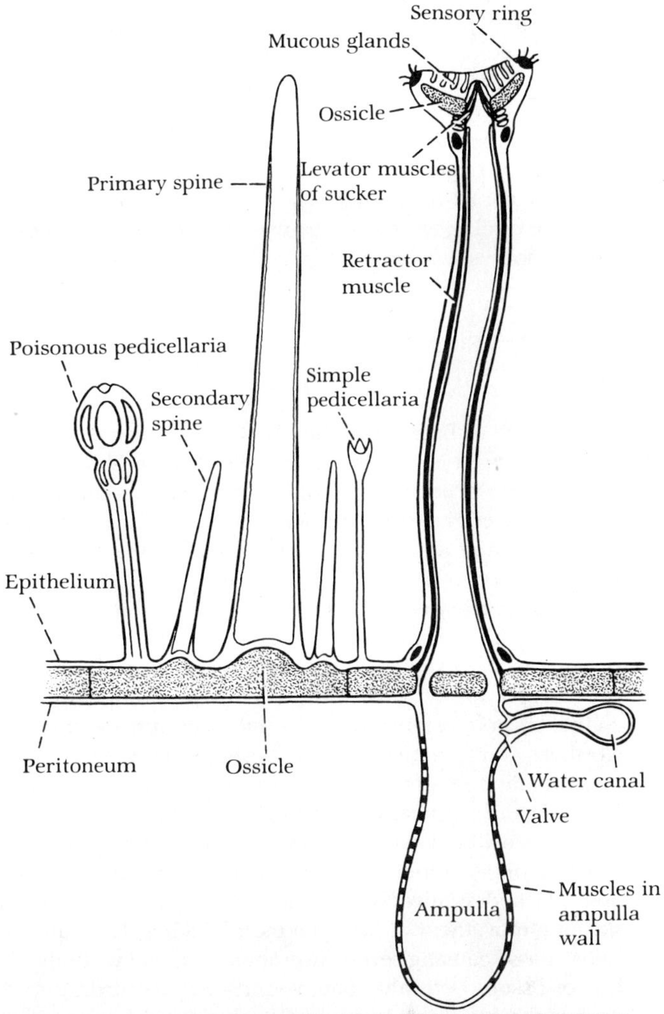

Fig. 83-3. Diagrammatic section through the body way of a sea urchin, showing one ambulacral and one interambulacral ossicle and associated structures. (From R.D. Barnes. *Invertebrate Zoology* [2nd ed.]. Philadelphia: Saunders, 1968.)

Treatment consists of cleaning the wound and irrigation with copious amounts of saline. All foreign particles must be removed. Wounds should not be sutured. Prophylactic antibiotic therapy is controversial. Antibiotic therapy is probably best withheld until there is evidence of wound infection.

Phylum Echinodermata

The phylum Echinodermata includes the starfish, sea urchins, and sea cucumbers. Of the 80 species venomous to humans, the majority are found in tropical waters. The calcareous spines of urchins encountered off American coasts do not contain poison glands. However, between the spines are small pincer-like organs called *pedicellariae,* which serve as venom organs (Fig. 83-3). Traumatic injury by penetration of the spines usually occurs without envenomation. Spines easily pierce the skin and may penetrate wet suits and sneakers. The brittle spines break off readily in the wound. Clinically, penetration is accompanied by intense pain followed by redness, swelling, and an aching sensation. Complications include tattooing of the skin, secondary infection, and granuloma formation if the spine is left in situ.

Treatment includes removal of all spines as completely as possible. If spines break off in the wound, debridement should be performed with local anesthetic under aseptic conditions. Irrigation of the wound with a 20-gauge needle attached to a 30-ml syringe is helpful in cleaning the wound. Systemic antibiotics should be used for secondary infection. No antidote is available.

MARINE VERTEBRATES

Sharks

The chance of being assaulted by a shark along the North American coast is roughly one in five million. However, clinicians who practice in coastal areas may be called on to manage a victim of these creatures because of the large number of sporting activities that take place in the ocean environment.

Most attacks are by the grey reef, great white, blue, and mako sharks. Factors increasing the risk of attack include swimming near sewer outlets, late afternoon and early evening hours, murky warm water, increased commotion, deep channels, and bright objects. Attacks of surfers along the Northern California coast are believed to be due to the misinterpretation of surfboard shapes in the water as elephant seals, part of the shark's usual diet.

The shark is usually not seen prior to the attack. Two types of bite wounds are described: (1) tangential injury, and (2) a definitive bite. Tangential injury is caused by slashing movement of the open mouth as the shark makes a "close pass" causing severe lacerations, incised wounds, and loss of tissue. Definitive bite wounds vary according to the part of the body seized by the shark. Most injuries involve only one or two bites and are confined to the extremities.

Hypovolemic shock due to extensive hemorrhage is the immediate threat to life in shark attacks. Bleeding should be controlled at the scene with direct compression, and intravascular volume should be replaced using crystalloid solutions until blood products are available. MAST devices may be used as an adjunct. The victim should be kept warm and given oxygen during transportation to an emergency department. Tetanus toxoid and tetanus immune globulin should be considered, and prophylactic penicillin in moderate doses (100,000–200,000 units/kg/day) is recommended.

Venomous Fish

There are at least 200 species of fish known to be venomous, including stingrays, scorpion fish, zebra fish, stonefish, weeverfish, toadfish, stargazers, ratfish, catfish, and surgeonfish. They are generally found in shallow water and around reefs, kelp beds, or coral. All are nonmigratory and slow swimming and are often buried in sand.

Stingrays

Stingrays are the single most important group of venomous fishes, accounting for an estimated 750 attacks per year in North America. These animals are found off all U.S. coasts and range in size from several inches in diameter to over 14 feet in length. Stingrays are bottom feeding fish and bury themselves in sand or mud of bays, shoals, lagoons, and river mouths. Envenomation occurs when an unsuspecting swimmer steps on the back of the animal and causes it to hurl its tail upward into the victim, a reflex defense response (Fig. 83-4).

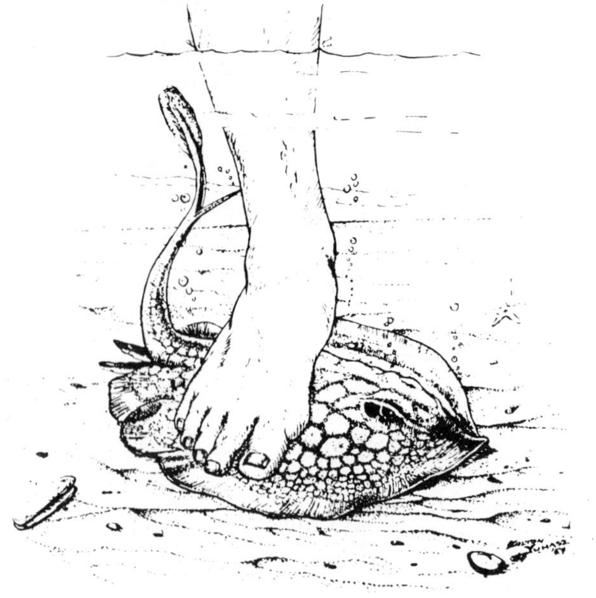

Fig 83-4. Stinging action of the round stingray. (From F.E. Russell, et al. Studies on the mechanism of death from stingray venom. *Am. J. Med. Sci.* 235:566, 1958.)

The venom is delivered by a serrated, retropointed, dentinal caudal spine located on the dorsum of the tail. The spines vary in length depending on the size of the ray. The spine is encased in an integumentary sheath that contains specialized secretory cells that contain venom. When the skin of the victim has been punctured by the barb, the integumentary sheath over the spine is ruptured, causing the venom to pass along the ventrolateral grooves into the wound. Laceration of the victim's tissue when the spine is withdrawn enhances absorption and distribution of the toxin. The venom is extremely heat labile. It contains at least 15 fractions, including serotonin, 5-nucleotidase, and phosphodiesterase. The toxin depresses medullary respiratory centers, interferes with the cardiac conduction system, and produces severe local pain.

The clinical manifestations are a result of the wound and the toxin. The wound produced by the stingray barb is a combination of puncture and laceration. Wounds vary in length from 3.5 to 15.0 cm. The sting is followed immediately by pain, which spreads from the site of injury and reaches its greatest intensity within 90 minutes. Generalized symptoms include syncope, weakness, nausea, vomiting, diarrhea, anxiety, sweating, and muscle fasciculations of the affected extremity. Generalized cramps, hypotension, cardiac arrhythmias, and death may occur. The wound has a jagged edge, which may be discolored and subsequently necrose. Remains of the integumentary sheath may be retained and may contaminate the wound.

Management of the scene includes irrigating the wound with cold salt water or sterile saline if available. Flushing can help remove much of the venom. Bleeding should be controlled with direct pressure. On arrival in the emergency department, any remnants of the integumentary sheath seen in the wound should be removed. The extremity should be placed in hot water (38–46°C) for 30 to 90 minutes. After soaking, the wound should be explored and further debrided. Pain may be relieved by meperidine (1–2 mg/kg). Tetanus prophylaxis should always be considered. Antibiotics are best reserved for wounds that become secondarily infected.

Scorpaenidae

Eighty species found in the Scorpaenidae family include the zebra fish, scorpion fish proper, and the stonefish. The venom apparatus consists of a number of dorsal, anal, and pelvic spines, covered by integumentary sheaths containing venom glands lying within anterolateral grooves. The venoms are unstable compounds between 50,000 and 800,000 daltons in weight.

The clinical signs and symptoms are essentially the same, varying among the species in degree only. Severe pain at the site of the wound is the first and primary clinical sign for all species. The wound and the surrounding area become ischemic and then cyanotic. Paresthesia and paralysis of the extremity may occur. Other clinical signs include nausea, vomiting, hypotension, tachypnea proceeding to apnea, and myocardial ischemia with electrocardiographic (ECG) changes.

MANAGEMENT. Treatment involves irrigating the wound with salt water or sterile saline. This is followed by immersion of the injured extremity in hot water (40°C) for 30 to 60 minutes or until the agonizing pain is completely relieved. Meperidine hydrochloride (1–2 mg/kg) may be required for pain. Patients should be monitored carefully for cardiotoxic effects and respiratory depression. Antivenin is available only for the stings of the stonefish of Australia and may be obtained from local zoos or aquariums. The initial dose depends on the number of puncture wounds the victim has received (1 ampule/2 wounds IM).

POISONING FROM INGESTION OF MARINE ORGANISMS

A variety of marine organisms are poisonous when ingested. Paralytic and neurotoxic shellfish poisoning account for all reported outbreaks of shellfish poisoning and ciguatera and scombroid fish poisoning account for 99 percent of vertebrate fish poisoning. Identification of the ingested organism is most helpful in establishing the diagnosis. All foods and beverages ingested should be evaluated. Identification on clinical findings may be difficult since many toxic marine ingestions share clinical manifestations. This is due in part because ciguatra and paralytic shellfish poisoning are caused by toxins that block voltage-gated sodium channels in myelinated and nonmyelinated nerves.

Shellfish

Mussels, clams, and crabs may be poisonous when these filter feeders have ingested toxic unicellular dinoflagellates. It is not known how the toxin accumulates or concentrates in the shellfish, but it does not affect them adversely. When the concentration of these dinoflagellates in the water are greater than or equal to 20,000/cubic mm, red, yellow, green, or blue tides are produced. It is at these times of the year that toxic levels in the shellfish are at their highest. The toxin is one of the most lethal known; minimum lethal dose is 1 to 4 mg, and there is a case fatality rate of 1 to 10 percent.

The toxic effects are due to direct depressant action on cardiac conduction leading to bundle branch block and decreased conduction of peripheral nerves, producing a curare-like effect.

The signs and symptoms of shellfish poisoning may be gastrointestinal, allergic, or paralytic. Gastrointestinal symptoms are most common and are probably due to bacterial pathogens rather than toxic tissues. Symptoms include nausea, vomiting, diarrhea, and abdominal pain usually within 8 to 12 hours after ingestion and lasting up to 48 hours. Allergic symptoms include erythema, swelling, urticaria, pruritus, and, in sensitive individuals, generalized edema and respiratory distress. Paralytic symptoms and signs are due to the toxin. These include paresthesia, distorted sensory and proprioception, weakness, headache, salivation and perfuse perspiration, decreased deep tendon reflexes, and bradycardia. Symptoms may progress to cardiac failure, respiratory paralysis, and death. The first 12 hours are critical, with survival past this period usually associated with a favorable prognosis.

No antidote is available. Treatment is supportive. Antihistamines, sympathomimetics, and, possibly, corticosteroids are indicated for the allergic symptoms. For the paralytic symptoms, oxygen, assisted pulmonary ventilation, and digitalization for cardiac abnormalities may be necessary.

Ciguatoxin or Ciguatera Poison

Ciguatera poisoning is found in more than 400 species of fish, many of which are edible, including barracudas, groupers, sea bass, snapper, jacks, surgeonfish, and parrot fish. It is the most commonly reported poisoning from vertebrate fish. The toxin is produced by a marine dinoflagellate, *Gambierdiscus toxicus,* which attaches itself to blue-green algae and is concentrated in fish tissues in the progression up the food chain. Little is known about the toxin but that it is heat stable and has anticholinesterase-like activity.

Clinical symptoms generally occur within 6 hours after ingestion, with the majority occurring within 12 hours. At least 180 manifestations can occur. Gastrointestinal symptoms usually occur and, when present, include nausea, vomiting, diarrhea, and abdominal cramps. When gastrointestinal symptoms occur, they precede the neurologic symptoms. Neurologic symptoms include pain and weakness in the lower extremities, arthralgias, circumoral paresthesia, hot and cold reversal, headache, myalgia and paresthesia in the extremities, ataxia, ptosis, and cranial nerve palsies. Neurologic symptoms may last from a few days to weeks. Cardiovascular signs and symptoms include hypotension and bradycardia.

There is no known antidote, and therapy is supportive. Atropine is necessary for symptomatic bradycardia (0.01 mg/kg), and intravenous fluids and dopamine infusion are given for hypotension. Although other drugs have been given to patients with ciguatera fish poisoning, the results have been variable and none have proven efficacy under controlled clinical trials.

Scombroid Poisoning

Scombroid poisoning is the second most common poisoning from vertebrate fish. The poisoning is due to inadequate preservation of mackerel-like fish such as tunas, skipjack, and bonitas. The toxin is due to the bacterial breakdown of endogenous histidine in the fish flesh to histamine and saurine.

Symptoms occur minutes to hours after ingestion and are related to severe histamine-mediated reaction. Symptoms include erythema, giant urticaria, pruritus, nausea, vomiting, abdominal cramps, watery diarrhea, bronchospasm, and hypotension. Symptoms tend to be self-limited, lasting 8 to 10 hours.

To prevent absorption of histamine, emesis should be induced if vomiting and diarrhea have not occurred spontaneously. Treatment consists of cimetidine, 300 mg intravenously (pediatric dose 20 mg/kg) over 5 to 30 minutes. This gives immediate and complete resolution of symptoms. Subcutaneous injections of epinephrine or intramuscular or intravenous antihistamines may also be used.

SELECTED READING

General

Auerbach, PS. Natural microbiologic hazards of the aquatic environment. *Clin Dermatol* 5:52, 1987.

Auerbach, PS, et al. Bacteriology of the marine environment: Implications for clinical therapy. *Ann Emerg Med* 16:643, 1987.

Ennik, F. Death from bites and stings of venomous animals. *West J Med* 133:463, 1980.

Halstead, BW. *Poisonous and Venomous Marine Animals of the World.* Princeton: Darwin Press, 1978.

Marine Invertebrates

Auerbach, PS. Hazardous marine animals. *Emerg Med Clin North Am* 2:531, 1984.

Baden, HP. Injuries from sea urchins. *Clin Dermatol* 5:112, 1987.

Beeching, N, and Morgan, HV. Sea urchin granuloma of the toe. *Practitioner* 226:1567, 1982.

Burnett, JW, and Calton, GJ. Venomous pelagic Coelenterates: Chemistry, toxicology, immunology and treatment of their stings. *Toxicon* 25:581, 1987.

Burnett, JW, et al. Local and systemic reactions from jellyfish stings. *Clin Dermatol* 5:14, 1987.

Burnett, JW, Calton, GJ, and Morgan, RJ. Venomous sea urchins. *Cutis* 38:151, 1986.

Burnett, JW, Rubinstein, H, and Calton, GJ. First aid for jellyfish envenomation. *South Med J* 76:870, 1983.

Halstead, BW. Coelenterate (Cnidarian) stings and wounds. *Clin Dermatol* 5:8, 1987.

Marine Vertebrates

Baldridge, HD, and Williams, J. Shark attack: Feeding or fighting? *Multi Med* 134:130, 1969.

Bitseff, EL, et al. The management of stingray injuries of the extremities. *South Med J* 63:417, 1970.

Grainger, CR. Sting ray injuries. *Trans R Soc Trop Med Hyg* 79: 443, 1985.

Halstead, BW, and Vinci, JM. Venomous fish stings (Ichthyocanthotoxicoses). *Clin Dermatol* 5:29, 1987.

Kizer, KW. Marine envenomations. *J Toxicol Clin Toxicol* 21:527, 1983.

Russell, FE. Stingray injuries: A review and discussion of their treatment. *Am J Med Sci* 226:611, 1953.

White, JAM. Shark attack in Natal. *Injury* 6:187, 1976.

Wingert, WA. Envenomation by Poisonous Arthropods and Marine Animals. In VC Kelley (ed), *Practice of Pediatrics.* Philadelphia: Harper & Row, 1985.

Ingestion of Marine Organisms

Hughes, JM, and Merson, MH. Current concepts: Fish and shellfish poisoning. *N Engl J Med* 295:1117, 1976.

Lange, WR. Ciguatera toxicity. *Am Fam Phys* 35:177, 1987.

Morris, JG, et al. Clinical features of ciquatera fish poisoning. *Arch Intern Med* 142:1090, 1982.

Sims, JK. A theoretical discourse on the pharmacology of toxic marine ingestions. *Ann Emerg Med* 16:1006, 1987.

84. Dysbarism

MOUNTAIN SICKNESS AND OTHER DISORDERS AT HIGH ALTITUDE

Stefan Goldberg
Robert Schoene

HISTORICAL PERSPECTIVES

People have lived as high as 17,000 feet in the Andes and the Himalaya for thousands of years. Those who resided permanently at high altitude adapted and did well, whereas low altitude residents were rarely exposed to the physiologic stresses of moving into the rarefied atmosphere of the earth's highland regions. Except for some transcontinental trading, in times past, people moved very little from one altitude to another. Recently, however, with increasing travel, for economic and military reasons at first, then for recreation, more people have sojourned to higher regions and have suffered the consequences of relatively rapid ascents to high altitude.

Isolated descriptions of mountain sickness date at least as far back as 2000 years when Too Kin, a government official of the Western Han Dynasty, included a description of mountain sickness in a travel report to his emperor, as described by Gilbert: "Next, one comes to Big Headache and Little Headache Mountains, as well as Red Earth and Swelter Hills. They make a man so hot that his face turns pale, his head aches, and he begins to vomit. Even the donkeys and swine react this way." According to Houston, in 1500, Mirza Mohammad Haidar, a trader who traveled in Asia from Tashkent to Tibet wrote another description of mountain sickness. He described the symptoms that he felt and that he observed in his fellow travelers, including nausea, breathlessness, sleeplessness, paroxysmal nocturnal dyspnea, peripheral edema, mental status changes, and sometimes death. He noticed that only sojourners were affected, whereas the Tibetans were unscathed by these problems. Gilbert describes how in 1590, Father Jose d'Acosta, a Jesuit priest, also reported the adverse consequences of traveling to high altitude. He wrote in graphic detail about the physical discomforts suffered by members of his company traveling high in the mountains of Peru. He even speculated that he and his fellow travelers became ill because "the element of the aire there is so subtle and delicate . . . the breathing of man requires a more gross and temperate aire." These early travelers were describing illnesses that are peculiar to the higher regions of the earth: acute mountain sickness (AMS), high altitude pulmonary edema (HAPE), and high altitude cerebral edema (HACE).

Houston writes that during the Renaissance, travelers and scientists learned more about the atmosphere and the effects of ascent to regions of low atmospheric pressure. In 1648, Florin Perier, a French scientist, first demonstrated the drop in barometric pressure on ascent to high altitude when he carried a mercury barometer to the summit of the Puy de Dome (3468 ft). Through the course of the following century,

Mayow, Lavoisier, and Priestley, among other scientists in Western Europe, discovered and described oxygen. Paul Bert simulated high altitude with experiments on humans in partially evacuated steel chambers and was associated with the flight of the Zenith in 1875. This famous hot air balloon rose to over 26,000 ft, resulting in the hypoxic death of two of the three scientists aboard.

With the increasing popularity of recreational mountaineering in the nineteenth century, more people made rapid ascents to high altitude and suffered the consequences thereof, as Houston describes. Dramatic accounts were written by the famous mountaineers Edward Whymper in the Alps and Edward Fitzgerald in the Andes. J. S. Haldane conducted research at the top of Pikes Peak (above 14,000 ft) in Colorado in 1911, where a train took large numbers of tourists. He compared the scene "to that on the deck or in the cabin of a cross-channel steamer in rough weather" with tourists in obvious distress, lined up at the rail holding their heads and vomiting.

Climbers and others making rapid ascents to the high mountains in this century experienced illness at high altitude, including specific syndromes of severe neurologic and pulmonary illness. Ravenhill, the physician at a mining camp at 15,000 ft in Peru, called these syndromes *nervous and cardiac puna.* In 1960, Charles Houston published the first modern description of high altitude pulmonary edema and attributed it to noncardiac causes. Pulmonary symptoms were previously diagnosed and treated as acute congestive heart failure or pneumonia. Modern descriptions of mountain sickness include those of Singh et al. and Hackett et al. The article by Hackett et al., based on observations of trekkers in the Mount Everest region of Nepal, was accompanied by an editorial that poetically alludes to several aspects of this disease in its title: "See Nuptse and die."

EPIDEMIOLOGY

Most mountain sickness in the world occurs in resort and recreation areas where large numbers of people travel rapidly from sea level to altitudes over 8,000 ft and spend several days, often engaging in strenuous activity. At Colorado ski areas, for example (8,000 to 9,000 ft base altitudes), 12 to 17 percent of all skiers develop mountain sickness, which results in $50 to $70 million each year in lost revenue to the tourist industry. At higher altitudes, the incidence increases. Among climbers of Mt. Rainier (14,410 ft), the incidence rate is 67 percent. Overall, there is also a small but significant mortality from severe mountain sickness. In the early 1970s, 10 of 500 trekkers per year who visited the Everest region of Nepal (14,000 to 18,000 ft) died of HAPE and HACE. Currently, about 5,000 trekkers per year visit the same region, and one or two of them die of HAPE or HACE. The tremendous improvements in public awareness and understanding of mountain sickness in the last 2 to 3 decades have led to this dramatic decrease in mortality from severe mountain sickness.

CLINICAL PRESENTATION

Case 1

During a cross-country ski trip from Aspen, Colorado (7900 ft), over a 12,000 ft pass, a 21-year-old college student developed dyspnea, weakness, and cough. These symptoms worsened the following day to the point that he could not proceed. His companion left him in a tent and returned late the next day with help. The student was alert, "desperately dyspneic on the slightest exertion," and coughing severely. He was evacuated to the nearest hospital, where he was cyanotic and dyspneic and had diffuse rales but a normal cardiac examination, with a pulse of 96 beats per minute. Chext x-ray film showed a diffuse infiltrate, right greater than left, and a normal cardiac silhouette. He also had a low-grade fever and a mild leukocytosis. He was treated with penicillin, supplemental oxygen, and an oral diuretic. No diuresis occurred, but he improved rapidly and was symptom-free within 36 hours of admission.

Case 2

A physically fit, 35-year-old surgeon from the East Coast flew to a Colorado ski area for a one-week vacation. During his first night at 8,000 feet, he was restless and slept poorly. He arose early the following morning with a severe global headache, mild nausea, no appetite for breakfast, and very little urine output. The headache improved to a dull ache, and the nausea resolved after moving about his condominium for an hour. Trying to keep up with his local friends, he started skiing on strenuous, difficult runs. He was soon exhausted and complaining of severe headache, nausea, and malaise. He returned to his condominium, where he took aspirin and rested for 2 days before his headache, nausea, and sleeplessness resolved and his appetite returned to normal. He resumed skiing, this time starting on moderate slopes.

Case 3

An American member of an expedition to Makalu (27,790 ft) in Eastern Nepal developed 2 days of mild symptoms of a viral illness that had previously afflicted most other members of the expedition, just prior to his successful summit bid. He then noticed a cough and uncharacteristic fatigue while climbing to the summit. He descended 8,000 feet the same day to camp 2 at 20,000 feet, where his cough worsened and he had no appetite for dinner. The two climbers who went to the summit and descended with him felt well. He soon developed respiratory distress. His respiratory rate was 40 breaths per minute, his pulse was thready at 110 beats per minute, and he had diffuse crackles and mild wheezing. He was treated overnight with supplemental oxygen and felt improved by morning. He was then strong enough to descend to base camp, where symptoms of an upper respiratory infection persisted for several more days. He had never experienced mountain sickness during many previous climbs, including one to the summit of Mt. Everest (29,028 ft). He had also been tested in a physiology laboratory, where he was found to have a very strong ventilatory response to hypoxia, which is thought to be protective against mountain sickness.

The first case was described by Houston in his seminal article in 1960, "Acute pulmonary edema of high altitude." The full presentation and discussion clearly establish that this and other cases he included were episodes of pulmonary edema that were unrelated to infection, pulmonary embolism, or heart failure. His case is typical of the rapid progression, potentially fatal outcome, and rapid resolution of HAPE that can be achieved with appropriate treatment. It also typifies the most common clinical setting of mountain sickness: young, otherwise healthy people getting sick at moderate, easily accessible altitudes. Although the percent incidence of mountain sickness becomes much greater at higher altitudes, most of the mountain sickness in the world occurs at the altitude of major mountain recreation resorts.

The second case is an example of one of the most common scenarios of AMS. A young, healthy, active man developed typical symptoms a few hours after arriving at 8,000 feet directly from sea level. His symptoms worsened through the night but improved in the morning during quiet activity at home to the point of being tolerable. They worsened again during strenuous exercise, and he was fortunate not to develop severe mountain sickness. Progression to severe mountain sickness may have been more likely at a higher altitude or if he had stubbornly ignored his symptoms, as many people do, and continued to exercise vigorously in spite of them. He recovered with the conservative treatment that is usually adequate—rest and mild analgesics. After 2 days of rest and acclimatization, he was able to resume skiing, this time making sure he tolerated moderate exertion before progressing to more strenuous activity.

The third case may be one of a respiratory infection increasing susceptibility to the development of mountain sickness in a person who had previously performed well at extreme altitude.

SIGNS AND SYMPTOMS

Symptoms of AMS include headache, lassitude, insomnia, anorexia, and nausea. Associated symptoms include decreased urine volume and peripheral, especially periorbital, edema. Headache is the most common symptom, although its absence does not rule out mountain sickness from the differential diagnosis. A mountain sickness headache typically occurs a few hours after arrival at a new altitude and is typically most severe upon awakening in the morning. All these symptoms can be due to other illnesses, but in the setting of an ascent to high altitude, they should be treated like mountain sickness. Because of its wide diversity of presentations, any illness in this setting should initially be considered to be mountain sickness. Physical examination is usually normal but may reveal tachycardia, mild tachypnea, and peripheral edema.

HAPE starts with mild shortness of breath, which is notable for being worse than that suffered by other members of the patient's party who have experienced the same exertion. A dry cough also occurs early and may be associated with normal auscultation of the lungs. Cyanosis is typical. Many asymptomatic sojourners to high altitude develop rales and an accentuated second heart sound, so these findings may not be helpful. In a study of 200 trekkers at 14,000 feet in Nepal by Hackett and Rennie, rales were found in 45 subjects, or 23 percent. Eight, or 18 percent, of these subjects had no symptoms of mountain sickness. Listening for rales is an important aid in following the patient's progress. Tachycardia is usually associated with pulmonary edema, although it is a nonspecific finding. Increasing anxiety is also common, although this symptom may be masked by the lethargy of HACE or extreme fatigue. Findings of worsening pulmonary edema are increasing tachypnea and a cough that is productive of clear, then pink frothy sputum. Neurologic findings may also develop due to severe cerebral hypoxia or concomitant HACE. If possible, oxygen saturation should be measured and a chest x-ray should be obtained. Oxygen saturation is substantially lower than normal for any given altitude in subjects with HAPE. The chest x-ray typically shows irregular, patchy, interstitial infiltrates, often initially in the right middle lobe, then spreading to a more diffuse pattern, with a normal cardiac silhouette.

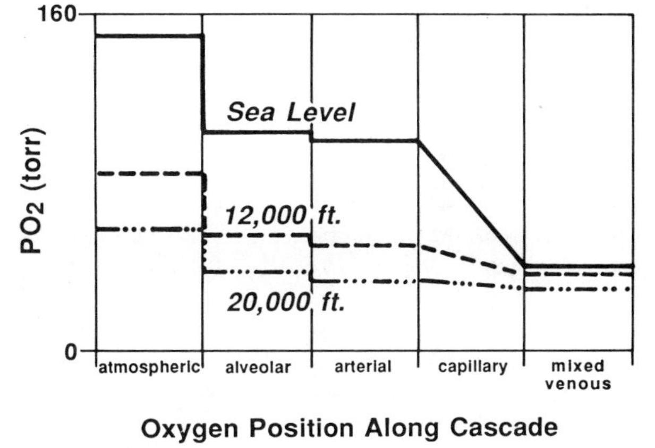

Fig. 84-1. The oxygen cascade.

HACE is diagnosed in sojourners in the appropriate setting who develop any neurologic signs or symptoms, most commonly ataxia, confusion, and severe headache. Other common features are memory loss, bladder dysfunction, persistent nausea and vomiting, irrational behavior, and severe lassitude that can progress to coma and death. Papilledema and retinal hemorrhages may be present but are not always helpful because they also occur in asymptomatic people at high altitude. Signs and symptoms are often obvious; they can also be elicited by tests of cerebellar function, such as heel-to-toe walking and finger-to-nose touching, and a mental status examination.

PATHOPHYSIOLOGY

Oxygen Cascade

A brief review of the process of gas exchange from air to tissue may help facilitate an understanding of the pathophysiology of altitude-related illness. The partial pressure of oxygen (PO_2) falls in a stepwise fashion with each stage in its passive transport from ambient air to the mitochondria. This progressive decline in partial pressure is called the *oxygen cascade* (Fig. 84-1). Adaptation to a hypoxic environment depends on optimizing the transfer of oxygen at each of these steps.

PO_2 falls 47 mm Hg during passage from the atmosphere to the alveoli due to mixture with water vapor and 5 to 10 mm Hg during diffusion of oxygen into pulmonary capillary blood. At sea level, this first drop in the oxygen cascade goes from 150 to 100 mm Hg. At high altitude, the ambient PO_2

Table 84-1. Resting ventilation and arterial blood gas values, measured during a simulated 40-day ascent of Mt. Everest in a chamber in seven subjects ("Operation Everest II")*

Altitude (ft)	Barometric pressure (mm Hg)	Partial pressure of inspired oxygen (mm Hg)	Minute ventilation (liters/min)	pH	Partial pressure of carbon dioxide (mm Hg)	Partial pressure of oxygen (mm Hg)	Oxygen saturation (%)
0	760	150	11.0 ± 1.0	7.43 ± 0.04	33.9 ± 3.5	99.3 ± 9.3	97.6 ± 0.1
15,000	429	80	14.6 ± 2.7	7.46 ± 0.02	25.0 ± 2.2	52.4 ± 4.0	84.8 ± 4.0
20,000	347	63	20.9 ± 6.3	7.50 ± 0.04	20.0 ± 2.8	41.1 ± 3.3	75.2 ± 6.0
26,500	282	49	36.6 ± 7.9	7.53 ± 0.03	12.5 ± 1.1	36.6 ± 2.2	67.8 ± 5.0
29,029	240	43	42.3 ± 7.7	7.56 ± 0.03	11.2 ± 1.7	30.3 ± 2.1	58.0 ± 4.5

*Values are mean ± standard deviation.

Source: Modified from J. R. Sutton, et al. Operation Everest II: Oxygen transport during exercise at extreme simulated altitude. *J. Appl. Physiol.* 64:1309, 1988.

is lower (Table 84-1), resulting in a lower inspired PO_2. An increase in alveolar ventilation resulting in lower $PACO_2$ and higher PAO_2 is the first response of the body to acute exposure to high altitude.

The next step is the transfer of oxygen from alveolar air to the blood. The efficiency of this step depends on the pressure gradient across the alveolar-capillary membrane, the diffusion coefficient of that membrane, capillary blood volume, the surface area for gas exchange, the affinity of oxygen and hemoglobin, and the transit time of blood through the pulmonary capillaries. In the hypoxic environment of high altitude, alveolar PO_2 is decreased, decreasing the diffusion pressure gradient. The diffusion capacity of the alveolar-capillary membrane probably remains constant during a sojourn to high altitude, although native residents may have higher values. Pulmonary capillary blood volume and ventilation/perfusion matching have been shown to increase with increasing altitude. Increased cardiac output and hypoxic pulmonary vasoconstriction, which increase pulmonary artery pressure, improve the homogeneity of blood flow in the lung. Increased perfusion of well-ventilated areas of the lung, especially at the apices (which are relatively underperfused under resting conditions at sea level), increases the gas–blood interface and improves ventilation/perfusion matching. Furthermore, because of the pressure gradient from air to blood, the transit time of blood through pulmonary capillaries at sea level, at rest, is 3 times more than adequate for complete equilibration of oxygen at the alveolar-capillary membrane. Even with the increased cardiac output of maximal exercise, the transit time is almost always sufficient. At high altitude, the combination of a lower pressure gradient and the higher cardiac output stimulated by hypoxemia and exercise prevents full equilibration.

The final drops in PO_2 occur at the capillary where oxygen diffuses across the membrane into the cytoplasm and then into the mitochondria. Structural and biochemical changes may occur during acclimatization to maximize the efficiency of this process.

Acclimatization

The mechanisms that protect oxygen delivery and other physiologic functions develop with time at high altitude. The first and possibly most important of these is hyperventilation. Hypoxemia is sensed by the carotid body, which then sends an afferent signal along the carotid sinus nerve to the central respiratory centers. Minute ventilation increases, first due to increasing tidal volume, then due to increasing respiratory rate. Even though hyperventilation is blunted by the acute respiratory alkalosis it produces (through a negative feedback control mechanism), it continues to increase over several weeks, and alkalemia persists. A diuresis of bicarbonate partially compensates for the respiratory alkalosis, but other mechanisms may contribute to the increasing and persistent elevation of alveolar ventilation.

Individuals with a low hypoxic ventilatory response (HVR) and consequently lower arterial oxygen saturation have a higher than normal incidence of mountain sickness. People with brisk ventilatory responses to hypoxia tend not to develop mountain sickness and to have more success climbing to extreme heights. This tendency is not absolute, and other factors may be more important, but it is the only factor related to acclimatization that has been found to show some possible predictive value for success at high altitude.

Transient changes in lung mechanics also develop on acute exposure to high altitude. Decreased compliance and vital capacity develop, suggesting that pulmonary interstitial fluid increases on initial exposure to high altitude. These changes resolve in a few days with normal acclimatization, but they increase in sojourners who develop HAPE.

Hemoglobin concentration increases from the time of first exposure to hypoxia. Initially, the diuresis and dehydration of acclimatization and inadequate water intake cause hemoconcentration. Erythropoietin levels start to rise on the first day at high altitude, and erythropoiesis begins within the first few days. Erythropoiesis may improve oxygen transport at first, but polycythemia occasionally develops, although rarely in sojourners, with hematocrit levels sometimes greater than 60 percent. The typical peak hematocrit level of travelers to 14,000 to 18,000 feet is 50 to 55 percent. This may be the optimal level for oxygen delivery, above which increased viscosity, with impairment of blood flow in the microvasculature, may actually decrease oxygen delivery and cause other deleterious effects.

The oxygen-hemoglobin dissociation curve undergoes several changes with increasing altitude. Hypoxia induces production of increasing levels of 2,3-diphosphoglycerate (2,3-

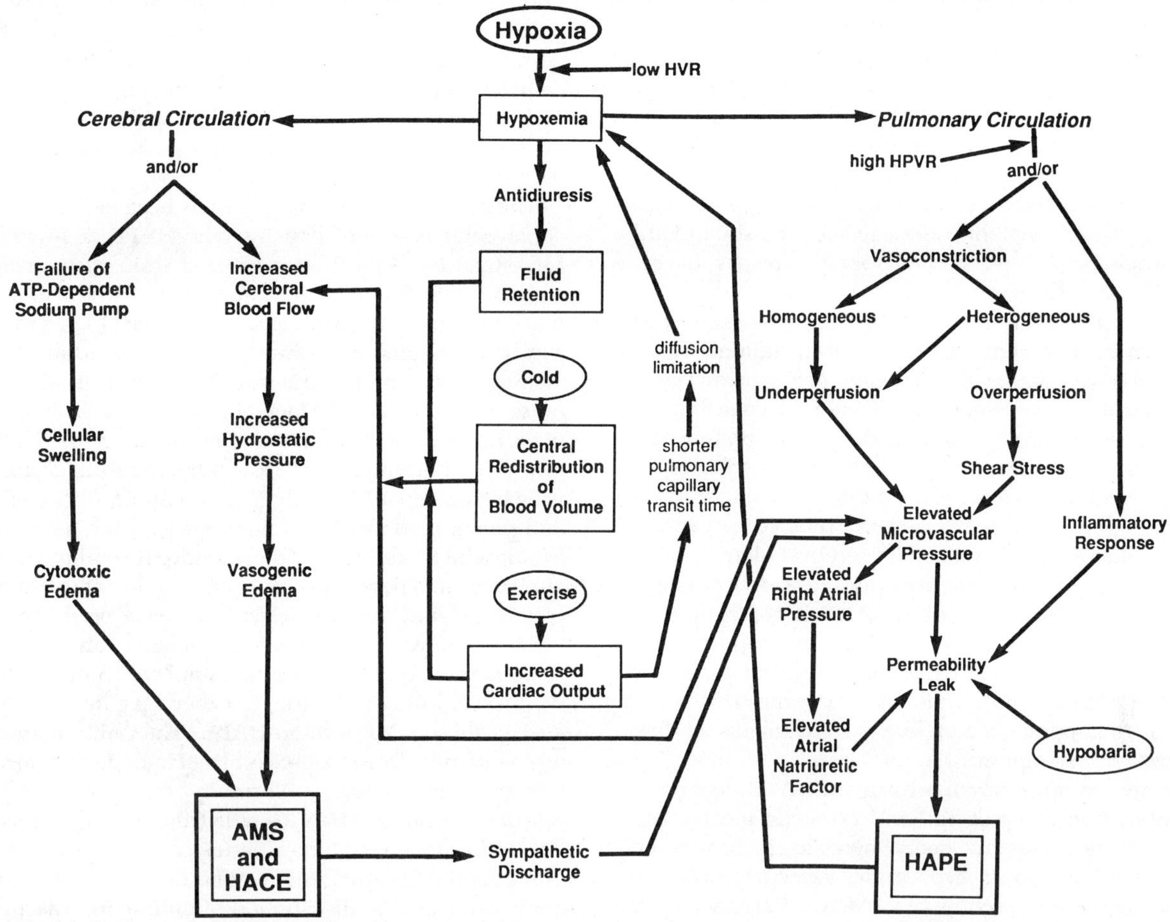

Fig. 84-2. Schema of possible pathophysiology of acute mountain sickness (AMS), high altitude cerebral edema (HACE), and high altitude pulmonary edema (HAPE). (HVR = hypoxic ventilatory response; HPVR = hypoxic pulmonary vascular response.)

DPG), which causes the curve to shift to the right, improving oxygen unloading at the tissue. At extreme altitude, however, in sojourners, the curve is shifted left, possibly due to a more potent effect of persistent respiratory alkalosis. This shift may facilitate loading of oxygen by hemoglobin in the pulmonary capillaries and may, in terms of improved oxygen delivery, more than offset the hindrance to off-loading in the tissues.

Changes also occur in tissue and cells. Relative capillary density may increase, probably due to a combination of capillary proliferation and recruitment and a decrease in skeletal muscle size. These changes decrease the diffusion distance from blood to cellular cytoplasm. Myoglobin concentration may increase, improving intracellular oxygen transport. Mitochondria also increase in number at high altitude, and their function seems to improve, resulting in improved oxidative capacity.

Maladaptation

The different forms of mountain sickness may all be parts of a spectrum of the same disease. AMS almost always precedes HACE and HAPE by hours or days, suggesting that it is simply a mild or early manifestation of mountain sickness. The symptoms of AMS are also similar to symptoms of cerebral edema from other causes, and several investigators have suggested that AMS is indeed a manifestation of mild HACE. HACE and HAPE often occur together, and each one may contribute to the pathogenesis of the other. In this section, we discuss AMS and HACE together, followed by HAPE (Fig. 84-2).

Acute Mountain Sickness and High Altitude Cerebral Edema

Symptoms of AMS usually develop 12 hours to 4 days after arrival in a hypoxic environment, even at altitudes as low as 8,000 feet, where arterial oxygen saturation is normally still greater than 90 percent. Some work has been done to distinguish between the effects of hypobaric and normobaric hypoxia, suggesting that the barometric pressure may play a role in pathogenesis. The time course of exposure is certainly a major factor, as it is well known that sudden or rapid ascent increases the likelihood of developing AMS and that gradual, staged ascent to high altitude is protective against it. Individual variation is also crucial, with some individuals showing greater susceptibility to developing AMS. Some possible mechanisms of this individual variation are discussed in the following paragraphs.

Fluid retention has been positively associated with the development of AMS. Singh, et al., and others demonstrated a marked diuresis in subjects who remained healthy after arrival at high altitude. Patients with AMS had lower urine output than fluid intake before and during their illness. They developed a diuresis (spontaneous or induced by furosemide) at the time of resolution of their symptoms. Hackett, et al., weighed trekkers arriving at 14,000 feet in Nepal and found weight gain in those who developed AMS and weight loss in those who remained healthy. In attempts to understand the mechanism of this response, vasopressin and aldosterone levels have been studied, but the results have, to date, been inconclusive.

Relative hypoventilation probably contributes to AMS. Lower than normal ventilation at a given altitude may be due to low HVR, or it may be secondary to a hypoxic ventilatory depression. Hypoventilation augments alveolar hypoxia, leading to greater hypoxemia and decreased oxygen transport. The development of HAPE likewise contributes to a widening alveolar to arterial oxygen difference and impaired oxygen transport. Hypoxemia and the relative hypercapnia of hypoventilation may also increase cerebral blood flow and lead to increased hydrostatic pressure and cerebral edema.

The role of brain blood flow in AMS is currently under active investigation. Brain blood flow is proportional to $PaCO_2$ and inversely proportional to PaO_2, but association of flow with AMS is controversial. Evidence has been contradictory in attempting to correlate measurements of brain blood flow with symptoms.

The increased intracranial pressure of HACE may be due to a combination of vasogenic and cytotoxic mechanisms. According to the vasogenic theory, hypoxic cerebral vasodilation predominates over hypocapnic vasoconstriction, resulting in increased cerebral blood flow. Exercise, by increasing cardiac output, and cold, by causing peripheral vasoconstriction and central redistribution of blood volume, may augment this flow, eventually overwhelming the integrity of the vascular endothelial junction, leading to the development of a leak of fluid from the intra- to extravascular space. Similar to severe hypertension, the resultant high intracranial pressure is associated with diffuse small hemorrhages and cerebral edema. HACE may also be partly cytotoxic in origin, with hypoxia-induced failure of the cellular adenosine triphosphate (ATP)-dependent sodium pump resulting in sodium and water accumulation within cells and cellular swelling. When endothelial cells are affected, the capillary lumen may be diminished, raising arterial pressure and decreasing perfusion. The finding of retinal hemorrhages could be due to either the cytotoxic or vasogenic mechanism and is likely to be a sign of similar hemorrhages occurring inside the brain. The beneficial effect of steroids in HACE supports the role of vasogenic edema; they have been shown to have little effect on models of cytotoxic edema.

High Altitude Pulmonary Edema

The pathogenesis of HAPE is partially understood. First, HAPE is a noncardiogenic form of pulmonary edema. Pulmonary capillary wedge pressure measurements are low or normal, and the cardiac silhouette on chest x-ray films is normal in patients with HAPE. Furthermore, there are no pleural effusions and no Kerley lines, in the presence of a patchy interstitial infiltrate, all of which are contrary to the findings in left heart failure. On auscultation, however, the pulmonic second heart sound may be accentuated, suggesting high pulmonary artery pressures, and right heart catheterization demonstrates that pulmonary hypertension is present. HAPE also usually resolves within hours of descent to low altitude, showing that any actual damage done to lung tissue is unlikely.

The nature of the edema fluid has been evaluated by bronchoalveolar lavage of patients with HAPE at 14,400 feet on Mt. McKinley. The fluid recovered from these patients included a very high concentration of cells, which were primarily alveolar macrophages, and a very high protein content, even higher than that found in the adult respiratory distress syndrome (ARDS), another form of noncardiogenic pulmonary edema. The lack of neutrophils, which predominate in early ARDS, suggests that the cause of HAPE is not primarily inflammatory. However, high-molecular-weight proteins, compatible with a permeability form of edema, and potent mediators of inflammation, such as chemotactic leukotriene B_4 and C_{5A}, and vasoactive thromboxane B_2 were also present. These findings suggest that inflammation does play a role and that the defect includes a permeability leak.

Several physiologic responses are associated with the development of HAPE. These phenomena occur in all people who travel to high altitude, but they may be more exaggerated in those who develop HAPE. The pulmonary vasculature constricts in response to alveolar hypoxia, raising pulmonary artery pressure. Normally, the hypoxic pulmonary vascular response (HPVR) redistributes pulmonary perfusion to improve ventilation/perfusion matching and thereby minimize hypoxemia. People who develop HAPE, however, may have a patchy distribution of pulmonary vascular reactivity, resulting in a heterogeneous distribution of areas of overperfusion with very high hydrostatic pressure and other areas of underperfusion. Their HPVR may also be more potent than that of people who do not develop HAPE. Furthermore, HAPE usually occurs in a cold environment and often after heavy exercise, two conditions that increase pulmonary vascular pressure and that may further compound the problems of overperfusion and high pulmonary artery pressure. The syndrome of reentry pulmonary edema may further support the role of HPVR in the pathogenesis of HAPE. In this situation, residents of high altitude who return from visits to lower regions have an increased incidence of HAPE. Their pulmonary arterial smooth muscle is hypertrophied from residence in a hypoxic environment; on return to that environment, sudden vasoconstriction may raise pulmonary artery pressure excessively and contribute to HAPE.

The positive fluid balance that is common in AMS may also contribute to increased pulmonary vascular volume and pressure. The increased right atrial pressure resulting from high plasma volume and high pulmonary vascular pressure may result in increased production of atrial natriuretic factor and a subsequent increased permeability leak from pulmonary vessels.

As discussed previously, one crucial physiologic response to high altitude is increased ventilation, the degree of which is partly governed by an individual's HVR. Low HVR has been associated with an increased incidence of HAPE and AMS. Low HVR at high altitude results in a relatively lower alveolar ventilation and greater alveolar hypoxia. More severe alveolar hypoxia accentuates pulmonary vasoconstriction and may contribute further to the marked pulmonary hypertension described previously.

HAPE may also be partly neurogenic in origin. HAPE and HACE often coexist clinically; autopsy studies of victims of clinical HAPE have shown pathologic evidence of HACE as well. Cerebral edema may result in a massive alpha-adrenergic discharge that causes generalized systemic vasoconstriction and a shift of blood into the relatively low resistance pulmonary circulation. This volume increase may contribute to the leak, whether it is hydrostatic or inflammatory. A "pulmonary edemagenic center" in the hypothalamus has been demonstrated in animal models of neurogenic pulmonary edema and may also be present in humans. Many questions remain concerning the relative contributions to HAPE of neurogenic, pressor, and inflammatory responses.

DIFFERENTIAL DIAGNOSIS

In the high mountain setting, mountain sickness may occur concurrently with hypothermia, hypoglycemia, dehydration, and exhaustion, whose symptoms may be similar to those of mountain sickness. These conditions should be included in the differential diagnosis. Other illnesses may also mimic or mask symptoms of AMS, such as respiratory infections, gastrointestinal illness, tension or migraine headache, carbon monoxide poisoning, and meningitis. In addition, pulmonary embolism may be confused with HAPE, and as discussed in the final section of this chapter, the risk factors for both problems are present in the mountain environment. In the appropriate setting, therefore, anyone with symptoms consistent with AMS should be treated for AMS while further observation and workup are undertaken to rule out other disorders.

EVALUATION

The most important aspect of the evaluation of a person who might have mountain sickness is a high index of suspicion in the appropriate clinical situation. People in a mountain setting must communicate with each other and be very sensitive to the possibility of the development of mountain sickness in themselves and their colleagues. The patient interview should focus on how the person is feeling and performing relative to other members of his or her party and to his or her level of fitness and previous performance in similar situations. AMS develops in a setting where shortness of breath, fatigue, and other physical ailments are normal occurrences. A person's symptoms are abnormal when they are worse than what should be expected in a given setting. Suspicion and early diagnosis may allow early treatment and recovery before the victim becomes moribund.

Other questions should determine the patient's sleeping altitude of the previous days, his or her level of activity, and any concurrent medical problems. Significant past medical history may include previous episodes of mountain sickness, medications, and preexisting cardiac or pulmonary disease. Some people have "threshold" altitudes above which they often develop mountain sickness. Sedatives and tranquilizers increase the likelihood of developing mountain sickness,

Table 84-2. Symptoms, prevention, and treatment of acute mountain sickness, high altitude pulmonary edema, and high altitude cerebral edema.

Illness	Symptoms	Prevention	Treatment
AMS	Headache, nausea, loss of appetite, sleeplessness, malaise	Staged ascent, time for acclimatization, avoidance of sedatives, medications:* acetazolamide (125–250 mg bid), dexamethasone (4 mg q6h)	Avoid further ascent, watch for progression to HAPE or HACE, descent if symptoms progress, mild analgesics, prochlorperazine for severe nausea or vomiting, acetazolamide or dexamethasone if symptoms are moderate to severe
HAPE	Inordinate shortness of breath, cough, cyanosis, tachycardia, rales	Treat AMS	Descent, supplemental oxygen
HACE	Severe headache, ataxia, confusion, slurred speech, hallucinations	Treat AMS	Descent, supplemental oxygen, dexamethasone

*Medical prophylaxis should be used only in situations of unavoidable rapid ascent (from sea level to over 8,000 ft, or gain in sleeping altitude of 3,000 ft in a day), or in people who have had previous recurrent AMS. Dexamethasone as prophylaxis should be reserved for people who are allergic to or intolerant of acetazolamide.

probably due to suppression of alveolar ventilation and decreased PAO_2. Some people mistakenly believe that acetazolamide, dexamethasone, or other drugs will, without fail, prevent them from developing mountain sickness. They then ascribe any symptoms they develop to other causes, avoid appropriate treatment, and may progress to develop HAPE or HACE.

Physical examination is less helpful than the interview. Vital signs should be obtained, and the skin should be examined for color, especially cyanosis, degree of moisture, and peripheral edema. Heart and lungs should be examined. Neurologic examination should be performed, focusing particularly on mental status and cerebellar signs. Details of the symptoms and physical findings in AMS, HAPE, and HACE are described under Clinical Presentation and are listed in Table 84-2.

MANAGEMENT

Prevention

The crucial factors in preventing AMS are slow rate of ascent, moderation in activities at the time of first arrival at high altitude, and attention to the possible development of symptoms. Anyone going from sea level to a sleeping altitude of 8,000 feet or more should either spend a night at an intermediate altitude on the way—for example, Denver (5,280 ft) on the way to a Colorado ski resort—or engage in only mild to moderate activity during the first day at that altitude. Excessive alcohol and any drugs that are respiratory depressants, such as sleeping pills, should be avoided at high altitude. Fluid intake should also be adequate to maintain production of copious, clear urine. At altitudes of 12,000 to 14,000 feet, physically active travelers may benefit from drinking 4 to 6 liters of fluid a day, to compensate for the high insensible losses that occur with exercise and hyperventilation and for the diuresis of acclimatization. For climbers or trekkers traveling above 10,000 feet, gain in sleeping altitude should be limited to 1,000 feet per day, although day trips can usually be made safely to higher altitudes. For trips above 14,000 feet, an extra night should be spent every 2,000 feet, starting at 12,000 feet. One should not climb to a higher sleeping altitude unless one feels 100 percent fit and well. This schedule prevents AMS in most people.

Some people, however, seem to have an altitude threshold above which they always develop AMS, no matter how slowly they gain altitude. These people may benefit from taking acetazolamide, 125 to 250 mg, 2 or 3 times a day, starting the day of ascent and continuing through the first few days at high altitude. Acetazolamide decreases the incidence of AMS. It is also useful for people who are members of rescue or military teams, who do not have time to acclimatize by slow ascent. Its beneficial effects may be due to carbonic anhydrase inhibition, causing a metabolic and respiratory acidosis. In the kidney, carbonic anhydrase inhibition causes increased renal excretion of bicarbonate and a subsequent metabolic acidosis. Carbonic anhydrase inhibition in red blood cells causes CO_2 retention in tissue and in venous blood, a respiratory acidosis that is not reflected by the arterial partial pressure of CO_2. Both acidoses stimulate ventilation, although probably only the renal effect is necessary for the prevention of AMS. Benzolamide, which selectively inhibits renal carbonic anhydrase, also aids acclimatization and prevents periodic breathing and oxygen desaturation during sleep. Low-dose acetazolamide, 5 mg/kg/day, is sufficient for selective renal carbonic anhydrase inhibition and may be adequate for prophylaxis of AMS, although higher doses, 250 to 500 mg 2 or 3 times a day, have been used in most studies. Decreased cerebrospinal fluid (CSF) production, and possibly decreased intracranial pressure, also occur with acetazolamide and may help explain its beneficial effects at high altitude. Its main danger is the false sense of security it instills in many people; it does not always prevent AMS and it may not prevent HACE or HAPE. It also causes benign paresthesias in many people, especially at higher doses, and causes carbonated beverages such as beer to taste metallic. Since it is a sulfonamide (nonbacteriostatic), it should not be taken by people who are allergic to sulfa drugs.

Dexamethasone, 4 mg every 6 hours, also decreases the incidence of AMS through mechanisms that are unclear. It does not, however, aid acclimatization. If taken as a prophylactic measure, it should be continued throughout the sojourn at high altitude. Dexamethasone may be better tolerated than acetazolamide because of its lack of immediate side effects, but it should be used with more caution. It may cause adrenal suppression and hyperglycemia during prolonged use. Because dexamethasone does not facilitate acclimatization, it is associated with a rebound worsening of symptoms if stopped suddenly. This risk is especially great on long remote trips, during which medications may be lost and replacement supplies may not be readily available. It is therefore recommended that dexamethasone be used only as treatment where improvement is necessary to aid descent.

Furosemide, 80 mg twice a day, was used successfully in a large Indian army study of prophylaxis of AMS during the 1960s, but most American authorities belive that the risk of severe dehydration is too great to recommend its use outside a medically controlled setting.

HAPE and HACE are usually prevented by not ascending or overexerting with symptoms of mild AMS and by descending if AMS symptoms worsen. A common sense approach usually prevents the development of severe mountain sickness.

Treatment

AMS usually improves with rest at the same altitude. Mild analgesics such as aspirin and acetaminophen are usually effective in treating mountain sickness headaches. Prochlorperazine suppositories are usually effective for the nausea or vomiting of AMS or HACE. Acetazolamide may be effective additional treatment. Much anecdotal experience supports its use in treating AMS, but it has never been proved to be effective by a good clinical trial. It may be especially useful if taken at night to treat the insomnia of AMS or the disordered sleep caused by Cheyne-Stokes breathing. In spite of its apparent usefulness in treating AMS and HACE, theoretic considerations suggest that acetazolamide may be contraindicated in HAPE.

Dexamethasone may also be useful, although it is recommended only for treatment of moderate or severe AMS or HACE. Its beneficial effect is rapid and may allow a sick, nonambulatory victim to improve and descend with little or no help.

HAPE and HACE require immediate descent of one thousand to several thousand feet, and patients usually respond completely within a day or two to this treatment, although HACE sometimes responds more slowly. Continuous oxygen treatment is the best currently available temporizing measure in lieu of descent, and it is often adequate definitive treatment of HAPE if available in sufficient quantity for 24 to 48 hours of continuous treatment. A continuous positive airway pressure mask, using 10 cm H_2O of expiratory pressure, has recently been tested on patients with HAPE. It improved arterial oxygen saturation, probably by increasing the ventilation/perfusion ratio, and may be another useful temporizing measure. Other medications such as furosemide, morphine, nitrates, nifedipine, and hydralazine have been used but should be considered experimental and may be dangerous. Dexamethasone is routinely used, up to 4 mg intravenously every 6 hours, for temporizing treatment of HACE. Glycerol and mannitol may be effective but have rarely been used in this situation. Most physicians consider their administration too difficult to perform safely in the field.

DISPOSITION

If standard preventive measures continue to be followed, a victim who recovers completely from AMS should be able to continue his or her scheduled activity without increased risk of redeveloping AMS. One who recovers from HAPE or HACE may be at increased risk of developing HAPE or HACE with reascent during the next few weeks. Some recovered victims of severe mountain sickness have returned within a few days to the altitude at which they became sick and have completed their climbs with no adverse consequences. Others have returned and developed even more rapid and fulminant illness.

OTHER HIGH ALTITUDE MEDICAL PROBLEMS

Peripheral Edema

Peripheral edema occurs twice as often in women as in men, although it is often seen in men. Periorbital edema is symmetric. Hands and feet also swell. The swelling usually resolves spontaneously, even during ascent, although a mild diuretic may hasten improvement. It is, however, associated with AMS, and the presence of peripheral, especially facial, edema indicates a need to look carefully for signs of mountain sickness.

High Altitude Retinopathy

Some people develop retinal hemorrhages above 14,000 feet—3.9 percent in Hackett's study in Nepal, with the incidence increasing at higher altitudes. They develop in one-third to one-half of climbers above 16,000 feet. Retinal hemorrhages are usually asymptomatic and resolve spontaneously within 2 weeks, although they are associated with an increased incidence of AMS. Blurred vision can occur if retinal hemorrhages develop over the macula. The cause is unknown but may be related to a microvascular hemorrhage. Other common asymptomatic findings are venous engorgement and tortuosity of retinal vessels. Transient blindness and blurred vision have also been reported, unrelated to hemorrhages, and may be due to cerebrovascular spasm, resulting in transient ischemic attacks (TIAs), or in regions of poor perfusion in the occipital cortex.

Periodic Breathing

Breathing in a Cheyne-Stokes pattern occurs in almost all sojourners to high altitude. It may disturb sleep by causing the sufferer to awaken frequently, gasping for air. These episodes usually improve or at least stop disturbing sleep during continued stay at high altitude, although, if they do not, acetazolamide taken at bedtime or breathing oxygen usually helps. The cause is probably related to oscillation between the ventilatory stimulation of hypoxia and the ventilatory inhibition of hypocapnea.

Thromboembolic Events

Young healthy climbers have sustained thrombotic events at high altitude, including TIAs, pulmonary emboli, and deep venous thrombosis, although the incidence is not known. A hypercoagulable state may develop at high altitude that may even contribute to the development of HAPE, although this relationship has not been conclusively demonstrated. However, other factors related to the physical hardships of the mountain environment, such as dehydration, polycythemia, cold, constrictive clothing, and venous stasis from periods of inactivity, may contribute to thromboembolic events.

Chronic Mountain Sickness

Chronic mountain sickness is most common in people who live at high altitude for prolonged stays. Its incidence is unknown. Symptoms, including headache, dizziness, lethargy, impaired memory, slow mentation, and sleeplessness, are primarily related to polycythemia. Like lowlanders with chronic hypoxia, these people also have pulmonary hypertension, cor pulmonale, plethora, and cyanosis. The hematocrit may exceed 75 percent. Treatment, in order of increasing practicality, includes moving to a low altitude, nighttime oxygen therapy, phlebotomy, and respiratory stimulants. Medroxyprogesterone acetate, 20 to 60 mg per day, and acetazolamide have been proved to improve oxygen saturation, decrease nocturnal breathing problems, and lower the hematocrit.

SELECTED READING

Historical Perspectives

Gilbert, DL. The first documented report of mountain sickness: The China or Headache Mountain story. *Resp Physiol* 52:315, 1983.

Gilbert, DL. The first documented discription of mountain sickness: The Andean or Pariacaca story. *Resp Physiol* 52:327, 1983.

Hackett, PH, Rennie, ID, and Levine, HD. The incidence, importance, and prophylaxis of acute mountain sickness. *Lancet* 2:1149, 1976.

Houston, CS. Acute pulmonary edema of high altitude. *N Engl J Med* 363:478, 1960.

Houston, CS. *Going Higher: The Story of Man and Altitude.* Boston: Little, Brown, 1987: Pp 3–65.

Ravenhill, TH. Some experiences of mountain sickness in the Andes. *J Trop Med Hyg* 20:313, 1913.

Singh, I, et al. Acute Mountain Sickness. *N Engl J Med* 280:175, 1969.

Epidemiology

Hackett, PH, and Rennie, D. Avoiding mountain sickness. *Lancet* 2:938, 1978.

Houston, CS. Incidence of acute mountain sickness. *Am Alpine J* 27:162, 1985.

Larson, EB, et al. Acute mountain sickness and acetazolamide. Clinical efficacy and effect on ventilation. *JAMA* 288:328, 1982.

Signs and Symptoms

Hackett, PH. *Mountain Sickness, Prevention, Recognition and Treatment.* New York: American Alpine Club, 1980. Pp 19–31.

Hackett, PH, and Rennie, D. Rales, peripheral edema, retinal hemorrhage, and acute mountain sickness. *Am J Med* 67:214, 1979.

Pathophysiology

Oxygen Cascade

Dawson, A. Regional pulmonary blood flow in sitting and supine man during and after acute hypoxia. *J Clin Invest* 48:301, 1969.

Dawson, A. Regional lung function during early acclimatization to 3100 m altitude. *J Appl Physiol* 33:218, 1972.
Dempsey, JA, et al. Effects of acute through life-long hypoxic exposure in exercise pulmonary gas exchange. *Resp Physiol* 13:62, 1971.
Gale, GE, et al. Ventilation-perfusion inequality in normal humans during exercise at sea level and simulated altitude. *J Appl Physiol* 58:978, 1985.
Haab, P, et al. Ventilation perfusion relationships during high altitude adaptation. *J Appl Physiol* 26:77, 1969.
Haldane, JS, Kellas, AM, and Kennaway, DM. Experiments on acclimatization to reduced atmospheric pressure. *J Physiol London* 53:181, 1919.
Hansen, TN, LeBlanc, AL, and Best, AL. Hypoxia and angiotensin II infusion redistribution lung blood flow in lambs. *J Appl Physiol* 58:812, 1985.
Sutton, JR, et al. Operation Everest II: Oxygen transport during exercise at extreme simulated altitude. *J Appl Physiol* 64:1309, 1988.
Sylvester, JT, et al. Components of alveolar-arterial O_2 gradient during rest and exercise at sea level and high altitude. *J Appl Physiol* 50:1129, 1981.
Vogel, JA, and Harris, CW. Cardiopulmonary responses of resting man during early exposure to high altitude. *J Appl Physiol* 22:1124, 1967.
Weiskopf, RB, and Severinghaus, JW. Diffusing capacity of the lung for carbon monoxide in man during acute acclimatization to 14,246 ft. *J Appl Physiol* 32:285, 1972.
West, JB. *Respiratory Physiology—The Essentials.* Baltimore: Williams & Wilkins, 1974.
West, JB, and Wagner, PD. Predicted gas exchange on the summit of Mt. Everest. *Respir Physiol* 42:1, 1980.

Acclimatization

Abbrecht, PH, and Littell, JK. Plasma erythropoietin in men and mice during acclimatization to different altitudes. *J Appl Physiol* 32:54, 1972.
Aste-Salazar, H, and Hurtado, A. The affinity of hemoglobin for oxygen at sea level and high altitude. *Am J Physiol* 142:733, 1944.
Banchero, N. Capillary density of skeletal muscle in dogs exposed to simulated altitude. *Proc Soc Exp Biol Med* 148:135, 1975.
Burton, MD, Johnson, DC, and Kazemi, H. CSF acidosis augments ventilation through cholinergic mechanisms. *J Appl Physiol* 66: 2565, 1989.
Faura, J, et al. Effect of altitude on erythropoiesis. *Blood* 33:668, 1969.
Gautier, H, Milic-Emili, J, and Miserocchi, NM. Pattern of breathing and mouth occlusion pressure during acclimatization to high altitude. *Respir Physiol* 41:365, 1980.
Gimenz, M, et al. Effects of altitude on myoglobin and mitochondrial protein in canine skeletal muscle. *Respiration* 34:171, 1977.
Heath, D, and Williams, DR. The Carotid Bodies. In D Heath and DR Williams (eds), *Man at High Altitude: The Pathophysiology of Acclimatization and Adaptation.* Edinburgh: Churchill Livingstone, 1977. Pp 60–74.
Hornbein, TF. The Relationship Between Stimulus to Chemoreceptors and Their Response. In RW Torrance (ed), *Arterial Chemoreceptors.* Oxford: Blackwell, 1968. Pp 65–68.
Jaeger, JJ, et al. Evidence for increased intrathoracic fluid volume in man at high altitude. *J Appl Physiol* 47:670, 1979.
Kellogg, RH. Effect of altitude on respiratory regulation. *Ann NY Acad Sci* 109:815, 1963.
Lakshminarayan, S, and Pierson, DJ. Recurrent high altitude pulmonary edema with blunted chemosensitivity. *Am Rev Resp Dis* 111:869, 1975.
Mansell, A, Poules, A, and Sutton, JR. Changes in pulmonary PV characteristics of human subjects at an altitude of 5366 m. *J Appl Physiol* 49:79, 1980.
Masuyama, S, et al. Control of ventilation in extreme altitude climbers. *J Appl Physiol* 61:500, 1986.
Moore, LG, and Brewer, GJ. Beneficial effect of rightward hemoglobin-oxygen dissociation curve shift for short-term high altitude adaptations. *J Lab Clin Med* 98:145, 1981.
Moore, LG, et al. Variable inhibition by falling CO_2 of hypoxic ventilatory response in humans. *J Appl Physiol* 56:207, 1984.
Ou, LC, and Tenney, SM. Properties of mitochondria from hearts of cattle acclimatized to high altitude. *Respir Physiol* 8:151, 1970.
Ou, LC, St John, WM, and Tenney, SM. The contribution of central mechanisms rostral to the pons in high altitude ventilatory acclimatization. *Respir Physiol* 54:343, 1983.
Pelligrino, DA, Musch, TI, and Dempsey, JA. Interregional differences in brain intracellular pH and water compartmentation during acute normoxic and hypoxic hypocapnia in the anesthetized dog. *Brain Res* 214:387, 1981.
Plum, F, and Posner, JB. Blood and cerebrospinal fluid lactate during hyperventilation. *Am J Physiol* 212:864, 1967.
Schoene, RB. Control of ventilation in climbers to extreme altitude. *J Appl Physiol* 53:886, 1982.
Schoene, RB, et al. Relationship of hypoxic ventilatory response to exercise performance on Mount Everest. *J Appl Physiol* 56:1478, 1984.
Severinghaus, JW, et al. Respiratory control at high altitude suggesting active transport regulation of CSF pH. *J Appl Physiol* 18:1155, 1963.
Sillau, AH, and Banchero, N. Effect of hypoxia on the capillarity of guinea pig skeletal muscle. *Proc Soc Exp Biol Med* 160:368, 1979.
Winslow, RM. Red Cell Function at Extreme Altitude. In JB West and S Lahiri (eds), *High Altitude and Man.* Bethesda: American Physiological Society, 1984. Pp 59–72.
Winslow, RM. High-Altitude Polycythemia. In JB West and S Lahiri (eds), *High Altitude and Man.* Bethesda: American Physiological Society, 1984. Pp 163–172.
Winslow, RM, Samaja, M, and West, JB. Red cell function at extreme altitude on Mount Everest. *J Appl Physiol* 56:109, 1984.

Maladaptation

Hackett, PH, et al. Acute mountain sickness and the edemas of high altitude: A common pathogenesis? *Resp Physiol* 46:383, 1981.
Sutton, JR, and Lassen, N. Pathophysiology of acute mountain sickness and high altitude pulmonary oedema: An hypothesis. *Bull Europ Physiopathol Respir* 15:1045, 1979.

AMS and HACE

Delamere, JP, and Jones, GT. Changes in renal function observed during a trek to high altitude. *Postgrad Med J* 55:487, 1979.
Fishman, RA. Brain edema. *N Engl J Med* 293:706, 1975.
Hackett, PH, et al. Vasopressin in Acute Mountain Sickness and High Altitude Pulmonary Edema. In W Brendel and RA Zinc (eds), *High Altitude Physiology and Medicine.* New York: Springer-Verlag, 1982. Pp 261–262.
Hamilton, AJ, Cymmerman, A, and Black, PMcL. High altitude cerebral edema. *Neurosurgery* 19:841, 1986.
Harber, MJ, Williams, JD, and Morton, JJ. Antidiuretic hormone excretion at high altitude. *Aviat Space Environ Med* 52:38, 1981.
Heyes, MP, and Sutton, JR. High altitude ills: A malady of water, electrolyte and hormone imbalance. *Semin Resp Med* 5:207, 1983.
Houston, CS, and Dickinson, JG. Cerebral form of high altitude sickness. *Lancet* 2:758, 1975.
Huang, SY, et al. Internal carotid and vertebral arterial flow velocity in men at high altitude. *J Appl Physiol* 63:395, 1987.
King, AB, and Robinson, SM. Ventilation response to hypoxia and acute mountain sickness. *Aerospace Med* 43:419, 1972.

Kogure, K, et al. Mechanisms of cerebral vasodilation in hypoxia. *J Appl Physiol* 29:223, 1970.

Mathew, L, et al. Chemoreceptor sensitivity and maladaptation to high altitude in man. *Eur J Appl Physiol* 51:137, 1983.

Moore, LG, et al. Low acute hypoxic ventilatory response and hypoxic depression in acute altitude sickness. *J Appl Physiol* 60:1407, 1986.

Reeves, JT, et al. Headache at high altitude is not related to internal carotid arterial blood velocity. *J Appl Physiol* 59:909, 1985.

Severinghaus, JW, et al. Cerebral blood flow in man at high altitude. *Circ Res* 19:274, 1966.

Wohns, RNW. High altitude cerebral edema: A pathophysiological review. *Crit Care Med* 9:880, 1981.

HAPE

Crosby, RL, et al. Elevated plasma atrial natriuretic factor and vasopressin in high-altitude pulmonary edema. *Ann Int Med* 109:796, 1988.

Dickinson, J, et al. Altitude-related deaths in seven trekkers in the Himalayas. *Thorax* 38:646, 1983.

Fred, HL, et al. Acute pulmonary edema of altitude: Clinical and physiologic observations. *Circulation* 25:929, 1962.

Gamble, JE, and Patton, HD. Pulmonary edema and hemorrhage from preoptic lesions in rats. *Am J Physiol* 172:623, 1953.

Goodman, WB, et al. Hemorrhagic pulmonary edema following stereotactic hypothalamic lesions in dogs. *Surg Forum* 27:472, 1976.

Hackett, PH, et al. Blunted Chemosensitivity and Hypoxic Ventilatory Depression in High Altitude Pulmonary Edema (abstract). In RR Sutton, CS Houston, and G Coates (eds), *Hypoxia. The Tolerable Limits.* Indianapolis: Benchmark Press, 1988. P 378.

Hirai, K, et al. Effects of hypobaria on lung fluid balance in awake sheep. *J Appl Physiol* 64:243, 1988.

Hyers, TM, et al. Accentuated hypoxemia at high altitude in subjects susceptible to high-altitude pulmonary edema. *J Appl Physiol: Respirat Environ Exercise Physiol* 46:41, 1979.

Hultgren, HN, et al. Physiologic studies of pulmonary edema at high altitude. *Circulation* 29:393, 1964.

Hultgren, HN, Grover, RF, and Hartley, LH. Abnormal circulatory responses to high altitude in subjects with a previous history of high altitude pulmonary edema. *Circulation* 44:759, 1971.

Hultgren, HN, and Marticorena, EA. High altitude pulmonary edema: Epidemiologic observations in Peru. *Chest* 74:372, 1978.

Levine, B, et al. Role of barometric pressure in pulmonary fluid balance and oxygen transport. *J Appl Physiol* 64:419, 1988.

Manohar, M, et al. Bovine regional blood flow during sojourn at a simulated altitude of 3500 M. *Respir Physiol* 58:111, 1984.

Reeves, JT, and Grover, RF. High-Altitude Pulmonary Hypertension and Pulmonary Edema. In Pn Yu (ed), *Progress in Cardiology.* Philadelphia: Lea & Febiger, 1975. 4:99–118.

Reynolds, RW. Pulmonary edema as a consequence of hypothalamic lesions in rats. *Science* 141:930, 1963.

Roy, S, et al. Haemodynamic studies in high altitude pulmonary oedema. *Brit Heart J* 31:52, 1969.

Schoene, RB. Pulmonary edema at high altitude: Review, pathophysiology, and update. *Clin Chest Med* 6:491, 1985.

Schoene, RB, et al. High-altitude pulmonary edema: Characteristics of lung lavage fluid. *JAMA* 256:63, 1986.

Schoene, RB, et al. The lung at high altitude: Bronchoalveolar lavage in acute mountain sickness and pulmonary edema. *J Appl Physiol* 64:2605, 1988.

Scoggin, CH, et al. High-altitude pulmonary edema in the children and young adults of Leadville, Colorado. *N Engl J Med* 297:1269, 1977.

Singh, I, Kapila, CC, and Rao, BDP. High-altitude pulmonary oedema. *Lancet* 1:229, 1965.

Staub, NC. Pulmonary edema due to increased microvascular permeability to fluid and protein. *Circ Res* 43:143, 1978.

Viswanathan, R, et al. Further studies on pulmonary oedema of high altitude. *Respiration* 36:216, 1978.

Viswanathan, R, Subramanian, S, and Radha, TG. Effect of hypoxia on regional lung perfusion by scanning. *Respiration* 37:142, 1979.

Wohns, RNW, and Kernstein, MD. The role of dilantin in the prevention of pulmonary edema associated with cerebral hypoxia. *Crit Care Med* 10:436, 1982.

Management

Bradwell, AR, Burnett, D, and Davies, F. Acetazolamide in control of acute mountain sickness. *Lancet* 1:180, 1981.

Cain, SM, and Dunn, JE II. Low doses of acetazolamide to aid accommodation of men to altitude. *J Appl Physiol* 21:1195, 1965.

Coudon, WL, and Block, AJ. Acute respiratory failure precipitated by a carbonic anhydrase inhibitor. *Chest* 69:112, 1976.

Ellsworth, AJ, and Larson, EB. A randomized trial of dexamethasone and acetazolamide for acute mountain sickness prophylaxis. *Am J Med* 83:1024, 1987.

Ferrazzini, G, et al. Successful treatment of acute mountain sickness with dexamethasone. *Br Med J* 294:1380, 1986.

Gray, GW, et al. Control of acute mountain sickness. *Aerospace Med* 42:81, 1971.

Greene, MK, et al. Acetazolamide in prevention of acute mountain sickness: A double blind controlled cross-over study. *Br Med J* 283:811, 1981.

Hackett, PH, et al. Dexamethasone for prevention and treatment of acute mountain sickness. *Aviat Space Environ Med* 59:950, 1988.

Johnson, TS, et al. Prevention of acute mountain sickness by dexamethasone. *N Engl J Med* 310:683, 1983.

Kronenberg, RS, and Cain, SM. Hastening respiratory acclimatization to altitude with benzolamide. *Aerospace Med* 39:296, 1968.

Maren, TH. Carbonic anhydrase: Chemistry, physiology, and inhibition. *Physiol Rev* 47:595, 1967.

Maren, TH. Benzolamide: A Renal Carbonic Anhydrase Inhibitor. In FE Karch (ed), *Orphan Drugs.* New York: Marcel Dekker, 1982. Pp 89–115.

Rock, PB, et al. Effect of dexamethasone on symptoms of acute mountain sickness at Pike's Peak, Colorado (4,300 m). *Aviat Space Environ Med* 58:668, 1987.

Schoene, RB, et al. High altitude pulmonary edema and exercise at 4400 meters on Mt. McKinley: Effect of expiratory positive airway pressure. *Chest* 87:330, 1985.

Senay, LC, and Tolbert, DL. "Effect of arginine vasopressin, acetazolamide, and angiotensin II on CSF pressure at simulated altitude." *Aviat Space and Environ Med* 55:370, 1984.

Swenson, ER, et al. The effects of benzolamide on sea level ventilatory drives and periodic breathing and oxygen desaturation during sleep at high altitude: Abstract. *Am Rev Respir Dis* 133 (Suppl):A201, 1986.

Swenson, ER, and Maren, TH. Acute mountain sickness (letter). *N Engl J Med* 320:1492, 1989.

Other High Altitude Medical Problems

Hackett, PH, et al. Cortical Blindness in High Altitude Climbers and Trekkers—A Report of 6 Cases (abstract). In JR Sutton, CS Houston, and G Coates (eds), *Hypoxia and Cold.* New York: Praeger Press, 1987.

Sutton, JR, Houston, CS, and Coates, G. (eds). *Hypoxia and Cold.* New York: Praeger Press, 1987.

Kryger, M, et al. Treatment of excessive polycythemia of high altitude with respiratory stimulant drugs. *Am Rev Resp Dis* 117:455, 1978.

Kryger, MH, and Grover, RF. Chronic mountain sickness. *Semin Resp Med* 5:164, 1983.

Lahiri, S, et al. Sleep and Periodic Breathing at High Altitude: Sherpa Natives versus Sojourners. In JB West and S Lahiri (eds), *High Altitude and Man.* Bethesda, MD: American Physiological Society, 1984.
Lubin, JR, et al. High altitude retinal hemorrhage: A clinical and pathological case report. *Ann Ophthalmol* 14:1071, 1982.
McFadden, MD, et al. High-altitude retinopathy. *JAMA* 245:581, 1981.
O'Brodovich, HM, et al. Hypoxia alters blood coagulation during acute decompression in humans. *J Appl Physiol* 56:666, 1984.
Turner, WA, et al. Carbon monoxide exposure in mountaineers on Denali. *Alaska Med* 30:85, 1988.
Wohns, RNW. Transient ischemic attacks at high altitude. *Crit Care Med* 14:517, 1986.

General

Hackett, PH. *Mountain Sickness: Prevention, Recognition and Treatment.* New York: American Alpine Club, 1980.
Hackett, PH, and Hornbein, TF. Disorders of High Altitude. In JF Murray and JA Nadel (eds), *Textbook of Respiratory Medicine.* Philadelphia: Saunders, 1988.
Houston, CS. *Going Higher: The Story of Man and Altitude.* Boston: Little, Brown, 1987.
Schoene, RB, and Hornbein, TF. High Altitude Adaptation. In JF Murray and JA Nadel (eds), *Textbook of Respiratory Medicine.* Philadelphia: Saunders, 1988.
Ward, MP, Milledge, JS, and West, JB. *High Altitude Medicine and Physiology.* Philadelphia: University of Pennsylvania Press, 1989.
West, J, and Lahiri, S (eds). *High Altitude and Man.* Bethesda, MD: American Physiological Society, 1984.
West, J. *Everest: The Testing Place.* New York: McGraw-Hill, 1985.

DIVING EMERGENCIES

Henry D. Unger

"There are old divers, and there are bold divers. But there are no old, bold divers."

Old diver's adage

In recent years, the diving community has seen dramatic growth. The National Underwater Accident Data Center (NUADC) estimates that there are 5.5 million recreational SCUBA divers certified since 1960. Roughly half of those are considered "active" (more than three dives per year), and the ranks swell annually with thousands of newly certified divers who have completed introductory courses.

As participation in recreational diving continues to increase, so do the numbers of diving-related accidents and pressure-related maladies (barotrauma). Data published by the NUADC in 1984 revealed a fatality rate of 2.33 per 100,000 divers. In 1988 the combined number of fatal and nonfatal accidents had reached 47 per 100,000. Presumably, because of underreporting and misdiagnosis, morbidity rates are magnitudes higher.

Emergency medicine must encompass in its core teaching the basics of hyperbaric physiology. Often, if not exclusively, it will be the emergency medicine physician whom the sport diver will first consult with symptoms referable to barotrauma. The onus is on the physician to understand and recognize diving pathophysiology, so that he or she can provide appropriate treatment or referral, or both. Failure to recognize a "trivial" complaint (i.e., monoarticular arthralgia in decompression sickness) can lead to a devastating outcome. Although it may not be within the scope of most medical facilities to provide definitive care to an acutely ill diver, early recognition of the disease state, emergency stabilization, and referral to a diving specialty center may be the difference between total recovery and needless morbidity and mortality.

PHYSICS AND PHYSIOLOGY OF DIVING

Essential to the understanding of diving medicine is a firm grasp of physics as it relates to the underwater environment. The basic concept common to all barotrauma is pressure.

Pressure is defined as a force per unit area. Its units of measurement include pound per square inch (psi), atmospheres (atm), and millimeters of mercury (mm Hg). Anything with mass exerts a pressure. A column of air one square inch in dimension extending from sea level to the theoretical "top of the atmosphere" weighs 14.7 lb. (equivalent to 760 mm Hg, or 1 atm). A column of salt water with identical mass would extend only 33 feet in height (Fig. 84-3). In practice, this means that as the diver descends in the ocean, every 33 feet of depth increases the ambient pressure by a factor of 14.7 psi, or 1 atm. Per foot of depth, the pressure increases by 0.445 psi. Since depth and pressure are related in a linear fashion, the ambient pressure can be calculated at any point in the dive.

There are three laws of physics—Boyle's, Dalton's, and Henry's—which describe the behavior of an ideal gas. These lay the groundwork for understanding dysbarism (pressure-related pathology).

Boyle's law states that in a closed system, the volume of a gas varies inversely with the ambient pressure. A balloon, fully inflated at the surface of the ocean, decreases in size when submerged (Table 84-3). When the balloon is inflated at depth, the reverse holds true; its volume will increase as it nears the surface. On a percentage basis, the largest volume changes are seen at shallower depths. Thus, the consequences of Boyle's law for the diver are most critical at depths less than 15 feet.

The diver has three air-filled spaces in his or her body. Each can present a problem on descent or ascent if one's anatomic structure is altered in a way that produces a closed system. Normally the middle ear, sinuses, and lungs all vent to ambient pressure via a contiguous respiratory tract. Local pathology (i.e., mucous plugging, blocked eustachian tube) can subject these spaces to volume changes in accordance with fluctuations in ambient pressure. Establishment of moderate pressure gradients on either ascent or descent between these spaces and the external environment can result in barotrauma. If the diver is unable to equilibrate on de-

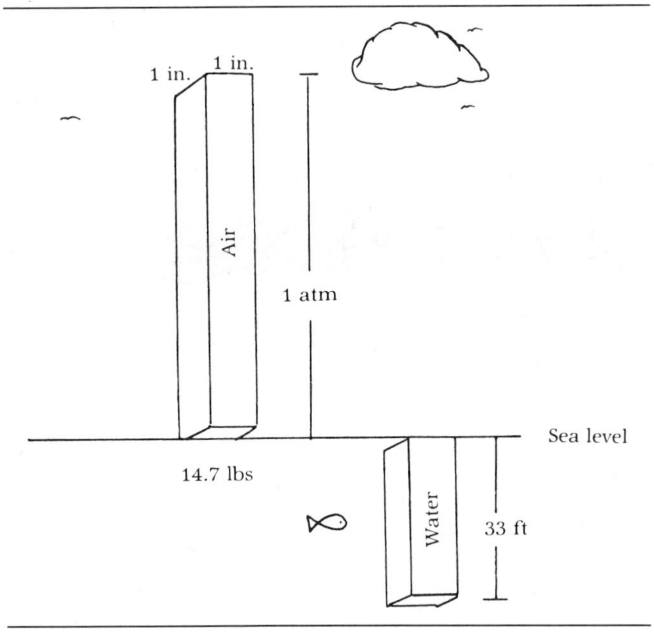

Fig. 84-3. One atmosphere pressure defined.

Table 84-3. Pressure volume relationships

Volume	Depth (ft)	Atmosphere	Pressure (psi)	Partial pressure (psi)
1	Sea level	1	14.7	Oxygen = 3 Nitrogen = 11.7
½	33	2	29.4	Oxygen = 6 Nitrogen = 23.4
⅓	66	3	44.1	Oxygen = 9 Nitrogen = 35.1

scent, the resulting compressive forces tend to "squeeze" the body compartments. On ascent, if the expanding gas is trapped, the local anatomy will be distorted, producing an overpressurization injury.

Although squeezes can occur in both the breathholding skin diver and the scuba diver on descent, it is solely the scuba diver who is at risk for overpressurization on ascent. Unlike the snorkeler, the scuba diver carries a self-contained breathing source. This tank is filled with compressed air at pressures approaching 3,000 psi. Attached to the cylinder is a regulator that provides air to the diver at the greatly reduced ambient pressure. This inspired air equilibrates throughout the body's spaces after it is inhaled. When the diver ascends in the water column, expanding volumes of this air must be allowed to vent to the regulator. If an anatomic blockage obstructs gas flow and prevents its escape, then the trapped portion of air increases in volume and causes damage to the adjacent tissues. This direct effect of pressure plays a significant role in the genesis of pulmonary barotrauma.

The indirect effects of pressure are caused by changes in the partial pressures and solubilities of different gases. In 1807, John Dalton wrote that the total pressure in a container is equal to the sum of the partial pressures (pp) of the constituent gases. The gas that the sport diver breathes is purified air. Regardless of depth, the breathing mixture remains constant: 79 percent nitrogen and 21 percent oxygen. Since the pressure of the air the diver breathes is equal to the ambient water pressure, it can be calculated knowing the depth. The following formula is used:

$$\text{Pressure} = [\text{depth (ft)} \times 0.445\ \text{psi}] + 14.7.$$

For example, at 33 ft, the total alveolar gas pressure is 29.4 psi (absolute). Nitrogen, accounting for 79 percent of the mixture, exerts a partial pressure of 23.2 psi. Oxygen accounts for the remaining 6.2 psi. Additional depth increases the partial pressures of the gases present but does not alter their ratio. As a consequence of their increased partial pressures, nitrogen and oxygen both produce toxic effects on the body.

The final gas law that directly impacts on the diver is Henry's law. It states that in a gas-liquid system, the solubility of gas is directly proportional to its partial pressure. Since the human body is largely composed of water, it follows that more gas will enter the fluid compartment as depth increases. The rate at which a gas will diffuse into the various tissues depends on the partial pressure, temperature, and the specific solubility for that gas in the particular tissue. The amount of gas that is absorbed is proportional to the duration of exposure.

If, after the tissue becomes saturated with gas, the ambient pressure is reduced beyond a critical point, the solubility of the gas will decrease and it will leave the liquid phase. This is analogous to the bubbling noted in a soda bottle when the cap is removed and the partial pressure of the dissolved carbon dioxide exceeds the partial pressure of CO_2 in the ambient air.

The dissolved gas that most affects the diver is nitrogen. Unlike oxygen, which is constantly metabolized, nitrogen is considered an inert gas. It is not metabolized and, consequently, accumulates in the body's tissues. If a given amount of nitrogen is dissolved in the body and the pressure is reduced beyond a critical point, it will leave solution in the form of bubbles. This pathologic state is known as the "bends."

DIRECT EFFECTS OF PRESSURE

Otologic Barotrauma

Middle Ear

The most common medical condition affecting the diver is middle ear barotrauma. It results when a pressure gradient develops between the outer and middle ear. Most often it is seen on compression, when water in the external ear canal causes inward displacement of the tympanic membrane (TM). Infrequently, the pressure gradient is reversed on ascent, tending to distract the TM. This is classified as a reverse ear squeeze.

Anatomically, the middle ear is a rigid, bony space with the eustachian tube (ET) serving as a conduit to ambient pressure. The tympanic membrane and the round and oval windows are the only distensible structures that can accommodate volume changes in accordance with Boyle's law

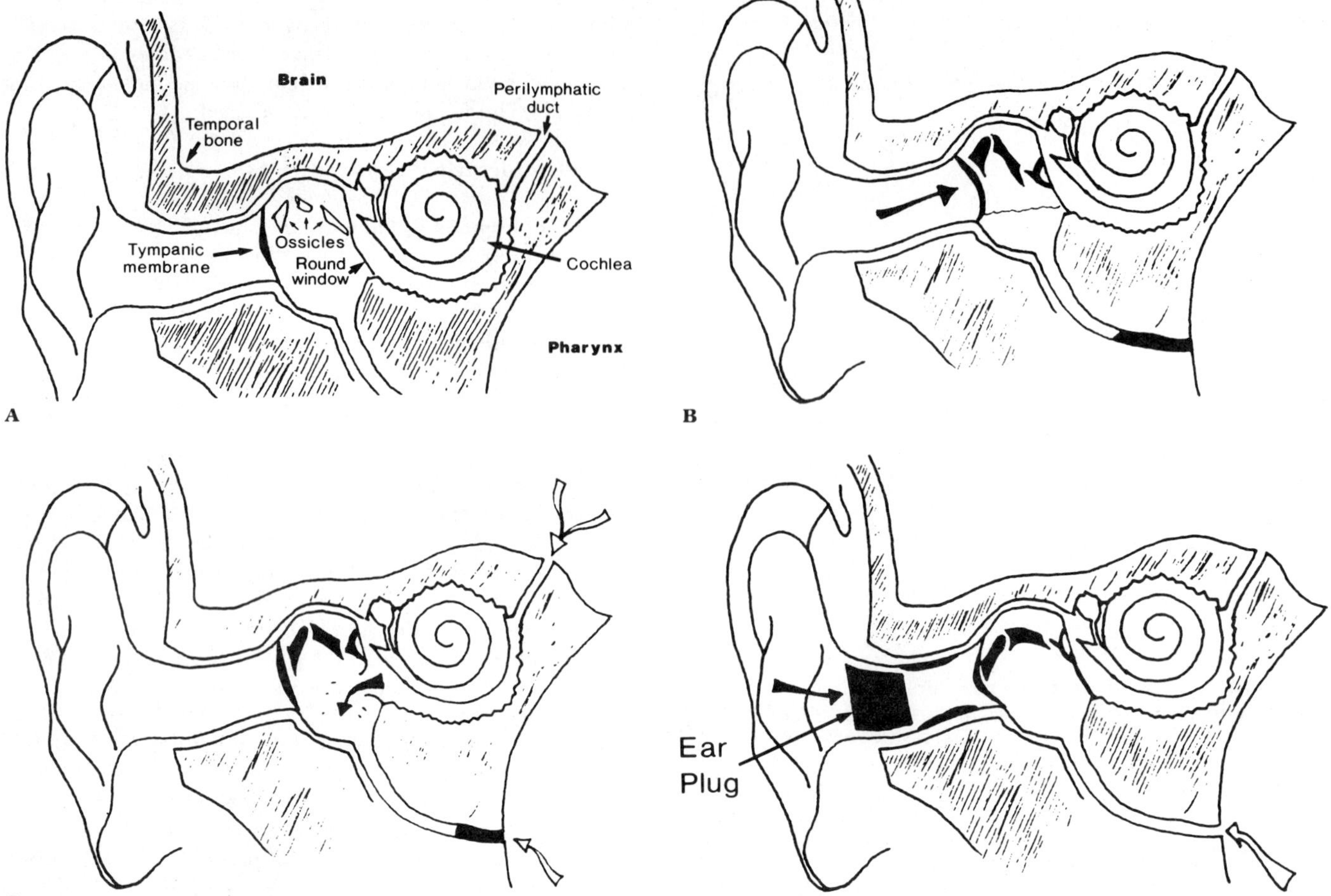

Fig. 84-4. A. Anatomy of the normal ear. Note the neutral position of the tympanic membrane when pressure is equilibrated. B. Middle ear squeeze. Arrow indicates water pressure. Note the tympanic membrane is retracted. The eustachian tube is blocked. C. Round window blow-out. Arrows indicate pressure gradient from CNS during Valsalva. Note the eustachian tube is blocked. D. External ear squeeze. Arrow indicates water pressure. Note swelling of the external canal and distention of the tympanic membrane. (Modified from J. C. Farmer and W. G. Thomas. Ear and Sinus Problems in Diving. In R.H. Straus [ed.], *Diving Medicine.* New York: Grune & Stratton, 1976.)

(Fig. 84-4A). The nasopharyngeal ostium of the ET is normally closed but can be manually opened by a variety of maneuvers, including yawning, swallowing, and a modified Valsalva maneuver known as the Frenzel. During descent, the diver repeatedly equilibrates pressure in the middle ear by forcing air through the patent ET. Obstruction of the orifice by local swelling (usually secondary to upper respiratory infection [URI]) leads to increasing negative pressure and an eventual middle ear squeeze.

In a thorough review of the subject, Farmer and Thomas describe the mechanics of the middle ear squeeze. At the surface, pressure in all three ear compartments (outer, middle, and inner) are equal. As the diver descends without equilibration, a pressure gradient is established. At a depth of 2.6 feet, the TM and the ossicles are displaced medially (Fig. 84-4B). The diver subjectively feels pain and a sense of fullness. A conductive hearing loss can result. Approaching 4 feet of depth without equalization of pressure causes "locking" of the ET ostium, preventing further equilibration. Rupture of the TM, resulting in severe vertigo, has been seen between 4 and 17 feet of depth.

Teed and Edmunds have described classification systems for evaluating middle ear barotrauma. Utilizing otoscopic findings, they divide ear squeeze into six categories. The spectrum of physical findings range from a normal TM to retraction and erythema of the membrane, fluid in the middle ear space, and, finally, blood in the middle ear or perforation of the TM. Farmer points out that these systems have limited clinical value and emphasizes instead the following classifications: (1) patients with symptoms (pain, conductive hearing loss) and no otoscopic findings, (2) symptoms with physical findings but without TM perforation, and (3) symptoms and perforation.

Treatment is dictated by the category in which the patient is placed. A diver with minor barotrauma (category 1) should receive systemic decongestants or topical nose drops, or both. Further diving should be restricted until all symptoms have resolved and the diver is able to "clear" or autoinflate his or her ears at the surface. Returning to depth while the squeeze is present can only exacerbate the situation.

A diver placed in category 2 will require a longer period of convalescence. At least 2 weeks will be necessary for resolution of symptoms. Treatment includes systemic and topical decongestants. Appropriate analgesia should be given. The use of prophylactic systemic antibiotics is controversial. Blood and serous fluid within the middle ear space provide an excellent culture media for bacteria. A high index of suspicion is warranted, and antibiotics should be utilized at the earliest signs of infection. Since pain is present in the absence of infection, fever and a purulent nasal discharge may be the only indicators of bacterial colonization. An intact TM precludes the use of topical antibiotics. Systemic treatment with ampicillin, erythromycin, or a cephalosporin is suggested. In an effort to decrease inflammation of the eustachian tube, many physicians advocate the use of nasally inhaled steroids (i.e., beclomethasone diprionate) or a 7 to 10-day course of oral prednisone. The diver should not return to the water until autoinflation can be performed.

Patients with perforated TMs should receive definitive care from an otolaryngologist. Historically, these divers describe difficulty equalizing, subsequent ear pain, followed by vertigo upon TM perforation. The water, cooler than body temperature, precipitates dysequilibrium as it layers against the inner ear. The episode is transient and resolves when the water approaches body temperature.

No otoxic solutions should be placed in the patient's ears. If blood and debris preclude visualization of the TM, a 1.5 percent hydrogen peroxide solution can be warmed to body temperature and used for irrigation. Once a perforated TM is identified, the ear should be kept dry and an ear-nose-throat (ENT) referral initiated. Prophylactic antibiotics are suggested by some physicians since contaminated water in the middle ear space can lead to infection. Return to diving will be dictated by the specialist but often is delayed until pneumatic otoscopy and audiographic studies are normal.

Rarely, a diver will suffer otologic barotrauma on ascent, commonly termed a *reverse ear squeeze.* Expanding volume in the middle ear can cause TM distention if venting via the ET is blocked. This occurs infrequently, since the nasopharyngeal ostium usually opens in response to the positive pressure. The condition is often unilateral, and transient vertigo results when asymmetric middle ear pressure stimulates the vestibular apparatus. The resulting *alternobaric vertigo* can be disabling to the diver if severe. A peripheral seventh nerve palsy has been seen in a number of these patients, possibly due to pressure effects on the vasa nervorum.

Examination of a reverse ear squeeze may reveal a bulging TM. If a squeeze is present from descent, concomitant changes in the appearance of the TM may be noted. Treatment is limited. Often slow decompression from the dive will allow for spontaneous equalization of pressures with resolution of pain and vertigo. The facial palsy is transient and resolves spontaneously. Persistent pain and decreased hearing may be treated with decongestants and analgesia.

Inner Ear

The inner ear interfaces with the middle ear via the round and oval windows. It is a fluid-filled structure and thus not compressible. However, it can sustain barotrauma secondary to pressure gradients across these distensible membranes (Fig. 84-4C). Edmunds, in 1974, described labyrinthine window ruptures. Two mechanisms of injury are postulated. The explosive mechanism suggests that an aggressive Valsalva maneuver increases intralabyrinthine pressure to some critical point above the relatively negative middle ear pressure. When a sufficient pressure gradient between the two spaces is reached, the round or oval window explodes and a fistula tract is formed. The implosive mechanism suggests that a successful Valsalva maneuver causes a rapid pressure increase in the middle ear space and subsequent inward rupture of the labyrinthine windows.

Regardless of the actual mechanism of injury, symptoms include roaring tinnitus and vertigo. On physical examination a sensorineural hearing loss will be uncovered. If an element of middle ear squeeze is present, a mixed hearing loss will be noted.

Definitive treatment is controversial and clearly calls for referral to an ENT specialist. Conservative versus exploratory tympanotomy are the available options. Initial management consists of bed rest with head elevation of 30 to 40 degrees. Any maneuvers that increase intracranial pressure and, hence, perilymphatic fluid pressure must be avoided.

The difficulty facing the emergency physician involves differentiating inner ear barotrauma from decompression sickness of the inner ear. This entity will be discussed in detail at a later point. It involves the evolution of nitrogen bubbles within the inner ear space. An accurate diagnosis is essential since treatment is different in each case.

The diagnosis of inner ear barotrauma is more likely when symptoms occur during the compression phase of the dive. A dive profile that does not suggest decompression sickness (i.e., shallow and of short duration) and symptoms and findings suggestive of middle ear squeeze all lend support to a diagnosis of inner ear barotrauma. In deep dives, with associated physical and historic findings of decompression sickness in other systems, inner ear bubble formation must be considered.

External Ear

Obstruction of the external canal by earplugs, tight-fitting thermal hoods, or cerumen can cause barotrauma of the outer ear. (Fig. 84-4D). A squeeze or overpressurization can occur, depending on the phase of the dive. Treatment includes removal of the obstruction and treatment of the middle ear pathology as outlined above. Divers are instructed to never dive with earplugs.

Paranasal Sinus Barotrauma

Barotrauma to the paranasal sinuses occurs when equalization is hampered on either ascent or descent. It is most commonly seen on descent and is associated with obstruction of the sinus ostia. Chronic infection, deviated septum, polyps, and mucous plugs have all been implicated as etiologic factors. The most common symptoms are pain followed by spontaneously resolving epistaxis. Most frequently, the pain is located in the frontal area (Farmer notes that the frontal sinus ostium is the longest and most tortuous), followed by ethmoid and maxillary locations. The pain is acute in onset and excruciatingly sharp in character. When involving the maxillary sinus, the pain can be misconstrued as an odontogenic problem. Often, severe pain on ascent will be spontaneously relieved when a large mucous/bloody clot is expelled from the nose, signaling removal of the obstruction and equalization of pressures.

Local reaction includes tissue edema with transudate into the sinus space. Overlying facial tenderness with mucosal thickening and air fluid levels on roentgenographic studies may be noted.

Use of systemic and topical decongestants is recommended. Often this will be sufficient, and symptoms will resolve over several days. Presence of a purulent discharge indicates the need for antibiotic therapy. Current recommendations include ampicillin or trimethoprim-sulfamethoxazole (TMP-SMX). The inflamed mucosal passageways may respond to a trial of a nasal steroid spray.

Dental Barotrauma (Aerodentalgia)

Although mentioned in all diving medicine texts, the occurrence of odontogenic pain secondary to barotrauma is rare. Expanding gas within the enamel confines of the tooth can theoretically lead to fracture on ascent. Definitive treatment requires dental referral, although emergent local anesthesia or nerve block will provide temporary relief.

Pulmonary Overpressurization Syndrome

Pulmonary overpressurization syndrome (POPS) represents a spectrum of diseases ranging from benign mediastinal emphysema to the potentially fatal arterial gas embolism. It has been the identifiable cause of death in the majority of diving fatalities.

In accordance with Boyle's law, if the diver does not allow expanding gas to vent the pulmonary tree on ascent, rupture of the alveolar membrane results. Experimentally, a transalveolar pressure of 80 mm Hg precipitates alveolar rupture. In linear measurements, this translates into a depth of 3.5 feet of salt water. The most common identifiable cause of POPS is a panicked emergency ascent, when the diver does not exhale during a rapid drop in ambient water pressure. Local airway obstruction can occur with bronchospasm, bullous disease, and scar tissue, which may lead to involuntary gas trapping.

The manifestations of POPS depend on the amount and location of escaping gas. Once alveolar rupture occurs, the gas tracks into adjoining tissues. Those alveoli surrounded entirely by other alveoli tend to vent their gas via the pores of Kohn into adjacent air sacs. Marginal alveoli, which rest on blood vessels, pleura, or connective tissue, vent gas into the pulmonary interstitium. Air escaping from these structures tracks along the perivascular sheaths towards the hilum. This collection of mediastinal gas (pneumomediastinum) may remain local or further dissect into adjoining tissues, producing subcutaneous emphysema, pneumoperitoneum, pneumothorax, or pneumopericardium. Air venting directly into the pulmonary veins can lead to a systemic air embolism.

Clinical manifestations depend on the amount and location of gas collection. In pneumomediastinum and subcutaneous emphysema, signs and symptoms are usually delayed several hours following the dive. In severe cases, they can be seen immediately upon surfacing. Chest pain (the most commonly reported symptom), dyspnea, and dysphagia have all been documented. Physical findings include voice change (tinny quality), crepitus in the soft tissues of the chest and neck, distant heart sounds, and mediastinal "crunch" (Hamman's sign). Cardiac tamponade from local gas dissection has been reported in the literature.

Treatment is conservative. In mild cases, rest and observation will be sufficient. In the event of severe symptoms such as airway compromise, recompression therapy is indicated. Supplemental oxygen and emergent airway management may be necessary until a decompression chamber can be reached. As a temporizing measure in the patient suffering respiratory embarrassment, a 14-gauge cannula placed superior to the suprasternal notch may assist in decompressing the neck and mediastinum. Airway control with an endotracheal tube may be required if extrinsic airway compression is severe.

Although most instances of pneumomediastinum and subcutaneous emphysema are mild and self-limiting, the prudent physician must be aware that they can be associated with more malignant forms of pulmonary barotrauma, such as systemic embolism. Pearson reviewed 199 cases of arterial gas embolism and found that 79 percent had associated mediastinal air.

Pneumothorax is an infrequent sequela of POPS. When present, it is likely to be bilateral, stemming from dissection of gas from the hilar region into the pleural space. A tension pneumothorax is seldom present, although with sufficient air leakage, ascent from a deep dive can produce one. Diagnosis and treatment of a pneumothorax from a diving-related incident are identical to diagnosis and treatment of a pneumothorax from a non–diving-related cause. Needle aspiration or tube thoracostomy is the preferred treatment. Although the physician must be alerted to other sequelae of pulmonary barotrauma, Pearson points out that only 5 percent of pneumothoraces are associated with arterial gas embolism.

The most severe form of pulmonary barotrauma is the arterial gas embolism. Gaseous emboli can migrate to the systemic circulation via one of two routes. Presence of a patent foramen ovale (incidence as high as 30% on postmortem examinations) can allow venous emboli to pass through to the left side of the heart. Return of gaseous emboli to the left atrium via the pulmonary veins provides the other pathway. The former route may play an important role in the genesis of decompression sickness, but it is the latter pathway that is the source of emboli in the case of pulmonary barotrauma.

Once in the systemic circulation, the emboli may travel to a multitude of locations. The two organs of most concern to the diver are the heart and brain. In dogs, it has been shown that the upright position tends to favor embolic migration to the cerebral circulation. Since the diver ascends in a head-up orientation, he or she is also at greater risk for cerebral emboli. Embolization to the brain will present with symptoms of stroke. When occlusion of the coronary circulation occurs, ischemia, arrhythmia, and cardiac arrest can result.

The hallmark of systemic gas embolization is the rapidity with which symptoms present following the dive. In a review of 116 cases of gas embolism, Leitch noted that the onset of symptoms occurred during ascent in 10 cases; 97 cases within 5 minutes of surfacing; and the remainder within 10 minutes. This historic feature is extremely important when trying to separate the later-occurring manifestations of decompression sickness from air embolism.

The neurologic manifestations include coma, confusion/disorientation, dizziness, monoplegia, asymmetric multiplegia, sensory changes, blindness/blurred vision, headache, deafness, seizures, loss of coordination, aphasia, nausea, and vomiting. Because of the cerebral location, findings tend to be either pure motor or pure sensory and are most commonly hemiplegic deficits. Although the presence of hemoptysis is classically included in this symptom list, Kizer points out that it occurred in less than 1 percent of cases that he reviewed.

Air embolism should be suspected in any diver suffering an acute neurologic deficit immediately following a dive. Decompression sickness and pulmonary barotrauma may have similar presentations and may be difficult to differentiate. In many cases, the disease states coexist. The history of the dive may aid the physician in determining which entity is present. Shallow dives (especially those under 33 feet in depth) and those of short duration tend to favor a diagnosis of pulmonary barotrauma. A table of "no decompression limits" developed by the U.S. Navy describes the maximum length of time a diver can remain at any given depth without suffering decompression sickness. This information can aid the physician in making a diagnosis; thus, a pertinent history of the patient should be elicited from accompanying divers.

The definitive treatment for air embolism is recompression therapy. The application of hyperbaric oxygen functions at many levels. In accordance with Boyle's law, the diameter of the emboli will decrease when recompressed. This allows for migration of the blockage to a more distal, it is hoped, less critical site. Breathing 100 percent oxygen increases the diffusion rate of the inert gases out of the bubble and increases the speed of bubble resolution. In an animal model, the observed response of the cerebral circulation to gaseous emboli is vasoconstriction followed by vasodilation. The resulting vasogenic cerebral edema is ameliorated by hyperbaric oxygen. Additionally, increased diffusion distances made possible by the elevated PO_2 reduces the hypoxic insult to the neuronal tissue.

Only a limited number of medical facilities have a recompression chamber. For assistance in determining the need for and the location of a recompression chamber, the Diving Accident Network (DAN) can be reached at 919–686–8111.

Once the diagnosis of air embolism is made, emergent treatment can be initiated by the physician. Arrangements for definitive therapy and transportation should be undertaken simultaneously. In the case of cardiac arrest, standard advanced cardiac life support (ACLS) protocol should be followed. Difficulty ventilating in the presence of pulmonary barotrauma should alert the physician to the possibility of a tension pneumothorax exacerbated by positive pressure ventilation. Appropriate measures should be taken.

The use of the Trendelenburg or Durant position (feet elevated, patient on left side) is advocated. Although some authors question its ability to protect from cerebral bubble migration, the head-down position will cause vasodilation and aid embolic migration to more distal sites. Unfortunately, this position tends to exacerbate existing cerebral edema. If used, the duration of time should be limited. Lying the patient supine will more than likely be adequate.

All patients should receive 100 percent oxygen. For all the previously mentioned reasons, its use is mandatory. Cardiac monitoring and intravenous access should be initiated immediately. Because of the concern for cerebral edema, the fluid load should be conservative. A dextrose, 2.5 percent, one-fourth normal saline solution is recommended.

Table 84-4. Pulmonary overpressurization syndrome

Classification	Etiology	Treatment
Subcutaneous emphysema	Air in subcutaneous tissues of neck	Observation
Mediastinal emphysema	Dissected air into the mediastinum	Observation
Pneumothorax	Hilar dissection of air into pleural space	Thoracostomy
Systemic air embolism	Emboli to coronary artery or cerebral circulation	Recompression

Adjunctive therapy includes the use of dexamethasone. A loading dose of 12 mg IV given immediately may be beneficial in reducing vasogenic cerebral edema. Loop and osmotic diuretics have been advocated by some physicians, although their application should be used in consultation with the physician providing the definitive therapy. Recently, the use of anticoagulants to limit clot propagation at the blood-bubble interface has been raised. Further research is required before recommendations can be made.

When the patient is stabilized, transport to the chamber must be initiated. Ground transportation is ideal. If it is necessary that the patient be transported by air, attention to cabin pressure is mandatory. Any reduction in ambient pressure will further increase emboli diameter. Either a low-flying helicopter or aircraft with the ability to pressurize its cabin should be used.

In general, the sooner that recompression therapy is given, the better the outcome. However, a delayed diagnosis should not lessen the vigor with which recompression therapy is sought. Cases of delayed compression with good clinical outcomes have been documented. When the patient is transported, a clearly documented history of the patient's dive must accompany the patient. Depth, duration, prior dives, and events surrounding the ascent should be included. All will be helpful in determining the hyperbaric therapy protocol (Table 84-4).

INDIRECT EFFECTS OF PRESSURE

Nitrogen Narcosis

As the partial pressure of nitrogen increases, so does its narcotic effect. The diver breathing compressed air will feel the untoward effects of nitrogen narcosis in excess of 125 to 150 feet. Delirium and impaired judgment and psychomotor skills have afforded this syndrome the nickname *rapture of the deep.* Martini's law, taught to neophyte divers, equates the effect of nitrogen on the diver to that of a dry martini on an empty stomach. Each additional 50 feet of depth, according to this law, is analogous to drinking another martini.

In and of itself, nitrogen narcosis is not dangerous. When the diver ascends, the effects immediately resolve (without a hangover). The concern is what the diver does while "under the influence" of nitrogen. Stories abound, ranging from the diver who "lent" his regulator to the mermaid to the diver who cut all his hoses (including the one that supplied air) because they were "in the way." It may be that unexplained cases of pulmonary barotrauma are somehow related to poor judgment secondary to nitrogen narcosis.

The effects of nitrogen under pressure can hamper the usefulness of support personnel in a recompression chamber when treating a patient. For professional divers who must work at depths in excess of 150 feet, a special mixture of gases is breathed that has replaced a portion of the nitrogen with helium.

Oxygen Toxicity

When the partial pressure of oxygen exceeds 30 psi, the risk of seizures is increased. This is an unlikely event for the recreational diver since this partial pressure will not be attained at less than 297 feet of depth. For more information, see the Hyperbaric Oxygen Therapy section of this chapter.

Decompression Sickness

In 1670, Sir Robert Boyle placed a snake in a vacuum. He wrote of his observations: "A viper furiously tortured, with a manifest bubble moving to and fro in the humor of its eye." Unbeknownst to the scientist, he had just reproduced a clinical state that would be responsible for the disability and death of thousands of divers in future years. By reducing the ambient pressure, Boyle had precipitated the formation of nitrogen bubbles within the tissues of the animal. Two hundred years later, miners exposed to rapid decompression after exiting from caissons filled with compressed air were observed to suffer severe joint pain and neurologic deficits. Returning the afflicted miners to the compressed air environment ameliorated the symptoms. Sufferers of *Caisson's disease* hobbled in pain and were derided by their fellow workers for ambulating in a manner similar to the affected posture of society women of the day. This style, the Grecian bend, was to become the origin for the most notorious diving disease, the bends.

The diver breathing compressed air is exposed to increased partial pressures of nitrogen. The established pressure gradient favors the saturation of the body's tissues with this inert gas. The total amount of dissolved nitrogen in any specific tissue is dependent on the duration of exposure, the partial pressure of the gas, and the specific characteristics of the tissue. After a 12-hour exposure at any depth, the tissues will become fully saturated and a steady state is attained.

When the diver ascends, the pressure gradient is reversed. The tissue compartment will begin to "unload" nitrogen. This is analogous to the soda bottle being uncapped where dissolved carbon dioxide leaves solution in the form of "bubbling" soda. If the diver ascends at a predetermined rate and makes scheduled interval stops during the ascent stage (decompression stops), the amount of bubble formation will be limited and no symptoms of decompression sickness will appear. If the guidelines are not followed, bubble nucleation can be severe and a myriad of symptoms can present.

The precise mechanisms governing bubble formation and subsequent tissue reaction remain obscure. Strauss suggests that joint pains originate from mechanical distention of the type 2 Ruffini corpuscles by bubble formation within the joint capsule. Hallenbeck, using a dog model, presents an elaborate explanation of the neurologic sequelae. His group proposes that bubble formation in the microcirculation with subsequent migration to the central venous system causes stasis in the large epidural venous complex. This resulting sludging allows the nitrogen bubbles to coalesce and produce obstruction with resulting infarct and ischemia. In addition to the mechanical effects of the bubbles, activity at the blood-gas interface activates the clotting system. Subsequent platelet aggregation, release of vasoactive amines, and fibrin deposition tend to propagate the obstruction.

Clinically, decompression sickness (DCS) is divided into five categories. Type 0 DCS includes those divers with cutaneous manifestations only. Pruritis and marbling of the skin reflect localized venous-lymphatic collections of gas. Type I DCS includes divers who present with joint pain only. Type II DCS includes more serious symptoms such as neurologic deficits and cardiopulmonary complications. Type III DCS is of the inner ear. Type IV DCS will not be discussed, but, for completeness sake, involves divers with aseptic osteonecrosis.

More than ninety percent of DCS cases are type I. The pain is periarticular and described as "aching." The shoulder is most commonly involved, followed by the remaining joints in the upper extremities, then the hips and knees. Movement tends to aggravate the pain; consequently, the joint is often held in a flexed position. If untreated, the joint becomes exquisitely painful over the ensuing hours. It has been noted that heat tends to exacerbate the pain; inflation of a blood pressure cuff around the joint may relieve the myalgia. Although these may be helpful diagnostic tools, the physician must not be quick to attribute joint pain to nonspecific causes in the diver. Most important, he or she should realize that 30 percent of type II divers also have arthralgias.

Type II involves the central nervous system (CNS) or cardiorespiratory systems, or both. Neurologic involvement can involve any part of the CNS, but the majority of cases tend to involve the spinal cord. Unlike barotrauma, which presents immediately on surfacing, the presentation of DCS is delayed. In a review by Dick, more than 50 percent of cases presented 1 or more hours after the dive. More than one-fourth occurred at least 6 hours following surfacing. In his review of 70 cases, most victims presented with a "warm, prickly paresthesia" in the affected limb, followed by numbness, weakness, and paralysis. It is generally accepted that the lower extremities are more frequently involved and deficits tend to be bilateral at a given cord level.

In a review of 935 cases of DCS, Rivera noted (in order of frequency) paresthesias, muscle weakness, vertigo, paralysis, visual disturbances, urinary retention, unconsciousness, personality changes, and seizures. Cord lesions can occur at multiple levels, yielding scattered findings. Radicular pain presenting as chest-back-girdle discomfort must be interpreted as a potential cord "hit." It is better to treat a diver for DCS who has a muscle strain than to miss dermatomal pain from the bends.

The lungs act as filters and efficiently trap nitrogen bubbles. It has been documented by Doppler ultrasonography that many divers who do not present with the clinical manifestations of bends still manifest bubble formation in the bloodstream following a dive. It is likely that the lungs collect these "silent" nitrogen bubbles and allow for their absorp-

Table 84-5. A comparison of decompression sickness and air embolism

	DCS	Air embolism
Etiology	Nitrogen bubbles	Air bubbles
Dive profile	Deep, prolonged, repetitive dive	Rapid ascents, breath holding
Symptom presentation	1–2 hr	Within 10 min of surfacing
Symptoms	Mixed motor and sensory hemiparaplegia	Pure motor-sensory hemiparesis
Emergency treatment	ACLS, rehydration, decompression	ACLS, limited fluids, decompression

Key: ACLS = advanced cardiac life suppport.

tion without producing symptoms. However, when a critical level of gas collection is reached, the pulmonary vasculature is overwhelmed. In severe cases of DCS, an increase in pulmonary vascular resistance, bronchospasm, and major alterations in the perfusion/ventilation relationship are noted. The diver suffers with severe chest pain, substernal burning, and shortness of breath. Referred to as the "chokes," in severe cases it can lead to hypoxia, shock, and death. If the patient has a patent foramen ovale, it is possible that the nitrogen bubbles can migrate to the systemic circulation and produce symptoms analogous to air embolism.

Type III DCS (inner ear decompression sickness) is the likely result of bubble formation within the perilymph-endolymph on ascent. Some animal studies have suggested the possibility of labyrinthine hemorrhage. Symptoms include vertigo, nausea, vomiting, and tinnitus on ascent or following decompression. There may be an associated hearing loss. It is important to evaluate the likelihood of DCS in such a patient so as to differentiate this inner ear lesion from barotrauma. Patients in the latter category will often yield a history of difficulty equalizing, otologic pain on ascent-descent, roaring tinnitus, and sudden onset of symptoms.

When attempting to differentiate DCS from air embolism, important historic factors can be of help (Table 84-5). Delayed symptom presentation favors the bends. An air embolism will seldom present after 10 minutes. A diver who has not exceeded 33 feet of depth has negligible risk for DCS. If the dive was well within the limits of time and depth as defined by the dive tables that most divers carry with them, DCS is less likely. A recent addition to the diver's repertoire of equipment includes portable decompression computers. Although these wrist-worn devices were designed to decrease the risk of DCS for the users, a significant number of divers have been "bent" while using them. Consequently, the physician cannot rule out DCS based on the dive computer's analysis. Increased depth, repetitive dives within a 12-hour period, obesity, alcohol, cigarettes, hypothermia, and dehydration tend to predispose to the bends. A thorough neurologic examination can aid in defining the pathology. In DCS, motor and sensory findings usually coexist, unlike the pure losses noted in gas embolism. Barotrauma tends to cause hemiplegia, in contrast to the paraplegia found from cord involvement in the bends.

A diver with type 0 DCS requires close observation and supplemental oxygen. If careful neurologic exminations remain normal, no further intervention is necessary. The definitive treatment of types I, II, III, and IV DCS is recompression therapy in a hyperoxic environment. As noted in the section on gas embolism, reduction of bubble size reduces the mechanical effects of embolic obstruction-distention on local anatomy. The use of hyperbaric oxygen versus compressed air has several advantages. It establishes a steeper pressure gradient between the nitrogen bubble and the surrounding environment. This favors more rapid inert gas washout. CNS edema, subsequent to tissue ischemia and vascular permeability changes, is ameliorated by elevated tissue PO_2. Another benefit of compression in oxygen is that no further nitrogen is absorbed during therapy itself.

Medical stabilization prior to recompression therapy is mandatory. Once the diagnosis of DCS has been made, an intravenous line should be established. Supplemental high flow oxygen should be administered. ACLS or ventilatory assistance should be given as needed. Simultaneously, calls should be placed to either the Diving Accident Network or the nearest chamber facility.

Hypovolemia secondary to generalized increased vascular permeability must be aggressively treated with crystalloid. The use of isotonic saline to maintain an adequate urine output is advised. The oral route for fluid replacement should be avoided.

Glucocorticoids may play a useful role inhibiting brain and spinal cord edema. Their anti-inflammatory actions may decrease local effects at the bubble-blood interface and also return vascular permeability to a more normal state. Recommendations include 100 mg hydrocortisone IV and 12 mg dexamethasone IM as an initial dose.

Research to evaluate the potential benefits of nonsteroidal anti-inflammatory drugs points to the use of aspirin. Although clinical studies are lacking, theoretically the drug should help by decreasing platelet aggregation. Recommendations range from 600 mg to 1 gm per day.

Anticoagulants have been suggested by some physicians as a method to inhibit the clotting process initiated at the bubble surface. With the risk of labyrinthine bleeding in the inner ear and the possibility of bleeding in an infarcted spinal cord, their use is not advocated at this time.

When planning transport to the recompression facility, one should bear in mind the need for low-level pressurized air evacuation or rapid ground systems. The patient should be either supine or in a slight Trendelenburg position.

Special mention should be made of flying after diving. Since commercial jetliners only compress their cabin to the equivalent of 8000 ft of altitude, a diver who has flown within 24 hours of diving is at risk of developing the bends. In 1988 DAN reported on 49 divers who developed symptoms of DCS while flying.

As in any disease state, the more rapidly that treatment is initiated, the better the outcome. If a patient presents with persistent symptoms days after a dive, therapy should still be initiated. Myers reports three patients treated successfully for DCS up to 1 week following exposure.

CONCLUSION

Awareness of diving pathophysiology will guide the physician toward successful diagnosis and treatment of the disease state. Because of the sport's popularity, the examining physician must always think to elicit a diving history when indicated. Often, as in the case of middle ear barotrauma, the symptoms and treatment will be straightforward. However, in the cases of DCS and air embolism, the clinical picture can be deceiving. If one keeps an open mind and includes these disease states in the differential diagnosis, appropriate care will be rendered.

SELECTED READING

Books

Strauss, RH (ed). *Diving Medicine.* New York: Grune & Stratton, 1976.

Shilling, CW, Carlston, CB, and Mathias, RA (eds). *The Physician's Guide to Diving Medicine.* New York: Plenum, 1984. Pp. 192–198, 223–269, 283–311, 316–327, 337–367.

Journals

Arthur, DC, and Margulies, RA. A short course in diving medicine. *Ann Emerg Med* 16:689, 1987.

Boettger, ML. Scuba diving emergencies: Pulmonary overpressurization accidents and decompression sickness. *Ann Emerg Med* 12(9):563, 1983.

Bove, AA. The basis for drug therapy in decompression sickness. *Undersea Biomed Res* 9(2):91, 1982.

Calder, IM. Dysbarism: A review. *Forensic Sci Int* 30:237, 1986.

Dick, PK, and Massey, EW. Neurologic presentation of decompression sickness and air embolism in sport divers. *Neurology* 35:667, 1985.

Edmonds, C, et al. Fistula of the round window in diving. *Trans Am Acad Ophthalmol Otolaryngol* 78:444, 1974.

Freeman, P, Tonkin, J, and Edmonds, C. Rupture of the round window membrane in inner ear barotrauma. *Arch Otolaryngol* 99:437, 1974.

Hallenbeck, JM, Bove, AA, and Elliot, DH. Mechanisms underlying spinal cord damage in decompression sickness. *Neurology* 25: 308, 1975.

Hills, BA, and James, PB. Spinal decompression sickness: Mechanical studies and a model. *Undersea Biomed Res* 9:185, 1982.

Kizer, KW. Corticosteroids in treatment of serious decompression sickness. *Ann Emerg Med* 10(9):485, 1981.

Kizer, KW. Delayed treatment of dysbarism: A retrospective review of 50 cases. *JAMA* 247:2555, 1982.

Kizer, KW. Diving medicine. *Emerg Med Clin North Am* 12(3):513, 1984.

Kizer, KW. Management of dysbaric diving casualties. *Emerg Med Clin North Am* 1(3):659, 1983.

Myers, RA, and Bray, P. Delayed treatment of serious decompression sickness. *Ann Emerg Med* 14(3):254, 1985.

Parell, GJ, and Becker, GD. Conservative management of inner ear barotrauma resulting from scuba diving. *Otolaryngol Head Neck Surg* 93(3):393, 1985.

Riveria, JC. Decompression sickness among divers: An analysis of 935 cases. *Milit Med* 129:314, 1966.

Strauss, MB, and Samson, RL. Decompression sickness: An update. *Phys Sports Med* 4(3):196, 1986.

Sykes, JW. Spinal cord decompression sickness: A review of the pathology and some new findings. *J R Nav Med Serv* 71:139, 1985.

Teed, RW. Factors producing obstruction of the auditory tube in submarine personnel. *US Nav Med Bull* 44:293, 1944.

Statistics

U.S. Underwater Diving Fatality Statistics 1983–1984, Report No. URI–SSR–86–18.

Report on 1988 Diving Accidents. Durham, NC: Divers Alert Network, 1989.

HYPERBARIC OXYGEN THERAPY

Michael Lucca
Henry D. Unger

Hyperbaric oxygen therapy (HBOT) a sophisticated technology that has seen its role expand beyond the realm of aquatic and aviation medicine into the domain of emergency medicine. It requires exposure of the entire body to increased atmospheric pressure while breathing 100 percent oxygen. New therapeutic applications have emerged that make this a desirable treatment modality (Table 84-6).

In this chapter, we focus on the use of HBOT in select disease states commonly encountered by the emergency physician. The history of hyperbaric medicine and its mechanisms of action will be reviewed. It will also mention the hazards of HBOT and the type of chambers available for treatment.

HISTORY

The clinical origins of hyperbaric medicine date back to 1662. Henshaw, a British physician, constructed a chamber called the "domicilium." It was equipped with a pair of organ bellow valves that could produce either hyper- or hypobaric conditions. A patient was placed in the chamber, and the "appropriate" environment was reproduced. Acute disorders were treated with hyperbaric conditions, and chronic diseases were exposed to low pressure. The results were mixed, with the latter group becoming abruptly cyanotic! Although the physiology was not understood, word of its limited success spread throughout Europe. Soon multiple chambers were constructed.

By the end of the nineteenth century, the popularity of hyperbaric therapy began to decline. It was not until 1918 that Dr. Orville Cunningham introduced HBOT into the United States. He often exaggerated his ability to cure disease with high-pressure oxygen. The American Medical Association attacked his claims and became an outspoken critic of HBOT. Soon he was forced to dismantle his first chamber facility. However, a patient who experienced a miraculous cure while under Dr. Cunningham's care convinced a wealthy friend to finance the building of another chamber. It was a hyperbaric hospital, measuring 64 feet in diameter, five stories in height, and housed 36 patients. It saw little use, and in 1936, hyperbaric treatments were discontinued. Dr. Cunningham had his license revoked and died in the late 1930s. The field of hyperbaric medicine entered its "dark age."

In the early 1950s, clinicians again became interested in hyperbaric medicine. Its true renaissance began with Dr. Boerema of Amsterdam, Netherlands. He explored the use

Table 84-6. Conditions treated with HBOT

Accepted conditions	Investigational indications
Air or gas embolism (acute)	Anaerobic and mixed aerobic, anaerobic brain abscesses
Carbon monoxide poisoning	Carbon tetrachloride poisoning
Acute smoke inhalation	Cerebrovascular accidents
Assumed carbon monoxide/ cyanide poisoning	Head injury
Crush injury	Fracture healing and bone grafting
Compartment syndrome	Hydrogen sulfide poisoning
Acute traumatic ischemias	Lepromatous leprosy
Acute cyanide poisoning	Meningitis
Decompression sickness	Multiple sclerosis
Enhancement of healing in selected problem wounds	Pyoderma gangrenosum
Diabetic wounds	Pseudomembranous colitis
Venous stasis ulcers	Radiation enteritis and proctitis
Decubitus ulcers	Radiation myelitis
Arterial insufficiency ulcers	Acute central retinal artery insufficiency
Exceptional blood loss (anemia)	Selected refractory mycoses
Gas gangrene	Sepsis (chronic), intra-abdominal abscesses
Necrotizing soft tissue infections	Sickle cell anemia crisis
Crepitant anaerobic cellulitis	Spider bites (brown recluse, loxsceles reclusa)
Progressive bacterial gangrene	Spinal cord injury
Necrotizing fasciitis	
Nonclostridial myonecrosis	
Fournier's disease	
Miscellaneous necrotizing infections in the compromised host	
Refractory osteomyelitis	
Radiation necrosis	
Osteoradionecrosis	
Soft tissue radiation necrosis	
Caries in radiated bones	
Selected refractory anaerobic infections: actinomycosis	
Skin grafts or flaps (compromised)	
Thermal burns	

of HBOT in the treatment of clostridial infections and wrote the classic article "Life Without Blood." In this paper he described the survival of profoundly anemic piglets in a hyperbaric environment. He showed that the pigs' entire oxygen needs could be met by the amount of oxygen physically dissolved in the plasma. Hemoglobin was no longer necessary for survival.

Extensive research conducted by the U.S. Navy in the 1950s and 1960s studied the effects of oxygen toxicity in humans. The continued interest in hyperbaric medicine led to the establishment in 1967 of the Undersea Medical Society (UMS). The Subcommittee on Hyperbaric Oxygen of the UMS was formed in 1976. Its role is to critically evaluate experimental and clinical applications of HBOT.

Table 84-7. Mechanisms of action of HBOT

Primary effects
Hyperoxygenation
Bubble reduction
Secondary effects
Vasoconstriction
Microbial effects
Bacteriostasis
Inhibition of toxin formation
Toxin deactivation
Antibiotic transport
Neovascularization
Leukocyte oxidative killing
Fibroblastic proliferation
Collagen formation
Osteoclast stimulation
Counterdiffusion
Barrier permeation

PHYSIOLOGY AND MECHANISMS OF ACTION

Hyperbaric oxygen therapy works by specialized scientific mechanisms (Table 84-7); therefore, its applications are specific. There are primary and secondary effects of high-pressure oxygen.

The hyperoxygenation effect is the most well-known mechanism of action. Under normobaric conditions, 97 percent of the oxygen is carried by hemoglobin in red blood cells, the remainder is dissolved in the plasma. As the partial pressure of ambient oxygen increases, the remaining 3 percent of the hemoglobin becomes saturated. Any additional oxygen must be physically dissolved in the plasma. The amount of gas that will enter this extracellular fluid is based on Henry's law. It states that the concentration of a dissolved gas equals the partial pressure of the gas multiplied by a solubility coefficient. At 3 atmospheres absolute (ATA) pressure, it is possible to reach an arterial oxygen pressure of 2,250 mm Hg. For each atmosphere of pressure, 2.3 volumes percent of oxygen is dissolved in solution. Therefore, 6.9 volumes percent of oxygen is dissolved in the plasma at 3 ATA (the working pressure for HBOT). As blood circulates through the capillary bed, 5 volumes percent is extracted. This is the A-VO_2 difference and accounts for the basal metabolic requirement of normal tissue. At 3 ATA, there is enough oxygen physically dissolved in the plasma to satisfy this basal need without utilizing any hemoglobin-bound oxygen. This is supported by the survival of Boerema's pigs.

Hyperoxygenation overcomes barriers. Edema, dead or devitalized tissue, and microcirculatory stasis all act to prevent oxygen from being delivered to tissues. Under hyperbaric conditions, the diffusion distance of oxygen is 2 to 3 times greater than in the normoxic environment. Since wound healing is dependent on adequate oxygenation, marginally ischemic tissue will benefit from increased oxygen diffusion. The enhanced oxygen delivery will promote neovascularization, fibroblastic proliferation, osteoclastic function, and leukocyte killing. All are essential in the wound-healing process.

Bubble reduction is another primary effect of hyperbaric oxygen. According to Boyle's law, the volume of a gas is

Table 84-8. Boyle's law: The volume of a gas is inversely proportional to its pressure at a constant temperature

ATA	Gas volume (%)
1	100
2	50
3	33
4	25
5	20
6	17

inversely proportional to its pressure. Exposure to hyperbaric oxygen will decrease the volume of gaseous emboli (Table 84-8) and allow for distal migration of any blockage. Iatrogenic air embolism and pulmonary barotrauma are amenable to this therapy.

The inhalation of 100 percent oxygen creates a steep diffusion gradient for the elimination of inert gases, such as nitrogen from air bubbles. The speed at which a gas embolus will be absorbed is proportional to the rate of gaseous diffusion. An air bubble composed of 80 percent nitrogen will diffuse quickly into an environment of 100 percent oxygen because the nitrogen gradient is quite steep (ambient $pN_2 = 0$). If placed in a compressed air environment, however, where the pN_2 is higher, the gradient is less and absorption rates are decreased. Therefore, treating the "bends" (systemic N_2 bubbles) and air emboli in hyperbaric oxygen not only provides for mechanical reduction in bubble size but also increased rate of absorption.

Vasoconstriction is a secondary effect of hyperbaric oxygen. Oxygen causes a 20 percent reduction in blood flow. However, because of the increased oxygenation of the plasma, the vasoconstriction does not compromise tissue oxygenation. The decreased blood flow will reduce tissue edema often seen as a consequence of crush injuries, traumatic ischemias, and burns.

APPLICATIONS

The Hyperbaric Oxygen Committee of the UMS determines the accepted indications for HBOT. It also categorizes conditions considered investigational (see Table 84-6). In this section, we discuss diseases frequently encountered by the emergency physician for which HBOT has proved beneficial.

Carbon Monoxide Poisoning

Carbon monoxide (CO) is a colorless, odorless, and tasteless gas produced by the incomplete combustion of organic material. Exogenous sources include cigarette smoke, automobile exhaust, fires, and poorly ventilated heating systems. Methylene chloride, a solvent used in paint strippers, is converted to CO endogenously.

In the United States, more than 1,500 people are killed each year by CO poisoning. In addition, most of the 10,000 fire-related deaths are due to the inhalation of toxic fumes that contain not only carbon monoxide but also cyanide and other toxic volatile gases.

Carbon monoxide inhibits the uptake, delivery, and utilization of oxygen. It rapidly produces tissue hypoxia, ischemia, and ultimately death. The affinity of hemoglobin for CO is 250 times greater than that for oxygen.

The formed carboxyhemoglobin (COHb), having decreased the pool of transported oxygen, causes a left shift of the oxyhemoglobin of dissociation curve. This results in reduced delivery of available oxygen to tissues.

Carbon monoxide affects the utilization of oxygen at the cellular level. It reversibly competes with oxygen for receptor sites on the cytochrome chain. By combining with C_3A oxidase, CO interferes with electron transport and cellular energy production. The heart and nervous system have the highest metabolic rates and thus are the most sensitive organs. Recent work suggests that CO may induce lipid peroxidation in cell membranes with subsequent neuronal death. This may play a role in the latent effects of CO poisoning.

The symptoms of CO poisoning range from headache, nausea, and irritability to angina, arrhythmias, myocardial infarctions, seizures, coma, and death. Delayed neurologic sequelae have been documented in patients exposed to CO days to weeks after the initial exposure. Subtle neurologic findings, including irritability, personality change, confusion, memory loss, and difficulty concentrating, have been reported. In a study by Myers and colleagues, 213 patients with CO poisoning were evaluated. One hundred thirty-one patients received HBOT and had no sequelae. Eighty-two patients were treated with oxygen at normal atmospheric pressure; 12.1 percent of these patients had clinically significant neurologic sequelae. Symptoms developed 1 to 21 days postexposure. After treatment with hyperbaric oxygen (HBO), the delayed symptoms resolved.

It has been current training for physicians to define treatment strategies based on measured COHb levels in patients with presumed CO poisoning. However, these levels often do not correlate with clinical findings. It is the amount of CO that is dissolved in the plasma that is responsible for producing symptoms. A high COHb level with little dissolved CO in the plasma will result in relatively few toxic symptoms.

The half-life of COHb breathing room air is 4 to 5 hours. Breathing 100 percent oxygen at normal atmospheric pressure decreases the half-life to 50 to 80 minutes. Exposure to 100 percent oxygen at 3 ATA results in a half-life of 23 minutes.

Patients requiring HBOT after CO exposure can be divided into several groups. The first group includes any patient with a history of chest pain, syncope, or mental status changes. Physical findings of hypotension, pulmonary edema, and cardiac ischemia referable to the exposure all require stabilization and emergent treatment. Patients with these findings should receive HBOT regardless of their measured CO levels.

The second population of patients requiring treatment are those who have minor symptoms (headache, dizziness, or blurred vision) with COHb levels less than 30 percent and who show no improvement after 4 hours of 100 percent oxygen in the emergency department.

Victims of CO exposure with levels exceeding 30 percent and no symptoms on initial presentation are at high risk for delayed neurologic sequelae. Most investigators believe that these patients should be treated. A neuropsychiatric test assessing psychometric function was designed by Myers. It

Table 84-9. Signs and symptoms of gas gangrene

Pain out of proportion to physical findings
Sense of heaviness or weight in the muscle
Tachycardia out of proportion to fever
Mental status changes
Low-grade temperatures
Bronze skin color with a thin brown exudate
Crepitance
Subcutaneous air on x-ray

can be helpful in evaluating those patients whose neurologic abnormalities are often subtle and missed on a routine physical examination.

Traumatic Ischemias

Traumatic ischemias are an indication for which HBOT has been approved by the UMS as an adjunct to surgical care. Often following extensive crush injuries, tissues are so severely injured that viability is questionable. Damage to blood vessels and the microcirculation is extensive. Red blood cell (RBC) sludging, resulting in decreased perfusion with subsequent ischemia and edema, increases tissue loss and risk of infection. If an intact vascular supply is present, HBOT can maintain adequate tissue oxygenation and decrease edema. The earlier that HBOT is initiated, the greater the likelihood that it will aid in limb salvage. It is best started within the first 4 to 6 hours after injury. However, it has proved beneficial when used up to 48 hours after injury.

It must be stressed that if vessel repair, debridement, or surgical decompression of a compartment syndrome is indicated, HBOT is *not* a substitute for these procedures. HBOT is an adjunct that may aid in increasing limb salvage or, if amputation is necessary, to minimize tissue loss. If surgery is delayed for any reason, HBOT may be given prior to surgery.

Gas Gangrene

Gas gangrene clostridial myonecrosis is a devastating infectious disease emergency. Although few cases are initially seen in the emergency department, early diagnosis is critical.

Clostridia perfringens (an obligate anaerobe) is responsible for most cases. Although initially thought to occur only after trauma, this infection has been seen postoperatively and has been associated with burns, skin infections, and intramuscular injections. A few cases of spontaneous myonecrosis in which no break in the skin could be found have also been reported. Following invasion of the wound by the clostridial organism, multiple exotoxins are released that are responsible for extensive tissue destruction and systemic toxicity. The two most important are the alpha and theta toxins. The alpha toxin, a lecithinase C, causes hemolysis and extensive tissue necrosis. The theta toxin is responsible for the cardiotoxic effects of clostridia. The incubation period varies from 6 hours to 3 days, and the onset of symptoms is acute. Table 84-9 summarizes the signs and symptoms of the disease.

Early in the disease there may be an absence of crepitance and subcutaneous gas on x-ray film. Some species of clostridia produce little or no gas. Gram stain of the drainage shows large gram-positive bacilli without spores and a scarcity of white blood cells (WBC).

Treatment must be started as soon as the diagnosis is suspected, since the disease progresses rapidly and any delay may be fatal. The overall management should be a combination of medical, sugical, and hyperbaric therapy. Antibiotics and surgical debridement are the cornerstones of treatment. The role of HBOT is adjunctive. It limits tissue necrosis and facilitates demarcation between viable and nonviable tissue at the time of surgery. HBOT inhibits toxin production and bacterial proliferation. Tissue partial pressures of oxygen above 300 mm Hg can be achieved at 3 ATA. Alpha toxin production is inhibited by a tissue oxygen tension above 250 mm Hg. The theta toxin is inactivated.

HBOT is given at 3 ATA for 90 minutes, 3 times a day in the first 24 hours. Thereafter, it is given twice a day for the next 4 to 5 days. The actual total number of treatments depends on the patient's response.

Decompression Sickness

Decompression sickness (also known as the "bends") is caused by nitrogen bubbles that have precipitated out of solution in the tissues. It afflicts divers who breathe compressed air and then surface without proper decompression steps. It is also seen in pilots suffering explosive decompression at altitude. Symptoms can be mild or severe, resulting in permanent neurologic disability or death. HBOT is the mainstay in the treatment of decompression sickness. See Diving Emergencies, earlier in this chapter, for a complete discussion of this topic.

Air Embolism

Air embolism is perhaps the most devastating condition that can affect divers. It occurs when a diver surfaces without exhaling, or air is trapped in the lungs secondary to local pathology. An emergency or panic ascent while diving is the most common precipitating factor to air embolism.

Air embolism may also be caused by direct trauma to the vasculature, either secondary to injuries or as a consequence of invasive medical procedures. More recently, air embolism has been reported to occur in patients who have experienced gunshot wounds to the chest. Orogenital sex in pregnant women also has been reported as a cause of air embolism. Air gains access to the venous system by entering the subplacental sinuses.

The initial treatment of air embolism consists of placing the patient in the left lateral decubitus position and immediate transport to a hyperbaric chamber. A more in-depth discussion of this topic can be found earlier in this chapter, in Diving Emergencies.

Problem Wounds

Although not an emergency problem, status ulcers are commonly seen in the emergency department. HBOT has proved useful in enhancing healing of selected problem wounds, especially in the diabetic patient.

Tissue oxygen tensions of 30 to 40 mm Hg are required

for neovascularization, fibroblastic proliferation, and WBC killing. The tissue oxygen tension in diabetic wounds is often poor, predisposing the wound to infection and hindering the healing process. HBOT is adjunctive therapy and must be combined with aggressive wound care and appropriate surgical debridement.

Burns

The use of HBOT in the treatment of burns remains controversial. The Committee on Hyperbaric Oxygen Therapy of the UMS believes that under a rigid protocol in a burn center, the use of HBOT is appropriate.

A study was done by Hart and associates at the Sherman Oaks Community Hospital Burn Center in California. In a randomized, controlled, double-blind study, they evaluated 191 patients with extensive burns ranging from 10 to 50 percent total body surface area. One hundred thirty-eight patients received HBOT; 53 patients did not. All patients received standard burn care therapy. Patients were treated within 24 hours of the injury. The mean healing time of the HBOT group was statistically different from the non-HBOT group (19.7 days versus 43.8 days, respectively). In those patients treated with HBOT, there was a 35 percent reduction of fluid requirements in the first 24 hours after admission.

HBOT in the treatment of burns is an adjunctive therapy to good burn care. It leads to decreased fluid requirements, reduces edema, improves flow through the microcirculation, helps decrease the conversion of partial- to full-thickness burns, and reduces the time of epithelialization. Also, patients with extensive burns often have had significant CO exposure. The role of HBOT in CO poisoning has been discussed previously.

INVESTIGATIONAL USES

There are numerous areas in which the use of HBOT is investigational (see Table 84-6). As with other treatment modalities, well-designed studies are needed to evaluate its efficacy.

An important experimental use is in the area of head injuries and cerebral edema. HBOT may have significant impact on the morbidity and mortality of these patients, especially when instituted by emergency physicians in the first few hours posttrauma.

Current therapy for increased intracranial pressure includes hyperventilation, fluid restriction, mannitol, and, occasionally, steroids. Because the brain is in a closed space, cerebral edema often leads to herniation and, ultimately, death.

The rationale for the use of HBOT is due to the vasoconstrictive effect of hyperoxia. There is a decrease in cerebral blood flow while maintaining tissue oxygenation. There have been reports of significant reductions of intracranial pressure. It is important to begin HBOT within 12 hours of the injury and always in conjunction with a neurosurgeon who will be ultimately responsible for the overall care of the patient.

HBOT is thought to be beneficial in spinal cord injuries for similar reasons. Like cerebral edema, spinal cord injuries are "compartment syndromes." Swelling occurs within a nonexpandable, rigid container ultimately resulting in neuronal death. HBOT has been found to be effective in experimental animals with nontransected spinal cord injuries when used within 4 hours of the time of injury.

Sickle cell crisis is an interesting area of HBOT research. Patients with this disorder often must come to emergency departments for pain relief. Hypoxia induces sickling of RBC, sludging of the microcirculation, and, ultimately, infarction. HBOT should resolve hypoxia, reduce microcirculatory stasis, and decrease pain. However, research has been hampered by the lack of an animal model of sickle cell anemia.

POSSIBLE COMPLICATIONS

A common problem associated with HBOT is the effect of pressure changes on air-filled cavities in the body. The sinuses and middle ear are most often affected. The ostium of the sinuses and the eustachian tube of the middle ear allow equalization of pressure with the atmosphere. As pressure is increased, air in these cavities becomes compressed. If access to the ambient pressure is blocked, fluid transudation occurs within the bony spaces. In the sinuses, this results in pain and is referred to as a *sinus squeeze.* In the ear, inward displacement of the tympanic membrane can cause pain and possibly rupture of the drum. Yawning, swallowing, or a Valsalva maneuver allows for equalization of pressure in the middle ear. Decongestants are often given to minimize risks of sinus and ear squeeze. For patients with continued difficulties, myringotomies or tympanostomy tubes can be placed prior to treatment.

High concentrations of oxygen can have toxic effects on the central nervous system. Grand mal seizures can occur, and although rare, the overall incidence is estimated to be between 1 in 2,000 and 1 in 5,000 treatments. It is more common at pressures above 3 ATA. No permanent neurologic sequelae have been noted, and seizures are terminated by changing the patient from oxygen to compressed air.

Pulmonary oxygen toxicity is well known with prolonged exposure to high concentrations of oxygen. However, because HBOT is given by intermittent exposure at 3 ATA or less, the incidence of clinically apparent pulmonary oxygen toxicity is negligible.

HBOT can produce progressive myopia in approximately 30 percent of patients treated for prolonged periods of time. It is usually transient and resolves spontaneously. HBOT accelerates the growth of preexisting cataracts. This effect is not reversible.

Pneumothorax and air embolism can be devastating potential complications of HBOT. If a patient holds his or her breath or if air trapping has occurred in the lungs while the pressure in the chamber is being reduced, alveoli can rupture with disastrous consequences. Slow decompression and good patient instruction minimizes these risks. In practice, pneumothorax and air embolism are rare complications.

CHAMBER TYPES

HBOT can be administered in either a monoplace or multiplace chamber. The multiplace chamber is a large steel con-

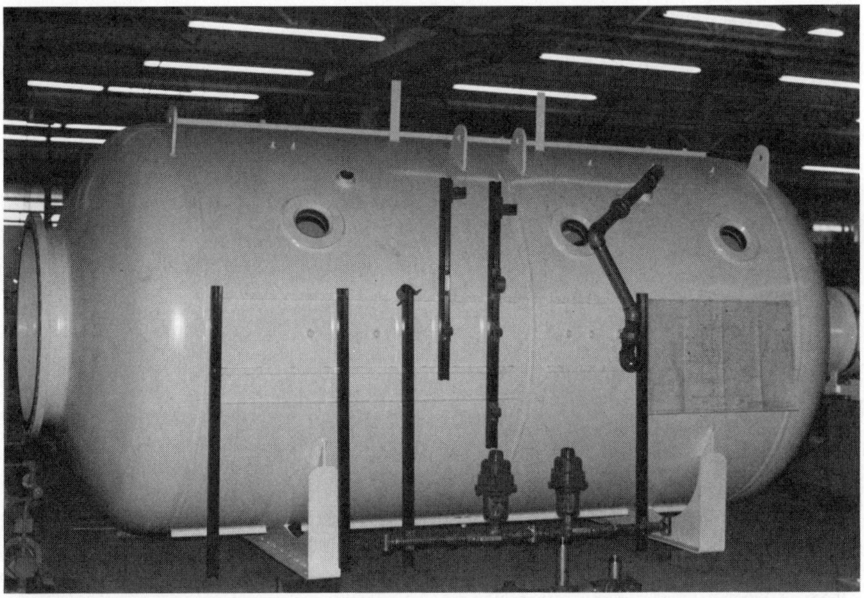

Fig. 84-5. Multiplace chamber capable of accommodating six patients. (Courtesy of Environmental Tectonics Corporation.)

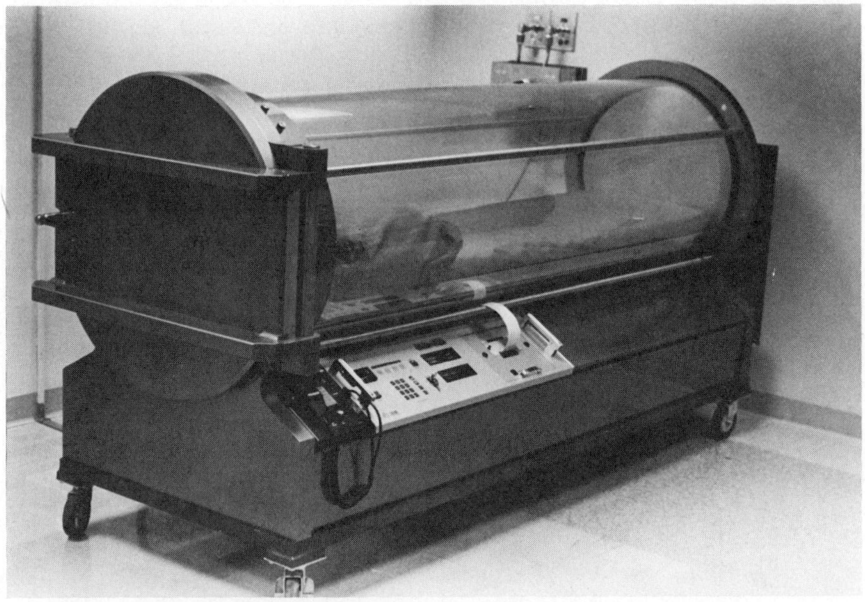

Fig. 84-6. Monoplace hyperbaric chamber suitable for compression to 3 ATA. (Courtesy of Environmental Tectonics Corporation.)

tainer that can accommodate numerous patients during each treatment (Fig. 84-5). The chamber is compressed with air, and the patients breathe pure oxygen by mask or hood. A specially trained chamber operator and inside chamber attendants are necessary for its operation. These facilities are costly to build and maintain. However, they allow hands-on patient care during treatment.

The monoplace chamber is small and relatively inexpensive (costing less than $100,000). It measures 7 feet long and 4 feet wide (Fig. 84-6). A hollow acrylic cylinder is encased by two steel bulkheads on each end. The entire chamber is compressed with oxygen. The vessel is large enough for the patient to lay supine in it. No masks or hoods are necessary. There is communication with the outside chamber operator by an intercom system. The patient can watch television or listen to music. Monoplace chambers do not require specially trained chamber operators because of their simplistic design.

Severely ill patients can be treated in a monoplace chamber. Patients on ventilators, with Swan-Ganz catheters, central venous lines, arterial lines, pneumothoraces, and intracranial pressure monitors, have all been treated in monoplace vessels.

The main disadvantage of the monoplace chamber is the lack of an inside chamber attendant. Access to the patient, neurologic examinations, suctioning, or resuscitation in the event of a cardiac arrest cannot be performed until the patient is decompressed and removed from the chamber. This can be accomplished rapidly if an emergency situation arises.

HBOT has a colorful past and a promising future. Well-defined indications based on sound physiological principles have made it a useful tool for the emergency physician. In select cases, it provides the standard of care.

HBOT is available at more than 200 institutions in the United States. As directed research and clinical studies are undertaken, the acceptance and availability of HBO facilities will increase.

SELECTED READING

Baroni, G, et al. Hyperbaric oxygen in diabetic gangrene treatment. *Diabetes Care* 10:81, 1987.

Bray, P, Myers, RA, and Cowley, RA. Orogenital sex as a cause of nonfatal air embolism in pregnancy. *Obstet Gynecol* 61:653, 1983.

Boerema, I, et al. Life without blood: A study of the influence of high atmospheric pressure and hypothermia on dilution of blood. *J Cardiovasc Surg* 1:133, 1960.

Cline, KA, and Turnbull, TL. Clostridial myonecrosis. *Ann Emerg Med* 14:459, 1985.

Davis, JC, and Hunt, TK (eds.), *Hyperbaric Oxygen Therapy* (3rd ed). Bethesda: The Undersea Medical Society, Inc., 1977.

Davis, JC, et al. Chronic non-hematogenous osteomyelitis treated with adjunct hyperbaric oxygen. *J Bone Joint Surg* 68-A:1210, 1986.

Hart, GB, et al. Treatment of burns with hyperbaric oxygen. *Surg Gynecol Obstet* 139:693, 1974.

Hart, GB, et al. Gas gangrene: A collection review. *J Trauma* 23:991, 1983.

Hart, GB, et al. Treatment of smoke inhalation by hyperbaric oxygen. *J Emerg Med* 3:211, 1985.

Murphy, BP, et al. Cerebral air embolism resulting from invasive medical procedures. *Ann Surg* 201:242, 1985.

Myers, RA, et al. Subacute sequelae of carbon monoxide poisoning. *Ann Emerg Med* 14:1163, 1985.

Norkool, DM, and Kirkpatrick, JN. Treatment of acute carbon monoxide poisoning with hyperbaric oxygen: A review of 115 cases. *Ann Emerg Med* 14:1168, 1985.

Nylander, G, et al. Reduction of postischemic edema with hyperbaric oxygen. *Plast Reconstr Surg* 76:596, 1985.

Olsen, KR. Carbon monoxide poisoning: Mechanisms, presentation, and controversies in management. *J Emerg Med* 1:223, 1984.

Strauss, MB. Chronic refractory osteomyelitis: Review and role of hyperbaric oxygen. *HBO Review* 1:231, 1980.

Strauss, MB, and Samson, RL. Decompression sickness: An update. *Physician Sports Med* 14:196, 1986.

Strauss, MB, et al. Delayed use of hyperbaric oxygen for treatment of a model anterior compartment syndrome. *J Orthop Res* 4:108, 1986.

Strauss, MB, et al. Reduction of skeletal muscle necrosis using intermittent hyperbaric oxygen in a model compartment syndrome. *J Bone Joint Surg* 65:656, 1983.

Strauss, MB, and Hart, GB. Crush injury and the role of hyperbaric oxygen. *Top Emerg Med* 6:9, 1984.

Sukoff, MH, and Ragatz, RE. Hyperbaric oxygenation in the treatment of acute cerebral edema. *Neurosurgery* 10:29, 1982.

Turnbull, TL, and Cline, KA. Spontaneous clostridial myonecrosis. *J Emerg Med* 3:353, 1985.

H. Occupational Exposures and Emergencies

85. Approach to the Patient with a Work-Related Emergency

Glenn Pransky

This chapter describes the social, regulatory, and legal context in which patients with occupational emergencies are seen, along with the resulting implications for the clinician. A practical approach to diagnosis and treatment is presented. Finally, resources for evaluating and treating these patients, as well as administrative issues for the physician in occupational practice, are discussed. The goal is to assist the emergency physician in making an important contribution to effective care and prevention of occupational injuries and illnesses.

EPIDEMIOLOGY

Occupational injuries and illnesses are serious medical and economic problems, directly affecting over five percent of all workers each year. In 1981, the estimated cost associated with work accidents was 32.5 billion dollars. These injuries caused over 12 percent of all deaths reported in the United States, and represented approximately 310,000 potential years of life lost before age 65.

Few data are available regarding the epidemiology of work injuries seen in emergency facilities. The National Institute of Occupational Safety and Health (NIOSH), in conjunction with the Consumer Product Safety Commission (CPSC), conducts surveillance in 66 representative hospital emergency departments in the United States, which participate in the National Electronic Injury Surveillance System (NEISS).

These data, as well as information from the National Health Interview Survey, suggest that 36 percent of all job-related injuries are treated in hospital emergency departments. Few of these patients are seen by specialists in occupational medicine. Age-specific incidence rates show that 16- to 24-year-old workers are at several times greater risk for job-related injuries than are older workers. Injury risk for men is twice as high as women, except in the older age groups. For younger workers, estimated monthly injury incidence is highest in summer and fall and lowest in winter. A number of factors contribute to these trends, including seasonal variation in employment levels, as well as demographic distribution by sex and age, favoring younger, male workers in the highest-risk occupations of construction, agriculture, and forestry.

Though this information provides an estimate of occupational injuries that occur each year, approximating the number of occupational illnesses that occur is more difficult, for several reasons. These illnesses do not generally lead to acute presentations to emergency departments, where data on incidence might be collected. Over 80 percent of injuries are compensated by insurers without contest, yet over 85 percent of occupational illnesses are initially denied by workers' compensation insurers as not being work related. These conditions are difficult to distinguish from non–work-related illnesses. As emergency practitioners rarely have had extensive occupational health training, recognition of linkage between illness and work may be limited. Identification of new work-related diseases has been the primary focus of modern occupational medicine.

Many more patients are seen with problems that are unrelated to work but decide to seek medical attention only because the condition is severe enough to interfere with employment. How many patients fit into this category is unclear. These visits may be triggered by the patient's need for medical treatment in order to return to work, or a requirement for certification of "disability" by employers, insurance companies, or government agencies.

THE CONTEXT OF WORK-RELATED EMERGENCIES

Unlike emergencies that occur outside of work, job-related emergencies are often the result of complex exposures or repetitive activities. These often result from the cumulative effect of stress on specific body structures over time and initially may not appear to be work related. Carpal tunnel syndrome is a typical example; it has an insidious onset after years of repetitive hand-intensive tasks, with apparently acute symptoms once the illness has fully developed. Treatment is likely to be ineffective unless the exacerbating work activities are modified.

Concerns about employer liability, lost wages, workplace modification, and even trade secrets can all arise in this setting. Over 50,000 hazardous chemicals are used in industry, with greater than 500 new chemicals added to this list each year.

Many physicians are concerned about the litigious nature of workers' compensation cases and fear depositions or court appearances. Others are mystified by the unique nature of reporting requirements or wish to avoid conflicts between employees' and employers' interests. As a result, physicians often avoid contact with the employer and provide patients with inappropriate work restrictions or unclear notes. The breakdown in communication between employer, physician, and employee is a source of friction between injured workers and employers even though the problem may have resulted from the physician's actions.

Workers' compensation is an insurance system designed to transfer some of the costs of occupational injuries and illnesses from employees to employers. Benefits include part of the injured worker's lost wages, most or all medical expenses, and reimbursement for rehabilitation, disfigurement, and death.

Workers' compensation first appeared in the United States early in this century. Previously, a worker who suffered an injury at work was forced to prove negligence of the employer in court to obtain compensation for lost wages and medical expenses. Few workers could amass the funds to finance the lawsuit or conclusively demonstrate that fellow employees were not also to blame (and therefore liable). As a result, an increasing number of injured workers and their families became destitute. This spurred the growth of unions to aid in these lawsuits, and employers, fearing more radical political action by workers, moved to join labor unions in creating a compromise insurance program.

The basic elements of workers' compensation programs have not changed since their inception. These systems are no-fault: If an injury occurs at work, the employer pays regardless of who is at fault. Workers give up the possibility of substantial awards by proving negligence in court for smaller, but predictable, reimbursement for a percentage of lost wages and medical and other expenses. Usually, injured employees receive two-thirds of lost weekly wages (up to a specified maximum amount) when unable to work. Employers gain the advantages of participating in a shared and limited-risk insurance system and lose some of their ability to refuse reimbursement to injured workers.

There are 50 distinct state workers' compensation systems, each with its own regulations, procedures, and payment schemes. In addition, there are three federally administered compensation programs, which cover federal employees, railroad workers, and longshoremen. The Veterans Administration benefits system is somewhat similar to workers' compensation. In each state, a regulatory agency sets rules for wage reimbursements and other payments, oversees private insurers who provide coverage for employers, and administers a mechanism for dispute resolution.

A key element of these systems is the legal definition of work related. This usually includes all injuries that "arise out of or in the course of employment." Thus, whether or not a worker is at fault, if an injury or illness occurs because of a workplace exposure or activity, it will be covered under this system. In addition, most medical problems that are aggravated or exacerbated by work are considered work related and are covered by the system. Consultants, employees who work on an irregular basis, real estate agents, and certain others are not covered in some states.

The legal definition of cause may be less exacting than the medical definition. A legal standard of proof is that a condition is work related if it is "more likely than not" that the condition would not have been present or would not have gotten worse had the work exposure not occurred. In most acute traumatic injuries (e.g., fractures or lacerations at work), the relationship with work is unquestionable and the system succeeds reasonably well at compensating the injured worker. In many disease cases, however, the relationship to work is less clear, and the demand on the physician is more complicated, with the chances for adversarial proceedings greater. Certain medical conditions that are difficult to substantiate by objective testing may not be covered under the law. For example, several states proscribe claims due to "stress" when the problem results from legitimate personnel actions.

For workers' compensation to provide benefits, medical documentation of work-related injury or illness must be given. Therefore, the physician's role is central in initiating workers' compensation payments. Most insurers will not provide reimbursement without medical documentation of injury and the relationship to work. For example, in Massachusetts, the workers' compensation law requires that physicians report the diagnosis, relationship to work, and prognosis for return to work to the insurer, the employee, and the state workers' compensation agency within 14 days of evaluating a patient.

Although medical information is important, all of these systems operate under administrative control. The laws in each jurisdiction specify what insurers, employers, and employees must do in the processing of claims. Employers or insurers must follow specific procedures if they wish to deny a claim, and opportunities for employees to appeal are provided. However, employees whose claims have been denied must frequently engage legal help, and benefits may be awarded only after considerable time and legal expense.

Certain terms are frequently encountered in workers' compensation. It is most important for the health-care provider to distinguish between impairment and disability.

Impairment is defined as the loss of function of an organ or part of the body compared to that which preexisted. Ideally, impairment can be defined and described in purely medical terms and quantified in such a way that a reproducible measurement is developed (e.g., severe restrictive lung disease with a total lung capacity of 1.6 liters).

Disability, on the other hand, is usually defined in terms of the impact of an impairment on societal or work functions. Thus, disability evaluation takes into account the loss of function (impairment) and the patient's work requirements. Disability determination requires knowledge of the patient's activities at work and understanding of a relationship between altered function after injury and decreased work capabilities.

A patient who cannot do any work because of an injury is *totally disabled.* If this person can work but has some limitations and cannot do his or her customary job, a *partial disability* exists. Most states provide for replacement of part of the difference between the lower wages associated with job tasks that a partially disabled worker can do and the wages before the injury. Whether the disability is partial or total, it is considered *temporary* so long as a complete resolution of the impairment is expected to occur. A *medical end result* has been achieved when no significant functional improvement is expected even though some minor medical progress occurs. Often, workers' compensation systems assume that if a condition has not changed substantially over a three- to five-year period, a medical end result has been reached, and a temporary (partial or total) disability is then legally considered as a *permanent disability.*

Most workers' compensation systems support the role of the treating physician in determining work-relatedness and the appropriate time for return to work. However, in the dispute resolution process, there is usually a provision for an *impartial medical examination.* This is often requested when insurer and employee have a difference of opinion regarding the work-relatedness of the condition or the extent of the disability. Physicians must remember that their evaluations are not the final determinants in awards for compensation; their information is only a part of the data used to make final decisions.

Outside of these legally mandated systems, many employees participate in *private disability plans* or have work rules that require provision of medical information. For example, workers may have additional disability insurance to supplement the limited payments available under workers' compensation. These insurance plans also require medical documentation of illness, impairment, disability, and prognosis. More often, the emergency physician encounters an employee who must bring documentation back to the employer to verify that he or she does indeed have an injury or illness that prevents work, or face disciplinary action. Thus, a proportion of workers who visit physicians do not desire additional medical treatment but wish to have the physician certify that their illness is temporarily disabling them from work.

In addition to workers' compensation agencies, several other regulatory agencies affect the workplace and may interact with the physician regarding injuries and illnesses. The Occupational Safety and Health Administration (OSHA), organized in 1970, is responsible for maintaining safe and healthful working conditions. OSHA inspects workplaces for violations of existing health and safety standards, holds hearings, and sets new standards for control of specific substances, conditions, or uses of equipment. The agency may act in a consultative rather than regulatory role with industry, providing assistance in resolution of deleterious occupational exposures, and may serve as a useful resource for the emergency physician. Local or state health and labor departments are also involved in workplace health and safety.

APPROACH TO THE OCCUPATIONAL EMERGENCY PATIENT

Despite a wide variety of presentations that bring workers into the emergency department, a number of common issues should always be addressed. The appropriate diagnosis of occupational injuries and illnesses entirely depends on an accurate occupational history. It is rare that laboratory testing or physical examination reveals occupational diagnoses not detected by a thorough history. At a minimum, each patient should be asked for a description of his or her current employment, amount of time at that job, type of work and work setting, and the circumstances in which the injury or illness occurred. Every worker should be asked about exposure to dust, chemicals, fumes, loud noise, or other hazards and about use of personal protective equipment (respirators, gloves, eye guards, hearing protection). The time course of the illness or injury in relation to occupational activities is very important; this can be the key to identifying an irritating or sensitizing substance in an extensive list of exposures that occur during the day. A basic understanding of the usual clinical course of the disease in question is important. For example, many workers with isocyanate-induced asthma may not develop symptoms while at the workplace but may have symptoms that are worse 6 to 18 hours after exposure. In contrast, workers with byssinosis (occupational bronchitis related to cotton dust exposure) may be worse on Monday mornings and gradually improve throughout the week. Symptoms that consistently improve during long weekends or vacations are often work related. Inquiries should always be made about whether current or previous coworkers have had similar symptoms.

In obtaining the occupational history, at a minimum the physician needs to know how the emergent condition of every working patient may affect ability to work. Some knowledge of the current job requirements and possible accommodations is necessary. More information is required to

Table 85-1. Elements of the full occupational history

Current job title
Current employer
Years at current employer
Brief job description
Hazards (noise, dust, chemicals, biological, physical, psychological)
Exposure controls (respirator, engineering controls, administrative)
Where meals are taken at work
Prior jobs and exposures
History of work-related or work-limiting illnesses
Hobbies and related exposures
Current illnesses and relation to work changes, exposures, vacations
Similar problems in coworkers
Unusual accidents or incidents, prior history of emergencies at work
Second or part-time jobs
Military service and related exposures

make a diagnosis of occupational disease, including most of the items listed in Table 85-1. Typically, the symptoms and signs are no different than nonoccupational versions of the same disease (such as asthma); several occupational diseases masquerade as common illnesses (Table 85-2). Therefore, the diagnosis of work-relatedness depends on a thorough occupational history. In all acute cases of dermatitis, neurologic or pulmonary disease, hearing impairment, back and joint symptoms, cancer, coronary artery disease, liver disease, and neuropsychiatric problems, all of these items should be asked. Though a full occupational and environmental history may be time consuming, it can be lifesaving.

Once occupational illness is suspected, more information about the workplace is needed. Acute injuries rarely present problems in identification of cause. Chronic problems that result from repetitive trauma may be more difficult. The identification of the chemical cause for occupational illness may be even more challenging. Readily available sources of data include material safety data sheets, basic reference texts, computerized data bases, poison control centers, consultants, coworkers, and union or management health and safety personnel. Use of this information is discussed in greater detail in Chap. 86. A few substances have characteristic odors or appearances; even fewer have pathognomonic biologic effects (Table 85-3). Again, diagnosis usually depends entirely on an accurate history.

Treatment of occupational injuries and illnesses is the same as for nonoccupational emergencies. If patients with work-related injuries ask for priority in triage, this is often because (unlike many other patients) they are also losing income while waiting and are concerned about other consequences of absence from work.

Follow-up care and disposition of occupational patients distinguish them from other patients. The four areas that the physician must address include return-to-work recommendations, follow-up care, prevention, and reporting.

Return-to-Work Recommendations

Most employers require certification that the patient can work after returning from the emergency department. Medical personnel often assume that the patient's limitations must be obvious; however, supervisors without medical experience are often reluctant to risk endangering the health of their employees. They erroneously assume that a physician who has briefly met a patient should be able to accurately determine exactly what that person can or cannot do, at a job that the physician has never seen.

In formulating recommendations, the physician seeks to balance a desire to maintain the patient's earning capacity and maximize the rehabilitative value of light duty against the potential adverse medical effects of returning to exposures that precipitated the illness. Extended disability, whether warranted or not, has serious social consequences, such as depression, alcoholism, family discord, and obesity. The ideal prescription for light duty should be based upon actual job descriptions or activities that the worker will do, including the length of time that the restrictions will be necessary. A brief call to employers or supervisors will usually be sufficient to determine if such light duty is available. These prescriptions are most useful when defined in terms of typical job actions such as pushing, pulling, sitting, stand-

Table 85-2. Occupational diseases that masquerade as other illnesses

Occupational disease	Similar non-occupational illness
Lead poisoning	Flu-like illness with gastrointestinal complaints (may mimic appendicitis)
Chronic solvent toxicity	Chronic alcoholism, dementia
Isocyanate sensitivity	Intrinsic asthma, dermatographism, urticaria
Mild carbon monoxide poisoning	Migraine
Industrial bronchitis	Viral bronchitis
Noise-induced hearing loss	Presbycusis
Mesothelioma	Pleurisy
Toxic hepatitis	Infectious hepatitis
Methylene dianiline bladder neuropathy	Benign prostatic hypertrophy
Metal fume fever	Influenza
Vibration-induced white finger	Raynaud's disease, scleroderma
Chlorine inhalation	Pulmonary edema
Beryllium lung disease	Sarcoidosis

Table 85-3. Occupational diseases with typical presentations

Disease	Presentation
Asbestosis	Characteristic chest x-ray
High-level lead toxicity	Lead lines, basophilic stippling of red blood cells
Carpal tunnel syndrome	Phalen's and Tinel's signs with median nerve palsy
Carbon monoxide poisoning (severe)	Cherry-red skin and mucosa
Pesticide poisoning (organophosphate)	Symptoms and signs of acetylcholinesterase blockade

Name ______________________________ Date ________

Job ____

Company ____________________________________

______ I have examined this patient, and in my opinion he/she can/cannot return to work

until ___/___/___ due to __________________________ (work-related diagnosis).

______ Able to return to work today without restriction.

______ Able to return to work today with the following restrictions.

______ Lifting up to ______ lbs ______ times/hr from (floor/table) height only

______ Bending to ______ ft off floor

______ Reaching overhead ______________________

______ Pushing/pulling: maximum ______ lbs force

______ Sitting ______ hrs/day

______ Standing ______ hrs/day

______ Machinery use: __________________________

______ Vehicle use: ____________________________

______ Other restrictions (chemicals, climate, inhalation, other activities or

exposures) ______________________________________

These restrictions will not be necessary after or will be reevaluated on ________________
(date)

Further medical evaluation will be at ______________________________________
(date) (doctor's office)

Please call at ______________________________ should you have any further questions.
(phone number of physician)

______________________________, MD ________________ (date)

Fig. 85-1. Return-to-work evaluation.

ing, lifting from floor or table, reaching, and limitations are specified regarding chemical or physical exposure. Reports are facilitated by a form as in Fig. 85-1.

Illegible or inadequate notes create the possibility of injury secondary to inappropriate job activities, or unnecessary disability and loss of income for the patient. Though this element of patient management is rarely time consuming, poor performance here can have marked effects in dissuading employers and workers from further referrals to the emergency physician.

Follow-Up Care

For workers who are seen in the emergency department at night or on weekends, getting information from employers regarding exposures or light duty, or arranging follow-up medical care, may not be possible at the time of the visit. Thus, a prompt referral is needed to a practitioner who will evaluate the patient during the day, when contact with employer or supervisor can be made. Many companies have standing relationships with physicians or occupational health nurses who are familiar with the workplace and can take an active role in the treatment, appropriate return to work, and rehabilitation of the patient. In most states, workers may choose whom they wish to see for follow-up care of an injury or illness. In any case, it is usually worthwhile to have some information given directly to the practitioner who has an ongoing relationship with and detailed knowledge of the company.

As patient advocates, health-care providers need to be

aware that depression is often a complicating factor in the patient with long-term disability. Patients frequently are financially and socially limited by their work incapacity, and social isolation frequently accompanies isolation from the workplace. Patients may be upset at how they have been handled by the "system," especially if benefits have been delayed or denied. They may be angry at the apparent insensitivity of their employer, insurer, or physician, and this anger often complicates their evaluation and treatment. Patients are often afraid of returning to the workplace where a serious injury has occurred, or they may be afraid of being dismissed once they have successfully returned to work. Being open to the complicated social, legal, and psychological state of disabled workers is an essential aspect of assisting their recovery. Appropriate referral for psychological diagnosis and treatment should be considered in every case of prolonged work incapacity.

Reporting

Reporting of medical information to workers' compensation insurers and employers often raises concerns regarding confidentiality and inappropriate use of information by nonmedical personnel. Most states mandate prompt reporting of diagnosis, work-relatedness, prognosis, and estimated return-to-work date to state agencies and to insurers by the health care provider. Medical documentation of a work-related injury is usually necessary before medical or wage reimbursement payments are released. Difficulties in gaining physician compliance have prompted states to consider fines for providers who fail to report this information in a timely manner. As with private health insurance, acceptance of a claim by a workers' compensation insurer usually implies authorization by the patient for a release of appropriate records. Thus, emergency physicians should write notes carefully, to ensure clear documentation of relevant issues. Non–work-related medical information should be placed on separate sheets, if possible, as there is no need for insurers or state agencies to receive these data. Notes that do not clearly discuss the evidence for relation to work can lead to reluctance of insurers to accept claims, unnecessary litigation, and delay in benefits for the worker, and, ultimately, a loss of reimbursement to the emergency department for medical services.

Prevention

When an emergency physician treats a child for ingestion of a few aspirins, reviewing safety issues with the parents may avert a lethal ingestion in the future. Prevention is also important with work-related injuries and illnesses. For each worker who is seen in the hospital, there may be many coworkers with similar, albeit less severe, problems. They have usually seen other practitioners, have not yet complained to a medical provider about their problem, or have not yet suffered the same consequences as the patient seen in the emergency department. Therefore, preventive efforts that reduce the risk of reinjury for one worker may often have a beneficial effect for many other workers. However, if the physician does not initiate preventive efforts, the injured worker is likely to return to work and, along with other workers, have a recurrence of the problem.

In determining what sorts of preventive efforts should involve the emergency physician, it is important to ask a few questions about the cause of the problem. Was it the result of usual activities, related to an emergency or breakdown of policy or equipment, or the result of coworker mistakes? What safeguards are in place to prevent this from happening; what ideas might the worker have? Is this a frequent occurrence and are others less severely affected or at similar risk? A potential strategy for prevention will usually become evident. However, in other instances, little information will be available, but the physician will have strong suspicions that some preventive action should be taken.

Several different activities should be considered to minimize an industrial hazard. Substitution with less hazardous materials or processes is ideal, as this eliminates the possibility of worker exposure. This may include substitution with a new chemical, a closed-tank system, better-maintained vehicles, or ergonomic tools. Engineering controls (ventilation, isolation of worker from hazard, change in process to decrease exposure) are often effective but still leave open the possibility of injury during maintenance or during equipment breakdowns. Job rotation divides hazardous exposure among more workers and seeks to decrease the individual exposure level of any single worker below a critical threshold. Use of personal protection devices (respirators, earplugs, gloves) requires worker cooperation, knowledge of use, periodic maintenance, and management support, and they are therefore less reliable than other measures. Worker education and safety policies also depend on worker performance and management support. Industrial hygiene monitoring seeks to document unhealthful areas of exposure, to identify a focus for preventive efforts. Biologic monitoring seeks to document early changes in worker health or evidence of adverse exposures related to the workplace but is rarely an effective means of prevention. Definitive answers regarding the best way to proceed may come from safety or industrial engineers, consultants, industrial hygienists employed by insurers or government agencies, or inspectors, but most come from workers themselves.

Industry personnel often initiate preventive activities if they are alerted to the problem by a physician. Though emergency physicians may not be familiar with workplaces or processes, brief consideration of possible strategies and review of these with the patient may help to formulate some preventive approaches. When experiencing difficulties in getting the interest of a company representative regarding a serious problem, one should not hesitate to call OSHA, state labor inspection agencies, or state or city public health officials. Careful documentation in the medical record of possible causes and potential preventive actions related to the injury or illness will aid in substantiating the need for action. Physicians should discuss these issues with patients before proceeding even though prompt action may be necessary to save lives. Patients should be aware that notifying regulatory agencies may jeopardize their jobs, despite legal sanctions against employers for firing workers who report unsafe conditions.

In dealing with workers' compensation, conflicts often arise in relation to medical disability determinations. Physicians are frequently uncomfortable when patients request certification of disability despite absence of objective evidence that the patient cannot work. Employers or insurers

A. Job title ______ Number of years here ______

Job description ______ Employer ______

Hazards (noise, dust, solvents, heat, cold, danger of injury)

______

Protective equipment (respirators, goggles, etc.)

______

Health problems in coworkers? (describe) ______

B. Previous jobs

	Job 1	Job 2	Job 3
Job title			
Company			
Job description			
Dates employed			
Hazards (dust, fumes, solvent, noise, heavy lifting)			
Associated illnesses			

C. Other hazardous exposures

Environment ______

Hobbies ______

Military ______

D. Current illness

Symptoms better on weekends/vacations? ______

Coworkers with similar problems? ______

Symptoms worse in relation to a particular exposure or activity? ______

______

Fig. 85-2. Work-related history sheet.

may attempt to manipulate the physician by suggesting that a condition was not work related, or by implying that a patient is mimicking an impairment. Since disability is not a healthful state and the legal system demands evaluation based on objective medical judgment, a generic stance of agreeing with patients or employers whenever faced with these issues is inadequate.

Several principles serve to limit these problems. Informing the patients regarding all concerns communicated by the employer or insurer helps avoid manipulation by either side. At times, insurance companies or lawyers are asking for a determination of permanency that seems to require a crystal ball. In many cases, the prognosis for functional improvement is uncertain. It is important to communicate uncertainty, both to the patient and to others involved with the case. Many emergency physicians avoid difficulties of prognosticating lengths of disability by certifying disability for a short period of time, after which return to work must be determined by the patient's primary care physician or a physician associated with the workplace. Either physician is more likely to be familiar with the job and the availability of modified work. Nevertheless, this approach does not fit every case. One may create undue hardship in patients with serious or obvious disability, who are required to make unnecessary visits to a primary physician only to obtain certification that they are unable to return to work. Judgment is necessary in this area.

Some familiarity with the state's workers' compensation system will aid in understanding situations and communicating with patients. For example, in many states, workers'

Date completed ________________

Completed by ________________

Company name ________________ Personnel director ________________

Address ________________ Safety director ________________

Phone number ________________ Company nurse ________________

Number of employees ________________ Hours available ________________

Shifts ________________ Company physician ________________

Product ________________ Hours available ________________

Union ________________

Union health and safety representative ________________

Brief description of process

____

____

Hazards and controls

____

____

Emergency preparedness on-site

____

____

Light duty? (yes/no) ________

How specified/What is available? ________________

Who to call to arrange/who receives note? ________________

Workers' compensation insurer ________________

Address ________________

Contact ________________

Fig. 85-3. Company information sheet.

compensation wage benefits do not begin unless five or more days of work have been lost; thus, requests for five rather than four days' absence due to injuries are frequently seen. Patients may not be aware that clearance for light duty usually allows partial continuation of wage replacement benefits, rather than forcing the patient to subsist on low wages. In all instances, the patient should be clearly informed that the physician's function in workers' compensation cases is to diagnose, treat, and appropriately recommend a return to work, not to act as an agent of the personnel department or as a legal adviser to the patient.

Occupational Medicine Education for the Emergency Physician

Occupational medicine education for the emergency physician is growing in importance as the scope of emergency practice expands. A number of annual courses are offered throughout the United States by the Educational Resource Centers, sponsored by NIOSH. These are designed to provide physicians with an intensive, one-week introduction to the basics of occupational medicine practice. Several periodicals focus on clinical practice issues in occupational medicine and complement the core texts in the field, so that a good basic knowledge can be acquired by reading alone: *State of the Art Reviews: Occupational Medicine, Journal of Occupational Medicine,* and *OM Newsletter.* See the Selected Reading list for recommended texts.

All physicians who regularly deal with occupational health issues should consider becoming well acquainted with the following skills:

1. Ability to take an accurate occupational history
2. Ability to recognize key features of occupational lead, solvent, carbon monoxide, or pesticide poisoning
3. Ability to recognize and deal with ethical issues in occupational health presentations
4. Ability to recognize information needed to establish work-relatedness in the state where the physician practices
5. Knowledge of appropriate role and planning necessary for emergency department participation in industry-specific disaster planning
6. Ability to interpret basic industrial hygiene information
7. Knowledge of basic ergonomic principles

Administration Issues

Encouragement of referrals from industry and promotion of worker confidence in medical care require an organization that is responsive to specific needs in the administrative area. Of course, prompt diagnosis, treatment, and appropriate reporting to companies and insurers are highly desirable. These are usually aided by development of forms that guide providers through the necessary steps in patient evaluation and formulation of recommendations. Examples are shown in Fig. 85-2 (brief work-related history sheet) and Fig. 85-1 (return-to-work recommendation sheet). A visit by a physician to a plant, with identification of a liaison person (company nurse, safety or personnel director, or union health and safety representative) can establish communication that will aid in resolving future problems. For each referral source evaluated by a physician, an information sheet, such as Fig. 85-3, should be developed that is available to all other providers. This helps in preparing return-to-work recommendations and in contacting the employer.

SELECTED READINGS

Burgess, WA. *Recognition of Health Hazards in Industry.* New York: Wiley, 1981.

Centers for Disease Control. Occupational injury surveillance—United States. *Morbid Mortal* 30:578–579, 1981.

Centers for Disease Control. Surveillance of occupational injuries treated in hospital emergency rooms—United States. 1982. *Morbid Mortal* 32:31ss–37ss, 1983.

Goldman, RH, and Peters, JM. The occupational and environmental health history. JAMA 246:2831–2836, 1981.

Kneip, TJ, and Crable, JV. *Methods for Biological Monitoring.* Washington: American Public Health Association, 1988.

Levy, BS, and Wegman, DH (eds). *Occupational Health* (2nd ed). Boston: Little, Brown, 1988.

National Safety Council. *Accident Facts.* Chicago: National Safety Council, 1982.

Zenz, C. *Occupational Medicine: Principles and Practical Applications* (2nd ed). Chicago: Year Book, 1988.

86. Hazardous Materials and Occupational Toxicologic Emergencies

Jay Himmelstein
Jerry Don Beavers

It has been estimated that over 50,000 chemicals are in daily use in the United States and that hundreds of new chemicals are introduced into commercial use each year. Toxicity data are available for fewer than 20 percent of these chemicals and in the majority of cases, no human toxicologic investigations have been pursued. There are no legal requirements for premarket testing for the human effects of industrial chemicals, as is the standard practice for pharmaceuticals. As the number of chemicals in our nation's workplaces and homes increases, the potential for exposure, absorption, and untoward health effects also increases. Chemical manufacture, transport, storage, and ultimate disposal of the wastes from toxic chemicals hold significant potential for human exposure. During the decade from 1973 to 1983, over 114,000 chemical spills were reported to the Department of Transportation's (DOT) Office of Hazardous Materials Transportation. These spills resulted in over 6,000 injuries and more than 200 deaths. In 1986 more than 4,000 workers were poisoned in the U.S. industrial setting.

Because workers and innocent bystanders will be seen in the emergency department for evaluation, decontamination, and treatment, all emergency departments should develop a system for managing chemically exposed patients. In this chapter we review the basics of occupational toxicology, including the principles of decontamination and clinical management based on the classes of chemical exposure and the acute local and systemic effects of the most commonly encountered workplace toxins. Also, an approach to disaster planning in relation to hazardous materials is outlined.

The underlying principles for managing occupational toxicologic emergencies are similar to those used in nonoccupational poisonings. Workplace poisonings differ from other intoxications in regard to likely routes of exposure, the spectrum of chemicals involved, the population at risk, and the resources for investigating the nature of the specific exposure.

In nonoccupational poisonings, accidental or intentional ingestion is by far the most common route of exposure. In occupational poisonings, however, ingestion is a rare cause of acute poisoning that occurs only when basic rules of hygiene are violated, such as eating at a work station where toxic chemicals might be used. More commonly, ingestion of industrial toxins, such as lead and other heavy metals, poses a risk of chronic, rather than acute, poisoning. In these cases no clear history of ingestion will be offered, and only a high level of suspicion will detect them.

The majority of poisonings in industry are related to exposures via inhalation or dermal absorption, and the physician must always be alert to the possibility of multiple routes of exposure. For example, a worker who describes being splashed with an organic solvent may experience a significant inhalation exposure in addition to the more obvious dermal exposure.

Most nonoccupational poisonings involve the use of pharmacologic agents (e.g., salicylates, tricyclic antidepressants) that have been well studied with regard to their human toxicity and treatment of overdose. In many cases, information from the patient or family members will quickly delineate the likely agent involved, and information on treatment approaches will be readily available. Occupational poisonings, on the other hand, commonly involve multiple exposures to substances that neither the patient nor the physician knows very much about. Even when the brand name of an industrially used chemical is available, little research may have been done on human toxicity, and even the sparse data available on industrial chemicals may not be readily accessible to the physician in an emergency situation. (See the following section on how to get more information about occupational exposures.)

Occupational poisonings commonly involve many workers from the same workplace and may involve rescue and clean-up personnel as well. In addition, the potential for mass exposure situations, such as occurred in Bhopal, India, makes it necessary to be prepared to respond to groups of victims from a single chemical incident. Therefore, the potential for mass chemical exposures, either from established industrial sites or from transportation incidents, should be considered in establishing local and regional disaster plans.

Despite the differences in routes of exposure, nature of offending chemicals, information sources, and potential populations at risk, the basic principles of treatment are the same for occupational and nonoccupational poisonings. The steps in evaluation and treatment include decontamination to prevent absorption and increase excretion, supportive treatment, treatment specific to the toxin (e.g., antidotes) and prevention of recurrence.

DECONTAMINATION

In general, initial decontamination procedures are most effectively carried out in the field before the patient arrives in the emergency department. Detailed field procedures for specific chemical exposures are described in Bronstein's *Emergency Care for Hazardous Materials Exposure* (see Selected Reading list). In this section we describe an approach to dealing with patients who are brought into the emergency department with residual contamination on their skin, mucous membranes, or clothing.

An area for decontamination should be designated and clearly identified where wet or otherwise contaminated clothing can be kept until it can be disposed of properly. The decontamination area should be outside the patient care area if the patient is in stable condition. The clothing should be removed by personnel who are wearing gloves made of butyl rubber or Viton, gowns, and masks. Contaminated clothing should be placed in a heavy plastic bag along with any brushes, towels, or other items used and disposed of as hazardous waste.

Once the clothing has been removed, the patient should be washed with tincture of green or other mild soap. A soft brush or sponge should be used, with care taken not to abrade the skin, as this can enhance absorption. The initial washing should be with cool water before one progresses to warm water, as warm water can enhance dermal absorption of some chemicals. Warm water can be used, however, if coexisting hypothermia is suspected. Special attention should be paid to nail beds, hair, and skin folds. In some cases in which particular glues or adhesives are involved, removal of the chemical may require the use of an appropriate solvent developed for this purpose. If ocular exposure is suspected, the eyes should be irrigated immediately with copious amounts of water or saline solution.

Ingestions can be removed by either emesis or nasogastric suction, with or without the use of activated charcoal and cathartics. For many chemicals, such as petroleum distillates and organic solvents, emesis is contraindicated due to the risk of aspiration and lipoid pneumonia. In rare instances excretion is enhanced by alkaline diuresis, dialysis, or other interventions.

SUPPORTIVE TREATMENT

As with other acute poisonings, primary attention must be given to maintenance of the airway and support for respiration and circulation. For the majority of exposures, treatment will be entirely supportive and will depend on the manifestations of the toxin in the patient under treatment. If the patient has inhaled a potent pulmonary irritant, for example, it is important to observe the patient for bronchospasm or delayed chemical pneumonitis. If these complications occur, standard treatment for bronchospasm or for aspiration pneumonia would be appropriate. The primary goal is to maintain adequate ventilation by whatever means necessary until the process resolves.

The physician's task beyond basic supportive care is to be aware of the potential complications associated with specific chemicals and exposure situations. In the next section, therefore, we review the most common chemicals and routes of exposure in order to familiarize the practitioner with basic approaches to treatment.

INHALATION EXPOSURES

Pulmonary Irritants

Acute responses to environmental toxins can range from simple upper-airway irritation manifested by cough and bronchospasm to full-blown adult respiratory distress syndrome (pulmonary edema). Many emergency exposure situations, such as chemical spills or fires, involve mixed chemicals in which the specific identity of the chemicals is not known. However, one can be certain that any significant exposure to combustion products will involve exposure to pulmonary irritants, and the full range of toxic complications, both acute and delayed, must be considered. For example, house fires frequently generate levels of acrolein, phosgene, and other combustion products, which may be associated with delayed pulmonary edema. If any indication of severe exposure is found in an unprotected situation, it would be wise to observe the patient for at least 24 hours for delayed pulmonary edema or severe bronchospasm.

A variety of exposure situations can lead to irritative damage to pulmonary tree or lungs. Physical factors such as extreme heat associated with fire or steam can cause local effects on the pulmonary tree that can exacerbate the effects of a pulmonary irritant. The major factors that determine the irritant effects of inhaled agents are water solubility and particle size.

In general, particles larger than 10 μ in effective aerodynamic diameter tend to deposit in the upper-respiratory tract. Particles less than 10 μ are considered to be respirable particles. Particles that are less than 1 μ have a high likelihood of diffusing across the alveoli, leading to systemic absorption and systemic health effects.

Toxic gases can adsorb onto particles and be distributed with these particles, or can penetrate the lung depending on their water solubility. Substances such as ammonia and hydrogen chloride, which are highly soluble in water, tend to deposit in the upper-respiratory tract and lead to irritation, with relatively little reaction in the lower airways. However, if the exposure is large enough, even a very soluble gas will penetrate to deeper portions of the lung. Less soluble substances, such as phosgene, deposit in the lower airways and do their damage at the alveolar level.

Some common examples of pulmonary irritants are listed in Table 86-1. Some of these irritant gases are discussed in more detail in Chap. 87. Supportive treatment for inhalation of respiratory irritants consists primarily of maintaining oxygenation. Oxygen should be administered by nasal cannula or mask in as high a concentration as necessary, and ventilation should be assisted as indicated. The patient may need to be admitted to the hospital and monitored for 24 to 48 hours for development of pulmonary edema or severe bronchospasm as well as the other potential complications of the specific agent(s) involved. Initial and frequent monitoring of arterial blood gases and chest x-ray should be used to detect any impending deterioration. Any pulmonary irritant is likely to be an eye irritant, so the eyes should be immediately flushed with at least one liter of normal saline. If the substance was also ingested and the patient is alert, 4 to 8 oz of water should be administered for dilution. Emetics should not be used. If pulmonary edema or bronchospasm develops, treatment is no different than for noncardiac pulmonary edema or bronchospasm of any other cause.

Asthmatic patients are more sensitive to pulmonary irritants than other individuals. Such exposures can trigger severe bronchospasm, even at relatively low levels. For instance, sulfur dioxide causes significant bronchospasm in asthmatics at less than one part per million whereas healthy individuals tolerate it well up to five parts per million. A history of exposure to pulmonary irritants should be sought in any patient who is seen in the emergency department with bronchospasm.

Table 86-1. Severe pulmonary irritants

Acrolein	Iodine
Ammonia	Ketene
Antimony	Maleic anhydride
ANTU	Methyl bromide
Beryllium and beryllium compounds	Methylene bisphenyl isocyanate
Boron trifluoride	Methyl iodide
Bromine	Methyl isocyanate
Butyl mercaptan	Methyl mercaptan
Cadmium dust/fume	Nickel carbonyl
Chlorine	Nitric acid
Chlorine dioxide	Nitroethane
Chlorine trifluoride	Nitrogen dioxide
1-Chloro-1-nitropropane	2-Nitropropane
Chloropicrin	Oxygen difluoride
Chromic acid and chromates	Ozone
	Paraquat
Chromium, metal and insoluble salts	Perchloromethyl mercaptan
	Perchloryl fluoride
Cotton dust, raw	Phosgene
Diazomethane	Phosphine
Diborane	Phosphorus trichloride
1,1-Dichloro-1-nitroethane	Phthalic anhydride
Dichloroethyl ether	Selenium hexafluoride
Diisopropylamine	Silicone tetrafluoride
Dimethylamine	Sulfur dioxide
Dimethyl sulfate	Sulfuric acid
Ethanolamine	Sulfur pentafluoride
Ethylene chlorohydrin	Tellurium hexafluoride
Ethyleneimine	Toluene-2,4-diisocyanate
Ethylene oxide	Tributyl phosphate
Ethyl mercaptan	Uranium (natural), soluble and insoluble compounds
Fluorine	
Hydrogen chloride	Vanadium pentoxide
Hydrogen fluoride	Zinc chloride fume
Hydrogen sulfide	

Source: N.H. Proctor, et al. *Chemical Hazards of the Workplace* (2nd ed.). Philadelphia: Lippincott, 1988.

Systemic Toxicity from Inhalation Exposures

Liquids that are used in the workplace frequently will have vapor pressures sufficient to cause measurable levels of contamination in room air. Even at relatively low levels in the air, the massive amounts of air exchanged with the environment on a daily basis make for a great potential for significant exposure in acute chemical spills and in normal workplace settings. For example, a young healthy worker has an alveolar ventilation of over 2,000 liters in a typical eight-hour work day doing light work. At a fairly typical exposure level of 10 parts per million of a solvent such as trichloroethylene, this would translate to 108 mg trichloroethylene presented to the alveoli. Under emergency conditions, in which the exposures are likely to be much higher, the potential exists for a significant exposure in the unprotected worker.

Inhaled toxins can be absorbed both at the alveolar level and through the mucous membranes of the airways. Consequently, any inhaled gas or particulate can potentially lead to systemic absorption. The site with the greatest potential for systemic absorption is the alveolus. The substances that are most likely to penetrate to the alveolar level are gases with low water solubility and particles of less than 5 to 10 μ in aerodynamic diameter. Gases with low water solubility tend to have high fat solubility, which increases absorption across the alveolar membrane. Inhaled particles may break up and be absorbed or may carry other agents adsorbed on their surface. For the sake of this discussion, inhalation exposures that lead to systemic toxicity are categorized as follows: organic solvents, asphyxiants, and other systemic toxins.

Organic Solvents

Organic solvents are probably the most ubiquitous chemicals in the industrial environment. They include petroleum distillates or synthetic hydrocarbons with or without halogens substituted onto their basic carbon-chain structure. The most commonly encountered solvents in the workplace are xylene, toluene, styrene, methylethyl ketone (MEK), and isopropanol. Also common are the halogen-substituted solvents 1,1,1-trichloroethane, tetrachloroethylene, trichloroethylene, and a large number of fluorinated species (Freons). A host of other ketones, aldehydes, esters, and alcohols are also used in industrial settings.

In general, organic solvents have high fat solubility, which makes them useful for removing grease and other contaminants from hard surfaces. This same property enables them to cross the alveolar membrane and blood-brain barrier. As a consequence, some of the commonly used industrial solvents have been used as anesthetic agents in animals and humans. They all can cause central nervous system (CNS) depression, euphoria, disorientation, confusion, and death. The CNS symptoms of organic solvents are similar to those of acute alcohol intoxication.

Many organic solvents have high vapor pressures and are therefore potentially hazardous when used in enclosed spaces. This is especially true of the halogenated solvents; many deaths have resulted from using Freon (a fluorinated solvent) to clean large tanks. These halogenated solvents are also potent cardiac sensitizers, and many deaths from glue-sniffing are thought to result from ventricular fibrillation rather than narcosis.

Exposure to organic solvents by inhalation or skin absorption, or both, is common. Workers with mild intoxication will complain of light-headedness and headaches that resolve with removal from exposure. Patients with more severe exposures may have giddiness, syncope, coma, or, occasionally, cardiac arrest. Treatment of the comatose victim is supportive until he or she regains consciousness. Treatment of the victim of cardiac arrest is restitution of normal cardiac rhythm by whatever means is required. Halogenated solvents such as trichloroethylene sensitize the myocardium to epinephrine, which should be avoided in the treatment of patients with such exposures. Chemical hepatitis has been associated with acute exposure to a number of industrially used solvents, of which carbon tetrachloride is the most well known. In all cases in which acute overexposure to solvents has occurred, liver function tests should be monitored. Treatment of ingested organic solvents is discussed in the chapter on hydrocarbon ingestions (see Chap. 156).

Chemical and Simple Asphyxiants

The term *chemical asphyxiant* refers to toxins that act by intefering with the metabolic processes involved in oxygen delivery. These substances can quickly cause death as a result of brainstem hypoxia and respiratory center depression. The classic example of this group is cyanide, which is the ion released in the body by hydrogen cyanide gas (HCN), cyanide salts, acetonitrile, and acrylonitrile. Cyanide causes cellular hypoxia by interfering with the cytochrome electron transport chain. HCN poisoning responds to a protocol that includes amyl nitrite, sodium nitrite, and sodium thiosulfate. Other examples of chemical asphyxiants include carbon monoxide (CO) and hydrogen sulfide (H_2S).

Table 86-2. Asphyxiants

Chemical asphyxiants
Acetonitrile
Acrylonitrile
Carbon monoxide
Cyanide (alkali)
Hydrogen cyanide
Simple asphyxiants
Acetylene
Argon, neon, and helium
Carbon dioxide
Dichloromonofluoromethane
Dichlorotetrafluoroethane
Ethane
Ethylene
Hydrogen
Liquid petroleum gas
Methane
Nitrogen
Propane
Propylene

Source: N.H. Proctor, et al. *Chemical Hazards of the Workplace* (2nd ed.). Philadelphia: Lippincott, 1988.

A variety of gases can act as *simple asphyxiants*, which cause hypoxia simply by displacing oxygen. This is more likely to occur with gases, such as carbon dioxide, that are heavier than air and gases with poor warning properties at high concentrations. Most irritant gases (e.g., ammonia) have good warning properties (e.g., low odor threshold, mucous membrane irritation), which allow conscious exposed individuals to escape before simple asphyxia can occur. The most hazardous simple asphyxiants, such as carbon dioxide (CO_2), have no significant warning properties. Examples of simple and chemical asphyxiants are given in Table 86-2.

Other Inhaled Toxins

Exposure to metal dusts and fumes can cause a wide variety of syndromes. Acute lead toxicity can result from inhalation of lead fume or dust and cause acute CNS toxicity. Likewise, arsenic, manganese, and mercury can cause systemic toxicity when they are inhaled as a fume or a particulate. Cadmium toxicity causes toxic nephrosis as well as pneumonitis. Fumes from molten zinc, copper, or magnesium can cause a unique entity called "metal fume fever," which consists of an acute flu-like illness with fever and rigors that resolves completely in 24 hours. This is usually found among welders and is quite common in that group. A similar syndrome called "polymer fume fever" is caused by the pyrolysis products of Teflon (tetrafluoroethylene resins), often due to smokers getting these resins on their cigarettes and then inhaling the pyrolysis products of the Teflon along with their cigarette smoke.

DERMAL EXPOSURES

The other common route of exposure in occupational and environmental settings is skin contact. Certain chemicals act directly on the skin, whereas others, including many pesticides and solvents, are absorbed through the skin into the bloodstream, where they may have toxic effects at distant sites.

Skin Irritants and Sensitizers

A great many industrial chemicals can lead to acute or chronic skin irritation, depending on the intensity of the exposure and the chemical reactivity. Chemicals that are particularly likely to cause skin irritation include organic solvents and corrosive chemicals. Atopic individuals and workers with preexisting skin disease may be particularly susceptible to irritation from industrial chemicals. In addition, many workplace chemicals act as sensitizers and can cause allergic contact dermatitis with even minute exposures. General principles of diagnosis and management of irritant and allergic dermatitis are covered in detail in Chap. 122.

Several workplace chemicals are associated with unusual dermatologic presentations or management considerations. Acids and alkalis of sufficient potency can cause severe chemical burns or ulcerations by denaturing the proteinaceous elements of the skin. Hydrofluoric acid (HF) is a uniquely dangerous acid. Even a small amount under the fingernail can lead to severe necrosis and sloughing of a fingertip despite the fact that no severe damage was initially suspected. The fluoride ion is very corrosive, necrosing soft tissue and decalcifying bone. It also attacks enzymes (of glycolysis) and cell membranes. The process of tissue destruction and neutralization of the HF is prolonged for days, unlike the situation with other acids, which are rapidly neutralized. For this reason any skin exposure to HF should be treated aggressively by decontamination, topical calcium gluconate gel, and local calcium gluconate injection in cases in which deep tissue injury, often indicated by severe pain, is suspected.

Because of their fat solubility, organic solvents will cause defatting of skin with chronic exposure, leading to an irritant dermatitis manifested by dryness, redness, and fissuring of the skin. Since organic solvents are ubiquitous and often used by workers to remove grease and oil from the hands, chronic hand dermatitis can result. Treatment primarily involves discontinuation of the exposure. Simple mineral oil removes grease from the hands very well and should replace solvents for this purpose. Moisturizing creams and lotions can be used to restore skin integrity, and appropriate gloves should be used when handling solvents. Many organic solvents are well absorbed through the skin and can cause systemic toxicity (see the following section).

Systemic Toxicity from Skin Exposures

Several chemicals can cause severe systemic toxicity after dermal absorption. Lipid solubility is the strongest determinant favoring skin absorption, whereas water-soluble substances penetrate very poorly. Other factors that affect skin absorption include the polarity of the solvent vehicle in which the chemical is dissolved, the state of hydration of the skin, skin temperature, pH, presence of surfactants, and the degree to which the substance directly disturbs skin integrity.

Some of the most common dermally absorbed toxins are pesticides such as chlordane, heptachlor, and pentachlorophenol. These substances are rapidly absorbed through the skin and can cause severe CNS toxicity, convulsions, and death within a short time. Phenol vapor is also primarily absorbed through the skin and can cause shock, coma, convulsions, and death. Pesticides can sometimes be absorbed by inhalation as well. Methylene chloride, a chlorinated organic solvent, can be dermally absorbed and causes cellular hypoxia when it is metabolized to carbon monoxide. Differing routes of absorption may affect the amount of chemical absorbed but do not alter the systemic effects of any given substance.

Table 86-3. Biological tests for occupational/environmental exposures

Substance	Assay	Half-life
Arsenic	Urine arsenic	2–24 hr
Benzene	Urine phenol Blood benzene	6–12 hr
Styrene	Urine phenylglyoxylic acid	8–24 hr
Toluene	Urine hippuric acid	8–24 hr
Chlorinated hydrocarbon solvents	Urine chloroacetate and similar compounds	0.5–8.0 hr
Carbon monoxide	Blood-carboxyhemoglobin	4 hr
Organochlorine pesticides	Blood, fat	1–20 mo
Lead	Blood lead	30 days
Polychlorinated biphenyl (PCB)	Blood PCB	Months–years
Organophosphate pesticides	Red blood cell cholinesterase	Days

USE OF THE LABORATORY

Laboratory testing can be useful in the emergency setting to establish an occupational diagnosis and can aid in confirmation of exposure or detection of unknown compounds, as well as in determining the therapeutic approach. Every emergency department physician should identify laboratory resources for determination of lead, zinc protoporphyrin, carboxyhemoglobin, and cholinesterase. Other laboratory measures of occupational contaminants that might be useful are listed in Table 86-3, along with information regarding how long the contaminants persist in detectable amounts after exposure. A few of these analyses can be obtained from clinical laboratories that perform routine testing, but most are available only in cooperation with a sophisticated laboratory that utilizes specialized techniques such as high-pressure gas-liquid chromatography with mass spectroscopy.

TOXIN-SPECIFIC TREATMENT

As with nonoccupational intoxications, specific antidotes are available for only a limited number of occupational poisons. These are summarized in Table 86-4. In the vast majority of cases, nonspecific therapy via removal from exposure,

Table 86-4. Antidotes for workplace toxins*

Agent	Antidote
Cyanide	Protocol of: 1. Amyl nitrite 2. Na nitrite 3. Na thiosulfate
Hydrofluoric acid	Ca gluconate topical or local injection
Arsenic	BAL IM
Lead	EDTA IV
Organophosphates	Protocol of: 1. Atropine 2. 2-PAM

*Package insert for the antidote or other reference should be consulted for exact indications and detailed management guidelines.
Key: BAL = British antilewisite; EDTA = ethylenediaminetetraacetic acid; PAM = pralidoxime.

decontamination, supportive care under observation, and treatment of complications will lead to successful recovery. The often futile search for a specific antidote should not be allowed to delay basic supportive care.

INFORMATION SYSTEMS

If patients or their companions do not know the identity of the agent in question, they may have or be able to describe a label or other information found on chemical containers or transportation vehicles. A variety of chemical labeling systems are in use. Labeling for chemicals in transport is governed by DOT regulations. These regulations require that chemicals being transported be labeled in the following ways: First, a hazard class–specific label or placard that uses symbols and key words to indicate the DOT hazard class; second, the chemical-specific four-digit United Nations (UN) identification number; and thirdly, a single-digit number indicating the UN hazard class number. (See Fig. 86-1 for example placard.) The DOT hazard classes are listed in Table 86-5. In addition, the driver who is transporting the chemicals is required to carry a shipper's manifest that specifically identifies the chemicals being carried. In cases in which placards are not available, the shipping manifest may provide necessary chemical information.

Labeling of chemicals in the workplace is governed by the Federal Hazard Communication Standard (Code of Federal Regulations 1910.1200), which requires that all storage containers in the workplace be labeled with the identity of the chemical as well as hazard and route-of-exposure information. Any labeling system that fits these requirements may be used. The employer is also required to keep a file of material safety data sheets readily available to the employee and his or her physician; these sheets must include the chemical identification (except when this is a trade secret) and basic toxicity and treatment information.

Once the chemical has been identified, a variety of information sources can be used to discover potential health effects and approaches to treatment. Poison control centers have expanded their data bases on industrial chemicals in recent years so that these centers may be a good source of information. As a result of the Hazard Communication Standard just described, material safety data sheets must now include an emergency number to be used by physicians

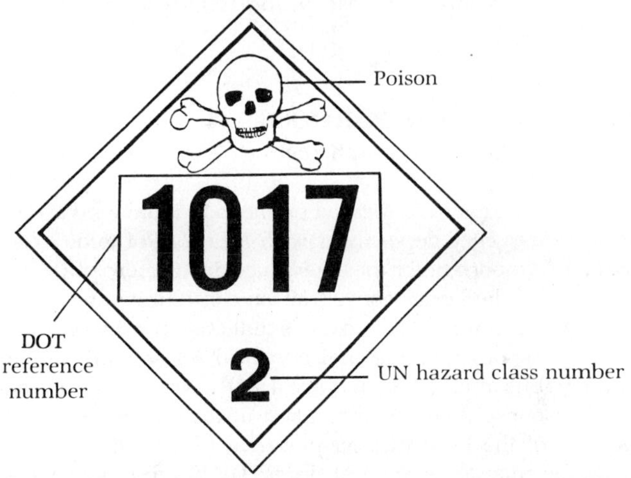

Fig. 86-1. Department of Transportation placard for chlorine. The number in the lower corner is the UN class or division number and does not correspond to the DOT class numbers in Table 86-5. The four-digit number is the UN identification number and may be displayed on the placard, label, or an orange panel located elsewhere on a tank truck. (From R.B. Leonard. Chemicals in transport: Be prepared. *Emerg. Med.* 16:19, 1984.)

Table 86-5. Department of Transportation hazard classes

1. Explosives
2. Flammable gases
3. Nonflammable gases
4. Combustible liquids
5. Flammable liquids
6. Flammable solids
7. Organic peroxides
8. Oxidizers
9. Irritants
10. Poisons
11. Etiologic agents (microorganisms and their toxins)
12. Radioactive agents
13. Corrosives

and others to get information regarding toxicity and emergency management. A number of other useful references are included in the Selected Reading list. One of these, *Emergency Care for Hazardous Materials Exposure* by Bronstein and Currance, is indexed by the United Nations identification number, the chemical name, and the DOT hazard classes. Through any one of these identifiers, the physician is quickly referred to one of 82 different guidelines, which have concise and up-to-date information on toxicity and management for the specific substance or hazard class.

Any exposure that might pose a continuing threat to the public at large should be reported to the local or state health department to assure that appropriate measures are taken to prevent continued exposure and to ensure appropriate medical triage. Contact with the employer should be made for work-site incidents, which suggest an ongoing hazard. If there is doubt that appropriate measures will be undertaken by the employer, it may be necessary to involve state occupational health authorities or the regional office of the federal Occupational Safety and Health Administration (OSHA).

PLANNING FOR HAZARDOUS MATERIALS EMERGENCIES

While this chapter has focused on the individual who arrives in the emergency department with a history of toxic exposure, it is important for the emergency department physician to consider the larger context of the community and its response to uncontrolled exposure situations. In the workplace or in transport, unintentional chemical releases are threats to the public at large that require a well-conceived and practiced response plan. Consideration of toxic releases should be part of the local disaster-planning process that coordinates the emergency medical system (EMS), fire, police, and civil defense intervention when disaster strikes.

First responders at the disaster scene need to make a rapid assessment of potential chemical exposures. A vital resource for this purpose is the 1987 *Emergency Response Guidebook*, published by the Department of Transportation (DOT Publication 5800.4). The guidebook allows quick identification of the chemical by the label or placard and the four-digit UN identification number. It gives concise first aid and site management guidelines. Following these guidelines will assure that decontamination is performed in the field, not in the emergency department. This book is small and inexpensive and should be in all EMS, fire, and other vehicles that may respond to such incidents. All emergency personnel should be aware of Chemtrec (phone number: (800) 424-9300), a nationwide hotline for toxic spills, sponsored by the Chemical Manufacturers Association, which can be especially helpful in determining the initial response to incidents that involve hazardous substances.

For hazardous materials incidents a plan is needed both for the site and the surrounding community. The site plan establishes clearly who is in charge at the scene and what personnel and equipment must be summoned. The decisions regarding isolation of the scene, extraction of victims, containment of material, and initiation of the community plan are made by the on-scene commander. These vary with the nature of the material, weather conditions, time of day, and other factors. The community plan addressed notification of the public, evacuation, and sheltering. An effective plan must be practiced. The disaster-response drills planned for the community should include chemical releases among the scenarios that the drills follow. A complete discussion of disaster planning is presented in Chap. 176.

SELECTED READING

Bronstein, AC, and Currance, PL. *Emergency Care for Hazardous Materials Exposure.* St. Louis: Mosby, 1988.

Casarett, LJ, and Doull, J. In CD Klaassen, MO Amdur, and J Doull (eds), *Toxicology, The Basic Science of Poisons* (3rd ed). New York: Macmillan, 1986.

Gosselin, R, and Smith, R. *Clinical Toxicology of Commercial Products* (5th ed). Baltimore: Williams & Wilkins, 1984.

Levy, BS, and Wegman, DH (eds). *Occupational Health* (2nd ed). Boston: Little, Brown, 1988.

NIOSH Pocket Guide to Chemical Hazards. US Department of Health and Human Services. DHHS (NIOSH) Publication No. 85-114, 1987.

Proctor, NH, et al. *Chemical Hazards of the Workplace* (2nd ed). Philadelphia: Lippincott, 1988.

Rom, WN. *Environmental and Occupational Medicine.* Boston: Little, Brown, 1983.

EMERGENCY TELEPHONE NUMBERS

CHEMTREC: A 24-hour chemical information hotline that is sponsored by the Chemical Manufacturers Association. CHEMTREC can be especially helpful in determining the initial response to hazardous substances, spills, and exposures. Telephone: 800-434-9300; international telephone: 202-483-7616.

National Pesticide Telecommunications Network: A 24-hour information hotline sponsored by the Environmental Protection Agency. This is a good first source for getting information about pesticide exposure and initial treatment. Telephone: 800-858-7378.

National Response Center: This hotline is sponsored by the U.S. Coast Guard, the Environmental Protection Agency, and the Department of Transportation. This center takes information on chemical releases and passes this information on to the local coast guard. This is *not* a good source for emergency medical information. Telephone: 800-424-8802.

Local and regional poison control centers: The list is updated yearly in *Emergency Medicine.*

87. Environmentally Caused Respiratory Disease

Peter J. Jederlinic

The unique role played by the lungs in gas exchange with the environment places them at increased risk for injury related to natural and manmade alterations in those gases. Affected patients are seen in the emergency department with a variety of respiratory syndromes and constitutional symptoms (Table 87-1). In some situations, the preceding circumstances, such as an industrial accident or fire, will suggest the cause. Alternatively, the absence of a clear precipitating work-related event results in the patient being diagnosed incorrectly with asthma or some other respiratory condition. Greater difficulty is encountered with the patient who has subacute or chronic respiratory symptoms and seeks attention for an acute exacerbation or worsening symptoms. Failure to elicit an environmental history will obscure the true cause, lead to an incorrect diagnosis and inappropriate therapy, and, moreover, result in continued exposure to the offending agent.

Although many environmental respiratory problems result from workplace exposure, inhabitants of communities located near industrial centers or mines or living along transit routes can also be affected, particularly when industrial accidents occur. The 1984 Bhopal disaster claimed an unconfirmed 10,000 lives after massive exposure to a cloud of methyldiisocyanate released accidentally from a nearby chemical plant. Natural disasters can have the same result, as seen in the asphyxiation of the entire population of a Nigerian village located on the shores of Lake Nios by a cloud of nitrogen gas released from the lake bed.

As modern man spends a greater portion of the day indoors, the health effects of indoor air pollution raise concern. By-products of materials used for furniture, walls, and insulation and poor ventilation of energy-efficient buildings result in exposure to a number of pollutants. These exposures occur in the home and office and can cause symptoms as nonspecific as cough or rhinitis. Tobacco smoking remains the major cause of indoor air pollution.

Specific knowledge of the patient's occupation helps determine whether or not symptoms are work related. For instance, the farmer is at increased risk for a number of acute respiratory distress syndromes, including farmer's lung, silo filler's disease, and occupational asthma, from several agents. Exposure to organophosphate insecticide can also affect the respiratory system. Coughing in a firefighter can represent occupational bronchitis, reactive airways dysfunction syndrome, or bronchiolitis obliterans after inhalation of toxic products of incomplete combustion. A careful history should attempt to elicit any recent change in the environment, such as installation of a new humidification or ventilation system, that could be implicated in an outbreak of *Legionella* or hypersensitivity pneumonitis.

Table 87-1. Key to the recognition of environmentally caused respiratory disease

Location	Clinical diagnosis	Major symptoms	Environmental causes	Key to recognition	Differential diagnosis
Upper airway	Rhinitis	Rhinorrhea Postnasal drip Throat clearing Cough	Toxic gases	Exposure history Work related	Allergic Vasomotor Coryza
	Sinusitis	Sinus drainage Headache Postnasal drip Throat clearing Cough	Toxic gases	Exposure history	Bacterial
	Pharyngitis	Throat pain Throat clearing Cough	Toxic gases	Exposure history	Strep throat Viral pharyngitis
	Laryngitis	Hoarseness Stridor	Toxic gases	Exposure history Recent spill	Viral
	Laryngospasm	Stridor Dyspnea	Chlorine Hydrogen chloride Sulfur dioxide	Exposure history Recent spill	Allergic Angioneurotic edema
Lower airway	Acute bronchitis (tracheobronchitis)	Productive cough Wheeze	Chlorine Phosgene Ozone Ammonia Sulfur dioxide	Exposure history	Bacterial Asthma
	Chronic bronchitis	Productive cough Wheeze Dyspnea	Hydrogen sulfide Chlorine Ozone Sulfur dioxide Vanadium/pentoxide	Chronic exposure history	COPD Chronic asthma
	Asthma	Cough Wheeze Dyspnea	Toluene diisocyanate Ammonia	Exposure history Recent onset	Atopic
Parenchyma and small airways	Bronchiolitis	Dyspnea Productive cough Wheeze	Oxides of nitrogen Sulfur dioxide Phosgene Organic dusts	Exposure history Recent spills	Viral Collagen-vascular disease Postpneumonia
	Pneumonia, acute	Dyspnea Cough Expectoration Cyanosis	Toxic gas Ammonia Chlorine	Massive exposure	*Mycoplasma* Tuberculosis ARDS (multiple causes)
	Pneumonia, chronic	Dyspnea Dry cough Weight loss	Asbestos Berylliosis Hypersensitivity reaction	Long latency Recurrent episodes	Idiopathic pulmonary fibrosis Sarcoidosis Tuberculosis
	Pulmonary edema ARDS	Dyspnea Cough Cyanosis Diaphoresis	Toxic gases Hydrogen chloride Hydrogen sulfide Ammonia Chlorine Oxides of nitrogen Sulfur dioxide Ozone Phosgene	Massive exposure	Cardiogenic ARDS (multiple causes)
Systemic	Viral syndrome	Fever Weakness Myalgia Cough	Polymer fume fever Metal fume fever Organic dust fever	New employee	Influenza
	Cardiopulmonary arrest	Unresponsive	Asphyxiants Toxic gases	Massive exposure Closed space	Cardiac cause

Key: COPD = chronic obstructive pulmonary disease; ARDS = adult respiratory distress syndrome.
Source: P.J. Jederlinic and R.S. Irwin. Acute Inhalation Injury. In Rippe, et al. (eds.), *Intensive Care Medicine* (2nd ed.). Boston: Little, Brown, 1991.

Familiarity with the past medical history and habits can direct evaluation along fruitful lines. A history of atopy is often present in persons in whom occupational asthma of the immunologic type develops. Cigarette smoking impairs mucociliary clearance and acts synergistically with other exposures to increase risk for disease.

The framework used to discuss environmental agents is by nature an arbitrary one. Frequently, a given agent will cause several syndromes, depending on the intensity and duration of exposure; short-term heavy exposure causes dramatic and acute symptoms such as pulmonary edema, while low-intensity long-term exposure leads to insidious onset of dyspnea after a prolonged latency, as with asbestosis. Problems also arise when the exposure is remote or past but symptoms persist. This problem is encountered with occupational asthma from toluene diisocyanate exposure. Symptoms of asthma persist indefinitely after one or several accidental exposures to this agent, which acts as a sensitizer.

Inhaled agents occur as gases—that is, in molecular form—or as particulates, which are further broken down into liquids in the form of mist or solids in the form of fumes. Large particles and droplets deposit in the nose and air passages while smaller particles reach and impact in the terminal bronchioles and alveoli. The smallest particles may not deposit at all but are still able to exert their effect.

ASPHYXIANTS

Simple asphyxiants include carbon dioxide (CO_2), nitrogen (N_2), and methane (CH_4), which are normally present in the atmosphere and can be fatal when present in increased concentration. Toxic asphyxiants are present in the atmosphere in minute amounts or are released by manufacturing processes or combustion, and these asphyxiate at low concentration. This group includes carbon monoxide (CO), hydrogen cyanide (HCN), acrylonitrile (vinyl cyanide), and hydrogen sulfide (H_2S) (Table 87-2).

Carbon dioxide accumulates in sealed or poorly ventilated areas, such as storage lockers, tanks, mines, and underwater caissons. Significant exposure causes dyspnea, hyperventilation, headache, diaphoresis, tachycardia, hypertension, and eventual loss of consciousness. Cardiac arrest follows shortly if oxygenation is not improved. Nitrogen is found in increased amounts in mines and, if present with increased amounts of carbon dioxide, causes significant reductions in ambient partial pressure of oxygen. Methane is a highly explosive asphyxiant gas released during breakdown of organic matter. It occurs naturally in the crust of the earth and is also present in mines. With modern mining methods and improved ventilation, the risk from these simple asphyxiants has been reduced.

Carbon monoxide is an odorless, colorless, tasteless asphyxiant that is ubiquitous. Its most important source is combustion, and it may be responsible for up to 80 percent of deaths caused by smoke inhalation. Other sources include cigarette smoke, motor vehicles, gas appliances, paint stripper, and solvents. Approximately 3,500 deaths are attributed to CO each year. Adverse health effects of chronic low-level exposure to CO occur in diseases with increased susceptibility to reduced oxygen transport–coronary artery disease, peripheral vascular disease, and chronic obstructive lung disease, and much of the data indicating an adverse effect in normals are considered to be inconclusive.

Cyanide is encountered in multiple settings: as inorganic salts (sodium and potassium) in metallurgy, electroplating, and photoprocessing; in the combustion of both natural (wood, silk) and synthetic polymers (nylon, polyurethane), including polyacrylonitrile with production of hydrogen cyanide and vinyl cyanide (acrylonitrile); and in suicides due to this agent.

Morbidity related to H_2S inhalation is minimal due to the characteristic "rotten eggs" odor that is appreciated at low concentration. Significant exposure and fatalities have occurred in industrial processes (sewage processing, petrochemical plants, and leather and rubber processing) and drilling where this gas is generated.

Pathophysiology

Simple asphyxiants work by displacing oxygen from inspired air (Table 87-3). The other agents discussed work via several other mechnisms. Carbon monoxide and H_2S alter the oxygen-carrying capacity of the blood by binding with hemoglobin to form carboxyhemoglobin (COHb) and sulfhemoglobin, respectively. Carbon monoxide binds reversibly to hemoglobin with an affinity 250 times that of oxygen, and COHb levels of 50 percent can be seen after a few minutes of exposure to 0.1 percent concentration. Furthermore, as the concentration of COHb increases, there is a leftward shift and flattening of the upper part of the oxygen dissociation curve as increased affinity of hemoglobin for oxygen at the remaining binding sites further reduces the amount of oxygen available to the tissues. Since the partial pressure of oxygen remains unchanged, breathlessness does not occur. Oxidative phosphorylation may be blocked as CO binds to cytochrome oxidase. Hydrogen sulfide also acts by poisoning the respiratory enzymes of the cell through binding to cytochrome oxidase, a method also characteristic of cyanide and acrylonitrile.

Cyanide binds to the cytochrome aa_3 complex, blocking the final step of oxidative phosphorylation and mitochondrial oxygen utilization. The tricarboxylic acid cycle is blocked and pyruvate is anaerobically converted to lactate, resulting in lactic acidosis.

Differential Diagnosis

The alternative diagnostic considerations for victims of asphyxiation are only entertained after rapid institution of emergency treatment, including cardiopulmonary resuscitation. Catastrophic conditions of cardiac and respiratory arrest, drug overdose, and intracranial hemorrhage, and the differential diagnosis of acute alteration in mental status and coma, all need to be considered, although the majority can occur with or be sequelae of the conditions being discussed.

Evaluation

Symptoms of hypoxemia accompany exposure to the simple asphyxiants and vary in severity depending on exposure intensity. These include breathlessness, tachycardia, headache and diaphoresis, bounding pulse, loss of consciousness, and cardiac arrest.

Table 87-2. Asphyxiant gases

Agent	Some sources	Uses	Form	TWA	IDLH	Effects	Pathophysiology	Treatment	Sequelae
Simple									
Carbon dioxide	Atmospheric 0.03–0.06%, combustion of organic material in oxygen, foundry work, mining	Carbonization, neutralizing, fire extinguishers, dry ice, refrigeration	Colorless, odorless, inert	5,000 ppm	50,000 ppm (5%)	Unconsciousness, asphyxia	Displaces oxygen	Oxygen supportive care	
Nitrogen	Atmospheric 78.09% from ammonia, decomposition of nitrogenous compounds, mining	Fertilizer, ammonia production, inert medium	Colorless, odorless, inert			Unconsciousness, asphyxia	Displaces oxygen	Oxygen supportive	
Methane	Decomposition of organics, mining, petroleum industry					Unconsciousness, asphyxia	Displaces oxygen	Oxygen supportive	
Toxic									
Carbon monoxide	Oxidation of hydrocarbons, combustion of organics in low oxygen, gas engine exhaust (1–10% of emissions), motor vehicles (55–60% of total), foundry work, refineries, distillation coal and wood, paint strippers	Reducing agent for metallurgy, industrial heating, gases	Colorless, odorless	50 ppm	1,500 ppm	(see Table 87-4) 10,000–40,000 ppm, death in minutes	Carboxyhemoglobin, carboxymyoglobin	High FIO_2, hyperbaric oxygen	Persistent memory deficit (43%)
Hydrogen cyanide	Almonds	Synthetic fibers, plastics, exterminating rodents, electroplating, steel industry	Colorless, water soluble, bitter almond smell	10 ppm	50 ppm	Weakness, headache, cherry-red color, confusion, asphyxia	Inhibits cytochrome oxidase and other enzymes, poisons cell respiration	Nitrate therapy, amyl nitrite (IV), thiosulfate (IV), cobalt EDTA (IM), hydroxycyanocobalamin	Chronic exposure dermatitis, motor weakness, headache
Vinyl cyanide (acrylonitrile)	Oxidation of ammonia and propylene	Synthetic fibers, plastics, resins, and rubber	Colorless, water soluble, faint odor	4 ppm	4 ppm	Slower than cyanide, weakness, dyspnea, cyanosis, burning throat, nausea, impaired judgment, convulsions, death	Inhibits cytochrome oxidase and other enzymes, poisons cell respiration		
Hydrogen sulfide	Decomposition of organics, mines, sewers, reacting iron sulfide with acid, petroleum products, synthetic materials	Analytic reagent production of sulfides, sulfuric acid, and organic sulfur	Colorless, water soluble, rotten egg odor	20 ppm	300 ppm	Green face and chest, unconsciousness, asphyxia, membrane irritation, diffuse rales, rhonchi, pulmonary edema; 10–500 ppm, slight poisoning, 500–700 ppm, moderate poisoning	Inhibits cytochrome oxidase	Oxygen supportive	Chronic bronchitis

Key: TWA = time-weighted average; IDLH = immediately dangerous to life and health; EDTA = ethalenediaminetetraacetic acid.
Source: P.J. Jederlinic and R.S. Irwin. Acute Inhalation Injury. In Rippe, et al. (eds.), *Intensive Care Medicine* (2nd ed.). Boston: Little, Brown, 1991.

Table 87-3. Methods of asphyxiation

Displacement of oxygen from inspired air
Nitrogen
Carbon dioxide
Methane
Altered oxygen-carrying capacity
Carbon monoxide → carboxyhemaglobin
Oxides of nitrogen → methemoglobin
Hydrogen sulfide → sulfhemoglobin
Poisoning of cell respiratory enzymes
Cyanide
Acrylonitrile
Hydrogen sulfide

Source: P.J. Jederlinic and R.S. Irwin. Acute Inhalation Injury. In Rippe, et al. (eds.), *Intensive Care Medicine* (2nd ed.). Boston: Little, Brown, 1991.

Carbon monoxide causes rapid loss of consciousness without adequate warning symptoms. Breathlessness is uncommon and cyanosis, previously thought to be an uncommon occurrence, is seen more frequently than the cherry-red skin color. Symptoms that reflect brain and myocardial impairment are most common with acute exposure. The high affinity of hemoglobin for CO causes even low-level exposures (0.5%) to have fatal potential (Table 87-4). Symptoms of cyanide exposure include headache, dizziness, tachycardia and tachypnea, nausea, chest and abdominal pain, confusion, and seizures. Victims give off a distinctive bitter almond odor, but its detection is unreliable and the correct diagnosis is better arrived at by the circumstances involved—for instance, suspicion of attempted suicide in a dentist or laboratory worker in conjunction with the finding of severe metabolic acidosis.

A careful baseline neurologic examination is helpful in excluding other causes of altered mental status and serves as a prognostic tool. Extrapyramidal signs and persistent cognitive and behavioral abnormalities have been reported in patients after recovery from CO poisoning. Crackles are present on auscultation in the case of severe exposure to H_2S, the result of pulmonary edema. Otherwise, abnormal physical findings may represent aspiration of gastric contents.

Arterial blood gas analysis helps alert the clinician to the possibility of CO or HCN exposure. In both cases metabolic acidosis is present while arterial oxygen tension is normal or near normal and saturation and content are reduced. A toxicology screen helps rule out other causes for these presenting symptoms. Carboxyhemoglobin levels are readily available and help to confirm the diagnosis in suspected cases (see Table 87-4). Levels less than 20 percent (mild exposure) are seen in patients who complain of headaches, tinnitus, dizziness, nausea, and slight behavioral abnormalities (see Table 87-4). With COHb levels from 20 to 40 percent (moderately severe exposure), patients can present in coma. A COHb level greater than 40 percent suggests a severe exposure and increases the risk of cardiac arrest. Continuous electrocardiographic monitoring is indicated.

Management

The principles of management for any asphyxiation include increasing inspired oxygen concentration, providing for cardiopulmonary resuscitation and support of the respiratory and circulatory systems, and treatment of complicating conditions such as burns, alcohol, and drug intoxication. Metabolic acidosis requires aggressive replacement therapy with sodium bicarbonate. Although simple, implementation of these measures can become complicated when the number of victims is large.

Table 87-4. Signs and symptoms seen with various carboxyhemoglobin concentrations

Carboxyhemoglobin concentration (%)	Signs and symptoms
0.3–0.7	None
2.5–5.0	Increased blood flow to vital organs, angina with less exertion
10–20	Headache, slight dyspnea, lethal to fetus and patients with severe cardiac disease
20–30	Nausea, increased headache, throbbing temples, flushing, decreased manual dexterity
30–40	Severe headache, vertigo, nausea, vomiting, weakness, irritability, impaired judgment, syncope
40–50	Syncope and collapse likely
50–60	Coma, convulsions, Cheyne-Stokes respiration
60–70	Depressed respiration and cardiac function, death possible
70–80	Weak pulse, slow respiration, central nervous system depression

Source: P.J. Jederlinic and R.S. Irwin. Acute Inhalation Injury. In Rippe, et al. (eds.), *Intensive Care Medicine* (2nd ed.). Boston: Little, Brown, 1991.

The two most important toxic asphyxiants, CO and HCN, call for special measures, which are better instituted when these intoxications are first suspected, without waiting to confirm the diagnosis. Early therapy with 100% oxygen is the most important measure in therapy for CO poisoning and is best delivered by an endotracheal tube in the unresponsive victim. Oxygen will reverse myocardial and cerebral ischemia and shorten the half-life of CO from 280 minutes breathing room air to 80 minutes with 100% oxygen. Further benefit can be achieved using hyperbaric oxygen, which decreases the half-life of CO to 25 minutes at three atmospheres and increases the amount of oxygen dissolved in blood. Some centers advocate use of 7% CO_2 with 93% oxygen, which will induce hyperventilation and further dissociate COHb. Hyperventilation also can be achieved by mechanical ventilation.

Hyperbaric oxygen (HBO) therapy has been shown to reduce morbidity and the development of neurologic sequelae in the CO-poisoned patient in some retrospective studies. The limited availability of HBO therapy limits its applicability. It has been suggested that comatose patients with high COHb levels (>40 percent COHb) should be treated at the initial facility if HBO is not immediately available until COHb falls to 5 percent. If coma or neurologic symptoms persist, such patients should be transferred to an HBO facility while receiving 100 percent oxygen.

Therapy for cyanide poisoning was previously based on

competition with cytochrome oxidase for cyanide. Intravenous or inhaled nitrites (amyl nitrite) form complexes with hemoglobin, resulting in methemoglobin production, which is subsequently converted to thiosulfate by thiosulfate transulfurase. Methemoglobin and cyanide complex to form cyanomethemoglobin, which then reacts with thiosulfate and is converted to nontoxic thiocyanate by transulfurase; sodium thiosulfate can be administered directly. Methemoglobin alters the oxygen-carrying capacity of the blood and contributes to tissue hypoxemia, although the risk of untreated cyanide poisoning is far greater. Newer therapies focus on the ability of cobalt to combine with cyanide. Hydroxycobalamine (vitamin B_{12}) is given intramuscularly but requires large doses. Dicobalt edetate, a chelated cobalt, is newer, more effective, less toxic therapy, which is also given intramuscularly. Care at the scene is important in survival, and inhaled amyl nitrite and dicobalt edetate can be given immediately while oxygen is administered and cardiopulmonary resuscitation instituted. Treatment for H_2S poisoning includes oxygen, supportive measures, and nitrites but not thiosulfate. Although nitrite therapy causes sulfmethemoglobin formation and increases excretion of oxidized sulfur, it delays excretion of sulfide, which is also toxic.

Disposition

Clinically significant asphyxiation and poisoning with CO (COHb level of 25 percent or greater) and HCN require admission to the intensive care unit for continuation of treatment. In victims who survive acute CO intoxication, long-term neurologic follow-up study and neuropsychological testing are indicated.

IRRITANT GASES

A variety of agents act as toxic irritants to the upper and lower respiratory tract, causing mucosal edema, mucociliary impairment, and diffuse alveolar damage, with pulmonary edema resulting from exposure to a high enough concentration (Table 87-5). Workers are exposed during industrial production and use. Other exposures occur in the home from cleaning solvents, pesticides, and other sources.

Ammonia (NH_3), a colorless, highly water-soluble gas, forms ammonium hydroxide in solution. The latter two properties make it highly irritating to the upper respiratory passages and mucous membranes, but it is capable of causing damage to alveoli when present in adequate amounts. Major uses include fertilizer production, chemicals, plastics, dye manufacture, and refrigeration. Up to three million workers are at risk of exposure, which most often occurs as the result of industrial accidents. Increased concentrations of ammonia in the environment are so irritating to the eyes and mucous membranes that the individual will attempt escape before significant pulmonary injury occurs.

Chlorine (Cl_2) is a heavy, very reactive gas, greenish-yellow under ambient conditions, with an unmistakable, pungent odor. Its density causes it to accumulate in dependent areas, and these sites should be avoided during its accidental release. Major industrial uses are in the production of alkali, bleaches, and disinfectants and in paper and textile processing. Most exposures occur during industrial spills. Approximately 15,000 workers are at risk, and a recent summary of exposures for 1986 compiled from 57 institutions by the Poison Control Center showed 3,174 exposures to chlorine gas, with an additional 673 exposures occurring in the home as the result of mixing household products. Hydrogen chloride (HCl) is much less toxic than chlorine gas and is used in the manufacture of fertilizer, dyes, textiles, and rubber. It is also released by thermal decomposition of polyvinyl chloride film.

One million workers are estimated to be at potential risk from exposure to oxides of nitrogen used in dye and fertilizer manufacture, during nitric acid use, in arc welding and braziering in poorly ventilated areas, in engraving, in metal work, in combustion of nitrogenous compounds including explosives, and in fresh silage. Gas stoves, tobacco smoke, and diesel fumes are commonly encountered sources of intense exposure to nitric oxide and nitrogen dioxide. Nitrous oxide (N_2O) is an anaesthetic agent. Nitric oxide (NO) is oxidized to nitrogen dioxide (NO_2, N_2O_4), which exists as an irritating, insoluble, heavy red-brown gas.

Phosgene ($COCl_2$) is a heavy, insoluble, colorless gas that imparts the smell of new-mown hay and hydrolyzes to form hydrochloric acid. It was responsible for the majority of fatalities from gas during World War I. Current uses in isocyanate, pesticide, dye, and pharmaceutical production, and exposure of firefighters, welders, and paint strippers to heated chlorinated hydrocarbons such as polyvinyl chloride place approximately 10,000 workers at risk. It is less irritating to eyes and mucous membranes than water-soluble agents and can be inhaled for prolonged periods without discomfort, thereby greatly increasing the risk of serious injury to the lower respiratory tract.

Sulfur dioxide (SO_2) is a colorless, heavy, irritating gas, highly soluble in water, with an identifiable pungent odor. A common atmospheric pollutant from combustion of coal and gasoline, it is also used in bleaching, refrigeration, paper manufacture, and other processes, exposing one-half million persons to potential risk. Ozone (O_3), another environmental pollutant, is an allotropic form of oxygen that is colorless, unstable, and reactive. Sources of exposure include arc welding, bleaching, high-flying aircraft, and waste treatment. With indoor levels in the home and office reaching 70 percent of outdoor levels, it is difficult to assess the population at risk.

Other agents require mention because they are ubiquitous and cause mild symptoms. Formaldehyde, a colorless, nonflammable, dense gas, was recognized as a hazard after extensive use of ureaformaldehyde foam insulation in homes. Industrial uses still include paper products, floor coverings, adhesives, and cosmetics. Exposure to cadmium as elemental metal, salt, dust, or more toxic vapor poses a risk to 2 million workers. Its volatility increases the risk to workers in or near heated environments. A variety of metal and electronics workers, welders, braziers, solderers, and painters are potentially exposed. Mercury is also dangerous in vapor form, with other exposures occurring to dust and salt forms. Nearly 1.1 million workers in metal manufacture; electronics; battery, drug, and dye manufacture; and other occupations are exposed. Vanadium pentoxide, a catalyst for various industrial processes, and residue of crude oil from various sources may affect approximately 174,000 workers. Osmium tetroxide, another acidic compound, is

Table 87-5. Toxic irritant gases

Agent	Sources	Uses	Form	Dose	Persons at risk (no.)	Pathophysiology	Effect	Acute	Chronic	Treatment
Ammonia	Combustion sources, wool, silk, nylon, melamine, polyurethane	Fertilizer production, chemical industry, pharmaceuticals, refrigerant, explosives, transport accidents, cleaning agents	Colorless, water soluble, sharp odor	50 ppm, TWA; 500 ppm, IDLH; 40–100 ppm, acute irritation in upper-respiratory tract; 700–1,700 ppm, inflammation	3 million	Forms ammonium hydroxide on contact with membranes	Liquefaction necrosis of membranes with sloughing, predominantly upper tract initially	Airway obstruction, pulmonary edema, bronchopneumonia	Tracheitis, bronchitis, bronchiectasis, small-airway disease, bronchiolitis, RADS	Oxygen observation, supportive airway maintenance, long-term follow-up study
Chlorine	Polyvinyl chloride, chlorinated acrylics	Bleaching agent in paper and textiles, disinfectant, polymers, solvents, pesticides, container leakages	Green-yellow, heavy, slight water solubility, pungent odor	1 ppm, TWA; 25 ppm, IDLH; 6–15 ppm, throat irritation; 30–90 ppm, coughing fits; 100–300 ppm may cause lethal damage; 1,000–3,000 ppm fatal after several breaths	15,000	Forms hydrogen chloride and free radical (O^-)	Affects entire respiratory tract, can be delay in effects after exposure	Airflow obstruction, pulmonary edema, ulcerative tracheobronchitis	Persistent airflow obstruction, RADS	Oxygen, observation, support, long-term follow-up
Hydrogen chloride	Polyvinyl chloride pyrolysis	Fertilizer, dye, textile and rubber manufacture, polyvinyl chloride, refining metal ore	Colorless, yellow, pungent odor	5 ppm, TWA; 100 ppm; IDLH; 4–10 ppm, burning throat			Upper airways and mucous membranes	Laryngospasm, atelectasis, pulmonary edema	Unknown	Oxygen, airway maintenance, observation, supportive
Oxides of nitrogen, nitrous oxide, nitrogen dioxide	Combustion of fabric and nitrocellulose films	Fresh silage, arc welding, combustion nitrogen polymers, chemical industry dyes and lacquers, mining, explosives, gas stoves	Red-brown gas, heavy, insoluble, irritating odor	5 ppm, TWA; 50 ppm, IDLH; 50 ppm, acute respiratory problems	1 million	Forms nitric acid, direct inflammation, peroxidation of lipids, impairs surfactant	Lower tract	Acute pulmonary edema	Bronchiolitis obliterans, chronic bronchitis, ?emphysema, persisting obstruction	Oxygen, observation, support, long-term follow-up study
Phosgene	Polyvinyl chloride combustion	Isocyanate production, pesticide, dye, and pharmaceutical products; polyvinyl chloride; carbon tetrachloride extinguishers	Colorless gas, heavy, prickling smell, mown hay, poor water solubility	0.1 ppm, TWA; 2 ppm, IDLH	10,000	Hydrolyzes to HCl and CO_2, sympathetic effects	Lower tract, delayed recognition, fluid shifts, necrosis and sloughing of mucosal surfaces, decreased lung volumes, decreased DLCO, hypoxemia	Atelectasis, acute pulmonary edema, acute bronchiolitis, ulcerative bronchitis	Air-trapping	Oxygen, observation, support, long-term follow-up study
Ozone	Photochemical smog, arc welding, high altitude	Oxidizing agent	Bluish gas, pungent odor, poor water solubility	0.1 ppm, TWA; 10 ppm, IDLH; 0.02–0.05 ppm, threshold; 2 ppm, acute symptoms	Diverse group	Powerful oxidizing agent, cholinergic effects	Lower tract, tolerance with chronic exposure	Acute pulmonary edema, asthma	?COPD	
Sulfur dioxide	Sulfur-containing compounds, wood, oil, etc	Combustion fossil fuels, smelting ores, paper manufacture, food preparation	Colorless gas, heavy, pungent odor, water soluble	5 ppm, TWA; 100 ppm, IDLH; 0.5 ppm, detectable; 6–10 ppm, irritation	500,000	Forms sulfate ($SO_3^{=}$) and bisulfite (HSO_3^{-})	Upper tract pulmonary vasoconstriction, extensive sloughing of mucosa, alveolar edema and hemorrhage	Laryngospasm, airway narrowing, pulmonary edema, bronchopneumonia, worsens asthma	?COPD, emphysema bronchiectasis, bronchiolitis obliterans	

Key: TWA = time-weighted average; IDLH = immediately dangerous to life and health; RADS = reactive airways dysfunction syndrome; DLCO = diffusing capacity.
Source: P.J. Jederlinic and R.S. Irwin. Acute Inhalation Injury. In Rippe, et al. (eds.), *Intensive Care Medicine* (2nd ed.). Boston: Little, Brown, 1991.

used to process tissue. These salts of vanadium and osmium are implicated in the development of bronchitis in exposed workers. Although paraquat is thought to cause problems by absorption through the skin, most accidents with this herbicide occur while it is being sprayed and inhaled, resulting in pulmonary fibrosis.

Pathophysiology

Accidental massive exposures to NH_3, Cl_2, HCl, oxides of nitrogen, $COCl_2$, SO_2, and some of the other irritant gases cause similar pathologic changes. Ammonia, sulfur dioxide, and hydrogen chloride have high water solubility and tend to be highly irritating to conjunctiva, mucous membranes, and upper air passages. Laryngospasm, bronchospasm, and mucous membrane necrosis ensue. Less soluble agents such as N_2O, O_3, and $COCl_2$ are able to penetrate deeper into the respiratory tree and cause damage at the alveolar level, resulting in pulmonary edema and bronchospasm. The absence of immediate irritant symptoms with these agents results in prolonged exposure. Chlorine has intermediate solubility and has effect throughout the respiratory tract, but exposure to a heavy concentration of any of these toxic agents causes diffuse involvement. In addition to solubility and concentration, the pH and chemical reactivity influence the amount of damage inflicted. Chlorine, HCl, SO_2, and $COCl_2$ are acidic, whereas O_3, Cl_2, and oxides of nitrogen are highly alkaline. Toxicity is enhanced if particulates are present (e.g., soot) that tend to carry irritants further down the airways. After acute exposure, residual damage to the respiratory system may occur in the form of reactive airways disease, asthma, bronchitis, bronchiolitis, or bronchiectasis. Most of our understanding concerning these agents is the result of accidents and controlled exposure to normal subjects.

The strong smell associated with NH_3 is present within minutes at 50 parts per million (ppm), and few persons are able to tolerate greater than 100 ppm without nasal stuffiness and irritating cough. The reaction of NH_3 with water on the mucous membranes, airways, and conjunctiva results in ammonium hydroxide formation and liquefaction necrosis with intense pain of affected areas, choking, cyanosis, aphonia, and suffocation. Death from asphyxiation can occur within one minute at high concentration (1,500 ppm). Findings within hours of acute exposure observed in fatal cases include edema, ulceration, necrosis, and sloughing of mucous membranes and airway mucosa, with airway obstruction due to laryngeal edema and plugging of airways by sloughed epithelium. Clinical bronchopneumonia and acute pulmonary edema are seen within 24 hours. Severe airway obstruction can take more than a year to improve. Long-term sequelae include bronchitis and bronchiectasis, and small airways disease, although bronchiolitis seems uncommon.

Chlorine is detectable at levels of 1 ppm. On contact with mucous membranes, HCl, hypochlorous acid (HOCl), and free oxygen radicals are formed, and much of the damage results from these last products. Shortly after initial exposure the ability to detect continued exposure is blunted, subjecting the victim to additional risk. After the onset of exposure, the individual experiences choking and coughing, which stop after removal from the exposure. The paucity of initial symptoms belies the true severity of the problem, and the patient may be inappropriately sent home from the emergency department. Slight wheezing and erythematous mucous membranes may be the only physical findings. If exposure is severe enough, death can result from laryngospasm or massive pulmonary edema. Hours to days after exposure, upper air passage edema, pulmonary edema, and exudative inflammatory bronchitis cause plugging of medium and small bronchi, leading to atelectasis. Development of stridor reflects upper-airway obstruction caused by nasal, pharyngeal, and laryngeal edema. Hypoxemia and hypercapnia occur secondary to these changes. Pulmonary edema and bronchopneumonia accompany peripheral airway obstruction. Changes subsequently revert to near normal but chronic airway problems persist.

Exposure to oxides of nitrogen at 50 ppm increases the risk of acute respiratory problems. Poor solubility results in a paucity of upper-tract and mucous membrane irritation and exposure may be inapparent because of this. Clinically, the response occurs in three phases: (1) Cough and dyspnea develop and are followed by pulmonary edema several hours later; (2) as pulmonary edema clears, slight dyspnea may be present for three to five weeks; (3) finally, an illness characterized by cough, dyspnea, and fever with nodular or patchy infiltrates progresses to chronic obstruction, and lung biopsy shows bronchiolitis obliterans. Molecular effects of N_2O include lipid peroxidation and impairment of surfactant activity. Most deaths occur during the acute phases.

Phosgene is only mildly irritating to the eyes and upper airways, increasing the risk of continued exposure. Dyspnea and dry cough develop and are followed by pulmonary edema. The increase in airway resistance after inhalation of low levels of ozone is abolished by atropine, suggesting an effect on the neural determinants of bronchomotor tone. Ozone also affects the lower respiratory tract, causing symptoms of chest pain, cough, and dyspnea. At 2 ppm, pulmonary edema is seen and fatalities have occurred at levels above 5 ppm.

Differential Diagnosis

The presentation of these disorders as a group is very distinctive and usually occurs in the setting of an industrial or transport-related accident. Patients are seen in acute respiratory distress with evidence for intense conjunctival and mucous membrane edema, erythema and ulceration, and laryngeal edema causing upper respiratory tract obstruction. The stridor may be associated with the clinical and roentgenographic picture of pulmonary edema, with bronchopneumonia occurring later. Anaphylaxis and angioneurotic edema with bronchospasm can appear similar, but severe mucous membrane inflammation and ulceration are not prominent features of these disorders.

Evaluation

The need for a careful history from rescue personnel, coworkers, witnesses, and plant managers cannot be overemphasized. This will help establish which agents are involved, relative concentrations, the site of exposure (closed space or outdoor), and duration. A description of symptoms and odors from those less affected is also useful, and exposures that occur as the result of industrial accidents will frequently involve groups of victims. Airway patency should be assured since laryngeal edema can lead to complete airway obstruction over several hours. Evidence of burn injury, skin lesions, and examination of eyes and mucous membranes allow some prediction of intensity of exposure and the likelihood of laryngeal obstruction. Auscultation of chest reveals crackles, rhonchi, and wheezing, depending on the time elapsed since injury. Arterial blood gas analysis should be obtained early and repeated as necessary to adjust oxygen therapy. A COHb level will assess simultaneous CO poisoning. Toxicology screening should be performed since this may shed light on why an accident occurred. A chest roentgenograph is indicated and the typical bat-wing distribution of cardiogenic pulmonary edema is a less likely finding than diffuse or patchy infiltrates of noncardiogenic pulmonary edema. Other findings include atelectasis, hyperinflation, and aspiration pneumonia.

Management

Exposures are minimized by worker education and by establishing and following certain safety guidelines. For instance, use of protective clothing and respirators in any situation that would require a worker to enter a storage tank to inspect or clean should be mandated. Disaster preparedness programs and drills can reduce the risk of workers in the event of an accident. Readily available emergency respirators and oxygen should be accessible in numerous sites in the workplace and workers should be fully aware of how to use these in an emergency. Basic life support training should be a part of these safety programs since it is frequently necessary to institute these measures at the scene.

The mainstay of management for any gas exposure is removal of the victim from the site of exposure by rescue workers using respirators and wearing protective clothing, and immediate administration of oxygen. Evidence for upper-airway obstruction secondary to edema and the need to control the airway in the unconscious patient are both indications for endotracheal intubation, emergency cricothyroidotomy, or tracheostomy. A large endotracheal tube ($>$8.0 mm inner diameter) is helpful for pulmonary toilet and for anticipated bronchoscopy to remove mucus plugs. Even when the development of respiratory distress is delayed, these measures may be required at a later time.

Exposure to Cl_2 and $COCl_2$ is accompanied by an initial period of well-being or minor distress followed several hours later by acute respiratory failure with clinical and roentgenographic evidence of pulmonary edema. These patients therefore will require prolonged monitoring in the emergency department before final disposition can be made. Treatment is otherwise largely supportive. Pulmonary edema is treated with oxygen and mechanical ventilation and positive end expiratory pressure therapy may be required. Bronchospasm is treated with inhaled and intravenous bronchodilators. Intravenous fluids are necessary because of fluid losses secondary to mucosal edema and sloughing and associated burn injury. Empiric antibiotics are not indicated and offer the disadvantage of selecting out resistant pathogens, but when convincing evidence for pneumonia exists their institution is not controversial. Corticosteroids should not be used in initial management and have been associated with a significant increase in mortality. Conversely, late complications such as airways disease or bronchiolitis are indications for their use. Complete pulmonary function testing should be obtained as soon as the patient is able since these results will form the basis for determining the degree of residual impairment.

Disposition

With acute massive exposure, victims will require admission to a respiratory intensive care unit, where they can be treated and closely monitored for increasing respiratory distress and mechanical ventilation can be instituted as needed. After discharge, long-term follow-up study with a pulmonary specialist will be necessary for monitoring of pulmonary function and treatment of complications.

INHALED AGENTS THAT CAUSE ACUTE SYSTEMIC REACTIONS

Several unrelated agents have been implicated in the development of a self-limited systemic illness, characterized as flu-like, in exposed workers. Causative agents fall into three groups (Table 87-6): fine powders of a variety of metal oxides, fluorocarbon polymer combustion products, and suspected endotoxin and mycotoxin contaminants of grains and cotton. The illness typically affects only new workers and may recur several times before tolerance develops, with no evidence for permanent or residual impairment.

Pathophysiology

All these disorders are characterized by development of a polymorphonuclear leukocytosis and fever several hours after inhalation of the agent. Respiratory symptoms of cough, chest discomfort, and dyspnea can occur. Polymorphonuclear leukocytes also localize to the airways. An increase in circulating pyrogen suggests that metallic oxides trigger release of endogenous pyrogen from circulating leukocytes. The inability to stimulate symptoms with commercial grades of pure metallic oxide indicates the need that they be freshly generated by welding, soldering, or some other physical action. Symptoms usually abate within 24 to 48 hours, and tolerance to repeat exposures occurs rapidly.

Temperature and reaction conditions determine which products are generated from combustion of fluorocarbon polymers. At extreme conditions they combust to hydrogen fluoride and carbon dioxide. Diffuse infiltrates resembling pulmonary edema have been observed on chest roentgenographs in some cases of high-level exposure; these have taken up to one week to clear. Tolerance is more difficult to demonstrate but is thought to occur.

Ubiquitous endotoxin induces cough, chest tightness, flu-like symptoms, and a polymorphonuclear leukocytosis when given to volunteers by inhalation, with symptoms that last for 24 hours. Physiologic studies show increased airway resistance. Dose-dependent pathophysiologic events include the ability to activate complement by the classic or alternate path and interaction with the cell membranes of neutrophils, endothelial cells, platelets, and macrophages, resulting in release of endogenous pyrogen and a variety of vasoactive mediators. Tolerance occurs but can be overcome by larger doses of endotoxin. Heavy mycotoxin exposure in silo work-

Table 87-6. Inhaled agents with systemic toxicity

Category	Agents	Occupation industry	Number exposed	Affected (%)	Form	Size (μ)	Clinical features: Acute	Clinical features: Chronic	Comments
Metal fume fever	Zinc oxide, zinc sulfide, copper, cadmium, magnesium, other metals	Alloy makers, braziers, electroplaters, galvanizers, welders, foundry workers, others	Indeterminate	20	Nascent oxides, fumes, fine powders	0.02–0.25	Chills, fever, cough, chest discomfort, leukocytosis	Tolerance	New workers
Polymer fume fever	Fluorocarbon, polymer combustion products, polytetrafluoroethylene, fluorinated ethylene, propylene	Fluorocarbon polymer fabrication, electronics industry, automotive industry, soldering, welding	5,000	86	Fumes	0.2–0.5	Chills, fever, cough, chest discomfort, leukocytosis, pulmonary edema	Tolerance	New workers, contaminated cigarettes
Organic dust fever	Bacterial endotoxin, mycotoxin	Cotton industry, mill workers, grain handlers	Indeterminate	50	Dust		Chills, fever, cough, chest discomfort, leukocytosis, acute interstitial lung disease	Tolerance, COPD, bronchiolitis obliterans	

Source: P.J. Jederlinic and R.S. Irwin. Acute Inhalation Injury. In Rippe, et al. (eds.), *Intensive Care Medicine* (2nd ed.). Boston: Little, Brown, 1991.

ers results in cough, mucous membrane irritation, and fever after several hours. Chest roentgenographs may show diffuse interstitial disease. Symptoms persist for up to one month and pathologic changes include acute inflammation of alveoli, terminal bronchioles, and interstitium. This disorder is distinct from hypersensitivity pneumonitis in that an immunologic response to fungi cannot be demonstrated. Tolerance in all of these illnesses develops as a result of increased ability to take up circulating pyrogen by an activated reticuloendothelial system.

Differential Diagnosis

Because of the mild and acute systemic nature of these reactions, the patient is inclined to treat it as a flu-like or viral illness and may not seek medical attention unless episodes are recurrent. The differential diagnosis includes viral infection and asthma.

Evaluation

The key to diagnosing these disorders is the work history, including recent hiring, job title, and substances encountered. The diagnosis should only be considered after exclusion of more common problems, such as upper or lower respiratory tract infection or asthma. A chest roentgenograph is indicated when there are positive findings on examination.

Management

Recognition that these disorders are self-limited may suggest little need for active management. However, their occurrence implies that a problem exists in the workplace and that steps should be taken to improve ventilation and worker protection.

ENVIRONMENTAL DISEASES OF THE AIRWAYS

The airways can be affected by extreme physical conditions such as heat or cold, by toxic agents based in part on water solubility and concentration, and via immunologic and nonimmunologic mechanisms. Three disorders represent the spectrum of environmental airways disease. These include occupational asthma (OA), the reactive airways dysfunction syndrome (RADS), and industrial or occupational bronchitis. The last of these is of more epidemiologic than practical significance. The entity of bronchiolitis has already been discussed in the section on toxic gases. It is estimated that 2 to 15 percent of asthma is related to workplace exposures. The rapid turnover of new workers in these occupations leads to an artificially low estimate of the true prevalence of asthma, known as the "healthy worker effect." Failure to recognize that an association exists between symptoms and workplace can result in progressive disease and disability in the patient and other exposed workers and prevent correction of the offending situation. Unlike other conditions that result from an acute exposure, OA may persist long after exposure has been discontinued.

Occupational asthma is defined as variable airway narrowing causally related to exposures encountered in the workplace to airborne dusts, fumes, vapors, and gases. Recognition requires that minimal criteria be met: symptoms consistent with asthma—cough, wheeze, dyspnea, and chest tightness; identification of the offending agent; proof that the suspect agent can cause asthma; spirometric evidence of airflow obstruction, including specific and nonspecific bronchoprovocative evidence of airways hyperreactivity; and finally, immunologic evidence, which may consist of demonstration of specific immunoglobulin E (IgE) and skin testing. Preexisting asthma should be considered as separate from OA since the former can be aggravated by a wide variety of industrial irritants. Sensitization to environmental agents is more likely to develop in those with atopy. The number of workers exposed to these agents is variable: 8 million farmers, animal handlers, and lumber workers; 250,000 bakers and beauticians; and 30,000 workers exposed to diisocyanates in the spray paint, plastics, and rubber industries.

The reactive airways dysfunction syndrome can be considered a form of inflammatory bronchoconstriction, usually resulting from a single or multiple accidental exposures to an irritating vapor, fume, or smoke, with symptoms that persist for years after exposure. The number at risk is probably as large as that for OA.

A number of factors predispose to the development of OA. Environmental determinants include poor ventilation, worker noncompliance with safety procedures, exposure to spills, and even the occurrence of a viral respiratory infection. Host factors include smoking, a history of atopy, and the presence of nonspecific bronchial hyperreactivity. Evidence suggests that smokers are more easily sensitized to some agents, and the majority of workers with red cedar asthma are lifelong nonsmokers. It is commonly assumed that bronchial hyperreactivity preexists in workers in whom OA develops, although the return of bronchial hyperreactivity to normal after discontinuation of exposure to the offending agent suggests that this may not be the case.

Pathophysiology

Bronchial hyperreactivity is an essential feature of asthma and can be reproduced by histamine or methacholine bronchoprovocation challenge. Any irritating agent can precipitate or aggravate airway obstruction in persons with a history of asthma, even in low concentration. This reaction is thought to occur via direct stimulation of irritant receptors in the bronchial submucosa, which are vagal in origin and can be blocked by atropine.

Accidental exposure to high concentrations of irritant gases, vapors, and combustion products results in inflammatory bronchoconstriction. Offending agents include Cl_2, fluorine, $COCl_2$, NH_3, and N_2O in gaseous form, and vapors of strong acids and organic solvents. In contrast to reflex bronchoconstriction, inflammatory bronchoconstriction occurs late, usually several hours after inhalation, reaches maximum severity in one week, and persists for up to several months. Airway obstruction in this setting also results from mucosal edema and epithelial sloughing as a direct effect of inflammatory mediator release. Persisting airways hyperreactivity can result from reinnervation of reepithelialized bronchial mucosa, altered smooth-muscle innervation, increased receptor affinity for acetylcholine, and increased epithelial permeability. These mechanisms are also a plausible explanation for the persisting bronchial hyperreactivity seen in RADS.

The dose-response relationship is characteristic of pharmacologic bronchoconstriction. These agents cause release of histamine, inhibit beta-adrenergic receptors, act as an anticholinesterase, or cause complement activation by the classic or alternate pathways with release of chemical mediators. At a high enough concentration, all exposed persons will demonstrate bronchoconstriction. Although nonspecific bronchial hyperreactivity may be present during exposure, this finding no longer persists when exposure ceases. Examples of pharmacologic bronchoconstriction include organophosphate insecticides, which precipitate airflow obstruction by their anticholinesterase action.

The majority of agents that cause OA do so by an allergic mechanism. They most often affect the person with a history of atopy. High molecular weight compounds from animal and plant sources are natural sensitizing agents and cause formation of specific IgE and IgG antibodies over weeks to months that can be demonstrated by skin tests and radioimmunoassay. These are reponsible for the immediate response seen during specific bronchoprovocation testing. Cross-reactivity of antigens exists within classes of agents.

The recognition of low molecular weight agents causing OA is burgeoning and includes inorganic and organic agents. Specific IgE may not be demonstrated to the agent alone, but when it is conjugated to serum protein it acts as a hapten and induces antibodies. It is clear that sensitization develops in workers exposed to diisocyanate weeks or months after initiating exposure, and thereafter an attack of bronchospasm can be induced by very low levels of the agent. Exposure to single or recurrent spills also plays a significant role in sensitization. Most patients with diisocyanate asthma have eosinophilia. Cross-reactivity exists to other diisocyanates. Diisocyanate-induced asthma persists long after exposure has ceased.

Differential Diagnosis

Symptoms and signs are consistent with a viral upper-respiratory infection, asthma, rhinitis, or bronchitis. Hypersensitivity pneumonitis (HP) is suggested in the patient who has onset of dyspnea in a characteristic exposure setting, but in HP the pulmonary response is predominantly an alveolitis with associated interstitial abnormality and granulomatous changes histologically, pulmonary function alterations are restrictive in nature, and immunologic findings are those of IgG precipitins and a cell-mediated reaction.

Evaluation

Since symptoms develop in most exposed persons within months of onset of exposure, duration of employment is important and exposure to spills or changes in the manufacturing process should be noted. The pattern of symptom development is helpful in diagnosis. Symptoms may improve dramatically over weekends and vacations, with maximal symptoms occurring the first day of the week. Other patterns include a progressive increase in symptoms through the week or a similar deterioration on each work day. After the environmental exposure is recognized, it becomes necessary to establish if there is a specific or nonspecific irritant effect. Also, a search for other known triggers for asthma should be undertaken. Other predisposing factors, such as smoking history and medications used, should be sought since beta-blocker or aspirin use can precipitate bronchospasm in some persons. Absence of wheezing on examination does not exclude OA. Determination of arterial blood gases and peak expiratory flows is only indicated as needed in the management of severe asthma or status asthmaticus. The total eosinophil count is elevated in some types of OA.

Pulmonary function studies demonstrate obstruction as measured by a reduction in forced expiratory volume in one second (FEV_1), in FEV_1 as percent of forced vital capacity (FEV_1/FVC%), and in peak expiratory flow. Normal studies do not exclude asthma and should be followed by nonspecific bronchial challenge with methacholine. Positive results on an inhalation challenge test offer further supporting evidence of asthma but do not confirm an environmental cause since a number of other conditions besides asthma can lead to positive test results. A negative challenge can result if the patient has left the workplace months earlier. When a return to the workplace is associated with conversion to a positive methacholine challenge, the result carries considerably more weight and documents that sensitization has occurred. The methacholine challenge test result helps determine how sensitive the patient will be to specific bronchial provocation testing with the suspected offending agent. The results of repeat methacholine challenge over time can be of use in following the response of OA to removal from the exposure. Several other nonprovocative methods can be used to follow the development of airflow obstruction in relation to the workplace. The patient can carry a portable peak flowmeter and make several determinations of peak flow during the day at work, in the evening and early morning, and over weekends and holidays. Alternatively, if malingering is suspected, spirometry can be measured by a qualified technician using a portable apparatus several times a day.

Classification of OA is based on pathophysiologic considerations (Table 87-7). Reflex bronchoconstriction is seen with exposure to cold air, exercise, noxious gases, and some inert particulates. Preexisting asthma is aggravated by these agents. Inflammatory bronchoconstriction results from most of the toxic asphyxiants discussed earlier and from solvents and fumes of a variety of volatile organic compounds found in household and industrial settings. Pharmacologic agents include cotton and related fiber dusts, organophosphate insecticides, plastic pyrolysis products, and diisocyanates.

The largest, most important, and best understood cause of OA consists of agents acting via an allergic mechanism. High molecular weight causes include proteins, polysaccharides, glycoproteins, and peptides derived from danders, excreta, feathers, marine animals, insects, grain, and plants during harvesting, processing, and a variety of industrial uses. A number of chemicals, including diisocyanates, anhydrides and other organic compounds, pharmaceuticals, metals and their salts, and fumes comprise low molecular weight agents that cause allergic-type OA.

With the appropriate agent, up to 5 or 10 percent of a given work force may be affected with OA. Occasionally, higher prevalences have resulted from abnormally high exposure intensity, poor ventilation, or unrecognized exposure. Examples include laboratory animal handlers, with a 30 percent prevalence of OA. The 4 to 5 percent prevalence of OA in workers exposed to Western red cedar or diisocyanates is more compatible with the prevalence of atopy in the general population.

Specific bronchoprovocation challenge may be indicated to study a previously unrecognized agent, to determine the causative agent in a complex environment, and on occasion for medicolegal purposes. The patterns of reaction—immediate, late, dual, and recurrent nocturnal—indicate that prolonged monitoring of spirometry is required after challenge is administered. Also, a control is necessary to be certain that the response is not merely a nonspecific one. The early or immediate response begins within minutes, peaks by 10 to 20 minutes, and resolves by 1 hour. The late response occurs 1 or more hours after exposure, peaks at several hours, and can last 24 to 48 hours. A dual response occurs with both early and late components and often a single agent, such as plicatic acid, can demonstrate any one of the three patterns in different patients. A prolonged late response that lasts weeks with a nightly decline in flow rates has occurred after challenge with toluene diisocyanate.

Allergy skin-prick testing is also useful for determining sensitization to suspected antigens and can help determine the dose of allergen for specific bronchoprovocation challenge testing. While high molecular weight agents can be used directly for skin testing, low molecular weight agents may require a carrier protein. Furthermore, many low molecular weight chemicals have a direct irritant effect and give confusing results. Specific IgE antibodies can be measured by radioallergosorbent test (RAST) and RAST inhibition or by enzyme-linked immunoabsorbent testing (ELISA) and have been demonstrated to both high molecular weight and low molecular weight protein conjugates. It should be emphasized that these tests only show sensitization that can occur in patients without respiratory symptoms and therefore lack specificity for OA.

Management

Treatment of acute asthma of any cause entails use of beta-sympathomimetics, theophylline, and corticosteroids and these measures have been discussed in Chap. 10. Once asthma is attributed to a specific environment, every effort should be made to remove the affected person from that exposure. This can be a complicated process that involves the physician, patient, union, management, and federal and state agencies. Economic exigencies may make it impossible for the worker to leave a job and increase the risk for development of chronic asthma. Although improving ventilation and production processes and the use of a dust mask or respirator may be of some help, these measures may be inadequate since the worker with OA is sensitized and reacts to a very low level of antigen. Although use of disodium cromoglycate and inhaled steroids may offer some control of symptoms, there is no evidence that they protect against the development of chronic asthma and fixed obstruction.

Table 87-7. Types of occupational asthma

Category	Examples (% prevalence)	Occupation	Mechanism	Onset	Durations	Comments
Reflex	Cold air Exercise Lactose powder	Refrigeration Athletics Pharmaceuticals	Direct effect on irritant receptors in bronchial submucosa	Immediate	Ceases after exposure discontinued	Aggravates preexisting asthma
Irritant	Ammonia Chlorine Solvents	Chemical industry	Chemical inflammation Mucosal edema Irritant receptor effect	Late	Prolonged (months)	RADS
Pharmacologic	Organophosphates	Farming	Acts as anticholinesterase	Immediate	Ceases after exposure	At high enough levels all exposed develop bronchoconstriction
	Cotton dust	Linen industry	Endotoxin mediated	Most severe at start of week		
Allergic High molecular weight	Biologic enzymes (66%) *Bacillus subtilis*	Detergent manufacture				Not from domestic use
	Animal products (30%)	Laboratory workers	Type I allergic reaction Positive skin tests Specific IgE	Immediate and late reactions	Ceases after exposure Remains sensitive	Rhinitis common
	Cereal flour (20%)	Bakers				Cross-reactivity among flours
Low molecular weight	Diisocyanates (10%)	Plastics		Weeks to months after exposure starts		Eosinophilia common
	Anhydrides (36%)	Epoxy resins	Type I allergic reaction Positive skin tests Specific IgE		Persists after exposure ceases	Cough syndrome Immediate rhinitis and asthma Late asthma and fever Pulmonary infiltrates
	Wood dusts (4%) Plicatic acid	Carpentry Sawmill		Late onset		More common in smokers

Key: RADS = reactive airways dysfunction syndrome.
Souce: P.J. Jederlinic and R.S. Irwin. Acute Inhalation Injury. In Rippe, et al. (eds.), *Intensive Care Medicine* (2nd ed.). Boston: Little, Brown, 1991.

Disposition

When OA is suspected as a potential cause for symptoms in the patient, a thorough evaluation is indicated and best carried out by a pulmonologist familiar with occupational disorders. After confirmation of the diagnosis, it is the patient's discretion to change his or her work situation and seek redress from his or her employer. This may require legal action and therefore the diagnosis must be certain. Long-term follow-up study is also required since patients with OA demonstrate persistence of asthma and nonspecific bronchial hyperreactivity long after exposure is discontinued.

HYPERSENSITIVITY PNEUMONITIS

In contrast to OA, HP results from an immunoglobic reaction to inhaled antigens, which affect the alveoli and interstitium of the lung. Causative agents are encountered in a variety of occupations and also result from indoor (home and office) exposure to antigens dispersed by contaminated humidification and climate control systems (Table 87-8). Implicated agents include organic compounds of the appropriate particle size, allowing them to be inhaled and induce alveolitis. Thermophilic actinomyces are a common cause of HP. They are responsible for farmer's lung, which occurs in farmers and dairy workers exposed to moldy hay and feedstuffs. Approximately 2.8 million workers are at risk, but the true incidence is difficult to establish since HP is usually diagnosed as some other condition. Bagassosis, mushroom worker's lung, and HP due to contaminated climate control systems are also caused by this class of antigens. Fungal antigens cause HP in cheese worker's lung, malt worker's lung, maple bark stripper's lung, paprika slicer's lung, sequoiosis, and suberosis. Animal antigens include amoebas, insects, animal excrement, and extracts. Chemical causes of HP include diisocyanates, phthalic anhydride, and trimellitic anhydride, although these more often cause OA. Some types of HP have unknown antigens but are associated with coffee dust, cereal grain, tap water, tobacco, sawdust, tea, and climate control systems.

Prevalence rates range from 3 to 15 percent, although altered cellular and humoral immunity are present in up to one-half of the population at risk. Specific examples of prevalence rate estimates for more common causes of HP are 0.9 to 9.6 percent for farmer's lung and 6 to 15 percent for pigeon-breeder's disease. Similarly, the prevalence of HP in populations exposed to contaminated air cooling systems ranges from 1 to 15 percent. The potential for chronic, progressive pulmonary disease exists with recurrent exposure to the offending antigen. Genetic factors, infection, and simultaneous exposure to other toxins may also play a role.

Table 87-8. Some causes of hypersensitivity pneumonitis

Agent	Source	Disease	Number at risk
Micropolyspora faeni	Moldy compost	Farmer's lung	2.8×10^6
Thermoactinomyces saccharii	Moldy sugar cane	Bagassosis	5×10^3
Thermoactinomyces vulgaris	Mushrooms	Mushroom worker's lung	6×10^3
Cryptostroma corticale	Moldy maple bark	Maple bark stripper's lung	
Aspergillus clavatus	Moldy malt	Malt worker's lung	1.8×10^3
Avian proteins	Avian droppings	Bird-breeder's lung	10^5
Diisocyanates	Spray paint, plastics	Isocyanate	9×10^3
Phthalic anhydride	Epoxy resins	Epoxy resin worker's lung	5.4×10^4

Source: P.J. Jederlinic and R.S. Irwin. Acute Inhalation Injury. In Rippe, et al. (eds.), *Intensive Care Medicine* (2nd ed.). Boston: Little, Brown, 1991.

Pathophysiology

The unifying features of agents that cause HP are their organic nature and ability, based on particle size, to penetrate the distal airways and alveoli, leading to development of alveolitis. Although serum precipitins (IgG) occur in the majority of symptomatic persons, they are also seen in large numbers of exposed asymptomatic persons and thus lack specificity. Current models invoke nonspecific stimulation by antigen of the alternative pathway of complement, resulting in increased vascular permeability, release of lysosomal enzymes and monokines, neutrophil chemotaxis, and activation of alveolar macrophages with release of enzymes and oxygen products, interleukin-1, and monokines. T- and B-lymphocyte recruitment results in further magnification of this cellular response and production of immune complexes.

Biopsy during the acute phase demonstrates infiltration of alveolar walls with neutrophils and some eosinophils, numerous intraalveolar macrophages, foreign body giant cells, and neutrophils. Later, the cellular infiltrate becomes more lymphocytic and includes plasma cells. Granulomas consisting of palisading epithelioid cells develop around areas of liquefaction necrosis. This initial reaction may vary in intensity based on the dose of antigen. Subsequent changes are influenced by the degree of sensitization, antigen dose, and frequency and number of exposures. With repeat exposures or chronicity, noncaseating granulomas are seen with greater regularity and the alveolar and interstitial infiltrates undergo organization (Table 87-9). Eventually, diffuse fibrosis and honeycombing result. Progressive bronchiolar involvement and organization result in bronchiolitis.

Differential Diagnosis

The presentation of acute HP with its constitutional and pulmonary symptoms suggests the diagnosis of pneumonia. HP's lack of a response to antibiotics and its recurrent nature are helpful in distinguishing these two disorders. In some instances HP is accompanied by wheezing and can be confused with asthma, and some antigens cause either of these disorders. Chest roentgenographic change consisting of interstitial and alveolar infiltrates and the restrictive pulmonary function changes of HP usually clarify the diagnosis.

Table 87-9. Clinical patterns of hypersensitivity pneumonitis

Pattern	Acute	Subacute	Chronic
Exposure	Intermittent	Intermittent but continuous	Continuous
Symptoms	Acute	Less obvious	Progressive and insidious
Onset	4–10 hr		
Peak	8–10 hr		
Pulmonary function	Restriction	Restriction Obstruction	Restriction Obstruction
Reversibility	Yes	Yes	No
Pathology	Alveolitis with macrophages	Noncaseating granulomas	Interstitial fibrosis
	Foreign body giant cells		Honeycombing, bronchiolitis obliterans

Source: P.J. Jederlinic and R.S. Irwin. Acute Inhalation Injury. In Rippe, et al. (eds.), *Intensive Care Medicine* (2nd ed.). Boston: Little, Brown, 1991.

Allergic bronchopulmonary aspergillosis is a form of hypersensitivity disease in which *Aspergillus* colonizes the airways and precipitins to this fungus are present in the blood. The presentation with difficult-to-control asthma, peripheral eosinophilia, and specific roentgenographic findings allows it to be distinguished from HP. When chronic changes have developed as the result of recurrent exposure to antigen, HP must be distinguished from other diseases that present as chronic interstitial lung disease. These include sarcoidosis and idiopathic pulmonary fibrosis. Peripheral, hilar, and mediastinal lymphadenopathy do not occur in HP. Differentiation requires demonstration of exposure to an agent known to cause HP or of precipitating antibodies, positive inhalation challenge to the agent, or lung biopsy demonstrating pathognomonic changes.

Evaluation

Clinical presentation of HP varies depending on intensity, duration, and recurrence of exposure. Brief intermittent exposure results in fever, chills, malaise, cough, and dyspnea within 4 to 10 hours, with severity of symptoms dependent on intensity of exposure. Fever can reach 40°C. On examination, patients appear acutely ill and chest auscultation demonstrates end-inspiratory crackles. Occasionally, an immediate, late, or dual bronchoconstriction response can be seen in atopic persons. With more continuous low-grade exposure, a subacute form of HP develops (see Table 87-9). Symptoms include productive cough, dyspnea, easy fatigue, and weight loss. Pulmonary function testing demonstrates restriction with decreased lung compliance. Hypoxemia results from alteration in ventilation-perfusion relationships. With long-term continuous or intermittent exposure, clinical features of pulmonary fibrosis predominate. Progressive restriction in association with obstruction and abnormal gas exchange lead to unrelenting respiratory failure and cor pulmonale even after exposure is discontinued.

A neutrophilic leukocytosis of up to 25,000/mm^3 with left shift is common; however, eosinophilia is rare. Erythrocyte sedimentation rate is elevated. Arterial blood gas analysis demonstrates mild to moderate hypoxemia and hypocapnia. Serum immunoglobulins are elevated and IgG precipitins can be demonstrated against the involved antigen; IgE is not elevated. Rheumatoid factor is often nonspecifically elevated. Skin testing with antigen is useful in some cases. Recently, bronchoalveolar lavage in patients with HP has shown a lymphocytic alveolitis with T cells predominating.

The chest roentgenograph in acute or subacute forms of HP can be normal, show a diffuse nodular or reticulonodular pattern sparing the costophrenic angles and apices, or reveal diffuse patchy infiltrates without associated adenopathy. In chronic HP, findings are those of pulmonary fibrosis, with reduced lung volumes, coarse linear or reticular interstitial infiltrates, and honeycombing.

Use of inhalation challenge with the suspected causative agent in HP may allow precise identification. In addition to following flow parameters after challenge, it is also useful to measure diffusing capacity and white blood cell count over time since these characteristically change in HP, whereas alteration in flow rates may not be demonstrated.

Management

Acute management of HP should include supplemental oxygen when hypoxemia is evident. Limited courses of corticosteroids may help speed resolution in acute and subacute forms, but in the chronic stage significant amounts of fibrosis may prevent a recognizable response. Reducing exposure to the offending agent is the most important measure and necessitates a change in occupation. Only this intervention can help prevent development of disabling pulmonary fibrosis. Less often, methods that improve air quality and remove the antigen from the environment are successful.

Disposition

Affected patients may require brief hospitalization unless symptoms and hypoxemia are mild. Unless the exposure situation is clearly recognized as a potential cause of HP, corticosteroids should be held pending confirmation of the diagnosis by a pulmonologist or allergist working in conjunction with occupational medicine and environmental engineers.

ACUTE INORGANIC DUST EXPOSURE

Inorganic dust exposures that cause respiratory disease usually do so after years have elapsed since onset of exposure. Such is the case with asbestos, silica, and beryllium. Several exceptions relate to acute, massive exposures to silica and beryllium and deserve mention since they constitute distinctive syndromes.

Acute silicosis has been reported in sandblasters and ceramics and silica flour workers. Heavy exposure to fine silica dust for several weeks can result in progressive severe dyspnea, cough, and fever. Chest roentgenograph shows diffuse nodularity and, in some cases, pulmonary edema. Severe hypoxemic respiratory failure that is refractory to therapy results in death.

After severe, intense exposure to beryllium during its commercial production or use in preparing alloys and heat-resistant ceramics, an acute pneumonialike illness can occur. Presenting symptoms include dyspnea, cough, and chest pain. Tachycardia, tachypnea, crackles, and cyanosis are accompanied by inflammation and ulceration of the mucous membranes, tracheitis, bronchitis, and alveolitis. Chest roentgenography shows pulmonary edema or patchy bronchopneumonia. Severe hypoxemia requiring oxygen therapy is present. In contrast to acute silicosis, acute berylliosis improves, although chronic berylliosis remains in some patients. Corticosteroids are advocated as part of acute therapy. Improved industrial hygiene in the United States has reduced the likelihood of these acute syndromes of inorganic dust exposure. Discussion of the chronic manifestations of these and other inorganic exposures is beyond the scope of this chapter.

SELECTED READING

Armstrong, CW, et al. An outbreak of metal fume fever. *J Occup Med* 25:886, 1983.

Bernstein, IL. Occupational asthma. *Clin Chest Med* 2:255, 1981.

Brooks, SM, Weiss, MA, and Bernstein, IL. Reactive airways dysfunction syndrome (RADS). *Chest* 88:376, 1985.

Burnett, WW, et al. Hydrogen sulfide poisoning: Review of five year experience. *Can Med Assoc J* 117:1280, 1977.

Chang-Yeung, M, and Lam, S. Occupational asthma. *Am Rev Respir Dis* 133:686, 1986.

Charan, NB, et al. Pulmonary injuries associated with acute sulfur dioxide inhalation. *Am Rev Respir Dis* 119:555, 1979.

Charan, NB, et al. Effects of accidental chlorine inhalation on pulmonary function. *West J Med* 143:333, 1985.

Churg, A, and Green, FHY. *Pathology of Occupational Lung Disease.* New York: Igaku-Shoin, 1988.

Dawson, SV, and Schenker, MB. Health effects of inhalation of ambient concentrations of nitrogen dioxide. *Am Rev Respir Dis* 120:281, 1979.

DoPico, GA. Occupational Lung Disease. In JBL Gee (ed), *The Rural Environment in Occupational Lung Disease* (vol 2). New York: Churchill Livingstone, 1984. Pp 141–181.

Dyer, RF, and Esch, VH. Polyvinyl chloride toxicity in fires: Hydrogen chloride toxicity in fire fighters. *JAMA* 235:393, 1976.

Epler, GR, and Colby, TV. The spectrum of bronchiolitis obliterans. *Chest* 83:161, 1983.

Flury, KE, Dines, DE, and Rodarte, R. Airway obstruction due to inhalation of ammonia. *Mayo Clin Proc* 58:389, 1983.

Galdston, M, et al. A study of the residual effects of phosgene poisoning in human subjects. I. After acute exposure. *J Clin Invest* 16:145, 1947.

Galea, M. Fatal sulfur dioxide inhalation. *Can Med Assoc J* 91:345, 1964.

Gee, JBL (ed). *Occupational Lung Disease.* Vol 2. In *Contemporary Issues in Pulmonary Disease.* New York: Churchill Livingstone, 1984.

Goldbaum, LR, Orellano, T, and Vergal, N. Mechanism of the toxic action of carbon monoxide. *Ann Clin Lab Sci* 6:372, 1976.

Golden, JA, Nadel, JA, and Boushey, HA. Bronchial hyperirritability in healthy subjects after exposure to ozone. *Am Rev Respir Dis* 118:287, 1978.

Graham, DL, et al. Acute cyanide poisoning complicated by lactic acidosis and pulmonary edema. *Arch Intern Med* 137:1051, 1977.

Haponik, EF, and Summer, WR. Respiratory complications in burned patients: Pathogenesis and spectrum of inhalation injury. *J Crit Care* 2:49, 1987.

Haponik, EF, and Summer, WR. Respiratory complications in burned patients: Diagnosis and management of inhalation injury. *J Crit Care* 2:121, 1987.

Horvath, EP, et al. Effects of formaldehyde on the mucous membrane and lungs: A study of an industrial population. *JAMA* 259:701, 1988.

Hunter, D. *The Disease of Occupations.* London: The English Universities Press, 1969.

Kriebel, D, et al. The pulmonary toxicity of beryllium. *Am Rev Respir Dis* 137:464, 1988.

Litovitz, TL, Martin, TG, and Schmitz, B. 1986 Annual Report of the American Association of Poison Control Centers National Data Collection System. *Toxicology* 5:405, 1987.

Merchant, JA, Boehlecke, BA, and Taylor, G. (eds). *Occupational Respiratory Disease.* US Department of Health and Human Services, 1986.

Montague, TJ, and MacNeil, AR. Mass ammonia inhalation. *Chest* 77:496, 1980.

Morgan, WKC, and Seaton, A. *Occupational Lung Diseases* (2nd ed). Philadelphia: Saunders, 1984.

Parks, WR. *Occupational Lung Disorders.* London: Butterworth, 1982.

Peters, WJ. Inhalation injury caused by the products of combustion. *Can Med Assoc J* 125:249, 1981.

Samet, JM, Marbury, MC, and Spengler, JD. Health effects and sources of indoor air pollution. Part I. *Am Rev Respir Dis* 136: 1486, 1987.

Samet, JM, Marbury, MC, and Spengler, JD. Health effects and sources of indoor air pollution. Part II. *Am Rev Respir Dis* 137: 221, 1987.

Schwartz, DA. Acute inhalational injury. *Occup Med:* State of the Art Reviews. 2:297, 1987.

Stewart, RD, et al. Rapid estimation of carboxyhemoglobin level in fire fighters. *JAMA* 235:390, 1976.

Summer, W, and Haponik, E. Inhalation of irritant gases. *Clin Chest Med* 2:273, 1981.

Terrill, JB, Montgomery, RR, and Reinhardt, CF. Toxic gases from fires. *Science* 200:1343, 1978.

88. Cumulative Trauma Syndrome

Rose H. Goldman

Persons with work-related musculoskeletal injuries frequently come to the emergency department for treatment. When the injury has resulted from acute trauma, the relationship to work is clearly seen. However, as noted earlier (see Chap. 85), when the injury has been caused by the accumulated effects of repetitive or stressful postures, the link to the job may not be so obvious. It is critical that the emergency physician identify the possible association to workplace factors, because treating a patient only symptomatically and then returning him or her to the same working environment can lead to the recurrence or worsening of the problem.

"Cumulative trauma syndrome," "repetitive motion disorders," and "overuse syndrome" refer to disorders associated with the overloading of particular muscle groups from repeated use or with the maintenance of constrained postures. These conditions typically develop over weeks, months, or years as a result of repeated actions. These overuse syndromes can involve tendons (e.g., de Quervain's disease), nerve entrapment (e.g., carpal tunnel syndrome), muscles (e.g., tension neck syndrome), or blood vessels (e.g., vibration white-finger disease or Raynaud's phenomenon of occupational origin). In addition to those disorders with specific physical findings on clinical examinations, workers in some occupations have elevated rates of complaints of pain in the upper extremity or neck that, as in some cases of low back pain, cannot be attributed to a specific anatomic source, yet can still lead to impairment and disability. The role of repetitive motions in the development of degenerative arthritis is still controversial.

Repetitive motions and strained postures occur in many workplace settings. For example, a data entry operator may perform 20,000 keystrokes per hour and a worker in a meat processing plant may produce 12,000 cuts with a knife each day. In performing a Beethoven sonata, a pianist may play thousands of notes within just a few minutes, in a manner that requires precision in the force and timing of joint flexion, extension, and rotation. Furthermore, a musician's hands and arms may undergo hours of constant repetition from intense practice sessions.

Some technological changes may have increased the incidence of work-related repetitive motion injuries. For example, Bammer has noted that using a video display terminal (VDT) may involve more rapid repetitive movements, static loading, and awkward body postures than using a simple typewriter. The computer's soft-touch keyboards allow users to attain much higher keystroke rates. In addition, elimination of nonkeying tasks when typing, such as changing paper, waiting for the carriage return, and using correction tape, also eliminates opportunities for variety in hand mo-

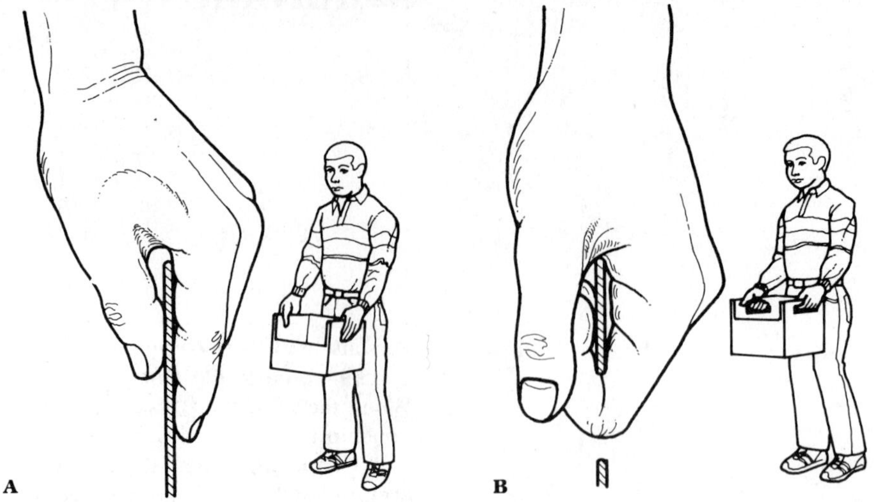

A B

Fig. 88-1. Three to four times as much muscle force is required to hold a container by pinching (A), than by using a power grip (B). (Adapted from T. J. Armstrong. Ergonomics and cumulative trauma disorders. *Hand. Clin.* 2:553, 1986.)

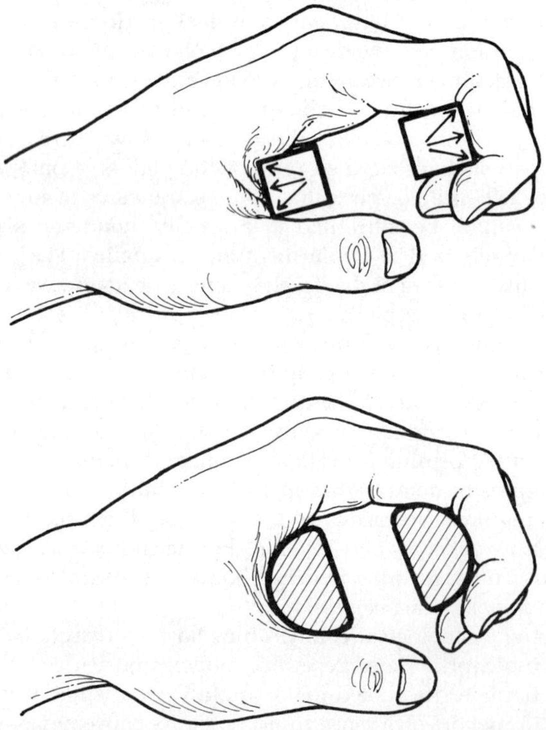

A

B

Fig. 88-2. A. Gripping objects with hard, sharp edges produces stress concentrations on the skin and on the underlying tendons. B. To avoid those stresses, objects that are held in the hand should be made from compliant materials and have well-rounded corners. (Adapted from T. J. Armstrong. Ergonomics and cumulative trauma disorders. *Hand. Clin.* 2:553, 1986.)

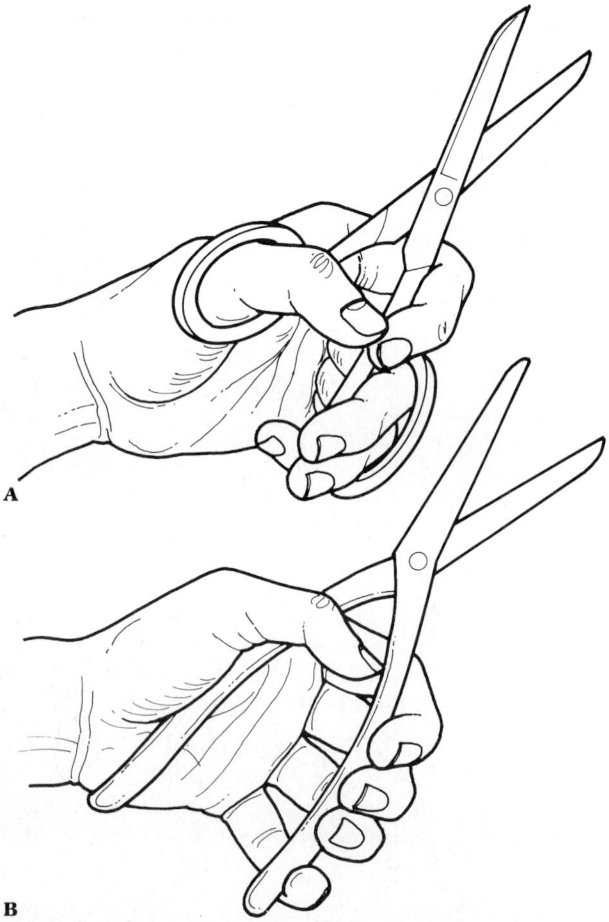

A

B

Fig. 88-3. A. Some types of scissors produce stress concentrations over the digital nerves. B. Scissors should have handles that have been designed to distribute forces only on the palmar surfaces of the fingers. (Adapted from T. J. Armstrong. Ergonomics and cumulative trauma disorders. *Hand. Clin.* 2:553, 1986.)

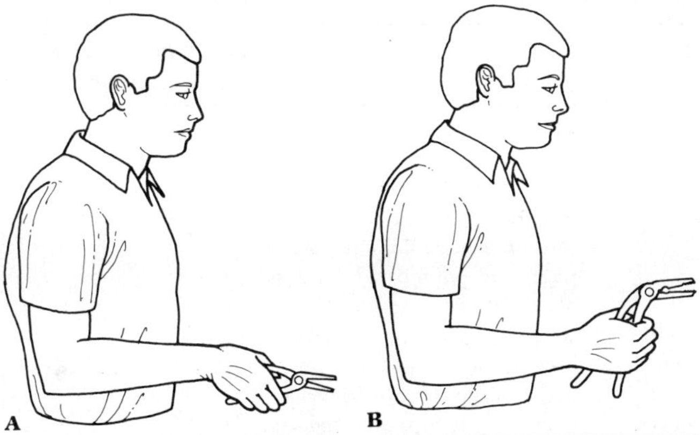

Fig. 88-4. A stress-saving principle is to bend the tool, not the wrist. A. Ulnar wrist deviation is required to hold the needle-nose pliers for bench assembly work. B. The wrist posture is improved by bending the handles of the pliers with respect to the chuck. (Adapted from T. J. Armstrong. Ergonomics and cumulative trauma disorders. *Hand. Clin.* 2:553, 1986.)

Table 88-1. Cumulative trauma disorders: Muscle-tendon unit

Disorder	Precipitating motions
Tenosynovitis Stenosing tenosynovitis of thumb abductors (abductor pollicis longus, extensor pollicis brevis) at that radiostyloid process (de Quervain's disease)	Repeated radial and/or ulnar deviations of the wrist, particularly in combination with forceful exertions of the thumb, e.g., combinations of firm grip with forearm roll as when using a screwdriver, wringing out a cloth, or using straight-nose pliers
Finger flexor tendons	Contraction of finger flexors with a flexed wrist
Finger extensor tendons	Ulnar deviation of the wrist with outward rotation, e.g., in VDT operators
Epicondylitis Lateral ("tennis elbow")	Use of wrist and finger extensors while elbow is extended; supination of the forearm; abrupt extensions of the elbow (e.g., tennis, pitching, tossing objects, lifting, and pushing up motions)
Medial ("golfer's elbow")	Use of wrist and finger flexors, forearm pronation
Rotator cuff tendonitis	Activities performed with the arms raised away from the sides, usually with rotation of the arm from the shoulder
Bicipital tendonitis	Motions like those that precipitate rotator cuff tendonitis; also constant or repetitive forward elevation of the arm at the shoulder
Tension neck syndrome	Prolonged unusual positions of the neck and head (e.g., in musicians, garment workers, VDT operators)

Fig. 88-5. Either tool redesign or work position can be used to reduce stressful body positions. A. Wrist flexion is required to use the pistol-shaped screw gun on a horizontal surface. Wrist posture can be controlled by using an inline handle (B) or by tilting the work surface vertically (C). (Adapted from T. J. Armstrong. Ergonomics and cumulative trauma disorders. *Hand. Clin.* 2:553, 1986.)

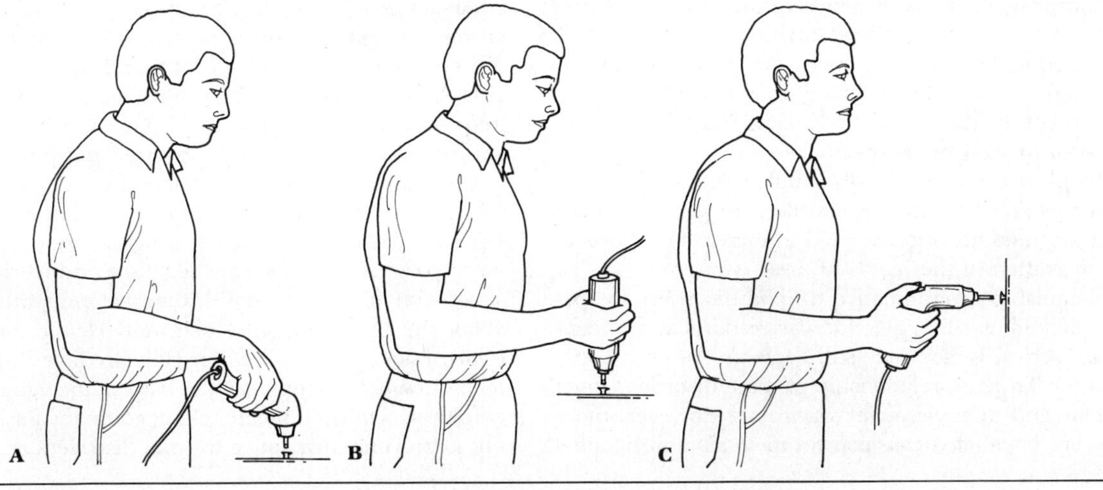

Table 88-2. Aggravating motions and occupations associated with median nerve injuries

Aggravating motions	Job tasks	Examples of high-risk occupations	Key signs	Site of damage: Nerve syndrome
Repeated forceful pronation accompanying forceful finger flexion	Writing Manipulating levers	Writer Assembly-line worker performing task on horizontal bench Cutter	Pain in the proximal forearm associated with pronation against resistance with tightly clenched fist; pain, disturbed sensation in radial side of palm and palmar side of first 3½ digits	Forearm: Pronator syndrome
Flexion-extension of wrist; additional stress when accompanied by pinching and gripping	Pulling cloth Milking cows Handling objects on conveyor belt with wrist flexed Pushing down ratchet, using screwdriver Hand weeding Using spray gun Knitting Scrubbing Playing stringed instrument with bow	Garment worker/stitcher Farmer Assembly-line worker Mechanic Gardener Painter Housewife Janitor Musician	Pain, paresthesias and numbness in thumb and first 2½ digits of hand; pain in wrist, hand, worse at night; weakness, atrophy of abductor pollicis brevis; weakness in precision grip Tinel's and Phalen's signs	Wrist: Carpal tunnel syndrome
Pinch-hand position	Grasping and tugging of fabric Assembling small parts Turning key Pinching motions	Production sewing or tailoring Electronics industry Locksmith		
Pressure against carpal tunnel	External pressure from poorly fitting gloves, wrist bands	Agricultural worker Mechanic Factory worker		
Pressure or pounding into pain	Pressing tool into palm; pounding safety lever or stamping machine	Painter (scraping) Carpenter (hand planing) Stable hand (using horsebrush) Time keeper Receipt processor	Weakness in precision grip; atrophy of opponens muscle Tenderness over nerve at distal edge of transverse ligament	Hand: Median nerve injury (oppenens branch)

Source: R. Feldman, R. H. Goldman, and W. M. Keyserling. Peripheral nerve entrapment syndromes and ergonomic factors. *Am. J. Ind. Med.* 4:661–681, 1983.

tions. These changes not only increase the number of the same repetitive movements but also increase static loading through the prolonged maintenance of the keying posture. Furthermore, using the additional function keys on the VDT keyboard frequently requires awkward posturing of the wrist and little fingers. These factors may contribute to the development of tendonitis of finger and wrist extensors, which is seen in VDT operators.

Technological advances in other industries, such as the use of laser scanners by grocery checkers, require awkward and repetitive motions and have led to increased reports of cumulative trauma in the hands of these workers.

The relationship of cumulative trauma disorders to specific work factors was first noted in case reports and uncontrolled case series, which may still serve as the only documentation for the work relationship of some disorders, such as ganglions and thoracic outlet syndrome. However, more recent studies have used case control methods and detailed job analyses to more definitively link repetitive motion disorders with specific job tasks in order to develop preventive strategies. For example, Armstrong and Chaffin compared garment workers with carpal tunnel syndrome to those who did not have this problem and found that the affected individuals used work methods that had a significantly higher frequency of forceful exertions, particularly flexion and extension with deviated wrist postures and pinching actions.

Cumulative trauma disorders are currently receiving wider recognition and attention than they did in the past. Upper-extremity cumulative trauma disorders have been found to be a major cause of lost time and workers' compensation claims in many hand-intensive industries. In October 1988, the Occupational Safety and Health Administration (OSHA) levied $4.33 million (later reduced to $990,000 in the settlement agreement), the largest fine against any single employer, against a meatpacking company for allegedly failing to prevent cumulative trauma disorders among employ-

Table 88-3. Aggravating motions and occupations associated with ulnar nerve injuries

Aggravating motions	Job tasks	Examples of high-risk occupations	Key signs	Site of damage: Nerve syndrome
Repetitive and sudden elbow flexion	Shoveling, hammering Lifting Manipulating handles of boring and punching machines	Carpenter Mail sorter Mechanic Construction worker Materials handler Assembly-line worker	Pain paresthesias, numbness in fourth and fifth fingers, lateral side of hand Inability to separate fingers or pick up small objects between thumb and index finger, loss of "power" grip, weak wrist flexor, "claw hand," atrophy of hypothenar and interosseous muscles	Elbow: Cubital tunnel syndrome
Repeated trauma or pressure to elbow at ulnar groove	Leaning on elbow at desk or workbench Working in tight places	Office clerk Telephonist Glass cutter Stone cutter Plumber Mechanic, bench assembly worker Truck or taxi driver		
Repeated blows or pressure to ulnar side of forearm	Kneading dough Pressing edge of desk or workbench	Baker Clerk, bench assembly or assembly-line worker Data entry clerk	Same as above	Forearm: Ulnar nerve injury
Pounding of object or pressure at base of hypothenar eminence	Using these tools: Pliers Plane Stapler Pneumatic drill Needle-nose pliers Garden shears Gripping handlebars Using hand as a hammer	Mechanic Carpenter City street repair person Gardener Cyclist	Disturbed sensation in ulnar-innervated fingers; tenderness over compression site; weakness, atrophy of ulnar-innervated muscles	Palm: Ulnar nerve injury (palmar branches)
Weakness of third and fourth lumbricales, all interossei		Electronics assembly worker Jeweler Machinist Repair worker	As above, but no sensory findings	Ulnar nerve injury (deep motor branch)

Source: R. Feldman, R. H. Goldman, and W. M. Keyserling. Peripheral nerve entrapment syndromes and ergonomic factors. *Am. J. Ind. Med.* 4:661, 1983.

ees. In December 1990, San Francisco passed a new ordinance that required businesses with at least 16 employees who work on VDTs for more than four hours per day to install flexible work stations and ergonomic equipment to reduce the potential for eye and wrist strain. This law is expected to affect 56,000 public and private businesses.

PATHOPHYSIOLOGIC ASPECTS

The factors of repetitiveness, forcefulness, mechanical stress, posture, vibration, low temperature, and unaccustomed work activities are consistently implicated in cumulative trauma disorders of the hand and wrist (Armstrong, 1986). A great number of repetitive motions create tissue changes that exceed normal mechanisms for recovery, thus leading to inflammation. In the case of sheathed tendons, overuse can exhaust the lubrication system, thus allowing friction to develop between the tendon and tendon sheath, leading to inflammation of the sheath, termed *tenosynovitis*. Chronic inflammation can then lead to hypertrophy of cells and thickening of the tendon sheath. Thickening of tendon sheaths can create undue constriction in snug compartments, such as the carpal tunnel, and cause compression of other structures, such as the median nerve. Chronic tenosynovitis can also lead to the development of fibrous tissue within the sheath, and a gradual constricture of the sheath, as seen in a trigger finger or de Quervain's disease. In nonsheathed tendons, such as those of the shoulder, repetitive motions or awkward postures can cause microscopic tears

Table 88-4. Aggravating motions and occupations associated with radial nerve injury

Aggravating motions	Job tasks	Examples of high-risk occupations	Key signs	Site of damage: Nerve syndrome
Pressure on upper arm (humeral area) Working in tight areas with arm against fixed structures	Carrying boxes on back Tourniquet around upper arm—"rifle sling palsy"	Porter Military recruit	Weakness in extension of wrist Weakness of triceps, biceps; sensation loss in dorsal area of hand	Upper arm: Wrist-drop syndrome
Repeated (or single) forceful supination-pronation of the arm; abrupt extension of the elbow	Hammering with a straight elbow; lifting with arms extended Throwing a screwball	Carpenter Builder Baseball pitcher	Inability to extend fourth or fifth finger; weak hand grip; tenderness along radial nerve in front of radial head; radial deviation on wrist dorsiflexion; no sensory signs	Elbow and forearm: Supinator syndrome Posterior interosseous nerve syndrome
Pressure on forearm Hyperextension of wrist, fingers	Carrying stones on forearm Organ playing	Brick layer Keyboard musician	Pain, alteration in sensation No weakness	Superficial radial nerve injury

Source: R. Feldman, R. H. Goldman, and W. M. Keyserling. Peripheral nerve entrapment syndromes and ergonomic factors. *Am. J. Ind. Med.* 4:661, 1983.

Table 88-5. Aggravating motions and occupations associated with brachial plexus syndromes

Aggravating motions	Job tasks	Examples of high risk occupations	Key signs	Site of damage: Nerve syndrome
Repetitive abduction and adduction movements of shoulder and arm Poor posture	Carrying heavy loads on shoulder Working overhead	Painter Welder Hiker Auto repair person	Bruit in infraclavicular area or damping of radial pulse with various maneuvers Hypertrophy of subclavius, pectoral muscles Intermittent vascular changes in hand, arm Numbness in 4th, 5th fingers	Shoulder: Thoracic outlet syndrome
Chronic pressure on shoulder	Carrying bag on shoulder	Letter carrier	Pain at lateral and posterior aspects of shoulder elicited by adducting extended arm passively across midline or by deep pressure in the region Restricted shoulder motion	Upper arm: Suprascapular nerve injury

Source: R. Feldman, R. H. Goldman, and W. M. Keyserling. Peripheral nerve entrapment syndromes and ergonomic factors. *Am. J. Ind. Med.* 4:661, 1983.

Table 88-6. Aggravating motions and occupations associated with peroneal, posterior tibial, and interdigital nerve injuries

Aggravating motions	Job tasks	Examples of high-risk occupations	Key signs	Site of damage: Nerve syndrome
Crouching Squatting Kneeling Repetitive flexion, extension of foot Crossing leg	Milking cows Fitting shoes Mining Repairing Operating a foot pedal Prolonged sitting	Farmer Shoe salesperson Miner Plumber Tailor Cyclist Executive, clerk	"Foot drop" Weakness in eversion of the foot and dorsiflexion of ankle; sensory loss along the distal, lateral aspect of the leg and dorsum of foot	Lower leg: Peroneal nerve injury
Prolonged walking or standing in shoes with little support	Working in store	Salesperson Barber Cash register operator	Tarsal tunnel syndrome Burning pain, tingling or numbness in toes, distal sole of foot; weakness in toe flexion; atrophy of abductor hallucis muscle	Posterior tibial nerve injury
Hyperextension of toes at the metatarsophalangeal joints	Kneeling	Electrician Plumber	Metatarsal pain with lancinating pain into third, fourth toes Point tenderness in region between metatarsal heads	Foot: Interdigital nerve injury

Source: R. Feldman, R. H. Goldman, and W. M. Keyserling. Peripheral nerve entrapment syndromes and ergonomic factors. *Am. J. Ind. Med.* 4:661, 1983.

to occur and individual tendon fibers to ravel and fray. As a result, the tendon becomes thickened and irregular and, as in the case of rotator cuff tendons, calcification can occur.

Dennett and Fry studied biopsy specimens of affected persons with overuse syndromes and demonstrated an increase in type I and a decrease in type II muscle fibers, hypertrophy of type II fibers, an increase in the internal nuclei count, and mitochondrial abnormalities. Type I fibers are smaller, with a high capacity for aerobic metabolism, and thus are good at sustaining low levels of exertion. They are termed "slow fibers" because they twitch with low peak tension and have a long rise time to peak tension. Type II (or fast fibers) rely more on anaerobic metabolism and have large peak tensions with a short rise time to peak tension.

Excessive force on structures of a limb also contributes to cumulative trauma. Force is exerted as fingers try to hold an object, such as a tool, and can relate to the weight, tightness of fit, or power setting of a tool. The force can be lessened by reducing the speed or torque setting of a tool. The amount of force exerted by the muscles on the tendons and fingers is also related to the posture of the hand. For example, less muscle force is required when objects are held in a power-grip posture; in contrast, four to five times as much muscle force is exerted to pinch objects with the fingertips (Fig. 88-1). In an effort to reduce forces on the soft tissues, handles of some tools have been designed to be held in a power grip rather than a pinch posture. Wearing gloves provides some protection from the cold but also decreases grip strength and requires more forceful exertion than an ungloved hand.

Mechanical stress is produced by hand-held tools with sharp edges or short handles (Figs. 88-2 and 88-3). The tool exerts as much force on the hand as the hand does on the tool. The use of such tools can contribute to the development of trigger finger or to digital neuritis. Pounding with the hand also produces mechanical stresses.

Work performed in awkward or static postures is another factor that contributes to cumulative trauma disorders (Figs. 88-4, 88-5). The level of mechanical stress produced by a muscle contraction varies with the posture of a joint. For example, contraction of the finger flexors exerts more stress if the wrist is flexed. Typing at a keyboard that is too high, with the forearm raised above the elbow, places extra stress on the tendons of the hand. Working with the arm elevated more than 60 degrees from the trunk is more stressful for the rotator cuff tendons than work performed with the arm at the trunk.

Segmental vibration can be transmitted to the hands and arms by using power tools, grinders, air guns, or jackhammers. Such localized vibration contributes to the development of Raynaud's phenomenon, although the mechanism is not clear.

RECOGNIZING WORK-RELATED CUMULATIVE TRAUMA DISORDERS

What questions can the emergency physician ask to provide clues of work-related cumulative trauma syndrome? First, one can inquire about work and home activities that involve the affected body part. It is usually helpful to ask the patient to perform (mime) the actual motions of the job. Take note of awkward positions or repetitions and whether those exertions and symptoms are consistent with the pattern seen with different types of tendonitis or entrapment neuropathies. (Refer to Tables 88-1 through 88-6 for assistance.) Ask about any recent changes on the job that might reveal precipitating factors, such as the use of a new tool or increased productivity demands (i.e., more overtime work and less breaks), or a change to a new assembly line. Some reminders concerning history and physical examination that are helpful toward making a diagnosis are found in Table 88-7.

By identifying potential precipitating factors (such as poor

Table 88-7. Symptoms and physical signs of work-related disorders of the upper limb and neck

Disorder	History	Physical examination
Wrist		
Carpal tunnel syndrome	Pain, tingling, or numbness in medial sensory distribution of the hand; nocturnal exacerbation; problems with dropping things	Positive Phalen's test; positive Tinel's test; thenar atrophy in severe cases; rule out pronator teres syndrome, cervical root syndrome
de Quervain's disease	Pain in anatomic snuffbox that may radiate up forearm; no history of radial fracture or wrist fracture	Rule out radial nerve entrapment; positive Finkelstein's test with sharp pain rather than just pulling sensation
Trigger finger	Finger locks in extension or flexion, requires assistance in unlocking; nodule on tendon	Nodule at base of digit palpable; locking in flexion or extension of digits
Ulnar nerve compression (Guyon canal syndrome)	Burning, tingling, or numbness in 4th and 5th digits; clumsiness in fine movements	Rule out cervical root disorder, rule out thoracic outlet syndrome; rule out cubital tunnel syndrome; decreased pinch strength; weakness on resisted abduction and adduction of digits; positive Tinel's sign at Guyon canal; positive Phalen's test in ulnar distribution
Tendinitis, tenosynovitis	Localized pain and swelling over muscle-tendon structure	Pain exacerbated by resisted motions; possibly fine crepitus on passive range-of-motion (ROM); no pain on passive ROM; pronounced asymmetric grip strength
Elbow/forearm		
Lateral epicondylitis (tennis elbow)	Pain at lateral epicondyle during rest or active motion of wrists and fingers	Pain on resisted extension of wrist with fingers flexed; no pain or limitation on full passive ROM; pain at epicondyle on palpation; pain on resisted radial deviation; rule out radial nerve entrapment
Medical epicondylitis (golfer's elbow)	Pain at medial epicondyle during rest or active motion of wrist and fingers	No pain on passive ROM; pain on resisted wrist flexion and resisted forearm pronation; pain at medial epicondyle on palpation
Olecranon bursitis	Pain and swelling at olecranon	No pain on passive or resisted ROM; swelling around olecranon on palpation (rule out rheumatoid arthritis)
Pronator teres syndrome	Burning pain in first 3 digits of hand and forearm	Increased pain in forearm by resisted pronation with clenched fist and flexed wrist (Mills's test); sensory impairment of thenar eminence; rule out carpal tunnel syndrome
Shoulder		
Rotator cuff tendonitis (mainly supraspinatus)	Dull ache generally localized to the deltoid area without neck or arm radiation; no symptoms of distal paresthesia; nocturnal exacerbation; the subject may note a "catch" on movement	Diffuse tenderness over the shoulder, especially over the humeral head and lateral to the acromion; if tenderness is localized, it is most often over the supraspinatus insertion; weakness is uncommon *Supraspinatus:* Shrugs shoulder on abduction, painful arc at 70–90 degrees; passive ROM normal; pain on resisted abduction *Infraspinatus:* Pain on resisted external rotation; painful arc *Subscapularis:* Pain on resisted internal rotation; painful arc; rule out rheumatoid arthritis (other joints affected bilaterally, diffusely full or swollen; decreased ROM in all directions, especially rotation and abduction)
Bicipital tenosynovitis	Pain localized to the bicipital groove area that may radiate to anterior aspect of the arm; no distal paresthesia; nocturnal exacerbation; the subject is able to use the forearm when the upper arm is held against the chest; the subject notes pain on abduction and rotation	Normal passive and active ROM; positive Yergason's test (resisted supination) or positive Speed's test (resisted wrist flexion)
Degenerative joint disease—acromioclavicular joint	Generalized aching shoulder pain exacerbated by motion; least difficulty in the morning but worse as the day progresses	Limitation is similar on active and passive ROM; most discomfort is with mild abduction; crepitus is common, tenderness on palpation directly over acromioclavicular articulation; pain is reproduced as arm is abducted more than 90 degrees; pain on shoulder shrug

Table 88-7. (Continued)

Disorder	History	Physical examination
Degenerative joint disease—glenohumeral joint	Pain is very diffuse and nocturnal	Tenderness to palpation along joint line; no deltoid or supraspinatus pain; passive ROM is full but painful; active ROM is retarded on flexion and extension (normal is 240 degrees in youth, 190 degrees at age 70; normal abduction in youth is 166 degrees, 116 degrees at age 70)
Thoracic outlet syndrome	Paresthesia usually in the ulnar distribution of hand and arm; pain and sensation of "weakness"; deep dull ache in arm and hand; problem holding small objects; nocturnal exacerbation common	Positive Adson's test; hyperabduction or costoclavicular test; decreased grip strength
Neck/scapula		
Tension neck syndrome (costoscapular syndrome)	Neck pain or stiffness, no history of herniated cervical disk, injury, or ankylosing spondylitis	Muscle tightness, palpable hardening and tender spots; pain on resisted neck lateral flexion and rotation
Cervical root syndrome	Pain radiating from the neck to one or both arms with numbness in the hand(s); exacerbated by cough	Limited passive and active ROM; radiating pain on passive motions; positive foraminal test; decreased pinprick in dermatome; absence of joint findings

Source: L. J. Fine and B. A. Silverstein. Work-Related Disorders of the Neck and Upper Extremity. In B. S. Levy and D. H. Wegman (eds.), *Occupational Health* (2nd ed.). Boston: Little, Brown, 1988. Pp. 358–370.

Table 88-8. Strategies for preventing cumulative trauma injuries

The physical strength required to perform a job should not exceed the strength capabilities of a potential employee.
Avoid postures or motions that place joints near the limits of their range of motion. Ideally, workstations and tools should be designed so that joints can be held in a neutral or near-neutral position. This is particularly important when high forces are exerted or when the frequency of a motion is high.
Pad areas where employees are likely to rest the elbows.
Select work gloves of proper size and thickness to avoid impaired gripping of tools or undue pressure over the carpal tunnel.
Avoid repeated gripping or "clothes wringing" motions.
Design the work space to provide proper surface height and distance from the workbench, or tilt the work piece so that awkward movements can be avoided.
Reduce task frequency (e.g., by rotating workers). This is particularly important when an employee is learning a new repetitive task.
Schedule regular rest breaks. This is particularly important when employees are compensated on a piece-rate or other incentive basis.
Design the job and tool handle so that tasks can be performed with straight wrists; avoid flexion, extension, or ulnar deviation.
Use tools of proper weight and balance; center of gravity of a tool should be aligned with the center of the grasping hand to reduce tendency of the tool to rotate and slip.
Use tools that take advantage of the strongest postures; pliers should be used instead of forceps for tasks in which high clasping force is required.
To avoid compression and trauma to small areas, the contact surface between tool and hand should be large. Avoid tools that press into the palm of the hand or against interphalangeal joints.

Source: Adapted from R. Feldman, R. H. Goldman, and W. M. Keyserling, Peripheral nerve entrapment syndromes and ergonomic factors. *Am. J. Ind. Med.* 4:661, 1983.

tool or work-station design or increased hours), the emergency physician can stimulate the company to consider prevention strategies, such as those listed in Table 88-8.

SELECTED READING

Armstrong, TJ. Ergonomics and cumulative trauma disorders. *Hand Clin* 2:553, 1986.

Armstrong, TJ, and Chaffin, DB. Carpal tunnel syndrome and selected personal attributes. *J Occup Med* 21:481, 1979.

Bammer, G. How technologic change can increase the risk of repetitive motions injuries. *Semin Occup Med* 2:25, 1987.

Dennett, X, and Fry, HJH. Overuse syndrome: A muscle biopsy study. *Lancet* 1:905, 1988.

Feldman, R, Goldman, RH, and Keyserling, WM. Peripheral nerve entrapment syndromes and ergonomic factors. *Am J Ind Med* 4:661, 1983.

Fine, LJ, and Silverstein, BA. Work-Related Disorders of the Neck and Upper Extremity. In BS Levy and DH Wegman (eds), *Occupational Health* (2nd ed). Boston: Little, Brown, 1988. Pp 358–370.

Lockwood, AH. Medical problems of musicians. *N Engl J Med* 320:221, 1989.

MacLeod, D. *Strains and Sprains.* Detroit: International Union, United Automobile, 1982.

Rowe, ML. The diagnosis of tendon and tendon sheath injuries. *Semin Occup Med* 2:1, 1987.

III. Acute Nontraumatic Disorders

A. Body Defense, Immunity, and Disorders of the Immune System

89. The Mechanisms of Immunity

GLOSSARY OF TERMS USED IN THIS CHAPTER

CD	Cluster designation. Internationally agreed on designation for cell surface proteins involved in the interaction of immune cells.
α protein chains	Designation given to one of the protein chains making up the T cell receptor.
β protein chains	Designation given to the second protein chain composing the T cell receptor. Forms a heterodimer with the α chain.
Monomer	Compound composed of a single protein unit.
Dimer	Compound formed by the combination of molecules.
Heterodimer	Compound formed by the combination of two different molecules.
Pentamer	Compound composed of five protein units.
Class I MHC molecule	A cell surface glycoprotein encoded by genes of the major histocompatibility complex. Expressed by all nucleated cells and platelets. Co-expressed with β-2 microglobulin. A recognition target for CD8-bearing T cells.
Class II MHC molecule	A cell surface glycoprotein encoded by genes of the major histocompatibility complex. Expressed by immune cells. A heterodimer composed of α and β chains. A recognition target for CD4-bearing T cells.
Ligands	Secreted mediators that activate cells through their capacity to interact with specific cell surface receptors.
Accessory (antigen-presenting) cells	Cells that internalize, denature, and present antigen to T lymphocytes. Essential co-factors for T cell activation.
Dendritic cells	Dedicated antigen-presenting cells located in the skin, lymph nodes, and spleen.
Autocrine	A secreted mediator that binds to and modulates the function of the same cell that secretes it.
Cytokine	Newly synthesized protein of the immune system involved in regulating immune interactions.
Lymphokine	Cytokine produced by lymphocytes.
Monokine	Cytokine produced by mononuclear phagocytes.

GENERAL HOST DEFENSE MECHANISMS

Lanny J. Rosenwasser
Larry Borish

The health of the individual is critically dependent on the appropriate regulation of the immune defenses. The immune system must be capable of launching an immune response to the enormous number of pathogens capable of assaulting the individual, both from the external and internal environment. The approximately 10^{12} proteins, carbohydrates, and lipids against which the immune system is capable of generating an immune response are termed *antigens*. Failure of the immune system is ultimately responsible for the infectious diseases and has an important role in the development of cancer. In addition to having to respond to the vast array of pathogens capable of causing disease, another requirement of the immune system is that it recognize and not respond to self. Breakdown of this self-tolerance is responsible for another class of human illnesses, the autoimmune diseases.

Immune responses are mediated by numerous carefully regulated cells and tissues of the immune system. These responses can be divided into two broad areas of reactivity. The *specific* immune system is responsible for the generation of antigen-specific factors of immune defense. This involves the continuous surveillance of the organism to distinguish self from foreign antigens. When a foreign antigen is identified, these components of the immune system are then responsible for the generation of an immune response specific for the offending antigen. The second area of reactivity of the immune system is *nonspecific*. These components are recruited by the specific factors, targeted toward the offending antigen, and mediate its ultimate elimination.

The major cell types of the immune system are lymphocytes, monocytes-macrophages, and granulocytes. Lymphocytes, cells with central nuclei, no granules, and abundant ribosomes, are divided into T lymphocytes, B cells, and non-T non-B cells. T lymphocytes are the "brain" of the immune system. Through their expression of receptors capable of binding virtually any antigen that can assault the individual, the T cell initiates the immune response. Equally important, the T lymphocyte determines what form the immune response to the antigen will take. This recruitment of the various potential effector arms of the immune system is subserved by a subclass of T lymphocytes, termed *T helper* cells. T helper cells recruit and activate monocytes-macrophages, which mediate target destruction in a form of immunity termed *cell-mediated immunity*. Monocytes and macrophages represent different degrees of maturity of the same cell. In addition to being the effector cell of cell-mediated immunity, monocytes-macrophages are also accessory cells, which are required for the optimal activation of T helper cells. T helper cells can alternatively recruit a second subclass of T lymphocytes, cytotoxic T cells, which are directly capable of lysing targets. B lymphocytes are the precursors of antibody-producing cells and their activation by T helper cells triggers the humoral immune response. Antibodies attach to targeted pathogens, rendering them susceptible to phagocytosis and destruction by monocytes-macrophages and granulocytes.

Neutrophils are the most important class of granulocytes and are the body's dedicated professional phagocytes. When targeted by antibody toward a pathogen, the pathogen is rapidly phagocytosed and destroyed by the neutrophil's vast array of toxic armaments. One type of humoral response potentially triggered by helper T cells involves the production of immunoglobulin E antibody. Immunoglobulin E production, with the subsequent activation of mast cells, eosinophils, and basophils, is the basis of allergy. Finally, T helper cells may be rendered nonresponsive to a given antigen, the basis of immune tolerance. Of the lymphocytes that are neither T nor B cells, the most important subclass is the natural killer cell. These NK cells do not require either previous sensitization or antibody to destroy targets but mediate the destruction of cancer cells or virus-infected cells through as yet unrecognized mechanisms.

In addition to circulating through the bloodstream and existing as isolated cells throughout the tissues of the body, immune cells are also organized into several immune organs. The thymus is responsible for the maturation of T (for "thymus-derived") lymphocytes. The precursors of T lymphocytes enter the thymus, where they mature into cells capable of recognizing and responding to foreign antigens. Simultaneously, T lymphocytes that may respond to self antigens are destroyed within the thymus. The maturation of B lymphocytes occurs with the bone marrow. The spleen is rich in B and T lymphocytes and is important both as a major site of antibody production and for the removal of pathogens from the circulation. Finally, both lymphocytes and monocytes-macrophages are carefully organized within the lymph nodes, where much of the processing of antigen and activation of the immune response within the body takes place. A more detailed description of each of these aspects of the immune system follows and a summary of the cells of the immune system is provided in Table 89-1.

Table 89-1. Cells of the immune system

Agent	Function
T lymphocytes	Activation via specific T-cell receptors Production of cytokines
Helper T lymphocytes	Activation of cell-mediated immunity, humoral immunity, allergy, or tolerance
Cytotoxic T lymphocytes	Destruction of target cells
B lymphocytes	Precursors of antibody-secreting cells
Monocytes-macrophages	Accessory cells for helper T-cell activation Destruction of target cells and pathogens Production of cytokines
Neutrophils	Phagocytosis and destruction of antibody-coated targets
Mast cells, basophils, eosinophils	Allergic immune responses

SELECTED READING

Nossal, G J. Immunology: The basic components of the immune system. *N Engl J Med* 316:1320, 1987.

LYMPHOCYTES AND MACROPHAGES IN CELL-MEDIATED IMMUNITY

Lanny J. Rosenwasser

The overall function of cell-mediated immunity is to provide the host with a defense against facultative intracellular mi-

Table 89-2. Tissue distribution and function of antigen-presenting cells

Cell	MHC class II expression	IL-1 production[d]
Mononuclear phagocytic		
Mononuclear phagocytes	+ + +[a,c]	+ + +[d]
Lining macrophages of the lymph node, spleen, and bone-marrow sinusoids	+ + +[a]	+ + +[d]
Alveolar macrophages (lung)	+ + +[a]	+ + +[d]
Kupffer cells (liver)	+ + +[a]	+ + +[d]
Freely migrating macrophages of the pleural and peritoneal cavities	+ + +[a]	+ + +[d]
Osteoclasts (bone)	+ + +[a]	+ + +[d]
Microglial cells (nervous tissue)	+ + +[a]	+ + +[d]
Type A synovial cells (joints)	+ + +[a]	
Macrophagelike		
Langerhans cells (epidermis)	+ + +[b]	+ +
Dendritic cells	+ + +[b]	—
Cells capable of antigen presentation		
B cells	+ + +[b,c]	+ +[d]
Thyroid epithelial cells	+ + +[a]	+
Islet cells (pancreas)	+ + +[a]	+
Endothelial cells	+ + +[a]	+ +[d]
Smooth-muscle cells	+ + +[a]	+ +
Type B synovial cells	+ + +[a]	+ +
Fibroblasts	+ + +[a]	+ + +
Epidermal keratinocytes	+ + +[a]	+ + +
Astrocytes	+ + +[a]	+ + +

[a]MHC class II antigen inducible by gamma IFN; variable level of constitutive expression.
[b]Constitutive MHC class II expression primarily.
[c]MHC class II inducible by IL-4.
[d]Inducible by appropriate cell activators (i.e., lipopolysaccharide).
Note: Membrane form of IL-1 reported.
Key: MHC = major histocompatibility complex; IL-1 = interleukin-1; IFN = interferon; + = present but not an important characteristic; + + = characteristic feature; + + + = important characteristic that is a critical component of functioning cell.

croorganisms. These organisms, which include mycobacteria, viruses, fungi, and parasites, are characterized by their capacity to not only survive but proliferate in the intracellular environment. This defense is primarily accomplished by the interaction of T lymphocytes with monocytes-macrophages.

ANTIGEN-PRESENTING CELLS

While critically important in determining the induction and form of an immune response, T helper lymphocytes are not capable of being directly activated by antigen. The immune response is only initiated when antigen is first processed and presented to the T helper cell by an antigen-presenting (or accessory) cell (APC). The most important APCs are cells of the mononuclear phagocytic series (monocytes-macrophages). Other cells that can function as APC include epithelial cells, blood vessel–derived endothelium, smooth-muscle cells, and B lymphocytes (Table 89-2). In addition, a specialized lymphoid cell, known as a *dendritic cell,* is prevalent in lymph nodes and the spleen and functions as a particularly efficient APC.

Antigen-presenting cells function by internalizing the antigen where it is denatured and proteolytically cleaved. The antigen receptor on T lymphocytes thus recognizes small (10–15 amino acid), linearized fragments of the original antigen. A second unusual feature of T helper cells is that they only "recognize" antigen when it is first noncovalently linked to class II major histocompatibility (antigen) complex (MHC) molecules. These molecules are evolutionarily related to both antibodies and T-cell antigen receptors and share with these molecules both a high degree of diversity and their capacity to bind antigens with high affinity. Thus, the combination of class II MHC molecules with noncovalently bound processed antigen induces T helper cell activation. This process is described in greater detail below.

Recognition of the role of MHC molecules as antigen-binding structures makes it easy to comprehend their role in both histocompatibility and as immune response–disease susceptibility genes. The T-lymphocyte antigen receptor readily binds MHC molecules and, in the presence of any associated foreign antigen, becomes activated. As two unrelated individuals are unlikely to share the same MHC molecules, transplantation results in the introduction of MHC mismatched molecules. These foreign MHC molecules will readily bind to the recipient's T-cell receptors but will be recognized as being foreign. An immune response will therefore develop without any need for antigen processing and, in the absence of immune suppression, rejection will soon result. MHC class II molecules also function as immune response genes insofar as the capacity to respond to an antigen is critically dependent on the binding affinity of the antigen for the individual's class II molecule. A strong immune

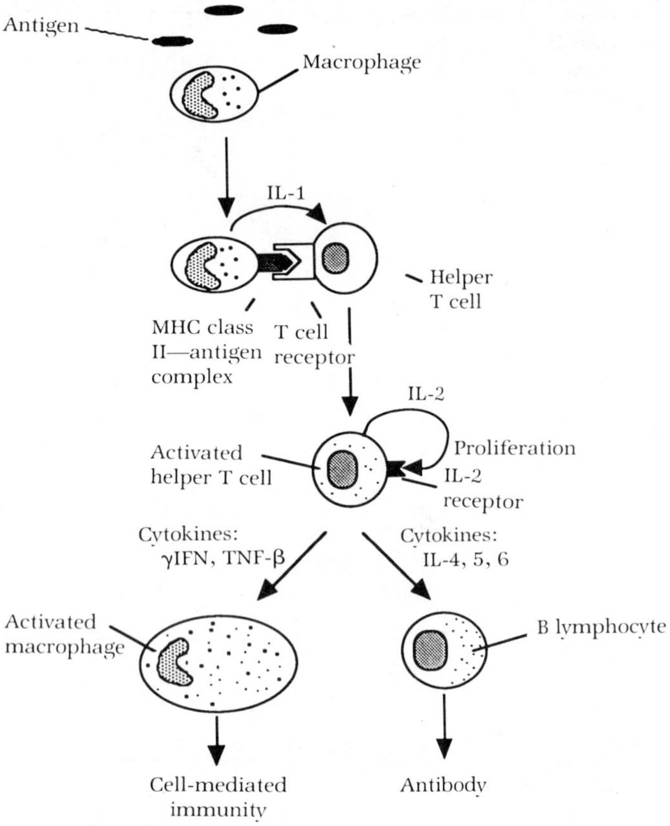

Fig. 89-1. Overview of cell-mediated immunity (see text for discussion). The products of activated helper T cells (cytokines) stimulate both B cells and macrophages, leading to antibody production and delayed hypersensitivity, respectively.

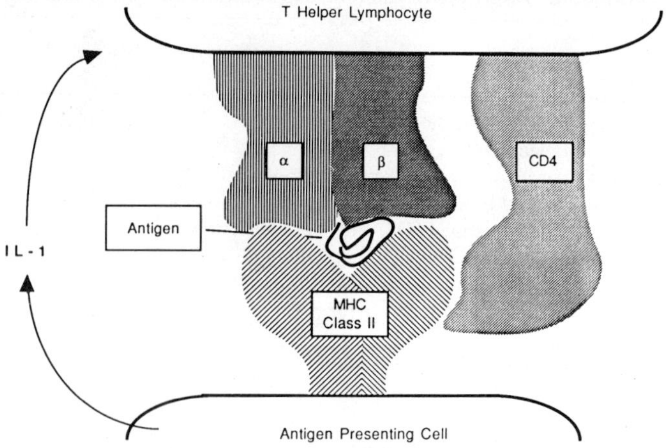

Fig. 89-2. Antigen presentation to T helper lymphocytes. Antigen is internalized by an antigen-presenting cell, where it is denatured, proteolytically cleaved, bound to a major histocompatibility complex (MHC) class II molecule, and expressed on the cell surface. It is this combination of MHC class II and antigen that is recognized by the T helper cell receptor. CD4 expressed by T helper cells also binds the MHC class II molecule and strengthens the binding affinity and stimulation provided by this interaction. Optimal activation of T helper cells requires the additional presence of a secreted mediator, generally interleukin-1.

response will develop in subjects whose MHC repertoire provides them with a high binding affinity, whereas little or no response will occur in the absence of antigen binding to class II MHC molecules. The failure to respond to an antigen secondary to the individual's lacking an MHC molecule capable of adequately binding to the antigen is the basis for the disease associations of MHC molecules.

A second function of antigen-presenting cells is the production of soluble immunoregulatory mediators. Only in the additional presence of these mediators will T lymphocytes be optimally activated and proliferate. Of these mediators, interleukin-1 is the most important; however, other mediators made by accessory cells, including interleukin-6, tumor necrosis factor α, and macrophage inflammatory protein(s), may also provide activation signals for T lymphocytes. These mediators are the subject of the next section of this chapter. The concept that activation of T lymphocytes requires the interaction with antigen presenting cells and soluble mediators is illustrated in Fig. 89-1.

T LYMPHOCYTES

T lymphocytes provide the most important regulatory component of the immune response and are involved in a wide variety of functions, including interactions with B cells to regulate the production and class of antibodies, the mediation of immune responses against transplants, the immune surveillance against neoplastic tissues, and activation of cell-mediated immunity. The maturation and differentiation of T cells involves the processing of precursor cells through the thymus. During this process, T cells acquire their specific antigen receptors. Antigen receptors are heterodimers composed generally of alpha and beta protein chains. During thymic development the antigen receptor is "educated" to only recognize antigen in association with self-MHC molecules (Fig. 89-2). At the same time, T cells that are capable of responding to self antigens, and thereby potentially capable of producing autoimmune diseases, are eliminated. Eventually, these cells leave the thymus and populate the peripheral blood, lymph nodes, spleen, and other secondary lymphoid organs.

A major technological advance that has enabled rapid progress in the understanding of T-lymphocyte biology has been the development of monoclonal antibodies specific for markers of the surface of these immune cells. By international consensus, as each new cell-surface marker is identified, it is given the designation *CD* followed by a specific number. Through the ability to sort purified populations of lymphocytes according to their expression of unique CD antigens, the function of several important lymphocyte subclasses has been identified. T lymphocytes are recognized by their surface expression of CD2 and CD3 markers. T helper cells are further characterized by their surface expression of the CD4 antigen. These CD4 cells are restricted in that they are only activated by antigen bound to class II MHC gene products (illustrated in Fig. 89-2). In the presence of appropriate stimulation, the T cells become activated. Gene activation in these stimulated T cells is followed by the secre-

Table 89-3. Classification of lymphocytes on the basis of cell-surface markers

Class	Cell-surface markers	Subsets	Restrictions	Functions
T cells	CD4+ CD3–T-cell receptor CD2+	Helper-inducer T cells	MHC restricted (class II)	Stimulate B cells to produce antibody; induce CD8+ cytotoxic T cells
	CD29–, CD45RA+	Naive T cells	MHC restricted (class II)	Activated in primary immune responses
	CD29+, CD45RO+	Memory T cells	MHC restricted (class II)	Stimulate secondary immune responses
	CD8+ CD3–T-cell receptor CD2+	Cytotoxic T cells	MHC restricted (class I)	Lyse antigen-bearing target cells
B cells	Surface Ig+ CD19+ CD20+	—	Antigen specific	Differentiate into antibody-producing surface Ig negative plasma cells or memory B cells
Natural killer cells	CD2+ CD16+ CD56+ CD3–, CD4–, CD8– T-cell receptor–	—	Non-MHC restricted	Kill tumor cells, virally infected cells

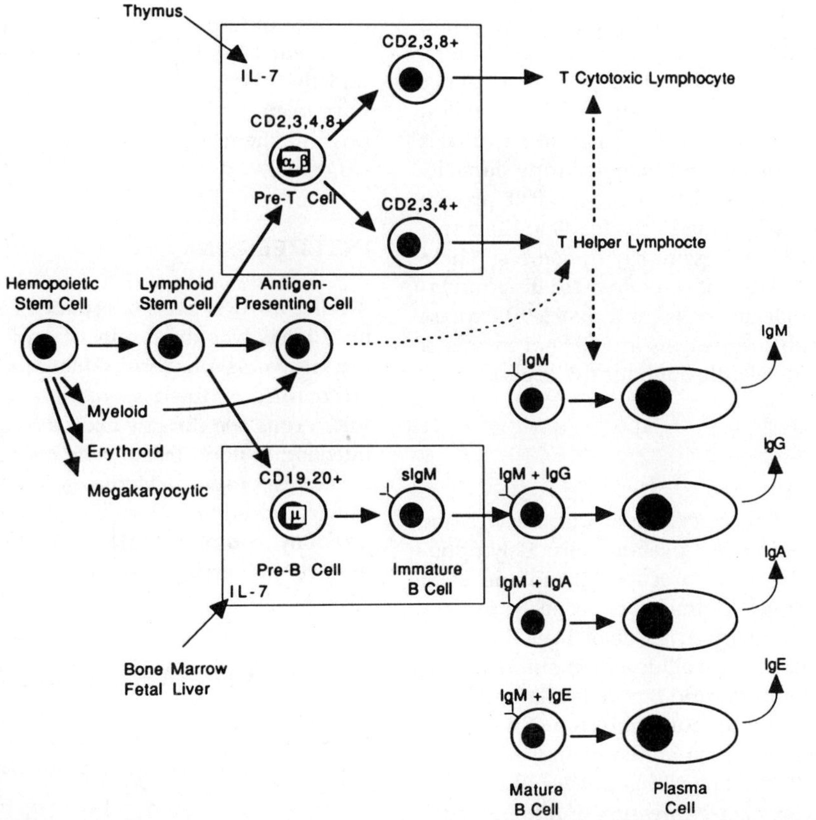

Fig. 89-3. Maturation of the lymphoid stem cell into T and B lymphocytes. T cell maturation occurs within the thymus and results in the production of T cell antigen receptor–expressing, CD2- and CD3-positive helper, or cytotoxic cells. B cell maturation occurs in the bone marrow or fetal liver and results in the development of surface immunoglobulin-positive, CD19- and CD20-positive B cells, the precursors of antibody-secreting plasma cells. (Maturation is represented by solid lines and helper function by dashed lines.)

tion of an array of new proteins, termed *cytokines,* as well as receptors for these cytokines. The cytokines stimulate the T cells to expand via clonal proliferation and regulate the form the ensuing immune response will take. Thus, cytokines are responsible for the recruitment and activation of monocytes-macrophages, B lymphocytes, cytotoxic lymphocytes, and so forth. A subset of the T lymphocytes that proliferate in response to antigen form memory T cells. These cells are characterized by the surface expression of the CD45RO and CD29 antigens and form the basis for the more rapid immune response that follows subsequent exposures to the antigen. These cells contrast with "naive" T lymphocytes, which express CD45RA but not CD29.

Circulating monocytes or resting tissue macrophages have only a limited capacity to phagocytose and kill targets. The terminal activation stage of cell-mediated immunity involves the secretion of several cytokines, including interferon-γ, which are macrophage activating factors. These cytokines mediate the recruitment of monocytes-macrophages into the site of inflammation followed by their activation into cells that are potent effectors of target-cell destruction.

CYTOTOXIC T LYMPHOCYTES

The second major subclass of T lymphocytes are the cytotoxic T cells. These cells are characterized by the surface expression of the CD8 antigen. They are critically important in the immune response against virus-infected cells. As new viral protein is synthesized by infected cells, these peptides are bound to class I MHC. As with class II MHC molecules, the class I molecules are evolutionarily related to antibodies and the T-cell receptor proteins and have a strong capacity to bind antigen. Expression of these class I–viral protein complexes on the surface of infected cells leads to their recognition by cytotoxic (CD8-expressing) lymphocytes. These cytotoxic cells are then capable of directly mediating target-cell destruction. As all nucleated cells (and platelets) express class I MHC molecules, this represents an efficient means of eliminating virus-infected cells throughout the organism.

B LYMPHOCYTES

The second major class of lymphocytes is B lymphocytes, the precursors of antibody-producing plasma cells. B lymphocytes are derived from the same precursor lymphoid stem cell as T lymphocytes. B-cell maturation occurs primarily within the bone marrow, although the fetal liver also provides an appropriate milieu for B-cell development. Differentiation of the lymphoid stem cell into B cells is characterized initially by the appearance within the cytoplasm of the heavy chain of immunoglobulin M (IgM) antibody and by surface expression of CD19 and CD20. Later stages of B-cell maturation are characterized by surface expression of IgM and subsequently additional subclasses of antibodies. As is discussed in a later section of this chapter, the differentiation of B lymphocytes into plasma cells is characterized by the disappearance of surface immunoglobulin and the active secretion of antibody into the circulation. The classification and functions of lymphocytes are summarized in Table 89-3 and in Fig. 89-3.

SELECTED READING

Kronenberg, M, et al. The molecular genetics of the T cell antigen receptor and T cell antigen recognition. *Annu Rev Immunol* 4:529, 1986.

Unanue, ER, and Cerottini, J-C. Antigen presentation. *FASEB J* 3:2496, 1989.

CYTOKINES, INTERFERONS, AND INTERLEUKINS

Lanny J. Rosenwasser

DEFINITION

Cytokines are nonimmunoglobulin proteins secreted by immune cells that have significant growth differentiation and activation function on contiguous or distant cells and tissues. Four major families of cytokines have been identified: interferons, colony-stimulating factors (CSFs), tumor necrosis factors (TNFs), and the interleukins. These mediators were first identified over 25 years ago and have been a source of great excitement and recent investigation. Through the application of the modern techniques of immunobiology, including monoclonal antibody production, long-term growth of lymphoid cells in vitro, and the use of recombinant deoxyribonucleic acid technology, the elucidation of the structure and the preparation of large quantities of these molecules have been made possible. These techniques have also made possible the use of these biologic response modifiers in clinical trials.

INTERFERONS

Among the first class of cytokines to be identified on a structural basis was the family of proteins with antiviral properties known as *interferons.* There are three classes of interferons defined on the basis of their cellular origin (Table 89-4). Interferons are directly toxic to virally infected cells, prevent infection of noninfected cells, and stimulate the antiviral immune response. Interferon-γ, in addition, is a potent macrophage activating factor, stimulating class II major histocompatibility complex (MHC) antigen expression, adherence, antigen processing, and antibody-dependent cellular cytotoxicity.

COLONY-STIMULATING FACTORS

While the homeostatic production of hematologic cells occurs without exogenous mediators, under conditions of in-

Table 89-4. Interferons

Interferon	Source
α	Monocytes
β	Fibroblasts
γ	T lymphocytes

Table 89-5. Colony-stimulating factors

CSF	Source	Product
Erythropoietin	Kidney	Erythrocytes
IL-3	T cells	Granulocytes Macrophages Platelets Mast cells
GM-CSF	T cells	Granulocytes Macrophages Platelets
G-CSF	Fibroblasts Endothelium	Granulocytes
M-CSF	Fibroblasts Endothelium	Macrophages
IL-5	T cells	Eosinophils

fection or stress the bone marrow can vastly increase its output. Numerous CSFs with varying sources and targets can stimulate hematopoiesis (Table 89-5).

TUMOR NECROSIS FACTORS

Tumor necrosis factors are a family of cytokines originally defined by their capacity to lyse cancerous cells in vitro and various transplanted cancers in vivo. TNFs represent two products, TNF-α and TNF-β, which are predominantly monocyte and lymphocyte derived, respectively. TNFs inhibit the enzyme lipoprotein lipase and mediate the cachexia associated with tumors and chronic infections (thus, the term *cachectin*). TNFs, in addition, are potent neutrophil and eosinophil activators, activate endothelial cells to permit the egress of inflammatory cells, and are endogenous pyrogens.

INTERLEUKINS

Another group of biologic response modifiers identified over the past years is a group of materials known as the *interleukins,* so termed because of their presumed ability to mediate lymphoid cell interactions (Table 89-6). This family of proteins all have unique spectra of biologic applications and might have significant clinical applications.

Interleukin-1 (IL-1) is actually a family of monokines (IL-1α and IL-1β) that mediate a wide range of immune and nonimmunologic functions. The more predominant form in humans is the neutral (pI–7.0) form, IL-1β. The IL-1α form is also secreted as a 17 kD glycoprotein, but with a pI of 5.0. Both of these forms of IL-1 bind to the same cellular receptor(s) with the same degree of specificity and affinity. Each form can successfully compete with the alternative form for receptors. The receptor is of high affinity (Ka = 10^{-10}) and is present on all cell types that can respond to IL-1. Some of the activities ascribed to IL-1 include the capacity to generate febrile responses, lethargy, lymphocyte activation, stimulation of the synthesis of acute-phase response proteins by the liver, B-lymphocyte growth, synovial cell secretion of prostaglandin E_2, protein catabolism within muscle cells, fibroblast proliferation, and bone and cartilage resorption.

Interleukin-2 was the first of the interleukin family to have its amino acid structure identified by gene cloning techniques. Interleukin-2 is a product made by T cells that promotes primarily T-cell growth. While other cells besides T cells, including natural killer cells, lymphokine-activated killer cells (LAK), B cells, and monocytes, have been identified as responding to IL-2, the major effect of this lymphokine is to promote the autocrine growth of T cells. T cells are activated by the combination of antigen plus class II MHC molecules and, for optimal stimulation, IL-1. In the presence of such appropriate stimulation, T cells begin to secrete IL-2 and express IL-2 receptors. Secreted IL-2 is then capable of binding to its receptor, resulting in T-cell proliferation. Interleukin-2 has major therapeutic potential as an immunostimulant, and it has been tried as a potential immune adjuvant in the immunodeficiency associated with cancer and acquired immunodeficiency syndrome. Interleukin-2 in very high doses is associated with the generation of lymphokine (IL-2)-activated killer cells. LAK cells in vivo have been useful in lysing a wide variety of metastatic cancers, which thus far have been refractory to standard chemotherapy. While toxic, this new form of immunologic intervention has generated a large amount of enthusiasm for the concept of immune intervention in cancer and immunodeficiency diseases.

Interleukin-3, or multi-CSF, is a member of the family of colony-stimulating factors. The term *multi-CSF* is derived from the wide range of activities of IL-3 on immature bone-marrow stem cells. Thus, IL-3 is capable of promoting the proliferation and differentiation of granulocytes, macrophages, megakaryocytes, and mast cells from a multipotential precursor. In mice, IL-3 is particularly effective in promoting the differentiation of mast cells, and long-term cultures of stem cells with IL-3 result in pure mast cell colonies. It is clear that other factors are involved in mast cell differentiation in humans, although IL-3 remains an important mast cell growth factor. Interleukin-3 alone, or in combination with other CSFs, has great potential in treating idiopathic or drug (e.g., chemotherapy)-induced cytopenias.

Interleukin-4, along with IL-5 and IL-6, was originally defined as a factor mediating T-cell–dependent B-cell growth and differentiation. Interleukin-4 was originally recognized by its capacity to costimulate proliferation of anti-immunoglobulin M (IgM)–activated B cells. Its spectrum of activities on B cells has been extended to include the abilities to enhance IgE production, the induction of class II MHC antigens, and the induction of low-affinity IgE receptors (FcεRII or CD23). Interleukin-4 is also a macrophage-activating factor, inducing class II MHC antigen and FcεRII expression and promoting ADCC. Interleukin-4, like IL-2, is a T-cell growth factor. IL-4 is both capable of and absolutely essential for IgE production. Thus, treatment of *Nippostrongylus basiliensis*–infected mice with anti–IL-4 antibodies totally abrogates their capacity to develop an IgE response. This combination of stimulating B cells to switch to the IgE isotype and stimulating expression of FcεRII on B cells and monocytes makes IL-4 of obvious interest to the allergist.

Interleukin-5 is a growth factor that directly stimulates the proliferation of B cells. Non-B–cell activities include the

Table 89-6. The interleukins

Interleukin	Other names	Function	Source
IL-1	Interleukin-1	Lymphocyte activation Fever, inflammation	MO
IL-2	Interleukin-2	Stimulates growth of T cells Costimulates B-cell differentiation	T cells
IL-3	Interleukin-3 Mast cell growth factor	Stimulates mast cell growth Multipotential hemopoietic cell growth factor	T cells
IL-4	Interleukin-4 B-cell stimulatory factor 1 B-cell growth factor I T-cell growth factor II Immunoglobulin E enhancing factor	Costimulates B-cell proliferation Stimulates limited T-cell growth Enhances IgE production Stimulates MHC class II expression on B cells and macrophages Costimulates proliferation of several hemopoietic progenitors	T cells
IL-5	Interleukin-5 T-cell replacing factor B-cell growth factor II Eosinophil differentiation factor	Stimulates in vitro antibody responses Costimulates B-cell growth Enhances eosinophil differentiation and activates mature eosinophils	T cells
IL-6	BSF-2 Hybridoma growth factor Hepatocyte stimulating factor (HSN) IL-HSN Interferon-β_2	Stimulates maturation and growth of activated B cells, plasma cells, and hybridomas	T cells Fibroblasts MO
IL-7	Lymphopoietin-1	Stimulates pre T and B cells	Thymic epithelia Bone-marrow stroma
IL-8	NAP MDNCF	Neutrophil activation and chemotaxis	MO
$MIP_{1\alpha}$ $MIP_{1\beta}$	nLD78 mTCA3	Neutrophil activation	MO
MIP_2	PF4 CTAP III β thromboglobulin	Neutrophil activation	MO

Key: MHC = major histocompatibility complex; MO = monocytes/macrophages; MIP = macrophage(-derived) inflammatory protein.

capacity to function as an eosinophilopoietin and to activate mature eosinophils. Interleukin-5 stimulates the cytotoxic capacity of mature $CD8^+$ T lymphocytes. The combination of stimulation of eosinophilia and generation of "primed" (hypodense) eosinophils is, again, suggestive of a role in allergic diseases. Increased IL-5 production has been associated with the hypereosinophil syndrome.

Interleukin-6 has almost as many activities as IL-1. It was originally recognized on the basis of its capacity to stimulate the terminal differentiation of B lymphocytes into immunoglobulin-secreting plasma cells. Interleukin-6 shares with IL-1 the capacity to mediate acute-phase protein synthesis from hepatocytes. It also synergizes with other CSFs to promote granulocyte-macrophage growth and differentiation.

Interleukin-7 is a recently cloned protein that functions in the thymus and bone marrow to promote the differentiation of lymphoid stem cells into T and B cells, respectively. Interleukin-8 is a monocyte-derived neutrophil chemotactic and activating factor. Closely related structurally to IL-8 are the macrophage-derived inflammatory proteins (MIP-1 and MIP-2), which also mediate polymorphonuclear neutrophil (PMN) chemotaxis. In addition, MIP-1 generates a PMN respiratory burst and degranulation.

T LYMPHOCYTE SUBTYPES

It is recognized that not all cytokines are produced by all T lymphocytes on activation, and several phenotypic subtypes of T helper (T_H) cells can be defined on the basis of their repertoire of cytokines. At least two subtypes of T_H cells have been defined in the mouse and human (Table 89-7).

T helper 1 cells, through their capacity to stimulate T-cell

Table 89-7. T helper subtypes

T_H1
Inteferon-γ
Interleukin-2
TNF β
T_H2
Interleukin-4
Interleukin-5
Interleukin-6
Both
GM-CSF
Interleukin-3

growth and macrophage activation, are particularly effective in cell-mediated immunity. T helper 2 cells stimulate IgE production, mast cell growth, FcϵRII expression, and eosinophilia, and are therefore of obvious importance in allergic diseases. Interferon-γ inhibits IL-4–mediated effects on B lymphocytes, and, thus, T_H1 cells should prevent allergic immune responses.

SELECTED READING

Cerami, A, and Beutler, B. The role of cachectin/TNF in endotoxic shock and cachexia. *Immunol Today* 9:28, 1988.

Miyajima, A, et al. Coordinate regulation of immune and inflammatory responses by T cell–derived lymphokines. *FASEB J* 2: 2462, 1988.

HUMORAL IMMUNITY AND COMPLEMENT

Larry Borish

ANTIBODIES

Antibodies (or immunoglobulins) are proteins that bind antigens and are the initial effector of humoral immunity. Approximately 25 percent of all plasma proteins are immunoglobulins (Ig). By binding to antigens, antibodies directly inactivate toxins and microorganisms, and, more important, direct cytotoxic effector cells to the antibody-bound targets. In addition, antibodies have potent proinflammatory activity through their capacity to mobilize a cascade of plasma proteins, termed *complement.*

Antibodies are the secreted product of plasma cells, which in turn are derived from B lymphocytes. B lymphocytes are derived from a lymphoid stem cell within the bone marrow. Mature B lymphocytes are distinguished by the presence of cell-surface immunoglobulin, usually IgM with or without the additional presence of IgD. B lymphocytes also express class II major histocompatibility complex antigens. This, with their capacity to use their surface immunoglobulin as an antigen receptor, makes B lymphocytes the most efficient antigen-presenting cell of the immune system.

Certain antigens, generally highly repetitive complex carbohydrates such as bacterial lipopolysaccharide, can directly stimulate B lymphocytes to secrete IgM. Most antigens, however, must be processed and "presented" to B lymphocytes to stimulate antibody secretion. Both the switching of antibody class from IgM (see later in text) and the stimulation of the proliferation of B lymphocytes and their differentiation into plasma cells is T lymphocyte dependent. This is accomplished by the secretion of several B-cell active cytokines by the T cells, including interleukins-2, 4, 5, and 6.

Defects in the maturation and differentiation of B lymphocytes are associated with immune deficiency. Patients most commonly have recurrent infections, with purulent bacteria affecting the sinopulmonary and gastrointestinal (GI) systems. These immune deficiencies are either congenital (X-linked agammaglobulinemia, Wiskott-Aldrich syndrome) or acquired (common variable immune deficiency, multiple myeloma).

ANTIBODY STRUCTURE AND DIVERSITY

Antibodies are markedly heterogeneous, as would be expected given their vast repertoire. Even antibodies directed against the same antigen represent dozens of different molecules, each with different molecular targets on the antigen. Thus, plasma from one person contains over a million different species of the Ig molecule. All Ig, however, share a basic subunit structure (Fig. 89-4). Antibodies are made up of two identical heavy and two identical light chains. The light chains are attached to the heavy chains by disulfide linkages, which together form the antigen combining site. The heavy chains are attached to each other by disulfide bonds. By electron microscopy, antibodies have the shape of a Y, with two antigen binding regions (Fab) attached via a hinge region to the stalk (Fc).

Unique amino acid sequences within the antibody combining site are responsible for their vast antigen-binding repertoire. This diversity of immunoglobulins is regulated by a family of Ig genes (Fig. 89-5). Each individual light chain and heavy chain of the Ig molecule is generated by the rearrangement of genetic information contained within the germ-line deoxyribonucleic acid (DNA). This rearrangement occurs during the differentiation of the lymphoid precursor into mature B lymphocytes. The germ-line DNA for light chains contains multiple gene segments within variable (V), joining (J), and constant (C) regions. Each final gene is assembled by the random selection of one of several V, J, and C region possibilities. In light chains, once a V-region gene has recombined with a sequence from the J region, a constant region gene is rearranged from the germ-line configuration. The resultant linear messenger ribonucleic acid molecule is then translated to the specific light-chain protein.

Fig. 89-4. Immunoglobulin structure. The immunoglobulin molecule consists of two identical heavy chains joined to each other and to two identical light chains by disulfide linkages. Variable regions within the light and heavy chains form the two antigen-binding regions. The heavy-chain constant region contains sites for Fc receptor and complement binding.

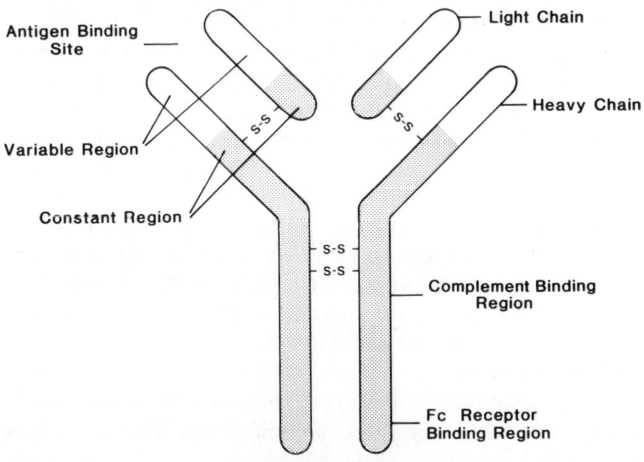

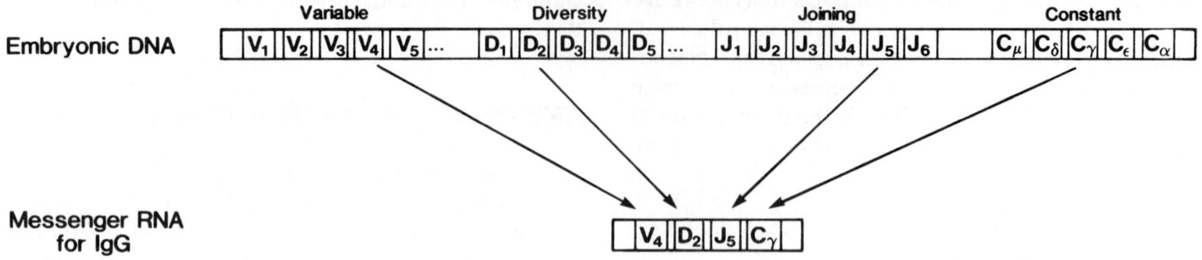

Fig. 89-5. Heavy-chain deoxyribonucleic acid (DNA) rearrangements. The embryonic DNA locus for heavy-chain genes consists of several hundred variable (V) gene segments, 10 to 20 diversity (D) segments, and 6 joining (J) genes. The constant region of the genome is formed by genes coding for the 5 heavy-chain classes (as well as 4 additional sequences for the gamma and alpha subclasses). During B lymphocyte development, mature DNA is generated by the random selection and approximation of individual gene segments from each of the V, D, and J regions and the deletion of the intervening DNA. Initially, the V-D-J sequences combine with the mu gene sequence to produce IgM heavy chains. During subsequent B lymphocyte maturation to plasma cells, there is a deletion of additional intervening DNA to produce IgG, IgE, and IgA heavy chains.

Heavy-chain DNA contains additional gene segments between the V and J regions, termed the *diversity (D) region.* In heavy chains, the initial stage of Ig gene maturation consists of the random selection and approximation of specific V, D, and J sequences. The genomic sequences for the constant region are arranged linearly (mu-delta-gamma-epsilon-alpha) after the V, D, and J regions. This confirmation permits the rearranged V-D-J genes to use different constant region genes in sequence as the immune response proceeds.

IMMUNOGLOBULIN ISOTYPES

Unique amino acid sequences within the Fc portion of the antibody define the class of heavy or light chain. The five different heavy chains (gamma, mu, alpha, delta, and epsilon) determine the five classes of antibody (IgG, IgM, IgA, IgD, and IgE, respectively). There are also four subclasses of the gamma isotype (gamma 1 through 4) and two subclasses of IgA (alpha 1 and 2).

Immunoglobulin G is the major immunoglobulin in the serum and circulates as a monomer. It readily crosses the placenta and is therefore responsible for neonatal immunity. Through Fc receptors on phagocytic cells, it is a potent opsonizer and is also capable of directly neutralizing toxins and viruses. It has a half-life of 23 days. There are different biologic activities within the subclasses. Only IgG1, IgG2, and IgG3, for example, bind complement, and only IgG1 and IgG3 adhere to phagocytic cells.

Immunoglobulin A is the second most prevalent serum immunoglobulin (15%). It primarily circulates as dimers held together by a J (joining) piece and is the predominant immunoglobulin in secretions (saliva, tears, respiratory mucus, GI tract, vaginal secretions, and breast milk). In secretions it is associated with the presence of a secretory piece that is produced by local epithelial cells and is responsible for the transit of the IgA from the serum into the secretions. Immunoglobulin A is highly resistant to proteolytic digestion, permitting it to survive intact in the gut. It functions in the absence of effector cells by binding to and neutralizing antigens and microorganisms, preventing their adherence to and invasion of the mucosal surface. In the gut IgA may also be important in limiting the absorption of dietary antigens. By itself, IgA does not opsonize. However, it can activate the alternative complement pathway, the products of which are opsonizers.

Immunoglobulin M represents 10 percent of serum immunoglobulins. It is present as monomeric IgM on the surface membrane of B cells or in a secreted pentameric form. Pentameric IgM is joined together by 5 J pieces and has 10 potential antigen binding sites. Immunoglobulin M is highly efficient at binding and activating the classical pathway of complement. It directly stimulates phagocytosis through the presence of Fc receptors on macrophages and is indirectly opsonic through its ability to activate complement. It is the only immunoglobulin produced by the uninfected fetus.

Immunoglobulin D is present in only trace amounts in the serum although in higher concentrations in the fetus. It functions primarily as a primitive receptor on the surface of immature B cells.

Immunoglobulin E is also present in the circulation in only trace amounts (0.004% of serum Ig). It avidly binds to basophils and mast cells, where it is the antibody that mediates atopic responses. The binding of antigen to mast cell–bound or basophil-bound IgE stimulates their degranulation, producing allergic reactions. Increased levels of IgE are present in allergic individuals. The role of IgE is uncertain; however, it may play a role in the defense against parasitic infections. Mast cell and basophil activation may also be important in inflammatory processes by increasing blood-vessel permeability and thereby facilitating the influx of serum proteins and effector cells to the site of inflammation.

NATURAL HISTORY OF IMMUNOGLOBULIN RESPONSES

The initial response to antigen is characterized by the occurrence of a lag phase of several days. This is followed by the appearance of increasing concentrations of IgM, which peaks at about 7 days. After this, IgG begins to be detected in the serum and reaches its peak at 10 to 14 days. After two weeks, the antibody titers begin to decline, with very little

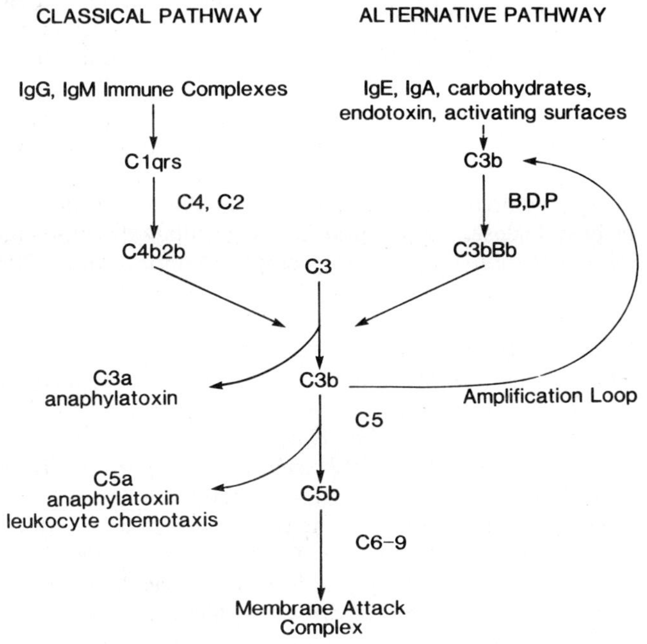

Fig. 89-6. The complement system. Complement activation occurs via the classical or alternative pathways. The classical pathway is activated by IgG- and IgM-containing immune complexes via C1, C4, and C2. Alternative pathway activation occurs when C3b is generated by activating substances or, as an amplification loop, by either complement pathway. C3b activates the final common pathway, leading to the generation of the membrane attack complex.

detectable after four to five weeks. Therefore, the presence of IgM to a pathogen suggests recent infection.

After a second exposure to the same antigen, both IgM and IgG appear in the serum without a lag phase and their levels quickly rise exponentially. Peak levels are much higher than with the primary response. The IgG response is greater and lasts longer than the IgM response. These antibodies also have greater affinity for the antigen and form more stable antigen-antibody complexes. The efficiency of the secondary response is due to the generation of "memory" B and T helper cells during the primary response, making them more available to respond on reexposure. This ability to evoke a secondary response is the basis for the efficacy of immunization in the prevention of infection.

THE COMPLEMENT SYSTEM

The humoral immune response is supplemented by a series of serum proteins that have regulatory, proinflammatory, and effector function. This series of 18 proteins, termed *complement (C),* has a crucial role in both the immune response to infection and in the generation of inflammation. The complement system is activated through a cascade of activating and regulatory proteins (Fig. 89-6).

There are two pathways of complement activation, the classical and alternative, both of which culminate in the activation of the final common pathway.

Classical Pathway

The classical pathway is activated by antigen-antibody complexes, which contain IgM or IgG (IgG1, IgG3, and, to a lesser extent, IgG2). C1 is a multimeric peptide, made up of C1q, C1r, and C1s subunits. C1q has six stems, each with a binding site for the antibody, and is bound to two C1r and two C1s molecules. Cross-linking of two of the C1q's exposes a proteolytic site on the C1r, which cleaves the proenzyme C1s into its active form. Enough IgG molecules must therefore be bound to a target to produce the statistical likelihood that two will be sufficiently approximate to cross-link two stems of C1q. This has been estimated to require approximately 800 IgG antibodies. Since IgM is a pentamer, one is sufficient to activate the classical pathway. Once activated, C1s cleaves both C4 and C2. C4 is cut into C4b, which binds covalently to the target-cell surface, and an inactive fragment, C4a. C2 is cleaved into a fragment, C2a, and C2b, which binds to C4b. C2a may have weak vascular permeability–inducing effects. The C4b2b complex is termed the *C3 convertase* and enzymatically fragments C3 into C3a and C3b. C3a is a potent mast cell degranulator. C3b binds to the target-cell surface adjacent to the C4b2b complex, this new complex becoming the C5 convertase.

Alternative Pathway

The alternative pathway does not require antibody for its activation and therefore has an important role in the initial, nonimmunologic defense against infection. Initial priming is required to produce a small amount of activated C3b. This is accomplished by the spontaneous degeneration of C3 into C3b. In addition, C3b generated via the classical pathway can activate the alternative pathway, producing an amplification loop. C3b binds factor B, which is then cleaved by factor D to form C3bBb and the fragment Ba. Ba is a weak stimulator of macrophage adherence. C3bBb is the C3 convertase of the alternative pathway. C3bBb cleaves C3, producing more C3b, which can bind more B, thereby amplifying and perpetuating the response. Factor P (properdin) augments this process by binding to and stabilizing the C3bBb complex. The combination of C3bBb and C3b produces the C5 convertase of the alternative pathway and terminal sequence activation.

C3b and its metabolites, C3bi and C3d, are recognized by specific receptors on numerous cell types. There are three classes of complement receptors (CR): CR1, CR2, and CR3, which recognize C3b, C3d, and C3bi, respectively. CR1 and CR3 are present on neutrophils, monocytes, and eosinophils, and promote adherence to and phagocytosis of opsonized targets. CR1 on erythrocytes clears C3b-coated immune complexes from the circulation. Thus, a deficiency of CR1 on erythrocytes is associated with the development of immune complex disease. CR1 is also present on B lymphocytes and glomerular podocytes, where its function is unknown. CR3 is found on large granular lymphocytes, where it may serve to enhance cytolysis of natural killer cell targets. CR2 on B lymphocytes and follicular dendritic cells promotes proliferation and antigen presentation. In addition, CR2 is the receptor for Epstein-Barr virus, the etiologic agent of infectious mononucleosis and some B-cell lymphomas. Finally, C3e, an additional breakdown product of C3, binds to an as yet uncharacterized receptor on neutrophils to stimulate their egress from the bone marrow.

Final Common Pathway

The C5 convertase generated by either pathway activates the final common pathway. Initially, C5 is cleaved into C5a and C5b. C5a (like C3a) is an anaphylatoxin, with the capacity to induce mast cell degranulation. In addition, C5a is a leukocyte activator. C5b sequentially binds C6, C7, and C8. This C5bC6C7C8 complex binds numerous molecules of C9. These C9's are inserted into the membrane, forming the "membrane attack complex." This complex produces a doughnut-shaped hole in the membrane and induces rapid lysis of the target.

Regulatory Protein

The activity of complement is regulated by a series of inhibitors. C1s is inactivated by C1 inhibitor (C1 INH). The C3 convertase of the classical pathway is inactivated by C4b binding protein (C4b-bp), which binds C4b and displaces C2b.

In the absence of regulatory proteins, the spontaneous generation of C3b from C3 or its stimulated generation by either pathway, with the subsequent amplification provided via the alternative pathway, would rapidly consume all of the terminal complement components. This regulation is provided by factors H and I. Factor H binds to C3b and blocks the binding of B to C3b and, if already bound, prevents its activation by D. Factor I inactivates C3b, producing C3bi. The C5 convertase (C3bC4b2b or C3bBbC3b) and C4b are also inactivated by I. Activation of the alternative pathway therefore only occurs as a consequence of the loss of inhibition. This occurs when C3 binds to cell surfaces that interfere with the binding of H to C3b. H normally has an affinity for C3b that is 100 times higher than that of B. Cell surfaces rich in the sugar sialic acid increase the affinity of C3b for H, while cells lacking sialic acid are activators. Most bacteria and all plants lack sialic acid. They are therefore excellent activators and will be lysed by complement even in the absence of antibody. Bacteria rich in sialic acid (group B *Streptococcus, Neisseria,* and *Escherichia coli*) resist nonimmune complement-mediated lysis and therefore are more pathogenic in neonates, who lack sufficient protective antibody. The alternative pathway is also activated through several other mechanisms, including IgA and IgE aggregates, lipopolysaccharides (endotoxin), complex carbohydrates (inulin), zymosan (yeast-cell walls), and cellophane (dialysis membranes).

Disorders of Complement Function

Several disorders have been ascribed to a deficiency in complement function. Individuals with C3, I, or H deficiency suffer from frequent infections with pyogenic organisms. The resultant immune deficiency may be as severe as that associated with immunoglobulin deficiency. Homozygous deficiencies of C5, C6, C7, C8, or C9 are associated with increased susceptibility to disseminated *Neisseria* infections.

A membrane protein that protects against the destruction of autologous cells by complement is decay-accelerating factor (DAF). DAF, like H, stimulates the dissociation of Bb from C3b. An acquired deficiency of DAF results in the complement-mediated hemolysis of erythrocytes in the disorder paroxysmal nocturnal hemoglobinuria.

Individuals with deficiencies of C1 INH, C1, C2, and C4 are unusually susceptible to rheumatic diseases. That they do not have a significantly increased susceptibility to infections demonstrates the adequacy of the alternative pathway for host defense. The classical pathway components are capable of solubilizing immune complexes and, through CR1 on erythrocytes, can clear immune complexes from the circulation. Loss of these functions may explain the increased risk for rheumatic diseases.

One form of membranoproliferative glomerulonephritis is associated with the presence of the "C3 nephritic factor," an antibody that binds C3bBb. This antibody develops spontaneously, stabilizes the C3bBb complex, and prevents factor H–mediated dissociation of Bb. Kidney failure occurs secondary to terminal complement activation within the kidney.

Hereditary angioedema (HAE) results from a deficiency in C1 inhibitor (C1 INH). HAE is characterized by recurrent attacks of angioedema involving the skin and the gastrointestinal and respiratory tracts. Death may occur secondary to laryngeal edema. Attacks are typically associated with severe abdominal cramps, vomiting, and watery diarrhea. Angioedema is not painful and is usually not accompanied by urticaria. Attacks often are induced by trauma (e.g., dental work) and typically last 48 to 72 hours. HAE was initially ascribed to the vasopermeability-inducing effects of C2a. More recently it has been shown that C1 INH also inhibits Hageman factor and kallikrein. These two enzymes are both involved in the kinin-forming system, suggesting that bradykinin may be the vasopermeability-inducing factor. Episodes of HAE can be prevented with attenuated anabolic steroids. There is no known treatment of attacks, which are self-limited after the complete consumption of C1 substrate. HAE is transmitted as an autosomal dominant disorder and is diagnosed on the basis of diminished serum C1 INH concentrations (5 to 30% of normal). Occasional patients (<20%) have normal levels of C1 INH by immunologic testing but have a dysfunctional enzyme. The concentration of the substrates of C1s, C4, and C2 are depressed between attacks and drop to negligible levels during attacks. The concentration of C1q is normal.

Recently, a group of patients has been described with an "acquired" form of HAE. These patients usually have either an underlying B-cell lymphoproliferative disorder or an immune complex disease. These diseases are associated with the increased turnover of C1q. This results in the consumption of C1 INH and secondary HAE. These patients are distinguished from those with congenital HAE by their diminished C1q concentrations.

SELECTED READING

Early, P, et al. An immunoglobulin heavy chain variable region is generated from three segments of DNA: V_H, D, and J_H. *Cell* 19:981, 1980.

Fearon, DT, and Austen, KF. The alternative pathway of complement—a system of host resistance to microbial infection. *N Engl J Med* 303:259, 1980.

Fearon, DT, and Wong, WW. Complement ligand-receptor interactions that mediate biological responses. *Annu Rev Immunol* 1:243, 1983.

Glass, DN, Fearon, DT, and Austen, KF. Inherited abnormalities of the complement system. In JB Stanbury, et al. (eds), *The Metabolic Basis of Inherited Diseases* (5th ed). New York: McGraw-Hill, 1982.

Milstein, C. From antibody structure to immunological diversification of immune response. *Science* 213:1261, 1986.

Reid, KBM, and Porter, RR. The proteolytic activation system of complement. *Annu Rev Biochem* 50:433, 1981.

GRANULOCYTIC PHAGOCYTES

Larry Borish

Phagocytic cells are critically important in the immune defenses against microorganisms and in inflammation. Thus, defective phagocytic cell function is associated with severe and recurrent infections and, conversely, phagocytic cells are generally the predominant cell type present at inflammatory loci. Polymorphonuclear leukocytes (PMN or neutrophils) are the most important phagocytic cells, but monocytes and eosinophils have phagocytic capacities.

Polymorphonuclear leukocytes are derived within the bone marrow from the pluripotential hematopoietic stem cell. The mechanisms that maintain basal neutrophil synthesis remain poorly understood. Under conditions of infection and stress, however, the bone marrow can significantly increase its capacity for the generation of neutrophils. Three factors have been characterized that stimulate enhanced PMN production: interleukin-3, granulocyte-macrophage colony stimulating factor (CSF), and granulocyte CSF, which act on progressively more advanced stages of PMN differentiation (Table 89-8).

Neutrophils (PMN) emerge from the bone marrow "programmed" to respond to stimulation in a highly reproducible, stereotypic manner. This activation involves a sequential, interdependent series of events: endothelial cell/matrix adhesion, chemotaxis, immune adherence, phagocytosis, degranulation, and the respiratory burst.

Adherence to endothelial cells is the initial event after PMN activation and must occur for PMN to emerge from the circulation. Furthermore, PMN migrate not by "swimming" but by adhering to and "crawling" along a surface. Adherence both to endothelial cells and to the intracellular matrix is mediated primarily by three glycoprotein receptors on the PMN surface membrane, which function as receptors for ligands on endothelial cells and the tissue matrix. Inflammatory stimuli induce PMN adherence by increasing their surface-membrane expression of adherence molecules. Recently, a series of patients were described whose neutrophils lack these receptors, resulting in defective adhesion and chemotaxis. These patients suffer from delayed umbilical cord separation, pus-free ("cold") abscesses, and frequent infections.

Neutrophils will respond to a concentration gradient of many mediators with directed migration (chemotaxis). These mediators include leukotriene B_4, the complement fragment C5a, platelet activating factor, neutrophil chemotactic factor of anaphylaxis, interleukin-8, and formylated bacterial peptides, such as formyl-methionyl-leucyl-phenylalanine (fMLP). Migration is accomplished by the contraction of actin filaments, which bind to actin-binding proteins on the surface membrane of the PMN and microtubules in the cell interior.

There is a close physiologic relationship between chemotaxis and degranulation. Thus, chemotaxis is associated with granule secretion along the leading edge. Neutrophils contain two classes of granules, named for the order of their appearance in the bone marrow: primary (or azurophilic) and secondary (or secretory). Primary granules contain myeloperoxidase, lysozyme, and several acid hydrolases and proteinases (Table 89-9). Secondary granules contain lysozyme, lactoferrin, collagenase, and vitamin B_{12} binding protein. The secondary granules combine with the surface membrane during chemotaxis. PMN need to recognize low concentrations of ligand, as might be present in the circulation, yet not be paralyzed by having their receptors saturated at the higher concentrations of chemotaxins present nearer the inflammatory locus. Degranulation not only releases granule contents into the extracellular milieu, but, more important, results in the insertion of granule membrane into the surface membrane. The secondary granule membrane contains receptors of fMLP, complement, and laminin (a matrix glycoprotein). Thus, degranulation that occurs during chemotaxis provides a continuous source of fresh unbound receptors at the leading edge of the PMN. This, in combination with the internalization of bound receptors, assures a constant supply of receptors, even across a large concentration gradient. In addition, the newly expressed re-

Table 89-8. Colony-stimulating factors

Factor	Source	Target
Interleukin-3	T lymphocytes	Pluripotential stem cell
Granulocyte-macrophage CSF	T lymphocytes	Colony-forming unit (CFU)–granulocytes/macrophages
Granulocyte CSF	Fibroblasts, endothelium	CFU-granulocytes

Table 89-9. Neutrophil granules

Primary granules	Secondary granules
Myeloperoxidase	Lysozyme
Lysozyme	Lactoferrin
Elastase	Vitamin B_{12} binding proteins
Cathepsin G	Cytochrome B_{558}
Collagenase	Collagenase
N-Acetyl-β-glucosaminidase	Complement type 3 receptors
β-glucuronidase	Formyl peptide receptors
β-Glycerophosphatase	Laminin receptors
α-Mannosidase	
Defensins	
Bactericidal/permeability-increasing peptide	

ceptors have a lower binding affinity for ligand and will therefore require a higher concentration for binding to occur.

Immune adherence is mediated by the immunoglobulins IgG1 and IgG3, through the Fc receptor, and the complement components C3b and C3bi, through complement receptors types 1 and 3, respectively. Immune adherence of appropriately opsonized targets is followed by their phagocytosis and degranulation of both granules into the newly formed phagolysosomes. Granule contents such as lysozyme, lactoferrin, cathepsin G, bactericidal/permeability-increasing peptide, and defensins are directly toxic to many pathogens. Additional granule components such as myeloperoxidase and cytochrome B558 are required for the optimal generation of respiratory burst products. Granule deficiency can be congenital (secretory granule deficiency syndrome) or acquired (e.g., severe burns, sepsis). Chédiak-Higashi syndrome is characterized by defective granule function. Histologically, these neutrophils contain giant granules, representing the product of uncontrolled fusion of granules. These diseases are all characterized by a diminished respiratory burst, decreased killing of pathogens, and defective directed migration.

The most potent PMN toxic function is mediated by the respiratory burst. The respiratory burst represents the sequential addition of electrons to molecular oxygen, resulting in the production of superoxide oxide, hydrogen peroxide, hydroxyl ion, singlet oxygen, and hypochlorous acid (Fig. 89-7). Hypochlorous acid, generated by the enzyme myeloperoxidase in the presence of hydrogen peroxide and halide ion, produces the irreversible halidization of target membranes. This is thought to be the predominant mechanism of PMN-mediated target destruction. However, myeloperoxidase deficiency, a relatively frequent occurrence, does not produce a severe immune deficiency, as any one or a combination of the other superoxide metabolites may be toxic to targets, and this defect is associated with a prolonged respiratory burst. The inability to initiate the respiratory burst, however, is associated with a severe immune deficiency, chronic granulomatous disease. Individuals with this disease suffer from frequent infections, most commonly with catalase-positive *Staphylococcus aureus.* Chronic infection leads to draining lymphadenopathy and granuloma formation. Catalase-negative organisms are unable to eliminate the hydrogen peroxide generated as a result of their physiologic oxidative processes. These organisms instead secrete hydrogen peroxide, which then serves as a substrate for the remaining sequences of the respiratory burst pathway, resulting in the pathogen's destruction.

The second major class of granulocytes are the eosinophils. Eosinophils are characterized by their large red-staining granules, which contain many toxic basic proteins and degradative enzymes. Eosinophils are characteristically found at sites of allergic immune reactions, such as in the lesions of atopic dermatitis, asthma, allergic rhinitis, and nasal polyposis. They are also characteristic features of the immune defenses against tissue-invading helminths, such as in schistosomiasis. Eosinophils secrete their toxic proteins and enzymes onto the surface of antibody-coated pathogens. They are therefore uniquely effective in the immune system's defense against these large nonphagocytosable targets. Their presence in allergic reactions may represent a failure of the organism to distinguish benign allergens from invading pathogens. Degranulation of eosinophils during allergic reactions represents a major component of the tissue damage associated with allergic diseases.

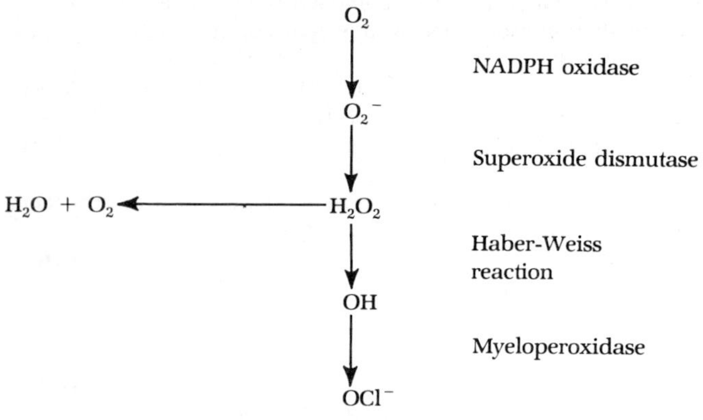

Fig. 89-7. The respiratory burst pathway.

The third class of granulocytes are the basophils. Basophils are characterized by the presence of metachromatic cytoplasmic granules. The core of the granule is made of heparin, which binds many vasoactive amines such as histamine. They are distinguished from mast cells (discussed below) by their multilobular nucleus and by the presence of relatively fewer granules. Basophils are circulating cells that may accumulate at the sites of inflammation, including allergic reactions. They are characteristic features of contact hypersensitivity reactions and allograft rejection responses.

In summary, the normal functioning of the phagocytic cell system maintains a large number of resting PMN in the circulation with the capacity to mobilize an even larger bone-marrow reserve. With the onset of infection or inflammation, there is a rapid influx of neutrophils into the inflammatory locus, where they activate their array of highly toxic, preformed granule components and newly generated, reactive oxygen metabolites.

SELECTED READING

Babior, BM. Oxygen-dependent microbial killing by phagocytes. *N Engl J Med* 298:659 and 298:721, 1978.

Fischer, A, et al. Deficiency of adhesive protein complex lymphocyte function antigen 1, complement receptor type 3, glycoprotein p150,95 in a girl with recurrent bacterial infections: Effects on phagocytic cells and lymphocyte functions. *J Clin Invest* 76:2385, 1985.

Gallin, JI. Neurotrophil specific granules: A fuse that ignites the inflammatory response. *Clin Res* 32:320, 1984.

Johnston, RB, Jr, and Baehner, RL. Chronic granulomatous disease: Correlation between pathogenesis and clinical findings. *Pediatrics* 48:730, 1971.

Malech, HL, and Gallin, JI. Neutrophils in human diseases. *N Engl J Med* 317:687, 1987.

Wade, BH, and Mandell, GL. Polymorphonuclear leukocytes: Dedicated professional phagocytes. *Am J Med* 74:686, 1983.

Wolff, SM, et al. The Chédiak-Higashi syndrome: Studies of host defenses. *Ann Intern Med* 76:293, 1972.

THE MAST CELL AND MEDIATORS OF THE IMMEDIATE HYPERSENSITIVITY REACTION

Larry Borish

Tissue mast cells and circulating basophils are the principal effector cells in the allergic response. Both are characterized by the presence of prominent cytoplasmic granules and high-affinity surface-membrane receptors for immunoglobulin E (IgE). When activated, mast cells and basophils secrete numerous vasoactive and inflammatory mediators, which are responsible for immediate hypersensitivity reactions.

MAST CELL AND BASOPHIL PHYSIOLOGY

Mast cells are readily identified with appropriate staining by the presence of approximately 1,000 granules and an ovoid nucleus. They are derived from bone-marrow precursors. Mast cell differentiation is dependent in part on T lymphocyte–derived cytokines, including interleukin-3, and also partly depends on local tissue factors. Mast cells are especially prevalent in the skin, gastrointestinal tract, and upper and lower respiratory tracts. Within these tissues, they appear chiefly in the loose connective tissue that surrounds blood vessels, nerves, and glandular ducts, and under epithelial, serous, and synovial membranes.

Basophils are circulating cells, although they are capable of migrating toward sites of inflammation. Thus, local accumulation of basophils has been demonstrated in allergic reactions, contact dermatitis, and tumors, and as part of the inflammation characteristic of transplantation rejection. Basophils comprise 0.5 to 1.0 percent of circulating leukocytes. They are bone marrow–derived granulocytes with a multilobed nucleus and contain approximately 80 granules per cell. Basophils are also distinguished from mast cells on the basis of the components of their granules and mediators released on stimulation.

Fig. 89-8. Cellular mechanisms of IgE-dependent mast cell activation. A. IgE molecules are bound to the surface of the mast cell via high-affinity IgE receptors. B. When two IgE molecules bind to antigen their receptors are brought into close proximity. This process results in the activation of phospholipase C.

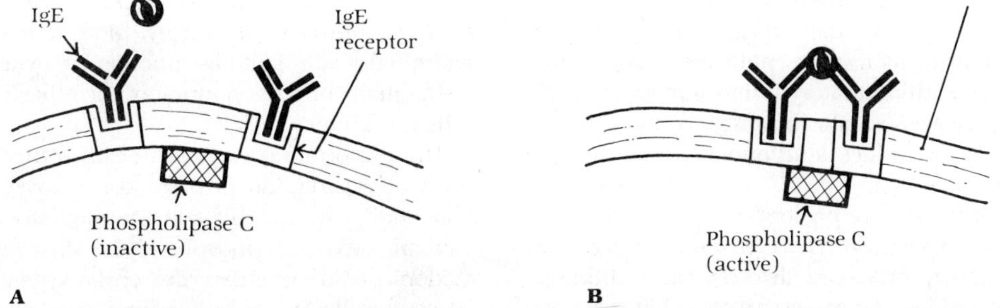

MECHANISMS OF MAST CELL ACTIVATION

Mast cell (and basophil) activation can be IgE dependent or IgE independent. Immunoglobulin E is present in minute amounts in the serum, where it has a half-life of two to three days. It is present in increased concentrations in the serum of allergic individuals. Fixed to the mast cell, IgE may be stable for years. Basophils and mast cells have between 10,000 and 500,000 IgE receptors, with receptor density related to serum IgE antibody concentration. To activate a mast cell, an allergen has to bind two adjacent IgE molecules on the surface, resulting in the cross-linking of the FcE receptors. The cellular mechanisms involved in mast cell degranulation are shown in Figs. 89-8 and 89-9. They are discussed in greater detail in Chap. 1.

The tendency of an individual toward the development of IgE responses to antigen is genetically controlled by genes that are different from those of the major histocompatibility complex. There is therefore a familial tendency toward the development of allergic diseases. Immunoglobulin E formation is under the control of both helper and suppressor T cells and can be regulated by soluble T-cell secreted factors. Interleukin-4, for example, stimulates IgE production, a process that is specifically inhibited by gamma interferon.

Numerous IgE-independent mechanisms can trigger mast cell activation. Complement activation generates the "anaphylatoxins" C3a and C5a, which degranulate mast cells. Aggregated IgE activates the alternative complement pathway. The generation of anaphylatoxins through this mechanism may be an important upregulatory pathway in IgE-mediated allergic diseases.

Mast cells degranulate in response to numerous inflammatory cell products. Lymphocytes secrete several histamine-releasing factors. Eosinophil-derived major basic protein triggers mast cell degranulation. Similarly, eosinophil peroxidase in the additional presence of hydrogen peroxide triggers histamine release. Both neutrophils and monocytes secrete products that activate mast cells. Mast cell degranulation is therefore a characteristic feature of most inflammatory processes.

Finally, important physiologic stimuli for mast cell secretion are the neuropeptides. Histamine release has been demonstrated after exposure to endorphins, substance p, gastrin, and neurotensins. These neuropeptides are important mediators of the "neuroimmune" system and may have roles in such conditions as intrinsic asthma and idiopathic urticaria.

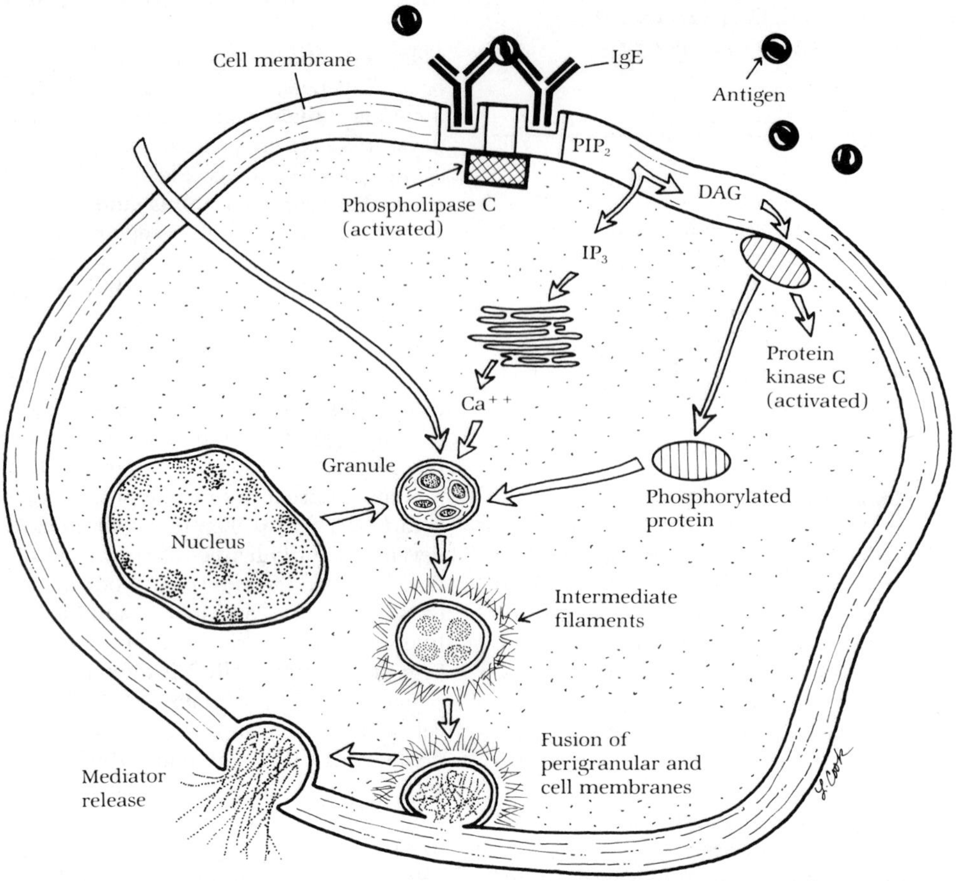

Fig. 89-9. Cellular mechanisms of mast cell degranulation. Activation of mast cell phospholipase C (see Fig. 89-8) results in the cleavage of phosphatidyl inositol (PIP_2) into two active moieties. Inositol 1,4,5-trisphosphate (IP_3) mediates the release of calcium from intracellular stores and to a lesser extent stimulates the influx of calcium from the extracellular environment. Diacylglycerol (DAG) activates the calcium-dependent enzyme, protein kinase C. Phosphorylation of an uncharacterized intracellular protein(s) initiates the movement of mast cell granules towards the cell surface. This movement is mediated by the activation of cellular contractile proteins termed microfilaments. At the cell surface, the perigranule membrane fuses with the cell surface membrane, after which the granules secrete their contents into the extracellular space.

MAST CELL MEDIATORS

Mast cells and basophil granules contain a number of potent preformed mediators, which are secreted within seconds of activation by either IgE-dependent or -independent mechanisms. In addition, other mediators are synthesized soon after activation (Table 89-10).

The most prevalent preformed mediator is histamine. Histamine induces increased vascular permeability and blood flow, causes contraction of the smooth muscles (such as the bronchioles and intestines), increases leukocyte motility, and stimulates irritant nerve receptors. The physiologic effects of histamine on these nerve receptors depend on the location of the degranulating mast cell. Thus, histamine release in the conjunctivae is associated with lacrimation, whereas histamine release in the nose produces sneezing, and histamine release in the skin causes itching. These irritant reactions have evolved as a means for the immune system to rid the body of invading pathogens. Mast cells also secrete preformed chemotactic factors for neutrophils and eosinophils, which contribute to the inflammatory infiltration that is present during allergic processes. The products of these newly recruited leukocytes can induce a secondary wave of mast cell degranulation.

Two important proteases are present within the mast cell granules, tryptase and Chymase. These enzymes may be important in inflammatory processes through their ability to degrade ground substance. Tryptase can also cleave C3, inducing a second wave of mast cell degranulation through the generation of the anaphylatoxin C3a. Tryptase activates other plasma cascade systems, including the clotting and kinin-generating systems. Chymase is a chymotrypsin-like enzyme and is a powerful angiotensin-converting enzyme.

The mast cell core is made of proteoglycans, either heparin or chondroitin sulfate. Heparin has both anticoagulant and anticomplement activity. Within the granule, heparin and chondroitin sulfates function as structural and binding components on which many of the other factors within mast cells are bound.

The important, newly synthesized mediators are derived from phospholipids through the activation of the enzyme phospholipase A_2. This enzyme mediates the release of arachidonic acid from phospholipids. Mast cells metabolize arachidonic acid by either the cyclooxygenase pathway, into prostaglandin D_2, or by the lipoxygenase pathway, into leu-

Table 89-10. Mast cell products

Mast cell product	Function
Preformed mediators	
Vasoactive mediators	
Histamine	Contraction of smooth muscle; bronchospasm Increase of vascular permeability Generation of prostaglandins Enhancement (H_1) or inhibition (H_2) of chemotaxis Increase of mucus production Stimulation of irritant (itch, sneeze) receptors
Adenosine	Inhibit platelet aggregation Enhance mast cell mediator release Constrict bronchial smooth muscles in asthmatics Inhibit neutrophil function (A_2) Coronary vasodilation and antiarrhythmic effects
Chemotactic mediators	
Neutrophil chemotactic factor(s)	Recruitment and activation of neutrophils
Eosinophil chemotactic peptide(s)	Recruitment of eosinophils
Enzymes	
Neutral proteases: tryptase, chymotrypsin (Chymase)	Complement and kinin activation Proinflammatory effects Degrade ground substance Angiotensin generation
Acid hydrolases: β-glucuronidase, β-hexosaminidases, arylsulfatase A	Inflammation Target (or innocent bystander) destruction
Proteoglycans	
Heparin, chondroitin sulfates	Anticoagulant Anticomplement activity Carrier substance for granule components
Newly formed mediators	
Platelet activating factor	Platelet activation and aggregation (serotonin, thromboxane A_2 release) Neutrophil and eosinophil recruitment and activation Vasodepression Bronchospasm Increase vasopermeability
Prostaglandin D_2	Bronchospasm Vasodepressor Increase polymorphonuclear leukocyte migration
Leukotrienes C_4, D_4, and E_4 (slow releasing substance of anaphylaxis)	Prolonged contraction of smooth muscle Increase vascular permeability Vasodepressor Vasodilatation Increase mucus production Depress cardiac function
Leukotriene B_4	Neutrophil chemotaxis

kotriene B_4, C_4, D_4, and E_4. Prostaglandin D_2 is a potent bronchoconstrictive agent and can cause wheal-and-flare reactions in human skin. It potentiates the random migration of neutrophils. Leukotriene B_4, a minor product of mast cells, is a potent chemoattractant for neutrophils. The primary metabolite of arachidonic acid by mast cells comes from the addition of the tripeptide glutathione to generate a family of molecules, termed *leukotrienes C_4, D_4, and E_4* (formerly the "slow releasing substance of anaphylaxis"). These leukotrienes cause slow onset and prolonged and strong contraction of bronchioles and other smooth muscles. In addition, they increase vascular permeability and enhance mucus secretion.

Platelet-activating factor (PAF) is a complex lipid generated from the addition of an acetyl moiety to lysophosphatidylcholine. Lysophosphatidylcholine represents the remnant of phosphatidylcholine that remains after the release of arachidonic acid by phospholipase A_2. PAF by itself induces vasopermeability and, when injected into the skin, causes a wheal-and-flare response. When inhaled it is a potent bronchoconstrictor and can induce long-term increases in bronchial hyperreactivity. As its name implies, PAF has the ability to induce platelet secretion and aggregation. Platelet activation is a feature of allergic diseases and results in the release of the vasoactive mediator serotonin and the proinflammatory lipid thromboxane A_2. PAF is both chemotactic for and an activator of neutrophils and eosinophils.

In summary, the activation of mast cells by allergen leads to the release of a series of vasoactive and pro-inflammatory mediators. These mediators produce a slowly evolving reaction that begins within 10 to 15 minutes with edema formation and subsequently produces an inflammatory infiltrate. The inflammatory response develops over several hours and is initially characterized by granulocytes, but later mononuclear cells predominate (Fig. 89-10). Symptoms resulting from mast cell degranulation depend on the location of the mast cell and include allergic rhinitis, urticaria, angioedema, allergic asthma, and anaphylaxis (see Chap. 90).

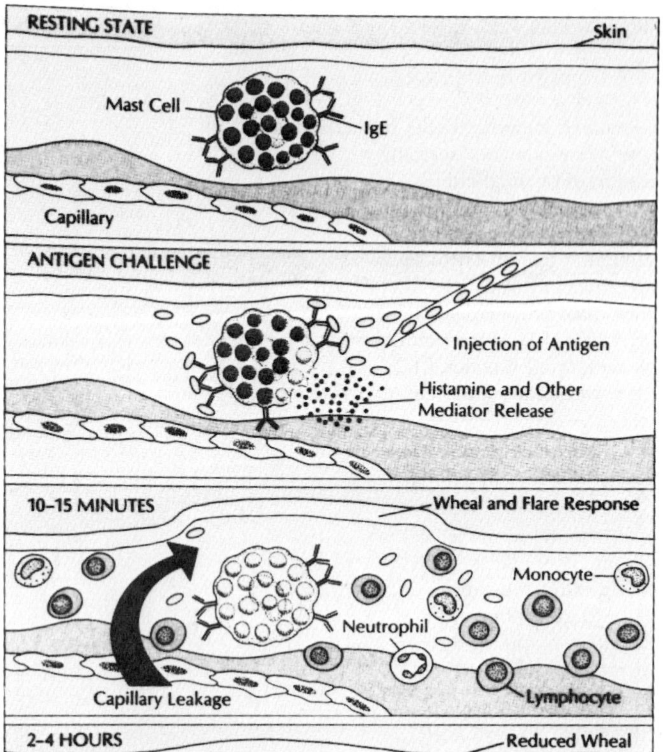

Fig. 89-10. Development of inflammation in allergic reactions. Antigen induces the IgE-dependent degranulation of mast cells. Vasoactive amines released from mast cells induce capillary leakage and neural reflexes, producing the wheal and flare response. Chemotactic and pro-inflammatory mediators that are also released by mast cells subsequently produce a characteristic inflammatory response. The initial infiltrate consists predominantly of monocytes, neutrophils, and eosinophils. Over the ensuing several hours, mononuclear cells begin to predominate and fibrin deposits are observed. (Reprinted with permission from R.F. Lockey. The imported fire ant: Immunopathologic significance. *Hosp. Practice* 25:109, 1990. Illustration by Ilil Arbel.)

REGULATION OF MAST CELL MEDIATOR RELEASE AND ACTIVITY

Mast cell degranulation can be regulated at several levels. The degree that a given mast cell degranulates depends on the amount of IgE bound to the cell, the affinity of the antibody for the allergen, and the amount of allergen. Degranulation can be modulated by the intracellular concentration of the regulatory nucleotide cyclic adenosine monophosphate (cAMP). Increased concentrations of cAMP inhibit mediator release. Histamine exerts a negative feedback control on its own release by increasing the intracellular concentration of cAMP. Many drugs used in the treatment of allergic diseases inhibit mast cell and basophil degranulation. Catecholamines (such as epinephrine) inhibit mast cell degranulation by stimulating cAMP production and reverse the effects of the mast cell mediators on target organs (by relaxing smooth muscles such as bronchioles). Sodium cromoglycate inhibits mast cell degranulation through a poorly understood mechanism. The mainstays of asthma therapy are methylxanthines (theophyllines), which, in addition to their other activities, inhibit mast cell degranulation by increasing cAMP.

Eosinophils attracted to the site of immediate hypersensitivity reaction may limit the severity of the allergic reaction. Their granules contain histaminase (which degrades histamine), phospholipase D (which degrades PAF), and other enzymes, which can metabolize various mediators. Superoxide produced by either the newly recruited eosinophils or neutrophils are potent inactivators of leukotrienes.

In summary, mast cells and basophils are potent effectors of immediate hypersensitivity disorders but are also activated in other inflammatory conditions. In allergy they can be stimulated through an IgE-dependent mechanism, but numerous additional mechanisms can also activate these cells. Through their preformed granule components and the rapid synthesis of additional mediators, mast cells and basophils stimulate not only increased vascular permeability and smooth-muscle contraction but also the influx and activation of leukocytes, with a resultant inflammatory response.

SELECTED READING

Feuerstein, G, and Hollenbeck, JM. Leukotrienes in health and disease. *FASEB J* 1:186, 1987.

Ishizaka, T, and Ishizaka, K. Activation of mast cells for mediator release through IgE receptors. *Prog Allergy* 34:188, 1984.

Metclafe, DD, Kaliner, M, and Donlon, MA. The mast cell. *CRC Crit Rev Immunol* 3:23, 1981.

Wasserman, SI. Mediators of immediate hypersensitivity. *J Allergy Clin Immunol* 72:101, 1983.

90. Clinical Manifestations and Management of Immediate-Type Hypersensitivity

ANAPHYLAXIS

Larry Borish

Anaphylaxis is the most dramatic and life-threatening of all allergic conditions, representing the clinical sequelae of the rapid systemic release of mediators from mast cells and basophils. It is generally the consequence of the injection, ingestion, or inhalation and systemic dissemination of a specific allergen. Anaphylaxis can range in severity from mild pruritus to irreversible hypotension or fatal respiratory insufficiency. Of documented cases of anaphylaxis, the mortality is 1 in 50. Thus, rapid diagnosis and intervention are critically important.

ETIOLOGY

A tremendously wide range of substances are capable of inducing anaphylaxis. In addition, these agents can induce mast cell and basophil degranulation by both immunoglobulin E (IgE)-dependent and -independent mechanisms. Mediators of IgE-dependent anaphylaxis include proteins, polysaccharides, haptens, and physical agents (Table 90-1). While virtually any food can cause allergic reactions, the most frequent offenders are eggs, peanuts, soy protein, milk, shellfish, fish, and wheat. Hymenoptera venom from the honeybee, wasp, yellow jacket, hornet, and fire ant is a frequent cause of anaphylactic episodes and results in 300 to 500 deaths in the United States per year. Therapeutic agents such as antibiotics (e.g., penicillin, cephalosporins, nitrofurantoin, tetracycline), hormones (insulin, adrenocorticotropic hormone, progesterone), chemotherapeutic agents (cyclophosphamide, L-asparaginase, cis-platinum, cytosine arabinoside), vitamins (thiamine, folic acid), chymopapain, and dextran can induce anaphylaxis. Administration of antiserum such as tetanus and diphtheria antitoxins, antithymocyte globulin, and anti–T-cell globulins can cause anaphylaxis. Systemic allergic reactions have been reported secondarily to human seminal plasma. Finally, cold-induced mast cell degranulation has been recognized to be an IgE-dependent process. Rapid cooling, such as can occur with swimming, may induce anaphylaxis in individuals prone to cold-induced urticaria.

It is increasingly recognized that there are numerous non–IgE-dependent mechanisms of mast cell and basophil degranulation (see Chap. 89) and that these mechanisms may be responsible for episodes of anaphylaxis (Table 90-2).

Table 90-1. IgE-mediated causes of systemic anaphylaxis in humans

Proteins	
Food	Egg, peanut, soy, milk, shellfish, fish, wheat
Antiserum	Tetanus and diphtheria antitoxins, antithymocyte globulin, anti-CD3
Hormones-enzymes	Insulin, adrenocorticotropic hormone, progesterone, chymotrypsin
Seminal plasma	
Venom	Hymenoptera
Allergen extract	Ragweed, grass, mites
Polysaccharides	Dextran
Haptens	
Antibiotics	Penicillin, tetracycline, nitrofurantoin, streptomycin
Chemotherapeutic agents	Cis-platinum, cyclophosphamide (Cytoxan), cytosine arabinoside, L-asparaginase
Vitamins	Thiamine, folic acid
Physical agents	
Cold induced	Swimming

Immune complex formation with secondary complement activation will result in the release of the anaphylatoxins C3a and C5a. This can occur during the administration of transfusions, immunoglobulin, plasma, or cryoprecipitate. Individuals may develop IgE antibodies against these products, but more commonly aggregates of immunoglobulins develop in these preparations that activate complement. Individuals with IgA deficiency (approximately 1 in 700 persons) are particularly prone to this complication. In these individuals IgG anti-IgA antibodies develop that rapidly form immune complexes on administration of blood products. (The presence of IgE anti-IgA antibodies has also been reported in some of these individuals and may contribute to the development of anaphylaxis.) Finally, complement activation with secondary anaphylaxis may occur secondary to exposure of blood to dialysis membranes.

Aspirin and other nonsteroidal antiinflammatory agents (NSAIDs) will induce anaphylaxis in as many as 1 percent of the population. No evidence has been found of an IgE antibody directed against these agents. Anaphylaxis entirely correlates with the ability of these agents to inhibit cyclooxygenase, the enzyme that converts arachidonic acid into the precursor of prostaglandins and thromboxanes. Anaphylaxis is thought to occur secondary to either the individual's dependence on prostaglandins (such as prostaglandin E_2) to protect against mast cell degranulation and bronchospasm, or to the shunting of arachidonic acid into the leukotriene pathway, with the increased production of these potent allergic mediators. Persons who are sensitive to either aspirin or an NSAID should avoid all agents within these classifications. These individuals, however, are generally able to tolerate acetaminophen, choline salicylate, and sodium salicylate. Alternatively, if the administration of aspirin or an NSAID is critical, desensitization has been reported to be safe and effective.

Numerous food additives have been proposed as mediators of anaphylaxis, including metabisulfites, tartrazine

Table 90-2. Non-IgE–mediated causes of systemic anaphylaxis in humans

Complement mediated	Transfusion reactions with IgA deficiency (also IgE), immunoglobulin, plasma, cryoprecipitate Dialysis membranes
Aspirin/nonsteroidal antiinflammatory agents	
Food additives	Sulfites, sodium benzoate, tartrazine, monosodium glutamate
Direct mast cell–releasing agents	Opiates, curare, tubocurarine, radiographic contrast agents, local anesthetics
Exercise	Can be associated with eating
Idiopathic	

(FD&C dye no. 5), benzoates, and monosodium glutamate. Deaths have been reported after exposure to these agents. Their mechanism of action has not been established but does not seem to require the presence of IgE antibodies.

Numerous other agents are known to mediate non–IgE-dependent mast cell degranulation and may result in anaphylaxis. These include opiates (morphine, codeine), radiographic contrast media, physical stimuli (exercise, heat, cold), local anesthetics (procaine, lidocaine), and muscle relaxants (curare and *d*-tubocurarine). Highly charged antibiotics, such as polymyxin B, are histamine-releasing agents. Finally, in many cases, no mechanism can be identified and the anaphylaxis is termed idiopathic.

DIAGNOSIS

Anaphylaxis is a clinically defined entity. Episodes are usually preceded by a feeling of generalized warmth and pruritus, and may be associated with a sensation of impending doom. Cutaneous involvement begins with erythema, which may develop into urticaria and angioedema. Respiratory distress may occur secondary to bronchospasm, with chest tightness, coughing, and wheezing. An important cause of anaphylactic death is laryngeal edema, which presents as pharyngeal pruritus, hoarseness, a sensation of tightness in the throat, dysphagia, or stridor, and eventually produces complete airway obstruction. Cardiovascular collapse manifests itself as light-headedness, loss of consciousness, and profound hypotension and, along with bronchospasm and laryngeal edema, is responsible for anaphylaxis fatalities. Vascular collapse results from the combined effects of hypovolemia (secondary to vascular leakage), peripheral vasodilatation, and the negative inotropic effects of anaphylactic mediators on the heart. Cardiac arrhythmias such as atrial tachycardias, atrioventricular block, and ventricular tachycardia and fibrillation may be present. Finally, gastrointestinal involvement during anaphylaxis can result in the development of nausea, vomiting, colic, and/or bloody diarrhea.

Anaphylaxis must be differentiated from other conditions that may imitate its manifestations. Especially important in the differential diagnosis are vasovagal reactions and food aspiration, which are readily distinguished by their associated bradycardia. In addition, anaphylaxis must be distinguished from myocardial infarction, cerebrovascular accidents, and seizure disorders. The most difficult differential diagnosis occurs in the clinical setting, where drug-induced anaphylaxis must be distinguished from either a complication of the underlying clinical syndrome or a toxic or idiosyncratic reaction to an administered agent. The presence of one or more symptoms within the spectrum of pruritic urticaria, throat tightness, respiratory insufficiency, or syncope with vascular collapse is diagnostic of anaphylaxis. Additionally, efforts should be made to identify the causative antigen. Frequently, it is possible to obtain a history of repeated exposures to the antigen with increasingly severe reactions and shortening of the latent period. For appropriate antigens, the presence of IgE antibodies may confirm the diagnosis (see later in text).

Laboratory findings associated with anaphylaxis are too nonspecific to aid with the diagnosis. These can include pulmonary hyperinflation on chest x-ray, electrocardiographic changes, and hemoconcentration. Mast cell mediators, such as histamine, tosyl-arginine methyl esterase, and prostaglandin D_2, can be measured in the serum or urine. Similarly, the release of chymotrypsin (chymase), platelet-activating factor, and heparin from mast cells is suggested by the presence of complement activation, platelet factor IV release, and prolongation of the partial thromboplastin time, respectively. None of these results can be achieved sufficiently quickly or is sufficiently specific to aid in the diagnosis.

The laboratory can be useful in documenting the etiologic agent responsible for mediating the anaphylactic episode. In addition, when there is confusion as to the pathophysiologic basis of an idiosyncratic clinical event, the documenting of allergy to an antigen to which the patient has recently been exposed, may establish the diagnosis of anaphylaxis. As with other IgE-mediated reactions, antigen-specific IgE can be identified through skin testing or the radioallergosorbent test (RAST), or by basophil histamine release. Skin testing is most reliable for penicillin and other beta-lactam antibiotics, local anesthetics, hymenoptera venom, insulin, heteroantisera, and other proteins such as pollens and foods. However, skin testing cannot be performed for several weeks after an anaphylactic episode, as a transient period of cutaneous nonreactivity may develop. Under these circumstances a diagnostic RAST (e.g., penicillin) may be diagnostic. Complement-mediated anaphylaxis can be diagnosed through the presence of circulating immune complexes or, in IgA-deficient individuals, IgG (or IgE) anti-IgA antibodies. For other non-IgE causes of mast cell degranulation (e.g., metabisulfite or aspirin allergy), the only reliable diagnostic test is graded oral challenge. This is a potentially dangerous procedure and should only be performed under carefully controlled circumstances.

TREATMENT

The treatment of anaphylaxis requires rapid intervention to maintain airway patency and blood volume. Prompt intubation and fluid replacement can be life saving. The treatment of choice in the initial management of anaphylaxis is epinephrine, which is administered subcutaneously in the dose of 0.1 to 0.5 ml of a 1 : 1,000 (1 mg/ml) solution. If practical, the epinephrine should be administered at the site of introduction of the allergen to delay absorption (e.g., with local anesthetics or hymenoptera). Application of a tourniquet proximal to the injection site is also appropriate in these cases. Except in individuals with severe vascular collapse, epinephrine should not be administered intravenously (IV), as this can cause a fatal arrhythmia or myocardial infarction. With honeybee stings, one should flick, not squeeze, the stinger from the site. Antihistamine therapy is totally inappropriate in the initial treatment of anaphylaxis, as it may mitigate symptoms of pruritus and urticaria while doing nothing to arrest the ongoing progression to a potentially life-threatening complication.

Respiratory complications can be treated initially with oxygen by controlled flow. Bronchospasm may require additional measures in addition to epinephrine, such as beta-adrenergic agents (e.g., albuterol by metered-dose inhaler or nebulizer) or methylxanthines (e.g., aminophylline, 0.9 mg/kg/hr). If effective oxygenation cannot be readily established, endotracheal intubation with assisted respiration is appropriate. Severe laryngeal edema may require a tracheostomy.

Hypotension is primarily the result of profound vascular leakage and is best treated with rapid, copious intravenous fluid replacement. As vascular dilatation may be a complicating factor, either levarterenol bitrate (2–8 μg/min) or dopamine (2–10 μg/kg/min) may be appropriate.

Hydrocortisone (100 mg), by intravenous push, is frequently administered as part of the initial therapy of anaphylaxis. While hydrocortisone will do nothing to reverse or mitigate the initial symptoms of anaphylaxis, it may shorten the duration of anaphylaxis or prevent a recurrence (see later in text).

A complication that is being recognized with increased frequency is the development of anaphylaxis in individuals who are receiving beta-blockers. Beta-blockers increase both the risk for the development of anaphylaxis, by making mast cells more susceptible to degranulate, and the severity of the ensuing anaphylaxis, by blocking responsiveness to catecholamine treatment. Thus, epinephrine is relatively ineffective therapy in persons who are taking beta-blocking drugs. Treatment in these individuals can include administration of atropine (0.6–1.0 mg intramuscularly); methylxanthines, intravenous isoproterenol (0.5–4.0 μg/min), or dopamine at sufficient doses may overcome the effects of beta-receptor blockade. The combined administration of H_1 (diphenhydramine, 50 mg IM/IV) and H_2 blockers (cimetidine, 300 mg IM/IV) may be helpful in these individuals. Finally, there is some evidence that glucagon (1 mg IM) may circumvent the effects of beta-blockers by stimulating fresh beta-receptor expression.

Protracted and recurrent symptoms are increasingly recognized as complications of acute anaphylaxis. Thus, in one study, 5 of 25 consecutive episodes of anaphylaxis were followed by a recurrence, which developed from 1 to 8 hours after the initial occurrence. In addition, 7 of 25 individuals had symptoms that persisted for 5 to 32 hours, despite appropriate initial therapy. These complications occurred irrespective of the cause of the anaphylaxis. Associations were reported with adrenal insufficiency, use of beta-blockers, oral administration of the offending agents, or the initial delayed onset of symptoms. For appropriate individuals, therefore, discharge from the emergency department should be delayed until it can be established that there is no risk for recurrence.

Clearly, the most important therapeutic intervention after treatment of anaphylaxis is prevention of subsequent episodes. An aggressive evaluation, as outlined previously, should be initiated to identify the etiologic agent. Patients can then be instructed to avoid exposure to the instigating agent (food, drug). Similarly, patients can be warned to avoid exercising after eating, swimming, to avoid exposure to seminal plasma, and so forth. Anaphylaxis to hymenoptera is an absolute indication for immunotherapy. Hymenoptera immunotherapy is more than 95 percent effective in preventing anaphylactic episodes after subsequent stings. If administration of a drug—for example, penicillin—is absolutely indicated for a life-threatening condition, rapid desensitization can be performed. If radiographic contrast media are required, hypersensitivity can be prevented through a pretreatment regimen consisting of prednisone, 50 mg (or equivalent) every six hours for four doses, ending one hour before the study, and diphenhydramine, 50 mg IM, and cimetidine, 300 mg IM, one hour before the study. Finally, individuals for whom a cause cannot be established or who have been inadvertently exposed to the agent should be instructed to carry with them and be able to self-administer epinephrine hydrochloride at the onset of the clinical symptoms of anaphylaxis.

SELECTED READING

Boxer, M, Greenberger, PA, and Patterson, R. Clinical summary and course of idiopathic anaphylaxis in 73 patients. *Arch Intern Med* 147:269, 1987.

Hunt, KJ, et al. A controlled trial of immunotherapy in insect hypersensitivity. *N Engl J Med* 299:157, 1978.

Jacobs, RL, et al. Potentiated anaphylaxis in patients with drug-induced beta-adrenergic blockade. *J Allergy Clin Immunol* 68:125, 1981.

Sheffer, AL. Anaphylaxis. *J Allergy Clin Immunol* 75:227, 1985.

Sheffer, AL, and Austen, KF. Exercise-induced anaphylaxis. *J Allergy Clin Immunol* 73:669, 1984.

Stark, BJ, and Sullivan, TJ. Biphasic and protracted anaphylaxis. *J Allergy Clin Immunol* 78:76, 1986.

Valentine, MD. Insect venom allergy: Diagnosis and treatment. *J Allergy Clin Immunol* 73:299, 1984.

Valentine, MD, and Lichtenstein, LM. Anaphylaxis and stinging insect hypersensitivity. *JAMA* 258:2881, 1987.

ALLERGIC ASTHMA

Larry Borish

The important role of allergies in the pathophysiology of asthma has become increasingly recognized and suggests unique approaches to the management of the disease. For years, many physicians have been reluctant to accept the importance of allergies to their patients' illnesses, except perhaps as a relatively unimportant secondary contributing factor. This reluctance derived from the failure to recognize the true pathophysiologic sequelae of allergen exposure, with the unfortunate misnaming of allergic diseases as "immediate hypersensitivity." Thus, while few physicians would fail to recognize the role of allergies in an individual who wheezes on exposure to cat dander and improves spontaneously with a change in environment, this pattern is clearly the exception for most asthmatics. Asthma is a chronic remitting and exacerbating disease, characterized by the presence of reversible airways obstruction and, most important, bronchial hyperreactivity. All of these features are consistent with the pathophysiologic consequences of allergen exposure.

PATHOPHYSIOLOGY

Bronchial hyperreactivity is recognized as the increased bronchospastic responsiveness of the airway to nonspecific bronchial irritants such as cold air, histamine, or methacholine. Such hyperreactivity is now thought to be the clinical correlate of bronchial airway inflammation. Thus, examination of the lungs of asthmatics reveals, in addition to bronchospasm and smooth-muscle hypertrophy, the presence of edema; large numbers of infiltrating eosinophils, neutrophils, and macrophages; and the sloughing of the respiratory epithelium, with its replacement by goblet cells. The resultant increased exposure of autonomic nerve endings contributes to the development of bronchial hyperreactivity.

Traditionally, bronchial hyperreactivity has been recognized to result from exposure to respiratory viruses (e.g., respiratory syncytial virus, parainfluenza viruses, and corona viruses) and toxins (e.g., ozone, thiocyanates) and possibly to occur congenitally. The concept that allergies can cause bronchial hyperreactivity was derived from studies with the inhalation of allergen by volunteers. For years it was recognized that virtually anyone with allergic rhinitis, when given a sufficient dose by nebulizer of an offending allergen, could develop a bronchospastic response. Recently, however, it was recognized that in as many as 50 percent of these patients a recurrence of their bronchospasm developed six to eight hours after the initial episode and that this recurrence was longer lasting, occasionally more severe, and more refractory to therapy than the initial episode. This late-phase response (LPR) was shown to correlate with the development of bronchial hyperreactivity. Thus, individuals with an LPR, but not those with just an immediate response, developed an increase in bronchial hyperreactivity, which preceded the LPR and persisted for as long as six weeks after the clinical study. Finally, it was shown that the LPR correlated with the development of airways inflammation, which could be recognized as the infiltration of bronchoalveolar lavage fluid by neutrophils, eosinophils, lymphocytes, and macrophages. These studies therefore demonstrate that exposure to an allergen is able to produce clinical and pathologic correlates of asthma—that is, chronic airway obstruction, inflammation, and bronchial hyperreactivity.

Natural exposure to an allergen will be very different from that in the laboratory. Most important, natural exposure represents a several-fold smaller dose of allergen. Under these conditions, an acute bronchospastic response to allergen may not be observed. It is reasonable to speculate, however, that the deposition of allergen in the airways can result in the generation of a localized, destructive inflammatory response. These inflammatory effects can persist for weeks after the exposure. Eventually, the cumulative effects of the deposition of allergenic particles throughout the airway will produce the pathophysiologic picture of asthma. Thus, allergic asthma can result even without any clinically apparent causative association with exposure to the allergen.

Several observations suggest that the ability of an allergen to produce an LPR and bronchial hyperreactivity is more than just an experimental artifact. The tendency to develop an LPR on experimental exposure to an allergen correlates with the development of clinical asthma on natural exposure. Similarly, mitigation of the LPR with immunotherapy correlates with clinical improvement.

Consideration of allergic mechanisms is therefore an important part of the evaluation of every patient with asthma. Several studies support the importance of allergies in naturally occurring asthma. Thus, in patients seen in an emergency department with asthma during pollen season, over 90 percent had significantly elevated immunoglobulin E (IgE) antibodies to the prevalent pollen. Even with perennial asthma, it was demonstrated that for individuals with IgE to a perennial indoor allergen (mite), avoidance therapy was effective in mitigating symptoms.

DIAGNOSIS

For many patients, the presence of allergic rhinitis or allergic conjunctivitis in association with asthma suggests an allergic mechanism. However, this may not always be true. The evaluation of any patient with asthma should therefore include both a detailed history and testing for the presence of IgE antibodies to aeroallergens. Seasonal asthma symptoms (even if they persist beyond the season) suggest pollen allergy. With perennial asthma, the presence of feathers, animals, moldy areas, and dust in the workplace or at home should be ascertained. The presence of chemical irritants and the adequacy of ventilation should also be elicited. The contribution of poorly ventilated "energy-efficient" buildings to the development of asthma has led to the recognition of the "sick building syndrome."

More obvious will be individuals in whom an acute asthmatic attack develops on exposure to allergen. This can occur either as a manifestation of anaphylaxis or with industrial exposures (discussed in detail elsewhere in this text). Of particular importance is the recognition of sulfite allergy as the basis for acute, postprandial, potentially life-threatening asthma. This seems to be a particular problem for individuals who already suffer from severe, frequently steroid-dependent asthma. A history of having recently ingested sulfite-containing foods (e.g., fresh salads, wine or beer, shrimp, potatoes) is highly suggestive. Recent Food and Drug Administration requirements to limit the use of sulfiting agents by restaurants and retail outlets should make this condition less frequent.

The diagnosis of allergy can be confirmed (or sometimes suggested) by the identification of specific IgE antibodies. This is best accomplished by skin testing using prick and then intradermal techniques with a battery of appropriate inhalant allergens. Prick tests, which are performed by pricking the skin and applying a drop of allergen, are less sensitive than intradermal techniques but may better correlate with clinical allergy. The intradermal technique is the more sensitive and may suggest relevant allergies missed by the prick test. Specific IgE can also be identified by the emergency physician via the radioallergosorbent test (RAST). This is the least sensitive technique but may be necessary in young children or in patients who either have severe skin disease or are receiving medications that can suppress skin tests (e.g., antihistamines, major tranquilizers, antinausea medications), or when skin testing is not readily available.

TREATMENT

The importance of recognizing the contributing role of allergies to an individual's asthma is critical, as this will suggest unique approaches to treatment. Clearly, the most effective treatment, and the one completely without the potential for side effects, is removal of the offending allergen. This is readily possible for foods, food additives, animals, and feathers. Even with perennial indoor allergens, such as dust mites, meticulous application of environmental measures can produce significant improvement in pulmonary function and number of disease-free days and a decline in bronchial hyperreactivity. For allergens that cannot be removed from the environment (especially pollens), immunotherapy may have an important role. While numerous investigations of the efficacy of immunotherapy in the treatment of asthma have been performed, most studies to date have been flawed by the failure to obtain appropriate control groups, inadequate sample size, inadequate dose of immunotherapy, or improper statistical methods. Despite this, the preponderance of evidence suggests the efficacy of immunotherapy using such allergens as ragweed, grass, dust mite, and cat.

The recognition of allergic asthma, with the institution of environmental measures and immunotherapy, therefore provides a unique role in the management of asthma. Whereas pharmacologic manipulations may provide symptomatic relief for asthmatics, only allergen avoidance and immunotherapy have the true potential to mitigate the underlying disease process.

SELECTED READING

Borish, L. The inflammatory theory of asthma. *Immunol Invest* 16:501, 1987.

Davies, D, et al. A trial of house dust mite extract in bronchial asthma. *Br J Dis Chest* 73:260, 1979.

Murray, AB, and Ferguson, AC. Dust-free bedrooms in the treatment of asthmatic children with house dust mite allergy: A controlled trial. *Pediatrics* 71:418, 1983.

Ohman, JL, Findlay, SR, and Leitermann, KM. Immunotherapy in cat-induced asthma. Double blind trial with evaluation of in vivo and in vitro responses. *J Allergy Clin Immunol* 74:230, 1984.

Platts-Mills, TAE, et al. Reduction of bronchial hyperreactivity during prolonged allergen avoidance. *Lancet* 2:675, 1982.

Pollart, SM, et al. Epidemiology of emergency room asthma in northern California: Association of IgE antibody to rye grass pollen. *J Allergy Clin Immunol* 82:224, 1988.

Warner, JO, et al. Controlled trial of hyposensitisation to *Dermatophagoides pteronyssinus* in children with asthma. *Lancet* 2:912, 1978.

ANGIOEDEMA AND URTICARIA

Lanny J. Rosenwasser

Urticaria is characterized by the appearance of pruritic, erythematous cutaneous elevations and swelling that blanch with pressure, indicating the presence of dilated blood vessels and edema. Histologic examination of urticaria, or hives, reveals dilatation of small venules and capillaries located primarily in the superficial dermis. Angioedema is essentially the same pathologic and pathogenetic alterations, but they occur deeper in the dermis and subcutaneous tissue. Angioedema is also distinguished from urticaria by the absence of erythema or pruritus. Pathophysiologically, the differentiation between urticaria and angioedema is somewhat artificial. The two represent an immunologic response in the skin that is mediated either by immunoglobulin E and mast cells or by other inflammatory cells, which are reacting to a stimulus in cutaneous blood vessels.

PATHOPHYSIOLOGY, DIFFERENTIAL DIAGNOSIS, AND EVALUATION

Major causes of urticaria and angioedema that should be considered when any patient is being evaluated include the possibility of reactions to drugs, foods, food additives, or natural salicylates. Rarely, inhalant allergens cause urticaria in the skin. Transfusion reactions, infections, insect stings, and other problems can also be associated with urticaria or angioedema. In addition, the two conditions can be a manifestation of more serious underlying disorders, including collagen-vascular diseases, cutaneous and systemic vasculitis, serum sickness, malignancy, thyroid disease, and other autoimmune processes. In one group of urticarias, known as "physical urticarias," the stimulus for their development depends on physical elicitation. This group includes cold, cholinergic (heat), pressure, vibratory, solar, and aquagenic urticarias, all of which are triggered by some physical manipulation of temperature or pressure to the skin.

Acute urticaria is extremely common, possibly affecting 10 to 20 percent of the general population at some time in their lives. It is most frequently a one-time disorder and very often a self-limited disorder caused by an allergic reaction to a food or drug. When patients are seen in the emergency department with acute urticaria or angioedema, an attempt should be made to provide an overview as to the possibility of a drug or food reaction or reaction to an infection or underlying disorder, but a serious or expensive evaluation should not be launched immediately. Rather, via arbitrary designation, when urticaria and angioedema exceed six weeks, they are then designated chronic; at this time a more intense workup should be initiated on the basis of identification of the potential causes outlined previously.

The initial evaluation that all chronic urticaria/angioedema patients should receive includes a history, a physical examination, a chest x-ray examination, complete blood tests, and sedimentation rate. Where appropriate, further evaluation for a number of other factors should be performed, including serology, antinuclear antibody and rheumatoid factor, protein electrophoresis (if sedimentation rate is elevated), stool examination for ova and parasites, thyroid function tests, hepatitis screen, renal and liver function tests, immune complex evaluation, and skin biopsy. In a situation in which physical urticaria is thought to potentially play a role, an attempt should be made to recapitulate the physical stimulus.

MANAGEMENT AND DISPOSITION

Therapy generally consists of supportive measures using H_1 antihistamines for relief of pruritus. The newer, nonsedating, long-acting antihistamines (e.g., astemizole, seldane) are particularly effective in urticaria. H_2-receptor antagonists (e.g., ranitidine, 150 mg PO bid, or cimetidine) are also effective in the treatment of chronic urticaria. While not displaying anti-urticarial efficacy by themselves, they have a synergistic effect when used in combination with H_1-receptor antagonists. Under some circumstances steroid treatment should be considered with severe urticaria and angioedema, if they include involvement of laryngeal edema or other systemic manifestations. One should hesitate to go beyond short bursts of steroid therapy for urticaria and angioedema because of the attendant side effects of long-term steroid administration and because of a rebound effect that can be seen as steroids are withdrawn. In individuals with recurrent angioedema and urticaria of an idiopathic nature that include potential airway involvement, the prescription of an injectable form of epinephrine (e.g., EpiPen, Ana-Kit) and chewable diphenhydramine hydrochloride (Benadryl) is strongly recommended.

SELECTED READING

Burrall, BA, and Huntley, AC. Urticaria and angioedema. *Clin Rev Allergy* 3:95, 1985.

Elias, J, Boss, B, and Kaplan, AP. Studies of the cellular infiltrate of chronic idiopathic urticaria: Prominence of T-lymphocytes, monocytes, and mast cells. *J Allergy Immunol* 78:914, 1986.

ALLERGIC RHINITIS

Lanny J. Rosenwasser

The term *rhinitis* is used to describe diseases that involve inflammation of the nasal mucosa and mucous membranes of the nasal and upper airway. This inflammation is associated with periods of nasal discharge, sneezing, and congestion that persist for longer than 30 minutes. The various causes of nasal obstruction and the symptoms of rhinitis include allergic and nonallergic rhinitis, vasomotor rhinitis, infection, foreign body, tumors, drugs, pregnancies, large adenoids, and a deviated septum.

PATHOPHYSIOLOGY, DIFFERENTIAL DIAGNOSIS, AND EVALUATION

The first distinction to be made in an emergency setting should be between infectious or purulent rhinitis and noninfectious, nonpurulent rhinitis. In infectious rhinitis, nasal secretions are predominantly cloudy, either yellow or green, with many neutrophils. Noninfectious rhinitis is characterized by relatively clear, watery, mucoid discharge that often contains eosinophils. The noninfectious group can be divided into seasonal allergic rhinitis (or hay fever), perennial allergic rhinitis, and perennial nonallergic rhinitis. The most important nonallergic rhinitis is known as *vasomotor rhinitis*. Its cause is thought to be an imbalance in autonomic nervous system control with parasympathetic dominance. However, more evaluation and research are required before this form of rhinitis will be totally understood.

In the emergency department, the evaluation of rhinitis requires a thorough history and physical examination, including an evaluation of the potential for an allergic cause to the rhinitic symptoms. Evaluation should proceed with a symptom diary and/or immediate hypersensitivity skin testing for pollens and other inhalant allergens of a seasonal and perennial nature. The possibility that the rhinitis is secondary to aspirin idiosyncrasy, food allergy or intolerance, or drug allergy should also be considered. Vasomotor rhinitis is generally evaluated on the basis of a history of atmospheric changes inducing the rhinitic symptoms. Rapid changes in temperature and humidity are very often associated with the triggering of symptoms via overstimulation of parasympathetic nerves. The presence of positive skin tests to relevant inhalant allergens and eosinophils in a nasal smear represents the most useful means of identifying allergic rhinitis. Treatment with histamine H_1 antagonists should be deferred until after skin testing is performed.

MANAGEMENT AND DISPOSITION

Topical corticosteroids and topical cromolyn sodium are of great value in the treatment of seasonal and perennial allergic rhinitis and should be the treatment of choice in most cases. The recent emergence of nonsedating H_1 antihistamines makes this approach attractive for relief of allergic rhinitis symptoms. Systemic corticosteroids should only be used in patients with extremely severe rhinitic symptoms or with marked obstruction due to polyposis. In certain circumstances, when allergen avoidance cannot be achieved and pharmacotherapy is limited due to toxicity or poor responsiveness, allergen-injection immunotherapy should be considered. Numerous studies have demonstrated the efficacy of this approach in the treatment of allergic rhinitis. In situations in which severe hyperplastic turbinates and polyps are identified, partial turbinectomy is sometimes considered. Generally, these rhinitic symptoms occur in association with sinus infection. Sinus surgery for relief of infection is therefore already a consideration.

A final point to be considered in the differential diagnosis of allergic rhinitis is the development of rhinitis medicamentosum secondary to the administration of over-the-counter sympathomimetic drugs. This condition is characterized by the swelling of the nasal membranes and symptoms of rhinitis that are perpetuated by the abuse of intranasal sympathomimetics. A period of withdrawal of these medications is generally associated with amelioration of this form of rhinitis, although occasionally the swelling is so severe that administration of topical steroids to enhance the shrinkage of the nasal passages is required.

SELECTED READING

Zeiger, RS, and Schatz, M. Chronic rhinitis: A practical approach to diagnosis and treatment: I. Diagnosis. *Immunol Allergy Pract* 4:17, 1982.

Zeiger, RS, and Schatz, M. Chronic rhinitis: A practical approach to diagnosis and treatment: II. Treatment. *Immunol Allergy Pract* 4:26, 1982.

91. Emergency Management of the Patient with Human Immunodeficiency Virus Infection

Jonathan E. Samuels
Gerald H. Friedland

EPIDEMIOLOGY

The first cases of what we now know as acquired immunodeficiency syndrome (AIDS) were described in 1981, with a report of a cluster of homosexual men in Los Angeles in whom unexplained *Pneumocystis carinii* pneumonia developed. Since that time, the etiologic agent of AIDS, human immunodeficiency virus, or HIV, has been discovered and routes of transmission and clinical manifestations have been well described. Tens of thousands of cases have been reported nationwide, with predictions of hundreds of thousands of new cases developing over the next decade. Regardless of the exact figures, it is clear that the AIDS epidemic will remain a problem of increasing magnitude for the foreseeable future. The emergency physician will need to be alert for both the type of patient likely to be infected with HIV and the clinical manifestations of HIV infection.

Epidemiologic information available regarding AIDS indicates that it is most prevalent in urban areas, especially the large coastal cities. The disease is more common in men than women and in persons who are black or Puerto Rican. The majority of cases occur in individuals in their twenties or thirties.

A survey of United States military recruits conducted during 1985 to 1986 revealed that the highest rates of HIV seropositivity occurred in persons from the following areas: New York City (especially Manhattan, the Bronx, and Brooklyn); the San Francisco Bay area; Washington, DC; northeastern New Jersey; Montgomery and Baltimore Counties, Maryland; Denver County, Colorado; and Travis County, Texas. The Centers for Disease Control *Morbidity and Mortality Weekly Report* (*MMWR*) data of new cases reported nationwide by state during 1988 show a somewhat similar pattern. States with the most new reported cases, in order of decreasing frequency, include: New York, California, Florida, New Jersey, Texas, Puerto Rico, and Illinois. Despite the predilection for certain areas, AIDS cases have been reported in all 50 states and in countries in all parts of the world. HIV-infected patients can be seen in emergency departments in any part of the country. The emergency department will often be the site where he or she will first come to medical attention.

The spectrum of emergency department presentations related to HIV infection can vary from the "worried well" noninfected patient to individuals with life-threatening respira-

Table 91-1. High-risk behaviors and groups at increased risk for HIV infection

1. Male homosexual contact
2. Intravenous (IV) drug use associated with needle-sharing
3. Prostitution
4. Heterosexual contact by a woman with a bisexual man, IV drug user, hemophiliac, or man from a country where heterosexual transmission of HIV is common, i.e., Caribbean and central African countries
5. Heterosexual contact by a man with a female prostitute, IV drug user, or woman from one of the aforementioned high-risk areas
6. Hemophiliacs
7. Recipients of blood transfusions or blood products before 1985, when mass screening of donated blood was instituted
8. Persons from countries where heterosexual transmission is believed to be the predominant mode of HIV transmission (see #4), who have had multiple sexual partners
9. Children born to mothers known to be at risk for infection with HIV

tory or neurologic emergencies. Historical data are crucial in determining the physician's level of suspicion of possible HIV infection. It can be uncomfortable for both the patient and the physician to deal with probing questions regarding sexual behavior and drug use. It is nevertheless crucial that these questions be explored, in a discreet and nonjudgmental way. This will facilitate the patient's privacy and increase the likelihood of obtaining a truthful answer. Infected persons may be unaware of the personal histories of their sexual contacts, and thus any sexually active person may be potentially at risk. Table 91-1 lists the categories of persons at increased risk of HIV infection.

PATHOPHYSIOLOGY

The immunologic derangement that occurs in AIDS is largely a result of depletion of CD4 helper-inducer lymphocytes. HIV selectively attacks these cells. This is believed to occur by attachment of gp 120, the major envelope glycoprotein of HIV, to a receptor on the surface of the CD4 lymphocyte. This receptor is most likely the CD4 molecule. The depletion of the CD4 lymphocyte render's the host progressively immunocompromised and susceptible to unusual opportunistic infections.

Human immunodeficiency virus is a ribonucleic acid (RNA)-containing enveloped retrovirus that possesses the enzyme reverse transcriptase. This enzyme uniquely enables HIV and related retroviruses to transcribe deoxyribonucleic acid (DNA) from viral RNA in infected cells. The DNA then becomes integrated into the host cell genome, where it may remain latent for long periods of time; alternatively, it may "turn on" and transcribe new viral RNA and new virions, resulting in destruction of the cell.

Certain populations of monocytes and macrophages express the CD4 antigen and can become infected with HIV. These infected cells are able to cross the blood-brain barrier, permitting HIV access to the nervous system. HIV has been implicated in various neurologic syndromes, including subacute encephalitis, aseptic meningitis, myelopathy, and peripheral neuropathy.

Polyclonal B-cell activation, associated with high levels of circulating immunoglobulins and poor antibody response to vaccines, is also associated with AIDS. This may be responsible for the frequent occurrence of serious bacterial infections in these patients.

CLINICAL MANIFESTATIONS OF AIDS VIRUS INFECTION

Primary HIV Infection

The initial infection with HIV, which results in seroconversion, has been associated with a mononucleosislike illness. Results from a recent study among homosexual men in Sydney, Australia, suggest that this occurs in between 53 and 93 percent of exposed individuals who become infected. The incubation period is generally between two and six weeks from exposure. Signs and symptoms can include fever, lymphadenopathy, truncal rash, arthralgias, headache, photophobia, diarrhea, sore throat, lymphadenopathy, depression, and irritability. An aseptic meningitis picture can also be present. Thrombocytopenia and lymphopenia can occur early in the illness, with lymphocytosis and an inverted CD4 : CD8 ratio during the recovery period. The latter phenomenon is due to an absolute increase in the number of circulating CD8 cells. The diagnosis of this entity depends on the documentation of a change in HIV antibody status from negative to positive. However, the diagnosis is likely with a compatible clinical syndrome in an individual at risk for HIV infection who has positive results on testing for HIV antibody, without documented seroconversion. Anti-HIV antibodies should be detectable two to six weeks after the onset of acute HIV illness.

Asymptomatic Carrier

Persons infected with HIV may be totally without symptoms and have normal results on physical examination and laboratory profiles. Some may have anemia, leukopenia, lymphopenia, or thrombocytopenia. They can remain asymptomatic for years, and during this time may transmit HIV infection via sexual or parenteral routes. Patients may or may not be aware of their serologic status and should be asked about this specifically when relevant. Persons at risk for HIV acquisition can be offered HIV testing after being counseled regarding the implications of a positive or negative result. Follow-up arrangements for posttest counseling should be arranged before discharge from the emergency department. Confidentiality of test results should be assured. Asymptomatic individuals may appear in the emergency department with mostly unrelated problems, such as trauma or other sexually transmitted diseases.

Persons who are known to be infected with HIV should be advised of known modes of transmission and reassured regarding lack of casual transmission of HIV—that is, that sharing of toilets, utensils, and towels and physical contact without exchange of secretions have not been associated with transmission of HIV. Persons who remain sexually active despite being HIV infected should be advised to use latex condoms in conjunction with the spermicide nonoxynol 9,

Table 91-2. Case definition for AIDS in adults[a]

1.	Candidiasis of the esophagus, trachea, bronchi, or lungs
2.[b]	Coccidioidomycosis, disseminated (at a site other than or in addition to lungs or cervical or hilar lymph nodes)
3.	Cryptococcosis, extrapulmonary
4.	Cryptosporidiosis with diarrhea persisting >1 month
5.	Cytomegalovirus disease of an organ other than liver, spleen, or lymph nodes
6.	Herpes simplex virus infection (mucocutaneous) persisting for >1 month, or any duration of respiratory or gastrointestinal involvement
7.[b]	HIV encephalopathy
8.[b]	Histoplasmosis, disseminated (at a site other than or in addition to lungs or cervical or hilar lymph nodes)
9.[b]	Isosporiasis with diarrhea persisting >1 month
10.	Kaposi's sarcoma
11.[b]	Lymphoma of B cell or other specified type
12.	Lymphoma of the brain
13.	*Mycobacterium avium-intracellulare* complex or *Mycobacterium kansasii* disease, disseminated (at a site other than or in addition to lungs, skin, or cervical or hilar lymph nodes)
14.[b]	*Mycobacterium tuberculosis* disease, extrapulmonary (with or without concurrent pulmonary disease)
15.	*Pneumocystis carinii* pneumonia
16.	Progressive multifocal leukoencephalopathy
17.[b]	Salmonella septicemia, recurrent
18.	Toxoplasmosis of the brain

[a]The diagnosis of AIDS depends on the absence of other coexisting immunodeficiency—i.e., long-term corticosteroid or other immunosuppressive therapy, certain hematologic malignancies, or other congenital or acquired immunodeficiency states.
[b]Positive HIV serology is required to confirm the diagnosis of AIDS.
Source: Adapted from Centers for Disease Control. Revision of the CDC surveillance case definition for acquired immunodeficiency syndrome. *MMWR* 36:15, 1987.

which is known to be virucidal. This is believed to greatly decrease transmission of the virus during sexual relations. Persons infected with HIV should not donate blood, other body fluids, or organs. They should be advised to inform their sexual partners of their status and also to inform health-care workers.

HIV-Related Illness

Persons with HIV infection who show signs and symptoms of illness but have not yet manifested AIDS-defining opportunistic infections or malignancies are categorized as having HIV-related illness. This has been referred to in the past as AIDS-related complex, or ARC. Signs and symptoms of HIV-related illness include the following:

1. Weight loss
2. Unexplained fevers or night sweats, or both
3. Chronic diarrhea without definite cause
4. Persistent generalized lymphadenopathy
5. Unexplained oral candidiasis
6. Oral hairy leukoplakia: raised white lesions with hair-like projections, characteristically on the lateral margins of the tongue; biopsy is required for definitive diagnosis
7. Chronic weakness or fatigue
8. Recurrent bacterial pneumonias
9. Uni- or multidermatomal herpes zoster infections

AIDS

This final stage of HIV infection is characterized by the development of clinical opportunistic infections or malignancies, or both. Most of the opportunistic infections that develop in patients with AIDS are caused by ubiquitous organisms of low virulence, which are known to establish latent infection in normal individuals. Additionally, common bacterial pathogens can cause serious infections in AIDS patients. Several malignancies, some formerly quite rare, herald the diagnosis of AIDS in the appropriate setting. Accepted criteria for the diagnosis of AIDS are shown in Table 91-2.

CLINICAL PRESENTATIONS OF PATIENTS WITH AIDS AND HIV-RELATED ILLNESS

Following is a review of the common and uncommon presentations of the major clinical syndromes, organized by organ system mode of presentation (Table 91-3). Diagnostic evaluations and initial therapy are suggested (Table 91-4), as well as guidelines to assist the emergency physician regarding the decision as to whether to admit patients to the hospital or discharge with outpatient follow-up study.

Respiratory

Pneumocystis carinii Pneumonia

Pneumocystis carinii pneumonia (PCP) is the most common opportunistic infection in patients with AIDS. It is the index diagnosis for approximately 60 percent of AIDS patients, and of the remainder, PCP will develop in a substantial proportion at some point in their illness.

A slowly progressive illness typically evolves over several days to weeks that is characterized by steadily worsening nonproductive cough and dyspnea accompanied by fever. Less frequently patients have chills, chest pain, and sputum production. Physical examination invariably reveals tachypnea, but rales may or may not be present. Chest x-ray findings can be variable but will most commonly show bilateral interstitial infiltrates involving the lower lobes or the entire lung fields. Alveolar, patchy, or unilateral infiltrates can occur. Early in the clinical course, patients may have normal chest x-rays. Rare cases have been reported in which patients have nodular or cavitary lesions or disease that is complicated by pneumothorax. Patients are generally hypoxemic or will show a significant decrease in arterial oxygen tension after exercising.

In patients with a compatible clinical story but normal chest x-ray, a positive gallium scan of the lungs will raise the diagnostic suspicion for PCP. In experienced hands, diagnosis can be made by cytologic examination of sputum in over 50 percent of cases. Induction of sputum can often be accomplished by the use of nebulized hypertonic saline. When this is not successful, bronchoscopy with transbronchial biopsy or bronchoalveolar lavage is often necessary to establish the diagnosis. In severely ill patients with hypox-

Table 91-3. HIV-related complications by major organ system involvement

Respiratory
Pneumocystis carinii pneumonia
Bacterial pneumonia
Tuberculosis
Mycobacterium avium-intracellulare
Cytomegalovirus pneumonia
Kaposi's sarcoma
Nonspecific interstitial pneumonitis
Other—i.e., cryptococcosis, histoplasmosis, coccidioidomycosis
Neurologic
Toxoplasmosis
Cryptococcosis
Central nervous system lymphoma
Tuberculosis
Progressive multifocal leukoencephalopathy
AIDS dementia, myelopathy, peripheral neuropathy
Gastrointestinal
Oral/esophageal candidiasis
Cryptosporidiosis and isosporiasis
Cytomegalovirus infection
Salmonellosis
Mycobacterium avium-intracellulare
"Slim" disease (HIV wasting syndrome)
Kaposi's sarcoma
Cutaneous
Kaposi's sarcoma
Herpes simplex and herpes zoster
Miscellaneous dermatoses
Ophthalmologic
Cytomegalovirus retinitis

emia, treatment should be instituted on clinical grounds, awaiting definitive laboratory diagnosis (see Table 91-4). Because of possible confusion with other diagnostic entities and the toxicity of therapeutic agents, it remains best to establish a definitive diagnosis even if empiric therapy has been instituted. Selected patients who are not severely ill and for whom careful medical follow-up can be arranged can be treated with antibiotics administered orally or parenterally on an outpatient basis.

Bacterial Pneumonia

Patients with AIDS have defects in humoral as well as cell-mediated immunity and are predisposed to infection with common bacterial pathogens. The most commonly implicated organisms are pneumococcus and *Haemophilus influenzae.* Bacterial pneumonia most often causes acute onset of fever, chills, pleuritic chest pain, cough productive of purulent sputum, and lobar or patchy infiltrates on chest x-ray. Pneumococcal bacteremia is significantly more common than in non-AIDS patients. Gram's stain of sputum usually reveals organisms and polymorphonuclear cells. Some cases may be clinically indistinguishable from *Pneumocystis carinii* pneumonia, with nonproductive cough and diffuse interstitial infiltrates. When the diagnosis is in doubt, it is desirable to institute empiric therapy for both bacterial pathogens (see Table 91-4) and *Pneumocystis carinii* pending results of sputum and blood cultures or bronchoscopy, or both. Selected patients with lobar infiltrates who are able to receive careful medical follow-up evaluation and are not severely ill can be treated as outpatients with orally administered antibiotics.

Tuberculosis

The number of reported cases of tuberculosis in the United States has been increasing since 1986, after over two decades of steady decline. The epidemic of HIV infection may be largely responsible. Latent tuberculosis may progress more frequently to cause clinical disease in the setting of HIV infection.

Tuberculosis is more common in patients of low socioeconomic status, which would include many intravenous (IV) drug users and Haitian immigrants. Patients will often complain of gradually worsening constitutional symptoms, such as anorexia with weight loss, fevers, chills, malaise, and night sweats. Cough productive of mucopurulent sputum is typical, but fever of unknown origin without localizing signs may be present. Chest x-ray findings differ significantly in HIV-infected patients from those of other patients with tuberculosis. Mediastinal or hilar adenopathy, or both, is common. Pulmonary infiltrates may assume a diffuse interstitial or miliary pattern or can be limited to the middle or lower lung fields. Typical upper-lobe infiltrates, cavitation, or normal chest radiographs occur in a minority of cases. Concurrent extrapulmonary disease or extrapulmonary involvement without lung disease is common, occurring in 37 to 72 percent of patients in various studies. Detection of acid-fast bacilli on smear or culture of sputum is an indication for the institution of empiric therapy for tuberculosis (see Table 91-4), as it generally takes several weeks to differentiate *Mycobacterium tuberculosis* from nontuberculous mycobacteria such as *Mycobacterium avium-intracellulare,* which is also commonly present in AIDS patients. The likelihood of acid-fast bacilli being detected in the setting of HIV infection, and ultimately yielding *M. tuberculosis* on culture, ranges from 2 to 60 percent in various studies and is more common in IV drug users and Haitian immigrants. It is sometimes clinically difficult to differentiate tuberculosis from *Pneumocystis carinii* pneumonia or other respiratory pathogens, and bronchoscopy with bronchoalveolar lavage or transbronchial biopsy may be necessary to make the diagnosis.

Pulmonary Mycobacterium Avium-Intracellulare

Mycobacterium avium-intracellulare (MAI) is often cultured from sputum but is generally not seen in tissue sections of lung. Its contribution to pulmonary symptomatology in the patient with AIDS is unclear, especially since it often coexists along with other opportunistic pathogens. There is no generally accepted effective therapy for MAI; however, when acid-fast bacilli are found on smear or culture of a respiratory specimen, the patient should be treated empirically for tuberculosis (see Table 91-4) until definitive culture results become available. A more detailed discussion of disseminated MAI infection is presented in the section on gastrointestinal (GI) presentations of AIDS.

Cytomegalovirus Pneumonia

Cytomegalovirus (CMV) can cause an interstitial pneumonia that is clinically indistinguishable from that caused by *Pneumocystis carinii.* Chronic nonproductive cough, dyspnea on exertion, and hypoxemia are present, with diffuse interstitial

Table 91-4. Suggested treatment regimens for HIV-related diseases

Disease	Drug	Dosage	Duration	Comments
Respiratory				
Pneumocystis carinii pneumonia*	Trimethoprim (TMP)/sulfamethoxazole (SMZ)	5 mg/kg TMP/20 mg/kg SMZ IV or PO q6–8h	14–21 days	After treatment course is complete, suppressive therapy should be instituted with either: 1. TMP/SMZ DS, 1 tablet PO bid or 2. Dapsone, 50 mg PO daily or 3. Aerosolized pentamidine, 300 mg via Respigard II nebulizer monthly.
	or			
	Pentamidine isethionate	4 mg/kg/day slowly IV (over 1 hr) or IM	14–21 days	
	or			
	Dapsone and	100 mg PO/day	14–21 days	
	TMP	5 mg/kg PO q6h		
	or			
	Pentamidine isethionate	600 mg via Respigard II nebulizer/day	14–21 days	
Bacterial pneumonia	Ampicillin or	1 gm IV q4h or 500 mg PO q6h		
	Cefuroxime or	1 gm IV q8h or 500 mg PO bid	10–14 days	
	Erythromycin	1 gm IV q6h or 500 mg PO q6h		
Tuberculosis	Isonicotinic acid hydrazide (INH) and	300 mg PO/day		
	Rifampin and	600 mg PO/day	Indefinite (may discontinue ethambutol and pyrazinamide if organism is INH sensitive)	
	Ethambutol and/or	15 mg/kg PO/day		
	Pyrazinamide and	25 mg/kg PO/day		
	Pyridoxine	50 mg PO/day		
Cytomegalovirus pneumonia	Ganciclovir (DHPG)	5 mg/kg q12h	14 days	
Pulmonary cryptococcosis, histoplasmosis, or coccidioidomycosis	Amphotericin	0.5–0.6 mg/kg IV/day	Administer total of about 2 gm over 8 weeks, then institute suppressive therapy with 50 mg IV once weekly	
Neurologic				
Toxoplasmosis	Pyrimethamine and	25–50 mg PO/day		
	Sulfadiazine and	1–2 gm PO q6h	Indefinite	
	Folinic acid	10 mg PO/day		
Cryptococcal meningitis	Amphotericin B	0.5–0.6 mg/kg IV/day	Administer total of 2 gm over about 8 weeks, then institute suppressive therapy with 50 mg IV once weekly, or Fluconazole 200–400 mg PO daily	
Central nervous system (CNS) lymphoma	Radiation therapy			
CNS tuberculosis	INH and	300 mg PO/day	Indefinite (may discontinue ethambutol and pyrazinamide if organism is INH sensitive)	
	Rifampin and	600 mg PO/day		
	Ethambutol and/or	15 mg/kg PO/day		
	Pyrazinamide and	25 mg/kg PO/day		
	Pyridoxine	50 mg PO/day		

Table 91-4. (continued)

Disease	Drug	Dosage	Duration	Comments
Gastrointestinal				
Oral candidiasis	Nystatin suspension	5 ml "swish and swallow" q6–8 h	Usually indefinite	
	or			
	Clotrimzaole troches	1 troche 3–5×/day	Usually indefinite	
	or			
	Ketoconazole	200 mg PO/day	Usually indefinite	
Esophageal candidiasis	Ketoconazole	200–800 mg PO/day	Indefinite	
Cytomegalovirus	Ganciclovir	5 mg/kg IV q12h	14 days, then suppressive therapy with 6 mg/kg/day IV 5 days per week, indefinitely	
Salmonellosis	Ampicillin	1 mg IV q4h	14 days, then suppressive therapy with 500 mg PO q6h	
	or			
	TMP/SMZ	5 mg/kg TMP with 25 mg/kg SMZ q6–8h	14 days, then suppressive therapy with TMP/SMZ DS, 1 tablet PO bid	
Mycobacterium Avium-Intracellulare infection	Ciprofloxacin and	750 mg PO BID	Indefinite except for amikacin, which should be given for only 1 month	
	Rifampin and	600 mg PO/day		
	Ethambutol and	15 mg/kg PO/day		
	Clofazimine and/or	50–100 mg PO/day		
	Amikacin	7.5 mg/kg IV/day		
Isosporiasis	TMP/SMZ	TMP, 160 mg/SMZ, 800 mg PO q6h		
Cryptosporidiosis	None			
Cutaneous				
Herpes simplex	Acyclovir	200–400 mg PO q4–6h or 5 mg/kg IV q8h	7 days	
Herpes zoster	Acyclovir	400–800 mg PO q4–6h or 10 mg/kg IV Q8H	7 days	
Ophthalmologic				
Cytomegalovirus	Ganciclovir	5 mg/kg q12h IV	14 days, then suppressive therapy with 6 mg/kg/day IV 5 days/wk	

*For patients with moderate to severe disease (i.e., $PO_2 \leq 75$ on room air), high-dose steroids should be administered (i.e., prednisone or its equivalent 40 mg bid).

infiltrates on chest x-ray. Patients will often have coexistent infection with other opportunistic pathogens, particularly *Pneumocystis carinii.* Bronchoscopy is generally required for diagnosis. Patients with positive CMV cultures from respiratory specimens without other identifiable pathogens may have CMV pneumonia, but this can also represent contamination with infected blood or saliva. The presence in lung tissue of pathognomonic cells with intranuclear cytomegalic inclusions is diagnostic. Treatment directed against CMV is available (see Table 91-4), but its efficacy in pneumonia is unproven.

Pulmonary Kaposi's Sarcoma

Kaposi's sarcoma (KS) of the lung has been reported in homosexual men with KS skin lesions. Patients may have extensive parenchymal and endobronchial involvement, causing dyspnea, fever, cough, and wheezing. Chest x-rays often show extensive interstitial or alveolar lesions, or both, with a nodular quality. Associated pleural effusion is common. Unlike patients with *Pneumocystis carinii* pneumonia, 50 to 70 percent of persons with pulmonary KS will have normal A-A gradients, often without postexercise oxygen desaturation. Bronchoscopic examination may show characteristic cherry-red endobronchial lesions. Curiously, attempts to confirm the diagnosis of pulmonary KS histologically from specimens of transbronchial biopsy, pleural biopsy, or pleural fluid cytology have often been unsuccessful. This has been achieved in one study only at autopsy.

Nonspecific Interstitial Pneumonitis

Nonspecific interstitial pneumonitis is a disease entity of unknown cause that has been well described and can produce cough, dyspnea, fever, and hypoxemia in AIDS patients. The clinical and radiographic appearance may be difficult to distinguish from that of *Pneumocystis carinii* or cytomegalovirus pneumonia. Symptoms tend to be milder, and about 50 percent of patients with nonspecific interstitial pneumonitis will have normal chest x-rays. Gallium scan is abnormal in the majority of cases.

Transbronchial biopsy or bronchoalveolar lavage demonstrates diffuse alveolar damage with increased numbers of macrophages, alveolar hemorrhage, or lymphoid aggregates, and no associated microbial pathogens. It is unclear whether this condition develops as a result of previous opportunistic infections, experimental therapy, or Kaposi's sarcoma. Nonspecific interstitial pneumonitis usually stabilizes or resolves without therapy, although it can recur.

Cryptococcosis, Histoplasmosis, and Coccidioidomycosis

Pulmonary cryptococcal disease is uncommon and may present as a subacute pneumonitis. Infiltrates, cavitary nodules, or effusion may be present on chest x-ray. Histoplasmosis generally occurs in persons from endemic areas, such as the Ohio River Valley and Puerto Rico. Coccidioidomycosis is endemic to the southwestern United States. These entities appear radiographically as a diffuse, interstitial fibronodular pattern that is virtually indistinguishable from tuberculosis. Bronchoscopy with biopsy is required for diagnosis. Treatment is outlined in Table 91-4.

Neurologic

Toxoplasmosis

Toxoplasmosis of the central nervous system (CNS) most commonly produces the symptoms of sudden onset of seizures, hemiparesis, headache, and decreased level of consciousness. Symptoms that occur in a minority of patients include fever, isolated visual and speech disturbances, ataxia, Bell's palsy, extrapyramidal movements, numbness, generalized weakness, dizziness, nuchal rigidity, nausea, vomiting, psychosis, and syncope. Patients with focal neurologic findings or other evidence of increased intracranial pressure (i.e., papilledema) should have computed tomographic (CT) examination of the head to rule out mass effect before lumbar puncture is attempted. Results of the CT scan will be abnormal in a majority of cases. Typically, single or multiple lesions can be seen, commonly with surrounding edema. Lesions will most commonly be hypodense or isodense and display ring-like or diffuse contrast enhancement. Rarely, results of CT examination will be normal, and in these cases magnetic resonance imaging should be considered. Cerebrospinal fluid (CSF) findings are not diagnostic since they can be entirely normal, or may show a few mononuclear cells with mildly elevated protein and normal glucose. Rare cases have been reported with large numbers of cells or hypoglycorrhachia. In a recent study the presence of *Toxoplasma* antibody (immunoglobulin G) was found in the CSF of 23 of 37 patients with biopsy-confirmed CNS toxoplasmosis, as opposed to none of 11 control subjects with AIDS alone. Serum *Toxoplasma* antibodies are found in a large proportion of the general population but may be helpful in excluding the diagnosis if absent. A fourfold rise in serum titer over time suggests the presence of active infection. The diagnosis of *Toxoplasma* encephalitis is usually presumed on the basis of clinical findings of focality and CT scan abnormalities.

When there is a high degree of suspicion of *Toxoplasma* encephalitis, it is appropriate to start empiric therapy (see Table 91-4). Clinical response is often prompt. Repeat CT scan should be planned in several days and brain biopsy should be considered if the patient's condition deteriorates or fails to improve after one week.

Cryptococcal Meningitis

Cryptococcal meningitis is frequently seen in AIDS patients. The clinical presentation is often subtle, with insidious progressive headache accompanied by fever, and occasionally nausea and vomiting. Some patients complain of a stiff neck, photophobia, and malaise. A minority have seizures or mental status changes with disturbances of vision or hearing. Computed tomographic examination of the head is most commonly normal, except in a few patients who may show hydrocephalus or lesions representing cryptococcomas. Cerebrospinal fluid most commonly is only mildly abnormal, showing a few mononuclear cells, elevated protein, and normal or depressed glucose. A few patients may mount a more vigorous pleocytosis. Patients with cryptococcal meningitis will have positive CSF and serum cryptococcal antigen titers. The India ink test will usually reveal encapsulated yeast forms, and culture of CSF will be positive in the great majority of patients. A large proportion of patients will have extraneural disease, with involvement of lungs, kidneys, skin, lymph nodes, liver, or other organs in addition to the CNS. Suggested therapy is outlined in Table 91-4.

Central Nervous System Lymphoma

Central nervous system lymphoma has been described in AIDS patients. Presenting symptoms have included subacute onset of progressive personality and behavioral changes, slurred speech, ataxia, apathy, headache, and seizures. Computed tomography generally will reveal single or multiple hypodense, diffusely enhancing lesions with mass effect. Diagnosis is made by brain biopsy. Treatment modalities are outlined in Table 91-4. Response to treatment is generally poor.

Central Nervous System Tuberculosis

Central nervous system tuberculosis in HIV-infected persons may have presenting symptoms of multiple cerebral abscesses, tuberculomas, or meningitis. It tends to be more common among intravenous drug users and recent immigrants from Haiti. The clinical presentation can include seizure, or gradual onset of steadily worsening headache and fever with altered mental status and neck stiffness. Computed tomographic examination may reveal ring enhancing lesions or hypodense areas, or it may be normal. Cerebrospinal fluid typically shows a lymphocytic pleocytosis with low glucose and elevated protein. Polymorphonuclear cells will predominate in a minority of cases and, rarely, there will be no cells. AFB stain of CSF will rarely reveal organisms, though CSF culture for mycobacteria should be positive, the yield increasing if large amounts of fluid (i.e., 10–20 ml), are sent for AFB culture. A past history of pulmonary tuberculosis, a positive purified protein derivative, or an abnormal chest x-ray suggests the diagnosis in the appropriate setting. Central nervous system tuberculosis can be confused with toxoplasmosis, and the decision to treat empirically should be based on the entire constellation of findings. When the diagnosis is unclear, as is often the case, brain biopsy should be considered. The finding of acid-fast bacilli in a specimen of CSF or brain tissue will almost invariably indicate the presence of *Mycobacterium tuberculosis*, as CNS infection with nontuberculous mycobacteria is rare. Suggested therapy is outlined in Table 91-4.

Progressive Multifocal Leukoencephalopathy

Progressive multifocal leukoencephalopathy (PML) is a demyelinating disease of the CNS caused by JC papovavirus. Presenting symptoms can include extremity weakness (hemiparesis or monoparesis), gait disturbance, visual loss, and cognitive dysfunction. Limb dysmetria and dysarthria can also occur. Computed tomographic scan will show nonenhancing, hypodense white-matter lesions, without mass effect in the majority of cases. Cerebrospinal fluid examination is nondiagnostic but may show an elevated protein and a few mononuclear cells. Definitive diagnosis can only be made by brain biopsy. Currently, no effective therapy is available for PML.

AIDS Dementia

AIDS dementia, also known as HIV encephalopathy or subacute encephalitis, is the most common CNS manifestation of AIDS. Patients with this condition have had HIV isolated from brain or cerebrospinal fluid, and the encephalopathy is believed to be caused by primary infection of the brain with HIV.

A slowly progressive subcortical dementia develops over several weeks to months. Apathy, mental slowness, confusion, memory loss, and psychotic behavior can occur. Signs and symptoms can include headache, nystagmus, spasticity, motor weakness, incontinence, hyperreflexia, and upgoing toes. Early in the illness, changes may be subtle. Behavioral symptoms can easily be mistaken for depression, obstinacy, or lack of intellect.

Computed tomographic examination of the head shows diffuse cerebral atrophy in about half of the cases of AIDS dementia. Cerebrospinal fluid may show an elevated protein with mildly depressed glucose and a few mononuclear cells. Diffuse, mild to moderate slowing can be seen on electroencephalography.

The clinical diagnosis of AIDS dementia should be made only after a thorough evaluation is pursued for other potentially treatable causes of neurologic dysfunction. The diagnosis of severe AIDS dementia is often associated with a survival of only a few months.

Other neurologic syndromes believed to be associated with HIV infection of neural tissue include myelopathy with spastic paraparesis and incontinence, peripheral neuropathy with painful distal dysesthesias and numbness, and cranial nerve palsies. There are anecdotal reports of neurologic improvement in these conditions with azidothymidine (AZT) therapy, although this treatment is not effective once far-advanced dementia has already occurred.

Gastrointestinal

Oral and Esophageal Candidiasis

Oral candidiasis is one of the most common clinical manifestations of HIV infection. Patients will often complain of feeling cracks or splits in the mouth. Lesions generally appear as patches of whitish curd-like material on the tongue, buccal mucosa, gingiva, or palate. Involvement may be diffuse or limited to one or two small lesions. The diagnosis should be confirmed by Gram's stain or potassium hydroxide smear of scrapings from affected areas, which will reveal pseudohyphae and budding yeast forms. One study showed that AIDS later developed in 59 percent of patients with unexplained oral candidiasis at a median interval of three months. Therapy is outlined in Table 91-4.

Many patients with oral thrush will also have esophageal candidiasis. This condition may be totally asymptomatic, or it may cause odynophagia, dysphagia, or retrosternal or upper-back pain. A presumptive diagnosis of esophageal candidiasis can be made in the patient infected with HIV who has microscopically documented thrush with odynophagia or dysphagia. Empiric therapy should be instituted in this setting (see Table 91-4). Except in cases of profound dehydration or malnutrition secondary to poor oral intake, most cases of esophageal candidiasis can be managed on an outpatient basis.

Barium swallow can reveal the characteristic "shaggy esophagus," although it can present as plaques, masses, ulcers, or strictures. Esophagoscopy will usually reveal white, plaque-like mucosal lesions, and definitive diagnosis can be made by examination of endoscopic brushings and biopsy specimens. Disease entities that can mimic *Candida* esophagitis include herpes simplex or cytomegalovirus infections and malignancies.

Cryptosporidiosis and Isosporiasis

Cryptosporidia and *Isospora* are related coccidial protozoans that can cause chronic diarrhea in patients with AIDS. Cryptosporidiosis is considerably more common than isosporiasis, and both conditions are diagnosed most frequently in homosexual men and Haitian immigrants. Patients with either condition may have frequent and voluminous watery diarrhea, cramping abdominal pain, weight loss, and dehydration for weeks to months. Fever, leukocytosis, and blood or leukocytes in the stool are uncommon. A peripheral eosinophilia can occur in isosporiasis. Diagnosis can be made by acid-fast staining of a thin smear of stool that has been fixed with methyl alcohol for one minute. Both parasites will stain bright red and are easily distinguished on the basis of size and shape. Isosporiasis responds readily to treatment (see Table 91-4). No effective treatment is currently available for cryptosporidiosis.

Cytomegalovirus Colitis

Gastrointestinal infection with CMV has been reported primarily in homosexual men. Its most frequent manifestation is colitis, although esophagitis, small-bowel infection, and rectal ulcers have been reported. The intensity of the diarrhea in patients with CMV colitis can vary from moderate to severe. Many patients will have several weeks of copious, watery diarrhea containing mucus or blood, with low-grade fever; 10 to 20 stools per day are not uncommon. Weight loss, cramping abdominal pain, and tenesmus may be present. The clinical syndrome is similar to that of ulcerative colitis, and sigmoidoscopy or colonoscopy with biopsy is required to make the diagnosis. Grossly, submucosal hemorrhage or ulcerations, or both, will be seen. Microscopic examination of biopsy specimens will reveal vasculitis with characteristic intracytoplasmic and intranuclear cytomegalic inclusions. A positive viral culture of stool or biopsy specimen for CMV is suggestive but not diagnostic, of this condition. In one series 73 percent of patients showed improvement with therapy (see Table 91-4).

Salmonella

Patients with defects in cell-mediated immunity are predisposed to infection with nontyphoidal salmonellae, and this is also true for patients with AIDS. The species most commonly implicated is *Salmonella typhimurium*. Symptoms include fever; rigors; watery, nonbloody, nonmucoid diarrhea; and abdominal pain. Bacteremic patients may have only high fever and no localized signs or symptoms. There is frequently an associated Coombs-positive hemolytic anemia. This disease in AIDS patients is characterized by a high rate of bacteremia (including breakthrough bacteremia while the patient is receiving antibiotics) and relapse after antibiotics are discontinued. Suggested treatment is outlined in Table 91-4.

Disseminated Mycobacterium Avium-Intracellulare Complex Infection

Disseminated infection with MAI is very common in AIDS patients. This infection was present in 60 percent of subjects in one autopsy series. The direct contribution of MAI to morbidity and mortality is unclear, as it often coexists with other opportunistic infections or malignancies; however, the presence of MAI is associated with a poor prognosis. One study showed an average survival after diagnosis of four months and another showed a maximum survival of seven months. It is uncertain whether patients die "with" this infection or "because" of it. The shortened survival may be related to extreme immunosuppression required for infection with this low-virulence organism, indicative of far-advanced HIV disease.

Clinically, MAI is characterized by weeks to months of high fevers, drenching night sweats, malaise, weakness, diarrhea with malabsorption, and progressive clinical deterioration. Pancytopenia may be present. Liver function tests are frequently abnormal, especially the alkaline phosphatase. Spontaneous remissions and exacerbations are common.

The diagnosis of AIDS is made when MAI is isolated from a deep organ other than lung or lymph node. Blood culture is the diagnostic procedure of choice, but special techniques are required for isolation. Organisms can also be obtained from bone marrow, liver, spleen, and GI tract. Organs are usually heavily infiltrated with organisms, with general absence of typical host response to mycobacteria. The presence of AFB on direct smear of stool is highly sensitive for disseminated infection. The significance of a positive stool culture with a negative smear is less clear.

There are anecdotal reports of combination drug therapy (see Table 91-4) resulting in lysis of fever and clearing of bacteremia in some patients, but as of yet no controlled data support treatment as a general recommendation. Since mycobacteria cannot be initially distinguished, the isolation or demonstration of AFB in a clinical specimen should prompt the institution of empiric antituberculosis therapy until final culture and identification are made.

Slim Disease

Slim disease, or HIV wasting syndrome, has been described primarily in African AIDS patients. Weight loss, cachexia, and chronic diarrhea without apparent cause are present in the setting of HIV seropositivity. Treatment is aimed at maintaining adequate hydration, nutrition, and electrolyte balance.

Gastrointestinal Kaposi's Sarcoma

The sites in the gastrointestinal tract most frequently affected by KS are the small intestine, stomach, and colon. Lesions can appear on the tongue or the oral mucosa. Presenting symptoms may include pain, obstruction, diarrhea, melena, perforation, and peritonitis. Microcytic hypochromic anemia can develop in patients with chronic blood loss.

The radiologic appearance of gastrointestinal KS may be similar to that of other malignancies or colitis. Endoscopy with biopsy is required for diagnosis.

Cutaneous

Kaposi's Sarcoma

Kaposi's sarcoma has been the index diagnosis in 35 to 46 percent of homosexual men with AIDS, but in fewer than 5 percent of AIDS patients in other high-risk groups. Some authorities believe that cytomegalovirus plays an oncogenic role in the development of KS. The extremely high incidence of cytomegalovirus infection in the homosexual population with AIDS may account for the predilection of this group for KS. The most common appearance of KS is violaceous macules or nodules, but the gross appearance of lesions can be quite variable and can mimic numerous other dermatologic conditions. Kaposi's sarcoma can appear anywhere on the skin as single or multiple lesions. The surface may be smooth, ulcerated, crusted, or keratotic. Biopsy is required to make the diagnosis.

It is estimated that 10 to 20 percent of patients with cutaneous KS have internal organ involvement. The lymph nodes, lungs, and GI tract are the sites most frequently affected.

Treatment modalities have included chemotherapy, radiation, and administration of interferon, with mixed results. Except in cases of extensive internal organ involvement, KS is generally not a direct cause of mortality in AIDS patients. Patients with KS lesions as their index diagnosis generally have a longer survival than those with other opportunistic infections or malignancies.

Herpes Simplex and Herpes Zoster

Herpes simplex virus (HSV) and herpes zoster infections in AIDS patients tend to be more frequent and more severe than those in immunocompetent hosts. Oral, genital, perianal, and cutaneous infections with HSV often begin with a sensation of tingling or numbness in the affected area, followed by the development of vesicles, which progress to shallow-based, clearly delineated ulcerations that are often painful. Oral infection with HSV can appear on the lip, palate, tongue, or in other locations in the oral cavity, and must be differentiated from nonherpetic aphthous ulcers, the treatment of which is quite different. Genital infection can be accompanied by tender inguinal adenopathy and dysuria. Anorectal involvement can produce tenesmus, constipation, and neurologic signs indicative of sacral plexus involvement (i.e., impotence, neurogenic bladder, and radiculopathy). Often, herpetic lesions are confused with decubitus ulcers.

Herpetic ulcerations in the normal host crust and heal over within 7 to 10 days. In AIDS patients chronic ulcerations often develop that can become superinfected. Nonhealing, cutaneous HSV infection for four weeks in the setting of HIV seropositivity fulfills the criteria for the diagnosis of AIDS.

Herpes zoster infection occurs frequently in persons with HIV infection. This condition (also known as shingles) begins as pain or tingling over a dermatomal distribution, followed by a localized erythematous papulovesicular rash and worsening pain. HIV-infected patients often have multidermatomal involvement, but generalized dissemination infrequently occurs. Lesions on the tip of the nose indicate involvement of the ophthalmic branch of the trigeminal nerve and should prompt immediate ophthalmologic consultation. Untreated, herpetic keratitis can result in permanent visual loss.

Definitive diagnosis of herpes simplex and herpes zoster can be made by culture, positive Tzanck stain, or biopsy. When there is a strong clinical suspicion, therapy should be started empirically (see Table 91-4). Persons without severe systemic illness can be treated on an outpatient basis.

Miscellaneous Dermatoses

Mild to severe seborrheic dermatitis is often seen in HIV-infected persons. Erythematous, scaling lesions, especially on the face, are present. Onychomycosis, with disfigurement and discoloration of one or many nails, is frequently seen.

Molluscum contagiosum, caused by a poxvirus, appears as round umbilicated papules, 1 to 3 mm in diameter. Individuals with HIV infection may have a few or hundreds of these lesions.

Histoplasmosis, and occasionally cryptococcosis, can have initial symptoms of skin lesions. Biopsy is required for diagnosis. Other dermatoses seen with HIV infection include acneform folliculitis, unusually severe psoriasis, and eosinophilic granuloma. These entities are significant in that they can provide an early clue to the presence of HIV infection when it might otherwise not be suspected.

Ophthalmologic

Cytomegalovirus Retinitis

Cytomegalovirus retinitis is estimated to occur in 15 to 40 percent of patients with AIDS. Affected individuals will complain of blurring or loss of vision, and both eyes will be affected in about half of these patients. Retinal lesions typically will first develop along the vascular arcades, with areas of dense white retinal necrosis, hemorrhage, exudates, and vasculitis. When this condition is left untreated, slow, steady progression to complete retinal destruction and blindness occurs. The inexperienced clinician may be unable to recognize CMV retinitis, and patients suspected of having this condition should be evaluated by an ophthalmologist.

CLINICAL EVALUATION OF SUSPECTED HIV INFECTION

The diagnosis of HIV infection is usually made on the basis of the previously described clinical syndromes. A history of high-risk behavior (see Table 91-1) should increase the clinician's suspicion of HIV infection. In the absence of a documented, major opportunistic infection or malignancy, any of the ARC-associated symptoms (see section on HIV-related illness), especially oral thrush, are important signs to remember. Unexplained anemia, leukopenia, and thrombocytopenia can occur in HIV-infected persons who are otherwise completely asymptomatic. Patients with advanced immunosuppression will have lymphopenia, low absolute numbers of CD4 lymphocytes, and an inverted ratio of CD4 to CD8 lymphocytes. Additionally, the presence of HIV infection can be documented by the detection of antibodies directed against HIV. Most commonly, serum is screened for HIV antibody with an enzyme-linked immunosorbent assay (ELISA) test and positive results are confirmed by Western blot analysis. The test should not be considered positive without Western blot confirmation.

Persons who undergo HIV testing experience severe psychological stress. Written informed consent should be obtained before testing, and information should be given to the patient regarding risk behavior (see Table 91-1) and risk reduction. This would include the consistent use of latex condoms in conjunction with the spermicide nonoxynol 9, which is known to be virucidal. Limiting numbers of sexual partners is extremely important. Referral to a social worker or community-based AIDS organization may be appropriate.

The HIV antibody test should only be employed for specific clinical indications, such as when trying to disentangle a clinical syndrome, or when the patient requests HIV testing. It is not considered appropriate to routinely screen all patients who come to the emergency department.

TREATMENT

Azidothymidine, or zidovudine (Retrovir), is the only drug that is currently approved for the treatment of HIV infection. It has been shown to prolong survival, decrease the incidence of opportunistic infection, and improve the general quality of life for many patients with AIDS and HIV-related illness. However, a significant incidence of toxic side effects is associated with the drug. These can include nausea and vomiting, insomnia, severe headache, myalgias, fevers, rash, lethargy, and agitation. Megaloblastic anemia severe enough to require transfusion and profound leukopenia may occur as side effects of chronic AZT therapy, but these complications have been reduced by revised dosage recommendations. Thrombocytopenia resulting from AZT use is extremely rare. Patients with symptoms of AZT toxicity should have the drug discontinued for several days or until symptoms abate, and then be restarted at a lower dosage. Transfusion is generally reserved for symptomatic individuals. Certain patients will have intolerable toxicity even when receiving low dosages of AZT.

PROGNOSIS

Many treatment modalities, especially the use of AZT and prophylaxis against *Pneumocystis carinii* pneumonia, have only recently come into widespread use. The extent to which these therapies will ultimately decrease morbidity and increase survival in patients with AIDS and HIV-related illness is yet to be determined.

Data derived from a population of homosexual men in San Francisco show that among asymptomatic individuals with HIV infection, AIDS will develop in approximately 50 percent over a 10-year period. Studies are currently under way to determine if AZT therapy can prevent or forestall progression to AIDS in these individuals.

Persons with AIDS who have Kaposi's sarcoma generally survive longer than those with CNS conditions. Among those who have *Pneumocystis carinii* pneumonia, average survival without AZT therapy or prophylaxis against recurrent *Pneumocystis* infection has been approximately one year. It is important to emphasize that duration of survival has improved with the introduction of better treatment modalities. It is anticipated that new therapies will become available in the near future.

TRANSMISSION TO HEALTH-CARE WORKERS

Cumulative studies of approximately 4,000 highly exposed health-care workers, including over 1,000 with a history of accidental needle-stick, showed 4 cases of HIV seroconversion, all following needle-stick accidents. Several additional cases of seroconversion or possible seroconversion have occurred after needle-stick or splash exposure. A study of over 1,000 dental professionals from the New York City area, most of whom had worked without gloves on patients from high-risk groups, found only 1 individual without other known risk factors who had antibodies to HIV. Thus, the risk of HIV acquisition in the health-care setting, while real, is small.

Since most persons with HIV infection are asymptomatic and the prevalence of infection in the United States is likely to increase, it can be anticipated that increasing numbers of persons infected with HIV will be seen in the emergency department for a wide range of HIV related or unrelated complaints. One study indicated an inability to predict in advance which patients seen in the emergency department will be carriers of HIV. Of 2,302 consecutive adult patients seen during a six-week period in an inner-city emergency department in Baltimore in 1987, 119 (5.2%) were seropositive for HIV. Only 27 of these 119 patients had symptomatic HIV infection. The remaining 92 patients, or 77 percent of the seropositives, had unrecognized HIV infection. It is thus important to observe blood and body-fluid precautions for all patients seen in the emergency department. This includes the wearing of gloves when drawing blood or coming in direct contact with blood or any body fluids. Phlebotomy on combative patients should be deferred. Engaging in conversation or other distractions should be avoided during invasive procedures. Meticulous attention should be paid to appropriate disposal of needles and other sharp objects. Needles should not be recapped. Protective eyewear, masks, and gowns should be worn only if splashes or aerosolization of blood or body fluids is anticipated. Spills should be carefully cleaned and disinfected with a 1 : 10 solution of household bleach. These measures will minimize the already low risk of occupational HIV infection without invoking unnecessary excessive measures for those patients perceived to be at high risk.

SELECTED READING

Ackerman, AB, and Gottlieb, G. Atlas of the Gross and Microscopic Features. In G Gottlieb and AB Ackerman (eds), *Kaposi's Sarcoma: A Text and Atlas.* Philadelphia: Lea & Febiger, 1988.

Amazon, K, and Rywlin, AM. Systemic Manifestations. In G Gottlieb and A B Ackerman (eds), *Kaposi's Sarcoma: A Text and Atlas.* Philadelphia: Lea & Febiger, 1988.

Barrio, JL, et al. *Pneumocystis carinii* pneumonia presenting as cavitating and noncavitating solitary pulmonary nodules in patients with the acquired immunodeficiency syndrome. *Am Rev Respir Dis* 134:1094, 1986.

Berger, JR, et al. Progressive multifocal leukoencephalopathy associated with human immunodeficiency virus infection. A review of the literature with a report of sixteen cases. *Ann Intern Med* 107:78, 1987.

Bishburg, E, et al. Central nervous system tuberculosis with the acquired immunodeficiency syndrome and its related complex. *Ann Intern Med* 105:210, 1986.

Bozette, SA, et al. A controlled trial of early adjunctive treatment with corticosteroids for *pneumocystis carinii* pneumonia in the acquired immunodeficiency syndrome. *N Engl J Med* 323:1451, 1990.

Burke, DS, et al. Human immunodeficiency virus infections among civilian applicants for United States military service, October 1985 to March 1986. *N Engl J Med* 317:131, 1987.

Centers for Disease Control. *Tuberculosis, Final Data—United States. MMWR* 36:817, 1986.

Centers for Disease Control. Cases of specified notifiable disease, United States, weeks ending June 4, 1988, and June 6, 1987. *MMWR* 37:347, 1988.

Chachoua, A, et al. 9-(1,3-dihydroxy-2-propoxymethyl) guanine (ganciclovir) in the treatment of cytomegalovirus gastrointestinal disease with the acquired immunodeficiency syndrome. *Ann Intern Med* 107:133, 1987.

Chaisson, RE, et al. Tuberculosis in patients with the acquired immunodeficiency syndrome. *Am Rev Respir Dis* 136:570, 1987.

Collier, AC, and Hansfield, H. Epidemiology. In G Gottlieb and AB Ackerman (eds), *Kaposi's Sarcoma: A Text and Atlas.* Philadelphia: Lea & Febiger, 1988.

Cooper, DA, et al. Acute AIDS retrovirus infection: Definition of a clinical illness associated with seroconversion. *Lancet* 1:537, 1985.

DeJarlais, DC, et al. Kaposi's sarcoma among four different AIDS risk groups (letter). *N Engl J Med* 310:1119, 1984.

De Lorenzo, LJ, et al. Roentgenographic patterns of *Pneumocystis carinii* pneumonia in 104 patients with AIDS. *Chest* 91:323, 1987.

Dreizen, S. Oral candidiasis. *Am J Med* Candidiasis Symposium 77:28, 1984.

Drew, WL, Buhles, W, and Erlich, KS. Herpesvirus infections (cytomegalovirus, herpes simplex virus, varicella-zoster virus). How to use ganciclovir (DHPG) and acyclovir. *Infect Dis Clin North Am* 2:495, 1988.

Eng, RHK, et al. Cryptococcal infections in patients with acquired immune deficiency syndrome. *Am J Med* 81:19, 1986.

Fiala, M, et al. Responses of neurologic complications of AIDS to 3′-azido-3′ deoxythymidine and 9-(1,3-dihydroxy-2-propoymethyl) guanine. I. Clinical features. *Rev Infect Dis* 10:250, 1988.

Fischl, MA, et al. Salmonella bacteremia as manifestation of acquired immunodeficiency syndrome. *Arch Intern Med* 146:113, 1986.

Fischl, MA, et al. The efficacy of azidothymidine (AZT) in the treatment of patients with AIDS and AIDS-related complex. A double-blind, placebo-controlled trial. *N Engl J Med* 317:185, 1987.

Fischl, MA, et al. Randomized controlled trial of reduced daily dose of zidovudine in patients with the acquired immunodeficiency syndrome. *N Engl J Med* 323:1009, 1990.

Gelmann, EP, et al. Combination chemotherapy of disseminated Kaposi's sarcoma in patients with the acquired immunodeficiency syndrome. *Am J Med* 82:456, 1987.

Gerberding, JL. Occupational health issues for providers of care to patients with HIV infection. *Infect Dis Clin North Am* 2:321, 1988.

Glaser, JB, et al. Recurrent *Salmonella typhimurium* bacteremia associated with the acquired immunodeficiency syndrome. *Ann Intern Med* 102:189, 1985.

Goddell, SE, et al. Herpes simplex bronchitis in homosexual men. Clinical, sigmoidoscopic, and histopathologic features. *N Engl J Med* 308:868, 1983.

Goodman, PC, Daley, C, and Minagi, H. Spontaneous pneumothorax in AIDS patients with *Pneumocystis carinii* pneumonia. *AJR* 147:29, 1986.

Gottlieb, MS, et al. *Pneumocystis carinii* pneumonia and mucosal candidiasis in previously healthy homosexual men. *N Engl J Med* 305:1425, 1981.

Greenspan, D, et al. Relation of oral hairy leukoplakia to infection with human immunodeficiency virus and the risk of developing AIDS. *J Infect Dis* 155:475, 1987.

Handwerger, S, et al. Tuberculosis and the acquired immunodeficiency syndrome at a New York City hospital. 1978–85. *Chest* 91:176, 1987.

Haverkos, HW. Assessment of therapy for *Toxoplasma* encephalitis. *Am J Med* 82:907, 1987.

Henderly, DE, et al. Cytomegalovirus retinitis and response to therapy with ganciclovir. *Ophthalmology* 94:425, 1987.

Hessol, NA, et al. The natural history of HIV infection in a cohort of homosexual and bisexual men: A decade of follow-up (abstract). Presented at the Fourth International Conference on AIDS, Stockholm, Sweden, 1988.

Ho, DD, Pomerantz, RJ, and Kaplan, JC. Pathogenesis of infection with human immunodeficiency virus. *N Engl J Med* 317:278, 1987.

Ho, DD, et al. Primary human T-lymphotropic virus type III infection. *Ann Intern Med* 103:880, 1985.

Ho, DD, et al. Isolation of HTLV-III from cerebrospinal fluid and neural tissues of patients with neurologic syndromes related to the acquired immunodeficiency syndrome. *N Engl J Med* 313: 1493, 1985.

Jacobs, JL, et al. Salmonella infections in patients with the acquired immunodeficiency syndrome. *Ann Intern Med* 102:186, 1985.

Jacobson, MA, and Mills, J. Serious cytomegalovirus disease in the acquired immune deficiency syndrome. *Ann Intern Med* 108:585, 1988.

Jeren, T, and Beus, I. Characteristics of cerebrospinal fluid in tuberculous meningitis. *Acta Cytol* 26:678, 1982.

Kaplan, LD, et al. Kaposi's sarcoma involving the lung in patients with the acquired immunodeficiency syndrome. *J Acq Imm Def Syn* 1:23, 1988.

Kelen, GD, Fritz, S, and Qaqish, B. Unrecognized human immunodeficiency virus infection in emergency department patients. *N Engl J Med* 318:1645, 1988.

Kiehn, TE, et al. Infections caused by *Mycobacterium avium* complex in immunocompromised patients. Diagnosis by blood culture and fecal examination, antimicrobial susceptibility tests, and morphological and seroagglutination characteristics. *J Clin Microbiol* 21:168, 1985.

Klein, RS, et al. Oral candidiasis in high-risk patients as the initial manifestation of the acquired immunodeficiency syndrome. *N Engl J Med* 311:354, 1984.

Klein, RS, et al. Low occupational risk of human immunodeficiency virus infection among dental professionals. *N Engl J Med* 318:1645, 1988.

Kovacs, JA, et al. Cryptococcosis in the acquired immunodeficiency syndrome. *Ann Intern Med* 103:53, 1985.

Levine, AE, et al. Development of B-cell lymphoma in homosexual men. Clinical and immunologic findings. *Ann Intern Med* 100:7, 1984.

Levine, MS, Macones, AJ, and Laufer, I. *Candida* esophagitis: Accuracy of radiographic diagnosis. *Radiology* 154:581, 1985.

Levy, RM, and Bredesen, DE. Central Nervous System Dysfunction in Acquired Immunodeficiency Syndrome. In M L Rosenblum, RM Levy, and DE Bredesen, *AIDS and the Nervous System.* New York: Raven, 1988.

Macphail, L, et al. HSV types in oral and pharyngeal ulcers in association with HIV infection. In Abstracts of the Fourth International Conference on AIDS, Stockholm, Sweden, 1988.

McArthur, JC, and Johnson, RT. Primary Infection with Human Immunodeficiency Virus. In ML Rosenblum, RM Levy and DE Bredesen (eds), *AIDS and the Nervous System.* New York: Raven, 1988.

Meduri, GU, et al. Pulmonary Kaposi's sarcoma in the acquired immune deficiency syndrome. Clinical, radiographic and pathologic manifestations. *Am J Med* 81:11, 1986.

Meiselman, MS, Cello, JP, and Margaretten, W. Cytomegalovirus colitis—report of the clinical, endoscopic and pathologic findings in two patients with the acquired immune deficiency syndrome. *Gastroenterology* 88:171, 1985.

Miller, RG, et al. Peripheral Nervous System Dysfunction in Acquired Immunodeficiency Syndrome. In ML Rosenblum, RM Levy, and DE Bredesen (eds), *AIDS and the Nervous System.* New York: Raven, 1988.

Mills, J. *Pneumocystis carinii* and *Toxoplasma gondii* infections in patients with AIDS. *Rev Infect Dis* 8:1001, 1986.

Pitchenik, AE, and Robinson, HA. The radiographic appearance of tuberculosis in patients with the acquired immune deficiency syndrome (AIDS) and pre-AIDS. *Am Rev Respir Dis* 131:393, 1986.

Pitchenik, AE, et al. Sputum examination for the diagnosis of *Pneumocystis carinii* pneumonia in the acquired immunodeficiency syndrome. *Am Rev Respir Dis* 133:226, 1986.

Polsky, B, et al. Bacterial pneumonia in patients with the acquired immunodeficiency syndrome. *Ann Intern Med* 104:38, 1986.

Potasman, I, et al. Intrathecal production of antibodies against *Toxoplasma gondii* in patients with toxoplasmic encephalitis and the acquired immunodeficiency syndrome (AIDS). *Ann Intern Med* 108:49, 1988.

Richman, DD, et al. The toxicity of azidothymidine (AZT) in the treatment of patients with AIDS and AIDS-related complex. A double-blind, placebo controlled trial. *N Engl J Med* 317:192, 1987.

Roberts, C. Coccidioidomycosis in acquired immunodeficiency syndrome. *Am J Med* 76:743, 1984.

Rothenberg, R, et al. Survival with the acquired immunodeficiency syndrome. Experience with 5833 cases in New York City. *N Engl J Med* 317:1297, 1987.

Saltzman, BR, et al. Factors that predict survival of AIDS patients:

Experience at a single New York City medical center (abstract). Presented at the Fourth International Conference on AIDS, Stockholm, Sweden, 1988.

Simberkoff, MS, et al. *Streptococcus pneumoniae* infections and bacteremia in patients with acquired immune deficiency syndrome, with report of a pneumococcal vaccine failure. *Am Rev Respir Dis* 130:1174, 1984.

Sindrup, JH, Lisby, G, and Weismann, K. Skin manifestations in AIDS, HIV infection, and AIDS-related complex. *Int J Dermatol* 26:267, 1987.

Small, CB, et al: Pulmonary cryptococcosis in AIDS patients (abstract). Presented at the 27th Interscience Conference on Antimicrobial Agents and Chemotherapy, New York, 1987.

Soave, R. Cryptosporidiosis and isosporiasis in patients with AIDS. *Infect Dis Clin North Am* 2:485, 1988.

Soave, R, and Johnson, WD. *Cryptosporidium* and *Isospora belli* infections. *J Infect Dis* 157:225, 1988.

Steigbigel, NH, and Friedland, GH. Acquired immunodeficiency syndrome. *Curr Ther Infect Dis* 2:94, 1986.

Suffredin, AF, et al. Nonspecific interstitial pneumonitis: A common cause of pulmonary disease in the acquired immunodeficiency syndrome. *Ann Intern Med* 107:7, 1987.

Sunderam, G, et al. Tuberculosis as a manifestation of the acquired immunodeficiency syndrome (AIDS). *JAMA* 256:362, 1986.

Tindall, B, Barker, S, and Donovan, B. Characterization of the acute clinical illness associated with human immunodeficiency virus infection. *Arch Intern Med* 148:945, 1988.

Tindall, B, Cooper, DA, and Donovan, B. Primary human immunodeficiency virus infection. Clinical and serologic aspects. *Infect Dis Clin North Am* 2:329, 1988.

Trier, JS, and Bjorkman, DJ. Esophageal, gastric, and intestinal candidiasis. *Am J Med* 77:39, 1984.

Wanke, C, et al. *Toxoplasma* encephalitis in patients with acquired immune deficiency syndrome: Diagnosis and response to therapy. *Am J Trop Med Hyg* 33:509, 1987.

Wheat, LJ, Salma, TG, and Zeckel, ML. Histoplasmosis in the acquired immunodeficiency syndrome. *Am J Med* 78:203, 1985.

Whimby, E, Kiehn, TE, and Armstrong, D. Disseminated *Mycobacterium avium-intracellulare* Disease: Diagnosis and Therapy. In JS Remington and MN Swartz, *Current Clinical Topics in Infectious Diseases* 7:112, 1986.

Wong, B, et al. Central nervous system toxoplasmosis in homosexual men and parenteral drug users. *Ann Intern Med* 100:36, 1984.

Young, LS, et al. Mycobacterial infections in AIDS patients, with an emphasis on the *Mycobacterium avium* complex. *Rev Infect Dis* 8:1024, 1986.

Zuger, A, et al. Cryptococcal disease in patients with the acquired immunodeficiency syndrome. *Ann Intern Med* 104:234, 1986.

B. Acute Hematologic Disorders

92. Acute Hematologic Emergencies

D. Gary Gilliland
David Rosenthal

ANEMIA

Anemia is not a disease but a manifestation of an underlying disorder that causes blood loss, increased red cell destruction, or decreased red cell production. It is defined in a clinical laboratory as a decrease in the hematocrit or hemoglobin level. The *hematocrit* is a volume measurement that estimates the red cell volume as a fraction of the total blood volume. A hematocrit of less than 40 percent in men or 36 percent in women indicates anemia. The *hemoglobin* is a concentration measurement and is usually expressed in grams per deciliter of blood. The range of values of normal hemoglobin in men is usually 14 to 18 gm/dl and in women is 12 to 16 gm/dl. Red blood counts (RBC) are not as accurate a guide in the diagnosis of anemia as are the hemoglobin and hematocrit because of variations in the hemoglobin content of individual red blood cells. For example, a patient with classic iron-deficiency anemia may have a normal number of red blood cells, but these cells will be smaller than normal (causing a decreased hematocrit) and contain little hemoglobin (producing decreased hemoglobin concentration).

There are three categories of anemia:

1. Blood loss: acute or chronic
2. Anemia of decreased red cell production
   a. Iron deficiency (microcytic anemia)
   b. Vitamin B_{12} or folate deficiency (macrocytic anemia)
   c. Bone-marrow infiltration or aplasia (normochromic, normocytic anemia)
3. Anemia of increased red cell destruction
   a. Loss of red cells through excessive bleeding (e.g., gastrointestinal, hematuria, trauma)
   b. Loss of red cells because of inherent red cell defects in the membrane, hemoglobin, or enzymes or because of environmental attacks on the red cells that shorten normal life span (e.g., hemolysis)

Evaluation of the Patient with Anemia

History and Physical Examination

Anemia may be recognized by the emergency physician because of patient complaints or the presentation. Fatigue, weakness, and increased respiratory or cardiac symptoms are nonspecific complaints and will vary depending on the severity and rapidity of onset of the anemia. Pallor, tachycardia, scleral icterus, and splenomegaly are findings that may alert the physician to anemia. When the hematocrit is reduced below 30 percent, the general symptoms are fatigue, exertional dyspnea, weakness, and dizziness. If the hemato-

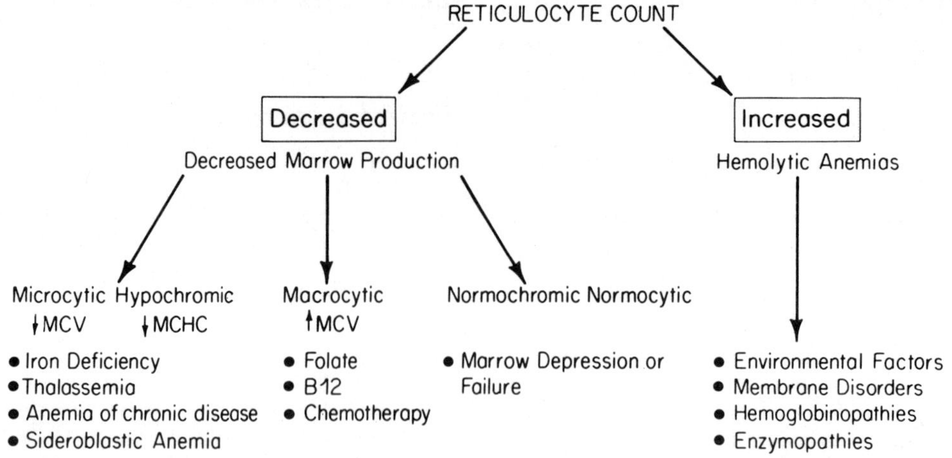

Fig. 92-1. Schematic approach to anemia based on the reticulocyte count, morphology, and indexes. (MCV = mean cell volume; MCHC = mean corpuscular hemoglobin concentration.)

crit is below 18 percent or the hemoglobin is less than 7 gm/dl dyspnea, tachycardia at rest, and a roaring sensation in the ears will usually develop. If anemia has developed gradually, the patient may be able to compensate sufficiently so that only minimal symptoms will be present even though the hemoglobin is less than 10 gm/dl. When it is below 7 gm/dl, all patients will have complaints regardless of the duration of the anemia.

If the anemia develops abruptly, as in acute blood loss or acute hemolysis, symptoms are related to loss of blood volume as well as to reduction of oxygen-carrying capacity. Significantly smaller decreases in red blood cell mass may produce symptoms that would not occur if the anemia developed gradually.

In the patient with acute blood loss, the hemoglobin and hematocrit measurements should not be used as the major or only guide in initial management, since these tests are not accurate indicators of total blood volume and do not change until after compensatory mechanisms restore intravascular volume. Fluid shifts between intravascular and extravascular compartments occur during the first four to eight hours after blood loss but can happen more rapidly when intravenous fluid replacement is used.

In patients with acute blood loss, postural changes in blood pressure and pulse or other evidences of shock are much more accurate indicators of the degree of blood loss. In the normal physiologic situation, blood pressure is slightly increased when the patient is standing. If blood volume has been lost abruptly, the blood pressure will decrease and the pulse rate will increase when the patient assumes a sitting or standing position. A decrease of more than 10 mm Hg in the systolic pressure or a rise in the pulse rate of 10 beats per minute or more indicates a significant loss of blood volume. Pallor, sweating, or possibly dizziness indicates a loss of at least 15 percent of the blood volume. A loss of 25 percent of the blood volume is suggested if postural hypotension is found in the range of 20 to 30 mm Hg. The loss is probably 50 percent or more if evidence of shock is seen when the patient is in the recumbent position.

Specific symptoms on history-taking and findings on physical examination may help to find the cause of anemia. Increased bruising or bleeding associated with significant postural hypotension suggests acute blood loss. Anemias of decreased production, such as iron-deficiency or vitamin B_{12} deficiency, also may have characteristic findings. For example, a sore beefy red tongue, cracking at the angles of the mouth (angular stomatitis), spooning of the nails, a craving for ice, and dysphagia strongly suggest severe iron deficiency. Lack of vitamin B_{12} can be suggested clinically by staggering gait, smooth tongue, or early graying of the hair. Many of the hemolytic anemias produce symptoms of scleral icterus or splenomegaly, or both.

Laboratory Evaluation

If acute blood loss has been excluded and the patient does not require urgent replacement of blood volume, the clinician should turn to the characterization of the anemia. Anemias can be classified both physiologically (decreased production vs increased destruction) and morphologically. They are characterized by the hemoglobin, hematocrit, red blood cell count, red blood cell indexes, reticulocyte count, and red blood cell morphology. The white blood cell count, white blood cell differential, and platelet count may add valuable clues in diagnosis.

The reticulocyte count, normally 1.0 to 1.5 percent, is an indirect measurement of bone-marrow function. It is decreased in anemias caused by lack of production of mature red cells and is increased in acute blood loss (hemorrhage or hemolysis). When the bone marrow is stimulated by a low hematocrit, at least a 48-hour lag is required before the reticulocyte count begins to rise. Figure 92-1 illustrates how the reticulocyte count aids a physician in determining whether the anemia is a result of decreased production (absolute decrease in the number of reticulocytes) or increased destruction or hemolysis (moderate to marked increase in reticulocytes).

By evaluating the red blood cell indexes and examining the peripheral blood smear, the decreased-production anemias can be further subclassified morphologically as hypochromic and microcytic, normochromic and normocytic, or macrocytic (see Fig. 92-1). When the complete blood count (CBC) is obtained from an automated counter, the indexes are automatically calculated. The mean cell volume (MCV)

Table 92-1. Red blood cell indexes

Index	Equation	Normal range
Mean corpuscular volume	$\frac{\text{Hematocrit} \times 10}{\text{RBC (in millions/mm}^3\text{)}}$	80–90 μm^3
Mean corpuscular hemoglobin	$\frac{\text{Hemoglobin (gm/100 ml)} \times 10}{\text{RBC (in millions/mm}^3\text{)}}$	27–31 pg hemoglobin per cell
Mean corpuscular hemoglobin concentration	$\frac{\text{Hemoglobin (gm/100 ml)} \times 100}{\text{Hematocrit}}$	32–36% (or gm hemoglobin per 100 ml RBC)

indicates size of the red blood cells and is the most accurate of the indexes (Table 92-1). A hypochromic, microcytic anemia would be characterized by a reduced MCV, mean corpuscular hemoglobin (MCH), and MCH concentration (MCHC); the peripheral blood smear should demonstrate small red blood cells with decreased hemoglobin (Fig. 92-2B). On a blood smear the normal red blood cell should be the size of the nucleus of an adult lymphocyte (Fig. 92-2B). An elevated MCV and the finding of large red blood cells in the peripheral blood smear would indicate a macrocytic anemia (Fig. 92-2C).

Microcytic, hypochromic anemias are most frequently caused by iron deficiency, which in adults is almost always a result of chronic blood loss (see Fig. 92-1). Less commonly in the United States, microcytic, hypochromic anemias are caused by thalassemia, chronic inflammatory disease, or sideroblastic anemia.

Macrocytic red blood cells in the presence of decreased reticulocytes suggest folate or vitamin B_{12} deficiency although it is not unusual for liver disease to cause this finding. Macrocytosis can also develop in patients who are receiving chemotherapy. In the presence of an elevated reticulocyte count, the MCV may be elevated and the cells appear large since young red blood cells (reticulocytes) are larger than old cells.

Normocytic, normochromic anemias can also be associated with a decreased reticulocyte count. The red blood cells that are produced are normal but are reduced in numbers because of marrow suppression or failure. Search for a diagnosis in these cases usually requires further investigative studies including bone-marrow examination.

Hemolytic anemia is suggested by the findings of decreased hematocrit and increased reticulocyte count in the absence of bleeding. Hemoglobin degradation in hemolytic anemia leads to indirect bilirubinemia, which causes the common clinical manifestation of jaundice. Associated changes produced by hemolysis include splenomegaly, increased serum lactate dehydrogenase, increased urinary urobilinogen, leukocytosis, and thrombocytosis. Polychromatophilic red blood cells are often seen in the peripheral smear. As red cells are destroyed in the circulation, free hemoglobin is released into the plasma. This can impart a pink-colored serum, small amounts of which can be measured in the laboratory using a spectrophotometer. Hemoglobinuria causes a brownish discoloration of urine.

The cause of the hemolytic anemia can be determined using the general scheme outlined in Fig. 92-3. Evaluation of the peripheral blood smear is the most helpful initial test in delineating the cause of hemolytic anemia. In evaluating the peripheral blood smear, the clinician should look for the presence of spherocytes (see Fig. 92-2D), target or sickle cells (see Figs. 92-2C, F), and schistocytes (see Fig. 92-2G). Spherocytosis suggests either an autoimmune hemolytic anemia or hereditary spherocytosis. As seen in the schematic approach in Fig. 92-3, the diagnostic test for immunohemolytic anemia is the direct Coombs' test, which detects the presence of either antibody or complement on the red blood cell surface. If Coombs' test is negative, an osmotic fragility test will help distinguish patients with hereditary spherocytosis from those with enzyme deficiencies that cause spherocytosis. Increased osmotic fragility would strongly suggest the diagnosis of hereditary spherocytosis. If the blood smear primarily shows normal red cells with rare spherocytes, enzyme deficiency may be the cause of the hemolysis. In glucose-6-phosphate dehydrogenase (G6PD) deficiency, "bite" cells may be noted on the blood smear. The two most common enzyme deficiencies, G6PD and pyruvate kinase, can be diagnosed by enzyme assays. G6PD deficiency is exacerbated by a variety of drugs (Table 92-2). A history for possible ingestion of these drugs should be obtained in an individual in whom an enzyme deficiency is suspected.

Target cells on blood smears are associated with abnormal hemoglobins, and sickle cells imply the diagnosis of sickle cell anemia. Hemoglobin electrophoresis or Sickle-dex test, or both, will detect most hemoglobinopathies. The appearance of schistocytes or helmet cells in a peripheral smear should suggest a traumatic or microangiopathic hemolytic anemia.

Microcytic, Hypochromic Anemias

Microcytic, hypochromic anemias have normal deoxyribonucleic acid (DNA) synthesis but disordered production of hemoglobin. Major causes include disordered iron metabolism, as in iron deficiency or anemia of chronic disease; disordered heme synthesis, as in sideroblastic anemias; and disordered globin synthesis, as in thalassemias. Microcytosis usually accompanies hypochromic anemia. Red cells on a smear thus appear small and pale. Laboratory values that correlate with this are decreased MCH, reflecting a low hemoglobin content, and MCV, reflecting a low red-cell volume.

Iron deficiency is a common cause of hypochromic anemia and should be documented with iron, total iron-binding capacity (TIBC), and ferritin levels. An iron:TIBC ratio of less than 10 percent in combination with low serum ferritin levels provide strong evidence for iron-deficiency anemia. If tests are not inclusive, a bone-marrow aspirate for stainable iron should be performed to delineate between iron-deficiency and sideroblastic anemia. Iron deficiency is often

concentration (MCHC)	Hematocrit	per 100 ml of RBC

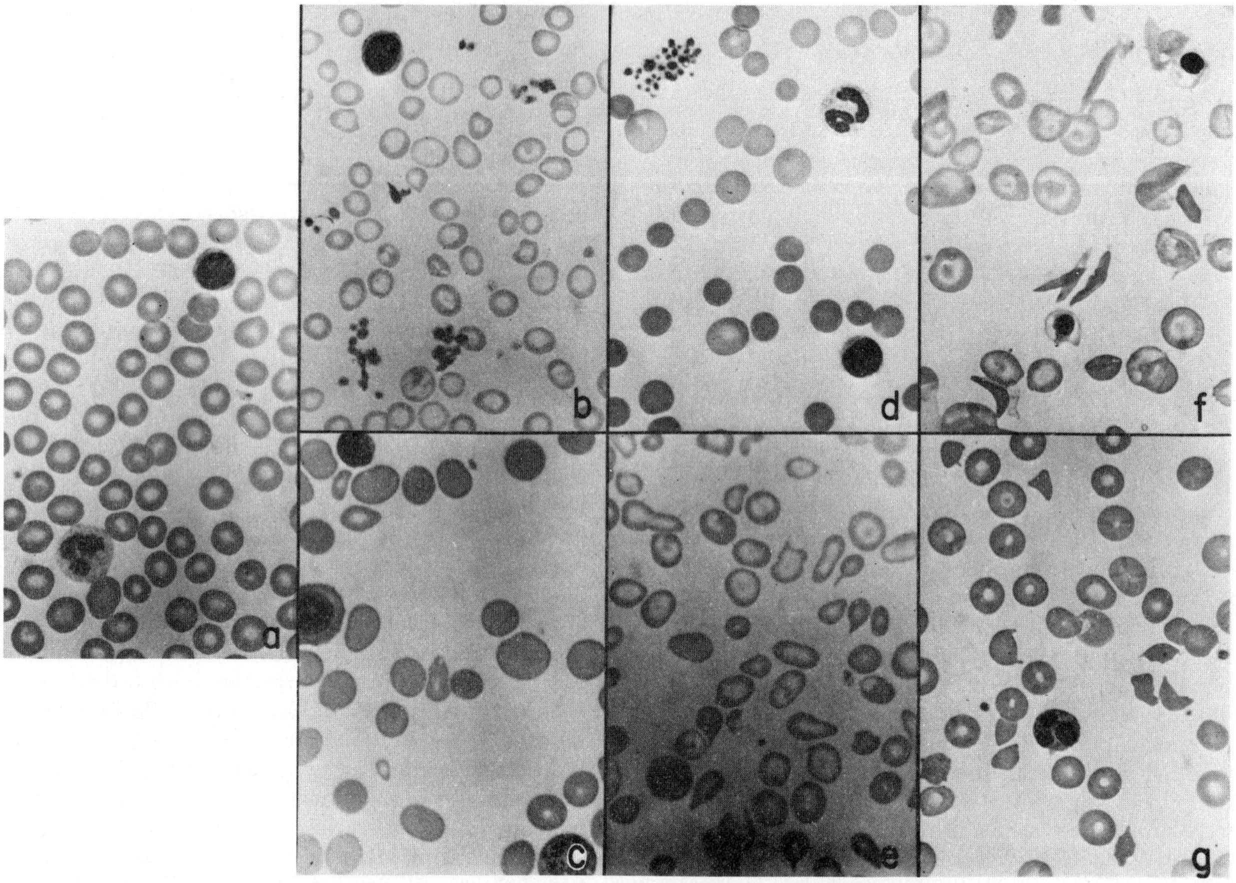

Fig. 92-2. Peripheral blood smears and their value in diagnosis. a. Normal. b. Hypochromia and microcytosis of iron deficiency. c. Macrocytosis of megaloblastic anemias. d. Spherocytosis. e. Target cells with hypochromia and microcytosis of thalassemia. f. Sickle cells and targets in sickle cell syndromes. g. Fragmented cells, schistocytes, helmet cells in microangiopathic hemolysis. (From D.S. Rosenthal. Problems Involving an Abnormal Blood Count. In W.T. Branch [ed.], *Office Practice of Medicine.* Philadelphia: Saunders, 1982. P 1030.)

the first indication of gastrointestinal bleeding. Blood loss that results in iron deficiency can be caused by hemorrhoids, diverticulosis, duodenal and gastric ulcers, ulcerative colitis, gastrointestinal neoplasms, and, in tropical areas, parasitic infection, especially hookworm.

Menstrual blood loss is a common cause of iron deficiency in women. Other less common causes of iron-deficiency anemia include frequent blood donation, hemoglobinuria, factitious anemia from self-induced blood-letting, and hereditary hemorrhagic telangiectasia. Iron replacement may be initiated when appropriate laboratory tests have been completed (e.g., ferrous gluconate, 324 mg, three times a day for one month followed by 324 mg every day). Reticulocytosis will occur within five to seven days, followed by gradual improvement in anemia. In rare cases, transfusion therapy may be necessary when anemia is severe and associated with serious clinical manifestations (such as myocardial ischemia, congestive heart failure, cerebrovascular insufficiency, or severe dyspnea).

Thalassemias are a heritable cause of microcytic, hypochromic anemia that are characterized by defective synthesis of either the alpha- or beta-globin chains or normal hemoglobin A (α_2,β_2). When these chains are not synthesized in coordinate fashion, production of normal $\alpha_2\beta_2$ tetramers is decreased. Erythropoiesis is thus ineffective, and cells are made that contain little hemoglobin and are often small and pale. Unbalanced synthesis can lead to precipitation of alpha or beta chains within the red cell, causing red cell survival to be short.

Molecular pathology of these disorders is highly heterogenous but has been extensively characterized. Unbalanced production of alpha- or beta-globin genes can be caused by structural gene deletions, unequal crossover events, or single nucleotide mutations in messenger ribonucleic acid (mRNA). Genetic defects that cause decreased alpha-globin production cause alpha-thalassemia; those that give rise to decreased beta-globin production cause beta-thalassemia. Beta-thalassemia is common in northwestern Africa and a

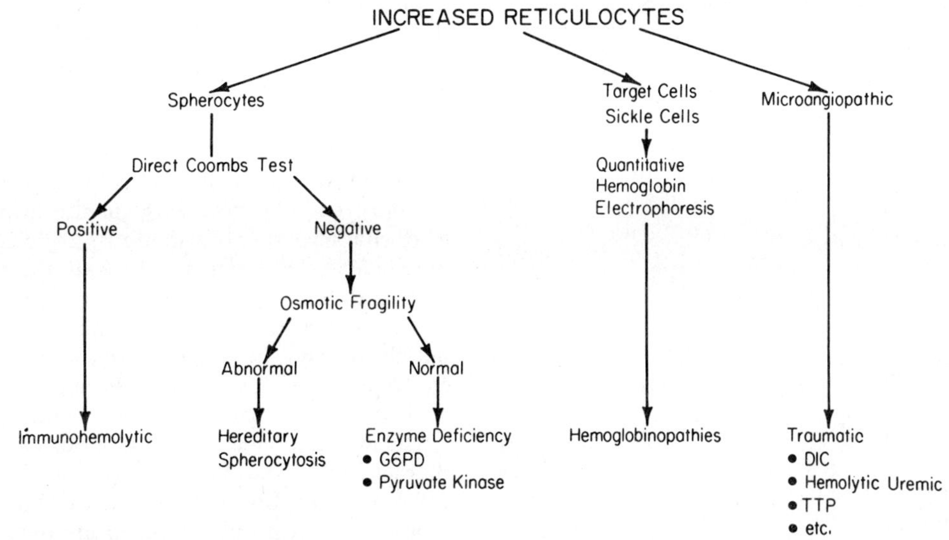

Fig. 92-3. Schematic approach to the workup and laboratory evaluation of hemolytic anemias. (DIC = disseminated intravascular coagulation; TTP = thrombotic thrombocytopenic purpura.)

Table 92-2. Agents and disorders associated with hemolysis in G6PD deficiency

Antimalarials	Antibacterials
Primaquine	Chloramphenicol
Quinacrine	Nalidixic acid
Chloroquine	Nitrofurantoin
Sulfonamides	Miscellaneous drugs
Sulfanilamide	Acetylsalicylic acid
Sulfapyridine	Acetophenetin
Sulfisoxazole	Methylene blue
Chemicals	Ascorbic acid
Benzene	Infections
Naphthalene	Hepatitis
Diabetic acidosis	

mild form affects 25 to 30 percent of black Americans. Beta-thalassemia also occurs in individuals from southeast Asia, where the frequency in some populations exceeds that of the normal genotype. Prevalence of thalassemia worldwide has been attributed to the protection it offers against malarial infection.

Beta-thalassemia is diagnosed through hemoglobin electrophoresis, which shows an increase in HbA_2, the minor hemoglobin of adults. Unfortunately, hemoglobin electrophoresis is not useful in diagnosing mild forms of alpha-thalassemia, and diagnosis relies on exclusion of iron-deficiency anemia, beta-thalassemia, and sideroblastic anemia in conjunction with a compatible ethnic origin.

No therapy is necessary for thalassemia heterozygotes. In fact, iron therapy is contraindicated in these individuals, since they do not respond and may become iron overloaded.

Sideroblastic anemias are disorders in which defective heme biosynthesis leads to anemia with decreased hemoglobin production. It is an acquired disorder in adults and can be idiopathic, drug related, or secondary to myelodysplastic syndromes. A bone-marrow biopsy will demonstrate less than 10 percent ringed sideroblasts and is required for diagnosis.

Perhaps of most importance in the acute setting are secondary sideroblastic anemias, which are caused by toxic effects of drugs on heme biosynthesis. Drugs that are commonly involved include antituberculous agents such as isonicotinic acid hydrazide (INH), chloramphenicol, and chemotherapeutic agents. Alcohol and chronic lead poisoning can also cause acquired sideroblastic anemias.

Defective heme biosynthesis in sideroblastic anemias leads to decreased hemoglobin production, with increased iron stores. During red cell maturation, surplus iron accumulates within mitochondria. The build-up of iron in mitochondria gives rise to unique arcs of Prussian blue–positive granules, creating an apparent ring around the nucleus. These ring sideroblasts are characteristic of the sideroblastic anemias and, when present in greater than 10 percent of bone marrow erythroblasts, are considered diagnostic.

Therapy in secondary sideroblastic anemias is directed toward removal of the causative agent. Occasionally, patients with sideroblastic anemia respond to pharmacologic doses of pyridoxine (vitamin B_6). When anemia is severe and symptomatic, transfusion therapy may be necessary. Iron is of no benefit and should be avoided in these individuals.

"Anemia of chronic disease" is a vague term applied to the hematologic syndrome that is seen in association with chronic inflammatory disease malignancy. The primary defect is lack of iron reutilization. The hematocrit shows a modest anemia, with levels rarely ranging below 30 percent. Other causes of anemias should be carefully excluded before this diagnosis is assigned.

Macrocytic Anemias

Macrocytic or megaloblastic anemias are commonly caused by folate or vitamin B_{12} deficiencies (Table 92-3). These are both essential cofactors for synthesis of DNA, so that a lack in one of these vitamins affects all cells in the body with rapid turnover rate, such as bone marrow and intestinal mucosal cells. Impaired DNA synthesis with normal RNA-directed synthesis of cytoplasmic components generates

Table 92-3. Common causes of megaloblastic anemia

Vitamin B_{12} deficiency
Dietary deficiency (vegans)
Deficiency of gastric intrinsic factor
Pernicious anemia
Gastrectomy
Intestinal malabsorption
Resected or diseased ileum
Competitive parasites/infections
Fish, tapeworm
Bacterial overgrowth
Folate deficiency
Nutritional
Impaired absorption (phenobarbitol, diphenylhydantoin, contraceptives)
Folate antagonists
Methotrexate
Increased demand
Hemolytic anemia
Pregnancy, infancy

progeny with excess cytoplasm and aberrant nuclear chromatin. This leads to morphologic characteristics of megaloblastic anemia, which can be seen in bone marrow aspirates and peripheral blood smears. Myeloid and erythroid cells in bone marrow have fewer divisions during development and result in cells that are large, appearing either as macrocytic red blood cells or hypersegmented polymorphonuclear leukocytes. Vitamin B_{12} and folate deficiency will also affect intestinal mucosal cells and may give class III or IV cytologies from gastric aspirates or Papanicolaou smears.

The most common cause of vitamin B_{12} deficiency is pernicious anemia, an acquired deficiency of gastric intrinsic factor. Most patients with pernicious anemia possess serum antibodies to the gastric parietal cell, which secretes intrinsic factor. Pernicious anemia may thus be an autoimmune disease. In association with megaloblastic anemia, vitamin B_{12} deficiency can also cause a neurologic syndrome, consisting of central nervous system irritability and depression, together with loss of position and vibratory sense in the hands and feet. Other causes of vitamin B_{12} deficiency include gastrectomy with loss of parietal cells, intestinal malabsorption either from resected or diseased ileum, competitive infections, or parasites. Rarely, vitamin B_{12} deficiency is caused by dietary deficiency. This is limited to vegetarians who abstain from eggs and milk (vegans). Although vitamin B_{12} deficiency is still rare in this population, it should be noted that offspring who are breastfed by mothers who are vegans can develop a severe megaloblastic anemia.

The most common cause of folate deficiency is dietary lack of the vitamin. Folate is present in leafy vegetables, meats, yeast, and dairy products but, since it is heat labile, overcooking can destroy the vitamin. Poor diet can lead to macrocytic anemia within six to eight weeks. In addition to dietary deficiency, folate can be decreased by interference with other medications, most commonly phenobarbitol, phenytoin (Dilantin), and contraceptives. Individuals with increased demand, including those with hemolytic anemias, pregnancy, and malignancies (especially myeloproliferative disorders), can also become folate deficient.

Clinical and Laboratory Presentation

High output failure with gradually progressive shortness of breath may be the presenting manifestation in patients with either folate or vitamin B_{12} deficiency. The skin may be lemon colored because of a combination of pallor and indirect bilirubinemia. A depapillated smooth tongue, slight splenomegaly, absence of olfactory sense, and absence of vibratory and position sense in the lower extremities are other characteristics of vitamin B_{12} deficiency. Physical signs in folic acid deficiency are those of a nutritional deficiency such as weight loss or cachexia. In a few patients with vitamin B_{12} deficiency, the neurologic symptoms may be more significant than the degree of macrocytic anemia. Rarely, a patient may have loss of vibratory and position sense because of vitamin B_{12} deficiency in the absence of anemia.

The anemia, often severe with decreased reticulocytes, is characterized by a macrocytosis and often accompanied by neutropenia or thrombocytopenia, or both. A bone marrow aspirate is necessary to confirm the diagnosis, and the patient should be referred immediately for this procedure. Morphologic changes in the marrow are diagnostic in megaloblastic anemia, but vitamin B_{12} and folate levels are required to differentiate the vitamin-deficiency state; blood samples to determine the levels should be obtained before any treatment is instituted. In vitamin B_{12} deficiency, a Schilling test may also be necessary to differentiate the cause of the deficiency. In this test orally ingested radioactive vitamin B_{12} will appear in the urine if intrinsic factor is present and the ileum is intact. If an abnormally low amount of radioactivity is present in the urine, the defect will be corrected in classic pernicious anemia by the simultaneous ingestion of oral intrinsic factor. Nonspecific abnormalities include increased serum lactic acid dehydrogenase (LDH) and indirect bilirubinemia.

Therapy

Patients are often started on both vitamin B_{12} and folate therapy. This practice arose because of concerns of exacerbating vitamin B_{12} deficiency (especially neurologic manifestations) with folate replacement alone. This complication is less likely now because of current rapid reporting of blood values. Patients should be treated with vitamin B_{12} and folate only if they are deficient in both. Recommended folate replacement is usually 1 mg a day orally, but individuals with active hemolysis may require as much as 5 mg a day. Vitamin B_{12} is given subcutaneously in a dose of 100 μg. Initially, and especially with combined vitamin B_{12} and folate, daily vitamin B_{12} injections are recommended for two weeks, and maintenance therapy is adequately accomplished by 100 to 1,000 μg subcutaneously monthly or bimonthly.

Prognosis

Therapeutic response in megaloblastic anemias is fairly rapid. Reticulocytes rise within three to five days, followed by a gradual increase in the hemoglobin and hematocrit as well as the white blood cell platelet counts. Complications can occur with treatment of older patients. Congestive heart failure can develop as a result of the abrupt increase in hemoglobin and hematocrit since, before therapy, volume expansion will have compensated for the gradually dropping red blood cell mass. Transfusions are usually withheld for the same reason unless oxygen-carrying capacity has been significantly impaired and produces problems, such as angina. With treatment, the serum potassium level can drop because of a sudden transfer of electrolytes into the intracellular space as therapy begins to stimulate DNA synthesis.

Abnormal gastric cytology or cervical Papanicolaou smears should be repeated after completion of therapy. An upper gastrointestinal series should be performed in any patient with persistently abnormal cytology because of the association of gastric neoplasm with pernicious anemia. In addition, because of the association of myxedema and hypothyroidism with megaloblastic anemias, routine thyroid studies should be obtained. Much of the evaluation of patients with macrocytic anemias can be initiated in the emergency department, with eventual referral to the specialist for marrow examination or therapy.

Hemolytic Anemia

Hemolytic anemia is defined as a falling hematocrit associated with increased reticulocyte count in the absence of bleeding. A cause for hemolytic anemia should be determined using the algorithms described previously. Causes of hemolytic anemias are diverse and include defects in the red cell membrane, immunologic destructions of red cells, genetic defects in glycolytic enzymes, Heinz body hemolytic anemia, abnormal hemoglobins, traumatic anemias, and anemias from infection of red cells. Table 92-4 gives a partial list of causes of hemolytic anemias.

Table 92-4. Causes of hemolytic anemias

I. Environmental factors
  A. Immunohemolytic anemias
    1. Idiopathic or primary
    2. Symptomatic or secondary
      a. Malignant lymphoproliferative disorders
      b. Chronic lymphocytic leukemia
      c. Other neoplasms
      d. Medications
      e. Systemic lupus erythematosus
      f. Other autoimmune disorders
      g. Infections (infectious mononucleosis, mycoplasmal pneumonia)
    3. Transfusion reactions—incompatibility
  B. Traumatic hemolysis (microangiopathic)
    1. Burns
    2. Disseminated intravascular coagulation
    3. Thrombotic thrombocytopenic purpura
    4. Malignant hypertension
    5. Metastatic carcinoma
    6. Abnormal prosthetic heart valve
    7. Hemolytic uremia syndrome
    8. March hemoglobinuria
  C. Infections
    1. Malaria
    2. Clostridia

II. Abnormalities of the red blood cell membrane
  A. Hereditary spherocytosis
  B. Paroxysmal nocturnal hemoglobinuria

III. Hemoglobinopathies
  A. Sickle cell anemia
  B. Thalassemias

IV. Red blood cell enzyme deficiencies
  A. Glucose-6-phosphate dehydrogenase deficiency
  B. Pyruvate kinase

Hemolytic Anemias Caused by Defects in Red Cell Membranes: Hereditary Spherocytosis

Hereditary spherocytosis is an autosomal dominant hemolytic anemia with spherocytosis, jaundice, and splenomegaly. It is almost invariably corrected by splenectomy. Severity of anemia will vary, and it can be asymptomatic and clinically silent for long periods. However, as with other hemolytic anemias, an aplastic crisis can be precipitated by any agent that causes marrow suppression, such as drugs and viral infections, among other causes. Other hereditary diseases that lead to increased hemolysis of red cells are rare and include hereditary elliptocytosis, acanthocytosis, stomatocytosis, and hereditary pyropoikilocytosis.

Hemolytic anemias can be caused by abnormal anaerobic glycolysis. Because mature red cells are completely dependent on glycolysis for generation of adenosine triphosphate (ATP) and self-survival, defects in any of the enzymes of the Embden-Meyerhof pathway will lead to decreased ATP synthesis and decrease cell survival with hemolysis. Enzymes that have been characterized as causing genetic deficiencies include pyruvate kinase, hexokinase, phosphofructokinase, aldolase, and phosphoglycerate kinase, among others. Although these disorders are relatively uncommon, they should be considered in a differential diagnosis of hemolytic anemias.

Heinz Body Hemolytic Anemias, Including G6PD Deficiency

Heinz body hemolytic anemia refers to the presence of a precipitated form of hemoglobin that can be seen with supravital staining of red cells. This represents precipitated hemoglobin due to oxidative damage. Hemolysis occurs presumably because dense, nondeformable Heinz body–containing cells are unable to pass through normal capillary beds. Drugs and chemicals that cause Heinz body hemolytic anemia are those that induce oxidative stress on the cell. These drugs overwhelm the ability of the red cell to generate reducing agents in the form of glutathione. Hemolysis due to oxidative stress can also be caused by a defect in the enzymes responsible for generating glutathione, including those in the hexose monophosphate shunt. By far the most common of these enzyme deficiencies is G6PD deficiency, which affects more than 100 million people, mostly black men. Most patients with G6PD deficiency do not ordinarily have chronic hemolysis but are susceptible to oxidant stress from drugs listed in Table 92-2. These include antimalarial agents, sulfonamides, sulfones, analgesics, antipyretics, and nitrofurans. In individuals of Mediterranean descent, hemolysis may be severe. In particular, devastating hemolysis can be caused by exposure to the fava bean.

Hemolytic Anemias Caused by Infections of Red Cells

Infection of red cells by protozoans is probably the most common cause of hemolytic anemia worldwide. Malaria has a prevalence of 300 million cases and is probably the most common protozoan infection of red cells. Malaria is transmitted by the bite of a female *Anopheles* mosquito, which also serves as reservoir for the organism. Malaria is caused by sporozoites from the genus *Plasmodium.* As was noted earlier, genetic mechanisms of resistance can include thalassemia, G6PD deficiencies, and hemoglobin S. Hematologic findings of malarial infection include anemia, reticulocytosis, spherocytosis, splenomegaly, and decreased red cell survival. Hemolysis with malaria is rarely associated with positive Coombs' tests and must be distinguished from immunohemolytic causes of hemolytic anemia.

Intravascular hemolysis, or so-called blackwater fever, is an unusual manifestation of falciparum malaria. Attacks are characterized by fulminant hemolysis with hemoglobinuria, jaundice, and hypovolemic collapse. Renal failure often occurs and mortality is approximately 20 to 30 percent. Blackwater fever is unlikely to be related to severe parasitemia. However, it is often seen after individuals who intermittently take quinine take another dose of this drug. There is no clear explanation for these attacks although they may have an immunologic basis.

Babesiosis is a relatively uncommon infection from the protozoan *Babesia,* which is seen in certain parts of North America. It is transmitted to humans by a tick. The sporozoite from *Babesia* penetrates the red cell membrane and generates characteristic ring forms and tetrads in red cells of affected patients. Hemolytic anemias caused by *Babesia* can be severe, with massive intravascular hemolysis. Other protozoan infections including leishmania and bacterial infections from *Bartonella bacilliformis* occur more rarely.

Immunohemolytic Anemias

In this class of anemias, red cell destruction is caused by antibodies directed against the red cell surface. Hemolysis occurs after attachment of antibody to the red cell surface. With antibodies of the immunoglobulin M (IgM) class, agglutination with complement activation causes red cell lysis. With antibodies of the IgG class, red cells are recognized and cleared by the reticuloendothelial system, with hemolysis usually in splenic tissue. These antibodies have classically been referred to as either "cold-acting antibodies," which are usually IgM, or "warm-acting antibodies," which are usually IgG. Autoimmune hemolysis from IgG can be idiopathic, drug induced by a wide variety of drugs, or associated with lymphoproliferative disorders and other diseases, including connective-tissue disorders and infection.

Sickle Cell Anemia

Sickle cell anemia is an inherited disorder of the hemoglobin molecule that can be associated with severe hemolysis. It results from a single amino acid substitution of valine for glutamic acid in the beta chain, causing the hemoglobin to become susceptible to polymerization in the deoxygenated state. Polymerization of hemoglobin inside red blood cells produces cells that are elongated and crescent in shape (sickle cells). As red blood cells sickle in vivo, they become rigid and do not easily pass through the microcirculation. Occlusion of the microvasculature by sickled cells produces the symptoms of sickle cell disease.

Patients who are homozygous for hemoglobin S (Hb S) develop sickle cell anemia with all of its clinical manifestations. Patients who are heterozygous for Hb S can be detected in vitro when their red blood cells are exposed to low oxygen tension; however, sickle trait does not usually produce any clinical disease. When Hb S trait is associated with some other hemoglobin abnormality such as hemoglobin C (Hb C) or thalassemia, a clinical picture indistinguishable from homozygous Hb S may be produced.

DIAGNOSIS. The signs and symptoms of sickle cell anemia may begin in an infant at approximately six months of age, when the normal switch from fetal hemoglobin to adult hemoglobin occurs. The disease produces both chronic and acute problems. Because the patient has a chronic hemolytic anemia, the manifestations of chronic anemia may be seen: cardiomegaly, chronic heart failure, pulmonary disease, and hepatomegaly. Except in infants, splenomegaly is not seen because of repeated splenic infarctions, resulting in a small fibrotic organ.

Many organ systems can be affected by sickle cell anemia. In infants and young children, the painful "hand-foot syndrome" (dactylitis) results from the vasoocclusion of nutrient arteries of the metatarsal and metacarpal bones. The child usually has painful swelling of hands and feet and bone infarction can develop. In the kidney, necrosis of the renal medulla can occur from hypoxia and hyperosmolarity. Decreased urine specific gravity (less than 1.010) is almost universal. Papillary necrosis can result in occasional episodes of gross hematuria and in rare cases of renal colic. In the eye, retinal infarcts and retinitis proliferans can occur. Aseptic necrosis and bone infarcts can result from vasoocclusive events in bone. Osteomyelitis, especially as a result of salmonellae, is not uncommon. Hepatocellular disease with persistent elevations of the serum glutamic oxaloacetic transaminase (SGOT) and LDH occurs with frequency.

Since hemolysis causes increased indirect bilirubinemia, patients with sickle cell anemia frequently develop calcium bilirubinate gallstones and obstructive jaundice. Central nervous system involvement can result in cranial nerve palsies, hemiplegia, blindness, aphasia, and occasionally coma or convulsions. Other troublesome complications include priapism and recurrent leg ulceration, rather than embolization. Pneumonia, especially secondary to pneumococcus, is a serious and not infrequent complication of sickle cell disease.

If the diagnosis of sickle cell disease has not been made previously, an evaluation of the blood smear may be satisfactory to make a diagnosis of a sickle cell syndrome so that therapy can be initiated. The presence of sickle cells in the peripheral blood smear is diagnostic. Recognition of sickle cell disease in the emergency department can be accomplished by the fairly reliable sodium metabisulfate method or by commercially available kits such as the Sickle-dex test. When a drop of red blood cells containing Hb S is mixed with a drop of reducing agent such as sodium metabisulfate on a glass slide, the cells will sickle and can be directly observed under the microscope after 15 to 30 minutes. The Sickle-dex test is based on the decreased solubility of the Hb S in high-phosphate buffer solutions. To make a definitive diagnosis of homozygous sickle cell disease and to distinguish it from the trait of the other sickle cell syndromes such as sickle cell thalassemia, hemoglobin electrophoresis is necessary.

Although the patient is susceptible to many acute problems, there are three common and debilitating sickle cell syndromes: painful crisis, aplastic crisis, and sickle lung syndrome. *Painful crisis* is a result of vasoocclusion of the microcirculation by sickled cells. Patients complain of a sudden pain in muscles, bones, chest, and abdomen. Many patients have typical crises in which their pain is located in the same place each time; however, pain can be located anywhere or in any combination of areas. Painful crises can be precipitated by situations in which hypoxia occurs. Crises can also be precipitated by fever, infection, dehydration, or acidosis. Although a precipitating event cannot always be determined, a thorough evaluation for a cause must be made, since the precipitating event must be rectified before the patient will recover from the crisis.

A patient who experiences painful crisis frequently has fever, leukocytosis, and tachycardia. Since these are the symptoms and signs associated with infection, it may be difficult to exclude infection as a precipitating event. A careful examination and appropriate cultures are mandatory. A leukocyte alkaline phosphatase (LAP), when available, may be a useful laboratory test. In general patients with sickle cell anemia have a low LAP score and will have an elevation of the score when infection is present. If a baseline LAP is available on the patient for comparison, this test can be particularly helpful.

The treatment of painful crisis in sickle cell anemia should be directed at correction of any precipitating event and relief of pain with analgesics; severe pain usually requires narcotics. A combination of meperidine (Demerol) and promethazine hydrochloride (Phenergan) is usually satisfactory. Good hydration is essential. Intravenous fluids should be administered to accomplish this; the amount depends on the degree of dehydration and the age and condition of the patient. Emergency therapies of questionable benefit include oxygen and alkalinization. There is no definite proof that oxygen benefits painful crisis; however, it generally does no harm and in the presence of cardiopulmonary disease or pneumonia it may be given liberally. Acidosis can result in precipitation of a painful crisis and, when present, should be corrected. When acidosis is not present, the use of alkalinization has not been shown to be of benefit. Transfusions are recommended if the crisis does not terminate within a reasonable period of time. When necessary, the patient should be transfused with packed red blood cells, which will reduce the patient's sickle cell concentration.

Aplastic crisis is a life-threatening complication of sickle cell disease. Because of ongoing hemolysis, most patients with sickle cell disease have reticulocyte counts that range from 5 to 15 percent. During an aplastic crisis, the reticulocyte count may drop to 0.5 percent or less. The hematocrit in this setting can rapidly drop from 25 to 30 percent down to 10 percent or less, which threatens the patient's survival. White cells and platelets are rarely suppressed; rather, there appears to be a selective deficiency in production of reticulocytes by erythroid precursors. Folate deficiency should be excluded as a cause of aplastic crisis (all patients with sickle cell disease should receive chronic folate therapy for ongoing hemolysis). Because aplastic crisis can be associated with painful crisis, patients with painful crisis should be monitored carefully for a decrease in reticulocyte count, which could presage a fall in hematocrit. Patients with aplastic crisis are treated by red cell transfusions. The key point in management is early recognition of aplastic crisis so that transfusion therapy can be initiated before severe morbidity or mortality occurs.

Sickle lung syndrome is characterized by fever, leukocytosis, pulmonary infiltrate, cough, and chest pain. The differential diagnosis includes bacterial pneumonia and pulmonary thromboembolism. Features that favor a diagnosis of pneumonia include age 25 years or older, rigors, upper-lobe disease, greater than 1,000 bands/μl, erythrocyte sedimentation rate greater than 20, neutrophils in sputum Gram's stain, and positive blood-sputum cultures. Features that favor infarction include lower-lobe disease, a clear chest roentgenogram at presentation, associated painful bony crisis, and mismatched ventilation-perfusion defect. Ventilation-perfusion studies are especially useful if a prior study in the patient is available, since many patients have recurrent episodes that cloud interpretation of these studies. Baseline ventilation-perfusion scans should be obtained in patients who have had an episode of pneumonia-infarction. Angiography should be avoided, since contrast dye can exacerbate pulmonary sickling. Antibodies for pneumonias should be given with consideration for common pathogenic organisms in sickle cell patients. In adults, *Staphylococcus aureus* and *Haemophilus* are more common than pneumococci. Pulmonary thromboembolus is treated with heparin.

PROGNOSIS. Often, the treatment of patients with sickle cell disease has only been by intermittent emergency department care, necessitated by crises, symptoms of anemia, or infections. It is important to recognize that the patient with sickle cell anemia needs coordinated and continued total care by physicians, nurses, and social workers, with the goal of preventing complications of the disease. With good supportive care, early therapy of crises, and hypertransfusion when needed, patients with sickle cell disease can live longer.

Microangiopathic Hemolytic Anemia

A variety of causes of microangiopathic hemolytic anemias are listed in Table 92-4. These include disseminated intravascular coagulation (DIC), malignant hypertension, disseminated carcinoma, thrombotic thrombocytopenic purpura, immunologic vasculitis, and mechanical cleavage such as that seen with mechanical valve prosthesis. When the peripheral smear suggests microangiopathic hemolytic anemia, a search should be initiated for the cause as many of the causes of this disorder can be life threatening.

Hemolytic anemia can be caused by cardiac prostheses, high pressure within the ventricles, and particularly a pressure gradient across the aortic outflow tract. Shearing of red cells by these mechanical forces is increased during exercise or any high cardiac output state. If the outflow track is narrowed, calcified, or altered by the presence of aortic valve prosthesis, hemolytic anemia can result. Less commonly, this type of anemia occurs after mitral valve replacement, particularly if there is regurgitant flow around the prosthesis or after unsuccessful valvuloplasty. Immediately after operation, hemolytic anemia is often mild or absent, but it may increase after discharge when the patient becomes more active and cardiac output increases.

Mild compensated hemolysis is a common finding in these patients, especially those with aortic valve prostheses. However, sudden onset of severe hemolysis and anemia almost certainly signifies significant prosthetic dysfunction and should be immediately investigated, as severe anemia in this group of patients can be life threatening. Patients with hemolytic anemia related to the prosthetic valve should receive supplemental iron to offset urinary losses of iron and hemoglobin.

DISSEMINATED INTRAVASCULAR COAGULATION. Intravascular coagulation leads to diffuse deposition of fibrin in the microvasculature, with subsequent vascular impediment to flow of red cells and fragmentation. DIC is most commonly caused by infection, obstetric complications, or disseminated carcinoma. However, it can also occur after transfusion, snake bite, heat stroke, burns, or hypothermia.

Infections. DIC is a common feature of septicemia induced by gram-negative bacteria. This is thought to be related to the presence of endotoxin, although consumptive coagulopathy can also be seen in infections from organisms that lack endotoxin. Endothelial cell injury can precipitate a cascade of coagulation, eventually leading to platelet aggregation and consumption. DIC associated with sepsis can be associated with hypoxia, acidosis, and shock, and prompt treatment of DIC and the underlying condition is imperative.

Obstetric Disorders. Abruptio placentae is commonly associated with DIC. The disorder is often related to shock from internal and external hemorrhage. DIC with thrombocytopenia contributes to the bleeding dyscrasia. Usually, it is rapidly improved by evacuation of the uterus. Therapy with fresh frozen plasma, platelets, and red cell transfusions may be warranted, but primary consideration should be given to treatment of the underlying disorder.

If pregnancy is complicated by *eclampsia* or severe preeclampsia, intravascular coagulation can also occur. This may be related primarily to hypertensive damage to arteriolar walls, but intravascular coagulation also contributes. Severe anemia and thrombocytopenia may be seen. Some patients benefit from heparin administration. However, immediate attention should be directed toward treatment of eclampsia.

Malignant Hypertension. Hemolysis in malignant hypertension is likely related to hypertensive damage to arterioles. It may be significant in malignant hypertension but rapidly resolves when blood pressure control is achieved.

Disseminated Carcinoma. DIC has been associated with disseminated carcinomas of lung, breast, and pancreas, and with acute promyelocytic leukemias. However, it may be seen in association with virtually any type of carcinoma. The combination of DIC and bone marrow involvement can cause severe anemia in these patients. It is possible that phospholipids released by tumor cells trigger thromboplastin release with resultant DIC. In addition, circulating microemboli can also contribute to injury of red cells. Treatment of DIC in this setting is difficult, usually because the underlying carcinoma is often advanced and not easy to treat. Heparin benefits some patients, but in many cases supportive transfusion therapy, fresh frozen plasma, and other supportive care are necessary. Long-term effectiveness of these treatments is minimal unless the underlying carcinoma can be effectively treated.

THROMBOTIC THROMBOCYTOPENIC PURPURA. Thrombotic thrombocytopenic purpura, a rare type of microangiopathic hemolytic anemia, is a disorder of young adults. Its hallmarks include microangiopathic hemolytic anemia and thrombocytopenic purpura, central nervous system crisis (e.g., stroke), fever, and renal failure. This combination of findings is seen in most patients with this disorder. Clinical manifestations include those of thrombocytopenia, with petechiae, ecchymoses, and gastrointestinal bleeding. Unusual central nervous system manifestations are thought to be related to thrombosis in the cerebral vasculature. The symptoms may wax and wane, and create unusual manifestations, including dysphasia, seizures, visual field defects, and hemiparesis. Renal dysfunction is also thought to be caused by thrombotic events in the microvasculature of the kidney and eventually can result in proliferative glomerular changes.

The cause of thrombotic thrombocytopenic purpura (TTP) is unclear. It may be immunologically mediated, and some have suggested that it is precipitated by drugs including oral contraceptives, viral infections, or immunologic vasculitis. Laboratory findings include those characteristic of hemolytic anemias. In contrast with DIC, the prothrombin time, reticulocytosis, hyperbilirubinemia, schistocytes, and increased LDH, as well as decreased hemoglobin, are often normal. The association of schistocytes, thrombocytopenia, and the clinical manifestations mentioned previously strongly suggests the diagnosis of TTP.

TTP is a rare disorder that was once universally fatal. Prognosis for untreated patients is less than 10 percent survival at one year; however, prompt recognition of this syndrome with initiation of appropriate therapy leads to long-term remissions in most patients. The mainstay of treatment of TTP is plasma exchange transfusion, which should be instituted as soon as possible after the diagnosis is confirmed. This should be continued on a daily basis until there is evidence of remission of clinical symptoms. Other therapies that have been used in conjunction with plasma exchange transfusion include aspirin and dipyridamole, as well as steroids. The benefit of these agents has been controversial. Because of the life-threatening nature of this disorder in young adults, these drugs are often given in conjunction with plasma exchange transfusion. There is no evidence that continued treatment with aspirin or other antiplatelet agents over the long term contributes to enduring remissions, and these agents should be discontinued after remission is obtained. In the emergency department the most important point is early recognition of the syndrome and prompt initiation of plasma exchange transfusion.

HEMOLYTIC-UREMIC SYNDROME. Hemolytic-uremic syndrome is closely related to TTP but usually affects infants and children. Renal manifestations are more severe and prevalent in children than in adults and central nervous system complications are less common. Treatment should focus on management of renal failure. Children with anuria for more than 24 hours with clinical signs of anemia should be considered for dialysis. Although many patients require dialysis, most will recover renal function with the appropriate therapy. Therapy remains controversial, with some success reported using antiplatelet agents. The value of heparin is less certain although plasma exchange transfusion, as with TTP, often provides marked improvement in hematologic renal function.

OTHER CAUSES. Other causes of microangiopathic hemolytic anemia include immune vasculitis, giant hemangiomas, exertional hemoglobinuria, severe burns, and hemolysis from toxins. Exertional hemoglobinuria is commonly seen in young athletes, such as marathon runners, who engage in prolonged athletic events. Episodes of hemolysis are usually transient and resolve with cessation of exercise; however, transient hemoglobinuria may be noted. Changing the type of shoe in some runners seems to help this process as red cells may be destroyed in blood that perfuses the soles of the feet. Burn patients show characteristic findings on peripheral smears, with very small spherocytes and spheroidal fragments accompanied by small, very irregularly shaped cells that are peculiar to severe burns. Treatment is aimed at the therapy of the underlying burn. Clostridial sepsis with *Clostridium perfringens* will cause severe intravascular hemolysis, which can be fatal. This complication can follow septic abortions, perforation of the gastrointestinal tract, or gangrenous tissue growth. Hemolysis, which can cause death within hours, is produced by the action of phospholipase on the lipid bilayer of the red cell. Fresh-spun blood plasma is deep red, and lysis may be observed to progress even in the tube. Therapy must be initiated immediately. Patients should be treated with transfusion and antibiotics and surgically treated as soon as possible to avoid death. Snake bites and spider bites can also cause modest hemolytic anemias, which are usually not life threatening and are self-limited.

HYPERVISCOSITY DISORDERS

When the blood becomes thick or viscous, secondary to elevations of the red blood cell mass (erythrocytosis) or to abnormal or increased levels of certain proteins (myeloma, Waldenström's macroglobulinemia, or cryoglobulinemia), symptoms such as lethargy, malaise, blurred vision, bleeding, thrombosis, delirium, and occasionally coma can develop. The onset can be acute or insidious but is often life threatening. These disorders can be recognized and evaluated in the emergency department, and therapy can be initiated there.

Polycythemia

Polycythemia is an increase in the red blood cell mass. It can be recognized by the results on hematocrit or hemoglobin testing. *Polycythemia,* and its synonym *erythrocytosis,* does not specify a specific disease entity but can be caused by a variety of conditions. As indicated in Table 92-5, a distinction can be made between relative and absolute polycythemia, as well as between primary and secondary polycythemia. Absolute polycythemia represents those diseases in which there is an absolute increase in the red blood cell mass. Relative polycythemia refers to conditions in which the red blood cell mass is normal but plasma volume is decreased, producing pseudopolycythemia. Primary polycythemia (polycythemia rubra vera) is one of the chronic myeloproliferative disorders, in which an elevated hematocrit occurs as a result of abnormal proliferation of all the marrow elements. It is not due to increased erythropoietin levels. Secondary polycythemia occurs as a response to increased amounts of erythropoietin. The secondary polycythemias can be further subclassified into those disorders that result from an appropriate increase in erythropoietin secretion (e.g., disorders associated with hypoxia) and those conditions in which erythropoietin is produced inappropriately (e.g., as from tumors or renal problems, or both).

Table 92-5. Classification of polycythemia

- I. Relative polycythemia
  - A. Stress
  - B. Dehydration
  - C. Diuretic therapy
  - D. Burns
- II. Absolute polycythemia
  - A. Primary—polycythemia vera
  - B. Secondary
    - 1. Decreased oxygen transport—appropriate erythropoietin stimulation
      - a. High altitude
      - b. Impaired ventilation
        - Chronic obstructive pulmonary disease
        - Pickwickian syndrome
        - Postural hypoxemia
      - c. Cardiovascular disorders
        - Cyanotic congenital heart disease
        - Septal defects
        - Fallot's tetralogy
        - Atrioventricular intrapulmonary aneurysms
        - Hemangiomas
      - d. Impaired hemoglobin function
        - Congenital methemoglobinemia
        - Congenital hemoglobinopathy with high oxygen affinity
        - Intense cigarette smoking
    - 2. Inappropriate erythropoietin production
      - Malignancy: kidney, hepatoma, adrenal, lung
      - Benign tumors: uterine fibroids, cerebellar, hemangioma, pheochromocytoma, Cushing's syndrome
      - Renal: cysts, hydronephrosis, Bartter's syndrome, transplantation

Relative Polycythemia

Relative polycythemia is a distinct and commonly encountered entity that is also referred to as "stress erythrocytosis." It is not a primary disease process and may be nothing more than a normal physiologic state in which the plasma volume is slightly decreased and the red cell mass is normal.

With stress erythrocytosis patients are often overweight, nervous, hypertensive, and prone to thromboembolic complications. The hematocrits rarely exceed 60 percent and usually range between 50 and 60 percent although other blood parameters are normal. Clinical manifestations of headache and itching are less severe than may be noted in patients with polycythemia rubra vera, and diagnosis may be distinguished only by red blood cell mass measurement and lack of splenomegaly. The complications are not hematologically related, and reduction of red blood cell volume by means of phlebotomy or chemotherapy is not appropriate. However, the hypertension may require aggressive management.

Secondary Polycythemias

The most common cause of secondary polycythemia is chronic hypoxemia secondary to chronic obstructive pulmonary disease. In some instances, the hemoglobin has been reported to be as high as 24 gm/dl and hematocrit as high as 75 percent. However, most patients with polycythemia as a result of chronic obstructive lung disease have hematocrits that do not exceed 57 percent and hemoglobins of 17 gm/100 ml or less.

Another cause of secondary polycythemia is cyanotic congenital heart disease. Hematocrits as high as 65 percent and hemoglobins greater than 20 gm/dl may be seen. The most common cardiac defects that produce these elevations are pulmonary stenosis, accompanied by interatrial or ventricular septal defect, complete transposition of the great vessel, Fallot's tetralogy, or persistent truncus arteriosis.

Some hemoglobin variants cause a shift in the hemoglobin-oxygen dissociation curve such that the hemoglobin molecule does not easily release oxygen to tissues, resulting in relative tissue hypoxia. Compensation by increase in the hemoglobin concentration or blood flow is the available mechanism to maintain oxygen delivery. It appears that the primary response is erythropoietin mediated.

Polycythemia can also occur secondary to inappropriate or nonphysiologic erythropoietin production—for example, as a result of tumors, renal cysts, or hydronephrosis. In some instances, after renal transplantation the hematocrit levels may be excessive and threaten kidney rejection.

CLINICAL PRESENTATION AND DIAGNOSIS. Hyperviscosity can occur as the hematocrit increases above 60 percent. Although the erythrocytosis may be compensating for chronic arterial hypoxemia, unduly increased blood volumes are undesirable. The optimal hemoglobin level in patients with cyanotic congenital heart disease and other chronically hypoxemic states is poorly defined. Cardiac function may be compromised because of both the load and viscosity of the blood. Ruddy cyanosis, headache, dizziness, roaring in the ears, thrombotic episodes, and bleeding are the major clinical findings.

Most patients with polycythemia can be evaluated as outpatients, but the workup can be started in the emergency department. The evaluation should be initiated with a complete history, physical examination, and a complete blood count including a platelet count. These studies may separate the secondary polycythemias from polycythemia rubra vera. After these initial studies, a hematologist should be consulted to determine the need for further study, such as a red blood cell mass or arterial blood gas determinations.

THERAPY. When a patient has symptoms of hyperviscosity or thrombotic or bleeding complications, urgent therapy may be required. Phlebotomy is the most rapid way to reduce the blood volume and symptoms. Later, appropriate investigations should be carried out to find the cause of the erythrocytosis. Prognosis depends on the underlying disorder.

Polycythemia Rubra Vera

Polycythemia rubra vera is a myeloproliferative disorder and results in many laboratory abnormalities in addition to erythrocytosis. Thrombocytosis, leukocytosis, elevated LAP activity, elevated levels of serum vitamin B_{12} and unsaturated B_{12} binding proteins, along with splenomegaly and pruritus, may be noted.

DIAGNOSIS. If erythrocytosis is accompanied by an increased red blood cell mass, a normal arterial oxygen saturation, and splenomegaly, the diagnosis of polycythemia rubra vera can be confirmed. The following laboratory abnormalities suggest the diagnosis: thrombocytosis, leukocytosis (in the absence of infection), elevated LAP activity, and elevated serum vitamin B_{12} and unsaturated vitamin B_{12} binding capacity.

Clinical symptoms of polycythemia rubra vera can be divided into those that are secondary to the increased red blood cell mass and increased blood volume (such as headaches, plethora, pruritus, dyspnea, and bleeding), those due to increased blood viscosity (such as paresthesias and thrombophlebitis), and those due to hypermetabolism (such as weight loss and night sweats). Angina and claudication are commonly elicited in the history, and arterial hypertension can occur frequently. Although paradoxical, hemorrhage and thrombocytosis are both complications of the disease. Bleeding can be caused by distention of veins and capillaries, by increased blood volume, or by abnormality of platelet function. Thrombosis can be related to increased blood viscosity, thrombocytosis, and perhaps abnormally increased platelet aggregation. Thrombosis can occur in peripheral blood vessels or cerebral and coronary vessels. Mesenteric and portal vein thromboses also occur but are less frequent.

THERAPY. Phlebotomy is usually performed gradually until the hematocrit falls into the 40 to 45 percent range. Thrombocytosis or other abnormalities such as painful splenomegaly may require further treatment with an antiplatelet agent or hydroxyurea. Hematologic consultation should be obtained to define these issues.

PROGNOSIS. Polycythemia rubra vera is a chronic myeloproliferative disorder with a fairly favorable long-term prognosis considering the elderly patients involved. Fatal complications include thrombotic episodes and a potential conversion to acute leukemia, aggravated by therapy with alkylating agents or radiation therapy.

Multiple Myeloma and Waldenström's Macroglobulinemia

Malignancies of the plasma cell and lymphocyte can also be associated with acute hyperviscosity symptoms. Waldenström's macroglobulinemia, multiple myeloma, and occasionally malignant lymphomas can be associated with high levels of serum immunoglobulins, causing an increase in plasma viscosity and, thus, impaired blood flow. Rouleau formations on the blood smear and moderate to marked increases in serum total protein ($>$8 gm/dl) may be the initial laboratory clues in suspecting these disorders. Although there are supportive as well as specific therapies for these disease entities, the acute viscosity symptoms are life threatening and deserve immediate attention and consultation.

DIAGNOSIS. Multiple myeloma is characteristically a disease of older individuals. Back or bone pain is usually accompanied by mild to moderate anemia, elevated sedimentation rate, osteolytic lesions, pathologic fractures, and osteoporosis. Diagnostic studies include a serum protein analysis, bone-marrow aspiration and biopsy, calcium level, and renal function studies. The viscosity problems, as well as hypercalcemia and hyperuricemia, may require urgent medical intervention.

Waldenström's macroglobulinemia occurs most frequently in older individuals and is less common than multiple myeloma. It is characterized by anemia, adenopathy, splenomegaly, an abnormal serum protein analysis, and a marrow infiltrated by a cell that morphologically is a cross between a plasmacyte and a lymphocyte ("plymphocyte"). Unlike myeloma, in this disorder osteolytic disease and bone pain are rare. The major symptoms are similar to those of lymphoma and related marrow replacement and viscosity secondary to the abnormal protein.

The hyperviscosity syndrome includes: (1) bruising, purpura, epistaxis, and bleeding from mucosal surfaces; (2) retinopathy with retinal hemorrhages, dilation, and segmentation of the retinal vein, and papilledema; (3) neurologic symptoms that may consist of weakness, fatigue, headache, anorexia, vertigo, transient paresis, nystagmus, and coma; and (4) hypervolemia that can result in distention of blood vessels with increased vascular resistance and cardiac failure. Although the diagnosis can be suspected by elevations in the serum protein levels, a diagnosis can be made by measurement of the serum viscosity. Symptoms do not usually develop unless the serum viscosity increases fourfold (relative to water).

THERAPY. The development of the hyperviscosity syndrome requires urgent therapy with intensive plasmapheresis to remove the abnormal protein. After hematologic consultation, chemotherapy to destroy the cells that are producing the proteins should be initiated. Although slow, plasmapheresis can be performed by repeated phlebotomies with reinfusion of the packed red blood cells. Only one unit can be safely removed at a time and brought to the blood bank for centrifugation and removal of the plasma, so that the remaining packed red blood cells can be retransfused. Each exchange can take up to one hour. More efficiently, plasmapheresis machines are available to allow multiple units of plasma exchange within one to two hours. If these machines are available, this is the preferred management of the condition.

PROGNOSIS. Although remissions are made possible by chemotherapy, multiple myeloma and Waldenström's macroglobulinemia are potentially fatal. Median survival of patients with myeloma is two to five years.

WHITE BLOOD CELL DISORDERS

The white blood cell count, like the sedimentation rate, is usually an indicator of underlying disease. As such it may increase or decrease with many stimuli.

Leukopenia and *leukocytosis* are general terms that refer to a reduction or an increase, respectively, in the total white blood cell count. In addition to the total white blood cell count, it is important to consider the differential diagnosis of neutropenia, neutrophilia, eosinophilia, lymphocytosis, monocytosis, and basophilia. Table 92-6 outlines the differential diagnosis of an abnormal white blood cell count. The two abnormalities of white blood cell count that are most commonly seen in the emergency room department are leukocytosis and neutropenia.

Table 92-6. Evaluation of an abnormal white blood cell count

I. Leukocytosis
   A. Neutrophilia
      1. Bacterial infection
      2. Inflammation, necrosis, or stress
   B. Lymphocytosis
      1. Viral infections
      2. Mononucleosis
      3. Pertussis
   C. Eosinophilia
      1. Allergic disorders
      2. Parasitic diseases
      3. Tumors, Hodgkin's disease
   D. Basophilia
      1. Myeloproliferative disorders
         a. Polycythemia rubra vera
         b. Myeloid metaplasia
         c. Chronic myelogenous leukemia
   E. Monocytosis
      1. Chronic infections
         a. Tuberculosis
         b. Subacute bacterial endocarditis
         c. Rickettsial
      2. Ulcerative colitis

II. Abnormal response
   A. Acute leukemias, lymphocytic, myelogenous
   B. Chronic leukemias, lymphocytic, myelogenous
   C. Polycythemia rubra vera
   D. Myeloid metaplasia with myelofibrosis
   E. Myelophthisic disorders

III. Neutropenia
   A. Infections
   B. Blood disorders
      1. Megaloblastic anemias, leukemias, aplastic anemias, hypersplenism
   C. Debilitated state or cachexia
   D. Chemicals
      1. Benzene
      2. Dichlorodiphenyltrichloroethane (DDT)
   E. Drugs
   F. Chemotherapy
   G. Irradiation
   H. Rare causes
      1. Cyclic neutropenia
      2. Familial neutropenia
      3. Chronic benign neutropenia
      4. Immune neutropenia

Leukocytosis

The most common cause of leukocytosis is infection. The evaluation and management of the patient with infection are discussed in Chap. 94.

Of the patients seen in the emergency department with leukocytosis, those with acute leukemia require urgent therapy because of bleeding or infection. Diagnosis requires evaluation of the blood smear and bone marrow by a hematologist. Treatment includes supportive measures and chemotherapy.

Chronic myelogenous leukemia can be confused with a leukemoid reaction. This differential diagnosis can be made by performance of an LAP. The LAP is low in chronic myelogenous leukemia and elevated in leukemoid reaction.

Neutropenia

Patients with neutropenia, especially those who have received chemotherapy, are frequently seen in the emergency department.

Diagnosis

Pathophysiologically, neutropenia can be secondary to decreased bone marrow production of the myeloid series, peripheral destruction of the cells, or increased use or loss of the cells to the tissues. Neutropenia is commonly seen secondary to chemotherapy for malignant diseases. It can be seen in patients with various types of infection but is most common with infections of viral cause. Neutropenia has also been seen with bacterial infections such as typhoid, rickettsial infections such as typhus or Rocky Mountain spotted fever, protozoan infections such as malaria, and overwhelming infections such as tuberculosis or septicemia, especially in a debilitated patient. Chemicals and drugs can induce neutropenia. Ionizing radiation, benzene, chemotherapy, antithyroid medications, anticonvulsants, and gold salts are commonly implicated. Neutropenia may accompany anemia and thrombocytopenia in aplastic anemia, megaloblastic anemia, refractory anemia, hypersplenism, and myelophthisic marrow disorders such as leukemia and lymphoma, or other tumors. In the absence of infection, drugs, or other associated hematologic problems, neutropenia can occur as an isolated problem. Black patients may normally have stable neutrophil counts of 1,500 or less per cubic millimeter. There are rare instances of congenital, familial, or acquired disorders such as cyclic neutropenia, chronic benign neutropenia, or immune neutropenia. Marrow examination is necessary since it may elucidate the cause of neutropenia.

Therapy

Patients with an absolute granulocyte count below 1,000 have a significantly increased susceptibility to infection, especially bacterial. Fever is a nonspecific finding, but when it is associated with stomatitis, pharyngitis, or bleeding, the possibility of severe granulocytopenia should be considered.

The patient with significant granulocytopenia with fever must be considered to have a life-threatening infection and should be treated as a medical emergency. The patient should be promptly evaluated for areas of specific infection, and all necessary cultures should be taken. The patient should then be immediately started on broad-spectrum antibiotics, preferably of bactericidal type; the cause of the granulocytopenia should be evaluated later.

BLEEDING AND THROMBOSIS

Normal Hemostasis

To understand the mechanisms of disorders that lead to the development of thrombosis or bleeding, it is necessary to understand normal hemostatic mechanisms. The normal sequence of events in clotting can be divided into (1) formation of platelet plugs, platelet release reactions, and generation of thrombin; (2) formation of fibrin clots; and (3) dissolution of the fibrin clot by way of the fibrinolytic system.

After a vascular injury, platelets are attracted to the site and will adhere to the exposed tissue. Figure 92-4 illustrates the normal coagulation schema. Activated platelets, as well as the damaged vessel wall, release substances that cause other platelets in the circulation to be attracted to the traumatic site, thus beginning the formation of a platelet plug.

As the platelet plug is being formed, exposed collagen from the damaged vessel activates Hageman factor (factor XII). Activated factor XII and its generated by-products stimulate the activation of the intrinsic clotting pathway, which eventually leads to the formation of thrombin. Small amounts of thrombin cause irreversible platelet aggregation and increase the platelet release reactions, promoting the formation of more thrombin. Thrombin can also be formed by the extrinsic clotting pathway through a tissue factor released from the damaged vascular endothelium.

Once thrombin has been formed, it attacks the fibrinogen molecule, converting it to fibrin, with release of two fragments, fibrinopeptides A and B. As fibrin is laid down, the hemostatic plug is strengthened and stabilized. Release of fibrinopeptide A initiates fibrin polymerization. With activation of factor XIII by thrombin, covalent cross-links are introduced between polymerized fibrin molecules, and the resultant clot becomes mechanically strong and able to withstand the trauma of other events within the vascular system.

Dissolution of the fibrin clot occurs by way of the fibrinolytic system. Plasminogen is incorporated within the clot, ready to be activated. The exposed endothelial cell serves as the activator during the laying down of fibrin. Fortunately, activation normally does not occur outside the clot, restricting the normal extent of fibrinolysis.

Clinical Evaluation of Bleeding Patients

In evaluating a bleeding patient, it should be remembered that localized processes such as a laceration, duodenal ulcers, and poorly sutured wounds, and not disorders of the hemostatic mechanism, account for most bleeding. However, certain bleeding manifestations may suggest the presence of a hemostatic disorder. The patient's past experience with surgery, trauma, and dental extractions is particularly helpful in this evaluation. A history of prior operation or trauma without bleeding is evidence against a hereditary hemostatic disorder but does not exclude the possibility of an acquired disorder. The history of easy bruising is difficult to evaluate but can be significant when the degree of bruising seems out of proportion to the trauma sustained. The development of large superficial ecchymoses or hematomas after minor trauma or a history of hemarthroses may be clues to an underlying coagulation disorder. Recurrent epistaxis and gingival bleeding are most commonly seen in patients with platelet abnormalities. Whenever historical clues to a hemostatic disorder are present, a history of drug intake, especially drugs that are known to affect hemostasis such as warfarin or aspirin, should be obtained. A positive family history of bleeding may help to define the abnormality.

In examining the patient it is important to search for a local cause to explain the bleeding or for evidence of associated diseases such as jaundice and liver disease that may explain the cause of the hemostatic disorder. The presence or absence of hepatomegaly, splenomegaly, lymph node en-

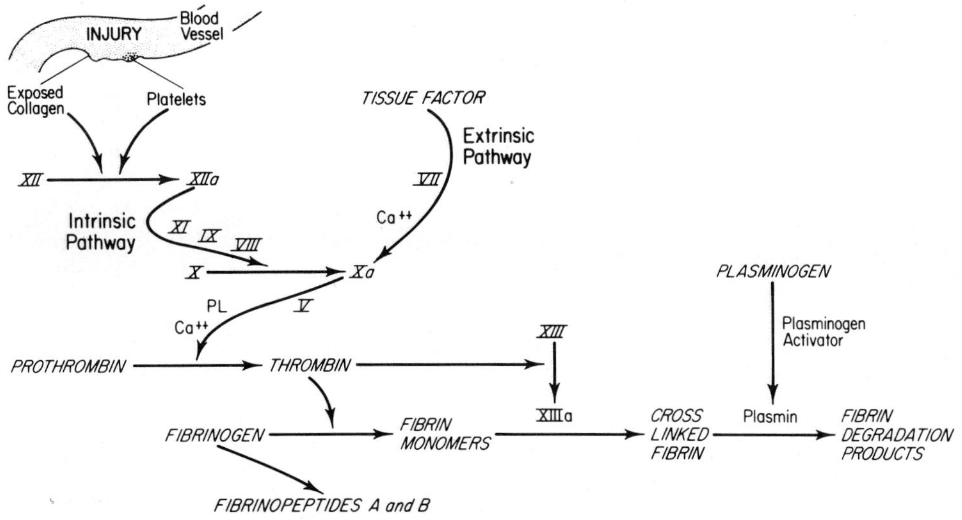

Fig. 92-4. Coagulation and fibrinolytic pathways after tissue injury. (PL = phospholipid; a = activated factor.) (From D.S. Rosenthal. Hematologic Oncologic Disorders and Heart Disease. In E.B. Braunwald [ed.], *Heart Disease.* Philadelphia: Saunders, 1980. P 1793.)

largement, and bone tenderness may be helpful in understanding the reason for a hemostatic disorder.

When bleeding is ongoing the patient will require initial management before turning to the laboratory to find a definitive diagnosis. The patient should be kept quiet and should not be exposed to any unnecessary trauma. Careful attention should be paid to problems, such as hypertension, that can lead to further bleeding. When the bleeding site is accessible, local pressure can be applied to control the bleeding, and local vasoconstriction, especially with the use of cold packs, may be of some value. When a hemostatic disorder is suspected, parenteral medication should not be given intramuscularly, unless essential, because of the possibility of causing the formation of intramuscular hematoma. Drugs such as aspirin and nonsteroidal antiinflammatory drugs (NSAIDs) that affect the function of platelets should be avoided. Table 92-7 outlines the clinical difference between the types of bleeding seen in patients with coagulation defects and those with platelet defects.

Laboratory Evaluation of Bleeding

The integrity of the clotting mechanism can be evaluated using various laboratory studies. Platelets are evaluated both numerically and functionally. Platelet function can first be screened by a simple bleeding time. Abnormal bleeding times can be further evaluated by platelet aggregation studies. Abnormalities of the intrinsic pathway can be detected by the activated partial thromboplastin time (PTT), whereas the extrinsic clotting pathway is screened by the prothrombin time (PT).

Platelet Count

Calculation of platelet number is usually performed by direct counting, similar to the white blood cell count, or by an

Table 92-7. Bleeding characteristics from platelet and coagulation abnormalities

Coagulation defect	Platelet defect
Intramuscular and deep hematomas	Petechiae, purpura
Hemarthrosis	Mucosal bleeding—e.g., epistaxis
Delayed onset of bleeding after trauma	Prolonged bleeding from minor cuts
Rebleeding late after initial episode	Widespread but especially located where capillaries are under hydrostatic pressure—e.g., legs
Hemorrhage from venipuncture site if firm pressure not maintained long enough	Superficial ecchymosis around venipuncture sites

automated cell counter. A quick but rough estimate of platelet number can be made on a peripheral blood smear by adding the number of platelets seen in each of five oil immersion microscopic fields and multiplying the sum by 2,000. Platelet counts normally range between 150,000 and 450,000 mm^3.

Bleeding Time

The bleeding time should be determined using commercially available templates to ensure reproducible results. The Ivy bleeding time (template method) is performed on the volar surface of the forearm while a blood pressure cuff inflated to 40 mm Hg is placed on the arm above the test site. A standardized puncture wound 1 mm deep and 9 mm long is made by the template blade, and the bleeding site is gently blotted with filter paper every 15 seconds until bleeding stops. With commercially available templates, the normal bleeding time range is three to nine minutes. A prolonged

Table 92-8. Laboratory evaluation—bleeding disorders

Platelets	Bleeding time	PT	PTT	Differential diagnosis	Diagnostic tests
↓	ND	nl	nl	ITP, drug sensitivity; bone marrow depression	Platelet antibody, marrow aspirate
↓	ND	abn	abn	DIC	Fibrinogen assays, fibrinogen split products, thrombin time
nl	abn	nl	nl	Platelet function defect, salicylates, uremia	Platelet aggregation, blood urea nitrogen (BUN), creatinine
nl	abn	nl	abn	von Willebrand's disease	Factor VIII assay, factor VIII antigen, platelet adhesiveness, ristocetin aggregation
nl	nl	abn	nl	Factor VII deficiency or inhibitor	Factor VII assay (nl plasma should correct PT if no inhibitor)
nl	nl	abn	abn	Factor V, X, II, I deficiencies as in liver disease or with anticoagulants	Liver function tests, F assays (could be a combined deficiency)
nl	nl	nl	abn	Factor VIII (hemophilia), IX, XI, or XII deficiencies or inhibitor	Individual factor assay (nl plasma should correct PTT if no inhibitor)
nl	nl	nl	nl	Factor XIII deficiency	Urea stabilizing test, factor XIII assay

Key: nl = normal; ↓ = decreased; abn = prolonged; ND = not done (when platelets ↓); F = factor; ITP = idiopathic thrombocytopenic purpura.

bleeding time indicates a defect in the formation of the platelet plug and can be caused by decreased numbers of platelets or abnormally functioning platelets. Since the bleeding time is affected by thrombocytopenia, obtaining a bleeding time does not add any additional information when the platelet count is less than 10,000. Platelet aggregation studies to evaluate the cause of an abnormal bleeding time are not reliable when the platelet count is less than 100,000.

Prothrombin Time
The PT measures the extrinsic pathway. An abnormally prolonged test suggests a deficiency in one or more of the following: factors V, VII, or X; prothrombin; or fibrinogen.

Partial Thromboplastin Time
The PTT tests the intrinsic pathway factors, including factors V, VIII, IX, X, XI, and XII; prothrombin; and fibrinogen.

This and the other three tests just described are readily available in all laboratories, and when they are performed as a screening evaluation for a bleeding disorder, they will be sufficient to detect over 95 percent of diagnosable bleeding dyscrasias. If an abnormality is found on the screening test, further evaluation is warranted and more specific tests can be performed to isolate the problem. Table 92-8 outlines the diagnostic possibilities if results of one or more of the tests are abnormal, as well as the next step that should be considered.

Platelet Abnormalities

Hemostatic disorders related to platelet abnormalities can be divided into quantitative and qualitative abnormalities. In quantitative disorders, bleeding occurs as a result of a decrease in platelet number. Qualitative disorders occur when the platelet number is adequate but function is abnormal. Both disorders should be associated with prolonged bleeding time.

Table 92-9. Drugs that induce thrombocytopenia

Thiazides, diuretics
Ethyl alcohol
Estrogen
Sulfa antibiotics
Diphenylhydantoin
Paraaminosalicylic acid (PAS)
Quinine
Quinidine
Digitoxin
Gold salts
Methyldopa

Patients who are thrombocytopenic or have abnormally functioning platelets are likely to complain of prolonged bleeding from superficial or minor cuts, easy bruisability, epistaxis, gingival bleeding, and menorrhagia. On physical examination petechiae, purpura, as well as gingival and mucosal membrane bleeding are found.

Thrombocytopenia
In general, major problems with hemostasis do not occur with platelet counts greater than 20,000, and patients with platelet counts over 50,000 should be able to undergo surgical procedures without excessive bleeding. If thrombocytopenia is established, the patient should be carefully questioned about the use of drugs associated with thrombocytopenia (Table 92-9). The next step in treating any thrombocytopenic patient is to request a hematologic evaluation and determine the need for bone marrow aspiration and therapeutic intervention. The thrombocytopenias can be

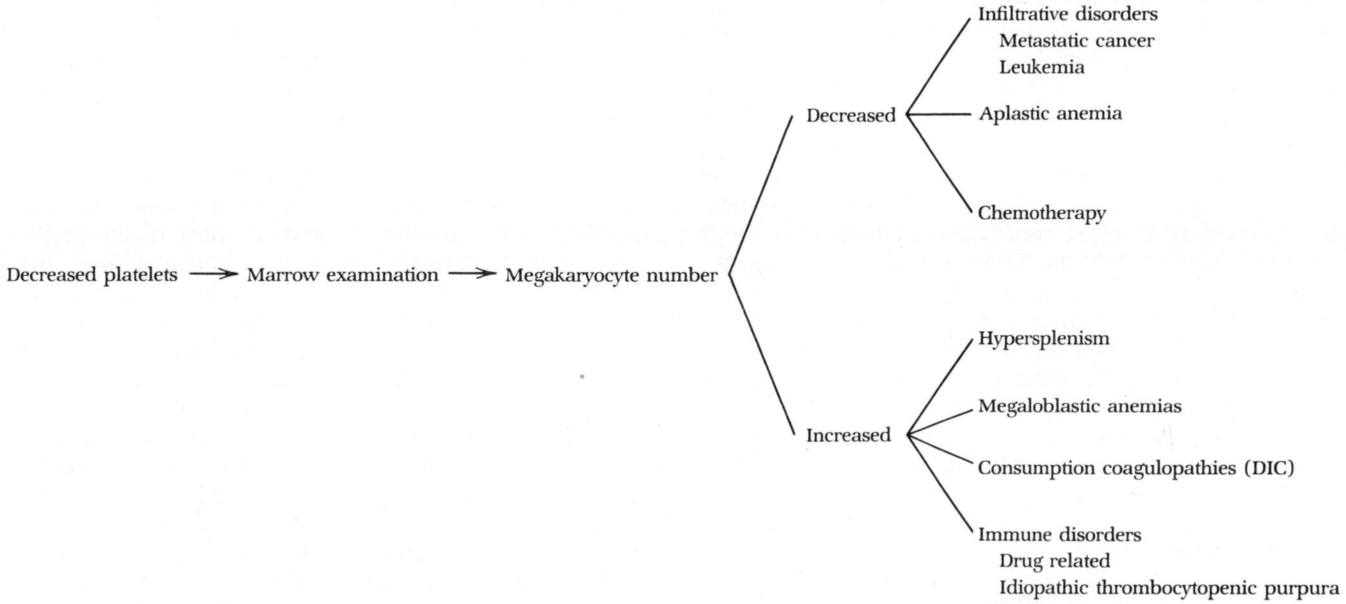

Fig. 92-5. Differential diagnosis of a decreased platelet count.

differentiated on the basis of the number of megakaryocytes in the marrow (Fig. 92-5).

TREATMENT. When the problem is lack of production of the platelets, platelet transfusion is usually the initial treatment of choice in the setting of active bleeding. For general purposes, the dose of platelet transfusion can be derived by anticipating an increase in platelet count of approximately $10,000/mm^3$ for each unit of platelet concentrate infused in the average-sized adult. In treating hemorrhage in thrombocytopenic patients, one should aim to increase the platelet count to approximately 50,000 to $100,000/mm^3$.

Treatment of thrombocytopenia secondary to peripheral destruction depends on the cause of the loss. Although platelet transfusion is not usually harmful, it may be totally useless. Careful questioning of the patient about possible use of associated drugs is of prime importance. If any drugs are implicated, they should be discontinued. Steroids are usually the initial therapy of choice in immune thrombocytopenic purpura (ITP), but splenectomy may be required in patients whose disease is refractory. Proper management in most cases requires hematologic consultation.

Disorders of Platelet Function

Disorders of platelet function are becoming more common, the increased incidence correlating with the availability of more reliable laboratory tests. These disorders are characterized by an abnormally prolonged bleeding time and can be classified as physiologic platelet defects (Table 92-10). When patients with aggregation defects require treatment for bleeding, they are given platelet transfusion with platelet concentrates, using the same guidelines as in thrombocytopenia.

Table 92-10. Platelet function defects

I. Decreased adhesiveness
  A. von Willebrand's disease
  B. Bernard-Soulier syndrome
II. Aggregation defects
  A. Thrombasthenia
  B. Storage pool syndrome
  C. Defective release reactions
    1. Uremia
    2. Dysproteinemias—myeloma, Waldenström's macroglobulinemia
    3. Drugs
      a. Aspirin and aspirin-containing drugs
      b. Chlorpromazine
      c. Diphenhydramine (Benadryl)

VON WILLEBRAND'S DISEASE. Von Willebrand's disease (VWD) is an autosomal dominant disorder that is one of the most common forms of mild bleeding. It is caused by plasma deficiency of factor VIII complex, which results in reduction of platelet adhesion to the vessel wall and is associated with a prolonged bleeding time. The factor VIII complex contains von Willebrand's factor (VWF) and antihemophilic factor (AHF). Because these factors circulate as a complex, VWD is associated with decreased factor VIII complex. Diagnostic laboratory tests, ordered by the specialty consultant, include an abnormal ristocetin aggregation, decreased factor VIII, and a decreased factor VIII antigen. These tests distinguish between type I VWD, which is caused by defective release of normal VWF from endothelial cells, and type II VWD, in which abnormal VWF is produced. There are wide variations in the severity of bleeding from patient to patient and even from time to time in the same patient. Most cases are mild and require no therapy. Patients are advised to avoid medications such as aspirin and NSAIDs. The treatment of choice for severe bleeding or major surgery is cryoprecipitate, which is a rich source of fibrinogen, factor VII, and VWF (as well as fibronectin and factor XIII). Commercial factor VIII concentrates are deficient in VWF and are not recommended.

Many patients with type I VWF, and some with mild type IIa, will respond to 1-deamino-α-D-arginine vasopressin (DDAVP), which appears to stimulate endothelial cell release of VWF. (DDAVP is also useful in treating patients with mild hemophilia.) For minor operations such as dental extraction, tonsillectomy, and hemarthroses, DDAVP is often adequate therapy. It should be avoided in patients with known type IIB VWD but used whenever possible in responsive individuals to avoid transfusion risks associated with cryoprecipitate. DDAVP should be administered 30 minutes before a planned procedure. Bleeding time, ristocetin aggregation, and VWF antigen should be monitored before and after DDAVP administration. Timing of further doses should be based on results of laboratory tests and clinical bleeding. A specialty consultation may be useful in these determinations. DDAVP has antidiuretic and mild pressor activity and these should be monitored during therapy.

Factor Deficiencies

Over 90 percent of patients with inherited coagulation disorders have classic hemophilia A (factor VIII deficiency). Christmas disease (hemophilia B or factor IX deficiency) accounts for another 9 percent, and hereditary factor XI, X, and VII deficiencies represent the remaining conditions.

Factor VIII and Factor IX Deficiencies (Hemophilia and Christmas Disease)

Factor VIII and IX deficiencies are X-linked recessive disorders, and about 25 percent of patients have no family history of a bleeding dyscrasia. The types of bleeding problems encountered are characteristically deep bleeding such as hematomas and bleeding into large joints (hemarthroses). As noted in Table 92-8, the PTT is prolonged, whereas the PT, platelet count, and bleeding time are normal. Specific factor assays are necessary to make a diagnosis.

TREATMENT. Factor levels relate to the severity of the bleeding (greater than 5% is mild, 1–5% moderate, and less than 1% severe). Therapy is required for spontaneous bleeding, trauma, surgery, and dental extractions. There are many commercially available factor VIII and IX preparations, as well as blood bank–prepared cryoprecipitate. The latter is more difficult to prepare and requires a larger volume for replacement, but it carries a lower risk of hepatitis.

All of the coagulation factors are measured in units. Each unit of a specific factor is defined as the amount of that factor in 1 ml normal plasma. To calculate the dose of factor to be administered, a 1 percent rise in factor level should be expected for each factor unit infused per kilogram of body weight. The concentrates have been assayed for the amount of factor present. With cryoprecipitate the amount of factor VIII present is usually 70 to 100 units per unit of cryoprecipitate. For a mild bleed, such as a simple joint bruise, a one-time infusion is sufficient to raise the factor level to 5 to 10 percent and to maintain it at that level for two to three days. For major surgical procedures, levels as high as 50 percent are needed for two to three weeks. Since factor VIII has a half-life of 12 hours, it is necessary to infuse it every 12 hours. Factor IX also has a half-life of 12 hours and, thus, it is necessary to infuse it every 12 hours. Factor IX has a half-life of 24 hours and can therefore be administered once a day.

Substantial progress has been made in developing factor VIII concentrates to minimize exposure risks for hepatitis and human immunodeficiency viruses (HIV). In the past factor VIII concentrates were obtained from pooled cryoprecipitate from thousands of donors and precipitated with organic solvents. New products include "dry" heat-treated factor VIII, "wet" pasteurized factor VII, and affinity purified factor VIII. Heat-treated product is obtained from HIV-negative donors (as with all blood products) and is heat treated. It is thought to be safe regarding HIV transmission, but carries risk for transmission of viral hepatitis. Pasteurized factor VIII (e.g., Humate-P) and affinity purified factor VIII (e.g., Monoclate, Hemophil-M) are substantially more expensive but thought to be free of HIV and hepatitis virus. Choice of factor VIII products in hemophiliacs should be based in part on prior exposure of the patient to these products.

Patients with severe hemophilia who receive frequent factor VIII replacement often develop inhibitors to factor VIII that impair function of the product. This can be circumvented in some cases by use of activated factor complexes. Specialty consultation is usually necessary in these cases to determine the most useful mode of therapy.

PROGNOSIS. Hematologic consultation should be requested early in the care of the patient with hemophilia, and long-term, close follow-up study is strongly recommended. Early treatment may prevent permanent joint damage. New programs of home care and self-care are available for these patients to limit the need for frequent emergency department visits.

Although factor VIII and IX deficiencies are the most commonly seen inherited disorders, patients with other factor deficiencies are occasionally seen in the emergency situation. Table 92-11 gives guidelines for therapy for inherited coagulation defects.

Acquired Bleeding Disorders

Liver Disease

Synthesis and degradation of many of the coagulation proteins take place in the liver. Most of these factors are the vitamin K–dependent factors. Impaired vitamin K function and liver failure will result in deficiencies of factors II, VII, IX, X, and V, and in severe cases fibrinogen decreases. Prothrombin time and PTT will both be abnormal because factors in both intrinsic and extrinsic pathways are affected. In addition, hypersplenism can cause thrombocytopenia.

In patients with liver disease, vitamin K should be administered in an attempt to improve the PT and PTT, but if the liver disease is severe, improvement may be only partial. It is not necessary to treat those patients with coagulation factors on a prophylactic basis, but when bleeding occurs it may be necessary to treat the patients with fresh or frozen plasma using 10 to 15 ml fresh or frozen plasma per kilogram of body weight.

Vitamin K Deficiency

Vitamin K deficiency causes decreased synthesis of the vitamin K–dependent coagulation factors (factors II, VII, IX,

Table 92-11. Summary of replacement therapy for inherited coagulation defects

Deficiency	Factor replacement	Dosage/kg body weight: Initial	Dosage/kg body weight: Maintenance per day
Fibrinogen	Plasma	25 ml	5–10 ml
(Factor I)	Cryoprecipitate	2–4 bags/10 kg	1 bag/kg every other day
Factor V	Fresh frozen plasma	15–25 ml	10 ml every 12 hr
Factor VII	Plasma	5–10 ml	5 ml four times a day
	Prothrombin complex	5–10 units	5 units four times a day
von Willebrand's	Fresh frozen plasma	Not necessary	10 ml
	Cryoprecipitate	Not necessary	1 bag/10 kg every 1–2 days
	DDAVP (type I)	0.3 μg	30 min before operation and every 12–24 hr
Factor IX			
Minor bleed	Fresh frozen plasma	30 ml	7 ml every 24 hr for 1–4 days
	Purified prothrombin complex	30 units	10 units every 24 hr for 2–4 days
Major bleed	Fresh frozen plasma	60 ml	28 units every 24 hours for 7–10 days
	Purified prothrombin complex	60 units	40 units every 24 hours for 7–10 days
Factor X (Stuart factor)	Plasma	10–15 ml	10 ml
Factor XI	Plasma	10–20 ml	5 ml
Factor XIII	Plasma	3–5 ml every 1–2 wk	Unnecessary
Factor VIII			
Hemophilia A			
Minor bleed	Purified factor VIII	Not necessary	1.25–1.75 bags/10 kg every 12 hr for 2–4 days
	Fresh frozen plasma	Not necessary	10–15 units every 12 hr for 2–4 days
	Cryoprecipitate	Not necessary	10–15 ml every 12 hr for 2–4 days
Major bleed	Purified factor VIII	3.5 bags/10 kg	1.75 bags/10 kg every 8–12 hr
	Fresh frozen plasma	30 units	10–15 units every 8–12 hr
	Cryoprecipitate	30 ml	15 ml every 8–12 hr

and X). It usually occurs in the setting of liver dysfunction, of abnormalities of vitamin K absorption from the intestinal tract, and with the use of coumarin anticoagulant drugs. Deficiency of vitamin K is manifest by elevation of the PT and PTT; however, in practice the PT is much more prolonged than the PTT.

When vitamin K deficiency is suspected, the most useful diagnostic test is a therapeutic trial of vitamin K. When 10 mg vitamin K is administered orally or parenterally (intramuscularly), the abnormal clotting study should return to normal within 12 hours.

Massive Transfusion

Blood stored at 4°C for 48 hours or more becomes deficient in factors V and VII and also in platelets. After transfusions of many units of stored blood, patients can become deficient in these factors on a dilutional basis. It usually requires 10 to 12 units of blood in a 24-hour period to dilute the patient's normal factors sufficiently to cause significant clinical problems. In most cases major trauma or surgery precipitates this degree of transfusion requirement; however, gastrointestinal hemorrhage or gynecologic or obstetric difficulties may also require massive transfusion.

Patients who are factor deficient from massive transfusion or coagulation studies will reveal abnormalities of the PT and PTT and a low platelet count. Factor deficiencies can be corrected with fresh frozen plasma and the thrombocytopenia can be corrected with platelet concentrates.

Disseminated Intravascular Coagulation

The sudden onset of diffuse hemorrhage in an acutely ill patient who arrives in the emergency department may be the result of DIC. This disorder results from aberrant release of substances that activate the coagulation system, leading to abnormal thrombin formation and eventual depletion of clotting factors with resultant bleeding. These patients may have one or more of the following: peripheral cyanosis, gangrene of the digits or tip of the nose, or diffuse hemorrhage in the skin, in the mucous membranes, and at venipuncture sites. Oliguria or anuria and neurologic difficulties are not uncommon. Many disorders have been associated with DIC; the most commonly encountered ones are listed in Table 92-12.

DIAGNOSIS. The clinical suspicion of DIC can be confirmed by laboratory studies. The peripheral blood smear may reveal microangiopathic red cells. The platelet count is decreased and the PT and PTT are both prolonged. In addition, fibrinogen is reduced, causing a prolonged PT, and fibrinogen breakdown products (fibrinogen split products) are formed, which contribute to a prolonged thrombin time.

TREATMENT. Treatment of DIC is directed against both the underlying disease and the resultant bleeding diathesis. These patients are usually acutely ill and require urgent therapy (e.g., treatment of septicemia, shock, acute obstetric catastrophe). If the primary disorder cannot be adequately treated, there may be little success in managing the DIC. If bleeding is minimal and the underlying disorder is being adequately treated, no therapy may be needed for the DIC. If, however, despite adequate treatment of the primary disorder, bleeding becomes a significant problem, hematologic consultation should be urgently sought regarding the use of fresh or frozen plasma and platelet transfusions, as well as

Table 92-12. Disorders associated with DIC

I. Pregnancy and delivery complications
   A. Abruptio placentae
   B. Amniotic fluid embolism
   C. Septic abortion
   D. Retained dead fetus
II. Infections
   A. Septicemia, especially with gram-negative organisms
   B. Meningococcemia
   C. Viral infections
III. Hemolytic transfusion reactions
IV. Metastatic carcinoma, especially prostate, pancreas, lung, stomach, and colon
V. Extensive tissue damage
   A. Massive trauma
   B. Heat stroke
   C. Burns
   D. Anoxia
VI. Anaphylactic drug reactions
VII. Acute leukemia, particularly promyelocytic leukemia
VIII. Surgical procedures
   A. Prostatic surgery
   B. Lung surgery
   C. Extracorporeal circulation

heparin. Heparin can prevent activation of the coagulation system by the underlying disorder. However, it can also increase bleeding and in general should not be used without replacements of platelets and coagulation proteins. When heparin is used the usual starting dosage is 500 to 1,500 units an hour, given as a continuous intravenous infusion. Heparin should be discontinued if bleeding increases. The course of the DIC should be followed closely, and frequent observations should be made of the coagulation parameters, including the platelet count, fibrinogen, PT, PTT, thrombin time, and fibrin split products. Improvement in the fibrinogen and reduction of the fibrin split products should occur within 24 hours of control of the DIC. The thrombocytopenia may persist for several days. Improvement of fibrinogen level or reduction of fibrin split products in the patient treated with heparin would be an indication for continuation of the drug.

PROGNOSIS. Since DIC is a result of an acute medical illness, prognosis depends almost entirely on the speed of the physician in handling the bleeding emergency, as well as the ability to treat the underlying disorder.

Fibrinolysis

Fibrinolysis usually accompanies DIC and rarely occurs as a primary disorder. Use of agents such as E-aminocaproic acid (EACA), which block fibrinolysis, can be dangerous in patients with DIC since they can lead to widespread and fatal thrombosis. Primary fibrinolysis has been associated with prostatic manipulation or cancer. In the latter instance, EACA may be indicated.

Hypercoagulable States

In addition to local injury or damage to vessel walls, several disorders are associated with abnormal increased clotting. Four mechanisms can lead to hypercoagulable states: abnormal blood flow and stasis, decreased concentration of clotting inhibitors, abnormal acceleration of platelet release and aggregation, and impaired clearance of activated clotting factors.

Abnormal blood flow or stasis is a contributing factor in thrombosis. Sickle cell disease, polycythemia, and hyperviscosity syndromes are good clinical examples. In addition, oral contraceptives have been repeatedly implicated in thromboembolic disease, in some cases associated with a shortened PTT and increased platelets.

Decreased inhibitors of coagulation proteins prevent the normal inactivation of these proteins and can cause thrombosis. For example, a deficiency of antithrombin III (AT III) activity has been reported in families with increased thrombosis. Antithrombin III is the principal factor responsible for inactivation of thrombin as well as factors X, XI, and XII. Antithrombin III deficiency is an autosomal dominant disease and may affect as many as 1 in 2,000 heterozygous individuals. (The homozygous state is apparently incompatible with life.) The most clinical manifestations of thrombosis are recurrent deep venous thrombosis and pulmonary embolism, but thromboembolism can occur in diverse and unusual sites. Screening PT and PTT can be shortened or completely normal. Serum levels of AT III are now available; heterozygous patients have AT III levels between 25 and 60 percent of normal. Protein C and protein S deficiency can also be associated with recurrent thromboembolism. Clinical manifestations and inheritance patterns resemble those for AT III deficiency. Protein C levels can be measured in the laboratory, but because it is a vitamin K–dependent protein, detection in patients who are receiving coumarin anticoagulants can be complicated. Initial therapy with heparin and long-term therapy with warfarin (Coumadin) are generally effective in these patients.

The so-called lupus anticoagulation is an immunoglobulin that inhibits activity of phospholipid in in vitro clotting reactions, which leads to prolonged PTT, and to a lesser extent PT. Although lupus anticoagulation prolongs PTT in vitro, it is clinically associated with risk of thrombosis.

Although most platelet aggregation defects are associated with bleeding, spontaneous aggregation has been reported to occur in disorders associated with thrombocytosis, such as polycythemia and essential thrombocytosis. Clearance of activated coagulation factors usually takes place in the liver and reticuloendothelial system, and occasionally cirrhosis and viral hepatitis impair the clearance mechanism and lead to widespread thrombosis.

ANTICOAGULATION TREATMENT. Anticoagulation is clearly beneficial in the treatment and prevention of thrombosis in the venous side of the circulation. Heparin and oral anticoagulants both have definitive roles in treatment, and platelet suppressive agents are currently being evaluated.

Heparin is the most useful drug available for prophylaxis and treatment of venous thromboembolism. The current recommended dosage for treatment of patients with acute thromboembolism is 30,000 units per day by continuous intravenous infusion or enough to keep the PTT at 1.5 to 2.5 times the control level. Studies have confirmed that a lower dose of heparin is effective prophylaxis against deep venous thrombosis in postoperative patients. If hemorrhage occurs

Table 92-13. Drug effect with coumarin derivatives

Potentiate	Antagonize
Phenylbutazone	Barbiturates
Salicylates	Other
Thyroid	Chronic alcohol
Other	Allopurinol
Acute alcohol	Cholestyramine
Anabolic steroids	Diuretics
Antibiotics	Glutethimide
Antiplatelet drugs	Nortriptyline
Clofibrate	Rifampin
Diphenylhydantoin	
Oral hypoglycemic agents	
Quinidine sulfate	
Sulfonamides	

with heparin therapy, protamine sulfate given at approximately milligram for milligram of heparin should correct the bleeding. The duration of action of heparin is about four hours. If bleeding occurs more than four hours after discontinuation of heparin, protamine is not required.

Oral anticoagulants, such as warfarin and its derivative, compete for vitamin K in the liver and interfere with the formation of factors II, VII, IX, and X. The primary indications for long-term therapy with these agents are venous thrombosis of the leg and pulmonary embolism after the patient has initially received heparin. In addition, warfarin is useful in prophylaxis in patients with significant mitral stenosis, especially patients with atrial fibrillation, with artificial heart valves, after an acute arterial embolic episode, or after hip surgery. The starting dosage of warfarin is 10 mg per day for three to four days and the usual maintenance dosage is 3 to 8 mg per day. Prothrombin times are usually kept at 1.5 to 2.0 times that of control.

Complications of anticoagulant therapy include significant bleeding or rethrombosis. Both can occur because of the addition or deletion of other medications to warfarin that potentiate or antagonize its action. Physicians should be aware of this combined drug effect. If the patient has to take any of the medications listed in Table 92-13, the physician should be alerted to any change in dosage schedule that may be necessary.

Warfarin overdose is best managed with fresh or frozen plasma transfusions. In general two units of fresh or frozen plasma will correct PT sufficiently to stop bleeding. Vitamin K in dosages of 10 to 25 mg is also effective parenterally, but it takes 12 to 24 hours to reverse the toxicity and it causes temporary resistance to further warfarin treatment.

Platelet suppressive agents such as aspirin, sulfinpyrazone, and dipyridamole are being tested in patients with valvular heart disease, prosthetic valves, cerebrovascular disease, threatened strokes, and coronary artery disease. Preliminary results are encouraging but not definitive.

SELECTED READING

Berlin, N I. Diagnosis and classification of the polycythemias. *Semin Hematol* 12:339, 1975.

Castle, W B, and Minor, G R. *Pathological Physiology and Clinical Descriptions of the Anemias*. New York: Oxford, 1936. P 2.

Handin, R I. Bleeding Disorders In W T Branch ed, *Office Practice of Medicine*. Philadelphia: Saunders, 1982. Pp 1049–1062.

Jones, P. Developments and problems in the management of hemophilia. *Semin Hematol* 13:375, 1977.

Kaplan, A P. Initiation of intrinsic coagulation and fibrinolytic pathways of man. *Prog Hemost Thromb* 4:127, 1979.

Nathan, D G, and Oski, F A. Hematology of Infancy and Childhood. In O Platt and D G Nathan (eds), *Sickle Cell Disease* (2nd ed). Philadelphia: Saunders, 1981. Pp 687–725.

Pirofsky, B. Clinical aspects of autoimmune hemolytic anemia. *Semin Hematol* 13:251, 1976.

Rosenthal, D S. Problems Involving an Abnormal Blood Count. In W T Branch (ed), *Office Practice of Medicine*. Philadelphia: Saunders, 1982. Pp 1027–1048.

Varat, M A, Adolphs, R J, and Fowler, N O. Cardiovascular effects of anemia. *Am Heart J* 83:415, 1972.

Williams, W J. Principles of Coagulation Tests. In W J Williams (ed), *Hematology*. New York: McGraw-Hill, 1972. Pp 1098–1104.

Williams, W J, et al. *Hematology* (2nd ed). New York: McGraw-Hill, 1977.

Wintrobe, M M. *Clinical Hematology* (8th ed.). Philadelphia: Lea & Febiger, 1982.

93. Principles of Emergency Transfusion Medicine

*Charles Huggins**

Blood in North America is collected from volunteer, unremunerated donors. Although some hospitals collect blood for transfusion, most blood is collected, separated into components, and tested by a regional blood center, which then distributes blood and its components to hospital transfusion services that in turn prepare the blood for the patient.

Each prospective blood donor is provided detailed information about the acquired immunodeficiency syndrome (AIDS) and its many signs or symptoms. Members of groups defined by the United States Public Health Service to be at high risk for human immunodeficiency virus (HIV) infection and their sexual partners are asked not to donate blood. After measurement of temperature, hemoglobin, pulse, and blood pressure, each donor undergoes a health history interview designed to identify conditions that might make blood donation unsafe for the donor, or the blood unsafe for the patient.

Donors are ultimately asked to sign a statement to the effect that they have read and understand the AIDS information, and that they are neither a member nor a sexual partner of a member of a "high-risk group." Potential donors are then asked to attest to the truth of their answers to the health questions and to authorize laboratory testing of their blood for the presence of antibodies to HIV.

Some potential donors may feel under social pressure to donate blood but are reluctant to admit potential high-risk behavior. In this situation a mechanism exists for "confidential unit exclusion" (CUE), in which the donor, after blood has been collected, can indicate in confidence whether or not the blood should be transfused.

The size of a normal blood draw is 450 ± 10% ml. Whole blood is rarely available for transfusion in much of the United States. Donated blood is usually separated shortly after collection into red blood cells, plasma, and platelet concentrate or cryoprecipitated antihemophilic factor. This separation of blood into its components permits the widest use of the different elements and allows optimum storage conditions for labile clotting factors in the plasma and the platelets. The expiration date for every blood component, which is stated on the container label, depends on the type of anticoagulant that was used and the storage conditions for the particular component. If blood or its components are issued and, for whatever reason, it is decided not to infuse them, the blood or components should be returned to the transfusion service as quickly as possible. If they are returned from the emergency department or a patient care floor longer than 30 minutes after issue, the blood or its components are discarded in case bacteria have multiplied.

*Deceased

LABORATORY TESTING ON DONATED BLOOD

All blood is typed for the ABO and Rh(D) blood group systems. The bag itself is labeled with this information. Serum from each donor is tested for the presence of unexpected antibodies against red cell antigens in other blood group systems. All blood is tested for hepatitis B surface antigen, anti-HIV-1, and anti-human T cell leukemia/lymphoma virus (HTLV)-I to detect transmitters of hepatitis B, HIV, and HTLV-I associated myelopathy or adult T-cell leukemia. A serologic test for syphilis is usually performed. Alanine aminotransferase (ALT) and hepatitis B core (HBc) antibody tests are performed as surrogate markers for non-A, non-B hepatitis (NANB). Serologic testing for hepatitis C virus (HCV), which can be detected in 80 to 90 percent of transfusion associated NANB, began in May 1990. Blood donors have had a positivity rate of approximately 0.7 percent. The current screening test for hepatitis C has a false-positive rate of approximately 60 percent. A true "confirmatory" test is not yet available, and all donors who test positively are permanently deferred at this time. Implementation of the hepatitis C screening test is expected to reduce the frequency of post-transfusion hepatitis by 85 percent. A multicenter study to determine the current incidence of post-transfusion hepatitis was being organized to begin in 1991. It is unlikely that the two NANB surrogate markers, the ALT and HBc antibody tests, will be eliminated because there is a potential that a surrogate test positive but HCV antibody negative donor could transmit hepatitis C. All of the above tests must be within normal limits, or negative, for blood to be considered suitable for transfusion. Blood units that fail to pass all tests are destroyed. To avoid clutter that might obscure essential information, the results of laboratory tests other than ABO and Rh grouping are not shown on the blood bag label. Blood banks or transfusion services can provide information about additional tests that may have been performed, as well as a *Circular of Information for the Use of Human Blood and Blood Components,* as required by federal law.

BLOOD SAFETY: TRANSMISSION OF INFECTIOUS DISEASES

Although the blood supply is as safe or safer than it has ever been, blood for transfusion must be considered *unavoidably unsafe* and must not be administered without a clear, urgent indication. The incidence of the most important transfusion-transmitted diseases varies in different parts of the world, but in the continental United States is approximately as follows:

Disease	*Incidence*
Non-A, non-B hepatitis	1/25–1/100
Hepatitis B	1/5,000–1/10,000
HIV infection	1/50,000–1/150,000

Non-A, non-B hepatitis is a high-frequency complication of transfusion. It is characteristically very mild or asymptomatic in the acute phase but is persistent in a large percentage of patients and can progress to chronic hepatitis, cirrhosis, and death or the need for liver transplantation. Hepatitis B tends to be clinically more severe than NANB in the acute phase, but most patients recover completely with only a small (±2–5%) percentage continuing as chronic carriers. Liver disease can progress in chronic carriers of hepatitis B to cirrhosis or primary hepatic malignancy. Because of the endemicity of hepatitis B in some areas of southern Europe, North Africa, the Middle East, and many parts of Asia, patients from these locations are frequently hepatitis carriers. Everyone who works in the field of emergency medicine should be tested for the presence of anti–hepatitis B antibodies, and if none are detectable they should receive hepatitis B immunizations.

Human immunodeficiency virus infection has been seen after transfusion of all blood components and blood derivatives except albumin or gamma globulin. Patients exposed to HIV via transfusion become infectious shortly after transfusion and remain so for the rest of their life. Infection with HIV ultimately leads to AIDS, although current studies indicate that prophylactic treatment with azidothymidine, or AZT (Zidovudine), or other antiviral agents can significantly delay progression from infection to the time of onset of AIDS.

Because of the very serious possible sequelae of blood transfusion, indications for transfusion must be very strict, and in no case should blood be transfused prophylactically. Crosby, in a prophetic editorial in 1958, wrote, "Thoughtless prescription of blood transfusion is playing Russian roulette with bottles of blood instead of a revolver. While the odds are in the physician's favor that nothing will go wrong, the patient takes the risk." Nothing could be more true today.

INDICATIONS FOR TRANSFUSION

Most hospitals require informed consent for transfusion. The patient should be told of the hazards of hepatitis and HIV infection. Alternatives to transfusion as well as the potential hazard of not being transfused should be described.

Red blood cell transfusions are indicated for rapid restoration of oxygen-carrying capacity secondary to acute blood loss. Blood transfusions are contraindicated for patients with anemia until studies have shown clearly that specific therapy—for example, iron, vitamin B_{12}, or erythropoietin—cannot be used specifically to correct the anemia. Otherwise normal patients, breathing room air, will seldom require blood transfusions if the hemoglobin is greater than 7 gm/dl or the hematocrit is greater than 21 percent. Clinical judgment must be used to guide transfusion therapy if the patient is bleeding actively or has widespread malignancy or other conditions that interfere significantly with oxygen transport to the tissues.

Red blood cells should only be transfused to increase oxygen-carrying capacity in patients who are anemic. Red blood cells are never indicated for volume expansion, to enhance wound healing, or to improve general "well-being."

Fresh frozen plasma is seldom appropriate for patients in the emergency department. It is indicated primarily for patients with bleeding plus significantly prolonged prothrombin time (PT) or partial thromboplastin time. Fresh frozen plasma should never be used for volume expansion. Crystalloid or colloid solutions, or both, can perform this latter function as well as or better than fresh frozen plasma and do not subject the patient to the inherent hazards of transfusion.

Fresh frozen plasma is only indicated to increase the level of clotting factors with a demonstrated deficiency. Patients with a prolonged PT secondary to long-term anticoagulation therapy should be allowed to normalize their PT off therapy or be given vitamin K_1 oxide rather than fresh frozen plasma unless there is a transcending indication for PT normalization. One should not transfuse fresh frozen plasma for volume expansion, as a nutritional supplement, or prophylactically with massive blood transfusion or after cardiopulmonary bypass.

Platelet concentrate should only be given to patients who are bleeding actively and are thrombocytopenic. Thrombocytopenia can be dilutional in massively transfused patients, can be due to decreased production in patients with leukemia, or can be caused by excessive destruction in patients with different forms of thrombocytopenic purpura.

Platelets should only be transfused to control or prevent bleeding associated with deficiencies in platelet number or function. Platelets should not be given to patients with immune thrombocytopenic purpura (ITP) unless life-threatening bleeding occurs. Patients with thrombotic thrombocytopenic purpura (TTP) should be given fresh frozen plasma. Platelets should not be used prophylactically with massive transfusion or after cardiopulmonary bypass.

TRANSFUSION REACTIONS

Reactions to blood transfusions can range from very mild to fatal. Urticarial reactions are the mildest, do not require termination of the transfusion, and can generally be managed with intramuscular or intravenous administration of 50 mg diphenhydramine (Benadryl).

Reactions to white blood cells, manifested by chills and fever, are seen most frequently in patients who have received blood previously or in women who have had multiple pregnancies. Because the symptoms of a febrile transfusion reaction can also be seen with the more serious hemolytic transfusion reaction, it is essential that the transfusion be stopped if symptoms arise. A posttransfusion reaction blood sample should be drawn and sent to the transfusion service along with the blood container. A urine sample should be sent to the laboratory to look for the possible presence of hemoglobinuria. The transfusion service laboratory will conduct a clerical check and review the blood groups of the pretransfusion cross-matching sample, the blood bag, and the posttransfusion sample. Reactions due to white cells in previously sensitized patients can be prevented effectively by administration of packed red cells passed through special leukocyte filters. Alternately, if leukocyte filters are not available, saline-washed or frozen deglycerolized red blood cells should be used.

Leukocyte filters and saline-washed or deglycerolized red cells should not be used routinely because of their significant added cost. They are indicated solely for patients who have had at least two previous febrile reactions.

Hemolytic transfusion reactions due to blood/recipient incompatibility almost invariably occur within the ABO blood group system and almost always are caused by clerical error in identification of the blood sample drawn for type and cross-match, the blood unit, or the intended recipient. So-called "mismatch" in the blood bank laboratory occurs very infrequently.

The symptoms of an acute hemolytic transfusion reaction include those of febrile reactions as described previously, as well as, back pain, burning in the arm through which the blood is infused, and, at times, a sense of impending doom. Hypotension is the rule, and bleeding secondary to disseminated intravascular coagulation (DIC) is frequently observed. The transfusion must be stopped, and the blood bag along with the postreaction samples described previously should be returned immediately to the transfusion service.

Red cell destruction from ABO incompatibility is normally intravascular with hemoglobinemia and hemoglobinuria. Red cell destruction in all other blood group systems is normally via extravascular removal of red blood cells by the spleen. In the latter case hemoglobinuria is the exception. Immunologic reactions between anti-A and anti-B antibodies and the A or B antigens on the incompatible erythrocytes activate the complement cascade, causing lysis of the red cells and DIC.

Hemoglobinuria due to a hemolytic transfusion reaction and hematuria due to bleeding into the urinary tract can be difficult to differentiate clinically. Urine in hemoglobinuria is translucent and is typically black in color (e.g., blackwater fever in malaria). Hematuria, on the other hand, is opaque, red, and, if the urine is centrifuged, will yield a "button" of red cells at the bottom of the tube. Hemoglobinuria, myoglobinuria, and hematuria will all give a positive test for occult blood on urinalysis.

Patients who have had a major hemolytic blood transfusion reaction should be kept well hydrated with crystalloid solutions. Urine output and central venous pressure should be monitored frequently to determine adequacy of hydration and to detect evidence of acute renal shutdown should this occur. Systemic heparinization or intravenous ethacrynic acid, or both, may be indicated if DIC is present, but consultation with a hematologist should be sought.

Incompatible transfusion reactions tend to be more severe in patients under general anesthesia than in conscious patients because the patient cannot participate in the blood identification routine, and the early symptoms of back pain and burning in the arm through which the transfusion is administered are masked. The incidence of fatal blood transfusion reactions is approximately 1 in 100,000, although the potential for a fatal reaction occurs much more frequently, possibly as often as one per 5,000 to 10,000 transfusions. According to federal law, fatal transfusion reactions must be reported to the United States Food and Drug Administration by the facility that did the cross-match. Such reporting must be made by telephone within 24 hours, with a full written report within seven days.

Blood refrigerators in emergency or operating rooms are very dangerous due to the ease with which a patient can be transfused inadvertently with blood intended for someone else.

PROTECTION AGAINST FATAL TRANSFUSION REACTIONS

When drawing blood for typing and cross-matching, a sample should be drawn from only one patient at a time. At the minimum the blood tube for cross-matching should have a permanent label affixed to it that includes the patient's full name, hospital identification number, and, ideally, date of birth and the name of the person who draws and labels the sample. One should be certain to obtain positive identification of the person from whom the cross-match sample is drawn. One should personally label the tube immediately; blood tubes should not be given to a clerk for labeling. The two most dangerous scenarios in the emergency department are those in which there are multiple "unknown white males" or multiple members of the same family injured in the same motor vehicle accident. Not only is name identification imperfect, but hospital unit numbers of those patients may differ by only one terminal digit.

When blood is drawn from patients on hospital floors for type and cross-match, the transfusion service will compare results on that sample with previous determinations of ABO and Rh group. If a blood group different from that found previously is identified, the transfusion service will request a new blood grouping sample because of the likelihood that a labeling error has taken place. In the emergency department, on the other hand, we usually do not have the luxury of having had the patient typed previously. It is imperative, therefore, that identification of blood samples drawn for cross-matching purposes in the emergency department have precise identification of the patient from whom the sample is drawn.

When blood is transfused it is optimum practice to have someone else (physician or nurse) review with you the identification and blood group appropriateness of the blood unit received from the transfusion service. The identity of the intended recipient should be verified by asking the patient to state his or her full name and date of birth. The identification wrist band should be checked to be certain that the name and unit number of the patient are correct. If someone other than yourself ordered the transfusion, make certain that a written order for transfusion has been given before you administer the blood.

ABO BLOOD GROUP COMPATIBILITY

The ABO blood groups consist of the four possible combinations of two blood group antigens, A and B. These antigens are integral parts of the red blood membrane. A person can have either A or B alone, both, or neither and thus would have an A, B, AB, or O blood type. Expected antibodies, anti-A or anti-B, will be present in the serum of individuals whose red cells lack the corresponding antigen. This relationship is illustrated in Table 93-1. It is not normal blood-banking practice to measure the strength of either antigens or antibodies in the ABO blood group system.

Table 93-1. Blood group antigens and antibodies

	Cells: antigen		Plasma: antibody	
Blood group	A	B	Anti-A	Anti-B
O	−	−	+	+
A	+	−	−	+
B	−	+	+	−
AB	+	+	−	−

Key: − = negative; + = positive.

ABO compatibility between donated blood and blood components and the recipient can be seen readily from Table 93-1. Whole blood, since it has the full complement of red blood cell antigens and plasma antibodies, must be ABO identical (O-O, A-A, B-B, AB-AB).

For practical purposes red blood cells lack plasma anti-A or anti-B antibodies and can be given to anyone who lacks plasma antibodies against the ABO antigens of the donated blood. Thus, group O red blood can be given to O, A, B, and AB patients; group A red blood cells can be given to A and AB patients; group B red blood cells can be given to B and AB patients; and group AB red blood cells can only be given to AB patients.

Plasma, on the other hand, can be given to patients whose red cells lack antigens against which the expected anti-A or B antibodies in the plasma might react. Thus, O plasma can be given to an O recipient; A plasma can be given to an A or O recipient; B plasma can be given to a B or O recipient; and AB plasma can be given to an O, A, B, or AB recipient.

It is customary practice to give whole blood or red cells of the same Rh group as the patient. It is also perfectly permissible to give Rh-negative red blood cells or whole blood to Rh-positive patients. In certain circumstances that will be described later, it is appropriate to give Rh-positive red cells to Rh-negative patients. Platelet concentrate and cryoprecipitated antihemophilic factor, because of the lack of A or B antigens and the small volume of plasma, can be given without concern to the ABO or Rh group of either the donor or recipient.

INDICATIONS FOR O-NEGATIVE BLOOD

There are virtually no indications for administration of un–cross-matched, group O, Rh-positive or Rh-negative blood. Patients who come to the emergency department with active bleeding are most in need of restoration of circulating blood volume, which can be accomplished most efficiently by rapid infusion of crystalloid solution. At the most, it will take between 5 and 10 minutes for the transfusion service to do ABO grouping on the patient, select ABO-compatible red cells, and complete the necessary paperwork.

UNEXPECTED ANTIBODIES

Expected antibodies, as already described, are anti-A and anti-B antibodies as appropriate for the patient's ABO blood group. Unexpected antibodies are directed against blood group antigens other than those within the ABO blood group system (e.g., Rh or Kell). Unexpected antibodies arise only in individuals who have been exposed to other blood group antigens by pregnancy or transfusion. Unexpected antibodies are found in the serum of only approximately 1 percent of the population and are present more frequently in women than men.

It is standard blood-banking practice to test all donated blood for the presence of unexpected antibodies. Whole blood or plasma that contains unexpected antibodies is not used for transfusion.

It also is standard blood-banking practice to test all blood samples from patients for the presence of unexpected antibodies. This process is called "antibody screening" and represents the term "screen" of "type and screen." If results of antibody screening are positive, the blood transfusion service will identify the antigen system against which the antibody is directed. If the patient needs blood, the service would then provide cross-match–compatible red blood cells that have been selected as lacking the antigen to which the patient has an antibody.

SWITCHING RH-NEGATIVE PATIENTS TO RH-POSITIVE RED CELLS OR WHOLE BLOOD

It is exceptionally bad blood-banking practice to allow supplies of Rh-negative red cells and whole blood or any ABO blood group to become exhausted. If this happened and a young girl or woman of childbearing age with active bleeding were transfused with Rh-positive blood because no Rh-negative was available, the patient could make an anti-Rh antibody that could cause hemolytic disease of the newborn in a future pregnancy.

If supplies of Rh-negative blood appear to be extremely low, it is perfectly acceptable blood-banking practice to give Rh-negative patients Rh-positive whole blood or red cells intentionally. If patients are intentionally switched from Rh-negative to Rh-positive, 50 to 70 percent of them will ultimately make an anti-Rh antibody, but it is hoped that the medical condition for which they were transfused will have been treated successfully by the time they do so. The best candidates for switching Rh types are men or women past childbearing age who have an acute process (e.g., ruptured abdominal aortic aneurysm), the outcome of which should be resolved in a relatively short period of time. These patients are preferred to patients (e.g., with leukemia) who may have a continuing need for transfusions over a long period of time. Since the apparent likelihood of forming an anti-Rh antibody is essentially the same whether an Rh-negative patient receives 10 ml or 20 liters of Rh-positive blood, it is best practice to switch Rh types early. The worst possible scenario would be to exhaust supplies of Rh-negative blood and then have to give the patient one unit of Rh-positive red cells. The transfusion service supply of Rh-negative blood would have been exhausted, and the patient who received the unit of Rh-positive red cells would be as likely to make an antibody as he or she would have if switched early.

OTHER ASPECTS OF EMERGENCY TRANSFUSION THERAPY

Packed red cells can be diluted with 0.9% sodium chloride to improve their flow characteristics. The need to dilute packed red cells now is substantially less than it was only a few years ago due to the widespread use by blood centers of additive solutions to dilute and biochemically modify the anticoagulated red cells to extend their shelf life. If the blood center used additive solutions, this can be determined by the presence of "AS-1," "AS-2," or "AS-3" on the blood bag label where it tells what anticoagulant was used. No medications or solutions other than 0.9% sodium chloride USP should be added to blood or red cells. Specifically, 5% dextrose-in-water should not be given before, in addition to, or following blood transfusion because the red cells may agglomerate and the large clumps can plug the intravenous device. Lactated Ringer's solution should not be added to blood because the calcium ions in it can cause the blood to clot.

All blood components must be filtered via an "inline" filter as they are administered. In the case of massive transfusion, it is frequently best to administer the blood via microaggregate blood filters.

A blood warmer placed inline between the blood bag and the patient may be useful to prevent hypothermia during massive transfusion. Warming of blood under a hot-water faucet, in a container of warm water, in a microwave oven, or by adding hot saline is not considered good clinical practice. Should blood be warmed to over 40°C, the red cells can become damaged or the plasma proteins can become poached. Red cells damaged by overheating can cause hemoglobinuria and lead to the false diagnosis that the patient had an ABO hemolytic transfusion reaction.

THE BLOOD TRANSFUSION SERVICE AS AN EDUCATIONAL RESOURCE

Blood transfusion services usually have a number of specialized publications and reference works. Any questions about transfusion therapy can be readily discussed with the medical director. If, by chance, the medical director cannot answer your questions, he or she will research the topic for you.

SELECTED READING

Circular of Information for the Use of Human Blood and Blood Components. American Red Cross, 1989.

Crosby, WH. Misuse of blood transfusions. *Blood* 13:1198, 1958.

Marx, JL. Wider use of AIDS drugs advocated. *Science* 245:811, 1989.

National Institutes of Health Consensus Conference. Fresh-frozen plasma: Indications and risks. *JAMA* 253:551, 1985.

National Institutes of Health Consensus Conference. Perioperative red blood cell transfusion. *JAMA* 260:2700, 1988.

National Institutes of Health Consensus Conference. Platelet transfusion therapy. *JAMA* 257:1777, 1987.

Index

Index

Note: Page numbers followed by f *indicate figures; those followed by* t *indicate tables.*